PRENTICE HALL NURSING

COMPREHENSIVE REVIEW FOR NCLEX-RN®

REVIEWS & RATIONALES

Mary Ann Hogan, MSN, RN
Clinical Assistant Professor
University of Massachusetts–Amherst
Amherst, Massachusetts

PEARSON
Prentice Hall
Upper Saddle River, New Jersey 07458

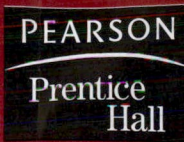

Library of Congress Cataloging-in-Publication Data
Hogan, Mary Ann, MSN.
Prentice Hall's comprehensive review for NCLEX RN / Mary Ann Hogan.
p. ; cm.
Includes bibliographical references and index.
ISBN-13: 978-0-13-119599-8
ISBN-10: 0-13-119599-9
1. Practical nursing—Examinations, questions, etc. 2. Practical nursing—Outlines, syllabi, etc. 3. National Council Licensure Examination for Practical/Vocational Nurses—Study guides. I. Title. II. Title: Comprehensive review for NCLEX-RN. III. Title: Review for NCLEX-RN.
[DNLM: 1. Nursing—Examination Questions. WY 18.2 H714pa 2008]
RT62.H583 2008
610.73076—dc22
2007000492

Notice: Care has been taken to confirm the accuracy of the information presented in this book. The authors, editors, and the publisher, however, cannot accept any responsibility for errors or omissions or for the consequences for application of the information in this book and make no warranty, express or implied, with respect to its contents.

The authors and the publisher have exerted every effort to ensure that drug selections and dosages set forth in this text are in accord with current recommendations and practice at time of publication. However, in view of ongoing research, changes in government regulations, and the constant flow of information relating to drug therapy and drug reactions, the reader is urged to check the package inserts of all drugs for any change in indications of dosage and for added warnings and precautions. This is particularly important when the recommended agent is a new and/or infrequently employed drug.

The authors and publisher disclaim all responsibility for any liability, loss, injury, or damage incurred as a consequence, directly or indirectly, of the use and application of any of the contents of this volume.

Publisher: Julie Levin Alexander
Assistant to Publisher: Regina Bruno
Editor-in-Chief: Maura Connor
Editorial Assistant: Mary Ellen Ruitenberg
Developmental Editor: Danielle Doller
Senior Managing Editor, Development: Marilyn Meserve
Managing Editor, Production: Patrick Walsh
Production Liaison: Anne Garcia
Production Editor: Jessica Balch, Pine Tree Composition
Manufacturing Manager: Ilene Sanford
Manufacturing Buyer: Pat Brown
Design Coordinator/Cover Designer: Mary Siener
Director of Marketing: Karen Allman
Senior Marketing Manager: Francisco Del Castillo
Marketing Specialist: Michael Sirinides
Media Product Manager: John J. Jordan
Media Project Manager: Stephen Hartner
Composition: Pine Tree Composition, Inc.
Printer/Binder: The Courier Companies
Cover Printer: Phoenix Color Corp.

Pearson Education Ltd., *London*
Pearson Education Australia Pty. Limited, *Sydney*
Pearson Education Singapore, Pte. Ltd.
Pearson Education North Asia Ltd., *Hong Kong*
Pearson Education Canada, Ltd., *Toronto*
Pearson Educatión de Mexico, S.A. de C.V.
Pearson Education—Japan, *Tokyo*
Pearson Education Malaysia, Pte. Ltd.
Pearson Education, Upper Saddle River, New Jersey

PEARSON
Prentice

10 9 8 7 6 5 4 3 2 1
ISBN-13: 978-0-13-119599-8
ISBN-10: 0-13-119599-9

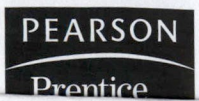

Contents

REVIEWS & RATIONALES

INTRODUCING: *PRENTICE HALL'S COMPREHENSIVE REVIEW FOR NCLEX-RN®*

This volume of the popular *Prentice Hall Nursing Reviews & Rationales* series is designed to serve as the ultimate study guide to prepare you for the NCLEX-RN® exam. It provides a comprehensive outline review of the essential content areas tested on the NCLEX-RN® exam, including critical areas such as management, delegation, leadership, decision-making, pharmacology, and emergency care. This book incorporates these topics throughout, and provides practice questions simulating the level of difficulty on the actual NCLEX-RN® exam.

The NCLEX-RN® exam is organized according to the categories and subcategories of client needs, integrating the concepts you learned in nursing school. While other books provide a review of nursing concepts, we integrate these concepts into the categories of client needs as they would be found on the actual NCLEX-RN® exam.

For example, in ***Prentice Hall's Comprehensive Review for NCLEX-RN®***, all of the concepts related to health problems commonly encountered in both medical–surgical and pediatric nursing are brought together in the body systems chapters in section 9 on Physiological Adaptation. Similarly, the important concepts while working with healthy individuals (such as growth and development, lifestyle management, health screening, age-related changes, nutrition, and healthy mothers and newborns) are brought together in the chapters in section 4 on Health Promotion and Maintenance. This unique organization allows you to study for specific sections of the test based on the results of any predictor tests for the NCLEX-RN® exam that you have taken.

WHAT YOU NEED TO KNOW ABOUT THE NCLEX-RN® EXAMINATION

The NCLEX-RN® licensing examination is a Computer Adaptive Test (CAT) that ranges in length from 75 to 265 individual (stand-alone) test items, depending on individual performance during the examination. Upon graduation from a nursing program, successful completion of this exam is the gateway to your professional nursing practice. The blueprint for the exam is reviewed and revised every three years by the National Council of State Boards of Nursing according to the results of a job analysis study of new graduate nurses practicing within the first six months after graduation. Each question on the exam is coded to a *Client Need Category* and an *Integrated Process.*

Client Need Categories

There are four categories of client needs, and each exam will contain a minimum and maximum percent of questions from each category. The *Client Needs* categories according to the NCLEX-RN® Test Plan effective April 2007 are as follows:

- **Safe, Effective Care Environment**
  - Management of Care (13–19%)
  - Safety and Infection Control (8–14%)
- **Health Promotion and Maintenance (6–12%)**
- **Psychosocial Integrity (6–12%)**
- **Physiological Integrity**
  - Basic Care and Comfort (6–12%)
  - Pharmacological and Parenteral Therapies (13–19%)
  - Reduction of Risk Potential (13–19%)
  - Physiological Adaptation (11–17%)

Integrated Processes

The integrated processes identified on the NCLEX-RN® Test Plan effective April 2007, with condensed definitions, are as follows:

- **Nursing Process:** a scientific problem-solving approach used in nursing practice; consisting of assessment, analysis, planning, implementation, and evaluation
- **Caring:** client–nurse interaction(s) characterized by mutual respect and trust and that are directed toward achieving desired client outcomes
- **Communication and Documentation:** verbal and/or nonverbal interactions between nurse and others (client, family, health care team); a written or electronic recording of activities or events that occur during client care
- **Teaching and Learning:** facilitating client's acquisition of knowledge, skills, and attitudes that lead to behavior change

More detailed information about this examination may be obtained by visiting the National Council of State Boards of Nursing website at **http://www.ncsbn.org** and viewing the *NCLEX-RN® Examination Test Plan for the National Council Licensure Examination for Registered Nurses.*[1]

PREPARING FOR THE NCLEX-RN® EXAMINATION

Study Tips

Using this book should help simplify your review. To make the most of your valuable study time, also follow these simple but important suggestions:

1. **Use a weekly calendar to schedule study sessions.**
   - Outline the timeframes for all of your activities (home, school, appointments, etc.) on a weekly calendar.
   - Find the "holes" in your calendar—the times in which you can plan to study. Add study sessions to the calendar at times when you can expect to be mentally alert, and then follow it!
2. **Create the optimal study environment.**
   - Eliminate external sources of distraction, such as television, telephone, etc.
   - Eliminate internal sources of distraction, such as hunger, thirst, or dwelling on items or problems that cannot be worked on at the moment.
   - Take a break for 10 minutes or so after each hour of concentrated study both as a reward and an incentive to keep studying.
3. **Use pre-reading strategies to increase comprehension of chapter material.**
   - Skim read the headings in the chapter; they identify chapter content.
   - Read the definitions of key terms, which will help you learn new words to comprehend chapter information.
   - Review all graphic aids (figures, tables, boxes); they are often used to explain important points in the chapter.
4. **Read the chapter thoroughly but at a reasonable speed.**
   - Comprehension and retention are actually enhanced by not reading too slowly.
   - Do take the time to reread any section that is unclear to you.
5. **Summarize what you have learned.**
   - Use questions supplied with this book and the ***NCLEX-RN® Test Prep CD-ROM*** to test your application of chapter content.
   - Review again any sections that correspond to questions you answered incorrectly or incompletely.

[1]National Council of State Boards of Nursing, Inc. NCLEX Examination Test Plan for National Council Licensure Examination for Registered Nurses. Effective April, 2007. Retrieved from the World Wide Web at https://www.ncsbn.org/RN_Test_Plan_2007_Web.pdf

Test-Taking Strategies

Every question in the book and on the accompanying CD-ROM provides test-taking strategies that enable you to select the correct answer by breaking down the question, even if you don't know the correct response. Use the following strategies to increase your success on nursing tests or examinations:

- Get sufficient sleep and have something to eat before taking a test. Take deep breaths during the test as needed. Remember, the brain requires oxygen and glucose as fuel. Avoid concentrated sweets before a test, however, to avoid rapid upward and then downward surges in blood glucose levels.
- Read each question carefully, identifying the stem, the four options, and any critical words or phrases in either the stem or options.
  - Critical words in the stem such as "most important" indicate the need to set priorities, since more than one option is likely to contain a statement that is technically correct.
  - Remember that the presence of absolute words such as "never" or "only" in an answer option is more likely to make that option incorrect.
- Determine who is the client in the question; often this is the person with the health problem, but it may also be a significant other, relative, friend, or another nurse.
- Decide whether the stem is a true response stem or a false response stem. With a true response stem, the correct answer will be a true statement, and vice-versa.
- Determine what the question is really asking, sometimes referred to as the issue of the question. Evaluate all answer options in relation to this issue, and not strictly to the "correctness" of the statement in each individual option.
- Eliminate options that are obviously incorrect, then go back and reread the stem. Evaluate the remaining options against the stem once more.
- If two answers seem similar and correct, try to decide whether one of them is more global or comprehensive. If the global option includes the alternative option within it, it is likely that the more global response is the correct answer.

HOW YOUR BOOK PREPARES YOU FOR SUCCESS ON THE NCLEX-RN® EXAMINATION

Prentice Hall's Comprehensive Review for NCLEX-RN® helps you prepare for the NCLEX-RN® exam in three ways:

1. Highlights critical concepts on the NCLEX-RN® Exam

One of the keys to your success on the NCLEX-RN® exam will be focusing your review on nursing concepts and interventions typically incorporated into the test questions. Your book has a few devices to help you familiarize with these topics so you can better manage your review time.

- **Memory Aid boxes** tie specific content from the review outline to the Test Plan and the latest Job Task Analysis. These boxes provide you with a quick review of content that is likely to be asked on the NCLEX-RN® exam.
- **NCLEX® Alert** identifies concepts that are likely to be tested on the NCLEX-RN® exam. Be sure to learn the information highlighted wherever you see this icon.

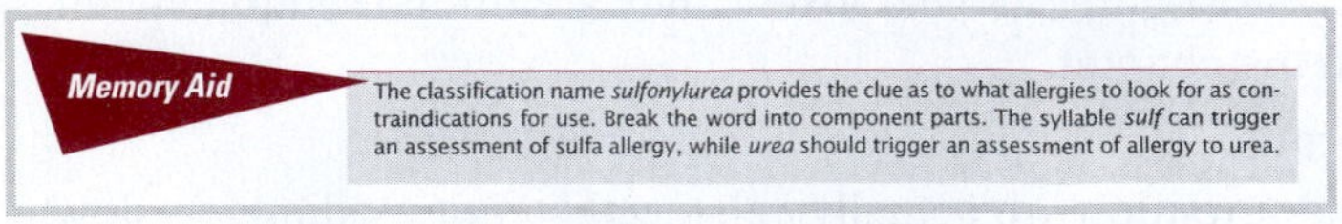
Memory Aid
The classification name *sulfonylurea* provides the clue as to what allergies to look for as contraindications for use. Break the word into component parts. The syllable *sulf* can trigger an assessment of sulfa allergy, while *urea* should trigger an assessment of allergy to urea.

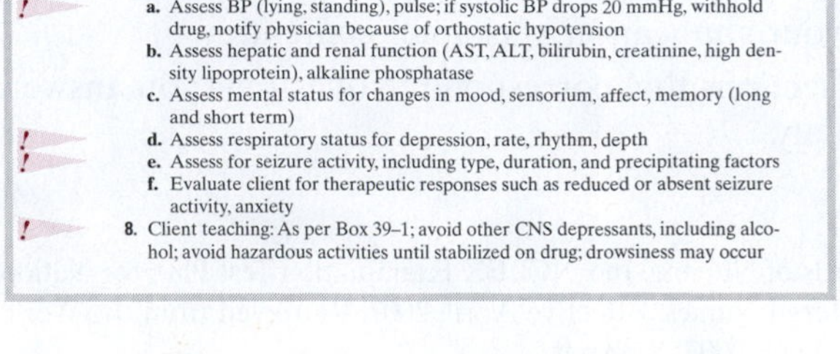

6. Side/adverse effects
   a. Dizziness, drowsiness, confusion, headache, fatigue, blurred vision
   b. Orthostatic hypotension, ECG changes, tachycardia, respiratory depression
   c. Constipation, dry mouth, rash, itching, neutropenia
7. Nursing considerations
   a. Assess BP (lying, standing), pulse; if systolic BP drops 20 mmHg, withhold drug, notify physician because of orthostatic hypotension
   b. Assess hepatic and renal function (AST, ALT, bilirubin, creatinine, high density lipoprotein), alkaline phosphatase
   c. Assess mental status for changes in mood, sensorium, affect, memory (long and short term)
   d. Assess respiratory status for depression, rate, rhythm, depth
   e. Assess for seizure activity, including type, duration, and precipitating factors
   f. Evaluate client for therapeutic responses such as reduced or absent seizure activity, anxiety
8. Client teaching: As per Box 39–1; avoid other CNS depressants, including alcohol; avoid hazardous activities until stabilized on drug; drowsiness may occur

Check Your NCLEX-RN® Exam I.Q. *You are ready for testing on this content if you can*

- Apply knowledge of expected actions and effects of neurological and musculoskeletal medications to client care.
- Correctly administer neurological and musculoskeletal medications to clients.
- Assess for side effects and adverse effects of neurological and musculoskeletal medications.
- Take appropriate action if a client has an unexpected response to a neurological or musculoskeletal medication.
- Monitor a client for expected outcomes or effects of treatment with neurological and musculoskeletal medications.

- **Check Your NCLEX-RN® Exam I.Q.,** found at the end of each chapter, provides an opportunity for you to assess your readiness for the NCLEX-RN® exam on the topics covered in the chapter.

2. Provides practice opportunities

Most faculty tell students they must practice thousands of questions before taking the NCLEX-RN® exam. This book provides you with thousands of questions so you can approach your practice review in a variety of ways.

- **Practice Test** sections provide a quiz at the end of each chapter to test your mastery of the concepts in that chapter.
- **Comprehensive Exam** at the end of the book contains 265 questions. This exam helps you build your endurance in case you have to answer questions for a long time in the real exam.

PRACTICE TEST

1. A client who is receiving phenytoin (Dilantin) to control seizures indicates an understanding of medication by making which of the following statements?
   1. "I need to take more of my Dilantin when I am having a stressful day."
   2. "I will be able to stop taking this medicine in about a year."
   3. "I will probably need to take this medicine all my life."
   4. "I will never have another seizure if I take this medicine."

2. A client with a history of seizures is admitted with a partial occlusion of the left common carotid artery. The client has taken phenytoin (Dilantin) for 10 years. When planning care for this client, it is most important that the nurse does which of the following?
   1. Obtains a history of seizure incidence
   2. Places an airway, suction, and restraints at the bedside
   3. Asks the client to remove any dentures
   4. Observes the client for increased restlessness and agitation

Comprehensive Test

1. A client exposed to *Mycobacterium tuberculosis* starts on chemoprophylaxis. The nurse provides what instruction to the client?
   1. "You will take a single drug such as isoniazid (INH) by mouth every day for 6 to 12 months."
   2. "You will be on at least two drugs effective against the tubercle bacillus for three months."
   3. "You will be on combination therapy in order to prevent development of drug resistance."
   4. "You will need to learn to give yourself subcutaneous injections."

2. The nurse delegates an unlicensed assistive person (UAP) to assist a client with a clean urinary catheterization procedure. The client had formerly been able to do the procedure but because of arthritis, he has been unable to perform the catheterization. Although the UAP has done this procedure before, which of the following must the nurse emphasize to the UAP?
   1. Let the client do most of the procedure and report the expected output.
   2. Report immediately any unusual observations, such as bleeding.
   3. Complete in proper order the steps of the procedure.
   4. Perform health teaching while performing the procedure.

3. The client is in the operating room for a surgical procedure. The nurse in the operating room is monitoring the physiological integrity of the client. Which of the following activities is most appropriate?
   1. Determine client satisfaction with care received.
   2. Assess client's emotional status.
   3. Monitor asepsis in the environment.
   4. Calculate fluid loss and its effects.

4. The clinic nurse is conducting health screenings. Which of the following client assessment findings indicates that client teaching is needed about the risk for stroke? Select all that apply.
   1. ____ Weight 205 lbs and height 5 feet 4 inches
   2. ____ Blood pressure 164/92 mmHg
   3. ____ Eats bran for breakfast daily
   4. ____ Smokes ½ pack cigarettes per day
   5. ____ Serum cholesterol level is 172 mg/dL

5. Which of the following actions would the nurse take to maintain medical asepsis when caring for a client with diabetes mellitus on the medical nursing unit who requires irrigation of a leg ulcer and insulin injections? Select all that apply.
   1. ____ Wash hands before and after client care.
   2. ____ Wear personal protective equipment during the dressing change.
   3. ____ Recap a needle after administering insulin.
   4. ____ Change the dressing for a diabetic ulcer using sterile gloves.
   5. ____ Wipe the rubber stopper on the insulin vial before withdrawing dose.

6. Laboratory test results indicate a client is in the nadir period that follows administration of a chemotherapy drug. Which drug should the nurse avoid administering to this client at this time?
   1. Acetaminophen (Tylenol)
   2. Ibuprofen (Motrin)
   3. Diphenhydramine (Benadryl)
   4. Guanefesin (Robitussin)

1419

- **NCLEX-RN® Test Prep CD-ROM** included with this book contains all 1,600 questions from the book, *PLUS* an additional 4,000 questions, to give you ample opportunities to practice NCLEX®-style questions and assess your readiness for the exam. Please see below for more information about the power of this CD-ROM.

3. Hones your test-taking skills

An important part of preparing for the NCLEX-RN® exam is understanding the questions asked and knowing how best to answer them. This book provides you with feedback to build these important skills.

- **Answers & Rationales** are provided following the Practice Test at the end of each chapter and on the CD-ROM. For every question, you will see a comprehensive rationale for the correct and incorrect choices, because it is important for you to understand why an answer option is correct or incorrect.
- **Test-Taking Strategies** are highlighted in the Answers & Rationales section of the book and on the CD-ROM. Since you cannot skip questions on the NCLEX-RN® exam, you need to learn how to select the correct answer even when you don't know what it is right away. These strategies break down each question and show you how to select the correct choice.
- ***Prentice Hall NursingNotes*** cards offer a quick review of testing strategies and frequently used information organized by the categories of client needs. These tear-out cards are designed to be useful in the clinical setting, when quick and easy access to information is so important.

ANSWERS & RATIONALES

1. **Answer: 4** The best method to improve communication with the client is to eliminate background noises that could interfere with hearing. The client should be approached from the front so as not to frighten him or her. The nurse should use normal pronunciation of words, speak in normal tones, and refrain from shouting, which is demeaning and not helpful.
Cognitive Level: Analysis **Client Need:** Physiological Integrity: Physiological Adaptation **Integrated Process:** Communication and Documentation **Content Area:** Adult Health: Eye, Ear, Nose, and Throat **Strategy:** The core issue of the question is the appropriate strategy for communicating with a client who is hearing impaired. Recall that clients rely on visual cues and can benefit from reduced background noise to aid in answering the question.

2. **Answer: 4** Ear pain is the most common symptom of otitis media that motivates clients to seek health care; secondary or associated symptoms include fever, nausea and vomiting, dizziness, and hearing impairment.
Cognitive Level: Analysis **Client Need:** Physiological Integrity: Physiological Adaptation **Integrated Process:** Nursing Process: Evaluation **Content Area:** Adult Health: Eye, Ear, Nose, and Throat **Strategy:** The critical words in the question are *most common,* which tell you it is necessary to prioritize the options in terms of the frequency of their occurrence. Use nursing knowledge and the process of elimination to make this

Analysis **Content Area:** Adult Health: Eye, Ear, Nose, and Throat **Strategy:** The core issue of the question is the ability to identify age-related changes in hearing in an ol
Use nursing knowledge and the process of elim
make a selection.

5. **Answer: 2** The client should avoid lying on the
following eye surgery in order to minimize ede
traocular pressure. Options 3 and 4 pose no risk
Option 1 is not a problem given the informatio
tion. Some clients with severe visual impairmen
health problems may need assistance to move
environment.
Cognitive Level: Analysis **Client Need:** Physiological
Physiological Adaptation **Integrated Process:** Nur
Implementation **Content Area:** Adult Health: Eye
and Throat **Strategy:** The core issue of the questi
teaching about safe and unsafe activities following cataract surgery. Recall that it is important to avoid positions in which gravity can lead to increased edema in order to make the correct selection.

6. **Answer: 1** When hearing loss is characterized by distortion of sounds, amplification of sound is of little help because it only increases the intensity of distorted sounds. The other options are incorrect.
Cognitive Level: Application **Client Need:** Physiological Integrity:

and Documentation **Content Area:** Adult Health: Eye, Ear, Nose, and Throat **Strategy:** The core issue of the question is the appropriate strategy for communicating with a client who is hearing impaired. Recall that clients rely on visual cues and can benefit from reduced background noise to aid in answering the question.

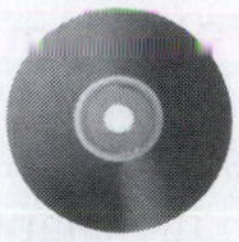

NCLEX-RN® Test Prep CD-ROM

For those who want to practice taking tests on a computer, the CD-ROM that accompanies this book contains more than 5,600 questions. It includes the practice test questions found in all chapters of the book as well as the final comprehensive exam questions. Plus, it contains 4,000 ***NEW*** questions to help you further evaluate your readiness for the exam and hone your test-taking skills. The CD-ROM allows you to choose from three operating modes—Study, Quiz, or Exam. These modes help you customize your practice according to what stage you are at in your NCLEX® exam preparation:

STUDY MODE allows you to practice answering a specific topic or topics in-depth and provides immediate feedback as you answer each question.

QUIZ MODE provides you with a 100-question quiz and offers feedback after you answer all the questions.

EXAM MODE provides you with a simulated NCLEX-RN® exam of 265 questions so you can practice pacing yourself to build your stamina so you can endure answering questions for a long period of time, just like the actual exam.

In all of the modes, you have the option of choosing questions randomly or selecting categories from the NCLEX-RN® Test Plan. For Quiz and Exam modes, you will receive a report showing how you scored, indicating your strengths and any areas in which you may need further practice. The CD-ROM includes alternate NCLEX® Test Items to give you valuable practice with different question types.

SHARE YOUR COMMENTS WITH PRENTICE HALL

Please let us know how this review book helped you prepare for the NCLEX® exam. We welcome your feedback so we can continue to develop this book and other resources to help students succeed in the classroom, in clinicals, and on the NCLEX® exam. Prentice Hall will share your comments with Mary Ann Hogan, the series editor and author of **Prentice Hall's Comprehensive Review for NCLEX-RN®.**
Send all comments to **nursing_excellence@prenhall.com.** Thank you in advance for sharing.

ABOUT PRENTICE HALL NURSING REVIEWS & RATIONALES SERIES

This popular series is the complete foundation for success within the classroom, in clinical settings, and on the NCLEX-RN® exam. Each topical volume offers a concentrated review of core content from across the nursing curriculum, while providing hundreds of practice questions and comprehensive rationales. The ***only*** review series offering a tear-out reference card and additional audio reviews, the complete series includes the following volumes:

- Anatomy & Physiology
- Nursing Fundamentals
- Nutrition and Diet Therapy
- Fluids, Electrolytes, & Acid-Base Balance
- Medical-Surgical Nursing
- Pathophysiology
- Pharmacology
- Maternal-Newborn Nursing
- Child Health Nursing
- Mental Health Nursing
- Physical Assessment
- Community Health Nursing
- Leadership & Management
- Comprehensive Review for NCLEX-RN®
- Comprehensive Review for NCLEX-PN®

Audio Reviews for Students On the Go

vango notes
Hear it. Get it.
www.vangonotes.com

Study on the go with **VangoNotes.** Just download chapter reviews from your text and listen to them on any mp3 player. Now wherever you are—whatever you're doing—you can study by listening to the following for each chapter of the Prentice Hall Nursing Reviews & Rationales Series:

- **Big Ideas:** Your "need to know" for each chapter
- **Practice Test:** A gut check for the Big Ideas—tells you if you need to keep studying
- **Key Terms:** Audio "flashcards" to help you review key concepts and terms

VangoNotes are **flexible;** download all the material directly to your player, or only the chapters you need. And they're **efficient.** Use them in your car, at the gym, walking to class, wherever. So get yours today. And get studying.

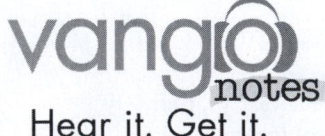

Acknowledgments

This book is a monumental effort of collaboration. Without the contributions of many individuals, this book and its CD-ROM would not have been possible. Thank you to all the contributors and reviewers who devoted their time and talents to this book. Their work will surely help students prepare for success on the NCLEX-RN® exam.

I owe a special debt of gratitude to the wonderful team at Prentice Hall Nursing for their enthusiasm for this project, as well as their good humor, expertise, and encouragement as the series developed. Maura Connor, Editor-in-Chief for Nursing, was unending in her creativity, support, encouragement, and belief in the need for this series. Danielle Doller, Developmental Editor, devoted many long hours to coordinating different facets of this project, and tirelessly and cheerfully encouraged our efforts as well. Her high standards and attention to detail contributed greatly to the final "look" of this book. Editorial Assistant, Mary Ellen Ruitenberg, helped to keep the project moving forward on a day-to-day basis, and I am grateful for her efforts as well. A very special thank you goes to the designers of the book and the production team, led by Anne Garcia, Production Editor, and Mary Siener, Designer, who brought the ideas and manuscript into final form.

Thank you to the team at Pine Tree Composition, led by Project Coordinator Jessica Balch, for the detail-oriented work of creating this book. I greatly appreciate their hard work, attention to detail, and spirit of collaboration.

Finally, I would like to acknowledge and gratefully thank my children, who sacrificed hours of time that would have been spent with them, to bring this book to publication. Their love and support kept me energized, motivated, and at times, even sane.

Mary Ann Hogan

About the *Author*

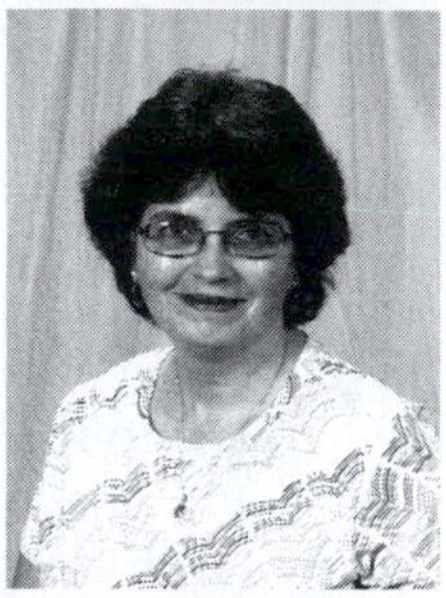

Mary Ann Hogan, MSN, RN has been a nurse educator for 25 years, currently as a Clinical Associate Professor at the University of Massachusetts, Amherst. She has taught in diploma, associate degree, and baccalaureate nursing programs. A former item writer for the CAT NCLEX-RN® exam, Ms. Hogan has been teaching review courses throughout New England for the last 15 years. She also has contributed to a number of publications in the areas of adult health, pharmacology, and fundamentals of nursing. She is a member of the American Nurses Association and Sigma Theta Tau, the International Honor Society for Nursing.

CONTRIBUTORS

Comprehensive Review for NCLEX-RN®

Kim Attwood, MSN
Moravian University
Bethlehem, PA
Chapter 20 Culturally Competent Care, Chapter 33 Blood and Blood Component Therapy

Denise Blais, MSN
St. Joseph's College
Rensselaer, IN
Chapter *29 Alternative and Complementary Therapies*

Jo Anne Carrick, MSN, RN, CEN
The Pennsylvania State University
Sharon, PA
Chapter *69 Basic Life Support*

Maureen Clusky, DNSc, RN
Bradley University
Peoria, IL
Chapter *7 Injury Prevention, Disaster Planning, and Protecting Client Safety*

Julie Eggert, MSN, PhD
Clemson University
Clemson, SC
Chapter *25 End of Life Care*

Latrell Fowler, RN, PhD
Florence Darlington Technical College
Florence, SC
Chapter *17 Promoting Healthy Lifestyle Choices*

Margaret Gingrich, RN, MSN
Harrisburg Area Community College
Harrisburg, PA
Chapter *34 Total Parenteral Nutrition, Chapter 47 Common Laboratory Tests*

Kathy Keister, PhD, RN
Miami University
Middletown, OH
Chapter *8 Preventing and Controlling Infection*

Virginia Lester, RN, MSN
Angelo State University
San Angelo, TX
Chapter *14 Lifespan Growth and Development, Chapter 28 Maintaining Function of Tubes and Drains, Chapter 48 Common Diagnostic Tests and Procedures, Chapter 49 Perioperative Care*

Donna M. Nickitas, RN, PhD, CNAA, BC
Hunter College
New York, NY
Chapter *6 Leadership and Management*

Lilli Raffeldt, RN, MA
Three Rivers Community College
Norwich, CT
Chapter *18 Age-Related Care of Older Adults*

Samir Samour, MSN, RN
Midlands Technical College
Columbia, SC
Chapter *32 Intravenous Therapy*

Kim Serroka, MSN, RN
Youngstown State University
Youngstown, OH
Chapter *15 Providing Immunizations*

Priscilla Simmons, EdD APRN, BC
Eastern Mennonite University
Lancaster, PA
Chapter *47 Common Laboratory Tests*

Nancy Wagner, MSN, RN
Youngstown State University
Youngstown, OH
Chapter *15 Providing Immunizations*

NCLEX-RN® Test Prep CD-ROM

Sharon Beasley, MSN, RN
Technical College of the Lowcountry
Beaufort, SC

Donna Bowles, MSN, EdD, RN
Indiana University Southeast
New Albany, IN

Barbara Carranti, MS, RN, CNS
Le Moyne College
Syracuse, NY

Rebecca Gesler, MSN, RN
Spalding University
Louisville, KY

Marilyn Greer, MS, RN
Rockford College
Rockford, IL

Kathleen Haubrich, PhD, RN
Miami University
Hamilton, OH

Judith Herrman, PhD, RN
University of Delaware
Newark, DE

REVIEWERS

Faculty

Mike Aldridge, MSN, RN, CCRN, CNS
The University of Texas at Austin
Austin, TX

Louise A. Aurilio, RNC, Ph.D., CNA
Youngstown State University
Youngstown, OH

Tatayana Bogopolskiy, ANRP
Florida International University
Miami, FL

Mary T. Boylston, RN, EdD
Eastern University
St. Davids, PA

Vera C. Brancato, EdD, MSN, RN, BC
Kutztown University
Kutztown, PA

Tracey Carlson, MSN, RNC
Kent State University
Kent, OH

Fang-yu Chou, RN,PhD
San Francisco State University
San Francisco, CA

Harvey "Skip" Davis, RN, PhD, CARN, PHN
San Francisco State University
San Francisco, CA

Peggy Davis, MSN, RN, CNS
The University of Tennessee at Martin
Martin, TN

Letty Chan Domingo, MSN, RN, CRNP, CEN
Temple University
Philadelphia, PA

Mary L. Dowell, PhD, RNC
University of Mary Hardin Baylor
Belton, TX

Marilyn S. Fetter, PhD, RN, CS
Villanova University
Villanova, PA

Julie Pearson Floyd, APRN, BC
The University of Tennessee at Martin
Martin, TN

Joni C. Goldwasser, RN, MSN, CEN
Radford University
Radford, VA

Rebecca Crews Gruener, RN, MS
Louisiana State Univ. at Alexandria
Alexandria, LA

Sandra Gustafson, MA, RN
Hibbing Community College
Hibbing, MN

Patricia K. Hawley, MEd
Ferris State University
Mecosta Osceola Career Center
Big Rapids, MI

Susan P. Holmes, RN, MSN, CRNP
Auburn University
Auburn, AL

Katherine M. Howard MS, RN, BC
Raritan Bay Medical Center
Perth Amboy, NJ

Barbara Konopka, MSN, RN, CCRN, CEN
Penn State University
Dunmore, PA

Darcus Margarette Kottwitz, MSN, RN
Fort Scott Community College
Fort Scott, KS

Sandra S. Meeker, RN, MSN
Central Texas College
Killeen, TX

Mary Pihlak, PhD, RN
University of Mary Hardin-Baylor
Belton, TX

Beth Hogan Quigley, RN, MSN, CRNP
University of Pennsylvania
Philadelphia, PA

Linda L. Rather, RN, MSN, MS
Neosho County Community College
Chanute, KS

Anita K. Reed, MSN, RN
Saint Joseph's College
Lafayette, IN

Linda Snell, DNS, WHNP-C
SUNY College at Brockport
Brockport, NY

Marianne F. Swihart, RN, MEd, MSN
Pasco-Hernando Community College
New Port Richey, FL

Patricia R. Teasley, APRN, BC
Central Texas College
Killeen, TX

Loretta Wack, RN, BSN, MSN
Blue Ridge Community College
Weyers Cave, VA

Gerry Walker, MSN, RN
Park University
Parkville, MO

Leanne M. Waterman, MS, APRN, BC, FNP
Onondaga Community College
Syracuse, NY

Dorothy Williams, MSN, RN
Baptist Health System
San Antonio, TX

Linda S. Williams MSN, RNBC
Jackson Community College
Jackson, MI

Kim C. Wright, MSN, RN
Amarillo College
Amarillo, TX

Student

Judy Armah
Villanova University
Villanova, PA

Katie Barlett
Auburn University
Auburn, AL

Jorge C. Castro
Florida International University
Miami, FL

Galina K. Ivanova
Northern Illinois University
DeKalb, IL

Mercedes Jimeńez
Florida International University
Miami, FL

Abby Parker
Case Western Reserve University
Cleveland, OH

The NCLEX-RN® Licensing Examination

1

In this chapter

Test Yourself

Are you ready for the NCLEX-RN® or course exams? Use the practice tests on the companion CD-ROM to check.

Passing the National Council Licensing Examination for Registered Nurses (NCLEX-RN®) is the last threshold you will cross after completing nursing school to enter the world of professional nursing. Congratulations, you are well on your way. Your star is rising! Although you may be nervous or even frightened about taking this test, you need to understand that it is not intended to be a barrier to keep you from finally achieving your goal. Rather, its purpose is to safeguard the public trust—to ensure that nurses caring for patients are minimally competent or safe for practice. When stated like that, it doesn't sound so bad, does it? Then why is the examination so often viewed as a hurdle to be jumped?

The answer partially lies in the construction of the test—it is not like other tests you often took in nursing school. This chapter helps you gain a greater understanding of the NCLEX-RN® exam, developed by the National Council of State Boards of Nursing (NCSBN). It reduces the fear of the unknown and thus reduces some of the anxiety that accompanies preparing for and taking this exam. Chapter 2 provides more information about how to deal with test anxiety and how to use effective test-taking strategies.

COMPUTERIZED ADAPTIVE TESTING: WHAT IS IT?

Computerized adaptive testing (CAT) is a method of test administration in which the computer randomly generates a test question from the test item pool and, after the first question, selects the next question based on your ability to answer the previous one. If the question is answered correctly, the next question is at a similar or higher level of difficulty. If the question is answered incorrectly, the next question is at a similar or lower level of difficulty. This process continues with each subsequent question. Because the questions are tailored to the individual, no two test takers will receive the same test. CAT also assures that anyone who takes the exam more than once never receives the same question twice within a prescribed period of time.

CAT explains why some people must answer the minimum number of questions (75) while others must take up to the maximum (265). In essence, successful test takers who can answer difficult questions will have a shorter but harder test, while those who can answer easier questions can expect a longer test.

A key difference between a tradional paper-and-pencil test and a CAT is that with CAT, each question must be answered in the order presented before the test taker can proceed to the next question. Thus, questions cannot be "skipped" to be returned to later. Although "forced" answering without the option to return to a question may be unnerving to the test taker who typically uses this strategy, it is actually beneficial. Why? Because in skipping and returning to questions, more answers are changed from correct to incorrect than are changed from incorrect to correct, according to student reports over time.

The overall goal of the CAT is to evaluate your ability to remain consistently above or below a predetermined passing standard. The computer will continue to select test items from the test bank until

- The requirements of the test plan have been met (see next section) and
- The computer has determined with 95% confidence statistically that your ability is either clearly above or clearly below the passing standard, or
- The maximum 265 questions have been answered, or
- The maximum time limit (6 hours) has been reached.

At this point, the computer will shut down and the examination is ended. Many test takers have mixed feelings at this time. Some are glad it is over, while others wish the computer would keep generating questions.

AN OVERVIEW OF THE NCLEX-RN® TEST PLAN

The test plan is designed to measure the knowledge, abilities, and skills needed by an entry-level nurse in order to practice safely and effectively (NCSBN, 2006). Each question in the test bank is written according to a two-part framework, including *Client Needs* and *Integrated Processes.* Each question is also written at a specific level of cognitive ability.

Cognitive Ability Level

Bloom's taxonomy for the cognitive domain of learning (Bloom et al., 1956, Anderson & Krathwohl, 2001) is used as the measure for coding the difficulty level of an individual test item in terms of its design. Four of the cognitive levels are knowledge, comprehension, application, and analysis. Because nursing is an applied human discipline that requires critical thinking and clinical decision making, most of the questions on the licensing exam for registered nurses are written at either the application or analysis levels (see Box 1–1 and Box 1–2 for samples). Thus, these questions are often more difficult than test questions on teacher-generated tests, which are more likely to contain a greater number of questions at the knowledge and comprehension level.

Client Needs

The framework for the test plan must identify nursing competencies that apply to all clients across all care settings. With this in mind, the NCSBN developed the test structure of Client Needs. There are four categories of Client Needs: *Safe Effective Care Environment, Health Promotion and Maintenance, Psychosocial Integrity,* and *Physiological Integrity.* Two categories—Safe Effective Care Environment and Physiological Integrity—are further divided into subcategories on the test plan. All test takers receive the same percentage of

Box 1–1

Sample Question Illustrating Application Cognitive Level

The nurse has an order to administer a daily dose of sodium warfarin (Coumadin) 5 mg by mouth. Prior to preparing this medication, the nurse would make note of which of the following results from the laboratory studies drawn at 0600 today?

___ **1.** Hematocrit (Hct) 42%
___ **2.** Hemoglobin (Hgb) 12.8 mg/dL
___ **3.** Partial thromboplastin time (PTT) 49 seconds
___ **4.** International normalized ratio (INR) 2.6

Answer: 4

A question written at the application level of difficulty requires you to consider nursing knowledge that is relevant to the question and use it to make a nursing judgment. In this question, the relevant nursing knowledge is that effectiveness of warfarin is evaluated by noting the results of the INR or prothrombin time (PT, which is not an answer choice in this question).

Box 1–2

Sample Question Illustrating Analysis Cognitive Level

The nurse on a medical nursing unit has been notified of an external disaster with an estimated 30 clients being brought to the emergency department. The nurse is asked to develop a list of clients on the unit that could be discharged. Which client would the nurse place at the top of the triage list for discharge?

___ **1.** A 39-year-old client who underwent laparoscopic cholecystectomy 24 hours ago and reports right shoulder pain rated as a 4 on a scale of 1 to 10.

___ **2.** A 54-year-old client with draining venous leg ulcer and a temperature of 100.8°F.

___ **3.** A 76-year-old client with chronic obstructive pulmonary disease with an oxygen saturation of 89% while wearing oxygen at 2 liters/minute.

___ **4.** An 82-year-old client who underwent pacemaker insertion 4 hours ago and whose cardiac monitor shows ventricular paced rhythm with no failure to capture.

Answer: 1

A question written at the analysis level of difficulty generally requires you to

➤ Consider multiple sets of information to make a nursing decision, and/or

➤ Make nursing judgments using ordinary nursing knowledge in unusual circumstances.

In this question, the nurse needs to use knowledge about which client is the most stable in order to make a decision. The situation is also unusual because nurses are not frequently involved in disasters in everyday nursing practice. Considering stability, you would not discharge first the client in option 3 (airway) or the client in option 2 (risk of infection). The client in option 4 still has potential for developing complications postprocedure, so you would discharge first the client in option 1 who had surgery 24 hours ago. Because it is a laparoscopic procedure, referred shoulder pain is expected, and the client could be taught effective pain management strategies.

questions from each category or subcategory in the test plan, regardless of the length of an individual test (see Table 1–1 ■). These percentages took effect April 2004, and the proposed test plan to take effect April 1, 2007 is unchanged from the 2004 test plan.

Safe Effective Care Environment

This category contains two subcategories: *Management of Care* and *Safety and Infection Control.* The *Management of Care* subcategory contains questions that evaluate your knowledge, skills, and ability to work effectively with the health care team to provide safe, integrated, and cost-effective care to clients (NCSBN, 2006). The *Safety and Infection Control* subcategory contains questions that evaluate your ability to protect the client, family, and health care team from infection and other health or environmental hazards (NCSBN, 2006). The topics included in each of these subcategories are outlined in Box 1–3.

Health Promotion and Maintenance

This category has no subcategories with the test plan effective April 2004. It contains questions that evaluate your ability to apply knowledge of growth and development to individual client situations as well as to promote optimal health and to participate in prevention and/or early detection of health problems (NCSBN, 2006). The topics included in this category are outlined in Box 1–4.

Table 1–1

Overview of the 2007 NCLEX-RN® Test Plan

Client Need Category/Subcategory	Percentage of Questions
Safe Effective Care Environment	
Management of Care	13–19%
Safety and Infection Control	8–14%
Health Promotion and Maintenance	6–12%
Psychosocial Integrity	6–12%
Physiological Integrity	
Basic Care and Comfort	6–12%
Pharmacological and Parenteral Therapies	13–19%
Reduction of Risk Potential	13–19%
Physiological Adaptation	11–17%

Box 1–3

Sample Topics for Safe Effective Care Environment

Management of Care

- Advance directives
- Advocacy
- Case management
- Client rights
- Collaboration with interdisciplinary team
- Concepts of management
- Confidentiality/Information security
- Consultation
- Continuity of care
- Delegation
- Establishing priorities
- Ethical practice
- Informed consent
- Information technology
- Legal rights and responsibilities
- Performance improvement (quality improvement)
- Referrals
- Resource management
- Staff education
- Supervision

Safety and Infection Control

- Accident prevention
- Disaster planning
- Emergency response plan
- Ergonomic principles
- Error prevention
- Handling hazardous and infectious materials
- Home safety
- Injury prevention
- Medical and surgical asepsis
- Reporting of incident/event/irregular occurrence/variance
- Safe use of equipment
- Security plan
- Standard/transmission-based/other precautions
- Use of restraints/safety devices

Psychosocial Integrity

This category also has no subcategories with the test plan effective April 2004. It contains questions that evaluate your ability to provide care to clients with either acute or chronic mental illness and to provide care that supports the emotional and psychosocial well-being of clients and families during stressful events (NCSBN, 2006). The topics included in this category are outlined in Box 1–5.

Box 1–4

Sample Topics for Health Promotion and Maintenance

- Aging process
- Ante/intra/postpartum and newborn care
- Developmental stages and transitions
- Disease prevention
- Expected body image changes
- Family planning
- Family systems
- Growth and development
- Health and wellness
- Health promotion programs
- Health screening
- High-risk behaviors
- Human sexuality
- Immunizations
- Lifestyle choices
- Principles of teaching/learning
- Self-care
- Techniques of physical assessment

Box 1–5

Sample Topics for Psychosocial Integrity

Abuse/neglect	Psychopathology
Behavioral interventions	Religious and spiritual influences on health
Chemical and other dependencies	Sensory/perceptual alterations
Coping mechanisms	Situational role changes
Crisis intervention	Stress management
Cultural diversity	Support systems
End of life care	Therapeutic communications
Family dynamics	Therapeutic environment
Grief and loss	Unexpected body image changes
Mental health concepts	

Physiological Integrity

This category has four subcategories: *Basic Care and Comfort, Pharmacological and Parenteral Therapies, Reduction of Risk Potential,* and *Physiological Adaptation* (NCSBN, 2006). The *Basic Care and Comfort* subcategory contains questions that evaluate your knowledge and ability to provide comfort and assistance during activities of daily living. The *Pharmacological and Parenteral Therapies* subcategory addresses your knowledge and ability to administer medications and parenteral therapies (e.g., intravenous therapy or blood transfusion therapy). The *Reduction of Risk Potential* subcategory addresses your ability to take action to reduce the likelihood that a client will develop a complication or health problem resulting from the current episode of care. The *Physiological Adaptation* subcategory addresses your ability to manage and provide care to clients with acute, chronic, or life-threatening physiological health problems. Topics included in each of these subcategories are outlined in Box 1–6.

Integrated Processes

The Integrated Processes category forms the second part of the structure of the test plan for the NCLEX-RN® examination. The four processes are the five-step nursing process (assessment, analysis, planning, implementation, and evaluation), caring, communication and documentation, and teaching and learning. Because these processes are considered foundational to nursing practice, they are integrated throughout the Client Need categories; however, there are no specific percentages attached to each.

TEST INNOVATIONS: ALTERNATE ITEM FORMATS

Alternate item formats were designed to provide ways, other than standard multiple-choice questions, to measure competence for entry-level nursing practice (NCSBN, 2004). As part of its own ongoing quality improvement program, NCSBN continually looks to the future to design, field test, and implement such innovative methods for assessing entry-level nurse competence. In so doing, NCSBN holds itself to the same high professional standards as other health-oriented organizations that hold the public trust. Alternate item questions may include the following:

- Hot spot (the candidate clicks on a specific area of an image or graphic to answer the question)
- Fill-in-the-blank (for example, the candidate types in a number after performing a calculation)
- Multiple response (the candidate clicks on as many responses as apply to the question)

Box 1-6

Sample Topics for Physiological Integrity Basic Care and Comfort

Basic Care and Comfort

Alternative and complementary therapies

Assistive devices

Elimination

Mobility/immobility

Nonpharmacological comfort interventions

Nutrition and oral hydration

Palliative/comfort care

Personal hygiene

Rest and sleep

Pharmacological and Parenteral Therapies

Adverse effects/contraindications and side effects

Blood and blood products

Central venous access devices

Dosage calculation

Expected outcomes/effects

Medication administration

Parenteral/intravenous therapies

Pharmacological agents/actions

Pharmacological interactions

Pharmacological pain management

Total parenteral nutrition

Reduction of Risk Potential

Diagnostic tests

Laboratory values

Monitoring conscious sedation

Potential for alterations in body systems

Potential for complications of diagnostic tests/treatments/procedures

Potential for complications from surgical procedures and health alterations

System-specific assessments

Therapeutic procedures

Vital signs

Physiological Adaptation

Alterations in body systems

Fluid and electrolyte imbalances

Hemodynamics

Illness management

Infectious diseases

Medical emergencies

Pathophysiology

Radiation therapy

Unexpected response to therapies

- Chart/exhibit (the candidate clicks on the "exhibit" button and then views information contained in three tabs to use in answering the question).
- Drag and drop/ordered response (the candidate uses the mouse to place in order a sequence of actions based on a client situation)

Alternate item formats are not found in any great number on the licensing exam. Currently, examinees are advised not to expect more than one or two of them per 100 questions, and some whose exam shuts off at 75 may not have any. These questions are scored as either correct or incorrect in the same way standard multiple-choice questions are scored. More information about alternate item format questions can be found on the Web site for the National Council of State Boards of Nursing at http://www.ncsbn.org. At least 200 alternate item format questions can be found in this book and on the accompanying CD-ROM to provide you with ample opportunity to practice these types of questions.

Remember that any question on the exam may contain a picture or graphic to use when answering the question. Multiple-choice questions that contain pictures or graphics are not necessarily alternate item format.

BEHIND THE SCENES: THE TEST DEVELOPMENT PROCESS

The test plan for the NCLEX-RN® examination is developed considering the content of Nurse Practice Acts in the various U.S. states and territories and the rules and regulations of the various boards of nursing. A practice (job) analysis study is also done every 3 years to assess what activities entry-level nurses perform in the clinical setting within the first 6 months after graduation. The study is large in scale and is rigorously carried out to ensure reliability and validity of results. The test plan is then modified after reviewing the results of the latest study and considering other data already mentioned.

In a separate process, the passing standard for the examination is also reviewed on a 3-year cycle in the same year that the revised test plan is approved. In April 2004, the passing standard was raised from −0.35 logits to −0.28 logits, a mathematical "line" above which the test candidate must remain to pass the exam. As an example, test takers who can answer difficult questions correctly remain easily above the line (and will thereby also take a shorter test). Those who can answer easier questions correctly can also pass as long as they remain above the line, but they must answer more questions to do so. The most important point is that as long as the computer is generating questions, it has *not* determined failure, so answer each question thoughtfully and carefully.

To ensure that the exam reflects current clinical practice, new test questions are continually added to the test bank, and outdated questions are discarded or modified. Once a question has been written, it is pilot tested during actual examinations. For this reason, 15 of the first 75 questions on any licensing examination do not calculate into the passing score. Because you will not know which questions they are, it is critical to answer all questions carefully.

New test items are written by a pool of people who volunteer their services as item writers. Item writers are extensively screened by the NCSBN and are registered nurses who hold a masters degree or higher; often they are nurse educators. A review panel (consisting of content experts who work in clinical settings) also looks at all questions developed by the item writers to ensure they reflect current nursing practice before being included in the test item pool.

REGISTERING FOR THE EXAM

The Registration Process

To be eligible to take the NCLEX-RN® examination following graduation, you must complete two processes simultaneously. The first is to apply for licensure to the Board of Nursing in the state or territory in which you wish to be licensed. The second is to register to take the licensing examination with the test service vendor, currently Pearson VUE.

Fill out the state licensure application completely and carefully, and be sure to submit the correct application fee (varies from state to state) in an approved form of payment. If the form is completed incorrectly, or if the proper fee is not enclosed using the correct form of payment, the application will be returned to you, which in turn will delay your ability to take the examination. After receiving your application, the Board of Nursing will determine your eligibility for licensure (based on state law) and notify the test service once you are authorized for admission to the licensing examination.

At the same time that you apply to a state Board of Nursing for licensure, you must register for the NCLEX-RN® examination with the test service. There is a separate registration fee for the test service. You can register on the Internet at the NCLEX® Candidate Web Site (http://www.pearsonvue.com/nclex). You can also register by mail or by telephone using the directions in the *NCLEX-RN® Examination Candidate Bulletin* obtained through your school of nursing or on the Web at http://www.ncsbn.org.

Once you are authorized to take the examination, an Authorization to Test (ATT) form will be mailed to you and also e-mailed to you if you included an e-mail address on your registration form. The ATT is valid for a time period specified by the Board of Nursing in which you seek licensure (average is 90 days, with a range of 60 to 365 days). Once you receive the ATT, you can schedule an examination appointment. If you don't receive an ATT within 4 weeks of registration, or if you lose the ATT card once it is sent, report this to the NCLEX® Candidate Test Service according to the directions in the *NCLEX® Examination Candidate Bulletin.*

Scheduling an Examination Appointment

After receiving the ATT, make the appointment for the exam right away, even if you do not plan to take it immediately. This will provide you with the greatest number of test dates and times to choose from. Remember that following graduation, there are many graduates seeking to fill the appointment slots, so popular time slots fill up quickly. Also, if you wait until your ATT card is almost ready to expire, the test center may not be as able to seat you easily. First-time applicants must be offered an appointment within 30 days of telephoning or e-mailing the test service; repeat candidates must be offered an appointment within 45 days.

Make sure you have an ATT form before you call or e-mail to schedule an appointment. It contains information needed to make the appointment, including your test authorization number, candidate identification number, and expiration date. Choose your test date carefully and be sure you have 6 hours available (the maximum length of the test).

If you need to change your appointment, you must call the test center at least 24 hours (1 full business day) in advance. For example, if your appointment is for Tuesday at 1:00 PM, you must call on or before 1:00 PM on Monday. For appointments scheduled on Saturday, Sunday, or Monday, you must call by the appropriate time on Friday.

THE TEST CENTER: WHAT TO EXPECT

Getting to the Test Center

Before the date of your appointment, take a test drive to the test center to become familiar with the route and parking availability. Do this at the same time of day you will be driving to your exam, which will give you an idea of traffic conditions and any road construction or other delays that may occur at that time of day. Tell family or friends who might accompany you on the actual test day that they will not be allowed to remain in the test center waiting area or to talk to you at any time during the examination.

Be sure to arrive at the test center 30 minutes prior to your appointment. If you do not, you may have to forfeit your appointment and reschedule it at a later date for an additional fee. The test service will report to the appropriate Board of Nursing any candidate who does not test on the date and time scheduled (due to late arrival or absence). Do not bring any textbooks or other study materials into the test center; these are prohibited and could lead to your dismissal from the test center or cancellation of your results.

Test Center Procedures

On arrival, you must present your ATT, a valid picture identification that has your signature, and a secondary form of identification that has your signature. It is critical that your name on the ATT and the picture identification match. You then must provide your signature. You will be photographed, and a digital fingerprint will be taken with a device that vaguely resembles a clip-on type of pulse oximeter probe.

A small storage locker will be provided for your use for personal belongings. Again, you are not allowed to bring books or study materials with you. It may be helpful to bring a small snack and/or drink in case you need to take a break during the test, but you may not bring them into the actual testing area.

The test administrator will provide you with a short orientation before escorting you to a computer terminal. After you are admitted to the testing area, the test administrator (proctor) will give you erasable note boards for your use during the test. They must remain in the room and will be collected after the test.

The Actual NCLEX-RN® Examination

The examination may take up to 6 hours to complete. This includes time needed for a short tutorial, a preprogrammed optional break after 2 hours, a second preprogrammed optional break after 3½ hours, and any unscheduled breaks that you choose. The computer alerts you when the preprogrammed breaks begin. If you take a break, you must leave the testing area and provide a fingerprint for readmission. All breaks count against your testing time. There is no minimum or maximum time that you must spend on each question, but maintaining a steady pace (averaging about one question every 80 seconds) over the course of the test will help to ensure that you do not run out of time. This is just an average, however; you may be able to answer some questions more quickly, and some may take longer. It is most important to do the best you can with each question that appears on the screen.

The first 75 questions of the examination will contain 15 questions that are being pretested (pilot tested). The computer may shut down at any time after 75 questions and up to 265 questions. Again, remember that as long as the computer is generating questions, you have not failed! Maintain concentration and give each question your full and thoughtful attention.

Some people are fearful that they will select an incorrect answer accidentally while taking the computerized exam. You do not need to worry about this. Once you select an answer, the computer will not generate another question until you click on "Next." Until you click the Next button, you are able to change your answer as many times as you wish. It is only when you click Next that the answer is finalized and a new question appears. A word of caution here: it is far more common to change the correct answer to an incorrect one because of self-doubt than to change an incorrect answer to the correct one. Change answers only for a good reason!

Once the computer shuts down, you will be given a brief computerized questionnaire about the testing experience. When you finish, the test administrator will collect the note boards and dismiss you from the test center.

GETTING THE RESULTS: WHAT NEXT?

You did it! You've taken the test, and you are probably both relieved and nervous at the same time. Your examination is scored twice (for quality control), once by the computer at the test site and again after the examination record has been transmitted to Pearson VUE, the test vendor (usually within 4 to 6 hours). The results are usually made available to the appropriate Board of Nursing in approximately 6 to 8 hours, and results are sent from the Board of Nursing to the candidates within 2 to 14 days.

In a majority of states and jurisdictions, an unofficial report of your result may be obtained for a fee 2 business days after the test at http://www.pearsonvue.com/nclex or by calling the NCLEX® Quick Results line at 1-900-776-2539 (1-900-77-NCLEX). Check the NCSBN Web site (http://www.ncsbn.org) to see whether the state in which you have applied for licensure utilizes this service. Do remember that results obtained in this way are unofficial and do not authorize you to begin practicing as a registered nurse. Only the official results from the Board of Nursing allow you to begin practice.

What if you did not pass? Don't give up hope! The Board of Nursing will send you a copy of your results, which will indicate the test plan areas in which you scored either "above the passing standard," "near the passing standard," or "below the passing standard." Talk to a trusted mentor (who is familiar with the NCLEX-RN® examination) and develop a study plan before retesting. Some of the finest nurses in practice did not pass on the first test, so stay focused on your goal.

How long will you have to wait to retest? The NCSBN has reduced the waiting period from 90 days to 45 days. Effectively, this means a candidate could take the test eight times in 1 year instead of four. To take advantage of this reduced waiting period, you must be applying for licensure with a participating board of nursing. At the time this book went to press, the following boards of nursing are *not* participating in the 45-day retake period for the NCLEX-RN®: California, Georgia, Guam, Montana, Oklahoma, Puerto Rico, South Dakota, Washington, and West Virginia. Check with your Board of Nursing as needed to verify the retake period. Contact information for the boards of nursing in all jurisdictions can be found on the Companion Web site for this series.

References

Anderson, L., & Krathwohl, D. (Eds.). (2001). *A taxonomy for learning, teaching, and assessing. A revision of Bloom's taxonomy of educational objectives.* New York: Addison-Wesley Longman.

Bloom, B., Engelhart, M., Furst, E., Hill, W., & Krathwohl, D. (1956). *Taxonomy of educational objectives: The classification of educational goals. Handbook I. Cognitive domain.* New York: David McKay.

National Council of State Boards of Nursing. (2006). Proposed 2007 NCLEX-RN® test plan. Presented at 2006 Annual Meeting of National Council of State Boards of Nursing, August 1–4, Salt Lake City, Utah.

National Council of State Boards of Nursing. (2004). *2004 NCLEX® invitational: Constructing the NCLEX® of the future.* Chicago, IL: Author.

National Council of State Boards of Nursing (2006). *Report of findings from the 2005 RN practice analysis: Linking the NCLEX-RN® examination to practice.* Chicago: Author.

National Council of State Boards of Nursing, Inc. Web site: http://www.ncsbn.org.

Test Preparation and Test-Taking Strategies

2

In this chapter

Test Yourself

Are you ready for the NCLEX-RN® or course exams? Use the practice tests on the companion CD-ROM to check.

Because you have successfully passed the courses in your nursing program, you have already demonstrated that you have acquired a set of test-taking skills. Some of you may say, "Yes, that's true for me," while others may say, "Wait a minute, I did pass, but I always struggle with tests. I'm not looking forward to the NCLEX-RN® exam at all!" This chapter helps you use the test-taking skills you currently have and build on them to increase your success on the NCLEX-RN® Licensing examination.

PHYSICAL AND PSYCHOLOGICAL PREPARATION FOR TEST-TAKING

Many nurses say that life during nursing school was a constant juggling act, trying to balance school schedules, study times, work responsibilities, and family and personal needs. However, life after graduation but prior to licensure doesn't automatically get much simpler. The school schedule is gone, but work schedules, study time, and family and personal needs are still part of your life.

One critical difference, though, is that you have achieved a great accomplishment—graduation! This alone shows that you have what it takes, and you must now focus on preparing in earnest for the licensing exam. A critical step in preparing for the exam is to regain the lost balance in your life, physically and mentally. Physical balance means getting back to basics and focusing on diet, rest and sleep, and exercise. Mental balance is achieved by creating a schedule in which you spend the right amount of energy at the right times doing the right things.

Diet

It's easy to give lip service to good nutrition, but it's another thing to follow through. Take time now to pay attention to what you eat and how you plan meals. This doesn't mean that you need to become a gourmet cook. Rather, get back to the basics of eating regular, balanced meals and nutritious snacks. Three small, light, and nutrient-packed meals will provide the fuel your body needs so much better than one large meal at the end of the day (when you're famished and more likely to eat anything you can chew and swallow). Choose snacks that are low in fat and light in calories. Make sure you have enough whole grains and fiber, and drink six to eight glasses of water per day. Cut back on caffeine and drinks with sugar, and keep alcohol intake low. Even after a few days, you should feel a difference in both your energy level and your ability to focus.

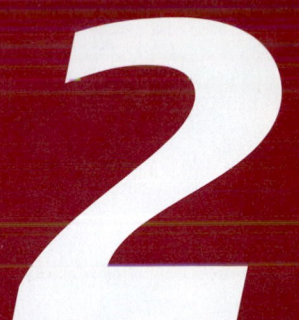

Rest and Sleep

This is another area of your life that probably got short-changed during nursing school. Most people know how many hours of sleep they need to feel rested, usually between 6 and 8 hours per night. Find out what is right for you, and indulge yourself in the sleep you need. Again, you will quickly reap the rewards of increased stamina, energy, and ability to concentrate.

Exercise and Diversional Activity

Most people have some form of physical activity or exercise that they enjoy. Exercise is not only good for the body, it's a stress reliever as well. Pick an activity that you enjoy (aerobic is even better!) and do it regularly. Aerobic exercise will increase your energy, provide a break from studying, and generally benefit your overall health. If you don't really like to exercise, try walking. It's healthy and can be adjusted to any distance and timeframe, depending on the schedule of your day.

Sometimes we all need mental relaxation, which is where diversional activities come into play. As you prepare for the licensing exam, take time to see a movie, go out to eat, visit with friends, or do something else that is fun and makes you happy. This gives you not only a physical break from studying but a mental one as well. Again, when you don't feel short-changed in another area of your life, you are more likely to focus better during your study time.

GENERAL STUDY AND PREPARATION TIPS

The Importance of Self-Assessment

There are two areas of self-assessment that will help you succeed on the NCLEX-RN® licensing examination. The first is to understand your preferred learning style(s), and the second is to understand your relative strengths and areas that need further development before you take the examination.

How Do You Learn Best?

The literature abounds with research about various learning styles, but this discussion focuses on how you use the senses for learning. If you are a visual learner (i.e., you learn best by seeing things), then form a mental picture of what you are studying or the scenario presented in the test question. Look carefully at pictures and diagrams. You may also enjoy reviewing materials on videotape. If you are an auditory learner, then use audiotapes, an MP3 player, or read material out loud as you do your review. You might enjoy listening to tapes while you are driving or doing errands. Keep in mind, though, that you will not be able to read questions aloud during the exam. If you are a kinesthetic learner, then you learn best by doing. You might find it beneficial to write things down as you study. For example, you might make flash cards with facts you find hard to remember. The simple act of writing may help you to retain the information better. You will also reap the benefit of having the flash cards handy to review when you have unexpected spare minutes in your schedule.

What Are Your Relative Strengths and Weaknesses?

Before you make a formal plan for NCLEX-RN® examination preparation, take a few minutes to honestly appraise your areas of relative strength. Write down in order from lowest to highest your areas of strength in nursing content blocks. An example is maternity, child health, psychiatric–mental health, medical surgical, and leadership. If you took any standardized tests that gave you results according to the Client Needs category of the NCLEX-RN® Test Plan, write down the areas from lowest to highest in terms of how you scored. An example might be Health Promotion and Maintenance, Psychosocial Integrity, Physiological Integrity, and Safe Effective Care Environment. This information will form the basis for a formal study plan.

Develop a Study Plan

To make an effective study plan, first determine a target date for testing. Then calculate the number of weeks you have for preparation. Many students take anywhere from 4 to 8 weeks to prepare, but this varies depending on the person's ability, perceived need for study, and availability of appointments near the target test date.

Create a calendar for those weeks that you plan to study. Block off one day per week that you will *not* devote at all to exam preparation. This will help ensure you keep that mental balance we discussed. Next, block off work schedules, appointments, and any other commitments you may have. The holes remaining in your calendar are the times that you have available for review and study. Plan to review approximately 2 hours per day or longer if you have the stamina and feel that you need the extra time. Actual preparation time may vary widely among graduates.

Map out what areas you will review over the course of weeks according to the lists you developed. Write into the calendar the areas to review, beginning with the areas in which you scored lowest and spacing the material out over the weeks you have available. Allow more time to review weaker areas, and less time for areas of identified strength. An advantage to this method is that you will concentrate your efforts most on the areas that need development, and if you run short on time, your areas of strength are the ones that have the least review.

Use this book to guide your review. This book was specifically designed to help you understand how the content blocks that you learned in school fit into the structure of Client Needs in the NCLEX-RN® Test Plan. On average, you should spend approximately one third to one half of your time initially reviewing content in the various chapters, with the other one half to two thirds of the time devoted to answering questions. As a rule, do not use class notes or reread your textbooks. Refer back to them only on an as-needed basis to clarify any areas of confusion or difficulty. Carefully read the answer rationales as well as the test-taking strategies to increase your retention and fine-tune your test-taking abilities. As you progess, you will spend less time on review and more on questions. Try to plan your review sessions for hours that you are normally alert.

Practice tests will also be an important part of your preparation. These are best scheduled on your days off when you have additional study time. In nursing school, your average tests were probably 50 to 100 questions in length. For the NCLEX-RN® examination, you may need to answer 265 questions. Because you can pass taking the maximum number of questions, it is important to have the stamina to answer each question well. To build your test-taking concentration and endurance, take a comprehensive review test once per week, increasing the number of questions each time. Try to work your way from 100 to 125, then to 150, and so on. Try to answer 265 consecutive questions at least a few times before your test date. Tests you took in nursing school prepared you to "sprint to the bus stop," but the licensing exam might be more like "running a marathon." You need to be able to stay strong and concentrate through the whole test. Your test might be only 75 questions, but it could go to 265. Be ready to go the distance! A sample calendar for exam preparation over a 6-week period of time might look like the plan outlined in Table 2–1 ■.

Create a Study Environment

Find a household area that is relatively free of foot traffic and external environmental disturbances, such as television, radio, and the like. Set this area up as your temporary study center. Turn off the telephone and cell phone if you need to. Also turn off any background Internet connection on your computer to avoid the "blinging" noises of instant messages and other pop-ups.

Before you begin a review session, make sure you have created an optimal "internal" study environment as well. Make sure you are not hungry or thirsty. Take a few minutes to relax and deep breathe to clear your mind; this will help you gather your attention for the task at hand and erase any non–test-related problems or issues that you cannot deal with right now anyway. Get focused and go to work! Plan to take a 10-minute break after each 50 to 60 minutes of concentrated review. This will serve both as a reward and as an incentive to go back to studying.

Stick to the Plan and What to Do When You Don't

Try hard to stick to your plan. If you get behind, it's not the end of the world, but review your calendar to see what the problem is. Was the calendar unrealistic, or did you not follow it? Rearrange your calendar if need be and figure out what you must do psychologically if procrastination is the problem. Remember, this period of time is an investment in yourself; do not use it poorly or throw it away! If you get very far behind, consider whether rescheduling the test is in your best interest.

Table 2-1 Sample 6-Week Exam Preparation Calendar

Sunday	Monday	Tuesday	Wednesday	Thursday	Friday	Saturday
6/5 Relax	6/6 (Work) Med-surg and Pharm	6/7 Med-surg, Pharm, and 100-question Phys Integ diagnostic test	6/8 (Work) Med-surg and Pharm	6/9 (Work) Med-surg and Pharm	6/10 (Work) Med-surg and Pharm	6/11 Med-surg, Pharm, and 150-question comprehensive test
6/12 Relax	6/13 (Work) Med-surg and Pharm	6/14 (Work) Med-surg and Pharm	6/15 Med-surg, Pharm, and 175-question comprehensive test	6/16 (Work) Med-surg and Pharm	6/17 (Work) Med-surg, Pharm, and 150-question final Phys Integ test	6/18 Wedding
6/19 Relax	6/20 (Work) Leadership or Fundamentals and 100-question SECE diagnostic test	6/21 (Work) Leadership or Fundamentals	6/22 (Work) Leadership or Fundamentals	6/23 (Work) Leadership or Fundamentals	6/24 Leadership and 200-question comprehensive test	6/25 Leadership or Fundamentals
6/26 Relax	6/27 (Work) Leadership or Fundamentals	6/28 (Work) Leadership or Fundamentals	6/29 Leadership and 150-question final SECE test	6/30 (Work) Maternity and 100-question HPM diagnostic test	7/1 (Work) Maternity	7/2 (Work) Maternity and 225-question comprehensive test
7/3 Relax	7/4 (Work) Maternity	7/5 Maternity and 150-question HPM final test	7/6 (Work) Psych and 100-question Psyc Integ diagnostic test	7/7 (Work) Psych	7/8 (Work) Psych	7/9 Psych and 150-question Psyc Integ final test
7/10 Relax	7/11 (Work) 250-question comprehensive test and review wrong answers	7/12 (Work) 265-question comprehensive test and review wrong answers	7/13 (Work) 265-question comprehensive test and review wrong answers	7/14 Relax; no review!	7/15 NCLEX-RN exam date	7/16 Relax and celebrate

Comprehensive = all test plan areas; HPM = Health Promotion and Maintenance; Med-surg = Medical-Surgical; Pharm = Pharmacology; Phys Integ = Physiological Integrity; Psyc Integ = Psychosocial Integrity; SECE = Safe Effective Care Environment

TEST-TAKING STRATEGIES

Read the Entire Question but Only the Question

Every test question contains all the information you need to know to answer the question. Each question contains three parts.

- The first part presents case-related information about the client in a few sentences or less.
- The second part asks you a specific question about the case provided. These first two parts are sometimes collectively called the question stem, although technically the second part is the stem.
- The third part of the question consists of the options. In a standard multiple-choice question, there are four options, labeled 1 through 4. You must select one of these as the answer. In an alternative item format question, the third part may require typing in numbers, clicking on a diagram, or arranging priorities. Incorrect options are often called distracters.

Box 2-1

The Core Issue of the Question

Sample question stem:
A 39-year-old female client is scheduled for discharge following right mastectomy with breast reconstruction. The nurse places highest priority on teaching the client which of the following points before discharge?

Sample reworded question stem:
What is the most important client teaching point for a client going home after mastectomy and breast reconstruction?

It is important to read every word in the entire question, one at a time. Do not speed-read the question, and do not read into the question anything that is not there. It is easy to read into questions based on your personal experience or the experience of others. Resist the urge to choose your answer based on real-world experiences. This exam represents the ideal world, and the case situation in the question may or may not closely resemble the one with which you have experience. For each question you answer, remember this is the ideal world in which the client in the question is your only client and you have all the supplies and materials you need to deliver care.

Reinterpret the Question to Identify the Core Issue

After you read the question stem but before you read the options, take a moment to reword the question in your head to help you identify the core issue of the question. The core issue is the specific skill, ability, or point of knowledge that is needed to make the correct answer selection. Identifying the core issue may prevent you from getting distracted by the options and subsequently making an incorrect choice. See Box 2–1 for an example of a reworded stem.

Focus on the Client in the Question

In most questions, the actual client presented is the subject of the question, but sometimes the essence of the question is really asking about a significant other, family member or friend, or even another health team member. As you read each question, deliberately determine who is the real client in the question, and choose the option that helps you to answer accordingly.

Find Critical Words in the Question

Critical words in the question help you to discriminate what you need to focus on while answering the question because they put the question into a specific context. The critical words may relate to time, probability, and sequencing of actions or priority setting, as shown in Box 2–2. Be sure to notice these words as you read, because they will help you to discard options that are incorrect answer choices.

Be Alert for Words That Are Red Flags

We do not live in an all-or-nothing world, and nursing practice is not an all-or-nothing endeavor. Watch for words that oversimplify the decision-making process in nursing practice. Examples of these words are *all, every, none, never, always, cannot, must not,* and *only.* You may recognize these words more quickly and easily as you practice more and more questions.

On the other hand, words that are not so extreme could indicate the option is correct. Options that contain words such as *often, usually, likely to,* and *probably* warrant closer examination because they could be part of a correct choice.

Box 2-2

Examples of Critical Words in a Question

Time: early, late, the day before, the day of, the day after, just prior to, immediately following, 1 hour after (or *x* hours after)

Probability: Most likely, least likely, at highest risk, at lowest risk

Sequencing of actions (priority setting): initial, first, last, immediately, highest priority, lowest priority, most appropriate, least appropriate

Identify Positive and Negative Words in Question Stems

Positive or negative words in the question stem help you determine whether to choose an option that is a true statement or one that is a false statement as it relates to the case situation. Many of the questions on the exam will be worded in the affirmative; fewer will use negative words. Consider the following examples, which ask about an identical core issue (discharge teaching information following tonsillectomy) but use positive and negative words that lead to entirely different answers:

- Positive: A 10-year-old child is being discharged to home following tonsillectomy. The nurse determines that the child's caregiver **understands** discharge teaching points after the caregiver makes which of the following statements?
- Negative: A 10-year-old child is being discharged to home following tonsillectomy. The nurse determines that the child's caregiver **needs further instruction** related to discharge teaching after the caregiver makes which of the following statements?

In the first example, the correct answer would be an option that is a true statement about a point of discharge teaching, while in the second, the correct answer would be the option that contains a false statement about a point of discharge teaching. Note how easy it could be to make an incorrect choice by missing the negative words "needs further instruction." Note also that the real client in this question is the child's caregiver, not the child who had surgery.

Eliminate Incorrect Options

Whenever you know an option is incorrect, immediately eliminate it as an answer choice. Sound easy? Yes, but sometimes it is easier said than done. For some questions, you will easily recognize one or more options as incorrect and eliminate them as possible choices. Each time you eliminate such an option, you increase the probability of ultimately choosing the correct answer. For example, if you don't know an answer and randomly choose from among four options, you have a 25% chance of getting the right answer. If you can eliminate one, leaving three to choose from, your odds of success are increased to 33%. If you can narrow down the choices to two options, you now have a 50% chance of making the correct choice. On the NCLEX-RN® examination, however, it is likely that more than one option or all of them may seem to be correct, so read on to the next section for more test-taking strategies.

Carefully Examine Options with Similarities

If you read a question to which you do not know the answer, look for similarities either between the stem and one option or between two of the options. Some possibilities are outlined below, with suggestions to guide your thought process.

Similarities Between the Stem and an Option

If the stem of the question and one of the options contain a similar idea, action, word, or emotion, then that option could be the correct answer. Consider this option carefully as you read all the options and prepare to make a selection.

Similarities Between Two or More Options

This could be a little trickier. If two or more options seem to have a similar idea, action, or response, examine them carefully. If they are essentially saying the same thing but using different words, then neither of them can be correct and you must eliminate them both (or all). If, however, they seem to be saying similar things but one option is more encompassing or global than the other option, it is possible that the more encompassing option is the correct answer choice. You can recognize the encompassing option because it contains the main thought of the other option plus some others within it. Reread the question and all viable choices to help you decide if this should be your selection. Examples of questions to which this strategy could apply are questions about communication processes, interdisciplinary care, or taking action in an emergency.

Recognize the Need to Prioritize

This is a very important test-taking strategy. Because many questions are written at the analysis level of difficulty, expect to get a reasonable number of questions in which all of the options are technically correct actions or responses. You must decide what is the best action or response for that client and situation. Questions such as these require you to engage in priority setting. Universal strategies for prioritizing in nursing are outlined in the following sections.

Maslow's Hierarchy of Needs

Examine the question and analyze if Maslow's Hierarchy of Needs theory applies. When a question or option seems relevant, recall that physiological needs (air/oxygen, water, food, sleep) come first, followed by safety needs. Secondary or psychosocial needs are addressed only after physiological and safety needs are met.

The ABCs: Airway, Breathing, and Circulation

This strategy is very straightforward. Airway takes priority, followed by breathing and then circulation. Remember that oxygen saturation could refer to either airway or breathing and that hypovolemia and hemorrhage relate to circulation.

Least Stable or Most at Risk for Complications

When choosing between which client to visit, assess, or care for first, remember that the correct answer is most likely to be the client that is the least stable of all clients presented or, if all are stable, then the one who is most at risk for developing a serious complication. These questions can be difficult to answer. To make the correct choice for such a question, you must understand up to four different client health problems and their significance, and you must understand principles of clinical decision making or triage. For this reason, it is very important to review the pathophysiology, nursing management, and client education for a wide variety of health problems.

Time/Scheduling

For some questions, priority setting may be guided by events that are time-bound. In questions that involve clients who have specific discharge times or have immediate preoperative or preprocedure status, consider whether the core issue of the question is caring for this client before other stable clients using time as the priority.

Assessment and Teaching

Some nursing activities cannot be delegated to other caregivers, such as licensed practical or vocational nurses (LPNs or LVNs), or unlicensed assistive personnel (UAPs). Priorities of care for the registered nurse include nursing activities such as assessing and teaching clients. These activities should not be delegated to other caregivers, whereas carrying out simple procedures and making routine observations can be delegated. Consider these elements when deciding priorities of care as they relate to delegation.

Use the Nursing Process Effectively

Assessment

Since assessment is the first step of the nursing process, consider when you read a question whether the correct answer is likely to focus on assessment. In general, when questions ask for your first nursing action, look to see how much data is presented in the case situation. If there is no data or just a single piece of data, the correct option is more likely to be an option that gathers more subjective or objective assessment data. If, on the other hand, you have a complete set of data presented to you, an option that reflects further assessment or assessment of a low-priority item is not as likely to be correct.

Analysis

Analysis questions require critical thinking and clinical decision making skills. These questions present physiological or psychosocial data in the case situation and ask you to interpret the information so you can take action based on the data or respond in a therapeutic way to the data. In any event, you need to draw the correct conclusions from the data in order to select the correct answer. Analysis questions are often difficult because they require interpretation of one or several pieces of data.

Planning

The planning step of the nursing process involves developing a plan of care, setting goals and/or establishing outcomes, and determining priorities of care. Because the plan must be communicated to others in the health care team, these questions may also involve interdisciplinary communication and collaboration.

Implementation

Questions that address the implementation step of the nursing process are action-oriented. They require you to supervise and delegate care; manage care; carry out interventions; teach clients; provide counseling; communicate with clients, families, and interdisciplinary team members; and document the outcomes of care. These types of questions are also often combined with priority setting, so again you need to use clinical decision making skills in selecting an option.

Evaluation

Questions that address this step of the nursing process require you to determine whether a client has met the expected outcomes of care. They may require you to determine any of the following:

- Whether the plan of care has been effective
- Whether a client has achieved the goals of care (returned to normal status or client's original baseline)
- Whether a client or family member understands how to care for a client following discharge (diet, activity, medications, and follow-up care)
- Whether the client has adequate knowledge of the underlying health problem
- Whether a health team member is performing care correctly
- Whether revisions to the plan of care are necessary

Because they involve clinical judgment and decision making, these questions are also more likely to be written at an analysis rather than application level of difficulty.

Strategies for Subsections of the Test Plan

Although there are many ways to write questions that address each part of the test plan, certain types of questions seem to naturally align with specific parts of the test plan. These types of questions include those utilizing communication and scientific principles and those addressing pharmacology.

Communication

Questions addressing communication have a natural affinity for the Psychosocial Integrity category of Client Needs. These questions require you to apply therapeutic communication skills. The correct answer will contain the most therapeutic statement, focus on the client's feelings, and/or assist the client to work toward therapeutic goals. Although communication strategies and communication blocks were part of your foundational nursing curriculum, they bear review and practice. Questions related to communication may have several options that seem similar in some ways, but different in others. You must be able to choose which one is *most* therapeutic. It is not uncommon for nursing graduates to say they either really like or really dislike communication questions.

Use of Scientific Principles

The use of everyday scientific principles is an all but unheard-of strategy for answering test questions. Yet, scientific principles play a key role in assisting you to answer some questions that are typically part of the Physiological Integrity category of Client Needs. Consider, for example, how gravity may affect your answers to questions about positioning clients, troubleshooting IV flow rate problems, and monitoring various tubes and drains. Consider how concepts of pressure affect your answers to questions about flail chest, mechanical ventilation, intracranial pressure, the Valsalva maneuver, stopping bleeding, and so on. If you visualize these options in terms of how they are affected by pressure, you may be able to eliminate one or more incorrect options.

Pharmacology

When answering questions related to pharmacology, look at both the generic name and the trade name provided. If you recognize the drug, use your knowledge about it to answer the question. If not, try next to determine what classification the medication belongs to by looking at the syllables in the name. For example, a medication that ends in *-mycin* is either an antibacterial agent or antitumor antibiotic. If you cannot determine the classification, try to look for hints in the case situation, such as the client's diagnosis. If none of these strategies work, look for other words in the question that provide clues.

Read the Memory Aid boxes contained in the pharmacology chapters in this book to learn common prefixes and suffixes that will enable you to recognize drugs more easily on sight. Also use general principles of medication administration, such as the following:

- Administer medications in the doses ordered without changing the dose or discontinuing the medication. You may need to withhold a single dose for a specific reason, such as withholding digoxin (Lanoxin) for a pulse rate of 48, or withholding metoprolol (Lopressor) for a blood pressure less than 90 systolic.
- Question an order if any part of the order is unclear.
- Look for endings such as XL, SR, and others that indicate a medication is sustained release. If present, do not crush or break the medication and do not allow the client to chew it.
- Do not take over-the-counter medications with a prescribed medication without checking with the physician first.
- Teach clients to avoid drinking alcohol while taking medications. This is especially true for medications that are central nervous system (CNS) depressants because alcohol also depresses the nervous system.

References

Katz, J., Carter, C., Bishop, J., & Kravits, S. (2004). *Keys to nursing success* (2nd ed.). Upper Saddle River, NJ: Prentice Hall.

National Council of State Boards of Nursing, Inc. (2006). *NCLEX-RN® examination. Test plan for the National Council licensure examination for registered nurses. Effective Date: April 2007.* Chicago, IL: Author.

National Council of State Boards of Nursing, Inc. (2004). *2004 NCLEX® invitational: Constructing the NCLEX® of the future.* Chicago, IL: Author.

National Council of State Boards of Nursing, Inc. Web site: http://www.ncsbn.org.

3 Test Preparation for International Nurses

Test Yourself

Are you ready for the NCLEX-RN® or course exams? Use the practice tests on the companion CD-ROM to check.

In this chapter

Although you are experienced and have been practicing as a nurse in your country of origin, it may feel as though you are starting all over again as you prepare for licensure in the United States. One set of concerns relates to completing all the requirements to be eligible for licensure in the United States. Another set relates to preparing for and passing the NCLEX-RN® Licensing Examination. This chapter explores your unique concerns and explains how this book can assist you in your preparation for the NCLEX-RN® exam. To help you meet eligibility requirements, contact the following sources:

- Commission on Graduates of Foreign Nursing Schools (COGFNS): this organization will help you obtain a COGFNS certificate, which is currently required by 42 state boards of nursing in the United States. A COGFNS certificate can be issued once the Commission reviews your original nursing program and your credentials and after you pass the COGFNS exam of general nursing knowledge and demonstrate proficiency in the English language by passing the Test of English as a Foreign Language (TOEFL). You can obtain free information and an application by calling 215-349-8767 or via the Internet at http://www.cgfns.org.
- International Commission on Healthcare Professions: This organization can assist you with information related to visa requirements and how to obtain one if you are already in the United States. Write the Commission at 3600 Market St., Suite 400, Philadelphia, PA 19104-2665 or call 215-349-6735. Other sources of this information are regional U.S. offices of the Immigration and Naturalization Service or the U.S. consulate or embassy in your country.

SCOPE OF NURSING PRACTICE

Depending on the country in which you work as a nurse, your current nursing practice may be similar to or very different from nursing practice in the United States. For example, nurses from India, the Philippines, Poland, and Great Britain all have very different backgrounds and experiences in nursing practice, and those differences vary by degree from nursing practice in the United States. One key area is the scope of nursing practice.

Nurses belong to a profession that self-regulates its practice through a variety of nursing organizations and state boards of nursing. There are well-defined standards of professional nursing practice for all areas of nursing. Because nurses are members of this profession, there is a high level of accountability by the individual nurse for his or her own nursing practice.

Nurses meet the individual needs of each of their patients or clients. Some clients need to have all of their physical care performed for them. Some need various degrees of assistance. Others are able to do self-care but need supervision for safety reasons. Whatever the required level of care, nurses meet that need.

Nurses are responsible for knowing about the health problems of clients and teaching them and their families how to manage their health problems at home. This means that, in addition to being knowledgeable about health problems, nurses have to know basic teaching and learning principles and use them effectively in practice.

Nurses have an important voice as members of the health care team. Nurses routinely communicate with other nurses, nursing supervisors, physicians, pharmacists, nutritionists and dietitians, respiratory therapists, physical and occupational therapists, social workers, and unlicensed assistive personnel. Communication is direct but respectful and includes acting as an advocate for the client if health needs are not being met by the current plan of care.

Nurses are holistic in their approach to clients. They are able to use communication skills to psychologically support the client and family, and they must also be comfortable working with highly technical equipment. For this reason, nursing practice in the United States is often considered both an art and a science.

Nurses play a key role in helping clients to stay healthy, not just helping them to recover from disease or injury. For this reason, health promotion (which commonly involves teaching) is also an important part of nursing practice.

Nurses are responsible for their own professional growth and seek opportunities to further their knowledge of nursing as it advances as a discipline through research. Nurses read books and journal articles, attend conferences, and use the Internet to help them stay abreast of new advances in nursing knowledge.

WORKING WITH A VARIETY OF CULTURES

In the United States there are people from many cultures. Part of the role of the nurse is to be competent in caring for people from a variety of backgrounds. This means not only respecting the culture of various clients but also understanding some of their key beliefs and changing the plan of care to accommodate culturally based customs and rituals when possible. Aspects of one's personal culture that tend to influence health include the amount of control one has over one's environment, physical and genetic differences, social environment, communication patterns, need for space, and orientation to time (Giger & Davidhizar, 2004). See Chapter 20 in this book for more information about delivering culturally competent care.

THERAPEUTIC COMMUNICATION

One of the key tools used by nurses practicing in the United States is communication. The special type of communication used in working with clients is called *therapeutic communication.* Nurses in the United States use eye contact while communicating with clients, which may be similar or different from the practice in your country of origin. Facial expressions and body language are also used to enhance the client's understanding of communication.

The content of communication between nurses and clients is client-centered and relates to the steps of the nursing process. The focus may be on obtaining health information from clients (assessment), goal-setting with clients about their care and its outcomes (planning), discussing how clients are experiencing or reacting to their care (implementation), and determining how effective the care was (evaluation). See Chapter 19 for more detailed information about therapeutic communication.

PHARMACOLOGY

Pharmacology may present special concerns for foreign-educated nurses. Not only do medications differ somewhat among countries but in some instances drugs that use the same names are entirely different medications! In the United States, nurses must possess significant knowledge about the medications being administered, how to safely administer them, and how to recognize and intervene if adverse effects are experienced. Nurses also teach clients about their medications and how to self-administer them. Because the body of knowledge for pharmacology is so large and keeps growing, see Chapters 30 through 46 for a review of this aspect of practice.

THE LICENSING EXAMINATION

The examination that you took to obtain your original nursing license may have been very different than the predominantly multiple-choice style used in the United States. The reason for this style of exam is that there are very large numbers of nurses who seek licensure each year. The use of computer-adaptive testing and multiple-choice questions is the quickest and most valid method currently available for determining that nursing school graduates are safe to practice. If you are not comfortable taking multiple-choice exams, read Chapter 2 carefully, and read it more than once if you have the need. Also, be sure to practice several hundred to thousands of questions to develop a sense of ease with this type of question. Also practice the alternate format styles of questions, which are being used in small numbers on the NCLEX-RN®examination. Use all of the tips and strategies presented in this book, and work with a mentor, if you have one, to help you succeed in the shortest possible time.

References

Giger, D., & Davidhizer, R. (2004). *Transcultural nursing: Assessment and intervention* (4th ed.). St. Louis, MO: Elsevier.

National Council of State Boards of Nursing. (2006). *NCLEX-RN® examination. Test plan for the National Council licensure examination for registered nurses. Effective Date: April 2007.* Chicago, IL: Author.

The NCLEX-RN® Examination Through the Candidate's Eyes

4

This chapter gives you an opportunity to hear directly from a few recent graduates who took the NCLEX-RN® licensing examination. Some basic questions were posed to them; the questions and their responses are outlined below. Each person has a unique perspective, and each one is valid, just as your own will be. Take and use what you can from them. They all wish you well! Thanks to the following graduates listed in alphabetical order, who shared their words of wisdom; I am thrilled that you are now my colleagues.

Veronica Baba, RN
Lisa Caparrotta, RN
Kerry Ferrara, RN
Meredith Hartlieb, RN
Jenny Massengill, RN

Test Yourself

Are you ready for the NCLEX-RN® or course exams? Use the practice tests on the companion CD-ROM to check.

What did you do to prepare in the months and weeks prior to the NCLEX-RN® exam, and how useful do you believe your strategies were?

RN 1, First-time pass at 75 questions: During the months prior to taking the exam, I took an NCLEX® review class offered at a local college. This class was one week long and it intensely went over as much of the nursing curriculum as possible. There were also test-taking strategies and NCLEX®-like questions throughout the course. Though not even a fraction of the stuff reviewed in the class was covered in the exam, I felt much more confident going into the exam. I also sat down almost every night two weeks prior to taking the exam, in a quiet room without distraction, and practiced NCLEX® questions. I would do a minimum of 100, working my way up to 265 (like you told us to!). This not only helped me prepare by getting accustomed to the type of questions that the exam might ask, it also helped me develop the stamina in case I had to answer all of the questions on the exam. I also would review with fellow new grads using flash cards. Because it was late spring, early summer, I would sit outside and have my friends or boyfriend quiz me. Now I'll be honest with you, I didn't go crazy with studying. I did study a lot, but not excessively. I took it easy, and I studied on my own time instead of scheduling it into my day. I tried to make it more enjoyable by studying with others. I'm the type of person that I would have stressed myself out if I tried to cover all of the material that I had learned in school. I covered all of the main areas, but definitely did not go over *everything.* I tried to be confident in the fact that I had just graduated from nursing school and would not have if I weren't adequately prepared for the exam.

RN 2, First-time pass at 75 questions: I prepared for the NCLEX® by taking a review course and doing the assignments. After graduation, I really began to give it my all by answering as many questions a day as possible. In the first weeks after graduation, I read the materials and answered questions in workbooks as well as on CDs. Then, for the last four weeks before the test, I focused on CDs mainly so that I could get used to the computer format of answering questions. I increased my tolerance for questions at one sitting and was finally taking 265 questions in one sitting two times a day. If it was an especially busy day, I would take 100-question computer tests three to four times a day. I actually got pretty fast. Using test-taking strategies helped so much.

RN 3, First time pass at 75 questions: I enrolled in an NCLEX® review course offered by my university that ran for the duration of my final semester, meeting one evening a week. Unfortunately for me, it required a significant commute following a full day at my internship site. I did not give the course the attention that I had hoped to when I signed up for it, and I often felt that I was lagging behind the other students in the course. However, it forced me to review the contents of my nursing program to some degree. Without this course, I am sure I would have procrastinated until after graduation to begin studying for the NCLEX®. I feel like it did give me a definite advantage in organizing my study schedule, reviewing topics, and primarily knowing how to read and interpret NCLEX®-type questions. After completing this course, I continued to review the NCLEX® review book, CD-ROMs, and some of my class notes.

RN 4, Second-time pass at 97 questions: The first time I studied for the test, I tried to memorize information rather than practice strategies and test-taking skills. When the test was getting closer, I realized it was very hard to recall so much information, so then I started practicing test-taking strategies. I was very stressed and let all of this studying workload overwhelm me. A number of family concerns also distracted me. After graduation, I spent a lot of time helping in the preparation of my brother's wedding. In addition, I worried about the inguinal hernia that my grandfather had, which would be repaired days after my test. I was also thinking about my own bright future and spending some time with my friends and not thinking about the test like I should have. When the time of the test came, I felt like there were many things I did not do that I should have.

The first test shut off at 131 questions, and I got a near passing average on all test sections. The second time (after a severe denial stage), I took time off to get ready again. This time I had the chance to gather my thoughts and do what I did not do the first time. I got away from all of my "friends," I did not compromise myself with too many activities, and I scheduled my studying time more thoroughly; [I learned] to be more assertive by saying, "No, I can't, I'm studying!"

I reviewed every system (not too much detail, just general overall concepts). Then I practiced all the test-taking strategies with the practice tests. With the strategies plus knowledge plus practice and perseverance, plus a lot of prayer, I finally felt confident to do it one more time. I took my test again, and this time it shut off at 97 questions and I passed!

RN 5, Third-time pass at 75 questions: To prepare for the NCLEX-RN® exam, I set up a schedule. Each day, I would read through a chapter or so and take notes on the topics that I felt were important or that I felt that I needed to learn more about. After each chapter, I would also do between 50 and 100 questions a night. When it became closer to the exam, I increased the number of practice questions I did each night. I also took a course in which there was a lot of repetition of the test-taking strategies during each class.

What was the actual testing center like? Did anything surprise you?

RN 1: Prior to the exam, I had gone to the testing center so that I would know how to get there, and I even went up to the office where the exam was held to be exactly sure of where it was. Walking in on the day of the exam, there were a lot of *nervous* future nurses. [The staff] asked for ID, a signature, and a fingerprint. It's probably the most tightly secured thing that I have ever done. You have to remove all outer clothing. I had a zip sweater on that I had to remove, as well as my watch—that surprised me. Then we were escorted into an exam room, fingerprinted before entering, and brought into a room that looked much like any computer lab, only with dividers between the computers. It was completely silent in the room other than the rapid mouse clicking and occasional sigh. During the exam, you are being video and voice recorded. There's a lot of tension in that room!

RN 2: The testing center was nice. The actual room that I took the test in was very comfortable, quiet, no distractions. The staff was very nice and friendly and seemed to understand how important this test was.

RN 3: The testing center was lacking in personality—that's for sure. It was very drab with a row of darkly colored cubicles, each containing one computer terminal for test-takers. They were relatively close to one another, which was a little distracting, but we were provided with earplugs to muffle the sounds of keyboards nearby. All of our belongings were secured in a locker in the reception area.

RN 4: At the test-taking center, the people were awesome. The test-taking center was very organized, professional, clean, and met all of my expectations. I would not say that anything surprised me except that I did not know I was going to be visually and audibly recorded at the computer station during the test.

RN 5: At the actual test center, the staff was very helpful and friendly. I only had to wait about 5 minutes from the time I walked in the door until I sat down at my computer. Having my own private section made me feel like I was the only one in the room.

How did you handle the stress of taking the exam and the waiting period until you received your results?

RN 1: Before the exam, I took a trial run to the exam location. This reduced the stress of having to worry about finding it on exam day. The night before the exam, I did nothing related to NCLEX®. I went out to eat with my boyfriend and went to see a movie. When I got home that night, I went over the instructions on what to bring with me and what to leave behind, gathered everything, including every form of ID I owned (not necessary by the way—a credit card and license is all they need), attempted to look over the NCLEX® one more time before having my book taken from me by my boyfriend, and went to bed early. The morning of the exam, I got up early, ate breakfast, took a long shower with some relaxing aromatherapy bath gel that my friend bought me to help me relax (I don't think that it worked, but I would have tried anything!), dressed in comfortable clothing, and went to the exam . . . trying to keep myself calm the whole way there.

During the exam, I tried to keep myself as calm as possible. If I found myself getting too anxious or worked up, I would stop what I was doing, close my eyes, and take some deep breaths. A nurse that I work with told me to picture a stop sign in my head, all of its details, and spell stop. I think that I did that once. I also found myself whispering, "It's okay, you can do this. It's only a test." I can only imagine what I must have looked like. In taking the exam, I tried not to focus too much on one question. I tried to read through it, maybe even twice at times, pick the answer that I thought was the absolute best in my mind (the most right out of all the possible answers), click next, and move on. At one point, about halfway through the exam, I found myself, in my mind, and maybe out loud at some point, swearing, as the questions seemed to blend together and none of the answers looked right. But again, I tried to calm myself down, focus, and pick the best possible answer. Sometimes the very next question seemed to give the answer to the one before that I had struggled with—but I tried to move past that one and focus on the one in front of me. Remember that there is no back button on the computer, so once you submit your answer, it's gone, move on. It took me about 45 minutes for the whole process, from start to finish. I answered the last question and then the dreaded blue screen came up. That was it. This test that I had prepared for for 4 years was done, just like that.

I think that I might have made it outside of the office before I started crying; I'm not quite sure. I did, though, cry the whole way home. I called my boyfriend and cried about how I had failed and how horrible I did on the exam. In my mind, there was no way that I could have passed it.

Now I may be a little more dramatic than most; I tried to carry on my normal life, but I didn't. I moped for two solid days, complaining about how I failed the NCLEX®, wanting in the worst way to call and reschedule the test so that I could take it again. I paid the $8 to find out early. I was so nervous to see the results that I had my friends find out the results while I waited in the other room, on the verge of hyperventilating or passing out or crying my eyes out. But then, there it was, on the computer screen, I passed! I was at work, where I worked as a nurse's aide and had been hired as a nurse pending [my passing] the NCLEX®, when I found out. So I found out there, and literally a minute later, my boss came down the hall and said, congratulations, gave me a hug, and called me into her office to go over my schedule to start orientation!

RN 2: I handled the stress prior to taking the test by putting all my nervous energy into test preparation, answering questions, and reviewing weak areas. I also planned fun outings with my kids and walked every night. Handling the waiting period for the test results—that was worse than preparing for the exam. I think I must have checked the Web site for my results 100 times a day! I just tried to distract myself by going to movies, going swimming, and keeping busy.

RN 3: I was okay once the exam began. I was a wreck the evening before and the morning of the exam. I was sure to get a good night's sleep and to get up early enough to have breakfast and get to the site in time. When the exam was in progress, I just focused on each question as best I could, took my time, but knew to move on if I was stuck and wasting time. I tried to pace myself to have time to complete all questions in the allotted time if that was my fate. Thankfully, it was not. I kept repeating in my mind, "remember your ABCs" and other tricks to pick the best answers. The waiting period was not too bad. I spoiled myself with a facial, massage, and lots of good food! I had a good feeling when I left the exam site, and it proved right, as I passed.

RN 4: I went to the gym almost every day, got myself on a healthy diet so I could have another goal on my mind, spent a lot of time with my family, went to church, and read the Bible. I focused on other very important things, like my health and soul.

RN 5: I handled the stress of taking the exam by listening to soothing music and trying to relax after studying before I went to bed. During the two days that I had to wait for my results, I kept busy. I got a massage and went out to dinner and a show.

What words of advice do you have for future graduates preparing for the NCLEX-RN® licensing exam?

RN 1: I recommend taking a review class. The instructor will review the basics and go over test-taking strategies. There is no way to know what will be on the exam, but taking the classes will at least give you the confidence to know that you have reviewed and have a basic knowledge of almost every area that could be covered. Also, do questions, questions, and more questions. It's just like anything. The more you practice, the better you become. If you can devote even 30 minutes a night to practicing, it will make you better prepared when it comes time to take the exam. I practiced with friends, both nursing and non-nursing. Make it fun, go outside, or practice with a group—anything to make yourself practice questions. Also, go over the rationales for the questions. This will help you understand why the correct answer is the best one.

Go to the site of the exam beforehand and make sure that you know exactly where the exam is. It reduces stress on exam day. Don't do anything NCLEX® related the night before the exam. Do something fun (and alcohol free) to relax and take your mind off of things. There is no use cramming the night before. It will just make you more stressed about the stuff that maybe you think that you haven't reviewed enough. On the morning of the exam, eat breakfast and give yourself extra time to get ready.

If you find yourself getting too stressed during the exam, take a minute and relax, breathe deeply, and do all of those relaxation techniques that they taught us in nursing school. It will only hurt you in the end if you let nerves get the best of you. Don't spend too much time on one question. If you are really unsure of the answer, read the question again. If that doesn't help, pick the best answer that you can, click next, and move on. Try to focus on the question in front of you, not the one before it, not the one to come. Answer the one on the screen and go to the next. So what if you got it wrong, there are still a bunch more questions to come, and you need to stay focused. Don't freak out if you go past 75. All it means it that you still have a chance to pass. One more question means one more passing answer.

Finally, and above all, *relax.* The NCLEX® is only a test. So much emphasis is placed on this exam when, in reality, it's just another test. Nursing school is challenging in itself. Have confidence in yourself. If you can make it through nursing school, then you can pass this test.

RN 2: The words of advice I can offer are to try to keep it in perspective—it is not the end of the world if you have to retake the exam. Just focus on getting used to answering as many questions as you can before the test.

RN 3: I think preparing for it during your final semester of nursing school and taking the exam shortly after graduation is the best course of action. That way the materials are all fresh in your mind, and having a target date motivates you to study.

RN 4: One, pray, or whatever works for you. Two, take all the time you need. Three, get away from all distractions (boyfriend, parties, friends). Four, exercise, diet, get pretty, *never* put yourself down. Five, enjoy leisure time (shopping, playing cards, video games, X-box, whatever). Six, last but not least, bring into the test *two baskets,* the first to *win* and pass that test, and the second to be *willing to try again,* because you are not the only one who is either going through this or has gone through this.

RN 5: I recommend a course to future graduates preparing for the NCLEX-RN® licensing exam. If for some reason you do not pass, it is not the end of the world. Don't give up. Reschedule and take it again. I feel that is does not reflect whether or not you are going to be a good nurse. You have already accomplished so much by graduating from nursing school. You already know the material. You just have to relax and take your time.

5 Legal and Ethical Nursing Practice

Test Yourself

Are you ready for the NCLEX-RN® or course exams? Use the practice tests on the companion CD-ROM to check.

In this chapter

Cross reference

Other chapters relevant to this content area are

Leadership and Management — Chapter 6

I. ETHICS, MORALS, AND VALUES

A. ***Ethics***

1. A branch of philosophy that seeks to utilize a body of knowledge to determine what is right or wrong
2. **ANA Code of Ethics for Nurses** !
   a. Developed by the American Nurses Association to provide guidance to nurses and protection for clients and families
   b. Guidelines delineate values and standards for professional practice
   c. Key elements include compassion and respect, commitment, advocacy, and **accountability** when working with clients, families, and communities, as well as responsibility to the profession

B. Morals

1. Personal philosophy based on what is right or wrong, good or bad
2. Applying ethics is practical way of putting morals into practice; leads to decision making and problem solving
3. Ethical considerations define morals essential to practice

C. Values

1. Are personally and professionally developed and based on philosophy and principles
2. Define actions and reactions to issues and problems
3. Provide guidance in determining actions; socialization and experiences help mold personal value system

II. ETHICAL PRINCIPLES AND DECISION MAKING

A. Ethical principles

1. Autonomy: freedom to make decisions that affect self and to take action for self; is self-governing; includes four basic elements of respect for others, ability to determine personal goals, complete understanding of choice, and freedom to implement plan or choice
2. Beneficence: to act in the best interest of others; to contribute to the well-being of others; includes client advocacy; has three major components: to promote good, prevent harm or evil, and remove harm or evil
3. Paternalism: acting in a fatherly or motherly manner; usually restricts client's autonomy and coerces decision making
4. Justice: fair, equitable, and appropriate treatment; resources are distributed equally to all
5. Fidelity: remaining faithful to ethical principles and ANA Code of Ethics for Nurses; keeping commitments and promises
6. Virtues: compassion, discernment, trustworthiness, and integrity; virtue ethics emphasize character of moral agent
7. Confidentiality: to maintain privacy of client and family; nondisclosure of data or personal information; is a component of ANA Code of Ethics for Nurses as well as HIPAA (Health Information Portability and Accountability Act)

Memory Aid

All interactions, even ordinary ones, between client and nurse utilize principles of ethical behavior. Memorize these principles to be able to engage in effective decision making as a nursing professional.

B. Ethical decision making

1. Nursing is based on ethics of care, including medical indications, client preferences, quality of life, and contextual factors
2. Nurses are required to make numerous ethical decisions every day; differences in clients' values, culture, and lifestyles often present nurses and other health care providers with ethical dilemmas
3. The perspective of principalism in ethics ignores the socioeconomic and cultural contexts and is too abstract to have practical application in clinical practice

III. LEGAL PARAMETERS OF NURSING PRACTICE

A. Practice of nursing must be done within confines of law; nurses must know law and parameters of nursing license

B. Legal limits of nursing are dictated by state and federal laws and guidelines and regulated by each state's Board of Nursing

1. Constitution: law of the land; defines structure, power, and limits of government; guarantees fundamental rights and liberty; other laws may not infringe on rights granted by Constitution
2. Statutory laws: laws enacted by legislative branch of government; includes licensing laws, guardianship codes, statutes of limitation, informed consent, living will legislation, protective and reporting laws; regulatory agencies are established through statutes
3. Common laws: judge-made law, derived from court decisions that establish a precedent by which other cases are judged
4. Administrative laws: laws made by administrative agencies such as a state board of nursing
5. Good Samaritan laws: designed to protect those who aid victims in emergencies; statutes vary among states; care rendered must be free of charge and done in good faith; will not protect nurse when there is gross negligence; once aid is offered, must stay with victim until stable or another provider with equal or greater training takes over

C. Licensure

1. Credential determined by state boards of nursing; qualifies individual to perform designated skills and services; requires completion of a nursing

curriculum that leads to successful passage of a licensing examination in order to be issued

2. **Nurse Practice Act** determines the scope of practice for a professional nurse in a specific state
   a. Establishes guidelines by which nurses can perform skills or services
   b. Is a set of state statutes (rules and regulations) that provide guidance to professional nurses
   c. Establishes educational, examination, and behavioral standards for nurses that protect public
   d. To enforce requirements, each state has a Board of Registration in Nursing to oversee implementation of Nurse Practice Act by nurses across care delivery settings

D. Sanctions against nursing license

1. Boards of nursing in state of licensure can deny, suspend, or revoke license to practice as registered nurse on basis of authority granted in state statute
2. Possible reasons for disciplinary action or sanction
   a. Unprofessional conduct
   b. Conduct that could negatively affect public health and welfare
   c. Accepting and carrying out assignments incorrectly or with insufficient preparation
   d. Physical or verbal abuse of client
   e. Breach of confidentiality
   f. Improper delegation of care that places client at risk for harm
   g. Failure to maintain accurate client record or falsifying client record
   h. Abandonment; leaving an assignment without proper notification and approval
   i. Failure to engage in continuing education activities as required by state statute

IV. LIABILITY IN NURSING PRACTICE

A. Liability: nurses are responsible and accountable for incorrect or inappropriate actions or inactions

B. *Negligence*: unintentional failure to act as a reasonable person in similar circumstance would act that results in injury to another; elements include the following

1. Duty: nurse has responsibility to care for and watch over client as a component of employment; duty indicates legal relationship between client and nurse
2. Breech of duty: nurse fails to complete this duty; this can include acts of commission (activities nurse did) or omission (activities nurse failed to do)
3. Injury occurred: client has suffered physical, emotional, or financial injuries
4. Proximate cause: there is a reasonably close causal connection between nurse's conduct and resulting injury
5. Actual loss or damage resulting from conduct

C. *Malpractice*: negligence by a professional; professional failure to carry out or perform duties that result in injury of another; scope of practice should be delineated in order to operate within it

1. Boundaries of malpractice are defined by statute, rules, and educational requirement
2. Malpractice is usually filed as a civil tort; a court finding of guilty usually results in restitution
3. Nurses may carry personal malpractice insurance to provide for restitution if malpractice occurs
4. Rarely are malpractice charges filed as criminal charges (in which a guilty verdict results in punishment, either jail or capital punishment)

D. Miscellaneous legal charges

1. Assault: threat of harm or unwanted contact with client that causes the client fear
2. Battery: a purposeful touching of client without that client's consent
3. Invasion of privacy: can result from violations of confidentiality
4. Fraud: deliberately deceiving client for purpose of unlawful gains

5. Defamation of character: sharing client information with a third party that results in damage to client's reputation; can occur in the form of slander (oral) or libel (in writing)
6. False imprisonment
   a. Prohibiting a client from leaving a health care facility with no legal justification
   b. Using chemical or physical restraints without satisfactory clinical evidence of need

! **E. Nursing activities to reduce risk of liability**

1. Practice within provisions of state Nurse Practice Act
2. Follow ANA Code of Ethics for Nurses and standards of professional practice
3. Treat every client with kindness and respect
4. Maintain confidentiality by not sharing client information with a third party without client's consent; do not share chart or medical record information without written client consent and then do so only in accordance with agency policies and procedures; see also next item
5. Avoid violations of HIPAA
   a. Protect client's personal identifying information (such as name, social security number, date of birth) and information about diagnosis or treatment
   b. Share information only with individuals involved directly in client's care, payment for care, and/or management of client's care
   c. Verify identity of persons asking for client information
   d. Dispose of confidential documents in accordance with agency policy (such as shredder, locked recycle bin)
   e. Keep contents of medical record out of public view
   f. Discuss client's care only in areas where conversation cannot be overheard
6. Document client assessments, interventions, and events factually and timely in medical record
7. Document on appropriate "against medical advice" forms when a competent client refuses care despite explanations about the benefits of that care
8. Maintain skills and knowledge base by completing continuing education programs
9. Recognize personal strengths and weaknesses; seek help when facing new experiences and job requirements

V. SAFEGUARDING CLIENT RIGHTS

A. Client rights

1. Patient's Bill of Rights communicates to clients and health care workers that clients are entitled to specific rights during care
2. Key rights include confidentiality (see previous discussion), informed consent, and others listed in following text that affect client self-determination

! **B. Informed consent**

1. A legal protection of client's right to choose type of care desired and make own decisions about health care
2. Required before care is provided except in an emergency situation or when client is unresponsive (assumption is that client would consent if able)
3. Must meet three requirements: client has mental capacity to consent; it is voluntarily done; and client understands treatment and information presented by provider of treatment
4. Information shared in process of obtaining consent consists of proposed treatment, procedure, surgery, or other care; associated risks and benefits; and alternatives to treatment; client has opportunity to ask questions and have them answered by provider of treatment
5. Obtaining informed consent is responsibility of physician or other health care provider performing treatment, procedure, or surgery
6. Nurses may witness signature of client on appropriate consent form validating that the client is actually the person signing the form and has no further questions; does not indicate provision of information by the nurse or understanding by the client

7. Occasionally clients do not want to hear details of planned procedures but do wish to consent to them; clients may waive right to informed consent, but waiver must be documented in medical record
8. Special considerations in informed consent
   a. If client is deemed by court of law incompetent to make informed decisions about health care, a court-appointed guardian makes these decisions
   b. Informed consent for minors is obtained from parent or legal guardian except in emergency situations, when minor is married or emancipated from parents, or with special needs for care, such as with sexually transmitted disease or pregnancy

Memory Aid

The chart of a typical hospitalized client could have up to three types of consents: the general consent for treatment signed at the time of admission, a consent for a surgical procedure or other type of invasive procedure, and a consent for anesthesia.

C. Privileged communication versus duty to disclose
1. Communications between clients and health care workers cannot be shared with others outside health care team (such as in court of law) unless client consents
2. Duty to disclose is health care professional's obligation to warn identified individuals if a client has made a credible threat to harm such individuals

! **D. Advance directives**
1. A document completed by a competent client outlining care desired should client become unable to make own decisions in the future
2. Advance directives provide guidance to the health care team and are followed if client's decision-making powers become impaired
3. Copy must be placed in medical record
4. Physician or other primary care provider is notified of advance directive so that orders can be written that are consistent with wishes of client

E. Health care proxy: a competent individual named by a client to have authority to make health care decisions on behalf of client during specified circumstances; may be designated at time of preparing advance directives

! **F. Organ/tissue donation**
1. Clients 18 years of age or older may choose to donate organs
2. Consent can be given through will, advance directive, or donor card
3. Decision can be made in advance when client is alive and competent or may be made at time of death by family
4. All 50 states utilize Uniform Anatomical Gift Act to procure cadaver organs for transplant
5. Transplant considerations
   a. Bereaved family must be approached with compassion by defined personnel in requesting a discussion on organ donation
   b. Goal is to assist those in need of transplant with organ necessary to prolong life
   c. Clinical death is defined as having no brain waves, no spontaneous breathing, and no superficial or deep reflexes
   d. Transplant team recovers organs after consent is obtained

VI. SAFEGUARDING LEGAL PROFESSIONAL PRACTICE

A. Physician orders
1. Determine prescriptive course of treatment for health care team; guide course of action for client and family
2. Typically includes orders for medications, diet, activity, diagnostic and laboratory testing, and procedures or treatments
3. Nurses must legally carry out physician's orders unless believed to be inaccurate
4. Nurse is obligated to question or clarify an order that is unclear or believed to be inappropriate
5. Physician's orders should be scrutinized for legibility and accuracy; when in doubt, they must be clarified with physician

B. Incident reports

1. Each agency develops a policy or protocol for reporting unusual or adverse events involving clients
2. Incident reports are communication tools designed to provide information to risk managers and administration about potential areas of exposure to liability; they may be used in legal cases
3. Incident reports are used to identify problems and develop solutions to prevent same incident from happening again
4. When completing an incident report, fill out form in accurate, complete, and factual manner
5. Do not place copy in client record or make reference to incident report in client record
6. Do record facts of incident in medical record

C. Risk management

1. A program designed to protect client and nurse from harm and protect organization from liability related to harm
2. A comprehensive risk management program includes organizational commitment to employee health and safety, a comprehensive worksite risk analysis, employee participation, and hazard prevention and control, including waste management

D. Reporting to external authorities or governing bodies

1. Nurses and physicians are required to report specific communicable diseases to the public health department
2. Nurses and physicians are also required to report evidence of crimes (such as homicide, suicide, inflicted injury such as stab or gunshot wounds, and abuse) to the police
3. Nurses need to confidentially report suspected chemical abuse by a coworker to supervisor; administration will notify the state board of nursing for investigation; treatment is the priority issue in this type of case
4. Under state and federal law, nurses as well as any other employee can report sexual harassment to supervisor or higher administration; consists of any unwelcome statements or behavior of a sexual nature
5. Unsafe working conditions need to be reported under Occupational Safety and Health Act (OSHA) regulations

VII. SPECIAL ETHICAL AND LEGAL CONSIDERATIONS IN PSYCHIATRIC MENTAL HEALTH SETTINGS

A. Client autonomy and liberty must be ensured by treatment in the least restrictive setting by active client participation in treatment

B. Voluntary admission occurs when a client consents to confinement in the hospital and signs a document indicating as much

C. Commitment, or involuntary admission, may be implemented on basis of being a danger to self or others; some states also have criterion of preventing significant physical or mental deterioration for involuntary admission

D. Competency is a legal determination that a client can make reasonable judgments and decisions about treatment and other significant areas of personal life

1. An adult is considered competent unless a *court* rules client incompetent; in such cases, a guardian is appointed to make decisions on client's behalf
2. Clients who are committed are still capable of participating in health care decisions

E. Clients in mental health settings do not relinquish right to informed consent because they have been admitted; may still accept or refuse specific aspects of treatment or care

F. Adherence to confidentiality is extremely important in practice of psychiatric mental health nursing

1. Federal rules apply to confidentiality regarding chemical dependence; staff members are not allowed to disclose any admission or discharge information
2. Some states require written consent before human immunodeficiency virus (HIV) tests may be performed; states have laws regarding when HIV test results or diagnosis of acquired immunodeficiency syndrome (AIDS) may be disclosed; this occurs regardless of psychiatric or nonpsychiatric health care setting

PRACTICE TEST

Check Your NCLEX-RN® Exam I.Q.

You are ready for testing on this content if you can

- Articulate ethical and legal issues in nursing practice that affect clients or families.
- Identify appropriate actions to promote ethical and legal nursing care.
- Evaluate the outcomes of interventions used to promote ethical and legal nursing care.
- Apply principles of confidentiality to client care situations.
- Identify actions to uphold client rights.
- Provide information to clients and families about advance directives.

PRACTICE TEST

1 A client is referred to a surgeon by the general practitioner. After meeting the surgeon, the client decides to find a different surgeon to continue treatment. The nurse supports the client's action, utilizing which ethical principle?

1. Beneficence
2. Veracity
3. Autonomy
4. Privacy

2 A nurse forgets to administer a client's diuretic and the client experiences an episode of pulmonary edema. This medication error would be considered negligence if it constituted which of the following?

1. The purposeful failure to perform a health care procedure
2. The unintentional failure to perform a health care procedure
3. The act of substituting a different medication for the one ordered
4. Failure to follow a direct order by a physician

3 A new graduate nurse orientee plans to show an adolescent client a video about self-injection technique. A staff nurse remarks, "I gave the client written literature yesterday, so the video probably isn't necessary." The nurse orientee proceeds with showing the video and discussing the skill with the adolescent after engaging in decision making related to which of the following?

1. Autonomy
2. Informed consent
3. Paternalism
4. Noncompliance

4 A client asks why a diagnostic test has been ordered and the nurse replies, "I'm unsure but will find out for you." When the nurse later returns and provides an explanation, the nurse is acting under which principle?

1. Nonmaleficence
2. Veracity
3. Beneficence
4. Fidelity

5 An individual has a seizure while walking down the street. During the seizure, a nurse from a physician's office is noticed driving past without stopping to assist. The individual sues the nurse for negligence but fails to win a judgment for which of the following reasons?

1. The nurse had no duty to the individual.
2. The nurse did what most nurses would do in the same circumstance.
3. The nurse did not cause the client's injuries.
4. The nurse was off-duty at that time.

6 The nurse is participating in a seminar about legal and ethical practice of nursing for continuing education credit. Which statement by a nurse best describes the relationship between law and ethics for the practice of nursing?

1. "The ethics of a discipline attempt to formulate and justify responses to moral dilemmas and may or may not be regulated by law."
2. "Laws dictate the ethics of nursing as they reflect societal choices about the ordering of relationships in society."
3. "Ethics represent the moral customs of an individual nurse; therefore, they cannot be regulated by the law."
4. "Ethical practice decreases the threat of a lawsuit, which is the primary source of legal influence on nursing practice."

7 A female client being treated in an outpatient setting for blood clots in the leg is taking anticoagulant medication. The client reports to her neighbor, a nurse, that she has a headache. The nurse offers the individual aspirin for the headache, which she takes. The client suffers a bleeding episode secondary to interaction between the aspirin and the anticoagulant. The legal nurse consultant interprets that which of the following elements of malpractice is missing from this case?

1. Breech of duty
2. Duty owed
3. Injury
4. Causation between nurse's action and injury

8 The client has decided to discontinue further treatment for cancer. Although the nurse would like the client to continue treatment, the nurse recognizes the client is competent and supports the client's decision using which of the following ethical principles?

1. Justice
2. Fidelity
3. Autonomy
4. Confidentiality

9 The physician orders a medication in a dose that is considered toxic. The nurse gives the medication to the client, who later suffers a cardiac arrest and dies. Which of the following consequences can the nurse expect?

1. The doctor, not the nurse, can be charged with negligence because the doctor ordered the dose.
2. The nurse and the doctor can dually be charged with negligence.
3. Because the nurse actually gave the medication, only the nurse can be charged with negligence.
4. Negligence will not be charged, as this event could happen to any reasonable person.

10 A nurse and teacher are discussing legal issues related to the practice of their professions. The teacher asks what is the primary purpose of the Nurse Practice Act in that state. The nurse replies that Nurse Practice Act is intended to do which of the following?

1. Accredit schools of nursing
2. Enforce ethical standards of behavior
3. Protect the public
4. Define the scope of nursing practice

PRACTICE TEST

ANSWERS & RATIONALES

ANSWERS & RATIONALES

1 **Answer: 3** Autonomy is the right of individuals to take action for themselves. Beneficence is duty to help others by doing what is best for them, whereas negligence is a legal term. Veracity is truthfulness. Privacy is the nondisclosure of information by the health care team.
Cognitive Level: Application **Client Need:** Safe Effective Care Environment: Management of Care **Integrated Process:** Nursing Process: Analysis **Content Area:** Fundamentals **Strategy:** The core issue of the question is the ability to interpret which ethical principle is operating in a given situation. Eliminate privacy first because it doesn't apply to the situation described. Eliminate beneficence and veracity next because they focus on an obligation of the nurse rather than on a right of the client.

2 **Answer: 2** Negligence is the unintentional failure of an individual to perform or not perform an act that a reasonable person would or would not do in the same or similar circumstances. Options 3 and 4 do not fit the description of the event, and option 1 is the opposite of option 2.
Cognitive Level: Application **Client Need:** Safe Effective Care Environment: Management of Care **Integrated Process:** Nursing Process: Analysis **Content Area:** Fundamentals **Strategy:** Options 1 and 2 are opposites, which is a clue that one of them may be correct. Choose option 2 over option 1 because it matches the description given in the stem of the question.

3 **Answer: 1** The nurse is exercising autonomy, the right to make one's own decision. Nurses who follow this principle recognize that each client is unique. In this situation, perhaps because of the developmental level, the nurse assessed that a video would be a better teaching-learning method than written literature. Paternalism restricts the freedom of the individual because another determines choices. Noncompliance occurs when an individual is fully aware of the consequences yet chooses the action anyway. Informed consent is providing agreement to undergo treatment following a description of a procedure with the risks, benefits, and alternatives explained.
Cognitive Level: Application **Client Need:** Safe Effective Care Environment: Management of Care **Integrated Process:** Nursing Process: Analysis **Content Area:** Fundamentals **Strategy:** Use the process of elimination. The correct answer is the one that supports the nurse's right to make decisions about his or her own practice.

4 **Answer: 4** Fidelity means to be faithful to agreements and promises. This nurse is acting on the client's behalf to obtain needed information and report it back to the client. Non-

maleficence is duty to do no harm. Veracity refers to telling the truth—for example, not lying to a client about a serious prognosis. Beneficence means doing good, such as by implementing actions (keeping a salt shaker out of sight) that benefit a client (heart condition requiring sodium-restricted diet). **Cognitive Level:** Application **Client Need:** Safe Effective Care Environment: Management of Care **Integrated Process:** Nursing Process: Implementation **Content Area:** Fundamentals **Strategy:** Use the process of elimination. The correct answer is the one that matches the description in the stem; that is, the nurse made a promise to a client and kept it, which constitutes fidelity.

5 **Answer: 1** The nurse must have a relationship with the client that involves providing care. The relationship is usually a component of employment. Options 2 and 4 are false. Option 3 is a true statement, but is not the one that applies to this case. **Cognitive Level:** Application. **Client Need:** Safe Effective Care Environment: Management of Care **Integrated Process:** Nursing Process: Analysis **Content Area:** Fundamentals **Strategy:** Use the process of elimination and nursing knowledge. The correct answer is the one that recognizes that the nurse was not in the role of employee at the time of the incident, removing the requirement of acting on the client's behalf.

6 **Answer: 1** Law is not the sole source of the ethical practice of nursing: numerous legal sources influence nursing practice. An individual should understand the ethics of a profession before becoming a member of that profession because those ethics may differ from personal ones. **Cognitive Level:** Analysis **Client Need:** Safe Effective Care Environment: Management of Care **Integrated Process:** Nursing Process: Evaluation **Content Area:** Fundamentals **Strategy:** Use the process of elimination and nursing knowledge to answer the question. The wording of the question tells you that only one answer can be correct.

7 **Answer: 2** In this situation, there was no nurse–client relationship. Although the neighbor offering the aspirin was a nurse, this action did not occur as a component of the nurse's employment. All of the other requirements were present. **Cognitive Level:** Analysis **Client Need:** Safe Effective Care Environment: Management of Care **Integrated Process:** Nursing Process: Evaluation **Content Area:** Fundamentals **Strategy:** Use the process of elimination. The wording of the question tells you that all of the options are requirements that must be met. Choose the one that focuses on the personal, not professional, relationship between the client and the nurse.

8 **Answer: 3** Autonomy refers to the right to make one's own decisions. Justice refers to fairness; fidelity refers to trust and loyalty; confidentiality refers to the right to privacy of personal health information. **Cognitive Level:** Application **Client Need:** Safe Effective Care Environment: Management of Care **Integrated Process:** Nursing Process: Analysis **Content Area:** Fundamentals **Strategy:** Use the process of elimination. The wording of the question indicates that only one option is correct and that you need to select the principle that is consistent with the circumstances in the question.

9 **Answer: 2** Nurses, along with physicians, can be charged with negligence for failing to recognize the incorrectly prescribed dosage of a commonly known drug. The other responses are incorrect interpretations of possible consequences. **Cognitive Level:** Application **Client Need:** Safe Effective Care Environment: Management of Care **Integrated Process:** Nursing Process: Analysis **Content Area:** Fundamentals **Strategy:** The wording of the question tells you that only one option is correct. Choose the response that holds both individuals accountable, since the nurse failed to question an incorrect dose.

10 **Answer: 3** A Nurse Practice Act serves to protect the public by setting minimum qualifications for nursing in relation to skills and competencies. One way it fulfills responsibility to protect the public is by defining the scope of nursing practice in that state. The state's board of nursing approves schools to operate but does not accredit them. It does not enforce ethical standards. **Cognitive Level:** Application **Client Need:** Safe Effective Care Environment: Management of Care **Integrated Process:** Nursing Process: Analysis **Content Area:** Fundamentals **Strategy:** Use the process of elimination and basic nursing knowledge to answer the question. The wording of the question tells you that only one option is a true statement.

Key Terms to Review

accountability p. 28
ANA Code of Ethics for Nurses p. 28
ethics p. 28
malpractice p. 30
negligence p. 30
Nurse Practice Act p. 30

References

American Nurses Association (2004). *Code for nurses with interpretative statements.* Kansas City, MO.

Coty, E. L., Davis, J. L., & Angell, L. (2000). *Documentation: The language of nursing.* Upper Saddle River, NJ: Prentice Hall.

Guido, G. (2006). *Legal and ethical issues in nursing* (4th ed.). Upper Saddle River, NJ: Prentice Hall.

Harkreader, H., & Hogan, M. (2004). *Fundamentals of nursing: Caring and clinical judgment* (2nd ed.). St. Louis, MO: Elsevier Science.

Kozier, B., Erb, G., Berman, A. J., & Burke, K. (2004). *Fundamentals of nursing: Concepts, process, and practice* (7th ed.). Upper Saddle River, NJ: Prentice Hall.

Thompson, I. E., Melia, M. M., & Boyd, K. M. (2006). *Nursing ethics* (5th ed.). Edinburgh: Churchill Livingstone.

ANSWERS & RATIONALES

Leadership and Management

6

In this chapter

Test Yourself

Are you ready for the NCLEX-RN® or course exams? Use the practice tests on the companion CD-ROM to check.

Cross reference

Other chapters relevant to this content area are

Injury Prevention, Disaster Planning, and Protecting Client Safety	Chapter 7
Coping with Stressors	Chapter 21

I. HEALTH CARE SETTINGS

A. Types of health care settings
1. Hospitals
2. Long-term care
3. Ambulatory
4. Home health care
5. Temporary service
6. Managed health care organizations

B. Types of managed care organizations
1. Health maintenance organization (HMO)
2. Preferred provider organization (PPO)
3. Point of service (POS)

C. Types of HMOs
1. Staff model
2. Independent practice associations
3. Group model
4. Network model

II. HEALTH CARE MANAGEMENT

A. *Health maintenance organizations (HMOs)*

1. A configuration of health care agencies that provide basic and supplemental health maintenance and treatment services to voluntary enrollees who prepay a fixed periodic fee without regard to either in-patient or out-patient services used
2. Formally established through federal legislation to reorganize health care services to reduce the rate of health care cost increases and control utilization of services
3. ! Geographically organized system that provides enrollees with an agreed-on package of health maintenance and treatment services
4. Types of HMOs
   - a. Staff model: physicians are HMO employees and are paid a salary
   - b. Independent practice associations: physicians maintain individual or group practices but contract with an HMO to serve enrollees for a negotiated fee
   - c. Group model: HMO contracts with a multispecialty group to provide enrollee services for a negotiated fee
   - d. Network model: HMO contracts with two or more IPAs, independent or group practices, to provide enrollee services at a fixed monthly fee per enrollee, called **capitation**

! **B. *Managed care***

1. A health care plan that brings together the delivery and financing function into one entity in contrast to a fee for service
2. The newest form of health care delivery; the objective is to restructure health care services to:
   - a. Enhance cost containment by decreasing unnecessary services
   - b. Maintain quality
   - c. Facilitate the management of patient care needs
   - d. Promote timely and appropriate care
3. Providers must submit written justification to request prior approval for diagnostic tests and interventions or to extend a client's length of stay
4. See Box 6–1, Key Objectives of Managed Care

! **C. Case management**

1. Organizes client care by major diagnoses and focuses on attaining predetermined client outcomes within specific time frames
2. Advantages
   - a. All professionals are equal members of team
   - b. Emphasis is on managing interdisciplinary outcomes
   - c. Promotes continuity of care
3. Disadvantage: requires essential baseline data be available to team members; role is still in process with job descriptions varying among institutions

D. Nursing care delivery systems

1. Functional nursing
   - a. Began in the mid-1940s
   - b. ! Client needs are defined by tasks to be allocated to RNs, LPNs, and unlicensesd assistive personnel (UAPs) and coordinated by a charge nurse
   - c. Advantages: efficient and effective at regularly performed tasks and financially advantageous for the organization
   - d. Disadvantages: fragmentation of care, absence of a holistic view of the patient, time-consuming communications, problems with follow-up

Box 6–1

Key Objectives of Managed Care

Cost containment	Administrative efficiency
Some forms of rationing	Contracting efficiency
Efficiency of care	Managing care
Less duplication	Appropriateness of care

2. Primary nursing
   a. Primary nurse designs, implements, and is accountable for the nursing care of clients with delegation of care to an associate nurse
   b. Care is given by primary nurse and associates
   c. Advantages include having a knowledge-based practice model; decentralization of nursing care decisions, authority, and responsibility to staff nurse; decrease in number of unlicensed personnel; enhanced family satisfaction with care; and high level of accountability
   d. Disadvantages are that it requires excellent communication between nurses, and continuity of care and accountability may be challenged; it is costly for institutions to hire highly skilled nurses
3. Team nursing
   a. Most common nursing care delivery system in the United States
   b. A team of nursing personnel provides total care to a group of clients
   c. Advantages are that it allows use of non-RN staff and coordination of activities requiring more than one person; team leader is a skilled practitioner; it is cost-effective for agency; and client satisfaction with care is increased
   d. Disadvantages are that communication is time consuming; continuity of care may be diminished, role confusion and resentment can occur, and the reporting mechanism is to only one person

E. *Shared governance* model of practice

1. Principles of shared governance include partnerships, equity, accountability, and ownership; the structure demands participation in ownership
2. Characterized by decentralized power sharing and decision making; interdisciplinary team building; activities and conferences; the priorities of the organization are accomplished through a series of committees
3. There is one representative for each committee from each nursing unit
4. Four committees generally set policies and address organizational issues
   a. Nursing practice
   b. Quality improvement
   c. Education (ensures continuing education requirements and staff competency)
   d. Management of the organization's service-specific areas such as general medical-surgical, maternal–child, critical care, intermediate care, and ancillary services such as employee and family health, radiology, and cardiac catherization
5. An overall coordinating council composed of a chairperson elected by nursing staff, a clinical nurse specialist, and four chairs of the housewide councils

III. ORGANIZATIONAL SKILLS

A. *Time management* allows the nurse to determine how best to prioritize client care, decide the outcomes, and perform the most important nursing intervention first

1. Time management is a set of skills that encourage and support the most effective and productive way to use time
2. Effective time management means becoming outcome oriented, not task oriented
   a. Identify long-term goals and divide them into achievable outcomes
   b. Write down all long-term goals and outcomes
   c. Goals and outcomes should remain fluid, flexible, and changeable to the situation at hand

B. Time management strategies for nurse leaders

1. The goal of time management should not be to find more time but to set a reasonable amount of time to spend on these roles and then use that time wisely
2. Managing time takes practice; keep asking throughout the day: *Is this what I want or need to be doing right now?* If the answer is yes, then keep doing it
3. Find a way to realistically and practically analyze your time, such as logging time for a week in 15-minute intervals; do it for a week and review your results to determine where time was well spent and where it was not

4. Spend time in areas where and on items for which you are needed rather than merely helpful
5. Learn the difference between *Do I need to do this now?* and *Do I need to do this at all?* (experienced nurses learn how to quickly answer this question when circumstances change on the nursing unit)
6. Delegate appropriately to others to free up time for priority items
7. Organize the work area and keep items where they belong so they will be easily found when needed
8. Look at stressors in personal life (over 24-hour day) and try to recognize and prevent their occurrence

C. Common symptoms of poor time management

1. Irritability and stress
2. Fatigue
3. Difficulty concentrating and forgetfulness
4. Disorganization and inability to complete tasks

D. How to organize nursing care shift responsibilities and activities

1. Arrange nursing care environment with efficient access to supplies, equipment, and client designated areas
2. Use previous shift's report to determine tasks and priorities
3. Develop a shift action plan that includes expected outcomes that are optimal and reasonable with a statement that includes by what time interventions will be completed
4. Make assignments indicating who will perform the interventions
5. Implement the shift action plan beginning with initial client care rounds
   a. Making client care rounds: a rapid assessment of information gathered
   b. Schedule treatments and monitoring: firm time commitment for treatments and monitoring
   c. Plan for appropriate equipment and supplies to be available for care
6. Evaluate outcomes and re-examine shift action plan
   a. Ask yourself if you achieved the optimal outcomes you set out to do; if not, why not?
   b. Determine if there were staffing problems or patient care crises
   c. Ask yourself if you set realistic outcomes, and if not, why not?
   d. Identify what you learned from this shift action plan and determine what you can apply in the future
   e. Make appropriate change when similar problems occur

IV. ESTABLISHING PRIORITIES OF CARE

A. Frameworks for determining priorities of client care (see Table 6–1)

1. ABCs: airway, breathing and circulation
2. Maslow's hierarchy of needs
3. Agency policies and procedures
4. Time
5. Client and family preferences
6. Care related to client acuity
7. Priorities in medication therapy

B. More stable versus less stable client

1. Attend to the least stable client first (whose condition is changing or deteriorating)
2. Clients who become unstable may have dramatic signs (such as bleeding, shock, or cardiopulmonary arrest) but could exhibit more subtle signs; watch for gradual trends in data, such as deteriorating vital signs, declining urine output, decreasing level of consciousness
3. When all clients are stable, attend first to the client who is most likely to become unstable or who is at risk for greatest complications because of the disease process

C. General client problems that usually indicate priority

1. Fresh postoperative clients (newly arrived on the nursing unit from postanesthesia care)

Table 6–1 Strategies for Priority Setting in Clinical Practice

Guiding Principles	First Priority	Second Priority	Third Priority
ABCs	Airway, breathing and circulation	—	—
Maslow's Hierarchy of Needs theory	Physiological (primary) needs: air, breathing, circulation, water, food (oxygen therapy, circulatory support, IV hydration, nutrition, critical lab values, treatment of pain)	Safety and security (primary) needs: prevention of falls, re-orientation to surroundings, abnormally high or low values that are not critical; may include some client teaching (e.g., insulin administration)	Secondary needs: activities and care that support "love and belonging," self-esteem (includes ability for self-care and self-management of health problem), and self-actualization; includes routine client teaching and psychosocial support
Policies and procedures	Activities governed by agency policy or procedure that involve strict timelines (e.g., restraints, falls, stat medications)	Activities governed by policy or procedure that directly affect client care (e.g., non-stat, regularly scheduled medications, dressings)	Activities not affecting patient care or that might be delegated to another (e.g., checking temperature of unit refrigerator, code cart check, emptying laundry bags)
Time	Clients with highly time-bound therapies (e.g., OR, stat x-ray); tasks that can be fully completed in less than 2 minutes if no competing priority present; necessary time-bound care for admission or discharge clients	Clients with scheduled therapies that need to be completed within a 2- to 4-hour window; routine client teaching	Clients with scheduled therapies that need to be completed once during the shift
Client and family preferences	Clients or families in physical or psychological distress	Clients or families with concerns about status or nursing care	Routine client and family preferences or requests
Care activities related to clinical condition of client	Life-threatening or potentially life-threatening occurrences (adverse changes in VS, change in LOC, potential for respiratory or circulatory collapse); often unanticipated	Activities essential to safety: life-saving medications and equipment that protect clients from infections or falls	Activities essential to the plan of care leading to outcomes of symptom relief or healing (that if omitted would slow client recovery; e.g., nutrition, positioning, ambulation)
Medication or IV therapy priorities	Medications that prevent or treat physiological distress (e.g., analgesics, updrafts, or inhalers); medications ordered more frequently (e.g., every 4 hours) because late medication delivery could affect next dose; IV therapy for hydration in clients who are NPO because of nonfunctional GI tract	Medications that prevent reoccurrences of symptoms of disease processes (e.g., digoxin, antibiotics); medications ordered once per shift; routine maintenance of IV therapy or heparin/saline lock care	Medications that maintain normal organ system functioning (e.g., stool softener); medications ordered daily or twice daily; site and dressing changes for IV therapy

2. Clients whose status has deteriorated from baseline (vital signs, level of consciousness, neurovascular status)
3. Clients exhibiting signs of shock (hypovolemic, hemorrhagic, cardiogenic, distributive)
4. Clients who have allergic reactions
5. Clients who have chest pain
6. Clients who have returned from diagnostic procedures and require temporary, more intensive monitoring, including assessing for complications
7. Clients who verbalize unexpected or unusual symptoms (such as new or suddenly increased acute pain, blurred vision, sudden weakness or paralysis)
8. Clients who have equipment or tubing malfunction or accident (such as disconnection of IV line, central line, chest tube; or alarms ringing on mechanical ventilator or cardiac monitor)

9. Lower priority clients are generally those whose main needs include teaching, which is not as time-bound unless individual circumstances indicate otherwise

V. DELEGATION AND SUPERVISION

A. Leadership and supervision

1. A critical job-related responsibility of the nurse leader is **leadership** or learning how to create a common **vision**, develop a big-picture mentality, and promote a sense of urgency; this responsibility influences workplace priorities and outcomes by
   - **a.** Connecting work objectives to the strategic plan
   - **b.** Ensuring that unit-based or clinical objectives support the common vision and ensure safe, high-quality care
   - **c.** Delegating authority to marshal and deploy scarce resources in order to manage all ongoing critical patient care situations
2. ! A **supervisor** is any individual having authority from the employer to hire, transfer, suspend, lay off, recall, promote, discharge, assign, reward, or discipline other employees
3. **Supervising** is the provision by the nurse leader of guidance or direction, evaluation, and follow-up of nursing personnel for accomplishment of a delegated nursing task
4. Supervisors are responsible for
   - **a.** A competent and disciplined staff
   - **b.** Clear directions and communication
   - **c.** Timely follow-up to ensure prompt execution of delegated activities and orders
   - **d.** Active listening skills
   - **e.** A thorough scope of technical knowledge of supervised work
   - **f.** Demonstrated fairness and respect toward all
   - **g.** Feedback for work well done and resolution of problems and conflicts

! B. *Delegation*

1. The use of nursing personnel to accomplish a desired objective through allocation of authority and responsibility; involves, as part of assigning work, asking another to do some aspect of client care
2. Delegation is
   - **a.** A complex process and a crucial management skill
   - **b.** Retaining accountability for the number and diversity of caregivers
   - **c.** Knowing the capacity and qualification level of each practitioner for doing the work
   - **d.** Accomplishing nursing tasks in the most efficient way using appropriate resources
   - **e.** Knowing the intricacy of the relationship among the nursing team, client, and environment
3. See Box 6–2 for suggestions on how to delegate
4. ! The National Council of State Boards in Nursing defines delegation as transferring to a competent individual the authority to perform a selected nursing task in a selected situation

Box 6–2

How to Delegate

1. Identify a suitable person for the task, who has the appropriate skill set.
2. Prepare the person. Explain the task clearly. Make sure that you are understood.
3. Make sure the person has the necessary authority to do the job properly.
4. Keep in touch with the person for support and to monitor progress while allowing sufficient time and opportunity to complete the task.
5. Retain responsibility for knowing the outcome of the delegation.
6. Praise and acknowledge a job well done.

C. Delegation of nursing assignments

1. Nursing care assignments are delegated based on knowing the competency of the delegatee, including the following
   a. Education level
   b. Knowledge level
   c. Skill level
2. Nurses must clearly identify the outcomes or expectations of each assigned nursing task or activity, including
   a. What is the standard of care
   b. Time frame for assignment completion
   c. Limitations regarding performance of task (see Box 6–3 for concepts that the nurse must consider to determine when to delegate)

D. Why nurses need to delegate

1. No one person can do everything
2. Delegation is the most efficient way to utilize appropriate resources
3. Delegation sparks the staff interest and prevents nursing staff from becoming nonproductive and ineffective
4. Delegation builds teamwork and encourages staff to discover those duties or tasks that best suit them and make them feel like they are part of the team regardless of their position
5. Nurse leaders can delegate authority but cannot delegate responsibility and therefore must ensure staff members are practicing in a competent manner

E. The nurse's top three *Do Not Delegate* tasks to nonprofessional staff (implementation is the only phase of the nursing process that may be delegated to nonprofessional staff)

1. The initial nursing assessment, the subsequent assessments, and those requiring professional judgment
2. The nursing diagnosis, nursing care goals, and progress plans
3. The interventions that require professional knowledge and skill, including client teaching

F. Components of delegation

1. Delegation is an essential skill required by all nurses who will transfer authority to perform a task or other clinical activities
2. The principles of delegation include the following
   a. Only authority, but not ultimate responsibility, can be delegated
   b. All delegated tasks must be clearly assigned and continuously clarified
   c. Know the job responsibilities of staff and what can and cannot be delegated
   d. Set clear parameters around how much authority is needed to accomplish the task; delegate just enough authority to accomplish the assigned task successfully
   e. Be sure the task that is delegated is completed as assigned
   f. Delegation requires ongoing follow-up and evaluation; obtain feedback on assigned tasks upon completion
3. For delegation to occur, there three important elements
   a. Delegator
   b. Delegatee
   c. Task or activity to be accomplished

G. The delegation process

1. Determine and identify the task and level of responsibility of each task
2. Evaluate the delegatee's fit with the assigned task

Box 6–3

Knowing when to Delegate

1. Nurse must understand the need to protect the client from potential for harm.
2. Nurse must understand the complexity of the task or delegated activity.
3. Nurse must understand how to solve problems and when innovation is necessary.
4. Nurse must be able to assess the unpredictability of the situation.
5. Nurse must be able to determine the level of interaction by the client.

3. Decide what level of supervision is needed and describe expectations
4. Reach agreement on performance and outcome
5. Provide continuous feedback—monitor performance and adjust accordingly

H. Barriers to delegation

1. Delegator barriers: the nurse sometimes does not delegate because of
   - **a.** A "do-it-myself" attitude
   - **b.** Inability to ask others
   - **c.** Inability to organize and manage
   - **d.** Feelings of uncertainty
   - **e.** Fear of competition
   - **f.** Fear of liability
   - **g.** Fear of loss of control
   - **h.** Fear of decreased job satisfaction
2. Delegatee barriers: the delegatee may resist and sometime refuse to accept delegated tasks because of
   - **a.** Inexperience
   - **b.** Incompetence
   - **c.** Disorganization
   - **d.** Irresponsibility
3. Situational barriers: the workplace itself may become a barrier in the process of accomplishing delegated tasks because of
   - **a.** Inadequate support
   - **b.** Hurried atmosphere
   - **c.** Hostile management

I. Advantages and disadvantages of delegation

1. Advantages
   - **a.** The delegator benefits by gaining more time (higher efficiency) to accomplish those activities that cannot be delegated to staff
   - **b.** The delegatee benefits by gaining new skills and abilities in accepting assigned tasks as well as an opportunity to demonstrate proficiency and self-confidence
   - **c.** General advantages to all include that it increases motivation, develops the skills of the nursing team, and allows for better distribution of work through the group; see Box 6–4, Advantages of Delegation
2. Disadvantages
   - **a.** Nurse leaders become ineffective delegators when tasks are not completed or are completed incorrectly; when he or she accepts a delegated task from a team member; or when he or she delegates too much authority or responsibility to team members

J. Inappropriate delegation

! 1. **Underdelegation**: the delegator does not think that team members can perform or complete an assignment or does not transfer full authority
   - **a.** It is crucial to develop team members who can provide complete and comprehensive patient care
   - **b.** If unable to perform tasks, team members must be directed and trained to reach the appropriate skill level

! 2. **Reverse delegation**
   - **a.** Team members requests that the nurse leader complete the task because of their inability or unwillingness to perform the designated task or procedure

Box 6–4

Advantages of Delegation

Positive aspects of delegation include

- ➤ Higher efficiency
- ➤ Increased motivation
- ➤ Development of skills of your team
- ➤ Better distribution of work through the group

b. Minimize reverse delegation with the use of competency-based orientation programs and in-service or staff development classes

! 3. **Overdelegation**: the delegator becomes overwhelmed by the situation and loses control by delegating too much authority and too much responsibility to the delegatee
   a. Tasks are delegated inappropriately; the nurse cannot successfully achieve work-related goals if overwhelmed by numerous requests
   b. Tasks that are beyond their scope of practice should not be delegated to unlicensed assistive personnel (UAPs)

! **K. Five rights of delegation**

1. The National Council of State Boards of Nursing (1995) defines the five rights of delegation as the following
   a. Right task
   b. Right circumstance
   c. Right person
   d. Right direction/communication
   e. Right supervision
2. See Box 6–5, The Essential Rights of Delegation
3. Registered nurses (RNs) retain the responsibility for caring for clients who require skilled assessment, whose status is changing or at risk for changing, and who require teaching
4. Licensed practical or vocational nurses (LPNs or LVNs) may be delegated the care of clients who are stable, but have higher levels of acuity or need performance of skills beyond the training of a UAP
5. LPNs and LVNs may collect data to report to the RN but are not responsible for the same level of client assessment that the RN conducts
6. Care of clients requiring routine nursing care and basic nursing procedures may be delegated to UAPs; nursing care activities that require ongoing assessment, interpretation, or clinical decision making that cannot be separated from the activity itself should not be delegated to a UAP

Box 6–5

The Essential Rights of Delegation

1. Right Task: Nurses determine those activities team members may perform. For each situation, the nurse must consider the client's condition, the complexity of the activity, the UAP's capabilities, and the amount of supervision the nurse will be able to provide.

2. Right Circumstances: The nurse evaluates the individual clients and the individual UAPs and matches the two. The nurse assesses the client's needs, looks at the care plan, and considers the setting, ensuring that UAPs have the proper resources, equipment, and supervision to work safely.

3. Right Person: The nurse follows organizational policies, which are congruent with state law, in determining the appropriate staff to which to delegate a nursing activity.

4. Right Direction and Communication: The nurse needs to communicate the acceptable tasks and activities. The nurse needs to clearly understand the organization's policies and procedures to carry out effective delegation.

   In turn, staff nurses need to direct UAPs' actions and communicate clearly about each delegated task. Nurses must be specific about how and when UAPs should report back to them. Nurses should feel comfortable asking, *Do you know how to do this? Where did you learn? How many times have you done it in the past? Where is your experience documented?*

5. Right Supervision and Evaluation: Nurse managers must ensure that each unit has adequate staffing and time, identify the task inherent to each staff role, and evaluate the impact of the organization's nursing service on the community. The delegating nurse then must supervise, guide, and evaluate the UAPs' task implementation. The nurse must ensure that UAPs meet expectations and must intervene if they aren't performing well.

VI. ASSIGNMENT-MAKING

!

A. Assignment-making process for delegating the duties and activities of client care to individual personnel
1. Give clear, concise directions
2. Delegate responsibility
3. Delegate authority for the performance of the care
4. RN retains accountability for the assignment
5. RN ensures that the education, skill, knowledge, and judgment levels of individual personnel are commensurate with the assignment

B. Assignment-making outcomes: once an assignment is made, RN must specify the following:
1. Expected outcome of the assignment
2. Time frame for completion
3. Limitations on the assignment
4. Feedback at the completion of the assignment

VII. INTERDISCIPLINARY CONSULTATION AND REFERRALS

A. *Interdisciplinary* describes situations in which various disciplines are involved in reaching a common goal, and each representative of a discipline brings to the situation his or her expertise

!

B. Interdisciplinary consultation requires
1. Cooperation, integration, and modification of efforts by contributing disciplines
2. Acknowledgment by participants to take into account the contributions of other teams members in making their own contribution
3. Understanding the intersecting lines of communication and collaboration that may emerge from these contributions

C. Interdisciplinary care team: works together with the client and family in planning care for the client from each team member's discipline-specific perspective
1. Discipline-specific perspectives are shared through staff conferencing and by consulting with each other
2. Collaboration helps team members gain new insights for addressing problems
3. Collaboration promotes development of a holistic plan for the client

D. Key components of the interdisciplinary care team
1. Team members understand, appreciate, and collaborate with other disciplines and providers
2. Team members make decisions about services in collaboration with the client and other discipline rather than dividing care decisions by discipline or setting
3. Team members have a thorough understanding of their own profession

E. *Consultation* involves communication with another nurse or health care professional (dietitian, pharmacist, for example) about an aspect of client care
1. This type of communication is facilitated in agencies who enjoy collaborative work relationships with other health team members
2. Nursing units that use interdisciplinary rounds on clients have created an environment that fosters this type of communication

F. Referrals: often nurses are integral in assisting and coordinating client care that requires referrals
1. The term referral may include any of the following definitions
   a. A formal process that authorizes an HMO member to get care from a specialist or hospital; most HMOs require clients to get a referral from their primary care doctor before seeing a specialist
   b. May be either an informal suggestion from one provider for the client to see another provider, or a formal process within managed care plans by which the primary care physician refers the client to specialists, hospitals, or other services
   c. The recommendation by a physician and/or health plan for a member to receive care from a different physician or facility
   d. A process in which a health care provider recommends that a client see a medical professional with advanced knowledge of a certain medical specialty or technique (such as heart disease or dermatology)

e. The process of sending a client from one practitioner to another for health care services; health plans may require a designated primary care provider (PCP) to authorize a referral in order for specialty services to be covered

2. In managed care, a health plan member must first contact his or her PCP to obtain medical services unless it's an emergency; together, the member and PCP decide if the member needs to see a specialist or obtain special services; this is also called *preauthorization*
3. A request by a PCP or other specialist to send a client to a specialist for consultation, diagnostic intervention, and/or treatment
4. In the acute care setting, nurses may have authority to refer clients for consultation by specific departments, such as dietary or wound care specialist; always follow agency policy for scope of RN referral ability in specific agencies

VIII. LEADERSHIP

A. Overview of leadership

1. Contemporary nursing leadership is about engaging people, building relationships, and influencing change; it is not only about formal titles, job duties, and functions
2. The terms leader, administrator, supervisor, and **manager** are sometimes used interchangeably; they are different but complementary
3. ! A **leader** is a person who possesses personal traits that enable her or him to personally move others constructively and ethically to positively impact the care of clients and families or to achieve a goal or vision
4. Leadership is
   a. The exercise of power, influence, and responsibility
   b. The attempt to change the behavior of another
   c. The art of getting others to want to do what one deems important
   d. Coping with change
   e. Mentoring others toward higher levels
   f. Flexible in varied situations

B. To be a leader, one must earn the respect and trust of another

1. Leadership is about learning to earn the respect and trust of others—otherwise, the leader will have no followers; gaining respect and trust involves
   a. Followers who exhibit extraordinary commitment and loyalty to their leader
   b. Followers who share a sense of stewardship and accountability toward their leader
   c. Leader who recognizes what type of followers he or she has and how to intervene accordingly
2. Types of followers
   a. Effective follower
   b. Alienated follower
   c. Yes follower
   d. Shy follower
   e. Passive-aggressive follower
   f. Independent follower
3. For followers to grow and flourish, the nurse leader must provide
   a. Personal attention: support and guidance in foreseeing problems and challenges
   b. Role modeling: encouragement of self-management, assessment, openness, and forthrightness
   c. Precepting: to assist, approach, and coach in a timely and appropriate manner
   d. Mentoring: to invest by sharing expertise and experience with others

C. Formal versus informal leadership

1. ! **Formal leadership** is bestowed upon a nurse by the organization and described in a job description; it provides for influence through
   a. Legitimate authority
   b. Power of position
   c. Ability to reward and punish

! 2. **Informal leadership** does not provide an official title in the organization but the informal leader can substantially influence others through
   a. Thoughtful and convincing ideas
   b. Knowledge
   c. Status
   d. Personal skills

D. Attributes of effective leaders
1. Consider their position a responsibility rather than a rank or privilege (see Box 6–6, Effective Leadership)
2. Desire strong associates and encourage them, push them, and glory in their success
3. Articulate the organization's vision in a manner that stresses the values of the followers
4. Involve followers in deciding how to achieve the organization's vision
5. Support followers' efforts to realize the vision by providing coaching, feedback, and role modeling and by recognizing and rewarding success
6. Do not blame others when things go wrong (and they sometimes do)

E. A nurse leader's first objective is to assist and support the professional clinical practice environment for nurses by
1. Putting clients first
2. Focusing on client safety
3. Enhancing care quality
4. Improving client care outcomes

F. Effective nurse leadership empowers nurses' participation in clinical decision making and the organization of clinical care systems through
1. Decentralized, unit-based programs or team organizational structures for decision making
2. Organization-wide or systemwide committee and communication structures that include staff nurse representation
3. Demonstrated leadership positions and roles for nurses in performance improvement of clinical care and the organization of clinical care systems
4. Review systems for nursing analysis and correction of clinical care errors and client safety concerns
5. Authority of professional nurses to develop and execute nursing care orders and actions and to control their practice

G. Leadership development and performance require learning a body of knowledge and using effective management, including the following core leadership skills:
1. Communication
2. Team building
3. Knowledge of health care economics
4. Financial accounting
5. Organizational management
6. Human resource management
7. Evidence-based outcomes

H. Theories of leadership and management
1. Trait theory
   a. Introduced during the early 1900s
   b. Focused on defining what leaders are
   c. Sought to identify inborn traits of successful leaders
   d. Attempted to specify a universal set of leadership characteristics

Box 6–6

Effective Leadership

Is a responsibility rather than rank and privilege.

Is knowing that when things go wrong, and often they do, leaders do not blame others.

Is acknowledging that leaders are ultimately responsible for their words and actions.

Is having strong and competent associates whom the leader encourages, coaches, and provides with ongoing evaluation and feedback.

   - **e.** Provided a benchmark by which most leaders continue to be judged
   - **f.** A menu of traits was developed, but no one trait or combination of traits were found to be optimal
   - **g.** Leadership traits are often classified into three categories: intelligence, personality, and abilities
   - **h.** Potential leaders possess and exhibit common traits such as dominance, aggressiveness, ambition, high need to achieve, self-confidence, tolerance of others' viewpoints, orderly thinking, flexibility, respect for others, and humility
2. Behavioral theories
   - **a.** Introduced in the early 1930s
   - **b.** Focused on the abilities and behaviors of leaders, including what leaders do
   - **c.** Personal traits provide only a portion of leader capacity
   - **d.** Leadership evolves through education, training, and life experiences
   - **e.** **Autocratic leadership**: based on belief that individuals are motivated by power, authority, and need for approval; an autocratic leader makes all the decisions, uses coercion and punishment, and is uncollegial
   - **f.** **Democratic leadership**: based on belief that individuals are motivated by internal drives and impulses, desire active participation in decisions, and desire to get the tasks done; democratic leadership promotes participation and majority rule for goal setting
   - **g.** **Laissez-faire leadership**: based on belief that individuals are motivated by internal drives and impulses, need to be left alone to make decisions about how to complete work; leader provides no direction or facilitation
   - **h.** **Bureaucratic leadership**: based on belief that individuals are motivated by external forces; leader trusts either followers or self to make decisions; relies on organizational policies and rules to identify goals and direct the work flow
   - **i.** Behavioral theory involves initiating structured behaviors that managers use to organize and define work goals, work patterns and methods, channels of communication, and roles
   - **j.** Behavioral theory includes consideration of behaviors that show mutual trust, respect, friendship, warmth, and rapport between the leader and followers
3. System 4 management model involves followers in decisions about their work, and this involvement becomes essential to effective leadership; leaders using this model have high level of confidence in followers, seek consensus in decision making, and share power with followers; four dimensions on increasing followers' level of involvement
   - **a.** Autocratic leaders have little trust in followers and exclude them from decision making
   - **b.** Benevolent leaders are kind to followers but still do not involve them in decision making
   - **c.** Consultative leaders seek employee advice about decisions
   - **d.** Participative or democratic leaders value employee involvement, teamwork, and team-building
4. The managerial grid leadership theory plots leadership styles into four quadrants of a two-dimensional grid (visualize a box with four squares in it) that illustrates the leader's concern for production or task (called structure) on one axis and concern for people (called consideration) on the other axis; results in five leadership styles
   - **a.** Impoverished: low concern for people
   - **b.** Authority: high concern for production, low concern for people and tasks
   - **c.** Country club: high concern for people, low concern for tasks
   - **d.** Middle of the road: moderate concern for both tasks and people
   - **e.** Team: high concern for both tasks and people
5. Contingency theories
   - **a.** Leaders adapt their style according to the situation
   - **b.** Leader behavior ranges accordingly, from authoritarian to permissive: crisis situations often require an authoritarian style to maintain command and

control; problem solving and consensus building call for a participatory style that encourages respect for followers' ideas and input and gains their commitment to the team

c. Leaders who base their leadership style upon the organizational environment, task to be achieved, and characteristics of their followers tend to be most effective; this is because their planned flexibility allows them to change styles as needed by the work environment

d. Two examples of contingency models are Fiedler contingency theory and situational leadership theory

6. Fiedler contingency theory
   a. Leadership effectiveness is related to how a leader's style (task-oriented or relationship-oriented) best matches the situation
   b. Fiedler cites three situational factors that impact leader effectiveness
      1) Manager–follower relationship (good to poor); if relations are good, the manager enjoys loyalty and support from the followers
      2) Task structure (high to low); whether or not the task is well defined or standard procedures are followed
      3) Manager power (strong to weak); the ability of the leader to use his or her legitimate power of position to reward or punish accordingly
   c. Task-leadership style is best used for high and low structured situations and relationship leadership style is more effective for weak to low situations
7. Situational leadership theory considers the follower's readiness and willingness to perform a designated task; leadership styles can be categorized according to the readiness and ability of the follower to perform the task
   a. Telling style (S1—high task, low relationship) is used for followers who are unable and unwilling to perform, or insecure about performing the assigned task
   b. Selling style (S2—high task, high relationship) is used for followers who are unable but willing to perform, or confident in performing the task
   c. Participating style (S3—low task, high relationship) is used for followers who are both able and willing to perform, and have confidence in performing the task
8. Quantum leadership theory: a contemporary theory in which the leader is viewed as an influential facilitator and followers assume an active role in decision making
   a. Leadership is a shared activity
   b. Information is freely disseminated to followers and clients
   c. Leaders are expected to be expert communicators and to possess strong interpersonal skills
   d. Followers are equitable and accountable partners in client care outcomes
   e. Quantum leadership evolves from concepts of chaos theory; reality is constantly shifting; levels of complexity are constantly changing; movement reverberates throughout the system; roles are fluid and outcome-oriented
9. Charismatic leadership
   a. Leaders possess powerful personal qualities, such as charm, persuasiveness, personal power, self-confidence, extraordinary ideas, and strong convictions
   b. Leader's personality arouses affection and emotional commitment
   c. Leader's personality drives and advances the vision, mission, and goals
10. **Transactional leadership**
   a. Built on the principles of social exchange
   b. Individuals engaged in social interactions expect to give and receive rewards
   c. Exchange process between leaders and followers is economic
   d. Leaders are most successful when they understand and meet the needs of followers
   e. Social exchange between leader and follower continues until the exchange of performance and reward is no longer valuable
   f. Uses incentives to enhance follower loyalty and performance
   g. Aimed at maintaining equilibrium or status quo

h. Performs work according to policy and procedures
i. Maximizes self-interests and personal rewards
j. Fosters interpersonal dependence

11. **Transformational leadership**
    a. Emphasizes interpersonal relationships
    b. Not concerned with the status quo
    c. Focuses on merging motives and values
    d. Generates followers' commitment to the leader's vision
    e. Fosters followers' inborn desires to pursue higher values and ideals
    f. Encourages followers to exercise leadership
    g. Inspires followers
    h. Uses power to instill a belief that followers can accomplish exceptional things
12. Relational leadership
    a. Acknowledges the importance of relationships as the cornerstone of effective leadership
    b. Connective relationships allow for better coordinated and integrated client care services in caring, noncompetitive manner
    c. Connective leaders encourage collaboration and interpersonal skills to broker alliances
13. Shared leadership
    a. Founded on the principles of empowerment, participation, and transformational leadership
    b. No one person or leader possesses all the knowledge and ability
    c. Elements of shared leadership include relationships, dialogs, partnerships, and understanding boundaries
    d. Different issues call for different responses
    e. Shared leadership allows for appropriate leadership to emerge in relation to current problems and issues as they arise
14. **Servant leadership**
    a. Focuses on desire to serve others and is based upon the principles of caring
    b. In the desire to serve, one can be called upon to lead—hence the name servant leadership
    c. A servant leader seeks to address others' needs as the priority
    d. Nurse leaders provide care and compassionate service to others

I. Desired leadership traits and competencies are the required knowledge, skills, and strategies that ensure leadership success; a nurse leader must possess some combination of the following traits and competencies:

1. Action orientation
    a. Uncovers and seizes opportunities when they arise
    b. Proceeds with extraordinary persistence and determination
    c. Champions initiatives beyond the scope of one's work
    d. Mobilizes resources and removes barriers
2. Team spirit focus
    a. Leverages the team's synergy to get results
    b. Uses the team to create a common culture
    c. Manages tensions inherent in the group process to forge innovative solutions
    d. Establishes a positive work climate, through personal actions, policies, and consistent signals, that nurtures enthusiasm and commitment in the team's mission
3. Command skills
    a. Inspires a high level of dedication to the mission
    b. Steadfastly maintains focus on goals in difficult situations
    c. Flexible in developing alternative methods of achieving goals
    d. Brings clarity and decisiveness in a crisis
4. Ethics and integrity
    a. Viewed as a highly credible and trustworthy person
    b. Stands up for what is right despite potential personal or business consequences

c. Creates and instills strong values and ethics within the health care organization
5. Interpersonal savvy
 a. Anticipates others' thoughts and reactions and responds accordingly
 b. Uses conflict as an advantage to create innovative solutions
 c. Forges and maximizes opportunities to build long-term productive relationships
 d. Enhances the workgroup dynamics through subtle methods of influencing
6. Vision and purpose management skills
 a. Creates a compelling and inspirational picture of the future
 b. Inspires others to dedicate themselves to achieve the vision
 c. Engages entire workgroup to achieve the vision
7. Ability to motivate and inspire others
 a. Engages in new and innovative ways of managing human and fiscal resources
 b. Recognizes and uncovers the full potential of team members by providing the needed resources, coaching, experiences, and other professional development opportunities
 c. Develops future leaders and talent for key positions within the organization
 d. Gives team members the opportunity and latitude to make key decisions to resolve problems
8. Problem solving skills
 a. Makes breakthrough decisions based upon analysis, wisdom, experience, and judgment
 b. Frequently sought out by other nurses for advice and solutions
 c. Suggests highly creative solutions to difficult problems
 d. Considers the impact of global, cultural, geographic, political, and regulatory factors in making decisions
9. Results orientation
 a. Goes beyond what's expected to achieve objectives
 b. Anticipates potential problems and develops contingency plans to overcome them
 c. Demonstrates strong commitment and drive to achieve results
 d. Delivers results that consistently improve client care outcomes
10. Strategic agility
 a. Adapts strategies and plans to address the impact of health care trends and issues on the team or health care organization
 b. Sees connections and patterns that are often not recognized as important by others

IX. MANAGEMENT CONCEPTS AND SKILLS

A. Management process

1. A manager is an individual employed by the organization who is responsible and accountable for efficiently accomplishing the goals of the organization
2. These responsibilities include
 a. Effectively accomplishing the goals of the organization
 b. Coordinating tasks and integrating resources
 c. Using the functions of planning, organizing, supervising, staffing, evaluating, and negotiating
 d. Clarifying the organizational structure
 e. Evaluating client care outcomes and providing feedback
 f. Coping with complexity

B. Functions of management process: planning, organizing, leading, and controlling

1. Planning and setting a direction
 a. Sets goals and decides the course of action through an inductive process
 b. Gathers data and looks for patterns
 c. Builds relationships and links to help explain issues, goals, expectations, and so on
 d. Creates visions and strategies for the organization's future
2. Organizing and aligning people
 a. Identifies work to be accomplished and goals to be achieved

b. Hires the right person for the right work
c. Creates interdependence by getting people to move in the same direction
d. Delegates authority by talking to anyone who can help implement the vision and strategies, as well as to those who can block implementation
e. Coordinates the work of others

3. Leading and getting others to believe the message
a. Influences others to get the job done
b. Keeps the message clear
c. Communicates with integrity and trustworthiness
d. Molds the culture and maintains morale
e. Insists on consistency between words and deeds

4. Controlling
a. Sets standards for accomplishing the organization's goals and activities
b. Determines means to measure performance and makes sure that quality lapses are spotted immediately
c. Evaluates performance
d. Provides feedback

X. MANAGING CHANGE

A. Change is making something different than it was; in many instances, the outcome remains the same, but the process is changed

B. Types of change
1. Personal change: voluntary change with the goal of self-improvement
2. Professional change: deliberate change with the goal of improving professional ability or status, or both
3. Organizational change: mandated change with the goal of improving the organization's efficiency

C. Change process: *planned change* involves a natural process that should be used as a guide for implementing change
1. Assessment: identifying the problem or opportunity that necessitates change
2. Data collection and analysis: gathering structural, technological, and personnel information and documenting the effects of these elements on the process
3. Strategic determination: identifying possible solutions, barriers, strategies
4. Change is often purposeful and usually is implemented to solve problems that affect nurses at work
5. Change is used to alter behavior of individuals and groups within the organization

D. Forces of change
1. Driving: those forces that facilitate change because they push toward the desired direction
2. Restraining: those forces that impede change because they push in the opposite direction
3. Change occurs because these forces shift the balance
4. Three-step process
a. Unfreezing: the reasons for making a change are given in a way to make the change desirable
b. Moving: the planned change is put into action
c. Refreezing: the new goal becomes established as an expected outcome
5. Attention is aimed at increasing driving forces, decreasing restraining forces, or both

E. Planned change is for low-level complexity change
1. It is easier to accept because it usually is a choice and has a deliberate process
2. It is not a coercive act or an accident
3. Planned change
a. Is being very structured
b. Is being stable in nature
c. Happens in increments
d. Proceeds sequentially and directionally
4. In contrast, high-level change is more fluid, more complex, and occurs in rapidly changing environments

F. Recognizing resistance

1. Individuals are often resistant to change because they are
   - a. Afraid of disorder
   - b. Upset by interruption of daily routine
   - c. Fearful of losing job
   - d. Fearful of losing power
   - e. Fearful of losing resources
2. Positive aspects of resistance
   - a. Change agent must be focused, ready to clarify information, and able to keep interest high
   - b. Resistance creates energy and movement
3. Negative aspects
   - a. Wears down supporters
   - b. Hard to stay focused among the constant challenges

G. Handling resistance

1. Be sure to communicate—often
2. Be clear and accurate
3. Be open and flexible
4. Acknowledge the negative consequences of resistance
5. Acknowledge the positive consequences of change
6. Maintain close contact and keep resisters involved
7. Promote trust, support, and confidence
8. Keep the energy moving—create disturbances
9. Monitor the politics of change
10. Develop good diagnostic skills and the ability to adapt the leadership style to the situation and the change
    - a. Allow participants to verbalize their concerns
    - b. Explain the rationale for change
    - c. Allow emotions to be expressed
    - d. Give information frequently
    - e. Help individuals cope with the change

H. Strategies to become a successful change agent

1. Present a clear and concise vision of the change
2. Set up ongoing meetings with team members to monitor the change process
3. Formulate a timeline and make team members accountable for their tasks
4. Keep all stakeholders and key individuals informed about the change and its progress
5. Be positive even in the face of resistance
6. Be alert for gossip, rumors, and inaccurate information about the change
7. Know the formal and informal leaders involved in supporting and implementing the change
8. Be confident and trust your own abilities in being a change agent

XI. PERFORMANCE IMPROVEMENT AND QUALITY ASSURANCE

A. History of quality assurance (QA)

1. Emerged in health care in the 1950s as an inspection approach to ensure minimum standards of care existed in health care institutions
2. Emphasized "doing the right thing" and was seen as punitive and not proactive toward preventing problems before they occurred
3. Is a program that focuses on clinical aspects of the provider's care, often in response to an identified problem

B. Total quality management (TQM)

1. Began in the manufacturing industry with W. Edwards Deming, Joseph Juran, and Japanese corporations in the 1950s
2. Focuses on customer satisfaction rather than on doing it right, but incorporates principles of QA
3. Integrated into health care delivery the 1980s

! **C. Definition of quality**
1. Meeting or exceeding the expectations of customers
2. Meeting and exceeding standards
3. Achieving planned outcomes

! **D. Quality management principles**
1. TQM
   a. Customer/client focus: recognizing customers and their needs
   b. Total organizational involvement: all organizational members are involved in the process
   c. Use of quality tools and statistics for measurement: decisions are supported by data
   d. Identification of key processes for improvement to continually do thing better for continuous quality improvement (CQI)
2. See Box 6–7, Ways to Enhance Quality Nursing Care

! **E. Components of quality management**
1. Comprehensive quality management plan
2. Structure, process, and outcome benchmarks
3. Performance appraisals
4. Intradisciplinary assessment and improvement
5. Interdisciplinary assessment and improvement

F. Methods of quality management in health care
1. Nursing audits
2. Peer review
3. Utilization review
4. Outcomes management

G. Measuring outcomes

! 1. **Indicators** are a measurement or flag used as a guide to monitor, assess, and improve the quality of client care, support services, and organizational functions affecting client outcomes

Box 6–7

Ways to Enhance Quality Nursing Care

1. **Seek to provide nursing care with the outcome of a continuous healing relationship.** Nursing care is responsive at all times (24 hours a day, every day), and access to nursing care should be provided over the Internet, by telephone, and by other means in addition to face-to-face visits.
2. **Provide nursing care based on patient needs and values.** The nursing care should be designed to meet the most common types of needs as well as to respond to individual patient choices and preferences.
3. **Remember that the client is the source of information.** Clients are given the necessary information and the opportunity to exercise the degree of control they choose over health care decisions that affect them.
4. **Nursing care requires shared knowledge and the free flow of information.** Clients have access to their own nursing and medical information and to clinical knowledge. The health team communicates effectively and shares information with clients and their families.
5. **Nurses use evidence-based decision making.** Clients receive care based on the best available scientific knowledge.
6. **Safety is a key feature in all aspects of nursing care.** Clients are kept safe and are protected from injury caused by the care system. Reducing risk and ensuring safety requires all nursing team members to pay greater attention to systems that help to prevent errors.
7. **Nurses anticipate client needs.** The nurses anticipate client needs rather than simply react to events.
8. **Nurses understand the essential need to cooperate with other clinicians.** Nurses and other clinicians actively collaborate and communicate to ensure an appropriate exchange of information and coordination of care.

! 2. Nurse-sensitive indicators are measurements of client care that are sensitive to nursing interventions, such as
   - a. Maintenance of skin integrity
   - b. Pressure ulcer prevalence rate
   - c. Pressure ulcer incidence rate
   - d. Fall injury rate
   - e. Medication incident rate
   - f. Restraint utilization rate
   - g. Client satisfaction for pain management
   - h. Client satisfaction with overall nursing care
   - i. Nurse satisfaction
   - j. Failure to rescue

H. Types of indicators

! 1. Structure indicator: describes characteristics of the setting that support and have an impact on care (e.g., availability of approved least restraint devices on a unit, RN-to-client ratio)

! 2. Process indicator
   - a. Measures an activity that is carried out to care for clients
   - b. Focuses on the nature and amount of care nurses provided during the hospital stay (e.g., rate of clients on fall prevention program, nurse satisfaction)

! 3. Outcome indicator
   - a. Describes the client's status at the defined time following care interventions
   - b. Measures the result of nursing care and process (examples: pressure ulcer prevalence rate, fall injury rate)
   - c. Measurement of nursing outcomes are key indicators to show impact of nursing care on positive client outcomes; indicators that most reflect the effect of nursing care are staff mix, total nursing care hours provided per patient day, pressure ulcers, client falls, client satisfaction, nosocomial infections, and nurse satisfaction

XII. RESOURCE MANAGEMENT

A. Resource management is determining the use of human and physical resources, which includes a variety of key activities:

1. Deciding to hire employees to fill these needs
2. Recruiting and training the best employees
3. Ensuring they are high performers
4. Dealing with performance issues
5. Ensuring your personnel and management practices conform to various regulations
6. Managing your approach to employee benefits and compensation, employee records, and personnel policies

B. Staffing and supervision are two of the most critical functions of a manager; each includes various other activities as well

! 1. Staffing can be viewed as a standard measure that quantifies nursing time and is measured by nursing care hours per day, or the nursing time available daily to each client

2. A full-time equivalent (FTE) is a measure of the work commitment of a full-time employee who works 40 hours a week, or 80 hours in a 2-week period
3. Hours worked and available for nursing care are called productive hours; nonproductive hours are designated as benefit time and include vacation, sick time, and educational time
4. A measurement tool used to describe the nursing workload for specific clients or a group of clients over hours worked is called a client classification system
5. A plan that identifies how many and what kind of staff are needed by shift and by unit is called a staffing pattern; staffing is a process that involves the following:
   - a. Deciding what human resources are needed, ideally in terms of knowledge, skills and abilities regarding specified roles, jobs and tasks (ideally these roles

are determined on the basis of strategic planning and defined in terms of competencies and/or job descriptions)
   - **b.** Recruiting the necessary human resources (sourcing, placing ads, etc.)
   - **c.** Considering outsourcing to hire outside expertise
   - **d.** Screening job candidates (interviewing, testing, etc.)
   - **e.** Selecting candidates (via job offers)
   - **f.** Equipping new hires (via orienting, training, facilities, assignments, etc.)

6. ! Supervision is the process of overseeing the productivity and progress of employees who report directly to the supervisors, often with use of direct reports, and also involves the following
   - **a.** Mutually setting goals with direct reports
   - **b.** Supporting conditions for their motivation
   - **c.** Observing performance and giving feedback and other forms of guidance
   - **d.** Conducting regular performance reviews
   - **e.** Addressing performance problems
   - **f.** Ensuring sufficient rewards

C. Level of supervision

1. First-level supervisors supervise entry-level employees
2. Middle managers supervise first-level supervisors
3. Chief executives supervise middle managers

D. Functions and activities of supervisors

1. Conducting basic management skills (decision making, problem solving, planning, delegation, and meeting management)
2. Organizing their department and teams
3. Noticing the need for and designing new job roles in the group
4. Hiring new employees
5. Training new employees
6. Employee performance management (setting goals, observing performance and giving feedback, addressing performance issues, firing employees, etc.)
7. Conforming to personnel policies and other internal regulations

! **E. Cost effectiveness**

1. Change in managed care plans has created the necessity to apply more accurate costing methods in the health care industry
2. Prior to the early 1980s, most health care providers operated on a retrospective payment basis, which based reimbursement on the cost of providing health care services
3. Medicare made a switch to a prospective service plan, which based payments on the client's diagnosis (coded in a reimbursement formula called Diagnosis Related Group, or DRG) and not on the cost of the services provided
4. In the 1990s, managed care plans refined DRGs further by making fixed payments, or capitations, for each member
5. Because hospitals and clinics must maintain costs below the capitation payments received in order to be profitable, it has become increasingly important for proper costing methods to be employed for better decision making

F. Cost containment

1. A primary concern of hospitals and other health care organizations, cost containment requires sound management practices, which include effective and efficient decision making using standardized, accurate, and timely operational management information, such as that provided by implementation of management information systems (MIS) Guidelines and workload measurement systems (WMS)
2. The MIS Guidelines are the national standards used to support the collecting, reporting, and use of financial and statistical data
3. Standardized information improves the quality and comparability of data for management planning, budgeting, monitoring, and evaluation
4. Through integration of official and statistical data, information is available to measure resource utilization and activity expenditure

5. The WMS are a key component of the MIS Guidelines that quantify the volume of activity provided by a specific service
   a. The use of standard definitions enhances the validity of a WMS; a reliable and valid nursing WMS is a key source of information
   b. WMS identify all activities of a nursing unit associated with clinical and nonclinical activities
   c. The collection of service activity statistics (e.g., inpatient days, visits) and caseload status statistics (e.g., new referrals, inpatient admissions, discharges) supplement workload
   d. Measuring the workload, service activity, and caseload status statistics gives a good indication of the amount and kind of service provided by a specific unit
   e. Data collected from WMS are used to develop indicators (ratios of financial and statistical data that help managers to plan, monitor, and evaluate performance); the use of indicators allows nurse managers to monitor variances between budgeted and actual results, determine the cause, and decide on corrective action
   f. Indicators provide nurse managers with the ability to explain the utilization of human and financial resources in quantifiable terms (e.g., cost of nursing care per inpatient day, workload units per visit, etc.)

G. Safety and quality of care

1. Directly related to the number and mix of direct care nursing staff
2. Nurse staffing levels and skill mix make a difference in the outcomes of clients; when there are more nurses, there are lower mortality rates, shorter lengths of stay, better care planning, lower costs, and fewer incidents
3. When health care facilities had more registered nurses per adjusted inpatient days, postoperative complications such as urinary tract infections, pneumonia, and blood clots in the legs were decreased
4. Increased registered nurse staffing is directly related to decreases in shock, upper gastrointestinal bleeding, decreased hospital length of stay, and fewer hospital-acquired infections such as urinary tract infections and pneumonia

H. Staff education

1. Organizational and individual excellence is best attained by training, development, and educational activities that build upon individual strengths and are forward looking; responsibility for performance and development lies jointly with the individual staff member and the health care organization
2. The individual staff member's responsibilities are to
   a. Take ultimate responsibility for his or her career
   b. Seek and use opportunities for development
3. The nurse leader's responsibilities are to
   a. Discuss development needs with individual staff member
   b. Influence performance with coaching and support
   c. Provide feedback on performance and potential for career development
4. The organizational responsibilities are to
   a. Identify human resource requirements
   b. Formulate and assign job roles
   c. Provide definitions and guidelines on performance expectations
   d. Establish training and development to advance levels of academic, technical, and administrative effectiveness in the organization

Check Your NCLEX-RN® Exam I.Q.

You are ready for testing on this content if you can

- Describe the various health care settings
- Monitor time management priorities
- Assist in assignment-making
- Request interdisciplinary consultation and referrals
- Provide effective leadership and management to nursing care personnel
- Demonstrate effective leadership strategies
- Describe the management process
- Effectively delegate nursing activities
- Apply the principles of change
- Incorporate performance improvement into clinical nursing practice
- Apply cost-effective measures to nursing practice

PRACTICE TEST

1 The nurse manager notes that several key organizational changes are about to begin, but staff morale is low on the nursing unit. How can the nurse leader best prepare the staff for the upcoming changes while maintaining the support of the frontline nursing staff?

1. Be willing to instill a deep-seated sense of ownership in the organization's work.
2. Use command-and-control behaviors to determine the priorities and manage supervision responsibilities.
3. Willingly share information and communicate to all frontline nursing staff within the organization.
4. Create a culture of workforce behaviors that includes having the right to act in the best interest of the organization.

2 A nurse is working in an organization that has a shared governance model. The nurse would assign priorities of the organization via which of the following mechanisms?

1. A decentralized decision-making model
2. A series of councils
3. A joint practice committee who decides the policies and procedures
4. An assigned-leadership council that establishes priorities of the organization

3 The nurse manager learns that the unit expenses have exceeded the budget allowance by $600,000 for the first half of the fiscal year. The nurse manager would use which of the following processes to most effectively prioritize client care activities and control the cost of care?

1. Decision-making process
2. Management process
3. Time management process
4. Total quality management process

4 A nurse is getting restless in the current position and is ready to apply for a middle-level manager position. A job is posted for a manager who would be responsible for directing and supervising several nursing personnel assigned to the surgical division of an acute care hospital. The nurse concludes that this position is at which level in the organization?

1. First-line manager
2. Director
3. Vice president of patient care services
4. Chief nurse executive

5 A female staff nurse on the unit asks the charge nurse to complete the wound care and dressing change on an assigned client because she finds wound care distasteful. The nurse manager would counsel the nurse about which of the following subjects?

1. Reverse delegation
2. Overdelegation
3. Underdelegation
4. Incomplete delegation

6 The emergency department just received a Homeland Security grant from the local department of health. It is the nurse manager's responsibility to determine how the funding should be allocated for staff training and equipment needs. The nurse manager considers that which leadership style would most effectively establish appropriate budgetary priorities?

1. Autocratic
2. Democratic
3. Laissez-faire
4. Bureaucratic

7 A staff nurse on the clinical excellence committee must prepare an in-service on delegation for nursing staff. In preparing the presentation, the nurse includes which explanation of how delegation impacts the safety and quality of client care?

1. It prevents nursing staff from becoming nonproductive and ineffective.
2. It gets the assigned nursing tasks done in the most efficient way, utilizing appropriate resources.
3. It gives nursing tasks to staff who can best understand the goal to be met.
4. It is a way to make the nursing staff feel as though they are part of the team.

PRACTICE TEST

8 A client on the medical surgical unit begins to code. The assigned registered nurse and the charge nurse are at lunch. The newly hired nurse manager begins to direct the resuscitation efforts until the code team arrives, using which of the following as the basis of power in this situation?

1. The staff's acceptance of direction
2. The manager's intelligence
3. The manager's formal position or rank
4. The manager's expertise and experience

9 A registered nurse who has been in practice for 6 months is due for the first performance evaluation. In preparing for the evaluation, the nurse should look to which standard against which to evaluate personal performance during the first 6 months of employment?

1. ANA standards of care
2. The state nurse practice act
3. The written job description
4. The organization's standard of clinical care

10 The registered nurse must delegate care of an assigned client to an unlicensed assistive person (UAP) for the shift. Which of the following clients would be best to delegate to the UAP?

1. A client who would benefit from talking about the recent death of her husband
2. A client with a Foley catheter and nasogastric feedings who is on bedrest
3. A client with an ostomy who has persistent problems with leakage
4. A client who was transferred from the critical care unit 3 days ago and is ambulatory

11 Which of the following tasks would not be appropriate for the registered nurse to delegate to licensed practical nurses (LPNs) or unlicensed assistive personnel (UAPs)?

1. Instructing the LPN to reinforce teaching of the RN's assigned clients prior to discharge
2. Assigning UAPs to complete vital signs and document and report information on any changes in client status to the RN
3. Asking the UAP to assess and evaluate the client response to IV pain medication
4. Instructing the LPN to remove a dressing from a postoperative client's abdominal wound

12 Nurse leaders have an obligation to find new ways to deliver needed nursing care services within new payment structures and cost-cutting strategies. What measures can the nurse leader take in an acute care setting to reduce the cost of health care?

1. Ask the nursing staff for suggestions to reduce waste.
2. Implement a quality improvement program to improve client outcomes and satisfaction.
3. Increase nurse–client ratios to reduce the cost of client errors.
4. Increase usage of unlicensed assistive personnel (UAP).

13 The charge nurse on the night shift reports that the narcotic count is incorrect. The nurse has already spoken to the staff nurse believed responsible for the incorrect count and has reason to believe that substance abuse by the nurse is the cause. If substance abuse by the staff nurse proves to be the cause of the incorrect count, what is the most appropriate next step?

1. Recount the narcotics with the staff nurse and take disciplinary action.
2. Ask the staff nurse to leave the unit immediately and report the incident to the American Nurses Association.
3. Complete an incident report, report findings to the pharmacy, and notify nursing administration.
4. Submit the findings to the Council on Nursing Practice.

14 The nurse manager has the responsibility to transfer or delegate to competent staff the authority to perform a selected task in a selected situation. Which of the following statements would be important for the nurse manager to make when delegating a responsibility?

1. "I am appointing you to be our unit's representative on the newly formed bioterrorists task force."
2. "I do not have the time for or interest in the monthly ethics committee meeting, so you will represent me."
3. "I am assigning you to do the performance evaluation on the unit's 10 UAPs. I am too busy working on the capital budget for next year to complete them myself."
4. "I chose you to attend the discharge planning meeting today because it seems you have the lightest assignment."

15 A quarterly audit is now due to assess the implementation of an electronic medical record system for client documentation on your unit. As the nursing unit representative who supervised the adaptation of this documentation system, how can the nurse determine if nursing staff members have accepted this change of the electronic medical record?

1. The nursing staff uses the electronic medical record daily in routine documentation.
2. The nursing staff verbalizes knowledge of the need for the electronic record but still choose to hand-write nursing notes into the clients' charts.
3. The nursing staff uses the electronic record sporadically to monitor clients' progress.
4. The nursing staff likes the electronic record because they believe it saves them time.

16 As a member of the hospital quality improvement team, the nurse has been asked to evaluate the quality of nursing care on the unit. The nurse has decided to ask the nursing staff for assistance in this endeavor. Which of the following would be appropriate to ask the nursing staff to do?

1. Track the number of supplies used by clients on the unit.
2. Document the time spent on direct client care.
3. Administer a client and family satisfaction survey.
4. Assess clients and report acuity daily.

17 As the registered nurse (RN) accountable for the delegation of nursing care activities for the shift, what must the nurse consider in determining the appropriate use of an unlicensed UAP?

1. The amount of support the RN can provide
2. The complexity of the nursing tasks
3. The amount of time the UAP will need to provide total client care
4. The capability of the UAP to perform client care assessment

18 A staff nurse decides to attend a continuing education class on the use of advanced technology in health care delivery. The nurse manager should interpret this participation in staff development and continuing education as which of the following?

1. A waste of time because CEU credits are not a mandate for promotion or relicensure
2. Not important because advanced technology is too expensive and only drives up the cost of health care without increasing direct client care
3. Essential to nursing care because advanced technology impacts several facets of health care delivery
4. Only important for nurse managers because they allocate the unit's resources for the use of advanced technology in client care

19 Authority occurs when a person has been given the right to delegate, based on the state nurse practice act, and also has official power to delegate from the health care organization. Which characteristic of a nurse manager could undermine this authority in the workplace?

1. Being confident in directing the work of others to accomplish their assignments
2. Being unsure of the scope and amount of authority given
3. Changing management style based on the situation and the needs of the staff
4. Easily accepting responsibility and accountability for actions

20 As a newly appointed charge nurse, the nurse has decided to assess the skills and competencies of all new nursing personnel assigned to your unit. What can the nurse do to help these new personnel learn their job duties and responsibilities?

1. Ask other nurses to keep an eye on the newly assigned staff.
2. Assign a preceptor to any new member of the nursing staff.
3. Ask current nursing staff to point out the new personnel's weak areas after a staff meeting.
4. Let the new nursing personnel learn job duties and functions without nursing staff interference.

21 An RN is about to make first rounds after receiving an intershift report at 3 p.m. In what order should the RN see the following clients? Fill in the order below.

1. A 54-year-old client 4 hours post–cardiac catheterization who has mild discomfort at the access site
2. A client newly diagnosed with diabetes mellitus who needs reinforcement of sick day management guidelines
3. A client who arrived 30 minutes ago from the postanesthesia care unit
4. A client who is ready for discharge but will not have transportation to home available until 5 p.m.
5. A client with pneumonia who has received two doses of IV antibiotics and has an oxygen saturation of 93%

Answer: ______________________

ANSWERS & RATIONALES

1 **Answer: 1** The nurse leader must be willing to instill a deep-seated sense of ownership in the organization's work to address the challenges and opportunities presented within the health care organization. Options 2, 3, and 4 are incorrect. A command-and-control leadership style will not gain the support of the frontline nursing staff, nor will sharing information and creating a culture of "know how to act right." Frontline staff must believe that they have entrepreneurial opportunities and a stake in the organization's success. **Cognitive Level:** Application **Client Need:** Safe, Effective Care Environment: Management of Care **Integrated Process:** Nursing Process: Planning **Content Area:** Leadership and Management **Strategy:** Use the process of elimination. The core issue of the question is determining the most effective way to prepare staff for needed organizational changes.

2 **Answer: 2** In a shared governance model, there is decentralized power sharing and decision making. Options 1, 3, and 4 are incorrect. The assigned priorities of the organization are accomplished through a series of councils. An example of a council might be a joint practice committee or a leadership council, but these councils would not be assigned the sole responsibility of assigning the organizational priorities. **Cognitive Level:** Application **Client Need:** Safe, Effective Care Environment: Management of Care **Integrated Process:** Nursing Process: Planning **Content Area:** Leadership and Management **Strategy:** The core issue of the question is methods for assigning priorities within a health care system using a shared governance model. Use the process of elimination and knowledge of the characteristics of this model in making a selection.

3 **Answer: 2** The management process includes planning, organizing, coordination, and control. Option 1 is incorrect because management is the process of coordinating actions and allocating resources to achieve organizational goals. Option 3 and 4 are also incorrect. Time management is a set of skills that helps nurses to use their time in the most effective and productive way possible. Total quality management process is a systematic process to improve outcomes based on client or customer needs.
Cognitive Level: Application **Client Need:** Safe, Effective Care Environment: Management of Care **Integrated Process:** Nursing Process: Planning **Content Area:** Leadership and Management **Strategy:** The core issue of the question is the appropriate process that will assist with determining appropriate, cost-effective priorities of care. Use the process of elimination and nursing knowledge in making a selection.

4 **Answer: 2** A middle-level manager is called a director. Option 1 is incorrect because a lower-level managerial job is a firstline management position. Options 3 and 4 are incorrect because a nurse in an executive role is called a chief nurse executive or vice president of client care services.
Cognitive Level: Application **Client Need:** Safe, Effective Care Environment: Management of Care **Integrated Process:** Nursing Process: Analysis **Content Area:** Leadership and Management **Strategy:** The core issue of the question is knowledge of the various levels of nursing positions within a health care organization. Use this knowledge and the process of elimination in making a selection.

5 **Answer: 1** Reverse delegation occurs when a person with a lower rank delegates to someone with authority. In this instance, the nurse with a limited client assignment is delegating upward to a nurse who has responsibility for the entire nursing unit for that shift. Option 2 is incorrect because overdelegation occurs when the delegator loses control over a situation by providing the delegate with too much authority or responsibility. Option 3 is incorrect, since underdelegation occurs when full authority and responsibility are not transferred. Option 4 is incorrect because incomplete delegation occurs when the delegator delegates a task and then, due to fear or inexperience, removes the task either while it is being accomplished or before it is fully accomplished, leaving the delegate feeling frustrated.
Cognitive Level: Application **Client Need:** Safe, Effective Care Environment: Management of Care **Integrated Process:** Nursing Process: Implementation **Content Area:** Leadership and Management **Strategy:** The core issue of the question is knowledge of the various types of delegation. Use knowledge of delegation and the process of elimination to make a selection.

6 **Answer: 2** Democratic leadership is participatory, and authority is delegated to others. Option 1 is incorrect. Autocratic leadership involves centralized decision making with the leader making decisions and using power to command and control others. Option 3 is incorrect. Laissez-faire leadership is passive and permissive, and the leader defers decision making. Option 4 is incorrect. Employee-centered leadership focuses on the human needs of subordinates.
Cognitive Level: Application **Client Need:** Safe, Effective Care Environment: Management of Care **Integrated Process:** Nursing Process: Planning **Content Area:** Leadership and Management **Strategy:** Note the critical words *most effectively* in the stem of the question. This tells you that more than one option could be chosen but that one is better than the others for one or more reasons. Use knowledge of leadership styles to make a selection.

7 **Answer: 2** The main purpose of delegation is to get the job done in the most efficient way using appropriate resources. The job must be delegated to team members who can understand and accept the responsibility of what the goal is and how it is to be achieved. Options 1, 3 and 4 are incorrect. Delegation can promote interest and prevent team members from becoming bored, nonproductive, and ineffective. By finding the duties or tasks that best fit team members, the nurse leader can help them feel valuable to the team regardless of their position. Each team member wants to feel that he or she is making a difference in the well-being of the client.
Cognitive Level: Application **Client Need:** Safe, Effective Care Environment: Management of Care **Integrated Process:** Nursing Process: Implementation **Content Area:** Leadership and Management **Strategy:** The core issue of the question is basic knowledge

related to the activity of delegation. Use this knowledge and the process of elimination to make a selection.

8 **Answer: 3** The nurse leader derives her or his source of authority within the workplace directly from a formally appointed position or rank. Options 2, 3 and 4 are incorrect. Although the followers or subordinates must accept the nurse leader's orders, they do so because of official authority. A nurse leader's personality traits, such as intelligence, are helpful for gaining compliance for delegated tasks but are not a source of authority. A nurse leader's expertise and experience are essential for delegation, but true authority and accountability for delegated tasks come directly from the organizational authority of the assigned position.
Cognitive Level: Analysis **Client Need:** Safe, Effective Care Environment: Management of Care **Integrated Process:** Nursing Process: Implementation **Content Area:** Leadership and Management **Strategy:** The core issue of the question is what type of power is best utilized in an urgent or emergent situation. Use knowledge of different sources of power and the process of elimination to make a selection.

9 **Answer: 3** The best way that the nurse can effectively self-evaluate performance of his or her job is to compare individual performance against the written job description. Job descriptions help identify activities that each staff member may perform. The ANA standards of care help set the parameters for minimal standards and should be used as guidelines. Individual state boards of nursing identify the legal boundaries of nursing practice to safeguard the public. The state nurse practice act assists nurse leaders in knowing what tasks are within the scope of their state's nurse practice act and the scope of practice for their staff members. The job descriptions are designed to support the organization's work and aide in standards of performance.
Cognitive Level: Analysis **Client Need:** Safe, Effective Care Environment: Management of Care **Integrated Process:** Nursing Process: Evaluation **Content Area:** Leadership and Management **Strategy:** The core issue of the question is knowledge of appropriate reference points when preparing for employee evaluations. Use the process of elimination and knowledge that the job description provides specific direction for practice in an institution to make a selection.

10 **Answer: 4** Factors to consider when delegating care include complexity of task, problem-solving innovation required, unpredictability, and level of client interaction. The client in option 4 is best because this client is likely to be stable with a low level of unpredictability. The client in option 1 requires a high level of client interaction. The client in option 2 represents a more complex client. The client in option 3 represents a client who would benefit from problem-solving innovation.
Cognitive Level: Analysis **Client Need:** Safe, Effective Care Environment: Management of Care **Integrated Process:** Nursing Process: Planning **Content Area:** Leadership and Management **Strategy:** The core issue of the question is basic concepts that are useful when considering delegation to a UAP. Use this knowledge and the process of elimination to make a selection.

11 **Answer: 3** The decision to delegate should be consistent with the nursing process (appropriate assessment, planning, implementation, and evaluation). The person responsible for client assessment, diagnosis, care planning, and evaluation is the registered nurse. LPN functions include reinforcing teaching and removal of dressings. Assistive personnel may perform simple nursing interventions, but the registered nurse remains responsible for analyzing the data and the client outcome.
Cognitive Level: Application **Client Need:** Safe, Effective Care Environment: Management of Care **Integrated Process:** Nursing Process: Implementation **Content Area:** Leadership and Management **Strategy:** The core issue of the question is the knowledge related to delegation of nursing tasks. Options 1, 3, and 4 are all within the scope of responsibilities of the assigned nursing personnel. UAPs cannot practice nursing. They cannot be delegated to assess or evaluate responses to treatment.

12 **Answer: 4** The purpose for using UAPs in acute care settings is to control cost and free registered nurses from duties, primarily non-nursing duties. This allows time for registered nurses to complete assessments of clients and evaluate their potential response to treatments.
Cognitive Level: Application **Client Need:** Safe, Effective Care Environment: Management of Care **Integrated Process:** Nursing Process: Analysis **Content Area:** Leadership and Management **Strategy:** Choose option 4 because personnel costs are the highest burden placed on health care institutions. By using UAPs, many institutions decreased their personnel budget and reduced significant costs. Eliminate option 2 because most health institutions have implemented quality improvement programs to improve client satisfaction and reduce risk first and then to save costs as a secondary factor. Then eliminate option 3 because it is incorrect. Acute care hospitals have increased the nurse–client ratios.

13 **Answer: 3** An incident report must be completed because of the inaccurate narcotic count. Narcotics are controlled substances and fall under federal law and regulation. Both the pharmacy and nursing administration must be notified. If the staff nurse is found to be using a controlled substance, this finding must be reported to the state board of nursing. Individual state boards of nursing identify the legal boundaries of nursing practice, including disciplinary action, through nurse practice acts (which differ among the states). The American Nurses Association, through the Code of Ethics for Nurses, provides guidance to nurses and protection for clients and their families but does not have the authority to discipline nurses.
Cognitive Level: Application **Client Need:** Safe, Effective Care Environment: Management of Care **Integrated Process:** Nursing Process: Analysis **Content Area:** Leadership and Management **Strategy:** The core issue of the question is an understanding of the nature and purpose of professional nursing organizations and institutions. Each state board is responsible for the regulation of nursing and articulates the principles for delegation and disciplinary action. Options 1 and 2 represent actions that a nurse manager would have to take to protect the public good. The functions of professional nursing organizations do not include statutory laws but rather ethical codes of conduct for both nursing students and professional nurses. Option 4 refers to professional organizations like ANA who may

have a Council on Nursing Practice which strive to develop standards of practice for professional nurses.

14 **Answer: 1** A key behavior in delegating tasks is to provide the delegatee with a reason for the task. Option 2 is incorrect because the nurse manager should delegate a task for the right reason and not because the task is time consuming or undesirable. Option 3 is incorrect: delegating performance evaluations is inappropriate because they contain private and confidential information. This task is solely the responsibility of the nurse manager and cannot be delegated. Option 4 is incorrect because the delegatee should be assigned a task that meets his or her abilities.

Cognitive Level: Application **Client Need:** Safe, Effective Care Environment: Management of Care **Integrated Process:** Nursing Process: Implementation **Content Area:** Leadership and Management **Strategy:** The core of the question deals with the delegation process. Delegation is transferring to a competent individual the authority to perform the task.

15 **Answer: 1** When people accept change, they integrate it into their routines and the change is maintained. Verbalizing, mentally rehearsing the change before agreeing to a pilot or trial, or even trying out the change are not indications that an individual has accepted the change.

Cognitive Level: Application **Client Need:** Safe, Effective Care Environment: Management of Care **Integrated Process:** Nursing Process: Implementation **Content Area:** Leadership and Management **Strategy:** Resistance to change is expected. The best way to know whether change has occurred is to witness it. Through observing how staff members adapt to the change by integrating into daily nursing assignments, the nurse manager knows for sure that the change has been accepted. Options 2, 3, and 4 do not illustrate that true change has occurred: actions speak louder than words.

16 **Answer: 3** Patient satisfaction surveys are an important tool to monitor and evaluate patient and family needs. This information helps health care organizations meet those needs. Options 1, 2, and 4 are extremely helpful but do not improve patient satisfaction and outcomes. Tracking supplies, documenting nursing time, and reporting on patient acuity provides information that can be used in preparing a budget or unit staffing requirements.

Cognitive Level: Application **Client Need:** Safe, Effective Care Environment: Management of Care **Integrated Process:** Nursing Process: Planning **Content Area:** Leadership and Management **Strategy:** The core issue of the question is quality management. The purpose of quality management is to improve performance and meet client needs. The best way to assess client satisfaction is to ask the client directly. Established standards of practice, policies, and procedures safeguard clients and protect them from potential injury and harm. Quality management programs seek to ensure quality care and improve client satisfaction.

17 **Answer: 2** Assignment-making requires that the nurse assess the education, skill, knowledge, and judgment levels of the staff being assigned to the task. This means that the nurse must know the functions of all personnel in delegating tasks, including the appropriate use of a UAP and LPN. Option 2 requires that the nurse understand the complexity of the nursing task before delegating it. Option 1 is incorrect because it is not the support but the amount of supervision the RN can provide that must be considered. Option 3 and 4 are incorrect because the UAP cannot provide total nursing care nor perform a client care assessment.

Cognitive Level: Application **Client Need:** Safe, Effective Care Environment: Management of Care **Integrated Process:** Nursing Process: Analysis **Content Area:** Leadership and Management **Strategy:** The core issue of the question is the delegation process. The nurse must always assess the client situation first. Know the skills and comfort level of the person to whom you are delegating.

18 **Answer: 3** Staff education is essential to maintaining clinical competence and patient safety; therefore, options 1 and 2 are incorrect. Information technology is important to all nurses not just to nurse managers to organize and manage nursing and health care delivery. Option 4 is incorrect as well.

Cognitive Level: Application **Client Need:** Safe, Effective Care Environment: Management of Care **Integrated Process:** Nursing Process: Analysis **Content Area:** Leadership and Management **Strategy:** The core of the question is understanding the impact of advanced technology on patient care and its underlying costs. Use general nursing knowledge and the process of elimination to make a selection.

19 **Answer: 2** The manager must feel worthy of the authority granted, and self-doubt can undermine this authority. Self-doubt is shown by being unsure. Options 1, 3, and 4 are all positive characteristics and attributes of a good manager.

Cognitive Level: Application **Client Need:** Safe, Effective Care Environment: Management of Care **Integrated Process:** Nursing Process: Implementation **Content Area:** Leadership and Management **Strategy:** The core of the question is knowledge about having and using authority. Nurse manager's are given formal authority upon appointment to the position by the organization. It is critical that nurse managers accept this authority and learn how to apply the power that comes from the appointed position.

20 **Answer: 2** A preceptor is an experienced nurse who assists someone new in learning his or her job. Asking others to keep an eye on the new nurse does not assure learning. Pointing out weaknesses after a staff meeting does not help the orientee become aware of learning needs. Learning without interference does not assure correctly learning the unit's expectations.

Cognitive Level: Application **Client Need:** Safe, Effective Care Environment: Management of Care **Integrated Process:** Nursing Process: Analysis **Content Area:** Leadership and Management **Strategy:** The core issue of the question is knowledge about the skills and competencies of the nurse manager. A nurse manager at any level, including charge nurse, is responsible for meeting the organizational needs. In order to meet this objective, the nurse must ensure all personnel are fully competent to carry out their job duties and functions.

21 **Answer: 3, 5, 1, 4, 2** Priority setting can be implemented using a variety of models. The client who is postoperative should be seen first because the client is newly arrived on the unit and is at most risk of becoming unstable or experiencing a change in clinical condition. The client with pneumonia

should be seen next because the infection involves the airway, although oxygen saturation levels are higher than the critical value of 90% or less. The client who is 4 hours post–cardiac catheterization should be seen next to evaluate the site and conduct general assessment of the affected extremity. The client who will be discharged should be seen next to determine that there are no last minute needs or issues. The client who needs teaching should be seen last because this is not a physiological need.

Cognitive Level: Analysis **Client Need:** Safe, Effective Care Environment: Management of Care **Integrated Process:** Nursing Process: Planning **Content Area:** Leadership and Management **Strategy:** Determine which client is at most risk of becoming unstable to pick client 3, followed by assessing the client whose airway is potentially at risk (client 5). The client with the cardiac catheter could become unstable but has been on the unit for 4 hours, so this client can be seen third. The fourth client scheduled for discharge should be checked fourth, because of time—it will not take long to address any remaining issues or concerns. The client needing teaching will need the most time and can be planned for last.

Key Terms to Review

autocratic leadership p. 49
bureaucratic leadership p. 49
capitation p. 38
consultation p. 46
delegation p. 42
democratic leadership p. 49
formal leadership p. 47
health maintenance organization (HMO) p. 38
indicators p. 55
informal leadership p. 48
interdisciplinary p. 46
laissez-faire leadership p. 49
leader p. 47
leadership p. 42
managed care p. 38
manager p. 47
overdelegation p. 45
planned change p. 53
reverse delegation p. 44
servant leadership p. 51
shared governance p. 39
supervising p. 42
supervisor p. 42
time management p. 39
transactional leadership p. 50
transformational leadership p. 51
underdelegation p. 44
vision p. 42

References

Aiken, L. H., Clarke, S. P., Cheung, S. P., Sloane, D. M., & Silber, J. (2003). Educational levels of hospital nurses and surgical patient mortality. *Journal of the American Medical Association,* 290(12), 1617–1623.

American Association of Colleges of Nursing. (2002). *Hallmarks of the professional nursing practice environment.* Washington, DC: Author.

American Nurses Association. (2001). *Analysis of American Nurses Association staffing survey.* Washington, DC: Author.

American Nurses Association. (2001). *Code of ethics.* Washington, DC: Author.

American Nurses Association. (2000). *Nurse staffing and patient outcomes in the inpatient hospital setting.* Washington, DC: Author

Blais, K. K., Hayes, J. S., Kozier, B. & Erb, G. (2002). *Professional nursing practice: Concepts and Perspectives.* Upper Saddle River: NJ: Prentice Hall, pp. 75–76, 100.

National Council of State Boards of Nursing. *Delegation: Concepts and decision making process* (1995). Position Paper. Retrieved December 29, 2005, from http://www.ncsbn.org/public/regulation/delegation_documents_delegati.htm#thefiver.

Delegation of UAP Issues: Delegation Documents. Council of State Boards on Nursing. Retrieved December 29, 2005, from http://www.ncsbn.org/public/regulation/delegation_documents.htm.

Dessler, G. (2004). *Management: Principles and practices for tomorrow's leaders.* Upper Saddle River, NJ: Prentice Hall, pp. 185–188.

Finkelman, A. W. (2001). *Managed care: A nursing perspective.* Upper Saddle River, NJ: Prentice Hall, pp. 246–247.

Grohar-Murray, M. E., & DiCroce, H. R. (2003). *Leadership and management in nursing.* Upper Saddle River, NJ: Prentice Hall, pp. 172–182.

Hansten, R. I., & Washburn M. J. (2004). *Clinical delegation skills: A Handbook for professional practice,* 3rd ed. Sudbury, MA: Jones & Bartlett.

Institute of Medicine. 2001. *Crossing the quality shasm: A new health system for the 21st century.* Washington, DC: National Academy Press.

Joint Commission on Accreditation of Healthcare Organizations. (2002). *Health care at the crossroads: Strategies for addressing the evolving nursing crisis.* Chicago: Author.

Sullivan, E. J., & Decker, P. J. (2005). *Effective leadership and management in nursing,* 6th ed. Upper Saddle River, NJ: Prentice Hall, pp. 43–64, 100–120.

7 Injury Prevention, Disaster Planning, and Protecting Client Safety

Test Yourself

Are you ready for the NCLEX-RN® or course exams? Use the practice tests on the companion CD-ROM to check.

In this chapter

Cross reference

Other chapters relevant to this content area are

Preventing and Controlling Infection **Chapter 8**

I. ACCIDENT PREVENTION ACROSS THE LIFE SPAN

! **A. Infant safety is dependent on the actions of parents and infant caretakers; anticipatory guidance at well-baby check-ups is an opportunity for the nurse to educate parents**

1. Infants should be placed on the back after eating and while sleeping; this will not increase risk of aspiration (contrary to prior thinking) and will reduce risk of sudden infant death syndrome (SIDS)
2. Rapid changes in development and acquisition of new motor skills put infants at increased risk for injury from falls from tables, beds, high chairs, infant seats, and so on
3. Infants riding in a car should be placed in a rear-facing car restraint system in the back seat; the rear-facing restraint system should be used until the child is 1 year old and at least 20 pounds
4. Because of their inability to communicate, infants are at risk for burns from applications of heat to the skin, such as from a hot water bottle or other heated device
5. Infant furniture should be carefully selected with special attention to current safety standards
   - **a.** Infants may be trapped by crib slats spaced too far apart
   - **b.** Infants or young children may be poisoned by lead paint on antique furniture (normal serum lead level is < 10 mg/dL; lead level 10-19 mg requires environmental history; higher levels require treatment to reduce or prevent neurological deficits)

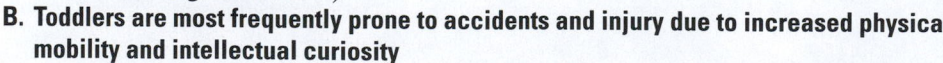

! **B. Toddlers are most frequently prone to accidents and injury due to increased physical mobility and intellectual curiosity**

1. Medications, cleaning supplies, and poisons should be in locked cabinets to prevent poisonings in the curious toddler; the poison control phone number should be readily available to the caregiver and posted on the telephone

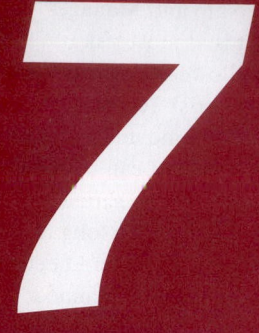

2. Car restraint systems for toddlers should be in the back seat and may be forward facing after the toddler has reached 1 year of age and 20 pounds; children should remain in car restraint systems until their shoulders are above the harness or their ears have reached the top of the seat; when a child outgrows the system, a booster seat with a lap/shoulder belt is required
3. Toddlers explore all objects with their mouths; assess toys for small parts; avoid giving foods such as hard candy, peanuts, and chewing gum to prevent choking and aspiration
4. Burns in toddlers occur as a result of chewing on electrical wires, pulling hot liquids from tables or stove tops, and touching space heaters; electrical outlets should be covered; handles of pans on stove tops should be facing inward
5. Drowning is one of the leading causes of death in toddlers; children should be accompanied at all times when in and around water in the bathtub, wading pool, or swimming pool

C. School-aged children are at risk for injury at home and in the community, as the school-aged child spends increased time away from the parent or caregiver

1. Pedestrian and bicycle safety must be taught and modeled to children at this age; bicycle helmets can prevent head injury to children biking, rollerblading, or skateboarding
2. Children under 12 years or under 4 feet 9 inches should be in the rear seat of a car with a lap/shoulder seatbelt; children should never be allowed to ride in the bed of a pickup truck or in an open, unsecured area of an automobile, such as a station wagon or van
3. School-aged children should be taught principles of fire safety; injury can occur from experimentation with matches, lighters, and fireworks; school-aged children can participate in implementing a school or home fire escape plan; teach to "stop, drop, and roll" if clothing catches fire
4. School-aged children should be taught principles of water safety; swimming lessons and life jackets are necessary for boating and swimming; children should never swim without adult supervision
5. Safety education for children should include playing in safe areas, avoiding strangers, recognizing unwelcome touch, and obeying traffic signals

D. Adolescent injury and death may be very violent in nature; newly found independence, feelings of invincibility and immortality, and access to motor vehicles can lead to accidents with injury

1. Courses in driver's education should be encouraged; seatbelt regulations should be role modeled and enforced by parents
2. Adolescents should be taught the dangers of alcohol and substance use
3. Adolescents may be injured in sports-related accidents; protective sporting gear should be encouraged for organized and impromptu sporting events
4. Water safety principles should be reviewed because adolescents can overestimate endurance when swimming
5. Adolescents benefit from information about sexual health, including information about sexually transmitted infections and pregnancy prevention (birth control)

E. Adult safety concerns can be related to the home, workplace, and leisure activities

1. Working adults should be encouraged to participate in occupational health programs offered in the workplace; musculoskeletal injuries are the most frequent workplace injury
2. Hazardous conditions and toxic substances may occur in the workplace; employees should be educated in **OSHA** (Occupational Safety and Health Administration) regulations and guidelines for use of safety devices and handling hazardous substances
3. Forty percent of deaths related to motor vehicle accidents are related to alcohol consumption; community programs that educate on hazards of drinking and driving should be implemented; other drugs that cause impairment pose similar risks

4. Firearms in the home may lead to accidental injury or death; all owners should attend firearm safety class; all firearms and ammunition should be stored in a locked cabinet
5. Residents in some neighborhoods may be at risk for crime and injury; assess for access to police and fire services
6. Residential fires account for the majority of fire-related injuries; all homes should have smoke detectors, a fire extinguisher in the kitchen, and a fire evacuation plan

F. Older adults may experience a decrease in strength, vision, hearing, and cognitive ability that could lead to accidents or injury; homes should be evaluated for safety hazards

1. Falls are the leading cause of accidents in older adults
   a. Stairwells should be well lit
   b. Rugs, runners, and mats should not be used
   c. Bathrooms and showers/tubs should have grab bars
   d. Furniture, floors, and passageways should be free of clutter
2. Modifications to the home may be necessary to accommodate safe use of wheelchairs or walkers
3. Clients taking some medications may have decreased cognitive abilities or impaired judgment; they should be encouraged to ask for assistance with activities of daily living
4. Neighbors, police, and fire officials should be made aware of older adults with disabilities living alone
5. Decrease in temperature regulation may increase the risk of hyperthermia or hypothermia; be careful with use of space heaters; be sure elders have fans or air conditioners in summer heat
6. Older adults may be prey to strangers and criminals who can inflict physical and financial injury; they should be cautioned against letting strangers into their homes or responding to telephone calls, e-mails, or letters asking for money or personal information
7. Motor vehicle accidents are of concern for older adults; frequent assessment of driving ability is required; loss of driving privileges can mean a loss of independence

II. ERROR PREVENTION IN HEALTH CARE SETTINGS

A. The Institute of Medicine has reported that people die in hospitals because of preventable medical errors; most errors are related to medications

1. Types of untoward medication events
   a. Medication error occurs when the wrong client, wrong medication, or wrong dose is given; it is also an error if it is given at the wrong time or by the wrong route
   b. **Adverse reaction** is an undesired effect of a prescribed medication, whether a side effect or a toxicity
   c. **Toxic reaction** is an effect that occurs when the prescribed medication dosage is excessive or poisonous to an individual; this may be due to client's size, health condition, or other medications being taken
   d. Side effects are actions or effects of drugs other than that desired
   e. **Idiosyncratic reaction** is an unusual response to a drug that may occur without relation to dose; the reaction may or may not reoccur if the medication is given again
   f. Hypersensitivity or allergic reactions may range from mild rashes to life-threatening anaphylaxis; this reaction will reoccur and could get worse with each subsequent exposure
2. Nursing interventions to prevent medication errors
   a. Know the medication administration system of the health care agency; follow the protocols
   b. Be familiar with medication resources at the institution

c. Ensure client information (e.g., heights, weights, allergies) is accessible to physicians, clinicians, and pharmacists
d. Verify medication orders; do not transcribe orders that contain unapproved or nonstandard abbreviations until clarified
e. Use standard hours and times for medication administration
f. Be familiar with side effects or possible adverse reactions; observe for these on an ongoing basis
g. Ask a nurse colleague to double check complex dosage calculations
h. Do not interrupt nurses giving medications; errors may be made because of interruptions during the administration process
i. Check client identification bracelet before administering medication; ask client to verbalize his or her name and date of birth according to agency policy; additional measures are needed with blood administration (see Chapter 33)
j. Double check medication when client questions appearance or dosage
k. Report and document any error or variation in the medication administration process

B. Allergies or an allergic response to an allergen can be life threatening for a client in the health care setting

1. Include a discussion of allergies in all health histories; ask about allergies to medications, food, tape, latex, or soap; document the type of reaction to the allergen
2. Allergies to seafood may alert the nurse to a potential allergy to iodine-based dyes used in radiologic procedures
3. Document all allergies on medical records, lab records, pharmacy records, client identification bracelet, and bedside nameplate

III. INJURY PREVENTION IN HEALTH CARE SETTINGS

A. Client safety can be at risk when admitted to a health care agency; assess risk factors for each client upon admission and identify methods to reduce the possibility of injury

B. Risk for falls is most common in infants and elderly clients; the nurse must administer a fall prevention program for those at risk

1. Assess ability to ambulate and transfer
2. Orient the client to the nurse call system and encourage use
3. Be sure the nurse call system is within reach
4. Keep bedside tables and chairs near the bed
5. Keep hospital beds in low position
6. Do not use full-length bed side-rails for confused clients; do not leave confused client alone—evaluate need for constant companion
7. Keep crib side-rails up when child is unattended
8. Encourage the use of nonskid footwear
9. Keep the room tidy and free of clutter
10. Use a bed or chair monitoring device if necessary for clients at risk for falls

C. *Restraints* are devices used to limit client mobility

1. Restraints can be physical or chemical
2. Purposes of restraints
   a. Reduce the risk of client injury from falls
   b. Prevent interruption of therapy such as traction or IV infusions
   c. Prevent a confused or agitated client from removing life support
   d. Reduce the risk of injury to others by an agitated client
3. There are legal implications related to the use of restraints because they limit client freedom
   a. A written order is needed to restrain a client
   b. Order must include the reason for restraint and the time period; PRN restraint orders are prohibited
   c. A nurse may apply physical restraints; however, physician/practitioner must evaluate client within an agency-prescribed time period, which may be as soon as 1 hour; verify hospital policy and follow it

! 4. Assess and document condition of a restrained client hourly; remove restraints, assess skin, and allow or assist client to reposition

5. Bed side-rails
   a. Are considered restraints
   ! b. Half or three-quarter rails may be better than full length rails for confused or agitated clients who may be injured climbing over rail; keep bed in the lowest position

! 6. Jacket, belt, or extremity restraints
   a. Apply only as specified by manufacturer; never tie them to a movable part of a bed or chair
   b. Use a half-bow knot for easy release when attaching the restraint to the bed or chair
   c. Check for adequate circulation when using restraints; maintain two finger widths between client and restraint

! 7. Try creative nursing measures to prevent use of physical or chemical restraints
   a. Orient client to surroundings
   b. Encourage family, friends, or a sitter to stay with client
   c. Keep confused clients near nursing station
   d. Provide confused clients with diversionary activities
   e. Maintain frequent toileting routine
   f. Reposition or ambulate frequently if appropriate
   g. Evaluate client medications for undesirable effects
   h. Use relaxation techniques such as music, aroma therapy, and books on tape

D. Seizure precautions protect client in case of seizure activity; clients are at risk for injury if they experience seizures

1. Explain purpose of seizure precautions
2. Pad head and side-rails of bed with blankets and linens to prevent injury
3. ! Keep suction and oxygen equipment near bed; use oxygen mask after seizure activity has ceased
4. ! Do not attempt to insert anything into mouth of client during seizure (bitestick, airway)

E. Fire safety

1. Preventive measures for hospital or agency
   a. Staff needs to be aware of safety precautions and fire prevention practices
   b. Know categories of fire and correct type of extinguisher to use for each
   c. Participate in practice fire drills and evacuation procedures
2. ! Use the acronym RACE to recall what to do in an actual fire:
   a. Remove clients from danger
   b. Activate the fire alarm
   c. Contain the fire
   d. Evacuate area (do horizontal evacuation if possible before vertical evacuation)

Memory Aid

Use the mnemonic RACE to remember in order the four steps to maintain client safety during a fire.
Remove clients from danger.
Activate the fire alarm.
Contain the fire.
Evacuate the area (horizontal evacuation should be done before vertical evacuation if possible).

3. Preventive measures for home
   a. Focus on teaching emergency phone numbers, maintenance of smoke alarms and fire extinguishers, importance of family fire drills, careful disposal of burning cigarettes and use of matches, grease fire prevention
   b. Teach precautions during an actual fire: close windows and doors to contain fire, cover nose and mouth with damp cloth when leaving a smoke-filled area, and stay as close as possible to the ground

F. Employee safety

1. Is the responsibility of each employee
2. Occupational Safety and Health Administration (OSHA), a federal agency, regulates the workplace to protect health of employees
3. **Bloodborne pathogen** exposure is a health hazard for many employees in a health care setting; OSHA has issued written standands that include recommendations from the Centers for Disease Control (**CDC**) regarding standard precautions (see also Chapter 8 on preventing and controlling infections)
   a. Standard precautions are techniques used with all clients to decrease risk of exposure to pathogens
   b. Gloves and face and eye protection will help protect health care workers from bloodborne pathogens
   c. Nurses may be required to have a vaccine for hepatitis B or sign a declination refusing the vaccine
4. The Needlestick Safety and Prevention Act was issued by Congress in 2000 to protect health care workers
   a. Nurses receive majority of needle and sharps injuries
   b. Do not recap needles and do not bend or break needles before disposal
   c. Ensure that sharps containers are in each client room and medication area
   d. Needle-free technology should be provided by employers
   e. Each health agency must have a needle/sharps injury protocol in case of injury; report all injuries and follow protocol for self-protection
5. Environmental infection control can protect employees and clients from exposure to pathogens; the U.S. Health and Human Services Centers for Disease Control and Prevention sets standards for infection control for health care agencies
   a. Employees may be annually tested for tuberculosis
   b. Laundry and medical waste are regulated by environmental infection control guidelines: laundry and items soiled with blood or body fluids must be identified by biohazard markers such as red bags
6. Latex allergy is a hazard for health care workers and clients
   a. Some individuals may have or develop an allergy to natural latex rubber products
   b. Latex rubber is used in many medical products but most frequently found in gloves used in health care settings
   c. Always ask clients about latex allergies; be sure latex-free gloves are available
   d. Provide a latex-free cart that includes latex-free tourniquets, IV tubing and IV supplies, and other items for clients with a latex allergy
7. Hazardous chemicals pose a safety threat in many areas of a health care setting
   a. Material Safety Data Sheets (**MSDS**) are OSHA-required informational handouts that describe any and all chemical agents in an employment setting
   b. Employees are required to be trained in the use of MSDS
   c. All chemicals are required to be properly labeled and have a corresponding MSDS
   d. Read and be aware of all information related to chemicals before handling or cleaning spills; examples of chemicals in a health care setting are antineoplastic agents (chemotherapy drugs), cleaning supplies, and pesticides
   e. In case of a chemotherapy drug spill, restrict the area of the spill and contact environmental services; if nurse must clean the spill, refer to the MSDS protocol on unit (see Box 7–1)

IV. INCIDENT REPORTS

A. An agency record of an accident or an unusual occurance

B. Agencies have specific forms to report accidents, falls, needle sticks, client infections, medication errors, or missing personal property

C. For the protection of client and nurse, it is vital to report all incidents

Box 7-1

Procedure for Chemotherapy Drug Spill

1. Restrict area of the spill.
2. Obtain a chemotherapy spill kit (gloves, gown, goggles, detergent, sponges, labeled container for disposal).
3. Use absorbent sponges to absorb spill.
4. Clean surface with designated cleanser.
5. Dispose of all supplies in approved container.
6. Wash hands.
7. Cleanse all skin exposed to chemotherapy agent—both client and staff.
8. Document the occurrence.

!

D. Procedure for incident reporting

1. Prevent further injury and provide care for client, visitor, or employee
2. Notify physician or practitioner immediately and take orders for interventions that may limit further harm
3. File report as soon as possible; the person filing the report may or may not be the person responsible for or involved in the incident
4. Identify client, visitor, employee, and all witnesses to the event
5. State objective facts of incident; do not draw conclusions or lay blame
6. Be specific—list name of medication or equipment involved
7. Document facts of incident in client's record also; do not document in client record that an incident report was filed
8. The policy for incident reporting is unique to each health care agency; review and follow specific agency policy for incident reporting

V. DISASTER PLANNING AND EMERGENCY RESPONSE

A. Disasters and emergencies are traumatic events that can affect an individual, family, community, or nation; nurses and health care providers are instrumental in disaster preparedness, disaster response, and client care in community and hospital settings

1. Disasters may be natural or man-made; disasters vary by predictability, frequency, preventability, imminence, and destructive potential
2. Natural disasters such as hurricanes and floods generally allow time for planning and evacuation; disasters such as earthquakes and tornados do not allow for evacuation but are predictable in certain parts of the country; residents and health care providers should be encouraged to prepare
3. Man-made disasters are usually less predictable; explosions, fires, airline accidents, radiation emergencies, bioterrorism, and toxic chemical releases occur randomly; however, plans can be made by health care providers and emergency response personnel to have trained resources to take action
4. The Federal Emergency Management Agency (FEMA) is a government agency that has a National Response Plan; it provides states and local communities guidelines for reporting threats and incidents and for assessment, response, and recovery during disasters; nurses are part of disaster planning and response at federal, state, and local levels
5. Purpose of disaster planning is to decrease community vulnerabilty and to assure available resources in the event of a disaster

B. Planning for any type of disaster must start with individuals and families; it is the role of the community health nurse to educate and guide citizens in preparedness

1. Families must have a communication plan; emergency phone numbers should be carried by all family members; establish a place to meet in an emergency
2. Be prepared to shut off all utilities in the home; water may be precious after a disaster; electricity and natural gas may pose a safety threat
3. A package of vital records should be readily available when evacuating a home; identification, health and immunization records, insurance policies, deeds, and cash or traveler checks would be needed during and after an evacuation

4. Identify special family needs; make an emergency kit; have extra medications and dietary requirements; have extra batteries for medical devices
5. Make plans for homebound pets; pets are not usually allowed in shelters; leave food and water; attach proper pet identification
6. Encourage family members to learn CPR and first aid

C. The Joint Commission on Accreditation of Hospitals *(JCAHO)* requires hospitals to have a disaster plan and to periodically practice response to plan

1. Plan should include policy and procedures for administration, nursing and patient service, medical staff, security, medical records, engineering, laboratory, radiology, as well as the following:
   a. Notification and communication of disaster
   b. Assessment of hospital resources
   c. Personnel recall system/transportation plan
   d. Establishment of a facility control center
   e. Maintenance of accurate records
   f. Communication and public relations
   g. Equipment and resupply
2. Nurses are responsible for knowing their role in disaster response and are part of committees that design and evaluate the hospital plan; nursing tasks during a disaster may include the following:
   a. Assess nursing unit for resources—staff, beds, and equipment
   b. Assess current clients for discharge in case of increased need of hospital/nursing services by high acuity/injured clients
   c. Activate staff recall plan
   d. Communicate with hospital disaster control center
   e. Assess disaster victims for extent of injury; this is called **triage**
   f. Render first aid
   g. Provide treatment based on protocols

D. Triage is a French word meaning "to sort"; in case of emergency, nurses may be asked to triage injured or ill clients to identify those in need of emergent, urgent, or nonurgent care

1. Primary survey focuses on airway, breathing, circulation, and neurological disability/deficits (ABCD)
   a. Clear and open the airway
   b. Assess for respiratory distress
   c. Assess quality of ventilation (rate, color, auscultate lungs)
   d. Check pulses for quality and rate
   e. Assess for external bleeding
   f. Take blood pressure
   g. Assess level of consciousness and pupillary response, weakness or paralysis of extremities

Memory Aid

Remember ABCD to recall the components of the primary survey for a victim of trauma: Airway, Breathing, Circulation, Disability (deficits).

2. The secondary survey is initiated after any lifesaving interventions have been implemented
   a. Measure and record a full set of vital signs
   b. Remove all of client's clothing
   c. Do a complete health history and physical examination
   d. Identify family members
   e. Administer comfort measures or pain medication if appropriate
3. After initial assessment, identify and label victims according to triage acuity system
   a. Priority I or emergent care is needed for victims who need immediate treatment, such as those with cardiac or respiratory distress, trauma and bleeding, or neurological deficits; these victims should be labeled with a red tag
   b. Priority II or urgent care is needed for victims who need treatment within 2 hours, such as clients with simple fractures, lacerations, or fevers; these victims should be labeled with a yellow tag and reevaluated every 30 to 60 minutes

c. Priority III or nonurgent care is needed for victims who need treatment that can wait for hours; those with sprains, rashes, and minor pain should be labeled with a green tag and reevaluated every 1 to 2 hours; an orange tag indicates a client who has a nonemergent psychiatric condition
d. Victims who are deceased should be labeled with a black tag and transported to designated temporary morgue

4. It is common to use the terms emergent, urgent, and nonurgent to describe a client's triage status if situation is not part of a disaster

Check Your NCLEX-RN® Exam I.Q.

You are ready for testing on this content if you can

- Identify client developmental and environmental factors that may lead to accidents or injury.
- Provide care and teaching to the client at risk for accident or injury.
- Protect the client who is at risk for injury.
- Utilize restraints safely, effectively, and only when necessary, such as when less restrictive measures are unsuccessful.
- Accurately identify situations requiring completion of an incident or unusual occurrence report
- Explain personal and professional actions to take for disaster preparedness.
- Effectively utilize triage concepts in an emergency or disaster situation.

PRACTICE TEST

1 The nurse determines a new mother is in greatest need of more education about infant care and safety when the mother states:

1. "I am pretty sure that I am going to breast-feed my baby."
2. "After feeding, the baby should be put on her tummy to prevent choking."
3. "Solid foods are not necessary during the baby's first 4 to 6 months."
4. "My baby will sleep frequently and should be awakened every 3 to 4 hours for feeding."

2 The result of a toddler's lead screening is 12mg/dL. The nurse should say which of the following to the mother at this time?

1. "His lab values are just fine."
2. "Have you noticed any blood in his stools?"
3. "When were his last immunizations?"
4. "Tell me about where you live."

3 When planning for discharge from the birthing center on the following day, the nurse learns that the father will drive the new mother and infant home. When teaching the new parents about infant restraint systems, the nurse should include that the restraint system be (select all that apply):

1. Forward facing
2. Rear facing
3. In the back seat
4. In the front seat
5. Of a bland or neutral color

4 Which of the following snacks should the nurse offer the hospitalized toddler?

1. Crackers
2. Peanuts
3. Grapes
4. Cereal bar

5 What is the best method for the nurse to use to encourage the use of bicycle helmets by school-aged children?

1. Advocate for legislation on helmet laws.
2. Teach parents to role-model helmet use while riding bicycles.
3. Verbally reprimand children who report not wearing helmets while riding.
4. Recommend the parents purchase stylish helmets to increase compliance.

6 A school nurse is planning a health class on accidents and injuries for a high school class. Which topic is most important to include?

1. Occupational-related injuries at work
2. Motor vehicle–related injuries
3. Fall-related injuries
4. Injury due to residential fires

7 The home health nurse is visiting an elderly client with diabetes mellitus. The nurse becomes concerned and implements safety education when which of the following occurs?

1. The neighbors bring a warm lunch to the elderly client.
2. The children install new air-conditioning units in the kitchen and bedroom.
3. The grandchildren fold laundry and place the baskets by the door to the bedroom.
4. The client stores the diabetic testing supplies on the kitchen table.

8 The nurse supervisor observes the new RN administering medications on the unit. The nursing supervisor concludes there is a risk for medication error when the nurse does which of the following?

1. Answers a physician's page while passing medications
2. Uses military time for documentation
3. Asks for help with a dosage calculation
4. Does not give a medication that the client questions

9 The nurse would ask a client scheduled for thyroid scanning about allergy to which of the following before the procedure?

1. Peanuts
2. Shellfish
3. Eggs
4. Meat tenderizer

10 The nurse prepares a dose of a medication ordered by the subcutaneous route and calculates the dose to be 4.5 mL. What is the first nursing action that the nurse should take?

1. Verify the written order.
2. Call the physician.
3. Call the pharmacist.
4. Ask another nurse to check the dosage calculation.

11 The nurse is restarting an IV line on a client known to have hepatitis B. Which precautions should the nurse use to protect against exposure? Select all that apply.

1. Hand washing
2. Gloves
3. Mask
4. Face shield
5. Gown

12 Which of the following medication orders should the nurse question?

1. Morphine sulfate (Morphine) 4mg IV every 3 to 4 hours as needed for pain
2. Ceftriaxone (Rocephin) IVPB every 8 hours
3. Furosemide (Lasix) 40 mg po daily
4. Metoprolol (Lopressor) 50 mg po twice a day

13 The nurse is aware that a confused elderly client is at risk for falls. Which of the following interventions would the nurse avoid using with this client?

1. Orient the client to the call light system.
2. Keep the hospital bed in low position.
3. Keep the full bed rails up at all times.
4. Assist with appropriate toileting every 2 hours.

14 The nurse has applied elbow splints on a confused client to prevent the client from removing the intravenous (IV) line. Which of the following interventions is required?

1. Document the appearance of the client's IV site every hour.
2. Remove the restraints every 8 hours.
3. Ask for a renewal of the physician's restraint order every 72 hours.
4. Assess and document client condition at least every hour.

15 A Code Red (fire) has been announced on the hospital unit. What is the nurse's first response?

1. Remove clients in danger from the fire.
2. Contain the fire.
3. Report the fire to other staff.
4. Extinguish the fire.

16 A client on the hospital unit has fallen. Place the following nursing interventions in order of priority.

1. Identify all witnesses.
2. Call the physician.
3. Assess and provide urgent care.
4. Notify the house supervisor.
5. Fill out the incident report.

17 Which of the following items would the nurse avoid documenting when a reportable incident has occurred?

1. Names of witnesses in the incident report
2. Nursing interventions in the medical record
3. Time the physician was called in the incident report
4. That an incident report was submitted in the medical record

18 Public health nurses have been activated to open a shelter due to an approaching hurricane. What most important items should families be encouraged to take to the emergency shelter?

1. Food and extra clothing
2. Cats and small dogs
3. Medication and vital records
4. Radios, televisions, and small personal electronics

19 A major portion of a construction project has collapsed. The emergency department (ED) has been notified that numerous victims are being transported to the ED. The first action of the ED nurses should be which of the following?

1. Assess the department for resources—staff, beds, equipment.
2. Implement the personnel recall system.
3. Discharge stable clients.
4. Set up a temporary morgue.

20 A young man is brought to the emergency department as one of the first victims of a motor vehicle accident that caused multiple casualties. The man is awake and alert. He has a fracture of his right tibia and several small lacerations on his face. How will the triage nurse categorize this client?

1. Priority 1 (red tag)
2. Priority 2 (yellow tag)
3. Priority 3 (green tag)
4. Priority 4 (black tag)

21 The nurse should explain to the mother of an 12-month-old infant that a forward-facing infant seat is safest once the infant weighs at least how many pounds? Fill in the number.

Answer: ______________

ANSWERS & RATIONALES

1 **Answer: 2** Infants should always be put to sleep on the back. Options 1, 3, and 4 are correct statements related to infant care and therefore pose no risk to the infant and no concern to the nurse.
Cognitive Level: Analysis **Client Need:** Safe, Effective Care Environment: Safety and Infection Control **Integrated Process:** Nursing Process: Evaluation **Content Area:** Child Health
Strategy: The wording of the question guides you to look for a false statement as the correct response. Use the process of elimination and nursing knowledge.

2 **Answer: 4** The lead value of 12mg/dL is high. Lead levels below 10mg/dL are acceptable. Levels of 10–19mg/dL require an environmental history. Levels above 20mg/dL require a full medical evaluation. Asking a question regarding the child's address is the first step in evaluating the environment. Older homes may have lead paint and lead in the plumbing. Option 1 is inaccurate because the level is high (not normal), and option 2 and 3 are unrelated to lead poisoning.
Cognitive Level: Application **Client Need:** Safe, Effective Care Environment: Safety and Infection Control **Integrated Process:** Nursing Process: Assessment **Content Area:** Child Health
Strategy: To answer the question it is required to know acceptable lead values. Option 4 is related to environmental assessment.

3 **Answer: 2 and 3** A child restraint system should always be in the back seat and rear facing. After a child is 1 year of age

and 20 pounds, the seat may be in the rear and front facing. Although bright colors are stimulating to an infant, the color of the system does not matter.
Cognitive Level: Application **Client Need:** Safe, Effective Care Environment: Safety and Infection Control **Integrated Process:** Teaching/Learning **Content Area:** Child Health **Strategy:** Option 3 and 4 cannot both be correct. Use the process of elimination and nursing knowledge of infant safety measures to make a selection.

4 **Answer: 1** Crackers are a soft consistency when chewed and swallowed. Toddlers can easily choke on small foods such as peanuts, popcorn, and grapes, and on firm consistency foods such as cereal bars.
Cognitive Level: Application **Client Need:** Safe, Effective Care Environment: Safety and Infection Control **Integrated Process:** Nursing Process: Implementation **Content Area:** Child Health **Strategy:** Option 1 is correct because it is unlike the other three options. Options 2, 3, and 4 are hard foods that do not dissolve in the mouth with the action of saliva.

5 **Answer: 2** Parent role models of behavior are the best method to develop good habits in children. The other options, although possibly valid (except option 3), are not the *best* answer.
Cognitive Level: Application **Client Need:** Safe, Effective Care Environment: Safety and Infection Control **Integrated Process:** Nursing Process: Planning **Content Area:** Child Health **Strategy:** The key word is *best.* All answers could be correct. Option 1 is a good idea but may not change behaviors. Option 3 is a negative behavior. Option 4 may be effective but is not realistic for all families.

6 **Answer: 2** Driving a car and having the independence to ride with friends is an important milestone for high school–aged adolescents. Some adolescents experiment with alcohol and drugs, putting them at increased risk for motor vehicle accidents. Option 1 is a risk for working adults, and options 3 and 4 are risk factors for the elderly.
Cognitive Level: Analysis **Client Need:** Safe, Effective Care Environment: Safety and Infection Control **Integrated Process:** Nursing Process: Planning **Content Area:** Child Health **Strategy:** Use knowledge of the principles of growth and development to aid in answering this question.

7 **Answer: 3** Laundry baskets that are set on the floor will pose a risk for falling for the elderly client. All hallways, floors, stairways, and furniture should be free of clutter. Neighbors bringing lunch and family controlling climate for the elderly client are good safety interventions. Keeping diabetic supplies on a kitchen table with easy access will facilitate diabetic testing.
Cognitive Level: Application **Client Need:** Safe, Effective Care Environment: Safety and Infection Control **Integrated Process:** Nursing Process: Assessment **Content Area:** Adult Health **Strategy:** Focus on the critical word *safety* and choose the option that poses a risk to the client. Recall that older adults are at increased risk for falls, so this should guide your thought process as you make a selection.

8 **Answer: 1** The nurse should never interrupt the process for administering medications. Errors are typically made when the nurse is interrupted. Military time is frequently used by institutions for documentation. The nurse should always ask for assistance with dosage calculations when in doubt. The nurse should never give a medication that a client questions. Always double check the order, dosage, and medication, and give the client an explanation.
Cognitive Level: Analysis **Client Need:** Safe, Effective Care Environment: Safety and Infection Control **Integrated Process:** Nursing Process: Analysis **Content Area:** Fundamentals **Strategy:** Review the process for medication administration to make the correct selection.

9 **Answer: 2** Iodine is used in many radiological procedures. Shellfish allergies may be an indicator of iodine allergy. The other options do not address this concern.
Cognitive Level: Application **Client Need:** Safe, Effective Care Environment: Safety and Infection Control **Integrated Process:** Nursing Process: Assessment **Content Area:** Fundamentals **Strategy:** Knowledge of radiological procedures must be applied. In addition, recall that allergy to iodine or shellfish commonly applies to radiological procedures.

10 **Answer: 1** If there is confusion related to a medication order, refer to and verify the original written order. Be careful to read abbreviations and dosage correctly. Asking another nurse or the pharmacist, or calling the physician are correct interventions, but not the first intervention, because the first step in the medication process is the writing of the order. Once that is verified, the nurse could choose any of the other options, which are correct.
Cognitive Level: Analysis **Client Need:** Safe, Effective Care Environment: Safety and Infection Control **Integrated Process:** Nursing Process: Implementation **Content Area:** Fundamentals **Strategy:** Think about the process involved in delivering a medication to a client. Recall that the order is first written, then filled by and delivered from pharmacy, then drawn up by the nurse, and then administered to the client. Begin with the first step—checking the order.

11 **Answer: 1, 2** Hand washing and gloves are the only precautions needed for starting an IV. Masks, face shields, and gowns are appropriate for procedures that may result in body fluids splashing.
Cognitive Level: Analysis **Client Need:** Safe, Effective Care Environment: Safety and Infection Control **Integrated Process:** Nursing Process: Planning **Content Area:** Fundamentals **Strategy:** Recall standard precautions and infectious disease precautions. Hand washing and use of gloves are appropriate for any procedure.

12 **Answer: 2** Option 2 does not have a medication dosage listed. All other options have required information for dispensing medications.
Cognitive Level: Application **Client Need:** Safe, Effective Care Environment: Safety and Infection Control **Integrated Process:** Nursing Process: Planning **Content Area:** Fundamentals **Strategy:** Read all options carefully. Apply the five rights of medication administration.

13 **Answer: 3** Full bed rails are a type of physical restraint. A confused client may attempt to climb over the rails, increasing the risk for fall and injury. The other options are positive interventions for reducing risk for falls.
Cognitive Level: Application **Client Need:** Safe, Effective Care Environment: Safety and Infection Control **Integrated Process:**

Nursing Process: Implementation **Content Area:** Fundamentals **Strategy:** Use the process of elimination and visualize the client in the question to select the option that could lead to client harm for a confused client.

14 **Answer: 4** The client should be checked at least hourly, and the nurse is required to document status. The IV site should be checked every hour, but documentation may be done only once per shift unless a problem occurs. Physical restraints impede a client's freedom, and thus their use needs to be ordered every 24 hours. Because restraints may also impede circulation, they should be removed according to agency policy, which is generally every 1 to 2 hours rather than every 8 hours. **Cognitive Level:** Application **Client Need:** Safe, Effective Care Environment: Safety and Infection Control **Integrated Process:** Nursing Process: Implementation **Content Area:** Fundamentals **Strategy:** Utilize knowledge of common policy and procedures for use of physical restraints. Always consider an answer that contains assessment as an option.

15 **Answer: 1** The primary responsibility of the nurse is client safety. Removing a client from danger should be the priority. Others can come to help contain or extinguish the fire. **Cognitive Level:** Analysis **Client Need:** Safe, Effective Care Environment: Safety and Infection Control **Integrated Process:** Nursing Process: Implementation **Content Area:** Fundamentals **Strategy:** Option one is client focused. The other options are fire focused. Remember the mneumonic RACE (remove, alarm, contain, extinguish).

16 **Answer: 3, 4, 2, 1, 5** The primary action of the nurse is emergency assessment and first aid. If the nurse contacts the nursing supervisor, there will be nursing help to contact the physician and speak with witnesses. After caring for the client and assessing the situation, the nurse is prepared to fill out the incident report. **Cognitive Level:** Analysis **Client Need:** Safe, Effective Care Environment: Safety and Infection Control **Integrated Process:** Nursing Process: Implementation **Content Area:** Fundamentals **Strategy:** Focus on the client first. Then obtain additional help, collect data, and do the paperwork last.

17 **Answer: 4** The medical record belongs to the client and should contain all of the facts related to the client and the incident. The incident report belongs to the hospital and should contain all of the facts and supportive data related to the client and the incident. The medical record should not refer to the incident report. **Cognitive Level:** Application **Client Need:** Safe, Effective Care Environment: Safety and Infection Control **Integrated Process:** Nursing Process: Implementation **Content Area:** Fundamentals **Strategy:** Use knowledge of policy and procedure regarding incident reports to analyze this situation.

18 **Answer: 3** Client medications and vital records are needed for a short or extended stay at an emergency shelter. Space is very limited in a shelter. There is no provision for storing food, and animals are not allowed. Loud electronic devices such as radios or televisions may cause disturbance between families or individuals. Electricity may or may not be available. **Cognitive Level:** Analysis **Client Need:** Safe, Effective Care Environment: Safety and Infection Control **Integrated Process:** Nursing Process: Planning **Content Area:** Fundamentals **Strategy:** Focus on the required items for a stay in the emergency shelter. A client's medications are the only provisions listed that emergency personnel may not be able to provide.

19 **Answer: 1** The nurses must first assess current emergency department resources. No decisions can be made without a comprehensive assessment, such as outlined in option 1. The other options are not as encompassing, and a comprehensive assessment is needed with a possible impending disaster. **Cognitive Level:** Analysis **Client Need:** Safe, Effective Care Environment: Safety and Infection Control **Integrated Process:** Nursing Process: Assessment **Content Area:** Fundamentals **Strategy:** Choose the option that is the most comprehensive or global of the option choices.

20 **Answer: 2** The client is awake and alert. He does not have overt signs of cardiac or respiratory distress. This client can wait for treatment for 1 to 2 hours. Check on his status every 30 to 60 minutes. Depending on the status of the other incoming casualties, this client may move up in priority. **Cognitive Level:** Application **Client Need:** Safe, Effective Care Environment: Safety and Infection Control **Integrated Process:** Nursing Process: Implementation **Content Area:** Adult Health: Musculoskeletal **Strategy:** Know the principles and protocols of triage. Eliminate priority I, which is always life-threatening, and option 4, which indicates death. Choose option 2 over 3 because fractures need attention within a few hours to reduce risk of complications.

21 **Answer: 20** The infant must weigh at least 20 pounds in order to be safe in a forward-facing infant seat and must be 1 year or older. **Cognitive Level:** Application **Client Need:** Safe, Effective Care Environment: Safety and Infection Control **Integrated Process:** Teaching/Learning **Content Area:** Child Health **Strategy:** Because this item is a standard, it is necessary to commit this information to memory. A quick way to remember this requirement is at that the number 20 is also the number of fingers and toes on an infant.

Key Terms to Review

adverse reaction p. 68
bloodborne pathogen p. 71
CDC p. 71
idiosyncratic reaction p. 68
JCAHO p. 73
MSDS p. 71
OSHA p. 67
restraint p. 69
toxic reaction p. 68
triage p. 73

ANSWERS & RATIONALES

References

American Academy of Pediatrics (n.d.). *For your family.* Retrieved April 24, 2005, from http://www.aap.org/family/carseatguide

Centers for Disease Control (n.d.). Retrieved May 21, 2005, from http://www.cdc.gov

Clark, M. J. (2003). *Nursing in the community: Caring for populations* (4th ed.). Upper Saddle River, NJ: Prentice Hall.

Consumer Product Safety Commission (n.d.). *Older consumers safety checklist.* Retrieved May 21, 2005, from http://www.cpsc.gov/CPSCPUB/PUBS/705.pdf

Deglin, J. H., & Vallerand, A. H. (2006). *Drug guide for nurses.* Philadelphia: FA Davis.

Federal Emergency Management Agency (n.d.). *Are you ready? Emergency planning and checklists.* Retrieved July 6, 2005, from http://www.fema.gov/areyouready/emergency_planning.shtm

Healthy People 2010 (n.d.). Retrieved April 24, 2005, from http://www.healthypeople.gov

Institute of Medicine of the National Academies (n.d.). Retrieved May 21, 2005, from http://www.iom.edu

Kozier, B., Erb, G., Berman, A., & Snyder, S. (2004). *Fundamentals of nursing: Concepts, process, and practice.* Upper Saddle River, NJ: Prentice Hall.

Lewis, S. M., Heitkemper, M. M., & Dirksen, S. R. (2004). *Medical surgical nursing: Assessment and management of clinical problems.* St. Louis, Missouri: Mosby.

Mothershead, J. L. (n.d.). *Disaster planning.* Retrieved March 12, 2005, from http://www.emedicine.com/emerg/topic718.htm

Otto, S. E. (2004). *Oncology nursing: Clinical reference.* St. Louis, Missouri: Mosby.

U.S. Department of Labor Occupational Safety and Health Administration (n.d.). *Bloodborne pathogens and needlestick prevention.* Retrieved March 12, 2005, from http://www.osha.gov

8 Preventing and Controlling Infection

Test Yourself

Are you ready for the NCLEX-RN® or course exams? Use the practice tests on the companion CD-ROM to check.

In this chapter

Cross Reference

Other chapters relevant to this content area are

Intravenous Therapy	Chapter 32
Total Parenteral Nutrition	Chapter 34
Perioperative Care	Chapter 49
Respiratory Disorders	Chapter 56
Oncological Disorders	Chapter 66
Communicable or Infectious Diseases	Chapter 68

I. STANDARD PRECAUTIONS

! **A. *Chain of infection* comprises six elements that must occur for infection to develop**

1. Etiologic agent: any pathogen capable of causing infection; causative agents include bacteria, virus, fungi, protozoa, rickettsiae, and helminths
2. Reservoir: favorable environment in which infectious organism grows and reproduces; reservoir may be animate (humans, animals, insects) or inanimate (food, water, soil, equipment); blood and the respiratory, gastrointestinal (GI), reproductive, and urinary tracts serve as reservoirs in humans
3. Portal of exit from reservoir: route by which microorganism leaves reservoir; portal of exit can be breaks in skin, the blood, and respiratory, GI, reproductive, and urinary tracts in humans
4. Method of transmission: mode by which microorganism is transferred from reservoir to host; transfer occurs by three mechanisms: direct transmission, indirect transmission, airborne transmission
   a. Direct contact involves physical transfer of causative agent from person to person; routes of direct transmission include touching, kissing, biting, and sexual intercourse; transmission can also occur through droplets when person talks, coughs, sneezes, or spits, but only when source is within 3 feet of susceptible host
   b. Indirect contact involves transfer from reservoir to susceptible host via either a vehicle or a vector; vehicle-borne transmission requires inanimate object to serve as mode of transmission; intermediary agent, such as an animal or insect, is required in vector-borne transmission

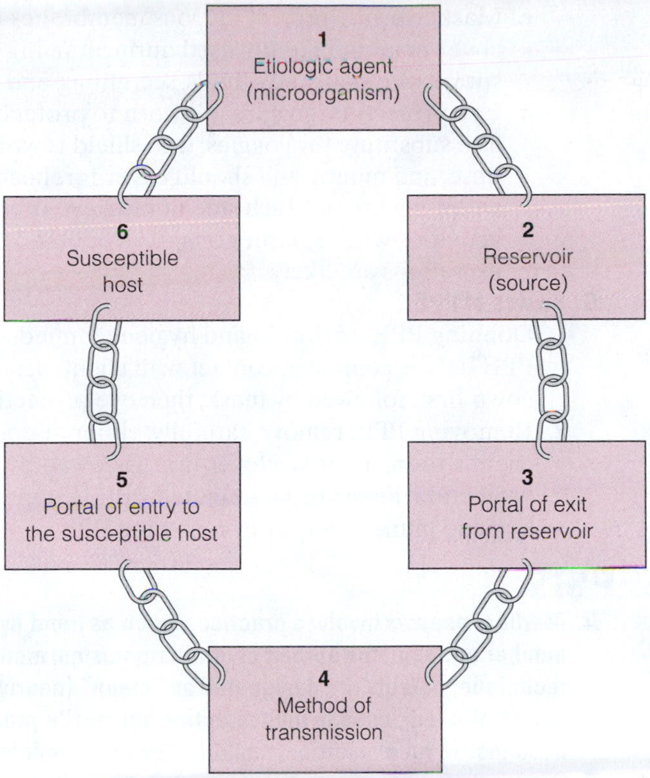

Figure 8–1

Links in the chain of infection.

Source: Kozier, Erb, Berman, & Snyder (2004).

c. Airborne transmission involves transport of droplet nuclei or dust bearing the infectious agent by air currents

5. Portal of entry to susceptible host: route by which infectious agent enters susceptible host; examples include breaks in skin and respiratory, GI, reproductive, and urinary tracts
6. Susceptible host: individual at increased risk for infection; infection occurs when infectious agent overwhelms host's defenses to resist infection (Figure 8–1)

! **B. *Standard precautions* represent first tier of Centers for Disease Control (CDC) guidelines for isolation precautions**

! **C. Standard precautions reduce risk of transmission of infection, protecting both health care providers and clients from recognized and unrecognized sources**

! **D. Always used in providing care to all clients regardless of medical diagnosis and regardless of setting**

E. Applies to blood, all body fluids, excretions, and secretions except sweat regardless of whether blood is visible or whether skin and mucous membranes are not intact

F. Includes hand hygiene and the use of *personal protective equipment (PPE)*

1. Hand hygiene: most effective way to prevent spread of microorganisms; perform before and after each client contact, immediately following exposure to blood and/or other body fluids and contaminated items, and before and after donning gloves; wash hands with plain (nonantimicrobial) soap and water or use waterless alcohol-based hand rub.
2. PPE is equipment worn by health care providers to prevent transmission of microorganisms and includes
   a. Gloves (clean, nonsterile): worn to protect health care provider's hands when exposure to blood, body fluids, secretions, excretions, and contaminated items is likely; used for touching mucous membranes and nonintact skin; change gloves if they become torn or heavily soiled, even between procedures on same client; avoid adjusting PPE or touching noncontaminated items with contaminated gloves; remove promptly after use and wash hands
   b. Gown: worn to protect health care provider's skin and clothing; used during procedures and care activities when splashing or spraying of blood, body fluids, secretions, and excretions is possible

c. Mask: worn to protect mucous membranes of nose and mouth; should fully cover nose and mouth; used during nursing care activities when splashes or sprays of blood, body fluids, secretions, and excretions can be expected
d. Eye protection: goggles are worn to protect eyes; do not use personal glasses as a substitute for goggles; face shield is worn to protect face, including eyes, nose, and mouth, and should cover forehead, extending below chin and wrapping around each side of face; eye protection is used during nursing care activities when splashes or sprays of blood, body fluids, secretions, and excretions are likely

G. Basics of PPE

1. Donning PPE: perform hand hygiene immediately before donning PPE; don PPE before coming in contact with client, usually outside client's room; don gown first, followed by mask, then eye protection, then gloves
2. Removing PPE: remove carefully, either at doorway or immediately outside client's room; remove gloves first, followed by mask, then gown, then eye protection; discard contaminated PPE in appropriate container; perform hand hygiene immediately after removing PPE

II. MEDICAL ASEPSIS

! **A. *Medical asepsis* involves practices, such as hand hygiene and use of PPE, to reduce the number and limit the spread of microorganisms; medical asepsis is also known as clean technique; objects are designated as "clean" (nearly free of microorganisms) or "dirty" (contaminated); used in implementing nonsterile procedures, such as taking vital signs, nasogastric tube insertion, and tube feeding administration**

B. Disposal of contaminated equipment and supplies is conducted in accordance with institution policies and procedures

1. Linens: handle soiled linen as little as possible in a manner that prevents exposure to health care provider's skin, mucous membranes, and clothing; contain soiled linens in a bag before removal from client's room
2. Dishes: no special considerations are needed; some facilities may use disposable dishes for convenience
3. Syringes, needles, and sharps: avoid recapping needles or detaching needles from syringes; dispose of items in a rigid, puncture-resistant container immediately after use
4. Equipment (thermometers, blood pressure equipment): dedicated equipment is used for clients with transmission-based precautions; discard single-use (disposable) items immediately after use in an appropriate manner; reusable (nondisposable) equipment must be cleaned and decontaminated before use with other clients
5. ! Lab specimens: place specimen in a leak-proof container with a biohazard label; container should be placed in a sealed plastic bag
6. ! Transportation of clients with infections: avoid transporting clients with infections to other parts of hospital; if transportation is necessary, take precautions to prevent spread of infection to others; an individual with respiratory infection should wear a mask; an individual with an infected wound should have wound covered; notify personnel in receiving department of client's infection

III. SURGICAL ASEPSIS

A. General principles

1. **Surgical asepsis** involves practices to maintain objects and areas free of microorganisms
2. Surgical asepsis is also known as sterile technique; objects are designated as "sterile" (completely free of microorganisms) or "nonsterile" (contaminated)
3. Used in implementing sterile procedures, such as intravenous therapy and urinary catheterization

! **B. Principles and practices of surgical asepsis are listed in Table 8–1**

Table 8–1 Principles and Practices of Surgical Asepsis

Principles	Practices
All objects used in a sterile field must be sterile.	All articles are sterilized appropriately by dry or moist heat, chemicals, or radiation before use. Always check a package containing a sterile object for intactness, dryness, and expiration date. Sterile articles can be stored for only a prescribed time; after that, they are considered unsterile. Any package that appears already open, torn, punctured, or wet is considered unsterile. Storage areas should be clean, dry, off the floor, and away from sinks. Always check chemical indicators of sterilization before using a package. The indicator is often a tape used to fasten the package or contained inside the package. The indicator changes color during sterilization, indicating that the contents have undergone a sterilization procedure. If the color change is not evident, the package is considered unsterile. Commercially prepared sterile packages may not have indicators but are marked with the word sterile.
Sterile objects become unsterile when touched by unsterile objects.	Handle sterile objects that will touch open wounds or enter body cavities only with sterile forceps or sterile gloved hands. Discard or resterilize objects that come into contact with unsterile objects. Whenever the sterility of an object is questionable, assume the article is unsterile.
Sterile items that are out of vision or below the waist level of the nurse are considered unsterile.	Once left unattended, a sterile field is considered unsterile. Sterile objects are always kept in view. Nurses do not turn their backs on a sterile field. Only the front part of a sterile gown (from the waist to the shoulder) and 2 inches above the elbows to the cuff of the sleeves are considered sterile. Always keep sterile gloved hands in sight and above waist level; touch only objects that are sterile. Sterile draped tables in the operating room or elsewhere are considered sterile only at surface level. Once a sterile field becomes unsterile, it must be set up again before proceeding.
Sterile objects can become unsterile by prolonged exposure to airborne microorganisms.	Keep doors closed and traffic to a minimum in areas where a sterile procedure is being performed because moving air can carry dust and microorganisms. Keep areas in which sterile procedures are carried out as clean as possible by frequent damp cleaning with detergent germicides to minimize contaminants in the area. Keep hair clean and short or enclose it in a net to prevent hair from falling on sterile objects. Microorganisms on the hair can make a sterile field unsterile. Wear surgical caps in operating rooms, delivery rooms, and burn units. Refrain from sneezing or coughing over a sterile field. This can make it unsterile because droplets containing microorganisms from the respiratory tract can travel 1 m (3 ft). Some agencies recommend that masks covering the mouth and the nose should be worn by anyone working over a sterile field or an open wound. Nurses with mild upper respiratory tract infections refrain from carrying out sterile procedures or wear masks. When working over a sterile field, keep talking to a minimum. Avert the head from the field if talking is necessary. To prevent microorganisms from falling over a sterile field, refrain from reaching over a sterile field unless sterile gloves are worn and refrain from moving unsterile objects over a sterile field.
Fluids flow in the direction of gravity.	Unless gloves are worn, always hold wet forceps with the tips below the handles. When the tips are held higher than the handles, fluid can flow onto the handle and become contaminated by the hands. When the forceps are again pointed downward, the fluid flows back down and contaminates the tips. During a surgical hand wash, hold the hands higher than the elbows to prevent contaminants from the forearms from reaching the hands.

Table 8-1 *(continued)*

Principles	Practices
Moisture that passes through a sterile object draws microorganisms from unsterile surfaces above or below to the sterile surface by capillary action.	Sterile, moisture-proof barriers are used beneath sterile objects. Liquids (sterile saline or antiseptics) are frequently poured into containers on a sterile field. If they are spilled onto the sterile field, the barrier keeps the liquid from seeping beneath it. Keep the sterile covers on sterile equipment dry. Damp surfaces can attract microorganisms in the air. Replace sterile drapes that do not have a sterile barrier underneath when they become moist.
The edges of a sterile field are considered unsterile.	A 2.5 cm (1 in.) margin at each edge of an opened drape is considered unsterile because the edges are in contact with unsterile surfaces. Place all sterile objects more than 2.5 cm (1 in.) inside the edges of a sterile field. Any article that falls outside the edges of a sterile field is considered unsterile.
The skin cannot be sterilized and is unsterile.	Use sterile gloves or sterile forceps to handle sterile items. Prior to a surgical aseptic procedure, wash hands to reduce the number of microorganisms on them.
Conscientiousness, alertness, and honesty are essential qualities in maintaining surgical asepsis.	When a sterile object becomes unsterile, it does not necessarily change in appearance. The person who sees a sterile object become contaminated must correct or report the situation. Do not set up a sterile field ahead of time for future use.

Source: Kozier, B., Erb, G., Berman, A., & Snyder, S. (2004). *Fundamentals of Nursing: Concepts, Process, and Practice* (7th ed.). Upper Saddle River, NJ: Pearson Education, pp. 655–656.

IV. TRANSMISSION-BASED PRECAUTIONS

A. *Transmission-based precautions* are measures to limit the spread of pathogenic microorganisms

! **B. *Airborne precautions***

1. Involves spread of infection through airborne droplet nuclei smaller than 5 microns, evaporated droplets that remain suspended in air for long periods of time, or dust particles containing infectious agent
2. Because microorganisms can be widely spread by air currents, special air handling and ventilation are needed
3. Examples of diseases include rubeola (measles), varicella (chicken pox), and tuberculosis
4. Use standard precautions and mask; use other PPE as appropriate for expected risk of exposure
    a. For tuberculosis, wear particulate respirator mask that is fit-tested to individual nurse
    b. For other airborne diseases such as rubeola or varicella, susceptible persons should not enter client's room; if entry is unavoidable, respiratory protection must be worn
    c. Individuals immune to rubeola or varicella do not need to wear respiratory protection
5. Place client in private, negative–air pressure room with 6 to 12 air exchanges per hour; air is discharged/vented to outdoors or undergoes high-efficiency filtration before being recirculated
6. If private room is not possible, client may be placed in room with another client (cohorted) who has an infection with same microorganism but no other infection
7. Client should remain in room with door closed
8. If transportation of client to other hospital departments is unavoidable, client should wear surgical mask
9. Visitors should wear mask appropriate to type of infection at all times

! **C. Droplet precautions**

1. Involves spread of infection by particle droplets larger than 5 microns that can be generated when client coughs, sneezes, talks, laughs, and so on

2. Examples of diseases include diphtheria (pharyngeal), mycoplasma pneumonia, rubella, pertussis, mumps, streptococcal pharyngitis, pneumonia, and scarlet fever
3. Use standard precautions; mask is required when providing care or if within 3 feet of client; use other PPE as appropriate
4. Place client in private room; if private room is not possible, client may cohorted with another client who has same infection but no additional infections
5. Client should remain in room; if transportation of client to other hospital departments is unavoidable, client should wear surgical mask; notify personnel in receiving department of client's infection
6. Door to room may remain open
7. Visitors should wear mask if within 3 feet of client and should try to maintain distance of 3 feet whenever possible

! **D. Contact precautions**

1. Involves spread of infection by contact with client or contact with items in client's environment
2. Examples of diseases include skin infections (scabies, pediculosis, herpes simplex or zoster), hepatitis A, and wound, GI or urinary infections, including those with multi–drug resistant organisms, such as **methicillin-resistant *Staphylococcus aureus* (MRSA)** and **vancomycin-resistant enterococcus (VRE)**
3. Use standard precautions; gloves are required; wear gown when contact with infected secretions is expected; use other PPE as appropriate for expected risk of exposure
4. Place client in private room; if private room is not possible, client may be cohorted with another client who has same infection
5. Door to room may remain open
6. Limit transportation of client to other hospital departments; infected wound should be securely covered; notify personnel in receiving department of the client's infection
7. Dedicate equipment for client care (such as stethoscope or sphygmomanometer) to a single client or cohort of clients; if such devices must be used to care for other clients, adequately clean and disinfect these devices first

E. Multiple precautions

1. A client is not limited to one set of transmission-based precautions; rather, precautions are implemented based on specific need
2. For example, a client with measles who has a wound infected with MRSA would require both airborne and contact precautions
3. Clients with severe acute respiratory syndrome (SARS) require the use of both airborne and contact precautions; SARS is a highly infectious viral infection that is transmitted by airborne respiratory droplets and by touching surfaces and objects contaminated with infectious droplets

Check Your NCLEX-RN® Exam I.Q. *You are ready for testing on this content if you can*

- Describe the chain of infection.
- Explain the principles of standard precautions.
- Correctly don and remove personal protective equipment.
- Distinguish between medical and surgical asepsis.
- Explain principles of medical and surgical asepsis.
- Compare and contrast transmission-based airborne, droplet, and contact precautions.
- Identify infectious diseases that require transmission-based precautions.

PRACTICE TEST

1 The nurse would do which of the following when washing the hands as part of medical asepsis before caring for an assigned client in an outpatient clinic?

1. Wash the hands with the hands held higher than the elbows.
2. Adjust the temperature of the water to the hottest possible.
3. Scrub the hands and nails with a scrub brush for 5 minutes.
4. Use a clean paper towel to turn the water off.

PRACTICE TEST

2 The nurse's forearm is splattered with blood while inserting an intravenous catheter. What action should the nurse take?

1. Wipe the blood away with an alcohol swab.
2. Wipe the blood away with a tissue.
3. Flush the forearm with hot water, letting the water flow from the elbow toward the fingers.
4. Wash the forearm with soap and water.

3 The nurse concludes that further teaching about standard precautions is needed when a family member of a client with acquired immunodeficiency syndrome (AIDS) states,

1. "I need to wear a mask when I visit."
2. "We can still hug one another."
3. "I don't need to use special dishes."
4. "My children cannot catch AIDS if they play a board game together."

4 The nurse would do which of the following to protect the client from infection at the portal of entry?

1. Place a sputum specimen in a biohazard bag for transport to the lab.
2. Empty a Jackson-Pratt drain, using sterile technique.
3. Dispose of soiled gloves in a waste container.
4. Wash hands after providing client care.

5 Which of the following actions by the nurse comply with core principles of surgical asepsis? Select all that apply.

1. Wash hands before and after client care.
2. Keep the sterile field in view at all times.
3. Wear personal protective equipment.
4. Add contents to the sterile field holding the package 6 inches above the field.
5. Consider the outer 1.5 inches of the sterile field as contaminated.

6 Which of the following precautions would the nurse implement when admitting to the nursing unit a client with herpes zoster?

1. Airborne precautions
2. Contact precautions
3. Droplet precautions
4. Neutropenic precautions

7 A client with tuberculosis asks the nurse if visitors will need to wear masks. What response by the nurse is most accurate?

1. "Everyone who enters your room must wear a mask to protect themselves from tuberculosis."
2. "Masks would not be necessary for visitors who have had tuberculosis before."
3. "It is less important for your family to wear masks, since they live in close contact with you."
4. "Only visitors who are at risk for tuberculosis need to wear a mask."

8 The nurse is leaving the room of a client who has methicillin-resistant *Staphylococcus aureus* (MRSA) microorganisms in a wound and the urine. Place the following personal protective equipment in order of removal.

1. Eye protection
2. Gloves
3. Mask
4. Gown

Fill in your answer below:

Answer: ____________________

9 A client with suspected severe acute respiratory syndrome (SARS) arrives at the emergency department. Which of the following physician orders should the nurse implement first?

1. Airborne and contact isolation
2. IV D_5NS at 100 mL/hr
3. Nasopharyngeal culture for reverse-transcription polymerase chain reaction
4. Sputum for enzyme immunoassay testing

10 In addition to standard precautions, which other type(s) of isolation precautions should the nurse use when caring for the client with severe acute respiratory syndrome (SARS)?

1. Droplet precautions
2. Airborne precautions and contact precautions
3. Contact precautions and droplet precautions
4. Airborne precautions

11 The nurse is changing an abdominal dressing on a client who has an infection spread by droplets. Which of the following pieces of personal protective equipment would the nurse use?

1. Clean gloves
2. Mask
3. Gown
4. Eye protection

12 A client with vancomycin-intermediate-resistant *Staphylococcus aureus* (VISA) is admitted to the nursing unit. What type of precautions should the nurse institute?

1. Standard precautions
2. Neutropenic precautions
3. Droplet precautions
4. Contact precautions

13 The nurse would formulate which of the following as the most appropriate goal for the client with droplet precautions?

1. The client will identify three ways to reduce the spread of infection.
2. The client will limit the risk of exposure to the causative agent.
3. The client will be taught how to take antimicrobial medication.
4. The client will understand how to protect other family members.

14 The nurse would implement which of the following as a requirement of care specific to the client who has tuberculosis?

1. Disposal of needles and syringes in a rigid, puncture-proof container
2. Handwashing after removing contaminated gloves
3. Wearing a gown if splashing is possible
4. A private room with negative air flow

15 The nurse would expect to institute transmission-based precautions for a client with which of the following?

1. Pneumonia caused by *Pseudomonas aeruginosa*
2. *Pneumocystis carinii* pneumonia
3. A sacral wound contaminated by *Escherichia coli*
4. A draining leg wound with methicillin-resistant *Staphylococcus aureus*

16 A client asks, "How did I get scarlet fever?" Which of the following would be the best response by the nurse?

1. "Scarlet fever is transmitted through sexual intercourse."
2. "You can get scarlet fever if you share contaminated needles or get a blood transfusion."
3. "Most people get it by eating contaminated food."
4. "You inhaled infected droplets in the air."

17 The nurse is assisting the client who has methicillin-resistant *Staphylococcus aureus* in collecting a clean-catch urine specimen. Which of the following protective equipment is unnecessary?

1. N95 particulate respirator
2. Gown
3. Eye protection
4. Sterile gloves

18 The nurse is preparing to irrigate a wound infected with vancomycin-resistant *enterococci.* Which of the following should the nurse wear?

1. Gloves, gown, and particulate respirator
2. Gloves and surgical mask
3. Gloves, eye protection, and particulate respirator
4. Gloves, gown, eye protection, and surgical mask

19 The nurse assigned to the respiratory care unit is working with four clients who have pneumonia. The nurse should assign the only remaining private room on the nursing unit to the client infected with which of the following organisms?

1. Penicillin-resistant *Streptococcus pneumoniae* pneumonia
2. *Pseudomonas aeruginosa* pneumonia
3. *Pneumocystis carinii* pneumonia
4. *Legionella pneumophila* pneumonia

20 The nurse is caring for a client with hepatitis A. Which of the following client statements indicates that teaching conducted by the nurse about disease transmission was effective? Select all that apply.

1. "We must avoid kissing."
2. "We can use the same bath towels."
3. "We must avoid eating with the same utensils."
4. "We must wear masks."
5. "No special precautions are needed."

ANSWERS & RATIONALES

1 **Answer: 4** Option 4 is correct because the faucet is considered contaminated. The hands are considered to be more contaminated than the elbows. Therefore, water should flow from least contaminated to most contaminated, eliminating option 1. Option 2 can result in burns to the nurse. Warm water removes less of the protective oils in the skin. Option 3 describes a surgical scrub.
Cognitive Level: Application **Client Need:** Safe, Effective Care Environment: Safety and Infection Control **Integrated Process:** Nursing Process: Implementation **Content Area:** Fundamentals **Strategy:** The core issue of the question is utilization of medical asepsis. Recall basic principles of care and use the process of elimination to make a selection.

2 **Answer: 4** Washing the skin with the combination of soap and water will remove the blood through mechanical friction. While alcohol can kill bacteria, it cannot kill viruses and fungi (option 1). Tissues would not adequately remove the blood (option 2). Hot water can burn the nurse, and water alone is inadequate in removing the blood (option 3).
Cognitive Level: Application **Client Need:** Safe, Effective Care Environment: Safety and Infection Control **Integrated Process:** Nursing Process: Implementation **Content Area:** Fundamentals **Strategy:** The core issue of the question is the most effective means of reducing the risk of bloodborne disease transmission after contact with the skin. Recall principles of medical asepsis and use the process of elimination to make a selection.

3 **Answer: 1** Standard precautions are used with all clients, regardless of the medical diagnosis. Clients with AIDS are not contagious, and family members are not required to wear protective equipment in a casual interaction.
Cognitive Level: Analysis **Client Need:** Safe, Effective Care Environment: Safety and Infection Control **Integrated Process:** Teaching/Learning **Content Area:** Fundamentals **Strategy:** The word *further* in the stem indicates the question is asking which statement indicates the family member does not understand standard precautions. Options 2, 3, and 4 are somewhat similar in that no special precautions are needed. Select option 1 by process of elimination.

4 **Answer: 2** Option 2 is an action aimed at interrupting the portal of entry link in the chain of infection. By using sterile technique, the nurse reduces the risk of introducing pathogens into the client's wound via the drain. Option 1 is an action that breaks the chain of infection at the reservoir link. Options 3 and 4 control the mode of transmission.
Cognitive Level: Application **Client Need:** Safe, Effective Care Environment: Safety and Infection Control **Integrated Process:** Nursing Process: Implementation **Content Area:** Fundamentals **Strategy:** Knowledge of the chain of infection is required. The portal of entry has to be a route whereby microorganisms can enter the client. Option 2 is the only choice in which that is possible.

5 **Answer: 2 and 4** Options 2 and 4 are core principles of surgical asepsis. Options 1 and 3 are core principles of medical asepsis. Option 5 is an incorrect principle of surgical asepsis. The outer 1 inch of a sterile field is considered contaminated.
Cognitive Level: Analysis **Client Need:** Safe, Effective Care Environment: Safety and Infection Control **Integrated Process:** Nursing Process: Implementation **Content Area:** Fundamentals **Strategy:** The core issue of the question is the ability to discriminate between medical and surgical asepsis and to choose correct interventions that support surgical asepsis. Use these principles and the process of elimination to make a selection.

6 **Answer: 2** Herpes zoster is caused by the herpes virus varicella zoster. It can be transmitted by direct contact with the client. It is not transmitted via droplets or air currents. Neutropenic precautions are not indicated because the client is not at risk for contracting an infection from the nurse or other individuals.
Cognitive Level: Application **Client Need:** Safe, Effective Care Environment: Safety and Infection Control **Integrated Process:**

Nursing Process: Implementation **Content Area:** Fundamentals **Strategy:** Herpes zoster is a viral skin infection. Specific knowledge of the types of transmission-based precautions is needed to select the correct answer. Eliminate options 1 and 3 because herpes zoster is not transmitted on air currents. Choose option 2 over 4 because neutropenic precautions are used with immunocompromised clients.

7 **Answer: 1** Tuberculosis is highly contagious and spread by inhalation of airborne droplets. Airborne precautions would be initiated, requiring everyone to wear a special particulate respirator fit-tested mask. Individuals who have had tuberculosis in the past can be re-exposed and develop the active form of the disease again.

Cognitive Level: Application **Client Need:** Safe, Effective Care Environment: Safety and Infection Control **Integrated Process:** Communication **Content Area:** Fundamentals **Strategy:** Look for similarities among the options in order to eliminate choices. Options 2, 3, and 4 are similar in that they suggest certain individuals would not be required to wear masks. Since they are similar and the opposite of option 1, they should be eliminated.

8 **Answer: 2, 3, 4, 1** Gloves are removed first because they would be most contaminated. The mask would be removed next, followed by the gown. Eye protection is removed last, followed by washing the hands.

Cognitive Level: Analysis **Client Need:** Safe, Effective Care Environment: Safety and Infection Control **Integrated Process:** Nursing Process: Implementation **Content Area:** Fundamentals **Strategy:** Remember that removal of PPE should occur in order of most contaminated to least contaminated items.

9 **Answer: 1** SARS is a highly contagious viral respiratory illness that is spread by close person-to-person contact. SARS is transmitted by airborne respiratory droplets and by touching surfaces and objects contaminated with infectious droplets. Instituting infection control measures would be the first priority of the nurse. This action would protect both health care workers and other clients in the emergency department. Then all other interventions can be safely implemented.

Cognitive Level: Analysis **Client Need:** Safe, Effective Care Environment: Safety and Infection Control **Integrated Process:** Nursing Process: Implementation **Content Area:** Fundamentals **Strategy:** The key words *implement first* indicate all of the answers are correct and the nurse needs to set priorities. The first priority is to implement measures that protect the client and/or nurse—option 1.

10 **Answer: 2** SARS is a highly contagious viral respiratory illness that is spread by close person-to-person contact. SARS is transmitted by airborne respiratory droplets and by touching surfaces and objects contaminated with infectious droplets. Personal protective equipment would include protective gowns, gloves, N95 respirators, and eye protection. Airborne precautions would also include placing the client in a private room with negative air pressure flow. The correct answer is option 2. Airborne and contact precautions would provide the necessary protection outlined above. Options 1 and 3 are incorrect. Droplet precautions would not protect the nurse who touches contaminated items. Droplet precautions do not provide a negative air pressure room. Option 4 is incorrect. Contact precautions alone would not provide adequate protection from airborne particles.

Cognitive Level: Analysis **Client Need:** Safe, Effective Care Environment: Safety and Infection Control **Integrated Process:** Nursing Process: Implementation **Content Area:** Fundamentals **Strategy:** Knowledge about SARS and its transmission is essential. Think about the signs and symptoms the client with SARS exhibits.

11 **Answer: 2** A mask is necessary for anyone within 3 feet of client with an infection spread by particle droplets. There is not enough information in the question to support the use of any other equipment.

Cognitive Level: Application **Client Need:** Safe, Effective Care Environment: Safety and Infection Control **Integrated Process:** Nursing Process: Implementation **Content Area:** Fundamentals **Strategy:** Look for PPE that provides adequate protection from an infection spread by droplet particles. Option 2 is the only choice that would protect the nurse from respiratory droplets.

12 **Answer: 4** Clients with antibiotic-resistant microorganisms must be isolated with transmission-based precautions. The organism is transmitted via close person-to-person direct contact and by touching contaminated surfaces and objects. Standard precautions are used with all clients, regardless of medical diagnosis. Reverse isolation is instituted for immunocompromised clients. This organism is not transmitted via droplet nuclei.

Cognitive Level: Application **Client Need:** Safe, Effective Care Environment: Safety and Infection Control **Integrated Process:** Nursing Process: Implementation **Content Area:** Fundamentals **Strategy:** The key words *vancomycin-intermediate-resistant* suggest the microorganism is difficult to eradicate, indicating it is highly contagious. Eliminate options 1 and 2. Select option 4 over 3, using nursing knowledge that *Staphylococcus aureus* is a microorganism that is commonly found on skin.

13 **Answer: 1** Option 1 is the only goal that is client-focused, specific, and measurable. Options 2 and 4 are client-focused but vague. Option 3 focuses on the nursing action of teaching.

Cognitive Level: Application **Client Need:** Safe, Effective Care Environment: Safety and Infection Control **Integrated Process:** Nursing Process: Planning **Content Area:** Fundamentals **Strategy:** Recall that criteria for writing an appropriate client goal is that the goal is client-focused, specific, and measurable. With this in mind, each of the incorrect options can be eliminated using the rationale provided above.

14 **Answer: 4** The client with tuberculosis can spread the infection by breathing and requires a private room and airborne precautions. Options 1, 2, and 3 are aspects of standard precautions that would be implemented with any client, regardless of medical diagnosis.

Cognitive Level: Application **Client Need:** Safe, Effective Care Environment: Safety and Infection Control **Integrated Process:** Nursing Process: Implementation **Content Area:** Fundamentals **Strategy:** The key words *specific care requirement* suggest that more than one answer may be correct or partially correct. Only option 4 is specific for the client with a diagnosis of tuberculosis.

15 **Answer: 4** Transmission-based precautions are required for all antibiotic-resistant microorganisms regardless of their mode of transmission. The other options indicate the need for medical and surgical asepsis in the care of the client but not the use of transmission-based precautions.
Cognitive Level: Application **Client Need:** Safe, Effective Care Environment: Safety and Infection Control **Integrated Process:** Nursing Process: Planning **Content Area:** Fundamentals **Strategy:** The key words *methicillin-resistant* in option 4 indicate a microorganism that is difficult to eradicate. Eliminate each of the incorrect options after visualizing each situation because they can be managed by use of standard precautions.

16 **Answer: 4** Scarlet fever is transmitted by particle droplets larger than 5 microns. Scarlet fever is not transmitted through sexual intercourse or the blood or by consuming contaminated food.
Cognitive Level: Application **Client Need:** Safe, Effective Care Environment: Safety and Infection Control **Integrated Process:** Communication/Documentation **Content Area:** Fundamentals **Strategy:** Begin by recalling that scarlet fever is transmitted by droplets. With this in mind, use the process of elimination to select the client situation that is compatible with the mode of transmission.

17 **Answer: 1** Methicillin-resistant *Staphylococcus aureus* requires transmission-based contact precautions. Eye protection would be worn to protect the mucous membranes of the eyes when splatters of body fluids or excretions are possible. A gown would be worn when the nurse is in direct contact with the client. Contact precautions require gloves. N95 respirators are needed when caring for the client with tuberculosis, so it is inappropriate for this scenario.
Cognitive Level: Application **Client Need:** Safe, Effective Care Environment: Safety and Infection Control **Integrated Process:** Nursing Process: Planning **Content Area:** Fundamentals **Strategy:** The critical word *unnecessary* suggests that all but one of the answers is correct. Using a process of elimination, look for the choice that identifies personal protective equipment that is not needed for contact precautions.

18 **Answer: 4** An infection with vancomycin-resistant *enterococci* requires transmission-based contact precautions. Since the nurse will be irrigating the wound and splatters of body fluids or exudates are possible, eye protection and surgical mask should be worn to protect the mucous membranes of the eyes, nose, and mouth. A gown would be worn when the nurse is in direct contact with the client. Contact precautions require gloves.
Cognitive Level: Application **Client Need:** Safe, Effective Care Environment: Safety and Infection Control **Integrated Process:** Nursing Process: Implementation **Content Area:** Fundamentals **Strategy:** Wound infections require contact precautions. Look for the option that identifies the correct PPE to be used with contact precautions. Options 1 and 3 are eliminated, since a particulate respirator is used with clients with tuberculosis, not those on contact precautions. Choose option 4 over 2 because the risk for splatters exists.

19 **Answer: 1** While each option contains "pneumonia," the causative agent is different for each. Option 1 includes a pathogenic microorganism that is difficult to treat and requires droplet precautions.
Cognitive Level: Application **Client Need:** Safe, Effective Care Environment: Safety and Infection Control **Integrated Process:** Nursing Process: Implementation **Content Area:** Fundamentals **Strategy:** Note the critical word *resistant* in option 1. This provides a clue that the infection is difficult to treat and requires specific additional infection control practices, in this instance droplet precautions. The pneumonias in options 2, 3, and 4 do not require droplet precautions.

20 **Answer: 1, 3** Hepatitis A is an infectious disease transmitted by the fecal–oral route. Standard precautions are mandatory. Contact precautions are instituted if the client is incontinent of stool. Family members should avoid close contact with the client. They should not kiss the client or use the same eating utensils and bath towels. Masks are not necessary because the disease is not transmitted by the respiratory tract.
Cognitive Level: Analysis **Client Need:** Safe, Effective Care Environment: Safety and Infection Control **Integrated Process:** Teaching/Learning **Content Area:** Fundamentals **Strategy:** The critical word *effective* indicates options that are correct are the ones that should be selected. Knowledge of how hepatitis A is transmitted is necessary. The fecal–oral route of transmission eliminates options 2 and 4. Options 1 and 3 are similar in that they limit close contact with the client, so they are both correct.

ANSWERS & RATIONALES

Key Terms to Review

airborne precautions p. 84
chain of infection p. 80
medical asepsis p. 82
methicillin-resistant *Staphylococcus aureus* (MRSA) p. 85
personal protective equipment (PPE) p. 81
standard precautions p. 81
surgical asepsis p. 82
transmission-based precautions p. 84
vancomycin-resistant enterococci (VRE) p. 85

References

Centers for Disease Control (n.d.). *Guideline for isolation precautions in hospitals.* Retrieved November 20, 2004, from http://www.cdc.gov/ncidod/hip/isolat/isolat.htm/

Elkin, M. K., Perry, A. G., & Potter, P. A. (2004). *Nursing interventions and clinical skills* (3rd ed.). St. Louis: Mosby, pp. 49–79.

Kozier, B., Erb, G., Berman, A., & Snyder, S. (2004). *Fundamentals of nursing: Concepts, process, and practice* (7th ed.). Upper Saddle River, NJ: Pearson Education, pp. 628–668.

LeMone, P., & Burke, K. (2004). *Medical-surgical nursing: Critical thinking in client care* (3rd ed.). Upper Saddle River, NJ: Pearson Education, pp. 227–229, 1101–1102.

Smith, S. F., Duell, D. J., & Martin, B. C. (2004). *Clinical nursing skills: Basic to advanced skills* (6th ed.). Upper Saddle River, NJ: Pearson Education, pp. 376–412.

Reproduction, Family Planning, and Infertility

9

In this chapter

Test Yourself

Are you ready for the NCLEX-RN® or course exams? Use the practice tests on the companion CD-ROM to check.

Cross reference

Other chapters relevant to this content area are

Uncomplicated Antenatal Assessment and Care	Chapter 10
Uncomplicated Labor and Delivery Care	Chapter 11
Uncomplicated Postpartum Assessment and Care	Chapter 12
Uncomplicated Newborn Care	Chapter 13
Complicated Antenatal Care	Chapter 50
Complicated Labor and Delivery Care	Chapter 51
Complicated Postpartum Care	Chapter 52
Complicated Newborn Care	Chapter 53

I. THE MALE AND FEMALE REPRODUCTIVE SYSTEMS

A. Female internal structures

1. Vagina: muscular, membranous tube with side walls covered with rugae that connect external genitalia with cervix and uterus; also called birth canal; provides a passageway for sperm when attempting conception, menstrual flow during menstruation, and fetus during childbirth
2. Cervix: neck of uterus, extends down into vagina; consists of fibrous tissue that distends during labor
3. Uterus: hollow muscular organ at superior end of vagina; also called womb; sheds endometrium with menstrual cycles and holds fetus during pregnancy; superior portion known as fundus; inferior portion ends in cervix
4. Fallopian tubes: connect each ovary with uterine body; ciliated to transport ovum or zygote; portion attached to uterus is the isthmus; middle section is the

ampulla; ends at ovary in funnel-shaped infundibulum, which has fingerlike fimbriae reaching toward ovary

5. Ovaries: almond-sized endocrine-functioning glands that secrete estrogen and progesterone; release one mature follicle and ovum during each menstrual cycle from menarche to menopause, except during pregnancy

B. Functions of female structures

! 1. Oogenesis: all oocytes are present at birth; meiosis leads to maturation of an individual ovum under influence of follicle-stimulating hormone (FSH); luteinizing hormone (LH) transforms follicle into corpus luteum, which maintains pregnancy through production of progesterone; ovaries produce estrogen and progesterone in both pregnant and nonpregnant states
2. Menstruation occurs if ovum is not fertilized and corpus luteum disintegrates; endometrium becomes ischemic as progesterone and estrogen levels drop in last week of menstrual cycle, leading to sloughing of myometrium
3. Conception occurs in fallopian tube when a 23-chromosome–containing spermatozoon enters a 23-chromosome–containing ovum and produces a 23-chromosome-pair–containing diploid zygote
4. Pregnancy: cleavage (rapid mitotic division of zygote) creates a blastocyst, which in turn becomes a multicellular solid ball of 16 cells (morula); further division leads to trophoblast stage, when it implants within endometrium
5. Secretion production: cervical secretions become stratified during ovulation to facilitate sperm transport toward ovum; endometrial secretions are rich in glycogen to nourish developing embryo until placental circulation is in place

C. Age-related changes of female reproductive system

1. Menses begin during puberty, stimulated by release of estrogen and progesterone
! 2. Menopause is characterized by 1 year of amennorhea and occurs on average at age 50; postmenopausal changes of reproductive tract include thinning and atrophy of external and internal structures

D. Male internal structures

1. Testes: two lobular, oval glands located within scrotum where spermatogenesis takes place via meiosis
2. Epididymis: tubelike duct arising from top of each testis and ending in vas deferens
3. Vas deferens: connects epididymis to prostate gland
4. Prostate gland: encircles urethra just below bladder, producing alkaline fluid that is released during ejaculation
5. Seminal vesicles: lobular glands located just superior to the prostate; produce seminal fluid that is secreted during ejaculation to support sperm metabolism and motility
6. Urethra: tube that passes through prostate gland and connects bladder and urethral meatus; also is passage for ejaculate
7. Semen: male ejaculate comprised of spermatozoa and glandular secretions; milky white in color; average volume from 2 to 5 mL

E. Functions of male structures

! 1. Spermatogenesis takes place in testes; spermatozoa then proceed through tubules of epididymis where motility and fertility develop, finally being stored in reservoir of epididymis
2. Ejaculation is a series of muscular contractions that release spermatozoa and seminal fluid through penis
3. Urination also takes place through urethra in the penis
4. Secretion production: prostate gland and seminal glands create a milky-white fluid that nourishes spermatozoa during and after ejaculation

F. Age-related changes of male reproductive system

1. Puberty is characterized by greatly increased serum levels of testosterone, which in turn stimulate elongation and thickening of penile shaft, spermatozoa production, and enlargement of testes and scrotum
2. Spermatozoa count, motility, and morphology begin to decrease in middle age
3. External organs atrophy in the elderly

II. FERTILITY

A. Female components

1. Primary infertility is that which occurs prior to ever having conceived; secondary infertility occurs after a pregnancy
2. Menstrual cycle: follicular phase is days 1 to 14 of cycle, incorporating menstrual phase (menses) and proliferative phase (beginning of endometrial thickening); variations in menstrual cycle length are caused by variations in length of follicular phase; luteal phase is days 15 to 28 of cycle and includes secretory phase (plush endometrium secretes glycogen in preparation for implantation of a fertilized ovum) and ischemic phase (beginning of endometrial breakdown when fertilization has not occurred); luteal phase is always 12 to 14 days in length
3. Ovulation: an ovum begins to mature during follicular phase as a result of FSH production; at onset of luteal phase, a blisterlike graafian follicle appears and enlarges on surface of ovary under influence of FSH and LH; ovum oozes out of follicle; ruptured follicle becomes the corpus luteum, which disintegrates if fertilization does not occur or creates progesterone if fertilization does occur; a body fat percentage of 14% or more is needed to support ovulation (caused by estrogen being stored in body fat); lower than 14% body fat will result in irregular menses or amenorrhea
4. Cervical mucus: becomes more plentiful, with a thinner and more stretchy consistency, and forms columns during ovulation to facilitate transport of sperm into uterus; cervical mucus production can be impeded by surgical treatments for abnormal Pap smears
5. Uterine structure: abnormalities result in unhealthy myometrium and fewer healthy places for an embryo to implant successfully; abnormalities include a septum (a fibrous, vertical, wall-like structure in center of uterine body), a unicornate uterus (one-sided, banana-shaped uterus), or a bicornate uterus (two banana-shaped uteri side by side, curving away from each other; may end at one cervix or have two cervices and vaginas)
6. Hormones
   - **a.** Estrogen: produced by ovaries, especially ovarian follicle during ovulation; responsible for development of secondary sex characteristics at puberty; peaks in follicular phase of menstrual cycle; inhibits FSH and LH production
   - **b.** Progesterone: secreted by corpus luteum; peaks during luteal phase; stimulates FSH and LH secretion; responsible for endometrial thickening
   - **c.** FSH: anterior pituitary hormone that matures one ovarian follicle each cycle
   - **d.** LH: anterior pituitary hormone that completes maturation of ovarian follicle; ovulation occurs 10 to 12 hours after LH peaks
7. Fallopian tube must be patent for sperm to reach ovum and for fertilized ovum to reach uterus; scarring can occur from an infection, such as a ruptured appendix during adolescence or **pelvic inflammatory disease (PID)**, an infection of uterus and fallopian tubes; cilia in fallopian tubes, which propel ovum toward oncoming sperm, have decreased motility in cigarette smokers, thereby decreasing fertility

B. Male components

1. Sperm production: at least 50% of sperm must have normal form to achieve optimal fertility; normal levels are greater than 20 million sperm per milliliter of ejaculate; at least 50% of sperm should have normal motion patterns; decreased sperm count and motility can be caused by increased scrotal temperature (from frequent hot tub or sauna use, tight clothing, or varicocele); heavy alcohol, marijuana, or cocaine use; trauma to the scrotum; mumps during adulthood; developmental factors; and cigarette smoking
2. Testosterone is primary hormone responsible for libido, sperm production, ability to have and maintain an erection, and ejaculation
3. Erections must be able to be maintained long enough for ejaculation to occur in vagina and near cervix for optimal fertility
4. Ejaculation must occur and contain sufficient numbers of normally formed and motile sperm to achieve fertility

III. INFERTILITY

A. Common diagnostic studies for infertility

1. **Basal body temperature (BBT)** or resting body temperature: obtained by woman taking her oral temperature each day prior to arising from bed and graphing results on a month-long graph; a sudden dip occurs on day prior to ovulation and is followed by a rise of 0.5 to 1.0°F, which indicates ovulation; this rise will remain until menstruation begins; **fertility awareness** includes monitoring BBT and cervical mucus changes to detect ovulation
2. Serum hormone testing: venous blood is drawn to assess levels of FSH and LH in infertile women, which are indicators of ovarian function
3. Postcoital exam: couple is instructed to have intercourse 8 to 12 hours prior to exam, 1 or 2 days before expected ovulation; a 10-mL syringe with catheter attached is used to collect a specimen of secretions from vagina; secretions are examined for signs of infection, number of active and nonmotile spermatozoa, sperm–mucus interaction, and consistency of cervical mucus
4. **Endometrial biopsy:** obtaining an endometrial tissue sample for examination; client is positioned on exam table in lithotomy position; provider inserts a vaginal speculum to visualize cervix; a paracervical block is first administered to decrease cramping and pain; a sample of endometrium is obtained; sample is then biopsied to check for a luteal phase defect (lack of progesterone)
   a. Preprocedure care should include assisting client (after undressing below waist and applying gown) onto exam table and advising client that she will feel crampy discomfort both during paracervical block administration and during the aspiration
   b. Postprocedure care should include providing sanitary napkins for client (vaginal bleeding will occur) and assessing client for a vasovagal response (sudden fainting caused by hypotension induced by vagus nerve stimulation) prior to arising from exam table
5. Hysterosalpingogram (HSG): detects uterine anomalies, such as septate, unicornate, or bicornate structures, and tubal anomalies or blockage; after the client is sedated or anesthetized, iodine-based radio-opaque dye is instilled through a catheter into uterus and tubes to outline these structures, and x-rays are taken to document findings
6. Laparoscopy: carried out under general or epidural anesthesia; abdomen is insufflated with carbon dioxide and one or more trochars are inserted into peritoneum near umbilicus and symphysis pubis; laparoscope is then used to visualize pelvic structures or perform surgical procedures
7. Male semen analysis: client ejaculates into a specimen container, and ejaculate is examined microscopically for number, morphology, and motility of sperm
8. Male and female partner: antisperm antibody evaluation of cervical mucus and ejaculate are tested for agglutination, an indication that secretory immunological reactions are occurring between cervical mucus and spermatozoa

B. Psychological factors associated with infertility

1. Many couples experience shame, guilt, blame, or the stages of grief when faced with a diagnosis of infertility as well as during treatment for infertility
2. The nurse should facilitate communication between the couple and provide information on resources for coping with infertility, such as support groups; professional counseling may be indicated for some couples

C. Collaborative management of infertility

1. Educational needs of infertile couple are extensive; and include the following:
   a. Performing various procedures (e.g., semen collection for analysis or postcoital exam)
   b. Understanding the meaning of results of tests and assessments
   c. Self-monitoring during medication administration
   d. Understanding how assisted reproductive technologies (ART) are performed
2. Hormonal therapy is used for induction of ovulation in preparation for in vitro fertilization; client and/or her partner must learn how to give subcutaneous and/or intramuscular injections

3. Medications such as clomiphene citrate (Clomid, Serophene) and single-dose hCG are used to achieve induction of ovulation in cases of anovulatory menstrual cycles (menstrual cycles without ovulation) or to achieve multiple ova prior to in vitro fertilization (see also Chapter 61); risks of ovulation induction include multiple births and ovarian hyperstimulation, which can result in enlarged ovaries, abdominal distention, pain, and occasionally ovarian cysts
4. Sperm washing for intrauterine insemination (IUI): client's ejaculate is centrifuged to concentrate the spermatozoa, which are then rinsed in saline to remove seminal fluid; spermatozoa are again centrifuged and then used for either in vitro or intrauterine artificial insemination
5. ! Intrauterine insemination is a form of **artificial insemination** whereby
    a. Sperm collected within 3 hours of coitus are inserted via a catheter into uterus
    b. Donor sperm may be used if male partner's sperm count or motility is low or for single women who desire to become pregnant
    c. Identity of sperm donor is kept confidential
6. **In vitro fertilization (IVF)**: multiple ova are harvested via a large-bore needle and syringe transvaginally under ultrasound guidance; ova are then mixed with spermatozoa, and up to four of resultant embryos are returned to uterus 2 to 3 days later; extra embryos can be frozen for later implantation; side effects include cysts on the ovaries, multiple births, and ovarian hyperstimulation
    a. Preprocedure care: instruct client to give synthetic FSH injections subcutaneously in abdomen, thigh, or upper arm to stimulate ova production for 5 to 6 days preprocedure; give sedation for ova retrieval procedure; observe client for about 2 hours after egg retrieval, and instruct to limit activity for next 24 hours
    b. Postprocedure care following embryo placement in uterus includes instructing client to have minimal activity for 24 hours; progesterone supplementation is commonly prescribed
7. Other specialized fertilization procedures
    a. Gamete intrafallopian transfer (GIFT): harvested ova and sperm are mixed and placed via large-bore needle and syringe under ultrasound guidance into ovarian end of fallopian tube
    b. Tubal embryo transfer (TET): in vitro fertilized embryos are placed into fallopian tube via large-bore needle and syringe under ultrasound guidance; performed 42 to 72 hours after egg retrieval
    c. Zygote intrafallopian transfer (ZIFT): ova fertilized in vitro are placed into fallopian tube via large-bore needle and syringe under ultrasound guidance; performed 18 to 24 hours after egg retrieval
    d. Micro-epididymal sperm aspiration (MESA) is a microsurgical technique to obtain a specimen of sperm from epididymis; done as an outpatient procedure under sedation and/or local anesthesia
    e. Percutaneous epididymal sperm aspiration (PESA) utilizes a small needle under local anesthesia to aspirate sperm from epididymis
8. Outcomes of infertility treatment include increased knowledge of couple about diagnostic studies, their infertility problems, and infertility treatment options; decreased anxiety regarding infertility; making an informed decision about pursuing or not pursuing treatment for infertility using open communication

IV. GENERAL CONSIDERATIONS IN FAMILY PLANNING AND CONTRACEPTION

A. Overview

1. Goal of family planning is to assist clients with reproductive decision making; enable client control in preventing pregnancy, limiting number of children, spacing time between children, and/or voluntarily interrupting pregnancy as desired
2. Legal issues related to family planning and contraception
    a. Laws pertaining to provision of contraceptives to minors without parental consent vary among states

b. Some states may require consent from client's spouse regarding sterilization and voluntary interruption of pregnancy
c. Because of potentially serious complications associated with many contraceptive methods, informed consent is obtained; document information provided and client's understanding of information

3. The mnemonic BRAIDED (see Memory Aid) may be useful to the nurse when counseling a client about family planning and contraceptive methods

Memory Aid

Use the mnemonic BRAIDED to recall important considerations regarding consent for contraceptive use:

B Benefits: information about advantages
R Risks: information about disadvantages
A Alternatives: information about other available methods
I Inquiries: opportunity for the client to ask questions
D Decisions: opportunity for client to make or change a decision
E Explanations: information about selected method and its use
D Documentation: information given and client understanding

V. NATURAL METHODS OF FAMILY PLANNING

A. Natural methods are safe, situational methods requiring increased self-awareness and self-control to be effective

B. Types of natural family planning methods

1. Abstinence is the practice of avoiding sexual intercourse
   a. Advantages: safe, free, and available to all clients; 100% effective in preventing pregnancy and sexually transmitted infections when consistently practiced; can be initiated at any time; encourages communication between partners
   b. Disadvantage: both partners must practice self-control
   c. Client education: teach alternative methods of obtaining sexual pleasure; provide positive feedback to clients who desire and maintain abstinence
2. Coitus interruptus (withdrawal)
   a. Requires male to withdraw penis from female's vagina when urge to ejaculate occurs and ejaculate away from external female genitalia
   b. Clients who choose this method must utilize self-control because the most pleasurable moment during sexual intercourse may coincide with time to withdraw penis
   c. Advantages: can be practiced at any time during menstrual cycle; is free
   d. Disadvantages: least reliable contraceptive method (80% effective with typical use); some pre-ejaculatory fluid (which may contain sperm) may escape from penis during excitement phase prior to ejaculation; at peak sexual excitement, exercising self-control may be difficult
   e. Client education: before intercourse male should urinate and wipe off tip of penis to decrease risk of introducing sperm into vagina; conception may occur if pre-ejaculatory fluid containing sperm enters introitus; a spermicide or postcoital contraceptive may be needed if female partner is exposed to sperm

VI. FERTILITY AWARENESS METHODS OF FAMILY PLANNING

A. Overview

1. These methods are based on an understanding of woman's ovulation cycle and timing of sexual intercourse
2. All methods attempt to identify period of female fertility and to avoid unprotected intercourse during that time period
3. Advantages: free, safe, and acceptable to couples whose religious beliefs (such as Roman Catholics) prohibit other methods; increases awareness of woman's body; encourages couple communication; can be used to prevent or plan a pregnancy
4. Disadvantages: requires extensive initial counseling and education; may interfere with sexual spontaneity; may be difficult or impossible for women with

irregular menstrual cycles; used alone, offers no protection against sexually transmitted infections; theoretically reliable but less effective in actual use

B. ***Calendar method***

1. Also known as rhythm method; based on assumptions that ovulation occurs 14 days (plus or minus 2 days) prior to next menses, sperm are viable for 5 days, and ovum is capable of being fertilized for 24 hours
2. Calendar method is least reliable of fertility awareness methods, 91% effective with perfect use, 75% effective with typical use
3. Client education: teach woman to maintain a menstrual calendar for 6 to 8 months to identify shortest and longest cycles; using first day of menstruation as first day of cycle, calculate fertile period by subtracting 18 days from length of the shortest cycle through length of longest cycle minus 11 days; counsel to avoid intercourse during fertile period

C. **BBT method**

1. Based on thermal shift in menstrual cycle, temperature drops just prior to ovulation, rises and fluctuates at a higher level until 2 to 4 days prior to next menses, then falls if no conception; 97% effective with perfect use, 75% effective with typical use
2. Client education
   - ! a. Teach client to take her temperature with a basal body thermometer, which shows tenths of a degree, and record findings on a temperature chart
   - ! b. Teach client to take her temperature each morning prior to getting out of bed or beginning activity
   - c. Counsel client to avoid intercourse on day temperature drops and for 3 days thereafter
   - d. Inform client that reliability of method can be affected by a decrease in BBT too small to detect, factors that may raise or lower the BBT (such as illness, stress, fatigue, consumption of alcohol the prior evening, or sleeping in a heated waterbed) and that intercourse just prior to drop in temperature may result in pregnancy

D. **Cervical mucus method**

1. Also known as ovulation or Billings method; based on cervical mucus changes that occur during menstrual cycle; effectiveness same as BBT method
2. Client education
   - a. Teach woman to assess her cervical mucus daily for amount, color, consistency, and viscosity
   - ! b. Counsel woman to avoid intercourse when she first notices cervical mucus becoming more clear, elastic, and slippery and for about 4 days after
   - c. Convey sensitivity as women who are uncomfortable touching their genitals may find this method unacceptable
   - d. Instruct client that cervical mucus can be affected by douches and vaginal deodorants, semen, blood and discharge from vaginal infections, antihistamine drugs, and contraceptive gels, foams, film, or suppositories

E. ***Symptothermal method***

1. The symptothermal method involves assessing multiple indicators of ovulation, recording findings and coital history on a menstrual calendar, then abstaining from intercourse during fertile period; effectiveness with perfect use is 98%, with typical use 75%
2. Client education
   - a. Instruct client to assess and record the BBT and condition of cervical mucus as primary indicators of ovulation
   - b. Teach client to become self-aware of and to record secondary indicators of ovulation: increased libido, abdominal bloating, midcycle abdominal pain (Mittelschmerz), breast or pelvic tenderness, pelvic or vulvar fullness, slight dilatation of cervical os, and softer cervix located higher in vagina
   - c. Counsel client to avoid unprotected sexual intercourse during fertile period
   - d. Teach client that this method provides no protection against sexually transmitted infections (STIs)

VII. MECHANICAL METHODS OF CONTRACEPTION

A. Overview

1. Provide a physical or chemical barrier to block sperm from entering the cervix
2. Some barrier devices are made from latex and should be avoided by those with latex allergies

B. *Male condom*

1. A sheath made of latex, plastic, or natural membranes, which is placed over an erect penis to collect semen; effectiveness is 97% with perfect use, 86% with typical use
2. Client education
   a. Check expiration date on package, and if it is past date, obtain another condom
   ! b. Avoid using oil-based lubricants, but contraceptive foam or water-based lubricants may be used
   c. Put on a condom by placing unrolled condom on tip of erect penis, leaving enough room at tip to collect sperm, then unrolling condom from tip to base of erect penis
   ! d. After intercourse, erect penis should be withdrawn from vagina while holding rim of condom to prevent leakage
   e. Inspect used condom for tears or holes because a break in integrity of sheath will decrease effectiveness
   f. Discard used condom in a disposable waste container; do not flush in toilet
3. Advantages
   a. Males can participate in contraception
   b. Sexual intercourse may be prolonged
   c. Condoms are available in a variety of sizes and styles at low cost
   d. Partners can participate in placing condom to enhance enjoyment
   e. All condoms except those made of natural skins offer protection against pregnancy and sexually transmitted infections; natural skin condoms have pores, which can allow passage of viruses and do not protect against STIs
4. Disadvantages
   a. Penis must be erect before placing condom
   b. To prevent spillage of semen, male must withdraw after ejaculating, while penis is still erect
   c. Condoms can rupture or leak, increasing potential for semen to escape into vagina
   d. Oil-based lubricants can decrease condom's effectiveness
   e. Condoms are for single use only
   f. Misplacement, perineal or vaginal irritation, or dulled penile sensation are possible

C. *Female condom*

1. A thin, polyurethane sheath with flexible rings at each end, which covers cervix, lines vagina, and partially shields perineum; effectiveness is 95% with perfect use, 79% with typical use
2. Client education
   a. Insert closed end of condom into vagina so ring fits loosely against cervix
   b. Have partner insert penis into open end leaving approximately 1 inch of sheath from flexible ring outside of introitus
   ! c. After intercourse, before woman stands up, condom should be removed by squeezing and twisting outer ring to close sheath while gently pulling it out of vagina
3. Advantages
   a. May be inserted up to 8 hours before intercourse
   b. Clients who are sensitive to latex can use female condom
   c. Both partners are protected against STIs during intercourse
   d. Female condoms are available without a prescription
   e. Use of lubricants will not decrease effectiveness
   f. Breast-feeding women can safely use condoms

4. Disadvantages
   a. May twist or slip during intercourse
   b. If penis is placed outside of condom, effectiveness is jeopardized
   c. Improper removal results in risk of ejaculate leaking out of condom
   d. Outer ring may irritate external genitalia
   e. High cost, noise produced with intercourse, or altered sensation are unacceptable for some couples
   f. Initially, insertion may be difficult or awkward

D. ***Spermicides***
1. Form a chemical barrier preventing pregnancy by killing sperm or neutralizing vaginal secretions and are available in a variety of forms, including creams, gels, melting suppositories, foaming tablets, aerosol foams, and vaginal contraceptive film
2. When used alone, effectiveness with perfect use is 94% and typical use 74%; when spermicides and other methods are combined, the contraceptive and antimicrobial benefits are increased
3. The most common spermicidal agents are nonoxynol-9 and octoxynol-9; allergic response is possible
4. Client education
   a. Apply spermicide inside vagina and close to cervix before penis is placed near introitus
   ! b. Spermicides must be applied with each act of sexual intercourse
   ! c. Onset of spermicidal action varies; when used alone effectiveness is no longer than 1 hour
   d. Contraceptive foams, creams, and gels are effective immediately
   e. Vaginal contraceptive film and suppositories become effective 15 minutes after insertion into vagina
5. Advantages
   a. No prescription is required to purchase spermicides
   b. Spermicides may be used alone, with a diaphragm, or with a condom
   c. Foams, gels, and suppositories may add additional lubrication and moisture
   d. The penis can remain in the vagina following ejaculation
   e. The method is safe for breast-feeding women
   f. A variety of forms offers clients additional choices in selecting a spermicide
6. Disadvantages
   a. May be irritating to one or both clients
   b. Some forms may be perceived as messy
   c. This method may interfere with spontaneity, as it is inserted before each act of intercourse and may require an interval of time before onset of action
   d. Does not protect against STIs if used alone without additional barrier method

E. ***Diaphragm***
1. A dome-shaped appliance made of rubber with a flexible rim that fits over cervix, is used with spermicidal cream or jelly, and prevents sperm from entering cervix; effectiveness with perfect use is 94%, with typical use is 80%
2. Client education
   a. Utilize models and visual aids when demonstrating insertion and removal of diaphragm
   b. Teach client proper insertion: apply about a teaspoon of spermicidal cream or jelly around rim and inside cup; squeeze sides of diaphragm together, insert through vagina, place side of device containing spermicide over cervix, and push upper edge under symphysis pubis
   c. Teach proper removal by grasping rim to dislodge from cervix and pulling down to remove through vagina
   d. Encourage client to practice insertion and removal when health care provider is present to check for proper placement in vagina
   ! e. Diaphragm remains effective if inserted up to 4 hours before sexual intercourse and should be left in place at least 6 hours after coitus

f. If diaphragm is placed more than 4 hours prior to intercourse or if coitus is desired again within 6 hours, a condom should be used or additional spermicide should be inserted into vagina without disturbing diaphragm
g. Remove at least once during a 24-hour period to decrease risk of toxic shock syndrome
h. Clean diaphragm with mild soap and water and inspect for tears, punctures, and thinning; avoid using oil-based lubricants, which weaken the rubber; replace diaphragm if any damage is observed
i. Dry device thoroughly, dust with cornstarch, and store in carrying case away from light and heat
j. Avoid use during the menstrual period or when abnormal vaginal discharge is present to decrease risk of toxic shock syndrome
k. Contact health care provider if experiencing any warning signs listed in Table 9–1

3. Advantages
   a. Using a diaphragm gives the woman control
   b. Provides some protection against STIs
   c. A partner may insert diaphragm if client has trouble with placement or as part of foreplay
   d. Contains no hormones and is safe for breast-feeding client
   e. Penis can remain inside vagina after ejaculation
4. Disadvantages
   a. Must be fitted by a qualified health care provider and replaced annually
   b. Refitting or replacement may be needed following pregnancy or a 15-pound weight gain or loss
   c. Some clients may have difficulty learning to correctly place diaphragm
5. Contraindications
   a. A history of urinary tract infections; pressure from diaphragm on urethra may interfere with complete emptying of bladder and increase risk of infection related to stasis of urine
   b. A history of toxic shock syndrome; if diaphragm is left in place for a long period of time, this may increase risk of infection

F. ***Cervical cap***

1. A small, thimble-shaped device made of soft rubber that fits over cervix, is held in place by suction, and acts as a barrier between sperm and cervix
2. Effectiveness is influenced by woman's childbearing history; effectiveness with perfect use for nulliparous women is 91%, with typical use is 80%; in parous women perfect use effectiveness is 74%, and typical use is 60%
3. Client education
   a. Teach client to apply spermicide inside cap
   b. Insert cap at least 20 minutes but not longer than 4 hours prior to intercourse
   c. May be left in place up to 48 hours
   d. Reapplication of spermicide with repeated intercourse is not needed
   e. Do not use cap during menstruation or if any abnormal vaginal discharge is present
   f. Contact health care provider if warning signs develop as previously described in Table 9–1
4. Advantages of cervical cap are similar to those of diaphragm
5. Disadvantages
   a. May be more difficult to fit because of limited sizes; some clients may have difficulty inserting and removing cervical cap
   b. Must be fitted by a qualified health care provider and should be replaced annually; clients must be rechecked for fit following pregnancy or a 15-pound weight gain or loss; effectiveness is reduced for parous women
   c. If device dislodges or slips during sexual intercourse, risk for contraceptive failure or acquiring a STI is increased
   d. Instruct client not to use cervical cap during menstruation or if any signs or symptoms of infection or inflammation are present

Table 9–1
Warning Signs and Symptoms Associated with Various Methods of Contraception

Method	Warning Signs and Symptoms
Cervical cap, diaphragm, and contraceptive sponge	Toxic shock syndrome Elevation of temperature >101.4°F Diarrhea and vomiting Weakness and faintness Muscle aches Sore throat Sunburn-type rash Difficult or painful urination Abdominal or pelvic fullness Foul-smelling vaginal discharge
IUD	Acronym **PAINS** **P**—Period late (pregnancy), abnormal spotting or bleeding **A**—Abdominal pain, pain with intercourse **I**—Infection exposure (STI), abnormal vaginal discharge **N**—Not feeling well, fever >100.4°F, chills **S**—String missing, shorter or longer than usually felt
Oral contraceptives	Acronym **ACHES** **A**—Abdominal pain **C**—Chest pain, cough, and/or shortness of breath **H**—Headaches, dizziness, weakness, or numbness **E**—Eye problems (blurring or change in vision) and speech problems **S**—Severe leg, calf, and/or thigh pain
Vasectomy	Fever >100.4°F Excessive pain Difficulty urinating Redness, swelling, bruising, drainage, or skin edges of the incision that are not closed Bleeding at the site
Tubal ligation	Fever >100.4°F Excessive pain Difficulty with defecation or urination Nausea or vomiting Redness, swelling, bruising, drainage, or skin edges of the incision that are not closed

G. *Contraceptive sponge*

1. A small, round polyurethane sponge containing nonoxynol-9 spermicide
2. Effectiveness in nulliparous women is 91% with perfect use and 80% with typical use; in parous women, perfect use effectiveness is 80%, and typical use effectiveness is 60%
3. Client education
   a. Moisten sponge with water prior to insertion into vagina to activate spermicide

b. Place concave side of sponge next to cervix for a better fit
c. Leave sponge in place for at least 6 hours after intercourse
d. Remove by pulling polyester loop on convex side of sponge downward and out of vagina
e. The sponge provides protection up to 24 hours and for repeated acts of intercourse
f. Leaving sponge in place for more than 24 to 30 hours should be avoided because of increased risk of toxic shock syndrome
g. Contact health care provider if warning signs develop as listed in Table 9–1

4. Advantages: same as for diaphragm; plus low cost
5. Disadvantages: some clients perceive sponge as bulky or awkward when in place, or uncomfortable during intercourse; effectiveness is reduced for parous women

H. ***Intrauterine device (IUD)***

1. The mechanism of action of IUD is unknown; contraception is achieved by immobilizing sperm and impeding their travel from cervix to fallopian tubes
2. Limited types of IUDs are available in United States
   a. ! The Progesterone T (Progestasert) is recommended for women who are allergic to copper; it must be changed annually
   b. The Copper T380A (ParaGard) is recommended for women who have at least one child; it can be left in place for 10 years; must be avoided for women with an allergy to copper
   c. Effectiveness with perfect use is 98.5% to 99.4%; typical use effectiveness ranges from 98% to 99.2%
   d. Preferred candidates for use include parous women in a stable monogamous relationship (low risk for STI) with no history of pelvic inflammatory disease (PID) and with healthy uterine anatomy; nulliparous women at low risk for STI or women with a history of PID who are in a stable monogamous relationship and have had a pregnancy since PID episode may also be considered on an individual basis
3. Client education
   a. Cramping or intermittent bleeding may occur for 2 to 6 weeks after insertion
   b. The first few menses after placement may be irregular
   c. Follow-up examination is suggested in 4 to 8 weeks
   d. ! Check for presence of string protruding through cervix by inserting a finger into vagina once a week for first month and then after each menstrual period
   e. ! Counsel client to contact health care provider if she is exposed to a STI or if warning signs known as PAINS develop, as listed in Table 9–1

Memory Aid

Use the mnemonics embedded in Table 9–1 to remember the warning signs for complications of selected contraceptive methods.

4. Advantages
   a. Are highly effective and provide continuous contraceptive protection
   b. Do not interact with medications
   c. Are a good contraceptive option for women who cannot use hormone contraceptives, are breast-feeding, or are smokers over 35 years of age
5. Disadvantages
   a. Must be inserted by a qualified health care professional
   b. Some women experience discomfort, bleeding, and cramping both during and between menses
   c. ! Client is at increased risk of pelvic infection for first 3 weeks following insertion
   d. Uterus may perforate during insertion
   e. May be expelled spontaneously
   f. Does not protect clients from acquiring STIs
   g. Adolescents rarely meet criteria for IUD insertion

VIII. HORMONAL METHODS OF CONTRACEPTION

A. *Oral contraceptives* (birth control pills) act by inhibiting release of an ovum, blocking cyclical release of gonadotropin-releasing hormone, and changing cervical mucus

1. Combined oral contraceptives contain both estrogen and progestin and are available in 21-day and 28-day packages; effectiveness with perfect use is 99.1%, with typical use is 95%
2. Progestin-only pill, also known as a mini-pill, does not contain estrogen, contains less progestin than combination pills, and may be used by lactating women, women with mild hypertension, and those who experienced side effects from oral contraceptives containing estrogen; perfect use effectiveness is 95.5 %, typical use effectiveness is 95%
3. Client education
   a. When starting oral contraceptives, begin pills on first Sunday after onset of menstrual period and take one pill at same time each day
   b. If a 28-day pack is prescribed or client is taking progestin-only pills, don't skip days between packages
   c. Clients using a 21-day pack should wait 7 days before starting next cycle of pills
   d. If one progestin-only contraceptive pill is missed at any time during cycle, take it immediately and take next pill at regular time; any time a pill is missed, use an additional method of contraception through end of that cycle
   e. If one combination oral contraceptive pill is missed at any time during cycle, take missed pill immediately and take next pill at the regular time, and no back-up method is needed; if two pills are missed during first 2 weeks, take two pills for next 2 days and resume taking pills on regular schedule; if two pills are missed during the third week, take one pill daily until Sunday, then begin a new pack on Sunday without missing any days; if three or more pills are missed at any time, take one pill daily until Sunday, then begin a new pack on Sunday without missing any days; if two or more pills are missed at any time, use a back-up method for 1 week or consider emergency contraception if unprotected intercourse occurs
   f. Observe for side effects of oral contraceptives, which can be estrogen related (such as thromboembolic disease, headache, fluid retention, and nausea) or progestin related (including acne, increased HDL cholesterol level, depression, and hirsutism)
   g. Contact health care provider immediately if warning signs develop, which are remembered using the mnemonic ACHES; see Table 9–1
4. Advantages
   a. Use of method is not directly related to act of sexual intercourse
   b. Menstrual periods are usually more regular and predictable
   c. Amount of menstrual flow and premenstrual symptoms are decreased
   d. Incidence or degree of iron-deficiency anemia may be reduced
   e. Are safe throughout reproductive years for women who do not smoke
   f. Noncontraceptive benefits include a decreased risk of ectopic pregnancy, fibrocystic breast disease, and ovarian and endometrial cancers; improvement of acne; and some protection against development of functional ovarian cysts
5. Disadvantages
   a. Risk of ectopic pregnancy is increased if client conceives while taking progestin-only pill
   b. Progestin-only pills are more likely to cause irregular bleeding or amenorrhea
   c. Offer no protection against STIs
   d. Clients need to remember to take a pill at same time each day
   e. Clients with preexisting medical problems may not be candidates for this method
   f. Oral contraceptives may decrease effectiveness of insulin and oral anticoagulants such as warfarin (Coumadin)
   g. Effectiveness of oral contraceptives may be decreased when taken with other drugs, such as phenytoin (Dilantin), carbamazepine (Tegretol), primidone

(Mysoline), topirimate (Topamax), griseofulvin (Grisactin), rifampin (Rifadin), ampicillin (Omnipen), and tetracycline (Achromycin)

! 6. Contraindications

a. Combined oral contraceptives should not be taken by women with a history of thromboembolic or cardiovascular disorders, breast cancer, or estrogen-dependent neoplasms

b. Combined oral contraceptives should not be used if woman is currently pregnant, lactating for less than 6 weeks, smokes more than 20 cigarettes per day and is over 35 years old, has headaches with focal neurological symptoms, is experiencing prolonged immobility or surgery on legs, or has hypertension higher than 160/100 or diabetes mellitus of 20 or more years duration with vascular disease

B. *Subdermal implants (Norplant)*

1. Consist of six silastic capsules containing levonorgestrel, a progestin, implanted subdermally into woman's upper inner arm during first 7 days of menstrual cycle; act by preventing ovulation and stimulating production of thick cervical mucus, which prevents penetration of sperm
2. Client education
   a. Inform client of possible side effects such as spotting, irregular bleeding, amenorrhea, weight gain, headache, fluid retention, mood changes, and depression
   b. Provide client with information regarding signs and symptoms of infection indicating need for postprocedure followup
3. Advantages: not user-dependent for effectiveness; perfect and typical use effectiveness is 99.95% in the first year, 98.9% cumulative over 5 years; provides continuous contraception not related to sexual intercourse; does not contain estrogen; effective within 24 hours and for up to 5 years
4. Disadvantages: requires minor surgery to insert and remove implants; may be visible under skin; irregular or prolonged menses may be unacceptable to client; cost may be prohibitive; offers no protection against STIs; slightly higher failure rates have been reported in women weighing more than 154 pounds in fifth year of use

C. Long-acting progestin injections

1. The injectable contraceptive hormone contains medroxyprogesterone acetate (Depo-Provera) 150 mg, a long-acting progestin that blocks the luteinizing hormone surge, prevents pregnancy by suppressing ovulation and thickens cervical mucus to prevent penetration of sperm with a perfect and typical use effectiveness of 97.7%
2. Client education
   a. Inform client of potential side effects such as menstrual irregularities, headache, weight gain, breast tenderness, and depression
   b. Follow 3-month injection regimen to maintain contraceptive effects; subsequent dose must be given 80 to 90 days after previous dose for continuous contraceptive protection
   c. Counsel client to contact health care provider if she experiences any warning signs of ACHES as identified in Table 9–1
3. Advantages: contraception is not related to sexual intercourse; safe for lactating women; does not contain estrogen; requires administration only every 3 months
4. Disadvantages: injection must be repeated within 80 to 90 days to maintain effectiveness; clients with cardiovascular disorders or breast cancer are not candidates for use; return of fertility may be delayed up to 1 year after stopping method

D. *Postcoital contraception*

1. Consist of measures that may be utilized when there is concern about pregnancy because of unprotected intercourse or when a contraceptive method fails
2. Postcoital contraception should be considered an emergency method and not be used by client on a frequent or regular basis

! 3. Methods of postcoital contraception should be initiated as soon as possible after unprotected intercourse or contraceptive failure; average reduction in pregnancy rates of 75% to 85%, with higher effectiveness if emergency contraception is initiated within 12 hours of unprotected intercourse

a. Oral contraceptives (MAP, or morning-after pills): initiate within 72 hours of unprotected intercourse or contraceptive failure
b. Insertion of an IUD
c. Mifepristone (RU 486): a progesterone antagonist that prevents implantation of a fertilized ovum; a 600-mg dose within 72 hours of unprotected intercourse or contraceptive failure is usually effective in preventing pregnancy

4. Client education
   a. Administration of oral contraceptives or insertion of an IUD may not be effective if client is pregnant
   b. The next menses can be expected about 5 days after last dose of oral contraceptives; if no bleeding occurs within 21 days, client should be evaluated for pregnancy
   c. Nausea and vomiting are common side effects of oral contraceptives unless an antiemetic has been given
   d. If postcoital contraception is sought repeatedly, reason for unprotected intercourse or contraceptive failure should be explored
   e. Counsel client regarding safer and more reliable methods of contraception for regular use
5. Advantages: offers an opportunity to prevent an unwanted pregnancy after forced sexual intercourse, mistake, or method failure; reduces anxiety about pregnancy prior to next menses; provides an opportunity to teach and counsel about reliable contraceptive methods for long-term pregnancy protection
6. Disadvantages: timing of next menses can be affected; amount of next menstrual flow increases in many women; provides no protection against STIs

IX. SURGICAL METHODS OF CONTRACEPTION

A. Overview

1. Surgical contraceptive methods: result in voluntary sterilization of male or female
2. Surgical consent: obtained after risks and benefits of specific method are explained

B. *Vasectomy*

1. During vasectomy, vas deferens is resected through small incisions made in each side of scrotum to block passage of sperm
2. Client education
   a. Procedure takes about 15 to 20 minutes and can be performed in a clinic setting under local anesthesia
   b. Client should refrain from driving immediately after procedure and arrange to have someone drive him home after discharge and remain with him for 24 hours postprocedure
   c. Rest with minimal activity for 48 hours; avoid strenuous activity for 1 week
   d. Avoid tub baths for 48 hours
   e. Wear a scrotal support to increase comfort
   f. Use ice packs intermittently to minimize discomfort and swelling
   g. Sitz baths can be used after 48 hours
   h. Contact health care provider if warning signs develop, as listed in Table 9–1
   i. Sterility is not achieved until semen is free of sperm, about 4 to 6 weeks or 6 to 36 ejaculations; until then, use another contraceptive method
   j. Two or three semen samples should be analyzed to verify sterility prior to resuming unprotected intercourse
   k. Semen should be rechecked at 6 and 12 months to verify stertility has been maintained
   l. Advantages: effectiveness rate is 99.85%; recovery time is short; simpler, safer, and more effective than female sterilization; complications are rare; sexual function is not affected; is cost-effective and convenient
   m. Disadvantages: although reversal is possible in some cases, this method is considered permanent; potential complications include adverse reaction to anesthesia, infection, bleeding, sperm granuloma, or spontaneous re-

anastomosis of vas deferens; fertility, in rare instances, may occur spontaneously due to recanalization of vas deferens

C. *Tubal ligation*

1. During a tubal ligation, fallopian tubes are accessed through two small incisions into abdomen and visualized using a laparoscope, then cut, tied, cauterized, or banded to block passage of sperm and prevent ovum from becoming fertilized
2. Effectiveness ranges from 99.2% to 96.3% depending on the method used; younger women have been reported to experience higher failure rates
3. ! Client education
   a. Procedure takes approximately 30 minutes and is performed under general or local anesthesia
   b. May need to restrict food and fluid intake for several hours prior to procedure, especially if general anesthesia is planned
   c. May experience pain for several days after procedure
   d. Avoid tub baths for 48 hours
   e. Avoid driving, lifting, and strenuous activity for 1 week
   f. Contact health care provider if warning signs develop, as listed in Table 9–1
4. Advantages: permanent and effective in preventing pregnancy; may be performed at any time (immediately after childbirth is optimal because uterus is enlarged and fallopian tubes are easy to identify); sexual function and spontaneity are not affected
5. Disadvantages: procedure requires outpatient surgery; potential complications include adverse reaction to anesthesia, infection, and bleeding; if pregnancy occurs after tubal ligation, risk of ectopic pregnancy increases; reversal of procedure may not be possible; occasional changes in menstrual pattern: posttubal ligation syndrome

Check Your NCLEX–RN® Exam I.Q. *You are ready for testing on this content if you can*

- Provide support to a client and partner during infertility assessment and treatment.
- Use knowledge from biologic and social sciences in discussions with clients contemplating contraception and family planning.
- Assess the client's readiness to use contraception.
- Determine the client's preferences for contraceptive methods.
- Describe risks and contraindications to selected contraceptive methods.

PRACTICE TEST

1 Which of the following statements indicates to the nurse that a couple is coping with the stress of infertility treatment?

1. "We are really trying to maintain a little romance in our relationship."
2. "My wife was so upset that she threw the syringe at me yesterday."
3. "My husband couldn't even have an erection when he was supposed to."
4. "We have two or three glasses of wine each night to help us relax."

2 The client has been diagnosed with Trichomoniasis vaginitis. The nurse explains during client teaching that this infection can affect fertility by

1. Utilizing the glycogen in vaginal secretions, leaving no nutrition for the spermatozoa.
2. Creating a blockage of the fallopian tubes that prohibits spermatozoa from reaching an ovum.
3. Decreasing the pH of the vaginal secretions, thereby destroying most spermatozoa.
4. Increasing the temperature inside the vagina, which decreases the motility of spermatozoa.

3 The nurse is concerned that which of the following viral infections, if experienced by an adult male, may cause infertility?

1. Varicella zoster
2. Rubella
3. Influenza
4. Mumps

4 Which of the following client statements indicates the need for additional teaching?

1. "I should come back for a postcoital test 1 to 2 days before I expect to ovulate."
2. "I should schedule my hysterosalpingogram for the week after ovulation."
3. "We should abstain for 14 days prior to coming back for the sperm penetration test."
4. "I should schedule my endometrial biopsy for the last week of my menstrual cycle."

5 What information does the nurse need to gather before scheduling a client's endometrial biopsy?

1. Usual length of menstrual cycle
2. Blood type and Rh factor
3. Presence of any metal implants
4. Last type of birth control used

6 The nurse is teaching a class in the community on common myths regarding fertility and infertility. Which of the following statements made by class participants indicates teaching has been successful?

1. "If my husband works out every day, he won't be able to make a baby."
2. "If we have intercourse standing up, we won't be able to conceive."
3. "If we have intercourse on the even days after ovulation, we will conceive a girl."
4. "If my husband sits in the hot tub every night, his sperm count will decrease."

7 The client couple is planning intracytoplasmic sperm injection, followed by intrauterine embryo transfer. Which of the following statements indicates that the nurse's teaching was effective?

1. "His sperm swim too fast for me to become pregnant."
2. "My eggs have thick walls and don't let his sperm in."
3. "Any extra embryos can be frozen for implantation later."
4. "We will have to wait several weeks to see if any eggs get fertilized."

8 The clinic nurse is interviewing a client couple for an initial infertility workup. Which of the following topics should the nurse plan to address?

1. Whether the couple has medical insurance
2. How infertility is affecting their lives
3. Whether the man has seafood allergies
4. Whether the woman works outside the home

9 The client is experiencing an inability to become pregnant after she has had one full-term pregnancy. The nurse should develop a plan of care for which health problem?

1. Primary infertility
2. Secondary infertility
3. Unexplained infertility
4. Combined factor infertility

10 The client has an obstruction between the uterus and the fallopian tubes. In obtaining a health history, the nurse collects information about which of the following that may have caused this problem?

1. Rubella infection prior to adolescence
2. Pelvic inflammatory disease caused by gonorrhea
3. Smoking two packs of cigarettes per day
4. Ingestion of 2 ounces of alcohol daily

11 Which of the following statements by the client could indicate a potential problem for the couple planning to use coitus interruptus?

1. "I really don't want to get pregnant right now, so we need a very effective method."
2. "I think I can always pull out before I ejaculate."
3. "We don't have any other sex partners."
4. "We want a contraceptive method that is inexpensive and completely natural."

PRACTICE TEST

12 Which of the following, if stated by the client, would indicate that teaching about cervical mucus changes as an indicator of ovulation has been understood?

1. "If my cervical mucus is yellowish and thick, I am probably fertile."
2. "The thin, clear mucus will block sperm from getting to my cervix."
3. "If my cervical mucus is thick and white, I will need to avoid intercourse or use a back-up method of contraception."
4. "If my cervical mucus is thin and stretchable, I am probably fertile."

13 The client who is married and has three children has come to the family planning clinic asking about a birth control method that is sanctioned by the Roman Catholic Church. She wants the most effective method possible. The nurse's best recommendation is which of the following?

1. Billings or cervical assessment method
2. Ovulation testing kit
3. Symptothermal method
4. Basal body temperature method

14 The client is interested in using female condoms and wants to know if there are any disadvantages. The nurse's best response would be:

1. "The female condom provides good protection against pregnancy but does not protect against sexually transmitted infections."
2. "The female condom may be difficult to insert and may be uncomfortable to both partners."
3. "The female condom is very effective; let me write you a prescription for some."
4. "The female condom is made of latex and should not be used when allergy is present."

15 Which of the following clients would be the best candidate for insertion of an intrauterine device?

1. A client who is married, has one child, and wants to get pregnant in about 6 months
2. A client who is unmarried, has no children, and has numerous sexual partners
3. A client who is married, has two children, and does not want more children for at least 3 years
4. A client who is unmarried, has one child, and has a history of pelvic inflammatory disease

16 The client, a 16-year-old female, has come to the clinic to discuss contraception because she has recently become sexually active. The client states that many of her friends are using spermicides and asks the nurse about their advantages and disadvantages. The nurse's best response would be:

1. "If you want an effective method, you should choose something else."
2. "It is a very convenient method and you will be able to insert the spermicide up to 4 hours before intercourse."
3. "Spermicides cause very few problems, and they are almost 100 percent effective."
4. "Spermicides may or may not be a good choice for you. They have a failure rate of about 21 percent and offer some protection against sexually transmitted infections."

17 In teaching a client about the risk of toxic shock syndrome associated with diaphragm use, the nurse should tell the client to do which of the following to decrease her risk?

1. Leave the diaphragm in place for 36 to 48 hours after intercourse.
2. Avoid using soap when cleaning the device.
3. Wear latex or rubber gloves when handling the device.
4. Seek treatment of any vaginal infection before reusing the device.

18 The client has come to the clinic to discuss use of a cervical cap for contraception. If determined by the nurse's assessment, which of the following would be a contraindication to use of the cervical cap?

1. History of blood clots
2. Age greater than 35 years
3. Abnormal Pap smear 6 months ago
4. Elevated liver enzymes

19 In teaching the client about factors that can decrease the effectiveness of oral contraceptives, which of the following should be included by the nurse?

1. Antibiotic use
2. Weight gain
3. Amenorrhea
4. Iron-deficiency anemia

20 In addition to prevention of pregnancy, oral contraceptives would provide benefits for a client with which of the following problems?

1. Pelvic inflammatory disease
2. Severe facial acne
3. Chloasma
4. Gallbladder disease

21 The client, who delivered her first child 2 days ago, is being discharged from the hospital. She is interested in a contraceptive method that is not associated with intercourse and will not interfere with lactation. The nurse concludes that which of the following probably would be the best method for this client?

1. Progestin-only oral contraceptives (mini-pills)
2. Female condoms
3. Diaphragm
4. Triphasic pills

22 Which of the following statements would indicate to the nurse that teaching was effective for the client who is to receive a Norplant subdermal implant?

1. "By the end of 5 years, the capsules will be absorbed by my body."
2. "If I get the Norplant implant, for 5 years I will have about the same risk of pregnancy as if I had surgical sterilization."
3. "I will need to wait until I am 18 to receive a Norplant implant."
4. "I will need to come to the clinic to have the implant reinserted every 3 months."

23 The nurse is preparing to administer an injection of Depo-Provera. Which of the following would result in safe and effective administration of this drug?

1. Check to see that it has been at least 8 weeks since the client's last injection.
2. Determine that the client's hemoglobin level is within normal range.
3. Using a 23-gauge needle, inject the medication into the deltoid muscle.
4. Check the client's medical record for a history of pelvic inflammatory disease.

24 In giving instruction to the client who is to receive Depo-Provera, the nurse should tell the client which of the following?

1. Like oral contraceptives, Depo-Provera increases the risk of venous thrombosis.
2. The most common side effect of Depo-Provera is amenorrhea or irregular uterine bleeding.
3. Depo-Provera has a higher failure rate than oral contraceptives.
4. Depo-Provera will interfere with lactation.

25 A client has been admitted as an outpatient for a tubal ligation. Following the procedure, the client should be told to expect which of the following?

1. Hot flashes and other hormonally associated symptoms
2. Heavier bleeding with menstruation
3. Possible pain for several days
4. Change in sexual function

ANSWERS & RATIONALES

1 **Answer: 1** Maintaining a healthy relationship is important during infertility treatments, which can be very stressful. Options 2, 3, and 4 may indicate ineffective coping strategies and warrant further investigation.

Cognitive Level: Analysis **Client Need:** Health Promotion and Maintenance **Integrated Process:** Nursing Process: Evaluation **Content Area:** Adult Health: Reproductive **Strategy:** Note a key word in the question is *coping.* Look for the option that indicates effective functioning or therapeutic communication with questions such as these.

2 **Answer: 3** Vaginal fluid pH is slightly alkaline, as is semen. Spermatozoa cannot survive in an acidic environment. Trichomoniasis vaginitis increases the acidity of the vaginal and cervical secretions, thus reducing the number of viable sperm.
Cognitive Level: Application **Client Need:** Health Promotion and Maintenance **Integrated Process:** Teaching and Learning **Content Area:** Adult Health: Reproductive **Strategy:** Look for the option that is a true statement and use knowledge of pathophysiology to eliminate incorrect distractors.

3 **Answer: 4** Mumps in adult males can cause permanent blockage of the vas deferens, contributing to or resulting in infertility. The other responses are incorrect.
Cognitive Level: Application **Client Need:** Health Promotion and Maintenance **Integrated Process:** Nursing Process: Analysis **Content Area:** Adult Health: Reproductive **Strategy:** Look for the option that exerts this effect and use knowledge of pathophysiology to eliminate incorrect distracters.

4 **Answer: 3** Sperm penetration test, which tests for the ability of sperm to penetrate an egg, should be performed after 2 to 7 days of abstinence.
Cognitive Level: Application **Client Need:** Health Promotion and Maintenance **Integrated Process:** Nursing Process: Evaluation **Content Area:** Adult Health: Reproductive **Strategy:** The wording of this question guides you to look for an incorrect statement as the correct answer to the question. Evaluate each option as to whether it is true or false. The false statement is then the correct answer.

5 **Answer: 1** The nurse needs to know the first day of the last normal menstrual period and the length of the menstrual cycle. Endometrial biopsy is performed on day 21 to 27 of the menstrual cycle to assess the endometrial response to progesterone and the degree of development of the luteal phase endometrium.
Cognitive Level: Application **Client Need:** Health Promotion and Maintenance **Integrated Process:** Nursing Process: Assessment **Content Area:** Adult Health: Reproductive **Strategy:** Eliminate option 3 first as irrelevant and then option 2 because excessive bleeding requiring transfusion is not expected. Use knowledge of the relationship between the menstrual cycle and the biopsy procedure to choose option 1 over 4.

6 **Answer: 4** Hot tubs, saunas, and tight underwear can raise the temperature of the testes too high for efficient spermatogenesis and lead to decreased sperm numbers and motility.
Cognitive Level: Analysis **Client Need:** Health Promotion and Maintenance **Integrated Process:** Nursing Process: Evaluation **Content Area:** Adult Health: Reproductive **Strategy:** The wording of this question guides you to look for a correct statement as the answer to the question. Evaluate each option as to whether it is true or false. The true statement is then the correct answer.

7 **Answer: 3** In vitro fertilization usually creates multiple embryos, of which up to four are implanted. Cryopreservation of excess embryos is common, and they can be implanted at a later date.
Cognitive Level: Analysis **Client Need:** Health Promotion and Maintenance **Integrated Process:** Nursing Process: Evaluation **Content Area:** Adult Health: Reproductive **Strategy:** The wording of this question guides you to look for a correct statement as the answer to the question. Evaluate each option as to whether it is true or false. The true statement is then the correct answer.

8 **Answer: 2** The psychological, cultural, and social ramifications of infertility can be extensive. You need to assess this area to ascertain if the couple needs assistance in coping with their infertility and treatment.
Cognitive Level: Application **Client Need:** Health Promotion and Maintenance **Integrated Process:** Nursing Process: Planning **Content Area:** Adult Health: Reproductive **Strategy:** Note the key word *infertility* and note also that this is a nursing assessment. With this in mind, eliminate option 1 as a non-nursing function and options 3 and 4 as not directly related to the topic.

9 **Answer: 2** Secondary infertility is the term for couples that have had one pregnancy but are unable to conceive again. Primary infertility describes the inability to conceive even once. Options 3 and 4 are not terms that are used when discussing fertility.
Cognitive Level: Analysis **Client Need:** Health Promotion and Maintenance **Integrated Process:** Nursing Process: Analysis **Content Area:** Adult Health: Reproductive **Strategy:** Eliminate options 3 and 4 first as terms that are not used, then choose option 2 over 1 because the couple has had one successful pregnancy.

10 **Answer: 2** Infectious processes of the reproductive tract such as PID may result in tubal scarring and therefore tubal blockage. Rubella infection in childhood usually results in the development of active immunity to the disease. Smoking and alcohol present health risks to the woman but not related to tubal patency.
Cognitive Level: Analysis **Client Need:** Health Promotion and Maintenance **Integrated Process:** Nursing Process: Analysis **Content Area:** Adult Health: Reproductive **Strategy:** The wording of the question guides you to look for an association between blockage in the reproductive system and a condition that is causally related to this. Recall that inflammation and infection can lead to scarring and obstruction in the body (which eliminates options 3 and 4). Choose option 2 over 1 because of the age in option 1 and the association of inflammation with option 2.

11 **Answer: 1** Because some semen is released before ejaculation, coitus interruptus has an 18% failure rate and would not be considered a very effective method for a couple wanting to avoid pregnancy.
Cognitive Level: Analysis **Client Need:** Health Promotion and Maintenance **Integrated Process:** Nursing Process: Assessment **Content Area:** Adult Health: Reproductive **Strategy:** The key words in the question are *potential problem;* they lead you to look for a statement that corresponds to a negative aspect of coitus interruptus. With this in mind, each incorrect option can be systematically eliminated.

12 **Answer: 4** Cervical mucus that is thin and clear indicates a rising level of estrogen and impending ovulation. Stretchability of the cervical mucus, or spinnbarkeit, is indicative of the fertile period and promotes motility of the sperm. Options 1 and 3 represent cervical mucus during the infertile period when sexual intercourse is unlikely to result in pregnancy.

Cognitive Level: Analysis **Client Need:** Health Promotion and Maintenance **Integrated Process:** Nursing Process: Evaluation **Content Area:** Adult Health: Reproductive **Strategy:** The key word *understood* indicates that the correct option is also a correct statement. Use knowledge of physical changes during ovulation to make a selection, or use logic to reason that sperm are more motile through thinner liquids than thicker liquids.

13 **Answer: 3** The symptothermal method combines cervical mucus and BBT measurements and results in a lower failure rate than single assessments of the fertile period. This method is completely natural and acceptable to the beliefs of this religious group. Ovulation testing kits do not give enough warning of ovulation to prevent pregnancy.
Cognitive Level: Analysis **Client Need:** Health Promotion and Maintenance **Integrated Process:** Nursing Process: Planning **Content Area:** Adult Health: Reproductive **Strategy:** Note the key word *best,* which indicates more than one option could be true. In this question, eliminate option 2 first as least timely, and choose option 3 over options 1 and 4 because option 3 is comprehensive and includes these other options.

14 **Answer: 2** Made of polyurethane, the female condom does not require a prescription but can be difficult to insert and cause discomfort. It is effective against both sexually transmitted infections and pregnancy.
Cognitive Level: Application **Client Need:** Health Promotion and Maintenance **Integrated Process:** Communication and Documentation **Content Area:** Adult Health: Reproductive **Strategy:** Eliminate option 3 first because only advanced practice nurses have prescriptive privileges and this is not relevant to the question. Use the key word *disadvantages* to focus your selection. Eliminate option 1 next because it is an effective barrier, and eliminate option 4 as a false statement.

15 **Answer: 3** Intrauterine devices are usually recommended for women who have been pregnant and are in a monogamous relationship so that they are at a low risk for sexually transmitted disease.
Cognitive Level: Analysis **Client Need:** Health Promotion and Maintenance **Integrated Process:** Nursing Process: Planning **Content Area:** Adult Health: Reproductive **Strategy:** Use knowledge of advantages and disadvantages of this birth control method to evaluate the options. Eliminate options 2 and 4 because of the risk for infection, and choose option 3 over 1 because the method is for long-term use, not short-term use.

16 **Answer: 4** Spermicides must be used within 30 minutes of intercourse, have a failure rate of 21%, and do offer some protection against sexually transmitted infections. Other key information needed is the sexual history of the client and her partner(s) to more accurately assess risk for STIs. Option 1 provides advice, which the nurse should not give. Options 2 and 3 are false statements.
Cognitive Level: Application **Client Need:** Health Promotion and Maintenance **Integrated Process:** Communication and Documentation **Content Area:** Adult Health: Reproductive **Strategy:** Note the key word *best,* which indicates more than one response may be partially or totally correct in terms of its content. Eliminate options 2 and 4 first as false statements, then choose option 4 over option 1 because it is true and it is a more therapeutic communication.

17 **Answer: 4** When using the device, the woman should wash her hands with soap and water, remove the device within 24 hours of intercourse, clean the device with soap and water, and seek treatment for vaginal infections before reusing the device.
Cognitive Level: Application **Client Need:** Health Promotion and Maintenance **Integrated Process:** Nursing Process: Implementation **Content Area:** Adult Health: Reproductive **Strategy:** The wording of the question indicates that the correct answer is an option that contains a true statement. Use nursing knowledge and the process of elimination to reject the incorrect options, which are false statements.

18 **Answer: 3** Long-term exposure to secretions, spermicides, and bacteria trapped inside the cap can result in abnormal Pap smear results. This client has a history of an abnormal Pap smear; cervical cap use could negatively impact this finding, and another method should be explored for this client. The other options have no relationship to use of the cervical cap.
Cognitive Level: Analysis **Client Need:** Health Promotion and Maintenance **Integrated Process:** Nursing Process: Planning **Content Area:** Adult Health: Reproductive **Strategy:** Note the key word *contraindication,* and use the process of elimination and nursing knowledge to select the option that would pose a risk to this client with regard to use of a cervical cap.

19 **Answer: 1** Antibiotic use can decrease the effectiveness of oral contraceptives. Oral contraceptives can help prevent iron-deficient anemia by decreasing menstrual blood flow. Weight gain and anemia are not related to the effectiveness of birth control pills.
Cognitive Level: Application **Client Need:** Health Promotion and Maintenance **Integrated Process:** Nursing Process: Implementation **Content Area:** Adult Health: Reproductive **Strategy:** Note the key phrase *decrease the effectiveness,* and use the process of elimination and nursing knowledge to select your answer. Recall as a general principle that medications can adversely interact, which is the basis for this question.

20 **Answer: 2** Oral contraceptives can reduce acne, result in signs and symptoms of early pregnancy including chloasma, and accelerate the progress of gallbladder disease. Birth control pills do not provide protection against STIs that can result in PID.
Cognitive Level: Analysis **Client Need:** Health Promotion and Maintenance **Integrated Process:** Nursing Process: Planning **Content Area:** Adult Health: Reproductive **Strategy:** This question is actually asking about secondary uses of oral contraceptives. Eliminate option 1 first because it is the least plausible. Eliminate options 3 and 4 next because they are aggravated by the use of oral contraceptives.

21 **Answer: 1** Oral contraceptives with a combination of estrogen and progestin are not recommended in the first 6 weeks of lactation. In addition, the long-term effects on the infant are not known. The use of female condoms and a diaphragm are associated with sexual intercourse. Progestin-only pills are safe for lactating women.
Cognitive Level: Application **Client Need:** Health Promotion and Maintenance **Integrated Process:** Nursing Process: Planning **Content Area:** Adult Health: Reproductive **Strategy:** Note the key phrase *not associated with intercourse,* which would lead

ANSWERS & RATIONALES

you to first eliminate options 2 and 3. Choose option 1 over 4 because progestin-only contraceptives are estrogen free and thus contain fewer hormones that a breast-feeding infant would be exposed to.

22 **Answer: 2** Norplant is a subdermal contraceptive implant that has about the same failure rate as surgical sterilization, is effective for 5 years, and must be surgically removed.
Cognitive Level: Analysis **Client Need:** Health Promotion and Maintenance **Integrated Process:** Nursing Process: Evaluation **Content Area:** Adult Health: Reproductive **Strategy:** The wording of the question indicates that the correct answer is an option that contains a true statement. Use the process of elimination and knowledge of contraceptive subdermal implants to eliminate the incorrect options.

23 **Answer: 3** The medication is administered intramuscularly every 80 to 90 days. Anemia, while important to the client's health, is not related to Depo-Provera use. The drug does not provide protection against sexually transmitted infections; counseling regarding the consistent use of condoms would be an effective intervention to prevent the reoccurrence of pelvic inflammatory disease.
Cognitive Level: Application **Client Need:** Health Promotion and Maintenance **Integrated Process:** Nursing Process: Implementation **Content Area:** Adult Health: Reproductive **Strategy:** The key words in the question are *safe and effective administration.* Eliminate options 2 and 4 first because they are unrelated to the question, and choose option 3 over 1 because it is true regarding administration of this drug.

24 **Answer: 2** The most common side effect of Depo-Provera is amenorrhea or irregular bleeding. With a failure rate similar to oral contraceptives, Depo-Provera does not interfere with lactation. Typically, the estrogen component of hormonal contraceptives is associated with thromboembolic disease; Depo-Provera contains only progestin.
Cognitive Level: Application **Client Need:** Health Promotion and Maintenance **Integrated Process:** Teaching and Learning **Content Area:** Adult Health: Reproductive **Strategy:** The wording of the question indicates that the correct answer is an option that is a true statement. Use medication knowledge and the process of elimination to make your selection.

25 **Answer: 3** Some clients report mild pain after the procedure, which is usually relieved with analgesics. Changes in menstruation, sexual function, or other hormonal symptoms are not typical.
Cognitive Level: Application **Client Need:** Health Promotion and Maintenance **Integrated Process:** Nursing Process: Implementation **Content Area:** Adult Health: Reproductive **Strategy:** The wording of the question indicates that the correct answer is an option that is a true statement. Use knowledge that this is a minor surgical procedure and the process of elimination to make your selection.

Key Terms to Review

artificial insemination p. 95
basal body temperature (BBT) p. 94
calendar method p. 97
cervical cap p. 100
contraceptive sponge p. 101
diaphragm p. 99
endometrial biopsy p. 94
female condom p. 98
fertility awareness p. 94
intrauterine device (IUD) p. 102
in vitro fertilization (IVF) p. 95
male condom p. 98
oral contraceptives p. 103
pelvic inflammatory disease (PID) p. 93
postcoital contraception p. 104
spermicide p. 99
subdermal implants p. 104
symptothermal method p. 97
tubal ligation p. 106
vasectomy p. 105

References

Bergman, R., Afifi, A., Miyauchi, R. Unicornate Uterus. *Virtual hospital: Illustrated encyclopedia of human anatomic variation.* Retrieved September 1, 2004, from the World Wide Web: http://vh.org/Providers/Textbooks/AnatomicVariants/AnatomyHP.html

Kozier, B., Erb, K., Berman, A., & Snyder, S. (2004). *Fundamentals of nursing: Concepts, process, and practice* (7th ed.). Upper Saddle River, NJ: Pearson Education.

Lowdermilk, D., & Perry, S. (2004) *Maternity and women's health care* (8th ed.). St. Louis, MO: Mosby, pp. 220–265.

Ladewig, M., London, M., Moberly, S., & Olds, S. (2006). *Contemporary maternal-newborn nursing care* (6th ed.). Upper Saddle River, NJ: Pearson Education, pp. 111–123.

Olds, S. B., London, M. L., & Davidson, M. (2004). *Maternal-newborn nursing and women's health care* (7th ed.). Upper Saddle River, NJ: Prentice-Hall, pp. 89–107.

Planned Parenthood Federation of America. Birth Control. Retrieved September 1, 2004, from the World Wide Web: http://www.plannedparenthood.org/bc/

ANSWERS & RATIONALES

Uncomplicated Antenatal Assessment and Care

10

In this chapter

Test Yourself

Are you ready for the NCLEX-RN® or course exams? Use the practice tests on the companion CD-ROM to check.

Cross references

Other chapters relevant to this content area are

Reproduction, Family Planning, and Infertility	Chapter 9
Uncomplicated Labor and Delivery Care	Chapter 11
Uncomplicated Postpartum Assessment and Care	Chapter 12
Uncomplicated Newborn Care	Chapter 13
Complicated Antenatal Care	Chapter 50
Complicated Labor and Delivery Care	Chapter 51
Complicated Postpartum Care	Chapter 52
Complicated Newborn Care	Chapter 53

I. ESSENTIAL CONCEPTS OF PREGNANCY

A. *Estimated date of birth (EDB),* or due date: can be determined by several methods

!

1. **Nägele's Rule:** take first day of last menstrual period, subtract 3 months, and add 7 days; this date is most accurate when woman remembers last menstrual period, has menses every 28 days, and was not taking oral contraceptives
2. **McDonald's method** uses uterine size to indicate gestational age by measuring, in centimeters, distance from symphysis pubis to top of uterine fundus
   a. This distance, **fundal height,** correlates well with number of weeks' gestation between 22 and 34 weeks
   b. Formula for calculating gestational age based on fundal height:

$$\frac{\text{distance in centimeters} \times 8}{7} = \text{total weeks of gestation}$$

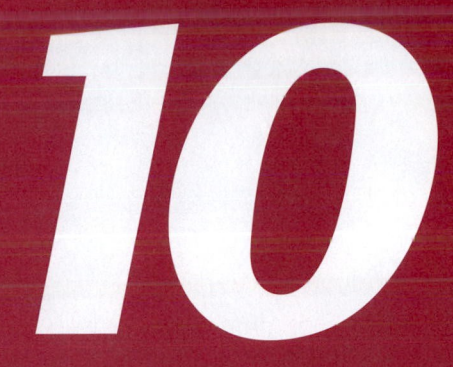

c. Prediction of EDB using this method can be affected by maternal height, irregular fetal growth, multiple gestation, and abnormal amounts of amniotic fluid

3. **Quickening,** feeling of fetal movement by mother, usually occurs between 16 and 18 weeks; because of wide range of times quickening is experienced, this method gives a less accurate EDB
4. Auscultation of fetal heart rate (FHR) can occur as early as 8 weeks' gestation using an ultrasonic Doppler device but is more commonly heard between 10 and 12 weeks; this variation can result in a less accurate date
5. Ultrasound examination estimates EDB when date of last menstrual period is unknown or uterine size is inconsistent with EDB calculated with Nägele's rule or McDonald's method

B. *Gravida* and *para*

1. Gravida and para are terms to describe a woman's childbearing history
2. Gravida is number of times woman has been pregnant
3. Para is number of infants delivered after 20 weeks gestation, born dead or alive; multiple births count as one delivery regardless of number of infants delivered
4. TPAL is a more detailed description of para

Memory Aid

Use the mnemonic TPAL to remember the detailed description of parity (para)
T number of **T**erm infants born after 37 weeks
P number of **P**reterm infants born between 20 and 37 weeks
A number of pregnancies that end in spontaneous or therapeutic **A**bortion prior to 20 weeks
L number of **L**iving children

II. SIGNS AND SYMPTOMS OF PREGNANCY

A. *Presumptive signs of pregnancy*

1. Subjective signs and symptoms that the woman reports (see Box 10–1)
2. May or may not be associated with pregnancy

B. *Probable signs of pregnancy*

1. Objective signs and symptoms noted by examiner (see Box 10–1)
2. May or may not be associated with pregnancy

C. *Positive signs of pregnancy*

1. Diagnostic signs and symptoms noted by examiner (see Box 10–1)
2. Can only be associated with pregnancy

III. NURSING CARE DURING FIRST PRENATAL VISIT

A. First prenatal visit

1. Determine why woman is seeking care; should include a complete health history and physical examination
2. History taking should include:
   a. Weight, nutrition, and exercise pattern
   b. Over-the-counter (OTC), prescription, and illicit drug use
   c. Allergies and potential teratogens
   d. History of surgery or present disease states, especially those with known implications for pregnancy, such as viral infections, diabetes, hypertension, cardiovascular disease, renal problems, and thyroid or bleeding disorders
   e. Gynecologic history including date of last Pap smear, previous infections, age at menarche, and menstrual, contraceptive, and obstetric histories
3. Physical assessment
   a. **Fetal heart rate** (FHR): fetal heart beats per minute, assessed by fetoscope (beginning at about 16 weeks) or by ultrasonic Doppler device (beginning at about 8 weeks); FHR is useful in determining gestational age and fetal well-being; fetal heart rate normally ranges from 120 to 160 beats per minute
   b. Fundal height, a measurement from symphysis pubis to top of uterine fundus (in centimeters), helps assess gestational age and fetal growth (see Figure 10–1 ■)

Box 10-1

Signs and Symptoms of Pregnancy

Presumptive Signs

amenorrhea

nausea and vomiting

fatigue

urinary frequency

breast changes

quickening

Probable Signs

Hegar's sign

McDonald's sign

enlargement of abdomen

pigmentation changes

abdominal striae

ballottement

positive pregnancy test

palpation of fetal outline

Positive Signs

fetal heartbeat

fetal movement palpable by the examiner

visualization of the fetus by ultrasound

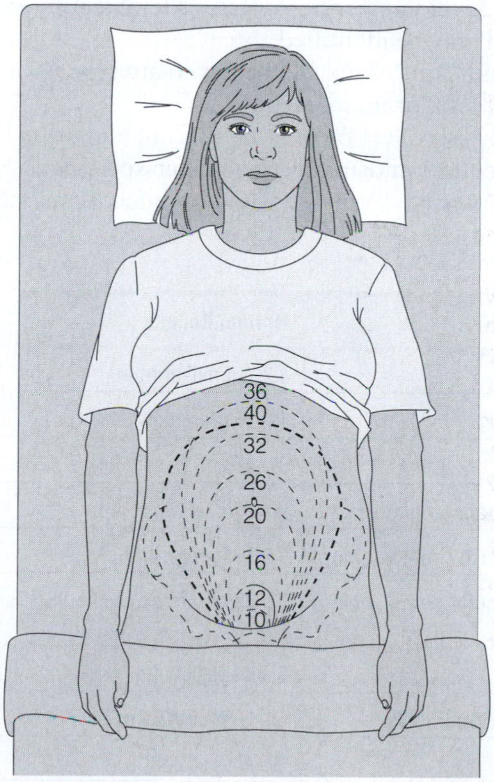

Figure 10-1

Fundal height changes during pregnancy.

!

c. Complete maternal physical examination includes vital signs; height and weight; thyroid; heart and breath sounds; and reproductive organs including pelvic musculature, size of uterus, and adequacy of pelvis for delivery

d. Laboratory assessment includes hematocrit and hemoglobin, blood type, Rh and irregular antibody, rubella titer, tuberculin skin test, renal function tests, urinalysis and culture, screening for sexually transmitted diseases, and Pap test; offer of HIV test (see section that follows)

!

4. Psychosocial assessment
   a. Emotions such as excitement, anxiety, and/or ambivalence about pregnancy
   b. Available support systems
   c. Stability and functional level of client's immediate and extended family
   d. Economic support adequate for housing, daily needs, and medical expenses
   e. Cultural preferences including practices to be used or avoided during pregnancy, preference of caregiver gender, and preferred support person(s)
5. Collaborative management
   a. Prepare client for physical exam by stating what to expect
   b. Provide information about prenatal care program, setting, and personnel
   c. Provide information about physiologic changes to be expected in pregnancy as well as danger signs to report
6. Outomes: client verbalizes knowledge of procedures for physical exam, future prenatal care, and expected changes related to normal and abnormal aspects of pregnancy

B. Laboratory and diagnostic testing during first prenatal visit

1. Testing done at initial visit can be analyzed for abnormal results; intervention can be implemented as soon as possible or at follow-up visits, as indicated
2. Complete blood count (CBC): provides information on hematologic system and other body systems; advantages include being inexpensive, easy to perform, and quickly available results; for individual tests, normal results, and changes in pregnancy, see Table 10–1 ■
3. Blood group and Rh typing
   a. Purpose: to determine client's blood group and Rh status so that fetus at risk for developing erythroblastosis fetalis or hyperbilirubinemia in neonatal period may be identified

!

   b. Significant results: mothers who are type O or Rh negative may require further fetal or infant testing
4. Urinalysis: collect fresh urine specimen in urine container; if culture is to be done, collect midstream, clean-catch specimen
   a. pH may be decreased with poor glucose metabolism and ketone acids in urine

Table 10–1

Complete Blood Count

Test	Normal Results	Changes in Pregnancy
RBC count	4.2–5.4 million/mm^3	5–6.25 million/mm^3
Hemoglobin	12–16 grams/dL	>11grams/dL
Hematocrit	37–47%	>33%
Mean corpuscular volume	80–95/cubic micrometer	none
Mean corpuscular hemoglobin	27–31/picogram	none
Mean corpuscular hemoglobin concentration	32–36 grams/dL packed RBCs	none
WBC count	5,000–10,000/mm^3	5,000–15,000/mm^3
Polymorphonuclear cells	55–70% of WBCs	60–85% of WBCs
Lymphocytes	20–40% of WBCs	15–40% of WBCs
Platelet count	150,000–400,000/mm^3	none until 3–5 days after delivery

b. Specific gravity may be increased with dehydration caused by excessive vomiting as seen in hyperemesis gravidarium
c. Color should be pale yellow to amber depending on foods ingested and concentration
d. Glucose reabsorption is impaired in pregnancy resulting in spilling of glucose in urine at a blood glucose level of 160 mg/dL
e. Protein may normally be found in urine during pregnancy at a level of trace to +1 using dipstick method; increased protein may indicate pregnancy-induced hypertension or preeclampsia
f. White blood cells (WBCs) or nitrites can indicate possible urinary tract infection, which can place client at risk for preterm labor
g. Casts, which are formed from clumps of materials or cells in renal distal and collecting tubules, form when urine is acidic and concentrated; can be associated with proteinuria and stasis in renal tubules
h. Ketones may indicate diabetes and hyperglycemia
i. Urine culture should be done to identify women with asyptomatic bacteriuria; greater than 10,000 bacteria/mL urine is indicative of urinary tract infection
j. Urine toxicology can screen for illicit drug use

5. TORCH infections: a group of infections caused by viruses and protozoa that cause serious fetal problems when contracted by mother during pregnancy; each letter represents a different infection: **T**oxoplasmosis, **O**ther infections (usually hepatitis), **R**ubella, **C**ytomegalovirus, and **H**erpes simplex virus; see sections that follow

6. Toxoplasmosis
a. Cause: infection with the toxoplasmosis protozoan
b. Transmission: development of infection in mother is associated with consumption of infested undercooked meat and poor hand-washing after handling cat litter; fetal infection occurs if mother acquires toxoplasmosis after conception and passes it to fetus via the placenta
c. Diagnosis: diagnosis is made by serologic testing; indirect fluorescent antibody test is most commonly used; IgG titers greater than 1:256 suggest a recent infection, whereas IgM titers greater than 1:256 indicate an acute infection
d. Maternal effects: flulike symptoms in acute phase
e. Fetal/neonatal effects: miscarriage is likely in early pregnancy; in neonates central nervous system (CNS) lesions can result in hydrocephaly, microcephaly, chronic retinitis, and seizures

7. Other infections, usually hepatitis virus
a. Cause: infection with the hepatitis A virus (HAV) or hepatitis B virus (HBV); HBV is most common in fetus
b. Transmission: HAV is spread by droplets or hands and is associated with poor hand-washing after defecation; transmission to fetus is rare but can occur; HBV can be transmitted to fetus via placenta, but transmission usually occurs when infant is exposed to blood and genital secretions during labor and delivery
c. Diagnosis: radioimmunoassay and enzyme-linked immunosorbent assay methods are used to detect HAV antibodies; elevated IgM antibody in the absence of IgG antibody indicates probable acute hepatitis; elevated IgG in the absence of IgM indicates a convalescent or chronic stage of HAV; HBV is detected through hepatitis B surface antigen (HbsAg)
d. Maternal effects: fever, malaise, nausea, and abdominal discomfort; may be associated with liver failure
e. Fetal/neonatal effects: preterm birth, hepatitis infection, and intrauterine fetal death

8. Rubella, sometimes called German measles or 3-day measles
a. Cause: infection with rubella virus
b. Transmission: infection is spread by droplet

c. Diagnosis: IgG antibodies to rubella are measured to determine client's rubella immunity status; a titer of 1:10 or greater indicates that woman is immune to rubella; a titer of 1:8 or less indicates minimal or no immunity
d. Maternal effects: fever, rash, and mild lymphedema
! e. Fetal/neonatal effects: miscarriage, congenital anomalies, and death

9. Cytomegalovirus (CMV)
a. Cause: exposure to the CMV
! b. Transmission: respiratory droplet, semen, cervical and vaginal secretions, breast milk, placental tissue, urine, feces, and banked blood; most common mode is respiratory droplet; workers in daycare centers, institutions for mentally retarded, and health settings are especially at risk
c. Diagnosis: a viral culture is most definitive diagnostic tool; CMV antibodies indicate a recent infection; a fourfold increase in CMV titer in paired sera drawn 10 to 14 days apart is usually indicative of an acute infection
d. Maternal effects: asymptomatic illness, cervical discharge, and mononucleosis-like syndrome
! e. Fetal/neonatal effects: fetal death or severe generalized disease with hemolytic anemia and jaundice, hydrocephaly or microcephaly, pneumonitis, hepatosplenomegaly, and deafness

10. Herpes simplex virus (HSV)
a. Cause: exposure to HSV
! b. Transmission: HSV type II is a sexually transmitted disease transmitted by exposure to vesicular lesions on penis, scrotum, vulva, perineum, perianal region, vagina, or cervix; infant is usually infected during exposure to lesion in birth canal; infant is most at risk during primary infection in mother
c. Diagnosis: viral culture is used for definitive diagnosis; serologic tests have a lower accuracy
d. Maternal effects: blisters, rash, fever, malaise, nausea, and headache
! e. Fetal/neonatal effects: miscarriage, preterm labor, or stillbirth; transplacental infection is rare but can cause skin lesions, intrauterine growth restriction (IUGR), mental retardation, and microcephaly
! f. Significant results: vaginal delivery is recommended if client has no visible lesions or prodromal symptoms; if visible lesions or prodromal symptoms are present, cesarean delivery is indicated

11. **Sexually transmitted infections (STIs),** also called sexually transmitted diseases or venereal diseases, are caused by bacteria, viruses, protozoa, or ectoparasites and include human papillomavirus (HPV), human immunodeficiency virus (HIV), group B streptococcus (GBS), syphilis, gonorrhea, and chlamydia; all sexual partners of clients with STIs should be contacted and treated, as indicated; see sections that follow

12. HPV
! a. Cause/transmission: sometimes called genital or venereal warts, HPV infection is spread through sexual contact; neonates can acquire infection during birth
b. Diagnosis: direct visualization of warts and confirmation by biopsy
c. Maternal effects: symptoms depend on viral strain causing infection but can include genital lesions, chronic vaginal discharge, pruritis, and cervical dysplasia; some strains are asymptomatic
d. Fetal/neonatal effects: juvenile laryngeal papillomata

13. HIV
! a. Cause/transmission: primarily through exchange of body fluids, including semen, blood, or vaginal secretions; neonatal transmission can occur transplacentally and is less likely if mother receives treatment during pregnancy; transmission can also occur by contact at time of delivery or through breast milk
b. Diagnosis: made with a reactive enzyme immunoassay (EIA) and a positive Western blot or immunofluorescence assay; the p24 antigen capture assay can diagnose neonatal HIV infection as early as 2 to 6 weeks after infection, detect HIV before seroconversion, and determine progression of AIDS; viral

cultures provide best diagnostic tool for neonates; but are expensive and require 4 to 6 weeks for results

c. Maternal effects: opportunistic diseases including *Pneumocystis carinii* pneumonia, candida esophagitis, and wasting syndrome; HSV and CMV infections are also common; fever, headache, night sweats, malaise, generalized lymphadenopathy, myalgias, nausea, diarrhea, weight loss, sore throat, and rash are associated with seroconversion

! d. Fetal/neonatal effects: asymptomatic at birth followed by opportunistic infections, immunodeficiency, failure to thrive, parotitis, lymphadenopathy, hepatosplenomegaly, fever, chronic diarrhea, dermatitis, thrush, and death

e. Test procedure: after explaining the test to the client, an informed consent must be obtained; clients may remain anonymous through the use of number identification

14. Group B streptococcus (GBS)

a. Cause/transmission: considered normal vaginal flora, found in 10% to 30% of healthy pregnant women; transmitted vertically from birth canal of infected mother to fetus

! b. Diagnosis: current recommendations are to screen all women at 36 to 37 weeks' gestation with a GBS culture

c. Maternal effects: preterm labor, chorioamnionitis, premature rupture of membranes, urinary tract infections, and postpartum infections

d. Fetal/neonatal effects: neonatal meningitis, sepsis, and septic shock; early onset GBS has a significant infant mortality rate

15. Syphilis

! a. Cause/transmission: caused by *Treponema pallidum,* a motile spirochete transmitted through microscopic abrasions in subcutaneous tissue; primarily transmitted via sexual intercourse, but may also be transmitted by kissing, biting, or oral–genital sex; transmission to fetus can occur via placenta at any time during pregnancy

b. Diagnosis: microscopic examination of primary and secondary lesion tissue; serology is used for diagnosis during latency and late infection; women should be screened at first prenatal visit and possibly again late in third trimester with VDRL (Venereal Disease Research Laboratories) or the RPR (rapid plasma reagin) test; if either is positive, diagnosis is confirmed with a fluorescent treponemal antibody absorption (FTA-ABS) test

c. Maternal effects: during acute stage, a chancre develops on skin near infection; second stage is marked by lymphadenopathy and rash on palms of hands and soles of feet; the latent stage, which can last up to 5 years, is asymptomatic; disease can progress to a tertiary stage that involves CNS, cardiovascular, and ocular signs and symptoms; infection can cause miscarriage or premature labor

! d. Fetal/neonatal effects: include CNS damage, hearing loss, or death

16. Gonorrhea

a. Cause/transmission: caused by *Neisseria gonorrhoeae,* an aerobic, gram-negative diplococci bacteria, transmitted by all types of sexual activity; neonates can acquire infection by exposure to bacteria in birth canal

! b. Diagnosis: all pregnant women should be screened at initial prenatal visit and at-risk women should be screened again at 36 weeks gestation; a Thayer-Martin culture of endocervix, rectum, or pharynx are completed for diagnosis

c. Maternal effects: sometimes asymptomatic but can cause purulent endocervical discharge, menstrual irregularities, pelvic or lower abdominal pain, and premature rupture of membranes

! d. Fetal/neonatal effects: preterm birth, neonatal sepsis, IUGR, and ophthalmia neonatorum, which can cause blindness

17. Chlamydia

a. Cause/transmission: the *Chlamydia trachomatis* bacteria is spread through sexual contact; Centers for Disease Control (CDC) recommends screening of asymptomatic, high-risk women

b. Diagnosis: cultures for chlamydia are expensive, require special transport and storage, and take up to 10 days
c. Maternal effects: although usually asymptomatic, infection can cause bleeding, mucoid or purulent cervical discharge, PID, or dysuria
! d. Fetal/neonatal effects: conjunctivitis, pneumonia, and ophthalmia neonatorum

IV. NURSING CARE DURING SUBSEQUENT PRENATAL VISITS

! **A. Frequency of follow-up prenatal visits**
1. Every 4 weeks during first 28 weeks' gestation
2. Every 2 weeks until 36 weeks
3. Every week until delivery

B. Collaborative management
1. Visits should include teaching as well as assessment of maternal and fetal well-being
2. Instruct mother concerning physical changes associated with pregnancy, such as quickening (first fetal movements felt) and colostrum production, as well as danger signs of pregnancy, presented in Table 10–2 ■
3. ! Assess for acceptance of pregnancy and adjustment to maternal role, changes from baseline measurement of vital signs, weight gain, nutritional status, and presence of glucose and/or protein in urine
4. Collect clean-catch urine specimen at each visit to assess for glucose, protein, nitrites, and leukocytes, which can indicate diabetes, pregnancy-induced hypertension, or infection
5. Assess maternal hemoglobin monthly for iron-deficiency anemia
6. ! Assess fetus at each visit for growth as measured by fundal height, movement, and heart rate
7. ! Blood levels of alpha-fetoprotein to screen for fetal neural tube defects should be assessed at 16 to 18 weeks; maternal blood glucose level should be assessed at 24 to 28 weeks to screen for gestational diabetes (see sections to follow)

C. Diagnostic tests during subsequent prenatal visits
1. **Alpha-fetoprotein (AFP)**
   a. During pregnancy, AFP leaks from fetus's body into amniotic fluid and is absorbed by the mother
   b. Peak levels of AFP are found in maternal serum at around 16 weeks; AFP in maternal serum is measured at 16 to 18 weeks
   ! c. Findings: increased maternal serum AFP levels may indicate neural tube defects or other body wall defects, threatened abortion, fetal distress, or death; decreased maternal levels of AFP may indicate trisomy 21 (Down syndrome) or fetal wastage

Table 10–2

Danger Signs in Pregnancy

Danger Sign	Possible Cause
Gush of fluid from vagina	Rupture of membranes
Vaginal bleeding	Abruptio placentae, placenta previa, bloody show
Abdominal pain	Premature labor, abruptio placentae
Temperature > 101°F	Infection
Persistent vomiting	Hyperemesis gravidarum
Visual disturbances	Hypertension, preeclampsia
Edema of hands and face	Hypertension, preeclampsia
Severe headache	Hypertension, preeclampsia
Epigastric pain	Preeclampsia
Dysuria	Urinary tract infection
Decreased fetal movement	Compromised fetal well-being

d. Interfering factors include multiple pregnancy and incorrect estimation of gestational age
e. Follow-up: abnormal levels of AFP may indicate a need for a triple-screen test, ultrasound, or assessment of AFP levels in amniotic fluid

! 2. **Triple-screen test**, an improved screening test for Down syndrome (trisomy 21), trisomy 18, and neural tube defects, includes AFP, human chorionic gonadotropin (hCG), and unconjugated estriol (UE3)
3. **Glucose tolerance test (GTT)** to screen pregnant clients for gestational diabetes; generally completed between 24 and 28 weeks gestation
   a. Test procedure: after test is explained to client, a 50-g oral glucose load is administered; time of day or time since last meal is not a factor; venous plasma glucose is assessed 1 hour after glucose load
   ! b. Findings: a level greater than 140 mg/dL is considered abnormal; abnormal results indicate a need for further testing
   c. Follow-up: clients with abnormal GTT results should be assessed with a 3-hour, 100-g oral glucose tolerance test to diagnose gestational diabetes
4. **Oral glucose tolerance test (OGTT)**
   a. Test procedure: client eats high-carbohydrate diet for 3 days before test; on day of test, she fasts for 8 hours (overnight), and a fasting serum glucose is obtained; following the fast, 100 grams of oral glucose is administered and glucose levels are assessed at 1, 2, and 3 hours
   ! b. Findings: gestational diabetes is diagnosed if two or more results are abnormal (see Table 10–3 ■); the results are borderline if one value is abnormal; with borderline results, the OGTT is repeated in 1 month
5. **Ultrasound:** sound waves with a frequency higher than 20,000 Hz produce a three-dimensional view and pictorial image to identify maternal and fetal tissues, bones, and fluids; screen for anomalies, assess fetal well-being, and establish gestational age; results can be used to decide whether to continue pregnancy or terminate because of fetal abnormalities
   ! a. Transvaginal ultrasound used primarily during first trimester; eliminates need for full bladder and gives clearer images in obese clients; some clients are embarrassed or uncomfortable with vaginal insertion of probe; contraindicated in clients with latex allergies as probe is covered with a latex condom-like sac
   ! b. Abdominal ultrasound provides a safe, noninvasive fetal assessment, but is best done when client's bladder is full; this can result in discomfort
   c. Viability is determined by assessment of fetal heart activity; this is possible at 6 to 7 weeks gestation with real-time echo scan; fetal death can be determined by absence of heart activity as well as scalp edema and maceration
   d. Gestational age can best be established during first 20 weeks' gestation because fetal growth rate is fairly consistent during this time; body part assessed is based on development; measurement of gestational sac is done at about 8 weeks, and crown-rump measurement is done at 7 to 14 weeks; with greater than 12 weeks' gestation, biparietal diameter (BPD) and femur length are measured
   e. Fetal growth is assessed by serial measurements of BPD and femur length; this information can assist the health care provider in distinguishing between IUGR and inaccuracy in dating of the pregnancy

Table 10–3
Abnormal Oral Glucose Tolerance Test Results

Time	Abnormal Result
Fasting	greater than 105 mg/dL
1 hour	greater than 190 mg/dL
2 hour	greater than 165 mg/dL
3 hour	greater than 145 mg/dL

Table 10-4

Childbirth Education Topics by Trimester

Trimester	Educational Topic
First	Physical and psychosocial changes of pregnancy Self-care in pregnancy Protecting and nurturing the fetus Choosing a care provider and birth setting Prenatal exercise Relief of common early pregnancy discomforts
Second	Planning for breast-feeding Sexuality in pregnancy Relief of common later-pregnancy discomforts
Third	Preparation for childbirth Development of a birth plan

D. Childbirth education

1. Childbirth classes provide information on pregnancy and childbirth to facilitate families in optimal decision making; topics should be timed to progress of pregnancy, as illustrated in Table 10–4 ■
2. In addition, classes can be planned for special groups such as grandparents, siblings, adolescents, and clients who will deliver by cesarean section
3. Exercise is an important topic for childbirth education; encourage women to participate in regular (three times per week) exercise during pregnancy
   a. Benefits of exercise include maintaining muscle tone and bowel function and having fewer complications during labor and delivery
   ! b. Exercises especially helpful for childbirth include pelvic tilt, partial sit-ups, Kegel exercises, and exercises to stretch inner thigh muscles
4. Classes on preparation for birth process provide information on selection of birthing method and relaxation techniques
   a. Commonly taught birthing methods include Lamaze, Kitzinger, and Bradley methods of prepared childbirth; see Table 10–5 ■ for a comparison of these methods
   ! b. Relaxation techniques commonly taught to be used in labor include touch, breathing, disassociation, and progressive relaxation
5. Classes geared toward knowledge needed after delivery include sessions on postpartum self-care, newborn care, infant stimulation, and infant safety needs

E. Management of common discomforts of pregnancy

1. Discomforts occur as a result of physiologic or anatomic changes of pregnancy; they differ from trimester to trimester
2. ! While not dangerous, they constitute a significant problem for client and present an opportunity for nursing intervention (see Tables 10–6 ■ and 10–7 ■)

V. PHYSIOLOGICAL CHANGES OF PREGNANCY

A. Reproductive

1. Uterus: during pregnancy takes on an ovoid shape and increases in capacity from 10 mL to 5 L; primarily caused by an increase in size of cells (hypertrophy) in

Table 10-5

Comparison of Common Birthing Methods

Method	Characteristics	Breathing techniques
Lamaze	Uses education about fetal growth and changes associated with pregnancy along with training in exercises that strengthen muscles used during labor and delivery to decrease fear and help the mother cope with the pain of labor	Patterned, paced
Bradley	Relies on partner or husband to coach the laboring woman; promotes relaxation through abdominal breathing and exercises	Primarily abdominal
Kitzinger	Prepares the woman for birth through the use of sensory memory and the Stanislavsky acting method to teach relaxation	Chest breathing with abdominal relaxation

Table 10-6

Management of Discomforts in Early Pregnancy

Discomfort	Management
Nausea and vomiting	Avoid strong odors Drink carbonated beverages Avoid drinking while eating Eat crackers or toast before getting out of bed Eat small, frequent meals Avoid spicy or greasy foods
Breast tenderness	Wear a well-fitting, supportive bra
Urinary frequency	Increase daytime fluid intake Decrease evening fluid intake Empty bladder as soon as urge is felt
Fatigue	Plan a rest period or nap during the day Go to bed as early as possible
Ptyalism	Use gum, mints, hard candy, or mouthwash
Nasal stuffiness/bleeding	Use cool air vaporizer

Table 10-7

Management of Discomforts in Late Pregnancy

Discomfort	Management
Heartburn	Eat small, frequent meals Avoid spicy or greasy foods Refrain from lying down immediately after eating Use low-sodium antacids
Constipation	Increase fluid and fiber intake Exercise Develop regular bowel habits Use stool softeners as needed
Hemorrhoids	Avoid constipation Apply topical anesthetics, ointments, or ice packs Use sitz baths or warm soaks Reinsert into rectum, if necessary
Backache	Practice good body mechanics Practice pelvic tilt exercise Avoid high heels, heavy lifting, overfatigue, and excessive bending or reaching
Leg cramps	Dorsiflex feet Apply heat to affected muscle Evaluate calcium-to-phosphorus ratio in diet
Varicose veins	Elevate legs Wear support hose Avoid crossing legs at the knee, restrictive clothing, and standing for long periods of time
Ankle edema	Practice frequent dorsiflexion of feet Avoid standing for long periods of time Elevate legs when sitting or resting
Faintness	Arise slowly Avoid prolonged standing Maintain hematocrit and hemoglobin
Flatulence	Avoid gas-forming foods Chew food thoroughly Establish regular bowel habits

response to estrogen, as well as distention caused by growing fetus; by end of pregnancy, uterus and its contents require up to one-sixth of total maternal blood flow

! 2. Cervix: under influence of estrogen, secretes mucus that forms a plug at opening of endocervical canal to limit bacteria entering uterus; increased blood flow to cervix results in **Goodell's sign** (softening of the cervix) and **Chadwick's sign** (bluish color of cervix during pregnancy)
3. Vagina: under influence of estrogen, vaginal mucosa thickens and connective tissue relaxes; vaginal secretions thicken and increase in amount during pregnancy; the pH is acidic, 3.6 to 6.0
4. Breasts: estrogen and progesterone cause breasts to increase in size and number of glands; **colostrum** (a thin bluish-white secretion high in protein and immune properties) is produced and may be expressed during last trimester

B. Cardiovascular

1. Cardiac output increases 30% to 40% over nonpregnant output with an increase in pulse of 10 to 15 beats/minute
2. Peak time for cardiac problems occurs around 28 weeks
3. Pulmonary and peripheral vascular resistance decreases 40% to 50%, resulting in a decrease in BP throughout first and second trimesters of pregnancy; in third trimester, begins to increase to prepregnant levels; postural hypertension may result as pregnant uterus presses on pelvic and femoral vessels, limiting blood return to heart

! 4. Vena cava syndrome results as gravid uterus compresses vena cava, causing decreased blood flow to right atrium and decreased BP
   a. Symptoms include pallor, dizziness, and clammy skin
   b. Problem can be prevented or treated by positioning woman on her left side or with a pillow under her right hip
5. Blood volume increases 45% over prepregnant levels
   a. Red blood cells (RBCs) increase 18% to 30% depending on degree of iron supplementation
   b. Plasma volume increases 50%
   c. The greater increase in plasma over RBCs results in physiologic anemia and is seen in a 7% decrease in hematocrit

C. Respiratory

1. Volume of air breathed increases 30% to 40% because of decreased airway resistance that occurs in response to progesterone
2. Intrathoracic volume remains unchanged even though enlarged uterus presses up on diaphragm, because rib cage flares and chest circumference increases

D. Neurologic: no known changes

E. Musculoskeletal

1. Relaxation of pelvic joints results in classic "waddling" gait often seen in pregnancy

! 2. Physiologic lordosis develops as curvature of lumbar spine increases to compensate for weight of gravid uterus; this can result in low back pain
3. Diastasis recti, separation of rectus abdominis muscle, can result as uterus enlarges

F. Gastrointestinal (GI)

1. During first trimester, human chorionic gonadotropin (hCG) increases and can cause nausea and vomiting

! 2. Increased progesterone levels relax smooth muscles, resulting in decreased peristalsis as noted by bloating, reflux of gastric secretions, and constipation; GI problems are worsened as gravid uterus presses on intestines
3. Constipation and increased pressure on blood vessels in rectum can result in hemorrhoids

G. Renal

1. In first trimester, gravid uterus presses on bladder, causing urinary frequency; relieved in second trimester by uterus moving into abdominal area; this problem returns in third trimester as presenting part presses on bladder

2. Glomerular filtration increases 50% during second trimester and remains elevated until delivery; kidneys may not be able to reabsorb all glucose filtered, resulting in glycosuria

H. Integumentary

1. In response to increased estrogen levels, some areas of skin have increased pigmentation; this is seen primarily in areas with increased pigmentation such as the areola, nipples, and vulva
   a. **Chloasma,** mask of pregnancy, is an increase in pigmentation on forehead and around eyes; it is seen most often in women of color and is aggravated by sun exposure
   b. **Linea nigra** is a darkly pigmented line that extends from umbilicus to pubic area
   c. **Striae gravidarum,** or stretch marks, appear as reddish streaks on trunk and thighs; result from stretching of connective tissue caused by increased adrenal steroid levels; while these generally change to a shiny gray-white color after delivery, they do not disappear
2. Sweat and sebaceous gland activity increases during pregnancy

I. Endocrine

1. Metabolism
   a. Average weight gain is 3 to 5 pounds in first trimester and 12 to 15 pounds in each following trimester
   b. Water retention occurs during pregnancy because of increased sex hormones and decreased serum protein
2. Hormones in pregnancy
   a. Secreted by trophoblast early in pregnancy, hCG stimulates progesterone and estrogen production; it is thought to support pregnancy and to cause nausea and vomiting in first trimester
   b. Human placental lactogen (hPL), also known as chorionic somatomammotropin, is an insulin antagonist that promotes lipolysis, resulting in increased amounts of circulating free fatty acids available for maternal metabolic use
   c. Estrogen and progesterone are produced by corpus luteum for first 7 weeks of pregnancy and then by placenta; estrogen stimulates uterine development to support fetal growth and stimulates ductal system of breast for lactation; progesterone maintains endometrium, decreases uterine contractility, stimulates development of breast acini and lobules, and causes relaxation of smooth muscle
   d. Relaxin, primarily made by corpus luteum, decreases uterine contractility, contributes to softening of cervix, and has long-term effects on collagen
   e. Prostaglandins, lipids that are found throughout female reproductive system, contribute to decrease seen in placental vascular system, and probably contribute to onset of labor

VI. NUTRITIONAL NEEDS

A. Factors affecting maternal nutrition requirements

1. Prepregnancy nutritional status: women who are underweight or overweight may need more or less calories respectively for adequate fetal weight gain
2. Maternal age: teenage mothers may need increased caloric intake to allow for maternal and fetal growth
3. Maternal parity: number of pregnancies and interval between them can affect nutritional needs

B. General principles of maternal nutrition

1. ! Healthy pregnant woman requires an additional 300 calories per day
2. ! Other nutritional requirements are increased during pregnancy, including protein, vitamins (especially folate), minerals, and trace elements; many health care providers recommend taking a prenatal vitamin supplement to ensure adequate intake and reduce risk of birth defects associated with folic acid (vitamin B_6) deficiency
3. ! Appropriate pregnancy weight gain averages 25 to 35 pounds for women with a normal prepregnant weight
   a. 10 to 13 pounds in the first 20 weeks
   b. About 1 pound per week after the 20th week

4. Maternal weight gain is distributed to a variety of structures, including fetus, placenta, and amniotic fluid (11 pounds); uterus (2 pounds); blood volume increase (4 pounds); breast tissue (3 pounds); and maternal stores (5 to 10 pounds)

C. Lactose intolerance

1. Results from insufficeint levels of lactase, an enzyme that breaks down lactose in dairy products into glucose and galactose (simple sugars)
2. ! Leads to nausea and vomiting, epigastric discomfort, abdominal cramping and distention, and loose stools
3. ! Lactase may be replaced by adding it as a liquid to milk or by chewing a tablet before ingesting milk products
4. Dairy products that may be better tolerated by client include cheese and yogurt, or milk products in cooked form
5. Lactose-free products are also available

D. Vegetarianism

1. Intake should include unrefined grains, legumes, nuts, fruits, and vegetables
2. ! Strict vegetarians (vegans) need to eat adequate amounts and combinations of proteins to be able to synthesize complete proteins; combinations should include whole-grain foods and legumes, nuts and legumes, and nuts and whole-grain foods
3. Ovovegetarians may add eggs to diet to help meet protein requirement
4. Lacto-ovovegetarians may use milk and eggs
5. ! All clients eating a vegetarian diet should take a daily supplement of vitamin B_{12} (cyanocobalamin)

E. Pica

1. A condition of eating items that are not foods or have no nutritonal value
2. Leads to iron-deficiency anemia
3. Commonly ingested substances are clay, dirt, and ice
4. Can affect all socioeconomic levels, although impoverished clients are more at risk

VII. PSYCHOSOCIAL NEEDS OF PREGNANCY

A. Role changes: occur as decisions are made concerning whether or not the mother will continue or return to work and who will meet household responsibilities

B. Anxieties: related to the birthing process, well-being of the mother and baby, and finances

C. Family strengths in coping with the psychosocial changes of pregnancy

1. Communication skills
2. Ability to resolve conflict and reach compromise
3. Willingness to seek and utilize support systems

D. Collaborative management

1. Discuss with client psychosocial processes that occur during pregnancy, such as role changes, anxieties related to well-being of mother and infant, and additional financial responsibilities
2. Explore family coping mechanisms, communication skills, and support systems

Check Your NCLEX_RN® Exam I.Q.

You are ready for testing on this content if you can

- Assess the physiological status of a pregnant client.
- Calculate an expected delivery date.
- Assess the psychosocial needs of a pregnant client.
- Assess results of maternal and fetal diagnostic tests.
- Provide antenatal care to a client.
- Provide instructions about self-care during the antenatal period.

PRACTICE TEST

1 The client has come to the clinic for her first prenatal visit. During the pelvic examination, the examiner indicates that the vaginal mucosa has a bluish color. The nurse documents this as a positive

1. Hegar's sign.
2. Goodell's sign.
3. McDonald's sign.
4. Chadwick's sign.

2 With regard to normal changes in the reproductive system during pregnancy, the nurse should teach the pregnant client about which of the following?

1. Vaginal secretions will increase and thicken.
2. Uterus will grow by adding many new cells.
3. Breasts will become red and hard.
4. Cervix will begin to dilate during the second trimester.

3 With regard to normal changes in the cardiovascular system during pregnancy, the nurse should teach the pregnant client that

1. Her pulse rate will decrease.
2. She may experience dizziness if she lays on her back.
3. She will have a decrease in red blood cells.
4. She may experience a feeling of fullness in her chest.

4 During a prenatal visit in the second trimester, which of the following, if reported by the client, would be a cause for concern?

1. Thirst and urinary frequency
2. +1 deep tendon reflexes
3. Constipation
4. Backache in the lower sacral area

5 The nurse is examining a client who is 12 weeks' gestation. The examiner would expect to find the fundus at which of the following locations?

1. 3 cm below the sternum
2. The level of the umbilicus
3. The level of the symphysis pubis
4. 3 cm below the umbilicus

6 When considering maternal serum alpha-fetoprotein testing for a client, the nurse would conclude that there is a contraindication for the test if the client

1. Is at 25 weeks' gestation.
2. Would not consider termination of the pregnancy.
3. Does not have a family history of neural tube defects.
4. Had an ultrasound at 8 weeks' gestation.

7 The nurse would formulate which of the following as a wellness-oriented nursing diagnosis for a client in the second trimester of pregnancy?

1. Anxiety related to lack of understanding about early prenatal physical changes
2. Beginning maternal–fetal attachment related to statements about perception of fetal movement
3. Promoting client safety
4. Knowledge deficit related to lack of preparation for labor and delivery

8 At the first prenatal visit, the client reveals that her last menstrual period began March 18. The nurse calculates her estimated date of delivery to be which of the following?

1. June 25
2. November 18
3. January 11
4. December 25

9 The nurse concludes by which of the following client statements that the pregnant client understands prenatal nutrition education?

1. "I understand that if I don't eat foods with folic acid, my baby will have birth defects."
2. "I understand that eating citrus fruits, especially oranges, will help me meet my need for folic acid."
3. "I understand that if my level of folic acid is low, it could cause my baby to have a neural tube defect."
4. "I understand that I should limit my intake of folic acid because it can build up in the liver and cause birth defects."

10 A pregnant client, who is a vegetarian, is concerned about her folic acid intake and asks the nurse to recommend some foods that she should include in her diet. Which of the following should the nurse recommend?

1. Peanuts
2. Hamburger
3. Bananas
4. Apple juice

PRACTICE TEST

11. The pregnant client has been started on an iron supplement. The nurse determines that the client understands possible side effects of therapy when the client states that the supplement may cause which of the following?

1. Red, raised rash
2. Gastric upset
3. Blood in the stool
4. Headache

12. The pregnant client has been started on an iron supplement. Which of the following information should be included by the nurse as a priority in her prenatal teaching about the iron supplement?

1. It should be taken 30 minutes after eating a full meal.
2. It is better absorbed if taken with a liquid containing vitamin C.
3. It will eliminate the need for prenatal vitamins.
4. It should be taken at the same time as the prenatal vitamin.

13. The pregnant client tells the nurse that she is lactose intolerant. When considering the recommendation of a calcium supplement, which of the following should be assessed?

1. History of kidney stones
2. Presence of leg cramps
3. Color of mucous membranes and conjunctiva
4. Resting heart rate

14. During the first prenatal assessment, the nurse discovers that the client has not had a second vaccination for measles, mumps, and rubella. The best plan for this client is to

1. Administer the vaccine during this visit.
2. Wait until the third trimester to administer the vaccine.
3. Administer the vaccine following delivery.
4. Omit the vaccine because these are childhood diseases not acquired by adults.

15. The pregnant client, who is 34 weeks' gestation, calls the prenatal clinic complaining of cramping pain in her abdomen. After the diagnosis of Braxton-Hicks contractions is made, the nurse should give the client which of the following recommendations?

1. "Go to bed and wait for your real labor to begin."
2. "Empty your bladder frequently and change positions if these contractions are bothering you."
3. "Avoid using your Lamaze breathing with these contractions because it might precipitate preterm labor."
4. "Just ignore these contractions; we will let you know if there is a problem."

16. The client, who is 37 weeks' gestation, is complaining of joint pain, especially in the lower back and pelvic area. The best response by the nurse is

1. "I'm afraid you are just going to have to put up with that for a few more weeks."
2. "Sleeping flat on your back may help with the pain."
3. "Aspirin taken every 3 to 4 hours will be the best thing to relieve this pain."
4. "It may help to apply a heating pad to the painful area for 15 to 20 minutes."

17. The pregnant client tells the nurse that she keeps hearing about someone called a "doula" but she isn't sure what a doula does. The nurse's best response is, "A doula

1. Eliminates the need for the father to be in the delivery room."
2. Will actually deliver the baby."
3. Will take the place of your labor and delivery nurse."
4. Will assist you with your Lamaze breathing during labor."

18. The pregnant client is trying to decide where she would like to give birth. She states she wants to be delivered by a nurse-midwife, doesn't want to move to several different rooms, and wants to be near pediatric services in case the baby has a problem. The nurse should advise her to consider which of the following birthing sites?

1. Home delivery
2. Freestanding birthing center
3. Traditional hospital setting with separate labor, delivery, recovery, and postpartum units
4. Hospital with combined labor, delivery, recovery, and postpartum (LDRP) rooms

19. In reviewing the chart of a prenatal client, which of the following would be considered by the nurse to be a probable sign of pregnancy?

1. Fetal heartbeat on ultrasound
2. Amenorrhea
3. Positive pregnancy test
4. Chloasma

20 The client is planning to breast-feed and asks the nurse what she should do to prepare. The nurse should advise the client to do which of the following?

1. Wash her nipples with water daily.
2. Apply lanolin daily in the last trimester.
3. Rub the nipples briskly with a towel twice a day.
4. Perform the pinch test daily.

21 The client has come to the clinic for her first prenatal visit and tells the nurse that she eats only vegetables. To assess for a problem related to this information, the nurse should assess what part of the complete blood count (CBC)?

1. Hemoglobin
2. Lymphocytes
3. Polymorphonuclear cell count
4. Platelet count

22 The nurse interprets that which of the following indicates a need for instruction to the pregnant client about avoiding infection with the rubella virus?

1. No history of having the disease
2. Rubella titer 1:12
3. Rubella titer 1:16
4. Rubella titer 1:8

23 Which of the following, if revealed to the nurse in a prenatal interview, would indicate an increased risk for exposure to cytomegalovirus?

1. Caring for a cat and litter box
2. Working at a day care center
3. Using IV drugs several years ago
4. Giving blood twice yearly

24 Which of the following, if found by the nurse during prenatal care, would indicate a need for delivery by cesarean section?

1. Positive herpes culture at the first prenatal visit; client asymptomatic at the time of delivery
2. History of genital herpes lesions; at the time of delivery, prodromal symptoms present but no lesions
3. Oral fever blisters at the time of delivery
4. Genital herpes lesion 1 month prior to delivery; no symptoms at the time of delivery

25 Follow-up for the pregnant client who is diagnosed with a sexually transmitted disease includes

1. Contacting and treating all sexual partners.
2. Delivery by cesarean section.
3. Amniocentesis for assessment of genetic damage.
4. Close monitoring of hematocrit and hemoglobin throughout pregnancy.

26 The nurse should plan for Group B streptococcus screening if the pregnant client meets which of the following criteria?

1. History of a sexually transmitted infection
2. 36 to 37 weeks' gestation
3. Has come in for her initial prenatal visit
4. Rash noted in the vaginal area

27 Which of the following, if reported to the nurse by a pregnant client prior to collection of a gonorrhea culture, would result in postponing specimen collection?

1. Recent diagnosis and treatment for herpes
2. Persistent vaginal discharge
3. Douching 3 days ago
4. Is currently menstruating

28 The client has come to the prenatal clinic complaining of repeated nausea and vomiting. The nurse would look to which of the following as providing the best information about client hydration status?

1. Hemoglobin
2. Platelet count
3. Urine specific gravity
4. IgG level

29 In taking a history from a pregnant client, which of the following would the nurse recognize as a risk factor for contracting sexually transmitted infection?

1. Report of anal intercourse
2. Use of oral contraceptives
3. Current monogamous relationship
4. Being 23 years old

30 In interviewing a pregnant client concerning sexually transmitted infections, the nurse should recognize which of the following as a barrier to client disclosure?

1. Nurse's use of a nonjudgmental attitude
2. Collecting information while the woman is still dressed
3. Use of only yes or no questions
4. Use of a culturally sensitive approach

ANSWERS & RATIONALES

1 **Answer: 4** Beginning around the fourth week of pregnancy, vasocongestion in the pelvic area results in a bluish color to the vulva, vagina, and cervix, known as Chadwick's sign. Hegar's sign is a softening of the lower uterine segment, Goodell's sign is a softening of the cervix, and McDonald's sign is an ease in flexing the body of the uterus against the cervix; none of these other signs involve color changes.
Cognitive Level: Analysis **Client Need:** Health Promotion and Maintenance **Integrated Process:** Nursing Process: Assessment **Content Area:** Maternal-Newborn **Strategy:** The key words in the question are *first prenatal visit* and *bluish color.* Use the process of elimination and knowledge of the changes in cervical mucosa in early pregnancy to make your selection.

2 **Answer: 1** During pregnancy, increased estrogen production results in an increased amount and thickening of vaginal secretions. The uterus grows by cell hypertrophy, not by adding more cells. Red and hard breasts or a cervix dilating during the second trimester are not normal findings.
Cognitive Level: Application **Client Need:** Health Promotion and Maintenance **Integrated Process:** Teaching and Learning **Content Area:** Maternal-Newborn **Strategy:** Note the key words *normal changes* during pregnancy. Eliminate options 3 and 4 first because they are abnormal. Use concepts of physiology to choose option 1 over option 2.

3 **Answer: 2** Pressure on the vena cava from the gravid uterus may cause a decrease in blood flow to the right atrium and result in a decrease in blood pressure. Dizziness is a symptom of hypotension. The pulse rate could stay the same or increase as the workload of the heart increases during the course of pregnancy. There is an increase in the number of red blood cells to meet physiological demand. Option 4 is not a cardiovascular change during pregnancy, although abdominal fullness occurs as the pregnancy progresses.
Cognitive Level: Application **Client Need:** Health Promotion and Maintenance **Integrated Process:** Teaching and Learning **Content Area:** Maternal-Newborn **Strategy:** Note the key words "normal changes," "cardiovascular," and "pregnancy." With these in mind, eliminate options 1 and 3 as incorrect. Choose option 2 over 4 by keeping in mind concepts of maternal and fetal circulation.

4 **Answer: 1** Urinary frequency usually disappears in the second trimester. Thirst and urinary frequency may be a sign of developing gestational diabetes and warrants further investigation. Deep tendon reflexes are assessed during a physical examination and are not reported to a health care provider by the client.
Cognitive Level: Analysis **Client Need:** Health Promotion and Maintenance **Integrated Process:** Nursing Process: Assessment **Content Area:** Maternal-Newborn **Strategy:** Note the key words *cause for concern,* which indicate that the correct answer will be an option that is an abnormal finding. Eliminate options 3 and 4 first, since they are typical complaints that may be associated with pregnancy. Choose option 1 over 2 by noting that option 1 is clearly abnormal and is also subjective data that is reported by the client.

5 **Answer: 3** By the twelfth week of gestation, the uterus should have increased in size to be palpable at the symphysis pubis. Factors affecting this finding include abnormal fetal growth or the presence of a multiple gestation.
Cognitive Level: Analysis **Client Need:** Health Promotion and Maintenance **Integrated Process:** Nursing Process: Assessment **Content Area:** Maternal-Newborn **Strategy:** To answer this question correctly, you must be familiar with expected physiological changes during pregnancy. Use nursing knowledge and the process of elimination to make your selection.

6 **Answer: 1** This test, which measures the level of maternal serum alpha-fetoprotein, is most sensitive between 16 to 18 weeks' gestation. However, it can be performed up to 22 weeks' gestation.
Cognitive Level: Analysis **Client Need:** Health Promotion and Maintenance **Integrated Process:** Nursing Process: Planning **Content Area:** Maternal-Newborn **Strategy:** Note the key word *contraindication.* This means the correct answer is an option that is a false statement. Use knowledge of the purpose of the test to eliminate each of the incorrect options.

7 **Answer: 2** Quickening usually begins around 16 weeks and results in enhanced attachment as the fetus becomes more real. Anxiety about early pregnancy changes would be more appropriate for the client in the first trimester. Knowledge deficit related to labor and delivery is an appropriate diagnosis in the third trimester. Promoting client safety is a nursing action, not a nursing diagnosis.
Cognitive Level: Analysis **Client Need:** Health Promotion and Maintenance **Integrated Process:** Nursing Process: Analysis **Content Area:** Maternal-Newborn **Strategy:** Note the key words *wellness-oriented nursing diagnosis* and *second trimester.* Eliminate options 1 and 4 because they are not wellness oriented, then eliminate option 3 because it is a nursing goal rather than a nursing diagnosis.

8 **Answer: 4** According to Nagele's rule, the estimated date of birth can be calculated by subtracting 3 months from the beginning date of the last menstrual period and then adding 7 days to that date.
Cognitive Level: Application **Client Need:** Health Promotion and Maintenance **Integrated Process:** Nursing Process: Analysis **Content Area:** Maternal-Newborn **Strategy:** Specific knowledge of Nagele's rule is needed to answer the question. Use

knowledge of this rule and mathematical/calculating ability to determine the appropriate due date.

9 **Answer: 3** Maternal folic acid deficiency has been linked to infant neural tube defects. Folic acid may be obtained from prenatal vitamin supplements as well as foods. The other responses contain incorrect statements and do not indicate understanding of prenatal nutrition.
Cognitive Level: Analysis **Client Need:** Health Promotion and Maintenance **Integrated Process:** Nursing Process: Evaluation **Content Area:** Maternal-Newborn **Strategy:** Note the key word *understands,* which indicates that the correct answer is also a correct statement. Eliminate option 4 first because water soluble vitamins do not accumulate in the liver. Eliminate option 1 next because of the words "will have." This implies a level of certainty that is unrealistic. Choose option 3 over option 2 because it is a true statement and because oranges are not an especially good source of folic acid.

10 **Answer: 1** Both peanuts and hamburger are good sources of folic acid, but since the client is a vegetarian, peanuts is a better recommendation. The other options do not contain significant amounts of folic acid.
Cognitive Level: Application **Client Need:** Health Promotion and Maintenance **Integrated Process:** Nursing Process: Implementation **Content Area:** Maternal-Newborn **Strategy:** Use the process of elimination and knowledge of nutrition to answer this question. Eliminate option 2 first because the client is a vegetarian, and eliminate options 3 and 4 because they are fruit or fruit products. Nuts are better sources of folic acid.

11 **Answer: 2** Iron supplementation can cause gastric distress, constipation, and diarrhea. They do not cause a red, raised rash (option 1), blood in the stool (option 3), or headache (option 4).
Cognitive Level: Analysis **Client Need:** Health Promotion and Maintenance **Integrated Process:** Nursing Process: Evaluation **Content Area:** Maternal-Newborn **Strategy:** Note that the wording of the question indicates that the correct answer is a true statement. Recalling that iron is associated with GI side effects will help you eliminate options 1 and 4. Recall that iron causes tarry stools, not bloody, to eliminate option 3.

12 **Answer: 2** Iron is absorbed best on an empty stomach (not after a full meal) and in the presence of vitamin C. It may or may not be taken at the same time as other vitamin supplementation. It does not replace the need for other vitamins.
Cognitive Level: Application **Client Need:** Health Promotion and Maintenance **Integrated Process:** Nursing Process: Planning **Content Area:** Maternal-Newborn **Strategy:** First eliminate option 3 because iron intake does not eliminate the need for other vitamins. Next eliminate option 1 because a full meal may decrease iron absorption. Choose option 2 over 4 by recalling the beneficial effect of vitamin C on iron absorption.

13 **Answer: 1** Increased calcium intake can lead to formation of kidney stones. A calcium supplement is not expected to affect leg cramps, color of mucous membranes and conjunctiva, or resting heart rate.
Cognitive Level: Analysis **Client Need:** Health Promotion and Maintenance **Integrated Process:** Nursing Process: Assessment **Content Area:** Maternal-Newborn **Strategy:** Recall that calcium is a salt, and use this information to recall that salts can form crystals, which can in turn lead to kidney stones.

14 **Answer: 3** The measles, mumps, and rubella vaccine contains live, attenuated virus and could cause disease and harm to the fetus during pregnancy. It should be given after delivery, and the woman should avoid conceiving for 3 months.
Cognitive Level: Analysis **Client Need:** Health Promotion and Maintenance **Integrated Process:** Nursing Process: Planning **Content Area:** Maternal-Newborn **Strategy:** Determine that the issue in this question is immunization safety during pregnancy. Eliminate option 4 first because it is totally incorrect. Next eliminate option 2 because it would not make sense to wait until late in the pregnancy to administer a vaccine. Note also that options 1 and 3 are opposites; choose option 3 over option 1, recalling the live attenuated viral nature of the vaccine.

15 **Answer: 2** Braxton-Hicks contractions are probably caused by stretching of the myometrium. They are usually relieved by position changes, frequent emptying of the bladder, resting in a lateral recumbent position, and walking or light exercise.
Cognitive Level: Application **Client Need:** Health Promotion and Maintenance **Integrated Process:** Communication and Documentation **Content Area:** Maternal-Newborn **Strategy:** The question addresses the issue of client teaching about Braxton-Hicks contractions. The wording of the question indicates the correct answer is a true statement. Eliminate option 3 because it is factually incorrect; breathing may decrease discomfort during contractions. Next eliminate option 1 as unnecessary. Choose option 2 because it is a correct statement, and it does not patronize the client as in option 4.

16 **Answer: 4** Heat may relieve pain caused by increased joint mobility resulting from hormonal changes. Aspirin (option 3) should be avoided in the last trimester because it increases bleeding time. Option 1 is not a therapeutic communication. Option 2 may not be helpful for maternal–fetal circulation because the gravid uterus may cause pressure on the great vessels in the abdomen. The client should lie on one side; often the left is advised.
Cognitive Level: Application **Client Need:** Health Promotion and Maintenance **Integrated Process:** Communication and Documentation **Content Area:** Maternal-Newborn **Strategy:** Use general knowledge of care during pregnancy to eliminate options 2 and 3. Next eliminate option 1 because it violates principles of therapeutic communication.

17 **Answer: 4** The doula is a trained professional who provides physical and emotional support during labor. A doula does not replace either the father or the labor and delivery nurse in the delivery room. The doula is not responsible for clinical tasks and will not deliver the baby.
Cognitive Level: Application **Client Need:** Health Promotion and Maintenance **Integrated Process:** Nursing Process: Implementation **Content Area:** Maternal-Newborn **Strategy:** Recall that the doula is an ancillary caregiver to eliminate options 2 and 3. Choose option 4 over option 1 because the father's presence in the delivery room should not be affected by a doula.

18 **Answer: 4** The LDRP room provides for all phases of the delivery process in one room with the added safety of full hospital services for both mother and infant that home delivery and a freestanding birthing center cannot provide.

Cognitive Level: Application **Client Need:** Health Promotion and Maintenance **Integrated Process:** Nursing Process: Planning **Content Area:** Maternal-Newborn **Strategy:** Match the client statement in the question to the option that has the best match. This will easily allow you to eliminate the incorrect options.

19 **Answer: 3** Probable signs of pregnancy are those that are detected by the examiner and are usually related to the physical signs of pregnancy. Amenorrhea and chloasma are reported by the client (presumptive signs) and can be caused by conditions other than pregnancy. Fetal heartbeat on ultrasound is a positive sign of pregnancy.
Cognitive Level: Analysis **Client Need:** Health Promotion and Maintenance **Integrated Process:** Nursing Process: Assessment **Content Area:** Maternal-Newborn **Strategy:** Specific knowledge of the different classifications of signs of pregnancy is needed to answer this question. If you recall that "probable" is the middle category, it may help you to eliminate option 1 (positive sign) and options 2 and 4 (possible signs).

20 **Answer: 1** Trauma and the use of substances other than water can cause nipples to crack during lactation. The pinch test is to determine if nipples are inverted and need only be done one time.
Cognitive Level: Application **Client Need:** Health Promotion and Maintenance **Integrated Process:** Nursing Process: Implementation **Content Area:** Maternal-Newborn **Strategy:** Use nursing knowledge to answer the question. It may also be helpful to recall general principles of skin care and avoidance of skin trauma, which helps eliminate each of the incorrect options.

21 **Answer: 1** The client who is not eating meat may have a problem with decreased iron intake, which could impact her hemoglobin level. Polymorphonuclear cells, lymphocytes, and platelets are unrelated to iron intake.
Cognitive Level: Application **Client Need:** Health Promotion and Maintenance **Integrated Process:** Nursing Process: Assessment **Content Area:** Maternal-Newborn **Strategy:** Recall that meat is rich in iron, which is needed for RBC production. Then recall that the hemoglobin level is affected by iron intake and iron stores. As an alternate strategy, eliminate each of the other options because they do not identify RBCs.

22 **Answer: 4** Rubella titer higher than 1:16 is indicative of immunity to rubella. Rubella is a mild illness, and the client may or may not be aware of past infection (option 1). A rubella titer of 1:8 or less does not demonstrate immunity, and avoidance of those with rubella infection is indicated. A level of 1:12 is midway between susceptibility and immunity, so a client with this level is not at greatest risk.
Cognitive Level: Analysis **Client Need:** Health Promotion and Maintenance **Integrated Process:** Nursing Process: Planning **Content Area:** Maternal Newborn **Strategy:** Use the process of elimination to omit option 1 first because it does not address a laboratory value and relies on patient history for accuracy. Use specific knowledge of the direction of titer values to choose the correct answer. In this case, the larger the number, the better the immunity.

23 **Answer: 2** Day care workers are frequently exposed to the virus. Exposure to cat litter can result in toxoplasmosis exposure. IV drug use increases the risk for HIV or hepatitis. Giving blood does not increase the client's risk.
Cognitive Level: Analysis **Client Need:** Health Promotion and Maintenance **Integrated Process:** Nursing Process: Analysis **Content Area:** Maternal Newborn **Strategy:** Use the process of elimination and knowledge of transmission of viral infections to answer this question. Eliminate option 4 first as unrelated to acquiring infection. Eliminate option 1 next because the organism in toxoplasmosis is not a virus. Choose option 2 over 3 because option 3 is transmitted by blood or body fluids.

24 **Answer: 2** Indications for cesarean section are presence of a herpes lesion or prodromal symptoms. If there are no herpes symptoms or lesions, a vaginal delivery is recommended.
Cognitive Level: Analysis **Client Need:** Health Promotion and Maintenance **Integrated Process:** Nursing Process: Analysis **Content Area:** Maternal-Newborn **Strategy:** Specific knowledge related to risk of delivery with herpes infection is needed to answer the question. Use concepts of time and direct contact with lesions to eliminate the incorrect options.

25 **Answer: 1** All partners have been exposed and should be made aware, tested, and treated as indicated. Cesarean section would be appropriate only if there were symptoms of a herpes lesion or prodromal symptoms. Genetic assessment and more than routine assessment of hematocrit and hemoglobin are not indicated.
Cognitive Level: Application **Client Need:** Health Promotion and Maintenance **Integrated Process:** Nursing Process: Implementation **Content Area:** Maternal-Newborn **Strategy:** Use knowledge of principles of communicable disease transmission to answer the question. The client in the question is actually the sexual partner(s), not the fetus.

26 **Answer: 2** Carrier status of Group B streptococcus is variable, so identification several weeks before delivery may not identify a woman who is positive at the time of delivery. The current recommendation is screening during the 36th to 37th week of gestation. Rash and history of STI do not alter this recommendation.
Cognitive Level: Application **Client Need:** Health Promotion and Maintenance **Integrated Process:** Nursing Process: Planning **Content Area:** Maternal-Newborn **Strategy:** Specific knowledge of the timing of prenatal assessments is needed to answer this question. Eliminate option 1 because of the word *history,* which does not necessarily imply a risk for an active problem. Eliminate option 4 as unrelated, and choose option 2 over 3 by considering the risk for exposure at the time of delivery.

27 **Answer: 4** Menstrual blood can affect the results of a gonorrheal culture. Douching within 24 hours can affect results, but diagnosis/treatment of herpes and persistent vaginal discharge would not affect the results, and therefore do not interfere with specimen collection.
Cognitive Level: Application **Client Need:** Health Promotion and Maintenance **Integrated Process:** Nursing Process: Planning **Content Area:** Maternal-Newborn **Strategy:** Use general knowledge of specimen collection procedures to answer the question. Visualize each option and choose the one that could physically alter the test results.

28 **Answer: 3** Urine specific gravity is a measure of the concentration of particles in the urine. Urine specific gravity rises when the client is dehydrated. Hematocrit would also rise when dehydrated, but is an indirect measure. Hemoglobin measurements are not as greatly affected. Platelet count and IgG levels are not affected.
Cognitive Level: Application **Client Need:** Health Promotion and Maintenance **Integrated Process:** Nursing Process: Assessment **Content Area:** Maternal-Newborn **Strategy:** Note the key word *best* in the question, which means that more than one value could be affected. Use knowledge of laboratory indicators of dehydration to eliminate options 2 and 4. Then choose option 3 over option 1 because it is a more direct measurement of fluid balance.

29 **Answer: 1** Because it frequently involves tissue trauma that facilitates invasion of pathogens, anal intercourse is considered a high-risk sexual behavior. As such, it could lead to contraction of an STI. The other factors listed here do not increase the client's risk for contraction of an STI.
Cognitive Level: Analysis **Client Need:** Health Promotion and Maintenance **Integrated Process:** Nursing Process: Analysis **Content Area:** Maternal-Newborn **Strategy:** Use knowledge of principles related to spread of infection to answer the question. Only option 1 directly relates to a link in the chain of infection.

30 **Answer: 3** Closed-ended questions are a barrier to communication in many nurse–client interactions. They are best used when trying to elicit very specific pieces of assessment data. Use of open-ended questions, framed in a culturally sensitive and nonjudgmental approach, tends to establish a trusting and open relationship with the client and enhance client disclosure. Conducting the interview with the client dressed may also increase overall client comfort and aid in client disclosure.
Cognitive Level: Application **Client Need:** Health Promotion and Maintenance **Integrated Process:** Communication and Documentation **Content Area:** Maternal-Newborn **Strategy:** Use general principles related to communication and history taking to answer this question. Application of these principles will easily help to eliminate each incorrect option.

Key Terms to Review

alpha-fetoprotein (AFP) p. 120
Chadwick's sign p. 124
chloasma p. 125
colostrum p. 124
estimated date of birth (EDB) p. 113
fetal heart rate p. 114
fundal height p. 113
glucose tolerance test (GTT) p. 121
Goodell's sign p. 124
gravida p. 114
linea nigra p. 125
McDonald's method p. 113
Nägele's rule p. 113
oral glucose tolerance test (OGTT) p. 125
para p. 114
positive signs of pregnancy p. 114
presumptive signs of pregnancy p. 114
probable signs of pregnancy p. 114
quickening p. 114
sexually transmitted infections (STIs) p. 118
striae gravidarum p. 125
TORCH infections p. 117
triple-screen test p. 121
ultrasound p. 121

References

Condon, M. (2004). *Women's health: An integrated approach to wellness and illness.* Upper Saddle River, NJ: Pearson Education, pp. 470–477.

Ladewig, M., London, M., & Davidson, M. (2006). *Contemporary maternal-newborn nursing care* (6th ed.). Upper Saddle River, NJ: Pearson Education, pp. 111–123.

Lowdermilk, D., & Perry, S. (2004) *Maternity and women's health care* (8th ed.). St. Louis, MO: Mosby, pp. 220–265.

Olds, S. B., London, M. L., & Davidson, M. (2004). *Maternal-newborn nursing and women's health care* (7th ed.). Upper Saddle River, NJ: Prentice-Hall, pp. 89–107.

Pagana, K., & Pagana, T. (1998). *Manual of diagnostic and laboratory tests.* St. Louis: Mosby, pp. 255, 372, 678, 862, 870–872.

11 Uncomplicated Labor and Delivery Care

Test Yourself

Are you ready for the NCLEX-RN® or course exams? Use the practice tests on the companion CD-ROM to check.

In this chapter

Cross reference

Other chapters relevant to this content area are

I. NURSING CARE OF THE LABOR AND DELIVERY CLIENT

A. Physiologic safety

1. The laboring client is actually two clients—mother and newborn
2. Nursing care focuses on physiologic safety of both

B. Psychological safety

1. Nursing care also focuses on pyschological safety of mother and includes consideration of fear, comfort, partner involvement, parental attachment to newborn, and past experiences
2. Primigravida women experience fear of unknown and often have longer labors
3. Multigravida women can expect a shorter labor with subsequent pregnancies but may have memories of perceived bad experiences from previous births

C. Maternal history: must be assessed for abuse, assault, and violence because these past experiences often manifest as extreme fear and tension during labor process or vaginal examinations

D. Cultural background

1. Must be assessed and understood in order to provide a safe and acceptable birthing environment for childbearing family
2. Some common nursing actions may be cultural taboos for a particular client and affect parents' view of child throughout life

E. Preparation for labor by client and her support person(s)

1. Can vary from formal prenatal education classes to information passed from generation to generation
2. Misconceptions of birthing process and expectations of sensations during birth can occur and should be addressed in a nonjudgmental manner that informs and supports birthing family

F. Electronic fetal monitoring

1. Provides computer-assisted auditory and visual assessment of fetal heart rate (FHR) and uterine contractions (UC)
2. FHR monitoring continuously records the fetus's heart rate on upper portion of monitor strip
3. External monitoring: an ultrasound transducer is placed over fetal back and detects movements of fetal heart; fetal or maternal movement and maternal obesity may interfere with obtaining a continuous reading
4. Internal monitoring
   a. An **internal fetal scalp electrode** is inserted through cervix (which must be at least 2 cm dilated with ruptured membranes) and attached to epidermis of presenting part providing a direct ECG of fetal heart
   b. Is unaffected by maternal obesity, maternal or fetal movement; thick fetal hair may prevent adequate insertion on a cephalic presentation
5. **Baseline fetal heart rate** is average heart rate between contractions; measured in beats per minute (bpm); normal range: 120 to 160; bradycardia: < 120; tachycardia: > 160
6. **Short-term variability:** change in rate between one fetal heart beat and the next; creates a jaggedness or zigzag appearance in baseline FHR; determined by interplay between fetal sympathetic and parasympathetic nervous systems; decreased by fetal tachycardia, prematurity, fetal heart and CNS anomalies, and fetal sleep; normal: 2 to 3 bpm; classified as present or absent and can be evaluated only by internal monitoring
7. **Long-term variability:** rhythmic fluctuations that occur 2 to 6 times per minute; determined by interplay between fetal sympathetic and parasympathetic nervous systems; increased by fetal movement and decreased by fetal sleep or hypoxia and subsequent acidosis; average or moderate: 6 to 25 bpm
8. Periodic changes in FHR are deviations from baseline separate from variability and occur in relationship to or independent of contractions
9. **Accelerations:** transient increases in FHR
   a. Nonperiodic (spontaneous): symmetric, uniform, not related to contractions, occur in response to fetal movement and indicate fetal well-being
   b. Periodic: occur with contractions and may indicate decreased amniotic fluid or mild umbilical cord compression
10. Decelerations are categorized as early, late, or variable
11. **Early deceleration:** decrease in FHR beginning at onset of a contraction and returning to baseline by end of contraction with nadir at acme
    a. Uniform shape inversely mirrors contraction
    b. Caused by fetal head compression; usually benign
    c. Nursing interventions include performing a vaginal examination to determine if fetus is descending in pelvis; if fetus is not descending, notify health care provider
12. **Late decelerations** begin after contraction starts, with nadir occurring after peak of contraction and returning to baseline after end of contraction
    a. Smooth, uniform shape that inversely mirrors contractions but late in onset and recovery
    b. Caused by uteroplacental insufficiency; always considered ominous
    c. Nursing interventions focus on maintaining oxygenation and include repositioning client to left lateral, administering oxygen by mask at 7 to 10 L/min, correcting hypotension through increased IV fluid rate or administration of medications, discontinuing oxytocin if being administered, and reporting to health care provider

13. **Variable decelerations** occur suddenly, vary in duration and intensity, vary in relation to contractions, and resolve abruptly
    a. Variable shape, usually U or V, with steep sides; may or may not be associated with contractions
    b. Caused by compression of umbilical cord
    c. Categorized as mild, moderate, or severe based on lowest FHR reading and duration of deceleration; repetitive, prolonged, or more severe decelerations with a slow return or overshoot to baseline are ominous and indicate fetal asphyxia
    d. Nursing interventions focus on relieving cord compression through repositioning client until improvement occurs, vaginal examination to detect prolapsed cord, and oxygen if decelerations are severe or uncorrectable
    e. Amnio-infusion, the instillation of warmed normal saline through an intrauterine pressure catheter, may be used to recreate cushioning effect on the umbilical cord during contractions that is normally provided by amniotic fluid
14. Uterine contraction monitoring documents contraction frequency, duration, and intensity; contractions are documented on lower half of monitor strip
    a. External monitoring: tocodynamometer is placed on maternal abdomen near fundus; accurate only for documenting contraction frequency and duration; affected by fetal or maternal movement, transverse or oblique lie, and maternal abdominal fat: a thin woman's mild contractions may look strong on monitor strip, while an obese woman's strong contractions may not be detected at all
    b. Internal monitoring is accomplished through an **intrauterine pressure catheter (IUPC),** a wire with pressure gauge on one end or a saline-filled tube, which is inserted through cervix and past presenting part into amniotic fluid in uterus; increase in intrauterine pressure is detected and measured in mm of Hg; cervix must be at least 2 to 3 cm dilated with ruptured membranes before an IUPC can be inserted

II. THE LABOR PROCESS

A. **Initiation of labor:** comes about from an interplay of factors, including distension of uterus causing irritability and contractility, and hormonal influence of prostaglandins, oxytocin, fetal cortisol, estrogen, and progesterone

B. **True versus false labor:** differentiated by cervical change: effacement and dilatation

C. **Factors of labor:** passageway, passenger, powers, and psyche

1. Passageway is maternal bony pelvis comprised of innominate bones (ilium, ischium and pubis), sacrum and coccyx
    a. False pelvis lies above pelvic brim, supports increasing weight of enlarging pregnant uterus, and directs presenting part into true pelvis below
    b. True pelvis consists of inlet, midpelvis, and outlet and represents bony limits of birth canal; adequacy of each part, measured as transverse and anterior–posterior diameters, must be sufficient to allow passage of fetus through passageway
    c. Four pelvic types are gynecoid, android, anthropoid, and platypelloid (see Table 11–1 ■); type of pelvis and its diameters influence descent of fetus, progression of labor, and type of delivery
2. *Passenger* refers to fetus
    a. **Attitude** is relationship of fetal parts to one another; normal attitude is flexion of neck, arms, and legs
    b. **Lie** is relationship of longitudinal axis of fetus to longitudinal axis of mother; vertex (head first) is most common, but breech (buttocks first), transverse (laterally across uterus), and oblique (diagonally across uterus) lies are possible
    c. **Presentation** is fetal part entering pelvis first; most common presentation is cephalic, but breech and shoulder can also occur
    d. **Position** is relationship of fetal presenting part to maternal pelvis; a three-letter notation is used to describe fetal position: see the memory aid box; the most common positions at delivery are ROA (right occiput anterior) and LOA (left occiput anterior)

Table 11-1
Pelvic Types

Pelvic Type	Incidence	Inlet	Midpelvis	Outlet	Implications for Birth
Gynecoid	50%	Round, adequate diameters	Round, adequate diameters	Wide transverse, long anterior–posterior diameters	Occiput anterior most common, NSVD favorable
Android	20%	Heart-shaped, angulated	Short anterior–posterior diameter	Short anterior–posterior diameter	Slow descent, arrest of labor, operative birth more common
Anthropoid	25%	Ovoid, long anterior–posterior diameter	Rounded, adequate diameters	Narrow transverse	Occiput anterior or posterior, NSVD favorable
Platypelloid	5%	Ovoid, wide transverse diameter	Rounded, wide transverse diameter	Wide transverse, short anterior–posterior diameter	Occiput posterior more common, NSVD not favorable

Memory Aid

Use the mnemonics in 2 and 3 to help remember fetal position:

1. **R** or **L**: **r**ight or **l**eft; direction that fetal presenting part of fetus faces
2. **AMOS: a**cromion process, **m**entum, **o**cciput, **s**acrum; the landmark of the fetal presenting part
3. **PAT: p**osterior, **a**nterior, **t**ransverse; the relationship of the landmark of the presenting part to the front, back, or side of the pelvis

e. **Engagement** occurs when largest diameter of presenting part reaches pelvic inlet and can be detected by vaginal examination; termed *floating* if it is directed toward pelvis but can easily be moved out of inlet; termed *ballotable* when presenting part dips into inlet but can be displaced with upward pressure from examiner's fingers; termed *engaged* if fixed in pelvic inlet and cannot be displaced

f. **Station** is relationship of presenting part to ischial spines of pelvis; measured in centimeters above (−1 to −5 station), at (0 station), or below (+1 to +4 station) the ischial spines (see Figure 11–1 ■)

3. Powers include the primary and secondary forces of labor
   a. Primary forces consist of involuntary contractions of uterine muscle fibers, which are stimulated by a pacemaker located in upper uterine segment
   b. Contractions consist of increment (building-up phase), acme (peak), and decrement (letting-up phase) and are followed by a resting phase (nadir) to facilitate uteroplacental–fetal reoxygenation
   c. Frequency of contractions is the time in seconds or minutes from onset of one contraction to onset of next
   d. Intensity is strength of contraction at acme, which can be palpated as mild, moderate, or strong; detected with a fetal monitor externally; or measured internally in mm Hg
   e. Duration is length of contraction measured in seconds from beginning of increment to end of decrement
   f. With each contraction, muscles of upper uterine segment shorten and exert longitudinal traction on cervix, causing **effacement,** the thinning and drawing up of internal os and cervical canal into uterine side walls; measured from 0 to 100 %; in primigravidas, effacement usually precedes dilatation; in multigravidas, effacement and dilatation normally occur simultaneously
   g. As uterus elongates with contractions, fetal body straightens and exerts pressure against lower uterine segment and cervix; **dilatation,** or opening of cervix, results, is measured from 0 to 10 cm, and allows for birth of fetus
   h. Secondary powers consist of voluntary use of abdominal muscles during second stage of labor to facilitate descent and delivery of fetus

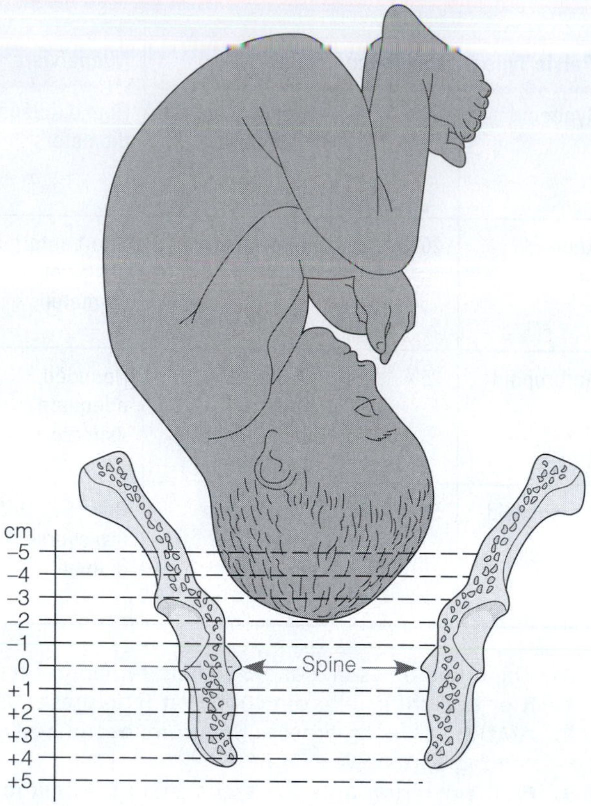

Figure 11-1

Stations of fetal descent measured in centimeters.

Source: Olds, S., London, M., Ladewig, P., and Davidson, M. (2004).

4. Psyche represents psychological component of childbearing; excitement, fear, perceived loss of control, and anxiety are common emotions during labor and birth process
   a. Extreme emotions such as fear will result in muscular tension, which can create more pain from friction between working uterus and tense abdominal muscles or impede descent of fetus when pelvic and perineal muscles are tense rather than relaxed when pushing
   b. Psyche can also be manifested physiologically as changes in maternal vital signs: increased blood pressure, pulse, and respiratory rates occur with fear, excitement, and anxiety
   c. Lack of knowledge and preparation for childbirth can negatively affect psyche

III. THE STAGES OF LABOR

A. First stage

1. Extends from onset of true labor to complete dilatation of cervix (0 to 10 cm) and is divided into three phases: latent, active, and transition
2. ! Latent phase
   a. 0 to 3 centimeters dilated, little descent occurs
   b. Contractions usually begin irregularly and become more regular, with increasing frequency and duration and intensity (from mild to moderate)
   c. Client is usually relieved labor has started; can recognize and express anxiety; may be happy, excited, and talkative; and changes position without reminder
   d. Average duration is 8.6 hours for nulliparas and 5.3 hours for multiparas
3. ! Active phase
   a. 4 to 7 centimeters dilated, effacement and descent are progressive
   b. Contractions usually every 2 to 3 minutes, 60 seconds in duration, and moderate to strong intensity
   c. Client is usually serious, intense, has a need for increased concentration, will answer questions in short phrases only between contractions; fatigue increases and woman becomes more dependent; pain increases, relaxation becomes more difficult, and woman may need reminders to change positions
   d. Average duration is 4.6 hours for nulliparas and 2.4 hours for multiparas

4. Transition phase
   a. 8 to 10 centimeters dilated, effacement is completed, and descent increases
   b. Contractions every 1½ to 2 minutes, lasting 60 to 90 seconds, strong intensity
   c. Client is working hard with intense concentration; gives one-word answers to questions only between contractions; anxiety increases, fears loss of control and abandonment, senses helplessness; relaxation is difficult as contraction time exceeds the resting phase; may experience intense low abdominal, pelvic, and rectal discomfort from fetal descent; nausea and vomiting are common; may need reminders to empty bladder and change position
   d. Average duration is 3.6 hours for nulliparas and 30 minutes for multiparas
5. Assessment upon admission: review medical, obstetric and prenatal history; labor status (contractions, vaginal examination if indicated), fetal status (heart rate, variability, periodic changes), status of membranes (intact or if ruptured, length of time and amount, color, odor), maternal vital signs, laboratory testing if ordered (Hgb and UA), desired birth plan including cultural considerations, preparation for childbirth, level of comfort and coping, and support system
6. Nursing assessments during first stage of labor
   a. Latent phase: BP, pulse, respirations q1h if normal; temperature q4h if normal or membranes intact and q2h if abnormal or membranes ruptured; contractions q30 min; FHR q1hr for low-risk women or q30 min if high-risk women or nonreassuring pattern
   b. Active phase: BP, pulse, respirations, temperature, contractions same as latent phase; FHR q30min for low-risk women or q15min for high-risk women or nonreassuring pattern; look for bloody mucus or "show" from cervical dilatation as active labor progresses toward transition
   c. Transition phase: BP, pulse, respirations q30min; temperature same as latent phase; contractions q15min, FHR q15min
7. Collaborative management
   a. Orient to environment, expected assessments, and procedures
   b. Encourage ambulation (if presenting part is engaged) unless contraindicated
   c. Provide comfort through frequent position change, effluerage, focal point, hydrotherapy, caregiver presence, therapeutic touch, sacral pressure, back rub, or administration of analgesia as requested by client and ordered by health care provider
   d. Encourage voiding q2h
   e. Monitor labor progress and fetal well-being
   f. Provide ice chips and clear liquids to prevent dehydration
   g. Teach, reinforce, or support use of relaxation, visualization, or breathing patterns
   h. Encourage rest between contractions
   i. Document in client record and provide continuing status reports to health care provider
8. Outcome is that client states she is able to cope with contractions; maternal and fetal well-being are maintained throughout labor

B. Second stage

1. Extends from complete dilatation of cervix to delivery of fetus; accompanied by involuntary efforts to expel fetus characterized by low-pitched, guttural, grunting sounds
2. Many women initially feel renewed energy because they can voluntarily work with contractions to push out fetus; over time can be exhaustingly hard work
3. Normal duration is up to 3 hours for nulliparas and up to 30 minutes for multiparas
4. **Cardinal movements** are adaptations that fetus undertakes to maneuver through pelvis during labor and birth; in most common presentation, occiput, movements occur in the following order:
   a. *Engagement* of the presenting part occurs
   b. *Descent* of fetus into pelvis
   c. *Flexion* of fetal head; (descent and flexion often occur simultaneously)
   d. *Internal Rotation* of fetal head must take place to accommodate maternal pelvis and occurs so that anterior–posterior (AP) diameter of fetal head (largest diameter of fetus) aligns with AP dimension of maternal pelvis

e. *Extension* of fetal head occurs as it comes under maternal symphysis pubis and emerges from vagina
f. ***R**estitution* occurs as fetal head turns 45 degrees to untwist neck after head has delivered
g. *External **R**otation* is viewed as head turns an additional 45 degrees as second-largest fetal diameter (lateral diameter of fetal shoulders) rotates into alignment with AP dimension of maternal pelvis
h. *Expulsion* occurs as the anterior shoulder slips beneath symphysis pubis, which facilitates delivery of body

Memory Aid

Use the following mnemonic phrase to assist in remembering the cardinal movements, using the first letter of each cardinal movement to begin a word: ***E**very **d**arn **f**ool **i**n **R**otterdam **e**ats **r**otten **e**gg **r**olls **e**veryday.*

5. **Crowning** is outward bulging and thinning of perineum and opening of vagina that occurs as fetal presenting part presses downward onto perineum and becomes visible prior to delivery; this process is slower in nulliparous client than in multiparous client
6. Nursing assessment
   a. BP, pulse, and respirations q5–q15min
   b. Contractions palpated continuously
   c. FHR q15min if low risk, q5min if high risk, and if nonreassuring pattern, monitor continuously
   d. Monitor fetal descent, cardinal fetal movements, and crowning
7. Collaborative management
   a. Position comfortably for pushing and birth; encourage rest and relaxation between contractions
   b. Comfort measures: cool cloth to forehead, support legs while pushing, provide encouragement to push
   c. Ice chips and clear fluids to prevent dehydration
   d. Empty bladder, straight catheter if bladder distended or unable to void
   e. Local infiltration of anesthetic agent for birth by health care provider
   f. **Episiotomy**: a surgical incision into perineum to enlarge vaginal opening; usually done during or just prior to crowning; medically indicated in presence of fetal distress, but often performed to prevent tearing of perineal tissues because lacerations have irregular edges and are more difficult to repair
   g. Types of episiotomy are midline episiotomy (1- to 3-centimeter incision straight back from vagina toward rectum), mediolateral (4- to 5-centimeter incision from vagina obliquely toward one buttock)
   h. Lacerations to perineum or surrounding tissues may occur during childbirth; see Box 11–1 for degrees of laceration; 3rd- and 4th-degree lacerations most commonly occur after midline episiotomy is performed
   i. Document in client record: time of birth, gender, position, nuchal cord if present, and medications administered
8. Outcome is that client copes with contractions and pushing; maternal and fetal well-being is maintained through delivery

C. Third stage

1. Extends from birth of newborn to delivery of placenta; average duration is 30 minutes for nulliparas and multiparas

Box 11–1

Degrees of Laceration

1st degree: involves only the epidermal layers; if no bleeding, may not need repair

2nd degree: epidermal and muscle/fascia involvement, which requires suturing

3rd degree: extends into the rectal sphincter

4th degree: extends through the rectal mucosa

2. Maternal assessment
   a. BP, pulse, and respirations q5min
   b. Uterine fundus maintains tone and contraction pattern to deliver placenta by decreasing surface volume of uterus and shearing placenta from uterine wall
   c. Monitor for signs of placental separation: uterus rises up in abdomen; uterine volume shrinks as a result of contractions creating a gush of blood vaginally as uterine contents are expelled; and as placenta is separating and beginning to be expelled, umbilical cord protrudes further from vagina and appears to lengthen
3. Fetal assessment
   a. **Apgar score:** quick method to assess fetal adaptation to extrauterine life; five criteria are scored at 1 and 5 minutes after birth with 0, 1, or 2 points given for each criteria (see Table 11–2 ■); Apgar scores of 8 or greater indicate need for minimal intervention (nasopharyngeal suction and oxygen near face); scores of 4 to 7 indicate need for oropharyngeal suctioning, tactile stimulation, and oxygen administration; scores of 3 or less indicate need for resuscitation
   b. Respirations: normally 30 to 60, may be irregular
   c. Apical pulse: 120 to 160, may be irregular
   d. Temperature: skin temperature above 97.8°F (36.5°C)
   e. Umbilical cord: normally two arteries and one vein
   f. Gestational age assessment: consistent with expected date of delivery
   g. Physical assessment: abbreviated examination is conducted to detect presence of visible congenital anomalies
4. Collaborative management
   a. Encourage mother to rest and relax while awaiting delivery of placenta
   b. Immediate care of newborn includes placing in a modified Trendelenburg position, suctioning nose and oropharynx (bulb syringe or DeLee mucus trap), providing and maintaining warmth (dry immediately with warm blankets, skin-to-skin contact with mother covered with warm blankets, radiant heat source, cap)
   c. Assist parents in seeing and holding newborn to begin attachment
   d. Document time of placental delivery, appearance and intactness of placenta, mechanism of placental expulsion, and estimated delivery blood loss (averages 250 to 500 mL)
   e. Administer oxytocic agent as ordered
   f. Consider cultural practices in disposal of placenta
5. Outcome is that mother and newborn experience a safe labor and birth

D. Fourth stage (immediate recovery phase)

1. Includes first 1 to 4 hours after delivery; this stage is actually part of postpartal period but client usually remains in birthing suite for nursing care
2. Assessment: BP, pulse, respirations, fundus, lochia and perineum per agency protocol; usually q15min for 1 hour; q30min for 2 hours; q60min for 1 hour
3. Collaborative management
   a. Episiotomy or lacerations are repaired
   b. Provide comfort: clean gown, warm blanket, position of comfort, ice to perineum if sutures or edema present, analgesia as requested and ordered
   c. Help parents to explore newborn and initiate breast-feeding if desired and if mother and baby are stable

Table 11–2
Apgar Scoring

	Color (Appearance)	Heart Rate (Pulse)	Reflex Irritability (Grimace)	Muscle Tone (Activity)	Respiratory Effort (Respirations)
0 Points	Blue, pale	Absent	Absent	Absent	Absent
1 Point	Blue extremities, pink body	< 100	Grimace	Some flexion of extremities	Slow, irregular
2 Points	Completely pink	≥ 100	Vigorous cry	Active motion	Good cry

d. Provide fluids and regular diet as tolerated; consider cultural preferences
4. Outcome is that maternal and newborn well-being are maintained; family unit is supported and participates in birth process as desired

IV. PAIN MANAGEMENT DURING BIRTH

A. **Analgesia and anesthesia:** can be given to decrease or eliminate pain during birthing process when nonpharmacologic methods of pain relief are ineffective

B. Type of analgesia or anesthesia

1. Determined by obstetric history of client, stage and phase of labor, rate of progression in labor, and preferences of client and health care provider
2. Regional differences in use of particular methods or medications exist

! C. **Nonpharmacologic methods of pain relief**

1. Position changes to decrease weight of fetus on area of most intense pain
2. Hydrotherapy by standing or sitting in a warm shower or reclining in a tub
3. Breathing techniques to prevent breath-holding and to facilitate oxygen and carbon dioxide exchange; use of a focal point for concentration
4. Relaxation through verbal instruction, massage, soft music, or therapeutic touch

D. **Pharmacologic methods of pain relief**

1. Analgesic agents decrease amount of pain perceived; goal is maximum pain relief with minimal risk for woman and fetus; must consider effect on woman, fetus, and contractions
2. ! All systemic drugs cross placental barrier in varying amounts; analgesia given too early may prolong labor and depress fetus; analgesia given too late may cause neonatal respiratory depression with no benefit to woman
3. Intravenous narcotics: nalbuphine hydrochloride (Nubain) and butorphanol tartrate (Stadol) most commonly used in active phase of first stage of labor
   a. Advantages: RN administration, rapid onset of pain relief, ease of administration, relatively short duration
   b. Disadvantages: may decrease contraction frequency and intensity, crosses placenta resulting in neonatal respiratory depression, short duration may not give adequate pain control during nulliparous or prolonged labor
   c. ! Nursing implications: Nubain is a narcotic agonist-antagonist and should never be given to a client with narcotic dependency or abuse as immediate withdrawal will occur that can stimulate seizures
4. Intrathecal narcotics: morphine sulphate (Morphine) or fentanyl citrate (Fentanyl) injected into L4–L5 or L5–S1 subarachnoid space
   a. Advantages: excellent pain control that occurs within several minutes, lasts several hours, rarely results in neonatal respiratory depression, easier and faster injection method for both provider and client than epidural
   b. Disadvantages: undesirable for rapidly progressing labor or transition phase; may eliminate urge to push; must be injected by anesthesia personnel; injection is uncomfortable; laboring client must hold very still during injections; spinal headache may occur from leakage of CSF through dura at injection site
   c. ! Nursing implications: monitor for common side effects, including nausea, pruritus, urinary retention, muscle spasms at site of injection
5. Lumbar **epidural block**: provides temporary and reversible loss of sensation by injection into area with direct contact to nervous tissue; needle and catheter introduced at L4–L5 or L5–S1 level; local anesthetic agents such as bupivacaine hydrochloride (Marcaine) or lidocaine hydrochloride (Xylocaine) injected; provides either regional analgesia or anesthesia depending on the dose injected
   a. Advantages: excellent pain relief, re-dosing possible, no neonatal respiratory depression results, may provide a few hours of postpartum pain relief as well as during labor and delivery
   b. Disadvantage: undesirable for rapidly progressing labor or transition phase; must be inserted by anesthesia personnel; usually causes numbness of lower extremities, limiting mobility; decreases contraction frequency and intensity; reduces or eliminates urge to push; relaxation of musculature below site of in-

jection often results in failure of fetus to accomplish internal rotation, necessitating an operative birth

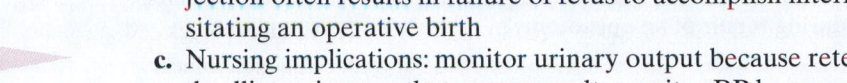

! c. Nursing implications: monitor urinary output because retention requiring indwelling urinary catheter may result; monitor BP because maternal hypotension commonly results from vasodilation; avoid supine position

6. **Paracervical block:** a type of regional anesthesia; local anesthetic agent injected into lateral aspects of cervix during active or transition phases
   a. Advantages: rapid onset of pain relief, no neonatal respiratory depression, can be administered during transition, relative ease of administration
   b. Disadvantages: systemic absorption of medication through vascular cervix, excessive bleeding from cervix, decreased or absent urge to push
   ! c. Nursing implications: FHR as bradycardia can result from systemic absorption
7. **Pudendal block:** local anesthetic agent injected into lateral vaginal walls near ischial spines to anesthetize pudendal nerve; administered during second stage in preparation for cutting and repairing an episiotomy
   a. Advantages: excellent anesthesia of perineum, rarely needs readminstration, provides a few hours of postpartum pain relief
   b. Disadvantages: must inject along presenting part, creating increased vaginal pressure and discomfort for client; eliminates urge to push
   ! c. Nursing implications: monitor client safety because decreased sensation in lower extremities affects mobility
8. Local infiltration: local anesthetic agents are injected into tissues of perineum to provide anesthesia for episiotomy incision or repair and suturing of lacerations
   a. Advantage: ease of administration, provides a few hours of postpartum pain relief
   b. Disadvantages: reinjection may be needed to obtain complete anesthesia with extensive lacerations or large episiotomies
   ! c. Nursing implications: loss of sensation may decrease urge or ability to urinate

Check Your NCLEX–RN® Exam I.Q. *You are ready for testing on this content if you can*

- Monitor the physiological status of a client in labor.
- Teach relaxation methods during labor.
- Assess fetal heart rate.
- Assist in delivery of a newborn.
- Provide effective support, teaching, and nursing care to a client in labor.

PRACTICE TEST

1 After walking for 30 minutes, the laboring client now has blood-tinged mucus on her underpad. Which of the following is the most appropriate interpretation by the nurse?

1. The fetus has had a bowel movement.
2. The amniotic sac has ruptured.
3. The client has fallen and sustained internal injury while walking.
4. The cervix is opening more rapidly.

2 After administration of an epidural block for labor analgesia, the client's blood pressure decreases from 130/75 to 90/50. The nurse should assist the woman to do which of the following?

1. Lie in a supine position.
2. Assume a semi-Fowlers position.
3. Empty her bladder.
4. Turn to the side to a left lateral position.

3 The client is in active labor and the nurse is taking an order from the health care provider for an opioid analgesic. The nurse verifies that the order is for which of the following priority routes for administration?

1. Intramuscular
2. Oral
3. Intravenous
4. Rectal

PRACTICE TEST

4 The nurse would question which of the following methods of pain relief during repair of an episiotomy?

1. Paracervical block
2. Epidural block
3. Pudendal block
4. Local infiltration

5 The nurse would use which of the following as the most accurate method to assess the frequency, duration, and strength of contractions of a woman in active labor?

1. Abdominal palpation
2. Tocodynamometer
3. Intrauterine pressure catheter (IUPC)
4. Client's description

6 A laboring client has recently had an intrathecal narcotic administered for relief of labor pain. The nurse determines that teaching has been effective when the client makes which statement?

1. "If I stay on the bedpan a little longer, I think I can urinate."
2. "I know my itching is from the intrathecal medication."
3. "The baby won't move as much now that I've had the intrathecal medication."
4. "I wouldn't be nauseated if I had received the intrathecal medication earlier."

7 The nurse concludes that the use of nonpharmacologic pain management techniques have been helpful to the client after observing which of the following?

1. Decreased short-term variability in the fetal heart rate
2. Increased maternal blood pressure and pulse
3. Decreased muscle tension in the arms and face
4. Increased frequency of contractions

8 The nurse's plan of care for the pain of a laboring client would incorporate which of the following concepts?

1. Childbirth pain is caused only by physical factors.
2. The expression of pain is universal.
3. Having the presence of a supportive partner eliminates pain.
4. Labor pain has physiologic and psychologic components.

9 The nursing care plan for a client with a prolonged latent phase of labor includes which of the following as a priority measure?

1. Encouraging rest and relaxation through the playing of soft music
2. IV hydration with either lactated Ringer solution or 5 percent dextrose
3. Continuous internal fetal monitoring of the fetal response to contractions
4. Measuring maternal blood pressure, temperature, and pulse every 15 minutes

10 The nursing plan of care for the client in early labor would include assessment of which of the following as a high priority at this time?

1. Cultural beliefs and practices
2. Maternal nutritional status
3. Reasons for selecting a nurse-midwife
4. Names the family has chosen for the infant

11 The client's fetal heart rate is 150 before the contraction begins. During the contraction, the heart rate falls to 110 and returns to baseline 30 seconds after the contraction ends. Which of the following is the priority nursing action in response to this finding?

1. Place the client into a semi-Fowler's position.
2. Administer oxygen by nasal cannula at 2 liters per minute.
3. Insert a Foley catheter and measure urinary output.
4. Place the client in left lateral position.

12 The fetal heart rate baseline is 145 beats per minute with short-term variability of 12 beats per minute. The nurse should take which of the following actions?

1. Notify the client's health care provider immediately.
2. Obtain an order to start an IV of lactated Ringer solution.
3. Reposition the client on her hands and knees.
4. Encourage continued use of breathing and relaxation techniques.

13 In planning care for the adolescent in labor, the nurse should address which of the following concerns?

1. Misconceptions of the functions of various body parts
2. The pregnant adolescent's nutritional needs
3. Reliability of her boyfriend as a support person
4. Appropriateness of names for her newborn that she has chosen

14 The fetal heart rate shows variable decelerations. Which of the following nursing actions could be implemented to decrease or eliminate this pattern?

1. Encourage the woman to relax in a warm shower.
2. Apply a fetal scalp electrode.
3. Assist the client into a supine position.
4. Begin an amnio-infusion of normal saline.

15 The laboring client is 8 centimeters dilated, 100 percent effaced, with vertex presenting at +2 station. The fetal heart rate gradually slows during each contraction, returning to baseline by the end of the contraction. The nurse concludes that which of the following is occurring?

1. The umbilical cord is becoming compressed.
2. There is uteroplacental insufficiency.
3. The fetal head is becoming compressed.
4. The fetus is moving between contractions.

16 A woman is admitted to the birthing unit. She is bearing down uncontrollably with contractions and says, "The baby is coming!" Which of the following is the priority action of the nurse?

1. Telephone the health care provider.
2. Put on gloves and prepare for immediate birth.
3. Obtain a medical and obstetric history.
4. Assess maternal vital signs and fetal heart rate.

17 The laboring client has begun to make guttural, grunting sounds during contractions. The nursing plan of care should now include which of the following?

1. Inspect the perineum to see if it is bulging outward.
2. Encourage the client's husband to go and eat now.
3. Teach the client about breast-feeding soon after delivery.
4. Assess the client's blood pressure and temperature.

18 A primigravida client is in the second stage of labor. The nurse determines that teaching has been effective when the client makes which of the following statements?

1. "I'll push two or three times and the baby will be born."
2. "It's not the baby, I have to have a bowel movement."
3. "I know I'll have to push a while. This is hard work."
4. "My doctor will come and pull the baby out now."

19 The newly delivered infant has been placed on the mother's abdomen. The priority nursing intervention for the newborn is to do which of the following?

1. Dry off the infant with blankets or towels.
2. Apply identification bracelets and obtain footprints.
3. Conduct a gestational age assessment.
4. Use the bulb syringe to clear the mouth and nose of mucus.

20 A laboring client's membranes spontaneously rupture. The first action of the nurse should be to do which of the following?

1. Assess the fetal heart rate.
2. Encourage the woman to ambulate.
3. Document the color, odor, and amount of amniotic fluid.
4. Prepare for imminent delivery of the newborn.

ANSWERS & RATIONALES

1 **Answer: 4** Bloody mucus is often called *bloody show* and becomes more profuse during the late active phase and into the transition phase of the first stage of labor and during the second stage of labor. Fetal bowel movements are not blood-tinged. Rupture of the amniotic sac would produce a clear watery fluid. There is no correlation of blood-tinged mucus during labor with injury sustained through walking. **Cognitive Level:** Analysis **Client Need:** Health Promotion and Maintenance **Integrated Process:** Nursing Process: Analysis **Content Area:** Maternal-Newborn **Strategy:** Note the key words *blood-tinged* and associate this with progression in labor. Recall that exercise such as walking hastens labor. Both of these concepts guides you to select option 4 as the answer.

2 **Answer: 4** Vasodilation occurs with epidural analgesia and anesthesia, which can result in hypotension. The client who is hypotensive after epidural administration should be turned to a left lateral position and have the IV fluid rate increased.

This will increase the circulation to the fetus and increase circulating volume, respectively.
Cognitive Level: Application **Client Need:** Health Promotion and Maintenance **Integrated Process:** Nursing Process: Implementation **Content Area:** Maternal-Newborn **Strategy:** The issue of the question is the appropriate action that counteracts a side effect of epidural analgesia. Recall that opioid analgesics often cause vasodilation, which can be counteracted by proper positioning. Eliminate options 2 and 3 first because they are not helpful; then choose option 4 over option 1 because option 4 assists both the mother and the fetus.

3 **Answer: 3** Narcotics given for pain relief in labor are most often given intravenously so that the medication will have a rapid onset and a relatively short half-life. This desired drug profile will provide maternal benefit while preventing neonatal respiratory depression.
Cognitive Level: Application **Client Need:** Health Promotion and Maintenance **Integrated Process:** Nursing Process: Planning **Content Area:** Maternal-Newborn **Strategy:** Use the process of elimination, choosing the route that will work rapidly but that hastens metabolism and excretion for the benefit of the fetus. With this in mind, eliminate options 1 and 4 first. Then choose option 3 over option 2 because the opioid analgesic is absorbed much more quickly intravenously.

4 **Answer: 1** Paracervical block is given during the active and transitional phases of labor to block the pain sensations of the dilating cervix. It has no effect on the perineum and would offer no analgesic effect during episiotomy repair. The other options affect the perineum and would offer analgesia during suturing of the episiotomy.
Cognitive Level: Analysis **Client Need:** Health Promotion and Maintenance **Integrated Process:** Nursing Process: Analysis **Content Area:** Maternal-Newborn **Strategy:** Specific knowledge of methods of pain relief during episiotomy care is needed to answer this question. Visualize each option, and make the selection that best fits with nursing knowledge.

5 **Answer: 3** Abdominal palpation will give limited information about uterine contractions, especially if the client is either very thin or obese. The client's description of the contractions will be influenced by her culturally based expression of pain as well as by her previous pain experiences and pain threshold. The tocodynamometer, or external uterine transducer, will detect the onset and end of contractions in most women but does not assess intensity of the contractions. Additionally, if the client is either very thin or obese, the fetal monitor tracing will either exaggerate the contractions or minimize them. Internal contraction monitoring through the use of an intrauterine pressure catheter will objectively measure the contractions in mm of Hg and is the most accurate method of contraction monitoring.
Cognitive Level: Analysis **Client Need:** Health Promotion and Maintenance **Integrated Process:** Nursing Process: Analysis **Content Area:** Maternal-Newborn **Strategy:** Note the key words *most accurate method* in the question, which tells you that more than one option may be partially or totally correct but that one option is best. Evaluate each option and make your choice based on the method (IUPC) that is closest to the source (fetus and uterus).

6 **Answer: 2** Women receiving intrathecal narcotics for labor analgesia often experience adverse effects such as urinary retention, nausea, vomiting, and pruritus (itching). A Foley catheter is routinely used to allow for urinary elimination. Fetal movement is not affected by intrathecal narcotics.
Cognitive Level: Analysis **Client Need:** Health Promotion and Maintenance **Integrated Process:** Teaching and Learning **Content Area:** Maternal-Newborn **Strategy:** Note the issue of the question, which is knowledge of adverse effects of intrathecal narcotics during labor. The word *effective* in the question tells you the correct answer is a true statement. Eliminate options 1 and 3 first as false statements. Choose option 2 over 4 because it reflects an accurate statement of side effects.

7 **Answer: 3** Objective signs of pain relief include decreased muscle tension as evidenced by unclenched fists; relaxed facial muscles and decreased grimacing, frowning, or creasing of the brow; and slightly lowered blood pressure, pulse rate, and respiratory rate. Frequency of uterine contractions would not be affected by relieving pain through nonpharmacological methods.
Cognitive Level: Analysis **Client Need:** Health Promotion and Maintenance **Integrated Process:** Nursing Process: Evaluation **Content Area:** Maternal-Newborn **Strategy:** The issue of the question is a satisfactory outcome of nonpharmacological methods of pain relief. With this in mind, use knowledge of general signs of pain relief to make your selection. Eliminate options 1 and 4 first because they are not evidence of pain relief, then eliminate option 2 because maternal blood pressure and pulse would decrease rather than increase with pain relief.

8 **Answer: 4** The pain of labor and childbirth has both physiologic and psychologic components. A support person's presence has been shown to decrease the perceived pain of childbearing. However, the expression of pain through nonverbal cues or verbalizations is highly culturally based (not universal), having been learned in early childhood.
Cognitive Level: Application **Client Need:** Health Promotion and Maintenance **Integrated Process:** Nursing Process: Planning **Content Area:** Maternal-Newborn **Strategy:** Note that options 1 and 4 are essentially the opposite of each other. When two options are opposites, often one of them is correct. Choose option 4 over option 1 because it is more comprehensive.

9 **Answer: 1** Prolonged latent phase of labor is defined as greater than 20 hours in primigravida women and greater than 14 hours in multigravida women. Encouraging rest and relaxation during this phase will help the client have enough energy to push effectively during the second stage of labor. Music is often used effectively to induce relaxation. Encouraging a well-rested client to ambulate will also facilitate the latent phase. Intravenous hydration is given to women who are unable to take oral fluids. Internal monitoring is indicated if labor is being augmented or induced, the amniotic fluid is meconium-stained, or there is evidence of fetal distress by external monitoring. During the first stage of labor, maternal vital signs are obtained every hour.
Cognitive Level: Application **Client Need:** Health Promotion and Maintenance **Integrated Process:** Nursing Process: Planning **Content Area:** Maternal-Newborn **Strategy:** Note the key word *priority* in the stem of the question. This tells you some or all

options may be partially or totally correct, but one is more important than the others. Eliminate option 4 first as unnecessary. Then eliminate option 3 because external monitoring may be equally effective. Choose option 1 over 2 because there is no indication that the client cannot tolerate fluids and also because of the key words *prolonged latent phase* in the stem of the question.

10 **Answer: 1** Cultural beliefs and practices are inseparable from the labor and birthing experience. The RN must include a cultural assessment as part of the admission of all laboring clients. Maternal hydration status would be indicated, but nutritional status is not indicated during the birthing admission. Choosing a nurse-midwife or physician is based on many factors, and the nurse's role is to follow the protocols of the appropriate care provider, not to be judgmental or question a client's decision. Asking about names can be a cultural taboo.
Cognitive Level: Application **Client Need:** Health Promotion and Maintenance **Integrated Process:** Nursing Process: Planning **Content Area:** Maternal-Newborn **Strategy:** Note the timeframe of *early labor.* With this in mind, eliminate options 2 and 3, which are no longer timely during labor. Choose option 1 over option 4 because it focuses on data that can assist the nurse to provide an individualized plan of care during labor.

11 **Answer: 4** Late decelerations are caused by uteroplacental insufficiency and are always ominous. To optimize uteroplacental blood flow and therefore fetal oxygenation, the client should be positioned on her left side. Oxygen is appropriate but would be administered via mask at 7 to 10 liters per minute. A Foley catheter is unrelated to the fetus's needs at this time.
Cognitive Level: Application **Client Need:** Health Promotion and Maintenance **Integrated Process:** Nursing Process: Implementation **Content Area:** Maternal-Newborn **Strategy:** Determine what the question is testing, which is uteroplacental insufficiency. With this mind, eliminate option 3 as unrelated and option 1 as potentially harmful. Choose option 4 over option 2 because it is more effective in increasing delivery of oxygen and blood flow to the fetus.

12 **Answer: 4** Normal fetal heart rate baseline is 120 to 160 beats per minute. Normal short-term variability is 6 to 25 beats per minute. This is a normal fetal heart rate tracing and requires continued support and assessment by the nurse. There is no indication to contact the health care provider, provide intravenous fluids, or position the client on her hands and knees.
Cognitive Level: Application **Client Need:** Health Promotion and Maintenance **Integrated Process:** Nursing Process: Implementation **Content Area:** Maternal-Newborn **Strategy:** The issue of the question is the ability to recognize a normal fetal heart rate and variability on fetal monitoring. Recall that a normal fetal heart rate is 120 to 160 to determine that at least the fetal heart rate is normal. You can then eliminate options 1 and 2. Choose option 4 over 3, understanding that the variability of 12 beats is acceptable.

13 **Answer: 1** The role of the nurse is to be informative, supportive, but never judgmental. Thus, the reliability of the boyfriend and the appropriateness of names chosen are not assessments that the labor and delivery nurse should perform. Because the client is in labor, it is too late to address nutritional needs of pregnancy. This might also be perceived by the client as judgmental behavior of the nurse. Adolescents commonly misunderstand the functions of their body parts and additional teaching may be needed so the adolescent client in labor understands how birthing will take place.
Cognitive Level: Application **Client Need:** Health Promotion and Maintenance **Integrated Process:** Nursing Process: Planning **Content Area:** Maternal-Newborn **Strategy:** The issue of the question is age-appropriate care of the adolescent during labor. Choose the option that addresses lack of knowledge. Eliminate option 2 because it is not timely. Option 4 does not address the client's current needs, and option 3 could create distance between the client and nurse, depending on the conversation.

14 **Answer: 4** Variable decelerations are caused by compression of the umbilical cord. The treatment for variable decelerations focuses on relieving the cord compression, which can be accomplished by either infusing saline into the uterus via an intrauterine pressure catheter or by repositioning the client to get the weight of the fetus off the portion of cord that is being compressed. Pregnant women are never placed in a supine position because the fetus will compress the vena cava, thus decreasing uterine blood flow. Taking a warm shower would be unlikely to affect fetal heart rate directly.
Cognitive Level: Application **Client Need:** Health Promotion and Maintenance **Integrated Process:** Nursing Process: Implementation **Content Area:** Maternal-Newborn **Strategy:** Specific knowledge of the meaning of variable decelerations is needed to answer this question. Eliminate options 1 and 3 because option 3 could adversely affect fetal circulation by position and because option 1 is ineffective in addressing variability. Choose option 4 over option 2 because it is an intervention rather than a means of obtaining an assessment.

15 **Answer: 3** Gradual decelerations that begin and end with contractions are early decelerations and are caused by fetal head compression. Variable decelerations result from umbilical cord compression and are characterized by a sudden drop from baseline during contractions with a sudden return to baseline as the contraction ends. Late decelerations are caused by uteroplacental insufficiency and are characterized by gradual decrease in the fetal heart rate after the contraction begins and gradual return to baseline after the contraction has ended. Fetal movement usually results in fetal heart rate accelerations.
Cognitive Level: Application **Client Need:** Health Promotion and Maintenance **Integrated Process:** Nursing Process: Analysis **Content Area:** Maternal-Newborn **Strategy:** Specific knowledge of the relationship between fetal monitoring results and the effect on the fetus is needed to answer this question. Rely on nursing knowledge and choose option 3 because the data indicates the changes occur during contractions, when the head would be compressed against the lower pelvic structures.

16 **Answer: 2** Delivery appears imminent and priority should be given to the safety of the woman and her newborn through a controlled and attended birth. Another person can be summoned to contact the health care provider and perform

assessments. The history provides helpful information but can be obtained at a later time.

Cognitive Level: Application **Client Need:** Health Promotion and Maintenance **Integrated Process:** Nursing Process: Implementation **Content Area:** Maternal-Newborn **Strategy:** The situation in the question is urgent and requires immediate action by the nurse. Eliminate options 3 and 4 because they are assessments, and choose option 2 over 1 because it addresses the immediate physiological and safety needs of the mother and fetus.

17 **Answer: 1** The second stage of labor begins when the cervix is completely dilated and pushing begins. Most women make a low-pitched, guttural, grunting sound when they push spontaneously. When the client begins to make these sounds, she is pushing. The nurse should immediately inspect the perineum for bulging and the appearance of the presenting part. If neither of these is occurring, the nurse should perform a vaginal examination to assess for complete dilatation of the cervix.

Cognitive Level: Application **Client Need:** Health Promotion and Maintenance **Integrated Process:** Nursing Process: Planning **Content Area:** Maternal-Newborn **Strategy:** The issue of this question is accurate interpretation of onset of the second stage of labor. Knowing that pushing is characteristic of this stage, eliminate option 2 first because it is important for the husband to be present at this time. Eliminate option 3 next because it is not timely. Choose option 1 over 2 because it addresses the status of the fetus during the pushing stage.

18 **Answer: 3** The average duration of the second stage of labor for primigravidas is 2 hours. Many women feel rectal pressure, as if they were having a bowel movement as the baby descends deeper into the pelvis. The use of vacuum extraction or forceps to assist delivery is not routine.

Cognitive Level: Application **Client Need:** Health Promotion and Maintenance **Integrated Process:** Teaching and Learning **Content Area:** Maternal-Newborn **Strategy:** The wording of the question indicates that the correct answer is a statement that is true. Use knowledge of the second stage of labor to systematically eliminate each of the incorrect options.

19 **Answer: 4** Although all of the nursing actions presented are important after delivery, clearing the airway is the highest physiologic need and ensures safe adaptation to the extrauterine environment.

Cognitive Level: Application **Client Need:** Health Promotion and Maintenance **Integrated Process:** Nursing Process: Implementation **Content Area:** Maternal-Newborn **Strategy:** The key word in the question is *priority,* which indicates that one intervention is more important than the others to be completed first. Eliminate options 2 and 3 first because physiological needs take priority, and choose option 4 over option 1 because it addresses the airway.

20 **Answer: 1** The nurse should immediately assess the fetal heart rate to detect changes, which may be associated with prolapse of the umbilical cord. Ambulation is appropriate if the fetal heart is determined to be within normal parameters and the presenting part is engaged. Documentation is important but is not the priority intervention. The membranes may rupture at any time during labor; preparing for delivery may not be indicated at this time.

Cognitive Level: Analysis **Client Need:** Health Promotion and Maintenance **Integrated Process:** Nursing Process: Planning **Content Area:** Maternal-Newborn **Strategy:** The key word in the question is *first,* which indicates that one intervention is more important than the others to be completed at this time. Choose the option that protects the fetus after membrane rupture, which allows you to eliminate options 2 and 3. Eliminate option 4 because delivery is not necessarily imminent.

Key Terms to Review

accelerations p. 135
Apgar score p. 141
attitude p. 136
baseline fetal heart rate p. 135
cardinal movements p. 139
crowning p. 140
dilatation p. 137
early deceleration p. 135
effacement p. 137
engagement p. 137
epidural block p. 142
episiotomy p. 140
internal fetal scalp electrode p. 135
intrauterine pressure catheter (IUPC) p. 136
late deceleration p. 135
lie p. 136
long-term variability p. 135
paracervical block p. 143
position p. 136
presentation p. 136
pudendal block p. 143
short-term variability p. 135
station p. 137
variable deceleration p. 136

References

Condon, M. (2004). *Women's health: An integrated approach to wellness and illness.* Upper Saddle River, NJ: Pearson Education, pp. 483–491.

Kozier, B., Erb, K., Berman, A., & Snyder, S. (2004). *Fundamentals of nursing: Concepts, process, and practice* (7th ed.). Upper Saddle River, NJ: Pearson Education, pp. 1133–1169.

Ladewig, M., London, M., & Davidson, M. (2006). *Contemporary maternal-newborn nursing care* (6th ed.). Upper Saddle River, NJ: Pearson Education, pp. 352–375.

Lowdermilk, D., & Perry, S. (2004). *Maternity and women's health care* (8th ed.). St. Louis, MO: Mosby, pp. 541–605.

McKinney, E., James, S., Murray, S., & Ashwill, J. (2005). *Maternal-child nursing.* (2nd ed.). Philadelphia: Elsevier.

Olds, S., London, M., Ladewig, P., & Davidson, M. (2004). *Maternal-newborn nursing and women's health care* (6th ed.). Upper Saddle River, NJ: Pearson Education, pp. 221, 473–489, 500–511, 560, 571, 665–667.

Uncomplicated Postpartum Assessment and Care

12

In this chapter

Test Yourself

Are you ready for the NCLEX-RN® or course exams? Use the practice tests on the companion CD-ROM to check.

Cross references

Other chapters relevant to this content area are

Reproduction, Family Planning, and Infertility **Chapter 9**
Uncomplicated Antenatal Assessment and Care **Chapter 10**
Uncomplicated Labor and Delivery Care **Chapter 11**
Uncomplicated Newborn Care **Chapter 13**
Complicated Antenatal Care **Chapter 50**
Complicated Labor and Delivery Care **Chapter 51**
Complicated Postpartum Care **Chapter 52**
Complicated Newborn Care **Chapter 53**

I. PHYSICAL CHANGES DURING THE POSTPARTUM PERIOD

A. *Involution*

1. Reduction in size of uterus after delivery to prepregnant size caused by uterine contractions that constrict and occlude underlying blood vessels at placental site
2. ! Table 12–1 ■ presents factors that slow or hasten this process during **puerperium,** the 6-week period after delivery

B. *Fundus*

1. Top portion of uterus is a palpable indicator of involution
2. If contractions of uterine muscle are interrupted, a **boggy uterus** results (one that is soft, relaxed) and is likely to cause hemorrhage

C. Lochia

1. ! Discharge of blood and debris following delivery; types include **lochia rubra, lochia serosa,** and **lochia alba**
2. Characteristics of lochia are shown in Table 12–2 ■
3. Should not contain large clots
4. Total volume is 240 to 270 mL, and daily volume gradually decreases
5. ! Amount may be increased by exertion or breast-feeding

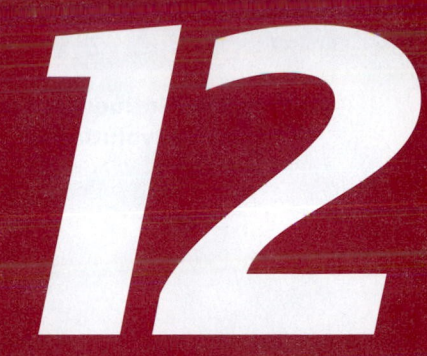

Table 12–1
Factors That Influence Involution

Factors That Enhance Involution	Factors That Slow Involution
Uncomplicated labor and delivery	Prolonged labor and difficult delivery
Breast-feeding	Anesthesia
Early ambulation	Grand multiparity
Complete expulsion of placenta and membranes	Retained placental fragments or membranes
	Full urinary bladder
	Infection
	Overdistention of the uterus

6. Pooling in uterus or vagina may occur while reclining, with increased bleeding upon arising
7. Unexplained increase in amount or reappearance of lochia rubra is abnormal

D. ***Afterpains***
1. Caused by intermittent uterine contractions following delivery
2. Occur in all women but are more painful in multiparous and breast-feeding women

E. **Cervix**
1. Soft, irregular, and edematous; may appear bruised with multiple small lacerations
2. Closes to 2 to 3 cm after several days, admits a fingertip after 1 week
3. Shape permanently changes after first delivery from round, dimplelike os of nullipara to lateral slitlike os of multiparous woman

F. **Vagina**
1. Smooth walls, edematous with multiple small lacerations
2. Client should be free from perineal pain within 2 weeks
3. Low estrogen levels postpartum lead to decreased vaginal lubrication and vasocongestion for 6 to 10 weeks, which can result in painful intercourse

G. **Abdominal wall**
1. Abdominal wall soft and flabby with decreased muscle tone
2. Striae, or stretch marks, that were red during pregnancy will fade to silver or white in Caucasian women; darker-skinned women will have darker striae that remain darker
3. **Diastasis recti,** separation of rectus muscles of abdomen, may improve postpartum depending on woman's physical condition, number of pregnancies, and type and amount of exercise

H. **Cardiovascular**
1. Returns to prepregnant state within 2 weeks

Table 12–2
Characteristics of Lochia

Type	Occurrence	Appearance	Composition
Lochia rubra	1–3 days	Dark red, bloody; fleshy, musty, stale odor that is nonoffensive; may have clots smaller than a nickel	Blood with small amounts of mucus, shreds of decidua, epithelial cells, leukocytes; may contain fetal meconium, lanugo, or vernix caseosa
Lochia serosa	4–10 days	Pink or brownish; watery; odorless	Serum, erythrocytes, shreds of degenerating decidua, leukocytes, cervical mucus, numerous bacteria
Lochia alba	11–21 days, may persist to 6 weeks in lactating women	Yellow to white; may have slightly stale odor	Leukocytes, decidual cells, epithelial cells, fat, cervical mucus, cholesterol, bacteria

2. Increase in blood volume by 40% during pregnancy is eliminated primarily by diuresis
3. First 48 hours postpartum pose the greatest risk of complications for clients with heart disease
4. Blood pressure should remain consistent with pregnancy baseline
5. Bradycardia of 50 to 70 beats per minute is common during first 6 to 10 days; tachycardia is related to increased blood loss, temperature elevation, or difficult, prolonged labor and birth
6. Increased fibrinogen continues for 1 week resulting in increased sedimentation rate and risk for thrombophlebitis
7. Increased white blood cells up to 30,000/mm^3 does not necessarily mean infection or may mask signs of infection; an increase of more than 30% in 6 hours indicates pathology
8. Decreased hemoglobin is related to the amount of blood loss during delivery; should return to prelabor value in 2 to 6 weeks depending on degree of decrease
9. Hematocrit increases by third to fifth day postpartum related to diuresis; a drop indicates abnormal blood loss

I. Urinary

1. Increased bladder capacity and decreased bladder tone lead to decreased sensation and increased risk of urinary retention and infection
2. Postpartum diuresis of 2,000 to 3,000 mL increases output in first 12 to 24 hours after delivery and accounts for a 5-pound weight loss
3. Increased glomerular filtration rate assists in diuresis
4. A full bladder displaces uterus, increasing risk of uterine atony and postpartum hemorrhage
5. Fluids are also lost through diaphoresis with increased perspiration most commonly occurring at night

J. Gastrointestinal

1. Hunger and thirst are common following birth
2. Risk for constipation increases because of decreased peristalsis, use of narcotic analgesics, dehydration and decreased mobility during labor, and fear of pain from having a bowel movement
3. Risk for hemorrhoids increases because of pressure from pushing during second stage of labor

K. Endocrine

1. Estrogen and progesterone levels drop rapidly after delivery of placenta
2. Menstruation usually resumes at 7 to 9 weeks for nonlactating women with 90% experiencing a menstrual period by 12 weeks; first cycle is usually anovulatory
3. Ovulation and menstruation return time is prolonged in lactating women and affected by length of time the woman breast-feeds and whether formula supplements are used; may vary from 2 to 18 months
4. Lactation
   a. Nipple stimulation leads to release of oxytocin from pituitary gland; this stimulates release of prolactin from pituitary gland, which causes production of milk and the **let-down reflex,** release of milk by contractions of alveoli of breast
   b. **Colostrum** is first milk secreted and is rich in protein and immunoglobulins
   c. Primary **engorgement** occurs on second or third day as supply of blood and lymph in the breast is increased and transitional milk is produced
   d. Mature milk is produced after 2 weeks and appears watery and slightly bluish in color, similar to skim milk

II. PSYCHOSOCIAL CHANGES DURING THE POSTPARTUM PERIOD

A. Phases of maternal adjustment

1. Taking-in phase
   a. First 3 days postpartum; needs to discuss labor and delivery
   b. Preoccupied with own needs; passive and dependent
   c. Touches and explores infant
2. Taking-hold phase

a. Third to tenth day postpartum
b. Obsessed with body functions
c. Rapid mood swings
d. Anticipatory guidance most effective now

3. Letting-go phase
a. 10 days to 6 weeks postpartum
b. Mothering functions established
c. Sees infant as a unique person

! B. ***Bonding*** (also known as attachment)
1. Process by which parents form an emotional relationship with their infant over time
2. Mother explores infant first with fingertips, then palms, and finally enfolding newborn with whole hands and arms
3. Holds infant in **en face** position, face-to-face position, about 20 centimeters apart and on same plane
4. Uses a soft, high-pitched tone of voice
5. **Engrossment** is father's absorption, preoccupation, and interest in infant shortly after birth, which can be stimulated by witnessing birth

! C. ***Postpartum blues:*** a maternal adjustment reaction
1. Transient depression usually occurs between second and third postpartum days and/or within first 2 weeks postpartum
2. Probably related to changes in hormone levels, fatigue, and psychological stress related to infant dependency
3. Experienced to some degree by a majority of women
4. Characterized by mood swings, anger, tearfulness, feeling let down, anorexia, and insomnia
5. Usually resolves spontaneously; may need evaluation for postpartum depression if symptoms persist or are severe

III. NURSING CARE OF THE POSTPARTUM CLIENT

A. General considerations with postpartum assessment
1. Evaluate prenatal and intrapartal history for risk factors
2. Provide privacy and encourage client to void prior to assessment
3. ! Position client in bed with head flat for most accurate findings
4. Proceed in a head-to-toe direction
5. Measure vital signs with woman at rest for better accuracy; will determine need or priority for other assessments
a. ! Temperature: above 100.4°F after first 24 hours may indicate an infection; may be elevated initially after delivery related to dehydration
b. ! Pulse: normal range postpartum is 50 to 80 beats per minute; report a rate greater than 100 to the health care provider
c. Respirations: normal range is 16 to 24 breaths per minute
d. ! Blood pressure: assess for orthostatic hypotension; monitor more closely if client has a history of preeclampsia
6. Women who experience operative procedures, cesarean delivery, or tubal ligation have both postpartum needs similar to those with vaginal births and needs of postoperative clients; monitor breath sounds and have client cough and take deep breaths

B. Postpartum assessment: use memory aids to remember nine components of assessment

Memory Aid

Use the mnemonic BUBBLE-HEB to aid in remembering the nine components of postpartum assessment:

B—Breasts
U—Uterus
B—Bladder
B—Bowel
L—Lochia
E—Episiotomy or perineal lacerations
H—Homan's sign
E—Emotional status
B—Bonding

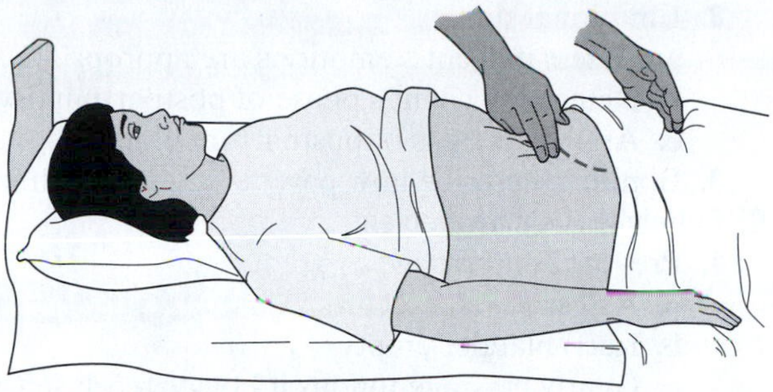

Figure 12–1

Measuring the descent of the fundus.

Source: Olds, London, & Ladewig (2000).

1. Breasts
   a. Determine if mother is breast- or bottle-feeding
   b. Palpate for engorgement or tenderness
   c. Inspect nipples for redness, cracks, and erectility if nursing
2. Uterus (see Figure 12–1 ■)
   a. Gently place nondominant hand on lower uterine segment just above symphysis pubis; dominant hand palpates top of fundus
   b. Determine uterine firmness, height of fundus, and position of fundus in relation to midline of the abdomen
   c. Correlate fundal location with expected descent of 1 centimeter each postpartum day
   d. Inspect any abdominal incisions, cesarean delivery, or tubal ligation, for REEDA: redness, edema, ecchymosis, discharge, and approximation of skin edges

Memory Aid

Use the mnemonic REEDA to remember components of an episiotomy/wound assessment:
R—Redness
E—Edema
E—Ecchymosis
D—Discharge
A—Approximation of skin edges

3. Bladder
   a. Client should void within 6 to 8 hours after delivery
   b. Assess frequency, burning, or urgency, which could indicate a urinary tract infection
   c. Evaluate ability to completely empty bladder
   d. Palpate for bladder distention if client's ability to void or complete emptying is in question
4. Bowel
   a. Assess for passage of flatus
   b. Inspect for signs of distention
   c. Auscultate bowel sounds in all four quadrants for postoperative clients
5. Lochia
   a. Inspect type, quantity, amount, and odor
   b. Correlate findings with expected characteristics of bleeding
   c. Cesarean-delivered women may have less lochia
6. Episiotomy or perineal lacerations
   a. Inspect perineum for REEDA (redness, edema, ecchymosis, discharge, approximation of skin edges)
   b. Inspect for hemorrhoids
7. **Homan's sign**
   a. Pain in calf upon dorsiflexion of foot is recorded as a positive sign and may indicate thrombophlebitis
   b. Inspect for pedal edema, redness, or warmth; if abnormal changes are present, assess pedal pulse

8. Emotional status
   a. Assess if client's emotions are appropriate for situation
   b. Determine client's phase of postpartum psychological adjustment
   c. Assess for signs of postpartum blues
9. Bonding: describe how parents interact with infant

C. Collaborative management

1. Prevent hemorrhage
   a. Assess for risk factors
   b. Keep bladder empty
   c. Gently massage fundus if boggy; teach self-massage of uterus
   d. Administer oxytocic medications if ordered: oxytocin (Pitocin), methylergonovine maleate (Methergine), ergonovine maleate (Ergotrate)
   e. Monitor for side effects of oxytocics if administered; hypotension with rapid IV bolus of Pitocin, hypertension with Methergine and Ergotrate
2. Promote comfort
   a. Apply ice to perineum 20 minutes on/10 minutes off for first 24 hours
   b. Encourage sitz bath, warm or cool, tid (three times a day) and prn (as needed) after first 12 to 24 hours
   c. Teach client to perform perineal care after every elimination: squirt or pour warm water over perineum; blot dry from front to back to prevent tissue trauma and contamination from anal area; apply clean perineal pad from front to back without touching surface that will be next to client
   d. Teach client to tighten buttocks, then sit and relax muscles
   e. Apply topical anesthetics (Dermaplast or Americaine spray) or witch hazel compresses (Tucks)
   f. Administer analgesics; acetaminophen (Tylenol), nonsteroidal antiinflammatory agents (ibuprofen), narcotics (codeine, hydrocodone, oxycodone)
   g. Utilize patient-controlled analgesia (PCA pump) as needed or morphine epidural for cesarean deliveries
   h. Monitor for side effects of morphine epidural if administered: late-onset respiratory depression (8 to 12 hours), nausea and vomiting (4 to 7 hours), itching (within 3 and up to 10 hours), urinary retention, and somnolence
3. Promote bowel elimination
   a. Encourage early and frequent ambulation
   b. Encourage increased fluids and fiber
   c. Administer stool softeners as ordered; suppositories are contraindicated if client has a third- or fourth-degree perineal laceration involving rectum
   d. Teach client to avoid straining; normal bowel pattern returns in 2 to 3 weeks
4. Urinary elimination
   a. Encourage voiding every 2 to 3 hours even if no urge is felt
   b. Catheterize as ordered for urinary retention; Foley catheter for 12 to 24 hours after cesarean delivery
5. Promote successful establishment of lactation and successful breast-feeding if desired
   a. Utilize well-fitting bra for continuous support of breasts
   b. Teach breast care, including no use of soap and air drying nipples after feedings
   c. Encourage nursing on demand every 2 to 4 hours, awakening during day and allowing to sleep at night
   d. Advise mother to nurse 10 to 15 minutes on first breast and until infant lets go of second; alternate breast used first and rotate positions
   e. Suggest football hold or side-lying position for mothers with cesarean delivery or tubal ligation to avoid discomfort caused by weight of infant on abdominal incision
   f. Provide help with positioning, latching on, and breaking suction when done nursing for women nursing multiple births
6. Promote successful suppression of lactation and successful bottle-feeding
   a. Utilize snug bra or breast binder continuously for 5 to 7 days to prevent engorgement

b. Avoid heat and stimulation of breasts
c. Apply ice packs for 20 minutes qid (four times a day) if engorgement occurs
! d. Encourage demand feedings every 3 to 4 hours, awakening during day and allowing to sleep at night

7. Explore impact of culture on feeding practices and support family choices as illustrated in Table 12–3 ■
    a. Amount of contact and degree of closeness between mother and newborn is often culturally determined
    b. Culture may influence how long breast-feeding continues
    c. Feeding practices vary across cultures
8. Promote rest and gradual return to activity
    a. Organize nursing care to avoid frequent interruptions
    b. Plan maternal rest periods when infant is expected to sleep
    c. Teach client to resume activity gradually over 4 to 5 weeks; avoid lifting, stair-climbing, and strenuous activity
    d. Simple postpartum exercises should be started, per orders, to strengthen muscles affected by childbearing; Kegel exercises tighten perineum by repeatedly attempting to stop flow of urine and then relaxing; raising chin to chest and doing knee rolls and buttocks lifts strengthen the abdomen
    e. Increased lochia or pain indicates overexertion; modify exercise plan
9. ! Promote adequate nutritional intake
    a. Encourage lactating mothers to add 500 kcal/day to prepregnancy diet; bottle-feeding mothers should return to prepregnancy diet
    b. Encourage fluid intake of 2,000 mL/day
    c. Continue administration of prenatal vitamins and iron, as ordered; iron is best absorbed in presence of vitamin C and may increase constipation
10. Promote psychological well-being
    a. Plan nursing care based on client's phase of psychological adjustment and degree of dependence/independence; provide choices whenever possible
    b. Encourage and support expression of feelings, positive and negative, without guilt
    c. Encourage client to tell story of her labor and birth to integrate expectations and fantasies with reality
    d. ! Provide recognition and praise for self- and infant-care activities
11. Promote family well-being
    a. Provide an environment that supports family unity and promotes attachment to the newborn
    b. ! Encourage rooming-in, presence of family members
    c. Assist parents in preparing siblings with realistic expectations of the newborn; involve siblings in infant care
    d. Teach parents that sibling regression is common
    e. ! Advise couple to resume sexual activity after episiotomy has healed and lochia has stopped, about 3 weeks after delivery; level of sexual interest and activity may vary, additional water-soluble lubrication may be needed, and breast milk may be released with orgasm

Table 12–3

Cultural Influences on Infant Feeding

Cultural Group	Infant Feeding Practice
North American and European	Exposing the breast is indecent; weaning is a sign of infant development
Hmong (southeast Asian)	Breast- and bottle-feeding may be combined; expressing or pumping breast milk is unacceptable
Mexican American, Filipino, Navajo, Vietnamese	Colostrum is not offered to the newborn
African-American	Plentiful feeding is emphasized; solids are introduced early
Muslim	Breast-feeding is encouraged to 2 years of age

f. Counsel couples regarding contraception before discharge, assist couple to select a method compatible with health needs and individual preferences; a diaphragm or cervical cap will need to be refitted following delivery; oral contraceptives containing estrogen may interfere with lactation

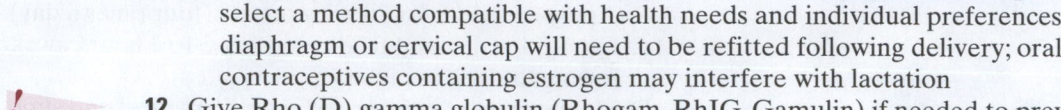

! 12. Give Rho (D) gamma globulin (Rhogam, RhIG, Gamulin) if needed to prevent Rh sensitization and future hemolytic disease of newborn
   a. Confirm woman is a candidate: Rh-negative mother not sensitized (negative indirect Coombs test), Rh-positive newborn not sensitized (negative direct Coombs test), and no known maternal allergy to globulin preparations
   b. Administer 300 mcg IM within 72 hours of delivery

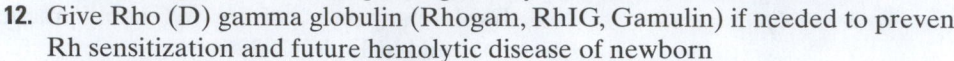

! 13. Give rubella vaccine to provide active immunity for mother and avoid fetal malformations if disease is contracted during a future pregnancy
   a. Confirm woman is a candidate: titer of less than 1:8 (not immune); no known allergy to neomycin
   b. Administer 0.5 mL subcutaneously prior to discharge
   c. If woman is a candidate for both Rhogam and rubella vaccine, delay rubella vaccine at least 6 weeks, and preferably 3 months, to avoid drug interaction and reduced rubella immunity
   d. Teach client to avoid pregnancy for at least 3 months following vaccination; vaccine contains live virus and can adversely affect fetus; side effects include burning and stinging at injection site, warmth and redness, mild symptoms of disease

! 14. Teach client postpartum warning signs to be reported
   a. Bright red bleeding saturating more than one pad per hour or passing large clots
   b. Temperature greater than 100.4°F
   c. Chills
   d. Excessive pain
   e. Reddened or warm areas of breast
   f. Reddened or gaping episiotomy, foul-smelling lochia
   g. Inability to urinate; burning, frequency, or urgency with urination
   h. Calf pain, tenderness, redness, or swelling

15. Outcomes are that assessment findings remain normal: maternal physical and psychological well-being is maintained, mother verbalizes or demonstrates techniques of self- and infant-care and shows positive signs of attachment with infant

Check Your NCLEX–RN® Exam I.Q.

You are ready for testing on this content if you can

- Perform a postpartum assessment.
- Assess the client for postpartum complications.
- Perform postpartum care.
- Provide postpartum discharge instructions.
- Incorporate cultural considerations into postpartum care.

PRACTICE TEST

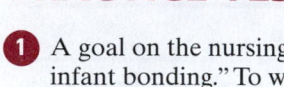

1 A goal on the nursing care plan is "to facilitate parent–infant bonding." To which of the following interventions should the nurse give priority in attaining this goal?

1. Provide assistance and encouragement with rooming-in.
2. Encourage the parents to join a new parent support group.
3. Keep the newborn in the nursery at night to allow the parents to rest.
4. Teach the parents infant-care skills to increase their confidence.

2 The nurse identifies that teaching has been effective when a postpartum client states, "When we bring the baby home, my 2-year-old

1. will be a great help."
2. may want to drink from a bottle again."
3. will decide he is ready to potty train."
4. may want to spend more time with his friends."

3 A postpartum client who delivered 3 hours ago states, "I feel all wet underneath." Which of the following should be the initial action of the nurse?

1. Determine when she last voided.
2. Ask the client to rate her pain on a 1 to 10 scale.
3. Perform perineal care.
4. Have the client roll over to assess her lochia flow.

4 After delivering a 9-pound 10-ounce baby, a client who is a gravida 5 para 5 is admitted to the postpartum unit. Priority nursing care for this client should be to:

1. palpate the fundus because she is at risk for uterine atony.
2. offer fluids, since multiparas generally dehydrate faster during labor.
3. perform passive range of motion on extremities because she is at risk for thromboembolism.
4. assess the client's diet because she is at risk for anemia.

5 Although a client initially wanted to breast-feed, she has now decided to bottle-feed her baby. The nurse concludes that teaching regarding breast care for this client has been effective when the client makes which of the following statements?

1. "I'll pump 2 to 3 times each day until my milk supply decreases."
2. "I'll rub lotion on my breasts if they are sore."
3. "I'll soak my breasts in a warm tub twice daily for the first week."
4. "I'll wear a snug bra continuously until my breasts are soft again."

6 When teaching a new mother how to breast-feed, the nurse should include which of the following interventions?

1. Wash the nipples with soap and water twice daily.
2. Begin nursing with the right breast at each feeding.
3. Slide a finger into the baby's mouth to break suction before removing from the breast.
4. Supplement the baby with formula every 12 hours until the milk supply is established.

7 The nurse is caring for a client who delivered vaginally 2 hour ago. The client's fundus is firm at 1 centimeter below the umbilicus and vital signs are stable. She received meperidine (Demerol) IV 4 hours ago for labor pain. The nurse should question which of the following new orders from the physician?

1. Sitz bath 20 minutes TID
2. Bathroom privileges
3. Regular diet
4. Rhogam for an Rh negative client

8 The nurse should notify the physician immediately with which of the assessment findings?

1. Three pea-sized clots passed 4 hours after delivery
2. Musty odor to lochia 48 hours postpartum
3. Scant amount of rubra lochia after cesarean delivery
4. Firm uterus with steady trickle of blood 2 hours after delivery

9 A client had a cesarean delivery 12 hours ago. Pain management includes a patient-controlled pump for the administration of Morphine (morphine sulfate). Which nursing diagnosis, if formulated for the client, is the highest priority?

1. Constipation
2. Ineffective family processes
3. Ineffective breathing pattern
4. Pain

10 Three hours after a vaginal delivery, the client complains of increased perineal pain. What should the nurse do first?

1. Assess the perineum.
2. Administer analgesia as ordered.
3. Apply ice to the perineum.
4. Perform perineal care.

11 The nurse notes that the postpartum client is Rh negative and her baby is Rh positive. Which maternal laboratory result should the nurse review next in determining if the client is a candidate for Rhogam?

1. Hemoglobin
2. Direct Coombs test
3. Indirect Coombs test
4. Bilirubin

PRACTICE TEST

12 A postpartum client's hemoglobin is 9.2 mg/dL after delivery, and she has been instructed to take an iron supplement at home. The nurse should include which of the following instructions when teaching the client about this medication?

1. Call the physician if your stools become black.
2. Take your iron with a glass of orange juice.
3. Don't drive a car while taking this medication.
4. Diarrhea is a common side effect of iron pills.

13 While assessing a postpartum client, the nurse extends the client's leg and dorsiflexes her foot. The client asks why the nurse is doing this. The nurses best response is that this maneuver:

1. evaluates for early signs of uterine infection.
2. assesses for the presence of a blood clot in the calf.
3. maintains joint mobility.
4. decreases uterine cramping when nursing.

14 The nurse is teaching a new mother how to breast-feed her infant. Which of the following interventions should the nurse plan to include in the teaching plan?

1. Place pillows under the baby's buttocks to elevate the hips while nursing.
2. Reposition the baby with the hips rotated away from the mother's abdomen.
3. Encourage the mother to use the football hold exclusively.
4. Provide positive feedback to the mother for correctly positioning the infant at the breast.

15 A new mother calls the clinic 4 days after delivery. She is breast-feeding and is concerned that her baby is not getting enough milk. What is the most important question for the nurse to ask this mother?

1. "How many wet diapers has your baby had in the last 24 hours?"
2. "Do you have any red or tender areas on the breasts?"
3. "Are your nipples sore or bleeding?"
4. "Do your breasts tingle when you begin nursing?"

16 A nurse is teaching a new mother how to care for herself after delivery. Which of the following statements should the nurse make during this discussion?

1. "Call your physician if you experience night sweats."
2. "Wait 1 week before resuming sexual intercourse."
3. "Change your perineal pad twice daily."
4. "Your diaphragm will need to be refitted."

17 A client's hemoglobin is 10.5 mg/dL. The nurse should encourage the client to include which of the following in her diet?

1. Whole wheat bread
2. Red meat
3. Yellow vegetables
4. Skim milk

18 A postpartum client asks the nurse how to strengthen her perineal muscles. The nurse teaches the client to do which of the following?

1. Trying to start and stop the flow of urine.
2. Bear down as though having a bowel movement.
3. Gently squeeze the uterus while pushing downward on the fundus.
4. Straighten the leg and point the toes toward the head.

19 The nurse notes the following maternal attachment behaviors. Which behavior indicates the need for further observation?

1. Talks to the baby during feedings
2. Holds the baby in the en face position
3. Does not pick up the baby when he or she cries to avoid "spoiling"
4. Refers to the baby as "my little angel"

20 In planning care for a postpartum client who delivered 2 days ago, the nurse should expect the client to do which of the following?

1. Ask questions about infant care.
2. Hesitate in making decisions.
3. Need help with hygiene and ambulation.
4. Request the baby be fed in the nursery at night.

ANSWERS & RATIONALES

1 **Answer: 1** Bonding occurs best when parents have direct and prolonged contact with their newborn in a supportive environment. Although the other answers may be appropriate, they would not be the priority in facilitating bonding.
Cognitive Level: Application **Client Need:** Health Promotion and Maintenance **Integrated Process:** Nursing Process: Implementation **Content Area:** Maternal-Newborn **Strategy:** The word *priority* in the stem of the question indicates that more than one or all options may be partially or totally correct. Identify the key issue as parent–infant bonding. Compare each option in terms of its ability to stimulate attachment, and then use the process of elimination to make a final selection.

2 **Answer: 2** Regression to previous behaviors is normal in young children when a new sibling is brought into the family. An example for a 2-year-old is drinking from a bottle again, which is characteristic of an earlier stage of growth and development. The other options represent items that are expected to happen in future growth and development, but would not be characteristic of the expected regression.
Cognitive Level: Analysis **Client Need:** Health Promotion and Maintenance **Integrated Process:** Nursing Process: Evaluation **Content Area:** Maternal-Newborn **Strategy:** Use knowledge of concepts related to growth and development to answer this question. Focus on the issue of the question, regressive behavior, to make the appropriate selection.

3 **Answer: 4** It is possible that a significant amount of lochia could pool beneath the client after delivery. The highest priority at this time is risk for hemorrhage, and this should be the initial assessment. Options 1 and 3 could then follow. Option 2 is irrelevant to the question as stated.
Cognitive Level: Analysis **Client Need:** Health Promotion and Maintenance **Integrated Process:** Nursing Process: Assessment **Content Area:** Maternal-Newborn **Strategy:** The key word *initial* in the stem of the question tells you that more than one or all actions are potentially correct, but one is better than the others. Focus on the ABCs (airway, breathing, and circulation) and on circulation and risk of hemorrhage to make your selection.

4 **Answer: 1** Uterine atony is the most common cause of early postpartum hemorrhage. This client is at greater risk for hemorrhage because she had an overdistended uterus with a large baby, and she is a grand multipara. Parity does not influence dehydration. The client may be at risk for thromboembolism, but there is no indication passive range of motion should be implemented rather than early ambulation. Nutritional assessment is important, but there is no indication the client is anemic and this action is not the priority for the client.
Cognitive Level: Application **Client Need:** Health Promotion and Maintenance **Integrated Process:** Nursing Process: Implementation **Content Area:** Maternal-Newborn **Strategy:** The key word *priority* in the stem of the question tells you that more than one or all actions are potentially correct, but one is better than the others. Consider that the core issue of the question is uterine atony and associated risk of hemorrhage. Then focus on the ABCs (airway, breathing, and circulation) and on the risk of hemorrhage to make your selection.

5 **Answer: 4** Mothers who are bottle-feeding should be encouraged to suppress milk production by wearing a snug bra or breast binder, applying cold compresses, and avoiding breast stimulation until primary engorgement subsides. Pumping the breasts and applying lotion to them (options 1 and 2) are forms of breast stimulation that should be avoided; option 2 is not helpful anyway. Applying heat via a warm bath (option 3) will also stimulate the breasts and should not be done.
Cognitive Level: Analysis **Client Need:** Health Promotion and Maintenance **Integrated Process:** Nursing Process: Evaluation **Content Area:** Maternal-Newborn **Strategy:** The core issue of the question is measures that will reduce breast stimulation and milk production. With this in mind, eliminate options 1 and 2 as mechanical stimulants, and then option 3 as a thermal stimulant.

6 **Answer: 3** It is important for a breast-feeding mother to break the infant's suction on the nipple before removing the baby from the breast. This will help prevent the nipples from becoming sore and the skin from cracking. The nipples should be cleansed with water after each feeding, but soaps can be harsh or irritating. The client should alternate between the right and left breasts for first use at each feeding. Milk production and supply is enhanced when no supplementation is used.
Cognitive Level: Application **Client Need:** Health Promotion and Maintenance **Integrated Process:** Nursing Process: Implementation **Content Area:** Maternal-Newborn **Strategy:** The wording of the question indicates that there is clearly one correct answer. Use nursing knowledge to systematically eliminate each incorrect option based on appropriate breast-feeding techniques.

7 **Answer: 1** Application of heat to the perineum 2 hours after delivery will cause vasodilation and increase the client's risk of edema and hematoma formation. Ice should be applied for the first 24 hours. Other interventions presented are appropriate.
Cognitive Level: Analysis **Client Need:** Health Promotion and Maintenance **Integrated Process:** Nursing Process: Implementation **Content Area:** Maternal-Newborn **Strategy:** The core issue of the question is knowledge of the effects of heat and cold on a client who is newly postpartum. Note the key word *question,* which tells you that the correct answer is an incorrect item. Eliminate each item that is an acceptable part of care and choose the option that increases the client's risk through application of heat instead of cold.

8 **Answer: 4** A steady trickle of blood in the presence of a firm uterus could indicate the presence of a vaginal or cervical laceration. The physician should be notified immediately so further evaluation can be initiated. The other findings are normal.

Cognitive Level: Analysis **Client Need:** Health Promotion and Maintenance **Integrated Process:** Nursing Process: Analysis **Content Area:** Maternal-Newborn **Strategy:** The key words *notify . . . immediately* indicate that the correct answer is an abnormal finding. From this point, use nursing knowledge and the process of elimination to make a selection. The words *steady trickle of blood* are also a strong clue that this is the correct answer.

9 **Answer: 3** This client is at risk for respiratory depression related to the administration of Morphine. For this reason, ineffective breathing pattern is of greatest concern. Remember airway, breathing, and circulation as priorities for patient safety and promoting maintenance of health. Constipation could also occur but is not as high a priority. Morphine should help to alleviate the pain and could have the next highest priority after begin certain that respirations are not affected. There is no basis in the question as stated for ineffective family processes.
Cognitive Level: Analysis **Client Need:** Health Promotion and Maintenance **Integrated Process:** Nursing Process: Analysis **Content Area:** Maternal-Newborn **Strategy:** The core issue of this question is knowledge of key adverse effects of opioid analgesics. Use this knowledge and the ABCs (airway, breathing, and circulation) to choose this over the other competing nursing diagoses.

10 **Answer: 1** The first step of the nursing process is assessment. Increased perineal pain in a client with a vaginal delivery could be a normal process as delivery anesthetics administered locally wear off. It could also indicate abnormal processes, such as the development of a hematoma. Assessment of this client is needed prior to intervention.
Cognitive Level: Analysis **Client Need:** Health Promotion and Maintenance **Integrated Process:** Nursing Process: Assessment **Content Area:** Maternal-Newborn **Strategy:** Analyze the question to determine that there is not enough information to guide nursing intervention. When more information is needed, an option that provides for further assessment is a good choice.

11 **Answer: 3** An indirect Coombs test assesses for the presence of Rh antibodies in the maternal blood. Direct Coombs test and bilirubin tests are conducted on the newborn. Hemoglobin is not a determinant for the administration of Rhogam.
Cognitive Level: Analysis **Client Need:** Health Promotion and Maintenance **Integrated Process:** Nursing Process: Analysis **Content Area:** Maternal-Newborn **Strategy:** The core issue of the question is the effect of an Rh-positive newborn on an Rh-negative mother. Use nursing knowledge to select the laboratory test that will directly evaluate the mother rather than the newborn.

12 **Answer: 2** Iron absorption is enhanced when taken with vitamin C, and orange juice is a good source of vitamin C. Darker colored stools and constipation (not diarrhea) are common side effects of iron administration. Iron should not cause impaired judgment or dizziness that would impair safety while driving.
Cognitive Level: Application **Client Need:** Health Promotion and Maintenance **Integrated Process:** Nursing Process: Implementation **Content Area:** Maternal Newborn **Strategy:** The core issue of the question is knowledge of administration and effects of iron as a supplement. Use the process of elimination to make the selection. Eliminate option 3 first because it is the least plausible, then eliminate options 1 and 4 based on knowledge of pharmacology.

13 **Answer: 2** Homan's sign is tested for by extending the leg and dorsiflexing the foot. This assessment is indicated in the postpartum because of the increased risk for thromboembolism. Sharp pain in the calf is a positive sign. Uterine infection would be indicated by fever, pain, and foul-smelling lochia. Joint mobility is best maintained by early ambulation. This sign has no effect on afterpains during breast-feeding.
Cognitive Level: Analysis **Client Need:** Health Promotion and Maintenance **Integrated Process:** Nursing Process: Assessment **Content Area:** Maternal-Newborn **Strategy:** The core issue of this question is proper identification of the purpose of testing for Homan's sign. Use this factual information to systematically eliminate each incorrect option. The wording of the question tells you that only one option contains a true statement.

14 **Answer: 4** The baby should be positioned with the head midline and with the abdomen toward the mother's abdomen. Positive reinforcement will facilitate the development of maternal competence and confidence in infant care.
Cognitive Level: Application **Client Need:** Health Promotion and Maintenance **Integrated Process:** Nursing Process: Planning **Content Area:** Maternal-Newborn **Strategy:** The core issue of this question is proper breast-feeding techniques. Use factual information to systematically eliminate each incorrect option. The wording of the question tells you that only one option contains a true statement.

15 **Answer: 1** Once the mother's milk comes in, typically after the third postpartum day, breast-fed babies should have 6 to 8 wet diapers each day. This would indicate the baby is getting enough milk. The other options address the mother, not the intake of the newborn. Red, tender areas or sore, bleeding nipples contribute to infection such as mastitis. Tingling is often used to describe the feeling mothers experience with the let-down reflex.
Cognitive Level: Analysis **Client Need:** Health Promotion and Maintenance **Integrated Process:** Nursing Process: Assessment **Content Area:** Maternal-Newborn **Strategy:** Analyze the question and determine that the core issue is how to evaluate whether an infant is getting sufficient milk intake while breast-feeding. Then systematically eliminate any option that focuses on the mother instead of the infant.

16 **Answer: 4** Diaphragms need to be refitted after each delivery and a change in body weight of greater than 10 to 15 pounds. Night sweats are common and need not be reported. Sexual intercourse can be safely resumed once the episiotomy is healed and the lochia stops in about 3 weeks. Perineal pads should be changed after each elimination.
Cognitive Level: Application **Client Need:** Health Promotion and Maintenance **Integrated Process:** Communication and Documentation **Content Area:** Maternal-Newborn **Strategy:** The core issue of this question is self-care and self-management following delivery. The wording of the question tells you that

the correct answer is a true statement and only one option contains a true statement. Use nursing knowledge to systematically eliminate each incorrect option.

17 **Answer: 2** A hemoglobin level of 10.5 is low and indicates anemia. Because of this, the client should eat foods high in iron, such as red meat. The other foods are important to a well-balanced diet but are not high in iron.
Cognitive Level: Analysis **Client Need:** Health Promotion and Maintenance **Integrated Process:** Nursing Process: Implementation **Content Area:** Maternal-Newborn **Strategy:** The core issues of the question are recognition of laboratory indicators of anemia and dietary treatment. Knowledge of both of these concepts are needed to answer the question. As a strategy, however, recall that hemoglobin contains iron; use this knowledge to make a dietary selection from the options presented.

18 **Answer: 1** Kegel exercises are designed to strengthen the muscles of the perineum. By alternately tensing and releasing the muscles of the perineum, as if to start and stop the flow of urine, muscle tone and strength is enhanced. Bearing down is the opposite type of exercise for this set of muscles. Options 3 and 4 are incorrect statements of technique.
Cognitive Level: Application **Client Need:** Health Promotion and Maintenance **Integrated Process:** Nursing Process: Implementation **Content Area:** Maternal-Newborn **Strategy:** The core issue of the question is specific knowledge of Kegel exercises. As a strategy, however, choose the option that helps to tighten the perineal floor, which is weakened by pregnancy and childbirth.

19 **Answer: 3** Establishing an emotional bond with the newborn includes responding to behavioral cues, attempting to provide comfort, and meeting the infant's needs. Holding the newborn and consoling the baby when he or she cries meets the infant's need for comfort and helps to establish trust. The other observed maternal behaviors are positive signs of attachment.
Cognitive Level: Analysis **Client Need:** Health Promotion and Maintenance **Integrated Process:** Nursing Process: Assessment **Content Area:** Maternal-Newborn **Strategy:** The wording of the question indicates that the correct answer is an option that is a questionable or abnormal behavior by the mother. Focus on the key word *attachment.* Use nursing knowledge to systematically eliminate incorrect options.

20 **Answer: 1** By the second to third postpartum day, mothers are moving into the taking-hold phase of adjustment and are eager to care for the baby and self independently. The other behaviors are characteristic of the taking-in phase, which occurs earlier and reflects greater dependence on the part of the mother.
Cognitive Level: Analysis **Client Need:** Health Promotion and Maintenance **Integrated Process:** Nursing Process: Planning **Content Area:** Maternal-Newborn **Strategy:** The core issue of this question is the progression of maternal behaviors in the days following delivery. The wording of the question leads you to understand that the correct option is a behavior that is customary or normal for that time period. Use nursing knowledge to make a selection.

ANSWERS & RATIONALES

Key Terms for Review

afterpains p. 150
boggy uterus p. 149
bonding p. 152
colostrum p. 151
diastisis recti p. 150
en face p. 152
engorgement p. 151
engrossment p. 152
fundus p. 149
Homan's sign p. 153
involution p. 149
let-down reflex p. 151
lochia alba p. 149
lochia rubra p. 149
lochia serosa p. 149
postpartum blues p. 152
puerperium p. 149

References

Condon, M. (2004). *Women's health: An integrated approach to wellness and illness.* Upper Saddle River, NJ: Pearson Education, pp. 492–495.

Ladewig, P., London, M., & Davidson, M. (2006). *Contemporary maternal-newborn nursing care* (6th ed.). Upper Saddle River, NJ: Pearson Education, pp. 728–770.

Lowdermilk, D., & Perry, S. (2004). *Maternity and women's health care* (8th ed.). St. Louis, MO: Mosby, pp. 607–680.

Olds, S., London, M., Ladewig, P., & Davidson, M. (2004). *Maternal-newborn nursing and women's health care* (7th ed.). Upper Saddle River, NJ: Pearson Education, pp. 424–429, 989–1043.

13 Uncomplicated Newborn Care

Test Yourself

Are you ready for the NCLEX-RN® or course exams? Use the practice tests on the companion CD-ROM to check.

In this chapter

Cross reference

Other chapters relevant to this content area are

Reproduction, Family Planning, and Infertility **Chapter 9**
Uncomplicated Antenatal Assessment and Care **Chapter 10**
Uncomplicated Labor and Delivery Care **Chapter 11**
Uncomplicated Postpartum Assessment and Care **Chapter 12**
Complicated Antenatal Care **Chapter 50**
Complicated Labor and Delivery Care **Chapter 51**
Complicated Postpartum Care **Chapter 52**
Complicated Newborn Care **Chapter 53**

I. IMMEDIATE CARE OF THE HEALTHY NEWBORN

A. Physical assessment

! 1. Vital signs
   - **a.** Heart rate: 120–160 beats/min, irregular, especially when crying, and possible functional murmur; may be as high as 170 when crying or below 120 when resting; count apical pulse for one full minute
   - **b.** Respirations: 30–60 breaths/min with short periods of apnea, irregular; cry is vigorous and loud; may be slightly elevated during crying, but over 60/min (tachypnea) 2 hours after delivery or less than 30/min (bradypnea) may indicate a problem; count for one full minute
   - **c.** Temperature: 36.5–37°C (97.7–98.6°F) axillary; stabilizes about 8 to 10 hours after birth; poor thermostability is related to heat loss via *convection* (loss to cooler air currents), *radiation* (indirect heat transfer from body to cooler surfaces), *evaporation* (from wet skin), and *conduction* (direct heat loss to cooler objects)
   - **d.** Blood pressure is 80/46; varies with changes in newborn's activity and blood volume; more accurate when newborn is resting

2. Pain assessment: intermittent crying not lasting more than 60 seconds, not high-pitched, quiets easily, and no tears noted

3. Collaborative management
   a. Maintain newborn on radiant warmer or in isolette with servocontrol to maintain skin temperature 36.5 to 37°C (97.5 to 98.6°F)
   b. Allow infant to assume a flexed position to decrease surface area of skin exposed to environment, thereby reducing heat loss
   c. Monitor axillary and skin probe temperature per institution's protocol
   d. Monitor respirations for tachypnea and skin color changes for mottling
4. Outcomes: at 2 hours of age newborn maintains axillary temperature of 97.7–98.6°F, heart rate of 120–160/min, respirations 30–60/min with no signs of distress, has pink skin color, and remains in flexed position

B. General assessment (performed in cephalocaudal or head to toe/tail manner)

1. Head
   a. One quarter of body size, molding of fontanels and suture spaces, round, and moves easily from left to right and up to down
   b. Frontal occipital circumference (FOC), measured around forehead and occipital area, is 32 to 37 cm (12.5 to 14.5 in.) or 2 cm greater than chest circumference
   c. Symmetric exception may be caused by birth trauma—that is, **caput succedaneum** (swelling of soft tissue under scalp that subsides within a few days) or **cephalhematoma** (collection of blood between cranial bone and periosteum; absorbs spontaneously in about 6 weeks)
   d. Anterior and posterior fontanels should be open, with posterior closing sooner (8 to 12 weeks) than anterior (by 18 months)
2. Hair: silky smooth, grows toward face, high above eyebrow, variations in texture depend on ethnic background
3. Face: symmetric movement
4. Eyes
   a. Clear blue/slate-gray or brown in color
   b. Pupils equal and reactive to light, blink reflex present, sclera is bluish white
   c. May have subconjunctival hemorrhage (small broken tiny capillaries on sclera, will disappear in few weeks)
   d. Edematous eyelids
   e. Lacrimal structures (tearing) functions at about 2 months
5. Nose: patent nares bilaterally, no discharge, may have flat bridge, sneezing done to clear nostrils
6. Mouth
   a. Symmetrical when cries, hard palate intact, uvula midline, reflexes present
   b. **Rooting reflex** (infant turns to side stimulated and opens mouth to suck); **sucking reflex** (when object placed in mouth or touches lips)
   c. May have **Epstein's pearls** (small white specks, inclusion cysts, on gum ridges), tongue not protruding
7. Ears: well-formed notch of ear on straight line with outer canthus of eye
8. Neck: short, freely movable, has **tonic neck reflex** or fencer position (when head is turned to one side, extremities on same side extend and extremities on opposite side flex)
9. Chest
   a. Clavicles straight and intact, barrel-shaped chest with bilateral expansion with inspirations
   b. Breath sounds clear
   c. Heart rate auscultated at border of left sternum extending left to midclavicle; regular rate and rhythm
   d. Point of maximum impulse (PMI) lateral to midclavicular line at third to fourth intercostal space
10. Breasts: nipples symmetrical, may have whitish discharge or supernumerary (extra small) nipples on chest surface
11. Abdomen
    a. Soft, dome-shaped, round, some laxness of muscles, moves with respirations
    b. Bowel sounds when relaxed

c. Umbilical cord is white, gelatinous with two arteries and one vein, clamped with no foul odor
d. Femoral pulses palpable and equal, no bulges or nodes along bilateral inguinal areas

12. Genitalia
 a. Male: pendulous scrotum with rugae, testes descended into scrotum, penis with urinary meatus at tip of glans on ventral surface of penile shaft
 b. Female: labia minora may have **vernix caseosa** (white, cheesy protective covering that decreases as gestational age increases) and smegma in creases, labia majora normally covers labia minora and clitoris, discharge (blood-tinged mucus or pseudomenstruation) may be present because of maternal hormones

13. Extremities and trunk
 a. Trunk: short, flexed, synchronized movement
 b. **Trunk incurvation** (Galant reflex): newborn lies prone, and when side is stroked, pelvis turns to stimulated side
 c. Hips: stable with no clicks or snaps upon movement
 d. To rule out hip dislocation, **Barlow's maneuver** adducts legs over hips and a snap is felt as femur leaves the acetabulum; with **Ortolani's maneuver,** the hip joint is abducted and lifted, and a click is felt as femur enters acetabulum
 e. Arms: equal in length with symmetrical movement; **grasp reflex** present, newborn grasps when object is placed in hand; nonmovement may indicate **Erb-Duchenne paralysis** or **Erb's palsy;** newborn inability to move upper arms or asymmetric Moro response may be caused by damage to fifth and sixth cervical roots of brachial plexus; five digits on each hand with normal palmar creases, nails present
 f. Legs: equal length, bowed, well-flexed, symmetric skin folds, peripheral pulses present
 g. Feet: creases on soles, may have "positional" clubfoot caused by intrauterine position but should be able to turn toward midline; **plantar grasp**—pressure on soles of feet elicits curling of toes; **Babinski reflex**—stroking sole upward and across ball of foot elicits fanning and extension of toes, disappears at 12 months
 h. Back: spine straight and flexible, may have small **pilonidal dimple,** a small dimple at base of spine but without connection to spinal cord
 i. Anus: patent, well-placed, may have meconium stool

14. Skin
 a. Color consistent with ethnic background, pink-tinged
 b. **Acrocyanosis:** bluish discoloration of hands and feet may be present
 c. May have mottling: lacy pattern of dilated blood vessels under skin caused by fluctuation of general circulation
 d. May have **milia**—obstructed secretions of sebaceous glands
 e. May have **Mongolian spots**—bluish pigmented areas on dorsal area of buttocks; most common in Asian, African, or Hispanic descent
 f. May have **lanugo**—downy, fine hair of fetus between 20 weeks and birth, noticeably found on shoulders, forehead, and cheeks
 g. May have Harlequin's sign—a deep red color over one side of body while other side remains pale; results from vasomotor disturbance

C. Gestational age assessment using Ballard tool

1. An assessment that evaluates six neuromuscular and six physical characteristics performed during first few hours after birth
2. A score of 1 to 5 is assigned to each characteristic and total score correlates to gestational age: that is, a term newborn given a score of 3 for each characteristic scores 18 for neuromuscular assessment and 18 for physical characteristics; total of 36 points correlates to 38+ weeks' gestation
3. The rating is then marked on a graph along with newborn's birth weight, length, and head circumference in order to classify newborn based on maturity and intrauterine growth

4. An overall rating below 10th percentile indicates infant is *small for gestational age (SGA);* between 10th and 90th percentile indicates infant is *appropriate for gestational age (AGA);* above 90th percentile indicates that infant is *large for gestational age (LGA)*
5. Determining ratings for each of subscores
   - **a.** Wear gloves when assessing newborn after birth prior to first bath
   - **b.** First evaluate observable characteristics without disturbing newborn, then proceed to characteristics that require more handling of infant
   - **c.** Maternal conditions such as gestational hypertension, diabetes, and maternal analgesia and anesthesia in intrapartal period may affect some gestational age components
   - **d.** Neuromuscular maturity: during first 24 hours, newborn nervous system is unstable; reflexes and assessments are dependent on his or her brain centers; results may be unreliable and need to be repeated in 24 hours
   - **e.** Physical maturity: not influenced by labor and birth and do not change significantly within first 24 hours after birth
   - **f.** Skin: opaque texture, few distinct larger veins, dry, some peeling
   - **g.** Lanugo: minimal, decreases as gestational age increases
   - **h.** Plantar surface: a reliable indicator of gestational age in first 12 hours of life; beginning at top of foot, creases should cover at least two thirds of entire foot surface
   - **i.** Breast: using forefinger and middle finger, gently measure breast tissue between them in millimeters; at term gestation, measurement should be between 5 and 10 mm; nipple should be raised above skin level
   - **j.** Eye/ear: eyes are open and clear; ears—when top and bottom of pinna are folded over each other, pinna will spring back quickly when released; upper two thirds of the pinna incurves
   - **k.** Male genitalia: testes descended, scrotum pendulous and covered with rugae
   - **l.** Female genitalia: labia majora increases as gestation increases and nearly covers clitoris at 36 to 40 weeks; at 40 weeks, majora cover labia minora and clitoris

II. PHYSIOLOGIC CHANGES

A. Cardiovascular

1. Expansion of lungs occurs with first breath; increases pulmonary blood flow and decreases pulmonary vascular resistance
2. Increased aortic pressure and decreased venous pressure present: clamping of umbilical cord increases vascular resistance, and aortic blood pressure increases
3. Increased systemic pressure and decreased pulmonary artery pressure occur because of loss of placenta; lung expansion increases pulmonary blood flow and dilates pulmonary vessels; pulmonary vascular beds open and perfuse other body systems
4. The **foramen ovale** (opening that previously connected right and left atria), functionally closes in about 1 to 2 hours and anatomically closes in a few weeks to 1 year, increasing left atrial pressure; some shunting may occur early in transition and with crying
5. The **ductus arteriosus** (in fetal circulation, an anatomic shunt between pulmonary artery and arch of aorta) closes, reversing blood flow, so now blood flows from aorta to pulmonary artery because of increased left arterial pressure
6. The **ductus venosus** closes (in fetal circulation, shunts arterial blood into inferior vena cava), thought to be related to severance of cord; results in redistribution of blood and cardiac output; closure forces perfusion of liver

B. Respiratory

1. Initial respirations are triggered by physical, sensory, and chemical factors
   - **a.** Physical: effort required to expand lungs and fill collapsed alveoli; changes in pressure gradient
   - **b.** Sensory: temperature, noise, light, sound

c. Chemical: changes in blood (decreased O_2 level, increased CO_2 level, decreased pH) as a result of transitory asphyxia during delivery

2. Newborn is an obligatory nose-breather, and any obstruction will cause respiratory distress; newborn's ability to maintain respiratory function is influenced by a large heart that reduces lung space and weak intercostal muscles, horizontal ribs and high diaphragm, which restrict space available for lung expansion
3. Collaborative care
   a. Monitor newborn's respirations for any signs of respiratory distress (increased rate, audible grunting, nasal flaring, retractions) per institutional protocol; normal limits are 30 to 60/min
   b. Monitor color of skin, oral area, and extremities for any signs of hypoxia
   c. Keep newborn on warmer for closer observation
   d. Keep infant NPO if respirations are above 60/min
   e. Maintain oral area free from mucus or emesis
4. Outcomes: newborn's respirations are within normal limits, color is pink, temperature stable with no signs of respiratory distress

C. Neurologic

1. Newborn's brain is a quarter the size of an adult's and myelination of nerve fibers is incomplete
2. Newborn exhibits uncoordinated movements, labile temperature regulation, poor control over musculature, easy startling, and tremors of extremities
3. Newborn reflexes are important indicators of normal development; these include **Moro reflex** (elicited by startling newborn; flexion of thighs and knees and fingers that fan, then clench as arms are thrown out then brought together) and previously discussed Babinski grasp, plantar grasp, sucking, and tonic neck reflexes
4. Periods of reactivity: pattern of behavior during first several hours after birth
   a. First period of reactivity: 30 to 60 minutes after birth; awake and alert; may display nursing and attachment behaviors with random diffuse movements
   b. Period of inactivity to sleep phase: activity diminishes, heart and respiratory rates decrease, and newborn enters sleep phase lasting from a few minutes to 2 to 4 hours; will be difficult to awaken
   c. Second period of reactivity: awakes from deep sleep, lasting 4 to 6 hours; close observation is required for changes in heart rate, respiration, and color

D. Musculoskeletal

1. Newborn should have full range of motion—when extremities are fully extended, they should return to a flexed position
2. Any variations should be further investigated

E. Gastrointestinal

1. Digestive enzymes are active at birth and can support extrauterine life by 36 to 38 weeks' gestation
2. Necessary muscular and reflex developments for transporting food are present at birth
3. Digestion of protein and carbohydrates is easily accomplished, but fat digestion and absorption are poor due to absence of pancreatic enzymes
4. Little saliva is manufactured until 3 months
5. An immature lower esophageal sphincter often leads to regurgitation or spitting up
6. **Meconium,** stool that contains bile, epithelial cells, and amniotic cells, is excreted within 24 hours in 90% of healthy newborns
7. Wide variations occur among newborns regarding interest in food

F. Genitourinary

1. Functioning nephrons are complete by 34 to 36 weeks' gestation
2. Glomerular filtration rate (reabsorption and filtration) is low; therefore, newborn may tend to reabsorb sodium and excrete large amounts of water
3. Decreased ability to excrete drugs and excessive fluid loss can lead to acidosis and fluid imbalance; uric acid crystals may cause a reddish stain in diaper

G. Hepatic

1. If mother's iron intake has been adequate, iron stores from mother are sufficient to carry newborn through fifth month of extrauterine life; iron supplements may be given after this age
2. Liver controls amount of circulating unconjugated bilirubin, a pigment derived from hemoglobin that is released with breakdown of red blood cells
3. ! Unconjugated bilirubin can leave vascular system and permeate other extravascular tissues (e.g., skin, sclera, oral mucous membranes), resulting in a yellow coloring termed jaundice or icterus
4. Because unconjugated bilirubin binds to albumin (protein) and is eliminated in stools, early and increased feeding may be encouraged to promote increased excretion of stool
5. Collaborative care
   a. Record intake (oral and parental) and output (weigh diapers) every 2 to 4 hours
   b. Monitor for adequate hydration; skin turgor, specific gravity with each voiding, noting quality and characteristics of urine
   c. ! Phototherapy; maintain "bili-mask" over eyes, check eyes for pressure from mask
   d. Monitor diaper area for skin breakdown and rash
6. Outcomes: newborn feeds every 2 to 3 hours with balanced intake and output; skin is elastic; oral mucous membranes are moist; urine is clear, straw-colored, and passes bili-stools 6 times in 24 hours; bili-mask positioned over eyes; diaper area is clean with no signs of skin breakdown

H. Integumentary

1. The more mature the newborn, the more mature the skin and more likely the newborn will be protected from heat loss and infection
2. Skin color depends on activity level, temperature, hematocrit levels, and race
3. Plethora is a ruddy (red) appearance and usually indicates a hematocrit greater than 65% and should be evaluated
4. ! A polycythemic infant should be monitored closely for signs and symptoms of cyanosis, respiratory distress, hypoglycemia, and jaundice
5. ! When infant cries, skin becomes bright red because of immature capillary system; acrocyanosis is common

I. Immune system

1. Of three major types of immunoglobulins (IgG, IgA, and IgM), only IgG crosses placenta; therefore, infants receive passive immunity from mother in form of IgG near end of gestation, or passive acquired immunity
2. Infants eventually produce antibodies (active acquired immunity) beginning at about 3 months, but IgA is missing from respiratory, urinary, and GI tract until approximately 4 to 6 months of age unless newborn is breast-fed or until infant produces antibodies himself or herself
3. Infants who are breast-fed receive antibodies from breast milk for as long as mother chooses to breast-feed and thereby receive protection from many infectious diseases, including influenza, mumps, and chickenpox
4. Use standard precautions and aseptic technique when caring for newborn; wear gown during care and prevent caregivers with infections from being assigned to newborns

III. NEWBORN NUTRITION

A. Nutrition guidelines

1. A well, healthy newborn needs 90 to 120 kcal/24 hr of nutrition and 140 to 160 mL/kg/24 hr of fluid intake
2. Weight gain is 4 to 8 ounces/week; weight doubles by 6 months of age, and triples by 1 year

B. Teaching guidelines for formula/bottle-feeding

1. Formula meets energy and nutrient requirements of newborn/infants, but does not have immunologic properties and digestibility of human milk

2. Standard formulas are available in three types
   a. Concentrated liquid: diluted with water at a 1:1 ratio
   b. Powder: mixed with water, usually 1 scoop to 2 ounces of water
   c. Ready-to-feed: can be poured directly into a bottle; must be refrigerated once opened and discarded after 24 hours
   ! d. The American Academy of Pediatrics (AAP) recommends that infants be given formula or breast milk until 12 months of age
   ! e. Soy formulas are available for infants who cannot tolerate cow's milk protein and lactose
3. Preparation of formula
   a. Aseptic sterilization: supplies are sterilized separately from formula by boiling in water for 20 minutes
   b. Terminal sterilization: formula is poured into unsterilized bottles and they are sterilized together for 25 minutes
   c. With sanitary conditions, bottles and formula are not routinely sterilized, but all equipment is cleaned thoroughly, including top of can of formula
   ! d. Formula may be warmed to room temperature in a container of warm water; bottles should never be warmed in a microwave; hot spots may develop and burn infant's mouth or throat; heating also changes nutritional composition of formula
4. Feeding techniques
   a. Hold infant close with head elevated
   b. Keep bottle tipped so that nipple remains full of formula
   ! c. Never prop bottle or put the infant to bed with a bottle in his or her mouth; propping can cause aspiration and middle ear infections
   d. Discard any formula left in bottle because of risk of bacterial growth

C. Teaching guidelines for breast-feeding

1. Influences on supply and demand (infant need)
   a. Maternal supply is related to frequency of feedings until about 3 to 4 weeks when the milk supply is well established; thereafter, critical factor for supply to meet demand is breast emptying
   ! b. Infants self-regulate their intake and control breast milk production by the degree to which they "empty" breast; a lactating breast is never "emptied" completely, but infant chooses how much to take
2. The suckling sequence and proper **latch-on**
   a. Nipple and areola are drawn into mouth enough for lips to cover 1 to 1.5 inches of areola
   b. Jaw should move up and down in a rhythmic motion during milk transfer; ears may wiggle; cheeks should be full and rounded, not sucked in
   c. Upper and lower lips should be flanged
   d. Tongue should be troughed—cup-shaped, beginning at bottom of mouth and extending over lower alveolar ridge; in this way, tongue draws nipple in and presses it against hard palate, forming a teat; tongue then humps up from back to front of areola in a rolling movement for milk transfer
3. ! Frequency of feedings: increasing frequency will not increase supply unless transfer of milk is successfully occurring; audible swallowing is best indicator of milk transfer; swallowing is more frequent as more milk is transferred
   a. Schedules should not be imposed on breast-feeding newborns because they have a stomach capacity of about 30 mL, and breast milk is more easily digested than artificial milk (formula)
   ! b. Breast-feeding infants should be fed when hunger cues are displayed: rooting, sucking on fists, clenched fists; these cues may be exhibited from 90 minutes to 3 hours after last feeding; crying is last sign of hunger
   c. Night feedings are necessary during first 6 to 8 weeks; fat content of breast milk is high in evening, which may help infant to consume more calories and therefore feel more satiated; infants who consume more calories during day may have longer stretches of sleep at night

4. Duration of feedings
   a. Research does not document common myth that limiting time at breast will minimize or prevent sore nipples; sore nipples are almost always caused by incorrect positioning at breast or poor latch-on
   b. Mothers should watch infant, not the clock; what the infant is doing at the breast is a better indicator of milk transfer than the time spent there
   c. Newborns/infants with different sucking styles take different amounts of time to complete a feeding, anywhere from 10 to 30 minutes; foremilk is milk that is produced and stored between feedings, looks like skimmed milk—bluish in tint—and usually has less fat content than hindmilk, which is produced during and released at end of a feeding and looks much richer, with a yellowish tint
   d. Signs of satiation are slowing of audible swallowing; pauses between sucking bursts; infant takes himself or herself off breast; hunger cues disappear; infant is relaxed, drowsy, sleeping
5. Good positioning for feeding is paramount for proper latch-on and effective suckling
   a. Body position for mother starts with good posture: straight back, pillows under arms (and under infant), feet touching floor or a footstool beneath her feet
   b. Hand position: in early weeks, breast should be supported with hand; use caution that fingers do not cover lactiferous sinuses or areola that infant needs to take into his or her mouth; later on, infant will be able to support breast after initial latch-on
   c. Cradle hold: infant is in chest-to-chest position, facing breast close enough to touch with nose and chin, with shoulder resting slightly lower on mother's forearm; mother's hand supports infant's buttocks, opposite hand supports breast
   d. Side-lying position: infant is lying alongside mother with a rolled-up blanket behind infant and a pillow behind mother to help maintain position; this position is suggested for nighttime feedings and mothers who had cesarean deliveries
   e. Football or clutch position: infant is positioned in mother's arm with his or her head, back, and shoulders in palm of hand; infant is tucked up under mother's arm, lining up infant's lips with nipple
6. Breast-feeding support is necessary for beginning and continuing breast-feeding
   a. Encourage use of breast-feeding support groups or telephone hotlines at hospitals
   b. Lactation consultants are trained and certified to provide assistance to breast-feeding mothers who experience problems
   c. La Leche League is an international breast-feeding support and information group, with local groups often meeting in neighborhoods
   d. Hospitals and birthing centers that subscribe to World Health Organization's (WHO) Baby Friendly Hospital promote "ten steps to successful breast-feeding" and stop distribution of breast milk substitutes (Box 13–1)

D. Outcomes

1. Infant gains 0.5 to 1 ounce per day, doubles weight by 6 months of age, and triples weight by 1 year of age
2. Infant has 8 to 10 wet or soiled diapers per day and is alert and responsive

IV. NURSING CARE OF THE HEALTHY NEWBORN

A. Eye prophylaxis after birth

1. May be done immediately after birth or delayed up to 1 hour (to allow eye contact that facilitates maternal newborn bonding); purpose is to prevent ophthamalia neonatorum, caused by *Neiserria gonorrhoeae* and *Chlamydia trachomatis*
2. Commonly used solutions are erythromycin (0.5%) and tetracycline (1%) ophthalmic ointment or drops

Box 13-1

Ten Steps to Successful Breastfeeding

Every facility providing maternity services and care for newborn infants should:

1. Have a written breast-feeding policy routinely communicated to all healthcare staff.
2. Train all healthcare staff in the skills necessary to implement this policy.
3. Inform all pregnant women about the benefits and management of breast-feeding.
4. Help mothers initiate breast-feeding within a half-hour of birth.
5. Show mothers how to breast-feed and how to maintain lactation even if they are separated from their infants.
6. Give newborn infants no food or drink other than breast-milk unless it is medically indicated.
7. Practice rooming-in—allow mothers and infants to stay together—24 hours a day.
8. Encourage breast-feeding on demand.
9. Give no artificial teats or pacifiers (also called dummies or soothers) to breast-feeding infants.
10. Foster the establishment of breast-feeding support groups and refer mothers to them on discharge from the hospital or clinic.

3. Silver nitrate (1%) solution is less commonly used because it can lead to chemical conjunctivitis and does not protect against chlamydia

B. Prevention of hemorrhagic disorders after birth

1. Newborn cannot synthesize own vitamin K until intestinal bacteria are present
2. Give prescribed vitamin K (Aqua-MEPHYTON) 0.5 to 1.0 mg IM in middle third of vastus lateralis muscle (lateral aspect) as a one-time dose

C. Screening for phenylketonuria (PKU)

1. Instruct mother that screening is done before hospital discharge and repeated in 7 to 14 days
2. ! Newborn should be taking breast milk or formula for 24 hours prior to screening so that there is sufficient protein intake

D. Bathing

1. Demonstrate and teach to parents care of infant prior to discharge as needed; provide ample time for new parents to practice skills
2. Plan bath for a time prior to feeding and ensure a warm room temperature
3. Gather all equipment, including mild soap
4. Principle of care is to bathe from cleanest area to dirtiest
   a. Clean eyes from inner canthus outward
   b. Use care when cleaning areas with skin folds, such as neck, axillae, genitals, and peri area
5. Instruct mother that bath time provides excellent opportunity for mother–infant interaction

E. Cord care

1. Keep cord clean and dry; cord clamp may be removed after 24 hours
2. Assess cord for discharge, odor, or swelling
3. Perform cord care according to agency protocol
4. Many variations of care exist, including triple dye and antimicrobial agents such as Bacitracin or 70% alcohol; cord care practices are based primarily on tradition rather than research; some recent evidence suggests alcohol may not aid in drying
5. ! Fold diaper down below cord stump to avoid covering it, folding diaper prevents contamination of area and enhances drying
6. ! Instruct mother to use sponge baths and avoid submerging cord in water until it falls off (in 7 to 14 days)
7. Assess for cultural practices related to umbilical cord care

F. Clothing

1. Instruct mother in how to swaddle (wrap) an infant to help maintain body temperature, provide a sense of closeness and security, and perhaps quiet a crying infant

2. Infant should be dressed in layers to avoid overheating or chilling
3. Infant's head should be covered in cool/cold weather to minimize heat loss when out of doors
4. Wash baby clothing separately from other family members' clothes in mild soap or detergent; rinse clothing twice to remove soap and residue and decrease possibility of rash

G. Circumcision care

1. Assess circumcision for signs of hemorrhage every 2 hours following procedure
2. Observe first voiding to evaluate urinary obstruction from penile edema or injury
3. Apply petrolatum and gauze following procedure and for first few diaper changes to reduce further bleeding unless Plastibell is used
4. Plastibell remains in place and should fall off within 8 days; no ointments or creams are used while in place, but may be used after it falls off; consult health care provider if it remains in place after 8 days
5. For either type of circumcision, a yellowish film indicates presence of normal granulation tissue
6. Use good hygiene measures to reduce risk of infection; report any signs of infection, including increased swelling, drainage, or absence of urine flow

H. Care of uncircumcised penis

1. Foreskin and glans are two layers of cells that separate fully between 3 and 5 years of age
2. Teach mother not to force foreskin back over glans for cleansing
3. Explain that when separation does occur, foreskin may be gently retracted daily for gentle cleansing with soap and water

Check your NCLEX–RN® Exam I.Q. *You are ready for testing on this content if you can*

- Assess the healthy newborn.
- Provide care to the healthy newborn.
- Assist the client in learning skills needed to perform newborn care.
- Evaluate client's ability to care for newborn.
- Provide discharge teaching about newborn care.
- Appreciate cultural differences related to aspects of newborn care.

PRACTICE TEST

1 A 6-hour-old infant passes an unformed, black, tarlike stool. The nurse should conclude that this is a

1. Meconium stool expected at this time.
2. Meconium stool expected at the time of birth.
3. Transitional stool expected at this time.
4. Transitional stool expected later.

2 Following delivery, the nurse would first assess which of the following two newborn body systems that must undergo the most rapid changes to support extrauterine life?

1. Gastrointestinal and hepatic
2. Urinary and hematologic
3. Neurologic and temperature control
4. Respiratory and cardiovascular

3 A newborn's father expresses concern that his baby does not have good control of his hands and arms. The nurse would explain which of the following concepts in a response to the client, using wording that the client can understand?

1. Neurologic function progresses in a head-to-toe, proximal to distal fashion.
2. Purposeful, uncoordinated movements of the arms are abnormal.
3. Mild hypotonia is expected in the upper extremities.
4. Asymmetric muscle tone is not unusual.

PRACTICE TEST

4 When caring for a newborn, the nurse must be alert for which of the following as signs of cold stress?

1. Decreased activity level
2. Increased respiratory rate
3. Hyperglycemia
4. Shivering

5 Which of the following physical assessment findings would be recorded as part of a newborn's gestational age assessment?

1. Umbilical cord moist to touch
2. Anterior and posterior fontanels non-bulging
3. Plantar creases present on anterior two thirds of sole
4. Milia present on bridge of nose

6 When planning client instruction on breast-feeding, the nurse includes that the amount of breast milk the mother produces is directly related to which of the following?

1. The effectiveness of the sucking stimulus
2. Her breast size
3. Her newborn's weight
4. Her nipple erectility

7 A healthy newborn was born at term. The first-time parents are very anxious. The mother asks why the baby's hands are clenched and why the baby's knees and elbows are bent. The nurse's response should include an explanation that

1. The baby's muscle tone will relax when he is stimulated appropriately.
2. Placing the baby in a supine position will decrease his flexed posture.
3. Parental anxiety causes the baby's tension and flexed posture.
4. Flexion is the normal position for the newborn.

8 Which of the following actions by a breast-feeding mother indicates the need for further instruction?

1. Holds the breast with four fingers along the bottom and thumb on top
2. Leans forward to bring her breast toward the baby
3. Stimulates the rooting reflex, then inserts the nipple and areola into the newborn's mouth
4. Checks the placement of the newborn's tongue before breast-feeding

9 A mother is anxious about her newborn. She asks the nurse why there are no tears when her baby is crying. The nurse's response incorporates the understanding that

1. The lacrimal ducts must be punctured to initiate tear flow.
2. Silver nitrate and antibiotic instillation at birth reduce tear formation for several days.
3. Exposure to rubella in utero can result in lacrimal duct stenosis.
4. Lacrimal ducts are nonfunctional until 2 months of age.

10 The nurse observes that when the newborn is supine and the head is turned to one side, the extremities straighten to that side while the opposite extremities flex. The nurse documents this as the

1. Tonic neck reflex.
2. Moro reflex.
3. Cremasteric reflex.
4. Babinski reflex.

11 The nurse anticipates that a newborn male, estimated to be 39 weeks' gestation, would exhibit which of the following characteristics?

1. Extended posture when at rest
2. Testes descended into the scrotum
3. Abundant lanugo over his entire body
4. The ability to move his elbow past his sternum

12 If a newborn does not pass meconium during the first 36 hours of life, which of the following is the most appropriate action by the nurse?

1. Observe the anal area for fissures.
2. Notify the physician.
3. Increase the amount of oral feedings.
4. Measure the abdominal girth.

13 During a physical assessment, the nurse palpates the newborn's hard and soft palate with a gloved index finger. The mother of the infant asks the nurse to explain what is being done to the infant. The nurse replies that this assessment is done to detect which of the following possible problems?

1. A shortened frenulum
2. Openings in the palate
3. A thrush infection
4. Adequacy of saliva production

14 A new mother asks the nurse, "Why are my baby's hands and feet blue?" The nurse explains that this a common and temporary condition known as which of the following?

1. Acrocyanosis
2. Erythema neonatorum
3. Harlequin color
4. Vernix caseosa

15 A new mother overhears a nurse mention "first period of reactivity" and asks the nurse for an explanation of the term. Which of the following statements would be best to include in a response?

1. "The period begins when the infant awakens from a deep sleep."
2. "The period is an excellent time to acquaint the parents with the newborn."
3. "The period is an excellent time for the mother to sleep and recover from labor and delivery."
4. "The period ends when the amount of respiratory mucus has decreased."

16 The nurse would suggest which of the following to the mother of a breast-feeding newborn as the best treatment for physiologic jaundice?

1. Switching permanently to formula
2. Giving supplemental water feedings
3. Increasing the frequency of breast-feeding sessions
4. Feeding the newborn nothing by mouth

17 In providing guidelines to follow when using concentrated formula for bottle-feeding, the nurse should instruct new parents to do which of the following?

1. Wash the top of the can and can opener with soap and water before opening the can.
2. Adjust the amount of water added according to the weight gain pattern of the newborn.
3. Make sure the newborn takes all the formula measured into each bottle.
4. Warm the formula in a microwave oven for a few minutes before feeding.

18 A new mother who is breast-feeding her infant asks the nurse, "What kind of stools will my baby have, and how many will there be during the next month?" Which of the following would be the best response by the nurse? "Your baby should have

1. One or two well-formed yellow-orange stools per day."
2. As many as 6 to 10 small, loose, yellow stools per day."
3. A well-formed brown stool at least every other day."
4. Frequent loose, green stools."

19 Which behavior by the postpartum client would indicate that the nurse's breast-feeding teaching has been effective?

1. Breast-feeds the infant every 4 hours
2. Allows the infant to breast-feed for 3 to 5 minutes from each breast on the day of delivery
3. Breast-feeds the infant every 2 to 3 hours, or on demand, whichever comes first
4. Supplements her breast-feeding infant with bottle feedings of glucose water

20 The nurse's admission assessment of a 3-hour-old newborn reveals all of the following findings. Which finding indicates a need for further assessment?

1. The newborn grasps the nurse's finger with his hand.
2. The newborn vigorously licks a nipple when it is placed in his mouth.
3. The newborn moves his pelvis towards stimulation on the same side of his spine.
4. The newborn moves his mouth toward the side of his face when it is gently stroked.

ANSWERS & RATIONALES

1 **Answer: 1** Meconium stools are tarry, black, or dark green and are usually passed within 8 to 24 hours of birth (option 1). It is unusual to pass meconium at birth unless there has been hypoxia or trauma (option 2). Transitional stools are thinner in consistency with a brown to green appearance and consist of part meconium and part fecal material. They are expected a few days later after food has been digested (options 3 and 4).
Cognitive Level: Analysis **Client Need:** Health Promotion and Maintenance **Integrated Process:** Nursing Process: Analysis **Content Area:** Maternal-Newborn **Strategy:** The core issue of the question is recognition and identification of meconium stool. The wording of the question indicates only one option is correct. Use nursing knowledge to make a selection.

2 **Answer: 4** To begin life, the infant must make the adaptations to establish respirations and circulation. These two changes are crucial to life. All other body systems become established over a longer period of time (options 1, 2, 3).
Cognitive Level: Analysis **Client Need:** Health Promotion and Maintenance **Integrated Process:** Nursing Process: Assessment **Content Area:** Maternal-Newborn **Strategy:** A key word in the question is *first,* which indicates more than one or all options may be partially or totally correct. The question requires you to set priorities for assessment. Use nursing knowledge and the ABCs to make your selection.

3 **Answer: 1** The newborn's body grows in a head-to-toe fashion; therefore, uncoordinated movements of the hands and arms are expected rather than abnormal (option 2). Mild hypertonia may be noted (option 3), and muscle tone should be symmetric (option 4). Diminished tone or asymmetric movement may indicate neurological dysfunction.
Cognitive Level: Analysis **Client Need:** Health Promotion and Maintenance **Integrated Process:** Nursing Process: Planning **Content Area:** Maternal-Newborn **Strategy:** The core issue of the question is discriminating between normal and abnormal motor movements of a newborn. Use knowledge of growth and development to make your selection.

4 **Answer: 2** When an infant is stressed by cold, oxygen consumption increases and the increased respiratory rate is a response to the need of oxygen. Additional signs of cold stress are increased activity level and crying (option 1), and hypoglycemia as glucose stores are depleted (option 3). Newborns are unable to shiver as a means to increase heat production (option 4).
Cognitive Level: Analysis **Client Need:** Health Promotion and Maintenance **Integrated Process:** Nursing Process: Assessment **Content Area:** Maternal-Newborn **Strategy:** This question is eliciting knowledge of manifestations of cold stress. The wording of the question leads you to look for a correct item. Make a connection between increased metabolic need (oxygen) from shivering and increased supply of oxygen (increased respiratory rate) to make a correct choice.

5 **Answer: 3** Plantar creases are part of the physical maturity rating on the gestational age assessment. Options 1, 2, and 4 may be observed but are not part of the gestational age assessment.
Cognitive Level: Application **Client Need:** Health Promotion and Maintenance **Integrated Process:** Nursing Process: Assessment **Content Area:** Maternal-Newborn **Strategy:** The key words in the stem of the question are *gestational age.* Eliminate options 1 and 2, which should be typical findings for all infants. From this point, use the process of elimination and nursing knowledge to choose option 3 over 4.

6 **Answer: 1** Prolactin and oxytocin, two hormones necessary for breast-milk production and let-down, are released from the stimulus of the newborn suckling. The mammary gland of each breast is composed of 15 to 20 lobes (where milk is produced and travels to the nipple) arranged around the nipple. Breast size is related to adipose tissue (option 2). Neither newborn weight (option 3) nor nipple erectility is directly related to breast-milk production (option 4).
Cognitive Level: Application **Client Need:** Health Promotion and Maintenance **Integrated Process:** Nursing Process: Evaluation **Content Area:** Maternal-Newborn **Strategy:** The wording of this question is straightforward and direct. Use nursing knowledge and the process of elimination to make a selection.

7 **Answer: 4** The full-term infant exhibits greater than 90-degree flexion of the extremities and clenched fists. Stimulation will not relax the muscle tone (option 1). Placing in a supine position will not decrease the flexed position (option 2), and parental anxiety does not cause the flexed position (option 3).
Cognitive Level: Analysis **Client Need:** Health Promotion and Maintenance **Integrated Process:** Nursing Process: Analysis **Content Area:** Maternal-Newborn **Strategy:** The core issue of the question is a communication that includes a rationale for musculoskeletal status of the newborn. Use knowledge of growth and development and the process of elimination to answer the question.

8 **Answer: 2** The newborn should be brought to the breast, not the breast to the newborn; therefore, the mother would need further demonstration and teaching to correct this ineffective action. Options 1, 3, and 4 are correct actions for successful breast-feeding.
Cognitive Level: Application **Client Need:** Health Promotion and Maintenance **Integrated Process:** Nursing Process: Implementation **Content Area:** Maternal-Newborn **Strategy:** Note the key words *further instruction.* This tells you that the correct answer has incorrect information in it. Evaluate the truth of each option presented, and select as the correct answer the option that contains false information.

9 **Answer: 4** The cry of the newborn is tearless because the lacrimal ducts are not usually functioning until the second month of life. Lacrimal ducts are naturally patent and not punctured (option 1). Neither silver nitrate nor antibiotics will reduce tear formation (option 2). Exposure to rubella is not known to cause stenosis of the lacrimal duct (option 3).
Cognitive Level: Application **Client Need:** Health Promotion and Maintenance **Integrated Process:** Nursing Process: Assessment

Content Area: Maternal-Newborn **Strategy:** The core issue of this question is physical growth and development of the newborn. Eliminate option 1 first as obviously incorrect. Use knowledge of growth and development to choose option 4 over options 2 and 3, which are incorrect statements.

10 **Answer: 1** The tonic neck reflex, or the fencing position, refers to the position the newborn assumes when supine with the head turned to one side. The extremities on that side will extend, and the extremities on the opposite side will flex. The Moro reflex occurs when the newborn is startled and responds by abducting and extending arms with fingers fanning out and the arms forming a "C" (option 2). The cremasteric reflex refers to retraction of testes when chilled or when the inner thigh is stroked (option 3). The Babinski reflex refers to the flaring of the toes when the sole of the foot is stroked upward (option 4).
Cognitive Level: Application **Client Need:** Health Promotion and Maintenance **Integrated Process:** Nursing Process: Assessment **Content Area:** Maternal-Newborn **Strategy:** The core issue of this question is knowledge of the normal reflexes of a newborn. Use knowledge of growth and development and the process of elimination to make a selection.

11 **Answer: 2** A full-term male infant will have both testes in his scrotum, with rugae present. Good muscle tone results in a more flexed posture when at rest (option 1) and inability to move his elbow past midline (option 4). Only a moderate amount of lanugo is present, usually on the shoulders and back (option 3).
Cognitive Level: Application **Client Need:** Health Promotion and Maintenance **Integrated Process:** Nursing Process: Assessment **Content Area:** Maternal-Newborn **Strategy:** The core issue of this question is knowledge of physical findings of an infant according to gestational age. First note that the infant is 39 weeks, which is a term infant. Eliminate option 3 because of the word "abundant." Then use knowledge of physical growth and development of the newborn to eliminate each of the other incorrect options.

12 **Answer: 4** The first meconium stool should be passed within the first 24 hours after birth; if not, the abdominal girth should be measured to evaluate distention and the possibility of obstruction. The presence of anal fissures will not prevent the passage of a meconium stool (option 1). Notifying the physician will not provide more information (option 2). Increasing the amount of feedings will not provide more information, and if there is an obstruction, will complicate that problem (option 3).
Cognitive Level: Analysis **Client Need:** Health Promotion and Maintenance **Integrated Process:** Nursing Process: Implementation **Content Area:** Maternal-Newborn **Strategy:** Note the key words *not* and *first 36 hours.* This tells you that there is a problem with the infant's gastrointestinal status. From there, make a selection that gathers more assessment data. Eliminate option 1 as obviously incorrect. Eliminate option 3 because increased feedings would not be given if a problem is suspected. Choose option 4 over 2 because a physician is called when there is a composite set of data, not one assessment item.

13 **Answer: 2** The hard and soft palates are examined to feel for any openings, or clefts. The frenulum is a ridge of tissue found under the tongue and usually does not affect sucking (option 1). A thrush infection is usually visible as white patches adhering to the mucous membranes and does not need to be felt (option 3). Saliva is normally scant and can be observed (option 4).
Cognitive Level: Application **Client Need:** Health Promotion and Maintenance **Integrated Process:** Nursing Process: Assessment **Content Area:** Maternal-Newborn **Strategy:** The question seeks to detect knowledge of the underlying rationales for newborn assessment. Use knowledge of physical assessment to eliminate incorrect options to make a final selection, noting the correlation between the words "palate" in both the stem of the question and the correct option.

14 **Answer: 1** Acrocyanosis is a bluish discoloration of the hands and feet and may be present in the first few hours after birth but resolves as circulation improves. Erythema appears as a rash on newborns, usually after 24 to 48 hours of life (option 2). Harlequin color results as a vasomotor disturbance, lasting 1 to 20 seconds, which is transient in nature and not of clinical consequence (option 3). Vernix caseosa is a cheese-like substance that protected the newborn's skin while in utero (option 4).
Cognitive Level: Application **Client Need:** Health Promotion and Maintenance **Integrated Process:** Nursing Process: Analysis **Content Area:** Maternal-Newborn **Strategy:** Note the key words *new mother* in the stem of the question to determine that the infant is a newborn. From there, use the process of elimination and knowledge of newborn physical assessment findings to make a selection.

15 **Answer: 2** The first period of reactivity lasts up to 30 to 60 minutes after birth. The newborn is alert, and it is a good time for the newborn to interact with parents. The second period of reactivity begins when the newborn awakens from a deep sleep (option 1). The amount of respiratory mucus may still be noted during this period (option 2). Mothers may sleep and recover during the newborn's sleep state (option 3).
Cognitive Level: Application **Client Need:** Health Promotion and Maintenance **Integrated Process:** Communication and Documentation **Content Area:** Maternal Newborn **Strategy:** Note the key words *first* and *reactivity* in the stem of the question. This leads you to interpret that this will be the first time the infant is quite alert, which could then lead you to select the option that maximizes interaction between mother and infant after birth.

16 **Answer: 3** Physiologic jaundice is best treated by more frequent feedings to increase stooling and the excretion of bilirubin. Switching to formula undermines the mother's feeling of her ability to provide nutrition for the newborn and may result in too early weaning (option 1). Supplemental water may lead the infant to take less breast milk, delay the breast-milk supply, and cause the bilirubin level to increase (option 2). Withholding food from the newborn will provide inadequate nutrition and cause bilirubin levels to increase (option 4).

Cognitive Level: Application **Client Need:** Health Promotion and Maintenance **Integrated Process:** Nursing Process: Implementation **Content Area:** Maternal Newborn **Strategy:** The core issue of the question is what interventions a new mother can use to decrease physiologic jaundice. Eliminate options 1 and 4 first because they are extreme options (the words *permanently* in option 1 and *nothing* in option 4). Choose option 3 over 1 because it reduces jaundice. Choose option 3 over option 2 because it the provides nutrition, not just hydration, for the newborn infant.

17 **Answer: 1** The top of the can and can opener should be washed with soap and water to remove microorganisms. The concentrate is mixed with an equal amount of water (option 2). Forcing an infant to finish a bottle after he seems satisfied may cause regurgitation and lead to infant obesity (option 3). Warming the bottle in the microwave can cause "hot spots" and burn the infant's mouth (option 4).
Cognitive Level: Application **Client Need:** Health Promotion and Maintenance **Integrated Process:** Nursing Process: Implementation **Content Area:** Maternal Newborn **Strategy:** The core issue of the question is proper methods and techniques for bottle-feeding an infant. Note the words *to instruct,* which tells you that the correct option is also a true statement. Use the process of elimination and nursing knowledge to make a final selection.

18 **Answer: 2** Breast-fed infants will have 6 to 10 small, loose, yellow stools per day during the first few months. Options 1 and 3 are incorrect in number and consistency of stool, and option 4 is incorrect with regard to color. Meconium may have a greenish color to it, but it is not a permanent color.
Cognitive Level: Application **Client Need:** Health Promotion and Maintenance **Integrated Process:** Communication and Documentation **Content Area:** Maternal-Newborn **Strategy:** The core issue of the question is normal bowel elimination patterns for a newborn infant who is breast-feeding. A simple way to remember this is to remember that they are yellow, liquid, and frequent. Eliminate options 1 and 3 first because they are formed, and eliminate option 4 next because meconium stools do not last for a month.

19 **Answer: 3** Breast-feeding the infant every 2 to 3 hours or on demand will stimulate hormone production which will, in turn, stimulate breast-milk production and the let-down reflex. Breast-feeding every 4 hours may result in a decreased or delayed milk production (option 1). Allowing the infant to breast-feed only 3 to 5 minutes does not allow enough time for the milk-ejection reflex to occur and may not allow for the let-down of the hindmilk, which contains a higher fat content (option 3). Supplementing with glucose water may cause nipple confusion in the infant and will decrease the infant's demand for breast milk, thereby decreasing supply (option 4).
Cognitive Level: Analysis **Client Need:** Health Promotion and Maintenance **Integrated Process:** Nursing Process: Evaluation **Content Area:** Maternal-Newborn **Strategy:** Note the key word *effective* in the question, which indicates that the correct response is also a true statement. Read each option and eliminate the incorrect ones because they are false statements. Use knowledge of breast-feeding methods and techniques to guide your response.

20 **Answer: 2** The expected response for the sucking reflex is that the newborn will suck the object placed in his mouth, not lick it. Option 1 is the expected response for the grasp reflex. Option 3 is the expected response for the trunk incurvation (Galant) reflex. Option 4 is the expected response for the rooting reflex.
Cognitive Level: Analysis **Client Need:** Health Promotion and Maintenance **Integrated Process:** Nursing Process: Assessment **Content Area:** Maternal-Newborn **Strategy:** The key words *further assessment* indicate that the correct answer is an option that contains abnormal or questionable data. The core issue is knowledge of newborn physical assessment data. Use the process of elimination and nursing knowledge to make your selection.

ANSWERS & RATIONALES

Key Terms to Review

acrocyanosis p. 164
Babinski reflex p. 164
Barlow's maneuver p. 164
caput succedaneum p. 163
cephalhematoma p. 163
ductus arteriosus p. 165
ductus venosus p. 165
Epstein's pearls p. 163
Erb-Duchenne paralysis (Erb's palsy) p. 164
foramen ovale p. 165
grasp reflex p. 164
lanugo p. 164
latch-on p. 168
meconium p. 166
milia p. 164
Mongolian spots p. 164
Moro reflex p. 166
Ortolani's maneuver p. 164
pilonidal dimple p. 164
plantar grasp p. 164
rooting reflex p. 163
sucking reflex p. 163
tonic neck reflex p. 163
trunk incurvation p. 164
vernix caseosa p. 164

References

Condon, M. (2004). *Women's health: An integrated approach to wellness and illness.* Upper Saddle River, NJ: Pearson Education, pp. 493–494.

Ladewig, P., London, M., & Davidson, M. (2006). *Contemporary maternal-newborn nursing care* (6th ed.). Upper Saddle River, NJ: Pearson Education, pp. 728–770.

Lowdermilk, D., & Perry, S. (2004) *Maternity and women's health care* (8th ed.). St. Louis, MO: Mosby, pp. 220–265.

Olds, S., London, M., Ladewig, P., & Davidson, M. (2004). *Maternal-newborn nursing and women's health care* (7th ed.). Upper Saddle River, NJ: Pearson Education, pp. 424–429.

Lifespan Growth and Development

14

In this chapter

Test Yourself

Are you ready for the NCLEX-RN® or course exams? Use the practice tests on the companion CD-ROM to check.

Cross reference

Other chapters relevant to this content area are:

Providing Immunizations Chapter 15
Promoting Healthy Lifestyle Choices Chapter 17
Age-Related Care of Older Adults Chapter 18
End of Life Care Chapter 25
Pediatric Dosage Calculation and Medications Chapter 31
Maternal and Newborn Medications Chapter 35

I. INTRODUCTION TO GROWTH AND DEVELOPMENT

A. Patterns of growth and development

1. Each individual displays definite predictable patterns of growth and development that are universal and basic to all human beings
2. Individual differences: although the sequence is predictable, rates of growth vary, and variation exists in the age at which individuals reach developmental milestones
3. Directional trends: growth and development follow a specific pattern
   a. **Cephalocaudal development:** process by which development proceeds from head downward through body toward feet (head to tail)
   b. **Proximodistal development:** process by which development proceeds from center of body outward to extremities (near to far)
   c. **Differentiation:** development from simple operations to more complex activities and functions

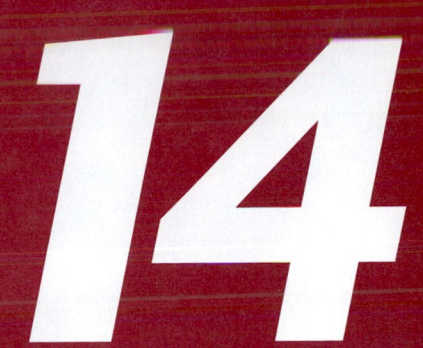

4. Sequential trends: an orderly sequence; each individual normally passes through every stage
    a. Each stage is affected by preceding stage and affects those stages that follow
    b. **Critical periods:** time period in which individual is especially responsive to certain environmental effects; sometimes called sensitive periods
    c. Positive and negative stimuli enhance or defer achievement of a skill or function

B. Factors influencing development

1. Genetics: a family history of diseases may be inherited by unique genes that are linked to specific disorders; chromosomes carry genes that determine physical characteristics, intellectual potential, and personality
2. Nutrition: greatest influence on physical growth and intellectual development; adequate nutrition provides essentials for physiologic needs, which promote health and prevent illness
3. Prenatal and environmental factors: includes nutritional status in utero and exposures in utero such as alcohol, smoking, infections, drugs, environmental exposures, such as radiation and chemicals, also influence growth and development of the developing child
4. Family and community: a stimulating family environment helps individual reach his or her potential; family structure and community support services influence environment in process of growth and development
5. Cultural factors: customs, traditions, and attitudes of cultural groups influence growth and development regarding physical health, social interaction, and assumed roles

II. GROWTH AND DEVELOPMENT THEORIES

A. Stages of Piaget's theory of cognitive development

1. Sensorimotor (birth to 2 years)
    a. Infant learns about world through senses and motor activity
    b. Progresses from reflex activity through simple repetitive behaviors to imitative behaviors
    c. Develops a sense of "cause and effect"
    d. Language enables child to better understand the world
    e. Curiosity, experimentation, and exploration result in the learning process
    f. Object permanence is fully developed
2. Preoperational (2 to 7 years)
    a. Forms symbolic thought
    b. Exhibits **egocentrism**—inability to understand another's position or put himself or herself in the place of another
    c. Unable to understand conservation (e.g., clay shapes, glasses of liquid)
    d. Increasing ability to use language
    e. Play becomes more socialized
    f. Can concentrate on only one characteristic of an object at a time (centration)
3. Concrete operational (7 to 11 years)
    a. Thoughts become increasingly logical and coherent
    b. Able to shift attention from one perceptual attribute to another (decentration)
    c. Concrete thinkers: view things as black or white, right or wrong, no in between or gray areas
    d. Able to classify and sort facts, do problem solving
    e. Acquires conservation skills
4. Formal operations (11 years to death)
    a. Able to logically manipulate abstract and unobservable concepts
    b. Adaptable and flexible
    c. Able to deal with contradictions
    d. Uses scientific approach to problem solve
    e. Able to conceive the distant future

B. Stages of Erikson's theory of psychosocial development

1. Trust vs. mistrust (birth to 1 year)
    a. Task of first year of life is to establish trust in people providing care

! b. Mistrust develops if basic needs are inconsistently or inadequately met

2. Autonomy vs. shame and doubt (1 to 3 years)
   a. Increased ability to control self and environment
   b. Practices and attains new physical skills, developing autonomy
   ! c. Symbolizes independence by controlling body secretions, saying "no" when asked to do something, and directing motor activity
   d. If successful, develops self-confidence and willpower; if criticized or unsuccessful, develops a sense of shame and doubt about his or her abilities
3. Initiative vs. guilt (3 to 6 years)
   a. Child explores physical world with all senses, initiates new activities, and considers new ideas
   ! b. Initiative is demonstrated when child is able to formulate and carry out a plan of action
   c. Develops a conscience
   d. If successful, develops direction and purpose; if criticized, leads to feelings of guilt and a lack of purpose
4. Industry vs. inferiority (6 to 12 years)
   a. Middle years of childhood displays development of new interests and involvement in activities
   b. Learns to follow rules
   c. Acquires reading, writing, math, and social skills
   ! d. If successful, develops confidence and enjoys learning about new things; if compared to others, may develop feeling of inadequacy; inferiority may develop if too much is expected
5. Identity vs. role confusion (12 to 18 years)
   a. Rapid and marked physical changes
   b. Preoccupation with physical appearance
   c. Examines and redefines self, family, peer group, and community
   d. Experiments with different roles
   ! e. Peer group very important
   f. If successful, develops confidence in self-identity and optimism; if unable to establish meaningful definition of self, develops role confusion
6. Intimacy vs. isolation (early adulthood)
   a. Depends on strong sense of self-accomplishment in adolescence
   ! b. Extends beyond sexual relations to broader view of psychosocial intimacy with a partner, parents, children, or friends
   c. Searches for continuity, regularity, or unity in meaningful relationships rather than for relationships with little commitment
7. Generativity vs. stagnation (middle adulthood)
   a. Includes a sense of productivity
   b. Reaches and attains goals
   c. Engages in critical self-review
   ! d. Lack of achievement of developmental goal leads to stagnation and self-absorption
8. Ego integrity vs. despair (older adulthood)
   a. Honest acceptance of life that has passed and current stage of life
   b. At peace with self
   ! c. Includes achieving an identity apart from work, acceptance of bodily changes without preoccupation, and acceptance of death

III. PRENATAL DEVELOPMENT

! **A. Physical growth and development (see Table 14-1 ■)**

! **B. Highlights of development of concern to parents**

1. Fetal heart begins to beat at 4 weeks
2. All body organs formed by 8 weeks
3. Fetal heart sounds heard by Doppler device at 8 to 12 weeks
4. Gender can be seen and has appearance of baby at 16 weeks

Table 14–1 Overview of Fetal Development by Gestational Age

Age	Length & Weight	Neurological and Musculoskeletal Systems	Cardiovascular and Respiratory Systems	Gastrointestinal and Genitourinary Systems	Endocrine, Integumentary and Immune Systems, Eye/Ear
2–3	2 mm crown-to-rump (C-R)	Groove forms along middle back; neural tube forms from closure of groove	Blood circulation begins; tubular heart begins to form in 3rd week; nasal pits form	Liver begins to function; kidneys begin to form	***Endo:*** thyroid tissue forms ***Eyes:*** optic cup and lens pit formed; pigment in eyes ***Ears:*** auditory pit closes
4	4-6 mm C-R; 0.4 grams	Anterior neural tube closes to form brain; posterior closure forms spinal cord; limb buds noted	Tubular heart beats (28 days); primitive RBCs circulate	Oral cavity forms; primitive jaws present; esophagus and trachea begin to divide; stomach forms; esophagus and intestine become tubular; pancreatic/liver ducts forming	***Eyes:*** primitive eye is present ***Ears:*** primitive ear is present
6–7	**6 wks:** 12 mm C-R **7 wks:** 18 mm C-R	**6 wks:** Brain became differentiated with cranial nerves present at week 5; bone rudiments present; primitive skeleton forming; muscle mass begins to develop; skull and jaw ossification begins	**6 wks:** Heart chambers present (atrial division at 5 weeks); blood cell groups identifiable; trachea, bronchi, lung buds present **7 wks:** Fetal heartbeats detectable; diaphragm separates abdominal/thoracic cavities	**6 wks:** Oral/nasal cavities and upper lip formed; liver starts to form RBCs; embryonic sex glands appear **7 wks:** Tongue separates; palate folds; stomach in final form; bladder and urethra separate from rectum; sex glands become testes or ovaries	**6 wks:** ***Ear:*** formation of external, middle, and inner ear continues **7 wks:** ***Eyes:*** optic nerve formed, eyelids present, lens thickens
8	2.5-3 cm C-R; 2 grams	Digits formed; skeletal cells differentiate further; ossification begins in cartilaginous bones; muscle development in head, trunk, and limbs allows some movement	Development of heart and fetal circulation complete	Lip fusion complete; rotation in mid-gut; anal membrane has perforated; external male and female genitalia appear similar until end of 9th week	***Ear:*** external, middle and inner ear assuming final forms
10	5-6 cm crown-to-heel (C-H); 14 grams	Neurons appear at caudal end of spinal cord; brain has basic divisions; nail growth begins in fingers/toes	By 9th week RBCs produced in the liver	Lips separate from jaw; palate folds fuse; developing intestines are enclosed in abdomen; bladder sac formed; testosterone physical characteristics at 8-12 wks (males)	***Endo:*** Islets of Langerhans differentiated ***Eyes:*** lids fused closed
12	8 cm C-R; 11.5 cm C-H; 45 g	Clear outline of miniature bones (12-20 wks); process of ossification established; involuntary muscles in viscera appear	Lungs acquire definitive shape	Mouth palate completed; muscles in gut appear; bile secretion begins; liver produces most of RBCs	***Skin:*** delicate, pink ***Endo:*** thyroid secretes hormones; insulin present in pancreas ***Immune:*** lymphoid tissue in thymus gland
16	13.5 cm C-R; 15 cm C-H; 200 g	Teeth begin to form hard tissue for central incisors	Fetal heart tones audible with feto scope at 16-20 weeks	Hard and soft palate differentiating; gastric and intestinal glands developing; intestines start to collect meconium; kidneys assume shape and organization; able to note sex	***Skin:*** scalp hair appears; body has lanugo; visible blood vessels beneath transparent skin; sweat glands developing ***Eyes, ears, nose:*** formed
20	25 cm C-H; 435 g (6% fat)	Spinal cord myelination begins; teeth begin to form hard tissue for canine and first molar (lateral incisors at 18 wks); lower limbs have final relative proportions	Fetal heart tones audible; primitive respiratory-like movements begin; iron is stored in the blood; bone marrow important	Fetus sucks and swallows amniotic fluid; peristalsis begins	***Skin:*** lanugo covers entire body; brown fat and vernix caseosa begin to form ***Endo:*** iron is stored; bone marrow functioning, fetal antibodies detectable ***Immune:*** fetal IgG levels detectable
24	28 cm C-H; 780 g	Brain appears mature; teeth begin to form 2nd molars	Resp. movements occur (24-40 wks), nostrils reopen, alveoli appear and begin to produce surfactant, gas exchange possible	Testes descend into inguinal ring (males)	***Skin:*** reddish and wrinkled ***Immune:*** IgG at mature levels ***Eyes:*** structurally complete
28–32	**28 wks**: 35 cm C-H; 1200-1250 g **32 wks**: 38-43 cm C-H; 2000 g	**28 wks:** Nervous system begins regulation of some bodily processes **32 wks:** More reflexes present	Viability is reached at 26-27 weeks; if born now, intensive care is needed to support respirations	Testes descend into inguinal canal and upper scrotum (males)	**28 wks:** ***Eyes:*** eyelids open ***Skin:*** adipose tissue begins to accumulate; eyebrows and eyelashes develop
36–40	**36 wks**: 42-48 cm C-H; 2500-2750 g **40 wks**: 48-52 cm C-H; 3200+ g (16% fat)	**36 wks:** Ossification centers present in distal femur	**38 wks:** Lecithin-sphingomyelin (L/S) ratio approaches 2:1 (less risk of respiratory distress from inadequate surfactant if born)	**36 wks:** small scrotum with few rugae (males), final descent of testes into upper scrotum (36-40 wks), labia majora/minora equally prominent (females) **40 wks:** rugous scrotum (males); labia majora well-developed and cover the smaller labia minora and clitoris (females)	**36 wks:** ***Skin:*** pale, lanugo disappearing, hair fuzzy/wooly, few sole creases, increased vernix caseosa (36-40 wks) ***Ears:*** lobes soft with little cartilage **40 wks:** ***Skin:*** smooth, pink; vernix in skinfolds, silky hair, lanugo on shoulders and upper back, nails extend to tips of digits, creases cover sole ***Ears:*** lobes firmer, increased cartilage

5. Heartbeat heard with a fetoscope and mother feels movement (quickening); assumes a favorite position in utero; head hair, eyebrows, and eyelashes present at 20 weeks
6. Weighs approximately 1 lb 10 oz and activity is increasing; fetal respiratory movements begin at 24 weeks
7. Surfactant needed for breathing at birth is formed, and baby is two thirds final size at 28 weeks
8. Fingernails and toenails formed and subcutaneous fat appears; baby appears less red and wrinkled at 32 weeks
9. Baby fills uterus and gets antibodies from mother at 38 to 40 weeks

IV. INFANT GROWTH AND DEVELOPMENT

A. Neonatal period (birth to 1 month)

1. General appearance: newborn's head is one quarter of body length; is top heavy with short lower extremities
2. Weight: 6 to 8 lb; gains 5 to 7 oz (142 to 198 grams) weekly for first 6 months
3. Height: 20 in. (50 cm); grows 1 in. (2.5 cm) monthly for first 6 months
4. Head circumference: 33 to 35 cm (13 to 14 in.); head circumference is greater than chest circumference

B. Growth during infancy (1 to 12 months)

1. Weight: doubles birth weight in 6 months; triples birth weight in 1 year
2. Height: increases 50% by 1 year
3. Head growth is rapid; brain increases in weight 2.5 times by 1 year
   - a. Head circumference exceeds chest circumference
   - b. Posterior fontanel closes at 2 to 3 months
   - c. Anterior fontanel closes by 12 to 18 months
4. Reflexes present at birth
   - a. Moro: startle reflex elicited by loud noise or sudden change in position
   - b. Tonic neck: elicted when infant lies supine and head is turned to one side; infant will assume a "fencing position"
   - c. Gag, cough, blink, pupillary: protective reflexes
   - d. Grasp: infant's hands and feet will grasp when hand or foot is stimulated
   - e. Rooting: elicited when side of mouth is touched, causing infant to turn to that side
   - f. Babinski: fanning of toes when sole of foot is stroked upward
5. Reflexes that appear during infancy
   - a. Parachute: involves extension of arms when suspended in prone position and lowered suddenly
   - b. Landau: when infant is suspended horizontally, head is raised
   - c. Labyrinth righting: provides orientation of head in space
   - d. Body righting: when caregiver turns hips to the side, the body follows
6. Gross motor development: developmental maturation in posture, head balance, sitting, creeping, standing, and walking
   - a. Gains head control by 4 months
   - b. Rolls from back to side by 4 months
   - c. Rolls from abdomen to back by 5 months
   - d. Rolls from back to abdomen by 6 months
   - e. Sits alone without support by 8 months
   - f. Stands holding furniture by 9 months
   - g. Crawls (may go backward initially) by 10 months
   - h. Creeps with abdomen off floor by 11 months
   - i. Cruises (walking upright while holding furniture) by 10 to 12 months
   - j. Can sit down from upright position by 10 to 12 months
   - k. Walks well with one hand held by 12 months
7. Fine motor development: use of hands and fingers to grasp objects
   - a. Hand predominantly closed at 1 month
   - b. Desires to grasp at 3 months
   - c. Two-handed, voluntary grasp at 5 months

d. Holds bottle, grasps feet at 6 months
e. Transfers from hand to hand by 7 months
f. Pincer grasp established by 10 months
g. Neat pincer grasp (e.g., picks up raisin) with thumb and finger by 12 months

8. Sensory development
   a. Hearing and touch well developed at birth
   b. Sight not fully developed until 6 years; differentiates light and dark at birth; prefers human face; smiles at 2 months
   c. Usually searches and turns head to locate sounds by 2 months
   d. Has taste preferences by 6 months
   e. Responds to own name by 7 months
   f. Able to follow moving objects; visual acuity 20/50 or better; amblyopia may develop by 12 months
   g. Can vocalize four words by 1 year
9. Nutrition
   a. Human breast milk is the most complete and easily digested
   b. Commercially prepared iron-fortified formulas used for bottle feeding closely resemble the nutritional content of human milk; recommended for first 12 months
   c. Solids are introduced no sooner than 6 months to avoid exposure to allergens
   d. Iron-fortified rice cereal is introduced first because of its low allergenic potential
   e. Eruption of deciduous "baby" teeth by 5 to 6 months; lateral incisors erupt first; increase in drooling and saliva; slight elevated temperature may be associated with teething
   f. Gradual weaning from breast to bottle to cup during second 6 months of infancy
   g. Juices may be introduced, diluted 1:1 at 6 months; preferably given by a cup
   h. Introduction of fruits, vegetables, and meats (one food each week is recommended to identify any allergy)
   i. Junior foods or chopped table foods introduced by 12 months
   j. No more than 32 oz formula per 24 hours should be given to infants, to avoid iron-deficiency anemia
10. Safety
   a. Infants up to 20 lb (9 kg) should be restrained in a rear-facing car seat in middle of back seat of car
   b. Keep side-rails of crib up
   c. Never leave infant unattended on table, bed, or in bathtub
   d. Check temperature of bath water, formula, foods
   e. Avoid giving bottles at naps or bedtime (may cause dental caries)
   f. Parents should learn injury prevention, including aspiration of foreign objects (buttons, toys, peanuts, hotdogs), suffocation (plastic bags, strangulation), falls, poisonings, and burns (electric cords, wall outlets, radiators, pots and pans on stoves)
11. Play (solitary)
   a. Provide black/white contrasts for premature and newborn infants
   b. Hang mobile 8 to 10 inches from infant's face
   c. Provide sensory stimuli (bath water) and tactile stimuli (feel of various shapes of objects), large toys, balls
   d. Expose to environmental sounds: rattles, musical toys
   e. Use variety of primary-colored objects during infancy
   f. Place unbreakable mirror in crib for infants to focus on their face
   g. Provide toys that let infants practice skills to grasp and manipulate objects
   h. Vocalization provides pleasure in relationships with people (smiling, cooing, laughing)

V. TODDLER GROWTH AND DEVELOPMENT

A. Period from 1 to 3 years of age

B. Weight: growth rate slows considerably; weight is four times the birth weight by 2½ years

C. Height: at 2 years, height is 50% of future adult height

D. **Head circumference:** 19½ to 20 in. (49 to 50 cm) by 2 years; increases only 3 cm in second year; achieves 90% of adult-size brain by 2 years

E. **Anterior fontanel closes by 18 months**

F. **Gross motor development:** still clumsy at this age
1. Walks without help (usually by 15 months)
2. Jumps in place by 18 months
3. Goes up stairs (with 2 feet on each step) by 24 months
4. Runs fairly well (wide stance) by 24 months

G. **Fine motor development**
1. Uses cup well by 15 months
2. Builds a tower of two cubes by 15 months
3. Holds crayon with fingers by 24 to 30 months
4. Good hand-finger coordination by 30 months
5. Copies a circle by 3 years

H. **Sensory development**
1. Binocular vision well developed by 15 months
2. Knows own name by 12 months; refers to self
3. Follows simple directions by 2 years
4. Identifies geometric forms by 18 months
5. Uses short sentences by 18 months to 2 years
6. Remembers and repeats 3 numbers by 3 years
7. Able to speak 300 words by 2 years

I. ***Object permanence* is knowledge that an object or person continues to exist when not seen, heard, or felt**

J. **Ritualistic behavior is exhibited during toddler period; *ritualism* is toddler's need to maintain sameness and reliability; provides sense of comfort**

K. **Nutrition**
1. Growth slows at age 12 to 18 months; thus appetite and need for intake decrease
2. Toddlers are picky, ritualistic eaters
3. Avoid more than 32 oz formula/day to prevent iron-deficiency anemia
4. Avoid large pieces of food such as hot dogs, grapes, cherries, peanuts
5. Able to feed self completely by 3 years
6. Deciduous teeth (approx. 20) are present by 2½ to 3 years
7. Teach good dental practices (brushing, fluoride)

L. **Safety**
1. Continue to use car seat properly; children 20 to 40 lb should be in a forward-facing position in back seat of car, with harness straps at or above shoulders
2. Supervise indoor play and outdoor activities
3. Teach that use of ipecac for accidental ingestions is no longer recommended
4. Teach injury prevention
   a. Childproof the home environment: stairways, cupboards, medicine cabinet, outlets
   b. Suffocation: plastic bags, pacifier, toys, unused refrigerators
   c. Burns: ovens, heaters, sunburns; check water and food temperature
   d. Falls: stairs, windows, balconies, walkers
   e. Aspiration/poisonings: medications, cleaners, chemicals; store harmful substances out of reach

M. **Play (parallel)**
1. Begins as imaginative and make-believe play; may imitate adult in play
2. Provide blocks, wheel toys, push toys, puzzles, crayons to develop motor and coordination abilities
3. Toddlers enjoy repetitive stories and short songs with rhythm

VI. PRESCHOOL GROWTH AND DEVELOPMENT

A. **Period from 3 to 5 years of age**

B. **Weight:** growth is slow and steady; gains 4 to 5 lb/year

C. **Height:** increases 2 to 3 in/year

D. Motor development

1. Skips and hops on one foot by 4 years
2. Rides tricycle by 3 years
3. Throws and catches ball well by 5 years
4. Balances on alternate feet by 5 years
5. Knows 2,100 words by 5 years
6. Increased strength and refinement of fine and gross motor abilities

E. Nutrition

1. Similar to toddlers' eating patterns
2. Demonstrates food preferences: likes and dislikes
3. Influenced by others' eating habits
4. Caloric requirement: 90 kcal/kg/day
5. Reinforce good dental hygiene: regular exams, brushing, fluoride, less concentrated sugar

F. Safety

1. Belt–positioning booster seat can provide safety when child reaches 40 lb weight; should include use of lap and shoulder belts
2. Able to learn safety habits
3. Teach injury prevention
   a. Traffic safety
   b. Strangers
   c. Fire prevention/safety
   d. Water safety; drowning

G. Play (associative)

1. Enjoys imitative and dramatic play
2. Imitates same-sex role in play
3. Provide toys to develop motor and coordination skills (tricycle, clay, paints, swings, sliding board)
4. Parental supervision of television
5. Enjoys sing-along songs with rhythm

VII. SCHOOL AGE GROWTH AND DEVELOPMENT

A. Period from 6 to 12 years of age

B. Weight: steady, slow growth; gains approximately 5 lb/yr

C. Height: increases 1 to 2 in/year; boys and girls differ little at first, but by end of this period girls gain more weight and height compared to boys

D. Motor/sensory development

1. Bone growth faster than muscle and ligament development
2. Susceptible to greenstick fractures
3. Movements become more limber, graceful, and coordinated
4. Have greater stamina and energy
5. Vision 20/20 by 6 to 7 years; myopia may appear by 8 years

E. Nutrition

1. Risk of obesity in this age group
2. Identify those above 95th percentile and below 5th percentile in weight and height on plotted growth charts
3. Requirement of 85 kcal/kg/day
4. Tendency to eat "junk" foods, empty calories
5. Secondary sex characteristics begin at 10 years in girls; 12 years in boys
6. Loses first deciduous teeth at age 6; by age 12 has all permanent teeth, except final molars

F. Safety

1. Incidence of accidents/injuries less likely
2. Teach proper use of sports equipment
3. Discourage risk-taking behaviors (smoking, alcohol, drugs, sex)
4. Introduce sex education
5. Teach injury prevention
   a. Bicycle safety

b. Firearms
c. Smoking education
d. Hobbies/handicrafts

G. **Play (cooperative)**
1. Comprehends rules and rituals of games
2. Enjoys team play, which helps instill values and develop sense of accomplishment
3. Enjoys athletic activities such as swimming, soccer, hiking, bicycling, basketball, baseball, football
4. Provide construction toys: puzzles, erector sets, small interlocking blocks
5. Good eye–hand coordination: interested in video and computer games (needs monitoring and time limits with this activity)
6. Enjoys music, adventure stories, competitive activities

VIII. ADOLESCENT GROWTH AND DEVELOPMENT

A. **Period from 13 to 18 years of age**

B. **Weight:** rapid period of growth causes anxiety; girls gain 15 to 55 lb (7 to 25 kg); boys gain 15 to 65 lb (7 to 29 kg)

C. **Height:** attain final 20% of mature height; girls: height increases approximately 3 in/year, slows at menarche, stops at 16 years; boys: height increases 4 in/year, growth spurt approximately at 13 years, slows in late teens

D. **Puberty**
1. Related to hormonal changes
2. Apocrine glands become active; adolescent may develop body odor
3. Appearance of acne on face, back, trunk
4. Development of secondary sex characteristics: girls experience breast development, menarche (average age 12½ yrs), pubic hair; boys experience enlargement of testes (13 years), increase in scrotum and penis size, nocturnal emission, pubic hair, vocal changes, possibly gynecomastia

E. **Nutrition**
1. **Growth spurt:** brief period of rapid increase in growth
2. "Hollow leg stage": appetite increases
3. Nutrition requirements: 60 to 80 kcal/kg/day which equates to approximately 1,500 to 3,000 kcal/day (11 to 14 yrs) and 2,100 to 3,900 kcal/day (15 to 18 years)
4. At risk for fad diets; food choices influenced by peers
5. Require increased calcium for skeletal growth
6. Continue emphasis on prevention of caries and good dental hygiene
7. Final molars erupt at end of adolescent period; orthodontia common dental need

F. **Safety**
1. Accidents are leading cause of death: motor vehicle accidents (MVA), sports, firearms
2. Provide drug and alcohol education
3. Provide sex education
4. Discourage risk-taking activities
5. Adolescents may display lack of impulse control, reckless behaviors, sense of invulnerability
6. Teach health promotion: breast self-exams (BSE), self-testicular exams
7. Teach injury prevention
   a. Proper use of sports equipment (protective gear)
   b. Diving, drowning
   c. Provide driver's education
   d. Use of seat belts
   e. Violence prevention
   f. Crisis intervention (stress, depression, eating disorders)
   g. Provide information about the risks of body piercing
8. Reinforce rules when necessary

G. **Play/activities**
1. Enjoy sports, school activities, peer group activities (movies, dances, eating out, music, videos, computers)
2. Interest in heterosexual relationships common

IX. ADULT GROWTH AND DEVELOPMENT

A. Consists of young adulthood (18–35 years), middle adulthood (36–64 years), and older adulthood (65 years and older)

B. See Chapter 18 for discussion of needs of older adults

! **C. Weight:** stabilizes in adulthood, although risks of overweight and obesity may apply to individuals based on lifestyle and eating habits

D. Height: stabilized

E. Young adulthood generally considered to be healthiest time of life

F. Physical strength, coordination, endurance, and speed of response are at maximal levels

G. Nutrition

1. Nutrient needs influenced by activity level and body size
2. Nutritional needs increase during pregnancy and lactation
3. Decreased fat intake, and increased intake of fruits, vegetables, and fiber recommended to promote healthy lifestyle (see Chapter 17)

! **H. Safety**

1. Accidents, injuries, and acts of violence are frequent causes of death
2. Injury prevention methods similar to those for adolescence and include proper use of safety and sports equipment, seat belts, and reduction of personal risk behaviors

! **I. Leisure activities**

1. Should include healthy form of exercise at least 3 times per week (see Chapter 17)
2. May take a wide variety of forms depending on personal interests
3. Leisure activities should be encouraged for personal enjoyment and as means to reduce stress

X. CHILD'S REACTION TO ILLNESS AND HOSPITALIZATION

A. Infants and toddlers

1. Parent–child relationship is disturbed
2. Unpredictable routine of hospital promotes feelings of distrust
3. Infants and toddlers experience **separation anxiety,** which is distress behavior observed in young children between ages of 6 and 30 months, when separated from familiar caregivers; separation anxiety peaks around 15 months
4. Stages of separation anxiety include protest (child appears sad, agitated, angry, inconsolable, watches desperately for parents to return), despair (child appears sad, hopeless, withdrawn; acts ambivalent when parents return), and detachment (child appears happy, interested in environment, becomes attached to staff members; may ignore parents)
5. ! Goal of nursing interventions is to preserve child's trust
   - a. Reassure child that parents will return
   - b. Provide "rooming in" to encourage parent–child attachment
   - c. Have parents leave a personal article, picture, or favorite toy with child
   - d. Maintain usual routine and rituals, whenever possible
   - e. Allow choices, whenever possible, to return control to parent and child
6. ! Responses to pain
   - a. Infants will have increases in blood pressure and heart rate and decrease in arterial oxygen saturation
   - b. Harsh, tense, or loud crying
   - c. Facial grimacing, flinching, thrashing of extremities
   - d. Toddlers will verbally indicate discomfort ("no," "ouch," "hurts")
   - e. Generalized restlessness, uncooperative, clings to family member
7. ! **Regression:** use of behavior that is more appropriate to an earlier stage of development, often used to cope with stress or anxiety
   - a. Result is lack of control, frustration, possible return to bottle feeding, temper tantrums, incontinence
   - b. Help parents to understand changes in behavior; avoid punishment

B. Preschoolers

1. Major fears
   - a. Mutilation: has general lack of understanding of body integrity
   - b. Intrusive procedures: will misinterpret words, has active imagination

2. Very egocentric and present-oriented
3. Perceives illness as punishment; associates own actions with disease; may believe hospitalization is punishment for bad behavior
4. Some degree of separation anxiety still exists; may become uncooperative, develop nightmares, become withdrawn or aggressive
5. Nursing interventions
   a. Encourage parents to participate in child care
   b. Allow child to express feelings
   c. Give simple explanations; avoid medical terminology
   d. Provide **therapeutic play** (planned play techniques that provide an opportunity for children to deal with their fears and concerns related to illness or hospitalization)
   e. Allow child to manipulate and play with equipment
   f. Maintain trusting relationship with parents and child; allow time for questions
   g. Praise child, focus on the desired behavior, give rewards (stickers)
6. May show signs of regression to toddlerhood (such as loss of bowel and bladder control)
7. Response to pain
   a. All children have a major fear of needles; preschoolers will deny pain to avoid an injection
   b. Restlessness, irritability, cries, kicks with experiences of pain
   c. Able to describe the location and intensity of pain

C. School-aged children

1. Major fears
   a. Pain and bodily injury
   b. Loss of control
   c. Fears often related to school, peers, and family
2. Ask relevant questions, want to know reasons for procedures, tests
3. Have a more realistic understanding of their disease
4. Become distressed over separation from family and peers
5. Nursing interventions
   a. Communicate openly and honestly; explain rules
   b. Clarify any misconceptions
   c. Encourage child's participation in care to maintain sense of control and independence
   d. Provide visiting for siblings and peers
   e. Use age-appropriate therapeutic play to provide an opportunity for children to deal with their fears and concerns related to illness or hospitalization
   f. Art therapy to assist child to express feelings
   g. Provide explanations; use visual aids such as diagrams, models, and body outlines
   h. Praise child; focus on the desired behavior
6. Response to pain
   a. Able to describe pain; concerned with disability and death
   b. Girls express pain more often than boys do
   c. Demonstrate overt behaviors: biting, kicking, crying, and bargaining
   d. Cues to pain: facial expression, silence, false sense of being "okay"

D. Adolescents

1. Major fears
   a. Loss of independence
   b. Loss of identity
   c. Body image disturbance
   d. Rejection by others
2. Separation from peers is a source of anxiety
3. Physical appearance has major influence on how adolescents perceive themselves
4. Behaviors exhibited by loss of control: anger, withdrawal, uncooperativeness, power struggles
5. Reluctant to ask questions; questions competency of others, will verify answers from more than one individual to determine if others are being truthful

6. Often believe they are invincible, nothing can hurt them, resulting in risk-taking and noncompliant behaviors
7. Nursing interventions
   a. Involve adolescent in plan of care
   b. Support relationships with family and peers
   c. Provide consistent and truthful explanations; can use abstract terms
   d. Accept emotional outburts
   e. Promote communication between adolescents and their parents
8. Response to pain
   a. Associates pain with being different from peers
   b. May exhibit projected confidence, conceited attitude; withdraws, rejects others
   c. Increased muscle tension and body control
   d. Understands cause and effect; able to describe pain

XI. CHILD'S REACTION TO DEATH AND DYING

A. Infants and toddlers

1. Both lack an understanding of concept of death
2. Infants react to loss of caregiver with behaviors such as crying, sleeping more, and eating less
3. Aware someone is missing; may experience separation anxiety
4. Toddlers may develop fearfulness, become more attached to remaining parent, cease walking and talking

B. Preschoolers

1. View death as temporary and reversible
2. Magical thinking and egocentricity lead to belief that dead person will come back
3. View death as a punishment; believe bad thoughts and actions cause death
4. First exposure to death is frequently death of a pet
5. Common behaviors: nightmares, bowel and bladder problems, crying, anger, out-of-control behaviors
6. Preschoolers will ask a lot of questions, may display fascination with death

C. School-aged children

1. View death as irreversible, but not necessarily inevitable
2. By age 10, understand death is universal and will happen to them
3. May believe death serves as a punishment for wrongdoing
4. May deny sadness, attempt to act like an adult
5. Common behaviors: difficulty with concentration in school, psychosomatic complaints, acting-out behaviors

D. Adolescents

1. View death as irreversible, universal, and inevitable
2. Seen as a personal but distant event
3. Develop a better understanding between illness and death
4. Sense of invincibility conflicts with fear of death
5. Common behaviors: feelings of loneliness, sadness, fear, depression; acting out behaviors may include risk-taking, delinquency, suicide attempts, promiscuity

E. Adults (see Chapter 25, "End of Life Care")

Check Your NCLEX-RN® Exam I.Q.

You are ready for testing on this content if you can

- Describe expected physical, cognitive, psychosocial, and moral stages of development.
- Assess the developmental stage of a client.
- Plan appropriate nursing care based on client's developmental stage.
- Modify nursing care based on developmental stage of client.
- Evaluate achievement of developmental milestones.

PRACTICE TEST

1 The charge nurse is developing plans to reduce the stress of a hospitalized, chronically ill 8-year-old child. Coping for this child will be improved if the nurse arranges for the child to

1. be allowed 24-hour open visitation with peers.
2. receive care specifically designed for a school-aged child.
3. avoid making any decisions while hospitalized.
4. have all tutoring postponed until discharge.

2 A mother brings her 15-month-old son to the clinic. During the a nursing assessment, the mother makes the following comments. Which comment merits further investigation?

1. "My son cries sometimes when I leave him at his grandparents' house."
2. "My son always takes his blanket with him."
3. "My son is not crawling yet."
4. "My son likes to eat mashed potatoes."

3 An inexperienced mother is playing with her 8-month-old in the playroom. The nurse has taught the mother about toys that are developmentally appropriate for the child. The nurse will conclude that teaching has been successful when the mother selects which type of toy?

1. A set of blocks
2. A wagon
3. A puzzle with large pieces
4. A rattle

4 The nurse is caring for a 7-year-old child scheduled for surgery in the morning. While conducting preoperative teaching, the nurse would choose which of the following visual aids to enhance the child's learning about the perioperative experience?

1. Videotapes
2. Colorful brochures
3. Dolls and puppets
4. A visit from the surgeon

5 A mother has brought her 4-year-old child for Denver II testing for routine assessment of social and physical abilities. The child refuses to complete the testing. What should the nurse do?

1. Refer the child to a specialist.
2. Explain that the child is developmentally delayed.
3. Complete the test as scheduled.
4. Reschedule the testing for another day.

6 The parents of a 16-month-old ask when they should begin toilet training. Which of the following should be included in a response by the nurse?

1. When the child walks well and shows signs of being dry for longer periods
2. When the child is able to sit alone without support
3. When the child enters preschool
4. When the child has a dry diaper throughout the night

7 The grandparents of a 2½-year-old ask what would be an appropriate toy to buy their grandson. Which of the following should the nurse recommend?

1. A play telephone
2. A 54-piece puzzle
3. A paint-by-number set
4. A musical mobile

8 The nurse working in a pediatric nursing unit of a hospital utilizes the concept that therapeutic play helps a child during illness. At which of the following times would the nurse avoid the use of therapeutic play?

1. During preoperative teaching
2. At bedtime
3. Before a diagnostic test
4. When the child is stressed

9 The nurse discusses the risk of aspiration with the parents of an 18-month-old. The nurse recommends the parents avoid giving their child which of the following food items to minimize this risk?

1. Oranges, crackers, and applesauce
2. Apples, fruit juice, and raisins
3. Cherries, peanuts, and hard candy
4. Cheerios, toast, and bananas

PRACTICE TEST

10 The pediatric nurse is a guest speaker for general health teaching in a prenatal class. In discussing factors that promote positive growth and development, the nurse stresses that the most important factor is

1. nutrition.
2. social income.
3. exposure to secondary smoke.
4. ethnic background.

11 The nurse working in a sexually transmitted infection (STI) clinic of the city health department gives a tour to a group of student nurses. A student notes that the clinic population consists largely of teenagers. The nurse explains to the group that adolescents are at a greater risk for contracting STIs because of which of the following factors?

1. The immune system of an adolescent is immature.
2. Untreated urinary tract infections will develop into an STI.
3. Adolescents are risk-takers and believe they are invincible.
4. Adolescents often lack parental supervision.

12 The nurse working in a sexually transmitted infection (STI) clinic uses communication skills to assess clients and to provide health education. When developing rapport with a new adolescent client, it is important for the nurse to do which of the following?

1. Consistently give honest information.
2. Have the parents present if at all possible.
3. Use jargon when communicating with the adolescent.
4. Allow the adolescent to smoke if desired during the conversation.

13 The Denver Developmental Screening Test has shown a 6-month-old infant is delayed in gross motor development. Activities by the nurse aimed at helping the child attain appropriate developmental levels would include which of the following?

1. Encouraging the child to stand
2. Talking to the child and playing music
3. Pulling the child to a sitting position or propping the child in a sitting position
4. Encouraging the child to hold a rattle or playing patty-cake with him or her

14 A child is delayed in language skills. Which of the following would be the most appropriate nursing diagnosis for this child?

1. Social isolation
2. Impaired parenting
3. Impaired verbal communication
4. Altered sensory-perception (auditory)

15 The nurse needs to obtain a height on a 3-year-old child as a part of routine health screening. To obtain an accurate measurement, the child at this age should do which of the following?

1. Be measured in a recumbent position
2. Remove shoes and stand upright with head erect
3. Stand with his or her feet wide apart
4. Face the wall as he or she is measured

16 The nurse admitting four children to the hospital unit learns that none of the parents will be staying with the children. The nurse would be most concerned with adjustment to hospitalization and separation from parents in the infant or child of which age?

1. 2 months old
2. 13 months old
3. 8 years old
4. 14 years old

17 A toddler is admitted for severe anemia, which is found to be dietary in nature. To increase iron in the diet as a means of promoting healthy growth and development, the nurse recommends to the parents that they:

1. Limit milk to no more than 32 oz/day.
2. Increase fat-soluble vitamins in the diet.
3. Include grains and legumes in the daily intake.
4. Limit foods that are high in protein in the daily caloric requirement.

18 The mother of a neonate states she is concerned about her relationship with the infant. She states the baby goes to anyone and doesn't seem to care if she is present or not. The nurse explains that prior to developing a dependence on the mother, the infant must develop which of the following?

1. Ritualistic behavior
2. Egocentrism
3. Conservation
4. Object permanence

19 The nurse discusses swimming pool safety with the parents of 4-year-old twins. Which statement identifies that more instruction is needed?

1. "We remove all toys from the pool area when not in use."
2. "The twins wear flotation devices when they are in the pool by themselves."
3. "Our children are enrolled in swimming classes."
4. "We always tell the twins not to run by the pool."

20 The nurse prepares to transport a sedated 3-year-old from the pediatric unit to the endoscopy department. Taking into consideration the child's developmental stage and safety, how should he or she be transported to the area?

1. Wagon
2. Wheelchair
3. Crib
4. Gurney (cart)

ANSWERS & RATIONALES

1 **Answer: 2** Age-specific care is care that most closely meets the needs of the hospitalized child at any age. Although visitation of peers is important, open visitation is usually recommended only for family members. Mutual decision making is beneficial for the child and family. Depending on the status of the child's illness and resources available, tutoring may be recommended.
Cognitive Level: Application **Client Need:** Health Promotion and Maintenance **Integrated Process:** Nursing Process: Planning **Content Area:** Foundational Sciences: Growth and Development **Strategy:** Use the process of elimination. Critical words in the stem are *8-year-old,* which leads you to look for an option that matches the needs of a child of this age group.

2 **Answer: 3** Children crawl or pull their body along the floor by their arms by 8 to 10 months. This is a growth and developmental milestone during infancy. For a 15-month-old child, the inability to crawl is an abnormal finding, and it should be referred to the pediatrician for follow-up. It is a normal response for the infant to cry when left with others. Infants often become attached to security items, such as a blanket. Toddlers begin to display food preferences.
Cognitive Level: Analysis **Client Need:** Health Promotion and Maintenance **Integrated Process:** Nursing Process: Analysis **Content Area:** Foundational Sciences: Growth and Development **Strategy:** Use the process of elimination and knowledge of growth and development to answer the question. The correct answer is the option that indicates that the child is not meeting developmental milestones.

3 **Answer: 1** Objects that can be grasped and banged together, such as blocks, are most appropriate for an 8-month-old child. Such play with blocks develops manipulation skills. Pleasure is experienced from the feel and sounds of these activities. A wagon or large-piece puzzle may be used by preschoolers and toddlers; rattles are recommended for infants (1 to 6 months).
Cognitive Level: Application **Client Need:** Health Promotion and Maintenance **Integrated Process:** Nursing Process: Evaluation **Content Area:** Foundational Sciences: Growth and Development **Strategy:** Use the process of elimination and knowledge of growth and development to answer the question. The correct answer is the one that matches the physical development level of the child with the skills ability needed to use the toy.

4 **Answer: 3** The use of dolls may decrease a child's anxiety and fear if the nurse uses such aids to explain what is expected. Brochures and videotapes are useful with explanations to adolescents. A visit from the surgeon is informative primarily with the parents.
Cognitive Level: Application **Client Need:** Health Promotion and Maintenance **Integrated Process:** Nursing Process: Implementation **Content Area:** Foundational Sciences: Growth and Development **Strategy:** Use the process of elimination and knowledge of growth and development to answer the question. The core issue of the question is the most effective method of teaching to use with a school-aged child.

5 **Answer: 4** There are many reasons why a child would be uncooperative, including fatigue, illness, and fear. In order to get accurate results, the test should be rescheduled for another day, and the child should not be forced to undergo testing that day. The child's behavior does not indicate developmental delay, and there is no evidence at this time that the child needs a specialist.
Cognitive Level: Analysis **Client Need:** Health Promotion and Maintenance **Integrated Process:** Nursing Process: Implementation **Content Area:** Foundational Sciences: Growth and Development **Strategy:** Use the process of elimination and knowledge of growth and development to answer the question. Keeping in mind that the 4-year-old may be trying to assert independence and control, each of the incorrect options may be eliminated as less than optimal responses by the nurse.

6 **Answer: 1** Children must have the physical and developmental capabilities to begin toilet training. They should be able to stand and walk well, pull pants up and down, recognize the urge to urinate or defecate, and be able to wait until they reach the potty chair.
Cognitive Level: Analysis **Client Need:** Health Promotion and Maintenance **Integrated Process:** Nursing Process: Planning **Content Area:** Foundational Sciences: Growth and Development **Strategy:** Use the process of elimination and knowledge of growth and development to answer the question. The core issue of the question is physical and mental readiness for toilet training. The wording of the question tells you that one answer is better than each of the others.

7 **Answer: 1** Imitative behaviors teach the toddler new skills. Toddlers enjoy such toys as a play telephone. Manipulation of toys develops both gross and fine motor abilities in this period. Paint-by-number sets and complex puzzles are recommended for school-aged children. Musical mobiles are appropriate for infants.

Cognitive Level: Application **Client Need:** Health Promotion and Maintenance **Integrated Process:** Nursing Process: Implementation **Content Area:** Foundational Sciences: Growth and Development **Strategy:** Use the process of elimination and knowledge of growth and development to answer the question. The core issue of the question is knowledge of appropriate play items for a toddler.

8 **Answer: 2** Play is not recommended at bedtime. A quiet and calm environment will promote sleep. Play is a very effective teaching intervention. It is often used before surgery and diagnostic tests to enhance understanding of these events. Play is therapeutic to help the child express feelings during stressful times.

Cognitive Level: Application **Client Need:** Health Promotion and Maintenance **Integrated Process:** Teaching and Learning **Content Area:** Foundational Sciences: Growth and Development **Strategy:** Use the process of elimination and knowledge of growth and development to answer the question. The core issue of the question is that therapeutic play must be used at appropriate times and in appropriate ways to be effective.

9 **Answer: 3** Toddlers chew well but may have difficulty swallowing large pieces of food. Young children cannot discard pits (such as from cherries). Firm foods such as peanuts and hard candies are easily aspirated, while softer ones, such as cereal or raisins, are better tolerated.

Cognitive Level: Application **Client Need:** Health Promotion and Maintenance **Integrated Process:** Teaching and Learning **Content Area:** Foundational Sciences: Growth and Development **Strategy:** Use the process of elimination and knowledge of growth and development to answer the question. The core issue of the question is knowledge of the physical abilities of the child to swallow foods at various ages.

10 **Answer: 1** Nutrition is the greatest influence on growth and development because diet supplies the nutrients needed to sustain physiological needs and for bodily growth, which then influences overall development. Other factors such an income and exposure to secondary smoke indirectly affect health, while ethnic background has significant influence on culturally based habits but not necessarily on biological growth and development.

Cognitive Level: Analysis **Client Need:** Health Promotion and Maintenance **Integrated Process:** Nursing Process: Implementation **Content Area:** Foundational Sciences: Growth and Development **Strategy:** Use the process of elimination and knowledge of growth and development to answer the question. The core issue of the question is knowledge of priority factors affecting overall growth and development.

11 **Answer: 3** Adolescents often think no harm can come to them, which places them at high risk for injury or disease from dangerous behaviors. The adolescent's immune system is well developed. Urinary tract infections do not cause sexually transmitted infections. Not all adolescents lack parental supervision.

Cognitive Level: Analysis **Client Need:** Health Promotion and Maintenance **Integrated Process:** Nursing Process: Implementation **Content Area:** Foundational Sciences: Growth and Development **Strategy:** Use the process of elimination and knowledge of growth and development to answer the question. The core issue of the question is characteristics of adolescent growth and development.

12 **Answer: 1** Nurses are credible sources of information, support, and encouragement that can help adolescents cope with challenges. To develop trust, honest and accurate information must be given to the client. The adolescent should be given the choice to have his or her parents present because of the nature of the health problem, but treatment for STIs can be given without parental consent. The client should not smoke during discussions with the nurse for general health reasons.

Cognitive Level: Application **Client Need:** Health Promotion and Maintenance **Integrated Process:** Communication and Documentation **Content Area:** Foundational Sciences: Growth and Development **Strategy:** Use the process of elimination and knowledge of growth and development to answer the question. The core issue of the question is knowledge that honest communication builds trust in a therapeutic relationship, regardless of the client's age. A concept that also applies is knowledge related to issues of informed consent for an adolescent.

13 **Answer: 3** The infant at 6 months should have head control and is working on sitting without support. Pulling the child to a sitting position allows the neck muscles to support the head. Propping the child in a sitting position helps to develop self-righting behaviors. It is too early to worry about standing. Talking to the child promotes language development. Handling a rattle is fine-motor behavior.

Cognitive Level: Analysis **Client Need:** Health Promotion & Maintenance **Integrated Process:** Nursing Process: Planning **Content Area:** Foundational Sciences: Growth and Development **Strategy:** Use the process of elimination and knowledge of growth and development to answer the question. The core issue of the question is the abilities of a 6-month-old infant.

14 **Answer: 3** The best nursing diagnosis is the one that directly relates to the lack of language skills. With this data, there is no evidence of hearing disability (option 4). There is insufficient data in the question to determine whether social isolation or parenting behaviors play a role in the language delay (options 1 and 2). Because a nursing diagnosis describes health promotion and health patterns that nurses can manage, the diagnosis of impaired verbal communication also gives the best guidance for appropriate nursing interventions.

Cognitive Level: Analysis **Client Need:** Health Promotion and Maintenance **Integrated Process:** Nursing Process: Analysis **Content Area:** Foundational Sciences: Growth and Development **Strategy:** Use the process of elimination and knowledge of growth and development to answer the question. Note the linkage between *language* in the stem of the question and *verbal communication* in the correct answer.

15 **Answer: 2** It is recommended that the child's height be measured with a stadiometer. The correct procedure is to have the child remove his or her shoes and stand erect facing the

ANSWERS & RATIONALES

examiner, holding the head erect. Shoulders, buttocks, and heels should touch the back of the wall.

Cognitive Level: Application **Client Need:** Health Promotion and Maintenance **Integrated Process:** Nursing Process: Implementation **Content Area:** Foundational Sciences: Growth and Development **Strategy:** Use the process of elimination and knowledge of growth and development to answer the question. The correct answer is the one that incorporates proper technique based on the developmental level of the child.

16 **Answer: 2** The 13-month-old will suffer from toddler hospitalization reaction, which is primarily related to separation from the parents. The 2-month-old has not recognized object permanence and will not suffer from the hospitalization as long as his or her needs are met in a consistent fashion. The 8-year-old and the 14-year-old are accustomed to separation from parents and working with new adults.

Cognitive Level: Analysis **Client Need:** Health Promotion and Maintenance **Integrated Process:** Nursing Process: Assessment **Content Area:** Foundational Science: Growth and Development **Strategy:** Use the process of elimination and knowledge of growth and development to answer the question. The core issue of the question is recognition of the client that is most at risk for separation anxiety from parents during hospitalization.

17 **Answer: 1** Excessive milk consumption should be discouraged, especially more than 1 liter/day (32 oz), since it is a poor source of iron. Fat-soluble vitamins will not increase absorption or utilization of iron. Although grains and legumes are good sources of nutrients, they are not especially high in iron. Foods high in protein should be encouraged, and especially food proteins of animal origin and organ meats, such as liver.

Cognitive Level: Application **Client Need:** Health Promotion and Maintenance **Integrated Process:** Teaching and Learning **Content Area:** Foundational Sciences: Growth and Development **Strategy:** Use the process of elimination and knowledge of nutrition, growth, and development to answer the question. The correct answer is the one that would either decrease the intake of iron-poor foods or increase the intake of iron-rich foods.

18 **Answer: 4** Object permanence is the knowledge that an object or person continues to exist when not seen, heard, or felt. The baby will not attach to a single person, even the mother, until he or she is aware of the mother's existence. Options 1, 2, and 3 do not address this phenomenon.

Cognitive Level: Application **Client Need:** Health Promotion and Maintenance **Integrated Process:** Nursing Process: Teaching and Learning **Content Area:** Foundational Sciences: Growth and Development **Strategy:** Use the process of elimination and knowledge of growth and development to answer the question. The core issue of the question is knowledge that a young infant has not developed an awareness of object permanence.

19 **Answer: 2** Flotation devices are not a substitute for supervision by an adult. Young children should never be left unattended in a swimming pool. Options 1, 3, and 4 all describe appropriate parental behaviors to support safety in the area of swimming pools.

Cognitive Level: Analysis **Client Need:** Health Promotion and Maintenance **Integrated Process:** Nursing Process: Evaluation **Content Area:** Foundational Sciences: Growth and Development **Strategy:** Use the process of elimination and knowledge of growth and development to answer the question. The critical words *need further instruction* guide you to choose the option that represents a safety hazard to 4-year-olds using a pool.

20 **Answer: 3** Toddlers should be transported in a high-top crib with siderails up to ensure safety. The sedated toddler is at risk for falls. A wagon, wheelchair, or gurney will not eliminate the risk of fall injury to a sedated toddler.

Cognitive Level: Application **Client Need:** Safe Effective Care Environment: Safety and Infection Control **Integrated Process:** Nursing Process: Planning **Content Area:** Foundational Sciences: Growth and Development **Strategy:** Use the process of elimination and knowledge of growth and development to answer the question. The correct option is one that prevents the child from slipping out of the transport device while under sedation.

ANSWERS & RATIONALES

Key Terms to Review

cephalocaudal development p. 177
critical periods p. 178
differentiation p. 177
egocentrism p. 178
growth spurt p. 185
object permanence p. 183
proximodistal development p. 177
regression p. 186
ritualism p. 183
separation anxiety p. 186
therapeutic play p. 187

References

Ball, J., & Bindler, R. (2006). *Pediatric nursing: Partnering with children and families.* Upper Saddle River, NJ: Pearson Prentice Hall.

Edelman, C., & Mandle, C. (2006). *Health promotion throughout the lifespan* (6th ed.). St. Louis: Mosby.

Jarvis, C. (2004). *Physical examination and health assessment* (4th ed.). St. Louis: Elsevier Science.

Hockenberry-Eaton, M. & Wilson, D., (2007). *Wong's nursing care of infants and children* (8th ed.). St. Louis: Elsevier Science.

15 Providing Immunizations

Test Yourself

Are you ready for the NCLEX-RN® or course exams? Use the practice tests on the companion CD-ROM to check.

In this chapter

Cross references

Other chapters relevant to this content area are

Preventing and Controlling Infection	Chapter 8
Uncomplicated Newborn Care	Chapter 13
Lifespan Growth and Development	Chapter 14
Promoting Healthy Lifestyle Choices	Chapter 17
Maternal and Newborn Medications	Chapter 35
Communicable or Infectious Diseases	Chapter 68

I. OVERVIEW OF IMMUNIZATIONS

A. Definition: a *vaccine* is a suspension of live, usually *attenuated* or activated microorganisms (e.g., bacteria, viruses, or rickettsiae) or fractions of microorganisms administered to induce immunity and prevent infectious disease or sequelae

B. Purpose of vaccines

1. To produce immunity against various diseases in children and adults
2. By introducing an antigen (a foreign substance that triggers an immune system response) into the body in the form of an immunization, a person produces antibodies against a specific disease
3. A vaccine produces **active immunity** in which antibody production is stimulated without causing clinical disease
4. **Passive immunity** can be conferred with use of immune globulins, in which antibodies to offending organism are already formed; it is also conferred via breast milk to breast-fed infants

C. Information resources: Immunization schedules, vaccines, infectious and communicable diseases

1. Recommended Childhood and Adolescent Immunization Schedule United States, 2006 (see Figure 15–1 ■); available at http://www.cdc.gov/nip/recs/child-schedule-bw-press.pdf
2. American Academy of Pediatrics (AAP) Red Book: Report of the Committee of Infectious Diseases (updated each year)
3. Centers for Disease Control (CDC) Web site: http://www.cdc.gov/nip
4. Advisory Committee on Immunization Priorities (ACIP)
5. CDC Morbidity and Mortality Weekly Report (MMWR)
6. *Journal of Pediatrics*

D. Potential nursing diagnoses associated with immunizations: see Box 15–1

E. General nursing considerations for vaccine administration

1. Provide a written vaccine information statement to client or caregiver and obtain written consent prior to administration
2. Strictly follow manufacturer's directions on storage, reconstitution, and administration of any vaccine
3. Place refrigerated vaccines on a center shelf to maintain stable temperature and avoid interfering with vaccine potency; do not store on a shelf on refrigerator door
4. Check manufacturer expiration date on single-dose or multidose vial or single-use ampule prior to administration; if a multidose vial is used, follow manufacturer's directions; some vials may be used for 30 days after initial use but must be relabeled with newer expiration date; follow agency policy and manufacturer's directions
5. If more than one vaccine is given at one time, draw up in different syringes and administer in different sites
6. Use age-appropriate techniques to reduce discomfort in a child receiving an immunization; see Box 15–2
7. Vaccines that must be given into muscle are administered into vastus lateralis muscle (optimally) in newborns and in deltoid muscle of arm for children and older infants; avoid using dorsogluteal site
8. Document on immunization record the day, month, and year of administration; vaccine manufacturer, lot number, and expiration date; route and site of administration; and name, title, and work address of person who administered dose
9. If an adverse reaction to an immunization occurs, complete a Vaccine Adverse Event Report (VAER) form and report severe reactions to National Vaccine Injury Compensation Program, U.S. Department of Health and Human Services, in accordance with federal law

II. HEPATITIS B VACCINE *(SEE TABLE 15–1 ■)*

A. Hepatitis B virus (HBV)

1. Hepatitis B is an infection of the liver caused by the HBV, which is transmitted in blood or body secretions
2. A series of three (3) injections prevent HBV infection

B. Administration technique

1. Store vaccine in center shelf of refrigerator at 2° to 8°C (35–46°F); do not freeze vaccine
2. Ask if there have been any previous immunization reactions
3. Vaccine will appear cloudy; shake prior to withdrawing; note strength and expiration date of vaccine prior to administering
4. An infant born from a HbsAg+ mother should also receive hepatitis B immune globulin (HBIG) at same time in a different site using new needle and syringe

C. Precautions

1. Give second dose at least 1 month after first dose
2. Give third dose at least 2 months after second dose and at least 4 months after first
3. Do not give third dose to infants younger than 6 months of age, because this could reduce long-term protection

DEPARTMENT OF HEALTH AND HUMAN SERVICES • CENTERS FOR DISEASE CONTROL AND PREVENTION

Recommended Childhood and Adolescent Immunization Schedule UNITED STATES • 2006

Vaccine ▼ Age ▶	Birth	1 month	2 months	4 months	6 months	12 months	15 months	18 months	24 months	4–6 years	11–12 years	13–14 years	15 years	16–18 years
Hepatitis B[1]	HepB	HepB		*HepB[1]*			HepB				HepB Series			
Diphtheria, Tetanus, Pertussis[2]			DTaP	DTaP	DTaP		DTaP			DTaP	Tdap		Tdap	
Haemophilus influenzae type b[3]			Hib	Hib	*Hib[3]*	Hib								
Inactivated Poliovirus			IPV	IPV		IPV				IPV				
Measles, Mumps, Rubella[4]						MMR				MMR		MMR		
Varicella[5]							Varicella				Varicella			
Meningococcal[6]								Vaccines within broken line are for selected populations	MPSV4		MCV4		MCV4 MCV4	
Pneumococcal[7]			PCV	PCV	PCV	PCV			PCV		PPV			
Influenza[8]						Influenza (Yearly)					Influenza (Yearly)			
Hepatitis A[9]										HepA Series				

This schedule indicates the recommended ages for routine administration of currently licensed childhood vaccines, as of December 1, 2005, for children through age 18 years. Any dose not administered at the recommended age should be administered at any subsequent visit when indicated and feasible. ■ Indicates age groups that warrant special effort to administer those vaccines not previously administered. Additional vaccines may be licensed and recommended during the year. Licensed combination vaccines may be used whenever any components of the combination are indicated and other components of the vaccine are not contraindicated and if approved by the Food and Drug Administration for that dose of the series. Providers should consult the respective ACIP statement for detailed recommendations. Clinically significant adverse events that follow immunization should be reported to the Vaccine Adverse Event Reporting System (VAERS). Guidance about how to obtain and complete a VAERS form is available at **www.vaers.hhs.gov** or by telephone, **800-822-7967**.

■ **Range of recommended ages** ■ **Catch-up immunization** ■ **11–12 year old assessment**

1. **Hepatitis B vaccine (HepB).** ***AT BIRTH:*** **All newborns** should receive monovalent HepB soon after birth and before hospital discharge. **Infants born to mothers who are HBsAg-positive** should receive HepB and 0.5 mL of hepatitis B immune globulin (HBIG) within 12 hours of birth. **Infants born to mothers whose HBsAg status is unknown** should receive HepB within 12 hours of birth. The mother should have blood drawn as soon as possible to determine her HBsAg status; if HBsAg-positive, the infant should receive HBIG as soon as possible (no later than age 1 week). **For infants born to HBsAg-negative mothers**, the birth dose can be delayed in rare circumstances but only if a physician's order to withhold the vaccine and a copy of the mother's original HBsAg-negative laboratory report are documented in the infant's medical record. ***FOLLOWING THE BIRTHDOSE:*** The HepB series should be completed with either monovalent HepB or a combination vaccine containing HepB. The second dose should be administered at age 1–2 months. The final dose should be administered at age ≥24 weeks. It is permissible to administer 4 doses of HepB (e.g., when combination vaccines are given after the birth dose); however, if monovalent HepB is used, a dose at age 4 months is not needed. **Infants born to HBsAg-positive mothers** should be tested for HBsAg and antibody to HBsAg after completion of the HepB series, at age 9–18 months (generally at the next well-child visit after completion of the vaccine series).
2. **Diphtheria and tetanus toxoids and acellular pertussis vaccine (DTaP).** The fourth dose of DTaP may be administered as early as age 12 months, provided 6 months have elapsed since the third dose and the child is unlikely to return at age 15–18 months. The final dose in the series should be given at age ≥4 years.
   Tetanus and diphtheria toxoids and acellular pertussis vaccine (Tdap – adolescent preparation) is recommended at age 11–12 years for those who have completed the recommended childhood DTP/DTaP vaccination series and have not received a Td booster dose. Adolescents 13–18 years who missed the 11–12-year Td/Tdap booster dose should also receive a single dose of Tdap if they have completed the recommended childhood DTP/DTaP vaccination series. Subsequent **tetanus and diphtheria toxoids (Td)** are recommended every 10 years.
3. ***Haemophilus influenzae*** **type b conjugate vaccine (Hib).** Three Hib conjugate vaccines are licensed for infant use. If PRP-OMP (PedvaxHIB® or ComVax® [Merck]) is administered at ages 2 and 4 months, a dose at age 6 months is not required. DTaP/Hib combination products should not be used for primary immunization in infants at ages 2, 4 or 6 months but can be used as boosters after any Hib vaccine. The final dose in the series should be administered at age ≥12 months.
4. **Measles, mumps, and rubella vaccine (MMR).** The second dose of MMR is recommended routinely at age 4–6 years but may be administered during any visit, provided at least 4 weeks have elapsed since the first dose and both doses are administered beginning at or after age 12 months. Those who have not previously received the second dose should complete the schedule by age 11–12 years.
5. **Varicella vaccine.** Varicella vaccine is recommended at any visit at or after age 12 months for susceptible children (i.e., those who lack a reliable history of chickenpox). Susceptible persons aged ≥13 years should receive 2 doses administered at least 4 weeks apart.
6. **Meningococcal vaccine (MCV4).** Meningococcal conjugate vaccine (MCV4) should be given to all children at the 11–12 year old visit as well as to unvaccinated adolescents at high school entry (15 years of age). Other adolescents who wish to decrease their risk for meningococcal disease may also be vaccinated. All college freshmen living in dormitories should also be vaccinated, preferably with MCV4, although **meningococcal polysaccharide vaccine (MPSV4)** is an acceptable alternative. Vaccination against invasive meningococcal disease is recommended for children and adolescents aged ≥2 years with terminal complement deficiencies or anatomic or functional asplenia and certain other high risk groups (see *MMWR* 2005;54 [RR-7]:1-21); use MPSV4 for children aged 2–10 years and MCV4 for older children, although MPSV4 is an acceptable alternative.
7. **Pneumococcal vaccine.** The heptavalent **pneumococcal conjugate vaccine (PCV)** is recommended for all children aged 2–23 months and for certain children aged 24–59 months. The final dose in the series should be given at age ≥12 months. **Pneumococcal polysaccharide vaccine (PPV)** is recommended in addition to PCV for certain high-risk groups. See *MMWR* 2000; 49(RR-9):1-35.
8. **Influenza vaccine.** Influenza vaccine is recommended annually for children aged ≥6 months with certain risk factors (including, but not limited to, asthma, cardiac disease, sickle cell disease, human immunodeficiency virus [HIV], diabetes, and conditions that can compromise respiratory function or handling of respiratory secretions or that can increase the risk for aspiration), healthcare workers, and other persons (including household members) in close contact with persons in groups at high risk (see *MMWR* 2005;54[RR-8]:1-55). In addition, healthy children aged 6–23 months and close contacts of healthy children aged 0–5 months are recommended to receive influenza vaccine because children in this age group are at substantially increased risk for influenza-related hospitalizations. For healthy persons aged 5–49 years, the intranasally administered, live, attenuated influenza vaccine (LAIV) is an acceptable alternative to the intramuscular trivalent inactivated influenza vaccine (TIV). See *MMWR* 2005;54(RR-8):1-55. Children receiving TIV should be administered a dosage appropriate for their age (0.25 mL if aged 6–35 months or 0.5 mL if aged ≥3 years). Children aged ≤8 years who are receiving influenza vaccine for the first time should receive 2 doses (separated by at least 4 weeks for TIV and at least 6 weeks for LAIV).
9. **Hepatitis A vaccine (HepA).** HepA is recommended for all children at 1 year of age (i.e., 12–23 months). The 2 doses in the series should be administered at least 6 months apart. States, counties, and communities with existing HepA vaccination programs for children 2–18 years of age are encouraged to maintain these programs. In these areas, new efforts focused on routine vaccination of 1-year-old children should enhance, not replace, ongoing programs directed at a broader population of children. HepA is also recommended for certain high risk groups (see *MMWR* 1999; 48[RR-12]1-37).

The Childhood and Adolescent Immunization Schedule is approved by:
Advisory Committee on Immunization Practices www.cdc.gov/nip/acip • American Academy of Pediatrics www.aap.org • American Academy of Family Physicians www.aafp.org

Figure 15-1 **Recommended Childhood and Adolescent Immunization Schedule 2006**

UNITED STATES • 2006

Recommended Immunization Schedule for Children and Adolescents Who Start Late or Who Are More Than 1 Month Behind

The tables below give catch-up schedules and minimum intervals between doses for children who have delayed immunizations. There is no need to restart a vaccine series regardless of the time that has elapsed between doses. Use the chart appropriate for the child's age.

CATCH-UP SCHEDULE FOR CHILDREN AGED 4 MONTHS THROUGH 6 YEARS

Vaccine	Minimum Age for Dose 1	Minimum Interval Between Doses			
		Dose 1 to Dose 2	Dose 2 to Dose 3	Dose 3 to Dose 4	Dose 4 to Dose 5
Diphtheria, Tetanus, Pertussis	6 wks	4 weeks	4 weeks	6 months	6 months[1]
Inactivated Poliovirus	6 wks	4 weeks	4 weeks	4 weeks[2]	
Hepatitis B[3]	Birth	4 weeks	8 weeks (and 16 weeks after first dose)		
Measles, Mumps, Rubella	12 mo	4 weeks[4]			
Varicella	12 mo				
Haemophilus influenzae type b[5]	6 wks	**4 weeks** if first dose given at age <12 months **8 weeks (as final dose)** if first dose given at age 12-14 months **No further doses needed** if first dose given at age ≥15 months	**4 weeks**[6] if current age <12 months **8 weeks (as final dose)**[6] if current age ≥12 months and second dose given at age <15 months **No further doses needed** if previous dose given at age ≥15 mo	**8 weeks (as final dose)** This dose only necessary for children aged 12 months–5 years who received 3 doses before age 12 months	
Pneumococcal[7]	6 wks	**4 weeks** if first dose given at age <12 months and current age <24 months **8 weeks (as final dose)** if first dose given at age ≥12 months or current age 24–59 months **No further doses needed** for healthy children if first dose given at age ≥24 months	**4 weeks** if current age <12 months **8 weeks (as final dose)** if current age ≥12 months **No further doses needed** for healthy children if previous dose given at age ≥24 months	**8 weeks (as final dose)** This dose only necessary for children aged 12 months–5 years who received 3 doses before age 12 months	

CATCH-UP SCHEDULE FOR CHILDREN AGED 7 YEARS THROUGH 18 YEARS

Vaccine	Minimum Interval Between Doses		
	Dose 1 to Dose 2	Dose 2 to Dose 3	Dose 3 to Booster Dose
Tetanus, Diphtheria[8]	4 weeks	6 months	**6 months** if first dose given at age <12 months and current age <11 years; otherwise **5 years**
Inactivated Poliovirus[9]	4 weeks	4 weeks	IPV[2,9]
Hepatitis B	4 weeks	8 weeks (and 16 weeks after first dose)	
Measles, Mumps, Rubella	4 weeks		
Varicella[10]	4 weeks		

1. **DTaP.** The fifth dose is not necessary if the fourth dose was administered after the fourth birthday.
2. **IPV.** For children who received an all-IPV or all-oral poliovirus (OPV) series, a fourth dose is not necessary if third dose was administered at age ≥4 years. If both OPV and IPV were administered as part of a series, a total of 4 doses should be given, regardless of the child's current age.
3. **HepB.** Administer the 3-dose series to all children and adolescents <19 years of age if they were not previously vaccinated.
4. **MMR.** The second dose of MMR is recommended routinely at age 4–6 years but may be administered earlier if desired.
5. **Hib.** Vaccine is not generally recommended for children aged ≥5 years.
6. **Hib.** If current age <12 months and the first 2 doses were PRP-OMP (PedvaxHIB® or ComVax® [Merck]), the third (and final) dose should be administered at age 12–15 months and at least 8 weeks after the second dose.
7. **PCV.** Vaccine is not generally recommended for children aged ≥5 years.
8. **Td.** Adolescent tetanus, diphtheria, and pertussis vaccine (Tdap) may be substituted for any dose in a primary catch-up series or as a booster if age appropriate for Tdap. A five-year interval from the last Td dose is encouraged when Tdap is used as a booster dose. See ACIP recommendations for further information.
9. **IPV.** Vaccine is not generally recommended for persons aged ≥18 years.
10. **Varicella.** Administer the 2-dose series to all susceptible adolescents aged ≥13 years.

Report adverse reactions to vaccines through the federal Vaccine Adverse Event Reporting System. For information on reporting reactions following immunization, please visit www.vaers.hhs.gov or call the 24-hour national toll-free information line 800-822-7967. Report suspected cases of vaccine-preventable diseases to your state or local health department.

For additional information about vaccines, including precautions and contraindications for immunization and vaccine shortages, please visit the National Immunization Program Website at www.cdc.gov/nip or contact 800-CDC-INFO (800-232-4636) (In English, En Español — 24/7)

Box 15–1

Potential Nursing Diagnoses with Immunizations

- Risk for ineffective breathing pattern related to possible laryngeal edema secondary to hypersensitivity to vaccine
- Altered comfort related to side or adverse effects of immunization
- Risk for impaired skin integrity related to vaccine response
- Deficient knowledge related to immunization schedules and recordkeeping
- Ineffective health maintenance related to cultural beliefs regarding routine immunization

4. People who have had a life-threatening allergic reaction to baker's yeast (yeast used for baking bread) or to a previous dose of hepatitis B vaccine should not receive this vaccine
5. People who are moderately or severely ill when scheduled to receive vaccine should be rescheduled to a later date

D. Contraindications

1. People who have had a life-threatening allergic reaction to baker's yeast (yeast used for baking bread)
2. People who have had a serious reaction to a previous dose of hepatitis B vaccine including anaphylaxis
3. People who have liver abnormalities

E. Side effects/adverse reactions

1. Common side effects include: pain or redness at injection site; headache; photophobia; altered liver enzymes; fever
2. Rare serious side effects including anaphylaxis; see Box 15–3 for treatment

III. DIPHTHERIA, TETANUS AND PERTUSSIS VACCINES *(SEE TABLE 15–2 ■)*

A. Diphtheria, tetanus, and pertussis

1. Diphtheria is an acute, contagious infection that can cause respiratory obstruction
2. Tetanus, referred to as lockjaw, can cause muscle spasms and rigidity over entire body; ultimately obstructs breathing; death occurs in 1 out of 10 cases
3. Pertussis, referred to as whooping cough, can lead to respiratory distress, pneumonia, seizures, brain damage, or death
4. Diphtheria, tetanus toxoids, and pertussis vaccines are examples of **inactivated vaccines,** (or **killed vaccines**), which confer a weaker response than a live virus and require regular booster injections
5. Current available vaccines include DTaP (tetanus, diphtheria, and acellular pertussis) for children receiving initial five-injection immunization series from ages 2 months to 4 to 6 years, Dtap (diphtheria, tetanus, and acellular pertussis) booster one time only for adolescents ages 11 through 18 years and adults 19 to 64 years, and Td (tetanus, diphtheria) booster every 10 years thereafter

Box 15–2

Reducing Discomfort from Immunizations

Reduce pain and anxiety associated with injections by using the following techniques:

- Determine feasibility of parent applying Emla cream to the site for an hour before the injection to numb the area
- Ensure use of correct needle size
- Distract child (e.g., by blowing bubbles or spinning a pinwheel)
- Apply site pressure for 10 seconds before the injection
- Use a coolant spray immediately before the injection
- Obtain the assistance of another provider and give two injections simultaneously in different extremities

Adapted from Ball, J., & Bindler, R. (2003). *Pediatric nursing: Caring for children* (3rd ed.). Upper Saddle River, NJ: Pearson Education, p. 391.

Table 15-1

Hepatitis B Vaccine

Recommended Age	Dosage	Route
For infant whose mother is HbsAg + Within 12 hours of birth 1–2 months 6 months	0.5 mL	Intramuscular
For infant whose mother is HbsAg – Birth–2 months 1–4 months 6–18 months or Birth–2 months 1 month after first dose 6 months after the first dose	0.5 mL 0.5 mL	Intramuscular Intramuscular
For older child, adolescent, or adult First dose anytime Second dose 1–2 months after first dose Third dose 4–6 months after first dose or Adolescents 11–15 years may only need two (2) doses of hepatitis B vaccine separated by 4–6 months (Consult health care provider)	≤ 19 yrs: 0.5 mL ≥ 20 yrs: 1.0 mL 1.0 mL	Intramuscular Intramuscular

Box 15-3

Actions to Take for Anaphylaxis

To be prepared for potential vaccine-induced anaphylaxis:

1. Keep epinephrine 1:1000 and resuscitation equipment immediately available
2. Administer once order obtained for epinephrine 0.01 mL/kg per dose
3. Repeat every 10 to 20 minutes until symptoms subside or other emergency care interventions are initiated
4. Expect to use supportive measures such as oxygen, vasopressors, and other interventions as needed (American Academy of Pediatrics, 2000)

Adapted from Ball, J., & Bindler, R. (2003). *Pediatric nursing: Caring for children* (3rd ed.). Upper Saddle River, NJ: Pearson Education, p. 391.

Table 15-2

Diphtheria, Tetanus, and Pertussis Vaccines

Vaccine	Recommended Age	Dosage	Route
DTaP	2 months 4 months 6 months 15–18 months 4–6 years	0.5 mL	Intramuscular
Tdap	11–12 years 13–18 years for 1 dose if received Td at age 11–12 19–64 years for 1 dose if received Td for previous booster	0.5 mL	Intramuscular
Td	Every 10 years	0.5 mL	Intramuscular

6. The rationale for introduction of Tdap booster is rise in pertussis infections in adolescents, especially those who go to college and live in crowded conditions with exposure to large numbers of people; Tdap is also recommended for adults, especially those who work with infants less than 12 months of age (who are at high risk for pertussis-related complications and death)

B. Administration technique

1. Store vaccine in body of refrigerator at 2° to 8°C (35–46°F) on center shelf; vaccine should not be frozen
2. It may be given at same time as other vaccines
3. Encourage use of same brand for all doses; ask about previous reactions to immunizations
4. Vaccine will appear cloudy; shake prior to withdrawing; if clumps cannot be re-suspended, do not use
5. Preferably administer in vastus lateralis muscle for nonwalking infants

C. Precautions

1. Anyone who is moderately or severely ill at time of vaccine should wait until they recover; people with minor illnesses, such as a cold, may be vaccinated
2. Aspirin-free pain reliever is recommended if fever or pain at the injection site occurred after previous dose of DTaP; administer for a period of 24 hours according to package instructions or advice from health care provider
3. Delay for 1 month after immunosuppressive therapy
4. Delay if immune serum globulin has been administered within 90 days

! **D. Contraindications**

1. Life-threatening reaction to a previous dose of DTaP
2. Seizure, inconsolable crying for 3 hours or more, or fever greater than 105°F after previous vaccine

! **E. Side effects/adverse reactions**

1. Serious: anaphylaxis, seizure, inconsolable crying for 3 hours or more, or fever greater than 105°F; lowered level of consciousness; and permanent brain damage (rare)
2. Common: redness, pain, swelling, and nodule at injection site; fever up to 101°F; drowsiness and fussiness; anorexia within two days of injection

IV. *HAEMOPHILUS INFLUENZAE* TYPE B (HIB) VACCINE *(SEE TABLE 15–3 ■)*

A. *Haemophilis influenzae*

1. *H. influenzae* type B was the most common cause of meningitis in children older than 1 month of age
2. Hib conjugate vaccine protects against a number of serious diseases such as meningitis, epiglottitis, pneumonia, sepsis, and septic arthritis

B. Administration technique

1. Store vaccine on center shelf in body of refrigerator at 2° to 8°C (35–46°F); vaccine should not be frozen
2. It may be given at same time as other vaccines
3. Depending on what brand of Hib is used, child may not need a dose at 6 months of age; consult health care provider
4. Children older than 5 years of age generally do not need Hib vaccine; some children with special health needs such as sickle cell anemia, HIV/AIDS, cancer treatment, or bone marrow transplant may need vaccine
5. Encourage use of same brand for all doses, since some brands require three doses while other brands require four doses

Table 15–3 ***Haemophilus Influenzae* Type B (Hib) Vaccine**

Recommended Age	Dosage	Route
2 months 4 months 6 months 12–15 months	0.5 mL	Intramuscular

6. Ask about previous reactions to immunizations
7. Preferably administer in vastus lateralis muscle

C. Precautions
1. Children with minor illnesses may receive immunization
2. Moderately or severely ill children should not be immunized until they recover from illness

D. Contraindications
1. Prior anaphylactic reaction
2. Severe reaction to previous dose (rare)

E. Side effects/adverse reactions
1. Serious: anaphylaxis (rare)
2. Common: pain, redness or swelling at site

V. INACTIVATED POLIO VIRUS VACCINE (IPV) *(SEE TABLE 15–4 ■)*

A. Poliomyelitis
1. A disease caused by a virus that affects the central nervous system (CNS); enters body through mouth; may not cause serious illness, but can cause paralysis, respiratory complications, and death
2. Polio vaccine begun in 1955 in the United States; the live oral polio vaccine no longer recommended for use in the United States
3. IPV is a trivalent vaccine that contains all three forms of polio
4. IPV is an inactivated vaccine, or killed vaccine, which confers a weaker response than a live vaccine, necessitating frequent boosters

B. Administration
1. Store in body of refrigerator at 2° to 8°C (35–46°F); do not freeze
2. Clear, colorless suspension; do not use if it contains particulate matter, becomes cloudy, or changes colors

C. Precautions
1. Prior to immunization, ask if child has any allergies to neomycin
2. Also assess for allergy to streptomycin or polymyxin B

D. Contraindications
1. Anaphylactic reaction
2. Anyone who is moderately or severely ill at time of vaccination should wait until they recover; people with minor illnesses, such as a cold, may be vaccinated

E. Side effects/adverse reactions
1. Serious: anaphylaxis
2. Common: elevated temperature 1 to 2 weeks after immunization; redness or pain at injection site; noncontagious rash; joint pain; irritability

VI. MEASLES, MUMPS, RUBELLA (MMR) VACCINE *(SEE TABLE 15–5 ■)*

A. Measles (rubeola), mumps (parotitis), rubella (German measles)
1. Infectious and communicable diseases in children that are vaccine-preventable; rubella is generally a mild disease but presents a major risk of spontaneous abortion, stillbirth, fetal death, and other anomalies for fetus during first trimester of pregnancy
2. MMR vaccine is a **live, attenuated vaccine** created from a live organism grown under suboptimal conditions to produce a live vaccine with reduced virulence

Table 15–4	Recommended Age	Dosage	Route
Inactivated Polio Vaccine	2 months 4 months 6–18 months 4–6 years	0.5 mL	Subcutaneous

Table 15-5
Measles, Mumps, Rubella Vaccine (MMR)

Recommended Age	Dosage	Route
12–15 months 4–6 years	0.5 mL	Subcutaneous

B. Administration
1. Store in center shelf of body of refrigerator at 2° to 8°C (35–46°F); do not freeze
2. Reconstituted solution is clear yellow; keep refrigerated and away from light; discard if unused within 8 hours; store diluent at room temperature or refrigerate
3. Table 15–5 lists recommended ages; however, second dose can be given at any age as long as it is at least 28 days after first dose
4. Those who have not received a second dose at 4 to 6 years of age should receive second MMR at scheduled visit at age 11 to 12 years

C. Precautions
1. College students are at greater risk due to increased exposure; ensure they have received a second MMR dose
2. ! Inform adolescent girls to avoid pregnancy for at least 3 months after immunization
3. MMR vaccine may be allowed for some infected with HIV; consult health care provider
4. Wait at least 3 to 11 months after administration of immune serum globulin or blood products before giving MMR vaccine
5. Thrombocytopenia or history of thrombocytopenic purpura

! **D. Contraindications**
1. Allergy to neomycin, gelatin, or eggs
2. Severely impaired immune system due to malignancy, immune deficiency disease, immunosuppressive therapy
3. Avoid administering a live-virus immunization during pregnancy and in women likely to become pregnant within 3 months

! **E. Side effects/adverse reactions**
1. Serious: anaphylaxis; encephalopathy; thrombocytopenic purpura; chronic arthritis
2. Common: elevated temperature 1 to 2 weeks after immunization; redness or pain at injection site; noncontagious rash; joint pain
3. Measles vaccine can cause a false-negative tine (TB) result

VII. VARICELLA VACCINE (VARIVAX) *(SEE TABLE 15–6 ■)*

A. Varicella (chicken pox)
1. A common childhood disease, usually mild, can lead to severe skin infection, scars, pneumonia, brain damage, or death
2. Varicella immunization is a live, attenuated vaccine used to stimulate immunity
3. The vaccine prevents chicken pox, or if the child has been vaccinated and gets the disease, it will be usually very mild, resulting in a faster recovery

B. Administration
1. Frozen at 5°F; store in center shelf of body of refrigerator at 2° to 8° (35–46°F) up to 72 hours before reconstitution; once reconstituted, must be used within 30 minutes or discarded; do not refreeze; keep diluent at room temperature
2. Individuals 13 years or older who have not had the disease require two doses 4 to 8 weeks apart
3. May use as postexposure if given within 3 to 5 days

C. Precautions
1. ! Instruct females of childbearing age to avoid pregnancy for 3 months after immunization

Table 15-6
Varicella Vaccine

Recommended Age	Dosage	Route
12–18 months	0.5 mL	Subcutaneous

2. Varicella vaccine is *not* recommended for those infected with HIV
3. Wait at least 3 to 11 months after administration of immune serum globulin or blood products before giving varicella vaccine

D. Contraindications

1. Allergy to neomycin or gelatin
2. Active, untreated TB
3. Pregnancy
4. Immunodeficiency or receiving immunosuppression therapy
5. Moderate or severe febrile illness

E. Side effects/adverse reactions

1. Serious: anaphylaxis
2. Common: pain or redness at injection site; fever up to 38.8°C (102°F) in children, up to 37.7°C (100°F) in adults, lasting for 1 week; varicella-like rash at injection site; irritability

VIII. PNEUMOCOCCAL CONJUGATE VACCINE (PCV) *(SEE TABLE 15–7 ■)*

A. Pneumoccocal infections

1. Heptavalent pneumococcal conjugate vaccine (PCV) is recommended to prevent and decrease severity of pneumococcal infections caused by *Streptococcus pneumoniae*
2. *Streptococcus pneumoniae* is the leading cause of bacterial meningitis in the United States
3. PCV is recommended for all children 2 to 23 months of age

B. Administration

1. Store in center shelf of body of refrigerator at 2° to 8°C (35–46°F); do not freeze
2. Clear, colorless, or slightly opalescent liquid

C. Precautions

1. It is highly recommended for children in day care
2. Also recommended for children with immunosuppression, pulmonary or cardiac illness, diabetes, sickle cell anemia, or asplenia

D. Contraindications

1. Hypersensitivity to diphtheria **toxoid**
2. Severe illness and anaphylaxis to a previous dose

E. Side effects/adverse reactions

1. Severe: anaphylaxis
2. Common: soreness, swelling, redness at injection site; mild to moderate fever; irritability; drowsiness; restlessness; sleep; decreased appetite; vomiting and diarrhea; rash or hives

IX. HEPATITIS A (HEP A) VACCINE *(SEE TABLE 15–8 ■)*

A. Hepatitis A

1. Serious liver disease caused by hepatitis A virus (HAV), which is found in stool of infected persons; usually spread by close personal contact and sometimes eating food or drinking water contaminated by HAV
2. Hep A vaccine can be given for postexposure prophylaxis against hepatitis A
3. Hep A vaccine is an inactivated, or killed vaccine
4. Immune globulin and Hep A vaccine can be given at same time in different sites

B. Administration

1. Store in center shelf of body of refrigerator at 2° to 8° (35°–46°F); do not freeze

Table 15–7

Pneumococcal Conjugate Vaccine (PCV)

Recommended Age	Dosage	Route
2 months 4 months 6 months 12–15 months	0.5 mL	Intramuscular

Table 15-8
Hepatitis A (Hep A) Vaccine

Recommended Age	Dosage	Route
2 doses given after age 24 months; two doses should be administered 6 months apart	≤ 18 yrs: 0.5 mL ≥ 19 yrs: 1.0 mL	Intramuscular

2. Do not restart series no matter how long since previous dose
3. May give with all other vaccines
4. Can be combined with hepatitis B vaccine (Twinrix); follow package instructions

C. Precautions

1. High incidence areas include Alaska, Arkansas, Arizona, California, Colorado, Idaho, Missouri, Montana, New Mexico, Nevada, Oklahoma, Oregon, South Dakota, Texas, Utah, Washington, Wyoming
2. Other high-risk populations include Native Alaskans, Native Americans, Pacific Islanders, persons with chronic liver disease, those who receive clotting factor concentrates, homosexual or bisexual males, and users of IV and illicit drugs

D. Contraindications

1. Moderate or severe illness warrants delaying administration of vaccine
2. Safety of hepatitis A vaccine for pregnant women is not yet known; risk is thought to be low

E. Side effects/adverse effects

1. Serious: anaphylaxis (rare)
2. Common: soreness at injection site, headache, loss of appetite, fatigue

X. INFLUENZA TRIVALENT INACTIVATED VACCINE (TIV)

(SEE TABLE 15-9 ■)

A. Influenza

1. Vaccine is also referred to as a flu shot, this is an inactivated or killed vaccine
2. Vaccine provides protection against strains of influenza; protection begins 2 weeks after administration and lasts 1 year
3. Close contacts of healthy children aged 0 to 23 months should receive influenza
4. An intranasal form of the influenza vaccine, a live, attenuated vaccine, is acceptable for children ages 5 and older

B. Administration

1. Store in center shelf of body of refrigerator at 2° to 8°(35–46°F); do not freeze
2. Administer in the fall and repeat yearly
3. Give two doses 4 weeks apart for children younger than 12 years; one dose for those older than 12 years

C. Precautions

1. Recommended for those undergoing immunosuppressive therapy
2. Recommended for those taking chronic aspirin therapy (e.g., for rheumatoid arthritis or Kawasaki disease)

D. Contraindications

1. Allergy to eggs
2. Anaphylaxis
3. Administration of live virus through intranasal route not appropriate for children with chronic illness (asthma, heart or renal disease, diabetes, immunosuppressed)

E. Side effects/adverse reactions

1. Serious: allergic reaction (rare)
2. Common: redness, soreness, swelling at injection site; fever; aching

Table 15-9
Influenza Trivalent Inactivated Vaccine (TIV)

Recommended Age	Dosage	Route
6–23 months of age ≥ 24 months of age with risk factors	0.25 mL	Intramuscular
≥ 3 years	0.5 mL	

Table 15–10 Meningococcal Vaccines

Vaccine	Recommended Age	Dosage	Route
Meningococcal polysaccharide vaccine or MPSV4 (Menomune)	2 years and older with asplenia	0.5 mL	Subcutaneous
Meningococcal conjugate vaccine or MCV4 (Menactra)	11–12 years and unvaccinated adolescents at high school entry or college freshman	0.5 mL	Intramuscular

XI. MENINGOCOCCAL VACCINES *(SEE TABLE 15–10 ■)*

A. Meningococcal infection

1. A serious respiratory infection that can result in critical illness such as meningitis, disseminated intravascular coagulopathy (DIC), shock, or death
2. This vaccine provides protection against *Neisseria meningitides*

B. Administration

1. Recommended for children 2 years and older with terminal complement deficiencies and asplenia
2. Recommended for 11 to 12 year olds, unvaccinated high school freshmen and unvaccinated freshman college students, military recruits, and those traveling to certain countries where there is added risk for exposure
3. Administer subcutaneous injection in anterolateral fat of thigh in young children or posterolateral fat of upper arm for older children and adults; administer intramuscular injection in large muscle

C. Precautions: the duration of protection is unknown

D. Contraindications: safety with pregnancy has not been established

E. Side effects/adverse reactions

1. Serious: anaphylaxis
2. Common: redness or tenderness at site

Check Your NCLEX-RN® Exam I.Q.

You are ready for testing on this content if you can

- Assess a client's or family's knowledge of immunization schedules.
- Assess a client's or family's immunization status.
- Administer correctly prescribed immunizations.
- Teach a client or family about prescribed immunizations.
- Identify contraindications to immunizations and other precautions.
- Respond appropriately when a client experiences side effects, adverse effects, or allergy to an immunization.

PRACTICE TEST

1 A newly adopted 8-year-old child is brought to the pediatric immunization clinic to begin the hepatitis B immunization series. Before providing the immunization, the nurse inquires about any known history of allergy to which of the following?

1. Aminoglycoside antibiotics
2. Mold
3. Baker's yeast
4. Egg yolks

2 A mother brings her infant into the immunization clinic for the final hepatitis B vaccine. After picking up the vial of vaccine to draw up the dose, the nurse notes that it is cloudy. Which of the following actions should the nurse take?

1. Warm the vaccine under running water.
2. Discard the vaccine and contact the supplier of the vaccine.
3. Shake the vial gently and draw up the vaccine for administration.
4. Calculate the pediatric dosage before drawing it up, since the vaccine is intended for adult usage.

PRACTICE TEST

3 The nurse who is preparing to draw up a dose of vaccine notices that a vial of DTaP vaccine on the countertop does not have a date recorded for when it was opened. Which of the following actions should the nurse take?

1. Use the vaccine but explain to the caregiver that the site may be quite tender.
2. Discard the vaccine according to agency's policy.
3. Contact the supervisor because this is reportable to the state Board of Public Health.
4. Use the vaccine just for the day and then discard it.

4 A parent brings a 3-year-old child to the immunization clinic for a DTaP vaccine. During the interview, the mother indicates the child is just finishing a tapered dose of prednisone for a chronic respiratory problem. Which of the following actions should the nurse take?

1. Delay the vaccine administration for 1 month after the medication is completed.
2. Provide the child with the vaccine as scheduled.
3. Cleanse the injection site with sterile saline instead of alcohol and administer the vaccine.
4. Keep the child in the clinic for 30 minutes after administration to assess the child's response.

5 A child is brought to the pediatric ambulatory clinic with a runny nose and a low-grade fever. He is scheduled to receive the MMR (measles, mumps, and rubella) and DTaP (diphtheria, pertussis, and tetanus toxoid) vaccines. What should the nurse do at this time?

1. Get special permission from the physician to administer the vaccine.
2. Defer both vaccines until the child is well.
3. Administer the vaccines as scheduled.
4. Administer the DTaP vaccine but defer the MMR.

6 A pediatric client is scheduled to receive a dose of MMR (measles, mumps, rubella) vaccine. The nurse would question the order to give the dose at this time if which of the following was noted during the short history obtained on intake?

1. Recent upper respiratory infection
2. Weight loss of 3 pounds during the last month
3. History of allergy to neomycin or gelatin
4. Local reaction to previous dose

7 The mother of a child who has been exposed to chicken pox calls the pediatric clinic for advice. The triage nurse who answers the telephone would inquire about which of the following before responding to the mother's request for information?

1. The child's exposure and immune status
2. Whether the child has had a rubella vaccination
3. The age, height, and weight of the child
4. The relationship of the person to whom the child was exposed

8 A 9-year-old client is brought to the pediatrician's office for a varicella virus vaccine. Before preparing the dose of the vaccine, the nurse asks the mother whether the child has:

1. received any blood products recently.
2. any allergies to milk.
3. an allergy to penicillin.
4. undergone removal of the spleen.

9 A child stepped on a rusty nail and is brought to the emergency department. If the child was not adequately immunized against tetanus according to the immunization schedule, what would the emergency department nurse anticipate will be ordered to treat this child?

1. Diphtheria, tetanus, and pertussis vaccine
2. Tetanus immune globulin
3. A broad-spectrum antibiotic
4. Tetanus toxoid

10 A 2-month-old client is seen in the pediatric clinic for a well-baby checkup. The nurse anticipates that which of the following routine immunizations will be administered at this time? Select all that apply.

1. Inactivated poliovirus vaccine (IPV)
2. Diphtheria, tetanus and acellular pertussis (DTaP)
3. Haemophilus influenza B conjugate vaccine (Hib)
4. Measles, mumps, and rubella (MMR)
5. Varicella zoster

11 A nurse is preparing to draw up a dose of *Haemophilus influenzae* type B (Hib) vaccine for a pediatric client. The nurse knows that the vial is acceptable to use after noting which of the following expected coloration of the fluid in the vial?

1. Pale yellow
2. Light pink
3. Clear
4. Slightly brown tinged

12 The pediatric clinic nurse has just administered a dose of *Haemophilus influenzae* type B (Hib) vaccine to a child. The nurse explains to the parents that they can expect which of the following local reactions following the injection?

1. Mild to moderate fever
2. Pain or redness at site
3. Irritability
4. Decreased appetite

13 The nurse has an order to give an infant a dose of inactivated poliovirus vaccine (IPV). The nurse would do which of the following prior to administering the medication to ensure the dose is safe and effective?

1. Take dose that has not expired from a box on the shelf in the medication room.
2. Assess prior to dose for allergy to neomycin, streptomycin, or polymixin B.
3. Gently agitate the cloudy white solution before drawing up.
4. Select a proper size muscle for injection.

14 The neonatal nurse is providing anticipatory guidance to the mother of a newborn infant. When discussing immunization schedules, the nurse explains that the first dose of inactivated poliovirus vaccine (IPV) is given at what age?

1. 1 week
2. 1 month
3. 2 months
4. 4 months

15 The nurse has conducted client teaching with the parents of a client who received a dose of heptavalent pneumococcal conjugate vaccine (PCV). The nurse evaluates that the parents understand the information presented if they state that which of the following symptoms is most important to report promptly to the health care provider?

1. Mild fever
2. Drowsiness
3. Decreased appetite
4. Rash with hives

16 The public health nurse is administering inactivated hepatitis A (Hep A) vaccine to clients at risk. The nurse determines that, according to statistics regarding incidence, a client from which of the following cultural groups should have highest priority to receive the vaccine?

1. A Native American client
2. A Jamaican American client
3. An African American client
4. A European American client

17 A child with cardiac disease has been recommended to receive the yearly influenza vaccine. The nurse would schedule the child to receive the vaccine at the routine visit scheduled in which of the following months?

1. January
2. April
3. July
4. October

18 A 6-year-old child with asplenia is receiving the meningococcal vaccine. The nurse explains to the child's mother that the vaccine should be effective for how many years?

1. 1
2. 2
3. 5
4. 10

19 A nurse working in an immunization clinic ensures at the beginning of each workday that which of the following priority medications is available and within the expiration date?

1. Lidocaine hydrochloride (Xylocaine)
2. Epinephrine (adrenalin)
3. Acetaminophen (Tylenol)
4. Ibuprofen (Motrin)

20 The mother of a pediatric client does not have a record of the child's immunizations. Which of the following initial nursing diagnoses would the nurse choose?

1. Powerlessness
2. Noncompliance
3. Ineffective health maintenance
4. Deficient knowledge

21 The pediatric nurse is seeing a 2-month-old infant in the outpatient clinic for routine immunizations. The nurse should select which of the following immunization teaching sheets to give to the mother prior to preparing the immunizations appropriate for this visit? Select all that apply.

1. Varicella
2. Diphtheria, tetanus, and acellular pertussis (DTaP)
3. Measles, mumps, and rubella (MMR)
4. *Haemophilus influenzae* type b (Hib)
5. Inactivated polio (IPV)

ANSWERS & RATIONALES

1 **Answer: 3** A history of an allergic reaction to baker's yeast would be a contraindication to receiving this series of immunizations. Aminoglycoside antibiotics, mold, and egg yolks do not pose any risk to the client for allergy to the vaccine.
Cognitive Level: Analysis **Client Need:** Health Promotion and Maintenance **Integrated Process:** Nursing Process: Assessment **Content Area:** Pharmacology: Immunological **Strategy:** Specific knowledge of contraindications to hepatitis B vaccine is needed to answer this question. Use the process of elimination, and review this content area if needed.

2 **Answer: 3** It is normal for the solution in the vial to appear cloudy. The nurse should gently shake the vaccine and then draw it up for administration. It is unnecessary to discard it or to notify the manufacturer. Warming the solution will not affect the cloudiness.
Cognitive Level: Application **Client Need:** Health Promotion and Maintenance **Integrated Process:** Nursing Process: Implementation **Content Area:** Pharmacology: Immunological **Strategy:** Specific knowledge of the nursing considerations for hepatitis B vaccine is needed to answer this question. Use the process of elimination, and review this content area if needed.

3 **Answer: 2** The vial should be discarded according to agency policy. Administering the vaccine does not protect the safety of the client, and it is unnecessary to report this particular incident to the state Board of Public Health.
Cognitive Level: Application **Client Need:** Health Promotion and Maintenance **Integrated Process:** Nursing Process: Implementation **Content Area:** Pharmacology: Immunological **Strategy:** The core issue of this question is safe handling of vaccinations. Use principles of general medication preparation to make a selection.

4 **Answer: 1** The dose should be delayed for 1 month following any type of immunosuppressive therapy, such as prednisone. The other actions do not protect the client or uphold safe administration procedures for immunizations.
Cognitive Level: Application **Client Need:** Health Promotion and Maintenance **Integrated Process:** Nursing Process: Implementation **Content Area:** Pharmacology: Immunological **Strategy:** Use the process of elimination. Recall that immunizations affect the immune system and that steroids such as prednisone suppress the immune system to make the correct selection.

5 **Answer: 3** The immunizations should be administered as scheduled. They would be withheld for clients who are immunosuppressed or have moderate to severe febrile illnesses. The presence of a runny nose and low-grade fever is not a contraindication according to the literature.
Cognitive Level: Application **Client Need:** Health Promotion and Maintenance **Integrated Process:** Nursing Process: Implementation **Content Area:** Pharmacology: Immunological **Strategy:** The core issue of the question is contraindications to administering scheduled immunizations. Use the process of elimination, and take time to review these immunizations if needed.

6 **Answer: 3** A contraindication to MMR vaccine is a history of allergic reaction to neomycin or gelatin. Minor illnesses and history of local reaction to a previous dose are not contraindications. Weight loss is irrelevant to the question.
Cognitive Level: Application **Client Need:** Health Promotion and Maintenance **Integrated Process:** Nursing Process: Implementation **Content Area:** Pharmacology: Immunological **Strategy:** The core issue of the question is knowledge of contraindications to MMR vaccine. Use the process of elimination to make a selection, keeping in mind that both neomycin and gelatin are reasons to withhold the dose.

7 **Answer: 1** The nurse would inquire about the nature of the exposure and the client's immune status. Chicken pox can be fatal in immunocompromised children, such as those who are undergoing steroid therapy, chemotherapy, and those who have other illnesses. If warranted, the varicella zoster immune globulin can be given up to 4 days after exposure to those with no history of chicken pox or prior exposure. Exposure to rubella (a different disease), height and weight of the child, and the person to whom the child was exposed are irrelevant as priority items in protecting the health of the child.
Cognitive Level: Analysis **Client Need:** Health Promotion and Maintenance **Integrated Process:** Nursing Process: Assessment **Content Area:** Pharmacology: Immunological **Strategy:** The core issue of the question is knowledge of indications for use of varicella zoster immune globulin. Use the process of elimination and general concepts of immunity to answer the question.

8 **Answer: 1** Contraindications to varicella virus vaccine include allergy to neomycin or gelatin, immunosupression, or administration of immune serum globulin or blood products in the last 3 to 11 months. A history of spleen removal and allergies to penicillin or milk are irrelevant to safe use of this vaccine.
Cognitive Level: Application **Client Need:** Health Promotion and Maintenance **Integrated Process:** Nursing Process: Assessment **Content Area:** Pharmacology: Immunological **Strategy:** The core issue of the question is knowledge of contraindications for use of varicella vaccine. Use the process of elimination and general concepts of immunity to answer the question.

9 **Answer: 2** When there is accidental exposure and inadequate vaccination, passive immunity with tetanus immune globulin is indicated for immediate protection from the bacterial spores in the nail. Options 1 and 4 provide active immunity and option 3 (broad-spectrum antibiotic) is inadequate.
Cognitive Level: Application **Client Need:** Health Promotion and Maintenance **Integrated Process:** Nursing Process: Planning **Content Area:** Pharmacology: Immunological **Strategy:** The core issue of the question is the ability to discriminate situations requiring active immunity and those requiring passive immunity. Use the process of elimination, and take time to review this information if needed.

10 **Answer: 1, 2, 3** The IPV, DTaP, Hib, and PCV vaccines are all scheduled to be given at 2 months of age. The MMR is given at 12 to 15 months, and again at 4 to 6 years. The varicella zoster vaccine is given at 12 to 18 months.

Cognitive Level: Application **Client Need:** Health Promotion and Maintenance **Integrated Process:** Nursing Process: Planning **Content Area:** Pharmacology: Immunological **Strategy:** The core issue of the question is knowledge of routine immunization schedules for a 2-month-old infant. Use general knowledge of immunization schedules and the process of elimination to make your selections.

11 **Answer: 3** The solution used for Hib vaccine is clear and colorless. MMR and varicella vaccines are a clear yellow in color. No vaccines are pale pink or brown, although some are cloudy.
Cognitive Level: Application **Client Need:** Health Promotion and Maintenance **Integrated Process:** Nursing Process: Analysis **Content Area:** Pharmacology: Immunological **Strategy:** The core issue of this question is the ability to determine safe appearance of vaccines before administration. Use nursing knowledge and the process of elimination to make a selection.

12 **Answer: 2** The parents should be taught to expect pain and redness at the site as possible local reactions. Fever, irritability, and decreased appetite are common side effects of the heptavalent pneumococcal conjugate vaccine (PCV).
Cognitive Level: Application **Client Need:** Health Promotion and Maintenance **Integrated Process:** Teaching and Learning **Content Area:** Pharmacology: Immunological **Strategy:** Use the process of elimination. One strategy to determine local reaction is to evaluate the options in terms of how confined they are to the site of injection. The incorrect responses are systemic in nature.

13 **Answer: 2** Before administering a dose of IPV, the nurse should assess for allergy to neomycin, streptomycin, or polymixin B. The solution should be kept in the refrigerator and should be clear and colorless. The dose is administered by the subcutaneous route.
Cognitive Level: Application **Client Need:** Health Promotion and Maintenance **Integrated Process:** Nursing Process: Implementation **Content Area:** Pharmacology: Immunological **Strategy:** The core issue of this question is the ability to administer IPV safely. Use nursing knowledge and the process of elimination to make a selection.

14 **Answer: 3** The first dose of IPV is given at 2 months, with subsequent doses at 4 months, 12 to 18 months, and 4 to 6 years, for a total of four doses. The other options do not match the acceptable timeline for administration of this vaccine.
Cognitive Level: Application **Client Need:** Health Promotion and Maintenance **Integrated Process:** Nursing Process: Implementation **Content Area:** Pharmacology: Immunological **Strategy:** The core issue of this question is the ability to administer IPV safely according to its recommended schedule. Use nursing knowledge and the process of elimination to make a selection.

15 **Answer: 4** Although mild to moderate fever, drowsiness, and decreased appetite are some of the side effects of PCV, the most important one to report to the health care provider is rash with hives. This likely indicates an allergic reaction, which could progress to anaphylaxis if left untreated.
Cognitive Level: Analysis **Client Need:** Health Promotion and Maintenance **Integrated Process:** Nursing Process: Evaluation **Content Area:** Pharmacology: Immunological **Strategy:** The core issue of this question is the highest priority teaching regarding PCV. The critical words in the stem of the question are *most important* and *promptly,* which tells you that more than one or all options may be technically correct. Use nursing knowledge, the ABCs, and the process of elimination to make a selection.

16 **Answer: 1** High-risk populations are found in specific states, all of which are west of the Mississippi River. Native American and Native Alaskan clients are the cultural populations at highest risk.
Cognitive Level: Analysis **Client Need:** Health Promotion and Maintenance **Integrated Process:** Nursing Process: Planning **Content Area:** Pharmacology: Immunological **Strategy:** The core issue of this question is the client population at highest risk for developing hepatitis A. Use general knowledge regarding this vaccine to make a selection. You can also use knowledge that hepatitis A is contagious and that Native Americans tend to live in groups to help you choose this option over the others.

17 **Answer: 4** The influenza vaccine is administered annually in the autumn, especially during October, November, and into December. The other months do not correlate with administration times that would prevent development of influenza during the winter months.
Cognitive Level: Application **Client Need:** Health Promotion and Maintenance **Integrated Process:** Nursing Process: Planning **Content Area:** Pharmacology: Immunological **Strategy:** The core issue of the question is the timing of the annual dosage of influenza vaccine. Use knowledge of the epidemiology of the disease to choose the month prior to when flu season occurs.

18 **Answer: 3** Meningococcal vaccine is indicated for children older than 2 years with asplenia. The vaccine duration is 5 years if the client is older than 4 years at the time of immunization. If the client is younger than 4 at the time of initial immunization, it should be repeated after 1 year.
Cognitive Level: Application **Client Need:** Health Promotion and Maintenance **Integrated Process:** Teaching and Learning **Content Area:** Pharmacology: Immunological **Strategy:** Specific knowledge related to the meningococcal vaccine is needed to answer the question. Take time to review this material if needed, and use the process of elimination in making a selection.

19 **Answer: 2** Epinephrine is the priority medication to have on hand if a client should experience hypersensitivity reaction/anaphylaxis following a dose of an immunization. Lidocaine is given for cardiac dysrhythmias, while acetaminophen and ibuprofen are peripheral CNS analgesics.
Cognitive Level: Analysis **Client Need:** Health Promotion and Maintenance **Integrated Process:** Nursing Process: Planning **Content Area:** Pharmacology: Immunological **Strategy:** The core issue of the question is knowledge that anaphylaxis is a potentially life-threatening consequence of immunization. Use the process of elimination, choosing the answer that is an emergency drug associated with reducing allergic response.

20 **Answer: 4** Initially, the nurse would be prudent to choose deficient knowledge. After explaining to the mother the rationale for and importance of maintaining vaccination records, other nursing diagnoses such as noncompliance

ANSWERS & RATIONALES

may apply. The other nursing diagnoses listed are inappropriate in this instance.

Cognitive Level: Application **Client Need:** Health Promotion and Maintenance **Integrated Process:** Nursing Process: Analysis **Content Area:** Child Health: Immunological **Strategy:** Use general nursing knowledge to make a selection after focusing on the critical word *initially* in the stem. In this case, the correct option gives the mother the benefit of the doubt about the reason for lack of immunization schedule maintenance.

21 **Answer: 2, 4, 5** Diphtheria, Tetanus and acellular pertussis (DTaP), *Haemophilus influenzae* type b (Hib), inactivated polio vaccine (IPV), and the pneumococcal conjugate vaccine (PCV) are the routine immunizations scheduled for the 2-month well-child visit. The MMR is given first at 12 to 15 months, and the varicella can be given at or anytime after 12 months.

Cognitive Level: Analysis **Client Need:** Health Promotion and Maintenance **Integrated Process:** Nursing Process: Implementation **Content Area:** Pharmacology: Immunological **Strategy:** The core issue of the question is knowledge of vaccinations that are due at a 2-month well-child visit. Use the process of elimination, recalling that MMR and varicella cannot be given before 12 months of age.

Key Terms to Review

active immunity p. 194
attenuate p. 194
inactivated vaccine p. 198
killed vaccine virus p. 198
live, attenuated vaccine p. 202
passive immunity p. 194
toxoid p. 203
vaccine p. 194

References

American Academy of Family Physicians. http://www/aafp.org.

American Academy of Pediatrics. http://www/aap.org.

Ball, J. & Bindler, R. (2006). *Child health nursing: Partnering with children and families.* Upper Saddle River, NJ: Pearson Prentice Hall.

Centers for Disease Control and Prevention. (2006). *Recommended childhood and adolescent immunization schedule.* Atlanta: CDC. Retrieved June 18, 2005, at http://www.cdc.gov/nip/recs/child-schedule-bw-press.pdf.

Hockenberry, M., & Wilson, D. (2006). *Wong's nursing care of infants and children* (8th ed.). St. Louis: Mosby.

Lowdermilk, D., & Perry, S. (2004). *Maternity and women's health care* (8th ed.). St. Louis: Mosby.

Olds, S., London, M., Ladewig, P., & Davidson, M. (2004). *Maternal-newborn nursing and women's health care* (7th ed.). Upper Saddle River, NJ: Pearson Education.

ANSWERS & RATIONALES

Health and Physical Assessment

16

In this chapter

Test Yourself

Are you ready for the NCLEX-RN® or course exams? Use the practice tests on the companion CD-ROM to check.

Cross reference

Another chapter relevant to this content area is
Lifespan Growth and Development **Chapter 14**

I. HEALTH HISTORY OF THE ADULT

A. Overview

1. A **health history** is a collection of data about client's present and past health status; using communication skills and interviewing techniques, it gathers **subjective data** while allowing opportunity to develop a therapeutic relationship with client
2. Sources of data
   a. Primary: client, who is best source of data unless confused, too young, or too ill to participate in interview
   b. Secondary: family members, caregivers, support people; old medical or other health records; and results of laboratory and diagnostic tests
3. Principles of history taking
   a. Provide privacy
   b. If client is tired or ill, ask most critical questions first
   c. Immediately document data in chart; do not keep any data on a loose piece of paper
   ! d. Maintain confidentiality
   e. Plan an appropriate timeframe: may require up to 1 hour or longer; allot enough time to take health history to avoid missing pertinent data; pace interview so as not to overtire client
   f. Gain trust: approach client and family in a professional manner; explain rationale for interview; tell the client to alert you right away if he or she becomes ill during interview; use therapeutic communication skills
   ! g. Note nonverbal cues about client's demeanor, posture, and overall appearance: physical indicators include cleanliness, body odor, personal grooming, hygiene, client's eye contact; signs of physical discomfort include diaphoresis, tremors, grimaces, and continual changes in position; signs of client stress include tears, skin blotching, nervous movements, inability to concentrate, arms

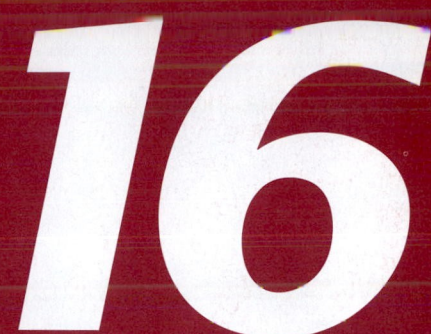

folded, diaphoresis; if client wants to end interview, respect this request and terminate interaction

h. Assess client's reliability: use proper terminology or words that indicate an understanding of health status; offer pertinent information about health status; do not change data reported; refer to previous ailments and treatment associated with illness; is oriented to person, place, time, and event; family members present concur that the data is accurate

i. Use an interpreter if there is a language barrier

j. Conduct interview in a logical, orderly manner; focus discussion by asking open-ended questions first regarding most important issues, then pertinent follow-up questions; use closed-ended questions (yielding yes-no responses) to clarify previous statements or to ask for specific additional information; clarify any discrepancies

B. Health history components

1. Format used may vary slightly depending on age of client and associated developmental considerations and reason for visit (routine care or an acute problem)
2. Biographical data includes name, address, telephone number, gender, marital status, religion, occupation, health insurance information, and possibly name and contact information for primary care physician and/or nurse practitioner
3. Chief complaint (problem or reason for which client is currently seeking treatment)
4. ! Symptom analysis, getting data about each of the following:
   a. Location: be as specific as possible regarding part(s) of the body involved
   b. Quantity: sometimes referred to as *severity* or *intensity;* whenever possible, use a numerical rating scale (0 to 10) or some type of visual analog scale; frequent examples of symptoms assessed this way are pain and dyspnea
   c. Quality: description of symptoms using various adjectives such as *burning, stabbing, pressure;* some disorders tend to be described in similar ways by clients, which can aid in diagnosing current problem
   d. Setting: location of client when symptom(s) began and a description of events going on at that time
   e. Timing or chronology: notation of when symptom first began; slow onset versus sudden; constant versus intermittent; whether symptom disturbs client's sleep
   f. Aggravating or alleviating factors: factors that make symptom worse or better (such as eating, resting, use of medication, among others)
   g. Associated factors: other symptoms that accompany primary symptom (such as diaphoresis or shortness of breath with chest pain)
5. Previous state of health and physical capabilities and how current symptoms have impacted physical, emotional, and psychosocial functioning
6. ! History of present illness (useful if problem has occurred more than once)
   a. When symptoms originally started
   b. How frequently exacerbations occur and whether onset is gradual or sudden
   c. Medications and/or other therapies used to treat problem and their degree of success (or lack of success)
7. Past health history: sometimes called *past history* or *medical history;* includes the following:
   a. Other possible health problems; some agencies use a checklist to obtain this information; focused (more detailed) assessment can be done on areas that are still currently problematic; clients commonly seek treatment for one health problem while having an active history of others, called comorbidities, that require ongoing management
   b. ! Childhood and adult immunizations and date of last tetanus prophylaxis; may also include influenzae vaccines
   c. Childhood illnesses such as measles, mumps, rubella (German measles), rubeola, chickenpox, rheumatic fever, scarlet fever, streptococcal infections, or other major illnesses

d. Prior hospitalizations, including dates, reasons (includes accidents and injuries as well as illnesses), surgical procedures, outcomes, and any complications experienced (such as reactions to anesthesia or blood products)

! **e.** Allergies: medication (reaction and symptoms, includes prescription, over-the-counter, and herbal products), food, seasonal (and their treatment), allergy to dyes used in diagnostic procedures (often assessed by asking about allergy to iodine or shellfish)

f. Pregnancy history and menstrual history as appropriate for female clients

! **g.** Current medications: prescribed dose, rationale, and duration of drug therapy; date and time of last dose; over-the-counter medications; herbal remedies; home remedies; complementary or adjunctive health care (if so, have client explain remedies used and effects)

8. Family health history

a. Identification of overall state of health of parents and relatives: any significant and chronic illnesses, cause of death, and age at time of death

b. Family health history can highlight genetically transmitted traits or disorders; keep in mind that ethnic background also plays a role in risk of developing certain disorders

c. Establish whether there is a history of hereditary disorders such as coronary heart disease, diabetes mellitus, stroke, high blood pressure, cancer, obesity, arthritis, bleeding disorders, or mental health disorders

! **d.** Helps to focus appropriate efforts on disease prevention and health promotion to lessen client's risk in an area; for example, cardiac health and healthy living

9. Personal/social history: includes social data and lifestyle assessment

! **a.** Diet: foods eaten on a typical day; number of meals and snacks; who shops and cooks; food preferences and patterns based on culture and/or religion; usual fluid intake; intake of caffeine (such as coffee, tea, cola)

! **b.** Activity and exercise: type, frequency, and duration of exercise; ability to perform activities of daily living (ADLs), including eating, bathing, elimination, dressing, grooming; ability to move about at will (locomotion)

c. Sleep and rest: usual number of hours of sleep, sleep problems, and effectiveness of any remedies used

! **d.** Tobacco use: number of packs per day (cigarettes) and number of years of smoking; type, frequency, and duration of use for other tobacco products

e. Substance use: amount, frequency, and duration of alcohol or recreational drug use

f. Living arrangements: location, type of dwelling, number of stairs to climb, home safety information, ability to access neighborhood or community resources

g. Family relationships or friendships: who is/are support person(s) in times of need; effects of illness on client and family roles and relationships (dynamics); identification of next of kin

h. Psychological data: major lifestyle changes or stressors experienced and how client dealt with them; client's usual coping patterns; general communication style and ability; appropriateness of verbal and nonverbal behavior; whether client is seeing a mental health professional; significance of current illness to client; effect of current illness on self-esteem or body image

i. Occupation: presence of occupational hazards, such as exposure to carcinogens (e.g., asbestos, other chemicals); distance and length of time client commutes to work each day and associated concerns; amount of time missed from work due to illness; history of a need to change jobs because of illness

j. Travel: out of country, when and length of time; military service abroad

k. Health resources used: current and past use of physicians (general and specialists), dentists, folk healers; satisfaction with care; accessibility to care

10. Review of systems (ROS): used to obtain subjective data in a medical model; nursing assessments often use a nursing model instead of the ROS, such as Gordon's 11 functional health patterns, Orem's self-care model, or Roy's adaptation model; health care agencies generally have a specific form to gather this data (forms may blend gathering of subjective data [history] and **objective data** [physical assessment or examination])

a. Skin: skin disease (eczema, psoriasis, hives), changes in moles, skin dryness or moisture, itching, bruising, rashes or other lesions, changes in hair or nails, sun exposure

b. Head: headaches, dizziness (vertigo) or fainting (syncope), head injury

c. Eyes: vision problems (blurring, blind spots, reduced acuity), double vision (diplopia), glaucoma, cataracts, eye pain, redness, discharge or watering, swelling, method of vision correction being used

d. Ears: hearing loss, hearing aid use, tinnitus, vertigo, earaches, infections, discharge and characteristics

e. Nose/sinuses: frequency and severity of colds, sinus pain or obstruction, discharge, nosebleeds, allergies, reduced sense of smell

f. Mouth/throat: pain or lesions in mouth (or tongue), toothaches, change in sense of taste, frequency of sore throats, bleeding gums, dysphagia, hoarseness, history of tonsillectomy, frequency of dental care and presence of any dental prostheses

g. Neck: pain, mobility, enlarged or tender lymph nodes, goiter, lumps or other swelling

! **h.** Breasts: history of breast disease or surgery, pain, lumps, rashes, nipple discharge, knowledge and performance of breast self-examination (BSE); date of last mammogram

i. Axilla: rash, lumps, tenderness, or swelling

! **j.** Respiratory: history of lung disease (tuberculosis, pneumonia, asthma, bronchitis, emphysema), shortness of breath (amount and triggering factors, such as activity level), wheezes/other noises associated with respiration, cough, sputum production (color, amount, and if relevant, timing), pain associated with breathing, hemoptysis, and exposure to pollutants or other inhaled toxins

! **k.** Cardiovascular: history of heart disease, murmur, hypertension, or anemia; chest pain (precordial or retrosternal, radiation, and other pain characteristics); dyspnea on exertion (specify amount); orthopnea, paroxysmal nocturnal dyspnea (PND); edema, nocturia

l. Peripheral vascular: discoloration of extremities (especially feet and ankles; note whether associated with activity); coolness, numbness, or tingling of lower limbs (note relationship to activity and time of day); history of intermittent claudication, ulcerations, thrombophlebitis, or varicose veins

m. Gastrointestinal (GI): appetite, nausea and vomiting, constipation or diarrhea, frequency of bowel movements and whether any recent changes, tarry or bloody stools, history of rectal conditions (such as hemorrhoids), food intolerances, dysphagia, heartburn, pyrosis (upper-GI burning with sour eructation), indigestion, abdominal pain (with or without eating), history of GI disorder, antacid use, and prescribed diet

n. Urinary: frequency, urgency, or dysuria; nocturia; polyuria or oliguria; characteristics of stream (narrowed, hesitancy, straining); cloudy urine or hematuria; incontinence; history of urinary disorder (renal disease or calculi, urinary tract infections); pain in back, flank, suprapubic area, or groin

o. Male genital: lumps, hernia, penile lesions or discharge, pain in testicles or penis, knowledge and performance of testicular self-examination (TSE), sexual health practices (contraceptive method and prevention of sexually transmitted diseases)

p. Female genital: menstrual history (age of menarche, last monthly period, duration of cycle, premenstrual pain, intermenstrual spotting or metrorrhagia, dysmenorrhea, amenorrhea, menorrhagia), vaginal itching or discharge, age at menopause, menopausal manifestations, postmenopausal bleeding, last Pap test and gynecological exam, sexual health practices

q. Musculoskeletal: joint pain, stiffness, or swelling; history of arthritis or gout; limited movement, noise with joint movement, obvious deformity; muscle pain, weakness, or cramping; difficulty with gait or activities; back pain or stiffness, history of back pain or disease; use of mobility aids and satisfaction with ability to perform ADLs

r. Neurologic: weakness, tics or tremors, paralysis, problems with coordination, paresthesias (numbness and tingling), recent or distant memory disorder, nervousness, mood changes, history of depression or other mental health problem, hallucinations, history of stroke, fainting or blackouts, seizure disorder

s. Hematologic: easy bruising or bleeding, swollen lymph nodes, history of blood transfusion and reactions, exposure to radiation or other toxins

t. Endocrine: history of diabetes, thyroid disease, adrenal disease, abnormal hair distribution, change in skin (pigmentation, texture), excessive sweating, relationship between appetite and weight, hormone therapy

II. HEALTH HISTORY OF THE CHILD

A. Overview

1. Provides opportunity to observe parent–child interactions
2. Principles are same as for an adult health history

B. Demographic and biographical information: similar to adult with addition of child's nickname, ages of child, siblings, parents

C. Reason for seeking care

1. Sometimes called *chief complaint*
2. May be wellness- or illness-oriented
3. Record in words of informant, parent, or child

D. History of present illness

1. Symptom analysis as previously described for adult client
2. Parents' perceptions of illness versus child's perception, if applicable

E. Past medical history

1. Birth history
   a. Length of pregnancy
   b. Mother's health and access to prenatal care
   c. Medications taken during pregnancy and any alcohol, tobacco, or street-drug use
   d. Duration of labor and type of delivery
   e. Apgar scores, if known
   f. Birth weight, length, head circumference
   g. Postnatal health problems
   h. Feeding: formula, including type, or breast-fed, including length of time
2. Past illnesses
3. Hospitalizations, injuries, accidents, or surgeries
4. Allergies: medication, food, or environmental
5. Immunizations including boosters
6. Habits and behaviors: sleep; discipline; socialization; exercise or activity; behavior issues; wellness behaviors; use of alcohol, drugs, nicotine, or caffeine; sexuality issues
7. Medications taken regularly: prescription, over-the-counter, home or folk remedies
8. Developmental data
   a. Age at which child achieved specific developmental milestones, including first held head erect, first rolled over, first sat unsupported, first steps, first used words appropriately, bowel and bladder control
   b. Current developmental performance measured by a screening tool such as Denver II, if known
   c. Academic performance if in school
9. Nutritional data
   a. Consider adequacy in terms of age
   b. Timing and frequency of meals and snacks
   c. Ethnic or cultural considerations in food choices
   d. Use a 24-hour diet recall or food frequency record to assess adequacy of diet
10. Family history
    a. Primarily for purpose of discovering potential or actual hereditary or familial diseases in the child or parents

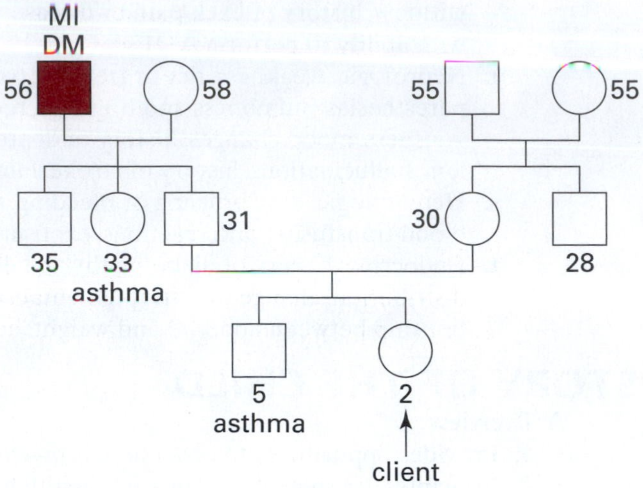

Figure 16–1

Sample genogram for a child. The child's brother has asthma, a paternal aunt has asthma, and the paternal grandfather died having myocardial infarction (MI) and diabetes mellitus (DM).

Source: *Hogan, M. & White, J. (2003).* Child health nursing. *Upper Saddle River, NJ: Prentice Hall, p. 33.*

b. Includes a **genogram** (pictorial representation of family tree) that includes hereditary diseases, ages and causes of death, and chronic conditions (see Figure 16–1 ■)

c. Family structure: immediate and extended members of family; previous marriages, divorces, separations, or deaths of spouses

d. Home and community environment: type of dwelling, sleeping arrangements, safety features, relationships with neighbors

e. Occupations and education of family members, including work schedules

f. Cultural and religious traditions, including language spoken at home

g. Family function: interactions and roles; power, decision making, and problem solving; communication; and expression of feelings and individuality

11. Review of systems

a. Includes a specific review of each body system

b. Begin with a broad question about child's overall health

c. Integument: pruritus, rashes (including location), acne, bruising, hair growth or loss, disorders or deformities of nails

d. Head: headaches, dizziness or injuries

e. Eyes: visual problems (bumping into things, squinting, blurred vision, holding books close or sitting close to television or computer), rubbing eyes, eye infections, glasses or contact lenses

f. Ears: earaches (frequency and treatment), evidence of hearing loss (needing to repeat requests, loud voice) previous hearing testing

g. Nose: history of nosebleeds, constant or frequent runny or stuffy nose, problems with sense of smell

h. Mouth: mouth breathing, dental visits, tooth-care habits (brushing, flossing), toothaches

i. Throat: sore throats, difficulty swallowing, choking, hoarseness or voice problems

j. Neck: stiffness or problems moving; difficulty in holding head erect

k. Chest: breast enlargement or development, breast self-examination for adolescents

l. Respiratory: frequency of colds, coughing or wheezing, difficulty breathing, sputum production, history of pneumonia or tuberculosis (TB), last TB test date

m. Cardiovascular: cyanosis or fatigue on exertion; history of heart murmurs, anemia, or rheumatic fever; blood type if known

n. Gastrointestinal: nausea or vomiting, jaundice, change in bowel habits, diarrhea, constipation

o. Genitourinary: pain on urination, unpleasant odor to urine, enuresis, testicular self-examination for adolescents

p. Gynecological: date or age of menarche, date of last menstrual period, pain on menstruation, vaginal discharge, last Pap smear and contraceptive use if sexually active

q. Musculoskeletal: weakness, clumsiness or lack of coordination, back or joint pain, muscle pain or cramps, abnormal gait or posturing or spasticity, history of fractures or sprains, usual activity level
r. Neurological: history of seizures, speech problems, nightmares or fears, dizziness or tremors, learning disabilities or problems with attention at home or school

12. Review of psychosocial systems
   a. Family composition: family members in home and their relationship to child, marital status of parents, parents' educational level, persons participating in care of child, recent changes or crises in family
   b. Financial resources: family members' employment status or occupation, health insurance coverage
   c. Home environment: safe play area; well or community water supply; availability of heat, electricity, and so on; transportation; neighborhood safety issues
   d. Child care arrangements: day-care resources needed/available, school attended
   e. Daily living habits: peer relationships; sleep, rest, activity patterns; social activities; self-esteem and body image
   f. Child's temperament

III. PREPARING FOR PHYSICAL EXAMINATION

A. Equipment needed

1. Basic equipment for a brief physical assessment includes blood pressure cuff, clean disposable gloves, drape, penlight, stethoscope, tape measure, thermometer, watch with a second hand, and weight scale
2. Additional equipment for a complete physical examination includes cotton ball, doppler, goniometer, hammer, lubricant, nasal speculum, near vision charts, neurologic hammer, ophthalmoscope, otoscope, reflex hammer, skin calipers, Snellen visual acuity chart, strabismoscope, tongue depressor/blade, tuning fork, tympanometer, and vaginal speculum; the nurse generalist may not conduct these aspects of exam but may need to set up exam room

B. Promoting comfort during physical assessment

1. Provide a comfortable room and minimize distractions
2. Ensure client privacy
3. Provide adequate lighting and normalize room temperature

IV. TECHNIQUES OF PHYSICAL EXAMINATION

A. Inspection

1. Utilizes observation to obtain important information about a client's state of health; also includes sense of smell
2. Ensure adequate lighting to visually inspect body without distortions or shadows; lighting can be sunlight or artificial
3. Items to assess using skill of inspection
   a. Overall appearance
   b. Demeanor, eye contact
   c. Interactions with other health care professionals and family
   d. Skin color, hair, nail beds, skeletal deformities
   e. Clothing appropriate for weather conditions
   f. Congruence of verbal and nonverbal behavior
   g. Sense of smell: any odors

B. Palpation

1. A physical assessment technique that utilizes touch to obtain important information about a client's state of health
2. Uses sensation of touch and pressure of hands and fingers to determine masses, elevations, temperature, organ position, and any abnormal findings
3. Ulnar surfaces of hands and fingers are most common areas used for palpation; hands should be warm and gentle; wear gloves as appropriate to area being examined

4. Can be light (1 cm in depth) or deep (4 cm in depth) depending on area of body being examined; nurse controls amount of pressure; deep palpation should occur after light palpation; most nurses use light palpation during physical examination, while deep palpation is used during a complete physical conducted by primary care provider

C. Percussion

1. A skill in which finger of one hand touches or taps a finger of other hand to generate vibration, which in turn produces a specific, diagnostic sound; sound changes as practitioner moves from one area to next
2. Sounds can be classified as tympanic, hyperresonant, resonant, dull, or flat; further description and examples of percussion notes can be found in Table 16–1 ■

D. Auscultation

1. ! Place stethoscope over bare skin to eliminate alterations in sound caused by clothing
2. Listen to sound, duration, pitch, and intensity
3. ! Must isolate sounds; if client has a large amount of chest or back hair, wet hair to flatten it and diminish extra sounds
4. Allot enough time to listen carefully to produced sounds; if in doubt, consult another health care professional for a second opinion

V. PHYSICAL EXAMINATION OF THE ADULT

A. Various purposes of physical assessment

1. Full examination by health care provider as part of wellness screening (annually or as recommended)
2. Full history and physical assessment done at time of hospital admission
3. Head-to-toe assessment at beginning of shift for hospitalized clients
4. Focused or body system–specific assessments that may be done frequently (more than once per shift, such as every 4 hours)

B. Vital signs

1. Temperature: average is 37°C or 98.6°F (normal range 35.8°C to 37.3°C or 96.4°F to 99.1°F); varies slightly depending on age, time of day, phase of menstrual cycle, exercise level, and method of measurement (rectal measures 1° higher than oral, axillary measures 1° lower than oral); measure using oral, rectal, axillary, or otic (tympanic membrane) route
2. Pulse: average is 68 to 78 beats per minute (bpm) in adult with a range of 60 to 100
   a. Radial: count the rate and rhythm and note amplitude
   b. Apical: listen for a full minute and compare to radial pulse; place stethoscope on chest at fifth intercostal space, midclavicular line (5ICS, MCL)
   c. Rhythm should be regular; if pulse is irregular, assess whether rhythm is regularly irregular or irregularly irregular and alert health care provider
3. Respiration: normal rate in adult is 12 to 20 breaths/minute; count rate, rhythm, and depth of respiration; note comfort level as client breathes; normal respirations are relaxed, silent, automatic, and regular
4. Blood pressure (BP): normal range is 100/60 mmHg to 130/85 mmHg in adult; varies with age, gender, weight, exercise, emotion, stress, and diurnal rhythm (early morning low and late afternoon/early evening high)
   a. Have person sit or lie down with arm supported at heart level; allow a 5-minute rest period with no activity, smoking, eating, or drinking before measuring BP

Table 16–1 Percussion Notes

Tone	Quality	Pitch	Example
Tympany	Drumlike	High	Gastric bubble
Resonance	Hollow	Low	Healthy lungs
Hyperresonance	Booming	Very loud	Emphysemic lung tissue
Flatness	Very dull	High	Muscle, bone
Dullness	Thudlike	Soft to moderate	Liver, spleen, heart

! **b.** If there is a question about BP, wait 1 to 2 minutes before taking it again to avoid falsely high diastolic readings

c. If unable to hear BP, take a palpated BP by placing index finger over brachial artery, inflating cuff, deflating cuff while palpating, and noting when pulsation disappears; only systolic pressure is noted and recorded as palpated

d. If client has poor circulation, BP may be faint; in this case or if BP cannot even be palpated, it is wise to use a doppler to hear sounds; note systolic pressure only and record as a doppler BP

C. Height and weight

1. Height: using a balance scale, raise headpiece on measuring pole and align it with the top of head while client is shoeless, standing erect, and looking forward
2. Weight: use platform scale if client can stand without assistance; special electronic scales and bed scales are also available if needed
3. ! Use professionally authorized charts to determine if client's height and weight fall within normal limits for age; also compare readings to client's own previous measurements

D. General appearance

1. Includes client's grooming and attire and personal hygiene
2. Includes gait and posture, general body build, and behavior

E. Mental status

1. A short mental status exam is often done during health history interview; assess client for overt signs of mental distress, crying, sullen demeanor, appropriate comments for situation
2. ! Four key areas of functioning

a. Appearance: as noted in previous section

b. Behavior: level of consciousness (LOC), awake, alert, aware of and responding to internal and external stimuli; lethargic and drowsy, stuporous, or unresponsive (use Glasgow coma scale for additional information); facial expression, speech (quality, pace, articulation of words, word choice); aphasia (receptive/Wernicke's, motor/expressive/Broca's, global), mood and affect

c. Cognition: orientation (to time, place, person, and events), attention span, recent memory, remote memory, new learning (four unrelated words test), judgment

d. Thought processes: includes thought content (logical, consistent), client's perceptions (reality-based, congruent with others), and absence/presence of suicidal thoughts/ideation

Memory Aid

Remember the four key areas of mental status (appearance, behavior, cognition, and thought processes) by using the abbreviation ABCT.

e. The Mini-Mental State Exam (Folstein) may be used to gather this data; requires 5 to 10 minutes to administer; highest score is 30 (average people score 27)

f. A full mental status examination may be done if indicated, and other tests can be added to gather data when problems exist (brain lesions or cerebrovascular accident, aphasia, mental illness, memory changes, alcoholism, and others)

F. Integument

1. Skin provides first layer of protection for body, protecting against infection and trauma and preventing fluid loss; it also regulates body temperature, provides sensory perception, produces vitamin D, excretes sweat and impurities, and is a barometer of emotions
2. Inspection of skin

a. Assess skin for color; look at entire body, including areas that are not usually exposed

! **b.** Daylight is best light to detect jaundice (yellowing of skin, sclera); use good lighting for best illumination; flashlights/penlights are also very helpful for general inspection

c. Scan body for color, texture, tone, distribution of lesions, skin symmetry, differences between body areas, evidence of rashes or eruptions, hygiene
d. Inspect body for color; compare areas that are exposed to sun and those that are not
e. Assess moles (pigmented nevi) for defining features such as symmetry, elevation, color, and texture
f. Normal findings: range of skin color varies from person to person; color should be uniform; sun-exposed areas will be darker; calluses appear yellow; nevi (moles) can be normal findings
! g. Abnormal findings: color changes in moles (could indicate cancerous changes); pale, shiny skin of the lower extremities (may indicate decreased peripheral circulation or diabetes mellitus); localized hemorrhages into cutaneous tissues (petechiae less than 0.5 cm in diameter or purpura more than 0.5 cm in diameter) that appear purple-red (could indicate injury, steroid use, or vasculitis)

3. Palpation of skin
   a. Feel skin for moisture, temperature, texture, turgor, and mobility; pinch skin to test turgor; skin should immediately return to normal but will be altered if edema or dehydration is present
   b. Normal findings: skin should be cool to warm, dry, and smooth under normal conditions; in stressful situations, skin may feel cool and clammy; assess skin by touching bilaterally and comparing findings
   ! c. Abnormal findings: lesions (provide descriptions of size, shape, color, texture, elevation/depression, pedunculation, exudates, configuration, location, and distribution)
4. Inspection of nails
   a. Inspect for color, contour, texture, configuration, symmetry, and cleanliness
   b. Nails offer a quick assessment of individual and cleanliness; note whether they are clean and well-manicured, bitten down, yellow and tobacco-stained; color should be pink with a brisk capillary refill (less than 3 seconds) when depressed (blanch test)
   c. Normal findings: nail plate is smooth and flat or slightly convex; nail base angle is 160 degrees
   d. Abnormal findings: white bands can indicate melanoma; white spots can indicate cuticle manipulation or trauma; yellow can indicate psoriasis, fungal infections, and chronic respiratory diseases; diffuse darkening can indicate malaria medication, candidal infection, hyperbilirubinemia, or chronic trauma; a green-black color can indicate pseudomonas infection or nail bed trauma (subungual hematoma)
5. Palpation of nails: should be hard and smooth with uniform thickness
   a. Squeeze nail; if it separates from nail bed, can indicate psoriasis or trauma
   b. A clubbed boggy nail can indicate infection with candida or pseudomonas

G. Head and neck

1. Inspection
   a. Head should be erect and still with symmetrical facial features
   b. Assess structure, conjunctiva, sclera, cornea, and iris of each eye
   c. Assess position, alignment, skin condition, and external meatus of ear
   d. Inspect external nose
   e. Inspect inside of mouth and throat (mucosa, tongue, teeth and gums, floor of mouth, palate, uvula)
   f. Assess for tics, spasms, lesions, and facial paralysis
   g. Neck should be symmetrical without masses
2. Palpation: palpate from front to back, assessing for smoothness and symmetry of cranium, scalp, and hair; palpate temporal artery; palpate salivary glands; palpate temporal artery and temporomandibular joint; palpate maxillary and frontal sinuses; push on tragus of ear for tenderness; palpate thyroid gland (for size, shape, tenderness, and presence of nodules)—stand behind client and use two fingers of each hand on sides of trachea, then displace trachea to left and

ask client to swallow (thyroid should feel smooth, small, and free of nodules); palpate for midline position of trachea
3. Inspect and palpate cervical lymph nodes
4. Special testing
   a. Eyes: test visual fields (confrontation), extraocular movements, pupil size, equality, roundness, and response to light and accommodation (PERRLA); check ocular fundus (with an ophthalmoscope) for red reflex, condition of optic disc, blood vessels and background of retina; may be documented under neurological exam
   b. Ears: use an otoscope to inspect the ear canal and tympanic membrane (should be movable, intact, and pearly white-gray in color); use tuning fork to do Rinne and Weber tests to check for bone and air conduction in hearing (see section on neurological exam for further information); may be documented under neurological exam
   c. Nose: use a nasal speculum to check the nasal mucosa, septum, and turbinates

H. Breasts and axillae

1. With client in a sitting position, inspect breasts for symmetry, contour, and shape; should be rounded, generally symmetrical
2. Look for areas of discoloration, hyperpigmentation, dimpling or retraction, swelling or edema; should be uniform in color, smooth, and elastic
3. Detect any areas of retraction by asking client to do three maneuvers: raise arms above head, push hands together with elbows flexed, and press hands down on hips
4. Observe areola for size, shape, symmetry, color, general surface characteristics, lesions or masses; should be round or oval, and color may vary among individuals, from light pink to dark brown
5. Inspect nipples for size, shape, position, color, and presence of any discharge or lesions; should be round, everted, and equal in size
6. Palpate axillary, subclavicular, and supraclavicular lymph nodes using palmar surface of the fingertips in the following four areas: edge of greater pectoral muscle in the anterior axillary line, thoracic wall in midaxilla, upper portion of humerus, anterior edge of latissimus dorsi muscle in posterior axillary line
7. Palpate breast for masses and tenderness, using one of the following three patterns: hands-of-the-clock, spokes-on-a-wheel, concentric circles; there should be no masses or tenderness
8. Palpate areola and nipples for masses; there should be none

I. Chest

1. Lungs
   a. Use standard thoracic landmarks when performing respiratory assessment
   b. Inspection: note overall appearance, nutritional status (dyspnea can impair oral intake), ability to breathe, respirations (bradypnea, tachypnea, shortness of breath, dyspnea), contour and movement of chest (should be symmetrical); note presence of retractions and the color of skin, nail beds, and lips
   c. Palpation: assess posterior aspect of chest for masses, bulges, muscle tone, subcutaneous emphysema (crepitus), and areas of tenderness
   d. Palpation: assess respiratory expansion by placing hands on eighth to tenth ribs (posterior); place thumbs close to vertebrae; slide hand medially and grasp a small fold of skin between thumbs; ask client to take a deep breath; thumbs should move evenly away from vertebrae during inspiration; note any delay in expansion
   e. Palpation: assess tactile fremitus (a palpable vibration that transmits sounds via patent bronchi to lung parenchyma and chest wall) by placing ulnar surface of hand or balls of fingers (palmar base) on outer chest wall; ask client to speak words "ninety-nine" or "blue moon"; begin palpating at lung apices and work from one side to other moving down posterior chest (but not over scapula); vibration should be equal on both sides in any location; decreased fremitus occurs with conditions that obstruct transmission of vibrations (pleural effusion, pneumothorax, and others); increased fremitus occurs with

consolidation or compression of lung tissue (such as in extensive lobar pneumonia with patent bronchus)

f. Percussion: have client lean forward slightly; begin by percussing over apex of left lung; then move hands systematically and compare percussion notes lobe to lobe and side to side; to determine excursion, locate 7th intercostal space and percuss downward along scapular line to diaphragm; mark line where resonance changes to dullness; have client take a deep breath and hold; mark second line; distance should be between 3 and 6 cm

! **g.** Auscultation: use flat diaphragm of stethoscope to listen systematically to posterior and anterior chest; begin posteriorly and listen from apices (at C7 level) to bases (at about T10), and laterally from axilla to 7th or 8th rib; normal sounds include bronchial, bronchovesicular, and vesicular; compare findings side to side while working downward over posterior chest (see Table 16–2 ■ for description of various adventitious breath sounds); note location, quality, and time of occurrence during respiratory cycle

h. Other abnormal findings during auscultation include bronchophony (ask client to repeat words "ninety-nine"; if heard clearly, indicates lung density in that area); egophony (ask client to say "ee-ee-ee-ee" during auscultation; sound changes to a long "aaaa" sound in areas of consolidation or compression); whispered pectoriloquy (ask client to say "one-two-three" during auscultation; sound will be faint yet clear and distinct with small amounts of consolidation); pleural friction rub (sounds like a grating, creaking, or groaning noise, often more noticeable on inspiration, and may be heard over inflamed areas of parietal and visceral pleura)

i. Repeat entire assessment process with anterior chest

2. Neck vessels

! **a.** Palpate carotid arteries *one at a time* in area medial to sternomastoid muscle; avoid area higher in neck to prevent stimulating baroreceptors and triggering bradycardia from vagus nerve stimulation; note contour and amplitude of pulse and compare findings side to side

b. Auscultate over carotid arteries for bruits using bell of stethoscope; sound should be absent; if bruit present, note whether it sounds like a buzzing, swishing, or blowing sound; bruit indicates turbulent blood flow from obstruction (i.e., atherosclerotic narrowing of carotid vessel)

c. Assess jugular vein distention (head of bed at 30 degrees; turn head slightly away; highest pulsation should be no more than 1.5 inches above sternal notch

3. Heart

a. Inspection: general appearance of client and color of skin and nail beds; observe for symmetry of movement, anatomical defects, retractions, pulsations, and heaves; locate point of maximal impulse (PMI) if visible (usually at the apex, 5th intercostal space, midclavicular line)

b. Palpate PMI (not visible in all clients) with ball of hand, then fingertips; next assess for abnormal pulsations in the sternoclavicular, aortic, pulmonic, tricuspid, and epigastric areas; palpate for thrills (over areas of turbulent blood flow)

! **c.** Auscultate in predetermined sequence (see Figure 16–2 ■) for S_1, S_2, extra heart sounds (S_3 and S_4) and murmurs; see Table 16–3 ■ for heart sounds;

Table 16–2

Adventitious Breath Sounds

Sound	Characteristics	Timing and Occurrence
Crackles (coarse)	Popping, frying sound; moist, low-pitched	Inspiration, some expiration
Crackles (medium)	Not as loud as coarse crackles	Middle of inspiration
Crackles (fine)	Noncontinuous, popping, high-pitched	End of inspiration
Rhonchi or gurgles	Continuous, low-pitched, prolonged	Expiration
Wheezes	Continuous, high-pitched, musical	Inspiration and/or expiration
Pleural friction rub	Low-pitched, dry, grating	Inspiration and/or expiration

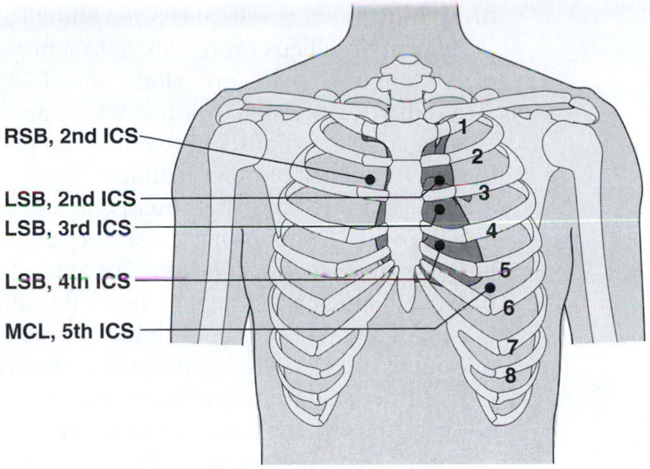

Figure 16-2

Sites for auscultation of the heart. Aortic valve area: RSB, 2nd ICS; pulmonic valve area: LSB, 2nd ICS; tricuspid valve area: LLSB, 4th ICS; mitral valve area: left MCL, 5th ICS

place client in three positions for complete assessment: lying on back with head of bed at 30 degrees, sitting up, and lying on left side; use the diaphragm of the stethoscope (to detect higher pitched sounds) and then bell (to detect lower pitched sounds)

Memory Aid

Moving from left to right and top to bottom (as when reading), remember the location of valvular heart sounds by remembering **A**ll **P**atients **T**ake **M**eds (**A**ortic, **P**ulmonic, **T**ricuspid, **M**itral). These sounds are best heard "downstream" from the actual flow of blood through the valve, giving their unique auscultatory locations.

d. Percussion: can be done to locate cardiac border, where sound changes from resonance to dullness; not often performed because chest x-ray is used to determine cardiac size

J. Abdomen

1. Preparation: ask client to empty bladder before exam; position client supine with a small pillow under head; bend client's knees or place a pillow under them; expose abdomen fully; place client's arms at sides or across chest (not over head because it tenses abdominal muscles); warm examiner's hands and stethoscope and ensure that fingernails are short; keep room warm to prevent chilling; use distraction techniques as needed
2. Inspection: four quadrants for contour, symmetry, bumps, bulges, or masses; note skin color (redness, jaundice) and condition (striae, scars), umbilicus, hair distribution, and any pulsations or movements of abdomen

! **a.** A bulge may indicate a distended bladder or hernia; look at shape and contour

Table 16-3

Heart Sounds

Sound	Location	Description	Character	Significance
S_1	Apex	Lub	Low-pitched and dull	Closure of mitral and tricuspid valves
S_2	Base	Dub	Shorter, more high-pitched than S_1	Closure of pulmonic and aortic valves
S_3	Apex	"Ken-tuck-y"	Low-pitched	Ventricles filling rapidly
S_4	Tricuspid or mitral areas	"Ten-ness-ee"	Occurs just before S_1 after atrial contraction	Increased resistance to ventricular filling
Pericardial friction rub	Left sternal border	Grating, leathery	Muffled, high-pitched, and transient	Pericardial inflammation

b. Midline umbilicus: to assess for umbilical hernia, have client lift arms over head; if umbilicus protrudes, hernia may be present
c. Abdominal movements: slight, wavelike movements are normal, especially in a thin person; visible rippling waves may indicate obstruction

! 3. Auscultation: must auscultate before palpation and percussion to avoid increasing the frequency of bowel sounds
a. Place diaphragm of stethoscope lightly against skin in right lower quadrant, where bowel sounds are most frequent (location of ileocecal valve)
b. Listen in a clockwise fashion for at least 2 minutes
c. Note character and quality; normal sounds are high-pitched and gurgling at a rate of 5 to 34 times per minute
d. Sounds are classified as normal, hypoactive (heard infrequently), or hyperactive (loud, high-pitched, more frequent than normal)
e. Use bell of stethoscope for vascular sounds over iliac, aortic, renal, and femoral arteries; listen for bruits, venous hums, and friction rubs

4. Percussion: do not percuss if abdominal aortic aneurysm is present or suspected
a. Detects size and location of abdominal organs
b. Percuss in all four quadrants
c. Tympany indicates an area of empty stomach or bowel
d. Dullness is normally heard over liver (used to estimate size), kidney, full bladder, and feces-filled intestines

5. Palpation: with warm hands, palpate lightly (about 1 cm deep with four fingers positioned close together) using a rotary motion in all areas to assess skin surface and superficial musculature; then repeat sequence deeply (about 4 to 6 cm) to determine size, shape, position and tenderness of organs
a. Light palpation helps detect superficial masses and fluid accumulation; a normal finding is an abdomen that is soft and not tender
b. Deep palpation can identify masses, tenderness, pulsations, organ enlargement (liver, spleen, kidneys); usually done by primary care provider or advanced practice nurse
c. If a mass is found, note its location, size, shape, consistency (hard, firm, or soft), type of surface (smooth or nodular), mobility, pulsatility, and tenderness
! d. If a mass is noted to be pulsatile, stop palpating in that area to avoid rupture
! e. Identify rebound tenderness: if an area is tender to light palpation or if client reports pain in an area, move hand to an area away from painful site, and position hand perpendicular (at a 90-degree angle) in relation to abdomen; push down slowly and deeply and then lift up quickly; normally there is no pain or tenderness, but if present (often severe and accompanied by muscle rigidity), it indicates peritoneal inflammation, possibly appendicitis or peritonitis from another disorder
f. Abdominal pain: indicates possible ulcers, intestinal obstruction, cholecystitis, peritonitis
g. Ascites: use a tape measure at fullest site on abdomen, usually at or near umbilicus
h. Inguinal area: palpate each groin for femoral pulse and inguinal nodes

K. Extremities

! 1. Inspect bilaterally for symmetry, skin characteristics, and distribution of hair; hair loss, thin shiny skin, and thickened toenails in older adults are called trophic changes and are often caused by decreased circulation from peripheral arterial disease resulting from atherosclerosis
2. Palpate peripheral pulses; in upper extremities, includes radial and ulnar pulses; in lower extremities, includes popliteal, dorsalis pedis (DP), and posterior tibial (PT) pulses
! 3. Palpate the skin for pretibial or other edema and to note temperature of extremities; compare side-to-side bilaterally
4. Separate toes and inspect them

L. Musculoskeletal

1. Inspect each joint for size, contour, masses, and deformity; measure any discrepancies in extremity (leg) length
2. Palpate each joint for musculature, bony articulations, and crepitation; assess for heat, swelling, or tenderness
3. Test range of motion (ROM) of joints of upper extremities (shoulders, elbows, wrists, and fingers) and lower extremities (hips, knees, ankles, and toes); describe any physical limitations; if less than full ROM is present, a goniometer may be used in a full exam to measure joint angles more precisely
4. Note the size, tone, and any involuntary movements of major muscle groups; compare findings bilaterally
5. Test strength of major muscle groups that control joints in upper and lower extremities by asking client to resist attempts to put joint through ROM; grading scale ranges from grade 0: no contraction to grade 5: full ROM against gravity and full resistance
6. ! Test ROM in spine by asking client to bend forward and touch toes (flexion should be 75 to 90 degrees with no curvature side to side; if curvature present, suspect and further assess for scoliosis), bend sideways (35 degrees of flexion normal), bend backward (hyperextension of 30 degrees normal), and twist shoulders from one side to other (rotation of 30 degrees bilaterally normal)
7. ! Straight leg-raising (with knee straight) should not be painful; if it is, suspect herniated nucleus pulposus (in intervertebral disk)
8. Note any musculoskeletal pain present during assessment; pain description should be very specific
   a. Bone pain: pain unrelated to movement unless fracture is present, deep, aching, and continuous; it also causes insomnia
   b. Muscle pain: cramps or spasms with possible relationship to posture or movement; tremors, twitches, or weakness may be manifested; muscle tension may produce referred pain
   c. Joint pain: joint may be tender to palpation; referred pain can be present; nerve root irritation may produce radiculitis (pain is distal); mechanical joint pain is worse with movement and worsens throughout day

M. Neurologic

1. Assess cranial nerves; see Table 16–4 ■ for a summary of normal and abnormal findings
   a. Olfactory nerve (CN I): not tested routinely but use items with different smells (alcohol, coffee, vanilla, peppermint, etc.) to detect abnormalities in sense of smell; test one nostril at a time if performed; sense of smell generally diminishes with aging
   b. Optic nerve (CN II): test visual acuity with Snellen chart, test visual fields by confrontation, and use an ophthalmoscope to examine fundus of eye (refer back to section G on examination of head and neck)
   c. Oculomotor, trochlear, and abducens nerves (CN III, IV, VI): assess pupils for size (in mm), equality, roundness, reactivity to light, and accommodation (PERRLA); assess extraocular movements by asking client to visually follow a finger through cardinal fields of gaze; observe for nystagmus (rapid back-and-forth oscillating movements of eyes in a horizontal or vertical plane, rotary direction, or combination)
   d. Trigeminal nerve (CN V): assess motor function by palpating temporal and masseter muscles while asking client to clench teeth and by trying to separate jaws by pushing down on chin; assess sensory function by touching client's face bilaterally in three divisions of nerve (ophthalmic, maxillary, and mandibular) and asking client to say "now" when face is touched with a wisp of cotton; test corneal reflex if necessary (may be omitted in a screening exam) by lightly touching cornea with a wisp of cotton brought in from the side of client's face
   e. Facial nerve (CN VII): test motor function by asking client to smile, frown, close eyes tightly (while examiner tries to keep them open), lift eyebrows,

Table 16–4

Cranial Nerve Assessment

Cranial Nerve(s)	Assessment	Normal	Abnormal
CN I	Smell	Can identify common substances	Difficulty detecting common substances
CN II	Visual acuity	Able to read; visual fields intact	Visual field defects
CN III, IV, VI	Extraocular movements, elevation of eyelids, pupil constriction	Can elevate eyes, PERRLA, eyeball movement present	Drooping of the eye, ptosis, unequal pupils
CN V	Sensory: corneas, nasal and oral mucosa, facial skin Motor: jaw and chewing muscles	Sensory: able to detect both sharp and dull sensations when face touched with pointed or blunt object Motor: clenches teeth while palpating temporal and masseter muscles	Inability to feel or identify facial stimuli; muscle weakness Pertinent disorder: trigeminal neuralgia
CN VII	Sensory: taste on anterior portion of tongue Motor: facial muscles	Sensory: can discriminate sweet, sour, and salty tastes Motor: facial symmetry present at rest and when frowning and smiling	If neurological impairment, entire side of face could be immobile Pertinent disorders: Bell's palsy, stroke
CN VIII	Hearing and equilibrium	Cochlear (hearing): • Whisper test: client can repeat what was said • Weber test: sound lateralizes equally • Rinne test: sound heard normally twice as long by air conduction (AC) as bone conduction (BC) Vestibular (equilibrium): normal balance, absence of nystagmus	Whisper: sensorineural hearing loss Weber: Sound lateralizes to bad ear with conductive hearing loss or to good ear with sensorineural hearing loss Rinne: AC equal to or less than BC with conductive hearing loss; AC-to-BC ratio normal but reduced overall with sensorineural hearing loss Vestibular: problems with gait or balance; presence of nystagmus
CN IX, X	Swallowing, salivating, taste perception, voice quality	Client swallows; gag reflex present; with tongue depressor against posterior pharynx, client says *ahh;* movement of soft palate and uvula present	Soft palate does not rise; deviation of soft palate and uvula, no gag reflex, dysphagia, hoarseness, taste abnormalities
CN XI	Strength of sternocleidomastoid muscles and upper portion of trapezius	Client shrugs shoulders with equal strength bilaterally	Drooping shoulders, asymmetric muscle contraction
CN XII	Tongue movement in swallowing and speech	Tongue protrudes in midline; client pushes tongue into cheek against resistance from examiner	Tongue atrophy and fasciculation, deviation

puff cheeks, and show teeth; test sensory function (not done routinely) by asking client to identify salty, sweet, or sour solutions applied to tongue

f. Acoustic or vestibulocochlear nerve (CN VIII): use voice test (whispered words from 1 to 2 feet away) to determine hearing ability; do the Weber test by placing a vibrating tuning fork on midline of skull and asking whether sound is heard equally in both ears or is better in one ear than the other; do Rinne test by placing a vibrating tuning fork on client's mastoid process and asking client to indicate when sound disappears; quickly invert tuning fork and place vibrating end near ear canal and ask client to indicate when sound is no longer heard

g. Glossopharyngeal and vagus nerves (CN IX and X): using a tongue blade, note pharyngeal movement when client says "ahh" or yawns; watch for uvula and soft palate to rise in midline and for tonsilar pillars to move medially; test gag reflex by touching posterior pharyngeal wall with tongue blade; note voice quality (should be smooth with no straining)

h. Spinal accessory nerve (CN XI): ask client to rotate head forcibly against resistance applied to other side of chin; ask client to shrug shoulders against resistance (all findings should be equal bilaterally); examine sternomastoid and trapezius muscles for size

i. Hypoglossal nerve (CN XII): inspect tongue; ask client to protrude tongue (should stay in midline); ask client to say words such as "light, dynamite, tight" to determine that lingual speech (the letters l, t, d, n) is clear

2. Assess motor system: inspect and palpate muscles as described in previous section

3. Assess cerebellar function

a. Observe gait after asking client to walk 10 to 20 feet, turn, and return to starting point; efforts should be rhythmic, smooth, and without effort; step length should be about 15 inches (heel to heel); next ask client to walk heel-to-toe in a straight line (should be able to do this and maintain balance)

! **b.** Romberg test: ask client to stand with feet together and arms at sides, close the eyes, and hold this position for 20 seconds; client should be able to maintain posture with minimal to no swaying, but stand close by to catch client if he or she falls

c. Other tests of cerebellar function include hopping on one leg; rapid alternating movements test (patting knees with palms of hands and then back of hands quickly or touching each finger to thumb, one hand at a time), finger-to-finger test (touching examiner's finger and then own nose); finger-to-nose test (touching own nose with eyes closed after stretching out arm); and heel-to-shin test (placing heel of one foot on other knee and running it down leg to heel); these movements should be done smoothly or in a straight line, depending on test

4. Assess sensory system

a. Requires client to be alert, cooperative, have an adequate attention span, and be in a comfortable position

b. Test client's ability to discriminate light pain (with a sharp object such as a pin) and touch (with a dull object such as a cotton wisp or pencil eraser), to detect temperature (warm water versus cold), vibration (placement of a vibrating tuning fork on various points of body), stereognosis (recognition of objects placed in hand while eyes are closed), graphesthesia (ability to determine a number traced on palm of hand) with eyes closed, two-point discrimination (ability to detect two separate stimuli, generally varies depending on area of body; fingertips are most sensitive at 2 to 8 mm; upper arms, thighs, and back are least sensitive at 40 to 75 mm)

5. Assess deep tendon reflexes using a reflex hammer

a. Have limb relaxed and muscle partly stretched; strike reflex hammer on insertion tendon of biceps (C5 to C6), triceps (C7 to C8), brachioradialis (C5 to C6), quadriceps or "knee jerk" (L2 to L4), and Achilles or "ankle jerk" (S1 to S2)

b. Reflexes are graded on a scale of 0 to 4 with 0 being absent and 4 being brisk or hyperactive; a rating of 2 is normal

6. Assess superficial reflexes
   a. Abdominal (upper T8 to T10; lower T10 to T12): stroke skin with a smooth object from one side of abdomen toward midline; abdominal muscle contracts on side of stimulus (ipsilateral response) and umbilicus deviates toward stroke; perform at both upper and lower end of abdomen
   b. Cremasteric reflex (L1 to L2): lightly stroke inner aspect of thigh of a male client with a reflex hammer or tongue blade and watch for elevation of ipsilateral testicle
   ! c. Plantar reflex or Babinski reflex (L4 to S2): use same object to stroke upward on lateral sole of foot and across ball of foot; normal (negative) response in adult is flexion of toes and possibly whole foot; an abnormal or positive response (which is normal in infants) is dorsiflexion of big toe and fanning of other toes

N. Genitals/rectum

1. Perianal region
   a. Don gloves and spread buttocks to visualize site
   b. Inspect for hemorrhoids, blood, fissures, scars, lesions, rectal prolapse, discharge
   c. Palpation: rectal exam is done by an experienced or advanced practice nurse; purpose is to palpate for rectal masses and assess stool for blood
2. Male genitalia
   a. Inspection: hair distribution in pubic region; penis (note presence of dorsal vein; urethral meatus appears slitlike; note bumps, blisters, redness, lesions, and masses; assess underlying skin after moving pubic hair); scrotum should be loose, wrinkled, with deeply pigmented pouch at base of penis; two compartments house testicles (oval, rubbery, suspended vertically and slightly forward in the scrotum); may appear asymmetrical because left testicle has a longer spermatic cord
   b. Palpation: use thumb and first two fingers; area is sensitive to gentle compression; penis should feel smooth, semifirm, and nontender; testicles should feel smooth, rubbery, and moveable with no nodules, lumps, swelling, soreness, masses, or lesions
3. Female genitalia
   a. Inspect external genitalia: mons pubis, labia majora, labia minora, clitoris, vagina, urethra, and Skene's and Bartholin's glands; with gloved hands, spread labia and assess urethral meatus; should be a pink, slitlike midline opening; labia majora and minora should be moist and free from swelling, lesions, discharge, and unusual odors
   b. Palpate external genitalia: spread labia and palpate; should feel smooth
   c. Internal genitalia examination and rectovaginal palpation are usually done by an advanced practice nurse, not a nurse generalist

O. Postexamination responsibilities

1. Provide tissues or assist client to cleanse lubricant/secretions as needed
2. Remove drape
3. Allow client opportunity or assistance to get dressed
4. Leave client in comfortable position
5. ! Document data clearly and immediately; compare findings to established norms and to previous findings; note specimens obtained during examination
6. ! Handle specimens collected during screening in a manner consistent with standard precautions; label specimens completely and send to laboratory with requisition attached according to agency policy

VI. PHYSICAL EXAMINATION OF THE CHILD

A. General considerations

1. Developmental level of child is most important consideration for a successful assessment (see Table 16–5 ■)
2. ! Use terms understandable to and appropriate for child and parents; encourage active participation of child or parents when possible; reassure child throughout examination

Table 16–5 Age-Specific Approaches to Physical Examination

Age	Approach
Infant	Child lying flat or held in parent's arms Use distraction with older infant Assess heart, pulse, lungs, respirations while quiet, then head to toe Eyes, ears, and mouth near end Check reflexes as body parts are examined Moro reflex last
Toddler	Minimal contact initially Allow to inspect equipment Assess heart and lungs while quiet, then head to toe Eyes, ears, and mouth last
Preschool	Allow to inspect equipment Head to toe if cooperative Same as toddler if uncooperative
School age	Respect privacy and explain procedures Head to toe with genitalia last
Adolescent	Explain proceedings and proceed as for school-age child

3. Allow child to become familiar with examiner prior to beginning examination
4. ! Save distressful or intrusive parts of examination for last
5. ! Prepare child and parents for new or painful procedures
6. Examine child in a comfortable and secure position

B. Methods of restraint !

1. May be necessary with infants, toddlers, or uncooperative children
2. When examining eyes, ears, nose, or throat, examiner may need to have a parent or other adult hold child supine with arms extended alongside head
3. "Hug" method has child sit on parent's lap with legs to one side and one arm tucked under parent's arm while parent holds other arm securely; child's legs may need to be held between parent's legs to prevent kicking
4. Ask another adult for assistance if parent is distressed and cannot help

C. Growth measurements

1. Plot results on growth charts; length/height to age, weight to age, length to weight
2. ! Overall pattern of growth is more important than any single measurement
3. ! Use 5th and 95th percentiles for determining which children are outside normal limits
4. Length/height
   a. Recumbent length (birth up to 36 months) with child supine and legs extended; use a horizontal measuring board; avoid using a tape measure because readings are often inaccurate; extend an infant's legs to obtain true length because infants tend to flex legs while at rest
   b. Use crown-to-heel measurement
   c. Children older than 2 or 3 years may stand shoeless as straight as possible
   d. A wall-mounted ruler can be used to measure height of small children if they have difficulty standing erect on a scale
5. Weight
   a. Weigh naked infant lying or sitting; measure infants on a platform-type balance scale; ensure calibration by noting that beam is balanced when weight is set to zero
   b. Weigh older children on upright scale dressed only in underpants or light gown
6. Head circumference
   a. ! Measure at every physical assessment for infants and toddlers under 2 years; always measure head circumference of child suspected of having a neurological problem or developmental delay
   b. Is best indication of brain growth
   c. Place measuring tape (paper or nonstretching tape) over most prominent part of occiput and just above supraorbital ridges

d. Make three measurements and take average as number to record
e. Percentiles should be comparable to child's height and weight
f. Head circumference exceeds chest circumference until between 1 and 2 years of age

7. Chest circumference
a. Is usually measured at birth and during early infancy
b. Place measuring tape at nipple level with child supine
c. Take measurement midway between inspiration and expiration
d. Head and chest circumference should be approximately equal between 1 and 2 years of age
e. During childhood, chest circumference exceeds head circumference by 2 to 3 inches

D. Vital signs (see Table 16–6 ■)

1. Temperature
a. Rectal, axillary, skin, or tympanic when assessing infants
b. Oral route may be used in children over 4 years of age
c. Use rectal only when necessary because of discomfort and intrusiveness
d. May be altered by exercise, crying, stress, or environmental conditions

2. Pulse
a. Newborn average is 120 bpm (range of 70 to 190) and decreases with increasing age
b. Try to take with child at rest, sleeping, or lying quietly
c. Take an apical pulse for children younger than 2 years and a radial pulse in children over 2 years of age
d. Count for one full minute
e. May be altered by anxiety, activity, pain, crying, medications, or disease
f. Record rate, rhythm, quality, and amplitude

3. Respirations
a. Try to take while child is at rest, sleeping, or lying quietly
b. Measure in infants and young children by observing abdominal movements; measure in older children by observing rise and fall of chest
c. Record rate, rhythm, and quality
d. May be altered by anxiety, activity, medications, fever, or disease

4. Blood pressure
a. Measure annually in children over 3 years of age
b. Select cuff width that covers 75% of length of upper arm
c. Cuff should encircle arm circumference without overlapping
d. Use Doppler or electronic device for infants
e. May be altered by anxiety, activity, crying, medications, or disease

Table 16–6

Normal Vital Signs for Infants and Children

Age	Average Pulse	Average Respirations	Average Blood Pressure
Newborn	120	35	73/50
1 year	120	30	90/56
2 years	110	25	91/55
4 years	100	25	92/55
6 years	100	22	96/57
10 years	90	20	100/61
14 years			
Female	85	16	114/65
Male	80	16	114/65
18 years			
Female	75	16	120/70
Male	70	16	120/70

E. General appearance

1. Cumulative, subjective impression of a child's physical appearance, nutrition status, behavior, hygiene, personality, posture and body movement, interactions with parents and nurse, speech and development
2. Observe **facies** (facial expression and appearance of child) for clues about illness, pain, fear, and so on

F. Skin, hair, and nails

1. Inspect and palpate
2. Skin: note color, texture, temperature, moisture, turgor, edema, rashes, or lesions
   a. **Mongolian spots:** bluish colored areas common on buttocks or lower back of dark-skinned infants; they disappear with age
   b. Storkbites, café au lait stains, or port-wine stains are common birthmarks
   c. Bruises in various stages or unusual locations or circular burn areas may indicate child abuse
   d. Acne vulgaris may be present in adolescents
3. Hair: observe for color, distribution, characteristics, quality, infestations, and texture
4. Nails: note color, texture, shape, and condition; clubbing frequently indicates pulmonary disease

G. Head, neck, and cervical lymph nodes

1. Inspect and palpate head, neck, and lymph nodes
2. Head: note shape and symmetry
   a. Anterior fontanel: closes by 12 to 18 months
   b. Posterior fontanel: closes by 2 months
   c. Infant should be able to hold head erect by 4 months of age
   d. Newborn skull may show molding from birth process or flattening from repeated lying in same position
   e. Note symmetry by having older child make faces
3. Neck and lymph nodes: note size, mobility, swelling, temperature, and tenderness
   a. Thyroid is difficult to palpate in infants because of thick neck
   b. Palpate submaxillary, sublingual, and parotid glands
   c. Observe trachea for midline placement
   d. Determine mobility of neck

H. Mouth, throat, nose, and sinuses

1. Inspect mouth, nose, and throat, and palpate sinuses
2. Mouth and throat
   a. Examine last in young children; is intrusive and may provoke fear
   b. Note tooth eruption, condition of gums, lips, teeth, palates, tonsils, tongue, and buccal mucosa
   c. Deciduous teeth erupt by about 6 months of age; all 20 appear by about 30 months
   d. Teeth begin to fall out at about 6 years when permanent teeth erupt; this progresses until all 32 teeth erupt by late adolescence
   e. Tonsils may normally be enlarged, atrophying to stable adult size by late adolescence
3. Nose and sinuses
   a. Inspect structure, patency of nares, discharge, tenderness, and any color or swelling of turbinates
   b. Percuss and palpate sinuses of children over age 3; sinuses of infants and young children not palpable

I. Eyes

1. Inspect external eye
   a. Note position, slant, epicanthal folds, eyelid placement, swelling, discharge, color of sclera and conjunctiva, redness, eyebrows, and lashes
   b. Epicanthal folds are normal in Asian children, suggestive of Down syndrome in others
   c. Outer canthus should be in line with tip of pinna

2. Visual acuity tests
   a. Include Snellen letter chart for school-age children, Snellen symbol chart (E chart) for preschool age, Faye symbol chart (pictures) for preschool age
   b. Visual acuity difficult to assess in infants; tested by observing infant's ability to fixate and follow objects
   c. Should be able to differentiate colors by 5 years
3. Extraocular muscle tests
   a. Cover-uncover test: cover one eye and have child look at object; observe uncovered eye for movement; remove cover and observe that eye for movement
   b. ! Eye movement during cover-uncover test may indicate **strabismus** (lack of eye muscle coordination), which can lead to **amblyopia** (blindness caused by weak eye muscle)
   c. Hirschberg test: shine light on cornea while child looks straight ahead; light should reflect symmetrically in center of both pupils
   d. Unequal reflection may indicate strabismus
4. Ophthalmoscopic examination
   a. Same procedure as for adults but save until last; may require restraint or distraction; done by primary care provider or advanced practice nurse
   b. Expected finding: pupils equal, round, and reactive to light and accommodation (PERRLA); red reflex should be present
   c. ! Permanent eye color by 9 months

J. Ears

1. Inspect and palpate external ear for placement, discharge, and lesions
2. Inspect internal ear with otoscope
   a. Save until last; this usually requires restraint in infants and young children
   b. ! With infants, pull pinna down and back because canal is short and straight; with older child and adult, pull pinna upward and back
   c. Observe for **cerumen** (earwax), foreign bodies, or discharge
   d. ! Tympanic membrane should be pearly gray to light pink with landmarks visible
   e. Tympanic membranes redden during crying
   f. May assess mobility of tympanic membrane with pneumatic otoscope; tympanic membrane should move with pressure
3. Hearing acuity
   a. Tested in infants by noting reaction to loud noise
   b. Newborns exhibit Moro (startle) reflex and blink eyes
   c. Older children may be tested with whispered voice
   d. ! Audiometry testing of all children should be done before they enter school

K. Thorax and lungs

1. Inspect shape of thorax and respiratory rate, depth (deep or shallow), quality (effortless, difficult, or labored), and rhythm (regular or irregular)
2. Palpate back or chest for respiratory movement and **fremitus** (conduction of voice sounds through respiratory tract)
3. Percuss lungs; hyperresonance is normal in infants and young children because of the thinness of chest wall; begin with anterior lung from apex to base with child lying or sitting
4. Auscultate lungs
   a. ! Encourage deep breathing in children by having them blow a pinwheel, cotton ball, or other readily available object
   b. Breath sounds may seem louder or harsher because of thin chest wall
   c. Use bell and diaphragm of stethoscope to hear both low and high pitched sounds
   d. Evaluate breath sounds for noise, grunting, snoring, and so on
5. Inspect and palpate breasts
   a. Newborns may have enlarged or engorged breasts due to influence of maternal hormones
   b. ! Breast exam and teaching of breast self-exam for adolescents

L. Heart

1. Inspect and palpate precordium for heaves and apical impulse

2. Perform early in exam because quiet child and environment are essential
   a. Apical pulse at 4th intercostal space (ICS) until age 7; then apical pulse at 5th ICS after age 7
   b. Apical pulse to left of midclavicular line (MCL) until age 4; just lateral to left MCL from 4 to 6 years; and at left of MCL by age 7
3. Auscultate heart sounds
   a. Rate (should be regular and same as radial pulse), rhythm (should be even and regular); note quality (clear as opposed to muffled), and intensity (should not be heavy or pounding)
   b. Note that sinus arrhythmia (rate that speeds up with inspiration and slows with expiration) is common in children
   c. Evaluate for presence of murmurs
   d. Sounds are louder, higher pitched, and of shorter duration in infants and children

M. Abdomen

1. To promote relaxation and cooperation, have child place one hand beneath examiner's, use age-appropriate distraction, or use conversation focused on topic of interest to child; inspect shape
   a. Abdomen is prominent when standing and supine in infants and children until age 4; abdomen is somewhat prominent when standing but flat when supine after age 4
   b. Scaphoid abdomen indicates malnutrition or dehydration
   c. Umbilicus should be pink without redness or discharge
   d. Umbilical hernias fairly common, especially in African American children
2. Auscultate bowel sounds in same manner as for adults
3. Palpate for masses or tenderness; principles are same as for adults; advanced practice nurses are more likely to do deep palpation to outine organs; palpate for inguinal or femoral hernias

N. Genitalia

1. Always wear gloves during examination
2. Assess development of secondary sexual characteristics with Tanner's Sexual Maturity Rating Scale
3. Male
   a. Inspect penis and urinary meatus; foreskin should be retractable by 3 months
   b. Redness, discharge, or lacerations in young children may indicate abuse
   c. Inspect and palpate scrotum and testes to determine if both are descended
   d. In young children, testicle may withdraw into inguinal canal because of cremasteric reflex; block cremasteric reflex in infants by beginning palpation at inguinal ring and moving down to scrotum
   e. Check for inguinal hernias by having child blow or bear down
4. Female
   a. Inspect external genitalia for evidence of discharge or redness, which may indicate abuse in young children
   b. Internal examination for sexually active adolescents, or at age 16 to 18

O. Anus and rectum

1. Inspect for patency in infants
2. Skin should be smooth and free of lesions
3. Internal exam not done unless symptoms suggest a problem

P. Musculoskeletal

1. Inspect neck, extremities, hips, and spine for symmetry, increased or decreased mobility, and anatomical defects
   a. Extremities should be warm, mobile, with pulses strong and equal bilaterally
   b. Newborn's feet may be turned in but can be manipulated to normal position without resistance
   c. True deformities do not return to normal position with manipulation and include metatarsus varus (forefoot turned in), talipes varus (adduction of forefoot and inversion of entire foot), talipes equinovarus or clubfoot (adduction of forefoot, inversion of entire foot, and pointing downward of entire foot),

medial tibial torsion (entire foot turned in while knee remains straight), medial femoral torsion (entire leg turned in with foot)

2. Assess for congenital hip dislocation
   a. Assessed until about 1 year
   b. Use Ortolani's maneuver (with infant supine, flex infant's knees while holding your thumbs on mid-thighs and fingers over greater trochanters; abduct legs, moving knees outward and down toward table); note click if dislocation present
   c. Use Barlow's maneuver: (with infant supine, flex infant's knees while holding your thumbs on mid-thighs and fingers over greater trochanters; adduct legs until thumbs touch)
   d. Gluteal folds should be equal, hips abduct easily, and legs should be of same length
3. Assess spine and posture
   a. Newborn spine is flexible and rounded
   b. Cervical curve develops by 3 to 4 months; lumbar curve develops by 12 to 18 months
   c. Healthy toddler has **lordosis** (exaggerated curvature of lumbar spine)
   d. Check for **scoliosis** (lateral curvature of spine) in adolescent girls by looking at spine as child is bent over with knees straight
4. Assess gait, joints, and muscles
   a. Observe unobtrusively during history; joints should have full range of motion, and muscles should be equally strong bilaterally
   b. Toddlers have wide-based gait and are usually bowlegged
   c. Children ages 2 to 7 are often mildly knock-kneed
   d. Scissoring gait in which thighs cross over each other with each step is common in cerebral palsy

Q. Neurologic

1. Integrate into overall assessment as much as possible; assess child over 2 years the same as adult
2. Newborn and infant assessment
   a. Observe symmetry of spontaneous movements, appearance, positioning, posture, and responsiveness to parents and environment
   b. Assess level of consciousness, behavior, adaptation, and speech
3. Autonomic infant reflexes
   a. Rooting reflex: touch infant's lip or cheek, and infant should turn head toward stimulation and open mouth; should disappear by 3 to 4 months
   b. Sucking reflex: infant should suck vigorously when gloved finger inserted into infant's mouth; disappears by 10 to 12 months
   c. Palmar grasp reflex: pressing fingers against palmar surface of infant's hand produces grasp strong enough to pull infant to sitting position; disappears by 3 to 4 months
   d. Plantar grasp reflex: touching ball of foot causes toes to curl downward tightly; disappears by 8 to 10 months
   e. Tonic neck reflex: with infant supine, turn head to one side; arm and leg on side to which head is turned will extend and opposite extremities will flex; appears at about 2 months and disappears by 4 to 6 months
   f. Moro reflex, also called startle reflex: when a loud noise is created, infant flexes and abducts legs, laterally extends arms, forms a "C" with thumb and forefinger, and fans other fingers; is immediately followed by anterior flexion and adduction of arms; disappears by 3 months
   g. Babinski reflex: while holding infant's foot, stroke up lateral edge across ball; positive reflex is fanning of toes; some infants have normal adult response of flexion of toes; either response should be symmetrical bilaterally; disappears within 2 years
   h. Stepping reflex: holding infant upright with support under arms, let feet touch a surface and infant appears to take steps in a walking motion; disappears by 2 months

4. Presence of reflexes beyond expected times indicates CNS problem
5. Cranial nerves and deep tendon reflexes are same as for adults
6. Hand preference develops during preschool years
7. Observe for "soft" neurologic signs, gray area between normal and abnormal, those things that may change with maturation
   a. Short attention span, easy distractibility
   b. Impulsiveness
   c. Poor coordination
   d. Language and articulation problems
   e. Problems with learning, especially reading, writing, and arithmetic

Check Your NCLEX-RN® Exam I.Q.

You are ready for testing on this content if you can

- Assess a client's perception of health.
- Describe expected physiological status based on age.
- Conduct a physical assessment appropriate to the age of the client.
- Use critical thinking when interpreting data gathered during health and physical assessment.

PRACTICE TEST

1 While palpating the sternal aspect of the client's thorax, the nurse discovers a sensation that feels like rubbing hairs between the fingers. Upon auscultation, an additional finding is a sound similar to a crackling, popping noise. The probable cause of this finding is which of the following?

1. Pneumocystis pneumonia
2. Pneumothorax
3. Hemothorax
4. Hemodilution

2 After assessing the client's pupils with a penlight for reaction, roundness, symmetry, and accommodation, the nurse can document normal findings as which of the following?

1. PARL
2. PERRLA
3. PRLE
4. PLRAE

3 The nurse would use which of the following tests to evaluate a client's motor ability and function as part of a neurological assessment?

1. Glasgow coma scale
2. Abdominal reflex
3. Babinski test
4. Romberg test

4 The nurse notes unexpectedly during a routine screening examination that the client has a thready pulse. In what other way could this finding be documented?

1. A 2+ pulse
2. Pulse rate irregular and forceful
3. Pulse difficult to palpate and easy to obliterate
4. Pressure with the index finger causes pulsation

5 To assess the intensity of a client's pain during a health history, the nurse could ask the client to do which of the following?

1. Identify the location.
2. Rate the pain on a scale of 1 to 10.
3. Identify the methods the client uses to control the pain.
4. Disclose how long the pain has persisted.

6 The nurse performs the Rinne test during a physical examination. This test will provide information that may contribute to which of the following nursing diagnoses?

1. Impaired physical mobility
2. Impaired thought processes
3. Impaired swallowing
4. Altered sensory/perception: auditory

PRACTICE TEST

7. The nurse would plan to do which of the following as a high priority during a routine health assessment?
   1. Teach the client about ways to maintain health and wellness.
   2. Identify all areas of pathology.
   3. Use humor if the client is anxious.
   4. Explore the client's family relationships.

8. When documenting the findings of the health history, the nurse should do which of the following?
   1. Wait until the client has left the area.
   2. Write the findings immediately on the appropriate form.
   3. Abbreviate the data whenever possible to save time.
   4. Ask the client to confirm that the documentation is accurate.

9. The nurse plans to do which of the following using the skill of inspection during a health assessment?
   1. Use eyes, ears, and sense of smell to make observations.
   2. Look at one side of the body first, then the other.
   3. Leave all prepared supplies on a nearby table.
   4. Spend a significant amount of time completing this portion of the exam.

10. The nurse would document which of the following pieces of information obtained using the skill of percussion?
    1. An area of upper-right quadrant density
    2. An area of ecchymosis on the flank
    3. An area of dryness on the skin of the legs
    4. An area of weakness in the right lower extremity

11. A client tells the nurse during the health history, "I feel jumpy all over since using my new respiratory inhaler." Which of the following questions would be most appropriate for the nurse to ask next?
    1. "Do you also feel sweaty when this happens?"
    2. "Why are you using a respiratory inhaler?"
    3. "Can you tell me what you mean by jumpy?"
    4. "What helps you to get over this feeling?"

12. When asking a client newly admitted to the hospital about dietary history, which of the following questions would be most important?
    1. "What time of day do you eat each meal?"
    2. "Do you eat alone or with family members?"
    3. "How often do you eat meals at restaurants?"
    4. "Do you have any dietary restrictions?"

13. Which of the following statements made during a client interview represents a value judgment by the nurse?
    1. "I think your weight loss of 50 pounds was beneficial to your health."
    2. "Why did you decide to stop taking your blood pressure pill?"
    3. "Can you tell me how many alcoholic drinks you have each night?"
    4. "How can you afford to smoke if you're currently unemployed?"

14. An elderly client has experienced Wernicke's aphasia following a cerebral vascular accident (CVA). The nurse would expect the client to have difficulty with which of the following activities?
    1. Reading the newspaper
    2. Reciting the alphabet
    3. Spelling his or her last name
    4. Chewing solid food

15. Which of the following is the most important data for the nurse to obtain regarding the family history of a client?
    1. Quality of emotional support provided by family
    2. Dates of immunizations and vaccines received
    3. Number and ages of client's siblings
    4. Major diseases of close family members

16. When assessing a preschool-age child's mouth, how many deciduous teeth should the nurse expect to find?
    1. Up to 10
    2. 11 to 15
    3. 16 to 20
    4. Up to 32

17 Which area is it important for the nurse to assess in an infant that does not need to be assessed in an older toddler?

1. Gag reflex
2. Nares
3. Head circumference
4. Tympanic membranes

18 When assessing a child for strabismus, the nurse should select which of the following eye tests?

1. The Snellen eye chart
2. The cover-uncover test
3. An ophthalmoscope exam
4. The convergence test

19 When taking the history of a 7-year-old, what question might the nurse ask the child that would help detect vision problems?

1. "How are you doing in school?"
2. "Do you have any problems seeing at night?"
3. "Do you have any problems with glare?"
4. "What color is your shirt?"

20 When assessing the heart sounds of a 10-year-old, the nurse notices that the rate varies with inspiration and expiration. The nurse determines that which of the following actions is most appropriate?

1. Discuss a referral to a cardiologist for further workup.
2. Question the child about caffeine intake.
3. Do nothing, as this is a normal finding.
4. Schedule an electrocardiogram following the exam.

21 When preparing to assess the vital signs of an infant, the nurse should make a decision to use which sequence?

1. Measure temperature, pulse, and respirations at the end of the exam.
2. Measure respirations, pulse, and temperature in that order.
3. Measure vital signs after the infant becomes familiar with the nurse.
4. Measure blood pressure before other vital signs.

22 Which of the following would be of concern to the nurse when assessing the hearing of a 6-month-old?

1. Babbling quietly
2. Failure to say "da-da"
3. No response to interesting sounds
4. Absence of Moro reflex

23 To assess the tympanic membranes of a 4-year-old, the nurse should pull the pinna in which direction?

1. Up and back
2. Down and back
3. Up only
4. Back only

24 When assessing a 1-month-old infant, the nurse finds a head circumference of 32 cm and a chest circumference of 30 cm. The nurse should draw which conclusion about this data?

1. Consider this normal.
2. Reevaluate the findings in 2 weeks.
3. Expect the chest circumference to be larger than the head circumference.
4. Report the finding to the physician.

25 When assessing a 6-week-old infant, the nurse should plan on assessing the Moro reflex at what point in the examination?

1. At the very beginning of the exam
2. Before assessing vision
3. When the infant is sleeping
4. At the end of the exam

ANSWERS AND RATIONALES

1 **Answer: 2** Subcutaneous emphysema or crepitus is caused by pneumothorax. This condition consists of air introduced into the tissue from another condition, such as pneumothorax. Pneumocystis pneumonia is an opportunistic infection often experienced by individuals who are HIV-positive; hemothorax refers to blood in the chest, and hemodilution is associated with fluid overload of the vascular system.
Cognitive Level: Analysis **Client Need:** Health Promotion and Maintenance **Integrated Process:** Nursing Process: Analysis **Content Area:** Fundamentals **Strategy:** The core issue of the question is identification of subcutaneous emphysema and the ability to correlate this finding with common causes. Rely on knowledge of abnormal physical assessment findings and associated pathophysiological conditions to eliminate the incorrect options.

2 **Answer: 2** The correct abbreviation for pupils that are equal, round, and responsive to light and accommodation is PERRLA. The other options represent incorrect abbreviations. It is important for nurses to document using agency-approved abbreviations to avoid misinterpretations and to enhance communication among caregivers.
Cognitive Level: Application **Client Need:** Health Promotion and Maintenance **Integrated Process:** Communication and Documentation **Content Area:** Fundamentals **Strategy:** Use knowledge of physical assessment techniques of the eye to answer the question. Recall that the first observation is whether pupils are equal (symmetry), which will help you to choose the option that has an E near the beginning of the abbreviation.

3 **Answer: 4** The Romberg test is done when the nurse asks the client to stand with eyes closed and feet together. There should be minimal swaying for up to 20 seconds. A positive Babinski test in adults indicates upper motor neuron disease of the pyramidal tract. The Glasgow coma scale assesses the client's level of consciousness. The abdominal reflex, if absent, may indicate a disease of the upper and lower motor neurons.
Cognitive Level: Application **Client Need:** Health Promotion and Maintenance **Integrated Process:** Nursing Process: Assessment **Content Area:** Fundamentals **Strategy:** The core issue of the question is basic knowledge of physical examination techniques. Use this knowledge and the process of elimination to make a selection.

4 **Answer: 3** A weak, thready pulse is one that is difficult to palpate and easily diminished by slight pressure. A 2+ pulse indicates one that is easily palpable and normal. A forceful pulse and a pulsation felt with pressure from the index finger may be labeled as "full" or "bounding."
Cognitive Level: Application **Client Need:** Health Promotion and Maintenance **Integrated Process:** Nursing Process: Implementation **Content Area:** Fundamentals **Strategy:** The core issue of this question is knowledge of how to document an abnormal finding in a clear and objective manner. First eliminate option 1, which is a normal finding. Use the process of elimination to select the option that most clearly matches the data in the question.

5 **Answer: 2** The nurse seeks to identify the intensity of the pain by asking the client to rate the pain on a scale of 1 to 10 with 1 indicating a slight nagging pain and 10 indicating an excruciating pain. Some of the other components of the assessment would include the location (option 1), duration (option 4), and methods that the client has used to control the pain (also called alleviating factors, option 3).
Cognitive Level: Application **Client Need:** Health Promotion and Maintenance **Integrated Process:** Nursing Process: Assessment **Content Area:** Fundamentals **Strategy:** The key word in the question is *intensity.* Correlate this word with degree or strength of the pain to choose option 2 as the answer.

6 **Answer: 4** The Rinne test involves the examiner using a tuning fork to compare air conduction to bone conduction related to transmission of sound. Mobility, thought processes, and swallowing are not assessed with this examination.
Cognitive Level: Application **Client Need:** Health Promotion and Maintenance **Integrated Process:** Nursing Process: Assessment **Content Area:** Fundamentals **Strategy:** The core issue of this question is the ability to correlate the Rinne test with the ear, and then to choose the nursing diagnosis that affects either hearing or balance (functions of the ear). Use the process of elimination to make your selection.

7 **Answer: 1** As the nurse performs the health assessment and focuses on various systems, time can be spent educating the client about achieving and maintaining wellness. The nurse should have a professional, caring approach and avoid in-depth focus on pathology. The focus of routine examinations is not to explore client–family relationships.
Cognitive Level: Application **Client Need:** Health Promotion and Maintenance **Integrated Process:** Nursing Process: Assessment **Content Area:** Fundamentals **Strategy:** Note the key term *high priority* in the question. This means that some or all of the other options may be partially or totally correct, and you must choose the most important item. Note also the key word *routine,* which implies the client is healthy. With this in mind, the highest priority is to maintain and promote health and wellness.

8 **Answer: 2** The information extrapolated from the health history should be documented in the client's medical record in a timely manner. If the nurse does not write the information down, the data could be forgotten or omitted from the record. The nurse should not wait until the client has left the area to document information unless there is an emergency. Standard abbreviations should be used in the chart. Asking the client to review the documentation is not required.
Cognitive Level: Application **Client Need:** Health Promotion and Maintenance **Integrated Process:** Nursing Process: Assessment **Content Area:** Fundamentals **Strategy:** The wording of the question tells you the correct answer is a true statement. Use the process of elimination, recalling that prompt documentation helps prevent omissions and errors at a later time.

9 **Answer: 1** Inspection of a client can offer many clues about the overall state of health and can include all data gathered through the senses. The nurse should compare each side of the body for symmetry prior to inspecting the next system (option 2). Equipment such as a tongue blade, otoscope, or tape measure can be used during inspection but does not necessarily need to be prepared ahead of time (option 3). The time required depends on the client's condition and the nurse's skill level (option 4).
Cognitive Level: Application **Client Need:** Health Promotion and Maintenance **Integrated Process:** Nursing Process: Assessment **Content Area:** Fundamentals **Strategy:** The core issue of the question is the skill of inspection. Choose the option that reflects principles of visual assessment. Eliminate options 3 and 4 because of the words *all* and *significant amount of time.* Choose option 1 over 2 using knowledge of physical assessment techniques.

10 **Answer: 1** Percussion is a method of touching and tapping that the nurse uses to assess areas of density. The notes of percussion differ in various regions of the body. The thorax and abdomen are usually assessed. Percussion can detect numbness, pain, or abnormal masses.
Cognitive Level: Application **Client Need:** Health Promotion and Maintenance **Integrated Process:** Nursing Process: Assessment **Content Area:** Fundamentals **Strategy:** Recall that percussion involves tapping to detect tissue density that correlates with major organs and masses. With this in mind, eliminate options 3 and 4 because they refer to the legs. Choose option 1 over option 2 because option 2 is obtained using vision, not touch.

11 **Answer: 3** The nurse is employing the communication technique of clarifying in order to fully understand the client's subjective complaint. After understanding the client's perception of this side effect, the other questions would be appropriate.
Cognitive Level: Analysis **Client Need:** Health Promotion and Maintenance **Integrated Process:** Communication and Documentation **Content Area:** Fundamentals **Strategy:** The core issue of this question is appropriate use of therapeutic communication techniques. Note the word *next* in the question that tells you that all of the questions may be asked, but one is more important to determine first. With this in mind, choose the option that seeks to find out more about the client's symptom. The other questions can then follow.

12 **Answer: 4** The client may have restrictions based on a medical condition (e.g., low-sodium for heart disease), food allergies (e.g., shellfish), or religious convictions (e.g., abstaining from pork if Jewish). The nurse must note these restrictions and communicate with the nursing and dietary staff in order to avoid a potentially harmful occurrence. The other questions are pertinent for a dietary history but would not lead to a physiologic alteration if changed while hospitalized.
Cognitive Level: Analysis **Client Need:** Health Promotion and Maintenance **Integrated Process:** Nursing Process: Assessment **Content Area:** Fundamentals **Strategy:** Note the key words in the question are *dietary history* and *most important.* These tell you that the answer is the option that has a high priority, although some or all of the questions may be asked of the client. Select the option that impacts the diet the client will receive in the hospital. The others could be asked based on need or as the basis for later dietary teaching.

13 **Answer: 4** How a client spends income, even on an unhealthy habit, is not necessary for the nurse to know in order to provide effective care. Option 1 would be considered appropriate in an initial interview as a means for the nurse to provide acknowledgment and positive reinforcement for a lifestyle change that resulted in a potentially improved health status. Options 2 and 3 would be common questions used to inquire about a client's behavior.
Cognitive Level: Analysis **Client Need:** Health Promotion and Maintenance **Integrated Process:** Nursing Process: Analysis **Content Area:** Fundamentals **Strategy:** The core issue of the question is communication techniques that force the nurse's values on the client and thus reduce the likelihood of open communication between client and nurse. Imagine you are the client and choose the option that is most likely to have an adverse effect on your willingness to communicate with the nurse.

14 **Answer: 1** Wernicke's aphasia is the inability to understand verbal or written words. Impairment is located in the posterior speech cortex in the temporal and parietal lobes. Based on the information provided, the client should be able to speak, spell, and eat with this type of neurological deficit.
Cognitive Level: Application **Client Need:** Health Promotion and Maintenance **Integrated Process:** Nursing Process: Analysis **Content Area:** Fundamentals **Strategy:** Specific knowledge of the types of aphasia is needed to answer this question. Use nursing knowledge and the process of elimination to make a selection.

15 **Answer: 4** Major diseases such as diabetes, hypertension, arteriosclerosis, and cancer often have a genetic disposition and put the client at greater risk for developing them. The number and ages of siblings is a component of the family history, as well as inquiring about the client's support network. Vaccines and immunizations would be covered in the section known as past history.
Cognitive Level: Application **Client Need:** Health Promotion and Maintenance **Integrated Process:** Nursing Process: Assessment **Content Area:** Fundamentals **Strategy:** Note the words *most important* in the stem of the question. This tells you that some or all of the options are data that you might wish to obtain but that you must prioritize to choose the option that represents the most essential piece of data. First eliminate option 2 because it does not relate to the family. Choose option 4 over options 1 and 3 because it has the greatest potential impact on physiological health status.

16 **Answer: 3** Children get the first of 20 deciduous teeth between the ages of 6 months and 5 years. Permanent teeth begin to erupt about the age of 6 as deciduous teeth fall out. All 32 permanent teeth are usually erupted in late adolescence.
Cognitive Level: Application **Client Need:** Health Promotion and Maintenance **Integrated Process:** Nursing Process: Assessment **Content Area:** Fundamentals **Strategy:** Specific knowledge of physical growth and development is needed to answer this question. Use nursing knowledge and the process of elimination to make a selection.

17 **Answer: 3** The single most important measure of brain growth in infants is head circumference, so it should be measured at every assessment.
Cognitive Level: Application **Client Need:** Health Promotion and Maintenance **Integrated Process:** Nursing Process: Assessment **Content Area:** Fundamentals **Strategy:** The core issue of the question is determining an assessment that discriminates between infants and older toddlers. Use specific knowledge of infant and toddler physical growth and development and the process of elimination to make a selection. Recall that in infants the anterior and posterior fontanels close at specific times. Then recall that while one or both fontanels are open, head circumference could increase beyond normal growth if there is a problem with cerebrospinal fluid production. Once closed (as with toddlers), this data is not useful for this purpose.

18 **Answer: 2** The cover-uncover test assesses coordination of eye muscle movement. In strabismus, one muscle is weaker and the eye wanders rather than focusing forward. Undetected and untreated strabismus can lead to amblyopia.
Cognitive Level: Application **Client Need:** Health Promotion and Maintenance **Integrated Process:** Nursing Process: Assessment **Content Area:** Fundamentals **Strategy:** The core issue of the question is assessment of strabismus. Use specific knowledge of physical assessment procedures and the process of elimination to make a selection.

19 **Answer: 1** By the time a child is 7 years old, the nurse can appropriately ask questions of the child. A 7-year-old would not be expected to have problems with night vision or glare and should know colors. Problems in school could be a sign of vision problems and warrants a thorough visual assessment.
Cognitive Level: Analysis **Client Need:** Health Promotion and Maintenance **Integrated Process:** Nursing Process: Assessment **Content Area:** Fundamentals **Strategy:** Note the key words in the question are *vision problems.* Recall that children are more likely to have myopia (nearsightedness) than problems with night vision or glare. With this in mind, eliminate options 2 and 3. For the same reason, choose option 1 over option 4, which could be negatively affected by the child's reduced ability to read a blackboard or other materials in the classroom.

20 **Answer: 3** An irregular heart rate that increases with inspiration and decreases with expiration is a sinus arrhythmia, which is common in children. It requires no action on the part of the nurse. Further evaluation is not necessary (options 1 and 4), and an assessment of caffeine (such as in carbonated beverages) is not indicated.
Cognitive Level: Analysis **Client Need:** Health Promotion and Maintenance **Integrated Process:** Nursing Process: Assessment **Content Area:** Fundamentals **Strategy:** Note that a core issue of the question is the age of the child, which is 10 years. With this in mind, correlate the heart sounds described with normal growth and development findings. After determining that this is a normal finding, eliminate each of the incorrect options.

21 **Answer: 2** Vital signs in an infant are best taken when the infant is quiet early in the exam. Counting respirations by observing the abdomen is least intrusive, followed by the heart rate and temperature.
Cognitive Level: Analysis **Client Need:** Health Promotion and Maintenance **Integrated Process:** Nursing Process: Assessment **Content Area:** Fundamentals **Strategy:** Note that the client in the question is an infant. Recall that vital signs may be affected by activity such as crying. With this in mind, select the order or sequence that creates minimal disturbance for the infant.

22 **Answer: 3** A 6-month-old should be able to babble as well as localize sounds by turning head toward sounds. Failure to turn toward sound is an indication that further hearing assessment is necessary. The Moro reflex should not be present in a 6-month-old, and an infant that young would not be forming words yet.
Cognitive Level: Analysis **Client Need:** Health Promotion and Maintenance **Integrated Process:** Nursing Process: Assessment **Content Area:** Fundamentals **Strategy:** Note the key word *concern* in the question. This tells you the correct answer is an option that contains a questionable or abnormal finding. Use knowledge of growth and development and physical assessment techniques (option 4) to make a selection.

23 **Answer: 1** The auditory canal of children over age 3 is like that of adults, narrower and more curved; therefore, the pinna should be gently pulled up and back.
Cognitive Level: Application **Client Need:** Health Promotion and Maintenance **Integrated Process:** Nursing Process: Assessment **Content Area:** Fundamentals **Strategy:** Use specific knowledge of anatomy of the child and knowledge of physical assessment techniques to systematically eliminate each of the incorrect options.

24 **Answer: 1** The normal head circumference of a full-term infant is 32 to 38 cm, about 2 cm greater than the chest circumference. In the toddler, both measures are about equal; after the age of 2, the chest circumference exceeds that of the head.
Cognitive Level: Analysis **Client Need:** Health Promotion and Maintenance **Integrated Process:** Nursing Process: Assessment **Content Area:** Fundamentals **Strategy:** Use specific knowledge of growth and development of the infant to systematically eliminate each of the incorrect options. Recall that the measurements "cross over" at about age 2 when the head becomes smaller in circumference than the chest.

25 **Answer: 4** The Moro reflex is also known as the startle reflex, and it may cause the infant to cry. For this reason, it should be performed at the end of the exam.
Cognitive Level: Application **Client Need:** Health Promotion and Maintenance **Integrated Process:** Nursing Process: Assessment **Content Area:** Fundamentals **Strategy:** Use basic knowledge of infant responses and specific knowledge of the Moro reflex to systematically eliminate each of the incorrect responses.

Key Terms to Review

References

Harkreader, H., & Hogan, M. (2004). *Fundamentals of nursing: Caring and clinical judgment* (2nd ed.). St. Louis, MO: Elsevier Science.

Jarvis, C. (2004). *Physical examination & health assessment* (4th ed). St. Louis, MO: Elsevier Science.

Kozier, B., Erb, G., Berman, A., & Snyder, S. (2004). *Fundamentals of nursing: Concepts, process, and practice* (7th ed.) Upper Saddle River, NJ: Pearson Education.

17 Promoting Healthy Lifestyle Choices

Test Yourself

Are you ready for the NCLEX-RN® or course exams? Use the practice tests on the companion CD-ROM to check.

In this chapter

Cross reference

Other chapters relevant to this content area are

Meeting Nutritional Needs **Chapter 26**

I. SUN EXPOSURE AND SKIN INTEGRITY

A. Sun exposure damages skin

! 1. Most harmful ultraviolet rays occur between 10 a.m. and 2 p.m.
2. Whether sunny or overcast, daylight hours allow damaging rays to affect skin integrity
3. Ultraviolet rays can penetrate loosely woven fabrics and harm skin underneath clothing
4. Individuals who work or do recreation outside almost daily are particularly at risk for sun damage to skin: farmers, carpenters, fishermen, golfers
5. Exposure to chemicals may increase risk of skin damage: miners, asbestos and arsenic workers

B. Important points in health education to prevent skin cancer

1. Babies and children under age 6 and individuals with light complexion are at highest risk for skin damage
2. Immunosuppressed clients have increased risk for skin cancers
3. There is a genetic link to melanoma
4. Limit sun exposure during middle of day
! 5. Use sunscreen with solar protection factor (SPF) of 15 and higher
! 6. Reapply sunscreen every 2 to 3 hours when outside
7. Daily use of sunscreen on exposed face, ears, and hands decreases risk
! 8. Wide-brimmed hats offer extra protection to head and neck
9. Apply sunscreen liberally to scarred skin, which is more vulnerable to damage
10. Preventing severe sunburns in early childhood is key to skin integrity and reducing risk of skin cancer later in life
11. Skin cancers can occur and recur in any age adult, so inspect bare skin, using two mirrors to inspect front and back of body to allow for early discovery

II. BREAST SELF-EXAMINATION

A. General concepts

1. Both men and women can get breast cancer
2. It is important to perform breast self-examination (BSE) monthly (both males and females)
3. Clients need to see health care provider for regular check-ups
4. Women over age 40 need annual mammography testing
5. Female clients should begin BSE at time of first gynecological exam, about age 20
6. Nurse's role is pivotal in educating females and males that BSE is important

B. Procedure

1. Focus on palpating consistency of breast tissue
2. Perform procedure 5 to 7 days after menses for female; for men and post-menopausal women, perform exam on same day of each month; associate it with a specific date, such as the first of month
3. Look at breasts in mirror, arms by side, over head, and on hips
4. Lie down and palpate each breast with opposite hand while other arm is under head, flattening out breast tissue
5. Palpate under axilla as well as nipple region (both males and females)
6. Feel breasts by pressing tissue firmly against chest wall, each region from outer to inner, with a circular or "corn-rows" approach
7. Once a baseline of "normal" is felt, each client will better understand changes to report to practitioner; report changes from personal baseline immediately for further evaluation
8. Menses, breast-feeding, and pregnancy enlarge the breast tissue naturally, and tissue feels more lobular
9. Clients who have cysts in breasts must carefully perform BSE to detect changes from personal baseline, which need to be reported

III. TESTICULAR SELF-EXAMINATION

A. General concepts

1. Males most at risk for testicular cancer are under age 40
2. The normal testicle is smooth and uniform in consistency
3. Normally, one testis is larger and hangs lower in the scrotum

B. Procedure

1. Once monthly, males should perform testicular self-examination (TSE), preferably during a warm shower when testicles are relaxed and may be soapy
2. Using one hand to displace penis, grasp testis with dominant hand, placing fingers beneath and thumb on top of testis to palpate it
3. Roll gently between thumb and fingers, feeling for any abnormality
4. Palpate testis, epididymis, and spermatic cord on each side
5. Report any nodules or lumps to physician as soon as possible
6. Report symptoms of testicular swelling, painless testicular swelling, or dragging sensation in scrotum

IV. EXERCISE

A. Regular *aerobic exercise,* such as walking, jogging, or cycling, at least three days weekly is important to cardiovascular, respiratory, and musculoskeletal systems; aerobic exercise is rhythmic, uses major muscle groups, and is maintained for a prolonged period of time

Memory Aid

Choose aerobic exercise over other forms when the goal is general health, because it increases circulation and respiration and burns calories for better weight control.

B. Client can monitor most appropriate level of exercise by monitoring pulse and speaking ability

1. If exercise is strenuous enough that individual cannot speak without breathlessness, it is too vigorous

2. Exercising to specific target heart rates may be prescribed as part of a health-promoting exercise plan
3. To calculate target heart rate, first determine maximum heart rate by subtracting client's age from 220; then, calculate target heart rate by subtracting client's resting heart rate from his or her maximum heart rate

C. Principles for instruction in exercise to promote good health and deter progressive complications of heart and musculoskeletal diseases

! 1. Fast walking is effective aerobic exercise, when performed daily, to strengthen all muscles, including heart, and to keep bones strong
2. Inability to talk due to short breaths can mean excessively strenuous exercise
3. Walking fast enough to increase heart rate is recommended as effective in maintaining cardiovascular function, with less stress on knees than jogging
4. Client can increase energy level and ability to deal with stress by exercising for 30 minutes or more three to five times weekly
5. Whenever instructing parents of young children, stress importance of including regular exercise as a lifelong habit
6. Walking or weight-bearing exercises help to prevent osteoporosis because of force exerted on long bones
! 7. Anyone with a chronic illness such as diabetes or hypertension should consult a nurse practitioner or physician before beginning a rigorous physical exercise routine
8. Cautions for clients with health problems should include: start slowly, monitor body's response to exercise, and take medication and fluids before exercise

V. NUTRITION

A. General concepts

1. Nutrition is an essential parameter of health and is essential in preventing some diseases and complications of diseases
2. Nutritional intake is foundation for body's building up and growing, as well as for all healing processes
3. A balanced diet for adults and children consists of protein, carbohydrates, and fruits and vegetables, with little fat
4. A general guideline to follow: if a lunch plate is half covered with fruit and vegetables, one fourth protein and one fourth bread, with a serving of milk and very little fat, it will likely be "balanced"

Memory Aid

To easily remember the components of a balanced diet, visualize a circle divided into quadrants (fourths). Put fruits and vegetables in two, protein in one, and complex carbohydrates in one. Add milk to this picture and the meal is balanced!

! 5. Six ounces of grains, 2.5 cups vegetables, 2 cups fruit, 3 cups milk products, and 5.5 ounces of meat and beans are recommended for adults daily in MyPyramid
6. Eating a variety of foods helps individuals to gather all essential vitamins and nutrients in a balanced proportion
! 7. Sodium should be limited in quantity to 2 grams daily
   a. Cooking with other seasonings such as lemon, liquid smoke, pepper, and other spices is advised to limit sodium intake
   b. Limit salt to what is naturally found in foods, especially for clients with hypertension or cardiac and renal disease
   c. Canned vegetables, soups, and tomato sauces may contain almost one gram sodium per serving
   d. Do not assume that salt substitutes are acceptable; these are often high in potassium, which could be contraindicated for clients with renal disease or who take potassium-sparing diuretics; clients should consult health care provider before using them
8. Fresh and frozen vegetables and fruit have more available nutrients than canned and highly processed foods

9. Color indicates freshness and usually more available nutrients, so recommend undercooking and retaining color, not overcooking vegetables
10. See also Chapter 26 for detailed information about nutritional needs of clients

B. Principles to guide nutrition instructions for disease prevention

1. Heart-healthy eating refers to consuming a low-fat, low-sugar, and balanced diet, which includes more than five fruits and vegetables daily and limits red meats
2. The ADA diet is recommended for clients with diabetes or with hypoglycemia because it controls the release of insulin by limiting glucose
3. Quickly accessible foods usually have more fat and sugar than adults can use in a day, and they add excess calories, which becomes fat
4. Sweets, like fats, should be limited in quantity for all ages; sugary foods provide ready glucose, increase insulin production, but do not sustain the body's energy
5. Vegetarians may choose to eat dairy products; strict vegetarians may not eat any eggs, cheese, or dairy products; alternative protein sources include soy milk, tofu, dry beans, and nuts; watch for B_{12} deficiencies with individuals who avoid all meats
6. Many colorful orange and green vegetables have vitamins A, C, D, E, and K and serve as anti-aging antioxidants to the cells of the body, especially the skin
7. Eating leafy green vegetables interferes with anticoagulant therapy by increasing vitamins D or K
8. Eating more frequent and smaller meals or snacks, such as three meals and two snacks, is healthier for most adults than eating three large meals
9. Water is needed to move nutrients through and flush waste products from body; about 8 glasses daily promotes hydration, prevents constipation, and aids in digestion; as a general rule, drink 1 milliliter (mL) for each calorie consumed, so for a 2000 calorie diet, at least 2000 mLs of water should be taken daily
10. Folic acid is an important element to childbearing-age female
11. Extra iron is needed during pregnancy and usually is added in a daily vitamin
12. Females need additional calcium after menopause
13. Daily calcium intake is important, especially for women and children; calcium is essential for bone growth; women who are prone to osteoporosis should supplement with 1500 milligrams daily, including vitamin D for uptake of calcium
14. Foods high in calcium include dairy products, green vegetables, salmon canned with bones, sardines, tofu, and molasses

C. See also Chapter 26 for additional information on meeting client's nutritional needs

VI. ALTERNATIVE HEALTH CARE PRACTICES

A. General concepts

1. Herbs should be used with medical supervision
2. Alternative and homeopathic health care practices can be helpful in symptom relief, and with guidance from a trained nurse practitioner or holistic medical provider, allow healing for individuals who choose this route
3. Caution individuals to not abandon traditional prescription medicines nor to replace all medicines with herbs without the guidance and monitoring of a physician or nurse practitioner
4. Individuals taking warfarin (Coumadin) or any other anticoagulants must avoid use of over-the-counter herbs such as garlic, ginseng, ginger, primrose oil, dong quai, and grape seed extract because of interactive effects
5. Certain vitamins—A, D, E, K—are fat-soluble and require healthy liver function to use; otherwise toxicity can result

B. Summary of specific key points

1. Echinacea is used to increase immunity and to treat colds and infections, but it is not intended or effective for daily use over long periods of time; persons with AIDS, lupus, arthritis, or any autoimmune disorders should not take echinacea
2. Individuals need to consult practitioners before adding herbal supplements such as St. John's Wart to treat depression when already on prescription medications; such therapy is generally contraindicated

3. Ginseng and ginkgo are commonly taken by individuals who wish to improve cognition, and both cause drug interactions; persons who take these herbs regularly need to be monitored for drug interactions and cross-toxicity and for altered bleeding times
4. See also Chapter 29 on Alternative and Complementary Therapies for detailed discussion of specific herbs

VII. HEALTH SCREENING

A. Routine health screenings are recommended for early detection of disease; in addition, health screenings provide an opportunity to do health-related preventive teaching

B. General guidelines for health screenings for adults are presented in Table 17-1 ■

C. General guidelines for health screenings for children are presented in Table 17-2 ■

D. Specific points related to health screening

1. Children need to be screened at least annually for first 6 years of life; nurses can monitor growth patterns, emotional and social skills, as well as motor and sensory (eye and ear) functions during routine physical examinations and interactions with child and parent or caregiver
2. Premature infants need screening exams for deficits earlier and are more likely to experience developmental delays and motor and visual deficits
3. At age 4, arrange for child to begin annual dental checks and to have at least a baseline eye exam
4. The Denver Development Assessment is commonly used annually from infancy to age 6
5. Height and weight are charted annually and serve as screening for obesity
6. If muscle function, vision, or hearing is abnormal, exams may be done during infancy and several times yearly for follow-up and interventions
7. Hemoglobin assessment at any age is a common screening blood test for nutrition and general health

Table 17-1

Unified Screening Recommendations for Adults*

Target Group	Type of Screening	Beginning Age	Frequency
Men and Women	Blood pressure measurement	20	Each regular health care visit, at least every 2 years
	Body mass index (BMI) measurement	20	Each regular health care visit
	Blood cholesterol test	20	At least every 5 years
	Blood glucose (sugar) test	45	Every 3 years
	Colorectal screening	50	Every 1 to 10 years depending on test used
Women	Clinical breast exam (CBE)	20	Every 3 years; yearly after age 40; may be modified by individual provider according to risk
	Mammography	40	Yearly
	Papanicolaou test	20	Yearly
		30	Every 1 to 3 years, depending on test used and individual risk
Men	Prostate-specific antigen test and digital rectal exam	50	Variable according to individual risk and pros and cons of testing

*Developed collaboratively by the American Cancer Society, American Diabetes Association, and American Heart Association

Source: Adapted from information at http://www.cancer.org/docroot/PED/content/PED_12_1_Recommended_Health_Screenings_from_ACS-ADA-AHA.asp

Table 17-2

Health Screening Recommendations for Children*

Type of Health Screening	Frequency
Well-child exam	Birth, 1, 2, 4, 6, 9, 12, and 15–18 months, age 2, 3, 4, 5, 6, 8, and annually age 10 to 17 years
Blood pressure	Age 3, 4, 5, 6, 8, and annually age 10 to 17 years
Vision	Age 3, 4, 5, 6, 8, 10, 12, 15 years
Hearing	Age 4, 5, 6, 8, 10, 12, 15 years
Hereditary metabolic screening	Birth to 1 month
Lead screening	As needed
Hemoglobin and hematocrit	12 months and as indicated; may be annually for females during adolescence
Urinalysis	Age 5, in adolescence, and when indicated

*Summary of recommendations from U.S. Preventative Services Task Force, American Academy of Pediatrics, American Academy of Family Physicians, and Centers for Disease Control and Prevention; condensed on 06/18/05 from http://www.pciinsurance.com/pdf/2004%20Highmark%20Preventive%20Schedule.pdf

8. A complete blood count (CBC) gives information about development of all blood cells
9. Urinalysis and blood glucose testing is advised for obese children
10. Teenagers need to be screened for sexually transmitted diseases if sexually active
11. Other health screening to include for teens: blood pressure, heart murmurs, Pap smears for females who are sexually active, testicular exams for males, eyes, dental, hemoglobin testing
12. ! Height and weight should be documented annually for adolescents, and they should be monitored for obesity or anorexia
13. Chest x-rays may be necessary for smokers to establish lung function
14. Young adults who are college-bound (especially 20 to 30 years of age) need to continue with updating immunizations: tetanus, hepatitis, meningitis, and tuberculosis; this is important because of contact with larger numbers of people and possibly more crowded living conditions
15. Screenings for young adults include Pap smears for abnormal cell growth, height and weight to monitor for obesity, blood testing for normal blood cells and glucose, blood pressure, chest x-rays, and female mammograms
16. ! Adults over age 40 need to have annual screenings or self-exams to detect heart disease, cancer, hypertension, or other risks for chronic diseases such as diabetes
17. If at higher than normal risk for breast or colon cancer, begin annual screening exams earlier than for the general population and adhere to recommended frequency of exam
18. If at average risk and over 40, screen for cancer every 2 years with mammograms, and at every visit check feces for occult blood; consider a colon or sigmoid endoscopy exam every 5 years for polyps leading to colon cancer as recommended by health care provider
19. After age 60, screening should address changes related to aging: skin changes, bone density and osteoporosis, height (decreases due to bone loss), motor function and balance
20. Emotional well-being should be addressed as retirement and lifestyle changes occur
21. Health screening throughout life should include the following:
    - **a.** Hearing, vision, and all sensory functions
    - **b.** Safety for living and functioning in home/work environment
    - **c.** Emotional adjustments to life stage and world surroundings
    - **d.** Nutritional status, in excess or deficits
    - **e.** Ability to seek help and manage health; independence

PRACTICE TEST

VIII. GENETIC COUNSELING

A. Prenatal genetic counseling

1. In prenatal clinics, a common reason for genetic counseling referrals is an abnormal alpha-fetoprotein screening
2. As a neural tube defect, spina bifida usually results from a multifactorial inheritance
3. Down syndrome can be diagnosed with true genetic testing and amniocentesis, and genetic links determined, as can cleft lip and palate
4. Marfan syndrome, sickle cell disease, and heart murmurs can be diagnosed and other family members tested, with follow-up counseling for future family planning

B. Nurses' role in genetic counseling

1. Nurses must consider total picture of health and well-being, not merely risks of a genetic disorder
2. New information about genetic predispositions may not be welcome information, or may be rejected at first
3. ! Ask for written permission to share and communicate this information with spouse and other providers
4. Coordinate genetic health care with relevant community and national support resources
5. ! Offer support to clients and families throughout genetic counseling process

C. Role of heredity in child-and adult-onset health problems

1. Cancer, heart disease, and diabetes can be assessed as having familial or genetic tendencies
2. Certain eye diseases that lead to blindness and brain dementia can also be linked to genetic traits

Check Your NCLEX–RN® Exam I.Q. *You are ready for testing on this content if you can*

- Identify health-promotion activities for individuals relative to nutrition and exercise.
- Describe risks, screening, and prevention measures for skin cancer, breast cancer, and testicular cancer.
- Explain commonly used herbal remedies and alternative therapies.
- Utilize health education principles that guide client teaching about health management.

PRACTICE TEST

1 The nurse selects which of the following as the most appropriate dietary menu items for a client with iron-deficiency anemia?

1. Salad with lettuce, fruit, and nuts
2. Roast beef and broccoli
3. Lasagna with tomato sauce and steamed carrots
4. Mixed green salads topped with tuna fish

2 When discharging a client on oral anticoagulant therapy, the nurse would include further teaching for the client who has a lifestyle that includes which of the following?

1. Growing green vegetables
2. Walking one mile a day
3. Living in a rural setting
4. Spending most of the time alone

3 The chronic renal failure client states, "I don't eat red meat." After further discussion with the client about what foods are acceptable, the nurse would recommend which of the following meal choices to the client?

1. Noodle casserole and canned peas
2. Steamed cabbage with rice
3. Milk and chicken soup with crackers
4. Baked white fish and fresh carrots

4 The nurse is most concerned with providing further teaching for the client with diabetes who does which of the following?

1. Drinks orange juice each morning
2. Eats an apple and cheese before going to bed
3. Buys canned fruit instead of fresh because it is cheaper
4. Eats six meals per day

5 The nurse explains to a client who has had all molars removed that he will likely be allowed which of the following foods added to the diet by the third postoperative day?

1. Bacon and eggs
2. Pancakes and eggs
3. Cereal and milk
4. Gelatin and applesauce

6 When the nurse assesses the intake of a vegetarian client's health and dietary patterns, which finding does the nurse conclude is most likely to negatively affect health status?

1. Use of vitamin B_{12} supplements
2. Intake of milk and dairy products
3. Genetic tendency toward lactose intolerance
4. Reports of problems with vision

7 Which of the following clients is most at risk for skin cancer?

1. An 80-year-old farmer who wears a cap when working
2. A 20-year-old lifeguard at the lake who wears sunscreen
3. A baby underneath a large beach umbrella
4. A teenager who wears a ski outfit when skiing

8 During a health fair at a public recreational park, the nurse providing cancer health risk information answers several questions for clients who use ultraviolet light tanning salons. Which piece of information is most important to include?

1. Tanning from ultraviolet light is safer than sunshine.
2. Skin damage from ultraviolet light is more likely than from indirect sunlight.
3. Using sunscreen will prevent skin cancers, even in tanning beds.
4. Using tanning beds without clothing contaminates skin and leads to infections.

9 When giving postoperative care to a 30-year-old male client, the nurse discusses cancer risks. The client states, "I have never heard of testicular exams." The nurse should include which of the following priority interventions in the plan of care?

1. Teach the client to see a physician for a yearly testicular examination.
2. Assist the client to set up a calendar of dates to perform self-testicular exams.
3. Allow the client to verbalize fears related to cancer risk.
4. Encourage a high-fiber diet to decrease the risk of testicular cancer.

10 When a client comes into the emergency department (ED) with complaints of constipation and abdominal pain, which of the following would be the most common risk factors to assess for?

1. History of diverticulitis or diverticulosis
2. Dietary and exercise patterns
3. Nutritional intake of proteins and fatty acids
4. Level of nutrition understanding and laxative abuse

11 When teaching a 30-year-old male about testicular exams, the nurse recognizes more education is needed when he states:

1. "I will perform self-exams monthly and see my practitioner yearly."
2. "In the morning after a shower is the best time for testicular exam."
3. "The smooth texture of the testicle and spermatic cords can be easily felt."
4. "If one testicle rides up into my lower abdomen during sleep, this is normal, but I need to do the exam when it is descended."

12 The ambulatory care nurse working with adolescent and young adult male clients determines that the client most at risk for testicular cancer is which of the following?

1. Client whose father had colon cancer
2. Baseball catcher who wears supportive gear during sports activities
3. Teenager who swims daily on a swim team
4. Twenty-year-old with one undescended testicle

PRACTICE TEST

13 The nurse is participating in a health promotion fair. When discussing aerobic exercise, the nurse should include which of the following points?

1. Exercise should be done a minimum of 5 days per week.
2. Fast walking is a good form of aerobic exercise.
3. If one cannot talk when exercising, then the appropriate level of energy is being used.
4. Each exercise session should last for at least 45 minutes, and preferably 60.

14 A postmenopausal client is just learning to do breast self-examination (BSE). To aid in remembering to perform the procedure, at which of the following times should the nurse recommend that the client perform BSE?

1. Weekly just before grocery shopping
2. On a random day once each month according to convenience
3. Once a month on a standard day that that the client can remember
4. Just prior to each 6-month check-up for another health problem

15 A school nurse has finished conducting a teaching session with high school girls about breast self-examination (BSE). The nurse concludes that the information was learned correctly when one of the girls states to do the exam at which of the following times?

1. Once per month when the client thinks she is ovulating
2. On the first day of each month
3. Seven days after menstruation begins
4. On the first day of the menstrual cycle

16 An older adult female client has osteoporosis. In counseling the client about the best form of exercise, the nurse would recommend which of the following?

1. Swimming
2. Jogging
3. Cycling on a stationary bicycle
4. Walking

17 The nurse working in a prenatal clinic concludes that genetic counseling would be most important for the client who has a family history of which of the following disorders?

1. Coronary heart disease
2. Sickle cell anemia
3. Type II diabetes mellitus
4. Hypertension

18 A 20-year-old female sees the health care provider for her first adult physical examination. The nurse anticipates that which of the following screening measures will be done at this visit as a baseline for further reference? Select all that apply.

1. Body mass index (BMI) measurement
2. Blood glucose level
3. Clinical breast exam (CBE)
4. Mammography
5. Serum cholesterol level

19 A 4-year-old client is coming to the health care provider's office for a well-child visit. Which of the following routine screenings does the nurse plan? Select all that apply.

1. Blood pressure
2. Vision
3. Urinalysis
4. Lead screening
5. Hearing

20 Which of the following symptoms that are important to report would the nurse include in teaching about manifestations of testicular cancer? Select all that apply.

1. Painless swelling of scrotum
2. Dull pain in scrotum
3. Nodules in between testes and cord
4. Dragging sensation in scrotum
5. Reddened rash over affected testicle

ANSWERS & RATIONALES

1 **Answer: 2** With iron-deficiency anemia, it is important to select dietary items that are high in iron to counteract the deficit. Red meat tends to be high in iron, as do some green, leafy vegetables. Although options 1 and 4 contain salad greens (and therefore are green, leafy vegetables), the other components of these meals are not as high in iron. Lasagna and carrots (option 3) are not as high in iron as the other choices.

Cognitive Level: Analysis **Client Need:** Health Promotion and Maintenance **Integrated Process:** Teaching and Learning **Content Area:** Foundational Sciences: Nutrition **Strategy:** The critical words *most appropriate* indicate that more than one option may contain iron, but you must pick the total meal selection that is best. Recall that iron is found in red blood cells to help focus on a dietary item such as red meat. Recall that green vegetables are also helpful to confirm your selection. Thus, option 2 is the only option that contains two good sources of dietary iron.

2 **Answer: 1** The oral anticoagulant drug is sodium warfarin (Coumadin), and its action can be limited by excessive intake of foods containing vitamin K. Since green, leafy vegetables are high in vitamin K, the nurse needs to counsel this client about the possible antagonistic effect of these foods with the medication. Walking, rural living, and spending time alone pose no particular risk to the client.

Cognitive Level: Analysis **Client Need:** Health Promotion and Maintenance **Integrated Process:** Nursing Process: Planning **Content Area:** Pharmacology: Cardiovascular **Strategy:** The core issue of the question is oral anticoagulant therapy. With this in mind, review each option for an item that will have either an antagonistic or additive medication effect. Choose option 1 because it could lead to antagonistic effect.

3 **Answer: 4** The client in renal failure needs balanced nutrition, and fish is often acceptable to clients who do not eat red meat. Option 3 is less appropriate because crackers are not nutrient-dense foods. Options 1 and 2 contain high amounts of sodium or potassium, which are not helpful to the client in renal failure.

Cognitive Level: Analysis **Client Need:** Health Promotion and Maintenance **Integrated Process:** Nursing Process: Planning **Content Area:** Foundational Sciences: Nutrition **Strategy:** Focus on the two core issues in the question: the client is in renal failure, and the meal choice must be acceptable to the client who does not eat red meat. Eliminate meal choices that contain meat and/or high amounts of salt and potassium, which must be limited because of renal failure.

4 **Answer: 4** The client who has diabetes needs to have regular meals that are evenly spaced throughout the day and may need to supplement meals with snacks. Eating six meals per day is excessive and could lead to inadequate glucose control. Options 1 and 2 pose no risk as long as they are in the client's meal pattern. Option 3 is acceptable as long as the client ensures that the fruit is packed in water instead of syrup.

Cognitive Level: Analysis **Client Need:** Health Promotion and Maintenance **Integrated Process:** Nursing Process: Planning **Content Area:** Foundational Sciences: Nutrition **Strategy:** Use principles of general dietary planning and calorie control to answer the question. Remember not to "read in" information into the question or the options, especially option 3.

5 **Answer: 2** By the third postoperative day, the suture lines from the teeth extraction should be beginning to heal, and the client should be able to manage soft foods. With this in mind, option 2 provides the client with carbohydrates and a protein source for healing in a soft form. Options 1 and 3 contain items (bacon and cereal, respectively) that could be scratchy and irritate the suture lines. Option 4 would be appropriate the day after surgery while the suture lines are still new.

Cognitive Level: Application **Client Need:** Health Promotion and Maintenance **Integrated Process:** Nursing Process: Implementation **Content Area:** Foundational Sciences: Nutrition **Strategy:** Keep in mind principles of healing and principles of nutrition needed for healing to make a selection. The correct option is the one that combines appropriate nutrients and a soft form that can be tolerated by the client.

6 **Answer: 4** Problems with vision may be attributed to vitamin deficiency, especially vitamin A. This finding could adversely affect the client's health status and requires follow-up by the nurse. Options 1 and 2 will not adversely affect health status. Option 3 has a lesser chance of adversely affecting health status, since it is a familial risk and not a personally identified problem.

Cognitive Level: Analysis **Client Need:** Health Promotion and Maintenance **Integrated Process:** Nursing Process: Assessment **Content Area:** Foundational Sciences: Nutrition **Strategy:** Use knowledge of components of a balanced diet to eliminate options 1 and 2. Choose option 4 over 3 because actual problems take priority over potential problems.

7 **Answer: 1** The older adult client has more years of living to increase risk of skin cancer from exposure to the sun. In addition, the farmer wears a cap, but no mention is made of protectant sunscreens or long-sleeved shirts and pants. The clients in options 2, 3, and 4 have lesser risk because there are physical barriers to the sun identified in each option: sunscreen, umbrella, and ski outfit.

Cognitive Level: Analysis **Client Need:** Health Promotion and Maintenance **Integrated Process:** Nursing Process: Assessment **Content Area:** Adult Health: Integumentary **Strategy:** First recall that exposure to ultraviolet light is a risk for skin cancer. Use the process of elimination while considering which option provides the least sufficient barrier to exposure to ultraviolet light to make your selection.

8 **Answer: 2** Ultraviolet light exposure greatly increases risk of skin cancer, both basal cell and melanoma types. While direct sunshine contains ultraviolet light, the amount is decreased in indirect light. The use of suncreen can reduce the risk of cancer but not "prevent" it. Option 4 is a global statement that may or may not be true depending on the disinfectant methods used.

Cognitive Level: Analysis **Client Need:** Health Promotion and Maintenance **Integrated Process:** Nursing Process: Implementation **Content Area:** Adult Health: Integumentary **Strategy:** The core issue of the question is which option provides the most accurate and important information about ultraviolet light exposure. Eliminate options 3 and 4 first because they are not necessarily correct all of the time, and choose option 2 over option 1 because option 1 is false.

9 **Answer: 2** The priority for this client is to learn and begin to perform testicular self-exam on a monthly basis. Option 1 is insufficient in timeframe, and a physician does not need to perform the screening. Options 3 and 4 are positive but general measures and do not target the immediate need of the client for information related to detecting testicular cancer.

Cognitive Level: Application **Client Need:** Health Promotion and Maintenance **Integrated Process:** Nursing Process: Planning **Content Area:** Adult Health: Oncology **Strategy:** Use the process of elimination and knowledge of cancer risk to make a selection. Note that the question and both options 1 and 2 refer to testicular examination, which gives a clue that one of them may be correct. Choose option 2 over 1 for frequency and accuracy of the statement.

10 **Answer: 2** Two common and key factors that increase risk of constipation are a diet that is low in fiber and fluids and inadequate exercise to stimulate bowel motility, which could lead to impaction and abdominal pain. Option 1 is partially correct; diverticulitis is something to assess for but is not as frequently an etiology as inadequate exercise and low-fiber diet. In addition, diverticulosis does not give rise to signs and symptoms. Upon diagnostic workup, the client's symptoms could be attributed to diverticulitis, but this is not as frequently found as constipation as an etiology. Options 3 and 4 are general assessments that are either irrelevant to the client's complaint (option 3) or too vague to be correct for this question (option 4).

Cognitive Level: Analysis **Client Need:** Health Promotion and Maintenance **Integrated Process:** Nursing Process: Assessment **Content Area:** Adult Health: Gastrointestinal **Strategy:** Note the critical words *most significant* in the stem of the question. This tells you that more than one option is likely to be correct and that you must choose the best option, which in this case is the most frequent cause.

11 **Answer: 4** It is not normal to have one testicle that does not remain descended into the scrotal sac. The client needs to see a primary care provider for this health problem. Each of the other statements related to testicular self-exam (TSE) are true.

Cognitive Level: Analysis **Client Need:** Health Promotion and Maintenance **Integrated Process:** Nursing Process: Evaluation **Content Area:** Adult Health: Oncology **Strategy:** The critical words in the stem of the question are *more education is needed,* which tells you that the correct answer is an incorrect statement. Use the process of elimination and knowledge of TSE.

12 **Answer: 4** Testicular cancer is most likely to affect late adolescent and young adult males. An undescended testicle is one risk for testicular cancer. The client who wears protective gear is not at increased risk, nor is the client who swims. A familial history of colon cancer does not increase specific risk of testicular cancer because colon cancer occurs at a different site.

Cognitive Level: Analysis **Client Need:** Health Promotion and Maintenance **Integrated Process:** Nursing Process: Analysis **Content Area:** Adult Health: Oncology **Strategy:** Use the process of elimination, focusing on the core issue of the question, which is risk factors for testicular cancer.

13 **Answer: 2** Each client should exercise at least 3 days per week for a minimum of 30 minutes in order for exercise to be effective. Fast walking is a good form of aerobic exercise. If one cannot speak when exercising, it is too strenuous and should be decreased in speed or amount.

Cognitive Level: Application **Client Need:** Health Promotion and Maintenance **Integrated Process:** Teaching and Learning **Content Area:** Adult Health: Cardiovascular **Strategy:** The core issue of the question is characteristics of effective aerobic exercise. Use the process of elimination and remember "3-30," which is the frequency in days and the minutes per session, to rule out some distracters. Choose walking as an extremely effective exercise as the correct answer.

14 **Answer: 3** The client needs to perform BSE once per month, on the same day each month. The client is encouraged to associate performing BSE with another monthly activity, such as paying bills, or to do it on the same calendar date each month (such as the first). The other statements represent incorrect timeframes.

Cognitive Level: Application **Client Need:** Health Promotion and Maintenance **Integrated Process:** Teaching and Learning **Content Area:** Adult Health: Oncology **Strategy:** Use the process of elimination and note that the core issue of the question is frequency and timing of BSE. Because the client is postmenopausal, look for the monthly option that is not associated with menses (as none are in this question).

15 **Answer: 3** BSE should be performed once per month, 1 week after beginning menstruation. At this time, the breasts are least likely to be tender and/or swollen from the effects of hormones. At ovulation and menstruation, hormonal changes are likely to interfere with accurate palpation of breast tissue. Performing the exam on the first of the month is recommended for postmenopausal women who do not need to be concerned with changes in hormone levels associated with the timing of the menstrual cycle.

Cognitive Level: Analysis **Client Need:** Health Promotion and Maintenance **Integrated Process:** Teaching and Learning **Content Area:** Adult Health: Oncology **Strategy:** The core issue of the question is knowledge that accurate BSE results depend on the exam being done without the interference of hormonal factors that could alter the results or make the BSE difficult to perform. With this in mind, each of the incorrect options can be eliminated using the influence of hormones as a guide.

16 **Answer: 4** Although all of the exercises listed are aerobic and therefore beneficial, the older adult client with osteoporosis needs to select an exercise that has a weight-bearing component and yet does not stress the joints. Such an activity will

ANSWERS & RATIONALES

help to retain calcium in bone and reduce the rate of bone loss to osteoporosis. Walking is an aerobic exercise that does not stress the joints of the legs. Swimming and stationary cycling are not weight-bearing exercises. Jogging could harm the knee and ankle joints and is not a preferred method of exercise for this client.
Cognitive Level: Application **Client Need:** Health Promotion and Maintenance **Integrated Process:** Nursing Process: Implementation **Content Area:** Adult Health: Musculoskeletal **Strategy:** The core issue of the question is the type of exercise that is appropriate for a client with osteoporosis and who is an older adult. With this in mind, eliminate swimming and stationary cycling as nonweight-bearing, and eliminate jogging as increasing stress on joints in the leg.

17 **Answer: 2** Sickle cell disease has an onset in childhood. This makes it the priority for genetic counseling. The other disorders listed (coronary heart disease, type II diabetes, and hypertension) are adult-onset problems and therefore have lower priority.
Cognitive Level: Analysis **Client Need:** Health Promotion and Maintenance **Integrated Process:** Nursing Process: Analysis **Content Area:** Child Health: Cardiovascular **Strategy:** Note that the stem of the question contains the critical words *most important*. This means that all of the options may represent conditions for which some genetic counseling may be useful, but you must select the option that has highest priority. Use age at onset as a means of making your selection.

18 **Answer: 1, 3, 5** A body mass index (BMI) measurement is done at age 20 and at each health visit. Serum cholesterol levels are started at age 20 and are recommended every 5 years. Blood glucose screening is recommended to begin at age 45 unless there is evidence of higher risk for diabetes. Colorectal screening begins at age 50 and is done every 1 to 10 years depending on method used. Clinical breast exam is done starting at age 20 and may be done every 3 years or more frequently depending on risk. Mammography is done yearly starting at age 40.
Cognitive Level: Analysis **Client Need:** Health Promotion and Maintenance **Integrated Process:** Nursing Process: Analysis **Content Area:** Adult Health: Oncology **Strategy:** Specific knowledge of frequency of recommended health screenings is needed to answer the question. Use the process of elimination, and review this content area if needed.

19 **Answer: 1, 2, 5** Blood pressure and vision screening are started at age 3 and continue with each visit. Hearing screening begins at age 4. Lead screening would only be done on an as-needed basis for a 4-year-old. Hemoglobin and hematocrit are done at 12 months and as needed (which may be annually for females during adolescence). Urinalysis is done at age 5, in adolescence, and otherwise only as indicated.
Cognitive Level: Application **Client Need:** Health Promotion and Maintenance **Integrated Process:** Nursing Process: Analysis **Content Area:** Child Health: Eye and Ear **Strategy:** Specific knowledge of frequency of recommended health screenings is needed to answer the question. Use the process of elimination, and review this content area if needed.

20 **Answer: 1, 2, 3, 4** Painless swelling of scrotum, dull pain in scrotum, nodules between testes and cord, and dragging sensation in scrotum are signs of testicular cancer. A reddened rash or feeling of wetness in the scrotum are not applicable to this diagnosis but should be followed up for general health reasons.
Cognitive Level: Analysis **Client Need:** Health Promotion and Maintenance **Integrated Process:** Nursing Process: Assessment **Content Area:** Adult Health: Oncology **Strategy:** Specific knowledge of manifestations of testicular cancer is needed to answer the question. Use the process of elimination and review this content area if needed.

Key Terms to Review

aerobic exercise p. 243 **prenatal genetic counseling** p. 248

References

Harkreader, H., & Hogan, M. (2004). *Fundamentals of nursing: Caring and clinical judgment* (2nd ed.). St. Louis, MO: Saunders.

Kozier, B., Erb, G., Berman, A., & Snyder, S. (2004). *Fundamentals of nursing: Concepts, process, and practice* (7th ed.). Upper Saddle River, NJ: Prentice Hall.

Potter, P., & Perry, A. (2005). *Fundamentals of nursing* (6th ed.). St. Louis, MO: Mosby, Inc.

Taylor, C., Lillis, C., & LeMone, P. (2005). *Fundamentals of nursing: The art and science of nursing care* (5th ed.). Philadelphia, PA: Lippincott, Williams & Wilkins.

18 Age-Related Care of Older Adults

Test Yourself

Are you ready for the NCLEX-RN® or course exams? Use the practice tests on the companion CD-ROM to check.

In this chapter

Cross reference

Other chapters relevant to this content area are

Lifespan Growth and Development	Chapter 14
Promoting Healthy Lifestyle Choices	Chapter 17

I. NEED FOR CARE

A. Older adults are the fastest growing population in the United States; subgroups of this age group have been identified

1. Young-old: 65–74 years
2. Old: 77–84 years
3. Old-old: 85–100 years
4. Elite old: over 100 years

B. As age increases, threats to health and need for assistance with daily care and health-related care increase

C. The majority of people 65 or older live in their own homes; only 5% of older adults live in a nursing home; retirement communities are changing the pattern of housing for older adults

D. Biological aging occurs at a loss of about 0.5% of maximum function per year, starting at age 35; most organ systems have large reserves, so detrimental effects are not noticed

E. Diseases that used to kill or disable middle-aged adults are reduced because of modern health practices and knowledge, with increase of degenerative diseases of old age being seen; chronic illnesses are seen more frequently in older adults (see Box 18–1)

F. Disuse is a core problem; it is estimated that 2% of the decline per year can be accounted for by simple disuse: "use it or lose it"

G. Preventative strategies related to health practices, nutritional intake, and exercise can slow the aging process (see also Chapter 17)

! **H. Health care practitioners need skill to assist clients in promoting healthy lifestyle choices and to be able to differentiate between "normal aging" and indicators of underlying conditions/symptoms of disease**

Box 18-1

Most Frequently Occurring Conditions in Adults 65 Years and Older, 2000–2001

Hypertension: 49.2%	Cancer: 20%
Arthritis: 36.1%	Sinusitis: 15.1%
Heart disease: 31.1%	Diabetes: 15%

From U.S. Department of Health and Human Services. Administration on Aging. *Portfolio of Older Americans 2003.*

II. AGE-RELATED PHYSIOLOGICAL CHANGES

A. Basic principles of physical aging

1. Rates between people vary; not year-specific
2. Each organ ages at a different rate within the same person
3. Toxic compounds called free radicals damage cellular proteins and eventually cause cell mutation and senescence
4. Physical aging presents differently in different cultures and environments
5. The aging process can be slowed
6. Important to differentiate normal aging from illness

B. Specific system changes and related health promotion activity

1. Skin
   - ! **a.** Subcutaneous tissue loss and dermal thinning leads to a loss of moisture, wrinkles, sagging, decreased perspiration, increased risk of heat stroke, inability to respond to heat and cold rapidly, skin pallor, and slowed healing processes
   - **b.** Increase in **lentigines** (brown age spots)
   - **c.** Hair thins and loses pigment on the scalp and pubic and ancillary areas but increases in male ears and female upper lip areas
   - **d.** Nail growth slows, and nails may become thicker
   - ! **e.** Skin tissue is more fragile, with fewer elastic fibers, decreasing skin turgor and increasing vulnerability to tears and pressure ulcers; caution clients about effects of sun
   - ! **f.** Use mucous membranes to assess potential anemia and fluid volume deficit
   - **g.** Sebaceous glands secrete less sebum, causing dryness and itching
2. Sensory and perceptual changes
   - **a.** Visual acuity changes; ocular changes in cornea, pupil, and lens lead to farsightedness and inability of lens to accommodate (**presbyopia**); there is increased sensitivity to glare and decreased ability to adjust to light or darkness because of slower constriction and dilation of pupils; there is also increased difficulty in differentiating colors because of changes in rods and cones
   - ! **b.** There is an increased need for light and use of glasses; night lights may be needed
   - ! **c.** Because decreased vision increases risk of falls, high-gloss wax should not be used on floors; safety strips should be placed on first and last steps
   - **d.** Cataracts may develop; eyelids lose elasticity
   - **e.** Arcus senilis is often seen because of deposits of calcium salts and cholesterol; it appears as a gray-white ring or partial ring surrounding limbus or outer edge of iris
   - **f.** Dry eyes often develop because of inability of goblet cells in conjunctiva to secrete mucin
   - **g.** Clients need to have regular ophthalmic exams
   - ! **h.** Older adults may have difficulty driving in darkness
   - ! **i.** Auditory acuity changes; ear canal narrows with calcification of ossicles and increased cerumen, resulting in progressive hearing loss (**presbycusis**)
   - ! **j.** Older adults have particular difficulty hearing high-pitched tones and words that begin with consonants, especially *sh, th, wh;* they will not hear "Swish this around your mouth" accurately if they cannot see the speaker's face; shouting does not help clients to hear
   - **k.** Ears should be cleaned of cerumen; if hearing aids are used, batteries and use should be reviewed regularly

! l. Olfactory bulb decreases, leading to an inability to smell and discriminate odors (**anosomia**); housing for older adults therefore should include working smoke alarms to detect fires

! m. Gustatory buds decrease on the tongue, causing decline in ability to taste; sweet sensation is especially affected; avoid the use of extra sugar and salt to satisfy desire; explore alternatives

! n. Touch sensation changes with reduced ability to sense heat and cold; monitor temperature of liquids to avoid injuries, monitor extremities for wounds which may go unnoticed because of decreased sensation, and beware of the myth that older adults do not experience pain

3. Neurological
   a. Conduction speeds of neuron firing and transmission decrease; may have decreased sensations and slowed response time that will impact safety, driving, and decision making
   b. Actively participating in mind exercises (learning new things, crossword puzzles, reading) has been shown to slow changes; assist client to incorporate exercise into lifestyle
   c. Memory retrieval is slower, and there is a decrease in vigilance, but intelligence and behavior does not change; older adults are capable of learning new health-related information, but may need more processing time
   d. Sleep stage 2–4 will shorten, leading to a decrease in deep sleep and physiologic and psychological rejuvenation; monitor perception of sleep, immune system, and mood/cognition state; promote healthy sleep rituals (e.g., quiet restful environment, no stimulants before bedtime, go to bed only when tired)
   ! e. **Proprioception** (sensation about the body's movement and position) decreases, so achieving balance or changing position may be difficult; demonstrate safe changes of position; incorporate safety devices and clear walkways in living spaces
4. Musculoskeletal
   a. Muscles **atrophy** (decrease in size and physiologic activity) so that there is a decrease in strength and stamina; more strength is lost in legs than arms; encourage regular exercise
   b. Joints stiffen because of deterioration of joint cartilage
   ! c. Intervertebral disks atrophy, resulting in a loss of height of 1 to 3 inches; bone demineralization may lead to **osteoporosis** and increased risk of fractures
   d. Encourage weight-bearing exercise, intake of calcium and vitamin D; walking is beneficial
   e. Monitor functional activity levels
5. Pulmonary
   a. Chest wall becomes rigid, thoracic muscles weaken, and ciliary activity decreases, so there is less efficient lung expansion, exchange of oxygen/carbon dioxide, effective coughing, and foreign body capture
   ! b. Teach effective coughing and deep breathing
   c. Practice healthy hygiene because of increased susceptibility to infection; encourage appropriate vaccine administration; sputum specimen collection may require suction technique
   ! d. Delivery and diffusion of oxygen to tissues decreases so that dyspnea is experienced after moderate, stressful activity; teach pacing of activities between periods of rest and throughout the day instead of clustered together
6. Cardiovascular
   a. Heart size remains the same unless there is pathology
   ! b. Cardiac output and stroke volume decrease, especially during increased demands, so there is a decreased stress response
   c. Shortness of breath on exertion and pooling of blood in extremities may occur
   d. Help client to incorporate pacing into activities of daily living (ADLs) and instrumental activities of daily living (IADLs)
   e. Valves stiffen so that murmurs are heard; know baseline so that disease-related abnormalities can be detected

f. Conductivity is altered, so there are more ectopic beats; assess apical heart rhythm and rate for a full minute
g. Vessels are less elastic, resulting in higher blood pressure; orthostatic hypotension may occur, and there is decreased perfusion to vital organs
h. Monitor client BP according to latest guidelines; assess perfusion to and resulting function of vital organs
i. Palpate peripheral pulses; use Doppler for measurement if needed
j. Instruct not to make sudden position changes to avoid orthostatic hypotension because of altered physiology or effect of many medications taken for chronic health problems, such as hypertension

7. Renal
   a. Nephrons decrease in function related to senescence and decreased arterial blood flow; monitor for output of at least 30mL/hr
   b. Glomerular filtration rate (GFR) decreases, which may lead to inadequate excretion of drug metabolites
   c. Creatinine clearance decreases; monitor for nephrotoxic medication adverse effects
   d. Urine concentration ability and conservation of water is decreased; urinary urgency and frequency may occur related to enlarged prostate in men or decreased perineal muscle support and urinary sphincter strength in women
   e. Bladder capacity decreases
   f. Incontinence is *not* part of normal aging; it occurs related to pathology
   g. Residual urine and nocturnal frequency may occur; teach client to credé bladder
   h. Monitor for urinary infection (new-onset confusion may be sign in older adults) and for restful nights (lack of nocturia); refer for treatment if needed
8. Gastrointestinal
   a. Thirst sensation decreases; monitor intake to prevent fluid deficit, especially if older adult takes diuretics or is in a hot environment
   b. Usually the system that stays healthy overall but generates the most complaints from older adults
   c. Swallowing time is delayed, and epiglottis does not completely cover trachea unless older adult is in a 90-degree position
   d. Monitor swallowing; have client sit upright when eating or drinking; gag reflex may diminish
   e. Gingivitis/periodontal disease often leads to loss of teeth and is caused by poor nutrition and inadequate oral care
   f. Saliva secretions lessen, so breakdown of carbohydrates may be decreased
   g. Intra-abdominal strength decreases; gastric acid and enzymes decrease, and absorption time is slower; monitor for reflux and vitamin deficiencies
   h. Intestinal walls are weakened, and there is a slower neural transmission and resulting decrease in peristalsis; observe for constipation and incontinence; caution against inappropriate use of laxatives because of risk of dependence
9. Endocrine
   a. TSH and thyroxin are reduced; slowed basal metabolism, dry skin, and thin hair are characteristic of hypothyroidism in young adults but normal manifestations in older adults with no history of disease
   b. Insulin levels increase, but insulin sensitivity decreases; observe for signs and symptoms of hypoglycemia or hyperglycemia, depending on client condition
   c. Alteration in hormone regulation decreases ability to respond to stress
10. Genital
   a. Prostate enlarges in men (usually benign); decreased sperm production occurs; encourage regular health checkups and PSA testing
   b. Vaginal changes in women occur because of diminished secretion of hormones; alkaline pH leads to vaginal dryness and atrophy; there may be a need for increased foreplay and use of a water soluble lubricant; encourage regular gynecologic exams; monitor menopausal changes; estrogen is not routinely prescribed
   c. For both genders, assess sexual activity and safe sex practices

11. Immune
   a. Thymus decrease in cell production with resulting decline in cell-mediated immunity and decreased T-cell functioning
   b. Monitor for signs and symptoms of infection and/or altered cell production
   c. First sign of infection in an older adult may be a fall; temperature pattern may be lower than for younger adult with the same infection
   d. Autoimmune response may not be associated with disease; monitor for changes in soaps or detergents if older adult develops unknown allergic rash
   e. Outbreaks of shingles occur if the varicella virus is reactivated while the older adult's immune system is weakened, *not* if they come in contact with new cases of chicken pox

III. AGE-RELATED PSYCHOSOCIAL CHANGES

A. Role and relationship transitions occur; adaptation is critical to positive aging

B. Maintain independence in as many activities as possible

C. According to Erikson (1963), everyone has specific developmental stages and tasks to fulfill within a chronological timeframe; in the 8th and last stage of life, Erickson stated, older adults review their life to establish beliefs of integrity or despair

1. Erikson and Peck (1968) identified discrete tasks of old age that must be addressed in order to establish integrity:
   a. Ego differentiation versus work role preoccupation; adults are no longer defined by work; satisfaction is found in other activities
   b. Body transcendence versus body preoccupation; adults care for themselves but do not spend all of their energy caring for the body; they see meaning in illness and death
   c. Ego transcendence versus ego preoccupation; adults focus on humanity outside of themselves; "I" is not as important; volunteerism for a greater good may be seen
2. Erickson's (1986) reframed work: ego integrity is tinged with some regrets, wisdom is balanced with frivolity, and letting go is balanced with hanging on; an adult comes to terms with life as it has been lived and derives sustenance from the past but is active in the present and plans for the future; reminiscence and life review are effective tools to encourage ego integrity

D. Other key changes

1. Balance is found in solitude and social interactions; adults who adapt develop a capacity for aloneness and the ability to enjoy his or her own company (not to the exclusion of significant others but in preparation for loss and death); old and new friendships are still valued; communication problems (vision, hearing, and withdrawal) may detract from finding this balance
2. Grandparenting has become an important role in the 21st century; some grandparents are the primary caregivers today; communication clarification is important
3. Retirement may be unattainable for some and undesirable for others; financial needs, resources, and loss of health insurance benefits may deter retirement, as may perceived loss of prestige, friends, and self-satisfaction; the years of retirement are increasing, so transition counseling or mentoring may be needed
4. Widowhood is more difficult for young-old during the adaptation process; transitions for all include stages that span 5 years
   a. First stage (reactionary): early responses of disbelief, anger, inability to communicate, searching for mate; interventions: support, reduce expectations
   b. Second stage (withdrawal): occurs in the first few months with depression, physiologic vulnerability, insomnia, unpredictable waves of grief; interventions: protect against suicide and involve in support groups
   c. Third stage (recuperation): occurs in the second 6 months with periods of depression and feelings of personal control beginning to return; interventions: support usual lifestyle patterns while assisting to explore new possibilities
   d. Fourth stage (exploration): occurs in the second year with new ventures but vulnerability during holidays, anniversaries, birthdays; interventions: prepare widow or widower for feelings during special times; support new roles

e. Fifth stage (integration): occurs in the fifth year with a healthy resolution of grief; interventions: assist individual to share own pattern of growth

E. **Stressors of aging**

1. ! Include loss of people or pets or driver license, abandonment, acute and chronic pain, sensory changes, medications, caregiving of a demented spouse, illness, hospitalization, lack of protection when frail, fear of senility, abuse and neglect, housing and home maintenance, relocation, institutionalization, fear of loss of independence, and fear of death or dying alone
2. Encourage recognition of fears and reinforce positive coping methods; monitor for inappropriate coping: alcoholism, withdrawal, contemplation of suicide
3. Role transitions from worker to retiree/volunteer and spouse to widow require looking at former roles differently; to the extent these are accepted and "at the right time," older adults can transition smoothly

F. **Intimacy and sexuality**

1. Continue to be critical at any age; touch is important to all; watch for touch deprivation; use of therapeutic touch and massage may enhance health
2. ! Sexually transmitted diseases are not exclusively young people's diseases; safe sex practices should be followed
3. Sexual dysfunction counseling, if needed, is multidimensional; use of medications to promote erections requires education related to safety
4. Privacy is needed in residential settings for marital sexual relations; health care workers need to evaluate own feelings regarding sexuality in older adults

G. **Many organizations promote positive aging adaptation**

1. AARP (American Association of Retired Persons)
2. Meals on Wheels
3. Local senior centers
4. Area agencies on aging
5. Churches

IV. MEDICATION CONSIDERATIONS

A. **Medication use is further affected by finances, ability to acquire medications, advertisements, and motivation and health of clients; fragmented care and lack of communication among prescribers can lead to *polypharmacy* (prescriptions for multiple medications written by multiple prescribers and possibly filled at more than one pharmacy); this can lead to adverse drug interactions and possible toxicity**

B. ! **Nurse may be only caregiver who knows all prescribed and over-the-counter medications and herbs that a client uses; this makes it critical for nurses to administer, educate, monitor for therapeutic effects and adverse effects, prevent and treat toxic effects, and advocate for appropriate and affordable medication use**

C. **Pharmacokinetics determines concentration of medication in body**

1. Absorption: aging alone affects oral drug absorption minimally but may be reduced with intramuscular delivery
2. ! Metabolism: liver size and hepatic blood flow decrease with advanced age so that drugs that undergo a first-pass effect are affected by age; disease states of the liver and circulation to liver will affect metabolism; drugs such as propranolol and lidocaine exhibit decreased metabolism and increased bioavailability
3. ! Distribution: decreased circulation to skin, muscles and fat results in slower and lower concentrations in these tissues; increased overall body fat and decreased lean body mass and water may change movement of medications; healthy older adults show little change in plasma binding proteins but lowered albumin levels in disease states can result in increased normal and adverse effects; note that some disease states (cancer, arthritis) which elevate protein binding capacity, decrease the effectiveness of some medications
4. ! Excretion: aging reduces renal medication excretion with decreased glomerular filtration rate, renal plasma flow, tubular function and reabsorptive capacity; creatinine clearance rates are calculated and some drug dosages are calculated by lean body weight versus ideal body weight

D. Pharmacodynamics

1. Aging changes some receptor sites thereby increasing susceptibility to some adverse effects; older adults are very sensitive to anticholinergic side effects of drugs as well as orthostatic hypotension
2. Older adults tend to have more adverse effects related to increased chronic problems and greater number of drugs taken

E. Medication usage

1. Older adults may take lower dosages of drugs especially when starting a drug regimen; therapeutic window narrows with age
2. "Start low, go slow."
3. Adverse effects are often atypical and may include falls, incontinence, **delirium,** (acute onset confusion) depression, sedation, urinary retention
4. Use brown bag method to take adequate history of medications taken
5. Review whether medications are taken as prescribed
6. Confirm that clients can see what they are taking
7. Pills should not be crushed if enteric coated
8. Antihypertensive should be taken as ordered even if blood pressure is within normal range
9. Diuretics should be taken during early waking hours so that effective sleep can occur
10. Medications that have hypotensive or sedative effects may be best taken at bedtime
11. Review all prescriptions if client takes more than five to eight medications; primary prescriber reviews necessity of all drugs
12. Altered electrolytes such as potassium or sodium may exacerbate toxic effects of electrolyte and adverse effects of drugs; if a client is taking spironolactone and a diet high in potassium, toxic potassium levels could occur
13. Mental status changes may be a side effect of a medication; diazepam, clonidine, digoxin, levodopa, and isoniazid have caused delirium and confusion in many older adults
14. Monitor for oto-and nephrotoxicity; assess urinary output and ringing in ears, especially in older adults receiving aminoglycosides or high doses of aspirin
15. Monitor for sexual changes; decreased sexual desire seen with antipsychotics, SSRIs, ketoconazole; priapism or prolonged painful erection is a surgical emergency that is associated with sildenafil, alprostadil, trazodone, and antipsychotics
16. Drug allergies may occur; take history especially of penicillin, cephalosporin, erythromycin, gentamicin, sulfa, nonsteroidal anti-inflammatory drugs, opiates, anesthetics; and contrast medias, their usage, and reactions
17. Changes in diet can impact medication; increased green vegetables counteract anticoagulant effects of warfarin; iron is not absorbed when calcium is taken at same time; decreased fluid intake, especially during hot weather, may lead to fluid volume deficit and increased sensitivity to orthostatic effects of beta blockers
18. Food–drug interactions must be reviewed; do not give dairy products with ciprofloxacin or tetracycline because drug will chelate with food; amiodarone, lovastatin, and busprione levels increase dramatically when taken with grapefruit juice
19. Monitor where medications are stored; nitrates must be stored in a dry, dark area; expiration dates must be adhered to

F. Common medications considered inappropriate for older adults

1. Analgesics: propoxyphene (Darvon) and combination products, meperidine (Demerol)
2. Hypnotics: diazepam, barbiturates except phenobarbital (Luminal)
3. Antiplatelet: dipyridamole (Persantine)
4. Anticoagulant: ticlopidine (Ticlid)
5. Antihypertensive: methyldopa (Aldomet)
6. Any medication with a highly anticholinergic profile
7. Garlic and ginkgo may increase risk of bleeding

V. OLDER ADULT ABUSE AND NEGLECT

A. Abuse is willful infliction of pain or injury physically, psychologically, financially, or socially

1. Examples include confinement, willful deprivation of services, verbal assaults, theft, mismanagement of belongings, demand to perform undesirable tasks, and physically injurious acts
2. Exploitation is illegal or improper use of an older adult's resources
3. ! Individuals at risk are those who are dependent because of health issues such as altered mental status, sensory deficits, or immobility
4. History of family violence and caregiver stress also increase risk of abuse

B. Neglect is lack of provision of services necessary for health

1. Self-neglect occurs when older adult chooses not to uses services that would promote health
2. If legally competent, an older adult has the right to refuse care

! **C. Assessment of abuse and neglect may reveal:**

1. Bruises, cuts, burns
2. Sprains, fractures, dislocations
3. Inconsistent history about injuries
4. Untreated medical problems
5. Improper use of medication
6. Malnutrition, dehydration, or both
7. Inappropriate dress, hygiene, drowsiness, or social interactions
8. Pulling away or expression of fear when touched
9. Excessive attachment to caregiver

D. Care includes:

1. Continued assessment
2. ! Reporting to appropriate agencies as mandated by each state
3. Involvement with protective services
4. Referral to appropriate resources and treatment for dysfunctional families

VI. COMMON PROBLEMS IN OLDER ADULTS

A. Nutrition

1. Assessment
   - **a.** Food patterns and preferences
   - **b.** Symbolism of food: sociability, security, and reward
   - **c.** Health screen for malnutrition
   - **d.** Dentition efficiency and oral hygiene
   - **e.** Taste and sensory changes influence choices; taste bud receptors decrease, especially for sweet and salt; olfactory receptors atrophy, decreasing taste ability further; visual changes affect presentation, while touch proprioception is altered too
   - **f.** Decreased thirst sensation and satiety
   - **g.** BMI, height and weight, ideal body weight; a BMI of 20 to 24.9 is considered healthy
   - **h.** Lab work: related to potassium levels, hemoglobin and hematocrit ranges, pre-albumin and albumin values
   - **i.** ! Disease and functional profile: any disease can cause poor food intake and weight loss for older adults; lactose intolerance is becoming more prevalent; arthritis may prevent use of regular forks, spoons, knives, and cups
   - **j.** Common nutritional problems include hypercholesterolemia, weight loss, protein malnutrition, osteoporosis (low bone density), obesity; see also Chapter 26
   - **k.** Income and food acquisition patterns may change
   - **l.** ! Clients at highest risk for decreased nutritional health: live alone, have many medications, have a history of dementia or depression, are institutionalized
2. Plan/implementation
   - **a.** Decrease total fats and saturated transfat
   - **b.** Control calories
   - **c.** Increase fluids to 30mL/kg body weight or 1 to 2 liters per day if not on fluid restriction

d. Increase whole grains and fiber intake
e. Limit intake of sodium and sugar; 2300 mg or 1 teaspoon per day (current recommendation for sodium); canned and processed foods contain large amounts of sodium; use substitute flavor enhancers but beware of potassium content of salt substitutes if client takes potassium-sparing diuretics or has renal disease
f. Use supplements if vitamins or minerals are needed; this allows for 100% of RDA if client is unable to eat right, has an illness that affects absorption, is on a restricted diet, or takes medications that alter appetite or nutrient absorption; assess calcium, iron, zinc, folic acid, and vitamins A, B_6, C, and E because they are frequently inadequate in an older adult's diet
g. Incorporate ways to promote enjoyment of food, such as setting different table areas and eating with another; learn to savor foods; if alcohol is used, do so in moderation; include cultural preferences in diet
h. Increase physical activity; walking is an efficient exercise, but increased exercise can be done in a chair too
i. Refer to a nutritionist if BMI is below 20 or above 25, there is prolonged limited food intake in quality or quantity, there is a limited knowledge of and motivation to comply with nutritional plan
j. Refer to a nutritionist and specialist for disorders requiring nutritional intervention: elevated lipid profile, osteoporosis, malabsorption, uncontrolled diabetes, obesity, congestive heart failure and other cardiac conditions, advanced renal or liver disease, prolonged high doses of chemotherapy or radiation
k. Refer to Meals on Wheels if preparation and acquisition of food is not easily done
l. Teach sources of nutrients, and potassium (potato, banana, fortified orange juice) and reinforce with written or pictorial materials
m. Investigate food-storage practices for hygienic safety; recommend nonperishable food items such as boxes of dry skim milk, peanut butter, canned tuna, dried fruit, fresh seasonal fruit, tea if refrigeration is limited
n. In the health care settings, adhere to Joint Commission on Accreditation of Healthcare Organization (JCAHO) standards: screen for nutritional risk, provide intervention and counseling, provide food and nutrition products, prescribe nutritional supplement products, and monitor response to nutritional care plan

B. Urinary incontinence

1. Incontinence is not part of normal aging but a disease process or functional change
2. Prevalence is 40% of hospitalized clients, 60% of clients in long-term care facilities, 25% of older adults in the community
3. Assessment is critical so that treatment can be started
4. Continence requires functional status in lower urinary tract, cognitive ability, dexterity in mobility, usable toileting environment, and motivation
5. Causes of transient incontinence include delirium; restricted mobility, retention; infection, inflammation, impaction; polyuria, pharmaceuticals; use the pneumonic DRIP to remember these causes

Memory Aid

D—delirium
R—restricted mobility, retention
I—infection, inflammation, impaction
P—polyuria, pharmaceuticals

6. Adverse effects of urinary incontinence include physical, psychological, and economic consequences
   a. Physical: odor, discomfort, skin problems, urinary tract infections, falls
   b. Psychosocial: embarrassment, isolation, depression, need for nursing home care
   c. Economic: nursing home costs and national effect on Medicare and Medicaid
7. Types of persistent urinary incontinence include stress, urge, overflow, functional, and neurogenic

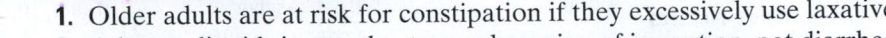

8. Treat according to cause and promote regular toileting schedules (such as every 2 hours), spacing fluids over day but not at night to avoid nocturia, and administering diuretics during early part of day

C. Constipation versus diarrhea

1. Older adults are at risk for constipation if they excessively use laxatives
2. A brown liquid ring on sheets may be a sign of impaction, not diarrhea

D. Vision and hearing

1. Visual problems associated with aging include presbyopia, dry eye, cataracts, glaucoma, diabetic retinopathy, and macular degeneration; see Chapter 64 for a discussion of these health problems
2. Hearing problems associated with aging include presbycusis, cerumen impaction, and possibly tinnitus; see Chapter 64 for a discussion of these health problems

E. Impaired skin integrity

1. Skin loses elasticity with the aging process
2. Decreased mobility also increases risk of pressure ulcer development in those who are ill or injured and have further reduction in mobility from baseline (see chapters 27 and 63 for further discussion of health problems related to skin)

F. Impaired mobility

1. Can occur as a consequence of chronic health problems such as arthritis, neuromuscular disorders, or osteoporosis leading to fractures, or because of acute illness, injury, or surgery (such as with hip and knee replacement or other surgery)
2. May occur because client is afraid of falling; impaired mobility can lead to increased risk for falls; see Table 18–1 ■ for risk factors for falls in older adults
3. May require use of assistive devices (mobility aids) such as a cane or walker

G. Dehydration

1. Assessment is critical because older adults are at risk for dehydration
2. Mucous membranes provide indication of hydration
3. Use abdomen or forehead to assess for skin turgor; tenting is a normal, age-related change on hand and is not a reliable indicator of dehydration
4. Delirium (a reversible, acute confusional state that must be evaluated) is frequently caused by dehydration and may accompany urinary tract infection; it often goes undiagnosed in older adults, and client is labeled cognitively impaired
5. See Chapter 54 for a detailed discussion of dehydration or deficient fluid volume

H. Depression

1. Older adults are at risk for depression related to multiple losses in their lives
2. It is important to differentiate between depression, delirium, and **dementia** (impairments in memory, abstract thinking, judgment and personality); see Table 18–2 ■
3. For detailed discussion, see Chapter 22 on mental health disorders

Table 18–1
Fall Risk Factors

Intrinsic Age-Related Changes	Intrinsic Disease-Related Changes	Extrinsic Risk Factors
Gait (step length and height)	Orthostatic hypotension	Floor surface: waxed, scatter rugs, tears in carpeting
Gait (symmetry and path)	Dehydration	Steps uneven, without hand rails
Balance when sitting	Cardiac arrhythmias and anemias	Edges and curbing without contrasting colors
Balance when standing	Urinary tract and other infections	Dim lighting, bright lights that cause glare
Balance when turning	Osteoporosis and fractures	Bathrooms without grab bars and seats
Stability	Hypoglycemia	High-heeled shoes
Cognition	Seizures, TIA, CVA, adverse effects of medication, delirium	Clutter

PRACTICE TEST

Table 18–2

Comparisons of Delirium, Dementia, and Depression in Older Adults

	Delirium	Dementia	Depression
Onset	Acute	Gradual	Sudden or gradual
Duration	Brief, resolve underlying cause	Years	Weeks to years
State of Consciousness	Disoriented	Alert	Self-absorbed
Behavior	Difficulty with attention and concentration	Personality changes, labile, easily agitated	Apathetic, feelings of worthlessness, vague somatic complaints
Ability to Follow Instructions	Unable to do tasks	Tries hard to follow and do with gradual loss of abilities	Able to, but does not do tasks
Mental Ability	Fluctuations in memory and orientation, disorganized thinking	Impaired memory, gradual loss of knowledge, language, and judgment	Selective memory loss
Ability to cure	Reversible	Irreversible	Reversible

Check Your NCLEX–RN® Exam I.Q. *You are ready for testing on this content if you can*

- State basic principles related to aging.
- List physical changes of aging and implied health promotion activities.
- Differentiate normal physical aging changes from indicators of illness.
- Discuss psychosocial issues of aging and how to promote healthy adaptation.
- Identify common problems, safety issues, and required health promotion teaching.

PRACTICE TEST

1 A nurse is teaching a class about aging at a senior citizen center. The nurse would know that a client needed further instruction if he or she made which of the following statements?

1. "Through nutrition and exercise, we can modify the rate of aging."
2. "Free radicals influence the quality of growing old."
3. "Some of the physical changes within our bodies are the result of disuse."
4. "Deterioration of body systems occurs at the same rate."

2 The nurse assesses that a 75-year-old client has lentigines and presbycusis. When planning care for this client, the nurse should do which of the following?

1. Refer the client to an oncologist and ophthalmologist.
2. Ask the nursing assistant to use water soluble creams and turn on all the lights.
3. Look and speak to the client so that he or she can see the nurse's lips.
4. Adjust the temperature and lighting of the room.

3 The nurse prepares to teach a class about normal aging changes to a group of nursing assistants. The nurse should select which of the following techniques as most appropriate?

1. Demonstrate use of incontinence pads for clients who become incontinent of urine.
2. Teach crutch walking because of high risk for falls and fractures in older adults.
3. Discuss a case study in which an older adult with an infection had a temperature of 98°F.
4. Show how to use a blood glucose monitoring device and how to disinfect it because of increased incidence of diabetes.

4 A nurse evaluates that the care plan related to normal physiologic changes has been effective for a 70-year-old client if he says,

1. "I have more sebaceous gland activity."
2. "I have lost some of my social support systems."
3. "I have an increased need for sleep."
4. "I have less joint cartilage than I used to."

5 After conducting a physical assessment, the nurse would conclude that a 75-year-old client's ability to maintain personal safety would be most adversely affected by declining function in which of the following systems?

1. Cardiovascular
2. Respiratory
3. Sensory
4. Integumentary

6 A 75-year-old woman with a pathological fracture of the arm asks, "How did I get a broken bone?" The nurse most appropriately responds by saying that which of the following is the most probable reason for the fracture?

1. Decreased mobility
2. Osteoarthritis
3. Scoliosis
4. Osteoporosis

7 Which nursing intervention would be most appropriate to meet safety needs when caring for an older adult with sensory changes?

1. Assist in preparing a bath because the client may not be able to determine the intensity of heat.
2. Use care when administering an injection because older adults experience more pain.
3. Massage with additional pressure because tactile perception of older adults is diminished.
4. Use minimal touch with an older adult because touch will feel uncomfortable.

8 The nurse explains to children of aging parents that it is important to remember that most older adults

1. require help with making all important decisions.
2. like a family role and need to be with grandchildren often.
3. should be supported in their desire to remain independent.
4. must be protected from injury at all times.

9 After teaching a driving safety education program for the old-old, a nurse should recognize which of the following as evidence of a favorable response by an older adult when driving?

1. Keeping the inside of the car warm at all times because of the loss of subcutaneous fat and resulting decreased tolerance to cold
2. Not turning his or her head to look to the left or the right because the older adult's response time is slower
3. Driving at a speed that matches the flow of traffic to facilitate increased response time
4. Driving during the day to increase use of vision capabilities

10 A nurse teaches an older adult client about misuse of medications. Which of these observations would indicate that the teaching was effective?

1. Combining prescribed medications with over-the-counter ones
2. Having prescriptions from different physicians
3. Using someone else's medications
4. Taking medications on time and, if a dose is missed, taking the next one on time

11 Which of these instructions, if included in the care plan for an older adult who has "leaking urine," would be most effective in strengthening pelvic muscles?

1. When coughing, bear down in the standing position.
2. Percuss the lower abdomen for dull sounds, indicating a distended bladder.
3. Observe for fullness immediately after urinating.
4. Stop the stream of urine during the middle of urination.

12 A nurse has selected a transparent film dressing for a stage 2 pressure ulcer. The nurse will change the dressing

1. every 8 hours.
2. when there is a change in color.
3. every 72 hours.
4. when the edges roll up and exudate leaks.

13 Which clinical manifestation would be significant when assessing the skin of an 85-year-old client?

1. Ecchymoses on both forearms
2. Cherry hemangiomas across the anterior and posterior trunk
3. Tenting of the skin on the back of the hands
4. Nevi on the neck and forehead

14 An older adult client is admitted to an extended care facility for follow-up care of a total hip replacement. The nurse assesses a BMI of 20, lackluster hair, and pallor. Which laboratory assessments will the nurse review to obtain the most sensitive information about the client's current nutritional status?

1. Serum albumin
2. Total cholesterol
3. Prealbumin
4. Complete blood cell count and differential

15 On admission, a 78-year-old client states he uses laxatives three times a week for constipation. The nurse would respond:

1. "As people age, they need laxatives to stimulate defecation."
2. "Eat a balanced diet if you use laxatives."
3. "Long-term use of laxatives can cause constipation."
4. "Please use laxatives two times a week at night."

16 The care plan for a client who has severe osteoporosis should include which intervention to prevent injury?

1. Administer vitamin D and calcium as ordered.
2. Use a lift sheet to reposition the client.
3. Place the client in a high Fowler's position to promote lung expansion.
4. Position pillows on the client's left side when in the side-lying position.

17 Which of these assessment findings in an older adult client should alert the nurse to an increased risk of falls?

1. Decreased bone density
2. Increased bone prominence
3. Kyphotic posture
4. Cartilage deterioration

18 The nurse is irrigating the ears of an older adult man with a cerumen impaction. The nurse would stop the procedure if

1. the man became nauseated.
2. the irrigating fluid did not return.
3. cerumen and fluid are expelled.
4. the man says he can't hear as well.

19 An older adult client is receiving the third unit of packed red blood cells in the last 8 hours. One hour into the third transfusion, the nurse observes the patient's distended neck veins. What is the next action the nurse would take?

1. Document the observation.
2. Measure the amount of PRBCs left in the bag.
3. Slow the infusion.
4. Assess the patient's pulse and blood pressure.

20 A nurse is assessing an older adult client who is at risk for shock. The nurse will effectively assess for cyanosis on the

1. sclera of the eyes.
2. oral mucous membranes.
3. skin of the forehead.
4. nail beds of the fingers or toes.

ANSWERS & RATIONALES

1 **Answer: 4** Options 1, 2, and 3 are true statements. Each physiologic system of a person ages at a different rate.
Cognitive Level: Application **Client Need:** Health Promotion and Maintenance **Integrated Process:** Nursing Process: Implementation **Content Area:** Foundational Sciences: Growth and Development **Strategy:** The key phrase *needs further teaching* tells you to look for an incorrect choice.

2 **Answer: 3** Lentigines (brown age or liver spots) represent normal aging of the skin. Presbycusis also occurs in normal aging. These changes do not require medical attention or interventions for vision or temperature.
Cognitive Level: Application **Client Need:** Health Promotion and Maintenance **Integrated Process:** Nursing Process: Planning **Content Area:** Foundational Sciences: Growth and Devel-

opment **Strategy:** When answering questions, look for all parts of the answer to be correct.

3 **Answer: 3** A normal body temperature of an older adult person may range from 96.5° to 99°F (35.9°–37.3°C). Therefore, a temperature of 98.6°F (37°C) may signify a fever in an older person. Incontinence is not a normal age-related change. Not all older adults have altered mobility needs, and those who do are more likely to use a cane or walker than crutches (which are used for injury). Use of blood glucose devices is generic or related to a diagnosis of diabetes and is not specifically related to normal aging changes.
Cognitive Level: Analysis **Client Need:** Health Promotion and Maintenance **Integrated Process:** Nursing Process: Planning **Content Area:** Foundational Sciences: Growth and Development **Strategy:** Eliminate choices that do not correlate to all parts of the question as well as those choices that have incorrect information.

4 **Answer: 4** With normal aging, there is loss of cartilage and joint fluid. Overall wear and tear does occur. Sebaceous glands are less active, and older adults sweat less. There is a decreased need for sleep, with shorter REM and non-REM sleep cycles. Social support may decrease with deaths and fewer resources but does not relate to the question of physiologic needs.
Cognitive Level: Analysis **Client Need:** Health Promotion and Maintenance **Integrated Process:** Nursing Process: Implementation **Content Area:** Foundational Sciences: Growth and Development **Strategy:** Read all choices, eliminating incorrect ones.

5 **Answer: 3** With normal aging changes, there is a decrease in vision, hearing, touch, smell, and taste. These changes can lead to falls, inability to leave a situation when called to do so, inability to distinguish temperature with resulting burns, inability to smell smoke in a fire, and inability to taste contaminated food. These changes can have a major impact on the safety needs of an older adult.
Cognitive Level: Analysis **Client Need:** Safe, Effective Care Environment: Safety and Infection Control **Integrated Process:** Nursing Process: Planning **Content Area:** Foundational Sciences: Growth and Development **Strategy:** When answering questions related to development and aging, distinguish between normal development, which affects all, and illness, which affects some.

6 **Answer: 4** Osteoporosis, a decrease in bone density, makes the older adult more prone to pathological fractures. Decreased mobility, osteoarthritis, and scoliosis do not cause pathological fractures. Scoliosis is a curvature of the spine, usually diagnosed in adolescents.
Cognitive Level: Application **Client Need:** Physiologic Integrity: Physiological Adaptation **Integrated Process:** Nursing Process: Implementation **Content Area:** Foundational Sciences: Growth and Development **Strategy:** Correlate the best reason with the choice.

7 **Answer: 1** Because of loss of skin receptors, the older adult has an increased threshold to pain, touch, and temperature. When feeding or bathing, remember that the older adult may be unable to distinguish hot or cold or to determine the intensity of heat. The older adult may feel less pain than younger adults and complain of only pressure or a minor sensation. The older adult, however, is the only one who can identify if they have pain or not. An older client's sensory perception is less acute than that of younger adults, so when giving a massage, less pressure is needed. Everyone, and especially the older adult, needs touch.
Cognitive Level: Analysis **Client Need:** Safe, Effective Care Environment: Safety and Infection Control **Integrated Process:** Nursing Process: Planning **Content Area:** Foundational Sciences: Growth and Development **Strategy:** Imagine giving the stated care to assist in choosing the correct answer.

8 **Answer: 3** Promoting independence is a basic nursing principle. Older adults thrive on independence, even with limitations. Older adults make their own decisions and do not appreciate others making decisions for them. Although some older adults cherish a family role, this is not necessarily the wish of every older adult. Remaining active is important for older adults; unnecessary protection from injury is inappropriate.
Cognitive Level: Application **Client Need:** Psychosocial Integrity **Integrated Process:** Nursing Process: Implementation **Content Area:** Foundational Sciences: Growth and Development **Strategy:** Usually, the word *all* denotes an incorrect choice.

9 **Answer: 4** Driving at night requires caution because accommodation of the eye to light is impaired and peripheral vision is diminished. Keeping the inside of the car warm at all times is not a significant issue when driving during the day or in warm climates. Reflexes are slowed for older adults; thus, caution in driving should be emphasized for this group.
Cognitive Level: Analysis **Client Need:** Health Promotion and Maintenance **Integrated Process:** Nursing Process: Evaluation **Content Area:** Foundational Sciences: Growth and Development **Strategy:** The phrase *favorable response* cues you to look for the desired outcome.

10 **Answer: 4** Taking medications on time and, if a dose is missed, taking the next one on time indicates proper self-administration. Misuse of medications by older adults include combining prescribed and over-the-counter medications; having prescriptions from different physicians and failing to tell each doctor what has previously been prescribed; and taking someone else's medications.
Cognitive Level: Analysis **Client Need:** Health Promotion and Maintenance **Integrated Process:** Nursing Process: Evaluation **Content Area:** Foundational Sciences: Growth and Development **Strategy:** The phrase *would indicate teaching was effective* means the choices will have three incorrect outcomes and one desired outcome, which will be the correct choice.

11 **Answer: 4** Interrupting the flow of urine assists the external urethra to contract and strengthens pelvic floor muscles. Other actions involve assessment activities.
Cognitive Level: Application **Client Need:** Physiologic Integrity: Physiological Adaptation **Integrated Process:** Nursing Process: Planning **Content Area:** Foundational Sciences: Growth and Development **Strategy:** Distinguish choices related to actions, assessment, implementation, and correlate to answers.

12 **Answer: 4** Transparent film dressings on a clean, noninfected wound can be left in place for days, until the seal is broken, exudate leaks out, or the edges roll up. Older adults are at risk for skin breakdown. A nurse needs knowledge of what dressings are chosen and when they are changed.
Cognitive Level: Application **Client Need:** Physiologic Integrity: Physiological Adaptation **Integrated Process:** Nursing Process: Implementation **Content Area:** Fundamental Skills **Strategy:** Consider the choices; when there are similarities, some choices can be eliminated.

13 **Answer: 1** Ecchymoses are not the result of aging.
Cognitive Level: Application **Client Need:** Health Promotion and Maintenance **Integrated Process:** Nursing Process: Assessment **Content Area:** Foundational Sciences: Growth and Development **Strategy:** The phrase *would be significant* indicates abnormality, so that is the choice you are looking for.

14 **Answer: 3** Prealbumin is a sensitive indicator of changes in nutritional protein status. Serum albumin can provide data about visceral protein stores but has a relatively long half-life and may not accurately reflect recent protein losses. Prealbumin can also alert the nurse to clients at risk for pressure ulcer development.
Cognitive Level: Application **Client Need:** Physiologic Integrity: Reduction of Risk Potential **Integrated Process:** Nursing Process: Assessment **Content Area:** Foundational Sciences: Growth and Development **Strategy:** Apply knowledge from other areas to choose the correct answer.

15 **Answer: 3** The gastrointestinal system is the system that most older adult clients have complaints about, yet it remains the healthiest system over time with proper diet and care. Prolonged use of laxatives can lead to dependence on them for stimulation of defecation and can actually lead to uncontrollable defecation.
Cognitive Level: Application **Client Need:** Physiologic Integrity: Pharmacological and Parenteral Therapies **Integrated Process:** Nursing Process: Implementation **Content Area:** Foundational Sciences: Growth and Development **Strategy:** Choosing the correct response requires use of nursing knowledge, not reliance on myths.

16 **Answer: 2** Severe osteoporosis causes bone density loss, which can result in pathologic fractures when the client is moved. A lift sheet can reduce the risk. The other choices do not address this safety issue.
Cognitive Level: Application **Client Need:** Health Promotion and Maintenance **Integrated Process:** Nursing Process: Implementation **Content Area:** Foundational Sciences: Growth and Development **Strategy:** Narrow your choices to the question asked.

17 **Answer: 3** Posture changes shift the center of gravity in an older adult client and put the client at risk for falls. The other conditions increase the risk of injury if a fall occurs but not the risk of falling.
Cognitive Level: Application **Client Need:** Safe, Effective Care Environment: Safety and Infection Control **Integrated Process:** Nursing Process: Assessment **Content Area:** Foundational Sciences: Growth and Development **Strategy:** Read the question carefully and use similarities in the question stem and the answer to make a selection.

18 **Answer: 1** Motion receptors can be stimulated with instillation of large amounts of fluid. Nausea or vomiting would be stimulated. Relief will occur if the irrigation procedure is stopped.
Cognitive Level: Application **Client Need:** Physiologic Integrity: Physiological Adaptation **Integrated Process:** Nursing Process: Implementation **Content Area:** Foundational Sciences: Growth and Development **Strategy:** The correct choice is the only answer that does not involve the ear or irrigation procedure directly.

19 **Answer: 3** Older adult patients are at risk for developing fluid overload during fluid therapy, especially when receiving multiple units of PRBCs. The infusion rate should be slowed to as low as possible to prevent worsening of the problem. Then assess the vital signs.
Cognitive Level: Analysis **Client Need:** Physiologic Integrity: Reduction of Risk Potential **Integrated Process:** Nursing Process: Implementation **Content Area:** Foundational Sciences: Growth and Development **Strategy:** Visualize care to determine first, second, third, and fourth action order.

20 **Answer: 2** Assessing cyanosis on older adult clients can be difficult, especially if they have darker skin. Fingernails and toenails can have ridges, fungal infections, and yellowing. The oral mucous membranes are the site where cyanosis and pallor are most obvious.
Cognitive Level: Application **Client Need:** Health Promotion and Maintenance **Integrated Process:** Nursing Process: Assessment **Content Area:** Foundational Sciences: Growth and Development **Strategy:** Answering this question requires use of critical thinking. Information given in reference to anemia and fluid volume teaches use of mucous membranes for assessment. Focus on the word *cyanosis* in the stem of the question, and recall age-related changes to aid in selecting an answer.

Key Terms to Review

anosomia p. 256
atrophy p. 256
delirium p. 260
dementia p. 264
lentigines p. 255
older adult abuse p. 261
osteoporosis p. 256
polypharmacy p. 259
presbycusis p. 255
presbyopia p. 255
proprioception p. 256

References

Ebersole, P., Hess, P., & Luggen, A. (2004). *Toward healthy aging: Human needs and nursing response* (6th ed.). St. Louis, MO: Mosby.

Kozier, B., Erb, G., Berman, A., & Snyder, S. (2004). *Fundamentals of nursing: Concepts, process, and practice* (7th ed.). Upper Saddle River, NJ: Prentice Hall.

Lehne, R. (2004). *Pharmacology for nursing care* (5th ed.). St. Louis, MO: Saunders.

Meiner, S., & Lueckenotte, A. (2006). *Gerontologic nursing* (3rd ed.). St. Louis, MO: Mosby.

Ulrich, S., & Canale, S. (2005). *Nursing care planning guides for adults in acute, extended, and home care settings* (6th ed.). St. Louis, MO: Elsevier.

ANSWERS & RATIONALES

Therapeutic Communication and Environment

19

In this chapter

Test Yourself

Are you ready for the NCLEX-RN® or course exams? Use the practice tests on the companion CD-ROM to check.

Cross reference

Other chapters relevant to this content area are

Culturally Competent Care **Chapter 20**

I. OVERVIEW OF COMMUNICATION

A. Characteristics of effective *communication*

1. Occurs when there is an exchange of information, ideas, attitudes, and emotions; therefore, successful communication occurs when message intended is message received
2. A basic skill in providing health care to clients; occurs between nurse and other health care providers as well as between nurse and health care consumers (clients)
3. Nurse needs to understand those basic elements of communication that tend to promote accurate dissemination of information as well as those that may inhibit successful communication so that client receives effective health care

B. Elements of communication (see Box 19–1)

C. Levels of communication

1. Intrapersonal: *intra-* is a prefix meaning within; occurs within oneself and happens constantly; involves thinking about a message before it is sent, interpreting it, and evaluating it (self-talk)
2. Interpersonal: *inter-* is a prefix meaning between; refers to communication occurring between people and involves sending and receiving a message and **feedback**
3. Public communication: involves sending a message to a group of people for dissemination of information; it generally does not require feedback

D. Forms of communication

1. Communication occurs both verbally and nonverbally in a therapeutic relationship; purposeful communication between nurse and client is often termed **therapeutic communication**
2. ! The nurse needs to be aware of communication chosen to ensure message sent is message received; must also be aware of own nonverbal body language and physical boundaries, such as client's personal space
3. ! **Verbal communication:** use of words that are either spoken or written
   a. Therapeutic rapport: verbal communication can be facilitated by a trusting relationship between nurse and client in which client believes that nurse

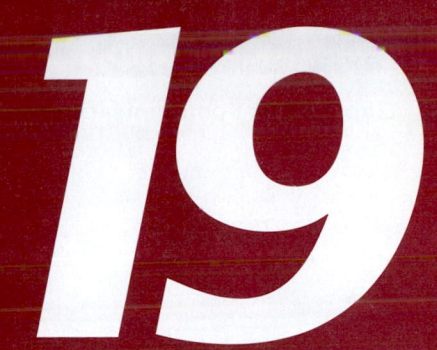

Box 19-1

Elements of Communication

1. Sender: initiates the communication in order to convey information, thoughts, ideas, or feelings to another; encodes the information by selecting the signs and symbols used in the communication (language, word selection, voice intonations, gestures, etc.).
2. Message: the information to be communicated; includes the codings (vocabulary, tone of voice, body language, and way the message is transmitted); effective communication occurs when the message intended is the message received.
3. Channel: the vehicle used to convey the message using any of the five senses; for example, written documentation (sight), oral communication (hearing), and therapeutic touch; it is important to use the correct medium to send the message, such as writing a message for a hearing-impaired client to ensure the message intended is the message received.
4. Receiver: the person or group that the message is intended for, also called the *decoder* of the message; perceives or interprets the message.
5. Environment: the physical, cultural, and social conditions in which the information is transmitted; sometimes called the *context* of the communication.
6. Feedback: sometimes called *response;* requires that the receiver respond to the message communicated by the sender; the response may be verbal or nonverbal and helps to determine whether communication was effective or ineffective.

cares about client's well-being and wants to assist client in meeting health-related goals

b. Pacing: rhythm and speed with which verbal message is sent; pace of a message may indicate interest, disinterest, or anxiety, among other emotions

c. Intonation: pattern of pauses and accents or stresses when sending a message can reflect an underlying mood of sender, such as anger, boredom, excitement

d. Clarity and brevity: clear, brief messages are more likely to be interpreted correctly than vague and lengthy messages; clarity of a message is influenced by congruence between verbal and nonverbal behavior

e. Timing and relevance: messages should be delivered when client is interested in receiving them, and content of message must be of interest to client at time communication takes place

!

4. **Nonverbal communication:** communication that occurs without use of words; often referred to as body language

a. Facial expression: can either convey or mask emotions; cautiously interpret eye and facial movements and validate impressions with further assessment before drawing final conclusions; some facial expressions are universal, such as a smile for happiness and a frown for displeasure

b. Eye contact: can be influenced by cultural norms; avoiding eye contact may be culturally appropriate or can indicate other feelings, such as embarrassment or lack of interest in communicating

c. Gestures: can convey urgency of a client's message or can be a coping response when client cannot express an urgent message quickly enough using words; some gestures (such as a wave of the hand) have almost universal meanings, while others are culture-specific; gestures can also be used as signals when a client cannot communicate with words

d. Posture and gait: can indicate a client's physical well-being, self-concept, and mood; an erect posture and a steady purposeful gait generally indicate a sense of well-being; slouching or a shuffling, slow gait may indicate depressed mood, presence of Parkinson's disease, or that client is physically tired or uncomfortable; validate with client any impressions gained from observing his or her posture and gait

e. Territoriality and personal space: all people, clients and nurses alike, have a physical zone around body that is considered an extension of self and that should not be entered by others; size of the space can vary considerably among cultures and individuals; the type of relationship one has with an individual also affects desired personal space; other forms of body language are often used as signals to indicate when someone has violated personal space (such as taking a step back)

f. Personal appearance: can be a general indicator of self-esteem, social status, emotional status, culture or other group association; selection of clothing is often highly personal; hygiene may be influenced by physical ability, emotional status, mental illness, energy level, and time; be careful not to judge clients based on personal appearance

! **E. Effective communication techniques (see Box 19–2)**

1. It is important for nurses to maintain appropriate boundaries as part of therapeutic communication
2. Nurses should also understand they cannot always be aware of how others perceive or misperceive messages they intended to convey; developing a sense of self-awareness and checking client's understanding of messages is critical to good communication
3. The same principles that are useful in communicating with clients are also useful when communicating with signficant others, families, and even other health care personnel

Memory Aid

The answers to communication questions are those that utilize therapeutic communication techniques while avoiding the use of communication blocks.

! **F. Communication techniques (blocks) to avoid**

1. Communication techniques to avoid are those that discourage further communication from client to nurse and/or place client's feelings on hold
2. Self-disclosure
   - **a.** Involves relating to a client by communicating a personal experience to client that focuses relationship on the nurse
   - **b.** Example: if a client is having difficulty adjusting to a changed body image following amputation, it is not helpful for nurse to state how he or she would feel if faced with a similar problem
   - **c.** A therapeutic helping relationship should be client-centered and goal-directed

Box 19–2

Effective Communication Techniques

Acknowledging: gives nonjudgmental recognition to a client for a certain behavior or contribution, or indicates attention to and care of the client.

Clarifying: asks for additional information to ensure understanding of the message sent; a statement like "Would you tell me more about what you have just said?" indicates that understanding the client's message is important to the nurse.

Focusing: focuses the client on information that is pertinent and helps the client expand on that information; this technique directs the client toward information that is important.

Giving information: provides specific information to a client either with or without the client's request.

Offering self: offers the nurse's presence without attaching any expectations or conditions on the client's behavior during that time.

Restating or paraphrasing: ensures the nurse understands the message sent; utilizing this technique, the nurse repeats the main thought of the message sent.

Reflecting: redirects the content of a client's message back to the client for further thought or consideration.

Summarizing: may be used at the end of an interaction to identify material discussed; it helps to sort out relevant from irrelevant information.

Using silence: allows for quiet time without conversation for several seconds or minutes to allow for reflection about the discussion that just occurred, to reduce tension, or to gather thoughts about how to proceed.

3. Inattentive listening
   a. Blocks communication by indicating that client's needs are not important
   b. A nurse who is thinking about other things when providing care to a client might unintentionally convey this to client; if this happens, nurse could be perceived as distracted or uncaring
4. Overuse of medical jargon
   a. Confuses clients and indicates nurse is not interested in ensuring health care information is understood
   b. Example: if nurse asks client how many times he or she has voided and client does not understand meaning of word *void,* client may not know how to respond to nurse
5. Giving personal opinions (approval, disapproval) or offering advice
   a. Should be avoided; may give impression that a person is closed to new ideas or to open discussion
   b. In a helping relationship, nurses assist clients to manage their own lives and problems and to formulate their own ideas and plans
   c. Examples of giving personal opinions or advice include "I wouldn't do that" or even simple statements such as "That's a good plan" or "That approach may not be a good idea"
6. Prying or probing techniques
   a. These may be helpful in limited circumstances, such as when seeking specific health-related information or to clarify a client's statement; this is particularly true in mental health settings
   b. If there is no health-related use for information obtained by probing or prying questions, this is a nontherapeutic communication; in such instances, the client may provide information to satisfy nurse's curiosity and the nurse's questions are inappropriate
   c. If a client shares with nurse that a problem was not discussed with primary care provider and nurse asks why not, it may place client in a defensive position
   d. Asking for information not pertinent to client's health status violates client's right to privacy
7. Changing the subject
   a. Blocks therapeutic communication by indicating that client should not continue to talk about previous topic; this leads conversation to only those areas that nurse wants to discuss
   b. Example: if a female client asks if her breast will be removed because of a tumor, and nurse asks if she has had a bowel movement since admission, this implies nurse's unwillingness to discuss client's concern
8. Challenging the client or being defensive
   a. Creates a power struggle between client and nurse and does not foster open and honest communication
   b. Avoid questions that contain words *why* or *why not,* which can create distance between client and nurse
9. Providing false reassurance
   a. Does not contribute to open and honest communication
   b. Can break bond of trust between client and nurse
10. Communicating with clients who have special needs (Box 19–3)

II. THERAPEUTIC NURSE–CLIENT RELATIONSHIPS

A. A *therapeutic relationship* is a nurse–client interaction that focuses on client needs and is goal-specific, theory-based, and open to observation or scrutiny by other members of health care team

B. Phases of therapeutic relationship

1. Pre-interaction phase
   a. Occurs prior to initial contact with a person and is similar to planning stage before an interview
   b. Any information that nurse has related to client is organized and analyzed prior to contact with client; during this phase, nurse prepares for initial contact

Box 19-3

Communication with Clients with Special Needs

Difficulty hearing

- To ensure that effective communication occurs with a client who is hearing impaired, stand or sit near client and speak clearly and slowly using a low-pitched voice.
- The environment should have adequate lighting and be quiet and free from distractions.
- Use therapeutic communication techniques to ensure that the message sent is the message received.
- Use writing, if necessary, to enhance communication with a client who is hearing impaired.
- Avoid using a loud voice when speaking to a client who is hearing impaired.

Difficulty seeing

- Ensure the environment has adequate light.
- Ensure that the quality of the spoken word matches the message communicated.
- Remember the visually impaired person may not be able to use nonverbal cues to help interpret the message.

Mute or unable to speak clearly

- When communicating with a client who is unable to speak clearly, has an artificial airway, or is mute, encourage the client to write a response or utilize word boards or pictures to ensure effective communication.
- Utilize the therapeutic technique of clarification or paraphrasing as needed to assist in communication.

Cognitively impaired

- Ensure the language is simple, concise, and spoken slowly and calmly.
- Allow adequate time for the client to process the information.
- Use environmental cues to convey the message to the client; for instance, hold a toothbrush in view while asking if the client would like to brush his or her teeth.

Unresponsive

- Use touch along with the spoken word and try to elicit a response from the client.
- Ask a closed question such as "Can you hear me?" and observe for nonverbal cues that may indicate the client has received the message to try to obtain a response.
- Speak to the client in a manner that assumes the client can hear every spoken word; avoid having conversations about the client's status or that are irrelevant to the client at the bedside.

Non-English-speaking clients

- Seek an interpreter fluent in the client's primary language if the client does not speak English; until an interpreter is available, communication must take place through nonverbal means.
- Use pictures, environmental cues, and body language to communicate with a client who speaks a different language.

! **2.** Orientation phase
   - **a.** May also be called introductory phase or pre-helping phase
   - **b.** Nurse and client get to know one another and develop a degree of trust
   - **c.** Three processes occur during this phase: opening the relationship, clarifying the problem, and structuring and formulating the contract for what will be accomplished during relationship

! **3.** Working phase
   - **a.** Includes exploring and understanding thoughts and feelings, along with facilitating client's work and taking action
   - **b.** Skills required during this phase are empathetic listening and understanding, respect, genuineness, concreteness, and confrontation

c. Client **transference,** an unconscious process of displacing feelings for significant people in past onto nurse in present relationship, can occur in this phase; **countertransference** is nurse's emotional reaction to clients based on feelings for significant people in past
d. At completion of this phase, client makes decisions and takes action, while nurse provides information and collaborates with and supports client

! 4. Termination phase
a. Primary goal of termination phase of therapeutic relationship is to review client's progress and plans for immediate future after reaching goals
b. May be difficult for both nurse and client; to reduce feelings of loss and ambivalence, it may be helpful for nurse to summarize relationship and to make follow-up phone calls to help client transition to independence
c. Nurse should prepare client for termination phase early in communication process

C. Components of a therapeutic relationship
1. Physical component of relationship includes all procedures and technical skills that nurses provide for clients
2. Psychosocial component involves qualities such as positive regard, nonjudgmental attitude, acceptance, warmth, empathy, and authenticity
3. Spiritual component is feeling of connectiveness with clients and respect for diversity of spiritual needs among clients
4. Power component includes beliefs about external and internal locus of control
a. A client with a strong internal locus of control tends to believe that he or she is able to make own decisions and can influence own health; this client may experience more positive health outcomes
b. A client with a strong external locus of control tends to believe that other people and events heavily affect his or her health and related decisions, and may perceive himself or herself as somewhat powerless; this client may have less positive health outcomes unless appropriate support people and services are in place

D. Principles of a therapeutic relationship
1. Nurse delivers care that is holistic and comprehensive of current client needs and priorities
2. Nurse respects client's uniqueness, with consideration given to cultural and spiritual beliefs, values, and practices that provide comfort, support, and hope during illness
3. Nurse fosters open and honest communication that focuses on client's needs and feelings
4. Nurse values empathy, respect, and genuineness in interactions with client
5. Nurse is able to set limits when necessary to foster client progress and growth
6. Nurse promotes client independence by assisting the client to utilize internal resources (such as personal strengths and problem-solving skills) as well as community resources

III. TEACHING AND LEARNING AS THERAPEUTIC COMMUNICATION

A. Purposes of client teaching
1. Maintenance and promotion of health and prevention of illness
a. Examples include providing information about immunization requirements, nutrition, and exercise; offering parenting and prenatal classes
b. Generally these programs are aimed toward groups of people with a health care need and are designed to disseminate information and skills needed for clients to develop positive health practices
2. Restoration of health
a. These programs are intended for clients with an active health problem and focus on cause, condition, and treatment
b. An example of this type of client teaching is insulin administration for a client who has new onset type 1 diabetes

3. Coping with impaired functioning
   a. This type of client teaching centers around providing instruction to an individual who has not made or cannot make a complete recovery
   b. An example is a client who modifies activities of daily living because of a lower limb amputation

B. Domains of learning

1. Cognitive learning involves acquiring and using knowledge; for instance, when teaching a parenting class, nurse provides information on developmental stages of children; when applying that knowledge to toilet training child, parent is learning in **cognitive domain**
2. Affective learning occurs when a client changes unhealthy attitudes or feelings and values; a parent who accepts and understands that children have specific developmental stages and may not become toilet trained until after age 2 is learning in **affective domain**
3. Psychomotor: learning to complete a physical act is learning in the **psychomotor domain;** for example, the nurse may role-play with a parent an appropriate dialogue to use if a toddler refuses to use toilet or appropriate assistance and supervision to provide while child is using toilet

C. Factors that influence client learning

1. Motivation
   a. Motivation is desire to learn
   b. Important to learning is that client recognizes need to learn a new behavior
   c. Nurses can assist a client in solving problems and identifying needs that may increase his or her desire to learn
2. ! Health beliefs
   a. A client's health beliefs may or may not be congruent with information being taught
   b. Nurse may assist a client by showing a cause-and-effect relationship between positive and negative health practices; for example, if cardiac client does not believe that smoking will affect his or her cardiac status, individual is unlikely to change behavior
   c. Nurses need to assess a client's health beliefs in order to develop beneficial teaching plans
   d. Nurses must understand that a client's health care beliefs may not change, despite concentrated efforts, because of multiple psychological, cultural, and environmental factors
3. Psychosocial adaptation to illness
   a. Psychosocial adaptation to illness describes transition from a healthy, independent state to an illness state
   b. Successful adaptation or acculturation to illness depends on client's emotional makeup
   c. ! It is important for nurse to understand that a client is unlikely to learn new health-related behaviors when he or she is not ready or motivated to learn or is experiencing problems unrelated to his or her health
   d. Nurse should regularly assess how a client is adapting
4. Active participation
   a. Active participation by client in teaching and learning process makes learning more meaningful
   b. ! Nurse needs to assess a client's learning needs and to involve client in learning process to encourage active participation
5. Literacy level and educational level: ability of client to read materials provided and understand spoken word
6. Developmental level affects ability to understand health problem and learn information needed for self–management
7. Individual learning style: learning is enhanced when nurse uses instructional methods that match client's preferred learning style

D. Basic teaching principles

1. Set priorities: rank client's learning needs according to importance; involve client in ranking needs because learning is more likely to occur when needs perceived by client are met
2. Use appropriate timing; for example, a client with diabetes is more likely to successfully self-administer insulin immediately after watching a video than if he or she waits until next morning
3. Organize materials: learning occurs from simple to complex; organize material in this manner to allow learner to assimilate information more readily
4. Promote and maintain learner attention and participation: keep environment physically comfortable and free from distractions; involve client actively in learning process to facilitate assimilation of information; ensure that information is personally relevant to client; provide opportunity for client feedback
5. Build on existing knowledge: assess client's knowledge of subject before teaching; when nurse builds on client's existing knowledge, material becomes more personal to client and enhances learning; it also increases learner's confidence in material
6. Select appropriate teaching methods
   a. Discussion: one-on-one formal or informal instruction allows client to set pace of learning and engage in verbal exchange with nurse; promotes customized learning for client
   b. Question and answer: meets needs of clients for specific pieces of information as requested by client; often beneficial as a follow-up to other teaching methods
   c. Role-play, discovery: allows client to simulate real-life situations and apply new knowledge or skills in an artificial or "safe" setting; helps to build client's confidence in newly acquired knowledge and skills once feelings of shyness, embarrassment, or awkwardness are worked through
   d. Computerized instruction: can include CAI (computer-assisted instruction) or interactive computer programs (using touch-screen technology); allows client to regulate pace of instruction and possibly direct nature of material presented next (interactive programs)
7. Use appropriate teaching aids: teaching aids are useful supplements to instruction if they are well-selected according to content and client's learning style; may include visual aids (drawings, charts, models, printed materials), audiotapes, films or videotapes, programmed instruction, games, and others
8. Provide teaching related to developmental level
   a. Infant: immunizations, infant safety, nutrition, rest/sleep patterns, and sensory stimulation; assess parents' learning needs and provide instruction accordingly; complete client teaching when infant is calm and happy to minimize parents' distraction
   b. Toddler: accident prevention, toilet training, dental hygiene, and appropriate play activities; toddlers fear pain and separation from parents; parent teaching for a hospitalized toddler includes participation in care, purpose of care plans, and developmental regression that can occur because of hospitalization
   c. Preschooler: accident prevention, dental health, nutrition, cognitive stimulation, and sleep patterns; assist hospitalized preschooler by using visual, tactile, and auditory images to decrease a toddler's fear of procedures; therapeutic play or using dolls or puppets to demonstrate procedures before they are done is also helpful to child
   d. School-aged child: dental hygiene, safety measures, promotion of physical fitness, and hygiene measures to prevent spread of infection; provide concrete examples and explanations of procedures to help child understand health care; encourage child to identify his or her own learning needs; therapeutic play may assist child to learn
   e. Adolescent: effects of drugs and alcohol, sexually transmitted diseases, reducing risk of injury (e.g., motor vehicle accidents, sports), and nutrition information; actively involve adolescent in learning to help him or her assimilate information provided; client contracting and peer education also promote learning

! f. Young to middle-aged adult: importance of routine health tests and screening, sun protection measures, importance of nutrition (especially adequate protein and calcium intake), and exercise to maintain health; evaluate client's learning needs and determine learning needs that client believes are important to maintain his or her health

! g. Older adult: importance of exercise in maintaining joint mobility, nutritional information (including caloric and fluid requirements), and fall prevention information; ensure there is adequate lighting and use large print if necessary for client who is visually impaired; for hearing impaired client, use written teaching materials and visual aids

IV. THERAPEUTIC ENVIRONMENTS

A. A therapeutic environment is one in which environment is manipulated or created to help restore or promote physical and mental health

B. See Box 19–4 for practice settings in which therapeutic environments are integral to care

1. Physical space may be designed with attention to color, layout, and aesthetic appeal, including artwork
2. Aids to memory or cognition, such as clock and white boards in room identifying names of caregivers for day, may be used in hospital or long-term care environments

C. Nursing interventions commonly used during care in a therapeutic environment

1. Health promotion and maintenance
2. Assessment and evaluation
3. Case management
4. Provision of a therapeutic milieu
5. Education of clients about factors that influence mental health and mental illness
6. Promotion of self-care and independence
7. Administration and monitoring of psychobiological treatment regimens
8. Crisis intervention and counseling
9. Engaging in social and community mental health efforts

D. *Milieu* therapy

1. Provides a therapeutic and safe environment in which client is free to express thoughts and feelings; this is particularly employed in mental health settings (see also Chapter 22)
2. Clients interact, share frustrations, and learn to relate to others in honest and constructive ways under supervision and assistance of mental health professionals
3. Norms for client behavior on unit to foster safety of all clients and staff are made known to clients; when clients act in a manner inconsistent with these norms, such as being verbally or physically aggressive with other clients or staff, staff sets limits with client and may enforce sanctions that are known to client in advance
4. Individual client growth is often achieved through group meetings in which focus may be learning social skills, problem solving, setting goals, or otherwise effecting positive self-change

Box 19–4

Practice Settings That Utilize a Therapeutic Environment

- Psychiatric hospitals
- Community mental health centers
- General hospitals
- Community health agencies (e.g., home health, primary-care centers, homeless clinics)
- Outpatient services
- Senior centers and daycare centers
- Schools
- Prisons
- Emergency and crisis centers

5. A prime tenet of group therapy is that all group members are valued and contribute to overall functioning of group

Check Your NCLEX-RN® Exam I.Q. *You are ready for testing on this content if you can*

- Utilize communication techniques appropriately and effectively.
- Determine accurately the components of a therapeutic relationship and how to maintain one.
- Create an environment conducive to client teaching, including preparation of the teaching plan.

PRACTICE TEST

1 The nurse has explained a therapeutic diet to a client. To ensure learning occurred, the nurse should do which of the following?

1. Repeat the details of the diet once or twice more.
2. Listen to comments from the client.
3. Ask another nurse to verify the client understands the diet.
4. Refer the client to a nutritionist.

2 A nurse is trying to establish whether a client who appears unconscious can communicate. Which of the following would be the best approach for the nurse to use?

1. Ask open-ended questions.
2. Ask the client to blink once or twice in response to questions.
3. Observe for facial grimaces during verbal stimuli from the nurse.
4. Assess for response to painful stimuli.

3 A client who is legally blind has been admitted to the cardiac unit. Which of the following actions by the nurse would be best to promote adjustment to the environment?

1. Speak slowly and in a low-pitched voice while facing the client.
2. Post a sign on the door indicating the client is blind.
3. Explain unit noises and physical surroundings.
4. Give clear, concise, simple instructions to the client.

4 The home care nurse has asked the client to demonstrate self-injection technique. In doing so, the nurse is primarily attempting to determine which of the following?

1. The number of home visits that will be required.
2. Other support services the client will need.
3. The quality of the client-teaching plan.
4. The client's ability to perform the skill.

5 Which of the following would be the most appropriate time for the use of confrontation as a therapeutic technique in communication with an assigned client?

1. When a good relationship exists and the client's anxiety level is low
2. During periods when the client is noncompliant
3. After the client has had time to reflect on his or her behavior
4. Immediately after a negative behavior has occurred

6 Which of the following teaching strategies should the nurse choose as being most likely to be effective when providing health instruction to an adolescent client?

1. Lecture format
2. Professionally made videos
3. Client contracting
4. Role play

7 A nurse is evaluating a client's ability to change the surgical dressing before discharge. During the demonstration, the nurse notices the client has not performed the procedure correctly. The most appropriate action of the nurse would be to do which of the following?

1. Immediately change the dressing again to demonstrate correct technique.
2. Praise the client for aspects of the procedure done accurately and correct the client's mistakes.
3. Praise the client for steps completed correctly and refer the client to home care for follow up.
4. Explain kindly that the procedure was performed incorrectly and have the client repeat the procedure.

8 When beginning to present information about heart disease to a client newly diagnosed with heart disease, which of the following is most important for the nurse to do first?

1. Find out what the client knows or has heard about the disorder.
2. Consult with the physician to determine content based on individual severity of disease.
3. Have a family member or significant other present who can reinforce diet and exercise tips.
4. Proceed from simple to complex concepts when discussing pathophysiology.

9 During the nursing assessment of an elderly female client, the nurse enhances communication by doing which of the following?

1. Speaking loudly and using many gestures
2. Interviewing the client quickly to conserve the client's energy
3. Interviewing the client with family present to verify responses to questions
4. Restating terms or phrases in different ways if the client does not understand

10 The nurse would use which of the following statements when trying to encourage a client to express her feelings and allow the nurse to genuinely respond to those feelings?

1. "You mentioned that you broke your leg last year. Can you tell me more about how that happened?"
2. "You shared with me a lot of information about your history of depression. It sounds as though medication alone may not be controlling your symptoms as you hoped."
3. "You mentioned that your back pain has never gone away since your surgery. How difficult has it been to adapt to having pain during everyday activities?"
4. "You told me that you have had asthma since you were 11 years old and that medication therapy requires adjustment every 8 to 10 months or so. Is that right?"

11 Which of the following is the best approach for a nurse to use to encourage a client to express feelings and to develop increased awareness about what those feelings are?

1. Challenge the client
2. Offer reassurance
3. Suggest coping strategies
4. Offer empathy

12 While talking with a client, the client tells the nurse, "You are just like my mother; you don't trust me or like me. You and she wish I were dead." The nurse interprets this statement as indicating which of the following processes?

1. Psychosis
2. Countertransference
3. Transference
4. Projection

13 The nurse is preparing to explain an upcoming procedure to a 72-year-old, English-speaking Latino client. The nurse determines that the best way to verbally communicate with this client is to

1. Speak quickly and avoid eye contact, which could be perceived as threatening.
2. Speak slowly and provide brief and simple explanations.
3. Get an interpreter or family member to interpret for the nurse as needed.
4. Give very complete explanations of all information.

14 The nurse observes a client who is fidgeting, wringing the hands, and has body tenseness and a wrinkled brow. What is the best way for the nurse to interpret these nonverbal cues?

1. Say, "You look tense. Can you tell me if something is making you afraid or nervous?"
2. Ask, "You look upset. Would you like some medication to help you become more calm?"
3. Say, "You look worried. Is something bothering you?"
4. Ask, "Why are you so nervous and jumpy?"

PRACTICE TEST

15 A nurse floating to the nursing unit learns during inter-shift report that a client suffered disfiguring injuries in an accident a week ago. What is the best way for the nurse to prepare for the first encounter with this client?

1. Learn about the client's support systems (family, friends, religion).
2. Obtain the specifics of the disfigurement to better control first reactions by the nurse.
3. Review all medications and treatment procedures prior to meeting the client.
4. Have all supplies and equipment ready to be able to provide efficient care.

16 The nurse enters a client's room to obtain an admission history, moves the chair to the top of the bed by the client's head, and sits down to better hear the client. The client draws back and moves to the opposite side of the bed. What is the best response by the nurse?

1. Move the chair a foot or two away from the bed and observe the client's response.
2. Say, "I will come back later when you are ready to talk to me."
3. Ignore the behavior and continue with the interview, observing the client for depression.
4. Lean over and touch the client to convey reassurance.

17 The nurse who has a heavy work assignment for the day due to high client census sees that a client is crying. Which of the following would be the best way for the nurse to convey a willingness to be with the client for support?

1. State, "Let's talk while I change your colostomy bag."
2. Ask, "Would you like to talk?" from the doorway, and go in if the client says yes.
3. Pull up a chair, sit down, and state, "I see something is bothering you. Do you want to talk?"
4. State, "I'll be back later and we can talk about what is troubling you at the moment."

18 A client asks about a new diagnostic test with which the nurse is unfamiliar. What is the best nursing response?

1. "I don't know much about that procedure, but I will find out and bring you information about it."
2. "The technicians in the radiology department will explain the procedure to you when you go for the test."
3. "It is your doctor's responsibility to explain that procedure to you. Would you like me to telephone the doctor?"
4. "I can't explain that now, but I'll get back to you later after all the morning medications are distributed."

19 A client can understand only minimal English, and no interpreter is available. What alternative measures can the nurse use to enhance communication?

1. Speak loudly to the client.
2. Use a paper and pencil to write questions and information.
3. Use pictures and nonverbal cues to communicate.
4. Speak more slowly and face the client.

20 A client has been on the nursing unit for a few weeks because of complications after surgery, including the need for extensive wound care. During the last dressing change before discharge to home with home health services, the client becomes angry with the nurse and says, "You don't have to be so careful. I'm being sent home anyway!" Which of the following responses by the nurse would be therapeutic? Select all that apply.

1. "I hear frustration or perhaps anger in your voice. Can you tell me more about how you are feeling right now?"
2. "Many people who have been in the hospital for an extended period have mixed feelings about going home. Can you tell me how you are feeling about discharge?"
3. "It sounds as though you are nervous about going home, but the wound care nurse who will see you also uses excellent technique. I'm sure your wound will continue to heal."
4. "Just because you are going home doesn't mean that your wound doesn't still require strict technique during a dressing change. Do you have any questions about your wound care after discharge?"
5. "Do you have any concerns about what will happen after discharge that you would like to talk about?"

Answer: ______________________

ANSWERS & RATIONALES

1 **Answer: 2** It is important for the nurse to listen to the feedback given by the client to ensure the message sent was the message received. Repetition is important in the teaching process but does not evaluate clients' understanding (option 1). Options 3 and 4 are unnecessary as part of evaluation. **Cognitive Level:** Application **Client Need:** Psychosocial Integrity **Integrated Process:** Communication and Documentation **Content Area:** Fundamentals **Strategy:** The core issue of the question is determining the client response to teaching. In evaluation questions such as these, the correct option is likely to be one that focuses directly on the client.

2 **Answer: 2** To evaluate an unresponsive client's ability to communicate, it is best for the nurse to ask questions that will elicit a single act or response by the client. Option 1 is not appropriate for the client's condition. Options 3 and 4 may be noted during neurological assessment but do not relate to communication.
Cognitive Level: Analysis **Client Need:** Psychosocial Integrity **Integrated Process:** Communication and Documentation **Content Area:** Fundamentals **Strategy:** In communication questions such as these, the correct option is one that is client-focused and relates directly to communication. With this in mind, eliminate options 3 and 4 immediately, and choose option 2 over 1 because of its simplicity.

3 **Answer: 3** A client who is blind does not have the benefit of nonverbal cues to facilitate communication and understanding of the environment. It is important for the nurse to explain physical surroundings and noises because the client cannot determine these without the added benefit of sight. Options 1 and 4 are approaches that a nurse should use with a client who is hearing impaired. Placing a sign on the client's door encroaches on confidentiality.
Cognitive Level: Analysis **Client Need:** Psychosocial Integrity **Integrated Process:** Communication and Documentation **Content Area:** Fundamentals **Strategy:** In communication questions with a client who has loss of vision, the correct option is one that supplements vision impairment with verbal communication. Note the critical word *best* in the stem of the question, which indicates more than one response may be partially or totally correct.

4 **Answer: 4** A return demonstration specifically identifies the client's ability to perform a skill. The client's skill level may provide incidental information related to options 1, 2, and 4, but they are not the primary reasons for asking the client to demonstrate a skill.
Cognitive Level: Analysis **Client Need:** Psychosocial Integrity **Integrated Process:** Communication and Documentation **Content Area:** Fundamentals **Strategy:** Recall that to evaluate learning of a skill, which is in the psychomotor domain, the best option is the one that utilizes return demonstration. In this way, the nurse can verify that the client can perform the skill and also has an opportunity to provide additional feedback.

5 **Answer: 1** Confrontation should not be used as a therapeutic communication technique unless trust has been established in the nurse–client relationship. Because confrontation can be uncomfortable for the client, it is important for the nurse and client to have a trusting relationship as a foundation. The other options represent situations in which the nurse might like to use confrontation but that are not appropriate for this communication technique.
Cognitive Level: Application **Client Need:** Psychosocial Integrity **Integrated Process:** Communication and Documentation **Content Area:** Fundamentals **Strategy:** Note the critical words *most appropriate* in the stem of the question. This tells you that more than one option will be plausible and that you must choose one over the others based on what is most therapeutic for the client.

6 **Answer: 3** Client contracting provides adolescents with the ability to be involved in their care. Adolescents should be involved in planning and decision making regarding their need for information about their own health issues. Lecture, viewing a video, and role-play would not provide opportunity for feedback.
Cognitive Level: Analysis **Client Need:** Psychosocial Integrity **Integrated Process:** Communication and Documentation **Content Area:** Fundamentals **Strategy:** In teaching and learning questions in which communication is key, choose the option that provides for two-way communication between the client and nurse. Note the critical words *most likely to be effective* in the stem of the question, which tells you that more than one option is plausible and that you must choose based on knowledge of communication theory.

7 **Answer: 2** Praising the client for steps performed correctly provides positive reinforcement. In addition, explaining the client's mistakes reinforces the correct way to perform the procedure. For the nurse to redo the dressing decreases the client's confidence. Praising the client without correcting the mistakes gives feedback that the procedure was done correctly. Having the client repeat the procedure and stating it was done correctly without further guidance does not reinforce or assist learning.
Cognitive Level: Analysis **Client Need:** Psychosocial Integrity **Integrated Process:** Communication and Documentation **Content Area:** Fundamentals **Strategy:** Note the critical words *most appropriate* in the stem of the question. This tells you that more than one option is plausible and that you must choose based on knowledge of communication theory.

8 **Answer: 1** When presenting information to a client, it is important that the nurse find out what the client already knows, and then build on existing knowledge. It is not necessary to consult with a physician. It may be helpful to have family members present, but it is not the priority at the time of initial teaching. It is important when teaching to begin with basic concepts and progress to the complex after determining current client knowledge.
Cognitive Level: Analysis **Client Need:** Psychosocial Integrity **Integrated Process:** Communication and Documentation **Content Area:** Fundamentals **Strategy:** Focus on the critical word *first* in

the stem of the question. This tells you that more than one option may be correct and that a time sequence is involved. Recalling that assessment is the first step of the nursing process, choose an option that assesses the client's current level of knowledge before beginning instruction.

9 **Answer: 4** Restating the information in different ways may assist the elderly client in understanding. Increasing speech volume and gesturing (option 1) only further confuses the client. Older adults do better with a slower paced interview with frequent breaks to decrease exhaustion (option 2). Relying on the family (option 3) is not respectful of the older adult's autonomy.
Cognitive Level: Application **Client Need:** Psychosocial Integrity **Integrated Process:** Communication and Documentation **Content Area:** Fundamentals **Strategy:** The core issue of the question is how to communicate most effectively with an elderly client. The correct option is the one that focuses on the client, incorporates age-related needs, and does not incorporate ageism into the response.

10 **Answer: 3** The communication technique of reflection (option 3) occurs when the nurse directs feelings and questions back to the client to encourage elaboration. The nurse uses the technique of focusing (option 1) by asking questions to help the client focus on a specific area of concern. In summarizing (option 2), the nurse highlights important points of the conversation. The nurse uses restating (option 4) by repeating back to clients the main points or content of the conversation.
Cognitive Level: Analysis **Client Need:** Psychosocial Integrity **Integrated Process:** Communication and Documentation **Content Area:** Fundamentals **Strategy:** The core issue of the question is knowledge of the various types of therapeutic techniques, specifically one that utilizes reflection as a means of encouraging continued communication. Use this knowledge and the process of elimination to make a selection.

11 **Answer: 4** Empathy is the ability of the nurse to see the client's perception of the world. Challenging clients (option 1) forces them to defend themselves from what appears to be an attack by the nurse. False reassurance (option 2) is another way of telling clients how to feel and ignoring their distress. Advising (option 3) occurs when the nurse tells clients what to do, preventing them from exploring problems and using the problem-solving process to find solutions.
Cognitive Level: Application **Client Need:** Psychosocial Integrity **Integrated Process:** Communication and Documentation **Content Area:** Fundamentals **Strategy:** The core issue of the question is knowledge of the purpose and use of therapeutic communication techniques. Use this knowledge and the process of elimination to make a selection.

12 **Answer: 3** Transference is the unconscious process of displaying feelings for significant people in the client's past onto the nurse in the present relationship. Countertransference (option 2) is the nurse's emotional reaction to clients based on feelings for significant people in the nurse's past. Psychosis (option 1) is a state in which a client is unable to comprehend reality and has difficulty relating to others. Projection (option 4) is a defense mechanism in which blame for unacceptable desires, thoughts, shortcomings, and mistakes is attached to others in the environment.
Cognitive Level: Analysis **Client Need:** Psychosocial Integrity **Integrated Process:** Communication and Documentation **Content Area:** Fundamentals **Strategy:** The core issue of the question is knowledge of various processes that can occur during therapeutic communication. Eliminate options 1 (a disorder) and 4 (a defense mechanism) first. Choose option 3 over 2 because it is the client who has made the transference, not the nurse.

13 **Answer: 2** Taking into account the age and ethnicity of the client, it is helpful to speak slowly and provide short and simple explanations. Speaking quickly does not help the client understand the information presented. Eye contact is acceptable. There is no need for an interpreter based on the information in the question.
Cognitive Level: Application **Client Need:** Psychosocial Integrity **Integrated Process:** Communication and Documentation **Content Area:** Fundamentals **Strategy:** Note that some options have more than one part to them. In such questions, all parts must be correct for the option to be correct. Eliminate option 3 based on information in the stem. Eliminate options 1 and 4 because they are opposite of information in the correct option.

14 **Answer: 1** The core issue of the question is the communication by the nurse that is most likely to elicit further data from the client. With this in mind, option 1 provides a broad opening for the client. Option 2 places a judgment on the client's behavior. Option 3 begins by acknowledging the client's feelings, but then risks putting the client in a defensive position by asking, "Is something bothering you?" Option 4 also places the client on the defense.
Cognitive Level: Analysis **Client Need:** Psychosocial Integrity **Integrated Process:** Communication and Documentation **Content Area:** Fundamentals **Strategy:** The core issue of the question is how to apply general principles of therapeutic communication. In this question, the correct option is the one that is nonjudgmental, uses therapeutic communication techniques, and avoids communication blocks.

15 **Answer: 2** The nurse is more likely to exhibit therapeutic verbal and nonverbal communication by being aware of the extent of the client's disfiguring injuries. This will reduce the likelihood of surprise that can be seen in nonverbal behavior. The remaining options are also items that the nurse will do, but they are general to all clients and not particular to the client in the question.
Cognitive Level: Analysis **Client Need:** Psychosocial Integrity **Integrated Process:** Communication and Documentation **Content Area:** Fundamentals **Strategy:** The critical phrases in the stem of the question are *best way* and *first encounter.* The phrase *best way* indicates that more than one option is a true statement and more than one option may compete for priority. The phrase *first encounter* assists you to focus on the real core issue of the question, which relates to communication.

16 **Answer: 1** The client may have a need for increased personal space, which may account for withdrawing to the other side of the bed. However, cultural considerations cannot be ruled out by the information in this stem. With this in mind, the correct action by the nurse is to validate the reason for the client's behavior. This is what option 1 represents, an attempt

to determine whether increased need for personal space is the reason for the behavior. Option 2 punishes the client for the behavior by leaving the client alone. Option 3 is inappropriate because it does not acknowledge an unspoken need by the client. Option 4 would further invade personal space and is inappropriate until further data is gathered.
Cognitive Level: Analysis **Client Need:** Psychosocial Integrity **Integrated Process:** Communication and Documentation **Content Area:** Fundamentals **Strategy:** The core issue of the question is how to respond to a client's nonverbal behavior in a therapeutic manner. Choose the answer that validates the original data or impression, which is option 1. Eliminate options 2 and 3 because they are nontherapeutic and option 4 because it could worsen the situation.

17 **Answer: 1** The nurse has two competing priorities: the need to accomplish work on a busy shift and the need to address the psychosocial needs of a client in distress. Option 1 takes into consideration both of these factors. Option 2 creates psychological as well as physical distance between the nurse and the client because the question is asked from the doorway. Option 3 ignores the other workload of the nurse. Option 4 puts the client's feelings on hold.
Cognitive Level: Analysis **Client Need:** Psychosocial Integrity **Integrated Process:** Communication and Documentation **Content Area:** Fundamentals **Strategy:** The core issue of the question is the most therapeutic response to a client in distress. Note that the question also contains the critical words *best way,* which implies that the options will have greater or lesser degrees of correctness and that you must choose between them. Use the process of elimination and choose the option that takes into account all of the relevant information in the stem of the question.

18 **Answer: 1** Option 1 demonstrates honesty and openness between the client and the nurse. It also addresses the client's need for information. Options 2, 3, and 4 are incorrect because they put the client's information needs on hold and do not represent a candid response by the nurse. The correct answer to communication questions is the one that best acknowledges the client and utilizes therapeutic communication techniques.
Cognitive Level: Analysis **Client Need:** Psychosocial Integrity **Integrated Process:** Communication and Documentation **Content Area:** Fundamentals **Strategy:** Eliminate options 2 and 3 because they are similar in that they put the client's request on hold and divert the responsibility to someone else. Eliminate option 4 because it is not a totally candid response. Choose option 1 because it is the only one that incorporates all the information in the stem of the question with regard to the nurse's level of knowledge and the client's need to know.

19 **Answer: 3** Because the client does not speak English, the nurse must utilize nonverbal communication. With this in mind, option 3 is the one that takes this need into account. Options 1 and 4 are helpful when the nurse is working with a client who is hearing impaired. Option 2 would be useful for the aphasic client who has use of the dominant hand, such as after a CVA.
Cognitive Level: Application **Client Need:** Psychosocial Integrity **Integrated Process:** Communication and Documentation **Content Area:** Fundamentals **Strategy:** The core issue of the question is the best method for communicating with a client when there is a language barrier. Eliminate options 3 and 4 because they are similar with respect to the spoken word. Eliminate option 2 because it also relies on words that may not be in the client's vocabulary.

20 **Answer: 1, 2, 5** The correct answers to communication questions are those that utilize therapeutic communication techniques and avoid communication blocks. Options 1, 2, and 5 utilize these techniques, while options 3 and 4 use the communication blocks of false reassurance (option 3), challenging the client (option 4). Another block would be putting the client's feelings on hold.
Cognitive Level: Analysis **Client Need:** Psychosocial Integrity **Integrated Process:** Communication and Documentation **Content Area:** Fundamentals **Strategy:** Analyze each statement in terms of being a communication enhancer or blocker. Choose the ones that incorporate therapeutic communication techniques without having any components of communication blocks.

Key Terms to Review

affective domain p. 275
cognitive domain p. 275
communication p. 269
countertransference p. 274
feedback p. 269
milieu p. 277
nonverbal communication p. 270
psychomotor domain p. 275
therapeutic communication p. 269
therapeutic relationship p. 272
transference p. 274
verbal communication p. 269

References

Harkreader, H., & Hogan, M. (2004). *Fundamentals of nursing: Caring and clinical judgment* (2nd ed.). Philadelphia: W. B. Saunders.

Kozier, B., Erb, G., Berman, A., & Snyder, S. (2004). *Fundamentals of nursing: Concepts, Process, and Practice* (7th ed.). Upper Saddle River, NJ: Prentice Hall.

Potter, P., & Perry, A. (2005). *Fundamentals of nursing* (6th ed.). St. Louis, MO: Mosby, Inc.

Taylor, C., Lillis, C., & LeMone, P. (2004). *Fundamentals of nursing: The art and science of nursing care* (5th ed.). Philadelphia: Lippincott Williams & Wilkins.

20 Culturally Competent Care

Test Yourself

Are you ready for the NCLEX-RN® or course exams? Use the practice tests on the companion CD-ROM to check.

In this chapter

Cross reference

Other chapters relevant to this content area are

Reproduction, Family Planning, and Infertility	Chapter 9
Uncomplicated Antenatal Assessment and Care	Chapter 10
Uncomplicated Postpartum Assessment and Care	Chapter 12
Blood and Blood Component Therapy	Chapter 33

I. CULTURALLY COMPETENT CARE OVERVIEW

A. *Culture* defined

1. A complex whole, encompassing knowledge, beliefs, morals, laws, customs, and any habits acquired by members of society
2. Represents ways of perceiving, behaving, and evaluating world

B. Culture and nursing care

1. Madeleine Leininger's Theory of Culture Care Diversity and Universality includes concepts of culture care; delineated as preservation/maintenance, accommodation/negotiation, and repatterning/restructuring
2. People from various cultures have specific ways of behaving to protect health or to restore health after becoming ill
3. A prerequisite to delivering culturally competent care is to understand one's own personal cultural values and health beliefs
4. It is necessary to be respectful and understanding of client's culture if goal of culturally competent care is to be met
5. Communicate with clients of various cultures using purposeful strategies
   a. Assess fluency in English and make arrangements for an interpreter if needed; speak directly to client even if using an interpreter
   b. Be attentive to body language that might offend client
   c. Learn and follow how client wishes to be addressed
   d. Provide an environment for communication that respects habits regarding eye contact and amount of personal space
   e. Use language that is free of slang or currently popular jargon; use simple, straightforward sentences

f. If a client does not understand, rephrase sentence or question
g. Prior to giving written health teaching materials, even if written in client's primary language, assess reading ability; health literacy can affect ability to learn health information regardless of cultural background

6. Religious laws may influence dietary practices, which in turn may influence nursing care during times of illness (see Table 20–1 ■); common restrictions include pork and alcohol; fasting may be done on certain religious holidays; children, pregnant women, and those who are ill are usually exempt from fasting
7. Culturally based dietary preferences are lifelong habits and can significantly influence health as well as compliance with medically recommended dietary changes (see Table 20–2 ■)
8. Cultural beliefs about maintaining or restoring health may clash with those of health care provider; remain nonjudgmental and work with client to incorporate client's cultural health practices while assisting client to meet his or her health goals

II. CULTURAL CONSIDERATIONS FOR AFRICAN AMERICANS

!

A. Communication

1. English is primary language; may be called African American Vernacular English, or AAVE
2. Direct eye contact may be considered inappropriate
3. May use oculistics (eye rolling) in response to communications perceived to be inappropriate
4. May use silence in response to what is perceived as an inappropriate question
5. Verbal and nonverbal communication is integral in communication process

B. Time orientation

1. Tend to be present oriented rather than future oriented; thus, preventive health care may be difficult to implement or maintain
2. However, time orientation varies according to age, subculture, and socioeconomic status
3. May not be punctual for appointments if the needs of family or friends require immediate attention

Table 20–1

Dietary Practices of Selected Religions

Religion	Dietary Restrictions or Practices
Orthodox Judaism	Kosher dietary laws allow fish that have scales and fins, cloven-hoofed animals, and animals that eat vegetables or are slaughtered in a ritualistic manner. Milk and meat may not be combined in any way. Fasting during Yom Kippur (24 hours).
Roman Catholicism	Meat is prohibited on Ash Wednesday, and Fridays during Lent, including Good Friday. Fasting is done on Ash Wednesday and Good Friday and is optional during rest of Lent.
Russian Orthodox	Meat and dairy products are prohibited on Wednesdays, Fridays, and during Lent. Fasting occurs during Advent.
Buddhism	Vegetarianism for some sects. Alcohol and drug use is not favored.
Hinduism	Vegetarianism for some with beef and veal prohibited for all. Fasting rituals vary depending on god worshiped.
Islam	Meats that are prohibited include pork and meats not slaughtered as part of ritual. Drug and alcohol use prohibited.
Jehovah's Witness	Meats that are allowed have been drained of blood; no foods to which blood has been added are allowed.

Table 20-2
Preferred Foods of Various Cultures

Cultural Group	Preferred Foods
Mexican Americans	Corn, dried beans, and chili peppers are basic foods. Tortillas are used for bread (corn, sometimes wheat) Relatively small amounts of meat are used. Fruits such as papaya and mango are used in varying amounts (based on availability and price).
Hispanic/Latino Americans	Similar food pattern to Mexican diet. Rice and beans are basic foods. Dried codfish is a staple, but meat, milk, green and yellow vegetables are used less often. Viandas (starchy vegetables and fruits such as plantains and green bananas) are used, but other fruits are used in limited amounts.
Native American and Alaska Natives	Variable depending on region and local crops or game. Fish (Alaskan) and meat (Navajo), including game, chicken, pork, mutton, are daily staples. Other staples are bread (tortillas or fry bread, blue corn bread, corn meal mush), eggs, vegetables (corn, potatoes, green beans, tomatoes), and some fruit.
African Americans	Breads and cereals include biscuits, cornmeal mush or muffins or cornbread, cooked cereals with corn and oats. Eggs and cheese are used, but milk is not as popular (perhaps because lactose intolerance has greater prevalence). Preferred vegetables include leafy greens, okra, sweet potatoes, potatoes, corn, and a variety of beans, often served with rice. Pork, poultry, fish, and organ meats are often more popular than beef. Fried foods are popular.
Asian Americans	Varies to some extent based on region. Chinese: rice, vegetables cooked in wok, eggs, soybean products (tofu), small amounts of meat, green tea. Japanese: rice, soy products, and green tea (similar to Chinese); seafood, sushi, steamed vegetables, fresh fruit. Southeast Asian: rice, fresh fruits and vegetables, seafood, chicken, duck, pork, nuts, and legumes.
European Americans	Varies somewhat by country of origin but tends to include more red meat and carbohydrates as well as vegetables and fruits.

C. Social roles
1. Extended family is important
2. Strong sense of obligation to relatives
3. Value friendships
4. Many single-parent families, typically headed by females
5. Tend to have large family support systems
6. Religious affiliation common

! **D. Views of health and illness**
1. Body, mind, and spirit are integrated
2. Good health is result of good luck; thus individual has little impact on health status
3. Illness may be a punishment from God
4. Illness is related to an individual's harmony with nature
5. Emotional or personal problems can be resolved through use of a spiritualist who is called by God to heal
6. Voodoo may be considered a powerful cultural healer
7. Practitioners who use roots, herbs, oils, candles, and ointments may be used in healing process

E. Health risks
1. Lactose intolerance and lactase deficiency
2. Hypertension
3. Sickle cell anemia

4. Cancers, including breast, colorectal, esophageal, stomach, cervical, uterine, and prostate
5. Coronary heart disease
6. Coccidioidomycosis
7. Diabetes mellitus

F. Nursing considerations

1. Avoid **stereotyping** (an expectation that all people within same ethnic or cultural group are alike and share same beliefs and attitudes) and generalizing
2. Include family in medical care if desired by client
3. Allow for flexibility in scheduling appointments
4. Facilitate and encourage use of folk healers and spiritualists
5. Encourage family to bring traditional diet if medically acceptable

III. CULTURAL CONSIDERATIONS FOR ASIAN AMERICANS

A. Communication

1. Primary languages include Chinese, Japanese, Vietnamese, Korean, and English
2. May use silence to demonstrate respect for elders
3. May consider direct eye contact to be impolite or aggressive; may look away as nurse attempts to make direct eye contact
4. Unlikely to criticize or disagree with others verbally
5. Consider word "no" to be disrespectful
6. Nodding one's head or smiling does not always suggest agreement with what has been said

B. Time orientation: tend to be present oriented while highly regarding past

C. Social roles

1. Respect aging members of society
2. Family bonds are important; large extended family networks exist with devotion to tradition
3. It may be expected that daughters and daughters-in-law will care for older family members as their health declines
4. Structured and hierarchical family unit, with men and elders being greatly respected
5. Women are expected to be subservient to men
6. Loyalty to family members is expected and highly regarded
7. Education is highly valued
8. Religious affiliation common, including Taoism, Islam, Buddhism, and Christianity
9. Traditions are highly valued

D. Views of health and illness

1. Chinese concept of yin and yang is a metaphor for forces of nature being balanced to produce harmony
2. Illness is a state of disharmony or imbalance of yin and yang
3. Foods are associated with concept of yin and yang; for example, yin foods are cold, whereas yang foods are hot; cold foods and beverages are consumed for hot illnesses, and hot food and beverages are consumed for cold illnesses
4. Illnesses may be attributed to overexertion or to prolonged sitting or lying

E. Health risks

1. Thalassemia
2. Lactase deficiency
3. G6PD deficiency
4. Hypertension
5. Cancer, with stomach and liver more common sites
6. Coccidioidomycosis

F. Nursing considerations

1. Asian clients are likely to be quiet and compliant during illness, thus placing them at risk for not having needs met
2. Asian clients may wish to take medications with certain foods or beverages believed to promote correct balance for health
3. Asian clients often do not trust health care providers and wish to include traditional healers along with Western medicine practices

4. Asian clients may expect health care providers to be authoritative
5. Limit eye contact and physical touching; touch a client's head only with permission from client or parent
6. Encourage and facilitate family involvement in care
7. Clients of Chinese descent may expect nurse to intuitively know their disease process
8. Alternative therapies such as acupuncture and herbal remedies are widely used by people of Asian cultures

IV. CULTURAL CONSIDERATIONS FOR LATINO/HISPANIC AMERICANS

A. Communication

1. Primary languages include Spanish and Portuguese
2. May utilize code switching, which is systematic mixing of English and Spanish languages
3. Simpatia, a desire for smooth or harmonious interpersonal relationships, should be considered; it is characterized by courtesy, respect, and absence of critical or confrontational behavior; confrontational interaction is avoided
4. Eye contact reflects respect; in nurse–client relationship, eye contact may be expected of nurse, although it may not be reciprocated by client
5. Tend to be verbally expressive
6. May engage in small talk, which should be appraised as a method of establishing rapport
7. Nonverbal communication plays important role in client assessment and interaction

B. Time orientation: tend to be present oriented; however, time orientation varies according to age, subculture, and socioeconomic status

C. Social roles

1. Family is most valued institution and is a primary source of personal identification
2. While nuclear families are common, extended families may also exist
3. Father is likely to assume role of head of household and may be decision maker for family
4. Collective achievement tends to be valued more than individual achievement
5. Religion is important; Catholicism is prevalent

D. Views of health and illness

1. *Mal de ojo* (evil eye) is a childhood disease characterized by fitful sleep, crying, and diarrhea; a common belief among Latinos is that *mal de ojo* is caused by unconscious energy of an adult flowing into child when adult simply looks at child
2. Health is thought to be the will of God
3. *Curanderos,* folk healers, may be consulted
4. Health may represent a state of equilibrium in world, which is characterized by balance of hot, cold, wet, and dry; when an imbalance exists, treatment focuses on application of opposite quality

E. Health risks

1. Diabetes mellitus
2. Hypertension
3. Pernicious anemia
4. Childhood obesity

F. Nursing considerations

1. Clients may seek guidance from within family network rather than from health care providers; nurses should include family members in health care education when appropriate
2. Male family member may be decision maker for client
3. Modesty is important, and measures should be taken to protect client's privacy at all times; clients may prefer to have a health care provider of same gender
4. Use of alternative therapies is prevalent and should be explored when client enters health care system; if possible, facilitate continuation of such services
5. Encourage family to bring traditional diet if medically acceptable

V. CULTURAL CONSIDERATIONS FOR NATIVE AMERICANS

A. Communication

1. Native American group includes Alaskan natives (Eskimos/Aleuts) also; languages primarily include Navajo and English
2. Language involves tonal speech, the pitch of which is important
3. When shaking hands, Navajos tend to extend a hand and lightly touch hand of person they are greeting
4. May appear silent and reserved upon meeting strangers
5. As a sign of honor to ancestors, Navajos may state their clan and location of their home

B. Time orientation

1. Time exists in a three-point range, including past, present, and future
2. Viewed as being primarily present oriented, with some members being both past and present oriented

C. Social roles

1. Family oriented, with biological family being central social organization
2. Family includes all members of extended family
3. Family members work collaboratively to assure success of family unit
4. Male family members may be granted greatest respect and may make decisions for family
5. Extended family may care for hospitalized relative throughout duration of hospital stay
6. Religion guided by sacred myths and legends

D. Views of health and illness

1. Desire to be in harmony with environment and family
2. Health is not limited to body; it includes harmony with family, environment, livestock, supernatural forces, and community
3. Health and religion are considered to be connected; healing ceremonies are common; magic, religion, and folk medicine may all be used for healing; healers may be men or women
4. The Blessingway ceremony is practiced to remove ill health through use of stories, songs, rituals, prayers, sand paintings, and symbols
5. Navajo medicine men and women may be utilized, including diagnosticians, singers, and herbalists
6. Diagnosticians diagnose illness, singers perform healing ceremonies, and herbalists use herbs to treat those who have ailments

E. Health risks

1. Alcoholism and chronic liver disease
2. Accidents
3. Arthritis
4. Chronic lower respiratory diseases
5. Diabetes mellitus
6. Heart disease, including hypertension and myocardial infarction
7. HIV and AIDS
8. Influenza
9. Malignant neoplasms
10. Malnutrition caused by high rates of poverty
11. Maternal and infant deaths
12. Obesity
13. Suicide
14. Tuberculosis

F. Nursing considerations

1. When possible, accommodate client's request to attend healing ceremonies held outside of hospital
2. Respect client's desire to be in harmony with environment whenever possible
3. Incorporate all medically acceptable practices into client's plan of care

4. Following birth, the umbilical cord may be buried near a place or an object that symbolizes parents' hope for child's future
5. Encourage active participation of family in client's care

VI. CULTURAL CONSIDERATIONS FOR EUROPEAN AMERICANS (CAUCASIAN)

A. Communication
1. English is primary language
2. Eye contact is valued and shows interest and respect
3. Body language is important in communication process
4. Facial expression tends to be utilized as part of communication process
5. Handshake is utilized for formal greetings
6. Personal space tends to be required during communication

B. Time orientation
1. Considered to be future oriented
2. Adhere to schedules and timeframes

C. Social roles
1. Nuclear family is predominant
2. Extended family plays important role
3. Religion is important, with a variety of denominations existing
4. Encourage children to develop their personal sense of identity
5. Subscribe to Protestant work ethic values, which stress importance of planning for future
6. Individual goals may take precedence over those of family

D. Views of health and illness
1. Health is considered absence of disease or illness
2. Utilize Western health care system

E. Health risks
1. Cardiovascular disease
2. Obesity
3. Diabetes mellitus
4. Breast cancer
5. Thalassemia

F. Nursing considerations
1. Respect client's need for autonomy and personal space
2. Maintain eye contact with client
3. Include family members in health care decisions when appropriate and with client's approval
4. There is a resurgence in interest in homeopathic medicine

Check Your NCLEX-RN® Exam I.Q.

You are ready for testing on this content if you can

- Be respectful, interested in, and understanding of other cultures without being judgmental.
- Assess the impact of clients' culture or ethnicity when planning, implementing, and evaluating nursing care.
- Determine level of fluency in English and need for interpreter to aid in planning care effectively for clients with a language barrier.
- Consider client's culture when providing client teaching.
- Demonstrate cultural sensitivity when communicating with clients.
- Evaluate client understanding and acceptance of health-related recommendations.

PRACTICE TEST

PRACTICE TEST

1 While conducting an initial assessment of an infant, a home health nurse notices that he is wearing a soiled piece of braided yarn around his neck. Which action by the nurse is most appropriate?

1. Leave the yarn in place but wash it with a cloth and mild soap.
2. Ask about its significance and suggest that it be placed more safely on his body.
3. Explain that the yarn offers no benefit and ask the parents to remove it.
4. Remove the yarn because it is soiled and could lead to strangulation.

2 A Native American client who has a low-grade fever tells the nurse on the reservation that he will only use a sweat lodge to treat his illness. Which approach by the nurse would be most therapeutic?

1. Explain to the client that the sweat lodge is likely to worsen the fever.
2. Alert the physician and ask him or her to talk to the medicine man of the tribe.
3. Continue to monitor the client's status.
4. Ask the client's family to convince him not to use the sweat lodge.

3 A male nurse needs to check the vital signs and oxygen saturation level of a female client from a different culture. As he approaches, the client moves to the other side of the bed and draws up the blanket. What is the best nursing action?

1. Invite a family member to be present and to assist with the oxygen saturation reading.
2. Ask a female nurse to perform the procedures.
3. Perform the assessments without acknowledging her reaction because she will adjust over time to hospital procedures.
4. Before touching the client, explain the procedure and ask for permission to continue.

4 A nurse is caring for two clients who have had abdominal surgery. One client is of Hispanic heritage, who writhes in pain and moans when touched. The other is an Asian client, who appears calm and rarely complains of pain or discomfort. The nurse appropriately draws which conclusion from these observations?

1. The Hispanic client is exaggerating his pain.
2. The Asian client is not experiencing pain.
3. The two clients have different culturally influenced ways of coping with pain.
4. The Hispanic client may be exhibiting drug-seeking behavior.

5 A hospice nurse in a small Appalachian community is caring for a client at home who is an active member of his church. As death nears, the minister and several members of the congregation come together in the home for a "death watch." Which action by the nurse is most therapeutic?

1. Ask the minister to have church members come in scheduled time blocks to avoid overcrowding.
2. Observe the client's religious beliefs and allow the family and minister unlimited access to the client.
3. Allow the family and three other visitors at a time to stay with the client, but keep everyone else in the next room.
4. Explain that the watch will not be a problem as long as it does not conflict with medical care.

6 A home health nurse is assigned to an Asian American client who refuses to take the blood pressure medication prescribed by his physician. The client is using acupuncture treatments and does not believe in taking pills. How can the nurse best help this client?

1. Notify the physician of the client's health practices, and monitor his condition for an impending crisis.
2. Ask the supervisor to transfer the client to an Asian American primary nurse.
3. Advocate for the client's decision, and explain that pills may not help based on his beliefs.
4. Discharge the client and advise him to call if he wishes to obtain home care services at a later date.

7 The nurse is checking the dietary trays that have been delivered to the nursing unit. A client of Orthodox Jewish faith has received a tray containing a chicken dinner with vegetables, tea, and a carton of 2% milk. What action by the nurse is best?

1. Instruct the nursing assistant to deliver the meal tray after removing the tea.
2. Call the dietary department to send a tray without chicken.
3. Have the dietary department replace the entire meal tray.
4. Ask the client if lactose-free milk would be preferred.

PRACTICE TEST

8 An Asian American client will be undergoing a cardiac echogram in a week. While the nurse is explaining the procedure, the client repeatedly nods the head and smiles at the nurse. What conclusion about this behavior would be most appropriate for the nurse to draw?

1. The client does not speak English well but may be too embarrassed to share this information.
2. The client understands the procedure and is just waiting for the nurse to finish.
3. The client may not understand but is trying to hide this fact from the nurse.
4. The client may be trying to indicate politeness and a sense of harmony.

9 The nurse is caring for a Chinese client who subscribes to the yin and yang theory of treating illness. The client tells the nurse she has a "hot" illness. The nurse explains to the oncoming shift that the client will likely wish to consume which of the following in the diet to treat the illness?

1. Foods that are considered yang, or "hot"
2. Foods that are considered yin, or "cold"
3. More "hot" foods than "cold"
4. More "cold" foods than "hot"

10 A nurse is working with a group of postpartum women. Using culturally based practices as a guide, which of the following clients is at greatest risk for postpartum depression?

1. A Chinese client
2. A Hispanic client
3. A Hindu client
4. An American client

11 The nurse is caring for a Native American woman who has given birth. The nurse anticipates that the couple will make which request regarding the umbilical cord?

1. To have it burned
2. To have the blood drained from it
3. To take it home
4. To inspect it

12 The nurse has taken a position in an ambulatory clinic in a Hispanic neighborhood. The nurse would use knowledge of which of the following practices to provide culturally sensitive care to this population? Select all that apply.

1. Herbal medicines are just as important as Western medicines in treating illness.
2. Mourners are likely to be hired by a family to demonstrate grief after a death.
3. Staring at a client who is a child will help to prevent or ward off the "evil eye."
4. Depending on the specific illness, either hot or cold foods would be used in treatment.
5. The client may want a caregiver of the same gender to enhance privacy.

Answer: ______________________

ANSWERS & RATIONALES

1 **Answer: 2** The action that demonstrates cultural sensitivity is the one that inquires about the significance of the braided necklace while taking into account issues of client safety (in this case risk of strangulation). Option 1 addresses risk of infection but not safety, while options 3 and 4 fail to demonstrate any cultural sensitivity.
Cognitive Level: Application **Client Need:** Psychosocial Integrity **Integrated Process:** Communication and Documentation **Content Area:** Fundamentals **Strategy:** Use the process of elimination and basic principles of culturally sensitive communication to make a selection. Eliminate options 3 and 4 as least respectful, and choose the correct option because it addresses the priority need of safety.

2 **Answer: 3** The nurse should continue to monitor the client's status because the fever is low grade and considering that treatment consistent with the client's beliefs will probably be the most successful. The other responses fail to show cultural sensitivity in respecting the client's culturally based beliefs about health.
Cognitive Level: Application **Client Need:** Psychosocial Integrity **Integrated Process:** Communication and Documentation **Content Area:** Fundamentals **Strategy:** Use basic principles of therapeutic communication, client autonomy, and cultural sensitivity to make a selection. The critical words in the stem are *low-grade fever,* which tells you that the situation is not life-threatening or even an emergency. Avoid option 2 because it does not keep the responsibility with the nurse and option 4 because this action would violate a client's right to self-determination.

3 **Answer: 4** The response that shows cultural sensitivity is one that respects the personal boundaries for the client and asks permission to engage in care activities. There is no need for family or a female nurse to assist in these noninvasive procedures at this time without assessing first what the client's

issues may be. The nurse should also not ignore the nonverbal communication being sent by the client; this would not be therapeutic.
Cognitive Level: Application **Client Need:** Psychosocial Integrity **Integrated Process:** Communication and Documentation **Content Area:** Fundamentals **Strategy:** Use basic principles of therapeutic communication, client autonomy, and cultural sensitivity to make a selection. First note that the nature of the nursing care activities involved indicate that this is not a situation that requires assistance from family or other nurses. Choose an option that focuses directly on the client.

4 **Answer: 3** Pain is an experience that is more likely to be culturally influenced for clients. Hispanic or Latino clients are more likely to externalize their pain, while Asian clients and some European American clients tend to show few external signs. The best interpretation is one that does not judge the level of the client's pain without direct assessment (options 1 and 2) and that does not label the client unfairly (option 4).
Cognitive Level: Analysis **Client Need:** Psychosocial Integrity **Integrated Process:** Communication and Documentation **Content Area:** Fundamentals **Strategy:** Use principles of therapeutic, helping relationships and cultural sensitivity to evaluate each option. Keep in mind that the correct option will also be the one that is most respectful of the client.

5 **Answer: 2** Cultural practices near the time of death are important for clients and their families. The nurse should respect the client and family wishes, since medical care is ineffective at this point in time (option 4). Options 1 and 3 do not fully respect the needs of the client and those who are important in his life.
Cognitive Level: Application **Client Need:** Psychosocial Integrity **Integrated Process:** Communication and Documentation **Content Area:** Fundamentals **Strategy:** Recall that practices related to birth and death are highly culturally influenced. With this in mind, select the option that provides the greatest respect for the client and significant people in his life.

6 **Answer: 1** The nurse should notify the health care provider of the client's practices and should continue to monitor the client to promote safe management of his health problem. It is unnecessary to ask for a nurse of the same culture to be assigned. The nurse would not indicate that the medication would not work because of health beliefs. It would be punitive to discharge the client from services because of culturally based health practices.
Cognitive Level: Application **Client Need:** Psychosocial Integrity **Integrated Process:** Communication and Documentation **Content Area:** Fundamentals **Strategy:** Eliminate option 4 because it implies punishment of the client. Eliminate option 2 because the nurse is abandoning the client. Choose option 1 over option 3 because option 3 is a false statement.

7 **Answer: 3** The Jewish religion prohibits the ingestion of meat and dairy products during the same meal. The nurse should ask that the entire meal tray be replaced by the dietary department. It is unnecessary to remove the tea (option 1) or the chicken alone (option 2). Option 4 will not resolve the dietary issue.
Cognitive Level: Application **Client Need:** Psychosocial Integrity **Integrated Process:** Nursing Process: Implementation **Content Area:** Fundamentals **Strategy:** The core issue of this question is that milk and meat products cannot be consumed during the same meal for clients of the Jewish faith. Use the process of elimination and this knowledge to make a selection.

8 **Answer: 4** The client may be trying to demonstrate interpersonal harmony, which reflects a culturally based value. There is insufficient evidence to support any of the other interpretations listed.
Cognitive Level: Analysis **Client Need:** Psychosocial Integrity **Integrated Process:** Communication and Documentation **Content Area:** Fundamentals **Strategy:** Use the process of elimination and knowledge of Asian American cultural values to make a selection. Choose correctly by recalling that peace and harmony are highly valued by Asian American people. As an alternative strategy, eliminate each of the incorrect options by noting a lack of data in the stem that would be consistent with those statements.

9 **Answer: 2** Yin and yang provide for balance in the body according to this theory. Because yin foods are cold and yang foods are hot, the client needs to eat cold foods for a hot illness and hot foods for a cold illness. Options 3 and 4 are incorrect because the two types of foods are not mixed in treating illness.
Cognitive Level: Application **Client Need:** Psychosocial Integrity **Integrated Process:** Communication and Documentation **Content Area:** Fundamentals **Strategy:** The core issue of the question is knowledge of the yin and yang theory in Chinese culture. Interpret the concept of balance as meaning "opposites" when choosing descriptions of foods in relation to the description of the illness.

10 **Answer: 4** Because American women tend to be more autonomous and have fewer relatives who assist in the postpartum period, American women are more at risk for postpartum depression. Many non-Western cultures will have family involvement in the care of the mother and infant for up to 50 days after delivery. This prolonged support helps to prevent the new mother from feeling overwhelmed with new responsibilities or feeling abandoned.
Cognitive Level: Analysis **Client Need:** Psychosocial Integrity **Integrated Process:** Nursing Process: Analysis **Content Area:** Fundamentals **Strategy:** Use the process of elimination and knowledge of the social roles and support of various cultural groups to make a selection. Recall that American society generally tends to value autonomy and independence, which affects the nature of relationships in the postpartum period.

11 **Answer: 3** Following birth, the umbilical cord may be buried near a place or an object that symbolizes the parents' hope for the child's future. For this reason, the parents of the newborn are likely to request to take it home. The other options do not represent the cultural beliefs of Native Americans regarding the significance of the umbilical cord after birth.
Cognitive Level: Analysis **Client Need:** Psychosocial Integrity **Integrated Process:** Nursing Process: Planning **Content Area:** Fundamentals **Strategy:** Use the process of elimination and knowledge of the cultural practices surrounding childbirth to make a selection. If needed, take time to review key cultural practices of Native American clients.

12 **Answer: 1, 4, 5** In the Latino culture, herbal medicines are just as important as Western medicines in treating illness. Mourners would not be hired by a family to demonstrate grief after a death (that practice could occur in Korean culture). Staring at a child could cause the "evil eye" because of their inexperienced and vulnerable spirits. Depending on the specific illness, either hot or cold foods would be used in treatment. Males may be the typical decision makers regarding health care. The client may want a caregiver of the same gender to enhance privacy.

Cognitive Level: Application **Client Need:** Psychosocial Integrity **Integrated Process:** Nursing Process: Analysis **Content Area:** Fundamentals **Strategy:** The wording of the question tells you that the correct options will also be correct statements about the Latino American culture. Use the process of elimination and nursing knowledge related to culture to make a selection.

Key Terms to Review

culture p. 284
stereotyping p. 287

References

Harkreader, H., & Hogan, M. (2004). *Fundamentals of nursing: Caring and clinical judgment* (2nd ed.). St. Louis, MO: Elsevier.

Kozier, B., Erb, G., Berman, A. J., & Burke, K. (2004). *Fundamentals of nursing: Concepts, process, and practice* (7th ed.). Upper Saddle River, NJ: Pearson Education.

Nix, S. (2005). *William's basic nutrition and diet therapy* (12th ed.). St. Louis, MO: Mosby.

Potter, P., & Perry, A. (2005). *Fundamentals of nursing* (6th ed.). St. Louis, MO: Mosby.

Spector, R. (2004). *Cultural diversity in health and illness* (6th ed.). Upper Saddle River, NJ: Prentice Hall.

Coping with Stressors

21

In this chapter

Test Yourself

Are you ready for the NCLEX-RN® or course exams? Use the practice tests on the companion CD-ROM to check.

Cross reference

Other chapters relevant to this content area are

Therapeutic Communication and Environment Chapter 19
Mental Health Disorders Chapter 22
Dependency and Addiction Chapter 23
Crisis Intervention and Suicide Chapter 24
End of Life Care Chapter 25
Psychiatric Medications Chapter 36

I. COPING AND DEFENSE MECHANISMS

A. Coping behaviors

1. Influence a client's response to a stressful event
2. ! **Coping** (cognitive, physical, or emotional attempts to manage stress) implies that client is attempting to lower tension in order to manage situation effectively; both adaptive and maladaptive coping behaviors are typically manifested
3. **Adaptive coping** behaviors: ability to mobilize internal/external resources and sustain general homeostasis
4. **Maladaptive coping** behaviors: inability to mobilize internal/external resources; disorganization occurs; ineffective and destructive behaviors appear; general homeostasis is not preserved

Memory Aid

All clients attempt to exhibit coping behaviors. The key role of the nurse is to determine whether they are healthy (adaptive) or unhealthy (maladaptive) and to support healthy ones.

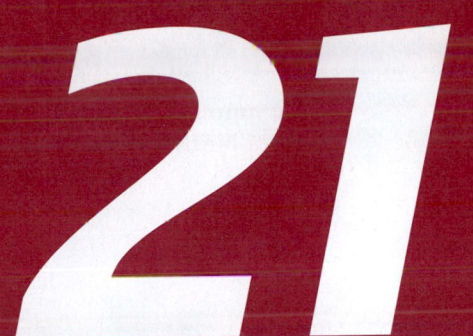

Table 21–1
Common Defense Mechanisms

Defense Mechanism	Description
Compensation	Making up for real or imagined weaknesses in one area
Denial	Refusing to acknowledge thoughts or impulses that are unacceptable to self
Displacement	Directing feelings about a person who is threatening to self to another person who is less threatening to self
Identification	Attempting to change oneself unconsciously for the purpose of resembling someone who is admired
Intellectualization	Using excessive reasoning ability to minimize or avoid feelings associated with distressing events or occurrences
Introjection	Incorporating the values and characteristics of another into oneself
Minimization	Refusing to acknowledge the importance or significance of one's behavior
Projection	Transferring unacceptable desires, thoughts, or internal feelings to another
Rationalization	Justifying unacceptable feelings or behavior by using faulty logic or by applying false but socially acceptable motives to the behavior
Reaction formation	Behaving or displaying attitudes that are exactly opposite of those that are felt
Regression	Reverting back to an earlier, less well-developed stage of functioning to deal with an uncomfortable reality
Repression	Using an unconscious process to block threatening or unacceptable thoughts, feelings, or desires to keep them from becoming conscious
Sublimation	Displacing energy associated with unacceptable needs or drives into more socially acceptable activities
Substitution	Replacing a highly valued but unobtainable or unacceptable object with a less satisfying but acceptable and available one
Undoing	Using words or actions to cancel out previous unacceptable thoughts or behaviors in an attempt to relieve guilt by making reparation

! **B. Defense mechanisms (see Table 21–1 ■)**
1. Strategies that assist client to protect own ego and reduce anxiety
2. Support appropriate use of defense mechanisms
3. ! Do not attempt to break down inappropriate defense mechanisms until other coping strategies are learned

II. COPING WITH ABUSE OR NEGLECT

A. Victims
1. Often present with depression
2. Describe feelings of powerlessness, dependency, or a sense of being trapped
3. Tend to have low self-esteem
4. Often do not recognize that they are victims
5. ! Frequently believe that they are to blame for abuse and that it would stop if client could do "better"

B. Abusers/perpetrators
1. Also have low self-esteem
2. May have been abused themselves during childhood
3. Depersonalize victims so as to feel entitled to engage in abuse
4. Tend to be self-absorbed, suspicious, and highly dependent on victim

C. Types of abuse/violence
1. Partner: cycle of physical or emotional threats and assaults by abuser followed by abuser remorse or attempts to make peace
2. Child: physical, emotional, or sexual
3. Elder: physical, emotional, sexual, or financial (lack of knowledge of finances and inability to pay bills while cognitively intact)

Table 21–2
Signs of Neglect

Child	Poor hygiene, presence of chronic hunger and inadequate weight gain, chronic fatigue, excessive school absences, and inadequate or lack of supervision
Elder	Poor hygiene and unkempt appearance, inadequate dress, absence of necessary physical aids (dentures, glasses, hearing aids), malnutrition, dehydration, skin tears

4. Abuse versus neglect: neglect is passive in nature, while abuse is active and purposeful

D. Assessment
1. Neglect: intentional or unintentional failure to care for victim (see Table 21–2 ■)
2. Abuse (see Table 21–3 ■)

E. Collaborative management (see also Chapter 7)
1. Report suspected abuse cases; this is part of mandatory reporting laws
2. Support client during physical assessment and treatment of physical injuries
3. Provide safe, nonthreatening environment for care

Memory Aid
Safety is always a key concern for victims of abuse.

4. Document assessments and client-reported events in an objective manner
5. Do not leave victim alone with abuser
6. Support coping mechanisms of victim
7. Encourage therapy for abuser, victim, and appropriate others (family)
8. Assess support systems of victim and abuser
9. Refer to appropriate community agencies for support
10. Assist with legal procedures as appropriate (police reports, restraining order/order of protection)
11. Child-specific interventions
    a. Avoid loud noises
    b. Position self to be at eye level with child when speaking
    c. Make no sudden movements
    d. Reassure child that he or she is a good person and is not to blame for abusive behavior

Table 21–3
Signs of Abuse

Type of Abuse	Child	Elder
Physical	Unexplained physical or thermal injuries Unusual apprehension, aggression, or withdrawal Withdraws from or is fearful of parents Does not cry when approached by strangers/caregivers	Skin tears Bruises that are multiple or in patterns (finger or hand prints) Burn injuries Lacerations or punctures Bone fractures
Emotional	Presence of repetitive motion habits such as sucking or rocking Psychoneurotic reactions Disorders of speech Difficulty with concentration or learning Suicidal behavior	Confusion Fear and apprehension Agitation Withdrawal from social activities Loss of interest in self Decreased appetite and weight
Sexual	Difficulty in sitting or walking Undergarments that are torn, stained, or bloody Pain, swelling, bruising, or bleeding in area of genitalia Change in usual routine, such as disruptive behavior or disrupted sleep Changes in school behavior, such as withdrawal from peers, truancy, or refusal to undress/change clothes for physical education classes	Difficulty in sitting or walking New onset genital infection Pain or bleeding in area of genitalia Undergarments that are torn, stained, or bloody

12. Elder-specific interventions
    a. Explore alternative housing that provides greatest freedom to client and least amount of disruption to routine
    b. Assist with exploring protection of finances

III. OVERVIEW OF PSYCHOLOGICAL ASPECTS OF MEDICAL ILLNESS

A. Factors influencing response to medical illness include developmental/lifespan level, personality type/behaviors, coping behaviors, precipitating stressors, support systems, and nature of illness

B. Developmental/lifespan issues: developmental stage at time of diagnosis of medical illness influences client's response to illness; in addition, illness can affect client mastery of a developmental/lifespan level, which further affects how client responds to illness

1. Early to middle adulthood
    a. Medical illnesses that occur when clients are in early to middle adulthood developmental/lifespan phase can interfere with intimacy, sexuality, and career goals
    b. An adolescent with a chronic illness is at high risk, and this may result in severe emotional stress, depression, anxiety, and possible suicidal ideation (see also Chapter 22)
2. Late adulthood: medical illnesses that occur when clients are in late adulthood developmental/lifespan phase can interfere with self-care and daily functioning, which may result in severe emotional stress

C. Personality traits: a client's predictable pattern of response to events; can be used to predict how client may respond to diagnosis of a medical illness, which then assists with planning care

1. Type A personality trait behaviors: might increase unhealthy responses to medical illness; these traits include rapid speech, irritability, rapid movements, time consciousness, difficulty relaxing, internalization of feelings, excessive dependence on approval of others, and low self-esteem
2. Type B personality trait behaviors: may contribute to healthy responses to medical illness and include easygoing manner, more "laid-back" in demeanor, relaxed and goal-directed behaviors
3. Behaviors that increase likelihood of occurrence of medical illness include pessimism, repression, limited/guarded social interactions, hostility, and despair
4. Behaviors that decrease likelihood of occurrence of medical illness include behaviors that are self-healing, energetic, questioning, humorous, inspirational, and that demonstrate good interpersonal skills

D. *Precipitating stressors*

1. Defined as events occurring prior to a medical illness that initiated a stress response consisting of physiological and psychological alterations
2. Precipitating stressors can influence a client's response to medical illness because client may already be in an emotionally compromised state prior to diagnosis of medical illness

E. Support systems: presence or absence of strong support systems influences a client's response to medical illness; strong family, friend, and community support systems can result in positive or negative responses

F. Nature of illness: a client's response to medical illness can depend on whether illness is an acute (or short-lasting) type, chronic (long-lasting) type, or terminal, life-ending type

1. Acute illness: sudden onset, may be caused by an accident or other fast onset type of illness
    a. Often results in crisis for client and family
    b. **Crisis** refers to an event in which client's regular coping mechanisms are inadequate
    c. Client may demonstrate a short attention span and a tendency to be unproductive and impulsive
2. Chronic illness: client must cope with illness that may be long-standing and debilitating in nature; this often results in ongoing stress for client and family; client often feels frustrated, hopeless, and fatigued

3. Terminal illness: a terminal illness diagnosis may place client and family in a crisis mode
   a. This type of illness continues to be extremely disruptive to client and family functioning
   b. Client often exhibits signs of anger, hopelessness/helplessness, and despair

IV. ASSOCIATED COMMON PSYCHOLOGICAL SYMPTOMS

A. Anger

1. Clients with a medical illness diagnosis typically demonstrate behaviors indicative of anger
2. These behaviors reflect feelings of helplessness and frustration about illness and effects it has on daily functioning
3. Behaviors likely to be exhibited include demanding types of action, loud verbalization, slamming of items, and social withdrawal

B. Depression

1. Clients with a medical illness diagnosis typically demonstrate symptoms of depression related to disruption of daily functioning
2. Signs associated with depression include feelings of helplessness/hopelessness, flat affect, poor eye contact, disrupted eating/sleeping patterns, absence of motivation and compliance, and a decreased energy level

C. Anxiety

1. Clients with a medical illness diagnosis typically demonstrate feelings and behaviors of anxiety
2. Anxious behavior reflects feelings of real or imagined threat to body image
3. Anxiety results in autonomic nervous system stimulation with increased heart rate, increased respirations, increased visual acuity, diaphoresis, shortness of breath, and restlessness

D. Helplessness/hopelessness

1. Clients with medical diagnoses typically demonstrate feelings of helplessness/hopelessness
2. Helplessness relates to feelings of powerlessness associated with being unable to change what is happening, while hopelessness relates to feelings of despondency and loss of optimism
3. This is reflected in feelings of loss of **control** (feeling that an event can be managed) and individuality and increased dependency on others

V. MEDICAL CONDITIONS CONTRIBUTING TO PSYCHOLOGICAL SYMPTOMS

A. Critical/acute illness: may occur without warning and immediately affect a client's daily functioning; clients typically experience feelings of loss of control, anxiety, helplessness, and anger

1. Cardiovascular illnesses
   a. Have been linked to occurrence of stress
   b. Include myocardial infarction, cerebrovascular accident, and hypertension
   c. Stress levels can influence course and/or outcomes of medical illness
2. Trauma
   a. May result from an accident or crime
   b. Behavioral and physiological responses occur and are demonstrated in client through social isolation, agitation, nightmares, and numbness
   c. Client typically struggles to control episodes of anxiety related to traumatic event
3. Surgery performed because of a critical or an acute medical condition may be disfiguring or incapacitating; surgical procedures can result in alterations of client daily functioning and changes in client's perception of self-image
4. Pain can accompany many acute illnesses; client's response is based on a need to protect oneself from harm

B. Chronic illness: produces long-term effects that client must cope with for a longer time; can be unpredictable in nature and require use of adaptive coping behaviors in an ongoing

manner; lower socioeconomic status increases risk of multiple ongoing health problems, and often reduced access to health care and financial resources to adhere to treatment plans

1. Pulmonary diseases
   a. Include disorders such as chronic obstructive pulmonary disease (COPD) and asthma
   b. Higher stress levels lead to increased secretions and airway spasms and result in increased episodes of breathing difficulties
2. Gastrointestinal (GI) diseases
   a. Irritable bowel syndrome, peptic ulcer, and ulcerative colitis are stress-influenced illnesses
   b. GI tract and autonomic nervous system are involved; increased acid and increased parasympathetic stimulation of lower bowel occurs and exacerbates symptoms when stress levels increase
3. Medical illnesses that result in chronic pain can have profound effect on clients and their adaptive and maladaptive coping behaviors; clients respond to pain in a psychological and physiological manner that requires them to continually attempt to adapt

C. Life-ending illnesses (see also Chapter 25)

1. HIV/AIDS: human immunodeficiency virus (HIV) and acquired immunodeficiency syndrome (AIDS) result simultaneously in a compromised immune system and occurrence of a psychiatric disorder; this further compromises health and well-being of client
   a. Assessment of clients with HIV disease is crucial because of occurrence of psychiatric symptoms/illness and enormous losses that client and family endure
   b. Psychosocial factors influencing occurrence of psychiatric symptoms/illness include fear that diagnosis will be shared with others, concern about stigma related to diagnosis, intimacy and sexual disruptions, and employment/insurance issues
   c. Symptoms of HIV and psychiatric illness overlap, especially with symptoms of depression and anxiety; these include fatigue, hopelessness/helplessness, weight loss, aching muscles, and diarrhea; other psychiatric symptoms specifically related to HIV/AIDS diagnosis include irritability, paranoia, psychosis, substance abuse, and suicidal ideation
   d. Cognitive changes related to HIV/AIDS diagnoses include dementia (chronic irreversible brain disorder associated with memory difficulties, impaired judgment, personality changes, and decline in physical appearance) and delirium (acute reversible brain disorder associated with inability to be attentive, cloudy consciousness, apathy, and bizarre behaviors)
   e. Interventions for clients with HIV/AIDS should include those that relate to AIDS dementia/delirium, changes in body image/self-esteem, imminent death, support of family/significant others, and management of pain
2. Other life-ending illnesses
   a. Dying client experiences feelings of helplessness and hopelessness
   b. In addition, feelings of depression, anger, and hostility are experienced
   c. Client's response to a life-ending diagnosis will be affected by coping skills, developmental/lifespan level, as well as spiritual, cultural, biological, and psychosocial factors
   d. Interventions for clients with a life-ending illness include use of empathy and compassion; a focus on aspects of client's life that were positive; spirituality assessment and reinforcement; support of family and significant others; allowing client dignity and control; and use of pain management

VI. ASSOCIATED PSYCHIATRIC SYMPTOMS

A. Psychosis is a disorder of organic or emotional origin characterized by gross impairment in reality testing

B. Psychotic symptoms that may be demonstrated in clients with selected medical illness diagnoses include evidence of delusions and hallucinations, thought process disruption, and difficulty in caring for oneself (see also Chapter 22)

1. Delusions may be persistent and recurrent; they are beliefs that are false but cannot be altered by reason or evidence
2. Hallucinations may be persistent and recurrent; they are defined as occurrences of a sight, sound, smell, taste, or touch when there is no external stimulus to corresponding sensory organ

VII. ASSESSMENT

A. Use various resources to collect psychological, biological, and social data

B. Consider subjective and objective symptoms, family/significant other reports, and diagnostic reports in assessment phase

C. Psychological assessment

1. Elicits clients' emotional reaction to medical illness diagnosis, coping abilities, and support resources
2. Perform a stress appraisal to identify source, number, and duration of stressors
3. Complete a full mental status examination if clients exhibit severe symptoms induced by stress
4. ! Complete a depression symptom assessment, noting time of initial symptoms, duration of symptoms, and physical appearance
5. ! Identify coping behaviors, including assessment of adaptive and maladaptive behaviors that reflect client's ability to identify problems and analyze feelings
6. Assess substance abuse/dependence, which is crucial in assessment phase because it can contribute to symptoms of depression, anxiety, hopelessness, helplessness, and eating/sleeping disruptions
7. Identify emotional stage of medical illness; plan interventions according to emotional stage
8. Theoretical stages of medical illness include the following (although individual clients may move forward and backward in these stages to some degree):
   a. Denial of medical illness and associated limitations
   b. Anger at loss of control and associated limitations
   c. Bargaining, with a plea for another chance and a seeking of new answers/treatments
   d. Depression when grieving occurs due to loss or anticipated loss
   e. Acceptance/adaptation when conflicts are resolved and client participates in care

D. Biologic assessment

1. This type of assessment is done to understand how stress might alter a client's internal body functioning
2. Biological changes can assist nurse with determining severity of an illness
3. Assess recent and past health conditions that may contribute to current level of physical and psychological functioning; recent and chronic illnesses alter client's immune system and raise susceptibility to additional health care problems
4. Conduct complete physical exam to reveal any physical conditions contributing to psychological symptoms; some medical illnesses will cause client to exhibit psychological symptoms that may be misdiagnosed as a mental health disorder
5. Complete a thorough neurological status exam to reveal current neurological state and any changes; findings will provide baseline level of functioning and may alert nurse to medical problems
6. Analyze laboratory results, which can provide insight into occurrence of psychological symptoms
7. ! Assess client's current abilities with physical functioning, activities, and exercise to identify baseline information from which to develop plan of care
8. ! Investigate sleep patterns, noting sleep disruptions such as inability to fall asleep, stay asleep, or a desire to sleep constantly; sleep disruptions may indicate either physiological or psychological problems
9. ! Complete a nutritional pattern assessment, noting disruptions such as lack of appetite, failure to enjoy previously enjoyable food, and overeating; eating disruptions can be indicative of either physiological or psychological stress
10. ! Complete a pharmacological assessment, noting medications that client is currently taking that could account for level of physical and psychological functioning

E. Social assessment

1. Explore family history, client lifestyle, life-changing events, and presence of social support systems (appraisal of networks that are supportive or not, negative or positive)
2. Explore recent life-changing events that may impact adaptation to current illness
3. Discuss client's lifestyle patterns as well as any potential impact of lifestyle choices on development and progression of disease
4. ! Note cultural practices for unique aspects that may indicate specific responses or need for special interventions
5. ! Assess family communication patterns, level of cohesion, flexibility, functioning, and general support
6. Explore community and support resources for availability of home services, mental health services, and other related services
7. Assess spiritual concerns; note traditional patterns or rituals, and inquire about other forms of spirituality that may be important to the client
8. Do an occupational assessment: determine whether client can continue in current occupation, either at present time or in future
9. Determine economic status, specifically whether there are finances to support current and future expenses

VIII. EMPOWERING STRATEGIES

A. Interventions

1. Collaborate with client and family members to develop a plan of care for client in which client response can be monitored; counseling and possibly psychotherapy may be appropriate
2. Interventions serve as foundation for all client care and are subject to change as client's condition changes
3. ! Specific interventions that exemplify empowering strategies
   a. Increase client control; provide opportunities for client decision making regarding care
   b. Engage in therapeutic interactions—empathetic listening
   c. Recommend psychotherapy when deemed appropriate to assist client with adaptation and support
   d. Assist with stress management—teach relaxation methods, imagery, biofeedback, exercise
   e. Reinforce current positive, adaptive coping behaviors
   f. Promote comfort and healing
   g. Utilize spiritual resources—provide opportunities for client to engage in spiritual traditions or rituals; offer resources related to complementary medicine if desired

B. Differential interventions for critical/acute versus chronic illnesses

1. ! Critical/acute illnesses typically result in abrupt interruption of a client's usual daily activities; this can precipitate a crisis stage if client perceives events as a threat to safety, self-esteem, or self-image
   a. Seek immediate ways to increase client's control
   b. Engage in therapeutic interactions with client and family; encourage verbalization of feelings
   c. Assist with immediate anxiety reduction through use of relaxation techniques
   d. Use firm, direct limit-setting to assist client with staying focused
2. ! Chronic illnesses typically require ongoing adaptation because long-term effects are unpredictable; chronic illnesses often deplete energy levels, support systems, coping reserves, and economic abilities, and may lead to suicidal ideation
   a. Increase self-care responsibilities as appropriate to preserve or facilitate functioning, self-esteem, and self-image
   b. Reward positive adaptive coping behaviors
   c. Reinforce existing support network and assist client with creating new links to support; identify support groups, self-help groups, and special interest groups

IX. EVALUATION/OUTCOMES

A. **Preservation of healthy physiological function**
B. **Disease process reduction/cessation:** client learns about illness and ways to decrease disease process, such as diet, exercise, and stress reduction activities
C. **Development/reinforcement/strengthening of adaptive coping behaviors:** this includes ability to express feelings related to the medical illness diagnosis and effects of the illness; it also includes productive interdependence of client with ongoing support systems, such as family and friends
D. **Participation in treatment/rehabilitation process**
E. **Optimal level of functioning**
F. **Independence in self-care**
G. **Development of functional support systems**
H. **Decreased anxiety**
I. **Evidence of an *internal locus of control***
   1. Clients who believe they have ability to decrease likelihood of illness or effects of illness have an internal locus of control and are less likely to experience symptoms of distress
   2. In contrast clients who have an external locus of control, who believe that forces outside them determine their lives, are less likely to believe they can control illness or manage stressors

Check Your NCLEX-RN® Exam I.Q.

You are ready for testing on this content if you can

- Assess clients experiencing stress.
- Support appropriate use of coping strategies and defense mechanisms for clients experiencing stress.
- Provide care to the abused client and family.
- Identify common clinical symptoms of psychotic disorders due to medical illness.
- Differentiate intervention strategies for clients experiencing critical acute illness and chronic illness.

PRACTICE TEST

1 A client diagnosed with a terminal illness states, "What's left for me? I feel hopeless." The nurse determines that which of the following would be the best response?

1. "Come on, it's not hopeless."
2. "Don't be so depressed."
3. "It must be difficult feeling as though there is no hope."
4. "I don't understand why you have to feel so bad."

2 The nurse observes that a client hospitalized with newly diagnosed heart disease is frequently crying and staying in the room. These actions should be noted during assessment by the nurse as identification of what behaviors?

1. Inappropriate
2. Psychiatric
3. Psychotic
4. Coping

3 The nurse would plan to include which of the following in a biological assessment of a client?

1. Laboratory test results
2. Feelings of anxiety about illness
3. Spiritual needs during illness
4. Prognosis

4 A client with a terminal illness states, "If I could only live until I can walk my daughter down the aisle at her wedding, I will donate all of my money to research." The nurse reports that the client is in which phase of the grief process?

1. Denial
2. Seeking
3. Bargaining
4. Resolution

PRACTICE TEST

5. A client diagnosed with a medical illness states, "I don't enjoy my food anymore." The nurse notes during the assessment phase that this statement indicates what kind of nutritional pattern?
   1. Eating disruption
   2. Eating disorder
   3. Bulimia
   4. Compulsive disorder

6. As part of the admission process, the nurse is conducting a social assessment of a client. The nurse should ask which of the following questions at this time?
   1. "What medications are you currently taking?"
   2. "Can you tell me what illnesses you have had in the past?"
   3. "Do you have any culturally based practices that you would like continued in the hospital?"
   4. "Do your brothers or sisters have any chronic illnesses?"

7. A client who has a diagnosis of a chronic illness states, "I'm so tired. I can't keep on like this every day." The nurse interprets that the feeling the client is expressing can be described as which of the following?
   1. Atypical
   2. Typical
   3. Pathological
   4. Resentful

8. The client hospitalized for 5 days with a medical illness says loudly, "Bring me my pain pills now!" The nurse concludes initially that the client's behavior is a
   1. Common response.
   2. Response that is inappropriate.
   3. Problem.
   4. Feeling of anger at the self.

9. The nurse notices that a client admitted with obstructive pulmonary disease has poor eye contact and has not been eating well. The nurse then looks for additional data that are consistent with which of the following?
   1. Hopefulness
   2. An eating disorder
   3. Anxiety
   4. Depression

10. In order to determine susceptibility to additional health problems in a client with medical illness, the nurse should ask about which of the following in the biological assessment?
    1. Past medications
    2. Recent illnesses
    3. Spiritual needs
    4. Cultural background

11. A client with a recent onset of multiple sclerosis is observed taking part in giving own care. The nurse interprets this behavior to be consistent with which of the following stages of adaptation?
    1. Acceptance
    2. Denial
    3. Compensation
    4. Indulgence

12. A client who underwent surgery for removal of a bowel tumor is exhibiting new onset of psychiatric symptoms. The nurse determines that the client should first have a thorough
    1. Psychiatric workup.
    2. Physical exam.
    3. Counseling session.
    4. Teaching session about the illness.

13. The nurse is assessing coping behaviors as part of the psychological assessment and wishes to address lifestyle factors that can contribute to depression. The nurse would ask the client about which of the following as a priority item?
    1. Occupation
    2. Substance abuse
    3. Number of siblings
    4. Level of income

14. In a client newly diagnosed with amyotrophic lateral sclerosis, an illness that leads to progressive loss of ability to perform activities of daily living, the nurse should anticipate that the client may react to the diagnosis using which of the following strategies in an attempt to cope?
    1. Denial
    2. Gambling
    3. Exercise
    4. Verbal abuse

15 The nurse observes a client and family interaction. Observed behaviors include anger, rigidity, and lack of support for one another. The nurse should consider this interaction as an assessment of which of the following family characteristics?

1. Recent life-changing events
2. Communication patterns
3. Lifestyle patterns
4. Community resources

16 A client with a medical illness tells the nurse that going to church is not a priority. Based on this information, the nurse should do which of the following?

1. Not mention religion again
2. Know that the client does not believe in God
3. Ask the client to come to church
4. Explore other spiritual patterns or rituals with the client

17 A client who was paralyzed from severe injuries sustained during an automobile accident continually attempts to do activities beyond capabilities. The most appropriate nursing diagnosis for this client would be which of the following?

1. Impaired adjustment
2. Anxiety
3. Anger
4. Impaired skin integrity

18 A client tells the nurse that acupuncture helps ease the pain of a terminal illness. The nurse should do which of the following?

1. Tell the client to stop the acupuncture.
2. Tell the client that it is illegal.
3. Understand that it is an appropriate intervention.
4. Understand that the client is not thinking clearly.

19 A client with inflammatory bowel disease has exacerbations when job responsibilities become heavy or there are family conflicts at home. The nurse determines that this client would benefit from instruction that focuses on which of the following?

1. How to keep feelings inside
2. Communication strategies
3. How to ignore stress
4. Stress management techniques

20 A client with chronic obstructive pulmonary disease (COPD) has given up smoking and spaces out activities over the course of the day. The nurse should respond by doing which of the following?

1. Say nothing about the behavior to avoid refocusing the client on the disease process.
2. Ignore the maladaptive behaviors.
3. Reward the adaptive coping behaviors.
4. Tell the client that adjustment was bound to occur over time.

PRACTICE TEST

ANSWERS & RATIONALES

ANSWERS & RATIONALES

1 **Answer: 3** Use of empathy in option 3 communicates understanding to the client and allows him or her to explore inner feelings of hopelessness. Options 1, 2, and 4 ignore and discount the client's feelings. These responses would not encourage the client to further explore his or her feelings with the nurse.
Cognitive Level: Application **Client Need:** Psychosocial Integrity **Integrated Process:** Communication/Documentation **Content Area:** Psychiatric/Mental Health **Strategy:** For questions involving nurse–client communication, choose the answer that is the most open-ended in promoting further communication and sharing of client's feelings.

2 **Answer: 4** Option 4 is correct because these actions indicate the client is attempting to cope with the situation in some way. Option 1 is incorrect because these actions may not be appropriate. Options 2 and 3 are incorrect in terms of the demonstrated behaviors.
Cognitive Level: Application **Client Need:** Psychosocial Integrity **Integrated Process:** Nursing Process: Assessment **Content Area:** Psychiatric/Mental Health **Strategy:** Consider that the client has just learned about diagnosis of a chronic illness. Reason that the client may engage in any number of behaviors, such as crying, to cope with the initial diagnosis.

3 **Answer: 1** Laboratory test results are part of biological assessment because they may provide insight into the occurrence of psychological symptoms. Options 2 and 3 do not relate to biological assessment, but to emotional and social assessments. Option 4 is not part of the assessment process, but rather is a prediction about the outcome of an illness.
Cognitive Level: Application **Client Need:** Psychosocial Integrity **Integrated Process:** Nursing Process: Assessment **Content Area:** Psychiatric/Mental Health **Strategy:** The critical word in the stem of the question is *biological.* With this in mind, select the option that deals most directly with physiological needs or parameters.

4 **Answer: 3** Bargaining is the stage in which the client attempts to bargain for more time. Denial (option 1) indicates the stage in which the client denies that he or she is terminally

ill. Seeking (option 2) reflects the stage in which a client seeks more answers and cures. Resolution (option 4) is the stage in which the client has come to terms with the illness.
Cognitive Level: Application **Client Need:** Psychosocial Integrity **Integrated Process:** Communication and Documentation **Content Area:** Psychiatric/Mental Health **Strategy:** The core issue of the question is ability to analyze a stage of grief by interpreting client comments. Use nursing knowledge and the process of elimination to make a selection.

5 **Answer: 1** Option 1 reflects the client's statement in that the client's normal eating pattern has been disturbed in some way. Options 2 and 3 reflect a more severe, true eating disorder diagnosis. Option 4 relates to a different psychiatric illness comprised of other behaviors.
Cognitive Level: Analysis **Client Need:** Psychosocial Integrity **Integrated Process:** Nursing Process: Assessment **Content Area:** Psychiatric/Mental Health **Strategy:** The core issue of the question is the ability to associate medical illness with the appropriate alteration in eating pattern. Use the process of elimination and nursing knowledge to make a selection.

6 **Answer: 3** Option 3 relates to social assessment and should be considered in terms of how a client might respond to the illness based on cultural background. Options 1, 2, and 4 relate to biological assessment.
Cognitive Level: Analysis **Client Need:** Psychosocial Integrity **Integrated Process:** Nursing Process: Assessment **Content Area:** Psychiatric/Mental Health **Strategy:** The core issue of the question is knowledge of the components of a social assessment. Use the process of elimination and focus on the option that takes into account the social habits or expectations of a client.

7 **Answer: 2** Option 2 is correct: it is typical of clients with a chronic illness to become tired and feel as though they can't continue on in this way. Option 1 is incorrect because atypical is the opposite of typical. Options 3 and 4 are incorrect labels.
Cognitive Level: Analysis **Client Need:** Psychosocial Integrity **Integrated Process:** Nursing Process: Analysis **Content Area:** Psychiatric/Mental Health **Strategy:** The core issue of the question is the nurse's ability to draw accurate conclusions about client statements in terms of coping with chronic illness. Use nursing knowledge and the process of elimination to make a selection.

8 **Answer: 1** Option 1 is correct because hospitalized clients often feel that things are out of their control and their frustration rises. Although the behavior may not be appropriate if it is disruptive, the nurse should first recognize that it is a common response. There is not enough data to support options 2, 3, or 4.
Cognitive Level: Analysis **Client Need:** Psychosocial Integrity **Integrated Process:** Nursing Process: Assessment **Content Area:** Psychiatric/Mental Health **Strategy:** The core issue of the question is the recognition that clients who are hospitalized may feel out of control and may express this feeling in ways that are not socially acceptable. Note the critical word *initially,* which indicates that more than one option may be partially correct but that one conclusion is more appropriate to draw first. Use nursing knowledge and the process of elimination to make a selection.

9 **Answer: 4** These symptoms are indicative of possible depression (option 4) and require further assessment. The observed behaviors do not indicate hopefulness (option 1), anxiety (option 2), or an eating disorder (option 3).
Cognitive Level: Analysis **Client Need:** Psychosocial Integrity **Integrated Process:** Nursing Process: Assessment **Content Area:** Psychiatric/Mental Health **Strategy:** The core issue of the question is the ability to recognize signs of depression in a client. Use nursing knowledge and the process of elimination to make a selection.

10 **Answer: 2** Recent illnesses should be considered when conducting a biological assessment to determine impact of these illnesses on current illness. Past medicines are not a primary concern related to biological assessment (option 1). Spiritual needs (option 3) and cultural background (option 4) are a part of social assessment.
Cognitive Level: Analysis **Client Need:** Psychosocial Integrity **Integrated Process:** Nursing Process: Assessment **Content Area:** Psychiatric/Mental Health **Strategy:** The core issue of the question is the ability to determine what elements to include in a biological assessment of a client. Use nursing knowledge and the process of elimination to make a selection.

11 **Answer: 1** Acceptance (option 1) indicates that the client is accepting limitations imposed by the illness and is attempting to help self as much as possible. A client would not be helping self if the stage was denial because there would be no awareness of need in the denial stage (option 2). Compensation (option 3) and indulgence (option 4) are not stages related to helping the self in medical illness.
Cognitive Level: Analysis **Client Need:** Psychosocial Integrity **Integrated Process:** Nursing Process: Evaluation **Content Area:** Psychiatric/Mental Health **Strategy:** The core issue of the question is the ability to determine the client's stage of adaptation to a chronic illness. Use nursing knowledge and the process of elimination to make a selection.

12 **Answer: 2** Option 2 is correct because physical illnesses can create psychiatric symptoms. Options 1 and 3 conclude that the origin of the client's symptoms are psychiatric in nature, and this conclusion is premature. Option 3 may or may not be appropriate for this client.
Cognitive Level: Application **Client Need:** Psychosocial Integrity **Integrated Process:** Nursing Process: Planning **Content Area:** Psychiatric/Mental Health **Strategy:** The core issue of the question is recognition that psychiatric symptoms may have a medical basis in a hospitalized client. Note the critical word *first,* which indicates that one action should be taken before some others.

13 **Answer: 2** Although occupation (option 1), number of siblings (option 3), and income (option 4) may be of interest when considering lifestyle, substance abuse is of primary interest as a maladaptive coping strategy and is also associated with depression.
Cognitive Level: Analysis **Client Need:** Psychosocial Integrity **Integrated Process:** Nursing Process: Assessment **Content Area:** Psychiatric/Mental Health **Strategy:** Note the critical word *depression* in the question. Review each option and choose the one that correlates best with depression, which in this case is substance abuse.

14 **Answer: 1** Denial (option 1) is most accurate because denial is a typical stage of grief related to loss. Options 2, 3, and 4 are isolated events that could possibly occur but would be based on individual client characteristics rather than anticipated general patterns of response.
Cognitive Level: Analysis **Client Need:** Psychosocial Integrity **Integrated Process:** Nursing Process: Analysis **Content Area:** Psychiatric/Mental Health **Strategy:** Note that the correct answer is one that is a more comprehensive and global option, while the other options contain specific items of behavior. This makes the correct option different from the others, and also recall that a global option is often correct.

15 **Answer: 2** The correct answer is option 2; communication patterns within the family should be assessed for flexibility and support. Option 1, recent life-changing events, relates to something occurring recently. Option 3, lifestyle patterns, refers to an overall way of living, and option 4, community resources, refers to support outside of the family.
Cognitive Level: Analysis **Client Need:** Psychosocial Integrity **Integrated Process:** Nursing Process: Assessment **Content Area:** Psychiatric/Mental Health **Strategy:** The core issue of the question is the nurse's ability to observe family behavior and interpret it correctly. Note the critical word *interaction* in the stem of the question and the word *communication* in the correct response.

16 **Answer: 4** Option 4 encourages the nurse to broaden the definition of spirituality and what this might mean to clients. Option 1 implies that communication should be closed, option 2 is not a correct assumption under the circumstances, and option 3 is inappropriate.
Cognitive Level: Application **Client Need:** Psychosocial Integrity **Integrated Process:** Nursing Process: Implementation **Content Area:** Psychiatric/Mental Health **Strategy:** The core issue of the question is the ability of the nurse to assess the spiritual needs of a client. Use nursing knowledge and the process of elimination to choose the option that asks a follow-up question during the interview process.

17 **Answer: 1** Option 1 refers to difficulty with adjustment to the current situation. Although options 2 and 3 might be occurring, it is not evident by the scenario described. Option 4 does not apply in this situation either.
Cognitive Level: Application **Client Need:** Psychosocial Integrity **Integrated Process:** Nursing Process: Analysis **Content Area:** Psychiatric/Mental Health **Strategy:** The core issue of the question is the ability of the nurse to critically analyze data and select the appropriate nursing diagnosis label. Use nursing knowledge and the process of elimination to make a selection.

18 **Answer: 3** Option 3 is correct because there is nothing wrong with complementary medicine, and it can be very helpful in coping with illness. Furthermore, it supports the client's right to autonomy and self-determination. There is no rationale for option 1, option 2 is inaccurate, and option 4 is a false assumption.
Cognitive Level: Application **Client Need:** Psychosocial Integrity **Integrated Process:** Nursing Process: Implementation **Content Area:** Psychiatric/Mental Health **Strategy:** The core issue of the question is the appropriate response to a client's choices about managing symptoms of chronic or terminal illness. The correct answer is the one that provides the greatest support to the client.

19 **Answer: 4** Option 4 relates to assisting the client with ways to effectively cope with stress, which may limit exacerbations of the disease. Options 1 and 3 are not healthy ways to cope with stress. Option 2 is not indicated by the information provided.
Cognitive Level: Application **Client Need:** Psychosocial Integrity **Integrated Process:** Nursing Process: Planning **Content Area:** Psychiatric/Mental Health **Strategy:** The core issue of the question is the ability to recognize the association between client stressors and exacerbation of the disease. Eliminate options 1 and 3 first as inappropriate, then choose option 4 over 2 because there is a clear association between client stressors in the stem and the words *stress reduction* in the correct option.

20 **Answer: 3** Option 3 is correct because a client's appropriate behavior should be acknowledged and reinforced. Option 1 is incorrect because the client is already living with the disease process and an attempt to avoid drawing attention to it is not reasonable. Option 2 is incorrect because the client's adjustment is not maladaptive. Option 4 is incorrect because it patronizes the client.
Cognitive Level: Application **Client Need:** Psychosocial Integrity **Integrated Process:** Communication/Documentation **Content Area:** Psychiatric/Mental Health **Strategy:** Use principles of communication to answer the question. The core issue of the question is recognition that the client has made an adaptation to medical illness and that this adaptation should be positively reinforced with the client.

ANSWERS & RATIONALES

Key Terms to Review

adaptive coping p. 295
control p. 299
coping p. 295
crisis p. 298
internal locus of control p. 303
maladaptive coping p. 295
precipitating stressors p. 298

References

Fontaine, K., & Fletcher, J. (2003). *Mental health nursing* (5th ed.).Upper Saddle River, NJ: Pearson Education.

Fortinash, K., & Holoday-Worret, P. (2004). *Psychiatric-mental health nursing* (4th ed.). St. Louis: Mosby.

Kniesl, C., Wilson, H., & Trigoboff, E. (2004). *Contemporary psychiatric-mental health nursing.* Upper Saddle River, NJ: Pearson Education.

Stuart, G., & Laraia, M. (2004). *Principles and practice of psychiatric nursing* (8th ed.). St. Louis: Elsevier Science.

Varcarolis, E. (2006). *Foundations of psychiatric mental health nursing: A clinical approach* (5th ed.). Philadelphia: W. B. Saunders.

22 Mental Health Disorders

Test Yourself

Are you ready for the NCLEX-RN® or course exams? Use the practice tests on the companion CD-ROM to check.

In this chapter

Cross reference

Other chapters relevant to this content area are:

I. OVERVIEW OF MENTAL HEALTH CONCEPTS

! **A. Assessment**

1. Appearance, behavior, and mood: grooming, relaxed state, confidence
2. Level of consciousness/sensorium: oriented to time, place, person; memory intact; able to think abstractly
3. Speech, content/thought processes, insight and judgment, self-perception
4. Stage of growth and development
5. Satisfaction of Maslow's hierarchy of needs (see Figure 22–1 ■)
6. Interactions with others: satisfying interpersonal relationships, ability to cope with stress, ability to trust
7. Risk factors for mental health problems: family history of mental illness, stressful life events, hormonal influence, weak or ineffective mental defense mechanisms
8. Poor support systems

B. Therapeutic management

1. Therapeutic communication techniques (see Chapter 19)
2. ! Therapeutic milieu and treatment modalities (see Table 22–1 ■)

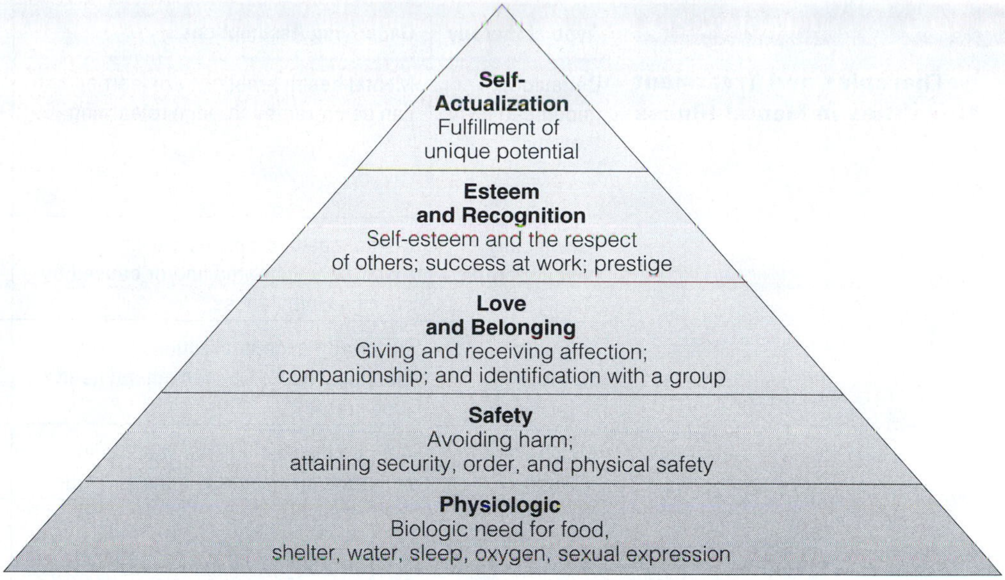

Figure 22–1

Maslow's hierarchy of needs.

Source: Maslow, A. (1962). Motivation and personality *(3rd ed.). Upper Saddle River, NJ: Pearson Education (as reproduced in Kniesl, C., Wilson, H., & Trigoboff, E. (2004).* Contemporary psychiatric-mental health nursing. *Upper Saddle River, NJ. Pearson Education, p. 36.).*

II. ANXIETY DISORDERS

A. Overview of Anxiety

1. **Anxiety:** a state of apprehension, dread, uneasiness, or fear of the unknown
2. Anxiety is an emotional, subjective response
   - **a.** Anxiety is commonly experienced by all human beings
   - **b.** Acute anxiety is also known as state anxiety
   - **c.** Chronic anxiety is also known as trait anxiety
   - **d.** Primary anxiety is related to psychological factors
   - **e.** Secondary anxiety is a response to a physical health problem
3. Fear: a reaction to a specific danger
4. Stress: a state of imbalance between demands placed on an individual and his or her ability to deal with these demands
5. Stressor: an internal or external event or situation that leads to feelings of anxiety
   - **a.** Physical illness, hospitalizations, and medical treatment
   - **b.** Person's perception of stressor leads to anxiety
   - **c.** Individuals evaluate stressors based on past experiences, social influences, and current resources
6. Burnout: a state of mental or physical exhaustion, or both, caused by excessive, prolonged stress
7. Anxiety can be a healthy adaptive reaction when it alerts client to impending threats
8. Anxiety is considered pathological when it is disproportionate to risks, continues after threat no longer exists, and/or interferes with functioning

! B. Levels of anxiety

1. Mild
   - **a.** Day-to-day tension
   - **b.** Person is alert, perceptual field is increased, learning is facilitated
   - **c.** Normal physiological responses
   - **d.** Positive affect
2. Moderate
   - **a.** Focus is on immediate concerns
   - **b.** Perceptual field is narrowed
   - **c.** Low-level sympathetic arousal occurs
   - **d.** Tension and fear are experienced
3. Severe
   - **a.** Focus is on specific details, and behavior is directed toward relieving anxiety
   - **b.** Perceptual field is significantly reduced, and learning cannot occur
   - **c.** Sympathetic nervous system is aroused
   - **d.** Severe emotional distress is experienced

Table 22–1

Therapies and Treatment Modalities in Mental Illness

Type of therapy	Underlying Assumptions	Summary of Treatment
Behavioral (modification) therapy	Mental health problems are learned and can be corrected through relearning	Operant conditioning (rewarding positive behavior to reinforce it); desensitization for phobias to slowly increase tolerance of objects perceived to be threatening
Biologically based therapies	Mental health problems are illnesses that may be inherited and/or caused by chemical imbalances	A variety of medications; electroconvulsive therapy (ECT)
Cognitive therapies	Distorted conceptualizations and dysfunctional beliefs lead to mental health problems	Reality testing; correcting distorted conceptualizations and dysfunctional beliefs by reinterpreting them
Activity therapy	A group task can set the stage to allow important group interactions to occur	Organized group activities that promote socialization and increase self-esteem
Family therapy	Mental health problems are family problems, not individual ones; in sick families, each member lacks a sense of "I"; the behavior of the sick member is seen as the cause of the problem but really serves a function in the family system	Unit of therapy is the entire family; develop a sense of self for each member; members learn new insights and coping behaviors
Group therapy	Relationships with others can be recreated and worked on with group members	Regular meetings are held with a leader to form a stable group; members learn new behaviors and coping skills during group work
Milieu therapy	A therapeutic environment aids in increasing self-awareness of feelings, sense of responsibility	Possible open wards, self-medication programs, token programs; client-planned group and social interactions
Play therapy	Children can express thoughts and feelings in play that they cannot verbalize; the child reflects his or her situation in family through interactions with and choice of toys, colors, activities (drawing)	A variety of toys are provided to facilitate interaction; play is observed; child is helped to work through problems through play
Psychoanalytical	Conflicts between id and ego parts of the personality lead to anxiety; ineffective or inappropriate defense mechanisms form to reduce anxiety	Interactions with therapist assist the client in recognizing unconscious thoughts and feelings, anxieties and defenses, and then in correcting them

4. Panic
   a. Dread and terror
   b. Details are blown out of proportion, personality disorganization, person fails to function
   c. Physiological arousal interferes with motor activities
   d. Overwhelming emotions cause regression to primitive or childish behaviors

C. General adaptation syndrome: an automatic physical reaction to stress mediated by sympathetic nervous system (SNS); three distinct stages are alarm, resistance, and exhaustion

1. Stress is viewed as a nonspecific body response to any demand
2. Alarm is initial response to a stressor
   a. As a result of hormonal activity triggering a fight-or-flight reaction (an automatic psychological state of high anxiety mediated by SNS), increased alertness is focused on immediate task or threat
   b. Level of anxiety is mild to moderate
3. Resistance occurs when body mobilizes resources to combat stress
   a. Body stabilizes and adapts to stress but functions below optimal level

b. Coping, efforts to manage specific demands that are appraised as threatening, and defense mechanisms, unconscious psychological responses designed to diminish or delay anxiety and protect the person, are used
c. Psychosomatic symptoms begin to develop
d. Level of anxiety is moderate to severe

4. Exhaustion occurs when adaptational resources are depleted
a. Results from inability to cope with overwhelming or long-lasting stress
b. Thinking becomes disorganized and illogical; may experience sensory misperceptions, delusions, hallucinations, and/or reduced orientation to reality
c. Level of anxiety is severe to panic
d. Physical illness and even death can occur if period of exhaustion is prolonged

D. Assessment

1. Because anxiety can contribute to organic illness, and organic illness can lead to anxiety, include physical assessment when assessing anxious individuals
2. Shame and fear may prevent individuals from disclosing anxiety
3. Assess anxiety using direct and specific questions (consider cognitive ability, level of education, and language)
4. ! Assess physical, affective, cognitive, social, and spiritual symptoms of anxiety
a. Physical signs include increased blood pressure, respiration, and heart rate; diaphoresis; dilated pupils; dyspnea or hyperventilation; vertigo or lightheadedness; blurred vision; urinary frequency; headache; sleep disturbance; muscle weakness or tension; anorexia, nausea, and vomiting
b. Affective symptoms include depression; irritability; apathy; crying; hypercriticism; feelings of guilt, grief, anger, worthlessness, apprehension, and helplessness
c. Cognitive symptoms include inability to concentrate, indecisiveness, inability to think and reason, lack of interest, and forgetfulness
d. Social symptoms include refusal to communicate or excessive communication, self-isolation, social withdrawal, and possibly suicidal ideation
e. Spiritual symptoms include feelings of hopelessness and despair, fear of death, and inability to find life meaningful

E. Therapeutic management

1. Assist in developing mental coping strategies
a. Include breathing exercises, guided imagery, meditation, listening to music, progressive muscle relaxation, recreational activities, crying, exercising, laughing, sleeping, diet and fluid intake, time management
b. ! Problem-focused coping is task-oriented and consists of assessing facts, developing goal, determining alternatives for coping, identifying risks and benefits of each alternative, selecting an alternative, implementing selected alternative, evaluating outcome, and modifying actions based on evaluation
c. Emotional-focused coping requires client to reinterpret meaning of situation and explore defense mechanisms (see Chapter 21)

2. Psychopharmacology
a. Common antianxiety agents (also known as anxiolytics or minor tranquilizers) used to treat anxiety are listed in Box 22–1 and discussed in Chapter 36
b. Benzodiazepines are most commonly used, but prolonged use can lead to dependency
c. Nonbenzodiazepine sedative-hypnotics are a new class of drugs used for short-term treatment of insomnia associated with anxiety; include zolpidem (Ambien) and zaleplon (Sonata)
d. Buspirone (Buspar) is a serotonin and dopamine agonist used in short-term treatment of anxiety
e. Beta blockers have a calming effect on central nervous system (CNS): propranolol (Inderal) is a beta blocker sometimes used to treat physical symptoms of anxiety, such as tremors and tachycardia
f. Antidepressants may be used to treat coexisting depression and insomnia associated with anxiety

Box 22-1

Common Antianxiety Medications

Benzodiazepines

Alprazolam (Xanax)

Chlordiazepoxide (Librium)

Clonazepam (Klonopin)

Diazepam (Valium)

Lorazepam (Ativan)

Oxazepam (Serax)

Serotonin and dopamine agonist

Buspirone (Buspar)

Beta blocker

Propranolol (Inderal)

3. Individual and **group therapy**
   a. Helps clients to discuss their feelings and problems with empathetic listeners
   b. Helps anxious individuals develop insight and rationales for feelings of anxiety
   c. Group therapy is an effective treatment modality for anxiety
   d. ! Guidelines for therapeutic nursing interventions to assist anxious clients are listed in Box 22–2
   e. Client education is an important intervention for anxious clients
4. Other useful therapies

Box 22-2

Guidelines for Therapeutic Nursing Interventions to Assist Anxious Individuals

- Be aware of own level of anxiety.
- Remain calm.
- Establish a trusting relationship.
- Protect and reassure the client.
- Structure the environment to eliminate stressors.
- Assessment of client's anxiety should be ongoing.
- Assess the client's use of caffeine, nicotine, and other stimulants.
- Assess the client for signs of depression and suicidal ideations.
- Help the client to identify stressors.
- Encourage the client to express feelings and explore sources of feelings.
- Help the client to examine cognitive processes and encourage positive self-talk.
- Help the client to maintain hope and find meaning in life.
- Support the client's use of effective coping mechanisms.
- Teach the client new coping behaviors.
- Provide opportunities for the client to practice new coping behaviors.
- Teach the client relaxation techniques.
- Encourage appropriate grooming, sleep, diet, recreational activity, and exercise.
- Facilitate the client's interactions with supportive significant others.
- Use role-playing to help the client rehearse appropriate reactions to stressors.
- Stay with clients who display high levels of anxiety.
- Refer the client to community resources.

a. Cognitive-behavior therapy helps individuals learn to identify stressors and plan responses to stressors

b. In cognitive restructuring, clients are encouraged to examine involuntary negative thoughts and to replace negative self-talk with more positive thoughts

c. Response prevention is a form of behavior modification used to teach clients with obsessive-compulsive disorder how to prevent compulsive behaviors associated with obsessive thoughts

d. Systematic desensitization is a form of behavior modification used to treat anxiety

e. Flooding, also known as implosion therapy, exposes client to imaginary or real-life stress-provoking stimuli for an extended period of time, and session is terminated when client's anxiety decreases

f. Thought-stopping involves such techniques as instructing client to shout "Stop!" or snap a rubber band placed on wrist when unwelcome thoughts occur

g. Other behavior modification techniques used to treat anxiety include modeling, shaping, token economy, role-playing, social skill training, aversion therapy, response prevention, and contingency contracting

F. Phobic disorders

1. Individuals with phobic disorders recognize that their **phobias** (fears of specific objects, activities and situations) are irrational
2. Avoidance of feared stimuli may drastically interfere with routine activities
3. Phobias

a. **Agoraphobia** (fear of being incapacitated by being trapped in an unbearable situation from which there is no escape) without panic attacks involves fear of places or situations such as crowds, standing in line, being on a bridge, and traveling in a plane, bus, train, or car

b. Social phobia is excessive fear of embarrassment and humiliation in public settings

c. Specific phobia involves unrealistic fear of a particular object or situation

4. Treatments include cognitive therapy and graduated exposure or desensitization; antianxiety medications may provide short-term relief of phobic anxiety
5. Nursing care includes accepting but not supporting phobia, exploring client's perceptions of threats, discussing feelings that may contribute to irrational fears, and identifying strategies for change

G. Generalized anxiety disorder (GAD)

1. Characterized by difficulty controlling unrealistic, excessive anxiety associated with common daily experiences
2. A continued high level of anxiety causes symptoms such as restlessness, irritability, fatigue, depression, difficulty concentrating, muscle tension, sleep disturbance, and feeling of helplessness
3. Symptoms interfere with normal daily activities
4. In an attempt to control symptoms, clients sometimes become dependent on alcohol or other substances
5. Generalized anxiety disorder has been successfully treated by a combination of cognitive therapy and relaxation training
6. Encourage clients with generalized anxiety disorder to rethink perceptions of stressor, recognize that some anxiety is a normal part of life, and learn new coping mechanisms
7. Benzodiazepines and buspirone are sometimes used to treat generalized anxiety disorders

H. Panic disorder

1. Characterized by recurrent panic attacks
2. Between panic attacks, client may have little or no debilitating anxiety or may suffer from chronic worry about future panic attacks
3. Onset of a panic attack is sudden, and source of anxiety may not be identifiable
4. Symptoms of panic attacks include a desire to escape, chest pain, chills or hot flashes, choking sensations, depersonalization, dizziness, nausea, palpitations, shortness of breath, sweating, trembling, and fear of loss of control and mental illness

5. Clients frequently associate their symptoms with physical illness and are concerned about death
6. Feelings of hopelessness, helplessness, and despair may lead to suicidal ideations
7. Agoraphobia is frequently associated with panic disorder
8. During panic attacks, nurse should remain calm, stay with client, offer reassurance, use short clear sentences, and reduce environmental stimuli
9. When level of anxiety is mild or moderate, explore possible causes of anxiety, teach signs and symptoms of escalating anxiety, teach and reinforce appropriate coping mechanisms and strategies
10. Benzodiazepines and antidepressants treat panic disorders

I. Obsessive-compulsive disorder (OCD)

1. Characterized by recurrent obsessive thoughts and uncontrollable compulsive behaviors that are irrational
2. Control of self, others, and environment is an important issue
3. Common **obsessions** (unwanted, persistent, intrusive thoughts, impulses or images related to anxiety) include thoughts about specific objects, contamination, questions, order, sex, aggressive feelings, and unacceptable impulses
4. Common **compulsions** (unwanted behavioral patterns or acts) include counting, praying, hand washing, repeating words, checking, and seeking assurance
5. Anxiety will increase if obsessive thoughts and compulsive behaviors are interrupted
6. Depression and/or substance abuse may occur as a complication
7. Treatments include relaxation and cognitive-behavioral techniques such as flooding and thought-stopping
8. Assist clients to identify situations that increase anxiety, explore meaning and purpose of thoughts and behavior, support client attempts to decrease obsessions and compulsions
9. Conduct teaching immediately following completion of a ritual when client anxiety is at its lowest
10. Selective serotonin reuptake inhibitors (SSRIs) are most effective somatic treatment for OCD
11. Electroconvulsive therapy (ECT) has been used to treat depressive symptoms associated with OCD

J. Posttraumatic stress disorder (PTSD)

1. Associated with exposure to an extremely traumatic, menacing event such as military combat, rape, assault, kidnapping, torture, incarceration, disasters, and life-threatening illnesses
2. Symptoms
   a. Apathy, social withdrawal and isolation, loss of interest in activities, and possible depression and hopelessness
   b. Restlessness, irritability, intrusive and unwanted memories of traumatic event, amnesia for certain aspects of trauma, nightmares, flashbacks, and occasional outburst of anger and rage
3. Denial, repression, and suppression are utilized as coping mechanisms
4. Provide a nonthreatening environment, encourage client to discuss traumatic event and associated feelings
5. Explore traumatic event; assess and acknowledge feelings of guilt, grief, and shame
6. Encourage and reinforce appropriate coping strategies, teach new coping strategies, and assist client in resuming regular activities
7. SSRIs, especially sertraline (Zoloft), seem to be somewhat effective in treatment of PTSD

III. MOOD DISORDERS

A. Overview

1. **Mood:** a prolonged emotional state that affects a person's life and personality
2. Change of mood is a normal and expected life occurrence; each individual feels a range of emotions, such as joy, happiness, sadness, depression, anger, and fear

3. **Affect:** an individual's present feelings and moods with verbal and nonverbal behavioral cues
4. *Mood disorders* are characterized by changes in mood that range from depression to elation
   a. **Major depression** (also called **unipolar disorder**) refers to a loss of interest in life and a mood that transforms from mild to severe and lasts at least 2 weeks; if uncontrolled, results in disturbances in eating, sleeping, and functioning at work, home, and/or school; withdrawal and decreased sociability; possible delusions and/or hallucinations with psychotic features if disorder progresses to severe depression
   b. **Dysthymic disorder:** a chronic disorder in which depressed mood fluctuates with a normal mood; symptoms are less severe than in major depression
   c. **Bipolar disorder** (also called manic-depressive disorder) is alternation of depression and elation; categorized as bipolar I disorder (one or more manic episodes and one or more depressive episodes), bipolar II disorder (less severe, has one or more *hypomanic* or mild mania episodes and one or more depressive episodes
   d. **Cyclothymic disorder:** mood disorder with mood changes between moderate depression and hypomania; lasts for at least 2 years; usually no sign of a normal range
   e. **Seasonal affective disorder (SAD):** depressed mood that occurs during fall and winter months; there is a direct correlation with light and production of melatonin
   f. **Schizoaffective disorder:** a combination of manifestations of schizophrenia and mood disorders; delusions, hallucinations, disorganized speech and behavior, communication difficulties, poor abstractions, passive social withdrawal, poor grooming and hygiene, poor rapport, and major depressive/manic symptoms or mixed symptoms, and possibly other physical or psychological disorders
   g. Fifteen percent of those who experience major depressive disorders die by suicide

B. Assessment

! 1. Conduct intake assessment of individuals (15- to 20-minute segments at one time)
   a. Individuals who have mood disorders do not have enough energy to talk or focus their attention for extended periods of time
   b. Clients with mania may not be able to sit still and concentrate because of elevated mood and flight of ideas
2. Bipolar disorders
   a. Characterized by moods alternating between episodes of depression and episodes of mania or hypomania
   b. Manic episodes are periods of elation during which there is an abnormally and persistently elevated, expansive, or irritable mood for at least 1 week and also includes at least three of the following: inflated self-esteem, decreased need for sleep, more than usual talkativeness, racing thoughts, distractibility, increase in goal-directed activity, and excessive involvement in pleasurable activities
   c. Hypomania is described as an elevation in mood with increases in activity but not as severe elation as in mania

! 3. Major depression
   a. Loss of interest in life and a depressed mood, which moves from mild to severe and lasts at least 2 weeks
   b. Depressed mood is present for most of day, nearly every day, as indicated by subjective (client reports) or objective (facial expression, appears tearful) signs and symptoms
   c. Markedly diminished interest or pleasure in all or almost all activities most of day, nearly every day (as indicated by subjective or objective signs and symptoms)

d. Significant weight loss or gain
e. Insomnia or hypersomnia
f. Psychomotor agitation or retardation nearly every day
g. Fatigue or loss of energy nearly every day
h. Diminished ability to think or concentrate, or indecisiveness, nearly every day
i. Social withdrawal
j. Recurrent thoughts of death; suicidal ideation with or without a specific plan or a suicide attempt

4. Dysthymic disorder differs from major depression in that it is a chronic, low-level depression; must have had depressed mood and at least three of these symptoms for most of the day, nearly every day, for at least 2 years: poor appetite or overeating; insomnia or hypersomnia; low energy; low self-esteem; poor concentration and difficulty making decisions; and feelings of hopelessness
5. Key characteristic differences between depressive disorder and bipolar disorders are noted in Table 22–2 ■

C. Therapeutic management

1. Risk for violence, self-directed related to depressed mood, feelings of worthlessness, hopelessness, and suicide ideation or plan
   a. Client's safety is nurse's first priority
   b. ! Danger for self-harm is more prominent as client begins to regain strength and hope; therefore, frequently assess client for levels of hopefulness or hopelessness and self-esteem, and be alert for signs and symptoms of thoughts or plan for suicide
   c. History of violence is *always* important in determining seriousness of client's present risk for self-harm
   d. Client often displays ambivalence or expresses sadness, dejection, hopelessness, or loss of pleasure or purpose in life
   e. Client makes overt attempts to harm self (e.g., hoards medications, performs self-mutilation, attempts to hang self)
   f. Assess for overt signs of hopelessness: refusal to eat, withdrawal from milieu, resistance to or refusal of medications; inability to see future for self; sudden giving away of possessions; refusal to sign a no self-harm contract
2. Risk for violence directed at others, related to poor impulse control and labile affect
   a. ! Client's safety is nurse's first priority; provide a safe environment, removing objects and barriers to prevent accidental or purposeful injury to self or others
   b. Help client to identify alternative behaviors that are acceptable to client and staff
   c. Encourage client, during calm moments, to recognize and identify antecedents or precipitants to agitation and loss of control
   d. Always give realistic and positive feedback and encouragement to client
   e. ! Decrease environmental stimuli when client is agitated; gradually increase environmental stimulation after agitation subsides
   f. Monitor client's ability to tolerate frustration and/or individual situations
   g. Offer alternatives when available (e.g., "There is no coffee available; how about a glass of juice?")
   h. Communicate with respect and a nonjudgmental tone
3. Ineffective individual coping related to lack of energy, inability to concentrate or make decisions
   a. Maintain activities of daily living (ADLs)
   b. Use a problem-solving approach
   c. ! Maintain a safe environment
   d. Observe client closely
   e. Encourage client to focus on strengths rather than weaknesses
   f. ! Encourage identification of individuals and systems that can support client
   g. Help client to learn strategies that will effect more positive thinking (cognitive, behavioral, imagery)
   h. Encourage client to express feelings and needs

Table 22–2

Assessment Findings in Major Depression and Mania

	Major Depression	Mania
Behavior	Progression from a decreased desire to engage in social, work, and school activities to an absence of participation in common activities of daily living; progressive loss of self-esteem, feelings of incompetence, decreased motivation; statements such as, "Why bother, I can't anyway" are common	Initially high energy and productivity with positive reinforcement from others; decreased ability to concentrate, make judgments, or engage in everyday activities; increasing frustration and irritability, shortened attention span, unrealistic self-confidence, and poor judgment, leading to inability to function; may engage in spending sprees, making foolish financial investments and/or high-risk lifestyle changes
Relationships	Withdrawal from personal and social activities and events	Unable to set boundaries; exhibits incessant talkativeness and gregarious behaviors that are often an embarrassment when they return to their normal range of mood
Affective characteristics	Sense of sadness that becomes increasingly pronounced; guilt that may be expressed as a vague concern or a specific issue: "I have so much to be thankful for, I shouldn't feel this way"; loss of emotional attachment evidenced by expressions of indifference toward family and friends; anhedonia, or a lack of pleasure	Mood ranges between cheerful and euphoric; in the presence of an external negative stimulus, can become irritable, argumentative, hostile, and even combative, then return to euphoria when negative stimulus is removed; absence of a sense of guilt; responds to others' feelings of hurt or anger with his or her own anger, laughter, or indifference; tries to participate in every activity/event available
Cognitive characteristics	Personal worth: presentation of self as a failure and totally incompetent; catastrophizes (exaggerates) life as a failure or personalizes comments by others; is self-critical and perfectionistic; anticipates disapproval from others; while in a depressed state: • Exhibits a decreased ability or even an inability for decision making • Has decrease in rate and number of thoughts • Perceives self as being ugly or unattractive • Has somatic delusions • Has hallucinations (15–25% of cases)	Personal worth: very grandiose belief about self; exhibits unwarranted positive expectations, is unable to see potential negative outcomes, and is irate if criticized by others; while in manic state of bipolar disorder: • Presents as easily distractible and impulsive • Has flight of ideas • Believes himself or herself to be very attractive • Exhibits delusions of grandeur • Exhibits hallucinations in approximately 15–25% of cases
Sociocultural characteristics	Loss of desire in sexual activities	Increase in sexual activity, even to promiscuity
Physiological characteristics	Either an increased or a decreased appetite; when in a severe state of depression, a decrease in appetite usually occurs; sleep can either be increased or decreased in mild to moderate depression; sleep is usually decreased in severe depression; constipation	Difficulty eating because of the inability to physically slow down or sit still; sleeps only 1 or 2 hours per night and is usually hyperactive when engaged in activities; constipation
Physical appearance	Unkempt appearance with little to no attention to hygiene	Bright clothing, frequent changes in clothing and an exaggerated presentation of the physical self

i. Inform family and friends that client may direct anger toward them but that he or she is learning more effective coping skills to deal with feelings

! j. Help client to gradually become involved with activities on unit

k. Encourage client to socialize as tolerated with staff, other clients on unit, and family members in a structured environment

4. Imbalanced nutrition, less/more than body requirements related to inappropriate nutritional intake to meet metabolic needs; lack of interest in eating/food or choosing nutritional foods; aversion to eating; dysfunctional eating pattern (e.g., eating in response to internal cues other than hunger)
   a. Client may have an aversion to eating because of paranoid thoughts, such as that food is contaminated or someone is trying to poison him or her
   b. ! Note common findings in manic states, including weight loss; easy distraction from eating; inability to sit through routine meals; wary or frightened appearance when offered food; physical signs of poor nutrition, dehydration, and electrolyte imbalances; hyperactive bowel sounds
   c. ! Offer small frequent feedings and frequent carbohydrate- and protein-rich snacks
   d. ! Offer nutritious finger foods and sandwiches
   e. ! Offer easy-to-carry drinks that are high in vitamins, minerals, and electrolytes
   f. ! Assess fluid and electrolyte status, especially sodium, potassium, and lithium levels
   g. Continually assess urinary output
   h. Assess daily bowel movements for frequency and consistency
   i. Assess for abdominal pain or discomfort
   j. ! Administer high-fiber foods unless contraindicated
   k. Clients with depression may demonstrate a nutritional pattern that relates more to their depressed mood, including lack of interest in eating, poor or no appetite, aversion to food, dysfunctional eating patterns, poor choices of food, recent weight loss or gain, poor muscle tone, pale conjunctivae and mucous membranes
   l. Monitor and record daily intake and output
   m. Explain to client importance of maintaining adequate intake of food and fluids to prevent malnutrition
   n. Determine client's daily caloric intake needs
   o. ! Monitor body weight
   p. Monitor laboratory studies (such as serum prealbumin, albumin, glucose, electrolytes, nitrogen balance)
5. Disturbed sleep pattern related to biochemical alterations (decreased serotonin) or psychological stress, lack of recognition of fatigue or need to sleep, hyperactivity
   a. In clients with mania, sleep disturbances can be evidenced by denial of need for sleep, changes in behavior and performance, increasing irritability, restlessness, and dark circles under eyes
   b. Identify environmental factors that might prevent or interrupt sleep
   c. Restrict intake of caffeine
   d. Offer small snack or warm milk at bedtime or when client is awake during night
   e. ! Encourage activities in morning and early afternoon, and restrict activities during evening and prior to bedtime
   f. Encourage routine bedtime relaxation techniques
   g. Administer medications as indicated
   h. Identify nature of sleep disturbance and variations from usual pattern (difficulty falling asleep, remaining asleep, or waking early and unable to return to sleep)
   i. ! Identify previous nighttime rituals that may have been effective and reestablish when possible
   j. Restrict evening fluids, and have client void before retiring
6. Spiritual distress related to a sense of no purpose or joy in life; lack of connectedness to others; misperceived shame and guilt

a. Allow client to express feelings and thoughts about religious doubt or fears of abandonment
b. Explore with client alternative or past effective religious or spiritual practice or ritual as an illness-prevention measure
c. Eliminate or reduce causative and contributing factors of illness if possible
d. Encourage client to discuss thoughts and feelings with clergy or chaplain when possible

7. ECT as treatment
   a. Useful for clients with severe depression who resist other types of treatment modalities, including medications such as tricyclic antidepressants (TCAs) and monoamine oxidase inhibitors (MAOIs)
   b. Involves application of pulses of electrical energy to forehead and temporal area of scalp, sufficient to cause a brief convulsion or seizure; usually carried out under anesthesia
   c. A series of ECT treatments is usually carried out over a short period of time
   d. Effects of ECT are usually very positive for treatment of depression
   e. Side effects are low and seem to be limited to short-term, temporary memory deficits; deaths have been reported in clients who undergo ECT, but they are infrequent; risks related to anesthesia are present
   f. Nursing care involves same principles as those used for client undergoing surgery or moderate (conscious) sedation; protect client's airway and provide for safety; monitor vital signs and provide explanations to client as needed
8. Antidepressant medications as treatment (see Chapter 36 for full discussion of antidepressant medications and lithium as treatment for mania)
   a. Tricyclic antidepressants (TCAs)
   b. Selective serotonin reuptake inhibitors (SSRIs)
   c. Monoamine oxidase inhibitors (MAOIs); avoid foods high in tyramine (see Box 22–3)
   d. Atypical antidepressants: bupropion (Wellbutrin), trazodone (Desyrel)
   e. Mood stabilizer medications: lithium carbonate, carbamazepine (Tegretol), and valproic acid (Depakote)
9. Group and individual therapies, including cognitive therapy, behavioral therapy, and interpersonal therapy for mild to moderate depression

Box 22–3

Foods to Avoid with Monoamine Oxidase Inhibitors

Foods to Avoid

- Aged cheeses: Roquefort, blue, brie, camembert
- Meats and fish: aged/cured
- Fruits and vegetables: broad bean pods, tofu, soybean extracts
- Alcohol: draft beer and chianti wine
- Other: sauerkraut, soy sauce, yeast extracts, soups (especially miso)
- Drugs: other antidepressant drugs; nasal and sinus decongestants; allergy, hay-fever, and asthma remedies; narcotics (especially meperidine); epinephrine; stimulants; cocaine; amphetamines

Consume with Caution

- Cheeses: mozzarella, cottage, ricotta, cream, processed
- Meats and fish: fresh chicken liver, meats, liver, herring
- Fruits and vegetables: raspberries, bananas, small amounts only of avocado, spinach
- Alcohol: wine
- Other: monosodium glutamate, pizza, small amounts only of chocolate, caffeine, nuts, dairy products
- Drugs: insulin, oral hypoglycemics, oral anticoagulants, thiazide diuretics, anticholinergic agents, muscle relaxants

10. Phototherapy
    a. A treatment that has been used effectively to lessen symptoms of recurrent SAD, because possibly exposure to *morning light* causes a circadian rhythm shift that regulates normal relationships between sleep and circadian rhythms
    b. Phototherapy treatment consists of a minimum of 2,500 lux of light usually administered on waking in morning; clients can be exposed for 30 minutes to several hours, depending on strength of light source
    c. An antidepressant effect is usually seen within 2 to 4 days and is complete after 2 weeks
    d. Maintenance treatment usually consists of 30 minutes of exposure each day; side effects are usually minimal
11. Evaluate achievement of short- and long-term goals for clients with mood disorders
    a. Remain safe and free from harm
    b. Verbalize suicidal ideations and contract not to harm self or others
    c. Verbalize absence of suicidal or homicidal intent or plan
    d. Establish a pattern of rest, activity, and sleep that enables fulfillment of role and self-care demands
    e. Describe information about his or her disorder, including triggers for relapse, preventive measures in place for relapse prevention, and medication use to control symptoms

IV. SCHIZOPHRENIA AND OTHER PSYCHOTIC DISORDERS

A. ***Schizophrenia:*** a syndrome characterized by difficulty in thinking clearly, knowing what is real, managing feelings, making decisions, or relating to others
1. Positive symptoms of schizophrenia are added behaviors not normally seen, such as delusions, hallucinations, loose associations, and overactive affect
2. Negative symptoms of schizophrenia are the absence of healthy behaviors; negative symptoms may include flat affect, minimal self-care, social withdrawal, and concrete thinking
3. People with schizophrenia may exhibit purposeless or ritualistic behaviors or even pace for hours on end; some have bizarre facial or body movements
4. Most common type of hallucination is auditory; next most common type is visual
5. Delusions are false beliefs that cannot be changed by logical reasoning or evidence; it is thought that they represent dysfunction in information-processing circuits between hemispheres of brain
6. People with schizophrenia frequently have ineffective social skills, which increases their sense of isolation
7. Neurobiological factors of schizophrenia include genetic defects, abnormal brain development, neurodegeneration, disordered neurotransmission, and abnormal brain structures
8. Psychiatric rehabilitation emphasizes development of skills and supports; considers client to be in control; and promotes choices, self-determination, and individual responsibility

B. ***Schizoaffective disorder:*** having clinical manifestations characteristic of both schizophrenia and a mood disorder, such as depression, mania, or a mixed episode
1. Client experiences symptoms of a mood disorder with one or more of the following:
    a. Delusions
    b. Hallucinations
    c. Disorganized speech
    d. Disorganized behavior
    e. Negative characteristics
2. Clients often have difficulty maintaining a job or functioning in school, experience problems with self-care, are socially isolated, and often suffer from suicidal ideation

C. ***Schizophreniform disorder:*** essential features of schizophrenia are present with the exception that duration is at least 1 month but less than 6 months

D. ***Other psychotic disorders***
1. Delusional disorder: presence of nonbizarre delusions (delusions that could possibly occur in reality) that persist for at least 1 month; no other manifestations of psychosis are noted

2. Brief psychotic disorder: presence of at least one positive symptom of schizophrenia with duration between 1 day and 1 month; existence or absence of any stressor should be noted
3. Shared psychotic disorder (*folie a deux*): a delusional system develops in context of a close relationship between two people who share a similar delusion
4. Substance-induced psychotic disorder: presence of hallucinations and delusions are a direct result of physiological effects of a substance
5. Psychotic disorder due to a general medical condition: presence of hallucinations and delusions are a direct result of general medical condition

E. Overview and classification of schizophrenia

1. Schizophrenia is one of a cluster of related psychotic brain disorders of unknown etiology
2. Schizophrenia is a combination of disordered thinking, perceptual disturbances, behavioral abnormalities, affective disruptions, and impaired social competency
3. ! Symptoms of schizophrenia
   a. **Delusional ideation:** a false belief brought about without appropriate external stimulation and inconsistent with individual's own knowledge and experience
   b. **Hallucinations:** false sensory perceptions that may involve any of five senses (auditory, visual, tactile, olfactory, and gustatory)
   c. Disorganized speech patterns
   d. Bizarre behaviors
4. At least two of these symptoms must be present for a significant portion of time during a 1-month period
5. Other manifestations include social impairment and cognitive impairment: subtypes of schizophrenia have similar features but differ in their clinical presentations
6. ! Generally, individual exhibits normal behavior early in life, experiences subtle changes after puberty, and experiences severe symptoms in late teens to early adulthood
7. Vast majority of individuals develop disorder in adolescence or young adulthood, with only 10% of cases first diagnosed in people over the age of 45
8. Current knowledge base on etiology of schizophrenia is uncertain; several types of factors have been identified as having a high correlation or association with development of schizophenia:
   a. Brain structure and functioning: structure, physiology, and neurotransmitters
   b. Genetic factors: increased risk if first-degree relatives also have disorder
   c. Psychological factors (stress does not cause but exacerbates disorder)
   d. Environmental factors: viruses and complications at labor and delivery

F. Critical essential features of each subtype of schizophrenia

1. Paranoid type
   a. ! Auditory hallucinations
   b. Preoccupation with one or more delusions usually of a persecutory nature
   c. May appear hostile or angry
2. **Catatonic** type
   a. ! Stupor (state of daze or unconsciousness) or extreme motor agitation
   b. Excessive negativism
   c. Inappropriate or bizarre body postures
   d. **Echolalia** (an involuntary, parrotlike repetition of words spoken by others) or **echopraxia** (a meaningless imitation of motions made by others)
3. Residual type
   a. Absence of prominent psychotic symptoms
   b. Social withdrawal and inappropriate affect
   c. Eccentric behavior
   d. Past history of at least one episode of schizophrenia
4. Disorganized type
   a. Disorganized speech
   b. Disorganized behavior
   c. Inappropriate or flat affect

5. Undifferentiated type
   a. Disorganized behaviors
   b. Psychotic symptoms (including delusions and hallucinations)

G. Assessment

1. Positive symptoms indicate a distortion or excess of normal functioning: they often occur as initial symptoms of schizophrenia and precipitate need for hospitalization;
2. Delusions—fixed false beliefs or ideas
   a. Paranoid type: individual believes others are out to get him or her; client may be hostile, suspicious, and aggressive
   b. Grandiose type: individual has excessive feelings of importance and power over others
   c. Religious type: individual has delusions that focus on a religious context
   d. Somatic type: individual has delusions fixed on an irrational belief about his or her body
   e. Nihilistic: client has delusions of nonexistence
   f. Persecutory: client has delusions that others are out to get or are plotting against him or her
   g. **Thought broadcasting:** individual believes that others can hear his or her thoughts
   h. **Thought insertion:** individual believes that others have ability to put thoughts in a person's mind against that person's will
   i. **Thought control:** individual believes that others can control a person's thoughts against that person's will
3. Hallucinations, usually auditory; visual is second-most common type
4. **Psychosis** is a disorderly mental state in which a client has difficulty distinguishing reality from his or her own internal perceptions
5. **Illusions:** inaccurate perception or misinterpretation of sensory impressions
6. Agitation or hostility
7. Bizarre behaviors (catatonic, etc.)
8. Association disturbances
   a. Echolalia or echopraxia
   b. **Clang associations:** rhyming words in a sentence that makes no sense
   c. Illogical thinking patterns
   d. **Neologisms:** inventing new words, which are meaningful only to that person
   e. **Word salad:** combining in a sentence words that have no connection and make no sense
9. Negative symptoms indicate a loss or lack of healthy functioning; they develop over time and hinder person's ability to endure life tasks; they include the following:
   a. Anhedonia: diminished ability to experience pleasure or intimacy
   b. Alogia: poverty of speech
   c. Anergia: lack of energy
   d. Avolition: lack of motivation and goals
   e. Ambivalence: inability to make a decision because of conflicting emotions
   f. Affect disturbances: blunted, flat, or inappropriate behavior; restricted emotion
   g. Ineffective social skills and social withdrawal
   h. Dependency
   i. Lack of self-care
10. Lack of ego boundaries
11. Concrete thought processes
12. Sleep disturbance

H. Nursing diagnoses and analysis

1. Impaired thought processes related to possible hereditary factors, delusional thinking, hallucinations, or inaccurate interpretation of environment
2. Anxiety related to inaccurate interpretation of environment, unfamiliar environment, repressed fear, or panic level of stress
3. Ineffective individual coping related to inability to trust, low self-esteem, or inadequate support systems

4. Social isolation related to lack of trust, regression to earlier level of function, delusional thinking, or past experiences of difficulty in interactions with others
5. Risk for violence, self-directed or directed toward others, related to lack of trust, panic-level anxiety, command hallucinations, delusional thinking, or perception of environment as threatening
6. Impaired sensory perception: auditory or visual related to hallucinations, delusional thinking, withdrawal into self, or perception of environment as threatening
7. Impaired verbal communication related to inability to trust, regression to earlier level of development, or disordered and unrealistic thinking
8. Self-care deficit (specify) related to withdrawal into self, regression to earlier level of development, or perceptual or cognitive impairment
9. Disturbed sleep pattern related to repressed fears, hallucinations, or delusional thinking
10. Chronic low self-esteem related to withdrawal into self, lack of trust, poor socialization skills, or chronic illness

I. Psychopharmacology (see Chapter 36)

1. Typical antipsychotics (traditional)
2. Atypical antipsychotics
3. Anti-parkinsonism (anticholinergics)

J. Individual and group interventions

1. ! Management of delusions and hallucinations
   - **a.** Establish a trusting, therapeutic relationship with client by being honest, supportive, and consistent
   - **b.** Encourage expression of feelings and thoughts
   - **c.** Assess for signs of delusions or hallucinations
   - **d.** Communicate with client using clear, direct statements
   - **e.** Provide an environment with a low degree of stimulation
   - **f.** Express to client an understanding of what he or she believes of delusion or hallucination but do not share in delusional belief or hallucination; do not argue with client
   - **g.** Provide reality testing and focus on reality
   - **h.** If client is experiencing a visual hallucination, provide a room with adequate lighting
2. General nursing considerations and interventions
   - **a.** Provide an environment that is safe for client and others
   - **b.** ! Avoid any physical contact or touching of client
   - **c.** ! Encourage client to verbalize feelings and thoughts openly
   - **d.** Utilize therapeutic communication techniques with client
   - **e.** Identify support systems for client
   - **f.** ! Assess for self-destructive behaviors and provide needed precautions
   - **g.** Provide for ADLs when client is not able to meet those needs
   - **h.** Provide opportunities for client that promote socialization and decrease isolation
   - **i.** Involve client in setting realistic goals in treatment plan
   - **j.** Provide daily living skills groups for client to participate in

K. Milieu therapy: a method of psychotherapy that controls environment of client to provide interpersonal contacts in order to develop trust, assurance, and personal autonomy

1. ! Provide for client's safety and safety of others in milieu
2. Provide a supportive, structured, and predictable environment
3. Collaborate with multidisciplinary team regarding client's plan of care
4. Collaborate with client and family regarding plan of care
5. Encourage client to participate in milieu groups and activities that promote socialization
6. Assist client with ADLs as needed, but encourage independence as client progresses

L. Family therapy

1. Involve family to determine use of appropriate community resources
2. Educate family about chronic illness of schizophrenia, implications, early signs and symptoms of relapse, disease management, medication management, and community support systems available

3. Provide an outlet for family to discuss their feelings and explore alternative effective coping skills

M. Evaluation and client outcomes

1. Remains free of harm and demonstrates absence of violence toward others
2. Reports cessation of hallucinations or delusional thought processes
3. Demonstrates increased socialization skills and decreased isolative behavior
4. Demonstrates appropriate affect and improved thought processes
5. Demonstrates improved speech patterns and congruent communication
6. Adheres to medication schedule as prescribed without adverse medication effects
7. Demonstrates effective coping patterns, including use of community resources

N. Evaluation and family outcomes

1. Can verbalize and identify early signs and symptoms of disease exacerbation, implications of schizophrenia as a chronic illness, and medication regimen
2. Can verbalize and identify signs and symptoms of EPS and neuroleptic malignant syndrome (NMS)
3. Can verbalize how and when to access emergency care services

V. PERSONALITY DISORDERS

A. Overview

1. Personality is composed of enduring patterns or traits that determine how individuals perceive, relate to, and think about environment and themselves; **personality traits** or patterns are reflected in how individuals cope with feelings and impulses, see themselves and others, respond to their surroundings, and find meaning in relationships
2. **Personality disorders** are diagnosed when personality patterns or traits are inflexible, enduring, pervasive, maladaptive, and cause significant functional impairment or subjective distress
   a. Reflect patterns of inner experience and behavior that differ from cultural expectations
   b. Result in problems in living rather than in clinical symptoms
   c. Clients frequently experience their personality patterns as natural or comfortable (**egosyntonic**) rather than painful or uncomfortable (**egodystonic**)
   d. If personality patterns are experienced as egosyntonic, clients rarely seek treatment because they tend to externalize cause of any functional impairment or subjective distress
   e. If personality patterns are experienced as egodystonic, clients are more likely to seek treatment to ease their distress
   f. Are coded under axis II disorders (personality disorders or mental retardation) using American Psychiatric Association's *Diagnostic and Statistical Manual of Mental Disorders, Fourth Edition Text Revision* (DSM-IV-TR) diagnostic criteria
   g. Frequently overlap: individuals may exhibit patterns or traits associated with more than one personality disorder
   h. Develop before or during adolescence and persist throughout life; symptoms may become less obvious by middle or old age
   i. May coexist with clinical disorders coded as axis I disorders (mood and thought disorders) using DSM-IV-TR
   j. Are organized into three diagnostic clusters, discussed in next sections
3. Characteristics of personality disorders are manifested in four areas
   a. Behavioral manifestations: include patterns of day-to-day behavior and impulse control
   b. Affective manifestations: include range, intensity, lability, and appropriateness of emotional response
   c. Cognitive manifestations: reflect how self, others, and events are interpreted
   d. Sociocultural manifestations: reflect interpersonal functioning
4. May result from limbic system dysregulation and CNS irritability, decreased levels of serotonin (5-HT), elevated levels of norepinephrine (NE) or abnormal levels of dopamine (DA); genetic factors may play a role

5. Other possible etiologies vary widely and include hostility toward self, trying to live up to perfectionistic standards, underdeveloped superego rules, inadequate parenting and unsatisfied basic needs, anxiety, social oppression, a changing societal value system, inability to manage family conflict, growing up in a multigenerational enmeshed family system and failure to individuate self, a chaotic and abusive environment, and possibly rigid gender-role stereotyping

B. Cluster A disorders (using DSM-IV-TR diagnostic criteria): characterized by odd or eccentric behavior

1. Paranoid personality disorder: pattern of distrust and suspiciousness such that others' motives are interpreted as malevolent
2. Schizoid personality disorder: pattern of detachment from social relationships and a restricted range of emotions
3. Schizotypal personality disorder: pattern of acute discomfort in close relationships, cognitive or perceptual distortions, and eccentricities of behavior

C. Cluster B disorders (using DSM-IV-TR diagnostic criteria): characterized by dramatic and erratic behavior

1. Antisocial personality disorder: pattern of disregard for and violation of rights of others
2. Borderline personality disorder: pattern of instability in interpersonal relationships, self-image, and affect, and marked impulsivity
3. Histrionic personality disorder: pattern of excessive emotionality and attention seeking
4. **Narcissistic personality disorder:** pattern of grandiosity, need for admiration, and lack of empathy

D. Cluster C disorders (using DSM-IV-TR diagnostic criteria): characterized by anxious and fearful behavior

1. Avoidant personality disorder: pattern of social inhibition, feelings of inadequacy, and hypersensitivity to negative evaluation
2. Dependent personality disorder: pattern of submissive and clinging behavior related to a need to be taken care of
3. Obsessive-compulsive personality disorder: pattern of preoccupation with orderliness, perfectionism, and control

E. Assessment guidelines

1. Since client probably does not perceive that a problem exists or believes that any problem is related to behavior of others, maintain sensitivity during interview process so client does not become guarded or defensive
2. Exercise professional judgment to protect client rights and to maintain confidentiality
3. ! Assess client's level of function in areas of affect, cognition, behavior (including impulse control), and sociocultural adaptation (interpersonal relationships)

F. Basic principles of nursing intervention

1. Recognize and accept that clients change or do not change; if patterns of behavior are egosyntonic, clients may lack motivation required to effect change
2. ! Help clients to see how behavior affects their lives to motivate them to develop a more adaptive lifestyle
3. Remember that personality traits are too ingrained to expect radical, long-term behavioral change; interventions should be based on short-term goals and focus on small steps designed to improve role functioning and decrease distress
4. Maintain hope for each client's improvement; all clients have potential for change
5. ! Identify own emotional responses when caring for clients diagnosed with a personality disorder because power struggles between staff members related to best treatment approach create staff divisiveness and a chaotic rather than structured milieu

G. Specific nursing management strategies: cluster-specific nursing interventions can be individualized for each client

1. ! Cluster A disorders (paranoid personality, schizoid personality, and schizotypal personality)
   a. Approach client in a gentle, interested, but nonintrusive manner

b. Respect client's needs for distance and privacy
c. Be mindful of own nonverbal communication because a client may perceive others as threatening
d. Gradually encourage interaction with others, if appropriate

! 2. Cluster B disorders (antisocial personality, borderline personality, histrionic personality, and narcissistic personality)
a. Be patient when clients display emotional and erratic behavior
b. Provide a consistent and structured milieu to avoid manipulation and power struggles
c. Safety is always first priority of care—protect clients from suicide and self-mutilation until they can protect themselves
d. Set limits as necessary to help clients maintain impulse control to protect themselves and others from injury
e. Engage in frequent staff conferences to prevent client's ability to play one staff member against another
f. Help clients recognize and discuss their fear of abandonment
g. Help clients recognize presence of dichotomous thinking or splitting, in which self and others are perceived as all good or all bad
h. Encourage direct communication to minimize attention seeking through use of dramatic, seductive behavior
i. Help clients who display a sense of entitlement to acknowledge needs of others

! 3. Cluster C disorders (avoidant personality, dependent personality, and obsessive-compulsive personality)
a. Point out avoidance behaviors and related losses and secondary gains
b. Provide problem-solving and assertiveness training to increase self-confidence and independence
c. Encourage expression of feelings to decrease rigidity and need for control
d. Help clients recognize any impairment or distress related to their need for perfection and control
e. Help clients acknowledge and discuss their sense of inadequacy and fear of rejection

H. Psychopharmacology

1. Antipsychotic agents may be prescribed on a short-term basis to alleviate psychotic symptoms associated with schizotypal or borderline personality disorders
2. SSRIs may be prescribed to diminish rapid mood swings and impulsive, aggressive, self-destructive behavior associated with borderline personality disorder
3. SSRIs may be prescribed to treat obsessive rumination associated with certain personality disorders (see Chapter 36)

I. Individual and group therapy

1. A decision for participation in individual or group therapy or both is based on a client's level of function and specific needs
2. Self-help groups may increase clients' self-awareness and assist them in coping with problems in living

J. Behavioral therapy

! 1. Impulse-control training is designed to support client safety by decreasing risk of suicide or self-mutilation through use of antiharm contracts, staff and client (self) monitoring, identifying triggers and patterns related to self-destructive behavior, and identifying alternative coping strategies

! 2. Setting limits discourages tendency to test and manipulate others
a. Involves establishing a structured environment with clear ground rules
b. Setting limits reflects three principles: limits must be clearly stated, necessary, and enforceable

3. Behavioral modification: social skills for clients who are helpless and dependent; goal is to increase coping skills and independent functioning
a. Assist clients to acknowledge feelings of helplessness and fear of becoming more independent
b. Explore clients' dichotomous thinking or tendency to see themselves as totally dependent or totally independent

c. Help clients identify what they would gain and lose by becoming less helpless
d. Engage clients in problem-solving exercises to increase their self-confidence
e. Provide assertiveness training
f. Take care not to be seen as a rescuer

4. Behavioral modification: social skills for clients who are socially isolative related to a fear of rejection; goal is to increase self-confidence
   a. Help clients acknowledge their fear of criticism and rejection
   b. Help clients identify what they would gain and lose by risking criticism and rejection
   c. Help clients identify interpersonal effects of social isolation and feelings associated with it
   d. Engage clients in problem-solving exercises to increase their self-confidence
   e. Provide assertiveness training
5. For clients who are socially isolated related to suspicion and mistrust of others, respect their need to be isolative while gradually encouraging interaction with others; if appropriate, help clients identify interpersonal effects of social isolation and feelings associated with them
6. For clients who seek out relationships with others through behavior that is attention seeking (dramatic, seductive) but superficial, help them to interact in a more direct fashion; help clients identify what they would gain and lose by communicating more directly
7. For clients whose relationships are based on manipulation, focus on their attempts at manipulation and help them to identify ways to interact in a more collaborative and less power-based manner; help clients identify what they would gain and lose by becoming less manipulative

K. Psychological comfort promotion—anxiety reduction

1. Encourage decision making to support a sense of competence and an internal locus of control; point out that an imperfect decision may be better than no decision and that many decisions can be remade
2. Some clients become perfectionistic to guard against anxiety of feeling inferior; explore their fear
3. Anxiety prevents some clients from asking for help because they fear rejection; help clients identify what they would gain and lose by asking for help

L. Evaluation and client outcomes

1. Be aware that realistic goals must reflect small steps to improve function and decrease subjective distress
2. Evaluate effectiveness of nursing interventions in relation to stated outcomes

VI. DISSOCIATIVE DISORDERS

A. Overview

1. Usually consciousness, memory, identity, and perception are integrated functions
2. In dissociative disorders, there is a sudden disruption in client's consciousness, identity, or memory
3. Defense mechanisms of dissociation and repression are used
   a. May experience considerable anxiety caused by expressed or fantasized forbidden wishes, often of sexual or aggressive nature
   b. May have considerable anxiety related to stressors or traumatic events
   c. Person does not consciously "decide" to dissociate
4. Physiological origins of "trance states" or dissociation
   a. Childhood trauma resulting in neurotransmitter and anatomical changes in brain
   b. Genetic predisposition to dissociate is hypothesized
5. Possible etiologies include traumatic experience (commonly accidents, natural disasters, assault) or severe physical, sexual, or emotional abuse; more easily induced if using psychoactive drugs (hallucinogens or cannabis)

B. Specific Disorders

1. **Dissociative amnesia:** a dissociative disorder in which client cannot remember important personal information and memory loss cannot be accounted for by ordinary forgetfulness

a. Client suddenly cannot recall memories: *localized amnesia* is loss of memory of a short time period (hours) after a disturbing event; *selective amnesia* is loss of memory of some, but not all, events; *generalized amnesia* is loss of memory of a whole lifetime of experiences (very rare); *continuous amnesia* is inability to remember successive events as they occur
b. Client with amnesia can recall other information, learn, and function coherently
c. Most common during wars and natural disasters
d. **Primary gain:** symbolic resolution of unconscious conflict that decreases anxiety and keeps conflict from awareness
e. **Secondary gain:** receipt of extra support and caring when experiencing an illness
f. Usually terminates abruptly
g. Special interventions: survivor support groups; gradual reconstruction of events through talking, listening, and reading others' accounts of the trauma

2. **Dissociative fugue:** a dissociative disorder characterized by client's suddenly leaving his or her usual place with no memory of some or all of past
a. Travels from usual environment
b. Unable to recall important aspects of identity and assumes new identity; old and new identities do not alternate; incomplete new identity; does not know information is forgotten
c. Usually lasts from hours to days, rarely months; considerable confusion when client returns to prefugue state
d. Often is a response to psychological stressors (war, family, marital)
e. Once client has returned to prefugue state, he or she has no memory of events during fugue
f. Special interventions: hypnosis, drug-facilitated interviews, support groups

3. **Dissociative identity disorder (DID):** a dissociative disorder characterized by two or more distinct personalities or identities (alters) in an individual person
a. An alter is a personality state or identity that recurrently takes over behavior of a person with DID; alters are personalities with different influences and power over one another; may represent different ages or genders
b. Each alter has relatively enduring pattern of perceiving, relating to, and thinking about self and environment
c. Alters each have different physiological responses and disorders (one alter may be myopic, while another is not)
d. Alters communicate with one another through "executive" alter
e. Some alters share "co-consciousness," aware of each other's experience and behavior; others are aware only of their own existence
f. "Switching" occurs by dissociating from one alter to another
g. **Host personality:** primary identity that holds person's name; is typically unaware of alters (anxiety-provoking aspects of personality), but alters are typically aware of host personality
h. Client "loses time" when alternate personality is present for a period of time: usually client is unable to give full account of childhood (few memories) because of dissociation; may appear forgetful and is often accused of lying
i. Mental status variations: marked variation in appearance from time to time; blinking, eye rolls, headaches, covering or hiding face, and twitches may occur when "switching" from one alter to another; marked variation in speech in brief periods of time; impaired insight, usually unaware of alters; may appear anxious or depressed
j. Associated with severe physical or sexual abuse during childhood and may be accompanied by many posttrauma symptoms (nightmares, flashbacks, hypervigilance), self-mutilation, suicidal or aggressive behavior
! k. Special interventions: institute no-harm contract and environmental safety if client is suicidal or is self-mutilating; meet and recognize alters and their unique experiences and needs; "map" personality system, noting characteristics of alters and co-consciousness; create emotionally safe environment for all alters; individual therapy with therapist skilled in working through trauma leading to integration (moving together of aspects of all identities); develop-

ment of new coping skills; family therapy with partners and children; hypnosis or drug-facilitated interviews (use is controversial because of possibility of remembering "too much, too soon" and being overwhelmed with anxiety)

4. Depersonalization disorder
   a. **Depersonalization:** feeling of detachment or separation from one's self, as if in a dreamlike state
   b. Client describes self as "detached from my body" or "being in a dream"
   c. Feels strange or unreal
   d. Able to function during experience
   e. Client may report distress about experiences and become depressed and anxious; often fears being "crazy"; feelings may be accompanied by **derealization,** a feeling that external world is unreal or strange
   f. Precipitated by stress and anxiety
   g. Most common in teenagers and young adults
   h. Special interventions: problem solving to reduce stress in general; stress-management techniques; "grounding" or focus on external environment

C. Assessment

1. Recounts trauma and/or severe stress
   a. Client acknowledges history of childhood abuse but often does not recall trauma
   b. Symptoms appear in adulthood after stressful event(s)
   c. Symptoms appear immediately or may be delayed for years
2. Extent of dissociation or amnestic symptoms varies widely with different dissociative disorders
   a. **Dissociation** is a defense mechanism in which experiences are blocked from consciousness so that affect, behavior, identity, memories, and/or thoughts are not integrated
   b. **Repression** is a defense mechanism in which thoughts and feelings are kept from consciousness
3. May report symptoms of depression or anxiety
4. Physical symptoms: headaches common with DID, but other dissociative disorders have no associated physical symptoms
5. Mental status examination
   a. Appearance: facial expressions and mannerisms may vary widely within one session or appearance may vary widely from day to day (DID)
   b. Mood: anxious, depressed; some clients have little mood change
   c. Memory: amnesia for events (variable extent)
   d. Perception: feelings of detachment from self or environment, feeling of physical change in body
   e. Insight: impaired, unaware of memory impairment

D. Nursing diagnoses and analysis

1. Disturbed personal identity related to threat to physical integrity, threat to self-concept, and underdeveloped ego
2. Anxiety related to traumatic experience
3. Ineffective individual coping related to childhood trauma, childhood abuse, low self-esteem, and inadequate coping skills
4. Disturbed sensory perception related to severe level of anxiety, repressed and decreased perceptual field
5. Impaired thought processes related to physical integrity and threat to self-concept
6. Powerlessness related to unmet dependency needs and fear of memory loss
7. Risk for self-mutilation related to response to increasing anxiety and inability to verbalize feelings

E. Nursing intervention strategies

1. Create safe, calm environment
   a. Mutually develop plan of care
   b. Prevent stressors that could elicit dissociation
2. Teach stress management and coping techniques
   a. Progressive muscle relaxation
   b. Physical exercise

c. "Grounding," or focus on external environment (what client can see and hear) rather than on internal feelings, thoughts, or sensations that can lead to "spacing out" (a lay term indicating lack of awareness of immediate environment)
d. Problem-solving strategies
e. Distraction
3. Discuss and explore traumatic event
4. Reconstruct memories through client's account and those of others
5. Educate about specific dissociative disorder
a. Relationship between anxiety and dissociation
b. Include family and significant others
6. Help staff and other clients to understand disorder (especially DID)
7. Plan for use of leisure time (anxiety often increases when client is alone without activities)

F. Psychopharmacology
1. Drug-facilitated interviews using thiopental sodium (Pentothal) or sodium amytal to recover memory
2. Antianxiety agents
3. Antidepressants for depression and antipsychotics for extreme agitation (if those symptoms are present)

G. Individual and group therapy
1. Hypnosis therapy to recover memories
2. Focus on emotional responses to trauma or stressors
3. Work through unacceptable impulses or behavior verbally
4. Refer to support groups
a. Parenting or occupational support
b. "Survivor" groups, particularly for natural disasters or abuse

H. Behavior modification
1. Teach cognitive techniques to promote positive self-statements
2. Reinforce stress management and coping strategies rather than dissociation

I. Evaluation and client outcomes
1. Client explains relationship between trauma, stress, anxiety, and dissociation, and can recall stressors and traumatic events with congruency
2. Client employs stress-management and positive coping behaviors, and actively seeks to solve problems
3. Client assumes or resumes social and occupational roles and uses leisure time constructively

VII. SOMATOFORM DISORDERS

A. Overview
1. **Somatoform disorders** are psychophysiological responses with amplified awareness of somatic stimuli caused by impaired CNS inhibitory function
2. Deficient communication between hemispheres of brain may impair ability to express emotions directly
3. Disorder is a defense against anxiety
a. A person expresses conflict and resultant anxiety through physical symptoms because being physically ill is socially acceptable, and client receives help and nurturance and has dependency needs met
b. Conflict does not have to be acknowledged
c. May consciously seek relief from physical symptoms or may unconsciously not want to give up symptoms because they decrease anxiety
4. Family dynamics
a. Family rules may prevent direct expression of conflict
b. Family may view physical illness as an acceptable way to avoid meeting otherwise required developmental tasks and role demands
c. Family may provide secondary gain
d. Symptoms may serve to control others or to stabilize relationships

! 5. Physical symptoms have no *organic basis;* that is, objective diagnostics tests usually do not reveal structural or functional changes

6. Somatoform disorders, in which there is no organic basis for physical symptoms, may or may not begin after a physical illness or injury
7. Culture influences physical expressions
   a. In some cultures, distress may be manifested in bodily symptoms, with psychological distress viewed as unacceptable
   b. Somatization is defined as a disorder primarily in Western societies
   c. Many culture-bound illnesses have little influence on role performance
8. Somatization disorders, characterized by multiple complaints of multiple body systems, are more prevalent in women than in men

B. Specific disorders

1. Somatization disorder
   a. Onset prior to age 30 with symptoms of several years duration
   b. Multiple physical complaints; must include four pain symptoms, two GI symptoms, sexual symptoms, and symptoms suggesting neurological disorders
   c. New symptoms often arise with increased emotional distress
   d. Lifestyle changes are evoked by physical illness, affecting occupational, family, and community relationships and self-care, and resulting in disability and inability to work, thereby leading to financial struggles
   e. Client seeks treatment for physical symptoms, occasionally for psychosocial complaints
   f. Special interventions: long-term medical management; treat physical symptoms conservatively, "matter-of-fact" approach; antidepressants if depressive symptoms present but no drug therapy for anxiety symptoms
2. **Conversion disorder**
   a. A somatoform disorder in which a motor, sensory, or visceral function is lost and about which client is usually indifferent
   b. Symptoms do not have an underlying organic cause
   c. Motor symptoms: mutism, paralysis, tremors
   d. Sensory symptoms: blindness, deafness, numbness
   e. Visceral symptoms: urinary retention, breathing difficulties, headaches
   f. Medically naïve clients have more implausible symptoms, which correspond to client's ideas of the problem but do not follow neurological pathways
   g. Clear, identifiable psychological factors (stress, conflict) are related to onset or exacerbation of symptoms
   h. Client's mood may be inappropriate for symptoms, and he or she may display little concern for symptoms (*la belle indifference*)
   i. Symptoms are often symbolically related to primary gain, such as glove anesthesia that prevents a student about to take comprehensive examination from being able to write or bilateral paralysis of lower extremities of man about to get married, preventing him from "walking down the aisle"
   j. Special interventions: nurse must treat symptom as "real" because client experiences it; use problem-solving approaches for dealing with conflicts and stressors
3. Pain disorder
   a. A somatoform disorder characterized by pain as dominant physical symptom
   b. Client seeks medical attention for severe, prolonged pain with no organic basis for pain
   c. Preoccupation with pain that is not controlled by analgesics
   d. Manifestations vary: low back pain, headache, chronic pelvic pain
   e. Historical relationship between stress, conflict, and initiation or exacerbation of pain; often follows physical trauma or injury; client usually refuses to consider psychological origin; diagnosis difficult because of personal and cultural differences in definition and expression of pain
   f. Commonly accompanied by depression, hopelessness, helplessness, anger, or irritability
   g. Special interventions: teach client about stress-tension-pain cycle; acupuncture, biofeedback training, transcutaneous electrical nerve stimulation (TENS); specific exercise programs, physical therapy; visualization and

relaxation training; pain management techniques (note: analgesics and antianxiety agents may be ineffective for pain, and addiction is possible)

4. Hypochondriasis

a. A disorder in which a physical symptom is interpreted as severe or life threatening, resulting in exaggerated worry
b. Physical symptoms may begin with sensitivity to vague physical sensations or mild physical symptoms that most people would not notice
c. Exaggerated worry and preoccupation with physical symptoms and sensations occur; often seeks information from clinicians or data sources to substantiate concerns
d. History of multiple visits to multiple practitioners, and concern persists despite negative findings and clinician reassurances
e. Accompanied by significant anxiety
f. Special interventions: teach rational interpretation of body sensations; assist resolution of family conflict about medical treatment and client distress; nonpharmacological treatment of anxiety

5. Body dysmorphic disorder

a. A somatoform disorder characterized by preoccupation with a defect in appearance, either an imagined defect or excessive concern over a minor anomaly
b. Causes significant distress or impairment in role function
c. Varies from flaws of face or head (complexion, hair thinning, asymmetry) to abdomen, extremities, or body shape/size
d. Client embarrassed about defects so may express them vaguely ("ugly," for example)
e. May frequently check defects, avoid reminders (removing mirrors), seek reassurances from others, or attempt to improve defect (exercise, surgery, cosmetics)
f. Often leads to social isolation
g. Disorder is persistent; client has repeated surgeries, dental work, or dermatological treatment for defects
h. Emotional distress may be severe enough to lead to depression and suicidal ideation
i. Special interventions: respect preoccupation; avoid challenging validity of client perceptions; focus on coping techniques; contract with client to increase social activities and relationships

C. Assessment

1. Onset is variable, depending upon disorder
2. Client has seen multiple care providers without relief of symptoms
3. Client sees problem as "physical" and denies psychological influences on symptoms
4. Primary gain: illness allows reprieval from responsibilities
5. Secondary gain: sick role allows for dependency needs to be met
6. Over time, client is increasingly socially isolated and physically inactive
7. Family may insist on client seeking assistance due to altered role performance
8. Mental status variations
    a. Depends upon type of disorder
    b. Appearance: ranges from deeply anguished to indifferent; may assume antalgic position
    c. Mood: depressed, anxious, or unaffected, or labile
    d. Thought: usually preoccupied with symptoms
    e. Insight: highly impaired, usually denying any stressors or minimizing reactions to stressful events; not "psychologically minded"
9. Physical symptoms
    a. Evaluate physical symptoms respectfully, thoroughly, and objectively
    b. Common organ system responses; see Table 22–3 ■ for specific symptoms
    c. Thorough health assessment including laboratory studies is necessary to rule out physical illness with organic basis or other mental disorders

Table 22–3

Specific Symptoms of Common Organ System Responses

Organ System	Specific Symptom
Cardiovascular	Fainting Hypertension Migraine headache Tachycardia
Musculoskeletal	Back pain Fatigue Tension headache Tremor
Respiratory	Bronchospasm Dyspnea Hyperventilation
Integumentary	Pruritis
Genitourinary	Difficulties in micturation Menstrual disturbances Sexual dysfunction

D. Nursing diagnoses and analysis

1. Ineffective individual coping related to severe level of anxiety, low self-esteem, regression to earlier level of development, and inadequate coping skills
2. Ineffective family processes related to detachment and inability to express feelings or to struggle for power and control
3. Ineffective denial related to threat to self-concept
4. Impaired social interaction related to fear of leaving neighborhood or home or to physical symptoms and disability
5. Disturbed body image related to low self-esteem and unmet dependency needs
6. Self-care deficit related to paralysis of body part; inability to see, hear, or speak; and pain or discomfort
7. Chronic pain related to severe level of anxiety and secondary gains from sick role

E. Specific nursing intervention strategies

1. ! Establish trusting, therapeutic relationship
   a. Avoid describing physical symptoms as "in client's head"
   b. Note that symptoms are not an attempt to get attention
   c. Recall that client does not create symptoms consciously or purposefully
   d. Accept reality of symptoms as client presents them, avoiding dispute
2. ! Client education
   a. Explain symptoms on a physiological level, using understandable and acceptable language
   b. Present current knowledge of mind–body interaction, emphasizing how stress and anxiety affect physiological functioning
   c. Teach methods to reduce physiological arousal, including relaxation techniques, visual imagery, self-talk strategies, and physical exercise (see Box 22–4)
3. Encourage verbalization of thoughts and feelings, life events, and stressors
4. Assist in problem solving specific conflicts or situations
5. Self-care strategies
   a. Modify exercise/activity plan to fit client's physical status
   b. Promote sleep and rest
   c. Promote healthy nutritional practices
   d. Teach day-to-day client management of symptoms
6. Encourage client to gradually resume expected work, family, and community roles commensurate with physical capabilities

F. Psychopharmacology

1. No specific psychotropic medications for somatoform disorders

Box 22-4

Tips for Teaching Relaxation Training

- Emphasize the relationship between stress and physiological arousal/symptoms.
- Note that relaxation techniques work by focusing attention to relaxation task, thus interrupting the preoccupation with symptoms, and decreasing physiological arousal, which negates physical symptoms of anxiety.
- To promote a sense of control, remind the client that he or she (not the technique) effects the change.
- Promote a daily return to physiological and psychological baseline to calm the mind and body through relaxation techniques, thus keeping general arousal low.
- Note that daily practice rather than episodic use builds skill level.
- Suggest additional techniques for use when client anticipates a stressful situation or finds himself or herself becoming anxious.
- Explain and teach a variety of techniques so that client can choose a technique that is acceptable and can be used in specific client environments.

2. Some evidence for use of antidepressants with pain and somatization disorders
3. Comorbid anxiety or depression treated symptomatically with anxiolytics and antidepressants
4. Medication for physical symptoms
   a. Give medications according to presentation of physical symptoms
   b. Encourage client to express thoughts and feelings experienced at time of discomfort
   c. Educate client regarding medication use, emphasizing provider–client collaboration to reduce self-adjustment of dosages

G. Individual and group treatment

1. Cognitive-behavioral approaches
   a. Identify self-statements and assumptions about stress, anxiety, and sick role
   b. Challenge irrational beliefs and self-statements regarding seriousness of illness, inability to cope, and/or mind–body relationships
   c. Provide accurate data to counter misinformation
   d. Encourage positive, self-coping statements
2. Groups for clients and families
   a. Discussion of mind–body relationships
   b. Forum for discussion and encouragement to talk out problems as a deterrent to physical symptoms
   c. Correct misinformation about origin of somatoform disorders
   d. Support for families and/or clients as roles shift during recovery
3. Supportive approaches
   a. Convey empathy: "This must be very trying for you"
   b. Convey respect: "I am impressed by how you have been able to do as much as you have, given how you feel"
   c. Explore with client ways to decrease isolation, improve role performance, and enhance self-esteem
   d. Focus on verbally expressing feelings and coping techniques rather than symptoms
   e. Keep discussion of symptoms brief and matter-of-fact, but without dismissal
4. Behavior modification
   a. In addition to cognitive behavioral approaches, engage client in self-modification to reward for engagement in treatment plan
   b. Teach family members to reinforce verbalization of stressors and life difficulties rather than symptoms

H. Evaluation and client outcomes

1. Identifies interaction of mind and body and effects of stress
2. Increases ability to verbalize thoughts and feelings, and conflicts and/or problems in situations and relationships
3. Employs self-help strategies: challenges irrational thoughts; corrects own misinformation; uses positive coping statements; engages in physical activity on regu-

lar basis; employs relaxation techniques or visual imagery; demonstrates sound nutritional practices, and resumes appropriate roles

VIII. COGNITIVE IMPAIRMENT DISORDERS

A. Overview

1. **Delirium:** an acute, usually reversible brain disorder characterized by clouding of consciousness (decreased awareness of environment) and a reduced ability to focus and maintain attention
   - ! **a.** Develops over a short period of time (usually hours to days) and tends to fluctuate during course of day
   - **b.** Evidence from history, physical examination, or laboratory findings suggests that disturbance is caused by direct physiological consequences of a general medical condition
   - **c.** Can be described as caused by general medical condition, substance intoxication, substance withdrawal, or multiple etiologies
2. **Dementia:** a chronic, irreversible brain disorder characterized by impairments in memory, abstract thinking, and judgment, as well as changes in personality
   - ! **a.** Chronic development of multiple cognitive deficits manifested by memory impairment and cognitive disturbances
   - **b.** **Aphasia,** inability to understand or use language
   - **c.** **Apraxia,** inability to carry out skilled and purposeful movement; inability to use objects properly
   - **d.** **Agnosia,** inability to recognize familiar situations, people, or stimuli; not related to impairment in sensory organs
   - **e.** Disturbance in executive functioning (i.e., planning, organizing, sequencing, abstracting)
   - ! **f.** Course is insidious and progressive, characterized by gradual onset and continuing cognitive decline
   - **g.** Cognitive deficits cause significant impairment in social or occupational functioning and represent a significant decline from previous level of functioning
   - **h.** Can be classified as Alzheimer's type (DAT), vascular dementia (formerly multi-infarct dementia), dementia due to other general medical conditions, substance-induced persisting dementia, or multiple etiologies
3. Amnestic disorders
   - **a.** Development of memory impairment characterized by inability to learn new information or inability to recall previously learned information
   - **b.** Can be transient (lasting for 1 month or less) or chronic (lasting for more than 1 month); can result from a general medical condition, substance abuse, or other cause
   - **c.** Cause significant impairment in social or occupational functioning and represent a significant decline from a previous level of functioning
4. Other cognitive disorders: mild neurocognitive disorder or postconcussional disorder

B. Etiologies

1. Regardless of specific cause, delirium, dementia, and other cognitive disorders result from an interference with cerebral blood flow and delivery of nutrients (e.g., oxygen, glucose, vitamins)
2. Associated medical conditions leading to reduced cerebral blood flow include cardiovascular and respiratory conditions, vitamin deficiencies, infections, endocrine and metabolic disorders, hepatic and renal failure, and trauma or tumors
3. Substances causing toxicity to the brain either by exposure to, high doses of, or withdrawal from substance can lead to cognitive disorders; these include a variety of prescribed medications as well as illegal drugs
4. Genetic or viral diseases can cause pathological changes or biochemical imbalances in the brain that interfere with cerebral blood flow (dementia of Alzheimer's type, Parkinson's disease, Huntington's disease, Pick's disease, Creutzfeldt-Jakob disease)

C. Assessment

1. Delirium has a sudden onset and an identifiable cause
   a. A thorough medical evaluation reveals abnormal lab results
   b. An electroencephalogram (EEG) confirms cerebral dysfunction
   c. More than one examination at different times of day detects fluctuations in level of consciousness
   d. Identify underlying cause of delirium and rule out other reasons for delirium (depression, anxiety, dementia, or personality disorder)
2. Presenting signs and symptoms of delirium
   a. Cyclic alternating periods of coherence with periods of confusion, specifically with disorientation that worsens at end of day, usually referred to as **sundown syndrome**
   b. Alternating patterns of hyperactivity (typical of drug withdrawal) to hypoactivity (typical of metabolic imbalance)
   c. Hyperactive behaviors: rambling, bizarre, incoherent, rapid, pressured, or loud speech; restlessness, picking at clothes or bed linen, irritability, euphoria; calling out for help, striking out at others, bizarre and destructive behavior, combativeness, anger, profanity
   d. Hypoactive behaviors: limited, dull patterns of speech; lethargy, apathy, withdrawn behavior; reduced alertness or awareness of environment
   e. Cognitive changes: disorganized thinking; diminished ability to focus attention, easily distracted; disorientation to time and place; impairment in recent and remote memory; visual or auditory hallucinations, frightening delusions
   f. Sleep pattern disturbances, including vivid and terrifying dreams or nightmares
   g. Predominant emotion is fear with a high level of anxiety
3. Dementia is a progressive disease and symptoms can be divided into four stages (Box 22–5)

D. Screening tools

1. Folstein Mini-Mental State Examination: an organic screening tool useful for differentiating dementia from functional states
   a. Total score of 30 points
   b. Score of 9–12 indicates a high likelihood of organic illness
2. Cognitive Performance Scale: a subscale from nursing home Minimum Data Set (MDS)
   a. Ranges from 0 (cognitively intact) to 6 (very severe cognitive impairment)
   b. Items assessed on MDS include comatose status, short-term memory, decision-making ability, making self understood, eating self-performance
3. Geriatric Depression Screening Scale (GDSS)
   a. Useful screening tool specifically developed for older adults to screen for possible depression (which can mimic dementia)
   b. A 15- or 30-item questionnaire with dichotomous yes or no answers; easy to administer in approximately 15 to 20 minutes; certain items are reverse-scored for more accurate assessment
   c. Results indicate absence of or mild depression (0 to 10), moderate depression (11 to 20), or severe depression (21 to 30) using the 30-item questionnaire

E. Differentiating between delirium and dementia

1. Delirium may coexist with dementia, making accurate assessment and appropriate treatment difficult; see Table 22–4 ■ for comparisons between delirium and dementia
2. Most prevalent primary dementia is Alzheimer's type, (occurs in 50% of older adults); vascular dementia resulting from narrowing of arteries affects 20% to 50% of older adults; less common forms of dementia stem from degenerative nervous system disorders (e.g., Parkinson's disease) and other pathological processes (e.g., AIDS dementia complex)

F. *Pseudodementia:* reversible disorder that frequently mimics dementia

1. Depression, (most common pseudodementia) is frequently misdiagnosed or overlooked in older adult; see Table 22–5 ■ for comparisons between dementia and depression

Box 22–5

Stages of Alzheimer's Disease

Stage 1

- Alzheimer's disease can be summarized as forgetfulness and loss of higher executive functions.
- Losses in short-term memory result in client losing things.
- Client compensates by using memory aids such as developing routines and using lists.
- Client is aware of problem and is concerned; he or she may be frightened by the confusion.
- Client may become depresssed, which worsens symptoms.

Stage 2

- Hallmark of Alzheimer's disease is confusion.
- Progressive short-term memory loss interferes with all abilities.
- Client experiences gaps in memory, which leads to confabulation (filling in memory gaps with imaginary information) in an attempt to hide the deficit.
- Client loses ability to carry out instrumental ADLs such as cooking, housekeeping, transportation, legal affairs, and money management.
- Client withdraws from social situations.
- Client exhibits declining personal appearance and may dress inappropriately for weather.
- Client exhibits lack of spontaneity in verbal and nonverbal communication.
- Client exhibits poor impulse control with frequent outbursts and tantrums, labile emotions, catastrophic reactions, or overreactions to minor stresses occur.

Stage 3

- Client loses ability to carry out ADLs in a typical order: bathing, grooming, choosing clothes, dressing, toileting.
- Client may exhibit wandering or aggressive behavior, hallucinations, delusions.
- Client may develop aphasia, which begins with the inability to find words and eventually limits the person to as few as six words.

Stage 4

- Hyperorality, the need to taste, chew, and examine any object small enough to be placed in the mouth.
- Perseveration phenomena, repetitive behaviors such as lip licking, finger tapping, pacing, or echolalia.
- Agraphia, the inability to read or write.
- Agnosia, the inability to recognize familiar situations, people, or stimuli
  1. Auditory agnosia is an inability to recognize familiar sounds such as a ringing doorbell or telephone.
  2. Astereognosia, or tactile agnosia, is an inability to identify familiar objects, such as a comb or pencil, when placed in the hand.
  3. Alexia, or visual agnosia, is an inability to identify a common object such as a toothbrush or telephone or its use by sight
- Hyperetamorphosis, the need to compulsively touch and examine every object in the environment
- Progressive motor deterioration, including inability to walk, sit up, or even smile
- Progressive decrease in response to environmental stimuli leading to total nonresponsiveness or vegetative state
- Severe decline in cognitive function, losing ability to recognize others or even self
- May scream spontaneously or be able to say only one word; frequently becomes mute

Table 22-4

Comparisons Between Delirium and Dementia

Delirium	Dementia
Onset is usually sudden; acute development	Onset is insidious and progressive; chronic development
Caused by temporary, reversible disturbance in brain function	Caused by irreversible alteration of brain function
Duration: hours to days	Duration: months to years
EEG: diffuse slowing of fast cycles related to state of excitement	EEG: normal or mildly slow
Disturbed attention, learning, and thinking, poor perception	Disorientation, impairments in judgment, abstract thinking, and learning
Impaired memory, both recent and remote	Impaired memory (recent memory affected before remote memory)
Orientation: fluctuates throughout day; periods of lucidity; sundown syndrome (worsens at night)	Progressively loses orientation to person, place, and time—loses time orientation first, then place, then person; sundown syndrome
Hallucinations, delusions, illusions	Change in personality; normal peculiarities are exaggerated: suspicious—paranoid, compulsive—rigid, orderliness
Labile affect	Labile affect; prone to apathy, depression, withdrawal, stubbornness in attempt to cope with surroundings and decreased abilities

2. Drug toxicity
3. Metabolic disorders
4. Infections
5. Nutritional deficiencies
6. Chronic lung disease and heart disease

G. ***Pseudodelirium:*** symptoms of delirium without any identifiable organic cause
   1. Symptoms may occur from psychosocial stress, sensory deprivation, or sensory overload (e.g., ICU psychosis)

Table 22-5

Comparisons Between Dementia and Depression

Dementia	Depression
Onset slow and progressive, difficult to pinpoint onset	Onset relatively rapid, can be traced to distressing event or situation
Recent memory is impaired; attempts to hide cognitive losses with confabulation	Readily admits to memory loss; other cognitive impairments may or may not be present; can recall recent events
Affect is shallow and labile	Depressed mood is pervasive
Attention and concentration may be impaired	Attention and concentration usually intact
Unable to recognize familiar people and places, may get lost easily, disoriented to time	Oriented to person, place, and time
Approximate "near miss" answers are common; tries to answer	"Don't know" answers are common; refuses to participate in activities and prefers to be left alone
Changes in personality (from cheerful and easy-going to angry to suspicious)	Personality remains stable
Struggles to perform ADLs; is frustrated as a result	Apathetic to performing ADLs, loses interest in appearance
Appetite and sleep patterns may not be affected	Changes in appetite, weight, and sleep pattern

2. A preexisting biochemical imbalance such as mood disorder, anxiety, schizophrenia, or dementia can make persons vulnerable to pseudodelirium

H. Nursing diagnoses and analysis

1. Priority nursing diagnoses for delirium
   - **a.** Acute confusion related to alcohol or drug abuse, medication ingestion, fluid and electrolyte imbalances, infection
   - **b.** Anxiety related to fear of cognitive and behavioral deficits
   - **c.** Impaired thought processes related to distractibility, decreasing judgment, memory loss, confabulation, delusions, hallucinations, illusions
   - **d.** Self-care deficit (bathing, hygiene, dressing, grooming, feeding), related to inability to sequence skills necessary to perform these tasks
   - **e.** Impaired verbal communication related to aphasia, agraphia, agnosia
   - **f.** Risk for injury or trauma related to aggressive behavior, labile emotions, impaired judgment, illusions, delusions, or hallucinations
   - **g.** Disturbed sleep pattern related to fear, anxiety, sundowning, agitation
2. Priority nursing diagnoses for dementia; all previously identified nursing diagnoses for persons with delirium, plus the following:
   - **a.** Ineffective family coping related to changing roles, physical exhaustion, financial problems
   - **b.** Risk for and/or caregiver role strain related to lack of respite resources or support from significant others, unpredictable illness course, insufficient finances, aggressive behavior or emotional outbursts of care receiver
   - **c.** Impaired sensory perception (visual, auditory, or tactile) related to biochemical imbalances for sensory distortion, agnosia, astereognosia, alexia
   - **d.** Disturbed self-esteem related to loss of independent functioning, loss of capacity for remembering, loss of capability for effective verbal communication
   - **e.** Risk for violence: self-directed or directed at others related to confusion, agitated state, suicidal ideation, delusions, hallucinations, illusions

I. Specific treatment modalities

! 1. Psychopharmacology
   - **a.** Cholinesterase inhibitors such as tacrine (Cognex) or donepezil (Aricept) can slow down progression of mild to moderate dementia
   - **b.** NMDA receptor antagonist memantine (Nemanda) antagonizes CNS receptors that may contribute to Alzheimer's disease
   - **c.** Antianxiety agents: lorazepam (Ativan), trazodone (Desyrel), buspirone (Buspar)
   - **d.** SSRIs, which are better tolerated in older adults than are TCAs; common SSRIs include fluoxetine (Prozac), paroxetine (Paxil), sertraline (Zoloft), and nefazodone (Serzone)
   - **e.** Atypical antipsychotic agents such as olanzapine (Zyprexa), quetiapine (Seroquel), and risperidone (Risperdal); use of haloperidol (Haldol), a potent neuroleptic, is controversial and has been known to cause tardive dyskinesia in older adults; small doses (0.5 mg) may help to regulate sleep

! 2. Behavior modification
   - **a.** Use physical restraints carefully and as a last resort; use sensor devices for client safety that alert staff when a client is out of bed or going outside
   - **b.** Use reality orientation (large-print calendars and clocks); discuss client's significant life events, family, work, or hobbies; avoid arguing about actual reality; communicate in a calm, quiet voice with simple, clear instructions

3. Group and individual therapies
   - **a.** "Review of life" therapy: discuss specific life transitions such as childhood, adolescence, marriage, childbearing, grandparenthood, and retirement; pets, music, and special foods can be used to evoke memories from client's past; share positive and negative feelings
   - **b.** Validation therapy: interacting with clients on a topic they initiate, in a place and time where they feel most secure; reflecting underlying feelings of concern (e.g., "You miss your husband. You must be feeling lonely here"); reality orientation is geared to person and place rather than to time

Box 22–6

Nursing Interventions for Clients with Cognitive Impairment

The following interventions should be incorporated into the care of confused clients:

- Provide simple, clear instructions focusing on one task at a time.
- Break tasks into very small steps.
- Speak slowly and in a face-to-face position when communicating with clients known to have a hearing loss. Shouting causes distortion of high-pitched sounds and can frighten the client.
- Allow the client to have familiar objects around him or her to maintain reality orientation and enhance self-worth and dignity.
- Discuss topics that are meaningful to the client, such as significant life events, family, work, hobbies, and pets.
- Refrain from arguing or convincing client that delusions are not real.
- Provide a simple, structured environment with consistent personnel to minimize confusion and provide a sense of security and stability in the client's environment.
- Encourage reminiscence and discussion of life review by sharing picture albums.
- Discuss family traditions and holidays, memories of school, courtship, dating rituals, favorite pets, and other past events.
- Encourage family/caregivers to express feelings, particularly frustration and anger.
- Provide a list of community resources and support groups available to assist in decreasing stress and role strain for the family/caregiver.

4. Milieu therapy (see Box 22–6)
   a. Special care units (SCU): environmentally designed and specifically programmed to serve needs of residents with Alzheimer's disease and related dementias
   b. ! Design components of SCU: safe, secure, specially adapted physical environment to accommodate wandering behavior inside and outside (circular design, secure walkway and patio); personalized rooms with own furniture and familiar belongings; clean, well-maintained, well-lit environment with windows; stimuli from birdcage, fish aquarium, or other pets; location adjacent to child daycare programs so that multigenerational interaction occurs
   c. Structured programs and activities that provide quality interaction between staff, residents, and families
   d. Caring staff: special training programs leading to certification for all levels of education (RN, LPN, CNA); consistent staffing pattern with stable personnel assignments

J. Evaluation and client outcomes

1. Client remains free of injury as evidenced by absence of falls, fractures, bruises, contusions, or burns
2. Client participates in self-care at optimal level with appropriate supervision and guidance
3. Client communicates basic needs using visual and verbal clues as necessary, and has minimal level in response to frustrating situations
4. Caregivers demonstrate adaptive coping strategies for dealing with stress of caregiver role
5. Client sleeps 5 to 7 hours per night and naps 1 to 2 hours per day, and maintains stable vital signs and weight

IX. EATING DISORDERS

A. Overview of eating disorders

1. Eating disorders are manifested by gross disturbance in a client's eating patterns
2. People with anorexia lose weight by dramatically decreasing food intake and sharply increasing amount of physical exercise
3. People with bulimia nervosa remain at near-normal weight and develop a cycle of minimal food intake, followed by binge-eating, and then purging

4. The two disorders have many features in common, and a person can alternate from one disorder to the other

B. Anorexia nervosa

1. Overview
   a. Life-threatening health problem because of fluid and electrolyte imbalance or starvation
   b. Client is preoccupied with food intake, fears obesity, and has a disturbed body image and self-concept
   c. Client eats minimal amounts of food, often in a rigid and regimented manner, such as eating only 3 bites of carrots or 2 mouthfuls of cereal; denies hunger
   d. Onset is often in teens and frequently associated with a major stressful life event
   e. Client is often an overachiever, seeks perfection, and experiences feelings of lack of control
2. Physical assessment findings
   a. Weight loss
   b. Electrolyte imbalances
   c. Vital signs: decreased body temperature, pulse, and blood pressure; cyanosis of extremities
   d. Gastrointestinal (GI): constipation, tooth and gum degeneration
   e. Skin: dry, scaly
   f. Neuromuscular/skeletal: numbness of extremities, bone deterioration
   g. Amenorrhea for at least 3 cycles
   h. Reports of sleep disturbances

C. Bulimia nervosa

1. Overview
   a. Preoccupation with food intake and body size, appearance
   b. Associated with low self-esteem and poor relationships with others
   c. Client engages in cycles of eating large amounts of low-nutrient food (binges), which may be done in secret, followed by purging through vomiting, laxatives, enemas, diuretics, or amphetamines
   d. Client experiences conflict between perceived loss of control and need to be in control, as well as guilt from binge–purge cycles; may exhibit mood swings
   e. Client is at risk for self-mutilating behavior and may have suicidal ideation or suicide attempts
2. Physical assessment findings
   a. Weight is often normal or near-normal
   b. Electrolyte imbalances
   c. Cardiovascular: cardiac disease, hypertension
   d. GI: tooth decay with loss of enamel (from vomiting), stomach ulcers, rectal bleeding, esophageal varices (vomiting), and possible rectal bleeding

D. Nursing diagnoses and analysis

1. Imbalanced nutrition: less than body requirements
2. Risk for deficient fluid volume
3. Risk for injury
4. Disturbed body image

E. Specific nursing intervention strategies

1. Clients with anorexia nervosa are typically treated in an eating disorders unit
2. Develop therapeutic, nonjudgmental relationship with client to foster sharing of precipitating factors to eating disorder and feelings about it
3. Support client during behavior modification, psychotherapy, support groups; encourage client to take any prescribed medications, such as antidepressants
4. Perform baseline and periodic assessments of nutritional status, including fluid and electrolyte balance and daily intake of food
5. For clients with severe malnutrition, refeeding protocols and tube feedings may be utilized
6. Form a contract with client regarding daily intake of food
7. Set a time limit for meals

8. Provide a pleasant environment for meals and observe client at meal times and following meals
9. Provide positive feedback for appropriate eating behaviors and goal attainment; token economy rewards system may be used
10. Record intake and output and daily weight (postvoid, same clothing, same time, same scale)
11. Monitor elimination patterns
12. Monitor and limit activity level (anorexia and bulimia)
13. Assess risk of suicide and implement suicide precautions as necessary

F. Evaluation and client outcomes

1. Client has normal or near normal nutritional status, gaining weight at rate of 1 to 2 pounds per week (anorexia nervosa), using newly learned eating behaviors regularly
2. Client is free of fluid and electrolyte imbalance and other complications of eating disorder
3. Client identifies and utilizes available support programs or services

Check Your NCLEX-RN® Exam I.Q.

You are ready for testing on this content if you can

- Assess for alteration in mood, judgment, and cognition in clients with a mental health problem.
- Assess for signs and symptoms of specific mental health problems.
- Assess the client's and family's reaction to diagnosis of an acute or chronic mental health problem.
- Help a client to adhere to the treatment plan for a mental health problem.
- Assess for change in a client's mental status and impaired cognition.
- Plan care for the client with an acute or chronic mental health problem.
- Provide client and family education about an acute or chronic mental health problem.
- Provide appropriate nursing care to a client undergoing electroconvulsive therapy.

PRACTICE TEST

1 A nurse has been told that a client's anxiety is at the panic level. The nurse would assess the client for which of the following?

1. Dizziness, palpitations, and nausea
2. Feelings of "butterflies" in the stomach
3. Feelings of fatigue and inability to remain awake
4. Obsessive thoughts and compulsive behavior

2 The nurse concludes that a client has agoraphobia after the client states a fear of which of the following?

1. Spiders
2. Being embarrassed in public
3. Leaving the home
4. Losing control

3 A nurse asks a client, "Have you ever felt a sudden, intense fear for no apparent reason?" When the client responds yes, the nurse would assess the client for other symptoms compatible with which of the following?

1. Agoraphobia
2. Obsessive-compulsive disorder
3. Panic disorder
4. Posttraumatic stress disorder

4 A client has just been told that another operation needs to be performed to correct a physical health problem. The client begins to cry and says, "I just can't take it anymore. Everything has gone wrong. I can't even think straight anymore." The nurse interprets that the client is in which stage of anxiety?

1. Alarm
2. Exhaustion
3. Fight-or-flight
4. Resistance

5 A nurse working with an extremely anxious client reports feeling short of breath, tense, restless, apprehensive, and nervous. The nurse would most appropriately draw which conclusion?

1. The client's anxious feelings have been transmitted to the nurse.
2. The client is probably becoming angry.
3. The client should be reassigned to a different nurse.
4. The nurse probably has a self-esteem disorder.

6 A client is going to begin electroconvulsive therapy (ECT). The nurse knows that ECT is usually prescribed for individuals who have major depression. The nurse prepares a teaching plan keeping in mind that clients with major depression

1. need to be treated with respect and dignity.
2. need to be brought to the treatment suite on a stretcher.
3. should have the procedure explained to them many times because they cannot understand or retain the information.
4. should not receive ECT.

7 The visiting nurse is at the home of a 52-year-old postoperative client. During his presurgical physical assessment, the client was diagnosed with type 2 diabetes mellitus. At that time, he also related that he was not sleeping well and had a decreased appetite. He reported that he lost his job of 34 years 3 weeks before the preoperative physical exam and was very angry. The nurse then asks the client additional questions to elicit data about possible

1. hypomania.
2. unipolar depression.
3. cyclothymia.
4. dysthymia.

8 Which would be the *safest* living environment for a client who inflicted harm on a family member earlier in the day?

1. In a local respite home
2. With a family member in another state
3. In an open-door seclusion room
4. In a closed-door seclusion room

9 Part of a discharge plan for a client on a psychiatric inpatient unit includes walking for half an hour 3 days per week to maintain cardiovascular health and decrease stress levels. The nurse includes this in the care plan as what type of nursing intervention?

1. Active
2. Performance
3. Preventive
4. Physical

10 A client has a diagnosis of bipolar disorder. The nurse is evaluating the client in a home environment after discharge from an inpatient unit 2 weeks ago. The nurse assesses the client for which of the following expected behaviors?

1. Euphoric and talkative presentation with nurse
2. Gregarious interactions with significant others
3. Quiet and evasive presentation
4. Calm, focused exchange of self-care information with nurse

11 A 21-year-old male college student has become increasingly suspicious of his professor and fellow classmates. He has accused the professor of conspiring with two other classmates to get him expelled from school. The client is admitted to a psychiatric unit after telephoning and threatening to kill the professor and his classmates. The client tells the nurse, "They are all out to get me expelled. I think they are even trying to kill me. I have to stop them." What would be the *most* appropriate response by the nurse?

1. "What makes you think they are out to get you expelled or to kill you?"
2. "I find it hard to believe that your professor and classmates are out to get you expelled or to kill you."
3. "It's not right to kill others even if they are out to get you expelled or want to kill you."
4. "Your professor and classmates are not out to get you expelled or to kill you. Let's look at the facts."

12 A client with schizophrenia is exhibiting delusions, hallucinations, minimal self-care, and hyperactive behavior. Which of the following would the nurse document as a negative symptom of schizophrenia?

1. Minimal self-care
2. Delusions
3. Hallucinations
4. Inappropriate affect

13 A client hears voices telling him that he is a terrible person who would be better off dead. Which of the following would be a *priority* nursing diagnosis?

1. Impaired verbal communication
2. Risk for violence, self-directed
3. Impaired sensory-perception
4. Impaired social interaction

PRACTICE TEST

14. A client living in an assisted living facility is taking conventional antipsychotic medications. One evening the nurse notices that the client is experiencing muscle rigidity, confusion, delirium, and has a temperature of 104°F. The nurse interprets these as symptoms of

1. dystonia.
2. akathisia.
3. neuroleptic malignant syndrome.
4. tardive dyskinesia.

15. A client states that he is able to receive radio waves from aliens because they placed a computer chip in his brain. The nurse would document this behavior as which of the following in the medical record?

1. A hallucination
2. Reality-oriented
3. An illusion
4. A delusion

16. The most appropriate outcome of care for a male client who has experienced a dissociative fugue is that the client will do which of the following?

1. Remember what occurred during his fugue state
2. Gain additional coping skills to deal with his current problems
3. Report no feelings of being detached from his body
4. State three positive aspects about himself

17. A client with dissociate identity disorder (DID) who has just been admitted with several fresh burns on her ankles and wrists is refusing to attend group therapy. What is the *priority* nursing diagnosis?

1. Self-care deficit
2. Impaired sensory perception
3. Risk for self-mutilation
4. Noncompliance

18. A client reports depersonalization experiences that have been frightening to him. Which of the following is the *most* therapeutic response by the nurse?

1. "It must be very scary for you. Tell me more about how they occur."
2. "Don't worry, you will always come back together."
3. "Being in the hospital must be very frightening."
4. "Let's focus on the stresses in your life."

19. Which of the following behaviors would indicate that care for a client who dissociates has been effective?

1. Client reports dissociative episodes to the nurse
2. Client seeks out social relationships
3. Client demonstrates three stress management techniques
4. Client is free from injury

20. A client with amnesia is hospitalized. What might the nurse expect to find during the *initial* assessment?

1. Confabulation of historical information
2. Gradual loss of memory over months
3. Disheveled appearance
4. History of severe stress

21. The nurse would look for which of the following characteristics in the behavior of a client diagnosed with obsessive-compulsive disorder (OCD)?

1. Dramatic/erratic
2. Odd/eccentric
3. Anxious/fearful
4. Rigid/critical

22. The nurse places highest priority on which of the following nursing interventions when caring for a client diagnosed with antisocial personality disorder?

1. Supporting the development of insight
2. Encouraging socialization
3. Maintaining consistent limits
4. Monitoring for suicidal ideation

23. The nurse looks for which of the following characteristics in a client diagnosed with a personality disorder?

1. Flexibility and adaptability to stress
2. A tendency to evoke some form of interpersonal conflict
3. A concomitant physical disorder
4. A desire for interpersonal relationships

24 Which of the following beliefs by the nurse as a member of the interdisciplinary team is most important to remember when developing a care plan for a client diagnosed with antisocial personality disorder?

1. Everyone involved in the client's care must agree with the diagnosis, goals, and plan.
2. The team leader must determine the diagnosis and treatment plan to insure accuracy.
3. The involvement of all team members in developing a nursing care plan is not necessary.
4. An unstructured rather than a structured treatment approach is usually beneficial.

25 The nurse is assessing a client with obsessive-compulsive personality disorder. Most of the client's cognitive content will be centered around which of the following?

1. The importance of rules and regulations
2. Global approaches to problem solving
3. Relationships with others
4. Preferred leisure activities

26 A client continues to have pain despite negative neurological findings. The nurse concludes that such pain is likely to continue because of which of the following?

1. Secondary gain
2. High endorphin levels
3. Structural changes of tissue
4. Derealization

27 A client has been eagerly preparing for his marriage. On the morning of the wedding, he is unable to move his legs. What would the nurse expect to find in the mental status examination?

1. Mood: depressed
2. Mood: anxious
3. Mood: blunted
4. Mood: la belle indifference

28 A female client with hypochondriasis discloses that she may decide to leave the psychiatric facility without completing her course of treatment and seek exploratory surgery. The nurse's *best* response is which of the following?

1. "If you decide to leave now, you will be committed against your will."
2. "You should not go until your doctor releases you. She knows what you need."
3. "Tell me more about your decision."
4. "Your surgery will just prove useless. Please stay."

29 A client who has had many different physical illnesses in the past few years is no longer employed, rarely does housework or shopping, and states that she "just can't seem to do anything." Which of the following is a *priority* nursing diagnosis?

1. Impaired home maintenance management
2. Fatigue
3. Powerlessness
4. Body image disturbance

30 The nurse evaluates that the plan of care for a client who suddenly lost her hearing (diagnosed as a conversion disorder) was effective if the client

1. resumed normal hearing.
2. began learning sign language.
3. was fitted for a hearing aid.
4. agreed to have a stapedectomy.

31 Which of the following approaches would be best for the nurse who is communicating with the cognitively impaired client?

1. Loud and precise
2. Simple and direct
3. As nonverbal as possible
4. Sign language

32 Which of the following evaluation criteria should the nurse give *first* priority to when planning the care of a client with dementia?

1. Preventing further deterioration
2. Finding suitable nursing home placement
3. Supporting family caregivers
4. Preventing injury

33 A client with suspected Alzheimer's disease is undergoing diagnostic workup. When the family asks the nurse the reasons for the "tests," the nurse responds that the diagnosis of Alzheimer's disease is usually based on which of the following?

1. Abnormal laboratory findings
2. A definitive CT scan
3. Physiological findings
4. Ruling out other causes for symptoms

34 The nurse writing a care plan for a client with dementia would include that the overall goal for nursing care is which of the following?

1. Reorient the client to reality.
2. Keep the loss of capacity for self-care to a minimum.
3. Assist the client with tasks of daily living.
4. Maintain adequate hydration and nutrition.

35 Which of the following nursing interventions would support optimal memory function for a client with dementia?

1. Develop stimulating and meaningful therapeutic activities.
2. Remind the client of forgotten events.
3. Orient the client to reality.
4. Restrain the client when agitated.

36 The nurse would conclude that a client with schizophrenia is exhibiting positive symptoms of the disorder after noting that the client does which of the following? Select all that apply.

1. Exhibits lack of energy
2. States he is a king
3. Repeats words the nurse says
4. Has a flat affect
5. Withdraws from other people

ANSWERS & RATIONALES

1 **Answer: 1** Subjective complaints of panic level of anxiety include choking or smothering sensation, dizziness, chest pain or pressure, and fear of loss of control and death. Feelings of "butterflies" in the stomach are seen in the fight-or-flight response. Feelings of fatigue and inability to remain awake may be seen in the exhaustion stage of the general adaptation syndrome. Obsessive thoughts and compulsive behaviors are common in obsessive-compulsive disorder.
Cognitive Level: Application **Client Need:** Psychosocial Integrity **Integrated Process:** Nursing Process: Assessment **Content Area:** Psychiatric–Mental Health **Strategy:** The core issue of the question is an ability to identify signs of panic in a client with anxiety. Use nursing knowledge and the process of elimination to make a selection.

2 **Answer: 3** Agoraphobia involves fear of being away from home and being alone in public places. Specific phobia involves unrealistic fear of a particular object or situation. Social phobia is excessive fear of embarrassment and humiliation in public settings. Fear of loss of control is common in most phobias.
Cognitive Level: Application **Client Need:** Psychosocial Integrity **Integrated Process:** Nursing Process: Assessment **Content Area:** Psychiatric–Mental Health **Strategy:** The core issue of the question is an ability to identify signs of agoraphobia in a client. Use nursing knowledge and the process of elimination to make a selection.

3 **Answer: 3** The onset of a panic attack is sudden, and the client may not be aware of the source of the anxiety. Agoraphobia is fear of being incapacitated by being trapped in an unbearable situation from which there is no escape. Obsessive-compulsive disorder is characterized by obsessive thoughts and compulsive behaviors. Posttraumatic stress disorder is associated with exposure to an extremely traumatic, menacing event.
Cognitive Level: Application **Client Need:** Psychosocial Integrity **Integrated Process:** Nursing Process: Assessment **Content Area:** Psychiatric–Mental Health **Strategy:** The core issue of the question is an ability to identify signs of panic disorder. Use nursing knowledge and the process of elimination to make a selection.

4 **Answer: 2** Because coping resources are depleted, the client can no longer deal with stressors. Stage of alarm is characterized by the fight-or-flight response, and increased alertness is focused on the immediate task or threat. Stage of resistance occurs when the body mobilizes resources to combat stress.
Cognitive Level: Application **Client Need:** Psychosocial Integrity **Integrated Process:** Nursing Process: Assessment **Content Area:** Psychiatric–Mental Health **Strategy:** The core issue of the question is an ability to differentiate stages of anxiety based on client presentation. Use nursing knowledge and the process of elimination to make a selection.

5 **Answer: 1** Anxiety in a client may be empathetically experienced by the nurse. It is imperative that the nurse recognize these symptoms. There is not enough data to support the client being angry. Even a nurse with high self-esteem is receptive to experiencing anxiety empathetically.
Cognitive Level: Analysis **Client Need:** Psychosocial Integrity **Integrated Process:** Nursing Process: Assessment **Content Area:** Psychiatric–Mental Health **Strategy:** The core issue of the question is the ability to determine the effect that an anxious client can have on the nurse. Use nursing knowledge and the process of elimination to make a selection.

6 **Answer: 1** The client always needs to be treated with dignity and respect. There is no reason to bring the client to the treatment suite on a stretcher (option 2), nor does the client usually need to have a procedure explained many times by the physician or the nurse (option 3). The client with major depression *can* receive ECT (option 4) if medication therapy is not effective.
Cognitive Level: Comprehension **Client Need:** Psychosocial Integrity **Integrated Process:** Nursing Process: Analysis **Content Area:** Psychiatric–Mental Health **Strategy:** The core issue of the question is the right of every client to be treated in a respectful manner. Use nursing knowledge and the process of elimination to make a selection.

7 **Answer: 2** The only possible correct answer is option 2. Hypomania is a mood of elation (option 1), while cyclothymia (option 3) is a disorder of at least 2 years' duration with episodes of hypomania, and dysthymia (option 4) is a depressive disorder of at least 2 years' duration.
Cognitive Level: Analysis **Client Need:** Psychosocial Integrity **Integrated Process:** Nursing Process: Analysis **Content Area:** Psychiatric–Mental Health **Strategy:** The core issue of the question is an ability to identify clients at risk for various forms of depression. Use nursing knowledge and the process of elimination to make a selection.

8 **Answer: 4** The client would be safest in a closed-door seclusion room (option 4) or in a locked unit (not an option here). The client would not have the continuous monitored care if he were in a respite home (option 1). He would have less safety or care in the home of a relative in another state (option 2). In an open-door seclusion room (option 3), the client could leave the area and harm others if there were distractions to the staff on the unit.
Cognitive Level: Analysis **Client Need:** Psychosocial Integrity **Integrated Process:** Nursing Process: Planning **Content Area:** Psychiatric–Mental Health **Strategy:** The core issue of the question is placement of a client who has harmed another. Use nursing knowledge and the process of elimination to make a selection. Keep in mind that the safety of the client and others around him or her is the first priority.

9 **Answer: 3** Options 1, 2, and 4 may be correct intervention terms, but option 3 is the most correct terminology for the nursing intervention described to prevent increased anxiety and stress.
Cognitive Level: Application **Client Need:** Psychosocial Integrity **Integrated Process:** Nursing Process: Planning **Content Area:** Psychiatric–Mental Health **Strategy:** The core issue of the question is the ability to determine various types of nursing interventions needed by a hospitalized client with a mental health problem. Use nursing knowledge and the process of elimination to make a selection.

10 **Answer: 4** The client who demonstrates a calm, focused exchange of information and self-care information would demonstrate control of the disorder, which is expected following discharge from an inpatient setting. The client in a manic state would present with the option 1 or 2 behaviors, while the client with depression would present as option 3 indicates.
Cognitive Level: Application **Client Need:** Psychosocial Integrity **Integrated Process:** Nursing Process: Assessment **Content Area:** Psychiatric–Mental Health **Strategy:** The core issue of the question is appropriate behavior exhibited by a client with bipolar disorder after treatment. Use nursing knowledge and the process of elimination to make a selection.

11 **Answer: 2** Voicing doubt about the delusions is the most therapeutic intervention. The client will continue to voice a delusion even though the evidence would suggest otherwise (option 1). A paranoid client cannot use logic to dispel delusions (option 3). Option 4 challenges the client's belief instead of voicing doubt. Providing evidence will not usually sway a paranoid client.
Cognitive Level: Analysis **Client Need:** Psychosocial Integrity **Integrated Process:** Communication and Documentation **Content Area:** Psychiatric–Mental Health **Strategy:** The core issue of the question is appropriate therapeutic communication techniques to use with a client who is paranoid. Use nursing knowledge and the process of elimination to make a selection.

12 **Answer: 1** Minimal self-care is a behavioral negative symptom of schizophrenia. A delusion is a cognitive positive symptom (option 2); hallucination is a perceptual positive symptom (option 3); and inappropriate affect (option 4) is an affective positive symptom.
Cognitive Level: Application **Client Need:** Psychosocial Integrity **Integrated Process:** Communication and Documentation **Content Area:** Psychiatric–Mental Health **Strategy:** The core issue of the question is an ability to discriminate between positive and negative signs of schizophrenia. Use nursing knowledge and the process of elimination to make a selection.

13 **Answer: 2** Client safety is a priority. Hearing voices (hallucination) is a sensory-perceptual alteration, but safety is a priority (option 3). There is not enough data to support the nursing diagnoses of impaired verbal communication (option 1) or impaired social interaction (option 4).
Cognitive Level: Analysis **Client Need:** Psychosocial Integrity **Integrated Process:** Nursing Process: Analysis **Content Area:** Psychiatric–Mental Health **Strategy:** The core issue of the question is an ability to set priorities for a client who experiences auditory hallucinations. Look for the option that puts client safety first. Use nursing knowledge and the process of elimination to make a selection.

14 **Answer: 3** Neuroleptic malignant syndrome (NMS) is a potentially fatal extrapyramidal symptom. Symptoms of NMS develop suddenly and include muscle rigidity, respiratory problems, and hyperpyrexia. Dystonia (option 1) and akathisia (option 2) are both extrapyramidal symptoms that are usually not fatal (option 1). Tardive dyskinesia symptoms include frowning, blinking, grimacing, puckering, blowing, smacking, licking, chewing, tongue protrusion, and spastic facial distortions, which can be socially disfiguring (option 4).
Cognitive Level: Analysis **Client Need:** Psychosocial Integrity **Integrated Process:** Nursing Process: Assessment **Content Area:** Psychiatric–Mental Health **Strategy:** The core issue of the question is an ability to identify signs of adverse medication effects

in a client being treated for psychosis. Use nursing knowledge and the process of elimination to make a selection.

15 **Answer: 4** A delusion is a false belief that cannot be changed by logical reasoning or evidence. A hallucination is the occurrence of a sight, sound, touch, smell, or taste without any external stimulus to the corresponding sensory organ; it is real to the client (option 1). The client is not exhibiting reality orientation (option 2). An illusion is a sensory misperception of environmental stimuli (option 3).
Cognitive Level: Application **Client Need:** Psychosocial Integrity **Integrated Process:** Communication and Documentation **Content Area:** Psychiatric–Mental Health **Strategy:** The core issue of the question is an ability to correctly identify the types of thought patterns expressed in a client's communications. Use nursing knowledge and the process of elimination to make a selection.

16 **Answer: 2** The client who gains coping skills reduces anxiety to a level at which dissociation is unlikely to occur. The client does not remember what occurred during the fugue state, nor does he experience depersonalization.
Cognitive Level: Analysis **Client Need:** Psychosocial Integrity **Integrated Process:** Nursing Process: Planning **Content Area:** Psychiatric–Mental Health **Strategy:** The core issue of the question is an appropriate outcome of care for a client who was in a dissociative fugue state. Use nursing knowledge and the process of elimination to make a selection, recalling that anxiety is usually the cause of the state, and therefore the answer points to an item that reduces anxiety.

17 **Answer: 3** Self-mutilation, not uncommon with DID clients, is identified in the assessment. The client remains at risk for injuring herself, producing tissue damage that provides tension relief. There is no intent to kill; however, the client will need to learn less damaging ways to obtain relief.
Cognitive Level: Analysis **Client Need:** Psychosocial Integrity **Integrated Process:** Nursing Process: Planning **Content Area:** Psychiatric–Mental Health **Strategy:** The core issue of the question is a priority nursing diagnosis. Questions such as these are frequently focused on safety. Use nursing knowledge and the process of elimination to make a selection.

18 **Answer: 1** This response demonstrates empathy and encourages the client to elaborate further about his experience. Options 2 and 3 dismiss the affective component or miss the point of the client's statement. Option 4 is helpful in making connections between events but is not the best response to the client's original comment.
Cognitive Level: Application **Client Need:** Psychosocial Integrity **Integrated Process:** Communication and Documentation **Content Area:** Psychiatric–Mental Health **Strategy:** The core issue of the question is a therapeutic response to a client who is experiencing depersonalizing events. Use nursing knowledge of therapeutic communication skills and use the process of elimination to make a selection.

19 **Answer: 3** The goal of care is to eliminate or reduce dissociative experiences, which can be accomplished in part by anxiety-produced stress–management techniques.
Cognitive Level: Analysis **Client Need:** Psychosocial Integrity **Integrated Process:** Nursing Process: Evaluation **Content Area:** Psychiatric–Mental Health **Strategy:** The core issue of the question is the ability to determine an appropriate outcome of care for a client who dissociates. Recall that anxiety plays a role in dissociation and choose the option that reduces anxiety.

20 **Answer: 4** Amnesia is precipitated by stress related to trauma or conflict. The amnesia occurs abruptly and there is no attempt to cover the memory loss. Confabulation, gradual loss of memory, and disheveled appearance are common in clients experiencing dementia.
Cognitive Level: Analysis **Client Need:** Psychosocial Integrity **Integrated Process:** Nursing Process: Assessment **Content Area:** Psychiatric–Mental Health **Strategy:** The core issue of the question is knowledge of expected assessment findings in a client with amnesia. Use nursing knowledge and the process of elimination to make a selection.

21 **Answer: 3** A client with OCD, a cluster C disorder, appears anxious or fearful. Individuals with a cluster A disorder appear odd or eccentric; those with a cluster B disorder appear dramatic or erratic. The category of rigid/critical does not reflect a diagnostic cluster.
Cognitive Level: Application **Client Need:** Psychosocial Integrity **Integrated Process:** Nursing Process: Assessment **Content Area:** Psychiatric–Mental Health **Strategy:** The core issue of the question is knowledge of expected behaviors that would be exhibited by a client with OCD. Recall that a client with this type of diagnosis is very ritualistic and therefore rigid. Use nursing knowledge and the process of elimination to make a selection.

22 **Answer: 3** In caring for clients diagnosed with antisocial personality disorder, it is important to maintain a structured and consistent environment to decrease their attempts to control the situation through manipulation. It is unlikely that they will develop insight as the causes of problems in living are externalized. They are frequently quite sociable and take advantage of others for personal profit. Suicidal ideation is not associated with this disorder.
Cognitive Level: Analysis **Client Need:** Psychosocial Integrity **Integrated Process:** Nursing Process: Implementation **Content Area:** Psychiatric–Mental Health **Strategy:** The core issue of the question is an ability to set priorities for a client who has an antisocial personality disorder. Use nursing knowledge and the process of elimination to make a selection.

23 **Answer: 2** Individuals diagnosed with personality disorders display either functional impairment or subjective distress. Frequently these problems in living are reflected in impaired interpersonal relationships. Flexibility and adaptability to stress (option 1) are incongruent with a diagnosis of a personality disorder. The presence of a physical disorder (option 3) has no relation to the diagnosis of a personality disorder. These individuals may or may not desire interpersonal relationships (option 4).
Cognitive Level: Application **Client Need:** Psychosocial Integrity **Integrated Process:** Nursing Process: Assessment **Content Area:** Psychiatric–Mental Health **Strategy:** The core issue of the question is knowledge of expected assessment findings regarding behavior style in a client with a personality disorder. Note that the type of disorder is not specified, so the answer is a global or general pattern. Use nursing knowledge and the process of elimination to make a selection.

24 **Answer: 1** Individuals diagnosed with antisocial personality disorder frequently try to play one staff member against the other in order to control their environment. It is imperative that staff present a unified, consistent, and structured approach to care to prevent this. Options 2, 3, and 4 are incorrect because they would result in lack of team unity and an unstructured approach to care.
Cognitive Level: Analysis **Client Need:** Psychosocial Integrity **Integrated Process:** Nursing Process: Planning **Content Area:** Psychiatric–Mental Health **Strategy:** The core issue of the question is core beliefs about the value and roles of the interdisciplinary team. Use nursing knowledge and the process of elimination to make a selection.

25 **Answer: 1** Individuals diagnosed with obsessive-compulsive personality disorder become overly involved in details such as rules and regulations related to a need to be perfect. As a result, they fail to see the big picture. Their relationships with others and participation in leisure activities are less important to them than is their devotion to work and productivity.
Cognitive Level: Application **Client Need:** Psychosocial Integrity **Integrated Process:** Nursing Process: Assessment **Content Area:** Psychiatric–Mental Health **Strategy:** The core issue of the question is knowledge of expected behavior styles in a client with OCD. Use nursing knowledge and the process of elimination to make a selection.

26 **Answer: 1** The continuance of pain is related to reinforcement of the symptoms, such as the caring responses of others, which give the client benefits that otherwise might not occur. There is no organic basis for the pain. High endorphin levels are associated with feelings of euphoria.
Cognitive Level: Analysis **Client Need:** Psychosocial Integrity **Integrated Process:** Nursing Process: Analysis **Content Area:** Psychiatric–Mental Health **Strategy:** The core issue of the question is knowledge of possible explanations of causation of pain in a client with no physical basis for pain. Use nursing knowledge and the process of elimination to make a selection.

27 **Answer: 4** The client with a conversion disorder is characteristically indifferent to the symptoms (*la belle indifference*) rather than being depressed, anxious, or blunted in affect.
Cognitive Level: Analysis **Client Need:** Psychosocial Integrity **Integrated Process:** Nursing Process: Assessment **Content Area:** Psychiatric–Mental Health **Strategy:** The core issue of the question is knowledge of expected assessment findings related to mood in a client with a conversion disorder. Use nursing knowledge and the process of elimination to make a selection.

28 **Answer: 3** Exploration of the client's decision is nonjudgmental and affirms the client's personal power. This reponse also helps the client understand connections in her own decision-making process.
Cognitive Level: Application **Client Need:** Psychosocial Integrity **Integrated Process:** Caring **Content Area:** Psychiatric–Mental Health **Strategy:** The core issue of the question is a therapeutic communication to a client with hypochondriasis. Use nursing knowledge of therapeutic communication skills and the process of elimination to make a selection.

29 **Answer: 3** Data indicates that the client perceives a lack of control over her situation. There is insufficient data to select any of the other nursing diagnoses.
Cognitive Level: Analysis **Client Need:** Psychosocial Integrity **Integrated Process:** Nursing Process: Analysis **Content Area:** Psychiatric–Mental Health **Strategy:** The core issue of the question is the ability to form an appropriate nursing diagnosis based on client assessment data. Use nursing knowledge and the process of elimination to make a selection.

30 **Answer: 1** When stressors and anxiety are decreased, there remains no need for conversion symptoms, and normal function resumes.
Cognitive Level: Analysis **Client Need:** Psychosocial Integrity **Integrated Process:** Nursing Process: Evaluation **Content Area:** Psychiatric–Mental Health **Strategy:** The core issue of the question is knowledge of appropriate outcomes of care for a client with a conversion disorder. Use nursing knowledge and the process of elimination to make a selection.

31 **Answer: 2** Verbal communication should be clear, concise, and unhurried. Shouting may be interpreted as anger; therefore, a pleasant, calm, supportive tone of voice should be used. The use of sign language or mostly nonverbal gestures would be frustrating to the client who may not understand what is being said.
Cognitive Level: Application **Client Need:** Psychosocial Integrity **Integrated Process:** Caring **Content Area:** Psychiatric–Mental Health **Strategy:** The core issue of the question is a therapeutic communication to a client with a cognitive impairment. Use nursing knowledge of therapeutic communication skills and the process of elimination to make a selection.

32 **Answer: 4** The most important area of concern identified by both family and staff is the safety of clients with dementia. The risk for injury is always present in clients with dementia, and as the disease progresses, the need for a safe and secure environment increases. The other options are appropriate for dementia but are not the first priority.
Cognitive Level: Application **Client Need:** Psychosocial Integrity **Integrated Process:** Nursing Process: Planning **Content Area:** Psychiatric–Mental Health **Strategy:** The core issue of the question is the ability to determine the appropriate priority of care for a client who has dementia. Focus on safety as an early priority whenever a client has a neurological impairment. Use nursing knowledge and the process of elimination to make a selection.

33 **Answer: 4** Alzheimer's disease is diagnosed by ruling out causes for the client's symptoms. The only definitive method of diagnosis is postmortem examination of brain tissue.
Cognitive Level: Analysis **Client Need:** Psychosocial Integrity **Integrated Process:** Nursing Process: Assessment **Content Area:** Psychiatric–Mental Health **Strategy:** The core issue of the question is methods of diagnosis for Alzheimer's disease. Use nursing knowledge and the process of elimination to make a selection.

34 **Answer: 2** Dementia is a progressive disease that causes the individual to lose the ability to perform tasks that were once familiar and routine. Self-care deficits involving many functional abilities occur to varying degrees. The most effective and respectful goals are those that allow the client to carry out as much self-care as possible. Option 2 is the most global goal that encompasses meeting needs for food, water, dressing, bathing, and so on.

Cognitive Level: Application **Client Need:** Psychosocial Integrity **Integrated Process:** Nursing Process: Planning **Content Area:** Psychiatric–Mental Health **Strategy:** The core issue of the question is the ability to set goals of care for a client with Alzheimer's disease. Use nursing knowledge and the process of elimination to make a selection.

35 **Answer: 1** Cognitive function will be supported by participation in meaningful activities that the client enjoys. Stimulating activities will also promote self-esteem and encourage the client to attain the highest level of cognitive function possible. Options 2, 3, and 4 could lead to frustration and more confusion.

Cognitive Level: Application **Client Need:** Psychosocial Integrity **Integrated Process:** Nursing Process: Implementation **Content Area:** Psychiatric–Mental Health **Strategy:** The core issue of the question is planning for a client with dementia that supports remaining memory function. Use nursing knowledge and the process of elimination to make a selection.

36 **Answer: 2, 3** Positive symptoms of schizophrenia are those behaviors that a client would not usually exhibit in everyday life, including delusion of being a king (option 2) or echolalia (option 3). Negative symptoms of schizophrenia are those that reflect the absence of what is normally seen in a person's behavior. These would include anergy (option 1), flat affect (option 4), and social withdrawal (option 5).

Cognitive Level: Application **Client Need:** Psychosocial Integrity **Integrated Process:** Nursing Process: Assessment **Content Area:** Psychiatric–Mental Health **Strategy:** The core issue of the question is the ability to discriminate between positive and negative symptoms of schizophrenia. Use nursing knowledge of these manifestations and the process of elimination to make a selection.

Key Terms to Review

affect p. 315
agnosia p. 335
agoraphobia p. 313
anxiety p. 309
aphasia p. 335
apraxia p. 335
bipolar disorder p. 315
body dysmorphic disorder p. 332
catatonic p. 321
clang association p. 322
compulsion p. 314
conversion disorder p. 333
cyclothymic disorder p. 315
delirium p. 335
delusional ideation p. 321
dementia p. 335
depersonalization p. 329
derealization p. 329
dissociation p. 329
dissociative amnesia p. 327
dissociative fugue p. 328
dissociative identity disorder p. 328
dysthymic disorder p. 315
echolalia p. 321
echopraxia p. 321
egodystonic p. 324
egosyntonic p. 324
group therapy p. 312
hallucination p. 321
host personality p. 328
hypochondriasis p. 332
illusion p. 322
major depression p. 315
milieu therapy p. 323
mood p. 314
narcissistic personality disorder p. 325
neologisms p. 322
obsession p. 314
personality disorder p. 324
personality traits p. 324
phobia p. 313
primary gain p. 328
pseudodelirium p. 338
pseudodementia p. 336
psychosis p. 322
repression p. 329
schizoaffective disorder p. 315
schizophrenia p. 320
seasonal affective disorder (SAD) p. 315
secondary gain p. 328
somatoform disorder p. 330
sundown syndrome p. 336
thought broadcasting p. 322
thought control p. 322
thought insertion p. 322
unipolar disorder p. 315
word salad p. 322

References

American Psychiatric Association (2000). *Diagnostic and statistical manual of mental disorders, fourth edition, Text Revision* (DSM-IV-TR). Washington, DC: American Psychiatric Association.

Carpenito, L. J. (2005). *Nursing diagnosis: Application to clinical practice* (11th ed.). Philadelphia: Lippincott, Williams, & Wilkins.

Fortinash, K., & Holoday-Worret, P. (2004). *Psychiatric mental health nursing* (3rd ed.). St. Louis: Mosby.

Kniesl, C., Wilson, H., & Trigoboff, E. (2004). *Contemporary psychiatric-mental health nursing.* Upper Saddle River, NJ: Pearson Education.

Stuart, G. W., & Laraia, M. T. (2004). *Principles and practice of psychiatric nursing* (8th ed.). St. Louis: Mosby.

Varcarolis, E. (2006). *Foundations of psychiatric mental health nursing* (5th ed.). Philadelphia: W. B. Saunders.

Dependency and Addiction

23

In this chapter

Test Yourself

Are you ready for the NCLEX-RN® or course exams? Use the practice tests on the companion CD-ROM to check.

Cross reference

Other chapters relevant to this content area are:

Coping with Stressors	Chapter 21
Mental Health Disorders	Chapter 22
Psychiatric Medications	Chapter 36

I. OVERVIEW

! **A. *Substance abuse* is purposeful but maladaptive pattern of substance use evidenced by recurring and significant adverse/harmful consequences of repeated use to self or others**

B. *Substance dependence* occurs when drug use is no longer under control and continues despite adverse effects; client develops tolerance and experiences withdrawal symptoms if use stops

! **C. Treatment focus is *abstinence* (voluntarily going without drugs), medications as appropriate, education, lifestyle change, and increasing self-awareness and personal growth**

D. Types and various diagnoses of addiction

1. Substance abuse disorder and **process addiction** syndrome are characterized by preoccupation with and compulsion to engage in an activity
   a. Substances: depressants (opiate, opioids, sedatives, hypnotics), stimulants (cocaine, amphetamines), cannabinoids and hallucinogens, inhalants
   b. Processes: eating disorders, compulsive gambling, compulsive sexual disorders, compulsive shopping/spending, compulsive Internet use, compulsive use of video games
2. Definitions associated with substance use disorders
   ! a. DSM-IV clinical syndromes: intoxication, withdrawal, abuse, dependence
   b. Substance dependence: a primary, chronic relapsing disease influenced by genetic, psychosocial, and environmental factors; characterized by continuous periodic impaired control over, preoccupation with, and use of substance despite adverse consequences; accompanied by distortions in thinking, most notably denial; inherent in definition are concepts of **tolerance, withdrawal, physical dependence,** and psychological dependence (American Society of Addiction Medicine)

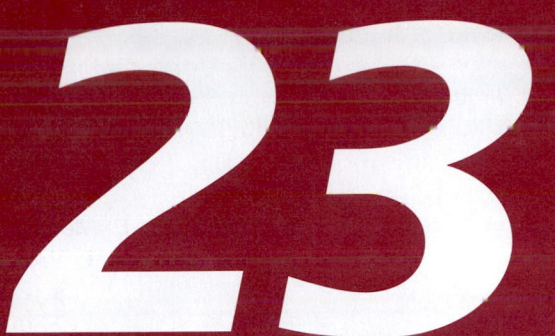

!

c. Addiction: an illness characterized by compulsion, loss of control, and continued pattern of abuse despite perceived negative consequences; obsession with a dysfunctional habit; dysfunctional patterns include patterns of alcoholism, drug abuse, misuse of tobacco, eating disorders, excessive gambling or spending, and certain compulsive sexual disorders (American Nurses Association and National Nurses Society on Addictions)

E. Medical theory of addiction: Jellinek four phases of alcoholism

1. Prealcoholic symptomatic phase
   - **a.** Distinct symptoms that the social drinker does not experience, such as drinking to cope with emotions
   - **b.** Lack of recognition that tension is caused by drinking
   - **c.** Phase lasts several months to 2 years
2. Prodromal phase
   - **a.** Begins drinking in secret
   - **b.** Gulps first few sips
   - **c.** Develops attachment to alcohol
   - **d.** Plans all social activities around access to alcohol
   - **e.** Develops tolerance (needing more alcohol to get the same effect)
   - **f.** Continues drinking despite negative consequences
   - **g.** Feels guilty about drinking
   - **h.** Becomes isolated and withdrawn
   - **i.** Experiences mood swings, and diminished self-esteem
   - **j.** Phase lasts 6 months to 5 years
3. ! Crucial phase
   - **a.** Beginning of disease process and psychological dependence
   - **b.** Intermittent loss of control ensues when drinking (uses more than intended)
   - **c.** Preoccupation with use develops
   - **d.** Use of defense mechanisms
   - **e.** Experiences craving triggers to use
   - **f.** Concern over drinking expressed by others
   - **g.** Anger, alienation of family and friends
   - **h.** Discontinues all nondrinking socialization, including friends who don't drink
   - **i.** Activities of daily living (ADLs) suffer; sleep, appetite, and energy problems are present
   - **j.** Family issues surface: alienation, anger, role and relationship problems
4. Chronic phase
   - **a.** Drinks to blackout, pass out, or become incapacitated
   - **b.** Cognitive, physical, emotional, health deterioration
   - **c.** Reverse tolerance may develop (less quantity than previously required to bring intoxication)
   - **d.** All areas of life are negatively affected, including family, career, and finances
5. Jellinek's theory can be applied to substance dependency and process addiction

F. Jellinek model applied to process addictions

1. Contact phase
   - **a.** Discover that engaging in addictive behavior is fun
   - **b.** Finds that it gives pleasure or reduces pain
2. Serendipitous phase: discovers that engaging in addictive behaviors helps person cope with distress
3. Instrumental phase
   - **a.** Consciously uses addictive behavior to cope with distress
   - **b.** Behavior becomes routine
4. ! Dependent phase
   - **a.** Unable to cope with life without engaging in addictive behavior
   - **b.** Experiences intermittent loss of control
   - **c.** Unable to stop despite negative consequences

II. ETIOLOGY

A. Addiction is a chronic brain disease evidenced by abnormalities in the neuronal activities of the brain reward system (BRS)

B. Process of BRS activation

1. All drugs affect cells in some way, either increasing or decreasing some cellular activities
2. Use of CNS-altering substances or engaging in addictive behaviors causes increased availability of dopamine, serotonin, and opioid peptides and facilitates dysregulation of other neurotransmitters (gamma-aminobutyric acid, glutamate, acetylcholine)
3. Short-term euphoric response is generated by this activity, which eventually leads to symptoms of addictive thinking, denial, and impaired control
4. Euphoric response engenders immediate and profound desire for readministration (**cravings** that are like psychological "hunger," triggers, and urges)
5. Positive, immediate short-term euphoria overshadows any long-term consequences associated with engaging in addictive behaviors
6. Continued use leads to development of tolerance
7. Experience of tolerance leads to increased dose and frequency of use
8. Physical dependence and withdrawal syndrome may develop
9. Psychological dependence develops

C. Genetic/biologic risk

1. No one specific marker is responsible for addictions—the more risk factors, the greater the risk for developing disease
2. Genetics: twins studies demonstrate a 30 to 50% vulnerability for addictions; daughters and sons of a parent with alcoholism have, respectively, a 3 and 4 times higher risk of addiction over those unaffected by alcoholism
3. Biology: intrapersonal genetic vulnerabilities leading to BRS abnormalities

D. Psychosocial risk

1. Personality traits: individuals with certain personality traits may be susceptible to reinforcing effects of engaging in addictive behaviors
   a. Antisocial: lack of responsiveness to people, places, and things in environment; persons with antisocial personality traits experience a positive response to psychoactive properties of engaging in addictive behavior
   b. Introversion: feelings of inadequacy or low self-esteem are mediated by euphoric effect of engaging in addictive behavior
   c. Impulsiveness: impulsivity is reinforced because of inability to anticipate impending negative consequences of use
2. Developmental failures: individuals who have lived with painful experiences are at risk to self-medicate or misuse their medication
   a. Abuse survivors—may experience disturbances in sense of self
   b. Lack of nurturance in childhood—may lead to an inability to self-soothe
   c. Coping skills deficit
   d. Positive coping skills may not have been learned in person's family of origin
   e. Learning positive coping skills may have been inhibited because of positive reinforcing effect of euphoria when using an addictive drug or behavior to cope with feelings

E. Dual disorders risk

1. Some individuals with a psychiatric disorder also have addiction
   a. Individuals with psychiatric disorders are at risk for developing addictive disorders
   b. Initially drugs and alcohol may be used to compensate for individual's lack of coping skills if he or she experiences depressive symptoms, anxiety, or recurrence of painful memories
   c. With continued use, addiction develops for individuals at risk
2. Individuals with addiction are at risk for developing psychiatric disorders
   a. Some individuals with addiction also have a psychiatric disorder

b. Substance use can induce development of psychiatric illness by affecting nucleus accumbens and ventral tegmental area (cognition, motivation, and learning) and neurotransmitter system (mood regulation)
c. Any one of a number of psychiatric disorders can develop
3. Individual with addictive disorders may be misdiagnosed because some disorders, such as anxiety disorders, depression, and chronic pain, mask addiction

Memory Aid

When a client has a problem with substance abuse or addiction, carefully screen for other mental health disorders as well, which may be comorbidities.

! 4. Individuals with dual diagnoses and who are intoxicated are at increased risk of suicide
5. Treatment for dual diagnoses is more successful if both illnesses are treated concurrently

F. Environmental risk

1. Social learning theory: use of addictive substances is a learned behavior
   a. Normalized behavior: engaging in addictive behavior is influenced by exposure to peer pressure, role models, societal norms
   b. Culture: engaging in addictive behaviors is influenced by culture; certain cultural groups have use patterns that put them at risk for developing addiction (such as Northern European, Native American)
2. Profession: health care professionals (HCPs) are at risk to develop addictive disorders because of high-stress, high-pressure jobs and exposure to substances
   ! a. Nurses are at risk for developing addictive disorders; nursing practice is impaired when individual is unable to meet requirements of professional code of ethics and standards of practice because of cognitive, interpersonal, or psychomotor skills affected by conditions of individual (psychiatric illness, excessive alcohol or drug use or addiction) in interaction with environment
   b. Risk factors for vulnerability: access to drugs, long hours, tremendous responsibility, job-related stress, family history of chemical dependence or mental disorder
   ! c. Signs and symptoms: increased irritability with clients and colleagues; mood swings; withdrawn or isolated and often wants to work night shift; avoids informal staff get-togethers; purposely waits until alone to sign out narcotics; late for work, misses work, offers elaborate excuses for missing work; work quality decreases; charting is illegible; signs out more narcotics than other nurses on unit
   d. System response: intervention and immunity from prosecution; in most states, there is opportunity for supportive intervention rather than loss of licensure if impaired nurse seeks treatment and strictly follows treatment and monitoring recommendations from Board of Nursing; if noncompliant, may lose nursing license

III. ASSESSMENT

A. Screening and assessment tools

1. CAGE: a positive answer for two of the following screening questions indicates need for further assessment
   a. Have you ever attempted to *Cut back* on your alcohol?
   b. Have you ever been *Annoyed* by comments made about your drinking?
   c. Have you ever felt *Guilty* about your drinking?
   d. Have you ever had an *Eye-opener* in the morning to calm your nerves?

Memory Aid

Use the initials of the CAGE questionnaire to trigger the memory of what each question refers to.

2. Michigan Alcoholism Screening Test (MAST)
3. Addiction Severity Index (ASI)

B. Nursing admission assessment data that focuses on use of mood-altering chemicals

1. Physical assessment/systems review
   - **a.** Blackout or lost consciousness: blacking out or passing out can be related to a person's use of alcohol or other substances
   - **b.** Changes in bowel movement: persons using alcohol and/or drugs frequently can experience changes in bowel movement; changes range from diarrhea caused by drinking to constipation caused by pain medications; withdrawal from narcotics can cause diarrhea
   - **c.** Liver problems: include manifestations of Wernicke's encephalopathy or Korsakoff's psychosis
   - **d.** Weight loss or weight gain: persons using alcohol or drugs regularly may experience weight loss or gain and/or poor nutritional balance
   - **e.** Experiencing stressful situation: stress can precipitate an increase in drinking; stress can also result from drinking or using drugs regularly
   - **f.** Sleep disturbances: persons using alcohol and/or other drugs experience a variety of sleep disturbances; an individual may start using alcohol to promote sleep, but once he or she develops tolerance, sleep is more difficult
   - **g.** Chronic pain: persons experiencing chronic pain may use drugs and/or alcohol to self-medicate
   - **h.** Concern over substance use: if friends and relatives worry about substance use, it is generally because a genuine problem exists
   - **i.** Cutting down on alcohol consumption (or drug use, prescription medication use, gambling, or addictive behavior): if one feels that he or she must cut down, it is usually because there are problems

Memory Aid

It is just as important to screen for psychosocial data as for physical assessment data during admission for treatment for addiction.

2. Personal family assessment: persons with positive family history are at risk for developing an addictive disorder
3. Substance use assessment: key elements
   - **a.** Identify type of substance used
   - **b.** Identify type of compulsive behavior
   - **c.** Pattern and frequency of substance use
   - **d.** Amount
   - **e.** Age at onset
   - **f.** Age of regular use
   - **g.** Changes in use patterns
   - **h.** Periods of abstinence in history
   - **i.** Previous withdrawal symptoms
   - **j.** Date of last substance use/compulsive behavior
   - **k.** Ask about each substance or behavior separately
   - **l.** Ranges of illicit drugs can be ingested into the body in numerous ways; remember that alcohol users may also use another substance
4. Medication assessment
   - **a.** Ask about pain-relief medications, laxatives, cold medications, sleep and/or stay awake medications, and/or anxiety/nerve control medications
   - **b.** Prescribed dose is now not enough to control pain or anxiety even though it might have helped at the beginning
   - **c.** Runs out of medication early and needs a refill early
   - **d.** Pain medication intended for physical pain is now used for emotional pain
   - **e.** Medication is used for dealing with "stress" or stressful events
   - **f.** More medication was taken than intended
   - **g.** Laxatives are used regularly because the pain medications cause constipation or because the individual has difficulty having bowel movements without use of laxatives
   - **h.** Cold tablets or cough syrup are taken more frequently than expected

5. Over-the-counter (OTC) or nutritional supplement assessment: use of any herbal, vitamin or OTC products to help with sleep, weight loss, staying awake, giving more energy, stabilizing mood and/or improving mood, or making client feel a certain way
6. Social history assessment: persons experiencing physical, sexual, or emotional abuse may medicate internal distress by using mood-altering substances
7. Laboratory value assessment: laboratory values that may be abnormal in substance abusers:
   a. Gamma glutamyl transferase (GGT)
   b. Serum glutamic oxaloacetic transaminase (SGOT) or aspartate aminotransferase
   c. Alkaline phosphatase (AK)
   d. Lactate dehydrogenase (LD)
   e. Mean corpuscular volume (MCV)
   f. Urine toxicology and blood screen for drugs of abuse
   g. Serum electrolytes

IV. PLANNING AND IMPLEMENTATION

A. Care of client while intoxicated

1. Focus is on safety
2. Interventions
   a. Maintain safe environment
   b. Orient to time, place, and person
   c. Maintain adequate nutrition and fluid balance
   d. Monitor for beginning of withdrawal signs and symptoms; note that, in general, drugs that depress the CNS lead to signs of CNS excitation during withdrawal, and drugs that are CNS stimulants lead to CNS depression during withdrawal
3. Outcome: client remains safe during periods of intoxication

B. Care of client experiencing withdrawal from psychoactive substances: focus is safe withdrawal process

1. Maintain safe environment
2. Create a low-stimulation environment
3. Monitor vital signs (especially increased blood pressure) and withdrawal symptoms, such as nausea/vomiting, tremor, paroxysmal sweats, anxiety, agitation, tactile disturbances, auditory disturbances, visual disturbances, headache or fullness in head, disorientation, and sensorium changes
4. Methadone is used to manage some clients who are opiate-dependent; may be initially prescribed for withdrawal but then client is maintained on certain daily dose; contrary to popular belief, many people who are maintained on methadone do well in recovery
5. Be careful in assessing client with chronic pain for withdrawal because some pain experienced is related to chronic pain and is not an acute withdrawal symptom
6. Even if female clients were initially screened for pregnancy, they should be screened later in episode of care to ensure that use of any medication potentially harmful to fetus is eliminated or minimized; alcohol is most harmful drug of all and is most harmful to fetus
7. Monitor for alcohol withdrawal delirium (formerly delirium tremens), psychotic symptoms, and suicide risk, and seizure risk
8. Administer withdrawal medication: anticonvulsants, benzodiazepines, sedatives, vitamins, or other medications as ordered; thiamine helps to prevent confusion (Wernicke's psychosis) and other mental status changes
9. Maintain adequate nutrition and fluid intake
10. Maintain normal comfort measures
11. Monitor for covert substance use during detoxification period
12. Provide emotional support and reassurance to client and family
13. Provide reality orientations and address hallucinations in a therapeutic manner
14. Advise client of depressive uneasy feelings and fatigue that usually occur during withdrawal

15. Begin to educate client about disease of addiction and initial treatment goal of abstinence
16. Outcomes are safe withdrawal from drugs and alcohol, client is oriented to reality, and begins to develop motivation for and commitment to abstinence and **recovery** (abstinence plus working a program of personal growth and self-discovery)

C. Nursing care during rehabilitative stages of abuse

1. Focus is on teaching about disease and recovery process and building on client's motivation for abstinence, lifestyle change, and recovery
2. Assist client to complete detoxification from all psychoactive substances; monitor for suicide and/or seizure risk
3. Promote abstinence from all psychoactive substances
4. Administer medications for enhancing abstinence, treatment of mood, anxiety, and/or thought disorders as applicable
5. Assist clients in putting structure and discipline back into their life
6. Facilitate hope
7. Teach disease and recovery dynamics
8. Teach about how disease has impacted roles and functions for individual and family
9. Provide therapeutic interaction/group counseling to:
   a. Process losses (i.e., loss of independence)
   b. Discuss memories and flashback
   c. Address shame and guilt
   d. Educate about disease/recovery
   e. Facilitate acceptance of illness
10. Teach and encourage practice of recovery skills
   a. Encourage daily commitment to sobriety and recovery
   b. Build and utilize sober support networks (i.e., Alcoholics Anonymous or other 12-step groups)
   c. Teach importance of honesty and making amends
   d. Encourage daily prayer or meditation
   e. Teach drink refusal skills and managing cravings
   f. Enhance coping, communication, and problem-solving skills
   g. Practice asking for help
   h. Recognize signs of impending **relapse** (return to addictive behavior): being hungry, angry, lonely, or tired; having thoughts about using but not telling anyone, slipping back into using old defensive mechanisms as opposed to honesty and openness
11. Help client to develop an emergency plan (a list of things client can do and people to call if he or she has urge to use or actually uses)

Memory Aid

Development of an emergency plan is high priority before discharge to home so that the client is better empowered to act on own behalf when the urge to abuse reoccurs.

12. Demonstrate how to utilize affirmations, slogans, and serenity prayer
13. Initiate random breathalyzers and urine drug screens to objectively assess for sobriety/substance use
   a. Breathalyzers are an inexpensive way to do random checks to see if individuals are coming into the program sober; because many clients have high tolerance, it is difficult to determine if they have been drinking
   b. Random urine drug screen test provides client with objective evidence of sobriety or use (urine collection procedure: instruct client not to turn on water or flush toilet until specimen is given to nurse)
14. Clients with anorexia nervosa or bulimia need to work with dietitian and primary case provider about increasing or decreasing (as indicated) caloric intake and discontinuing laxative use; they will need to increase daily water and fiber intake
15. Clients with multiple relapses who seem to have severe addiction may not have a goal of immediate total abstinence; their goals may be to increase number of

sober days within a specific period of time or reduce number of drinks ingested or money gambled at one sitting (harm reduction model; while not an ideal goal, it decreases risk of more serious consequences if someone is using lesser amounts of substances)

D. Treatment modalities and nursing interventions

1. Medical model: teach disease and recovery dynamics
2. Assist client in complying with treatment recommendations
3. Assist with dual diagnosis treatment
4. Detoxification, abstinence, medications
   - **a.** Disulfiram (Antabuse): usual dose is 250 mg/day; prevents breakdown of alcohol; person who drinks alcohol becomes very sick (flushing, weakness, nausea/vomiting); teach about monitoring for use of alcohol in products/food containing alcohol; can elevate liver enzymes
   - **b.** Naltrexone (ReVia): usual dose is 50 mg/day orally: prevents or diminishes cravings/euphoric effect of engaging in addictive substance use; can elevate liver enzymes
   - **c.** Antidepressant/antianxiety medications: enhance and stabilize mood and diminish anxiety; teach about decreased effectiveness of medication with use of psychoactive substances; discontinuation of medication should be gradual to prevent rebound effect or seizures
5. The 12-step model
   - **a.** Teach that there is no effective cure for addiction
   - **b.** Encourage 12-step involvement
   - **c.** Regular attendance at meetings diminishes ambivalence and promotes acceptance about never engaging in addictive behaviors again
   - **d.** Key elements of 12-step framework are acceptance, surrender, processing grief, higher power, and power of the group
6. Cognitive behavioral model
   - **a.** Develop and use positive coping skills
   - **b.** Implement specific skill training: assertiveness, drink refusal, problem-solving, cognitive restructuring, mood management, anger problems, social skills, listening and communication skills
   - **c.** Identify and change behaviors associated with addictive behaviors (i.e., going into liquor store to buy soft drinks)
7. Relapse prevention model
   - **a.** Identify situations and factors that contribute to relapse
   - **b.** Increase positive self-efficacy expectations about ability to achieve abstinence
   - **c.** Identify euphoric recall about engaging in addictive behavior, which can serve to keep someone actively engaging in addiction
8. Motivational enhancement and stages of change
   - **a.** Utilize various types of reflective listening and other specialized communication strategies to help build a client's commitment to change
   - **b.** Express empathy; ambivalence is a normal part of change process
   - **c.** Help clients develop discrepancy between the way they see themselves and the way they really are
   - **d.** Avoid getting into arguments over things, especially labels
   - **e.** Change strategies if resistance is encountered
   - **f.** Support client's self-efficacy
9. Assess client's stage of change and apply nursing interventions accordingly
   - **a.** Precontemplation: "We are blind to our problems"
   - **b.** Contemplation: "We are not ready to change"
   - **c.** Determination and preparation: "We are getting ready to change"
   - **d.** Action: "We are learning how to change; we are doing it"
   - **e.** Maintenance: "We make changes stick"

V. EVALUATION/OUTCOMES

A. Completes withdrawal process safely

B. Makes a commitment to sobriety, participates in treatment process

C. **Identifies consequences of substance use or addictive behaviors**
D. **Begins to practice some recovery behaviors while in treatment and identifies coping behaviors to address cravings, thoughts, and triggers to use or engage in addictive behaviors**
E. **Begins to accept having an addictive disorder and never being able to use safely or engage in addictive behavior again**

VI. DUAL DISORDER ISSUES

A. **Focus is on teaching that each disorder is an illness that requires co-occurring treatment and building on client's motivation for abstinence, remissions of mental illness, lifestyle change, and recovery process**
B. **Additional interventions**
   1. Discuss physiological aspects of mental illness, substance abuse, and interaction effects
   2. Teach that psychiatric medications are nonaddictive and can enhance recovery
   3. Medication teaching includes emphasizing that drinking or drug use will interfere with efficacy of psychiatric medication and that medication use and drinking should not mix

VII. FAMILY ISSUES

A. **Anger and alienation of substance dependent person**
B. **Teach disease dynamics**
   1. Family rules and communication
   2. Family members' dysfunctional behaviors and denial about addiction of family member
C. **Problematic coping skills**
D. **Mood adjustment problems**
! E. **Codependency and low self-esteem**
F. **Learn and practice recovery dynamics and skills**
   1. Include self-love and self-care
   2. Utilize support groups (i.e., Al-Anon)
   3. Establish healthy relationships and boundaries
   4. Engage in daily prayer or meditation
   ! 5. Improve coping and problem-solving skills
   6. Ask for help
   ! 7. Confront dysfunctional beliefs and learn how to change them
   8. Use affirmations, slogans, serenity prayer
G. **Processing anger, losses, and memories**
   1. Confront substance abuser about consequences of his or her use and how it affected family
   2. Process emotional distance between family members
   ! 3. Process loss of "helper/competent" role now that recovering family member is taking back some of his or her lost family roles

Check Your NCLEX-RN® Exam I.Q.

You are ready for testing on this content if you can

- Assess clients for signs of dependency or addiction.
- Assess reactions of clients and families to a diagnosis related to dependency or addiction.
- Counsel clients who have a substance-related disorder.
- Participate in providing therapy to a client with a disorder of dependency or addiction.
- Identify factors that could interfere with the recovery of a client from a substance-related disorder.
- Provide teaching about treatments, including support groups, for disorders of dependency or addiction.
- Assess and provide care to a client undergoing substance withdrawal or drug toxicity.

PRACTICE TEST

PRACTICE TEST

1. A client is transitioning to a less intensive level of outpatient treatment for addiction. The client statement that most reflects risk for relapse is:
   1. Dreaming about gambling or engaging in compulsive sex.
   2. Not feeling happy.
   3. Feeling hungry or tired.
   4. Keeping thoughts of using a secret.

2. What statement made by the mother of a recovering compulsive Internet user would indicate the need for more teaching?
   1. "My son is not going to enough 12-step meetings, he doesn't do his daily readings, and I don't think he is taking this seriously enough."
   2. "My daughter and I are going to go to Al-Anon for the first time because we realize we have been affected by my son's addiction."
   3. "I need to sign up for a meditation class for me because I get too preoccupied with what my son is or is not doing."
   4. "I still have a lot of anger about the relationship problems that occurred between my son and me as a result of his addiction."

3. The nurse observes a family visit on the unit and recognizes that the family is suffering with effects of addiction and codependence. What long-lasting interpersonal problems might the nurse expect family members to manifest?
   1. Lowered Self-esteem
   2. Impatience
   3. Frustration tolerance
   4. Being argumentative

4. A mother brings her daughter into the Emergency Department. She was at a party and danced for the last few hours. Now she is sweating and does not look well. The nursing assessment reveals temperature of 103°F, grinding the teeth, rapid weight loss. What should the nurse be most concerned about?
   1. Poor nutrition from excessive alcohol consumption
   2. Possible eating disorder
   3. Dehydration and electrolyte imbalance
   4. Flu with accompanying high fever

5. The nurse is completing an admission for a client with alcohol dependence. During the admission process, the client acknowledges occasional sexual performance problems. Then he says, "It's nothing a little alcohol can't fix." The nurse provides education about the effect of alcohol on sexual functioning by sharing that regular alcohol use causes which of the following?
   1. Increased desire and performance ability
   2. Headaches and the "too tired syndrome"
   3. Hyperarousal and premature ejaculation for men and anorgasmia for women
   4. Decreased desire and ability to perform

6. A physician just wrote an order for a client to take naltrexone (ReVia). What would be the greatest concern of the nurse while getting ready to administer this medication?
   1. The medication blocks the euphoric feeling from narcotics and alcohol.
   2. Whether the physician provided good medication teaching.
   3. The medication can precipitate withdrawal if the client is not completely detoxified.
   4. The client will not be able to experience pleasurable sensations.

7. You are conducting a daily nursing assessment on a client with gambling and alcohol addictions who is in the outpatient addiction program. As she checks in with you, she makes which of the following statements that reflects a need for more teaching?
   1. "I am going to have a night out with some friends at an area night club."
   2. "I felt like drinking, so I cleaned the house instead."
   3. "It is hard for me to make phone calls if I feel like using, but I did it last night."
   4. "I told my brother that I couldn't help him as much as I have in the past."

8 After completing a family session about addiction, a woman approaches the nurse and shares that as a mother, she will always have to bear the suffering of having a chemically dependent daughter who could relapse at any time. What would be important information to share about family recovery from addiction?

1. Family recovery can begin when the addictive behavior ceases.
2. Family recovery can begin even if active use continues.
3. Family recovery will fail if the recovering addict relapses.
4. Family recovery will be enhanced if the recovering addict attends several Alcoholics Anonymous meetings.

9 A married client with marijuana dependence has difficulty keeping her house clean because she spends a lot of time playing an entertaining game on the Internet. She also says that she waits until everyone goes to bed to start writing messages with sexual content online with another man. What are the nurse's concerns?

1. The Internet will cause her to break her marriage vows.
2. Her children won't bring any friends home because the house is messy.
3. She seems preoccupied with the Internet and is using poor judgment.
4. She is depressed and finds her marriage unfulfilling.

10 The nurse is educating parents about the purpose of laws that prohibit nicotine advertising on billboards within 1,000 feet of children in academic and social areas. In response to a question from the group, she shares that the law was designed to do which of the following?

1. Educate the general public about the hazards of smoking cigarettes.
2. Diminish the environmental risk to teens.
3. Diminish the effects of second-hand smoke.
4. Limit the free speech of children.

11 A new mother who bottle-feeds her infant comes in for her 6-week postpartum visit and talks about how depressed she is feeling. The health care provider prescribes an antidepressant for her. As the nurse delivering medication education, you assess the client's alcohol use patterns, and she shares with you that she has one to two drinks once or twice a week. You inform the client that she should not drink alcohol or use drugs in this situation because:

1. it will cause nausea and vomiting.
2. it will increase the effectiveness of the antidepressant.
3. it will decrease the effectiveness of the antidepressant.
4. it will cause increased blood pressure.

12 A cocaine-dependent client in recovery shares with the nurse that she has been using an over-the-counter sleep medication to help her get to sleep each night for the past 3 weeks. She gets defensive when the nurse raises concerns, stating emphatically that it is not addictive. How does the nurse respond to the client?

1. Validate how difficult it is to have a tough time sleeping and explain that nonaddictive medication can be abused if taken in larger doses or more frequency than recommended.
2. Acknowledge to the client that because the medication cannot be abused, it is not addictive. State there is a general concern that it could become a problem.
3. Confront her firmly and persistently because she is increasing the risk for developing addiction if she uses this medication too frequently.
4. Suggest she take some natural herbal sleep medication such as valerian or melatonin because they cannot cause any activation of the brain reward system.

13 As the nurse asks about sexuality during a nursing assessment, the client acknowledges that she has sexual problems. She shares that she has a masturbation compulsion and is trying to stop on her own but can't; she needs to know what she can do to stop. Based on her stage of change, the nurse should use which approach to care?

1. Help her to see that she has a serious problem.
2. Encourage her that she will feel better if she stops the compulsive sexual behavior.
3. Identify a date for her to stop her compulsive sexual behavior.
4. Review strategies to assist her to stop the compulsive sexual behavior.

14 The mental health nurse reminds clients who are learning about cross-addiction that there is a synergistic or addictive effect from using various kinds of chemicals together. The nurse uses which of the following as examples of combinations of chemicals that create this additive effect?

1. Drinking beer and smoking cigarettes
2. Drinking coffee and eating donuts
3. Drinking wine and taking a benzodiazepine
4. Drinking wine and coffee

PRACTICE TEST

15 A male client is saying he is "wired," feels like he is on "pins and needles," and is irritable. He says he stopped using alcohol abruptly. What is the nurse's next intervention in caring for this client?

1. Wait to see if any other symptoms occur in the next few hours and then report them to the physician.
2. Assess the time of his last drink and begin assessing signs and symptoms of alcohol withdrawal.
3. Assess the client for all current substance-use patterns, including time of last usage, and begin to assess for withdrawal.
4. Ask the physician to write an order for a stimulant medication to help prevent delirium tremens.

16 The nurse has coordinated a health fair for the church parish with four other nurses. The first nurse speaks about safe driving and includes that coordination and mental alertness are affected at a blood alcohol level of 0.04, even though many states have a legal limit of intoxication of 0.08 (formerly 0.10). When asked how many drinks per hour the average person needs to reach 0.08 intoxication level, the nurse would make which of the following replies?

1. A 4-ounce glass of wine if the individual has eaten recently
2. A 1- to 4-ounce glass of wine on an empty stomach
3. Three to five 4-ounce glasses of wine, depending on how recently food was consumed
4. Seven to eight 4-ounce glasses of wine, depending on how recently food was consumed

17 A nurse working in the addictions unit is stopped in the cafeteria by a coworker who states she is upset about something the nurse told to a client. The client understands that the nurse said, "If your drinking has created any problems for you, then you have addiction." The nurse clarifies that the statement was, "If you have the hallmark symptom of drinking, you have addiction." The nurse goes on to share which of the following as the hallmark?

1. Use despite negative consequences
2. Impaired control of use
3. Withdrawal
4. Tolerance

18 An orthopedic client who broke his ankle while drinking at a party is wondering if his drinking is "okay." He says he has never been arrested for driving intoxicated, nor has he experienced any health or relationship problems. He called in sick to work one time and drove intoxicated several times. Family information validates his self-report. The nurse concludes the client has an alcohol abuse problem on the basis of which of the following characteristics of this syndrome?

1. Drinking more than two drinks per occasion
2. The inability to stop drinking despite negative consequences
3. Drinking that causes an individual to pass out or experience a blackout
4. Drinking too much and too often with using poor judgment, and having negative consequences

19 The school nurse at the local high school is teaching a drug prevention class to teens. They don't think that cigarettes should be labeled a drug. The nurse explains that when dealing with addiction, the word "drug" means which of the following?

1. An illegal substance that activates the pleasure center
2. A substance that activates the pleasure center in the brain
3. A chemical that produces a pharmacological action when ingested
4. Any kind of pill that is broken down in the stomach by digestive action

20 A female student nurse visiting an outpatient addiction program is reviewing nursing care plans. She notices that there is one client with opiate addiction who takes methadone and will not be tapering off the medication. The student nurse asks the preceptor for the day about this. The preceptor responds that clients with an opioid addiction who are on methadone maintenance

1. are at high risk for using opiates.
2. are not really in recovery because they are still using a drug.
3. do fairly well in recovery as long as they are not using other drugs.
4. are exempt from having to participate in a 12-step program.

ANSWERS & RATIONALES

1 **Answer: 4** The problem with thoughts of using is keeping them a secret. When keeping things secret, the client is not telling the whole truth and is manipulating something. Engaging in secrets is reminiscent of using behaviors and can trigger using behaviors. It is natural to feel sad (option 2), hungry, or tired (option 3), and to have thoughts of using (option 1).
Cognitive Level: Application **Client Need:** Psychosocial Integrity **Integrated Process:** Nursing Process: Evaluation **Content Area:** Psychiatric-Mental Health **Strategy:** Use the process of elimination and nursing knowledge to answer the question. The wording of the question tells you that one answer is better than the others because it contains the key word *best.*

2 **Answer: 1** Checking on the compliance of a family member is an example of codependent behavior. The nurse would focus the teaching on helping the mother detach from her son and his recovery program and focus on her own well-being. Options 3 and 4 would indicate that she is trying to identify and deal with her feelings. Option 2 is an obvious healthy behavior.
Cognitive Level: Application **Client Need:** Psychosocial Integrity **Integrated Process:** Nursing Process: Evaluation **Content Area:** Psychiatric-Mental Health **Strategy:** The wording of the question tells you that only one answer is correct. Use knowledge of codependency to differentiate the problematic behavior from the other expected behaviors.

3 **Answer: 1** There are three communication rules learned in families in which addiction is present: don't talk, don't trust, don't feel. While these experiences cause anger, anxiety, or maladaptive coping, they can also contribute to the development of shame, depression, and low self-esteem. Without family healing, these problems can create much pain and suffering for all involved.
Cognitive Level: Application **Client Need:** Psychosocial Integrity **Integrated Process:** Nursing Process: Analysis **Content Area:** Psychiatric-Mental Health **Strategy:** The core issue of the question is underlying consequences to families when addiction is present. Use nursing knowledge and the process of elimination to make a selection.

4 **Answer: 3** The client most likely has used one of the "club drugs" or "rave drugs"; these drugs most often are a cross between a stimulant and a hallucinogen. Such drugs are used at dance parties and along with black lighting or strobe lights create a surreal experience. The stimulant effect of the drug causes users to grind their teeth. To avoid this, teens often use pacifiers to suck on. The combination of drug, dancing, and dehydration lead to dangerous body temperature increases, which must be addressed immediately. This client may also have an eating disorder, but that would not be the nurse's primary concern (option 2). Options 1 and 4 are incorrect.
Cognitive Level: Application **Client Need:** Psychosocial Integrity **Integrated Process:** Nursing Process: Analysis **Content Area:** Psychiatric-Mental Health **Strategy:** Note the stem of the question contains the critical words *most concerned.* This tells you that more than one option may be partially correct and that you must prioritize an answer. Correlate elevated body temperature and weight loss with fluid balance to choose option 3 as correct.

5 **Answer: 4** While most individuals believe that drugs of abuse enhance their sexual experience, the opposite is mostly true. The four kinds of sexual problems that commonly occur as the result of chemical use are anxiety about one's sexual performance; decrease or absence of sexual arousal; difficulties in reaching orgasm; and decrease or absence of pleasure in and/or intensity of orgasm.
Cognitive Level: Analysis **Client Need:** Psychosocial Integrity **Integrated Process:** Teaching and Learning **Content Area:** Psychiatric-Mental Health **Strategy:** The core issue of the question is the relationship between chronic substance abuse and sexual performance. Use the process of elimination and nursing knowledge to answer the question. The wording of the question tells you that only one option is correct.

6 **Answer: 3** Naltrexone is an excellent medication to treat alcohol or opiate dependence. It helps to prevent cravings and triggers to use, and it blocks the euphoric response if alcohol or opioids are ingested (option 1). The nurse should always evaluate the client's current knowledge level and provide education as needed (option 2). However, if the client is not completely detoxified from opiates, the use of naltrexone can precipitate withdrawal (option 3). Persons should be opiate-free for 7 to 10 days before starting this medication.
Cognitive Level: Analysis **Client Need:** Psychosocial Integrity **Integrated Process:** Nursing Process: Analysis **Content Area:** Psychiatric-Mental Health **Strategy:** Note the key words *greatest concern* in the question. This tells you that more than one option could be partially correct and that you must prioritize an answer. Use nursing knowledge related to this medication to choose the option in which the client is at greatest risk.

7 **Answer: 1** Recovering clients may tend to underestimate how difficult it will be to stay sober if they visit with friends who are still using or frequent old "hangout" places where they used to engage in addictive behaviors. In early recovery, clients are encouraged to detach from people, places, and things associated with their addiction. As the person gains sobriety and recovery, he or she may be able to re-engage, on a limited basis, with certain activities, such as being with friends who drink or celebrating an occasion at a bar. Options 2, 3, and 4 demonstrate positive coping measures and good management of potential triggers.
Cognitive Level: Analysis **Client Need:** Psychosocial Integrity **Integrated Process:** Nursing Process: Assessment **Content Area:** Psychiatric-Mental Health **Strategy:** The wording of the question tells you that the correct option is a statement that contains either a false statement or one that indicates the client is at risk. Choose option 1 over the others because it puts the client in an area where temptation is likely.

8 **Answer: 2** Addiction affects the entire family system; communication roles and boundaries. Some problems that individual family members experience are low self-esteem, guilt, shame, insecurity, and preoccupation with the chemically dependent family member. Families need treatment to facilitate their own healing. If they get involved in a treatment facility–operated family program, a spiritually centered family recovery program, or any of the family 12-step programs, active healing can take place whether the addict is using or not. Options 1 and 3 are incorrect. If the family is not engaged in its own treatment, it may not make any difference how many meetings the addicted member attends (option 4).
Cognitive Level: Analysis **Client Need:** Psychosocial Integrity **Integrated Process:** Teaching and Learning **Content Area:** Psychiatric-Mental Health **Strategy:** The core issue of the question is the family dynamics and impact on the family of a substance-using family member. Use nursing knowledge and the process of elimination to make a selection. The wording of the question indicates that only one answer is correct.

9 **Answer: 3** The client is spending a great deal of time on the Internet, which seems to be interfering with not only her parental relationships but also her relationship with her husband as well. If the client does not stop using marijuana and start practicing recovery, and if her Internet problems are not addressed, they are unlikely to "go away on their own" and her family problems may get worse (options 1, 2, and 4).
Cognitive Level: Application **Client Need:** Psychosocial Integrity **Integrated Process:** Nursing Process: Analysis **Content Area:** Psychiatric-Mental Health **Strategy:** Use the process of elimination and critical thinking skills to answer the question. The correct answer is one that is most comprehensive of all aspects of the problem described and does not place judgment on the client.

10 **Answer: 2** Environment and peer pressure play very strong roles in the development of addiction. Most smokers (90%) are addicted to nicotine by age 20. Although only 28 percent of the U.S. population smokes, the vast majority of new smokers are under age 18. The Federal Drug Administration (FDA) is trying to reduce smoking among children and teens by regulating tobacco advertisements near schools and youth centers. The rationale is that by restricting tobacco advertising to youths, the desire to smoke will be reduced. It is good for the public to be educated about the hazards of smoking, including second-hand smoke. This law does not specifically address option 1 and 3. Option 4 is part of the tobacco industry response to the proposed FDA regulation.
Cognitive Level: Analysis **Client Need:** Psychosocial Integrity **Integrated Process:** Teaching and Learning **Content Area:** Psychiatric-Mental Health **Strategy:** Use the process of elimination to answer the question. The correct answer is the one that reduces the exposure of children and teens to advertising about tobacco in locations that they tend to frequent, thereby diminishing the pressure to use.

11 **Answer: 3** Antidepressants regulate dysfunction in the neurotransmitter system, which results in mood equilibrium. Alcohol is a depressant that causes dysfunction in the neurotransmitter system, which can cause depression and/or anxiety. Use of alcohol or other mood-altering drugs while taking antidepressants is contraindicated.
Cognitive Level: Analysis **Client Need:** Physiological Integrity: Pharmacological and Parenteral Therapies **Integrated Process:** Teaching and Learning **Content Area:** Psychiatric-Mental Health **Strategy:** The core issue of the question is the interaction of a prescribed antidepressant with alcohol use. Recall that alcohol is a CNS depressant, which has an opposite effect of antidepressants. Use the process of elimination and general knowledge of drug interactions to make a selection.

12 **Answer: 1** Persons can experience tolerance or tolerance-like symptoms in response to taking certain OTC medications. OTC sleep medications or psychoactive sleep medications are meant for short-term use, no longer than 1 week consecutively (options 2 and 3). The FDA does not regulate herbal products, and it is difficult to know what dose to recommend or how the product might interact with the client. Sleep difficulties are often a problem for people in early recovery. Providing education on sleep hygiene and validating experiences proves helpful in addressing this problem (option 4).
Cognitive Level: Application **Client Need:** Psychosocial Integrity **Integrated Process:** Communication and Documentation **Content Area:** Psychiatric-Mental Health **Strategy:** Use the process of elimination and nursing knowledge to answer the question. Eliminate incorrect options because of the presence of "red flag" words *cannot* in options 2 and 4 and *firmly and persistently* in option 3.

13 **Answer: 4** The client acknowledges her problem and has tried to stop on her own; this puts her in the action stage. She is actively trying to change. The correct action of the nurse, then, is to assist. Option 1 demonstrates precontemplation; option 2, contemplation; and option 3, determination and preparation.
Cognitive Level: Application **Client Need:** Psychosocial Integrity **Integrated Process:** Nursing Process: Implementation **Content Area:** Psychiatric-Mental Health **Strategy:** The critical words in the question are *stage of change.* This tells you that the correct answer is the one in which the action of the nurse matches the stage of change represented by the client statements. Use the process of elimination and nursing knowledge to make a selection.

14 **Answer: 3** Alcohol and benzodiazepines are both depressants. Persons often use two drugs within the same class to enhance their effects. The capacity of other psychoactive substances within the same class of drugs to enhance the effect of the primary drug is called cross-tolerance. Options 1 and 4 are examples of combining a stimulant with a depressant, while option 2 has only a stimulant.
Cognitive Level: Application **Client Need:** Psychosocial Integrity **Integrated Process:** Nursing Process: Analysis **Content Area:** Psychiatric-Mental Health **Strategy:** The core issue of the question is knowledge that cross-addiction occurs between drugs in the same class. Use the process of elimination and knowledge of the categories of the chemicals in the options to make a selection.

15 **Answer: 3** Tactile disturbances are a symptom of alcohol dependence, and if the client reports stopping alcohol use

abruptly, he or she may be starting to experience withdrawal symptoms. However, the client may also have used and stopped other substances abruptly as well. The nurse must assess for other substances used. Multiple drug use is the rule more than the exception. Waiting (option 1) places the client at risk, and stimulants are not indicated (option 4). **Cognitive Level:** Application **Client Need:** Psychosocial Integrity **Integrated Process:** Nursing Process: Implementation **Content Area:** Psychiatric-Mental Health **Strategy:** The wording indicates that the core issue of the question is possible withdrawal. Use the process of elimination for options 1 and 4. Choose option 3 over option 2 because it is more comprehensive and includes option 2 within it.

16 **Answer: 3** It takes the average person 1 hour to metabolize 1 ounce of alcohol or a 4-ounce glass of wine. If three to five glasses of wine are consumed within an hour, the average person becomes intoxicated. Options 1 and 2 are insufficient, while option 4 is greatly excessive.
Cognitive Level: Analysis **Client Need:** Psychosocial Integrity **Integrated Process:** Teaching and Learning **Content Area:** Psychiatric-Mental Health **Strategy:** Use the process of elimination to answer the question. Eliminate options 1 and 2 first because they contain small amounts of alcohol and because they tend to be more rigid amounts. Recognizing that the question has the key words *average person,* choose option 3 over option 4 because it is more moderate and because it allows for individual variation, which options 1 and 2 do not.

17 **Answer: 2** Impaired control is the defining symptom that moves someone's use or abuse category to the dependence category. The symptom of "use despite negative consequences" fits in both the abuse and dependence category (option 1). Withdrawal (option 3) and/or tolerance (option 4) may or may not be present for someone who has dependence.
Cognitive Level: Analysis **Client Need:** Psychosocial Integrity **Integrated Process:** Communication and Documentation **Content Area:** Psychiatric-Mental Health **Strategy:** The core issue of the question is knowledge of hallmarks of alcohol abuse. Use the process of elimination and nursing knowledge to make a selection.

18 **Answer: 4** The behavior of drinking and driving fits in the abuse category as "recurrent substance use in hazardous situations." Option 1 is incorrect. Option 2 demonstrates the category of dependence. Option 3, "black out," is a symptom of intoxication.
Cognitive Level: Analysis **Client Need:** Psychosocial Integrity **Integrated Process:** Nursing Process: Assessment **Content Area:** Psychiatric-Mental Health **Strategy:** Use the process of elimination to make a selection, matching the client statements in the question with the conclusions in the correct option. The wording of the question tells you that only one option contains a correct statement.

19 **Answer: 2** Any substance, legal or illegal, that activates the pleasure center in the brain has the potential to cause dependence. Nicotine takes only 10 seconds to reach the brain. Nicotine causes both physical and psychological dependence.
Cognitive Level: Analysis **Client Need:** Psychosocial Integrity **Integrated Process:** Teaching and Learning **Content Area:** Psychiatric-Mental Health **Strategy:** Use the process of elimination and basic knowledge of addiction to make a selection. The wording of the question tells you that only one option contains a correct statement.

20 **Answer: 3** Methadone maintenance therapy seems to be an effective treatment regimen for a select population. Clients with heroin and/or other opiate addictions receiving oral methadone do not receive the euphoria associated with their drug of choice (option 1). The person on methadone maintenance who works a recovery program and is abstinent of all other mood-altering substances is in good recovery (option 2 and 4).
Cognitive Level: Analysis **Client Need:** Psychosocial Integrity **Integrated Process:** Teaching and Learning **Content Area:** Psychiatric-Mental Health **Strategy:** Use the process of elimination and basic knowledge of addiction to make a selection. The wording of the question tells you that only one option contains a correct statement.

ANSWERS & RATIONALES

Key Terms to Review

abstinence p. 351
craving p. 353
physical dependence p. 351
process addiction p. 351
recovery p. 357
relapse p. 357
substance abuse p. 351
substance dependence p. 351
tolerance p. 351
withdrawal p. 351

References

Boyd, M. (2005). *Psychiatric nursing: Contemporary practice* (3rd ed.). Philadelphia: Lippincott Williams & Wilkins.

Fortinash, K., & Holoday-Worret, P. (2004). *Psychiatric-mental health nursing* (4th ed.). St. Louis: Mosby.

Kniesl, C., Wilson, H., & Trigoboff, E. (2004). *Contemporary psychiatric-mental health nursing.* Upper Saddle River, NJ: Pearson Education.

Stuart, G., & Laraia, M. (2004). *Principles and practice of psychiatric nursing* (8th ed.). St. Louis: Elsevier Science.

Varcarolis, E. (2006). *Foundations of psychiatric mental health nursing: A clinical approach* (5th ed.). Philadelphia: W. B. Saunders.

24 Crisis Intervention and Suicide

Test Yourself

Are you ready for the NCLEX-RN® or course exams? Use the practice tests on the companion CD-ROM to check.

In this chapter

Cross reference

Other chapters relevant to this content area are

I. OVERVIEW OF CRISIS

A. Definition of *crisis*: experience of being confronted by a stressor with which individual is unable to cope and which he or she cannot resolve

1. Change or loss threatens individual's **equilibrium** (state of balance; a condition in which contending forces are equal)
2. Accompanying anxiety and tension make coping with this experience more difficult
3. Feelings of hopelessness and helplessness result in state of cognitive disorganization in which previous experience and coping fail to enable individual to problem-solve; **coping** is a conscious attempt to manage stress and anxiety; may be physical, cognitive, or affective
4. **Hopelessness:** a subjective state in which individual sees limited or no alternatives or personal choices available and is unable to mobilize energy on own behalf
5. **Helplessness:** a state that may arise when client has a condition in which he or she depends on outside sources for life support
6. Loss of equilibrium ensues
7. ! Crises are generally time limited, lasting from 4 to 6 weeks; during this time there is potential for either increased psychological vulnerability or personal growth

Memory Aid

A crisis cannot go on for extended periods; it lasts generally for 4 to 6 weeks.

! **B. Developmental phases of crisis**

1. Initial increase in tension as stimulus continues, and further discomfort is experienced

2. Failure to succeed in coping with stimulus while continuing to experience distress
3. Additional tension forces mobilization of internal and external resources directed at emergency problem-solving efforts; problem may be redefined or individual may resign himself or herself and give up certain aspects of a goal perceived to be unattainable
4. If problem remains unresolved and cannot be ignored, tension builds and major disorganization results

C. Characteristics of crisis

1. Stimulus is beyond client's usual experience
2. Previously developed coping mechanisms are ineffective
3. Anxiety, tension, and cognitive disorganization ensue
4. Client perceives threat to own integrity or established goals
5. ! Maturational crises involve normal life transitions that evoke changes in client's self-perception in role, status, and integrity

Memory Aid

Associate the term *maturational* with a crisis event that occurs as the client gets older.

6. ! Situational crises involve an external event that disturbs client's equilibrium (loss, change) and threatens consistency between self-behaviors and values or beliefs

Memory Aid

Associate the term *situational* with a crisis event that occurs unexpectedly to a single client.

7. ! Adventitious crises involve external events (such as natural disasters or other unpredictable catastrophic events) that are unpredictable and often engender fear, confusion, and loss of consistency with internalized beliefs or values and behavior; these may also be called community crises
8. Cultural crises accompany culture shock experienced by an individual adapting to a new culture or returning to his or her own culture after being assimilated into another culture

D. Balancing factors determining the client's response to crisis

1. The individual's perception of event
2. Past experience in coping with stress
3. Established coping strategies
4. Availability of support persons and other resources

Memory Aid

The better a client's coping strategies are in general, the better the client will be prepared to cope with a crisis.

E. Client goals for treatment

1. Remain free of self-harm
2. Identify specific problem
3. Verbalize feelings related to event
4. Analyze event or problem and express perceptions of it
5. Identify and seek help from support systems
6. Explore alternatives for coping with crisis
7. Participate in choosing an action plan
8. Implement an action plan
9. Experience less anxiety and tension
10. Verbalize enhanced self-esteem

II. NURSING PROCESS DURING CRISIS

A. Assessment

1. Identify history of presenting problem
   a. ! Focus on immediate problem, not on past history

   b. Determine client's perception of problem: how threatened is he or she?
   c. Assess client's cognitive appraisal; identify any faulty thinking
2. Identify current feelings
   a. Help client express current feelings
   b. Validate current feelings and help client to accept them
   c. Acknowledge that client ultimately makes own decisions
3. Assess coping mechanisms
4. Assess client's support systems
   a. Identify available resources in whom client trusts
   b. Identify spiritual and religious beliefs
5. Assess potential for self-harm
   a. Ask directly if client has had any thoughts of hurting or killing himself or herself; some clients engage in self-mutilation and do not want to die but do inflict self-harm, such as with razor blades or glass
   b. Use questions such as "Do you have thoughts of killing yourself?" and "Do you have thoughts of hurting yourself?"
   c. If the client has thought of harming or killing self, determine if client has made specific plans to accomplish this, which is a danger signal—the more specific the plan, the more likely it is that the client will carry it out
   d. Determine if client has means to harm or kill self (guns in house, access to medications with potential for overdose)
   e. Determine if client can contract with nurse to maintain safety; work with client to identify an action plan if suicidal ideation increases or client feels he or she will act on ideas to harm self

B. Planning and implementation for clients in crisis

1. Specific treatment modalities
   a. Mutual goal planning; often the nurse must use a directive approach
   b. Goals are set based on the assessment and nursing diagnoses
   c. Overarching goals include establishing relationship with client, identifying problem, identifying and reducing client's perceptual distortions, enhancing self-esteem, alleviating anxiety, promoting use of support systems (family and friends), reinforcing healthy coping, and validating client's ability to problem-solve
   d. Examine client's feelings that may block ability to cope adaptively
   e. Teach client how to ask for help from others
   f. Identify previously acquired adaptive coping strategies and help client modify and expand these coping strategies to new stress
   g. Teach and encourage use of expression of feelings, comfort strategies, and self-care activities
   h. Focus on problem resolution in a step-by-step, concrete way, first focusing on alternatives and then selecting and acting on appropriate ones

Memory Aid

Clients in crisis tend to be disorganized in their thinking. Use simple words and sentences, and give concrete, step-by-step instructions to facilitate effective communication.

   i. Consider involving client in a crisis group, which helps clients feel less isolated and engage in group problem solving to identify alternatives
   j. Involve family in crisis intervention because other members of family often experience crisis

C. Evaluation and outcomes for clients in crisis

1. Evaluation of outcomes is measured by comparing actual outcomes to goals of treatment and client response to nursing interventions
   a. The client will remain free of self-harm
   b. The client has clearly identified the problem
   c. Perceptual distortions have been identified and resolved
   d. The client verbalizes a stable sense of self-esteem and perceives ability to work on problem

e. Anxiety has been reduced by identification and implementation of effective coping strategies
f. Unhealthy coping mechanisms are identified and explored if client is willing
g. The client acknowledges his or her need for help and asks for help
h. The client identifies and verbalizes his or her feelings
i. The client demonstrates self-care behaviors
j. The client verbalizes an action plan
k. The client has begun to implement action plan

D. Potential for growth

1. Client identifies and practices new coping skills that may be useful in future in dealing with stressful and potentially traumatic events
2. Client verbalizes a renewed or enhanced sense of self-worth

III. PSYCHOPHARMACOLOGY AS TREATMENT DURING CRISIS

A. Treatment with pharmacologic interventions should not interfere with crisis intervention strategies such as crisis intervention

B. A crisis is not a psychiatric illness nor a prolonged condition; therefore, pharmacologic interventions are not interventions of choice

! **C. Pharmacologic agents may be used to treat target symptoms that interfere with client's ability to function but should *not* be used as a substitute for crisis intervention**

D. Anxiolytics such as alprazolam (Xanax), clonazepam (Klonopin), diazepam (Valium), and lorazepam (Ativan), may be used to treat anxiety, panic, and sleep disturbances that accompany a crisis; short term use is encouraged because of risk of dependence

E. Other agents, such as Zolpidem (Ambien) and Zaleplon (Sonata), may be used to manage insomnia

F. Neuroleptic medications: the atypicals, such as olanzapine (Zyprexa), risperidone (Risperdal), quetiapine (Seroquel), and typical agents such as haloperidol (Haldol), may be used to treat psychotic symptoms that emerge; however, psychosis does not commonly follow experience of a crisis unless client has a preexisting psychotic disorder

IV. ANGER AND AGGESSION

A. Assessment of other-directed violence

1. Violence is frequently, although not always, preceded by specific behaviors
   a. Increased activity or hyperactivity such as restlessness or pacing behaviors
   b. Verbal abuse, instigation of arguments, and use of profanity
   c. Change in amount of eye contact (greater or lesser)
   d. Visible signs of tension such as clenched fists or jaws, rigid facial expression or posture, talking or muttering to self
   e. Change in voice such as louder or softer, and possibly either faster or slower rate of speech
2. Key risk factors include a history of violent behavior and impulsivity on part of client
3. Precipitating events for violence in in-patient settings often include staff factors such as inexperience, controlling behavior, inability to set effective limits, and indiscriminate removal of unit privileges

B. Planning and implementation to deescalate violent client

1. Remain calm
2. Maintain client dignity and self-esteem
3. Identify client stressors and indications of stress presented by client
4. Assess what the client considers to be his or her need
5. ! Use calm and clear tone of voice and nonaggressive body posture
6. ! Keep large personal space between self and client and assess for personal safety; always stay positioned facing the client with an escape route to the back
7. Provide several options to client
8. Remain goal-oriented and avoid arguing with client
9. Use stepwise progression of interventions from least restrictive to more restrictive, according to client's behavior
10. ! Use time-outs when appropriate

11. Use seclusion and restraints as a last option when other interventions have failed; use least amount of restraint that is effective; if physical restraints are used, check circulation every 30 minutes and release one at a time every 2 hours and provide range of motion
12. Administer medications according to order or protocol
13. Provide debriefing session for staff to ventilate feelings immediately after event in which violence has occurred

C. Evaluation

1. Client is able to control own behavior
2. The safety of client, other clients, and staff is maintained

V. OVERVIEW OF SUICIDE

A. *Suicide:* intentionally and voluntarily taking one's life

B. Suicide is 11th leading cause of death among all age groups and third leading cause of death in those age 10 through adolescence (Boyd, 2005)

1. Whites are more likely than nonwhites to die from suicide
2. Men are three to four times more likely than women to commit suicide, and elderly are four times more likely than younger people to kill themselves
3. Gay teens are at increased risk of suicide

C. Adolescent and young adult suicide: suicide is third leading cause of death in adolescents and second-most common cause of death in college students; in past 25 years there has been a 25% increase in suicides among adolescents

D. Clients contemplating suicide often perceive themselves as isolated through physical distance or interpersonal discord; they often experience feelings of helplessness, loss of self-esteem with feelings of worthlessness, and hopelessness, the latter being most predictive of suicide

E. Often a desire to be free from pain or to be dead is accompanied by depression and anger

F. Warning signs that may indicate risk for suicidal ideations and self-injurious behavior include changes in personal habits such as appetite, sleep patterns, personal appearance, personality, use of alcohol and other drugs, as well as bodily complaints, self-deprecating comments, making wills, and giving away personal belongings

G. Academic and occupational warning signs include truancy and absenteeism, decline in academic or occupational performance, boredom, apathy, disruptive classroom or work behavior, and anger and hostility toward authority figures

H. Family and social relationship warning signs include decreased interactions with peers and friends; a change in people with whom client spends time, and either a decrease in or absence of romantic relationships

Memory Aid

Do not ignore warning signs of suicide; take action to further assess and intervene immediately, seeking help from other health care professionals as well.

I. The single-most predictive psychiatric disorder for suicide is presence of a mood disorder

J. Common myths of suicide

1. People who talk about suicide won't actually commit suicide
2. People who are serious about suicide will show warning signs or give clues
3. Young children do not commit suicide
4. An improvement in mood means risk for suicide is over
5. Only people who are depressed commit suicide
6. A written or verbal safety contract is a guarantee that client will not kill himself or herself

K. Conscious and unconscious suicidal intention

1. Conscious suicidal ideations include an awareness of client of potential outcomes or results of suicidal behavior, awareness of others' response to suicidal threats or attempts, awareness of lethality index of a chosen method, and awareness of rescue possibilities
2. Unconscious suicidal ideation may be more difficult to assess
   a. The desire to cause self-harm or self-destruction may be beyond client's conscious awareness

b. The client may engage in high-risk behaviors as a way of acting out unconscious desire to harm themselves (e.g., drinking and driving and engaging in potentially lethal activity)

c. Careful attention must be paid to direct and indirect ways in which client may be communicating unconscious suicidal ideations

VI. NURSING PROCESS FOR SUICIDAL CLIENTS

A. Suicide assessment

! 1. During initial assessment, question client about any thoughts or feelings related to harming or killing himself or herself; assessment includes determining suicidal ideations, how client has sought help, what kind of plan client has made and client's mental status, available support systems, and lifestyle

a. Ask questions like, "Have you had any thoughts about life not being worth living?"

b. Move from general to specific questions like, "Have you had any ideas about killing yourself?"

c. It is a false assumption that client will volunteer this information without being asked

d. The nurse must be comfortable asking these questions directly and in a matter-of-fact way

e. If client answers yes, ask client, "Have you thought of, or made any plans for, how you might harm or kill yourself?" (passive suicidal ideation is the presence of suicidal thoughts without a plan, in contrast to suicidal ideation with a plan)

f. Levels of lethality may be assessed, in part, based on answers to these questions; further assessment includes asking about access to means to self-harm, (e.g., do you have a gun in your home? Do you know how to use it?) and evaluating lethality of means (e.g., guns vs. pills)

g. Take a careful history of previous self-harming behaviors by asking client such questions as, "Have you ever tried to harm or kill yourself in the past?"

h. Assess also use of alcohol, drugs, and level of impulsivity

i. Complete a mental status assessment to determine such things as evidence of alterations in thought process, impulsiveness, perceptual distortions, insight, and judgment

j. Inquire about currently available support systems

2. Many people experience ambivalence about committing suicide; assessment of these ambivalent feelings is an important role of the nurse

3. Initially, clients may lack emotional or psychic energy to act on suicidal ideations as a result of some of negative or neurovegetative symptoms they experience

! 4. The nurse must be aware that a sudden sense of peace or wellness reported by client may indicate that client has sufficient psychic energy to carry out a suicidal act; this risk increases as client stabilizes on antidepressant medications

B. Goals for clients at risk for suicide

1. Remain safe and free of self-harm

2. Verbalize suicidal ideations and discuss these with nursing staff

! 3. Develop a safety plan with nursing staff and other members of treatment team that identifies steps to keep himself or herself safe, and ask for help before acting out a suicidal or self-harm thought

4. Verbalize a decrease in or absence of suicidal ideations

5. Verbalize a desire to live and reasons for living

! 6. Identify an aftercare plan following discharge from hospital that includes a commitment to follow up with psychotherapy and adherence to psychopharmacologic interventions

7. Identify a support system outside hospital

C. Nursing interventions to reduce risk of suicide (self-directed violence)

1. Inpatient treatment is indicated if client is felt to be at high risk for self-directed or other-directed violence

2. Inpatient interventions include providing a safe milieu in which client's ability to act out on suicidal ideations or other-directed violence is minimized

a. While client may be admitted to milieu voluntarily, unit is self-contained and doors are commonly locked; nursing staff regulate flow of traffic on and off unit

! b. Depending on degree of suicidal ideation and lethality assessed, place client on constant observation for first 24 hours or until degree of suicidal risk is lessened according to agency policy

! c. Place client on every-15-minute checks or every-30-minute thereafter, depending on agency policy

d. Maintain an awareness of client's whereabouts constantly

e. Develop rapport and foster a therapeutic relationship with client

f. On admission to unit, assess client's personal belongings and remove any items that could be used by client to harm himself or herself or others (drugs, potentially sharp objects, cords, shoelaces, belts, neck ties, lighters) and keep them in a safe place

! g. Keep unit free of materials that can be readily used by clients to harm themselves or others (e.g., metal or glass objects that may be altered to create a sharp edge, shoelaces, belts, electrical or call bell cords); keep windows locked and count silverware; check gifts and other items brought in by family members or friends for safety before they are given to client; let family members place belongings in locker before entering unit; scan all visitors with a metal detector prior to entering unit

Memory Aid

When a client is at risk for self-directed or other-directed violence, select answers to test questions that protect the safety of all: the client, other clients, and staff.

h. Work with client to develop a safety plan, and assess client frequently

i. Meet one on one with client to explore client's feelings and help client work toward re-engagement with significant others and fulfilling life activities

! j. Give suicidal client a roommate to reduce opportunity for solitude

k. Make sure that client swallows oral medications and is not holding medication in oral cavity (cheeking) to hoard for a later overdose

! l. Work with client's participation to identify an aftercare plan that includes a commitment on client's part to attend aftercare appointments, maintain contact with social support systems, and identify a safety plan with emergency contact numbers and an action plan should suicidal ideations return

m. Realize that despite use of all proper precautions, a client may still take own life after hospitalization (if unable to do so during); an ultimate decision to live belongs with client

n. Initiate debriefing session for staff members after client's suicide or any violent behavior to provide forum for staff to ventilate feelings

! **D. Evaluation and outcomes for clients comtemplating suicide; the client will:**

1. Remain safe and free from self-directed violence
2. Verbalize absence or decreased intensity and severity of suicidal ideations, with absence of plan and intent
3. Verbalize a desire to live and state several reasons for living
4. Agree to maintain a no-self-harm contract with nursing staff and other treatment staff for specified periods of time
5. Identify a safety plan that provides for asking for help before acting out should suicidal ideations worsen, intent reemerge, or unsafe feelings occur
6. Meet other goals incorporated in treatment plan relative to other problems identified

VII. PSYCHOPHARMACOLOGY AS TREATMENT TO PREVENT SUICIDE

A. Pharmacologic interventions used in presence of suicidal ideations are aimed at treating underlying mood disorder, other psychiatric disorder, or coexisting psychiatric disorders; see Chapter 36 for detailed information on these medications

B. Since there is a high correlation between mood disorders and suicide, adequate treatment of these mood disorders is essential in the overall treatment of clients at risk for suicide

C. Depressive disorders are treated with antidepressants

! **D. Because of relatively low risk of lethal overdose and relatively low side-effect profiles with use of selective serotonin reuptake inhibitors (SSRIs), these agents are often first-line drugs to treat depression that could lead to suicide**

1. Citalopram (Celexa)
2. Paroxetine (Paxil)
3. Fluoxetine (Prozac)
4. Sertraline (Zoloft)
5. Escitalopram (Lexapro)

! **E. While effective in treatment of depression, tricyclic antidepressants can be highly lethal in overdose and are not a first-line agent; when used, quantity dispensed at any one time should be kept at a minimum and may need to be managed by a family member; the tricyclics are:**

1. Amitriptyline (Elavil)
2. Clomipramine (Anafranil)
3. Desipramine (Norpramin)
4. Doxepin (Sinequan)
5. Imipramine (Tofranil)
6. Nortriptyline (Pamelor)
7. Trimipramine (Surmontil)

F. Other agents such as tetracyclics and atypical antidepressants are also helpful in treating depressive disorders and include:

1. Bupropion (Wellbutrin)
2. Nefazadone (Serzone)
3. Trazadone (Desyrel)
4. Venlafaxine (Effexor)
5. Mirtazipine (Remeron)
6. Duloxetine (Cymbalta)

! **G. Monoamine oxidase inhibitors (MAOIs) are useful occassionally in treating depressive disorders; however, serious drug and food interactions make these agents particularly challenging; they can be used if clients will comply with a tyramine-free diet (noncompliance can lead to hypertensive crisis); they are:**

1. Tranylcypromine (Parnate)
2. Phenelzine (Nardil)
3. Isocarboxazid (Marplan)

H. Bipolar disorders: characterized by cycling of moods with episodes of mania and depression and are also associated with suicide

1. They are treated with a class of drugs known as mood stabilizers:
   - **a.** Lithium
   - **b.** Valproic acid (Depakote)
   - **c.** Carbamazepine (Tegretol), lamotrigine (Lamictal), gabapentin (Neurontin) and topiramate (Topamax) as antiepileptic drugs
   - **d.** Olanzapine (Zyprexa), an atypical antipsychotic, which is associated with increased risk of metabolic syndrome

I. Clients with other psychiatric disorders are also at risk for suicide and may be treated with anxiolytics, neuroleptics, and other psychotropic agents

1. Any psychotropic medication can be dangerous in overdose, so a careful assessment must be made with proper client and family teaching about each drug (see Section III, Psychopharmacology as Treatment during Crisis)
2. Recall that clients may be at increased risk of suicide once medication takes effect and client has sufficient energy to act on suicide plan; assess client carefully and provide protective measures as needed

Check Your NCLEX-RN® Exam I.Q. *You are ready for testing on this content if you can:*

- Assess a client's coping mechanisms.
- Help a client to utilize and enhance coping mechanisms.
- Assess a client experiencing a crisis.
- Help a client to process the experience of a crisis.
- Explore social supports to aid a client in recovery from a crisis.
- Assess a client's risk of self-harm.
- Provide care to reduce the client's risk of harm to self or others.

PRACTICE TEST

1 When conducting an admission evaluation or an assessment of the client within the unit for the potential for violent or aggressive behavior, it is important for the nurse to

1. reassure the client that everything will be all right, and the staff will make sure nothing untoward happens.
2. reinforce that the client is solely responsible for his or her own actions and will experience the consequences of acting out.
3. explain that violence is not acceptable, and the staff will not allow the client to act out.
4. reassure the client that limited acting out will be allowed but only in a controlled setting.

2 When responding to clients who display the potential for violence, the nurse would use which of the following as the most restrictive intervention?

1. Meeting in a quiet room to reduce stimulation
2. Administering a PRN medication to reduce anxiety
3. Providing physical interventions, such as two-person escort out of a program area
4. Using restraints, such as a four-point restraint

3 Which of the following is the most important intervention by the nurse when a client does not respond to less restrictive interventions and is rapidly escalating toward violence?

1. Cease negotiation with client and implement plan of intervention to control client and provide safety.
2. Bargain with client to determine what can be done to prevent assaultive behavior.
3. Offer a PRN medication to reduce anxiety.
4. Ask client to move to a less stimulating, private area and spend some time alone.

4 After a staff member has been involved in a particularly violent episode with a client, debriefing should

1. occur after the staff has had the opportunity to calm.
2. take place immediately to facilitate processing of feelings.
3. not occur until the staff requests such intervention.
4. be done after a 3-day time-off period.

5 Which one of the following situations experienced by a client would the nurse document as a situational crisis?

1. Being in the middle of menopause
2. Recently being involved in an automobile accident
3. Being a survivor of a flood following a hurricane
4. Recently returning home from military duty after an armed conflict

6 Which of the following coping behaviors does the nurse expect to note in a client who encounters a situation in which there is a significant psychological threat and great personal vulnerability?

1. Finding inner strength to get through the crisis
2. Being more oriented toward mastery
3. Acting in a more self-protective manner
4. Being totally immobilized

7. A nurse is planning an intervention for a client in crisis who witnessed a violent crime. Which of the following is a key component of crisis intervention that the nurse should plan to utilize at this time?

1. Identify the client's maladaptive coping mechanisms.
2. Identify and support the client's coping patterns.
3. Assist the client in forgetting the crisis situation.
4. Teach the client to handle future crises.

8. The nurse developing a care plan for a client using crisis management principles would base interventions on which of the following primary tasks of crisis management?

1. Provide support.
2. Relieve anxiety.
3. Provide encouragement.
4. Foster independence.

9. An adult client is having difficulty coping with a new diagnosis of colon cancer. The nurse telephones the physician for an order for medication therapy to assist the client in coping with this crisis situation. The nurse anticipates an order for which of the following types of medication?

1. Haloperidol (Haldol)
2. Amitriptyline (Elavi)
3. Lorazepam (Ativan)
4. Valproic acid (Depakote)

10. The nurse working with the family of a client with suicidal ideations is asked if the medication the client is taking will prevent suicide. Which of the following would be the best response by the nurse?

1. "Clients who take their medication as prescribed are at decreased risk for suicide."
2. "Medication helps to treat an underlying mood disorder associated with suicidal thinking and therefore prevents suicide."
3. "Medication helps decrease the frequency and intensity of suicidal thoughts."
4. "The client has said that she would never try to hurt herself again; therefore, there is no need to worry."

11. A suicidal client with low self-esteem seems less lethargic today and agrees to participate in an occupational therapy program. To help make the session successful, the nurse should do which of the following?

1. Introduce the client to wood carving; show him how to safely use the carving and burning tools.
2. Stay away from the client in occupational therapy so that he is free to express himself.
3. Teach the client to macrame a plant hanger from jute rope and encourage him to work on it later in his room.
4. Structure his activity to help him complete one simple task, such as painting a picture.

12. A client has recently been admitted for depression and suicidal ideations with a plan to hang himself. The nurse assesses the client most carefully for risk for attempting suicide when

1. he is mute and unlikely to tell anyone.
2. he is ready to go home and afraid of leaving the hospital.
3. his family goes on vacation.
4. he begins to demonstrate clinical improvement.

13. Which of the following individuals is at greatest risk for suicide?

1. A 65-year-old African American male
2. A 70-year-old European American male
3. A 30-year-old Hispanic American female
4. A 16-year-old African American female

14. A client states that voices are telling him to hang himself. The nurse documents that the client is at risk for suicide on the basis of which of the following?

1. An intractable sense of hopelessness
2. Intolerable emotional pain
3. Delusions of grandeur
4. Command hallucinations

15 Which statement made by a client would indicate the highest risk for suicide?

1. "I know you've been worried about me. You won't have to worry too much longer."
2. "I think I've found a solution to my problem. I'm going to check it out with my doctor."
3. "I'm looking forward to the holiday season and the kids coming home from school. They will be a good distraction."
4. "Over the past week I have been hearing the voices that tell me to hurt myself less often."

16 A client who became violent on the psychiatric unit had restraints applied at 10:00. The nurse makes a note to release the restraint at no later than which of the following times?

1. 10:15
2. 11:00
3. 12:00
4. 14:00

17 A female client has been admitted to the psychiatric unit after spending 24 hours in the intensive care unit. Before the client's admission, she overdosed on 12 sertraline (Zoloft) tablets. Of the following nursing goals, which would be a priority on admission?

1. Assuring the client that someone is concerned about her
2. Protecting the client until she can protect herself
3. Teaching the client how to solve problems
4. Discussing the meaning of death

18 When interviewing a potentially violent or aggressive client, which of the following environmental factors is *most* important for the nurse to consider?

1. The interview should take place in a calm and quiet area to reduce stimuli.
2. Care should be taken to make sure that other staff do not interrupt.
3. Restraint devices should be in full view of the client to reinforce consequences for violent behavior.
4. The client should be told that violent behavior will not be tolerated.

19 A new nurse orientee asks why a client admitted to the psychiatric unit has been placed in seclusion. The nurse who is precepting the orientee explains that which of the following is a benefit of seclusion?

1. The reduced sensory input allows the client to regain control.
2. The unit can be managed with fewer staff.
3. Clients are encouraged to communicate with others.
4. Clients are forced to be responsible for themselves.

20 A 19-year-old female client recently admitted after attempting suicide becomes very dejected and states that life is not meaningful and no one really cares what happens to her. The nurse's best response would be which of the following?

1. "Of course people care. Your parents stayed with you in the ICU."
2. "Let's not talk about sad things. Why don't we go for a walk?"
3. "Can you write down a list of who does not care for you?"
4. "I care about you, and I am concerned that you feel so down."

21 The nurse has been working with a teenage female client who was in crisis after she was assaulted and robbed late one night when leaving a local mall at closing time. Which of the following outcomes indicates to the nurse that the client has achieved the expected outcomes of treatment? Select all that apply.

1. The client can talk about the incident without excessive distress.
2. The client states she will never shop at the mall again.
3. The client states a plan to choose parking spaces that are close to building entrances when possible.
4. The client is enrolling in a local self-defense class for women.
5. The client states she will go shopping only when she has someone available to accompany her.

ANSWERS & RATIONALES

1 **Answer: 2** Clients need to have communicated to them that they are in control of their own behaviors and that "acting out" will result in consequences. Reassuring the client that the staff will make sure nothing happens (option 1) takes away responsibility from the client. Just explaining that violence is unacceptable and not explaining to the client that he or she is in control (option 3) is nontherapeutic. Acting out is usually not allowed (option 4) because of safety of client and others.

Cognitive Level: Application **Client Need:** Psychosocial Integrity **Integrated Process:** Nursing Process: Implementation **Content Area:** Psychiatric-Mental Health **Strategy:** The core issue of the question is effective communication with a client at risk for acting out. Use the process of elimination and choose the option that provides accurate information to the client and holds the client accountable for his or her actions.

2 **Answer: 4** Preventing a client from free mobility is the most restrictive technique. Meeting in a quiet room (option 1) is the least restrictive and most therapeutic. Chemical restraint (option 2) and escorting a client (option 3) are restrictive but less so than full four-point restraint.

Cognitive Level: Analysis **Client Need:** Psychosocial Integrity **Integrated Process:** Nursing Process: Implementation **Content Area:** Psychiatric-Mental Health **Strategy:** Note the critical word *most* in the stem of the question. This tells you that you must order the interventions presented from least restrictive to most restrictive to enable you to choose correctly.

3 **Answer: 1** Once a client has escalated beyond least restrictive interventions, the nurse should plan for the next step. Bargaining (option 2) with a client is counterproductive and positively reinforces behavior. Offering a PRN medication (option 3) to reduce anxiety would occur after negotiation for least restrictive interventions is complete. Asking a client to take a time out (option 4) is a least restrictive intervention to which the client is not responding.

Cognitive Level: Application **Client Need:** Psychosocial Integrity **Integrated Process:** Nursing Process: Implementation **Content Area:** Psychiatric-Mental Health **Strategy:** The wording of the question tells you that more than one option may be partially or totally correct and that you must prioritize your answer. Choose the option that best protects the safety of all people in the environment, including other clients and staff.

4 **Answer: 2** Debriefing allows the staff an opportunity to ventilate feelings and to calm down (option 1). It should always occur, and all staff should be encouraged to participate (option 3). Debriefing following a violent episode should occur as soon as possible after the client and others are safe (option 4).

Cognitive Level: Application **Client Need:** Psychosocial Integrity **Integrated Process:** Nursing Process: Evaluation **Content Area:** Psychiatric-Mental Health **Strategy:** The core issue of the question is the need for staff to process personal feelings after an episode of violence occurs with a client. Use the process of elimination and knowledge that staff can be traumatized by these events to choose the correct option.

5 **Answer: 2** A situational crisis is one that occurs from external life events. An event involving normal stages of development (option 1) is a maturation crisis. A natural disaster (option 3) and an armed conflict (option 4) are examples of community crises.

Cognitive Level: Analysis **Client Need:** Psychosocial Integrity **Integrated Process:** Nursing Process: Assessment **Content Area:** Psychiatric-Mental Health **Strategy:** Use the process of elimination. The core issue of the question is the ability to differentiate among various types of crises and to document them appropriately.

6 **Answer: 3** When a person is threatened and perceives himself or herself to be vulnerable to a situation, coping behaviors are self-protective. Coping behaviors may be ineffective to provide strength (option 1). Coping during a crisis is oriented toward the immediate here-and-now, not mastery (option 2). Coping behaviors may or may not be immobilized (option 4).

Cognitive Level: Application **Client Need:** Psychosocial Integrity **Integrated Process:** Nursing Process: Analysis **Content Area:** Psychiatric-Mental Health **Strategy:** The core issue of the question is the expected response of a client to a threatening situation. Use knowledge of coping skills and the process of elimination to find the correct answer.

7 **Answer: 2** Assisting the client in identifying coping patterns and then supporting them is essential to managing a crisis. Identifying the client's maladaptive coping mechanisms (option 1) may be beneficial after identifying the client's strengths. Assisting the client to forget (option 3) is not a therapeutic intervention for crisis management. Teaching a client to handle future crises (option 4) is more appropriate once the current crisis has abated.

Cognitive Level: Application **Client Need:** Psychosocial Integrity **Integrated Process:** Nursing Process: Implementation **Content Area:** Psychiatric-Mental Health **Strategy:** The critical words in the question are *at this time*. This tells you that more than one option may be correct, but one of them is more timely than the others. Use nursing knowledge and the process of elimination to make a selection.

8 **Answer: 1** Providing support and guidance are the primary objectives of crisis management. The client's anxiety (option 2) may be needed in order for him or her to be energized to cope with the crisis; the goal is to achieve a manageable level of anxiety. Providing encouragement (option 3) and fostering independence (option 4) are important and may occur during crisis intervention, but they are not the primary task of crisis management.

Cognitive Level: Application **Client Need:** Psychosocial Integrity **Integrated Process:** Nursing Process: Planning **Content Area:** Psychiatric-Mental Health **Strategy:** The critical word in the question is *primary*. This tells you that more than one option may be correct, but one of them is more important than the others. Use nursing knowledge and the process of elimination to make a selection.

9 **Answer: 3** Short-acting antianxiety agents are most useful in helping a client to achieve an effective reduction in level of anxiety. Antipsychotics (option 1) should be avoided. Antidepressants (option 3) require some time to achieve therapeutic levels and are not useful in a crisis situation. Mood stabilizers (option 4) are not indicated.

Cognitive Level: Application **Client Need:** Psychosocial Integrity **Integrated Process:** Nursing Process: Analysis **Content Area:** Psychiatric-Mental Health **Strategy:** The critical words in the question are *crisis situation,* which tell you that the correct answer is a medication that will have a rapid onset of action and be effective in treating the client's reaction to the diagnosis of colon cancer. Use nursing knowledge and the process of elimination to make a selection.

10 **Answer: 3** Medications will help decrease the frequency and intensity of suicidal thoughts. Medication may treat the underlying cause of the suicidal ideation but does not necessarily reduce the risk for completing suicide. Medication does not prevent suicide; in fact, many times when clients regain their energy from medications, they are at an increased risk for completing suicide (options 1 and 2). A client may not be currently suicidal, but medications do not assure that they will not be suicidal in the future (option 4).
Cognitive Level: Application **Client Need:** Psychosocial Integrity **Integrated Process:** Communication and Documentation **Content Area:** Psychiatric-Mental Health **Strategy:** The critical word in the question is *best*. This tells you that more than one option may be partially correct, but one of them is better than the others. Use nursing knowledge and the process of elimination to make a selection.

11 **Answer: 4** A client who is just regaining his or her energy should be encouraged to do simple tasks, which will also promote the client's self-esteem. Suicidal clients are most at danger when they are feeling better and regaining their energy. Introducing the client to wood carving (option 1) and making a belt from rope (option 3) place the client at risk for self-harm. The nurse should encourage the client participate in the occupational therapy for self-expression (option 2).
Cognitive Level: Analysis **Client Need:** Psychosocial Integrity **Integrated Process:** Nursing Process: Implementation **Content Area:** Psychiatric-Mental Health **Strategy:** The core issue of the question is a safe activity for a client who is suicidal. The correct answer is the option that does not pose risk to the client or provide the client with the means to engage in self-harm.

12 **Answer: 4** Suicidal clients are at most risk when they begin to demonstrate improvement and have the energy to carry out suicide. A mute client who is not willing to share with others (option 1) is at risk for suicide but may be placed on constant observation. Being afraid to go home (option 2) may be a positive sign that the client is aware of the danger he may pose to himself. Vacation is a stressful time, and being left alone (option 3) would place the client at risk; however, it is well documented that clients are at greatest risk when showing signs of improvement.
Cognitive Level: Application **Client Need:** Psychosocial Integrity **Integrated Process:** Nursing Process: Planning **Content Area:** Psychiatric-Mental Health **Strategy:** The core issue of the question is recognition that the risk of suicide increases when a client begins to feel better, since the client now may have the energy to carry out a suicide attempt. Use the process of elimination and this knowledge to make a selection. The wording of the question tells you that only one answer is correct.

13 **Answer: 2** The group at highest risk for successfully completing suicide attempts are European American males over the age of 50 (white, male, older adult). The clients in options 1, 3, and 4 are not in high-risk groups.
Cognitive Level: Analysis **Client Need:** Psychosocial Integrity **Integrated Process:** Nursing Process: Assessment **Content Area:** Psychiatric-Mental Health **Strategy:** The core issue of the question is knowledge of high-risk groups for suicide. The wording of the question tells you only one answer is correct. Use nursing knowledge and the process of elimination to make a selection.

14 **Answer: 4** Voices telling a client to hurt himself or others are called command hallucinations. There is not enough data to support hopelessness (option 1), emotional pain (option 2), or delusions of grandeur (option 3).
Cognitive Level: Application **Client Need:** Psychosocial Integrity **Integrated Process:** Communication and Documentation **Content Area:** Psychiatric-Mental Health **Strategy:** The core issue of the question is correct interpretation of a client's symptoms. The wording of the question tells you only one answer is correct. Use nursing knowledge and the process of elimination to make a selection.

15 **Answer: 1** The client is communicating that he or she may not be around for the nurse to worry about. Creating a solution (option 2), expressing hope for the future and making plans (options 3), and decreasing frequency of voices (option 4) indicate that the client is experiencing a reduction in the risk for suicide.
Cognitive Level: Analysis **Client Need:** Psychosocial Integrity **Integrated Process:** Nursing Process: Evaluation **Content Area:** Psychiatric-Mental Health **Strategy:** The critical words in the stem of the question is *highest risk*. This tells you that more than one option may indicate risk, but one is stronger than the others. Use nursing knowledge and the process of elimination to make a selection.

16 **Answer: 3** Releasing restraints at least every 2 hours is a standard of care to prevent physical harm. Every 15 minutes (option 1) or hour (option 2) may be too often, and every 4 hours (option 4) is too long and may cause the client injury. In addition to the intervention described, the client's circulation should be checked every 30 minutes. Ensuring the client's safety and well-being are a priority.
Cognitive Level: Application **Client Need:** Safe Effective Care Environment: Safety and Infection Control **Integrated Process:** Nursing Process: Planning **Content Area:** Psychiatric-Mental Health **Strategy:** The core issue of the question is knowledge of safe care to a client who is in restraints. Use the process of elimination and nursing knowledge to make a selection, recalling that 30-minute circulation checks and 2-hour release times are standards of care.

17 **Answer: 2** Safety of the client is always a priority for clients who have recently attempted suicide. Options 1, 3, and 4 are all appropriate goals after safety has been assured.
Cognitive Level: Analysis **Client Need:** Psychosocial Integrity **Integrated Process:** Nursing Process: Planning **Content Area:** Psychiatric-Mental Health **Strategy:** The critical word in the stem of the question is *priority*. This tells you that more than one or all options may be correct actions for the client, but one is more important than the others. To aid in making a selection, recall that safety needs are high priority for clients following a suicide attempt.

18 **Answer: 1** The nurse should ensure that the interview be conducted in a quiet environment. Interruption should be kept to a minimum (option 2), but may not be possible to prevent. Intimidation of the client (options 3 and 4) is inappropriate.
Cognitive Level: Application **Client Need:** Psychosocial Integrity **Integrated Process:** Nursing Process: Implementation **Content**

Area: Psychiatric-Mental Health **Strategy:** The critical words in the stem of the question are *most important.* This is a clue that more than one option may be partially or totally correct, but one is more important than the others. Use nursing knowledge and the process of elimination to make a selection.

19 **Answer: 1** Decreasing sensory input may decrease the anxiety or anger and help the client regain control. Seclusion should never be used for staffing ratios (option 2). Communication with others (option 3) is part of milieu therapy. Seclusion takes away the client's responsibility temporarily (option 4).
Cognitive Level: Application **Client Need:** Psychosocial Integrity **Integrated Process:** Nursing Process: Implementation **Content Area:** Psychiatric-Mental Health **Strategy:** The core issue of the question is the benefit of seclusion as a therapy for a potentially violent client. Use nursing knowledge and the process of elimination to make a selection.

20 **Answer: 4** Option 4 provides the client with information that the nurse is concerned about her, which may ease her emotional pain. Telling the client, "Of course people care" (option 1) is false reassurance. Telling the client not to talk about sad things (option 2) invalidates and ignores the client's feelings. Option 3 may be seeking clarification but may also cause the client to feel she has to defend her position.
Cognitive Level: Analysis **Client Need:** Psychosocial Integrity **Integrated Process:** Communication and Documentation **Content Area:** Psychiatric-Mental Health **Strategy:** The core issue of the question is a therapeutic communication technique to use with a client who attempted suicide and is experiencing emotional pain. Use knowledge of therapeutic communication techniques and the process of elimination to make a selection.

21 **Answer: 1, 3, 4** The client demonstrates effective coping by being able to discuss the incident without excessive distress and formulating a realistic plan to prevent recurrence, which will reduce anxiety (parking closer to buildings and enrolling in self-defense classes). If the client states she will never shop at the mall again, or will go shopping only when accompanied, this shows unresolved anxiety and a nonadaptive approach that is likely to interfere with her lifestyle.
Cognitive Level: Analysis **Client Need:** Psychosocial Integrity **Integrated Process:** Nursing Process: Evaluation **Content Area:** Psychiatric Mental Health **Strategy:** The core issue of the question is knowledge of adaptive responses to crisis or near-crisis situations. Choose the options that demonstrate adequate coping, which are ones that are neither insufficient nor extreme in tone.

ANSWERS & RATIONALES

Key Terms to Review

coping p. 366
crisis p. 366
equilibrium p. 366
helplessness p. 366
hopelessness p. 366
suicide p. 370

References

Boyd, M. (2005). *Psychiatric nursing: Contemporary practice* (3rd ed). Philadelphia: Lippincott Williams & Wilkins.

Fontaine, K., & Fletcher, J. (2003). *Mental health nursing* (4th ed.). Upper Saddle River, NJ: Pearson Education.

Fortinash, K., & Holoday-Worret, P. (2004). *Psychiatric-mental health nursing* (4th ed.). St. Louis: Mosby.

Kniesl, C., Wilson, H., & Trigoboff, E. (2004). *Contemporary psychiatric-mental health nursing.* Upper Saddle River, NJ: Pearson Education.

Stuart, G., & Laraia, M. (2004). *Principles and practice of psychiatric nursing* (8th ed.). St. Louis: Elsevier Science.

Varcarolis, E. (2006). *Foundations of psychiatric mental health nursing: A clinical approach* (5th ed.). Philadelphia: W.B. Saunders.

25 End of Life Care

Test Yourself

Are you ready for the NCLEX-RN® or course exams? Use the practice tests on the companion CD-ROM to check.

In this chapter

Cross reference

Other chapters related to this content are:

Coping with Stressors — Chapter 21

I. GENERAL NEEDS NEAR END OF LIFE

A. There is no typical death

B. Quality end of life

1. Positive experience for client and family with accomplishment of personal goals, even with suffering and loss
2. Caregiver-led client advocacy with a meaningful and dignified death

! **C. Core principles guiding clinical policy and professional practice for end-of-life care**

1. Respect dignity of both client and caregivers
2. Be sensitive to and respectful of client's and family's wishes
3. Use most appropriate measures that are consistent with client's choices
4. Make alleviation of pain and other physical symptoms a high priority
5. Assess and manage psychological, social, and spiritual or religious problems
6. Offer continuity (client should be able to continue to be cared for, if so desired, by his or her primary care and specialist providers)
7. Provide access to any therapy that may realistically be expected to improve client's quality of life, including alternative or nontraditional treatments; ensure clients are not abandoned because of their choice
8. Provide access to palliative care and hospice care
9. Respect right to refuse treatment, as expressed by client or authorized surrogate
10. Respect physician's professional judgment and recommendations with consideration for both client and family preferences
11. Recognize that dying is a profoundly personal experience and part of life cycle
12. Encourage health care professionals to help ensure that their care environment provides quality care and accountability for performance
13. Promote clinical and evidence-based research on providing care at end of life

D. Issues of policy, ethics, and law

1. Ethical issues are influenced by personal values, religion, and culture
2. The principles of autonomy, privacy, and **veracity** are fundamental to nursing practice; veracity is determination to be truthful

3. **Beneficence, nonmaleficence,** and **justice** are basic ethical principles for end-of-life care; beneficence is ethical principle of doing good; nonmaleficence means "first, do no harm"; and justice is being fair
4. Client preferences or **advance directives (AD)** are based on the 1990 Client Self-Determination Act that directs agencies receiving Medicare and Medicaid to provide information about ADs; ADs allow clients to make decisions in advance about end-of-life care should they become unable to communicate their desires
5. **Euthanasia** is a controversial intervention that offers a deliberate end to life for persons with a terminal illness or intolerable suffering; the Code for Nurses and American Nurses Association's position statements state that nurses should not participate in euthanasia
6. A decision to withdraw food and fluids allows disease to progress to its natural end
7. Discontinuing life support is a difficult decision for health care providers because they have been educated to support life in all situations
8. Professional standards and guidelines have been developed and approved by American Nurses Association, the Hospice and Palliative Nurses Association, and National Hospice and Palliative Care Organization to guide end-of-life practices
9. Confidentiality allows client to feel secure that he or she can safely discuss sensitive matters regarding health care without fearing disclosure

II. PHYSIOLOGICAL CARE NEAR END OF LIFE

A. *Palliative care* focuses on assessing and treating symptoms while evaluating whether to deal with cause; palliative care is care of client whose disease is no longer responsive to curative treatment

B. Symptom management is important at end of life; nurses should focus on interventions that promote client advocacy, assessment of needs, pharmacologic and nonpharmacologic treatments, and client and family education

! 1. Fatigue
   - a. A subjective symptom that may be caused by the disease or may be psychological and/or treatment related
   - b. Treatment of disease-related causes, such as anemia, may alleviate fatigue
   - c. Fatigue may not be relieved by frequent rest periods, though an exercise program may decrease its severity

! 2. Pain
   - a. American Nurses Association position statement "Promotion of Comfort and Relief of Pain in Dying Clients" (1995) supports nurse in goal of adequate pain control, noting, ". . . increasing titration of medication to achieve adequate symptom control, even at the expense of maintaining life or hastening death secondarily, is ethically justified"
   - b. Nurse should feel comfortable with decision not to limit use of opioids and to provide pain relief without fear of respiratory depression
   - c. The usual course of death is for clients to become sleepy; however, this may not occur in a small cohort of clients who experience intractable pain; in this situation, sedation may be the only option
   - d. Nonverbal signs of pain include grimaces, moans, irritability or withdrawal; these signs need to be carefully monitored in noncommunicative clients

3. Depression
   - a. Frequently associated with a terminal illness, depression may be disease related or associated with other symptoms such as pain, or may be treatment related or psychological in origin
   - b. Assessment should include questions to rule out suicide intentions
   - c. Early diagnosis and intervention allow client to accomplish goals associated with a quality end of life
   - d. Interventions can include medication
   - ! e. Nonpharmacological approaches include life review, grief or psychiatric counseling as appropriate, and encouraging client to draw on previous successful coping mechanisms, such as use of faith

4. Delirium
   a. An acute state of disorientation without drowsiness; commonly accompanied by agitation
   b. Pharmacological treatments may diminish agitation
   c. Minimize stimulation by family or staff and intervene with relaxation or massage therapy
   d. Hydration may also be effective
5. Dyspnea
   a. Occurs frequently
   b. Elevating head of bed, providing oxygen as ordered, and teaching pursed lip breathing to keep airways open for a longer time may alleviate dyspnea
6. Nausea and vomiting
   a. Immediate treatment is the goal
   b. Identify underlying cause to adequately control this frustrating symptom dyad
   c. Nonpharmacological measures such as serving meals at room temperature, distraction, and avoiding strong odors may be helpful
7. Anorexia and cachexia
   a. Anorexia is a loss of appetite; cachexia is a general wasting and lack of nutrition seen with most terminal illnesses
   b. Causes can include symptoms of pain, nausea and vomiting, constipation, and other GI disruptions; metabolic changes due to inflammation and cytokine activity may also be contributing factors
   c. Depression and anxiety are also associated with loss of appetite
   d. Treatments such as chemotherapy can cause taste alterations
   e. Pharmacological interventions include appetite stimulants or anti-emetics
   f. Alcohol before meals can be a helpful nonpharmacological approach
   g. If odors are a problem, moving client away from kitchen at mealtimes might stimulate his or her appetite
8. GI alterations
   a. To prevent constipation encourage client to follow personal bowel regimen; encourage high-fiber intake with adequate fluids and stool softeners
   b. Differentiate between diarrhea caused by fecal impaction (rapid onset) and anal incontinence (twice a day)
   c. Malabsorption is associated with foul-smelling, fatty, pale stools
   d. Problems with skin integrity occur as circulation to periphery diminishes; encourage very gentle massage with emollients and position change at regular intervals

C. Prognosis

1. Exact time of death cannot be predicted
2. Some individuals instinctively know when it is time to die
3. The type and stage of disease, a person's will to live, and his or her wish to wait for a special event, person, or attainment of a goal can extend life
4. Suggested signs and symptoms of dying are a guideline and may occur out of order or may never occur
5. The process of dying is natural with a decline of physical processes and mental abilities; these changes can occur in a few minutes or hours or may develop over days or weeks prior to actual death

D. Physical symptoms of nearing death

1. Changes in neurological function with alteration in level of consciousness, confusion, disorientation, and/or delirium
2. Weakness and fatigue, which are enhanced by decline in food and fluid intake
3. Increased drowsiness and sleeping with diminished reaction
4. Decreased oral intake; it is rare for individuals to complain of hunger as death approaches; dehydration can promote comfort of dying client because of these effects:
   a. Increased ketone production, causing sleepiness, euphoria, and decrease in pain with accompanied decreased urinary output
   b. Diminished GI secretions and stimulation, resulting in less nausea and vomiting, abdominal distention, and hunger

c. Decreased generalized edema and possible shrinkage of edematous layer around tumor if tumor is present
d. Increased opioid peptide production, causing elevated endorphin levels, producing "natural" analgesia
5. Dehydration can also result in comfort concerns for client because of potential for "dry mouth"; feeding (including provision of fluids) is symbolic of nurturing; withholding intake suggests abandonment of client; provision of nutrition and fluid is considered "basic" care
6. Hypernatremia and uremia, resulting in clouding of consciousness
7. Smaller quantities of lung secretions
8. Decreased or lack of swallow reflex
9. Surges of energy
10. Terminal restlessness and/or agitation may be due to metabolic alterations close to end of life; these need to be distinguished from behavior change caused by untreated symptoms
11. Fever
12. Change in bowel elimination ranging from constipation to diarrhea
13. Incontinence of stool and/or urine

E. Imminent death

1. Signs and symptoms of imminent death should be communicated to and discussed with family and monitored by nurse
2. Teach family signs and symptoms so they understand client's impending death (see Box 25–1)

F. Postmortem care of body (see Box 25–2)

III. PSYCHOSOCIAL SUPPORT NEAR END OF LIFE

A. Communication with dying clients and families

1. Goals of communication focus on individualized needs of client and family; keeping communication lines open; and making certain nurse clearly understands expectations of clients, family, and plan developed by partners in care
2. ! Sensitive listening is a communication tool that encompasses mental, emotional, and physical presence of individuals
3. Physical limitations due to age, disease treatment, or progression need to be addressed with sensitivity
4. ! Fear of a variety of death-related issues can create barriers to communication at end of life; these can be due to lack of experience with topic, unresolved loss, concern about showing emotion or not knowing answers, and even worry that family/caregivers would be held responsible for client's death
5. Telling the truth is an important element when reinforcing bad news previously given by physician; building rapport, planning and organizing what will be said in understandable terms, and continuously identifying what client wants and needs to know are important nursing activities
6. ! Changes in roles of family members at end of life can cause altered family dynamics; family members may require assistance to work through these issues
7. ! Beliefs related to spirituality and organized religions are not necessarily the same; sensitivity to culture, ethnic values, and religion is important when discussing palliative care options or decisions with clients and family members (see Table 25–1 ■)

Box 25–1

Signs/Symptoms of Imminent Death

- ➤ Decreased urine output with darkening and/or abnormal colorations such as brown or red.
- ➤ Drop in body temperature, with cold and mottled extremities
- ➤ Vital sign changes, including systolic pressures below 70 and diastolic below 50; pulse is weak and difficult to locate
- ➤ Respiratory congestion, including respiratory bubbling with breathing pattern changes, with very rapid respirations and/or Cheyne-Stokes respirations
- ➤ Glassy eyes that are tearing and half open

Box 25-2

Care of the Body Postmortem

- Close the eyes and place dentures in the mouth.
- Clean the body of mucus, wound drainage, urine, and feces released at the time of death.
- Remove external tubing and drains.
- Bathe the body and pad any drainage areas.
- Pack the anal orifice with gauze.
- Align the body with hands folded across the chest or lap.
- Pull a sheet up to the neck to cover the body for viewing and then shroud after the family leaves.
- Keep the ID band in place; attach two more to the toe and outside the shroud.
- Document time of death, deposition of the body, and belongings.

8. Communication between interdisciplinary team members promotes accurate implementation of client's desires and end-of-life goals for their care; this is accomplished through well-documented medical records and daily communication among multiple team members

B. The dying child

1. End-of-life care provided by pediatric nurse includes working with dying child as well as with siblings, parents, and extended family and friends
2. Some families prefer not to tell a child that she or he has a terminal illness; however, children are often aware that they have a terminal illness even if it is not openly discussed; they are sensitive to subtle changes in the way staff and family members interact with them both interpersonally and during physical care
3. ! Respect parents' choices and decision making while assessing opportunities to encourage open communication between parents and child
4. Provide support and caring to client and family without taking away realistic need for hope
5. Be available to listen and talk, even if child chooses not to talk about disease

Table 25-1 Comparison of Diverse Religious Practices and Beliefs

	Hinduism	Islam	Judaism	Christianity	American Indian	Buddhism
Terminal Care		Do not prolong	Do not prolong	Varies	Traditional healers	
Drugs or blood	May refuse pain meds	Allowed	Allowed	Allowed, but Jehovah Witnesses refuse blood	Allowed	May refuse pain meds
DNR/advanced directives	Yes/varies	No/varies	Allowed	Allowed/varies	No/varies	Allowed
Autopsies		Restricted	Restricted		Restricted	
Organ donation			Restricted		Restricted	
Upon death		Family handles body	Burial society prepares body; body not left alone			
Bereavement	Reincarnation	Grief counseling may be intrusive	Active mourning supported	Public grieving	Grief counseling may be intrusive	Restrained
Burial	Cremation	No embalming	No embalming	Cremation or burial	Cremation or burial	Cremation or burial

Adapted from Sheehan, O. K. & Forman, W. B. (2003). *Hospice and palliative care: Concepts and practice.* Sudbury, MA: Jones & Bartlett Publishers, p. 192.

6. Consider developmental and educational level of child and interact with child accordingly
7. Be aware that a child may let the nurse know he or she no longer wants to talk about a topic by walking away, changing subject, shifting his or her posture, or with other verbal or nonverbal cues
8. Understand that just the presence of the nurse can be meaningful to a child and/or parents
9. Encourage all family members to care for child
10. Siblings often feel left out as parents focus on dying child
    a. Assess all children in family for acting out, negative behavior, or "perfect child" behavior
    b. Encourage parents to find resources and support people to take siblings to their extracurricular activities
    c. Allow siblings to verbalize feelings in a safe place without their feeling as though they are making their parents feel worse
11. Encourage a life review by getting family members and friends to discuss events that were meaningful (birthdays, vacations, anniversaries of grandparents, and special events)
12. Provide support to other family members, including grandparents, extended families through divorce and remarriage, and classmates

C. The dying older adult

1. Determine whether client has examined his or her own mortality before learning of impending death; elders may or may not easily accept idea of own death
2. Elders have less death anxiety with advancing age
3. Elders may find it easier to face their mortality if they:
    a. Philosophically accept what their life had to offer
    b. Have numerous experiences with death, including parents, friends, spouse, or children
    c. Learn to cope with personal losses
    d. Are able to recover emotionally between multiple deaths
    e. Believe death is a part of living
    f. Find support in religious beliefs and concept of life after death
4. Cultural aspects
    a. Many cultures view death and dying differently from the open and blunt Euro-American approach
    b. From a cultural perspective, it is important to talk with client and family about a designated decision maker, management of pain, and care of body after death (see again Table 25-1)

IV. FAMILY SUPPORT NEAR END OF LIFE

A. Theoretical tasks of grief

1. Models that assist nurses to work with clients and families who are grieving
    a. Psychodynamic models (e.g., Freud) address factors that can complicate grief, such as quality of relationship with deceased or mental health of any affected individuals
    b. Task models (e.g., Lindemann, et al.) identify steps individual must complete to deal with grief
    c. Stage models (Kubler-Ross) and family function models (Kissanne, et al.) suggest grief occurs within individuals and their families
    d. Table 25-2 ■ summarizes additional models of grief work

B. Assessment of grief should include the following

1. Distinguishing between **loss, grief, mourning,** and **bereavement** and relevant social, cultural, and religious characteristics; loss is absence of a possession or future possession; grief is emotional response to loss; mourning is external behaviors, rituals, and traditions; bereavement is a combination of grief and mourning
2. Differentiating between anticipatory, normal, complicated and disenfranchised grief

Table 25-2

Theoretical Tasks of Grief

Kubler Ross (1969)	Parkes (1987)	Bowlby (1980)	Worden's Tasks (1991)	Rando's Process of Bereavement (1993)
1. Denial 2. Anger 3. Bargaining 4. Depression 5. Acceptance	1. Alarm 2. Searching 3. Mitigation 4. Anger and guilt 5. Gaining a new identity	1. Numbing 2. Searching and longing 3. Disorganization and despair 4. Reorganization	1. Accept reality of the loss 2. Experience the pain of grief 3. Adjust to an environment without the deceased 4. Withdraw emotional energy and reinvest in another relationship	1. Recognize the loss and death 2. React to, experience, and express the separation and pain 3. Reminisce 4. Relinquish old attachments 5. Readjust and adapt to the new role while maintaining memories, and form a new identity 6. Reinvest

Source: Brown-Satlzman, K. (1998). *Transforming the grief process.* In R. Carroll-Johnson, L. Gorman, and N. J. Bush (Eds.), *Psychosocial nursing care: Along the cancer continuum.* Pittsburgh, PA: Oncology Nursing Press.

3. Identification of grief reactions, including stage, task, and factors affecting grieving process
4. Careful review of caregiver survivor to determine if he or she is maintaining nutritional status and self-care, sleeping, able to continue working, and sustaining family roles and social networks

C. Interventions and resources

1. Working with dying clients may require nurse to move through five stages of adaptation: intellectualization; emotional survival; depression; emotional arrival; and deep compassion
2. Education in end-of-life care provides nurse with tools to deliver competent and nurturing care to dying client and his or her family
3. Formal support systems need to be available to nurse for safe expression of feelings; these can include postclinical debriefing and ceremonies or programs that enable individuals to acknowledge and express their grief

D. Diagnosis of staff grief

1. Multiple losses within a brief period of time place an individual at risk for "bereavement overload" and dysfunctional grieving
2. Focusing on only physical needs and care of clients, avoiding emotion-laden conversations, or talking only about topics of comfort are indications a nurse may be experiencing **death anxiety** in which a nurse is overcome with fears about death
3. Awareness of feelings about and responses and reactions to death allows a nurse to provide sensitive caregiving to clients and families

Check Your NCLEX-RN® I.Q. *You are ready for testing on this content if you can:*

- Monitor the physiological status of a dying client.
- Provide effective physical, psychological, and spiritual support; teaching; and nursing care to a dying client and his or her family members.
- Identify how culture impacts end-of-life care.
- Differentiate between the needs of the dying child and the dying adult.

PRACTICE TEST

1 While the nurse is discussing a client's likely death with family members, one of the adult children inquires, "We plan on taking turns being here for now, but we all want to be here at the time of death. Is there any way we can tell when that time is close?" Which of the following is the nurse's best response?

1. "Often, people become lucid for about 15 minutes during the last hour before death. Watch for your [family member] to become more alert, with clearer eyes, and to look around, focus on faces, and clear his [or her] throat. Call the others in at that time."
2. "I wish I could tell you that there was a way to know. It could be minutes from now or another three days. One just never knows."
3. "The arms and legs become more bluish in color and are cool to touch. Breathing will become irregular and shallow and will change speed. Call me if you hear mucus in the throat. The pulse and blood pressure will decrease."
4. "You can expect the muscles to become rigid, with staring eyes and mouth closed. The head is pulled back with neck rigidity. Don't be alarmed when you hear a death rattle in the throat."

2 A 90-year-old client expresses a wish to die at home after being told that an esophageal stricture prevents swallowing. The client refuses a feeding tube. The family fully supports this decision. Which of the following would be most appropriate for the nurse to call?

1. Hospice care
2. The rabbi
3. An attorney
4. The medical examiner's office

3 The nurse is providing postmortem care for a client. Which of the following interventions would be appropriate prior to allowing the family to visit? Select all that apply.

1. Prepare the body to look as clean and natural as possible.
2. Keep the sheet over the client's face until the family is comfortably seated in the room.
3. Wear sterile gloves to pack the anal canal with gauze.
4. Remove the external tubes and drains.
5. Call the physician to verify the time of death before taking the body to the morgue.

4 A dying client's spouse is afraid to leave the client's room to get a meal in the cafeteria for fear the client will die while she is gone. There are no other family members or visitors present. The client is nonresponsive, pulse is irregular and bradycardic, and he has Cheyne-Stokes respirations. Which of the following represents the best course of action for the nurse?

1. Encourage the client's spouse to take a break and go to the cafeteria and eat. The client is nonresponsive and won't know she is gone.
2. Make arrangements for the client's spouse to receive a meal in the client's room.
3. Tell the client's spouse she will be called if there are any changes and ask a nurse aide to sit with the client while the wife is gone to the cafeteria.
4. Do not interfere with the spouse's decision.

5 The family of a client diagnosed with terminal cancer has been informed that he is not expected to live more than 2 months. Which of the following statements made by the family indicates to the nurse that the family understands the client's prognosis?

1. "Hospice nurses are going to help care for him at home until he gets better."
2. "Hospice nurses are going to help care for him until we learn how to provide the care."
3. "Hospice nurses are going to help care for him until he can take care of himself."
4. "Hospice nurses are going to help care for him to make him more comfortable."

6 A client's spouse is upset and crying because her husband is no longer taking liquids. She understands fluids can prolong his death but is most concerned that he will become dehydrated and feel uncomfortable. The nurse will formulate an answer addressing which ethical principle?

1. Justice
2. Beneficence
3. Nonmaleficence
4. Veracity

PRACTICE TEST

7 The nurse anticipates that which of the following clients newly diagnosed with a terminal illness is least likely to have difficulty facing his or her mortality?

1. A 71-year-old female whose grandson, sister, and best friend died over the past 6 months
2. A 59-year-old male who never married, is an only child, and whose parents are both healthy
3. A 70-year-old male who has planned his funeral and enjoys riding his motorcycle at high speeds in rural areas
4. A 68-year-old female who is an atheist

8 A client with terminal lung cancer is receiving total brain radiation therapy to control the tremors in hands due to multiple metastatic lesions. As the nurse assists him back to his wheelchair, he comments "I'm hoping this treatment will let me see my first tomato on the fourth of July." According to Kubler-Ross, this statement is an example of which stage of death and dying?

1. Denial
2. Bargaining
3. Anger
4. Depression
5. Acceptance

9 The Registered Nurse would intervene after hearing a Licensed Practical Nurse (LPN) make which of the following statements regarding a client with severe arthritis who is also newly diagnosed with a rapidly growing colorectal cancer?

1. "Even though it hurts a bit, your arthritic joints will become less stiff with gentle exercise."
2. "If we give more pain medication, will it stop his breathing?"
3. "He has a living will that says he does not want to be resuscitated."
4. "You have on a diaper so it's okay if you do not make it to the bathroom."

10 Based on Rando's process of bereavement, place in order the following statements indicating the steps of the process as experienced by a client regarding his father's death.

1. "This is the second anniversary of my father's death."
2. "My father was an alcoholic, so every Christmas I make certain that local AA groups have coffee and chocolates to help the members through the holidays."
3. "It was so much fun to rummage through the antique stores together."
4. "It's too difficult to be around his stepfamily, so I visit friends on vacation."
5. "The homestead has run down since his death. It was hard to drive past and see the lack of care in his vegetable garden."

11 A 46-year-old female client with a history of head and neck cancer was recently told she has multiple metastatic sites in her lung. The nurse is discussing the situation with the client and her sister. Which statement during the conversation reflects the ethical principle of justice?

1. "The staff will do everything possible to make your sister comfortable while she is in hospice."
2. "She told the doctor she did not want to lose her hair. It is not right that he coerced her into taking that experimental chemotherapy. Now she is bald and dying."
3. "Why did I have to get this terrible disease? I just want my life back."
4. "We have made special arrangements for her care at home. Now the doctor says she has to have more tests to see if there is cancer in her liver. Why? We know she's dying."

12 A 22-year-old hospitalized client with a recent diagnosis of acquired immunodeficiency syndrome (AIDS) says to the nurse, "The food on this breakfast tray is terrible. Why can't you people do even simple things well?" What is the nurse's best response?

1. "I know you are angry, but I cannot let you make me the object of your anger. I will send up the dietitian."
2. "This is not about breakfast. Tell me what you are really angry about."
3. "I understand you are angry. I'll shut the door and let you cool off."
4. "I hear a lot of anger in your voice that is quite normal and healthy. Do you want a new breakfast or do you want something else?"

13 While talking to adult children of a dying male client, the nurse finds them tearful, with ambivalent feelings toward the client. The client often expresses beliefs of a wasted life. The children say that their father often showed love but followed it with criticism, anger, damaging accusations, and emotional abuse. The nurse would suggest which of the following interventions that is most likely to be helpful at this time?

1. Listen to relaxation tapes before visiting each other. If negative feelings arise, listen to the tapes together.
2. Have a nurse present in the room at all times when a family member visits the client so that the nurse can intervene with conflict resolution if problems arise.
3. Assure the client and children that the past no longer matters; the only time that matters is the present and the future. Encourage the children to spend more time with their father.
4. Make a videotape of each adult child telling a story of a time when their father showed love, while the client tells of a special love for each child. Plan a time for them to watch it together.

14 A client questions the nurse about the difference between a living will and power of attorney. The nurse's best response is which of the following?

1. "The living will allows the client to indicate specific medical treatments to be omitted in the event of terminal illness, while durable power of attorney legally appoints another to make those decisions on the behalf of the client."
2. "A lawyer carries out a living will, while a designated family member or friend carries out advanced directives."
3. "In a living will, the client specifies medical treatments to be carried out should he or she be incapable of making decisions, while durable power of attorney allows the client to include both treatments to be carried out and treatments to be omitted in the event of terminal illness."
4. "The living will indicates when a client wishes life support to be discontinued, while durable power of attorney gives that power to another in the event of terminal illness."

15 The nurse working with a terminally ill client wishes to support the client's decisions concerning end-of-life care. To do this appropriately, the nurse should do plan to which of the following?

1. Be comfortable in assisting the client with euthanasia when requested to do so.
2. Ask another nurse to provide care if the client has a belief system that differs from the nurse's belief system.
3. Respect the client's wishes about death to the extent possible by law.
4. Encourage the client to request a do-not-resuscitate order because the client has been diagnosed with a terminal illness.

16 The terminally ill client asks the nurse for information about hospice care. The nurse would best respond by stating:

1. "Hospice care is home nursing care provided to terminal cancer clients."
2. "The client qualifies for hospice care at the time of diagnosis with a terminal illness."
3. "The main focus of hospice is to educate the client concerning treatment options and alternatives."
4. "Hospice regards dying as a normal part of life and provides support for a dignified and peaceful death."

17 The nurse concludes that which of the following would not be considered a sign of grief resolution in the bereaved client whose husband died a year ago?

1. Becoming future oriented when discussing details of everyday life
2. Considering the opinions of the deceased prior to making decisions about everyday life
3. Experiencing occasional waves of grief triggered by pictures or events
4. Sharing stories of good times that the client and her husband shared over the years

PRACTICE TEST

18 Which of the following nursing interventions would be most appropriate for the nurse to include in the care plan of a client with a nursing diagnosis of anticipatory grieving?

1. Hope instillation
2. Forgiveness facilitation
3. Medication management
4. Hypnotherapy

19 A client is dying, is in excruciating pain, and refuses anything for relief that alters his sensorium. The nurse checks the psychosocial data part of the client's medical record, expecting that which religion is most likely practiced by the client?

1. Islam
2. Judaism
3. Buddhism
4. Catholicism

20 Which of the following indicates to the nurse that a non-communicative client's pain is not well managed?

1. Crackles in the lung
2. Hyperactive bowel sounds
3. Unwillingness to eat without assistance
4. Constant restlessness and leg movement

ANSWERS & RATIONALES

1 **Answer: 3** Peripheral circulation decreases and shifts to the vital organs. The vascular system collapses, causing decreasing pulse and blood pressure. The gag reflex is lost, and mucus accumulates in the back of the throat. Respirations decrease in rate, and the rhythm is irregular. Muscle rigidity typically occurs after death. Vision is blurred. A lucid moment is not a pattern in death. It is difficult to pinpoint the exact time when death will occur, but the imminence of clinical death can be detected.

Cognitive Level: Application **Client Need:** Psychosocial Integrity **Integrated Process:** Teaching and Learning **Content Area:** Psychiatric-Mental Health **Strategy:** Note the issue of the question, which is knowledge of impending signs of death. The words *best response* in the question tell you it is a true statement and will be a priority in client care. Options 1 and 4 are inaccurate. Choose option 3 because option 2 does not provide information about the characteristics of impending death.

2 **Answer: 1** Hospice specializes in end-of-life care. A rabbi is an important person during the end of life, but there is not an immediate need to make this call. An attorney or medical examiner is not necessary at this time.

Cognitive Level: Application **Client Need:** Psychosocial Integrity **Integrated Process:** Nursing Process: Planning **Content Area:** Psychiatric-Mental Health **Strategy:** The key issue is that the client wishes to die at home. Option 1, hospice care, can be provided in the home at all times. The other options (the attorney or medical examiner) do not address the client's issue, which is 24-hour care in the home at the end of life.

3 **Answer: 1, 4** The body is to be handled with dignity at all times. Even though humor can alleviate stress, it is not appropriate at this time. Once the body is cleaned, all external tubes and drains are removed, the linen is freshened, the sheet is pulled to cover the client's shoulders. While gloves should be worn during postmortem care, sterility is not an issue. State laws and policies differ regarding the nurse's ability to declare death. Even if a physician is required to declare death, the time of death cannot be verified exactly and is not required prior to the family being allowed to view the client after death.

Cognitive Level: Application **Client Need:** Psychosocial Integrity **Integrated Process:** Nursing Process, Implementation **Content Area:** Fundamentals **Strategy:** Use the process of elimination to identify the options that contain inaccurate information. While some of the information is correct in options 3 and 5, there are elements that make those responses incorrect. For example sterile gloves are not necessary, although clean gloves are worn. The family can visit before the physician is called.

4 **Answer: 2** The signs and symptoms listed indicate death will occur soon and the spouse is fearful to leave the room at this time. Obtaining a meal for the client's spouse while she remains at the bedside and supporting her during the client's imminent death demonstrate knowledge of the dying process in addition to compassion and concern for the client and spouse.

Cognitive Level: Application **Client Need:** Psychosocial Integrity **Integrated Process:** Nursing Process: Implementation **Content Area:** Psychiatric-Mental Health **Strategy:** The key issue is the signs and symptoms of imminent death of the client and the spouse's desire to be with him when he dies. Options 1 and 3 would increase the spouse's anxiety if she were notified while she was absent. Option 4 is correct but does not include the support from the nurse exemplified in option 2.

5 **Answer: 4** Hospice care is provided to those clients who have 6 months or less to live. Hospice nurses are skilled in pain and symptom management as well as in emotional support to the dying clients and their families. Hospice care does not terminate once families learn to provide care (option 1), and a client in need of hospice services cannot be expected to resume self-care (option 3).

Cognitive Level: Application **Client Need:** Psychosocial Integrity **Integrated Process:** Nursing Process: Evaluation **Content Area:** Psychiatric-Mental Health **Strategy:** The core issue of the question is knowledge of the purpose and goals of hospice care. The other options indicate that the family expects improvement in the client's condition, which is not realistic.

6 **Answer: 3** This client situation acknowledges that while the lack of nutrition and fluids will produce ketones and cause somnolence to decrease the client's anxiety and promote overall comfort, the wife is more concerned about how dehydration might feel to her husband. Beneficence promotes doing good for the client, the focus of a quality death. Veracity and fairness are not considerations in this situation.
Cognitive Level: Application **Client Need:** Psychosocial Integrity **Integrated Process:** Caring **Content Area:** Fundamentals **Strategy:** The focus of this question is the ability to apply the ethical principles to end-of-life care. Eliminate options 1, 2, and 4 because they do not represent the principle of doing good.

7 **Answer: 3** People cope better when they accept what their life had to offer, have learned to cope with personal losses, have the time and ability to recover emotionally between multiple deaths, believe that death is a part of living, and have religious beliefs. Option 3 indicates the individual has planned for the future and believes that death is part of living. The client in option 1 is incorrect because this client has lost three people over a brief period of time (6 months). The client in option 2 is incorrect because he shows dependence, having never moved out of the home of his parents, who are both healthy. The client in option 4 is incorrect because individuals with religious beliefs are found to cope better.
Cognitive Level: Application **Client Need:** Psychosocial Integrity **Integrated Process:** Nursing Process: Assessment **Content Area:** Psychiatric-Mental Health **Strategy:** The focus of this question is knowledge of how older adults cope with a diagnosis of a life-threatening illness. Using the criteria outlined in the rationale, use the process of elimination to make the correct choice.

8 **Answer: 2** Clients go through multiple stages and tasks when they are dying. During bargaining, they "negotiate" to meet a life goal. The other stages are not consistent with the client's statement. Denial would be refusal to accept the diagnosis of terminal cancer. Anger and depression are natural reactions to anticipated loss. Acceptance is shown when the client has come to terms with the diagnosis and anticipated death.
Cognitive Level: Application **Client Need:** Psychosocial Integrity **Integrated Process:** Communication and Documentation **Content Area:** Psychiatric-Mental Health **Strategy:** This question focuses on Kubler-Ross's five stages of death and dying. The client statements on options 3 and 4 do not include reflections of anger or depression. Denial statements would show refusal to accept the diagnosis or pushing away the reality from consciousness. Option 5 indicates the client has accepted the need for treatment but has not accepted the reality of the extent of his disease.

9 **Answer: 4** Option 4 does not treat the client with respect and sensitivity and therefore is an example of maleficence. Option 1 provides a rationale for a therapy that may be uncomfortable. Options 2 and 3 advocate for the client.
Cognitive Level: Application **Client Need:** Psychosocial Integrity **Integrated Process:** Caring **Content Area:** Fundamentals **Strategy:** The critical word in the stem of the question is *intervene*, making the correct option the one that is physically or emotionally harmful. Option 4 can cause anxiety and distress to the client and is therefore the statement that potentially causes harm. Eliminate option 1 because it merely questions the rationale behind an intervention and option 2 because it tries to safeguard the client. Eliminate option 3 because it is a communication about client desires.

10 **Answer: 1, 5, 3, 4, 2** Rando's process of bereavement is to (1) recognize the loss and death, (2) react to experience and express the separation and pain, (3) reminisce, (4) relinquish old attachments, (5) readjust and adapt to the new role while maintaining memories and form a new identity, and (6) reinvest.
Cognitive Level: Analysis **Client Need:** Psychosocial Integrity **Integrated Process:** Nursing Process: Evaluation **Content Area:** Psychiatric-Mental Health **Strategy:** Remember the Six R's of Rando: recognize, react, reminisce, relinquish, readjust, and reinvest. They all begin with "re" and then the letters CAMLAI. A helpful memory aid could be Chocolate Always Makes Lads Act Icky.

11 **Answer: 1** The definition for the ethical principle of justice is "fairness." Option 2 reflects anger on the part of the family, while option 3 reflects anger on the part of the client. Option 4 demonstrates a concern that the client will suffer an injustice by enduring unnecessary tests.
Cognitive Level: Application **Client Need:** Psychosocial Integrity **Integrated Process:** Communication and Documentation **Content Area:** Fundamentals **Strategy:** Option 1 is the only statement indicating fairness in client care. Option 2 is coercion, and 4 is an ethical dilemma. Option 3 is an example of the stages of the grief process.

12 **Answer: 4** Anger is a common element to all the theories of grief and stages of dying. It is important to acknowledge the client's anger, help him or her identify the source of the anger, and offer choices or control when possible. It is important to be nonconfrontational (option 2), not to take the anger personally (option 1), and not to ignore the client's issue (option 3).
Cognitive Level: Application **Client Need:** Psychosocial Integrity **Integrated Process:** Nursing Process: Analysis **Content Area:** Psychiatric-Mental Health **Strategy:** Eliminate option 1 because it indicates the nurse is taking the statement personally and assuming what the client needs. Option 2 also makes an assumption but does address the anger. The anger is also addressed in the third option but does not encourage the client to share the source of the anger. For these reasons, options 2 and 3 should be eliminated also. The last option addresses the normalcy of the anger in this situation and encourages the client to engage in further conversation with the nurse.

13 **Answer: 4** Open communication with concrete evidence of emotional attachments assists in coping at the end of life. Option 4 provides concrete assurance in the presence of the loved ones. Relaxation tapes help with stress reduction but do not help with resolution of problems experienced by the family. Staffing needs do not permit a nurse to be with one client continually, and families require privacy as well. Assurance that the past no longer matters is an assurance lacking concrete properties.

Cognitive Level: Application **Client Need:** Psychosocial Integrity **Integrated Process:** Caring **Content Area:** Psychiatric-Mental Health **Strategy:** Use the process of elimination and address the client in the question. In this case, both the client and the adult children are the affected clients, so the correct option is one that benefits all of them.

14 **Answer: 1** A living will is written by the client and includes desires for use of different types of treatment in case of a life-threatening illness. A durable power of attorney is a legal document designating an individual to make legal decisions if the client is unable to make choices independently.
Cognitive Level: Application **Client Need:** Psychosocial Integrity **Integrated Process:** Teaching and Learning **Content Area:** Fundamentals **Strategy:** The core issue of the question is knowledge of a living will. The wording of the question indicates that the correct answer is a true statement. Systematically eliminate options 2, 3, and 4 because they are incorrect statements.

15 **Answer: 3** The nurse needs to consider the client's wishes while also acting within the law. Euthanasia constitutes illegal nursing practice in the United States at this time. To act ethically, the nurse should provide care to clients according to need, regardless of belief systems. Clients who are diagnosed with terminal illness may or may not be ready for do-not-resuscitate orders, depending on anticipated life expectancy, quality of current life, and psychosocial variables.
Cognitive Level: Application **Client Need:** Psychosocial Integrity **Integrated Process:** Nursing Process: Implementation **Content Area:** Fundamentals **Strategy:** Eliminate option 1 because it is illegal. Nurses need to provide unbiased care to all clients, regardless of conflicts with belief systems, so option 2 is also incorrect. Option 4 is incorrect because it may or may not reflect the client's preference at this time.

16 **Answer: 4** The focus of hospice is improving the quality of life and preserving dignity for the client in death. Hospice care may be provided by nurses, volunteers, or other members of the health care team in a variety of settings. It is available to any client who has a terminal illness with a life expectancy of 6 months or less.
Cognitive Level: Application **Client Need:** Psychosocial Integrity **Integrated Process:** Teaching and Learning **Content Area:** Fundamentals **Strategy:** Eliminate options 1, 2, and 3 because they represent incorrect definitions of hospice and do not accurately reflect the care provided. In addition, option 1 is insensitive.

17 **Answer: 2** Grief resolution requires letting go of the past and looking forward to the future. The client needs to be able to put the loss in perspective and engage fully and effectively in daily life as an independent person. In option 2, the client has not let go of the past because decisions are made in the present only through memories of preferences of the deceased. Options 1, 3, and 4 all indicate healthy grief resolution.
Cognitive Level: Application **Client Need:** Psychosocial Integrity **Integrated Process:** Nursing Process: Analysis **Content Area:** Psychiatric-Mental Health **Strategy:** The critical word in the question is not, which tells you the correct option is a statement that indicates inadequate coping with the loss or unresolved grief.

18 **Answer: 1** Hope instillation is often an effective intervention in dealing with anticipatory grieving. Option 3 deals with the symptom and not the actual problem. Options 2 and 4 are not appropriate because there is no evidence in the stem of the question to support their need.
Cognitive Level: Application **Client Need:** Psychosocial Integrity **Integrated Process:** Nursing Process: Planning **Content Area:** Psychiatric-Mental Health **Strategy:** The key words in the stem of the question are *anticipatory grieving.* Use the process of elimination to select the option that focuses on anticipated loss. Choose option 1 because of the word *hope* in the option, which relates to the word *grieving* in the question.

19 **Answer: 3** The Hindu and Buddhist religions require that believers are alert and mindful as they leave the life on earth and transcend to their next life. This requirement is not found in Islam or Catholicism.
Cognitive Level: Application **Client Need:** Psychosocial Integrity **Integrated Process:** Nursing Process: Planning **Content Area:** Fundamentals **Strategy:** Use the process of elimination. Only the religion identified in option 3 requires a state of being "mindful" and alert as their faithful transcend from life into death.

20 **Answer: 4** Knowledge of response to pain offers accurate and careful assessment of pain with earlier and more complete pain relief. It should include physical and emotional behaviors.
Cognitive Level: Application **Client Need:** Psychosocial Integrity **Integrated Process:** Nursing Process: Assessment **Content Area:** Fundamentals **Strategy:** Options 1 and 2 are due to inactivity from uncontrolled pain. Requesting assistance to eat is not an indication of pain, so option 3 is not a correct response.

Key Terms to Review

advance directives (AD) p. 381
beneficence p. 381
bereavement p. 385
death anxiety p. 386
euthanasia p. 381
grief p. 385
justice p. 381
loss p. 385
mourning p. 385
nonmaleficence p. 381
palliative care p. 381
veracity p. 380

ANSWERS & RATIONALES

References

American Geriatric Society Position Statement. *The Care of Dying Clients.* (2002). Retrieved December 29, 2004, from http://www.americangeriatrics.org.

American Nurses Association. (2003). *Position statement on pain management and control of distressing symptoms in dying clients.* Retrieved March 5, 2005, from http://www.ana.org/readroom/position/ethics/etpain.pdf.

American Nurses Association. (1994). *Ethics and human rights statement: Active euthanasia.* Retrieved March 5, 2005, from http://www.nursingworld.org/readroom/position/ethics/eteuth.htm.

Bednash, G., & Ferrell, B. (2000). *End-of-Life Nursing Education Consortium (ELNEC): Faculty Guide; Module 1, Nursing Care at End of Life.* American Association of Colleges of Nursing and City of Hope National Medical Center.

Bednash, G., & Ferrell, B. (2000). *End-of-Life Nursing Education Consortium (ELNEC): Faculty Guide; Module 2, Pain.* American Association of Colleges of Nursing and City of Hope National Medical Center.

Bednash, G., & Ferrell, B. (2000). *End-of-Life Nursing Education Consortium (ELNEC): Faculty Guide; Module 3, Symptom Management.* American Association of Colleges of Nursing and City of Hope National Medical Center.

Bednash, G., & Ferrell, B. (2000). *End-of-Life Nursing Education Consortium (ELNEC): Faculty Guide; Module 4, Ethical/Legal Issues.* American Association of Colleges of Nursing and City of Hope National Medical Center.

Bednash, G., & Ferrell, B. (2000). *End-of-Life Nursing Education Consortium (ELNEC): Faculty Guide; Module 5, Culture.* American Association of Colleges of Nursing and City of Hope National Medical Center.

Bednash, G., & Ferrell, B. (2000). *End-of-Life Nursing Education Consortium (ELNEC): Faculty Guide; Module 9, Preparation and Care for the Time of Death.* American Association of Colleges of Nursing and City of Hope National Medical Center.

Corless, I. B. (2001). Bereavement. In B. R. Ferrell & N. Coyle (Eds.), *Textbook of palliative nursing care.* New York: Oxford University Press. Hospice Client's Alliance. Retrieved December 29, 2004, from http://www.hospiceclients.org/hospice60.html.

Cotter, V. T., & Strumpf, N. E. (2002). *Advanced practice nursing with older adults: Clinical guidelines.* New York: McGraw Hill.

Egan, K. A., & Labyak, M. J. (2001). Hospice care: A model for quality end-of-life care. In B. R. Ferrell & N. Coyle (Eds.), *Textbook of palliative nursing care.* New York: Oxford University Press.

Karnes, B. (1986). *Gone from my sight: The dying experience.* New York: Dutton.

Kubler-Ross, E. (1969). *On death and dying.* New York: MacMillan.

Rando, T. A. (1984). *Grief, dying and death: Clinical interventions for caregivers.* Champaign, IL: Research Press.

26 Meeting Nutritional Needs

Test Yourself

Are you ready for the NCLEX-RN® or course exams? Use the practice tests on the companion CD-ROM to check.

In this chapter

Cross reference

Other chapters relevant to this content area are

Alternative and Complementary Therapies	Chapter 29
Total Parenteral Nutrition	Chapter 34
Common Laboratory Tests	Chapter 47

I. OVERVIEW OF NUTRIENTS

A. Proteins (macronutrients)

1. Composed of amino acids; required for proper growth and development; provide 4 calories/gram
2. Proteins may be complete, incomplete, or complementary depending on composition of amino acids
3. Essential amino acids cannot by synthesized by body and must be obtained in diet
4. High-quality proteins are found in meat, fish, poultry, eggs, and dairy products
5. Protein is needed for energy, growth, bodily repair, maintenance of fluid and electrolyte balance, and production of enzymes, hormones, and antibodies
6. Adult recommended daily allowance (RDA) for protein is 0.8 g/kg/day, which correlates to roughly 10% of total calories; additional protein may be required by infants, children, and pregnant or lactating women
7. Insufficient protein intake can lead to protein energy malnutrition; this is characterized by atrophy and wasting of muscle tissue

B. Carbohydrates (macronutrients)

1. Include starches, sugars (fructose, glucose, lactose, sucrose), and cellulose
2. Provide 4 calories/gram and are a key source of energy
3. Found in fruits, vegetables, milk, and grains
4. Promote normal metabolism, including fat metabolism, and prevent protein from being used for energy (protein sparing)
5. Insufficient intake results in protein and fat being used for energy

C. Fats (macronutrients)

1. Concentrated sources of energy, providing 9 calories/gram
2. Needed for proper absorption of fat-soluble vitamins
3. Stored in body to maintain body warmth and cushion or protect internal organs
4. Sources include animal products, egg yolks, organ meats (including liver), butter, cheeses, and various oils
5. Can be described according to their cholesterol content and whether they are saturated, monounsaturated, or polyunsaturated; in general, the more solid the fat, the higher the saturated fat content
6. Can lead to obesity, heart disease, and some cancers if taken in excess of bodily needs
7. Insufficient intake can result in increased risk of infection, skin lesions, amenorrhea, and cold sensitivity (insufficient fat stores)

D. Minerals (micronutrients)

1. Part of bones, cells, and hormones
2. Enhance cellular function and catalyze various bodily processes
3. Widely abundant in foods
4. Major minerals include calcium, sodium, potassium, magnesium, chloride, and phosphorus
5. Trace elements that are also needed include iron, iodine, copper, zinc, selenium, manganese, fluoride, chromium, and molybdenum
6. Minerals can also be obtained by supplementation, often in conjunction with a multivitamin

E. Vitamins (micronutrients)

1. Classified as water soluble (B and C vitamins), which are easily excreted from body, or fat soluble (vitamins A, D, E, K), which can be stored and cause toxicity if taken to excess
2. Used as catalysts of body functions, coenzymes in metabolic processes, for growth, collagen production, wound healing, hormone synthesis, and vision
3. See Table 26–1 ■ for summary of vitamin functions, food sources, and signs of deficiency or excess states
4. Vitamins can be obtained by diet alone, or with supplementation, either with or without minerals

II. GENERAL DIETARY GUIDELINES

! **A. Characteristics of healthy diet (U.S. Department of Agriculture [USDA] and U.S. Department of Health and Human Services [USDHHS])**

1. Emphasizes fruits, vegetables, whole grains, and fat-free or low-fat milk and milk products
2. Includes lean meats, poultry, fish, beans, eggs, and nuts
3. Is low in saturated fats, *trans* fats, cholesterol, salt (sodium), and added sugars

B. Individualized food guidance system: MyPyramid Plan (USDA)

1. A computer-generated, individualized daily food intake plan that considers age, gender, and physical activity (< 30 minutes, 30–60 minutes, or > 60 minutes/day); see Figure 26–1 ■, page 397
2. Components
   a. Grains: all foods made from wheat, rice, oats, cornmeal, and barley, such as bread, pasta, oatmeal, breakfast cereal, tortillas, and grits
   b. Vegetables: all fresh, frozen, dried, or canned vegetables or vegetable juices
   c. Fruits: all fresh, frozen, dried, or canned fruits or fruit juices
   d. Milk: all fluid milk products and foods made from milk that retain calcium content (yogurt and cheese, but not cream cheese, cream, or butter, which do not have significant calcium content)
   e. Meats and beans: lean meat, poultry, fish, eggs, peanut butter, beans, nuts, and seeds

C. Key recommendations for general public from USDA *Dietary Guidelines for Americans 2005* (USDA; www.healthierus.gov/dietaryguidelines)

1. Adequate nutrients within calorie needs

Table 26-1

Overview of Fat and Water Soluble Vitamins

Vitamin	Function	Food Sources	Deficiency	Excess
Thiamin (B_1)	Coenzyme	Pork, wheat germ, fortified cereals	Beriberi, Wernicke-Korsakoff syndrome	
Riboflavin (B_2)	Coenzyme	Milk, enriched grains	Ariboflavinosis	
Niacin (B_3)	Coenzyme	Peanuts, legumes, enriched grains	Pellagra (3 D's: dermatitis, diarrhea, dementia)	Flushing, abnormalities in blood sugar and liver function
Pantothenic acid (B_5)	Coenzyme	Meat, whole grains	Rash, fatigue	
Pyridoxine (B_6)	Coenzyme	Pork, organ meats, whole grains, wheat germ	Nutritional anemia	
Cobalamin (B_{12})	Coenzyme	Animal protein	Pernicious anemia	
Folic acid	Coenzyme	Orange juice, meat, leafy green vegetables	Nutritional anemia, neural tube defects	
Biotin	Coenzyme	Egg yolks, liver	Dermatitis	
Ascorbic acid (vitamin C)	Antioxidant, wound healing, hormone synthesis	Citrus fruits	Scurvy, bleeding gums	
Vitamin A	Vision, bone and tissue growth, immune and reproductive function	Animal foods, fruits, vegetables, fortified milk	Night blindness, xerophthalmia	Toxicity can result
Vitamin D	Calcium and phosphorus metabolism, PTH, kidney	Dairy products, fortified food sources	Rickets, osteomalacia	Toxicity can result
Vitamin A	Vision, bone and tissue growth, immune and reproductive function	Animal foods, fruits, vegetables, fortified milk	Night blindness, xerophthalmia	Toxicity can result
Vitamin D	Calcium and phosphorus metabolism, PTH, kidney	Dairy products, fortified food sources	Rickets, osteomalacia	Toxicity can result
Vitamin E	Antioxidant, immune function	Vegetable oil, peanuts, margarine	Hemolysis of RBCs	May interfere with vitamin K activity
Vitamin K	Blood clotting	Liver, and through intestinal synthesis	Hemorrhagic disease of the newborn, hemorrhage	Toxicity can result

a. Consume a variety of nutrient-dense foods and beverages from basic food groups while limiting intake of saturated and trans fats, cholesterol, added sugars, salt, and alcohol

b. Adopt a balanced eating pattern, such as the USDA MyPyramid or the Dietary Approaches to Stop Hypertension (DASH) eating plan

! **2.** Weight management

a. Balance calories from foods and beverages with calories expended

b. Prevent gradual weight gain over time by making small decreases in calories and increasing physical activity

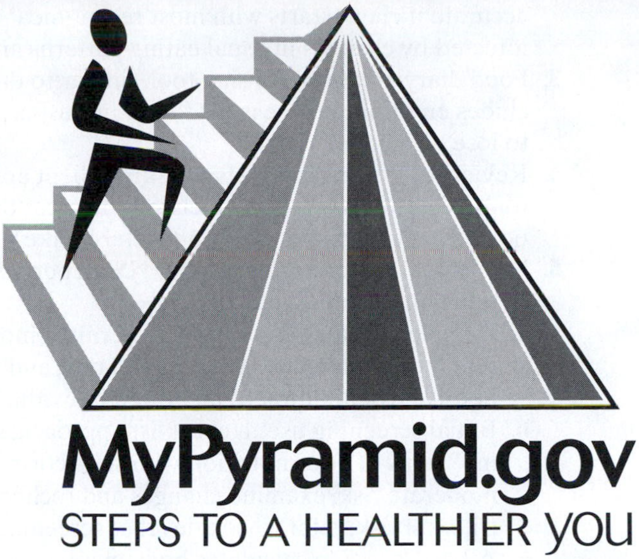

Figure 26–1

MyPyramid Plan replaces the Food Guide Pyramid for diet selection. Color bands from left to right indicate grains (orange), vegetables (green), fruits (red), milk (blue), and meat and beans (purple). Staircase emphasizes role of physical activity in health.

Source: USDA. Online: http://www.mypyramid.gov. Accessed 06/01/06.

3. Food groups to encourage
   - **a.** Eat sufficient fruits and vegetables while staying within energy needs (e.g., 2 cups of fruit and 2½ cups of vegetables per day are recommended for a reference 2,000-calorie intake, with higher or lower amounts as needed)
   - **b.** Eat a variety of fruits and vegetables from all five vegetable subgroups (dark green, orange, legumes, starchy vegetables, and other vegetables)
   - **c.** Eat three or more ounce-equivalents of whole-grain products per day; at least one half of grains should come from whole grains
   - **d.** Drink 3 cups per day of fat-free or low-fat milk or equivalent milk products
4. Fats
   - **a.** Consume less than 10% of calories from saturated fatty acids and less than 300 mg/day of cholesterol, and keep trans fatty acid consumption as low as possible
   - **b.** Keep total fat intake 20% to 35% of calories, with most fats coming from polyunsaturated and monounsaturated fatty acids, such as in fish, nuts, and vegetable oils
   - **c.** When selecting and preparing meat, poultry, dry beans, and milk or milk products, make choices that are lean, low-fat, or fat-free
   - **d.** Limit intake of fats and oils high in saturated and/or trans fatty acids, and choose products low in such fats and oils
5. Carbohydrates (CHOs)
   - **a.** Eat fiber-rich fruits, vegetables, and whole grains often
   - **b.** Use little added sugar or caloric sweetener when preparing food and beverages, such as amounts suggested by the USDA MyPyramid and the DASH eating plan
   - **c.** Practice good oral hygiene and consume sugar- and starch-containing foods and beverages less frequently to reduce risk of dental caries
6. Sodium and potassium
   - **a.** Take in less than 2,300 mg of sodium (approximately 1 teaspoon of salt) per day
   - **b.** Choose and prepare foods with little salt, while increasing potassium-rich foods, such as fruits and vegetables (provided no contraindication to potassium in diet, such as in renal failure)

III. ASSESSMENT OF NUTRITIONAL STATUS

A. Documented history

1. Dietary intake record: client records every food eaten and every beverage consumed during a set time (often a 1-week period); this record is then analyzed for nutrient content
2. 24-hour recall: dietary intake recording tool in which all foods and beverages consumed in last 24 hours are recalled either verbally or in writing; is most

accurate if client starts with most recent meal and works backwards; is greatly affected by changes in usual eating patterns and routines

3. Food diary: intake recording tool, similar to dietary intake record, but also includes emotions and reasons for eating; especially helpful for persons who want to lose weight
4. Review of systems: consists of asking client about each body system for symptoms of nutrition problems related to excess or deficiency (example: constipation as a result of low fiber and water intake)
5. Nutritional screening initiatives (NSIs): performed for special populations, such as pregnant women or elderly
   a. Provide a 3-step approach to determine individual's nutritional health, to assess those at increased nutritional risk, and then to provide a more comprehensive examination of identified individual with poor nutrition
   b. Initial screening uses a checklist approach; self-evaluation indicates "warning" signs of poor nutrition with self-scoring (0–2: recheck in 6 months; 3–5: moderate risk, examine changes and recheck in 3 months; 6 or more: high nutritional risk, refer to next level of screening)
   c. A level 1 screen calculates body mass index (BMI; see next section), evaluates eating habits, and assesses environment to determine risk level with referral to next screening if needed
   d. A level 2 screen incorporates anthropometric data (see next section), lab data, and clinical evidence with detailed assessment of eating habits, environment, functional status and mental/cognitive status
6. After diet history is completed, nutrient content can be determined through comparison of data collected with food composition tables or computerized diet analysis program

B. Anthropometric measurements

1. Height, weight, and body size are obtained and compared to a table of norms for reference; Metropolitan Life Insurance Table is commonly used; client is categorized as **underweight,** ideal weight, or overweight; does not take % of body fat or lean muscle into account
2. BMI: assesses relative weight for height; calculated by dividing weight in kilograms (2.2 pounds = 1 kg) by the square of height in meters (2.54 cm = 1 inch), or Weight ÷ $(\text{Height})^2$ = BMI; charts or nomograms may be used to calculate BMI (see Figure 26–2 ■)
   a. ! Provides a range to evaluate a healthy body weight ("healthy" range 18.5 – 24.9)
   b. ! A BMI lower than 18.5 reflects underweight status while BMI higher than 25 reflects excess weight (25–29.9 overweight or grade I obesity; 30–40 grade II obesity; > 40 grade III obesity)
   c. BMI silhouettes can be used as a visual tool with a client to determine both body image perception and recognition of body weight
   d. BMI does not reflect body composition, and individuals with greater muscle mass may appear to be overweight and yet not have increased body fat
   e. High or low BMIs correlate with clinical pathology and disease pathology
3. Basal metabolic rate (BMR): measures body's consumption of oxygen and therefore rate of calories burned during basic activities—a higher BMR indicates client can consume more calories without weight gain
   a. Lean muscle tissue mass most directly affects BMR; BMR decreases about 2% during each decade after maximum at age 30
   b. BMR increases with activity, stress, temperature, pregnancy, smoking, caffeine, stress, and during growth spurts
   c. BMR decreases with sleep, fasting, or starvation states and undernutrition
   d. ! Identification of BMR and typical activities/lifestyle is necessary to determine exact caloric requirements
4. ! Distribution of body fat is important in assessing health risk potential: central (truncal) **obesity** represents increased intra-abdominal fat and is associated with increased risk of disease

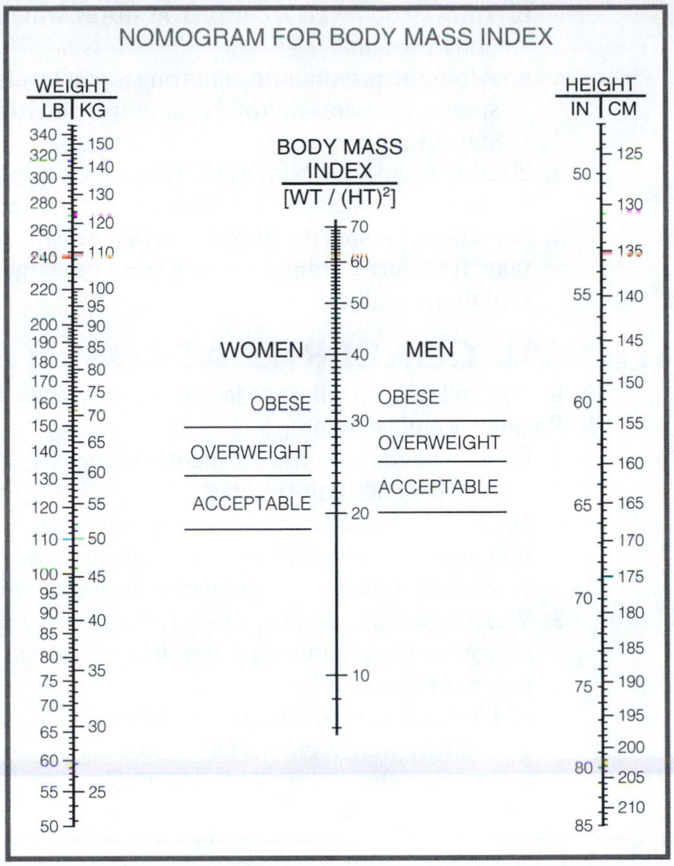

Figure 26-2

Body mass index nomogram plots height against weight to identify the BMI and determine weight status.

Source: Nutrition Screening Initiative, a project of the American Academy of Family Physicians, American Dietetic Association, and the National Council on Aging, Inc. Accessed 11/01/03 @ www.aafp.org/nsi.htm

a. Determination of waist circumference and/or hip–waist ratio correlates with "apple" versus "pear" body type and reflects risk pattern for disease ("apple" types are at greater risk than "pear" types)

b. The use of fat fold measurements as part of anthropometric data also helps determine distribution of body fat

5. Skin fold measurements using calipers provide an objective measurement of body fat stores and nutritional status

a. Triceps skin fold (TSF) is most commonly performed measurement using subscapular and suprailiac skin folds

b. Mid-arm circumference (MAC) provides information about muscle and fat stores and is used to calculate mid-arm muscle circumference (MAMC)

c. MAMC provides information about skeletal muscle mass and distinguishes differences in muscle and body fat

C. Laboratory and diagnostic measurements

1. Albumin levels: good overall indicator of nutritional status because of long half life (18–20 days); body stores and maintains normal levels until chronic malnutrition occurs (refer to Table 26–2 ■)

a. Prealbumin levels are a more sensitive indicator of nutritional status because of shorter half life and because they respond to short-term changes in protein stores

Table 26-2

Serum Albumin Levels

Category	Serum Albumin Level
Normal	3.5–5.5 grams/dl
Mild depletion	2.8–3.4 grams/dl
Moderate depletion	2.1–2.7 grams/dl
Severe depletion	less than 2.1 grams/dl

! b. Transferrin levels identify iron stores, which provides information on visceral body protein

! c. Albumin, prealbumin, and transferrin levels are used to evaluate clinical response in clients on total parenteral nutrition (TPN) and overall nutritional status in other clients

2. Total lymphocyte count (TLC) decreases as protein stores become depleted, which has implications for immune system function

! 3. Screening for specific nutrient deficiencies: hemoglobin levels reflect iron intake; transferrin transports iron from intestine into serum and drops more rapidly than albumin

IV. KEY NUTRITIONAL CONCERNS ACROSS THE LIFESPAN

A. Culture and religion influence food choices in times of health and illness; see Table 26–3 ■

B. Pregnancy and lactation

! 1. Calorie needs increase during pregnancy by about 300 calories/day and during lactation by 500 calories/day

2. Intake of a balanced diet is important, with attention to adequate intake of protein, folic acid, magnesium, iron, calcium, vitamin C, and B complex vitamins (especially folic acid to prevent neural tube defects)

! 3. Weight gain during pregnancy is based on prepregnant weight using BMI as a reference point (note variation in underweight classification from non-pregnant state)
   a. Underweight clients (BMI < 19.8) should gain 28 to 40 pounds
   b. Healthy weight clients (BMI 19.8–24.9) should gain 25 to 35 pounds
   c. Overweight clients (BMI 25–29) should gain 15 to 25 pounds

Table 26–3

Influences of Culture and Religion on Nutritional Status

Cultural or Religious Group	Practices and/or Issues*
African American	Traditional foods high in fat, cholesterol, sodium and low in calcium. Frying and adding fat to food is common. Obesity, cardiovascular disease, and diabetes are common.
Asian	Traditional diet is plant-based: low in fat, saturated fat, and cholesterol; rich in fiber and nutrients; may be high in sodium. High risk for osteoporosis.
Native American	Diet varies with region. Some use corn and other cultivated crop staples; many attempt to live off land. Widespread poverty and use of food assistance programs (food stamps, food distribution on reservations) exist in this group. Diabetes and obesity are common.
Hispanic (Mexican origin)	Traditional diet is vegetarian, high in complex carbohydrates, such as corn, beans, and squash. High levels of calories, fats (saturated in particular), and sugar are eaten. Fat and fatty methods commonly are used in food preparation. Obesity, diabetes, and high triglycerides are common.
Islam	No pork, birds of prey, alcohol, tea, or coffee are consumed. Fasting is common during certain religious events.
Christianity	Catholics eat no meat on Ash Wednesday or Fridays during Lent; fasting is common on some religious days. Eastern Orthodox practice some fasting. Mormons consume no coffee, tea, alcohol, or tobacco. Seventh Day Adventists generally are lacto-ovovegetarians. No coffee, tea, alcohol, or strong seasonings are consumed. Meals are at least 4 to 5 hours apart with no snacking between meals.
Judaism (those following strict dietary rules)	Only kosher meat and poultry—no pork, shellfish, or fishlike mammals—are eaten. Milk or dairy at the same meal with meat or poultry is forbidden. Separate utensils are required for preparing and serving meat and dairy.

*Although identified by a specific ethnic or religious group, practices vary with area of origin and sect. Not all individuals within these groups follow these practices or have these issues.

d. Obese clients (BMI > 29) should gain 15 pounds or less

4. Common symptoms that may affect nutrition
   a. Nausea and vomiting: consume CHOs before getting out of bed in morning; eat small, frequent meals; avoid foods with offensive odors; do not drink fluids with meals; avoid coffee, tea, and spicy foods; limit high-fat foods
   b. Heartburn: interventions are similar to above; wait at least 1 hour before reclining after a meal
   c. Cravings and aversions: avoid nonnutritive substances (pica) that replace essential nutrients and may interfere with their absorption; aversions are usually self-limiting
   d. Constipation: caused by iron intake, enlarging uterus, decreased physical activity, and possibly inadequate fiber and fluid; consume at least 8 glasses of water daily and increase fiber in diet

C. Infancy

1. Infants may be breast- or bottle-fed according to maternal preference; breastfeeding is accepted as preferred nutrition whenever possible
2. Weight doubles in first 6 months of life and triples by 1 year
3. Avoid giving cow's milk during first year (deficient in essential fatty acids, iron, zinc, vitamin E, and vitamin C); could lead to decrease in hemoglobin and hematocrit and possible intestinal bleeding
4. Fluoride supplements are generally prescribed for infants 6 months of age and older if water supply has less than 0.3 parts per million (ppm) fluoride
5. Do not add cereal to bottle because of risk of aspiration with stronger suck reflex needed
6. Do not give bottle containing milk, juice, or sweetened beverage before sleep to avoid nursing bottle syndrome (dental caries)
7. Start solid foods at 4 to 6 months of age to reduce risk of food allergies and because of immaturity of GI tract
8. Introduce one new food no more frequently than every 4 to 7 days to detect allergy; give only 1 to 2 teaspoons initially and increase over time
9. Cook foods well and cut into tiny pieces to reduce risk of choking; supervise during meals and avoid giving hard round foods such as grapes, peanuts, popcorn, hotdogs, and others
10. Avoid using honey because of risk of infant botulism

D. Childhood

1. Dietary needs differ among toddlers, preschoolers, and school-aged children; total energy needs increase with age, but calories per kilogram of weight decrease
2. Toddlers and preschoolers may have erratic and ritualistic eating patterns and strong food preferences, including food jags (preferring one or a few types of foods over all others); these place child at risk for nutritional deficiencies; provide a balanced diet over time if not at each meal
3. Facilitate nutrient intake in young children by not forcing child to eat, maintaining relaxed mealtimes, offering one new food with a favorite food, using child-sized portions, serving foods with mild flavors, and providing finger-foods
4. Encourage school-aged children not to skip breakfast; encourage regular meal patterns; nutrient stores for puberty are laid during this time
5. Encourage healthy after-school snacks rather than high-calorie and high-fat items found in fast foods; choose popcorn, fresh fruits and vegetables, peanut butter, cheese, nuts, eggs, and yogurt
6. Encourage adequate physical activity to reduce risk of childhood obesity
7. Daily intake of a multivitamin may reduce risk of vitamin deficiency from occasional erratic dietary patterns (such as from after-school and sports schedules)

E. Adolescence

1. Need for macro- and micronutrients significantly increases during this time
2. Male adolescent growth spurt begins at 12 to 13 years, peaks at 14, and continues until approximately 19 years
3. Female adolescent growth spurt begins at 10 to 11 years, peaks at 12, and continues until approximately 15 years

4. Adolescents frequently consume inadequate amounts of vitamin A, C, B_6, iron, calcium, zinc, and magnesium
5. Adolescents frequently engage in dieting; follow fad or restrictive diets; skip meals; snack on high-calorie, high-fat, or high-sugar foods; and eat more meals outside home (including fast foods); these eating patterns increase risk of calorie and/or nutrient deficiencies
6. Diet should be well–balanced with sufficient calories but eliminating empty, (nonnutritive) calories and high fat foods; vitamin supplements may be helpful
7. Eating disorders (anorexia nervosa, bulimia nervosa) or obesity may be of concern; see Chapter 22 for discussion of eating disorders

F. Adulthood (age 18–64 years)

1. Dietary needs include maintaining ideal body weight and maintaining balanced dietary intake
2. There is significant variation in metabolic needs based on age, weight, height, and physical activity; overall energy needs decrease during adulthood, although needs for selected nutrients may increase
3. Special nutritional concerns include stress (affects metabolic processes) and occupational influences (such as travel) that affect meal patterns and dietary intake
4. Poor nutritional habits through lifetime increase risk of cardiovascular disease, diabetes mellitus, cancer, and obesity
5. Take multivitamin and mineral supplements as needed and follow balanced meal plan and possibly therapeutic diet based on identified health problem(s)
6. Lose weight if indicated to reduce further health risks

G. Older adulthood (age 65 and older)

1. Caloric requirements continue to decrease
2. Nutrient absorption may be adversely affected because of chewing difficulties (periodontal disease, loss of teeth, dysphagia due to stroke or other neuromuscular disease), decreased peristalsis, and reduced secretion of digestive enzymes
3. Therapeutic diets may affect intake of calories and specific nutrients
4. Clients who have dysphagia from cerebrovascular accident (CVA) (stroke) will have dysphagia staged using videofluoroscopy and evaluated by speech and language therapist; diet will be prescribed as (1) pureed foods, (2) ground/minced meat, (3) soft/easy-to-chew foods, or (4) modified general diet; commercial thickeners for liquids will also be used
5. Prescribed medications may interact with specific foods or may cause side effects (nausea, vomiting, diarrhea, constipation, inactivation of nutrients) that affect nutritional health
6. Loss of family or friends may reduce socialization at mealtimes and provide for fewer opportunities for social eating
7. Those who have insufficient finances or rely on others to shop for food or prepare food are at risk for nutritional deficiencies
8. Thirst response declines with age and can lead to fluid and electrolyte imbalances
9. Common nutrient deficiencies in older adults include protein, fiber, total calories, iron, calcium, magnesium, and vitamins D, B_{12}, and B_6

V. PHYTOCHEMICALS AND NUTRITIONAL SUPPLEMENTS

A. Phytochemicals

1. Overview
   a. Nonnutrient chemical substances found in plants that correlate with health benefits in disease treatment and prevention
   b. *Functional foods* are food items (nutrients) that correlate with health benefits; this newer term is being used to assess therapeutic effects of foods that contain phytochemicals
   c. Nutraceuticals are natural products and consist of botanicals and phytomedicine; term is not currently recognized by FDA
2. Indications for use and availability
   a. Some phytochemicals function as antioxidants and have been found to be effective in preventing cancer (breast, lung, prostate, and stomach), cardiac

disease, osteoporosis, and macular degeneration, and in alleviating menopausal symptoms

b. Phytochemicals are found in plant sources (fruits and vegetables), whole grains, tea and soy products

c. Many foods contain several phytochemicals and therefore can exert multiple effects on many body systems

d. Increase fruits and vegetables in the diet (because they contain phytochemicals) by using them as main ingredients, snack items, and alternate food selections (try new choices in diet)

3. Types of phytochemicals (see Table 26–4 ■)

!

4. Health applications

a. Antioxidant function and cancer prevention ability have led to great interest and continued research in area of phytochemicals

b. "Natural" approach of including functional foods that provide phytochemicals can be incorporated into an individual's lifestyle

c. Phytochemicals are being used as part of therapeutic treatment in clients with cancer, CAD, and hypercholesterolemia

d. Dietitians can assist in selection of food products that contain phytochemicals

B. Nutritional supplements

1. FDA guidelines maintain specific requirements for products to be called a nutritional supplement

Table 26–4

Types of Phytochemicals

Phytochemical	General Information
Carotenoids	Found in colorful fruits and vegetables (green, orange, red and yellow) Chemical classification includes beta-carotene and lycopene (found in tomato products, sauces, and ketchup); function as both pro-oxidant and antioxidant Health benefits include retinal protection; decreased risk of CAD, lung, prostate, and breast cancers; enhanced immune effects in older adults
Indoles	Found in vegetables such as broccoli, cauliflower, cabbage, and kale Chemical classification includes organosulphur compounds; are members of cruciferous vegetable family Health benefits include hormone stimulation to make estrogen less effective (decreasing risk of nonhormone-dependent breast cancer) and protection against carcinogen development by influencing DNA enzyme activity
Isoflavones	Found in soy foods (tofu, soy milk, and soybean products) and black and green tea Chemical composition includes phenylpropanoids that include flavonoid group (also found in nuts, wine, and oregano) Health benefits include inhibition of cancer cell growth (breast, prostate, and endometrial), alleviation of menopausal symptoms, and prevention of osteoporosis by increasing bone density
Phenolic Acids	Found in coffee beans, fruits and vegetables, green tea, wine, and soybeans Chemical structure includes phenylpropanoids, which act as antioxidants and bind metals to promote excretion of carcinogenic substances Health benefits include decreased risk of certain cancers (skin, lung, and stomach) and effect on glycemic control
Terpones	Found in the oil of citrus peel and menthol Chemical structure includes isoprenoid Health benefits include protection against carcinogens
Phytoestrogens	Found in vegetables, plants, soybean, and whole-grain fruits and berries Chemical structure falls under phenylpropanoids and specifically includes isoflavones and lignans Health benefits include protection against cardiac disease, cancer (breast and prostate), and osteoporosis
Catechins	Found in teas Chemical structure includes phenylpropanoids; are rich in phenolic acid Health benefits include possible antioxidant activity, prevention of cancer, and antihypertensive effects

2. Nutritional supplements are products that contain vitamins, minerals, herbs, botanicals, amino acids, enzymes, extracts, or combinations of these
3. Also included in this category are **ergonomic aids** that include a variety of items used to enhance body performance and promote muscle growth
   a. Amino acids are often used to promote anabolism and maintain strength in the form of glutamine and branch chain amino acids (BCAA); protein is increased often to the level of 1.3 to 2 grams/day
   b. CHO loading (glycogen loading) consists of high glucose ingestion before intense exercise in order to increase glycogen stores and delay onset of fatigue
   c. Metabolic end products are often used as ergonomic aids (creatine and steroids) in body
4. Although many products claim to be ergonomic aids, clinical research does not support all claims; clients should consider each product's potential harm and/or available benefit prior to use

C. Indications for use and availability

1. Nutritional supplements are used to decrease risk of disease, support body's increased needs during growth and stress periods, and improve overall body functioning
2. Selected clients, who fall under at-risk categories due to life cycle concerns (pregnancy, lactation, or children), underlying disease states (illness, stress, or malabsorption), inadequate intake of nutrients (strict vegans or constant dieters), and/or clinical intervention that requires therapy, may need nutritional supplements
3. Supplements are available in several forms ranging from oral formulations (pills, liquids) to powders to incorporated food substances (such as power bars or energy beverages)

VI. THERAPEUTIC DIETS WITH ALTERED CONSISTENCY

A. Clear liquid diet

1. Provides adequate fluid/water, 500 to 1,000 kcal of simple sugars and electrolytes but is fiber free
2. Requires minimal digestion because there is no residue or fiber
3. Recommended for short-term use (1–2 days); can be used both before and after surgery or diagnostic procedures, during acute stages of illness, or as initial diet after significant period of GI inactivity/bowel rest
4. Consists of clear foods that are liquid at body temperature: gelatin, tea, coffee, bouillon, clear broth, popsicles, apple juice, carbonated beverages (no milk or milk products can be used or added to coffee or tea)

B. Full liquid diet

1. Provides water, calories, protein, vitamins and minerals, and dairy products (contains lactose) and is considered to be low in residue
2. Indicated for some clients who have difficulty chewing or swallowing, but not indicated for a client following a CVA (stroke)
3. Can be considered a transition diet (temporary diet as client progresses postoperatively or postprocedure from clear liquids to solids); is deficient in many nutrients and calories
4. Consists of all foods found on a clear liquid diet plus milk, juices, pudding, ice cream, soups, yogurts, all prepared liquid formulas (all foods that are liquid at body temperature)
5. Clients who are lactose intolerant may require lactose-free supplements to prevent clinical symptoms

C. Pureed diet

1. Provides essential nutrients in a chopped, ground, or pureed form for clients who are unable to chew or swallow
2. Can be used as a long-term diet—preparation of food items is deciding factor
3. Use of seasoning depends on individual client preferences
4. A blender or food processor is used to change foods into pureed or blended form for use in diet

5. Certain foods such as raw eggs, nuts, whole breads, fruits, vegetables, and foods containing seeds are not allowed

D. Dysphagia diet

1. Consists of thickened liquids provided to clients who have swallowing problems and are at risk for aspiration (such as post-CVA)
2. Thickening agents can be added to foods to maximize texture and help facilitate swallowing process
3. Dysphagia diet is a modification of soft diet with increased attention to liquid component to avoid possible aspiration
4. Stringy, raw, dry, and fried foods are not allowed on this type of diet because of potential aspiration
5. Foods considered to be small in size or hand held, such as popcorn, nuts, and small candies, should be avoided because of risk of aspiration
6. ! Position client to at least 30 to 45 degrees head elevation and monitor feedings during meals to decrease risk of aspiration and evaluate client's attempts at eating

E. Soft diet

1. Used for clients who have problems with chewing (dental problems, oral lesions, difficulty chewing or swallowing)
2. Includes food items that contain small amounts of seasoning and moderate fiber content but are easy to chew, digest, and absorb
3. Highly seasoned, fried, and high in fiber foods; nuts; coconuts; and foods that contain seeds are not included because they could cause GI upset
4. Can be used as a progressive or transition diet and is a modification of regular diet

F. Mechanical soft diet

1. Focuses on including all foods and seasonings in a form that it easily handled by client
2. Soft textured, tender, and chopped foods are included in diet
3. Can be used as a long-term diet or a transition diet
4. Is a modification of regular diet with attention to texture
5. Tough foods (seeds, nuts, and fruits with pits) are not included in this diet

G. Bland diet

1. Consists of foods that do not irritate the GI tract and that lead to less gas formation and reduced gastric acid stimulation
2. Avoids spicy or fried foods, pepper, alcohol, and caffeine–containing beverages
3. Is used for a wide variety of GI disorders, such as esophagitis, gastritis, inflammatory bowel disease

H. High-residue/high-fiber diet

1. Includes intake of 20 to 25 grams of fiber daily to add bulk to stool and speed rate of passage through GI tract
2. Used for clients with constipation, asymptomatic diverticular disease, and to treat alternating constipation and diarrhea of irritable bowel syndrome; stimulates peristalsis, promotes regularity, and maintains normal bowel function and elimination patterns
3. Fruits, vegetables, legumes, and whole grains are eaten in larger quantities or proportions in this diet
4. Additional benefits are improved regulation of serum cholesterol and blood glucose, which is useful to clients with heart disease and diabetes mellitus

I. Low-residue/low-fiber diet

1. Includes foods such as white bread, cereals, and pasta (high CHO)
2. Avoids raw vegetables, fruits (bananas allowed), whole grains, plant fiber, and seeds; limits intake of dairy products to 2 servings daily
3. Fried foods, pepper, alcohol, and heavily seasoned foods are restricted because of possible GI upset
4. Used for conditions in which GI inflammation or scarring has narrowed bowel lumen and food intake could contribute to obstruction, such as inflammatory bowel disease, partial bowel obstruction, enteritis, and diarrhea

VII. RESTRICTED OR ENHANCED DIETS

A. Carbohydrate-controlled

1. Assists in regulating serum glucose levels in conditions in which they rise and fall, such as in diabetes mellitus, hypoglycemia, dumping syndrome, galactosemia, and obesity
2. Utilizes a dietary exchange system (designed by American Dietetic Association and American Diabetes Association) that groups foods according to protein, CHO, and fat content per specified food serving
3. Includes complex CHOs for 55% to 60%, proteins for 10% to 20%, and saturated fats for less than 10% of total daily calories; also included recommended fiber intake of 20 to 35 grams/day
4. Gestational diabetes diet is a meal pattern that encourages adequate calories based on prepregnant weight status, frequent small feedings, and snacks throughout day to normalize postprandial glucose levels, maintain normal (euglycemic) levels throughout pregnancy, and prevent ketosis
5. ! Hypoglycemic diet consists of small feedings at frequent intervals to help normalize blood glucose levels; when episodes of hypoglycemia occur, ingest 15 gram CHO snack, recheck glucose in 15 minutes, and repeat if necessary (15/15 rule)
6. Carbohydrate counting is a means of controlling carbohydrate intake over a 24-hour period

B. Gastric bypass diet

1. ! Consists of eating small meals several times a day, drinking liquids between meals, and taking multivitamin supplements with an emphasis on nutrient-dense foods
2. Diet is low in fat and high in protein
3. Carbonated beverages, simple CHOs, and foods with high fiber and residue are restricted

C. Fat-controlled diet

1. Used to manage malabsorption, chronic pancreatitis, and gallbladder disease
2. Medium chain triglycerides (MCT) are utilized in diet because they are easily digested along with high intakes of CHOs and protein
3. High-fat foods are limited or omitted, (such as red meats and dairy products) and no additional fat is used in cooking process
4. Enzyme replacements may be necessary along with fat-soluble vitamin and mineral supplements
5. Foods that are high in oxalates are limited to prevent risk of kidney stone formation
6. Clients with hyperlipidemia (high cholesterol and/or triglyceride levels) should be placed on a low-saturated-fat diet (increase monounsaturated fats and small amounts of polyunsaturated fatty acids) with restricted sodium and hydrogenated food products
7. Clients who have cardiovascular disease, congestive heart failure, and posttransplant will have some form of fat-controlled diet as life-long dietary pattern

D. Protein-controlled diet

1. ! Used for clients with renal disease (renal failure, end-stage renal disease, dialysis, and transplant) or liver disease (liver failure, hepatic encephalopathy, cirrhosis, transplant, and hepatitis) because they are unable to handle protein load
2. Provides necessary protein to maintain nutritional status but does not result in excess wastes or metabolites of protein breakdown (usually 40–60 grams protein daily or 0.8 grams/kg of dry weight)
3. Depending on client's clinical condition, protein levels may be increased to account for metabolic response to dialysis and regeneration of liver tissue (1.5–2.0 grams/kg/day)
4. A minimum level of CHOs must be present in the diet (50–100 grams/day) in order to spare protein; protein intake must be high quality
5. Vitamin and mineral supplements may be indicated for clients who have liver failure
6. ! Restricts foods such as meat, fish, poultry, and dairy products; other foods need to be evaluated individually for protein content

Box 26–1

Gluten-Restricted Diet

- ➤ Foods included: cornmeal, corn flakes, popcorn, hominy, and potato chips
- ➤ Food substitutions: corn, potato, rice, soybean flour, and low-gluten wheat flour
- ➤ Foods to avoid: processed (commercially prepared) foods that include wheat flour extenders, additives, or stabilizers
- ➤ Foods to avoid: root beer, beer, and all products that contain identified grain sources (wheat, rye, barley, buckwheat, oats and malt)

E. Food allergy diet

1. Egg-free diet is used for clients who have a known sensitivity to eggs and restricts use of eggs and egg products
2. Many foods, such as cow's milk, eggs, fish, shellfish, nuts, soybean, and wheat, have allergic potential
3. Primary therapy is avoidance of the particular food item
4. Children often present with food allergies and certain diets (allergy I and allergy II) are used in sequence to identify potential food allergens by eliminating intake of potential food allergens in a controlled manner; these diets are used in a limited time frame because they are not nutritionally complete
5. Gluten-restricted diet (gluten gliaden–free diet) is used for clients who have celiac disease (malabsorption syndrome) and omits wheat, rye, barley, buckwheat, oats and malt (gluten proteins) from the diet (see Box 26–1)
   - **a.** Clinical manifestations resulting from inability to handle gluten protein are steatorrhea, diarrhea, weight loss, anemia, and edema formation caused by loss of nutrients
   - **b.** Lactose-intolerant clients must follow additional diet restrictions
6. Lactose-restricted diet is used for clients who have lactose intolerance (due to lactase enzyme deficiency) and may require lactase enzymes in diet to tolerate dairy products (see Box 26–2)
   - **a.** Primary lactose intolerance is more common among certain ethnic groups (African Americans, Asian, Hispanic, and Native Americans)
   - **b.** Secondary lactose intolerance is caused by another established disease process (such as infection) or medication (chemo agents that inhibit cell growth) that affect GI tract's ability to produce lactase
   - **c.** Clinical symptoms affect GI tract, resulting in gas, bloating, and diarrhea

Box 26–2

Lactose-Restricted Diet

- ➤ Foods included: aged cheese (hard) rather than soft cheese because hard cheese is lower in lactose due to aging process
- ➤ Yogurt can be included in the diet because of its bacterial action, and frozen yogurt may have even less lactose due to bacterial action and freezing process
- ➤ OTC products such as Lactaid are specific formulations used to assist clients who have identified lactose deficiency; these products are usually available in liquid or tablet form
- ➤ Special milk products formulated with Lactaid are available for use by lactose-intolerant clients (products of this type are usually sweeter than regular milk products)
- ➤ Individual tolerance is variable, and client is the best judge of how little or how much "lactose" they can handle without onset of clinical symptoms
- ➤ Check food labels for milk, milk solids, casein, and whey, which are sometimes used as additives and stabilizers in processed food products
- ➤ Check medication ingredients because lactose can be used as binders or fillers in certain formulations
- ➤ Lactose-restricted diets are often low in calcium, vitamin B_2 (riboflavin), and vitamin D, so additional nutrient supplements may be necessary to maintain optimal nutrient levels

7. Restriction and/or avoidance therapy is utilized to prevent or minimize food allergies

F. Purine-controlled diet

1. Indicated for clients who have gout, tumor lysis syndrome, or multiple myeloma, which all cause elevated uric acid levels
2. Excessive purine accumulation leads to an increase in uric acid, which is a normal end product of purine catabolism
3. ! Includes use of dairy products and restricts organ meats, anchovies, alcohol, and seafood

G. Sodium-controlled diet

1. Indicated for clients with hypertension, cardiovascular disease, heart failure, and conditions in which fluid restriction is beneficial (renal failure, cirrhosis, or liver failure)
2. Restriction ranges from mild (3,000–4,000 mg/day) to severe (500 mg/day)
3. ! It is important to evaluate food labels (sodium is a common preservative), medications, and restaurant dietary intake pattern for hidden sources of sodium
4. Clients using salt substitutes may be at risk for elevated potassium levels and should be evaluated for risk of hyperkalemia, especially if taking potassium-sparing diuretics, such as triamterene (Dyrenium)
5. ! Avoid table salt and using salt in cooking; meat and dairy products have physiological saline, while fruits tend to be lowest overall in sodium
6. See Box 26–3 for examples of high-sodium foods to avoid

H. Tyramine- and dopamine-restricted diet

1. Indicated for clients taking monoamine oxidase inhibitors (MAOIs, or antidepressants); foods containing tyramine affect drug action by blocking enzyme pathways and lead to release of norepinephrine, resulting in a hypertensive crisis
2. Tyramine is an intermediate product of amino acid metabolism formed in conversion of tyrosine to epinephrine and is found in many food items
3. Other amines, such as dopamine, are also restricted because excess accumulation can lead to similar hypertensive effects
4. ! Diet restrictions include aged cheese, chocolate, smoked fish, processed meats such as bologna, bananas, liver, fava beans, and large amounts of soy sauce
5. Foods that can be included are unfermented cheese (ricotta and cottage cheese) and small amounts of certain foods such as sour cream

I. Low-potassium diet

1. Used for clients who have renal failure or who are taking potassium-sparing diuretics
2. Potassium is abundant in many foods, but avoid foods outlined in Box 26–4, which are high in potassium
3. Reduce potassium content of vegetables by cooking and then draining cooking water; this method also reduces vitamin content of foods, however
4. In contrast, high-potassium foods may be encouraged for clients with normal renal function taking potassium-sparing diuretics

Box 26–3

Foods High in Sodium

Condiments: pickles, olives, nuts, meat tenderizers, commercial salad dressings, ketchup, soy sauce, Worcestershire and other sauces, monosodium glutamate (MSG), commercial mustard, table salt, and seasoned or buttered salts

Breads: commercial breads with salt added, salted crackers, potato chips, popcorn, pretzels, other salted snacks

Meats: smoked, cured, or processed meats (ham, bacon, hot dogs, luncheon meat, canned meats); all cheeses except cottage cheese and low-sodium cheese

Soups: canned or dehydrated soups, bouillon

Vegetables: sauerkraut, pork and beans, canned tomato or vegetable juices, hominy

Beverages: commercial milk, instant drink mixes

Box 26-4

Foods High in Potassium

Apricots	Oranges and orange juice
Avocado	Peanuts
Bananas	Potatoes (white or sweet)
Cantaloupe	Prune juice
Raw carrots	Spinach
Dried beans or peas	Tomatoes and tomato products
Dried fruits	Winter squash
Melons	

J. High-calcium diet

1. Indicated for clients with disease states that promote calcium loss and lead to bone demineralization (osteoporosis, osteopenia), endocrine abnormalities, and kidney failure
2. Good sources of calcium include milk and other dairy products; green leafy vegetables are adequate sources also

K. High-protein diet

1. The use of a high-protein diet has been indicated for burns, liver disease, and for athletes (1.2–1.6 grams/kg/day) to maximize endurance, according to current research evidence
2. Includes meat, fish, poultry, and dairy products and protein supplements

L. High-calorie diet

1. Indicated for clients with debilitating disease or need for tissue repair, including cancer, burns, stress, acquired immunodeficiency disease, and others
2. Should include added protein to preserve muscle mass
3. Includes use of nutritious snacks (milkshakes, puddings) between meals to increase calorie intake
4. Includes added use of sugars and possibly fats to increase overall calories

M. High-iron diet

1. Indicated for clients with anemia
2. Includes added sources of iron, such as meat (especially organ meats), egg yolks, leafy vegetables, whole wheat breads and products, legumes, and dried fruits

N. Vegetarian diets

1. Vegan (strict vegetarian): includes plant-based foods with no meat, fish, poultry, dairy products, or eggs
2. Ovovegetarian: no meat, fish, or poultry and no dairy products; eggs are allowed
3. Lactovegetarian: no meat, fish, poultry, or eggs; diary products are allowed
4. Ovolactovegetarian: no meat, fish, or poultry; diary products and eggs are allowed

VIII. ENTERAL NUTRITION

A. Overview

1. **Enteral nutrition** is a method of feeding clients who have a functioning GI tract but have chewing or swallowing difficulty or impaired upper GI tract function, leading to poor nutrient digestion, transport, and absorption
2. Feedings can be delivered orally or via tube placement

B. Indications for use

1. Short-term use via nasogastric tubes or oral route
2. Long-term use via enterostomy placed surgically or percutaneously

C. Administration

1. Continuous feedings occur throughout a 24-hour period at a prescribed flow rate and a total set volume using an infusion pump
2. Intermittent infusions occur over a time frame of 30 minutes (to mimic usual eating pattern) or more with a prescribed total set volume ranging from 250 to 400 ml of formula using an infusion pump or gravity

3. **Cyclic feeding** occurs over a period of several hours (prescribed flow rate and a set total volume using an infusion pump), usually at night as a transitional approach to healthy GI functioning
4. **Bolus feeding** occurs when there is a rapid delivery of a large amount of formula (preset volume 250–300 in a present time of 10 minutes or less) in a short time frame

D. Collaborative Management

1. Formula selection
   a. Characteristics of formula include protein classification, nutrient density, and amounts of residue and fiber; different osmolality of formulas available (isotonic and hypertonic)
   b. Client's underlying clinical condition influences selection of formula
   c. Elderly clients and newborns may be unable to tolerate large volume feedings and may require modification of treatment regimen in order to meet nutritional needs
2. ! Monitoring response to treatment
   a. Document weight status; document trends and communicate to health care team
   b. Monitor for expected weight gain and stabilization of visceral protein measurements (albumin, prealbumin and transferrin), TLC, BUN, creatinine, and other pertinent serum chemistries during therapy
   c. Dietitian will evaluate requirements for macronutrients and fluid requirements based on body weight calculations

E. Nursing responsibilities

1. ! Document baseline weight and daily weights thereafter to evaluate response to therapy
2. Inspect tube insertion site for signs of potential irritation or infection
3. ! Check tube placement prior to initiation of any feeding regimen or medication administration
   a. Aspirate to check for gastric contents
   b. Measure pH of gastric aspirant
   c. Use stethoscope to auscultate for "whoosh" caused by air placement in stomach if agency does not provide pH testing strips
4. ! Check for residual on all tube feedings (based on rate per hour) to prevent complications, and document response to therapy
   a. Residuals are often checked q 4 hours during continuous feedings
   b. When feedings are intermittent, check residual prior to instituting next feeding
5. If residual amount is greater than expected, rate of feeding will be decreased or held in order to prevent overload complications resulting from inadequate digestion
   a. In a continuous feeding checked every 4 hours, if residual is greater than or equal to the 1 hour rate, then feeding should be withheld and residual rechecked in 1 hour to determine if client is now able to tolerate feeding
   b. If the feeding is not on a continuous schedule, then if half of volume from previous feeding is remaining, then feeding should be withheld and residual rechecked in 1 hour as with a continuous feeding
   c. Adjustment of volume amount and/or method of feeding (bolus, continuous, cyclic, or intermittent) may be necessary based on residual findings
   d. Follow specific agency or provider guidelines if different from those listed above
6. Check pertinent labs, daily weight, and I&O to monitor response to clinical therapy
7. Communicate with other health care team members in order to meet individualized client goals
8. ! Refer to Box 26–5 for a listing of nursing interventions specific to enteral tube feedings
9. ! Be aware of potential complications of tube feedings (Box 26–6)

IX. PROBLEMS WITH WEIGHT CONTROL

A. Overview of obesity

1. Obesity: weight that is more than 20% above ideal body weight (IBW)

Box 26-5

Interventions for Enteral Tube Feedings

- Inspect formula for particulate matter and untoward appearance that might suggest chemical breakdown.
- Do not hang more than the documented amount of formula per hospital protocol per shift because doing so can lead to bacterial overgrowth and chemical breakdown.
- Change solution and tubing per hospital protocol to prevent risk of infection.
- Check placement of tube prior to any feeding, flush, or medication application to ensure patency.
- Flush tube with water per hospital protocol in order to prevent dehydration that can occur if only formula feedings are used as the sole fluid replacement.
- Include flush or irrigation used in the client's I&O.
- Position client to ensure patency and maintain head of bed at 30 degrees prior to and during feeding.
- Monitor pertinent labs per hospital protocol and document daily weights.
- Work with health care team members (dietitian and enterostomal therapist) to maintain nutritional balance and skin integrity.
- Incorporate concepts of altered nutritional status and body image in developing plan of care.

2. Caused by an excess of body fat; can exist in a person of normal weight
   a. Men: greater than 22% body fat in young men and greater than 25% body fat in older men
   b. Women: greater than 35% body fat
   c. Morbid obesity is generally more than 100% above ideal body weight and having an adverse effect on a person's health

Box 26-6

Complications of Tube Feedings

- Mechanical complications include clogged tube, tube dislodgment, and use of a malfunctioning infusion pump.
- Metabolic complications include dehydration, electrolyte imbalances, and altered blood glucose levels (usually hyperglycemia).
- Complications related to formula selection and client tolerance include diarrhea, cramps, abdominal distention, constipation, nausea, and vomiting.
- If client is experiencing diarrhea from enteral feedings, a decreased rate and volume of solution may be indicated. The feeding interval may need to be changed to allow client to absorb and process feedings.
- Check serum albumin levels because changes in colloid oncotic pressure can cause fluid shifting (greater amount of water in the bowel), which also can lead to diarrhea. Low serum albumin levels also represent a malnourished state with decreased intestinal enzyme action that can increase incidence of diarrhea.
- The formula may have to be switched to an isotonic formula or a less hypertonic formula to minimize risk of diarrhea from dumping syndrome.
- Dermatologic complications include irritation at feeding tube site (enterostomy) caused by leakage of formula feeding or in response to skin applications or dressings at site.
- Potential complications from medication instillation via tube include clogging of tube from incorrect medication form or formula-drug interactions.
- Monitor amount of feeding and fluid replacement (water) specified per shift and 24-hour totals to minimize risk of dehydration and maintain hydration.
- Clients who have nasogastric tube feedings may be at risk for aspiration due to positioning or decreased gastric emptying. Maintain adequate client position by elevating head of bed during feedings and check residuals.

3. Causes of obesity include genetic factors (Prader-Willi syndrome), but these are uncommon
4. Neuroendocrine causes of obesity include Cushing's syndrome, polycystic ovarian syndrome, hypogonadism, insulinoma, and growth hormone insufficiency
5. Most common cause is dietary; associated with high-fat diet and sedentary lifestyle
6. Some drugs promote obesity, such as estrogens, corticosteroids, antidepressants, antiepileptics, antihypertensives, nonsteroidal anti-inflammatory drugs (NSAIDs), and phenothiazines
7. Social factors such as loneliness, stress, depression, guilt, and boredom, as well as cultural views of obesity as desirable and a sign of prosperity, influence eating habits and development of obesity
8. ! Complications of obesity include hypertension, hiatal hernia, diabetes mellitus, hyperlipidemia, coronary artery disease, sleep apnea, cholelithiasis, osteoarthritis, back pain, and increased susceptibility to infection

B. Nursing assessment of obesity

1. Measure height and weight and compare to Metropolitan Life tables
2. A BMI of 30 or above indicates obesity; 25.0 to 29.9 indicates overweight status; 18.5 to 24.9 is normal; less than 18.5 is underweight
3. Assess fat distribution profile: "apple" (intra-abdominal/truncal obesity) and "pear" (hips and thighs) waist-to-hip ratio (greater than 1.0 in males and 0.8 in females) can help establish a diagnosis of obesity
4. Examine body type: endomorph (stocky), ectomorph (tall), and mesomorph (middle range), along with upper body (android) and lower body (gynecoid) categories
5. Calculation of body weight as a percentage of IBW, usual weight, and recent weight changes are determined to assist in clinical diagnosis
6. Complications of obesity or comorbid conditions are determined by measuring serum glucose, serum cholesterol, and lipid profile, and by electrocardiogram (ECG)
7. ! Obtain history of eating habits, duration of obesity, medications, cultural factors, 24-hour food recall, usual physical activity, and situations that trigger eating behavior
8. Assess methods used for previous attempts at weight loss

C. Therapeutic management of obesity

1. Diet therapy
   a. Developed collaboratively with client, health care provider, and dietitian
   b. Safe weight loss rate is 1 to 2 pounds per week; individual results may be higher at first and then slow over time; FDA indicates weight loss is effective if maintained for 2 years
   c. Goals of diet therapy are aimed at decreasing weight to a healthy level based on client's BMI, activity status, and basal energy expenditure (BEE)
2. Behavioral therapy: helps client to change daily eating habits and includes keeping a food diary, establishing exercise patterns, controlling external cues to eating behavior, and switching focus from physical appearance to health
3. Surgery is an option for morbidly obese individuals who do not respond to other methods of weight loss and have a BMI above 35 with additional health risks, or for anyone with a BMI above 40; operative procedures include gastroplasty (most common), intestinal bypass, maxillomandibular fixation, and esophageal banding; pre- and postoperative care is similar to that for other gastric surgeries
4. ! Exercise enhances weight loss and should be part of daily schedule; recommendations for a healthy lifestyle include at least 30 minutes aerobic activity per day; walking is recommended; plan activity appropriate for client considering physical and environmental limitations
5. Provide information about support groups such as Overeaters Anonymous and Weight Watchers
6. Medication/pharmacological intervention
   a. Drug treatment is controversial and is usually only suggested with BMI above 30 (or >27 with comorbidities) and in conjunction with diet and exercise modifications

b. Anorexic medications are commonly used to suppress appetite so client eats less and loses weight slowly over time; they are contraindicated during pregnancy and lactation and in clients with cardiac, hepatic, or renal disease
c. Amphetamines and antidepressants are controversial because of reported cases of toxicity and dependency

D. Client teaching related to obesity

1. Prescribed diet therapy and exercise
2. New food pyramid (MyPyramid) and portion sizes (e.g., a serving of meat is 3 oz and is about size of a deck of cards; a serving of dry breakfast cereal is 1 oz or 1 cup)
3. Symptoms of possible adverse effects of weight loss medications, such as chest pain, shortness of breath, insomnia, and nervousness

E. Overview of underweight status

1. An underweight client has a BMI below 18.5 with subsequent ill effects on health
2. Physical conditions caused by disease or medical treatments can lead to underweight status
3. (Failure to thrive) FTT infants do not meet expected growth curves and developmental milestones and are clinically malnourished; weight and height are below expected percentile; these infants start out underweight and become more underweight over time
4. Psychological conditions (anorexia, bulimia, and depression) can lead to decreased intake, poor nutrition, and underweight status
5. Loss of visceral protein stores (body storage) results in negative nitrogen balance
6. Underweight clients may have adverse health effects if further compromised by stress, injury, or infection

! **F. Therapeutic management of underweight status**

1. Increase calories and reestablish regular meal pattern to promote weight gain
2. Increase intake of foods with high nutrient density (highest kcal/food)
3. Calculate ongoing nutrient needs based on BEE and evaluation of pertinent lab work (albumin, pre-albumin, transferrin levels, and TLC) in collaboration with dietitian and healthcare provider
4. Refer to Box 26–7 for realistic eating plan to promote weight gain
5. Medication therapy: megestrol acetate (Megace) and dronabinol (Marinol) as appetite stimulants (useful in clients with cancer, HIV, and AIDS)

G. Overview of malnutrition

1. State of poor nutrition from either undernutrition or overnutrition
2. Includes protein-calorie malnutrition (PCM) or protein-energy malnutrition (PEM)
3. Healing is adversely affected because of loss of protein stores and essential and nonessential nutrients that are coenzymes in metabolic processes

Box 26–7

Realistic Eating Plans for Underweight Client

- Do not skip meals. It is important to start an eating pattern based on eating all scheduled meals.
- Increase portion sizes and add nutrient-dense foods to the eating plan. Now is the time to add new foods, taste new foods, and sample old foods.
- Drink fluids and make sure to include them as sources of energy by using fruit juices and milkshakes to add to dietary intake.
- Incorporate physical activity in order to maintain muscle tone, gain strength, and promote endurance.
- Supplemental feedings may be required via enteral or parenteral route to realize dietary goals.
- Reasonable weight gain expectations should be noted and weight gained over time is more likely to stay on than weight gained through daily forced feeding.
- Medications may be prescribed to boost appetite and stimulate weight gain. If the client is experiencing any nausea or other GI symptoms, additional medications may be prescribed to minimize these symptoms and promote an adequate eating pattern.

4. Immune function is compromised because of insufficient nutrients
5. Fluid shifts due to low protein levels can lead to third spacing (ascites as in Kwashiorkor) and edema states (dependent and or periorbital) because of electrolyte imbalances
6. Dermatologic changes include brittle hair that can fall out, nail changes (brittle with ridges), pruritus, and poor healing
7. Hormonal imbalances can develop, affecting neurological status (irritability, paresthesias, decreased reflex response), musculoskeletal status (decreased muscle tone, cramping, deformities), and cardiac status (altered blood pressure, murmurs, possible cardiac enlargement)
8. Clinical evidence of malnutrition: mouth sores, oral cavity changes, and decreased hydration status

H. Therapeutic management of malnutrition

1. Nutrient calculation by the dietitian uses BEE, BMI, activity level, and pertinent lab testing
2. A significant increase in caloric intake is required to effect weight gain (3500 calories per week for a 1-pound weight gain requires additional 500 calorie per day)
3. Supervised program to work toward achieving individual client goals
4. Supplemental feeding may be required via enteral or parenteral routes
5. Frequent feeding regimen may be utilized to prevent hypoglycemia and hypothermia, which can cause further tissue catabolism
6. Controlled regimen for children (not less than 80 calories/kg/day up to 100 or more) and for adults (30–40 kcal/kg/day) in order to meet nutritional goals
7. Document and trend pertinent labs and weight status and correlate with client's underlying medical condition

I. Weight cycling

1. "Yo-yo" effect is a weight loss/weight gain pattern that can lead to a higher weight than when diet therapy was started
2. This usually occurs with unrealistic weight goals and/or altered dietary patterns without benefit of activity or lifestyle changes
3. In order for weight control to be effective, a combination of dietary, lifestyle, behavioral, and activity changes, not merely changes in food intake, are necessary

Check Your NCLEX-RN® Exam I.Q.

You are ready for testing on this content if you can

- Apply knowledge of nursing procedures to the care of a client with nutritional needs.
- Assess nutritional status of client, including a diet history.
- Determine the impact of illness on nutritional status.
- Provide a special diet based on health problem and nutritional needs of a client.
- Provide dietary teaching according to client need.
- Provide nutritional supplements to clients as needed.
- Promote independence in eating.
- Check placement and patency of a client's feeding tube.
- Assess for side effects of enteral nutrition.
- Evaluate effectiveness of diet therapy on weight and overall nutritional status.

PRACTICE TEST

1 An adolescent client is competing in a long-distance running event. The nurse is teaching the client about eating for competition. The nurse explains that which of the following is an appropriate meal before the competition?

1. Sausages, eggs, biscuits, and gravy
2. Pancakes with fresh strawberries, orange juice, wheat toast, and fresh melon slices
3. Yogurt, milk fortified with dry skim milk powder, and protein bar
4. Cheese omelet, hash brown potatoes, bacon, and coffee

2 The nurse has completed a comprehensive health assessment of a Hispanic client. Some cultural food practices place the client at risk for cardiovascular disease. Which suggestion by the nurse is appropriate for this client?

1. "Try to stop eating so many complex carbohydrates."
2. "Try to bake some foods instead of frying them."
3. "Lean meats should replace the beans and nuts in your diet."
4. "Do not stop stewing meat and vegetables together; it is a healthy cooking method."

3 Which of the following dietary recommendations should the nurse include in the discharge instructions of a client diagnosed with coronary artery disease?

1. Limit intake of whole grains.
2. Limit intake of tuna.
3. Limit intake of soybean products.
4. Limit intake of egg yolks.

4 The nurse is planning discharge teaching for the client with gastroesophageal reflux disease (GERD). What dietary modification should be included?

1. Eat three meals and a bedtime snack.
2. Avoid intake of caffeine and alcoholic beverages.
3. Drink 12 to 16 ounces of water with each meal.
4. Lie down for 15 to 20 minutes after eating.

5 The nurse interprets that which of the following client behaviors reflects compliance with a 2-gram sodium-restricted diet?

1. Using only the two packets of salt found on the meal tray
2. Limiting milk to 1 cup per day
3. Avoiding use of salt in cooking
4. Using salt-free butter with meals

6 The nurse determines that a hypertensive client understands the DASH diet (Dietary Approaches to Stop Hypertension) when the client chooses which items from a sample menu used in dietary teaching?

1. Caesar salad, bread sticks, frozen yogurt
2. Grilled chicken sandwich, strawberries, and lettuce salad
3. Grilled cheese sandwich, canned pineapple, brownie
4. Chicken and vegetable stir-fry, rice, egg roll

7 A client who is recovering from partial- and full-thickness burns has been advanced to a general diet. Which foods should the nurse encourage the client to eat most often?

1. Meats, citrus fruits, milk
2. Vegetables, cheese, pasta
3. Milkshakes, salads, soups
4. Breads, cereals, yogurt

8 Which of the following client comments indicates to the nurse that more teaching is needed for the client experiencing dumping syndrome after gastric surgery?

1. "I should eat six small meals per day."
2. "I should not drink fluids with my meals."
3. "I should use honey or jelly instead of butter."
4. "I should lie down for 30 to 60 minutes after eating."

9 Which of the following dietary teaching statements would the nurse make to a client who has renal calculi?

1. "The presence of renal calculi is directly correlated to dietary intake."
2. "Decreasing calcium intake will prevent the formation of renal calculi."
3. "An increase in dietary protein can increase the likelihood of renal calculi."
4. "Reducing dietary intake of complex carbohydrates decreases formation of renal calculi."

10 A client with chronic obstructive pulmonary disease (COPD), who has been consuming more than 3,000 calories/day to gain weight, now reports increased breathing difficulty. The client states, "I thought that if I gained weight by eating more, I would feel better." How would the nurse respond to the client's concern?

1. "The increase in calories is not as important as an increase in the fat percentage in the diet."
2. "It is not necessary to increase caloric intake because medication therapy can be given to help with desired weight gain."
3. "An increase in both calories and carbohydrates can lead to increased respiratory effort and clinical symptoms that you are having."
4. "An increase in high-quality proteins will help correct the respiratory symptoms."

11 Which snack selection would be most appropriate for the nurse to make for a client with cancer who has stomatitis?

1. Peanut butter sandwich
2. Soft pretzels with salt
3. Tomato soup
4. Yogurt

12 A client who is lactose intolerant is recovering from a surgical procedure. What impact does the nurse expect this to have on progression of diet as tolerated?

1. The client will be able to progress from a clear to full liquid diet easily once bowel sounds and gag reflex return.
2. There is no impact with regard to diet progression because of lactose intolerance.
3. The client's diet can be progressed following a bowel movement indicating return of bowel activity.
4. The client's full liquid diet may have to be altered because this diet contains milk products.

13 A client is placed on enteral feedings via nasogastric tube to meet nutritional goals. Which of the following assessments should be included in a plan of care in order to maintain fluid balance?

1. Assess the skin area around the tube site.
2. Weigh the client every other day.
3. Maintain strict I&O and flush the tube once a day to ensure patency.
4. Irrigate the tube with water as ordered and include this fluid in total I&O.

14 Which of the following points would the nurse make when doing dietary teaching with a client placed on a fat-restricted diet because of significant cardiac history?

1. "This diet will be used temporarily to reduce saturated fat intake and cholesterol levels."
2. "All forms of fat should be restricted because of your significant cardiac history."
3. "No additional fat should be utilized when cooking or preparing foods."
4. "Ice cream can be included in the diet, although fat from butter and meat is excluded."

15 A client's mother wants to know why she should have her daughter follow an allergy I and II diet. How would the nurse reply to this mother's concern?

1. "This is a short-term therapy diet, and it will be over before you know it."
2. "This diet needs to be followed until your daughter grows out of her allergy phase."
3. "This diet sequence helps to both identify and eliminate potential allergens, making future diet selection choices easier."
4. "Allergy testing usually accompanies this type of diet pattern, and you should see an immunologist."

16 Which of the following items should the nurse encourage in the diet of a client diagnosed with celiac disease?

1. Oatmeal
2. Whole wheat toast
3. Beef barley soup
4. Cornflakes

17 Which of the following foods would the nurse suggest as an item from the lunch menu for a client taking a monoamine oxidase (MAO) inhibitor?

1. Smoked fish
2. Bologna sandwich
3. Cottage cheese
4. Salad with bleu cheese dressing

18 How would the nurse best respond to a client's statement, "I am always dieting, but I never seem to be losing weight"?

1. "Weight loss is only maintained if you really want to lose the weight."
2. "Dieting is a way of life, and compliance is required to maintain weight loss."
3. "By saying you are always dieting, it sounds like you need some assistance in attaining your weight loss goals."
4. "I need to know which type of the diet you are on because it may not be effective."

19 The nurse would encourage the client wishing to reduce risk of cancer to maintain adequate intake of which foods?

1. Meat and dairy products
2. Fruits and vegetables
3. Rice and beans
4. Milk and cheese

20 An athletic client states that he is thinking of using carbohydrate (CHO) loading to increase his performance. How should the nurse respond to this client?

1. Suggest the use of alternative ergonomic aids such as creatine or creatinine because they provide better results.
2. Discuss foods that are high in CHOs to assist the client in meeting his desired goal.
3. Ask the client what type of sport activity he is doing to see if this method would help.
4. Refer the client to a sports/nutritional specialist or trainer so that he can be properly supervised.

21 The nurse would consult with the physician about either advancing the diet or instituting parenteral nutrition if the client has been on a clear liquid diet for the maximum of how many days?

____

ANSWERS & RATIONALES

1 **Answer: 2** The diet before competition should be high in complex carbohydrates and low in fat and protein. Option 2 reflects the best selection to meet this dietary balance. All of the other options are high in fat and/or protein and would not be beneficial in terms of supporting athletic performance.
Cognitive Level: Application **Client Need:** Physiological Integrity: Basic Care and Comfort **Integrated Process:** Nursing Process: Planning **Content Area:** Foundational Sciences: Nutrition **Strategy:** The core issue of the question is knowledge that complex carbohydrates are beneficial before lengthy exercise. Use nutrition knowledge and the process of elimination to make a selection.

2 **Answer: 2** One characteristic of Hispanic diets is the high-fat preparation method used in cooking. Suggesting a new preparation method for a familiar food item would best help the client to begin changing cooking habits. Option 1 is incorrect—complex carbohydrates should not be eliminated because they are components of a healthy diet. Option 3 is incorrect—the Hispanic client would probably be unwilling to relinquish beans and nuts in the diet because these are considered staple food products. Option 4 is incorrect because stewing is considered a high-fat method of cooking because the fat from the meat does not drain off.
Cognitive Level: Application **Client Need:** Physiological Integrity: Basic Care and Comfort **Integrated Process:** Nursing Process: Implementation **Content Area:** Foundational Sciences: Nutrition **Strategy:** The core issue of the question is knowledge of methods of reducing fat in the diet. Use nutrition knowledge and the process of elimination to make a selection.

3 **Answer: 4** Egg yolks are high in cholesterol and should be limited to 2 to 3 per week. Dietary fiber, fish, and soybean products have been shown to lower blood lipids. Dietary fiber is necessary in the body to promote regulation of elimination patterns and to help lower blood lipids. Soybean products are a source of phytoestrogens and have been shown to be cardioprotective. Tuna is an excellent source of omega-3 fatty acids, which are helpful in protecting cardiac function and decreasing clot formation.
Cognitive Level: Application **Client Need:** Physiological Integrity: Basic Care and Comfort **Integrated Process:** Nursing Process: Planning **Content Area:** Foundational Sciences: Nutrition **Strategy:** The core issue of the question is knowledge of the components of a low-fat diet and that this is the diet required by clients with heart disease. Use nutrition knowledge and the process of elimination to make a selection.

4 **Answer: 2** Foods that decrease lower esophageal sphincter (LES) pressure should be avoided to reduce reflux symptoms; these include caffeine, alcohol, and chocolate. Clients should also avoid eating large meals, drinking fluids with meals, and eating at bedtime; they should remain upright for 1 to 2 hours after eating.
Cognitive Level: Application **Client Need:** Physiological Integrity: Basic Care and Comfort **Integrated Process:** Nursing Process: Planning **Content Area:** Foundational Sciences: Nutrition **Strategy:** The core issue of the question is knowledge of foods that lower LES pressure and increase risk of reflux in GERD. Use nutrition knowledge and the process of elimination to make a selection.

5 **Answer: 3** A 2-gram sodium-restricted diet requires use of no salt in cooking, no salt added at the table, avoiding high sodium foods, and limiting milk to 2 cups per day. Option 1 is incorrect—no salt can be added in this restricted diet. Options 2 and 4 are incorrect—1 cup of milk per day and the use of salt-free butter are requirements of a 1-gram sodium restricted diet.

lactase enzyme. Full liquid diets are based on milk and dairy products. If a client is known to be lactose intolerant, the diet will have to be adjusted to reflect lactose-reduced or lactose-free products in order to prevent GI irritation. Option 1 is incorrect—it does not reflect the added clinical condition of lactose intolerance but merely refers to progression of diet. Option 2 is incorrect because lactose intolerance does have an impact on diet patterns. Option 3 is incorrect because diet progression does not rely merely on the return of a bowel movement pattern.

Cognitive Level: Analysis **Client Need:** Physiological Integrity: Basic Care and Comfort **Integrated Process:** Nursing Process: Planning **Content Area:** Foundational Sciences: Nutrition **Strategy:** The core issue of the question is knowledge of concepts related to lactose intolerance. Use nutrition knowledge and the process of elimination to make a selection.

13 **Answer: 4** A client who is receiving enteral feedings via nasogastric tube can be at risk for dehydration caused by inadequate fluid intake. It is therefore important to irrigate the tube with water as ordered (before and after feedings or medication administration) and include these irrigations in the client's total I&O measurements. Option 1 is incorrect because although inspection of the skin surrounding the tube is necessary, it does not relate specifically to fluid balance. Option 2 is incorrect because clients are often weighed daily. Option 3 is incorrect because feeding tubes are not flushed only once a day.

Cognitive Level: Application **Client Need:** Physiological Integrity: Basic Care and Comfort **Integrated Process:** Nursing Process: Planning **Content Area:** Foundational Sciences: Nutrition **Strategy:** The core issue of the question is knowledge that a client receiving enteral feedings is at risk for dehydration if there are no sources of free water provided. Use nutrition knowledge and the process of elimination to make a selection.

14 **Answer: 3** A client with a significant cardiac history on a fat-restricted diet should not use additional fat during the cooking or preparation process. Option 1 is incorrect—a client with a significant cardiac history will require some form of fat control or restriction as part of a dietary pattern for the rest of his or her life. Option 2 is incorrect—fat is a necessary nutrient for the body. To deprive a client of all fat sources can lead to a clinical deficiency of essential fatty acids that can cause further problems for the client. Option 4 is incorrect because ice cream is considered a high-fat product. The client could have low-fat ice cream, yogurt, or sherbet to satisfy dietary needs.

Cognitive Level: Application **Client Need:** Physiological Integrity: Basic Care and Comfort **Integrated Process:** Teaching and Learning **Content Area:** Foundational Sciences: Nutrition **Strategy:** Use nutrition knowledge and the process of elimination to make a selection.

15 **Answer: 3** Allergy I and II diets are used in sequence to identify and eliminate potential food allergens. Option 1 is incorrect—even though this diet pattern is used over a short time period, this response does not address why it is necessary to follow the diet pattern. Option 2 is incorrect because it provides false and inaccurate information. Option 4 is incorrect—referral to an immunologist for allergy testing is not a required accompaniment to this dietary pattern. Referral to an immunologist for allergy testing may eventually be indicated if the client is found to have a multiple allergy profile.

Cognitive Level: Application **Client Need:** Physiological Integrity: Basic Care and Comfort **Integrated Process:** Communication and Documentation **Content Area:** Foundational Sciences: Nutrition **Strategy:** The core issue of the question is knowledge of the purposes of allergy I and II diets. Use nutrition knowledge and the process of elimination to make a selection.

16 **Answer: 4** Foods that contain gluten (wheat, oats, rye, and barley) are restricted for a client with celiac disease because of an inability to handle gluten protein. All of the other choices reflect items that cannot be used in a gluten-restricted diet.

Cognitive Level: Application **Client Need:** Physiological Integrity: Basic Care and Comfort **Integrated Process:** Nursing Process: Implementation **Content Area:** Foundational Sciences: Nutrition **Strategy:** The core issue of the question is knowledge that a foods containing wheat, rye, oats, and barley are restricted in celiac disease. Use nutrition knowledge about foods containing these grains and the process of elimination to make a selection.

17 **Answer: 3** A client taking MAO inhibitors has to avoid foods that are high in tyramine because it can lead to significant complications resulting in hypertensive crisis. Cottage cheese is an unfermented cheese that can be used in the diet. All of the other options reflect foods that are high in tyramine. Aged cheeses are not allowed on the diet.

Cognitive Level: Analysis **Client Need:** Physiological Integrity: Basic Care and Comfort **Integrated Process:** Nursing Process: Planning **Content Area:** Foundational Sciences: Nutrition **Strategy:** The core issue of the question is knowledge that clients taking MAOIs require a low-tyramine diet. Use nutrition knowledge of low-tyramine foods and the process of elimination to make a selection.

18 **Answer: 3** The perception of being in a state of "always dieting" can be problematic in terms of compliance and goal attainment because it can be viewed either as a restriction or as a form of punishment. Option 1 is not true: wanting to lose weight is not the only factor to consider; many other variables affect weight loss. While it is important to find out the type of the diet the client is on (or has been on), this knowledge doesn't address the main concern of the client regarding "always dieting" and yo-yo effect (weight cycling).

Cognitive Level: Application **Client Need:** Physiological Integrity: Basic Care and Comfort **Integrated Process:** Communication and Documentation **Content Area:** Foundational Sciences: Nutrition **Strategy:** The core issue of the question is identification of a client's need for assistance with weight control. Use nutrition knowledge and the process of elimination to make a selection.

19 **Answer: 2** Diets that are rich in fruits and vegetables have been proven to be effective in decreasing the risk of developing cancer because these foods contain phytochemicals. None of the other food groupings have been shown to decrease the risk of cancer.

Cognitive Level: Application **Client Need:** Physiological Integrity: Basic Care and Comfort **Integrated Process:** Nursing Process: Implementation **Content Area:** Foundational Sciences: Nutrition **Strategy:** The core issue of the question is knowledge of foods that contain protective chemicals against cancer development. Use nutrition knowledge and the process of elimination to make a selection.

20 **Answer: 4** When an athletic client is considering utilizing any ergonomic aid or supplement, trainers and/or nutritional specialists can monitor the client closely to establish a client baseline, provide education, and prevent potential complications related to therapy. Option 1 is incorrect because a nurse should not suggest an alternative ergonomic aid. The client needs a proper referral to an expert in the field. Option 2 is incorrect because it does not address the priority need—to make the referral. Although it is important to note what type of exercise the client practices, it is still more important to refer the client to the proper specialist who can assist in supervising an athletic treatment regimen.
Cognitive Level: Application **Client Need:** Safe Effective Care Environment: Management of Care **Integrated Process:** Nursing Process: Implementation **Content Area:** Foundational Sciences: Nutrition **Strategy:** The core issue of the question is appropriate anticipatory guidance to a client seeking to use nontraditional methods of nutrition for supplemental use. Use knowledge that this client requires special monitoring and the process of elimination to make a selection.

21 **Answer: 2** A clear liquid diet is recommended for short-term use (1–2 days). Therefore, the maximum is 2 days. It can be used both before and after surgery or diagnostic procedures, during acute stages of illness, or as an initial diet after a significant period of GI inactivity or bowel rest.
Cognitive Level: Application **Client Need:** Physiological Integrity: Basic Care and Comfort **Integrated Process:** Nursing Process: Implementation **Content Area:** Foundational Sciences: Nutrition **Strategy:** The core issue of the question is the length of time a clear liquid diet is appropriate. Use knowledge of clear liquid diet as a therapeutic diet to make a selection.

Key Terms to Review

bolus feeding p. 410
cyclic feeding p. 410
enteral nutrition p. 409
ergonomic aids p. 404
obesity p. 398
phytochemicals p. 402
underweight p. 398

References

Ball, J., & Bindler, R. (2006). *Child health nursing: Partnering with children and families.* Upper Saddle River, NJ: Pearson Education.

Dudek, S. (2005). *Nutrition essentials for nursing practice* (5th ed.). Philadelphia: Lippincott, Williams, & Wilkins.

Grodner, M., Long, S., & DeYoung, S. (2004). *Foundations and clinical application of nutrition* (3rd ed.). St. Louis, MO: Mosby.

Harkreader, H., & Hogan, M. (2004). *Fundamentals of nursing: Caring and clinical judgment* (2nd ed.). St. Louis, MO: Elsevier Science.

Kozier, B., Erb, G., Berman, A., & Snyder, S. (2004). *Fundamentals of nursing: Concepts, process, and practice* (7th ed.). Upper Saddle River, NJ: Pearson Education.

Nix, S. (2005). *Williams' basic nutrition and diet therapy* (12th ed.). St. Louis, MO: Elsevier Mosby.

Smith, S., Duell, D., & Martin, B. (2004). *Clinical nursing skills: Basic to advanced skills* (6th ed.). Upper Saddle River, NJ: Pearson Education.

Meeting Basic Human Needs

27

In this chapter

Cross reference

Other chapters relevant to this content area are

Meeting Nutritional Needs Chapter 26
Maintaining the Function of Tubes and Drains Chapter 28

Test Yourself

Are you ready for the NCLEX-RN® or course exams? Use the practice tests on the companion CD-ROM to check.

I. MEETING HYGIENE NEEDS

A. Functions of skin

1. Protection: body's first line of defense against microorganisms
2. Sensation: pain, temperature, and pressure
3. Temperature regulation
4. Excretion and secretion: of sweat (water, chloride, potassium, glucose, and urea) and sebum (an oily substance); acid pH of skin secretions inhibits bacterial growth

B. Skin care

1. Developmental changes: age and ability influence skin care practices
   a. A newborn requires only sponge baths, not tub baths; dry newborn immediately and wrap to prevent heat loss; shivering in newborns starts at a lower body temperature than in adults, and infants have greater body surface area for heat loss compared to adults
   b. A toddler depends on caregiver to provide care but may want to perform tasks (such as brushing teeth) independently
   c. An older adult who is frail may be dependent but may still be able to identify skin care preferences; excessive bathing can contribute to dry skin
2. Cultural considerations
   a. Hygiene practices vary considerably among different cultures; in some cultures, daily bathing is a ritual, while in others, a weekly routine is acceptable
   b. Other examples of differences are in use of deodorants and preference for tub or shower
   c. Some cultures are concerned with hot/cold imbalances as a cause of illness
   d. Bathing may be avoided with some body conditions; for instance, some cultures avoid bathing during menstruation and childbirth

! 3. Common skin problems requiring care
   a. Excessive dryness: flaky and rough skin may crack; may be accompanied by pruritus (itching)
   b. Abrasions: epidermis (superficial layer of skin) rubbed or scraped off
   c. Ammonia dermatitis (diaper rash): reddened skin that may be excoriated, caused by skin bacteria reacting to urea in urine
   d. Contact dermatitis: reddened skin accompanied by pruritus that may result in infection if scratched
   e. Erythema: redness of skin associated with rashes, infections, and allergic responses
   f. **Pressure ulcer**: an open skin lesion, often over bony prominences, caused by decreased circulation

C. Specific hygiene measures

1. Partial bed bath: client may do certain portions of bath as desired or as condition permits; includes only parts that may cause discomfort or odor if not washed
2. Complete bed bath: nurse washes client's entire body
3. Perineal care to genitalia and rectal area
4. Nail and foot care
5. ! Document observations such as general skin condition, reddened areas over bony prominences, irritation, and inflammation
6. Oral care: brushing and flossing teeth and denture care; document abnormalities such as irritated mucous membranes and ill-fitting dentures
7. Hair and scalp care: includes brushing and shampooing hair; personal habits and cultural influences affect hair care practices; clean hair limits microbe count, and groomed hair can increase general comfort level
8. Care of eyes, ears, and nose
   a. ! Eye care: wipe loosened secretions from inner to outer canthus; for unconscious client, use artificial tears every 2 hours or as ordered to reduce corneal injury
   b. Ear care: if cerumen (earwax) is visible, loosen it by retracting auricles downward, then remove with a damp washcloth
9. Care of removable prosthetic (artificial) eye: see Box 27–1
10. Promote client independence as much as possible during care
11. ! Document ability to bathe, feed, groom, and toilet self as indicators of functional ability; communicate this information to discharge planners, long-term or rehabilitation care centers, and home health nurses

D. Care of client's room environment

1. ! Keep area clutter-free
   a. Arrange furniture to avoid accidents; for example, no furniture in middle of room
   b. Remove unnecessary objects; keep obstacles out of walkways
2. Keep objects needed by client nearby; put necessary objects for daily hygiene and activities of daily living within reach (e.g., client's eyeglasses, cane, fluids, and call bell)
3. Control odors
   a. Provide good ventilation
   b. Remove and dispose of offensive waste products appropriately
   c. Use room deodorizers as necessary

Box 27–1

Care of an Eye Prosthesis

- Using gloves, exert slight pressure below eyelid to overcome suction and remove artificial eye
- Clean the socket and tissues around eye with moistened washcloth
- Clean artificial eye with warm normal saline and rinse
- To reinsert prosthetic eye
  - retract eyelids and exert pressure on supraorbital and infraorbital bones
  - hold prosthetic eye with index finger and thumb of the other hand and slip it gently into socket

II. MEETING OXYGENATION NEEDS

A. Summary of physiology of cardiovascular and respiratory systems

1. Heart serves as a system pump, moving blood through blood vessels to tissues and transports blood containing oxygen and nutrients to cells; wastes are collected for elimination
2. Respiratory system
    - **a.** Pulmonary ventilation, or breathing: inspiration (inhalation)—air flows into lungs; expiration (exhalation)—air moves out of lungs
    - **b.** Alveolar gas exchange: after alveoli are ventilated, diffusion of oxygen occurs from alveoli into pulmonary blood vessels
    - **c.** Transport of oxygen (O_2) and carbon dioxide (CO_2): O_2 is transported from lungs to tissues, and CO_2 is transported from tissues back to lungs; O_2 combines with hemoglobin in red blood cells (RBCs) and is then carried to tissues as oxyhemoglobin

B. Factors affecting oxygenation

1. Environment
    - **a.** Altitude: higher altitude increases respiratory and cardiac rate and respiratory depth
    - **b.** Heat: causes peripheral vessel dilation, increased blood flow to skin, and decreased resistance to blood flow; cardiac output (CO) increases, raising blood pressure (BP); rate and depth of breathing also increase
    - **c.** Cold: vasoconstriction occurs and BP elevates, decreasing cardiac action because of reduced need for oxygen
    - **d.** Air pollution: leads to symptoms such as coughing, choking, and difficulty breathing
    - **e.** Health status: healthy individuals have a sufficient O_2 supply to meet body's demands; in cardiovascular disease, O_2 transport is compromised; in respiratory disease, oxygenation of blood is affected
    - ! **f.** Narcotics: opioids such as morphine and meperidine (Demerol) decrease respiratory rate and depth by depressing respiratory center of medulla
2. Developmental factors affecting oxygenation
    - ! **a.** Premature infants: inadequate respiratory function is caused by immature lungs; stimulation of respiratory center of brain is immature; gag and cough reflexes are weak
    - ! **b.** Infants and toddlers have smaller airway passages, which contributes to obstruction by foreign objects such as peanuts, coins, and small toys; diseases such as cystic fibrosis and asthma lead to difficulty breathing and affect oxygenation
    - **c.** Because of exposure to infectious agents at school and play, upper respiratory problems are common in school-aged children
    - **d.** At puberty, heart and lungs increase considerably in size and heart rate drops
    - **e.** Aerobic capacity (ability to provide O_2 to body's organs) and CO show age-related changes during work or exercise starting at age 35 to 40; loss of blood vessel elasticity may contribute to hypertension, which affects oxygenation; atherosclerosis (plaque buildup in aterial walls) decreases blood flow, particularly to heart muscle
    - ! **f.** In older adults, chest wall becomes more rigid and lungs are less elastic, so more air is retained in lungs at expiration; cough effectiveness decreases; protective cilia become less effective, so older adults may be more prone to upper respiratory infections; decreased respiratory reserve increases risk for exercise intolerance; blood flow may be impaired because of hypertension, atherosclerosis, and obstructive lung disease
3. Lifestyle factors affecting oxygenation
    - **a.** Nutrition: high fat and salt intake may increase risk for heart disease, and inadequate diet can lead to anemia (insufficient RBCs)
    - **b.** Physical exercise: increases rate and depth of respirations and cardiac rate, thus increasing supply of oxygen in body
    - ! **c.** Smoking: nicotine increases heart rate, BP, and peripheral resistance; vasoconstriction occurs and decreases oxygenation to tissues

d. Substance abuse: alcohol is a respiratory depressant and slows respirations; long-term use increases BP and tendency for malnutrition and anemia

! **e.** Anxiety: in moderate and severe anxiety, client hyperventilates and arterial pressure of O_2 rises and pressure of CO_2 falls; client often experiences lightheadedness, numbness of fingers and toes; epinephrine and norepinephrine released under stress increase BP and cardiac rate

C. Alterations in respiratory functioning

1. **Hyperventilation:** reduced rate and depth of respirations
   - **a.** Causes: stress, increased CO_2 retention; metabolic acidosis may cause Kussmaul's breathing, a type of hyperventilation
   - **b.** Signs and symptoms: increased rate and depth of respiration
2. **Hypoventilation:** inadequate alveolar ventilation
   - **a.** Causes: alveolar collapse, airway obstruction, or side effect of some drugs
   - **b.** Signs and symptoms: inadequate alveolar ventilation; CO_2 retained in bloodstream; can lead to hypoxia

! 3. Hypoxia: inadequate amount of O_2 transported to tissues
   - **a.** Causes: diseases such as anemia, pulmonary edema, heart failure; drugs such as anesthetics
   - **b.** Signs and symptoms: rapid pulse; rapid shallow respirations, **dyspnea;** flaring of nostrils, restlessness; substernal or intercostal retractions; and cyanosis; in chronic hypoxia, client may experience fatigue and lethargy and have clubbing of fingers and toes

Memory Aid

Early respiratory symptoms are mild in nature, such as increasing respiratory rate and minimal amounts of mild dyspnea; later signs are more extreme in nature.

4. Cyanosis
   - **a.** Causes: severe anemia, respiratory tract obstruction, heart disease, cold environment; a very late indicator of hypoxia
   - **b.** Signs and symptoms: bluish discoloration of skin, nail beds, and mucous membranes

Memory Aid

Cyanosis is always a late sign, regardless of what the health problem is!

5. Pain: chest pain can impair breathing patterns and respiratory functioning
   - **a.** Causes: respiratory diseases such as pneumonia, pulmonary embolism, advanced bronchogenic carcinoma; and heart conditions, such as coronary artery disease, and angina
   - **b.** Signs and symptoms: complaints of pain that may be dull, aching, persistent or localized and radiating; discomfort accompanied by pallor, rapid or slowed breathing; anxiety; rapid heart rate
6. **Orthopnea:** (positional breathing discomfort associated with lying down)
   - **a.** Causes: respiratory and cardiac diseases, airway obstruction
   - **b.** Signs and symptoms: inability to breathe except when in a sitting or upright position; **dyspnea** (difficulty breathing progressing to air hunger) when in a reclining position
7. Wheezing
   - **a.** Causes: severely narrowed bronchus
   - **b.** Signs and symptoms: high-pitched, continuous musical, rasping, or whistling sounds heard during inspiration or expiration; does not clear with coughing
8. Cough: natural lung clearance mechanism to remove secretions
   - **a.** Causes: excessive sputum production; allergies; pulmonary diseases
   - **b.** Signs and symptoms: forced exhalation and clearing of airway passages
9. Hemoptysis
   - **a.** Causes: pulmonary infection, carcinoma of lungs, abnormalities of heart or blood vessels

b. Signs and symptoms: bright red, frothy blood from lungs mixed with sputum; initial symptoms include tickling in throat, salty taste, a burning or bubbling sensation in chest

D. Nursing interventions to promote oxygenation

1. Positioning: Fowler's position allows maximum chest expansion that eases respirations in clients with dyspnea; turn clients from side to side every 1 to 2 hours for alternate sides of chest to expand
2. Decrease anxiety: promote relaxation techniques, alleviate pain by using distraction or guided imagery
3. Deep breathing and coughing: helps to clear fluid from lungs and promote oxygenation
   a. Assume a comfortable position: sitting or lying position with knees flexed
   b. Place one hand on abdomen just below ribs
   c. With mouth closed, breathe in deeply through nose to count of three; concentrate on feeling abdomen rise
   d. Purse lips and breathe out slowly and gently; concentrate on feeling abdomen fall and tightening abdominal muscles; count to seven during exhalation
   e. Repeat several times (about 10 times initially) and gradually increase to 5 to 10 minutes 4 times a day
   f. For coughing: inhale deeply and hold breath for a few seconds, lean forward and cough rapidly, using abdominal, thigh, and buttock muscles (coughing is contraindicated in postoperative eye, ear, neck, or brain surgery or in other clients at risk for increased intracranial pressure)

Memory Aid

Airway and *breathing* are the A and B of ABC's. Assessments and interventions to promote these are high priority using Maslow's hierarchy of needs theory for prioritizing care.

4. Suctioning: oro/nasopharyngeal, tracheal
   a. See Box 27–2 for procedure, p. 426
   ! b. Take care during suctioning to limit time to 10 to 15 seconds because no O_2 exchange occurs during this portion of procedure; provide rest periods between suctioning to allow client to inhale oxygen
   ! c. Assess for dysrhythmias or cyanosis as grave indicators of inadequate oxygenation; hyperoxygenate before suctioning, between attempts, and when suctioning is complete
5. Chest physiotherapy: percussion, vibration, postural drainage (often done by respiratory therapist unless nurse is authorized and competent to perform); see Box 27–3, p. 427
6. ! Oxygen therapy: when oxygen therapy is used, follow safety precautions (see Box 27–4, p. 427)
   a. Check physician's orders and assess client's respiratory and cardiovascular status
   b. Explain procedure to client and place client in a semi-sitting position
   c. Set up O_2 equipment: attach flow meter to wall outlet or portable oxygen cylinder; fill humidifier with water and attach to base of flow meter
   d. Attach delivery system and tubing to flow meter; turn on O_2 at prescribed rate; see Table 27–1 ■ (p. 428) for types of O_2 delivery systems
   e. Assess client's respiratory and cardiovascular status regularly; check client's nares for irritation if cannula is used, facial skin if face mask is used; document observations
   f. Check flow of O_2 and level of water in humidifier regularly
7. Incentive spirometer
   a. Check physician's orders; assist client to a sitting or Fowler's position and explain procedure
   b. Assemble equipment; set marker at recommended volume goal
   c. Instruct client to place mouth tightly around mouthpiece
   d. Instruct client to inhale slowly and maintain a steady flow, like pulling through a straw; encourage client to raise and maintain flow rate indicator

e. Instruct client to remove mouthpiece but hold breath for 2 to 3 seconds and then exhale slowly through pursed lips

f. Have client repeat procedure a few times and then cough; encourage to use 5 to 10 times hourly; keep spirometer within reach of client

Box 27-2

Summary of Key Points for Suctioning

- ➤ Prepare equipment: portable or wall suction with tubing and collection container; sterile normal saline or water; sterile gloves; water soluble lubricant; Y-connector; sterile gauzes; disposal bag.
- ➤ Select appropriate sterile suction catheters, usually #12 to #18 for adults; #8 to #10 for children; and #5 to #8 for infants.
- ➤ Set pressure on the suction gauge.
  - For wall unit: adults: 100–120 mmHg; children: 95–110 mmHg; infants: 50 to 95 mmHg.
  - For portable unit: adults: 10 to 15 mmHg; children: 5 to 10 mmHg; infants: 2 to 5 mmHg.
- ➤ Explain procedure to the client. Position a conscious client in a semi-Fowler's or an unconscious client in a lateral position with head turned toward nurse.
- ➤ Don the sterile gloves, maintain sterility of the dominant hand, and connect sterile catheter to the suction.
- ➤ Measure distance between the client's nose and earlobe (approximately 13 cm or 5 in. for the adult) and mark position with the fingers of sterile gloved hand. Test pressure and patency by placing nondominant thumb or finger on port or open branch of the Y-connector.
- ➤ Hyperoxygenate the client with deep breaths or bag-valve-mask device.
- ➤ Lubricate catheter tip with sterile water or saline (or for nasopharyngeal suctioning, may use lubricant).
- ➤ Insert the catheter.
  - For oropharyngeal suctioning: pull tongue forward with gauze; introduce and advance catheter along one side of mouth into oropharynx.
  - For nasopharyngeal suctioning: introduce catheter through the nostril or naris and advance to the recommended distance.
  - For tracheal suctioning: insert during inhalation because epiglottis is open; continue to advance catheter to approximately 20 cm or until resistance is met; pull back slightly (expect client to cough during insertion).
- ➤ Do not apply suction while inserting the catheter.
- ➤ Apply nondominant gloved thumb or finger to the port to start suction and gently rotate catheter. Apply suction intermittently and release while withdrawing movements of catheter; Allow 20- to 30-second intervals between each suction and limit each suctioning to 10–15 seconds maximum.
- ➤ Oxygenate the client between suction attempts and at the completion of the procedure.
- ➤ For oropharyngeal suctioning, it may be necessary to suction secretions that collect in the buccal cavity.
- ➤ Clean catheter by wiping off secretions with sterile gauze; flush catheter with sterile water; relubricate and repeat suctioning until air passage is clear. Alternate nares for repeat suctioning. Encourage client to breathe deeply and cough between suctions.
- ➤ Provide nasal or oral hygiene. Dispose of equipment.
- ➤ Assess effectiveness of suctioning: observe respiratory rate, skin color, dyspnea, and level of anxiety. Document relevant information.

Box 27-3

Performing Chest Physiotherapy

Percussion or Clapping

1. Explain procedure to client.
2. Encourage client to breathe slowly and deeply.
3. Place client in comfortable sitting or side-lying position.
4. Cover area with a gown or towel.
5. Cup hands, alternately flex and extend wrists rapidly to percuss the affected lung segments for 1 to 2 minutes.

Vibration (vigorous or high-frequency quivering over chest wall used alternately with or after percussion)

1. Explain procedure to client and position comfortably.
2. Encourage client to breathe slowly and deeply.
3. Place hands one on top of the other with palms down.
4. During exhalation, tense hand and arm and, using mostly the heel of hand, vibrate or shake hands against client's chest.
5. Stop vibrating when the client inhales.
6. After each vibration, encourage client to cough and expectorate.
7. Vibrate five times over each lung segment.

Postural Drainage (use of gravity to drain secretions from respiratory tract)

1. Explain procedure to client.
2. Position client so that the head is lower than the chest (in prone position).
3. Place sputum container and wipes within client's reach.
4. Do percussion and vibration for 5 minutes and allow 5 minutes for drainage.
5. Encourage client to cough and expectorate.
6. Instruct client to turn to the other side, then to the supine position, and repeat procedure.
7. Assist client to a sitting position and offer mouth care.
8. Document observations.

Box 27-4

Safety Precautions During Oxygen Therapy

- Place cautionary signs reading, "No Smoking: Oxygen in Use" on the client's door, at the head or foot of the bed, and on the oxygen equipment.
- Instruct the client and visitors about the danger of smoking when oxygen is in use. If necessary, remove matches, lighters, and ashtrays.
- If oxygen therapy is used at home, instruct family members or caregivers to smoke only outside. If smoking is permitted, teach visitors to use smoking room.
- Avoid materials that generate static electricity, such as woolen blankets and synthetic fabrics; use cotton fabrics instead.
- Avoid use of volatile, flammable substances such as acetone in nail polish removers, alcohol, ether, and oils near clients using oxygen.
- Remove any friction type or battery operated gadgets, devices, or toys.
- Make sure electric devices such as radios, razors, and televisions are in good working order to prevent short-circuit sparks.
- Ensure that electric monitoring equipment and suction machines are properly grounded. Disconnect any ungrounded equipment.
- Personnel must know the location of fire extinguishers and be able to use them properly.
- Know location of oxygen meter turn-off valve.

Table 27–1

Types of Oxygen Delivery Systems

Nasal cannula	Has either single or double short prongs inserted into nostrils. Often uses flow of 1 to 6 L/min of a 23% to 42% oxygen concentration.
Oxygen mask	Most effective means of delivering oxygen. Can deliver concentrations up to 100%. Must fit well over the nose and mouth. Use only clean and uncontaminated plastic or other nonlatex masks to avoid hospital–acquired infection. May deliver either low or high concentrations of oxygen.
Simple face mask	Useful for short-term therapy (i.e., early postoperative period or when intermittent oxygen therapy is required). The flow rate is only 6 to 8 L/min at a low-oxygen concentration of 40% to 60%. Because mask is loose fitting and can leak, it is suitable for those with carbon dioxide retention. Also indicated for clients who cannot use a nasal cannula, such as those who have a nasal obstruction.
Partial re-breathing mask	A disposable, lightweight plastic face mask with a reservoir bag and a partial rebreathing valve. Commonly used by individuals who require oxygen. On expiration, conserves approximately one third of exhaled air. Because this air comes from trachea and bronchi (does not participate in gas exchange), it is rich in oxygen. To prevent the rebreathing of carbon dioxide, reservoir bag should deflate only slightly on inhalation. By this method, a concentration of 50% to 75% oxygen can be delivered at a flow rate of 8 to 11 L/min.
Nonrebreathing mask	Fits tightly over face. Usually made of rubber with a reservoir bag and a nonrebreathing valve. On inhalation, oxygen flows into bag and mask, and one-way valve prevents exhaled air from flowing back into bag. Expired air instead escapes through the one-way flap valve in the mask. Oxygen concentration is 80% to 100%, with flow adjusted to keep reservoir bag fully inflated. Used for short-term therapy, such as counteracting smoke inhalation. Prolonged use can cause discomfort because mask becomes warm and sticky.
Oxygen tent	Used rarely, but may be useful during infancy. Disadvantage is need to open canopy to monitor vital signs and provide care. Flow rate is 20 L/min at an oxygen concentration of 60% but is hard to control with intermittent opening by staff.
Plastic hoods	May be used to deliver oxygen to infants. Clear plastic head hood allows maintenance of either low or high concentrations of oxygen even during nursing care. A rate of 4 to 5 L/min is required to maintain oxygen concentrations and remove exhaled carbon dioxide.
Ventimask (Mix-O-Mask)	Originated from Venturi mask. Used for clients with chronic alveolar hypoventilation and carbon dioxide retention. Delivers exact low-flow concentrations of oxygen. Provides an air–oxygen mixture with the desired oxygen concentration. Size of orifice to mask determines concentration of oxygen—24% or 28%, 31%, 35%, and 40% with flow rates of 4, 6, 8, and 10 L/min, respectively. A thin elastic band holds Ventimask in position and tends to press into skin behind the ears; gauze padding under each side of elastic band alleviates pressure. Must be removed when client eats and may give client a feeling of being smothered.

III. MEETING THE CLIENT'S NEED FOR SLEEP

A. Physiology of sleep

1. Circadian rhythm: rhythmic repetition of patterns each 24 hours; sleep is a complex biologic rhythm; if a person's biological clock coincides with sleep–wake patterns, the person is in **circadian synchronization**
2. Sleep regulation: centers in lower portion of brain actively inhibit wakefulness, causing sleep
3. NREM (non–rapid eye movement): deep and restful sleep characterized by decrease in physiologic functions: BP and pulse decrease, skeletal muscles relax, basal metabolic rate (BMR) decreases, brain waves become slower; there are four stages of NREM
   a. Stage I: very light sleep; sleeper is relaxed and drowsy and feels a floating sensation; eyes roll from side to side; lasts only a few minutes
   b. Stage II: light sleep; sleeper is easily roused; pulse and respirations decrease slightly; lasts 10 to 15 minutes
   c. Stage III: medium-depth sleep; sleeper is less easily aroused; pulse, respirations, and other physiologic functions such as BP and temperature continue to fall; skeletal muscles are relaxed, reflexes diminished; snoring may occur
   d. Stage IV: called delta sleep; deepest sleep stage; sleeper is difficult to rouse and rarely moves; muscles are completely relaxed; dreaming may occur; may last about 30 minutes
4. REM (rapid eye movement) sleep: usually occurs every 90 minutes and lasts 5 to 30 minutes; active dreaming occurs and dreams are remembered; brain is highly active, and sleeper is difficult to rouse or may wake up spontaneously; REM and irregular muscle movements occur; muscle tone is depressed; heart and respiratory rates are irregular

B. Normal sleep requirements and patterns

1. Neonates: newborns sleep, on average, 16 to 18 hours per day, divided into about 7 sleep periods; most NREM sleep is spent in stages III and IV, and nearly 50% is in REM sleep
2. Infants: range of sleep is from 12 to 22 hours; periods of wakefulness increase with age; by 4 months, infants sleep through night and nap during day; at end of first year, they sleep about 14 of every 24 hours; half of time, infants have light sleep, and 20% to 30% is REM sleep
3. Toddlers: normal sleep–wake cycle established by 2 to 3 years; generally sleep for 10 to 12 hours, still require a midafternoon nap, but morning nap needs decrease; still 20% to 30% is REM sleep
4. Preschoolers: need 11 to 12 hours sleep but may fluctuate because of activity and growth spurts; older preschoolers do not need a nap; continue to have 20% to 30% REM sleep
5. School-age: most school-aged children sleep 8 to 12 hours without daytime naps; REM sleep decreases to about 20%
6. Adolescents: amount of time for sleeping declines, but adolescents still need 8 to 10 hours of sleep; changes in pattern occur for adolescents who need daytime napping
7. Young adults: generally, young adults require 7 to 8 hours, but because of lifestyle changes, they may have erratic sleep patterns
8. Middle-aged adults: sleep pattern established earlier is maintained, and middle-aged adult sleeps 6 to 8 hours/night; about 20% is REM sleep; duration of stage IV NREM sleep decreases
9. Older adults: sleep about 6 hours a night with about 20% to 25% REM and a marked decrease in stage IV NREM sleep; they awaken more frequently and have difficulty returning to sleep, so they experience less restorative sleep

C. Factors affecting sleep

1. Illness: when a person is ill, sleep requirement is increased; however, illness may cause pain, breathing difficulty, or discomfort with movement that interferes with sleep; elevated body temperature can cause a reduction in stages III and IV NREM and REM sleep

2. Drugs and substances
   a. Excessive alcohol disrupts REM sleep, although it may accelerate onset of sleep; individuals with tolerance to alcohol may have difficulty with sleep, and when drug effects wear off, may have nightmares
   ! b. Caffeine and amphetamines act as stimulants and interfere with sleep
   c. Nicotine has stimulating effect, and smokers have more difficulty falling asleep
3. Lifestyle: shift work may interfere with ability to adjust sleeping patterns; inactivity or boredom may contribute to sleep problems
4. Usual sleep patterns and excessive daytime sleepiness: individuals commonly refer to themselves as morning or night people; these are their sleep patterns; excessive daytime sleepiness may be caused by nighttime sleep deprivation
5. Emotional stress: anxiety makes it difficult for a person to fall asleep; depression may cause difficulty in falling asleep or premature awakening
6. Environment: any change in noise level may inhibit sleep—people are habituated to a certain noise; ventilation and environmental temperature can affect sleep
7. ! Various prescribed drugs: decongestants, narcotics, sedatives, beta-blockers, and antidepressants may cause drowsiness and may disrupt REM sleep
8. Exercise and fatigue: moderate exercise is conducive to sleep but, if excessive, may delay sleep; moderate fatigue may lead to a restful sleep
9. Food/calorie intake: weight loss is associated with reduced quantity of sleep, broken sleep, and earlier awakening; weight gain is associated with increased total sleep time, less broken sleep, and later waking

D. Overview of sleep disorders

1. Insomnia: inability to obtain an adequate amount or quality of sleep
   a. Can be initial (difficulty falling asleep), middle or intermittent (difficulty maintaining sleep because of frequent or prolonged waking), or terminal (early or premature awakening), which may be associated with depression
   ! b. Treatment is usually directed at developing new sleep-inducing and sleep-maintaining behaviors such as modifying environment or using relaxation techniques
2. Sleep apnea: periodic cessation of breathing during sleep; episode lasts from 10 seconds to 2 minutes, and incidence may range from 50 to 600 per night
   a. Suspected when person snores loudly, has frequent nocturnal awakening, and experiences excessive daytime sleepiness, fatigue, irritability, and personality changes caused by disrupted sleep
   b. Incidence of sleep apnea is high in elderly men
   c. Apnea is also common among obese clients
   d. Complications of prolonged sleep apnea may be increased BP, cardiac dysrhythmias, and left-sided heart failure
   e. Treatment is directed at cause: if obstructive, enlarged tonsils or adenoids may be removed
   f. Use of a nasal continuous positive airway pressure (CPAP) device may be effective
3. Narcolepsy: sudden wave of overwhelming sleepiness during day; person with narcolepsy may doze while involved in activities; treatment is with stimulants, such as amphetamines
4. Parasomnias: abnormal behavioral or physiologic events that are associated with stages of sleep and interfere with sleep; treatment consists of relaxation technique and sleep hygiene practices
   a. Somnambulism: sleepwalking that occurs in stages III and IV NREM sleep; it is episodic and occurs 1 to 2 hours after falling asleep; sleepwalker does not notice dangers such as stairs
   b. Sleeptalking: talking occurs during NREM sleep, before REM sleep
   c. Nocturnal enuresis: bedwetting, more common in male children over 3 years old; often occurs 1 to 2 hours after falling asleep, when rousing from stage III to IV of NREM sleep
   d. Nocturnal erections: both erections and emissions start around adolescence and occur during REM sleep
   e. Bruxism: clenching and grinding teeth during stage II NREM sleep

5. Sleep deprivation: syndrome in which individual's prolonged disturbance results in a decrease in amount, quality, and consistency of sleep
   a. REM sleep deprivation can be caused by alcohol, shift work, jet lag, or extended ICU hospitalization and can result in excitability, confusion, and emotional lability; delay procedures or medications when possible to avoid waking a client during REM sleep
   b. NREM sleep deprivation can be caused by same factors in REM deprivation, as well as by hypothyroidism, depression, sleep apnea, and age (common in elderly), and can result in withdrawal, excessive sleepiness, and hyporesponsiveness
   ! c. An individual who has both REM and NREM sleep deprivation may have difficulty with concentration, judgment, and attention; marked fatigue; and perceptual distortions

E. Health promotion to improve sleep

1. Environmental controls: ensure appropriate lighting, ventilation, and temperature; keep noise level to a minimum
2. ! Promote bedtime routines: respect client's customary rituals or routines to promote relaxation and encourage sleep; provide hygiene such as washing face, brushing teeth, and voiding; allow listening to music or praying, children's bedtime stories, or adults' conversations with their caregivers or family members if possible
3. ! Promote comfort: provide backrubs, change of linen/clothing, position for comfort; administer medications for pain to promote and help maintain sleep; listen to client's concerns to alleviate emotional stress and promote relaxation; avoid heavy meal 3 hours before bedtime, decrease fluid intake 2 hours before sleep, and avoid alcohol, caffeine, and heavily spiced foods
4. Promote activity: encourage adequate exercise during day to reduce stress, and a nonstrenuous activity prior to sleep
5. Pharmacological aids (sedatives and hypnotics)
   a. Medications should be used as a last resort and be taken prn (as necessary)
   ! b. Clients need to know desired and adverse effects of medications; medications vary in onset and duration; regular use may lead to drug tolerance and possibly to rebound insomnia

IV. MEETING URINARY ELIMINATION NEEDS

A. Healthy urinary function

1. Normal output of urine is 60 mL/hr or 1500 mL/day; should remain 30 mL/hr or higher to ensure continued healthy kidney function
2. Urine usually consists of 96% water
3. Solutes found in urine
   a. Organic solutes, including urea, ammonia, uric acid, and creatinine
   b. Inorganic solutes, including sodium, chloride, potassium, sulfate, magnesium, and phophorus
4. Table 27–2 ■ describes the characteristics of healthy urine as well as possible abnormal findings

B. Common abnormal assessment findings

1. Urgency: strong desire to void may be caused by inflammations or infections in bladder or urethra
2. Dysuria: painful or difficult voiding
3. Frequency: voiding that occurs more than usual when compared with client's regular pattern or generally accepted norm of voiding once every 3 to 6 hours
4. Hesitancy: undue delay and difficulty in initiating voiding
5. Polyuria: a large volume of urine voided at any given time
6. Oliguria: a small volume of urine or output between 100 and 500 mL/24 hr
7. Nocturia: excessive urination at night, interrupting sleep
8. Hematuria: RBCs in the urine

C. Common urinary elimination problems

1. Urinary retention: occurs when bladder emptying is impaired, urine accumulates, and bladder becomes overdistended; causes include prostatic hypertrophy,

Table 27-2

Characteristics of Normal and Abnormal Urine

Characteristic	Normal	Abnormal	Nursing Considerations
Amount in 24 hours (adult)	1200–1500mL	Under 1200 mL Over 1500 mL	Urinary output normally is approximately equal to fluid intake. Output of less than 30 mL/hr may indicate decreased blood flow to the kidneys and should be immediately reported.
Color, clarity	Straw, amber; transparent	Dark amber Cloudy Dark orange Red or dark brown Mucus plugs, viscid, thick	Concentrated urine is darker in color. Dilute urine may appear almost clear, or very pale yellow. Some foods and drugs may color urine (e.g., beets, phenazopyridine, phenytoin). Red blood cells in the urine (hematuria) may be evident as pink, bright red, or rusty brown urine. Menstrual bleeding can also color urine but should not be confused with hematuria. White blood cells, bacteria, pus, or contaminants such as prostatic fluid, sperm, or vaginal drainage may cause cloudy urine.
Odor	Faint, aromatic	Offensive	Some foods (e.g., asparagus) cause a musty odor; infected urine can have a fetid odor; urine high in glucose has a sweet odor.
Sterility	No micro-organisms present	Micro-organisms present	Urine specimens may be contaminated by bacteria from the perineum during collection.
pH	4.5–8	Under 4.5 Over 8	Freshly voided urine is normally somewhat acidic. Alkaline urine may indicate a state of alkalosis, urinary tract infection, or a diet high in fruits and vegetables. More acidic urine (low pH) is found in acidosis, starvation, diarrhea, or with a diet high in protein foods or cranberries.
Specific gravity	1.010–1.025	Under 1.010 Over 1.025	Concentrated urine has a higher specific gravity; diluted urine has a lower specific gravity.
Glucose	Not present	Present	Glucose in the urine indicates high blood glucose levels (>180 mg/dL) and may be indicative of undiagnosed or uncontrolled diabetes mellitus.
Ketone bodies	Not present	Present	Ketones, the end product of the breakdown of fatty acids, are not normally present in the urine. They may be present in the urine of clients who have uncontrolled diabetes mellitus, are in a state of starvation, or who have ingested excessive amounts of aspirin.
Blood	Not present	Occult (microscopic) Bright red	Blood may be present in the urine of clients who have urinary tract infection, kidney disease, or bleeding from the urinary tract.

Source: Kozier, B., Erb, G., Berman, A., & Snyder, S. (2004). *Fundamentals of nursing: Concepts, process, and practice* (7th ed.). Upper Saddle River, NJ: Prentice Hall, p. 1264.

surgery, medications such as anticholinergics, antidepressants, antipsychotics, antiparkinsonian agents, antihypertensives

2. Urinary tract infections (UTI): infectious process leads to inflammation in any portion of urinary tract
   a. Lower UTI: urethritis is inflammation of the urethra; cystitis is inflammation of urinary bladder, the most common UTI; prostatitis is inflammation of prostate gland

b. Upper UTI: pyelonephritis is inflammation of renal pelvis and parenchyma, functional portion of kidney tissue

3. Incontinence: involuntary urination
   a. Stress incontinence: involuntary loss of urine of less than 50 mL occurring with increased abdominal pressure through coughing, laughing, or lifting
   b. Reflex incontinence: involuntary loss of urine at predictable intervals when bladder reaches a specific volume
   c. Urge incontinence: involuntary loss of urine soon after a strong urge to void
   d. Functional incontinence: involuntary, unpredictable passage of urine
   e. Total incontinence: continuous and unpredictable involuntary loss of urine

D. Urinary diversion devices: ureterostomy is a surgical rerouting of urine from kidneys to a site other than bladder, usually when bladder is removed or diseased

1. Cutaneous ureterostomy: ureter is brought directly to skin surface to form a small stoma; disadvantages include that stomas provide direct access to microorganisms from skin to kidneys, small stomas may present difficulty in fitting pouches, stenosis of stomas may occur as a complication
2. Ileal conduit: a segment of ileum is separated from small intestine and formed into a pouch with open end brought out through abdominal wall to form a stoma; ureter is implanted into ileal pouch (see Figure 27–1 ■)

E. Common urinary tests

1. Urinalysis: macroscopic and microscopic analysis of urine to determine physical and chemical characteristics; findings include
   a. pH: indicates acidity or alkalinity, reflects ability of kidney to maintain normal H^+ ion concentration in plasma and extracellular fluid; normal pH is 4.5 to 8
   ! b. Specific gravity: reflects kidney's ability to concentrate or dilute or may reflect degree of hydration or dehydration; normal 1.010 specific gravity is to 1.025
   ! c. Glucose: normally negligible amounts; done to screen clients for diabetes mellitus and to assess pregnant clients for glucose tolerance
   ! d. Ketones: product of breakdown of fatty acids, not normally found in urine but present in clients with poorly controlled diabetes mellitus
   ! e. Proteins: not normally found in urine, but protein escapes if there is damage in glomerular membrane of kidney
   f. Occult blood: may be present in chronic renal failure
2. Urine culture/sensitivity: to identify infecting organism and most effective antibiotic; a clean-catch specimen or catheterized specimen is needed; culture requires 24 to 72 hours for organism growth and identification
3. Intravenous pyelogram (IVP) or intravenous urogram (IVU): intravenous (IV) injection of a radiopaque contrast media that concentrates in urine to facilitate visualization of kidneys, ureters, and bladder
4. Renal scan: radiotraces or isotopes injected IV to evaluate renal size, shape, position, and function or blood flow to kidneys; pictures are taken by a scintillation camera

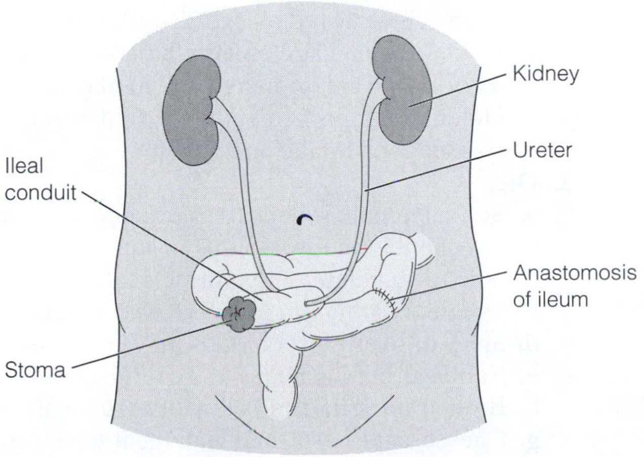

Figure 27–1

Ileal conduit as it is connected to abdominal organs.

Source: Kozier, B., Erb G., Berman, A., & Snydems. (2004). Fundamentals of Nursing; Concepts, process and practice *(7th ed.). Upper Saddle River, NJ: Pearson Education, p. 1283.*

5. Ultrasound: high-frequency sound waves are used to create ultrasonic images of urinary system
6. Cystoscopy: direct visualization of urethra and bladder with a cystoscope that is a self-contained optical lens system and provides a magnified illuminated view of bladder
7. Bladder scan at bedside: detects amount of urine in bladder to help determine need for voiding or straight catheterization; may be done by nurses or other personnel trained to use portable device

F. Teaching and health promotion for urinary elimination

1. Adequate hydration: daily intake of 1500 mL of measurable fluids recommended; if prone to development of stones or infections, increase fluid intake to 2000 to 3000 mL per 24 hours; if experiencing abnormal fluid losses, additional fluid intake is necessary
2. Personal hygiene: teach client to maintain cleanliness by washing perineal area with soap and water daily and after defecation; instruct female clients to wipe from front to back (urinary meatus toward anus) after voiding and discard after each wipe; for recurrent infections, avoid tub baths
3. Emptying bladder completely: regular exercise increases muscle tone that is important to maintain ability to contract detrusor muscle of bladder for complete emptying; abdominal muscle contraction assists in bladder emptying; teach **Kegel exercises**—contract perineal muscles and hold for a count of 3 to 5 seconds and relax; do ten contractions five times daily
4. Infection prevention measures
   a. Drink eight 8-ounce glasses of water daily
   b. Empty bladder at least every 2 to 4 hours while awake, avoiding voluntary retention; if client is incontinent, instruct to void according to a timetable rather than urge to void (bladder training), void at regular intervals (habit training), or supplement habit training by encouraging and reminding client to void (prompted voiding); instruct client to practice deep, slow breathing until urge to void diminishes
   c. For women: wear cotton briefs; cleanse perineal area from front to back after voiding and defecating; void before and after sexual intercourse; avoid bubble baths, feminine hygiene sprays, and douches
   d. Unless contraindicated: teach client to maintain acidity in urine by drinking at least two glasses of cranberry juice per day and avoiding excess milk products and sodium bicarbonate; vitamin C acidifies urine also
   e. Client should be able to identify symptoms and prevention measures of UTI and understand importance of reporting symptoms promptly

V. MEETING BOWEL ELIMINATION NEEDS

A. Factors that influence bowel elimination

1. Age
   a. Infants and toddlers: have immature control of bowel elimination; daytime control is achieved by age 2½ with toilet training
   b. School-age and adolescents: have similar bowel habits as adults; however, school-aged children involved in play may delay elimination
   c. Older adults: prone to constipation because of slowing of GI motility and decreased food intake and activity
2. Diet
   a. Sufficient bulk is needed to provide fecal volume
   b. If a client is on low-residue or low-fiber diet, there may be insufficient volume to stimulate reflex for defecation
   c. Irregular eating can interfere with regular elimination
   d. Spicy or overly sweet foods may cause diarrhea
   e. Cabbage, onions, beans and cauliflower are gas-producing
   f. Bran, prunes, figs, and alcohol have laxative effect
   g. Cheese, eggs, pasta, and lean meat have constipating effect

3. Position: normal bowel elimination is facilitated by thigh flexion (increases intrabdominal pressure) and a sitting position, which increases downward pressure on rectum; using a bedpan while in a supine position is not comfortable and does not facilitate defecation, so client needs to be placed in a semi-sitting position
4. Pregnancy: there is decreased intestinal secretion; colon is displaced upward, laterally, and posteriorly; peristaltic activity is decreased, causing constipation; later in pregnancy, venous pressure increases, causing hemorrhoids
5. Fluid intake: healthy elimination requires an intake of 2000 to 3000 mL/day; inadequate fluid intake or excessive fluid output may lead to hard feces
6. Activity: stimulates peristalsis; immobility, weak muscles from lack of exercise, or impaired neurologic functioning can lead to constipation
7. Psychological: anxiety or anger can increase peristalsis and lead to subsequent diarrhea; depression slows intestinal activity, resulting in constipation
8. Personal habits: if an individual continually ignores urge to defecate, water continues to be reabsorbed and feces harden; reflexes tend to be progressively weakened and may be lost
9. Pain: when pain or discomfort occurs upon defecation, client may suppress urge to defecate to avoid pain, thereby causing constipation
10. Medications: antidepressants, antipsychotic and antiparkinsonian agents, morphine, and codeine may cause constipation
11. Surgery and anesthesia: general anesthetics may cause a slowing of intestinal movement resulting in constipation; surgery in abdominal area that involves handling of intestines may cause cessation of intestinal movement (paralytic ileus) that lasts for 24 to 48 hours

B. Characteristics of normal stool

1. Color: varies from light to dark brown; foods and medications may affect color
2. Odor: aromatic, affected by ingested food and person's bacterial flora
3. Consistency: formed, soft, semisolid; moist
4. Frequency: varies with diet; once a day is a common pattern
5. Amount: varies with diet (about 100 to 400 grams/day)
6. Constituents: small amounts of undigested roughage, sloughed dead bacteria and epithelial cells, fat, protein, dried constituents of digestive juices (bile pigments), inorganic matter (calcium, phosphates)

C. Common bowel elimination problems

1. Constipation: abnormal infrequency of defecation and abnormal hardening of stools
2. Impaction: accumulated mass of dry feces that cannot be expelled
3. Diarrhea: increased frequency of bowel movements (more than 3 times a day) as well as liquid consistency and increased amount; accompanied by urgency, discomfort, and possibly incontinence
4. Incontinence: involuntary elimination of feces
5. Flatulence: expulsion of gas from rectum
6. Hemorrhoids: dilated portions of veins in anal canal causing itching and pain and bright red bleeding upon defecation

D. Diagnostic tests

1. Abdominal film: x-ray of abdomen taken with client in flat and upright positions
2. Upper GI barium swallow: fluoroscopic x-ray examination of esophagus, stomach, and small intestines after client ingests barium sulphate
3. Barium enema: fluoroscopic x-ray examination visualizing entire large intestine after client is given an enema of barium, which outlines structural changes such as polyps and diverticulitis
4. Endoscopy: use of a flexible tube (fiberoptic endoscope) to visualize GI tract; images produced are transmitted to a video screen
5. Upper endoscopy: a telescopic eyepiece is inserted through mouth; EGD—esophagogastroduodenoscopy
6. Lower endoscopy: a telescopic eyepiece is inserted through rectum—proctosigmoidoscopy

E. Health promotion for elimination problems

1. Constipation: increase fluid intake; instruct client to drink hot liquids and fruit juices, especially prune juice, and to eat foods high in roughage or fiber, such as raw fruits and vegetables, bran products, whole-grain cereals and bread
2. Diarrhea: encourage oral intake of fluids and bland foods; avoid spicy and fatty foods, alcohol, beverages with caffeine, and high-fiber foods
3. Flatulence: limit chewing gum, carbonated drinks, drinking straws, and gas-producing foods such as cabbage, cauliflower, beans, and onions

F. Bowel diversion ostomies: an ostomy is a surgical opening in abdominal wall for elimination of feces or urine; bowel diversion ostomies are classified according to status (temporary or permanent), anatomic location, and construction of stoma

1. Permanence: colostomies can be temporary (for traumatic injuries or inflammatory conditions) or permanent (birth defect or disease such as cancer)
2. Anatomic location (see Figure 27–2 ■): identifies site from which ostomy empties
   a. Ileostomy: distal end of small intestine (ileus)
   b. Cecostomy: first part of ascending colon (cecum)
   c. Ascending colostomy: ascending colon
   d. Transverse colostomy: transverse colon
   e. Descending colostomy: descending colon
   f. Sigmoidostomy: sigmoid colon
3. Construction of stoma
   a. Single: one end of bowel as opening
   b. Loop: a loop of bowel brought out into abdominal wall and supported by a glass rod or a plastic bridge; has two openings—proximal, or active, and distal, or inactive; usually performed as an emergency procedure and situated often in right transverse colon
   c. Divided: two separated stomas; opening from digestive end is colostomy and distal end is mucus fistula (bowel continues to secrete mucus)
   d. Double-barreled: proximal and distal loops are sutured together and both ends are brought out through the abdominal wall

G. Health promotion for clients with ostomies

1. For a client with a colostomy, dietary teaching needs to include information about:
   a. Foods that cause stool odor: asparagus, beans, eggs, fish, onions, garlic
   b. Foods that increase gas: cabbage, onions, beans, and cauliflower
   c. Foods that thicken stool: applesauce, bananas, rice, tapioca, cheese, yogurt
   d. Foods that loosen stool: chocolate, dried beans, fried foods, highly spiced foods, leafy green vegetables, raw fruits and vegetables
2. For a client with ileostomy, teaching to relieve food blockage should include:
   a. Drink warm fluids or grape juice if not vomiting
   b. Take a warm shower
   c. Assume a knee-chest position

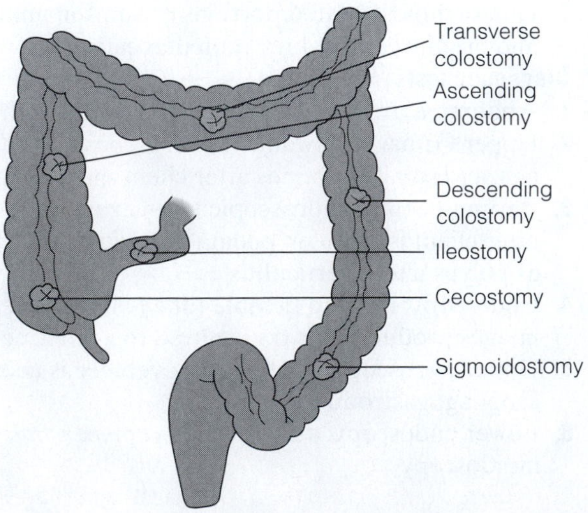

Figure 27–2

Locations of various bowel diversion ostomies.

Source: Kozier, B., Erb, G., Berman, A., & Snyder, S. (2004). Fundamentals of nursing: Concepts, process, and practice *(7th ed.). Upper Saddle River, NJ. Pearson Education, p. 1232.*

d. Massage peristomal area
e. Remove pouch if stoma is swollen and apply one with a larger opening
f. Eat a low-residue diet initially; avoid foods that cause blockage such as popcorn, nuts, cucumbers, celery, fresh tomatoes, figs, blackberries, and caraway seeds
g. Limit high-fiber foods and chew them well if eaten
! h. Know signs of blockage: abdominal cramping, swelling of stoma, and absence of ileostomy output for 4 to 6 hours

VI. MEETING SENSORY AND PERCEPTUAL NEEDS

A. Factors affecting sensation and perception

1. Numerous factors affect sensory function, including illness, developmental stage, medications, stress, and lifestyle
2. Illness may result in hospitalization; this change of environment may affect mentation, especially for older clients; mentation could result from an underlying disease process or simply a change in physical environment
3. Developmental stage affects sensory perception
   a. Infants have adequate sensory organs but have no mental concepts to understand sensory input
   b. As development occurs, person develops understanding of sensory input
   c. Adults have many learned responses to sensory cues; with aging, sensory input diminishes because of decreased sense organ functioning
4. ! Medications can affect both sensory function and awareness; many drugs decrease level of consciousness (LOC); others contribute to mental confusion; in older adults, polypharmacy may lead to drug interactions that cause decreased sensory functioning
5. Stress can be described as eustress or distress
   a. Eustress stimulates individual functioning; an example is a client who needs to lower cholesterol level and lose weight, and stress encourages client to avoid fatty foods
   b. Distress is presence of more stress that depresses individual functioning; anxiety tends to limit amount of sensory input a client can deal with effectively
   c. Illness and hospitalization can both cause distress; today, hospitals try to create aesthetic environments more conducive to healing, such as with bright and cheerful walls with beautiful pictures, carpeted floors, and an overall attempt to create a pleasant, "homelike" environment
6. Lifestyle influences sensory perception; one individual may thrive in a stimulating environment that may overwhelm others

B. Sensory and perceptual alterations

1. Three factors known to contribute to alterations in client behavior include (but are not limited to) sensory deprivation, sensory overload, and sensory deficits
2. **Sensory deprivation:** a lack of meaningful stimuli; actual amount of incoming stimuli is reduced because of either a decrease in environmental stimuli or impairment in one or more of client's senses; decreased sensory input can lead to disorientation over a period of time
   a. If client cannot derive meaning from environment, sensory deprivation may ensue; an example is a blind client who is admitted to hospital; client's environment has changed drastically because landmarks that were present at home are gone
   b. Changes in any kind of sensory input could lead to deprivation; an example is a person who has a visual impairment and loss of tactile perception because of a neurological illness; sensory deprivation can then lead to distortions in perception, which may affect client's ability to perceive environment correctly
   c. ! Risk factors that may lead to sensory deprivation include dysfunction of senses, medications, immobility, isolation, and language barriers
   d. ! See Box 27–5 for clinical signs and symptoms of sensory deprivation
   e. Hospital rooms have clocks, calendars, and sometimes boards that identify names of caregivers on that shift, all of which provide meaningful stimuli to hospitalized clients and promote orientation to surroundings

Box 27-5

Signs of Sensory Deprivation and Sensory Overload

Sensory Deprivation

- Excessive yawning, drowsiness, sleeping
- Decreased attention span, difficulty concentrating, decreased problem solving
- Impaired memory
- Periodic disorientation, general or nocturnal confusion
- Preoccupation with somatic complaints, such as palpitations
- Hallucinations or delusions
- Crying, annoyance over small matters, depression
- Apathy, emotional liability

Sensory Overload

- Increased muscle tension
- Fatigue and inability to sleep
- Irritability and restlessness
- Inability to concentrate
- Decreased problem-solving performance

3. **Sensory overload:** an increase in intensity of stimuli to levels beyond normal; it generally occurs when a person is unable to process amount or intensity of stimuli or when person is exposed to numerous stimuli that are not meaningful
   a. Increased internal stimuli (such as anxiety) and increased external stimuli (noise, equipment, multiple health care personnel) can lead to sensory overload
   b. Sensory overload leads to sleep deprivation, which reduces individual coping abilities; when overloaded with sensory stimuli, client may feel out of control; assess environment and recognize that sights and sounds familiar to health care worker may add to overload for client
   ! c. Contributing factors that add to overload could be pain, anxiety, and lack of sleep; incidence is increased in clients in intensive care units after 2 to 3 days
   d. Refer again to Box 27–5 for clinical signs and symptoms of sensory overload
4. **Sensory deficit:** impairment of both reception and perception of one or more senses; when loss of sensory function is gradual, individual compensates for loss; for instance, someone with impaired vision may decrease area in which they travel alone

C. Common sensory deficits

1. Visual: vision is an important sense because it allows people to interact with their environment
   a. People with visual impairment may wear glasses or contact lenses to correct refraction errors of lens of the eye
   b. Refraction errors include myopia (nearsightedness), hyperopia (farsightedness), and presbyopia (loss of lens elasticity results in inability to focus on close objects; occurs with aging, around age 45, and requires corrective lenses—"reading" glasses or bifocals)
   c. Cataracts: often seen after age 65; lens opacity blocks light rays and distorts and impairs visual field; surgical removal is often required as cataract progresses; see also Chapter 64
   d. Glaucoma: a painless blockage in circulation of aqueous fluid in eye that leads to an increase in intraocular pressure and possibly blindness; see also Chapter 64
   e. Diabetic retinopathy: leading cause of blindness among adults age 20 to 70; proliferative retinopathy or neurovascular disease occurs when ischemic retinal blood vessels bleed, causing vitreous hemorrhage; this hemorrhage can be repetitive and may lead to permanent visual loss
   f. Macular degeneration: degenerative changes in blood vessels arising in retina; macular blood vessels leak and damage macula; scarring occurs and

visual loss results; signs and symptoms are blurring and distortion of visual images; see also Chapter 64

2. Hearing: difficulty with hearing may make client feel isolated; it can interfere with health teaching and even increase client's risk of injury
   a. Conductive hearing loss results from interrupted transmission of sound waves through outer and middle ear; possible causes are a tear in eardrum (tympanic membrane); obstruction in auditory canal caused by swelling or other factors; degeneration of hammer, anvil, and stirrup from infection; or continuous low-sensory input
   b. Sensorineural hearing loss results from damage to inner ear, auditory nerve, or hearing center in brain from viral infection or ototoxic medications (whose names often end with *mycin*)
   c. **Presbycusis** is loss of hearing ability related to aging; gradual loss of hearing is more common in men than in women
3. Balance: with aging comes a gradual reduction of power and contraction of muscles; after age 50, there is a steady decrease in muscle fibers; often balance is impaired with this process as well; degenerative joint changes may occur, making movement more restricted
4. Taste: reduction in ability to taste can affect appetite and contribute to poor nutrition; if a corresponding loss of sense of smell occurs, client's appetite will also not be stimulated by aroma of food
5. Smell: in addition to its effect on client's appetite, loss of smell can be a safety issue; with decrease in smell, client will not be aware of a gas leak, for example
6. Touch: tactile deprivation can occur from a disease or an injury that leads to destruction of or damage to nerve cells
   a. Children born with myelomeningocele have damage to nerves below level of pathology; injuries that destroy nerves will have same effect; loss of tactile ability may contribute to safety issues; a client who has suffered loss of sensation in a part of body, for example, could easily be burned because he or she cannot feel pain
   b. Peripheral neuropathy interferes with innervation of peripheral nerves; with aging, diabetes, or arteriosclerosis, overall effectiveness of blood vessels decreases; superficial blood vessels constrict to divert blood to larger vessels; with constriction of peripheral blood vessels, peripheral nerve endings in constricted area suffer effects of decreased blood flow and neuropathy develops
   c. Multisensory deficit conditions: some conditions, such as stroke or "brain attack," cause damage to more than one sense and lead to ischemia in affected area of brain; results may be decreased mobility, decreased sensation, and/or paresis or paralysis of extremities, as well as aphasia, blindness or other visual impairment, or impaired swallowing

D. Promoting self-care

! 1. Screening and prevention: early detection of sensory deprivation is an important health-screening function
   a. Routine auditory testing is done at birth and during early school years
   b. Periodic vision screening of all school-aged children is done
   c. Health fairs often provide a means to screen a large number of healthy individuals
   d. Be aware of disease processes that can lead to sensory deprivation, and screen for symptoms to detect sensory problems early
   e. Teach health measures to protect sensory organs; encourage protective eye and ear gear; emphasize, especially to teenagers, risk of damage to ears from loud noises or music
   f. Teach clients general health measures such as regular eye and ear exams
   g. The Occupational Safety and Health Administration (OSHA) provides regulations and guidelines to limit hazards affecting senses to individuals in workplace; OSHA guidelines are carefully followed in health care settings also

2. Assistive aids: nurse assists clients with a sensory deficit by encouraging use of specific aids to support sensory function, promoting use of other senses, communicating effectively, and working to ensure client's safety
   a. ! Visual and hearing aids: give eyeglasses to clients upon awakening and assist in storage at bedtime; ensure that hearing aid is in place and functioning during daytime and prior to any explanations about care or treatment; see Box 27–6 for information on possible visual and auditory aids
   b. For clients with smell and taste deficits, nurse can supply diets that include a variety of flavors, temperatures, and textures that may stimulate taste buds
   c. Each client with a sensory deficit should be evaluated to determine appropriate assistive device
3. Communication
   a. Client with a sensory deficit is at risk for not accurately interpreting information shared during communication
   b. Convey respect to client and enhance his or her self-esteem
   c. A person with a hearing deficit needs to concentrate at all times during a conversation
   d. When speaking to a client with a hearing deficit, face client and speak directly to him or her without large numbers of people around; too many people in environment will be a distraction
   e. A client with visual deficits might misinterpret nonverbal clues during conversation
4. See Box 27–7 for further information about communicating with clients who have visual or hearing deficits

Box 27–6

Aids for Clients with Visual and Auditory Deficits

The nurse can help a client select aids that are appropriate for that client.

For Clients with Visual Deficits

- Prescription eyeglasses
- Proper lighting in rooms
- Shades on windows to reduce glare
- Large-print books
- Color-coded stove dials; the colors of blue and yellow are the easiest contrast
- Auditory books
- Seeing-eye dog
- Red-tipped cane or laser cane
- Magnifying glasses

For Clients with Auditory Deficits

- Hearing aids
- Closed caption service for television
- Telephone with amplifiers
- Flashing alarms in the home for fire, doorbells, and so on
- Cochlear implants
- Service dogs
- TDD phone
- Telephone with light that flashes when ringing
- Vibrating alarm clock
- Wireless page, phone, and e-mail service

Box 27-7

Communicating with Clients Who Have a Visual or Hearing Deficit

Visual Deficit

- Always announce presence and identify self by name when entering client room.
- Stay in the client's field of vision if vision loss is partial.
- Speak in a warm and pleasant tone of voice, but not with excessive loudness.
- Always explain what you will do before touching client.
- Explain sounds in environment.
- Indicate when conversation has ended and you are leaving the room.

Hearing Deficit

- Before initiating a conversation, move to a position where you can be seen or gently touch client.
- Decrease background noises (e.g., radio) before speaking.
- Talk at a moderate rate and in a normal tone of voice; shouting does not make voice more distinct and could make understanding more difficult.
- Address client directly; do not turn away during a remark or story; make sure client can see your face easily and that it is well lighted.
- Avoid talking with chewing gum or other substances in your mouth; avoid covering your mouth with your hand.
- Keep voice at about the same volume throughout each sentence, without dropping the voice at the end of each sentence.
- Always speak as clearly and accurately as possible; articulate consonants with particular care.
- Do not "overarticulate"; mouthing or overdoing articulation is just as troublesome as mumbling; pantomime or write ideas, or use sign language or finger spelling when appropriate.
- Use longer phrases, which tend to be easier to understand than short ones; also, word choice is important: "Fifteen cents" and "fifty cents" may be confused, but "half a dollar" is clear.
- Pronounce every name with care; make a reference to the name for easier understanding—for example, "Joan, the girl from the office" or "Talbots, the big store at the mall."
- Change to a new subject at a slower rate, ensuring that the client follows the change; a key word or two at the beginning of a new topic is a good indicator.

Adapted from Kozier, B., Erb, G., Berman, A., & Burke, K. (2004). *Fundamentals of nursing: Concepts, process, and practice* (6th ed.). Upper Saddle River, NJ: Prentice Hall, p. 949.

VII. SKIN INTEGRITY AND WOUND CARE

A. Healthy skin integrity

1. Layers of skin
   a. Epidermis: outermost layer made of stratified squamous epithelial cells; can be further divided into five layers; innermost layer is basal-cell layer responsible for replacing sloughed and damaged cells
   b. Dermis: second layer of skin composed of connective tissue; gives elasticity to skin; blood vessels, nerve fibers, glands, and hair follicles are embedded in this layer
   c. Subcutaneous tissue: consists of adipose tissue and provides support and blood flow to dermis
2. Skin glands: sebaceous glands, soporiferous glands, and cerumenous glands
   a. Sebaceous glands (within dermis) secrete an oily substance called sebum, made up of fats, cholesterol, proteins, and salts; function of sebum is to protect hair from drying; it also forms a protective film on skin that prevents excessive evaporation of water; sebum also inhibits growth of certain bacteria on skin

b. Soporiferous glands (sweat glands) produce a watery secretion; there are two types: apocrine (primarily found in skin of axilla and pubic regions; produce odor when decomposed by bacteria) and eccrine (chiefly found on palms of hands, soles of feet, and forehead; produce a watery discharge that helps cool body through evaporation)
c. Ceruminous glands secrete a thick, oily substance called cerumen, a waxy secretion of external ear (also known as earwax)

3. Skin alterations related to aging: overall health status, age, nutritional status, and energy and activity level play a role in maintaining client's skin condition; problems associated with skin alterations in elderly include:
   a. Epidermis thins and has a lower water content, leading to dry skin
   b. Elasticity and some of fatty cushion are lost, resulting in wrinkles and fragile skin
   c. Blood vessels in skin also become more fragile with aging, leading to easy bruising

B. Classification of wounds: a wound is a break in skin or mucous membrane resulting from physical means; may be superficial (affecting skin surface only) or deep (involving blood vessels, nerves, muscle, fascia, tendons, ligaments, and bones)

1. Wounds are classified according to continuity of surface they cover (tissue involved)
   a. An open wound is characterized by a break in skin and could be superficial or deep; examples are an abrasion, laceration, or puncture
   b. A closed wound is one in which there is no break in the skin; examples are a contusion and ecchymosis; these injuries may be caused by a blow or other type of trauma
2. Full and partial thickness refer to depth of injury and are used most frequently to describe burns
   a. Partial thickness involves entire epidermis, part of dermis; sweat glands and hair follicles are intact
   b. Full thickness involves epidermis and dermis, extending to subcutaneous tissue and possibly even to muscle and bone
3. Noninfected and infected wounds
   a. A noninfected or clean wound has not been invaded by pathogenic microorganisms; a clean wound heals without infection
   b. An infected wound or septic wound is one in which pathogenic microorganisms have invaded wound and clinical signs and symptoms of infection develop
4. Surgical wound: an intentional wound made by a surgeon for therapeutic purposes using a sharp cutting instrument; it is a clean wound that heals without infection
5. Pressure ulcers: lesions caused by unrelieved pressure, which also damages underlying tissues
   a. Contributing factors include immobility, fragile skin in older adults, moisture, malnutrition, shearing, and friction
   ! b. Assess individual client's relative risk using scales such as Braden scale or Norton scale (see Table 27–3 ■)
   c. Stage I: skin is intact, although nonblanching erythema will be noted; client may report tingling or burning; darker-skinned clients may have skin discoloration, warmth, edema, and induration or hardness as indicators
   d. Stage II: involves superficial, partial-thickness skin loss with blister or abrasionlike appearance; it may also look like a shallow crater
   e. Stage III: full-thickness skin loss; necrotic tissue will be seen in subcutaneous layer that extends down to (but not through) underlying fascia; ulcer will appear as a deeper crater with or without undermining of surrounding tissue
   f. Stage IV: continuation of stage III with damage to muscle, bone, and supporting structures such as tendons or joint capsule; undermining of tissue and sinus tracts may also be present

C. Wound healing

1. Three phases
   a. Inflammatory phase: serum and RBCs form a fibrin network of protein fibers in wound; blood flow increases to area; damaged tissue then heals; fibrin and other protein at wound surface dry out, forming a scab that seals skin in 3 to 4 days

Table 27-3 Pressure Ulcer Risk Assessment Scales

Norton Scale

Physical Condition		Mental Condition		Activity		Mobility		Continence	
Good	4	Alert	4	Walks	4	Full	4	Good	4
Fair	3	Apathetic	3	Walks with help	3	Slightly limited	3	Occasional incontinence	3
Poor	2	Confused	2	Sits in chair	2	Very limited	2	Frequent incontinence	2
Very poor	1	Stuporous	1	Remains in bed	1	Immobile	1	Urine and fecal incontinence	1
Total	___	Total	___	Total	___	Total	___	Total	___
Grand total = _____									

A score of 14 or less indicates a risk of pressure ulcer; a score under 12 indicates a high risk.

Braden Scale

Sensory Perception		Moisture		Activity		Mobility		Nutrition		Friction and Shear	
No impairment	4	Rarely moist	4	Walks frequently	4	No limitations	4	Excellent	4		
Slightly limited	3	Occasionally moist	3	Walks occasionally	3	Slightly limited	3	Adequate	3	No apparent Problems	3
Very limited	2	Moist	2	Chairfast	2	Very limited	2	Probably inadequate	2	Potential problem	2
Completely limited	1	Constantly moist	1	Bedfast	1	Immobile	1	Very poor	1	Problem	1
Total	___	Total	___	Total	___	Total	___	Total	___	Total	___
Grand total = _____											

Assign a score of 1 to 4 in each category. Total the score; if it is 18 or less, the client is at moderate or high risk for pressure ulcer development.
Source: Smith, S., Duell, D., & Martin, B. (2004). *Clinical nursing skills: Basic to advanced skills* (5th ed.). Upper Saddle River, NJ: Prentice Hall, p. 853.

b. Proliferative phase: fibroblasts grow to form granulation tissue (4 to 21 days), which is very friable, soft, and pinkish red in color because of new capillaries; next epithelial cells grow from edges; connective tissue then fills area and becomes a scar that is stronger than granulation tissue; when wound is extensive and requires excessive granulation tissue for closure, a large, uneven scar called a **keloid** forms

c. Maturation or remodeling phase (healing of the scar): often occurs by weeks 3 to 4, but can extend for 2 years after injury; characterized by reorganization of collagen fibers, wound remodeling, and tissue maturation; a fully healed wound has tensile strength of up to only 80% of preinjury state, making it more susceptible to future injury

2. Factors affecting wound healing

! a. Age: healthy children and adults heal faster than older clients; see Box 27–8 for factors that inhibit healing in older adults

! b. Nutrition: protein is needed to build new tissue; vitamin C helps maturation of fibrous tissue and enhances protein synthesis; undernourishment results in inadequate body stores of nutrients, while obesity tends to decrease blood flow to tissue and increase risk of developing infection

Memory Aid

Remember that foods containing protein or vitamin C are good choices for clients who have healing wounds.

c. Condition of tissues: wound contamination and infection slow healing process; organisms present in wound will compete with body cells for O_2 and nutrition
d. Efficiency of circulation: factors that restrict local blood supply to a wound (damaged arteries, edema of tissues, and dehydration) interfere with healing; anemia and blood dyscrasias may interfere with oxygen delivery to tissues; conditions such as diabetes and liver dysfunction can delay healing; individuals who participate in regular exercise tend to have better circulation and thus tend to heal faster; smoking may limit O_2 supply to tissues
e. Rest, anxiety, and stress: adequate rest of injured part will affect wound closure; anxiety and stress can stimulate release of hormones that slow healing
f. Medications: antiinflammatory drugs such as steroids and hormones slow formation of fibrous tissue and therefore impair healing

3. Wound closures
   a. **Primary intention:** characterized by return of tissues to a healthy state with minimal inflammation and little if any scarring; wound edges are well approximated and wound heals without infection
   b. **Secondary intention:** healing occurs when wound is extensive and edges cannot or should not be approximated; because of greater injury, more granulation tissue is needed to close wound; healing time is prolonged; secondary intention carries greater risk for infection and results in deeper, more extensive scarring
   c. Surgical interventions: sutures, staples, and clips are devices used to approximate wound edges; some sutures absorb and others must be removed; staples and clips are alternatives to suturing and are usually made of silver; these require removal in approximately 7 to 10 days
4. Complications that affect wound healing
   a. Hemorrhage: assess internal hemorrhage by distention in area of wound; external hemorrhage is evidenced by blood on dressing or leaking from dressing; if bleeding is severe, client may exhibit manifestations of shock; risk of hemorrhage is greater within first 48 hours; if pressure dressings do not successfully stop bleeding, surgical intervention may be necessary
   b. Infection: clinical signs and symptoms include redness, swelling, heat, and pain at site; purulent exudate (consisting of leukocytes, liquefied dead tissue debris, and dead and living bacteria) may be noted; client may be anorexic, nauseous, febrile, and have chills; physician will order a wound culture, and antibiotics will be administered after culture is obtained
   c. **Dehiscence:** accidental reopening of suture line (usually abdominal, but could occur with any wound) with tissue separation under wound; results from infected suture line or factors that impede wound healing; clients often "feel something giving way"; place client in bed with head of bed low to eliminate gravity and with knees bent to decrease pull on suture line; cover wound with large, sterile, wet saline dressings; notify surgeon immediately because repair of surgical site is necessary

Box 27-8

Factors Inhibiting Wound Healing in Older Adults

- Impaired blood flow to the wound from cardiovascular disease or diabetes
- Less flexible collagen tissue (may enhance damage from pressure, friction, and shearing)
- Reduced formation of antibodies and monocytes necessary for wound healing
- Nutritional deficiencies (may reduce red blood cells and leukocytes, negatively affecting oxygen delivery and the inflammatory response essential for wound healing)
- Slower rate of cell renewal

Adapted from Kozier, B., Erb, G., Berman, A., & Snyder, S. (2004). *Fundamentals of nursing: Concepts, process, and practice* (7th ed.). Upper Saddle River, NJ: Prentice Hall, p. 862.

! **d. Evisceration**: internal organs (viscera) protrude through incisional edges after dehiscence; contributing factors include infection, poor nutrition, failure of suture material, dehydration, and excessive coughing; treated in a manner similar to dehiscence

D. Wound assessment and management

1. Inspect wound and gently palpate surrounding area regularly
2. Note whether wound edges are approximated; as an incision heals, a healing ridge may be noted
3. ! Note presence and characteristics of any drainage from wound or on dressing; outline drainage on dressing, noting date and time
4. ! Observe for signs of infection: redness, swelling, increased tenderness, or disruption of wound edges; note body temperature and white blood cell count as other indicators
5. Purposes for dressing a wound
   - **a.** Absorb drainage
   - **b.** Splint or immobilize wound to provide rest
   - **c.** Protect wound from mechanical injury
   - **d.** Promote hemostasis
   - **e.** Prevent contamination
   - **f.** Provide mental and physical comfort for client
6. Purposes for maintaining a wound undressed
   - **a.** Eliminate conditions that favor growth of microorganisms
   - **b.** Allow for better wound observation and assessment
   - **c.** Facilitate bathing and hygiene
   - **d.** Avoid adhesive tape reaction
   - **e.** Avoid friction and irritation that destroy new epithelial cells
7. Wound irrigation: may be needed to cleanse or flush wound to enhance healing; normal saline and antibiotic solutions are most commonly used

E. Wound management products

1. ! Wound cleansers: all wounds need to be cleansed appropriately; in clean wounds where tissue is granulating, minimize any disruption of wound bed; wound should be cleaned gently and debris rinsed away with normal saline (see Box 27–9 for wound cleansing guidelines)
2. Dressings: a variety of dressing materials are available, each with different purposes; some are designed to provide barrier protection from contamination;

Box 27–9

Clinical Guidelines for Cleaning Wounds

- Use physiologic solutions, such as isotonic saline or lactated Ringer's solution, to clean or irrigate wounds. If antimicrobial solutions are used, make sure they are well diluted.
- When possible, warm the solution to body temperature before use.
- If a wound is grossly contaminated by foreign material, bacteria, slough, or necrotic tissue, clean the wound at every dressing change.
- If a wound is clean, has little exudate, and reveals healthy granulation tissue, avoid repeated cleaning.
- Use gauze squares. Avoid using cotton balls and other products that shed fibers onto the wound surface that can become embedded in granulation tissue and can act as foci for infection or stimulate foreign body reactions, prolonging the inflammatory phase of healing and delaying the healing process.
- Clean superficial, noninfected wounds by irrigating them with normal saline.
- To retain wound moisture, avoid drying a wound after cleaning it.
  - Hold cleaning sponges with forceps or a sterile gloved hand.
  - Clean wound in an outward direction.

Adapted from Kozier, B., Erb, G., Berman, A., & Snyder, S. (2004). *Fundamentals of nursing: Concepts, process, and practice* (7th ed.). Upper Saddle River, NJ: Prentice Hall, p. 880.

Table 27–4
Types of Dressings

Dressing Type	Description
Gauze	Plain or impregnated with an antimicrobial Packs and fills wound Absorbs drainage Used for full- and partial-thickness wounds with drainage May be applied dry, wet-to-moist, and wet-to-wet
Transparent	Adhesive membrane that is occlusive to liquids and bacteria Protects wound and promotes autolytic **debridement** (the removal of dead tissue from a wound) Impermeable to bacteria Op-Site and Tegaderm are examples
Composite dressing	Contains an absorbent pad and an adhesive covering Purpose is to absorb drainage Advantage is that it only has to be changed three times a week
Hydrocolloids	Adhesive made of gelatin Is occlusive to microorganisms and liquids and promotes absorption of wound exudates Enhances autolysis of necrotic tissue within wound bed Duo-Derm and Tegasorb are examples
Hydrogel	Water or glycerin is primary component of this nonadherent dressing Maintains moist wound surface and provides some absorption Permeable to oxygen and can fill dead spaces in a wound Secondary nonadhesive dressing may be required
Calcium alginates	Pad made of seaweed fibers Purpose is to absorb larger amounts of drainage
Exudate absorbers	Semipermeable polyurethane foam dressings that absorb large amounts of exudates while keeping the wound moist Nonadherent
Absorptive or filler dressings	Absorb moderate amounts of drainage Duo-Derm paste is an example

some may be impregnated with antibiotics; others are moist and aid in liquefying necrotic tissue; see Table 27–4 ■

3. Bandages are strips of cloth used to wrap a body part
   a. Made of gauze, which is light and porous, or of an elasticized material, which provides pressure to area
   b. Widths vary from 1 to 4 inches and are determined by body part to be wrapped
   c. Purposes include to anchor dressings, provide support to a body part, immobilize a body part, or promote circulatory return
   d. Apply bandage with body part in normal position
   e. Pad bony prominences
   f. Bandage from distal to proximal area to support blood return
   g. ! Use even pressure while applying bandage, especially when using elastic bandages that could impair circulation
   h. ! Inspect and palpate the area regularly—more frequently on a fresher wound, less frequently on an older wound; note neurovascular status of extremity (temperature, blanching, and sensation) and pain (evaluate for its cause)
4. Enzymatic debriding agent: an enzyme paste or solution, such as Elase, that is applied to necrotic tissue; enzyme digests necrotic tissue

VIII. MEETING NEEDS FOR MOBILITY

A. Common causes of immobility

1. Pain: reduces spontaneous movement in an attempt to decrease painful stimuli; will also cause client to decline to participate in rehabilitative activities, including coughing and deep breathing

2. Motor and nervous system impairment: disorders of musculoskeletal and nervous system can limit mobility; certain neurological diseases can cause muscles to become stiff or lose function
   a. Arthritis and amputations are examples of musculoskeletal conditions
   b. Multiple sclerosis and Parkinson's disease are neurological conditions that may render muscles unable to function normally
   c. Alterations in LOC and stroke (CVA) could also leave client immobile
3. Functional problems: some chronic conditions that limit supply of O_2 and nutrients or increase cardiac work affect activity tolerance, such as chronic obstructive lung disease, congestive heart failure, angina, and obesity
4. Generalized weakness
   a. With increasing age, muscle tone and bone density decrease; flexibility and reaction time slows; osteoporosis (demineralization of bone) begins to wear away bone; aging also affects posture, balance, and gait
   b. Chronic illness may also cause changes in body that affect client's energy level and his or her ability to be active
5. Psychological problems: emotional disorders such as depression or stress can impede a client's desire to be active
   a. Depression may reduce motivation and energy to participate in activities of daily living
   b. A client who is under prolonged stress can also be depleted of energy
   c. Fear may also prevent client from going outside or leaving home
6. Medically induced immobility
   a. Physicians may place their clients on bedrest or restricted activity to allow healing of body parts
   b. Orthopedic devices can also mandate immobility; traction, casts, splints, and braces can all lead to inactivity of some part(s) of body

! **B. Major complications of immobility**

1. Psychological effects: powerlessness and possible reduced self-esteem
2. Atrophy and contractures
3. Disuse osteoporosis
4. Pressure ulcers
5. Orthostatic intolerance (postural or orthostatic hypotension)
6. Deep vein thrombosis
7. Pneumonia
8. Decrease in peristalsis (paralytic ileus)
9. Kidney stones

C. Nursing interventions for impaired mobility

1. Explain benefits of exercise
   a. Improves tone and strength of muscles; also improves joint flexibility and range of motion
   b. Promotes good pulmonary ventilation, which prevents pooling of secretions in lungs and reduces risk of pneumonia
   c. Improves gastrointestinal motility and tone, thereby improving digestion and elimination
   d. Since exercise decreases bone loss of calcium, urine maintains acidity and thus decreases risk for renal calculi
2. Types of exercise
   a. Isometric: tension or resistance is produced in a muscle without a change in length of muscle; isometric exercises strengthen muscle groups that will be used later in ambulation; teach client to push or pull against a stationary object as a form of isometric exercise; muscles exercised are abdominal, gluteus, and quadriceps
   b. Isotonic: exercises that shorten muscle to produce contraction and active movement; there is no significant change in resistance during movement, so force of contraction stays stable; they increase muscle tone and maintain joint flexibility; using a trapeze to lift body or pushing body into a sitting position are examples of isotonic exercises for bedridden client

c. Passive range of motion: accomplished with assistance of a caregiver who supports client's body part while moving it
d. Active range of motion: exercises performed independently; these are isotonic exercises of each joint in body and can maintain or improve muscle strength; these exercises prevent deterioration of joint movement and subsequent contractures

D. Assistive ambulation device: crutches

! 1. Used to assist client in moving and ambulating; all crutches require rubber tips to prevent slipping on floors; various types of crutches are available (see Figure 27–3 ■)
   a. An axillary crutch is most frequently used type of crutch
   b. A Lofstrand or forearm crutch is used as a substitute for a cane; consists of a single tube of aluminum with a handle and a cuff for forearm; allows user to release hand bar because metal cuff maintains placement of crutch and prevents it from falling
   c. Canadian or elbow extensor crutch is used for client whose forearm extensor muscles are weak; it allows upper arm to provide stability to crutch

! 2. Measuring for crutches
   a. Measure client who is lying supine from anterior fold of axilla to heel of foot and add 1 inch (2.5 cm)
   b. Also measure placement of hand on crutch while client stands and adjust crutch so that it maintains elbow at a 30-degree angle
   c. With client standing erect, ensure that shoulder rest of crutch is 3 fingerwidths (2.5 to 5 cm, or 1 to 2 inches) below axilla

! 3. Safety with crutches
   a. Place rubber tip on end of crutch
   b. Teach client appropriate gait
   c. Prior to gait training, assist client in preparing for crutch walking by encouraging client to push body off the bed with hands and arms
   d. While utilizing crutches, have client bear weight on arms, not axillae, to avoid nerve damage to axillae caused by continued pressure

4. Gaits used for crutch walking: client's ability to bear weight and maintain balance determines choice of five gaits; client alternates body weight between one or both legs and crutches; see Box 27–10

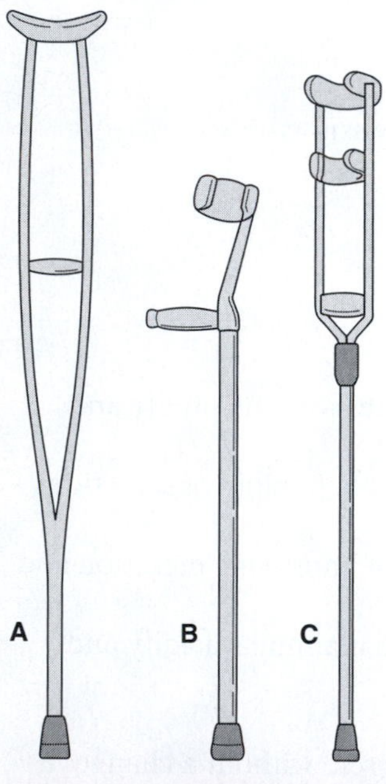

Figure 27–3

Three types of crutches: (A) axillary crutch; (B) Lofstrand crutch; (C) Canadian or elbow extension crutch.

Source: Kozier, B., Erb, G., Berman, A., & Burke, K. (2000). Fundamentals of nursing: Concepts, process, and practice *(6th ed.). Upper Saddle River, NJ: Prentice Hall, p. 1052.*

E. Cane: assists a client to walk with greater balance and support

1. Three types of canes
   a. Quad cane has four feet
   b. Tripod has three feet
   c. Straight cane
2. Canes are adjustable; length should allow elbow to bend slightly
3. Canes allow clients to ambulate faster and with less fatigue
4. Clients may use one or two canes; a single cane is used on unaffected side
5. A rubber cap is fitted at tip of cane to prevent slipping

F. Walker: provides more support than a cane

1. Useful for clients who have poor balance or cardiac problems or who cannot use crutches
2. Standard walker has four legs with rubber tips on feet and plastic grips for hands
3. Client must be allowed partial weight-bearing and must have strength in his or her wrists and arms
4. Client uses his or her upper body to propel walker forward
5. Two- or four-wheeled walker is useful for client who is too weak or not stable enough to move a walker by lifting it; some walkers have an attached seat to allow client to sit and rest as needed during walk
6. Walkers are height-adjustable

G. Other assistive devices

1. Hydraulic lift (e.g., Hoyer Lift): used for clients who are unable to stand and too heavy for health care workers to lift safely
2. Lift has three parts: sling, arm, and base; a pressure release valve is on base

Box 27–10

Crutch Walking Gaits

Four-Point Gait: Partial Weight-Bearing

1. The client must be able to bear weight on both legs.
2. It is the safest gait and provides three points of support at all times.
3. It requires constant shifting of weight and coordination of movement of legs and crutches.

Three-Point Gait: Requires One Leg to Be Able to Bear Weight of Entire Body

1. Non-weight-bearing on affected leg
2. Alternates between good leg and affected leg with both crutches

Two-Point Gait: Requires Partial Weight-Bearing on Both Legs

1. Client can move at a faster gait than with the four-point gait
2. Two points are used to support the body at all times
3. Crutch movement is similar to the swinging of the arms while walking

Swing-Through Gait: Weight-Bearing Gait that Requires Strength and Coordination

1. Client moves both crutches forward together
2. Then the client lifts his or her body weight and swings through

Swing-To Gait: Weight-Bearing on Both Legs

1. Similar to swing-through gait except body motion is only to level of crutches
2. Useful for clients with paralysis of legs and hips

3. Place sling under client: arm of device has a hook that attaches to sling; lift is raised to elevate client
4. Lift is then moved and aligned with chair; pressure release valve is released, and client is lowered to chair
5. Sling can be removed from hooks but left under client to facilitate returning client to bed

Check Your NCLEX–RN® Exam I.Q.

You are ready for testing on this content if you can

- Assist a client with personal hygiene needs.
- Evaluate a client's ability to perform activities of daily living.
- Plan nursing care to promote rest and sleep.
- Assess the elimination needs of a client.
- Provide care to a client to assist with urinary and bowel elimination.
- Take action to prevent complications of immobility.
- Assess a client's wound-healing status.
- Implement nursing measures to promote wound healing.
- Assess a client's need for assistive devices.
- Implement care for a client using an assistive device.

PRACTICE TEST

1 While completing a nursing assessment, the client states he is 70 years old, has a history of staphylococcus infections, increased intraocular pressure, and blurry vision. The nurse concludes that which item reported by the client is a risk factor for the development of cataracts?

1. History of staphylococcus infections
2. Increased intraocular pressure
3. Age of 70 years
4. Long complaint of blurry vision

PRACTICE TEST

2 A 92-year-old client is in the hospital. The client is very hard of hearing, and the nurse needs to do the admission interview. Which of the following should the nurse do when assessing the client?

1. Obtain a cotton swab to clean cerumen in the client's ear before beginning the interview.
2. Speak louder in the client's better ear after determining which has better hearing.
3. Lower the pitch of the voice and face the client during the interview.
4. Put new batteries in the hearing aid to ensure proper functioning.

3 A 72-year-old client has been in the ICU for the last 2 days. Which intervention would be the most appropriate in decreasing the risk for sensory deprivation?

1. Remove equipment from the room.
2. Explain all procedures and routines to the client upon admission.
3. Provide a clock and calendar in the client's room.
4. Provide the client with prolonged rest periods.

4 A client has a sprained ankle, and the nurse must apply an elastic bandage to provide support to the ankle. Which of the following actions should the nurse take during this procedure?

1. Wrap the bandage while stretching it from distal extremity to proximal.
2. Apply the bandage loosely around the extremity.
3. Apply heavy pressure with each turn of the bandage.
4. Start at the upper end of the extremity and work toward the distal end.

5 All of the following clients appear in the emergency room during one shift. The nurse would clarify with the physician the reason for an antibiotic order for a client with which of the following injuries?

1. Cat bite to the hand of an elderly client
2. Laceration from broken glass in a 6-year-old client
3. Stab wound in a 37-year-old client
4. Closed-fractured ankle in a 40-year-old soccer player

6 A client is on complete bed rest and is at risk for disuse syndrome. Which of the following client goals is appropriate?

1. The client has shorter periods of immobility.
2. The client remains free of contractures in lower extremities.
3. The nurse turns the client every 2 hours.
4. The nurse performs passive range of motion to lower extremities every 4 hours.

7 This is the first hospitalization for an adult client who, after being admitted 3 days ago, is now having trouble sleeping. The nurse also notes some confusion during waking hours. Which of the following would be the most appropriate nursing diagnosis for this client?

1. Ineffective health maintenance
2. Ineffective individual coping
3. Disturbed sensory perception
4. Disturbed sleep pattern

8 An 80-year-old client has been admitted to the nursing unit with Parkinson's disease. Which of the following activities would be most appropriate in preventing disuse syndrome?

1. Providing for the nutritional needs of the client
2. Promoting weight-bearing exercises
3. Encouraging 8 glasses of fluid in 24 hours
4. Turning and positioning every 2 hours

9 A client has a pressure ulcer on the left hip. The nursing staff has written a nursing diagnosis of Impaired skin integrity with a client goal of "skin heals by 6/12." Prior to June 12, the nurse evaluates progress on reaching this goal. Which statement is the best notation of progress toward the goal?

1. Turning every 2 hours and avoiding lying on left side
2. Wet to moist dressing changed every 4 hours
3. No additional areas of breakdown noted
4. Ulcer less reddened and granulation tissue noted on edges

10 In assessing a client who has been immobilized because of illness, the nurse would most likely document the client's muscles as which of the following?

1. Hypertrophied
2. Atrophied
3. Flexible
4. Hardened

11 A female client can move her right arm and leg but has hemiplegia on the left. The nurse instructs the nursing assistant to do which of the following exercises on the client's left side during care?

1. Active range of motion
2. Passive range of motion
3. Isotonic
4. Isometric

12 A client has weakness of the lower extremities and uses crutches for mobility. The nurse concludes the client needs further information about using crutches when the client does which of the following?

1. Uses the swing-to gait
2. Uses axillary crutches
3. Bears weight on the armpits
4. Has new rubber tips on the crutches

13 A male client suffered numerous types of wounds when he lost control of his motorcycle and was thrown onto the pavement. The client asks the nurse which wounds will scar more. The nurse's reply will be based on analysis that which of the following wounds would generally be least likely to scar?

1. A wound that heals by primary intention
2. A wound that heals by secondary intention
3. A wound that becomes infected
4. A wound to an extremity

14 A postoperative client tells the nurse that he developed dehiscence after his last surgery and wants to make sure it doesn't happen this time. In attempting to prevent dehiscence from occurring, the nurse's interventions would be aimed at doing which of the following?

1. Helping the client lose weight
2. Preventing vomiting
3. Administering antibiotics
4. Keeping the wound dry

15 An elderly postoperative client has an abdominal wound. Weeks after the surgery, the wound is still healing. The client asks the clinic nurse why the wound is healing so slowly. The nurse would explain that which of the following is one factor that negatively affects healing in the elderly?

1. Vascular changes decrease the blood flow to the wound.
2. Most elderly clients are overweight.
3. Decreased activity levels prevent blood from reaching the area.
4. Keloid formation prevents healing.

16 A young adult is admitted to the hospital for gallbladder surgery. The client is also diagnosed as having a vitamin C deficiency. The nurse places high priority on assessing this client for which development postoperatively?

1. Unusual muscle weakness
2. Mental confusion
3. Delayed wound healing
4. Ataxia upon ambulating

17 The nurse is assisting a client with a mobility problem in determining the appropriate assistance device. The client has no paralysis of the lower extremities, but the legs are very weak. Upper-body strength is also reduced. The nurse would suggest which device for this client?

1. Cane
2. Four-wheeled walker
3. Canadian or elbow extension crutch
4. Lofstrand crutch

18 The nurse is evaluating a client using a cane. Which assessment made by the nurse would indicate that the client is using the cane appropriately?

1. Client holds the cane with the hand on the stronger side.
2. Client holds the cane with the hand on the affected side.
3. Client moves the cane and the affected leg together.
4. The cane tip is made of aluminum to prevent slippage.

19 A client is at risk for the developing a pressure ulcer and is placed on a repositioning regimen. The client does not like to lie on his side and complains about the need to turn. To enhance compliance, the nurse uses which of the following most effective explanations?

1. "Turning will help you to maintain normal sensation in all skin areas under pressure."
2. "Excess pressure interferes with skin absorption of vitamin D."
3. "Staying in one position prevents proper heat loss from that area of the body."
4. "Changing position prevents tissue breakdown that could ultimately become infected."

PRACTICE TEST

20 The nurse is changing the dressing of a client who is 4 days postoperative with an abdominal wound. The nurse has changed this dressing daily since surgery. Today, the nurse notes increased serosanguineous drainage, wound edges not approximated, and puffy tissue protruding through the wound. The nurse concludes which of the following conditions exists?

1. Hemorrhage
2. Normal healing by primary intention
3. Normal healing by secondary intention
4. Evisceration

21 The nurse needs to conduct an admission interview with a 74-year-old client who is hearing impaired. Which of the following should the nurse do to enhance the client's ability to hear? Select all that apply.

1. _____ Position self to be within the client's line of vision.
2. _____ Dim the lights in the room.
3. _____ Overarticulate words.
4. _____ Turn down the television in the room.
5. _____ Talk at a moderate rate and with the same tone for all words.

ANSWERS & RATIONALES

1 **Answer: 3** Age above 65 is a risk factor for cataracts. Double vision, increased intraocular pressure, and blurry vision are signs of glaucoma. **Cognitive Level:** Application **Client Need:** Physiological Integrity: Basic Care and Comfort **Integrated Process:** Nursing Process: Assessment **Content Area:** Fundamentals **Strategy:** The core issue of the question is knowledge of factors that increase client risk for conditions affecting sensory perception. Use the process of elimination and nursing knowledge to make a selection.

2 **Answer: 3** Hearing loss, especially of upper-range tones, is common in the elderly. Speaking to the client slowly and in a lower-pitched voice while facing the client is the best means of communication. Options 1 and 4 are not helpful, and option 2 is unnecessary.
Cognitive Level: Application **Client Need:** Physiological Integrity: Basic Care and Comfort **Integrated Process:** Communication and Documentation **Content Area:** Fundamentals **Strategy:** The core issue of this question is the optimal choice for communicating with a client who is hearing impaired. Eliminate options 1 and 4 first as least helpful or unnecessary measures. Eliminate option 2 because it may not allow the client to see the nurse's face, which assists in determining words when a client is hard of hearing.

3 **Answer: 3** Providing the client with a clock and calendar helps the client to be oriented to time and date. These would be meaningful stimuli for the client and decrease the chance for sensory deprivation. It may not be realistic in an ICU to remove equipment from the room. Explaining all procedures and routines would increase the risk of overload. Giving the client prolonged rest periods would only increase the risk for deprivation.
Cognitive Level: Application **Client Need:** Physiological Integrity: Basic Care and Comfort **Integrated Process:** Nursing Process: Implementation **Content Area:** Fundamentals **Strategy:** The core issue of the question is nursing actions that can prevent the client from experiencing sensory deprivation. Use knowledge of basic nursing measures to help a client stay oriented to time, place, and person make a selection.

4 **Answer: 1** To prevent vascular impairment, proper application of elastic bandages is required. Wrapping distal to proximal is compatible with the flow of venous return. Wrapping the bandage evenly while stretching it ensures that there will be even tension applied to the extremity. Wrapping it loosely will not secure the bandage in place. Excessive pressure would cause circulation to be compromised.
Cognitive Level: Application **Client Need:** Physiological Integrity: Basic Care and Comfort **Integrated Process:** Nursing Process: Implementation **Content Area:** Fundamentals **Strategy:** The core issue of the question is knowledge of basic wound-care procedures. Use nursing knowledge of these procedures and concepts related to blood flow to make your selection.

5 **Answer: 4** A closed fracture has no break in the skin. A cat bite, a laceration, and a stab wound all impair skin integrity, which could lead to infection.
Cognitive Level: Analysis **Client Need:** Physiological Integrity: Basic Care and Comfort **Integrated Process:** Nursing Process: Implementation **Content Area:** Fundamentals **Strategy:** The core issue of the question is appropriate use of antibiotic therapy. Restate this question in the following way: "Which client is not at risk for infection?" Use the process of elimination and nursing knowledge to make the selection that poses little risk of infection.

6 **Answer: 2** Disuse syndrome is a result of prolonged immobility. Stating "the client remains free of contractures" describes in active terms the desired outcome for the client. The last two options describe nursing activities to meet the stated client goal. The nurse has no control over option 1.
Cognitive Level: Application **Client Need:** Physiological Integrity: Basic Care and Comfort **Integrated Process:** Nursing Process: Planning **Content Area:** Fundamentals **Strategy:** Recall that goal statements are indicators of what the nurse wants to happen as a result of care. With this general principle in mind, eliminate each of the incorrect responses because they are focused on the nurse or are beyond the nurse's control.

7 **Answer: 4** The client is in a new environment. Changes in environment bring about uncertainty, and the client may be unable to sleep or may sleep less well than at home. Although the client is confused, there is no other data presented that could be the cause, making disturbed sleep pattern a more appropriate selection than disturbed sensory perception. In

addition, disturbed sensory perception relates to one of the five senses. Ineffective health maintenance and ineffective individual coping are more global and not applicable to this client's situation.

Cognitive Level: Analysis **Client Need:** Physiological Integrity: Basic Care and Comfort **Integrated Process:** Nursing Process: Analysis **Content Area:** Fundamentals **Strategy:** The core issue of the question is the ability to draw correct conclusions about client assessment data and translate it to a nursing diagnosis. In this case, the original problem is sleeping, and the correct answer is one that focuses on this problem.

8 **Answer: 2** Weight-bearing exercise is the best approach to preventing disuse syndrome. Disuse syndrome occurs because the stresses of weight bearing are absent and the bone releases calcium. The other options list general nursing interventions that are not specific to weight-bearing.

Cognitive Level: Application **Client Need:** Physiological Integrity: Basic Care and Comfort **Integrated Process:** Nursing Process: Implementation **Content Area:** Fundamentals **Strategy:** The core issues of the question are the cause of disuse syndrome and nursing approaches that will minimize it. Use concepts of basic nursing care to answer the question.

9 **Answer: 4** Options 1 and 2 indicate nursing activities aimed at promoting healing. Option 3 refers to other areas of the body. Option 4 refers to the wound itself and is the best indication of the wound's current status.

Cognitive Level: Application **Client Need:** Physiological Integrity: Basic Care and Comfort **Integrated Process:** Communication and Documentation **Content Area:** Fundamentals **Strategy:** The core issue of the question is the type of documentation that best described progress toward wound healing. Questions such as these seek an answer that reflects an outcome rather than activities.

10 **Answer: 2** After immobilization, unexercised muscles will atrophy. The muscles would not be flexible or hardened. Hypertrophy is the opposite of atrophy.

Cognitive Level: Application **Client Need:** Physiological Integrity: Basic Care and Comfort **Integrated Process:** Communication and Documentation **Content Area:** Fundamentals **Strategy:** This question requires application of basic nursing knowledge to a client situation. Select the term that is a common finding in clients who are immobilized.

11 **Answer: 2** Passive range of motion is most appropriate because the client is unable to move that side of the body on her own. The other exercises require resistance on the part of the muscles on the left side, and the client is unable to do that.

Cognitive Level: Application **Client Need:** Physiological Integrity: Basic Care and Comfort **Integrated Process:** Nursing Process: Implementation **Content Area:** Fundamentals **Strategy:** The critical words in the question are *unable to move.* This indicates that the client has hemiplegia and is unable to actively participate in exercising the joints. The wording of the question tells you that there is only one correct answer.

12 **Answer: 3** The weight of the body should be borne on the arms, not the axillae. When clients allow the axillae to bear the weight of the body, they are at risk of developing crutch palsy, a nerve damage. The other options represent correct information about use of crutches, and therefore no further information is needed on those points.

Cognitive Level: Analysis **Client Need:** Physiological Integrity: Basic Care and Comfort **Integrated Process:** Nursing Process: Evaluation **Content Area:** Fundamentals **Strategy:** The core issue of the question is proper use of crutches. Keep in mind that improper use can lead to nerve injury, and select the option that puts the client at risk.

13 **Answer: 1** Primary intention healing occurs when the wound edges are well approximated; wounds that heal by secondary intention have edges that cannot be approximated. Scarring is greater for wounds that heal by secondary intention and those that become infected. The location of a wound has little to do with scarring.

Cognitive Level: Application **Client Need:** Physiological Integrity: Basic Care and Comfort **Integrated Process:** Nursing Process: Analysis **Content Area:** Fundamentals **Strategy:** The core issue of this question is knowledge of physiological wound healing. Use nursing knowledge and the process of elimination to make a selection.

14 **Answer: 2** Activities that are likely to lead to dehiscence include vomiting and coughing because they increase intraabdominal pressure. In addition, clients who are obese and those with poor nutrition are candidates for dehiscence. Since the client is already postoperative, encouraging weight loss at this time would not affect risk for dehiscence.

Cognitive Level: Application **Client Need:** Physiological Integrity: Basic Care and Comfort **Integrated Process:** Nursing Process: Planning **Content Area:** Fundamentals **Strategy:** The core issue of the question is knowledge of risk factors for dehiscence. Recall that dehiscence is most likely to occur when there is some type of stress on the incision line. Consider that vomiting puts sudden tension on the suture line to select it as the option that is most likely to be harmful to the client.

15 **Answer: 1** Vascular changes, such as atherosclerosis and atrophy of capillaries, impair blood flow to the wound. The other statements are false. Older adults are not necessarily overweight, although weight gain does tend to occur with increasing age. Decreased activity levels with aging does not diminish local blood supply to a healing wound. Keloid formation is an abnormal type of healing of a wound.

Cognitive Level: Application **Client Need:** Physiological Integrity: Basic Care and Comfort **Integrated Process:** Nursing Process: Implementation **Content Area:** Fundamentals **Strategy:** The core issue of the question is age-related changes that have a negative impact on wound healing. Use nursing knowledge and the process of elimination to make a selection.

16 **Answer: 3** Protein and vitamin C are necessary for building and maintaining tissues. A deficiency of vitamin C would prolong wound healing. The other options have nothing to do with vitamin C.

Cognitive Level: Application **Client Need:** Physiological Integrity: Basic Care and Comfort **Integrated Process:** Nursing Process: Planning **Content Area:** Fundamentals **Strategy:** The core issue of this question is the role of vitamin C in wound healing. Use nursing knowledge and the process of elimination to make a selection.

17 **Answer: 2** The client has bilateral weakness of the lower extremities, and the proper assistive device is one that will provide bilateral support. In this case, a walker provides the most support. Additionally, a four-wheeled walker does not require the client to lift the walker as steps are taken.

Cognitive Level: Analysis **Client Need:** Physiological Integrity: Basic Care and Comfort **Integrated Process:** Nursing Process: Implementation **Content Area:** Fundamentals **Strategy:** The core issue of the question is the assistive device that will provide the safest support to the client. The critical word *legs* in the stem of the question guides you to look for an option that provides bilateral support.

18 **Answer: 1** To provide maximum support and appropriate body alignment while walking, the cane is held in the hand on the stronger side. The tip of the cane should have rubber to prevent slipping.

Cognitive Level: Application **Client Need:** Physiological Integrity: Basic Care and Comfort **Integrated Process:** Nursing Process: Evaluation **Content Area:** Fundamentals **Strategy:** The core issue of the question is the proper use of a cane as an assistive aid. Use the process of elimination and basic nursing knowledge to make a selection.

19 **Answer: 4** Unless the skin loss is extensive, the skin will continue to absorb vitamin D and prevent the loss of heat from the body. Tactile stimulation can still occur with a wound. However, a loss of skin integrity places the client at risk for bacterial invasion and subsequent infection.

Cognitive Level: Application **Client Need:** Physiological Integrity: Basic Care and Comfort **Integrated Process:** Communication and Documentation **Content Area:** Fundamentals **Strategy:** The core issue of the question is knowledge of the functions of the skin and how pressure ulcers interfere with normal skin function. Use the process of elimination and basic nursing knowledge to make a selection.

20 **Answer: 4** Evisceration occurs when internal viscera protrude from an incision that is dehiscing. In this situation, the nurse notes changes in wound appearance such as increased serosanguineous drainage, edges lacking approximation, and the protruding viscera.

Cognitive Level: Analysis **Client Need:** Physiological Integrity: Basic Care and Comfort **Integrated Process:** Nursing Process: Analysis **Content Area:** Fundamentals **Strategy:** The core issue of this question is the ability to draw accurate conclusions about the status of a surgical wound. Use the process of elimination and basic nursing knowledge to make a selection.

21 **Answer: 1, 4, 5** The nurse should position herself or himself within the client's line of vision to enable the client to read lips during the conversation. It is good to decrease background noises that interfere with the client's ability to hear the nurse. It is also helpful to speak at a moderate rate and use the same voice tone throughout each sentence, not dropping the tone at the end of a sentence. The lighting should not be dimmed because doing so would interfere with the client's ability to read lips. Words should not be overarticulated; exaggerated, unnatural movement of the lips can distort words for the client who relies on lip reading to compensate for hearing loss.

Cognitive Level: Application **Client Need:** Physiological Integrity: Basic Care and Comfort **Integrated Process:** Communication and Documentation **Content Area:** Fundamentals **Strategy:** The core issue of the question is effective communication strategies with a client whose hearing is impaired. Remember that correct answers to questions such as these focus on enhancing the client's vision during communication and are moderate in overall approach (not excessive or insufficient).

ANSWERS & RATIONALES

Key Terms to Review

circadian synchronization p. 429
debridement p. 446
dehiscence p. 444
dyspnea p. 424
evisceration p. 445
hyperventilation p. 424
hypoventilation p. 424
Kegel exercises p. 434
keloid p. 443
orthopnea p. 424
presbycusis p. 439
pressure ulcer p. 422
primary intention p. 444
secondary intention p. 444
sensory deficit p. 438
sensory deprivation p. 437
sensory overload p. 438

References

Daniels, R. (2004). *Nursing fundamentals: Caring and clinical decision making.* Clifton Park, NY: Delmar Learning.

Harkreader, H., & Hogan, M. (2004). *Fundamentals of nursing: Caring and clinical judgment* (2nd ed.). St. Louis, MO: Elsevier Science.

Kozier, B., Erb, G., Berman, A. J., & Snyder, S. (2004). *Fundamentals of nursing: Concepts, process, and practice* (7th ed.). Upper Saddle River, NJ: Pearson Education.

Potter, P., & Perry, A. (2005). *Fundamentals of nursing* (6th ed.). St. Louis, MO: Mosby.

Smith, S., Duell, D., & Martin, B. (2004). *Clinical nursing skills: Basic to advanced skills* (6th ed.). Upper Saddle River, NJ: Prentice Hall.

Taylor, C., Lillis, C., & LeMone, P. (2005). *Fundamentals of nursing: The art and science of nursing care* (5th ed.). Philadelphia: Lippincott Williams & Wilkins.

Maintaining the Function of Tubes and Drains 28

In this chapter

Test Yourself

Are you ready for the NCLEX-RN® or course exams? Use the practice tests on the companion CD-ROM to check.

Cross reference

Other chapters relevant to this content area are

Meeting Nutritional Needs	Chapter 26
Perioperative Care	Chapter 49
Respiratory Disorders	Chapter 56
Renal and Genitourinary Disorders	Chapter 59
Gastrointestinal Disorders	Chapter 60

I. RESPIRATORY TUBES

A. Tracheostomy tube

1. Overview
   - **a.** Tracheotomy is a surgical procedure that creates an opening in trachea to establish a patent airway
   - **b.** A **tracheostomy** is an opening (stoma) that is surgically created
   - **c.** A variety of tubes can be inserted into a tracheostomy, depending on whether it is temporary or permanent, on length of anticipated use, on whether mechanical ventilation will be used, and on need to be able to speak while in place (see Figure 28–1 ■)
   - **d.** ! Variations in tubes include double-lumen or single-lumen (inner cannula or no inner cannula), cuffed or cuffless, and fenestrated or nonfenestrated (see Table 28–1 ■)
   - **e.** Clients who have permanent tracheostomies often use metal trach tubes, which are cuffless and have an inner cannula; can be used long-term with regular cleaning (example: Jackson tube)
2. Therapeutic management
   - **a.** Maintain head of bed elevated at least 30 degrees
   - **b.** ! Ensure that a manual resuscitation (Ambu) bag is at bedside at all times

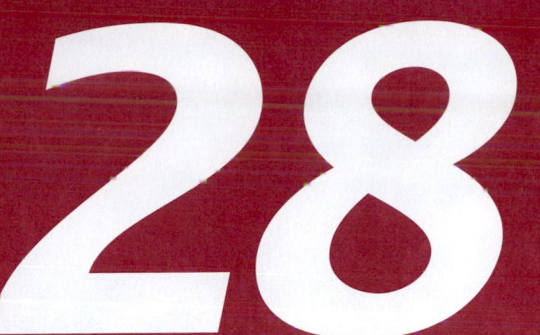

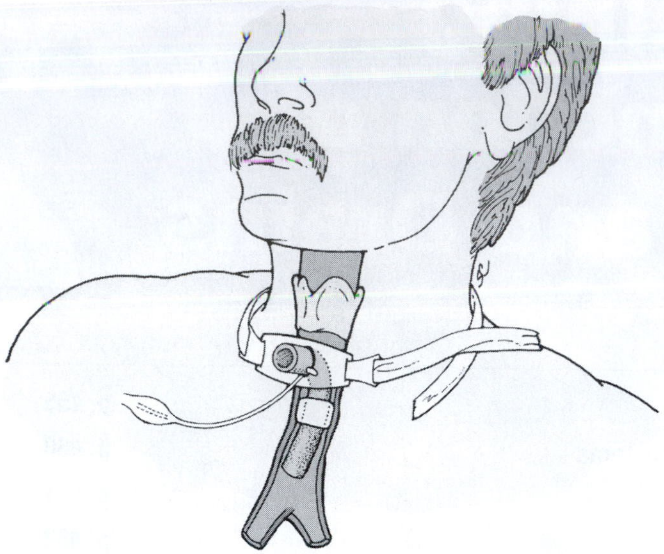

Figure 28–1

Tracheostomy tube in place.

Source: Smith, S., Duell, D., & Martin, B. (2004). Clinical nursing skills: Basic to advanced skills *(6th ed.). Upper Saddle River, NJ: Pearson Education, p. 911.*

c. Keep spare tracheostomy set of same size, obturator, and clamps at bedside for use if trach is accidentally removed
d. Ensure that air and oxygen flowing into airway is humidified; notify respiratory therapy if water bottle attached to oxygen flowmeter runs low
e. Encourage coughing and deep breathing to reduce risk of atelectasis and pneumonia
f. Perform respiratory assessments, including breath sounds, at regular intervals, minimally every 4 hours
g. Monitor and document trend of oxygen saturation and/or arterial blood gas results
h. Suction client as indicated by results of assessment (cough, noisy respirations, or adventitious breath sounds are indicators of need to suction); hyperoxygenate client before and after, suction for no more than 10 seconds at one time; assess nature of secretions (purulent secretions indicate infection)

Table 28–1

Comparison of Features of Tracheostomy Tubes

Feature	Present	Absent
Inner cannula (a removable inner tube within an outer tracheostomy tube that can be removed for cleaning)	Double-lumen tubes have both an inner cannula and an outer cannula; inner cannula allows for easy cleaning, especially with heavy secretions, and may be reusable or disposable (e.g., Shiley trach)	Single-lumen tubes have no inner cannula and may be used short term or in clients not anticipated to have copious respiratory secretions (e.g., Portex trach)
Cuff	Cuffed tube allows airway to be sealed to prevent air loss during mechanical ventilation or to prevent aspiration of saliva, gastric contents, or tube feedings; is inflated with air using syringe attached to pilot balloon	Cuffless tube is often selected for long-term use in clients who do not need mechanical ventilation and are at low risk of aspiration
Fenestration	Fenestrated trachs have holes in tube to allow air to flow between larynx and trachea; used frequently during weaning so client regains ability to breathe naturally; it allows client to speak	Nonfenestrated trachs have no holes and are ideal for clients on mechanical ventilation or who cannot speak

i. Assess stoma for redness or signs of infection; assess for and report subcutaneous emphysema (subcutaneous air, also called crepitus)
j. Perform tracheostomy care every 8 hours; use half-strength peroxide for cleansing site and inner cannula unless agency policy is different
k. Change tracheostomy ties daily or more often if soiled; have assistance to hold trach in place so client cannot cough trach out; if assistance is unavailable, place new ties before cutting and removing old ones to prevent client from coughing tube out
l. Monitor cuff pressures (if inflated) at least every 8 hours as indicated by agency policy (should not exceed 20 cm); see endotracheal tube section that follows for cuff inflation techniques
m. Provide for alternate means of communication (word or picture board, writing pad) if client cannot talk because of cuff inflation
n. If client has order for oral intake while trach is in place, inflate cuff to reduce risk of aspiration and sit client upright during meals and for 1 hour afterward as ordered
o. Before capping or plugging trach as final stage of weaning prior to trach removal, ensure that fenestrated trach is in use and that cuff, if present, is deflated

3. Complications (see Table 28–2 ■)
4. Accidental removal
a. If trach inserted was during previous 72 hours, use manual resuscitation bag to ventilate client while second nurse calls resuscitation or rapid response team
b. After 72 hours postplacement, extend neck and open stoma by grasping retention sutures or using curved clamp to spread tracheal tissue; insert obturator into trach tube, insert tube into trachea, remove obturator, ventilate with manual resuscitation bag, and assess air exchange and respiratory status; if unsuccessful or ineffective, call for resuscitation or rapid response team
5. Purposeful removal
a. Suction trachea and oropharyngeal area to remove any secretions
b. Ensure that cuff is deflated
c. Physician cuts sutures that hold tracheostomy in place and withdraws tube during exhalation
d. Place dry sterile dressing over stoma and tape gently in place
e. Stoma closes over next few days and leaves small scar

B. *Endotracheal tube* (see Figure 28–2 ■, p. 459)

1. Overview
a. An artificial airway that maintains airway patency and allows for client to receive mechanical ventilation; intended for short-term use, up to 10 to 14 days
b. Consists of a long tube with a universal adapter at proximal end for attachment to oxygen source or ventilator, inflatable cuff at distal end, and pilot balloon at proximal end for cuff inflation
2. Routes of insertion
a. Orotracheal insertion route allows for use of larger tube, rapidly restores airway, and reduces respiratory effort; disadvantages include discomfort to client, possible displacement through tongue movement, and occlusion from biting on tube; oral airway may need to be used
b. Nasotracheal route allows for use of smaller tube, prevents dislodgement by client's tongue, but increases respiratory effort; contraindicated with bleeding disorders, epistaxis, or nasal obstruction
3. Therapeutic management
a. To check placement after insertion, ventilate with manual resuscitation bag, assess that both left and right sides of chest rise and fall, and auscultate for bilateral breath sounds; if only right-sided chest movement and breath sounds are present, tube needs to be pulled back slightly from placement in right mainstem bronchus
b. Auscultate over epigastric area to ensure esophageal intubation did not occur; if it did, ventilation sounds will be louder over stomach than chest and

Table 28-2

Complications of Tracheostomy

Complication	Prevention and Therapeutic Management
Short term	
Tube displacement	Secure tube properly. Keep spare tube of same size at bedside. Do not allow client to pull at tube. Prevent traction on tube during care and avoid excessive tube movement.
Tube obstruction	Humidify oxygen. Suction as needed and note if secretions are becoming thick and viscous. Encourage client to cough and deep breathe. Keep inner cannula clean by doing trach care regularly as scheduled. Assess client for respiratory difficulty and/or newly increased peak pressure on mechanical ventilator. Prepare for rapid tube replacement in the event of obstruction caused by cuff prolapse over distal end of tube.
Long term	
Tracheomalacia (tracheal dilation and erosion caused by high cuff pressures)	Note whether trach tube has low pressure cuff for prevention. Monitor air volumes needed to keep cuff inflated and cuff pressures as per policy; identify and report increases. Assess for air leaks around cuff or lost tidal volume if mechanical ventilation is being used. Assess for aspiration of bits of food or fluids if client is allowed oral intake. Monitor for and report onset of bleeding caused by pressure. Progress client to use of uncuffed tube at earliest opportunity.
Tracheoesophageal fistula (abnormal connection between posterior wall of trachea and esophagus from high cuff pressure)	Similar to tracheomalacia above. Assess for coughing or respiratory distress while taking food or fluids. Administer supplemental oxygen by mask to treat hypoxemia. Prepare client for possible insertion of gastric or jejunostomy tube for feedings if pressure of nasogastric tube in esophagus was contributing factor.
Tracheal stenosis (tracheal lumen narrowing from scar formation secondary to cuff irritation)	Prevent by avoiding high cuff pressures and avoiding traction or pulling on tube. Observe for respiratory difficulty, increased coughing, inability to manage secretions, or difficulty in speaking after cuff deflation or trach tube removal. Prepare client for surgical dilation of trachea for definitive treatment as needed.
Tracheal-innominate artery fistula (erosion of lateral wall of trachea into artery caused by pressure from distal end of tube)	Prevent by keeping tube in midline position and avoiding traction on tube from any cause. Assess for pulsation of trach tube with each client heartbeat and notify physician immediately if it occurs. Note fresh bleeding at or through stoma and report immediately. Physician may remove trach tube immediately and apply direct pressure to blood vessel at stoma site. Prepare client for immediate life-saving surgical repair.

abdomen will rise and fall with ventilations; tube is removed immediately if this occurs

c. A carbon dioxide (CO_2) analyzer is frequently used to check proper placement in the trachea using advanced cardiac life support (ACLS) protocols

! d. Confirm placement by portable chest x-ray; distal tip of tube should be 1 to 2 cm above carina (point of bifurcation of right and left mainstem bronchi)

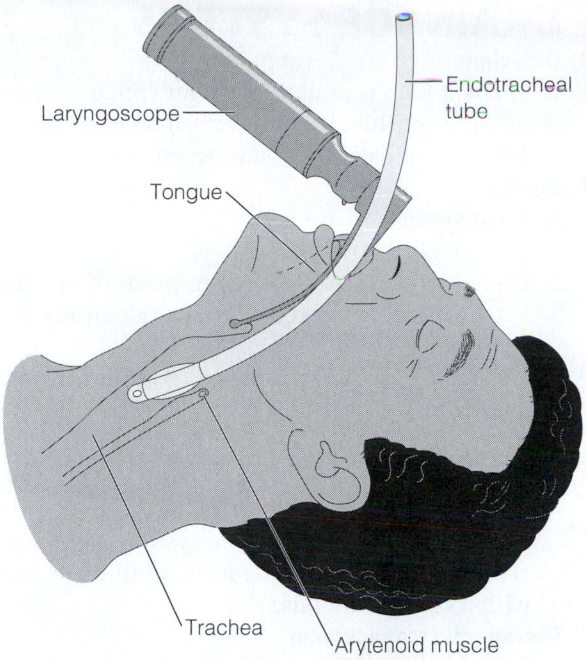

Figure 28–2

Endotrachael tube insertion assisted by laryngoscope.

Source: Lemone, P. & Burke, K. (2004). Medical surgical nursing: Critical thinking in client care (3rd ed.). Upper Saddle River, NJ: Pearson Education, p. 138.

e. Note position of tube by noting centimeter marking at lip line and then tape tube in place or use other securing device; monitor placement at least every 8 hours
f. Ensure manual resuscitation bag is kept at bedside at all times
g. Perform respiratory assessments every 4 hours and as needed; suction client as indicated by results of assessment as with tracheostomy
h. Inflate cuff using minimal occluding volume technique by injecting air into pilot balloon just until no air leakage sounds can be heard during inspiration with stethoscope placed over trachea
i. Inflate cuff using minimal leak technique by injecting air into pilot balloon until sealed and then deflating slightly so that no harsh sounds can be heard during inspiration but slight leak is heard at peak of inspiration
j. Insert oral airway if orotracheal route is used to prevent client from biting tube or displacing tube with tongue movement
k. Reposition orotracheal tube from one side of mouth to other daily with assistance of one other person; assess oral cavity for ulceration or necrosis
l. Provide oral care every 2 hours to prevent drying and cracking of lips and mucous membranes
m. Provide for alternative means of communication (word or picture board, writing pad)

4. Removal
   a. Suction endotracheal tube well, then suction oropharyngeal area
   b. Elevate head of bed to semi-Fowler's or high-Fowler's position as tolerated
   c. Cuff is deflated and client is asked to inhale; at peak inspiration, tube is removed
   d. Encourage client to cough and deep breathe to clear any residual secretions in pharyngeal area
   e. Apply oxygen as ordered
   f. Monitor client closely for first 30 minutes after extubation and continue to monitor frequently thereafter; notify physician if respiratory rate or effort show steady increase, oxygen saturation decreases, or respiratory distress occurs
   g. Teach client that sore throat and hoarse voice are common; monitor status and report hoarseness that doesn't improve over time, which may indicate damage to vocal cords

Cognitive Level: Application **Client Need:** Physiological Integrity: Basic Care and Comfort **Integrated Process:** Nursing Process: Analysis **Content Area:** Foundational Sciences: Nutrition **Strategy:** The core issue of the question is knowledge of the various degrees of sodium restriction in the diet. Use nutrition knowledge and the process of elimination to make a selection.

6 **Answer: 2** The DASH diet increases daily servings of vegetables and fruits, and recommends low-fat dairy foods and reduced intake of saturated fats and cholesterol. Option 1 reflects increased fats; option 3 represents increased fat, cholesterol, and sugar; option 4 reflects increased sodium content.
Cognitive Level: Application **Client Need:** Physiological Integrity: Basic Care and Comfort **Integrated Process:** Nursing Process: Evaluation **Content Area:** Foundational Sciences: Nutrition **Strategy:** The core issue of the question is knowledge that hypertensive clients should lose weight if necessary and restrict dietary intake of sodium. Use nutrition knowledge and the process of elimination to make a selection.

7 **Answer: 1** The client with burns needs increased amounts of protein and vitamins C and D until the wounds are completely healed. Option 1 reflects high-protein sources, an antioxidant source, and fortified milk that includes vitamin D and calcium. The other options do not reflect the necessary protein, vitamins, and mineral sources needed for the care of clients recovering from burns.
Cognitive Level: Application **Client Need:** Physiological Integrity: Basic Care and Comfort **Integrated Process:** Nursing Process: Implementation **Content Area:** Foundational Sciences: Nutrition **Strategy:** The core issue of the question is knowledge that increased protein and vitamins are needed for wound healing. Use nutrition knowledge about food sources of protein and vitamins and the process of elimination to make a selection.

8 **Answer: 3** Simple sugars and carbohydrates, including honey and jelly, increase the osmolality of the gastric contents and enhance movement of food out of the stomach. Therefore, these should be avoided by the client at risk for dumping syndrome. Six small meals per day, not taking fluids with meals, and lying down for 30 to 60 minutes after meals will help reduce the risk of dumping syndrome.
Cognitive Level: Analysis **Client Need:** Physiological Integrity: Basic Care and Comfort **Integrated Process:** Nursing Process: Evaluation **Content Area:** Foundational Sciences: Nutrition **Strategy:** The stem of the question has a negative wording, which tells you that the correct answer is an incorrect statement. Recall that sugars and concentrated carbohydrates should be avoided to help choose option 3 as the statement that is incorrect.

9 **Answer: 3** Increased dietary protein can lead to increased uric acid formation, which in turn lowers urinary pH and causes precipitation of uric acid stones. Clients should not exceed protein intake of 100 grams per day and should monitor purine content of foods. Option 1 is incorrect—factors other than dietary intake can cause stone formation, specifically alterations in urinary pH and the presence of metabolic disease. Option 2 is incorrect—there is no clinical evidence to suggest that decreasing calcium intake will prevent the formation of renal calculi; rather, research is showing that a high-calcium diet offers protection against stone formation. Even though most renal calculi are composed of calcium oxalate, it is the oxalate component that appears to cause the formation of stones. Option 4 is incorrect because increasing intake of complex carbohydrates is recommended to prevent renal calculi formation.
Cognitive Level: Application **Client Need:** Physiological Integrity: Basic Care and Comfort **Integrated Process:** Nursing Process: Implementation **Content Area:** Foundational Sciences: Nutrition **Strategy:** The core issue of the question is knowledge that protein sources can lead to uric acid formation and subsequent stone formation. Use nutrition knowledge and the process of elimination to make a selection.

10 **Answer: 3** Clients with COPD who overeat, in addition to consuming excess carbohydrates, have increasing difficulty with breathing because of excessive CO_2 levels that place additional stress on the lungs. The client should eat a proper diet and correct percentages of macronutrients to maintain adequate weight. In addition, chronic COPD is associated with PEM (protein-energy malnutrition), infection, and unintentional weight loss. Option 1 is incorrect—increased calories alone can lead to increased work of breathing. The percentage of fat in the diet may also pose a problem if the client is experiencing contributory disease or malabsorption. Option 2 is incorrect—merely providing medication therapy to stimulate weight gain does not address the problem of the obvious excess of calories that the client is consuming or that the client is experiencing difficulty breathing. Option 4 is incorrect because an increase in high-quality proteins will not help to correct the clinical symptoms.
Cognitive Level: Analysis **Client Need:** Physiological Integrity: Basic Care and Comfort **Integrated Process:** Communication and Documentation **Content Area:** Foundational Sciences: Nutrition **Strategy:** The core issue of the question is knowledge that excessive carbohydrate intake results in excess carbon dioxide production, which can be harmful to the client with COPD. Use nutrition knowledge and the process of elimination to make a selection.

11 **Answer: 4** A client who has stomatitis will have pain upon ingestion of food caused by the inflammatory process. Cool foods are often tolerated better than hot foods, as are soft, creamy products. Option 1 is incorrect—peanut butter is a thick, dense food that may irritate the mouth by sticking on mucous membranes and requiring more effort to swallow. Option 2 is incorrect—pretzels are high in salt, which may cause further irritation to the oral cavity. Option 3 is incorrect because tomatoes are high in ascorbic acid; even though they are in the form of a soup, they may cause irritation.
Cognitive Level: Application **Client Need:** Physiological Integrity: Basic Care and Comfort **Integrated Process:** Nursing Process: Implementation **Content Area:** Foundational Sciences: Nutrition **Strategy:** The core issue of the question is knowledge that clients with stomatitis need foods that are soft, nonirritating, and not hot. Use nutrition knowledge and the process of elimination to make a selection.

12 **Answer: 4** A client who is lactose intolerant has a difficulty handling milk and dairy products because of deficient

II. CLOSED CHEST DRAINAGE SYSTEMS

A. Overview

1. A **chest tube** is used to drain air (pneumothorax), blood (hemothorax), or large amounts of fluid (pleural effusion) from pleural cavity
2. Restores negative pressure to intrapleural space

B. Design

1. Most systems in use today have 3 chambers: collection, water seal, and suction (Figure 28–3 ■)
2. Collection chamber lies under point of attachment between tube and system and consists of marked columns (generally three) that indicate amount of drainage collected
3. Water seal chamber is filled to 2-cm marking during system setup; water allows air to escape system but not to reenter; water moves up and down in tube in this chamber with inhalation and exhalation to indicate patency
4. Suction control chamber allows use of suction to provide negative pressure to chest; negative pressure aids in reinflating lung more quickly by removing air, blood, pus, or effusion; some systems use "dry" suction, controlled by adjusting suction knob appropriate level, both types are connected to low wall suction with a connecting tube

C. Therapeutic management

1. Maintain occlusive dressing at chest tube insertion site; dressing is secured with large strips of wide tape or Elastoplast; dressing may be reinforced as needed but not changed
2. Secure all chest tube and suction tubing connections with tape
3. Keep collection apparatus below chest level to allow gravity to promote chest drainage; keep tubing straight to prevent dependent loops or obstructions
4. Milk chest tube to maintain tube patency *only if ordered;* milking chest tube can cause tissue damage
5. Chest tube is not to be clamped when client is mobile and is never clamped without a physician order; keep a clamp at bedside for use by surgeon if needed and as noted by agency policy and procedure
6. Monitor chest tube drainage at 1- to 4-hour intervals; report and document bright red blood, sudden increase in drainage, or consistent drainage greater than 100 mL/hour (physician may also specify volume to report)
7. Maintain 2-cm water level in water seal chamber; low water volume creates higher suction than may be desired, contributing to pleural tissue damage

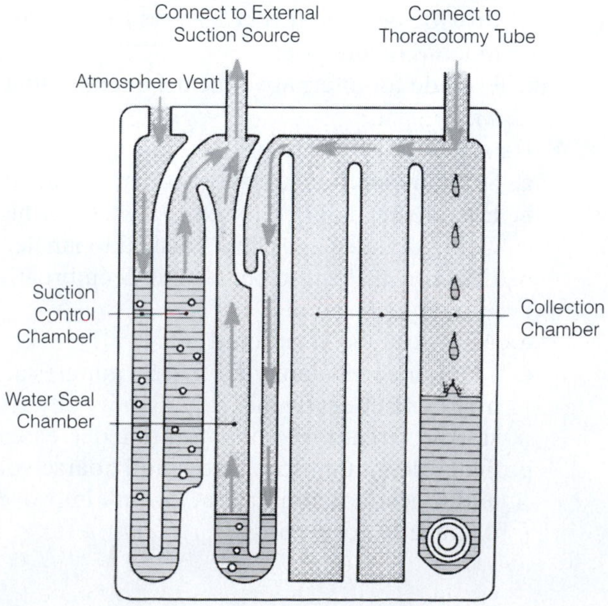

Figure 28–3

Disposable closed chest drainage system with three chambers: collection, water seal, and suction.

Source: Smith, S., Duell, D., S Martin, B. (2004). Clinical nursing skills: Basic to advanced skills *(6th ed.). Upper Saddle River, NJ: Pearson Education, p. 924.*

8. Assess for fluctuation in water seal chamber, which indicates tube is patent; lack of fluctuation may indicate tube obstruction, loop, or kink (requires correction) or may indicate full lung reexpansion (indicating tube is ready for removal); check client condition and timeframe to aid in diagnosis
9. Assess for bubbling in water seal chamber
   a. Continuous bubbling indicates an air leak in system and needs to be corrected; if leak is not found, notify surgeon of problem
   b. Intermittent bubbling with inspiration indicates drainage of air (pneumothorax) from pleural space and proper function of chest tube; continue with usual monitoring
10. Assess suction control chamber for correct amount of suction by either dial (dry suction system) or water level (fluid system); add sterile water if level is low (excessive wall suction can cause more rapid evaporation); remove excessive water by aspirating from rubber seal in chamber
11. Suction control chamber in system that uses water should have gentle, continuous bubbling as sign of proper function; vigorous bubbling will evaporate water but not increase suction, and lack of continuous bubbling will not harm client but will not provide suction that assists in clearing pneumothorax or hemothorax
12. Assess respiratory status, breath sounds, oxygen saturation, and comfort level every 4 hours or as indicated; assess that dressing is intact and check for and report subcutaneous emphysema
13. Change client position every 2 hours and encourage coughing and deep breathing
14. Anticipate that client may have frequent (up to daily) portable chest x-rays to monitor lung reexpansion
15. Keep occlusive dressing materials and sterile water at bedside for emergency use (petrolatum gauze, dry sterile gauze, wide adhesive tape)
16. If drainage system becomes damaged or broken, insert chest tube into sterile water to reestablish underwater seal and replace with new system
17. If chest tube is accidentally pulled out of chest, pinch skin together, apply occlusive dressing using materials noted above, and notify surgeon immediately
18. Chest tube removal
   a. Indicated when fluctuation stops in water seal chamber, chest x-ray shows full lung expansion, and client has returned to normal or baseline respiratory status
   b. Obtain suture removal set, petrolatum gauze, dry sterile gauze or Telfa gauze, and wide adhesive tape; premedicate client with oral medication 30 minutes prior to removal if possible
   c. Instruct client to take deep breath, hold breath (Valsalva) or exhale according to surgeon preference just prior to tube removal
   d. Open and prepare dressing materials just prior to removal of tube by physician; assist with application of dressing, and obtained follow-up chest x-ray if ordered
   e. Assess respiratory status post-removal

D. Heimlich valve

1. Used instead of chest tube for selected ambulatory clients who have pneumothorax or to treat tension pneumothorax
2. Valve allows air to escape from chest cavity during exhalation but closes during inhalation to prevent air from reentering pleural cavity

III. RENAL AND URINARY TUBES

A. Nephrostomy or ureteral tube

1. Position tube carefully (no kinks or compression) to maintain patency; do not clamp tube
2. Monitor and record urine output carefully; report output of less than 30 mL/hr or no drainage for 15 minutes or more
3. Never irrigate tube unless there is a specific order allowing it
4. Irrigate with a maximum of 5 mL volume and use strict surgical aseptic technique
5. Report and document immediately if irrigation fails to restore patency of tube

B. Indwelling urinary catheter

1. Insert using sterile technique; measure and record initial outflow amount and characteristics of urine
2. Properly position drainage bag below level of bladder and secure catheter to thigh to prevent traction of tube balloon against urethra and bladder neck
3. Measure and record outputs accurately
4. Provide routine catheter care using soap and warm water; follow standard precautions
5. Wash front to back for females; in males retract forekin if present, and return to original position after cleansing
6. Explain procedure to client just prior to removal; empty and record drainage, deflate balloon, and withdraw catheter while client exhales to reduce discomfort

IV. NASOGASTRIC TUBES

A. Overview

1. Inserted via naris to stomach for decompression of stomach and occasionally for enteral feeding
2. Commonly used tube is Salem sump, a double-lumen tube with air vent that allows for continuous (rather than intermittent) suction for gastric decompression
3. Much less commonly used tube is Levin tube, a single-lumen tube that requires use of intermittent suction (lack of air vent causes tube to collapse if continuous suction is used)

B. Insertion procedure

1. Sit client upright (high Fowler's position)
2. ! Place distal end of tube at tip of nose and measure to earlobe and then to xiphoid process to determine distance for tube insertion; apply tape to tube to indicate point at which to stop insertion
3. Lubricate distal 2 to 3 inches of tube with lidocaine gel or water-soluble gel according to policy (not petrolatum/oil-based lubricant, which could cause pneumonia if tube enters trachea)
4. Ask client to tilt head downward to close epiglottis and allow tube to enter esophagus
5. Insert tube into naris and advance upward and backward until resistance is met at back of nose; rotate catheter gently and advance into nasopharynx
6. ! Ask client to take sips of water if able while tube advanced gently into stomach
7. Stop tube insertion and pull back on tube if client coughs or chokes during procedure; when client's respiratory status returns to normal, continue insertion
8. Stop advancing tube once tape reaches naris; check placement as outlined below
9. Tape tube in place
10. Place tube to low continuous (Salem sump) or intermittent (Levin) suction for gastric decompression
11. Do not begin enteral feedings by nasogastric tube unless placement confirmed by chest x-ray (see Chapter 26)

C. Therapeutic management

1. Assess placement
   a. ! Chest x-ray is most reliable method of assessing tube placement
   b. ! Aspirate gastric contents using piston syringe and apply to strip of pH test paper (color indicating pH of 4 or less is consistent with gastric placement and pH of 6 or greater indicates intestinal placement); note that enteral feedings could alter pH and make this method less reliable
   c. Insert 5 to 10 mL air into tube while listening over epigastric area with stethoscope for "whooshing" or popping sound as air enters stomach; this method is less reliable than x-ray or gastric pH measurement
   d. ! Check placement every 4 hours after insertion
2. Assess residual prior to and regularly during enteral feedings (see Chapter 26 for details)
3. Irrigate tube with 30 to 50 ml water or saline as ordered to check tube patency; instill fluid using piston syringe and aspirate contents back; repeat if tube is

difficult to irrigate or sluggish; document fluid instilled and aspirated back on intake and output record

4. Assess naris for ulceration from pressure when changing tape daily; provide nose care by removing any crusted areas with moist swabs
5. Provide mouth care every 2 hours; presence of tube in nose leads to mouth breathing and dryness
6. Tube removal
   a. Check order and apply gloves
   b. Remove tape securing tube to nose
   c. Ask client to hold breath
   d. Withdraw tube smoothly over 3 to 6 seconds while coiling tube around hand for control
   e. Provide comfort care and document procedure

V. NASOENTERIC (INTESTINAL) TUBES

A. Overview

1. Miller-Abbott tube or Cantor tube is inserted nasally into stomach and passed into intestine via peristalsis assisted by tungsten weight at lower end of tube
2. Tube is secured to nose once final placement is reached and verified by serial abdominal x-rays
3. Suction applied to tube allows for bowel decompression and removal of accumulated intestinal secretions

B. Therapeutic management

1. Check physician order and institutional policy regarding tube advancement and removal
2. ! Wait until tube has reached final placement, as verified by x-ray (may take several hours), before securing to nose with tape
3. ! Maintain client position on right side to facilitate tube passage through pyloric sphincter of stomach into small intestine
4. ! Perform routine abdominal assessments and measure abdominal girth
5. Monitor and record amount and characteristics of tube drainage
6. Remove tube according to institutional policy and procedure
   a. Aspirate tungsten and air using 5-mL syringe
   b. Withdraw tube approximately 6 inches each hour or as prescribed
   c. Dispose of tungsten as per agency policy

VI. COMBINED ESOPHAGEAL AND GASTRIC TUBES

A. Overview

1. Exert pressure against or provide tamponade to bleeding esophageal varices
2. Contraindicated if client has history of esophageal surgery or has ulceration or necrosis of esophageal area
3. Airway management is an ongoing priority concern
4. ! **Sengstaken-Blakemore tube** has three lumens; one gastric lumen provides low intermittent gastric suction while round gastric balloon (in area of lower esophageal sphincter) and tubular esophageal balloon apply pressure against bleeding blood vessels
   a. Gastric balloon, if inflated first, and then esophageal balloon is inflated (25 to 45 mmHg pressure) if gastric balloon is insufficient to stop bleeding
   b. Traction is needed to maintain position of inflated balloons
   c. Check placement of tube by x-ray of chest and upper abdomen
   d. Prepare to insert nasogastric tube in opposite naris to suction secretions that accumulate above esophageal balloon in esophagopharyngeal area to prevent aspiration
5. Minnesota tube is similar to Sengstaken-Blakemore tube but has additional (fourth) lumen to drain secretions from esophagopharyngeal area, eliminating need for separate tube placement in this area

B. Therapeutic management

1. Position client upright for insertion

2. Check all balloons prior to insertion and label each lumen
3. Double clamp lumens to avoid air leaks
4. Keep head of bed raised after insertion
5. Obtain x-ray to verify placement
6. Release esophageal balloon pressure intermittently per agency policy to prevent esophageal injury from ulceration or necrosis
7. Keep scissors at bedside to cut tube to rapidly deflate balloons if respiratory distress occurs
8. Monitor for complications
   a. Continued bleeding: steady or increased bloody drainage from gastric suction port
   b. Esophageal rupture: upper abdominal and back pain, hypotension, tachycardia; report immediately: this is medical emergency

VII. TUBES FOR GASTRIC LAVAGE

A. Overview

1. Used to remove toxins from the stomach that occur as a result of drug or chemical poisoning or overdose
2. An **Ewald tube** is a large, reusable tube with a single lumen used for one-time rapid irrigation followed by aspiration of stomach contents
3. A Lavacuator tube has a lavage/vent lumen for irrigation and another lumen to provide continuous suction so that irrigation and suction can occur simultaneously

B. Therapeutic management

1. Determine that the poison is appropriate for removal by lavage prior to procedure
2. Substances that have probably already been absorbed or substances that must be dialyzed out would contraindicate the need for irrigation
3. Airway management is a priority because of risk of aspiration, especially with possible decreased level of consciousness depending on poison or substance overdosed

VIII. WOUND DRAINS

A. Closed wound drainage system

1. Consists of wound drain connected to electric suction apparatus or portable drainage suction (such as Jackson-Pratt drain or Hemovac drain)
2. Tube is sutured into place in surgery and attached to drainage reservoir
3. Measure and record drainage every shift; notify physician if drainage increases suddenly or becomes brighter red in color; drainage should decrease over time
4. Wear gloves when emptying reservoir; avoid touching drainage port to prevent infection
5. Reestablish suction after emptying by compressing device with one hand while cleansing drainage port with alcohol swab and then closing cap or plug before releasing pressure
6. Often removed between 3 and 5 days postop, so prepare to teach some clients how to empty and maintain system at home

B. Penrose drain

1. A surgical drain less commonly used but may be optimal when excessive serosanguineous or purulent drainage is expected
2. Usually inserted via a stab wound a few inches away from original incision to keep incision dry; drain is often 0.5 to 1.5 inches in diameter and up to 10 to 14 inches long
3. Advantage is preventing formation of abscesses because of excessive drainage
4. Drain may be pulled out or shortened by 1 to 2 inches each day as drainage lessens
5. Thick dressings, need for frequent dressing changes, and careful assessment of underlying skin are all priorities based on nature of drainage
6. Use of sterile technique is essential to prevent infection

Check Your NCLEX-RN® Exam I.Q.

You are ready for testing on this content if you can

- Use critical-thinking skills and scientific principles when caring for a client with a therapeutic tube or drain.
- Assess the client for patency and function of a therapeutic tube or drain.
- Monitor the progress of a client who has a therapeutic tube or drain.
- Teach the client and family pertinent information about a therapeutic tube or drain.
- Teach a client or family self-care of a therapeutic tube or drain as appropriate.

PRACTICE TEST

1 A client has returned to the nursing unit following a tracheostomy. The nurse would place highest priority on assessing which of the following?

1. Respiratory rate and breath sounds
2. Amount of oxygen ordered to be delivered
3. How long ago client received any pain medication
4. Status of tracheostomy dressing

2 The nurse is providing tracheostomy care to a client who had a tracheostomy performed 2 weeks ago. The client coughs the tube out of the trachea. Which of the following actions should the nurse take first?

1. Call aloud for help
2. Suction the stoma to remove residual secretions
3. Grasp and spread the retention sutures to open the stoma
4. Attempt to reinsert a new tracheostomy tube

3 The client has just had emergency intubation for respiratory distress. Immediately after endotracheal tube insertion, which of the following actions by the nurse is most appropriate?

1. Tape the tube securely in place
2. Assess for bilateral breath sounds
3. Call for chest x-ray to determine placement
4. Assure the client that alternative communication means will be provided

4 Which of the following respiratory assessment findings is of greatest concern to the nurse following endotracheal tube extubation?

1. Increased respiratory rate from 16 to 20
2. Scattered bilateral rhonchi
3. Expectoration of whitish yellow secretions
4. A harsh or crowing sound with inspiration

5 A client with a closed chest drainage system tries to get out of bed alone and disconnects the chest tube from the drainage system, which falls on the floor. Which of the following actions should the nurse take first upon entering the client's room?

1. Submerge the tube in sterile water or saline.
2. Set up and attach a new closed chest drainage system.
3. Assess the client's respiratory status.
4. Check the client's pulse and blood pressure.

6 Following chest tube insertion, the nurse notes gentle, continuous bubbling in the suction control chamber of the closed chest drainage system. Which of the following actions should the nurse plan to take at this time?

1. Document and continue to monitor the bubbling.
2. Add water to the suction control chamber.
3. Remove water from the suction control chamber.
4. Turn up the suction on the wall suction unit.

7 During routine chest tube assessment, the nurse notes the presence of continuous bubbling in the water seal chamber of the closed chest drainage system. The nurse suspects that which of the following has most likely occurred?

1. The client has developed a sudden new pneumothorax.
2. There is an air leak in the system.
3. The wall suction unit has been set to intermediate or high level instead of low suction.
4. The connections have been taped too tightly.

PRACTICE TEST

8 The client is scheduled for removal of a chest tube at 09:00. The nurse should take which of the following actions at approximately 08:30?

1. Call the radiology department for a telephone report of the morning chest x-ray findings.
2. Premedicate the client with an analgesic if it is ordered and can be given at this time.
3. Ensure that a suture-removal set and dressing materials are available.
4. Explain to the client the upcoming removal procedure.

9 The nurse has received a telephone order to irrigate a nephrostomy tube after notifying the physician that it has stopped draining. The nurse plans to use no more than how many milliliters to carry out this procedure safely?

1. 2 milliliters
2. 5 milliliters
3. 10 milliliters
4. 20 milliliters

10 The nurse should take which of the following actions when caring for a client with a nephrostomy tube?

1. Irrigate the tube every hour regardless of drainage.
2. Keep a clamp at the bedside.
3. Ensure the tubing is free of kinks.
4. Tape the drainage bag to the bedrail.

11 A nurse is assigned to a client with a nasogastric tube and is checking gastric pH to verify correct tube placement. The nurse determines that the tube is properly positioned after obtaining which of the following pH readings?

1. 4
2. 6
3. 7
4. 8

12 The nurse would use which of the following landmarks to correctly measure a client prior to nasogastric tube insertion?

1. Tip of nose, mandible, and sternal notch
2. Tip of nose, mandible, and xiphoid process
3. Tip of nose, earlobe, and sternal notch
4. Tip of nose, earlobe, and xiphoid process

13 A client with a partial bowel obstruction will have a nasoenteric tube placed by the physician later in the day. The nurse explains to the client that which of the following positions will be utilized following tube placement so it will migrate to the intended area?

1. Flat and on the left side
2. Flat and on the right side
3. Head of bed elevated and on the left side
4. Head of bed elevated and on the right side

14 The nurse enters the room of a client who underwent insertion of a nasoenteric tube for partial bowel obstruction the previous evening. The nurse notes that the tube is not taped at the nose. Which of the following actions is most appropriate at this time?

1. Call the physician immediately.
2. Tape the tube in place.
3. Note the finding on the client's flowsheet.
4. Call the radiology department to see if an abdominal x-ray has been done.

15 The nurse is about to receive an intershift report on a client who has a Sengstaken-Blakemore tube in place. The nurse expects that the client has which of the following health problems as the primary reason for tube placement?

1. Cirrhosis of the liver
2. Esophageal varices
3. Portal hypertension
4. Abdominal ascites

16 The nurse has just assisted with insertion of a Sengstaken-Blakemore tube. Before leaving the client's room, the nurse ensures that which of the following equipment is at the bedside in case of tube dislodgement?

1. Suction machine
2. Oxygen mask
3. Scissors
4. Laryngoscope

17 The nurse working in the emergency department learns that a client will be arriving who took an overdose of acetaminophen (Tylenol) a short while ago. The nurse should anticipate that which of the following tubes will be used to evacuate the client's stomach upon arrival?

1. Minnesota
2. Sengstaken-Blakemore
3. Ewald
4. Miller-Abbott

18 A client who took an overdose of a prescribed medication was treated with gastric lavage. The nurse assesses the client carefully for which of the following as a priority to detect possible complications of treatment?

1. Respiratory status and breath sounds
2. Heart rate and blood pressure
3. Skin color and body temperature
4. Urine output and peripheral edema

19 The nurse has emptied a Jackson-Pratt wound-drainage device and needs to reestablish suction to the tube. Which of the following actions should the nurse take to accomplish this objective?

1. Ensure the tubing has no kinks.
2. Squeeze the collection chamber.
3. Wipe the port with alcohol.
4. Close the cap on the device.

20 The nurse has received report on a client who underwent pelvic exenteration the previous day and has a Penrose drain placed in the lower abdomen. The nurse should take which of the following actions in the care of this wound drain?

1. Ensure that the drain always stays in the original position placed by surgeon.
2. Place only a few gauze dressings around the tube to allow for easier assessment.
3. Assess the abdominal skin for irritation or breakdown with dressing changes.
4. Notify the physician for moderate amount of drainage.

21 The nurse has an order to insert a nasogastric tube into the stomach of an assigned client. Place in order the steps that the nurse would follow to complete the procedure.

1. _____ Place distal end of tube at tip of nose and measure to earlobe and then to xiphoid process to determine distance for tube insertion.
2. _____ Insert tube into naris and advance upward and backward until resistance is met; rotate catheter gently and advance into nasopharynx.
3. _____ Sit client upright (high Fowler's position).
4. _____ Ask client to take sips of water if he or she is able while tube is advanced gently into stomach.
5. _____ Tape tube in place.

ANSWERS & RATIONALES

1 **Answer: 1** The status of the client's airway and breathing is of highest concern. Once the nurse has assessed the airway and breathing, then the amount of oxygen and dressing status can be assessed. Finally, the time lapse since any analgesic medication can be determined.
Cognitive Level: Analysis **Client Need:** Physiological Integrity: Basic Care and Comfort **Integrated Process:** Nursing Process: Planning **Content Area:** Adult Health: Respiratory **Strategy:** Remember the ABC's: airway, breathing, and circulation. In questions asking for a priority action, all options may be correct, and you need to select the option that is most important or timely. Remembering the sequence of airway, breathing, and circulation may help with questions that relate to respiratory or circulatory disorders or procedures.

2 **Answer: 3** The priority action of the nurse restores a patent airway. With this in mind, the nurse spreads the retention sutures to reopen the stomal area. The nurse then quickly calls aloud for help so assistance will arrive to aid in tube reinsertion. The nurse is not likely to suction the area at this time, and the nurse would reinsert a new tracheostomy tube if allowed by agency policy, since the tube has been in place for more than 72 hours.
Cognitive Level: Analysis **Client Need:** Physiological Integrity: Basic Care and Comfort **Integrated Process:** Nursing Process: Implementation **Content Area:** Adult Health: Respiratory **Strategy:** Remember the ABC's: airway, breathing, and circulation. The correct answer is one that directly affects the client's airway, which is opening the stoma. The other options are incorrect because they either are not the first action (options 1 and 4) or may not be done at all (option 2).

3 **Answer: 2** The first action by the nurse is to assess for bilateral breath sounds as an initial indication of correct tube placement. The nurse would next secure the tube and then call for chest x-ray to confirm tube placement. Once the client's airway and breathing have been attended to, then the nurse can assure the client about alternative communication means.
Cognitive Level: Analysis **Client Need:** Physiological Integrity: Basic Care and Comfort **Integrated Process:** Nursing Process: Implementation **Content Area:** Adult Health: Respiratory **Strategy:** Remember the ABC's: airway, breathing, and circulation. The correct answer is one that directly affects the client's airway, which is assessing for bilateral breath sounds. Because the question asks for the priority action of the nurse, the other actions must be systematically eliminated.

4 **Answer: 4** A harsh or crowing sound with inspiration indicates stridor, which is consistent with airway narrowing and edema following endotracheal tube removal. This is of

greatest concern because it could lead to upper respiratory obstruction. The nurse needs to notify the physician. The other options are of less concern, since clients may be expected to have secretions or some rhonchi immediately after tube removal. An increase in respiratory rate from 16 to 20 bears watching for trends but is still with normal limits.
Cognitive Level: Analysis **Client Need:** Physiological Integrity: Basic Care and Comfort **Integrated Process:** Nursing Process: Assessment **Content Area:** Adult Health: Respiratory **Strategy:** Note the critical words *of greatest concern*. This tells you that the correct option is the finding that is most abnormal. Use the process of elimination and knowledge of normal and abnormal physical assessment data to make a selection.

5 **Answer: 1** The priority action of the nurse is to submerge the tube in sterile water or saline to reestablish the underwater seal. This will prevent the client from sucking air through the chest tube into the pleural space during inspiration, thereby causing pneumothorax. After this initial action, the nurse would assess the client's respiratory status, set up a new system, and then check the client's full vital signs before reporting incident to the physician.
Cognitive Level: Analysis **Client Need:** Physiological Integrity: Basic Care and Comfort **Integrated Process:** Nursing Process: Implementation **Content Area:** Adult Health: Respiratory **Strategy:** Note the critical word *first* in the question. This tells you that more than one option may be technically correct but one is better than the others based on the client's status or the needs of the situation. Recall that an underwater seal is critical to chest tube functioning to select the correct option.

6 **Answer: 1** The nurse should document this normal finding and continue to monitor. Fluid addition or removal is based on fluid level, not on bubbling action of suction. The nurse should not turn up suction because the gentle bubbling indicates proper function, and increased suction could cause more rapid evaporation of water from chamber.
Cognitive Level: Analysis **Client Need:** Physiological Integrity: Basic Care and Comfort **Integrated Process:** Nursing Process: Planning **Content Area:** Adult Health: Respiratory **Strategy:** The wording of the question tells you that there is a single correct answer. Recall that gentle bubbling is normal to guide your answer. Use nursing knowledge about closed chest drainage systems and the process of elimination to make a selection.

7 **Answer: 2** Continuous bubbling in the water seal chamber most often indicates a leak or loose connection in the system, and air is being sucked continuously into the closed chest drainage system. If the client experienced a new large pneumothorax, there could be rapid bubbling, but this is not the most likely explanation. Turning up the suction on the wall unit would increase the bubbling in the suction control chamber, not the water seal chamber. Taping the connections too tightly is not a concern.
Cognitive Level: Analysis **Client Need:** Physiological Integrity: Basic Care and Comfort **Integrated Process:** Nursing Process: Analysis **Content Area:** Adult Health: Respiratory **Strategy:** The core issue of the question is the significance of finding continuous bubbling in the water seal chamber. Use the process of elimination and knowledge of closed chest drainage systems to make a selection.

8 **Answer: 2** The client should be premedicated approximately 30 minutes prior to chest tube removal if the client has an analgesic order and the medication can be given at this time. It is the physician's responsibility to determine the results of the daily chest x-ray. Obtaining equipment for removal and explaining the procedure to the client can be done earlier or later than the timeframe indicated.
Cognitive Level: Analysis **Client Need:** Physiological Integrity: Basic Care and Comfort **Integrated Process:** Nursing Process: Planning **Content Area:** Adult Health: Respiratory **Strategy:** The core issue of the question is what action is timely 30 minutes before chest tube removal. Analyze each option to determine whether each needs to occur at that time. Recall that analgesics are usually given approximately 30 minutes prior to a painful procedure to select the correct option.

9 **Answer: 2** The maximum amount of fluid that should be used to irrigate a nephrostomy tube is 5 milliliters. The nurse should also use strict aseptic technique to prevent infection of the renal pelvis as a result of the procedure.
Cognitive Level: Application **Client Need:** Physiological Integrity: Basic Care and Comfort **Integrated Process:** Nursing Process: Planning **Content Area:** Adult Health: Renal and Genitourinary **Strategy:** The core issue of the question is knowledge of appropriate volumes of fluid that should be used to irrigate tubes such as a nephrostomy tube. Eliminate the smallest and largest numbers as being least plausible. Choose 5 mL over 10 mL after visualizing the amount in the syringe and estimating the size of the renal pelvis. Memorize this number if the question was difficult.

10 **Answer: 3** The nurse should ensure that the tubing is free of kinks or other obstructions to urine flow. The tube is irrigated according to physician order only. The tube should never be clamped. Taping the drainage bag to the bedrail is dangerous because it could cause traction when the client moves in bed and become dislodged.
Cognitive Level: Application **Client Need:** Physiological Integrity: Basic Care and Comfort **Integrated Process:** Nursing Process: Implementation **Content Area:** Adult Health: Renal and Genitourinary **Strategy:** Use general principles of tube management to answer the question. Eliminate option 4 first as being hazardous. Eliminate option 1 next as being excessive. Choose option 3 over 2 knowing that the tubing should be kept free of kinks and that these tubes should not be clamped.

11 **Answer: 1** Gastric pH is acidic and readings should be 4 or less if the tube is placed properly in the stomach. The other options indicate placement in the intestine or higher up in the esophagus, since normal body pH is 7.35 to 7.45.
Cognitive Level: Analysis **Client Need:** Physiological Integrity: Basic Care and Comfort **Integrated Process:** Nursing Process: Analysis **Content Area:** Adult Health: Gastrointestinal **Strategy:** The core issue of the question is knowledge of pH readings that are consistent with placement of a nasogastric tube in the stomach. Use specific nursing knowledge and the process of elimination to make a selection.

12 **Answer: 4** The nurse correctly measures the distance from tip of nose to earlobe and then to the xiphoid process and

marks the tube at this length prior to insertion. The other options identify one or more incorrect landmarks.
Cognitive Level: Analysis **Client Need:** Physiological Integrity: Basic Care and Comfort **Integrated Process:** Nursing Process: Planning **Content Area:** Adult Health: Gastrointestinal **Strategy:** The core issue of the question is knowledge of how to properly measure a client for nasogastric tube insertion. Use specific nursing knowledge and the process of elimination to make a selection.

13 **Answer: 4** In order for the tube to migrate to the area of intestinal blockage, the tube must pass through the pyloric sphincter of the stomach. Recall that this tube has a weighted tip and thus gravity will affect its movement, as will peristalsis. Positioning the client with head elevated and on the right side will utilize gravity to help the tube migrate into the intestines. The other responses will lead to less effective tube movement.
Cognitive Level: Analysis **Client Need:** Physiological Integrity: Basic Care and Comfort **Integrated Process:** Teaching and Learning **Content Area:** Adult Health: Gastrointestinal **Strategy:** The core issue of the question is knowledge of proper client position following nasoenteric tube placement. Visualize tube movement using laws of gravity to aid in making a selection. Gravity should be a prime consideration as a possible influence whenever answering questions related to tube placement.

14 **Answer: 3** Nasoenteric tubes are not taped in place until they have migrated to proper position and been confirmed by x-ray. The nurse should note the assessment finding on the medical record. The nurse does not need to call the physician, and it is unnecessary to immediately determine the x-rays that are scheduled. It is completely unnecessary to notify the physician at this time.
Cognitive Level: Analysis **Client Need:** Physiological Integrity: Basic Care and Comfort **Integrated Process:** Nursing Process: Implementation **Content Area:** Adult Health: Gastrointestinal **Strategy:** The core issue of the question is knowledge that nasoenteric tubes are not taped until they have reached final position. Use specific nursing knowledge and the process of elimination to answer this question.

15 **Answer: 2** A Sengstaken-Blakemore tube is inserted to control bleeding from esophageal varices, which is the primary health problem of concern with use of this tube. The underlying health problem that causes the bleeding is portal hypertension, which is a complication of cirrhosis of the liver. Abdominal ascites may also accompany cirrhosis.
Cognitive Level: Analysis **Client Need:** Physiological Integrity: Basic Care and Comfort **Integrated Process:** Nursing Process: Analysis **Content Area:** Adult Health: Gastrointestinal **Strategy:** The core issue of the question is knowledge of the rationale for placement of a Sengstaken-Blakemore tube. Use knowledge of pathophysiology and the process of elimination to make a selection.

16 **Answer: 3** Scissors need to be kept at the bedside of a client who has a Sengstaken-Blakemore tube. If the tube becomes dislodged and the client cannot breathe, the nurse cuts the tube to allow the balloons to deflate and restore a patent airway. A suction machine and oxygen are generally helpful airway adjuncts, but they do not apply to this situation. A laryngoscope is used to insert an endotracheal tube but it does not apply to this question.
Cognitive Level: Analysis **Client Need:** Physiological Integrity: Basic Care and Comfort **Integrated Process:** Nursing Process: Planning **Content Area:** Adult Health: Gastrointestinal **Strategy:** The core issue of the question is knowledge that tube dislodgement can block the airway and that scissors are needed for rapid balloon deflation if this occurs. Use nursing knowledge and the process of elimination to make a selection.

17 **Answer: 3** An Ewald tube is a large-bore tube used to evacuate stomach contents rapidly following poisoning or overdose. Minnesota and Sengstaken-Blakemore tubes are used for clients with bleeding esophageal varices. A Miller-Abbot tube is a nasoenteric tube used to decompress the bowel with small bowel obstruction.
Cognitive Level: Application **Client Need:** Physiological Integrity: Basic Care and Comfort **Integrated Process:** Nursing Process: Planning **Content Area:** Adult Health: Gastrointestinal **Strategy:** The core issue of the question is knowledge of the use of various types of drainage tubes. Use nursing knowledge and the process of elimination to make a selection.

18 **Answer: 1** The risk of aspiration with gastric lavage is of concern to the nurse. For this reason, assessment of respiratory status, including respiratory rate and breath sounds, is of great concern. Other vital signs are also important as a measure of general condition but are not focused on detection of complications of this procedure. Urine output is of general concern, but peripheral edema is not a priority.
Cognitive Level: Analysis **Client Need:** Physiological Integrity: Basic Care and Comfort **Integrated Process:** Nursing Process: Assessment **Content Area:** Adult Health: Gastrointestinal **Strategy:** The core issue of the question is knowledge that gastric lavage can lead to aspiration as a complication. Use nursing knowledge and the process of elimination to make a selection.

19 **Answer: 2** The nurse should squeeze the collecting chamber to reestablish negative pressure and suction to the device. The nurse then wipes the port with alcohol before closing to reduce the risk of infection. The tubing should always be free of kinks to prevent obstruction.
Cognitive Level: Analysis **Client Need:** Physiological Integrity: Basic Care and Comfort **Integrated Process:** Nursing Process: Implementation **Content Area:** Adult Health: Integumentary **Strategy:** The core issue of the question is which action by the nurse will reestablish suction to a Jackson-Pratt wound-drainage device. Use nursing knowledge and the process of elimination to make a selection.

20 **Answer: 3** A Penrose drain allows free flow of abdominal drainage out of the abdominal cavity and onto thick layers of gauze dressings that are placed around the drain. It is used when moderate to large amounts of drainage are expected, as with extensive abdominal surgeries. The nurse should assess the skin for irritation and breakdown from contact with abdominal skin if dressing changes are not done on time or if an insufficient number of gauze dressings are

used around drain. The drain may be advanced over days for gradual removal. The surgeon does not need to be notified of moderate amounts of drainage because it is expected.
Cognitive Level: Application **Client Need:** Physiological Integrity: Basic Care and Comfort **Integrated Process:** Nursing Process: Planning **Content Area:** Adult Health: Integumentary **Strategy:** The core issue of the question is knowledge that this type of drain can cause skin irritation by nature of the volume of drainage. Use nursing knowledge and the process of elimination to make a selection.

21 **Answer: 3, 1, 2, 4, 5** The head of bed is raised first because airway and breathing are the priority. Next, the tube is measured for accurate length of insertion. The tube is then advanced past the nasopharynx. The client is then asked to take sips of water to help with tube advancement into the stomach. Finally, the tube is taped when placement is assured.
Cognitive Level: Application **Client Need:** Physiological Integrity: Basic Care and Comfort **Integrated Process:** Nursing Process: Planning **Content Area:** Adult Health: Gastrointestinal **Strategy:** The core issue of the question is knowledge of the insertion procedure for a nasogastric tube. Use nursing knowledge to arrange in sequence the steps that the nurse must take. Visualize the procedure to aid in answering the question.

Key Terms to Review

chest tube p. 460
endotracheal tube p. 457
Ewald tube p. 464
nasoenteric (intestinal) tube p. 463
Sengstaken-Blakemore tube p. 463
tracheostomy p. 455

References

Ball, J. & Bindler, R. (2006). *Child health nursing: Partnering with children and families.* Upper Saddle River, NJ: Pearson Education.

Black, J., & Hawks, J. (2005). *Medical surgical nursing: Clinical management for positive outcomes* (7th ed.). St. Louis, MO: Elsevier Science.

Corbett, J. (2004). *Laboratory tests and diagnostic procedures with nursing diagnoses* (6th ed.). Upper Saddle River, NJ: Pearson Education.

Harkreader, H., & Hogan, M. (2004). *Fundamentals of nursing: Caring and clinical judgment* (2nd ed.). St. Louis, MO: Elsevier Science.

Ignatavicius, D., & Workman, L. (2006). *Medical-surgical nursing: Critical thinking for collaborative care* (5th ed.). Philadelphia: W. B. Saunders.

Kozier, B., Erb, G., Berman, A., & Snyder, S. (2004). *Fundamentals of nursing: Concepts, process, and practice* (7th ed.). Upper Saddle River, NJ: Pearson Education.

LeMone, P., & Burke, K. (2004). *Medical-surgical nursing: Critical thinking in client care* (3rd ed.). Upper Saddle River, NJ: Pearson Education.

Lewis, S., Heitkemper, M., & Dirksen, S. (2004). *Medical-surgical nursing: Assessment and management of clinical problems* (6th ed.). St. Louis, MO: Elsevier Science.

Porth, C. (2004). *Pathophysiology: Concepts of altered health states* (7th ed.). Philadelphia: Lippincott Williams & Wilkins.

Smith, S., Duell, D., & Martin, B. (2004). *Clinical nursing skills: Basic to advanced skills* (6th ed.). Upper Saddle River, NJ: Pearson Education.

Alternative and Complementary Therapies

29

In this chapter

Cross reference

Other chapters relevant to this content area are

Promoting Healthy Lifestyle Choices Chapter 17
Culturally Competent Care Chapter 20

Test Yourself

Are you ready for the NCLEX-RN® or course exams? Use the practice tests on the companion CD-ROM to check.

I. NONPHARMACEUTICAL COMPLEMENTARY THERAPIES

A. Massage

1. Relaxes muscles and leads to release of lactic acid that accumulates during exercise
2. Stretches joints and relieves pain
3. Improves blood and lymph flow
4. Reduces anxiety and provides for relaxation and sense of well-being; enhances readiness for meditative state
5. When providing back massage, cover areas other than back to avoid chilling
6. Warm lotion before applying to back
7. ! Use combination of circular and long strokes on back, and continue massage for approximately 3 to 5 minutes using an unhurried manner
8. ! Assess skin during back massage and document findings and client response to massage
9. ! Use caution in massaging clients at risk for skin breakdown to prevent damage to skin and underlying tissue

Memory Aid

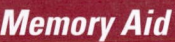

Massage is a basic touch therapy that many clients respond well to. Consider this therapy as an early choice for clients who are tense and cannot sleep.

B. Progressive relaxation

1. Reduces chronic pain and relieves stress by controlling bodily responses to anxiety and tension
2. Consists of tensing and then relaxing 7 major muscle groups
3. ! Leads to decreased oxygen consumption, muscle tension, metabolism, and vital signs (heart rate, respiratory rate, and blood pressure)
4. Should be done for minimum of 10 minutes
5. Assist client to assume correct posture, such as sitting with feet flat on floor (body parts supported, joints slightly flexed, and arms and legs uncrossed)

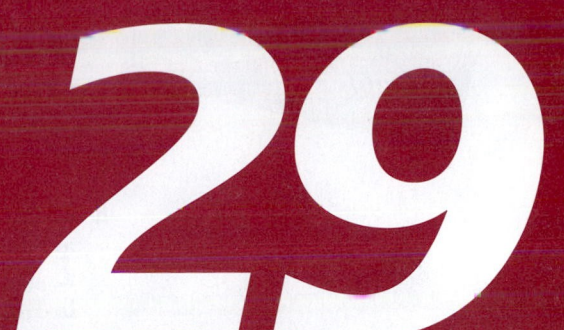

Memory Aid

Position clients properly before engaging in progressive relaxation. The body must be fully supported to prevent risk of fall or other injury.

6. Tense and release muscles in specific sequence (more than one sequence available):
   a. Right fist, left fist, then both fists
   b. Both fists and both arms
   c. Toes, then ankles, then knees
   d. Buttocks and groin
   e. Stomach and lower back
   f. Chest and upper back, then shoulders
   g. Forehead, then jaw
7. Use with deep breathing and statements of positive affirmation (e.g., "Let go of the tension") to enhance relaxation

C. ***Imagery***
1. Uses power of imagination to assist with physical, psychological, or spiritual healing
2. Often involves visualization but can also utilize other senses to create desired image
3. When imagery is assisted, it is called guided imagery
4. Consists of creating one or more of several types of images
   a. Healing a specific body part or increasing energy in a bodily area (body–mind)
   b. Destroying microorganisms or increasing local circulation (correct biologic)
   c. Being in a healed state (end state)
   d. Experiencing sense of unity, light, power, or spirituality (generalized healing)
   e. Connecting with higher levels of consciousness (transpersonal)

D. ***Meditation***
1. Produces combined state of deep peace and rest along with mental alertness
2. May or may not be associated with religious practice or prayer
3. Includes relaxation and focused attention; may focus on an object (concentrative meditation) or remain open to all stimuli (mindfulness meditation)
4. General guidelines
   a. Choose specific time (early morning or evening, at least 2 hours after meal) and comfortable, distraction-free environment
   b. Keep spine straight and body relaxed; may sit cross-legged on floor or be upright in straight-backed chair
   c. Close eyes and place palms on thighs
   d. Use deep breathing or relaxation exercises; focus on either breathing or selected mental image; let distracting thoughts drift out of mind without focusing on them
   e. Perform daily for 10 to 20 minutes at a time

E. ***Music therapy***
1. Often used in preoperative holding and cardiac units, birthing and counseling rooms, rehabilitation units, and for sleep induction
2. Used to alter ordinary level of consciousness, change mental focus, or change perception of time
3. Type of music chosen (classical, romantic, impressionistic, New Age, and others) depends on client preferences and goals of therapy
4. Choose music without words to enhance relaxation
5. Encourage clients to record preferred musical selections
6. Typical use is for approximately 20 minutes
7. Encourage client to let body respond to music spontaneously (such as relax muscles, lie down, hum, or clap)

F. **Humor and laughter**
1. Helps clients to establish relationships by decreasing social distance and placing people at ease
2. Helps to relieve anxiety or tension

3. Assists in relieving aggression or anger
4. Helps to facilitate learning if carefully planned
5. Laughter raises heart and respiratory rates and increases oxygen exchange and muscular tension
6. A relaxation phase follows laughter, which reverses these changes
7. Humor can stimulate endorphin production, which reduces pain
8. Has healing properties because it fosters positive emotions

G. ***Clinical aromatherapy***

1. Consists of controlled use of essential oils to achieve measurable outcomes
2. Used to improve mood and reduce stress, edema, acne, bruising, and allergies
3. Uses essential oils from plants that are inhaled, added to bath water, massaged into body, or applied as cold or warm compresses; over 300 oils currently in use
4. Oils vary in quality and are unregulated; caution clients to use carefully
5. Teach client to use only as directed; some oils, such as wintergreen and camphor, are toxic if inhaled
   a. Before using topical application of oil, test skin for allergies with a small amount of diluted oil
   b. Dilute essentials oils properly before applying to skin
   c. Do not use near eyes or internally
   d. Store in dark-covered bottles and keep away from light and heat
   e. Consult health care provider before using essential oils if pregnant; some are reported to bring on menstruation while others are reportedly useful in pregnancy and delivery

Memory Aid

Essential oils are chemicals. As such, they can be toxic. Use them cautiously after consulting with primary health care provider.

H. **Nurses' role**

1. Assess client's use of alternative therapies, such as those discussed in this section and other alternative therapies, such as acupuncture, massage therapy, or hypnosis provided by other practitioners
2. Communicate openly with client to build trust
3. Educate client about how to evaluate data sources, such as Internet or infomercials
4. Do not provide advice regarding use of alternative therapy regimens; instead, communicate data to primary care provider, who will collaborate with client

II. PRINCIPLES OF USING HERBS AS DIETARY SUPPLEMENTS

A. **General use**

1. Not intended for acute illness episodes or long-term therapy
2. Appropriate as adjunct to conventional Western therapies
3. Therapeutic effectiveness is slower than prescription medications; may take as long as several weeks, depending on the herb
4. Many herbs are available in multiple forms, including teas, extracts, tinctures, and capsules or tablets containing powdered or freeze dried forms of the herb
5. Most herbs are multipurpose, used, for example, as skin wash, gargle, compress, lotion, and eye bath
6. They are not intended to replace healthy lifestyle
7. Safe use in pregnancy and lactation is either contraindicated or unknown and may dry up breast milk during lactation; ginger may be an exception
8. Although they may be effective in children, herbs should be avoided in acute, sudden-onset illness
9. Many herbs interact with other herbs, food, and prescription medications

B. **Government regulation**

1. The Dietary Supplement Health and Education Act (DSHEA) of 1994 defines herbs as dietary supplements
2. Because they are not defined as medicines, herbs cannot be promoted with therapeutic claims but only with information about how they affect structure and function of human body

3. The Food and Drug Administration (FDA) does not regulate use of the herbs in the United States but approves certain herbs for their action on the body (how they affect structure and function); does not monitor herbs for quality, composition, or preparation
4. Formulations vary in their potency and recommended dosage, with frequent lack of consensus on dosing

C. Safety, labeling, and purity

1. Container labels must carry a disclaimer stating the FDA does not evaluate the product for treating, curing, or preventing disease
2. Labels should contain specific directions for dosing and use
3. Only the standardized extract, when available, should be used
4. Not all herbs have empirical support for their safety and efficacy
5. Much of the research and standardization originates in Europe, where use of herbs is popular, particularly in Germany
6. ! Many herbs contain toxic substances (e.g., arnica, belladonna, hemlock, lily of the valley, and sassafras)
7. Health care providers should report all adverse effects of herbs to the FDA

D. Nurses' role and client education

1. Obtain a complete history and physical before starting any therapy with herbs
2. Herbs are not effective for or to be used for acute illness or episodes
3. ! Herbs take longer to work than do prescription medications, usually weeks
4. Report use of all herbs to health care provider
5. ! Explain that client should start with one herb at a time, at lower than recommended doses, and closely monitor response
6. Teach client to know particular use, dosing, and safe administration of each herb and take only as directed
7. ! Herbs may cause allergic reactions and adverse effects; if one occurs, discontinue herb and report symptoms to health care provider
8. Become familiar with all herb–herb, herb–drug, and herb–food interactions
9. Client should purchase herbs from a reputable source and be aware of where and how the herb was processed, and should purchase standardized form of herbs if possible
10. Terms such as *natural* or *all natural* do not equate with safety or efficacy of herb
11. Become familiar with various names by which particular herbs are identified
12. Client should avoid use of herbs in pregnancy, lactation, and in children
13. Client should accurately assess advertising claims; few definitive clinical trials have demonstrated safety and efficacy of these agents
14. Nurses should continue to read new evidence that emerges from research in this field, such as studies funded by National Center for Complementary and Alternative Medicine
15. Nurses should refrain from recommending or endorsing any particular product or agent

III. SPECIFIC HERBAL SUPPLEMENTS

A. Bilberry (*Vaccinium myrtillus,* European blueberry, huckleberry, whortleberry)

1. Description
   a. Relative of blueberry and cranberry; shrub with small, sweet, black berries
   b. Active ingredients: anthocyanoside (antioxidant bioflavonoid), pectin (soluble fiber)
   c. Stabilizes collagen activity
   d. Prevents production and release of compounds that promote inflammation, such as histamine and prostaglandins
   e. Relaxes smooth muscle in vasculature
   f. Inhibits platelet aggregation
   g. Reduces permeability and strengthens capillary wall membrane
2. Uses
   a. ! Most commonly used for treatment of simple diarrhea

b. Prevention and treatment of eye disorders: diabetic retinopathy, night blindness, macular degeneration, glaucoma, cataracts
c. Diabetes mellitus
d. Antioxidant
e. Possible treatment of varicose veins, hemorrhoids

3. Precautions
a. May increase coagulation time
b. May interfere with iron absorption when taken internally
c. Use cautiously with acetylsalicylic acid (aspirin), anticoagulants, vitamin E, fish oils, feverfew, garlic, ginger, ginkgo
d. Contraindicated in pregnancy and lactation
e. Avoid long-term large doses; doses over 1.5 grams/kg/day may be fatal, and doses over 480 mg/day may be dangerous

B. Black cohosh (*Cimicifuga racemosa,* black snakeroot, bugroot, rattleweed, rattleroot, squawroot, cimifuga)

1. Description
a. Active ingredients: triperpenoid glycosides, isoflavenones, aglycones
b. Binds to estrogen receptors
c. Inhibits luteinizing hormone
d. Apparent estrogen-like activity

2. Uses
a. Primarily used for treatment of premenstrual syndrome (PMS), and postmenopausal symptoms
b. Promotes labor of pregnancy
c. Decreases blood pressure
d. Used to treat snake bites
e. Recommended uses by herbalists: dysmenorrhea, rheumatism, antispasmodic, astringent, diuretic, expectorant, sedative

3. Precautions
a. Contraindicated use with antihypertensives or hormone replacement therapy
b. May cause bradycardia, hypotension, joint pain
c. Contraindicated in lactation
d. Use in pregnancy only when birth is imminent to promote labor
e. Adverse side effects include nausea, dizziness, decreased pulse rate, and increased perspiration

C. Echinacea (*Echinacea purpurea,* snake root, purple or American cone flower, sampson root, black sampson, hedgehog, survey root)

1. Description
a. Member of daisy family, with 9 species
b. Active ingredients: polysaccharides, alkylamides, flavonoids, caffeic acid derivatives (echinacosides), essential oils, and others
c. Available in capsule, tablet, candle, glycerite, hydroalcoholic extract, fresh-pressed juice, lollipop, lozenge, tea, and tincture forms
d. Activates T lymphocytes and intensifies phagocytosis of macrophages
e. Stimulates tumor necrosis factor, interferon, and interleukin
f. Nonspecific stimulation of immune system
g. Stabilizes hyaluronic acid (a component of connective tissue) to protect cells and connective tissue from microorganism invasion and attack from free radicals
h. Inhibits lipoxygenase to reduce inflammation

2. Uses
a. Most common: prevention or reduction of symptoms of cold or influenza

Memory Aid

Recall that echinacea is an ingredient in some sore throat drops. This will aid in remembering that it is most effective if used early for colds and sore throats.

b. Boosts immune system and increases body's resistance to infection, particularly upper respiratory and urinary infection
c. Used to treat herpes simplex and Candida infection
! d. Topically: improves wound healing, provides antioxidant protection from ultraviolet A and B light rays

3. Precautions
! a. Not to be used in presence of autoimmune disease (e.g., HIV/AIDS, collagen disease, multiple sclerosis, tuberculosis), severe illness, or allergy to sunflower or daisy family
b. Not to be used with immunosuppressants (e.g., corticosteroids or cyclosporine)
c. Prolonged use (longer than 8 weeks) may cause hepatotoxicity and suppression of immune system
d. Not to be used with other hepatotoxicants (e.g., anabolic steroids, amiodarone, methotrexate, ketoconazole)
e. May influence fertility by spermatazoa enzyme interference
f. Many tinctures contain large amounts of alcohol
g. Contraindicated in alcoholism, children, pregnancy, and lactation
h. Adverse effects: allergic reaction and anaphylaxis

D. Feverfew (*Tanacetum parthenium,* bachelor's button, febrifuge plant, feather few, feather foil)

1. Description
a. Short, bushy perennial; member of daisy family; has yellow flowers and yellow-green leaves resembling chamomile
b. Active ingredients: sesquiterpene lactones, especially parthenolide, essential oils
c. Suppresses secretion of granules in platelets and neutrophils to inhibit platelet aggregation
d. May suppress production of prostaglandins (thromboxane, leukotriene)
e. Inhibits release of serotonin

2. Uses
! a. Principle use: prevention of recurrent migraine headaches, treatment of arthritis
b. Relief of menstrual pain
c. Asthma
d. Dermatitis, psoriasis
e. Antipyretic (promotes diaphoresis)

3. Precautions
a. Long-term studies not done
b. Contraindicated in pregnancy, lactation, and under age 2
c. Cross-allergy to ragweed
! d. Adverse effects: allergic reaction, lip and tongue swelling, mouth ulcers and loss of taste from chewing leaves, abdominal colic, palpitations, increased menstrual flow
e. Sudden withdrawal may cause post-feverfew syndrome (muscle aches, pain, and stiffness); taper off to discontinue
f. Other proven (conventional) remedies for relief of migraine should be used first; do not use feverfew while taking prescription drugs for headache
g. May interfere with blood-clotting mechanism; not to be used with anticoagulants such as aspirin, warfarin (Coumadin), bilberry, garlic, ginger, ginkgo
! h. Feverfew is known to cause rebound headaches

E. Garlic (*Allium sativum,* stinking root or rose, nectar of the gods, camphor of the poor, poor man's treacle, rustic treacle)

1. Description
a. Empirical support for effectiveness and use; most widely researched herb
b. Active ingredients (23 constituents): allicin (odorless, sulfur-containing amino acid), ajoene
c. Should be crushed or bruised to effectively convert various enzymes, protein, lipids, amino acids, and other ingredients to allicin
d. Allicin and ajoene not found in dried garlic but may be present if dried at low temperatures or taken in enteric-coated tablets

e. Inhibits platelet aggregation
f. Well-documented research shows that it reduces and inhibits metabolism of cholesterol
g. Increases bile acid secretion

2. Uses
a. Principle uses: reduces cholesterol (decreases triglycerides and low-density lipoproteins; increases high-density lipoproteins) and lowers mild hypertension
b. Reduces risk of stroke
c. Antibacterial, antiviral, antifungal
d. Anticancer properties
e. Lay use: antihelmintic, antispasmodic, diuretic, carminative (relieves flatulence), digestant, expectorant, topical antibiotic

3. Precautions
a. Avoid large amounts of garlic with ASA (aspirin), anticoagulants such as warfarin (Coumadin), and other herbs that affect coagulation (bilberry, feverfew, ginger, ginkgo)
b. May potentiate diabetes drugs
c. Adverse effects: contact dermatitis, vertigo, garlic breath or scent, hypothyroidism, GI irritation, nausea, and vomiting with large doses
d. Enteric-coated tablets containing powdered form may reduce bad breath but are not as potent as raw garlic
e. Contraindicated in pregnancy, GI (peptic ulcer and GERD) and bleeding disorders
f. Chronic use may lower hemoglobin levels
g. When used to decrease cholesterol levels, plan should be monitored by the health care provider

F. Ginger (*Zingiber officinal,* Jamaica ginger, African ginger, Cochin ginger, black ginger, race ginger)

1. Description
a. Green-purple flower resembling the orchid
b. Active ingredient: sesquiterpenes, aromatic ketones (gingerols), and volatile oils
c. Inhibits thromboxane production to enhance effects of anticoagulation
d. Inhibits leukotrienes and prostaglandins to produce anti-inflammatory and analgesic effect

2. Usage
a. Principle use: antiemetic; improves appetite
b. Diuretic, digestion aid; alleviates dyspepsia
c. Anti-inflammatory in treatment of rheumatoid arthritis and osteoarthritis
d. Relieves muscle pain
e. May reduce motion sickness and relieve vertigo

3. Precautions
a. Adverse effects: headache, anxiety, insomnia, elevated blood pressure, tachycardia, asthma attack, postmenopausal bleeding
b. Contraindicated in postoperative nausea in clients with increased risk of bleeding
c. Not to be used concomitantly with bilberry, feverfew, garlic, ginkgo, or other anticoagulants such as ASA (aspirin) or warfarin (Coumadin)
d. Severe overdose: possible CNS depression and cardiac arrhythmias
e. Excess of 6 grams/day results in gastric irritation and ulcer formation
f. Conflicting data related to safe use during pregnancy (relatively safe according to FDA); contraindicated in treatment of hyperemesis gravidarum

G. Ginkgo (*Ginkgo biloba,* GBE 761, GBE, GBX, Tebonin, Tebofortan, Ginkogink)

1. Description
a. Active ingredients: flavone glycosides, flavonoids, terpene lactones (such as ginkgolides and bilobalide)
b. Ginkgo biloba extract referred to as GBE
c. Flavonoids act as antioxidants by destroying lipid layer of cell membrane
d. Flavone glycosides produce mild platelet aggregation
e. Ginkgolides antagonize platelet-activating factor to decrease coagulation

f. Bilobalide increases cerebral circulation to improve tissue perfusion and increase memory
g. Protects brain from effects of hypoxia

2. Uses
   a. ! Cerebrovascular insufficiency and symptomatic relief of organic brain dysfunction to improve short-term memory loss
   b. ! Peripheral vascular disease (e.g., Raynaud's disease, intermittent claudication), varicosities
   c. Senile macular degeneration
   d. Treatment of age-related mental decline such as short-term memory loss and poor concentration
   e. Treatment of depression-related cognitive disorders
   f. Treatment of depression in older adults, particularly depression related to chronic cerebrovascular deficiency that does not respond to standard drug therapy
   g. Tinnitus

3. Precautions
   a. Effects may not be apparent for 4 to 8 weeks
   b. Not to be used concomitantly with bilberry, feverfew, garlic, ginger, or other anticoagulants, such as ASA (aspirin) or warfarin (Coumadin)
   c. ! Avoid use of unprocessed ginkgo leaves that contain allergens related to urushiol, the chemical responsible for the itch in poison ivy
   d. Crude, dried leaf or tea may not contain sufficient active ingredients to be effective
   e. Large doses my cause restlessness, headache, nausea, vomiting, diarrhea, dizziness, or palpitations
   f. Edible solid form sold in Oriental shops should be kept out of reach of children because seeds may cause seizures
   g. Avoid use in pregnancy, lactation, and children

H. Ginseng, Korean (*Panax ginseng,* American ginseng, Panaschinseng)

1. Description
   a. Active ingredients: triterpenoid saponin glycosides (ginsenosides, panaxosides)
   b. Possible effect on pituitary gland with action similar to corticosteroids
   c. Improves serum glucose, glycosylated hemoglobin (HbA_{1c}) and aminoterminalpropeptide concentrations
   d. Hypertensive effect with low doses, hypotensive effect with higher doses

2. Uses
   a. ! Most common: counteracts effects of physical and mental fatigue and improves stamina and concentration in healthy individuals
   b. Used to treat chronic hepatotoxicity related to alcohol and drug ingestion
   c. Improves body's ability to resist stress and disease; increases vitality
   d. Regulates blood pressure
   e. Improves psychomotor performance (attention, auditory reaction time); may reduce mood swings
   f. Regulates blood glucose levels in type 2 diabetes
   g. Aphrodisiac

3. Precautions
   a. Most side effects reported are related to excessive or inappropriate use
   b. ! Avoid concomitant use with stimulants, such as coffee, tea, cola
   c. ! May potentiate MAOI actions
   d. Adverse effects: insomnia, palpitations, pruritus, nervousness, euphoria

I. Ginseng, Siberian (*Eleutherococcus senticosus,* five fingers, tartar root, Western ginseng, seng and sang, Asian ginseng, Jintsam)

1. Description
   a. Active ingredients: eutherosides
   b. Pharmacologic actions not well understood
   c. Elevates lymphocyte count (T cells), boosts immune system

2. Uses
   a. Enhances physical and mental performance under stress
   b. Improves athletic performance
   c. Increases oxygen metabolism, work capacity, and exhaustion time in a variety of illnesses (e.g., atherosclerosis, diabetes, chronic bronchitis)
   d. Stimulates WBC production in clients undergoing antineoplastic therapy
3. Precautions
   a. Adverse reactions: hypertension, tachycardia, insomnia, and irritability
   b. Contraindicated in pregnancy, lactation, premenopausal women, hypertension, CNS stimulants, or with antipsychotic medications

J. Hawthorn (*Crataegus oxyacantha,* Mayblossom, Maybush, whitehorn, LI 132)

1. Description
   a. Small to medium tree of several species; leaves, flowers, berries (fruit) are used in standardized extracts
   b. Active ingredients: flavonoids, primarily procyanidins and proanthocyanidins
   c. Acts as antioxidant that decreases damage by free radicals to cardiovascular system by increasing levels of vitamin C intracellularly
   d. Increases coronary and myocardial circulation
   e. Decreases peripheral vascular resistance to decrease blood pressure
   f. Increases strength of myocardial contraction (positive inotropic effect) and decreases heart rate (negative chronotropic effect)
   g. Angiotensin-converting enzyme (ACE) activity that prevents the conversion of angiotensin I to angiotensin II, a potent vasoconstrictor
   h. Decreases total plasma cholesterol and low-density lipoprotein (LDL) levels
   i. Improves cardiac function in chronic angina clients and those with early congestive heart failure
2. Uses
   a. Treatment of mild hypertension
   b. Treatment of athero- and arteriosclerosis
   c. Treatment (prevention) of chronic angina: not intended for acute angina
   d. Treatment of early congestive heart failure
3. Precautions
   a. Contraindicated with concomitant use of prescription antihypertensives or nitrates
   b. Supervision of health care provider necessary for those with existing cardiac disease
   c. May interfere with digoxin pharmacodynamics and monitoring
   d. Adverse effects: nausea, fatigue, perspiration and cutaneous eruption of the hands, increased CNS depression and sedation
   e. Contraindicated in pregnancy and lactation

K. Milk thistle (*Silbyum marianum,* Mary thistle, Marian thistle, Lady's thistle, Holy thistle, silymarin, the "liver herb")

1. Description
   a. Tall plant, prickly leaves, milky sap, member of daisy family
   b. Active ingredients: silymarin and its component silybinin to act as hepatoprotectant
   c. Promotes glutathione production, a powerful endogenous antioxidant
   d. Binds to hepatocyte membrane and blocks uptake of toxins into liver cell
   e. Stimulates nucleolar polymerase A activity to promote new liver cell growth
   f. Stimulates regeneration of liver by stimulating protein synthesis
   g. Inhibits action of leukotriene by Kupffer cells
   h. Binds to site on liver cell membrane, blocking availability for attack from phalloidine, the toxin in death cap mushroom
   i. Stabilizes liver cell membrane by decreasing turnover rate of phospholipids

Memory Aid

Note that the words milk and thistle both contain the letters *l* and *i*, which may help you to associate this herb with the liver.

2. Uses
   a. Reduces hepatotoxicity related to psychoactive drugs such as phenothiazines
   b. Adjunct therapy in liver inflammation related to cirrhosis, hepatitis, and fatty infiltrate related to alcohol or other toxins
   c. Treatment of overdose of death cap mushroom
3. Precautions
   a. Insoluble in water, not to be taken in tea form
   b. Avoid alcohol-based extract in decompensated cirrhosis
   c. Cross-allergy to ragweed
   d. Adverse effects: loose stools, diarrhea in high doses
   e. Contraindicated in pregnancy and lactation
   f. Close monitoring by health care provider in presence of active liver disease

L. Saw palmetto (*Serenoa repens,* sabal, American dwarf palm tree, LSESR)

1. Description
   a. Shrublike palm tree with reddish-brown to black berries
   b. Active ingredients: saturated and unsaturated fatty acids and sterols from berries (liposterolic acid)
   c. Reduces action of 5-alpha-reductase enzyme that converts testosterone to dehydrotestosterone (DHT) in aging (effects similar to finasteride [Proscar] with fewer side effects)
   d. No effect on prostatic-specific antigen
   e. May reverse testicular and mammary gland atrophy
   f. May increase sperm production and increase sexual vigor
2. Uses
   a. Demonstrated effects through research: symptomatic treatment of benign prostatic hyperplasia (BPH)
   b. Helps initiate urine stream; decreases urinary frequency, residual volumes, nocturia, and dysuria; unclear whether actual prostatic size is reduced
   c. Lay uses: treatment of asthma, bronchitis, and gynecomastia
3. Precautions
   a. Long-term use with approximately 6 weeks for initial effects
   b. Insoluble in water; not to be taken in tea form
   c. Adverse effects: nausea, abdominal pain, hypertension, headache, diarrhea with large doses
   d. May interfere with iron absorption
   e. Supervision by health care provider necessary for diagnosed BPH
   f. Should not be used by pregnant or lactating women

M. St. John's wort (*Hypericum perforatum,* amber, goat weed, touch-and-heal, Johnswort, witch's herb, klamath weed, chassediable, devil's scourge)

1. Description
   a. Yellow perennial flower with red-pigmented leaves containing small black dots
   b. Active ingredient: hypericin from red-pigmented leaves, pseudohypericin and flavonoids, tannin, and others
   c. Inhibits reuptake of serotonin; actions not well determined or understood
   d. Low monoamine oxidase inhibitor (MAOI)
   e. Effects comparable to imipramine (Tofranil)
   f. Produces fewer side effects than prescription antidepressants
2. Uses
   a. Treatment of mild to moderate depression
   b. Not intended for treatment of suicidal ideation, psychotic behavior, or severe depression
   c. Possible antibacterial, antiviral, wound healing properties
3. Precautions
   a. Not to be used concurrently with prescription antidepressants, especially selective serotonin reuptake inhibitors (SSRI) or MAOIs or foods containing tyramine (such as aged cheese, smoked meats, liver, figs, dried or cured fish, yeast, beer, Chianti wine)

b. Not to be used concurrently with opioids, amphetamines, or OTC cold and flu preparations
c. May inhibit absorption of iron
d. Adverse effects (may continue for 2 to 4 weeks): GI distress, emotional vulnerability, fatigue, pruritus, weight gain, headache, dizziness, restlessness
e. May cause photosensitivity; avoid sun exposure, especially if fair skinned
f. May decrease digoxin levels
g. Contraindicated in pregnancy, lactation, and children

N. Valerian root (*valerian officinalis,* wild valerian, garden heliotrope, setwall, capon's tail, all-heal, Amantilla, Baldrian wurzel, benedicta)

1. Description
   a. Tall perennial with hollow stem, leaves, and white or red flowers
   b. Active ingredients: valepotriates and susquiterpine derivatives, valeric acid, valeranone, and others
   c. Binds weakly to gammaaminobutyric acid (GABA) receptor sites to decrease CNS activity, causing sedation with decreased side effects
   d. Action similar to benzodiazepines but nonaddicting and produces no morning hangover
2. Uses
   a. Sedative, reduction of anxiety
   b. Treatment of insomnia

Memory Aid

Remember that valerian is an ingredient often found in teas that are recommended for sleep.

   c. Adjunct therapy for benzodiazepine withdrawal
   d. Possible antispasmodic
3. Precautions
   a. Valepotriate (which may be carcinogenic) should be removed from final product
   b. Not to be used concurrently with other sedative or hypnotics, anxiolytics, or antidepressants
   c. May be used safely while operating machinery or car, although CNS effects should be monitored
   d. Sedation is not increased with alcohol use, although caution should be exercised
   e. Adverse effects: headache; mild, temporary upset stomach
   f. Adverse effects with overdose or long-term use (overdose with 2.5 grams): excitability, insomnia, cardiac dysfunction, blurred vision, hepatotoxicity, severe headache, morning headache, nausea
   g. May cause hepatotoxicity; monitor liver function and avoid use in hepatic dysfunction
   h. Extract contains 40% to 60% alcohol; avoid use in clients with alcoholism
   i. Contraindicated in pregnancy and lactation

Check Your NCLEX-RN® Exam I.Q.

You are ready for testing on this content if you can

- Identify appropriate uses of alternative and complementary therapies.
- Assess a client regarding need for alternative and complementary therapies.
- Teach a client about alternative and complementary therapy choices.
- Participate in providing alternative and complementary therapies to a client.
- Evaluate the outcomes of alternative and complementary therapies for a client.

PRACTICE TEST

PRACTICE TEST

1 Which of the following assessment data would prohibit the use of imagery with a client?

1. No previous history of using imagery techniques
2. States anxiety level of a number 6 on 0 to 10 scale
3. Client feels reluctant to close eyes for the imagery session
4. Client has a history of psychosis

2 The nurse has determined that music therapy may be appropriate for use with a client. Which of the following should the nurse consider when choosing the music? Select all that apply.

1. Choose only music with words.
2. Choose music that is 5 to 7 minutes in duration.
3. Allow the client to choose music of his or her choice.
4. Instruct the client to listen to the music and let the music take him or her wherever the music wants to go.
5. Ask the client not to analyze the music.

3 The nurse is using meditation with a client to help him decrease his pain. Which of the following factors is important to consider when using this type of therapy?

1. The type of meditation is best determined by the nurse or other health care provider.
2. Consideration of the client's condition, schedule, and personal preference is necessary when choosing a type of meditation.
3. The type of meditation used is based on whether it is taught in an inpatient or outpatient setting.
4. A certified meditation professional should be the one teaching the client how to perform meditation.

4 The client asks the nurse how humor therapy affects the client physiologically. The nurse responds that laughter has which effect(s)? Select all that apply.

1. Decreases heart rate and oxygen saturation.
2. Increases salivary immunoglobulin A (S-IgA).
3. Produces an antagonist response to stress hormones.
4. Decreases the immune response by decreasing T-lymphocytes.
5. Increases temperature set point in the brain.

5 The nurse decides to teach a client with hypertension the progressive relaxation response. Which instructions should the nurse give to the client when using this relaxation method?

1. Sit in an upright position with legs crossed.
2. Place sensors on the forehead to monitor physiological activity.
3. Contract and then relax all your muscles sequentially from head to feet.
4. Repeat a word or phrase forcefully with your breathing.

6 The nurse teaches the client about massage therapy. Which statement by the client demonstrates a correct understanding of the benefits of massage?

1. "Massage increases blood clot formation."
2. "Massage inhibits lymphatic drainage."
3. "Massage causes an accumulation of lactic acid as a result of the exercise."
4. "Massage stimulates circulation while causing relaxation."

7 You have been invited to talk to the Woman's Guild in your community about the cautions of aromatherapy. Which of the following would be correctly presented to the audience?

1. Aromatic oils are produced by a standard-quality formula.
2. The oils can be stored in any type of container.
3. The skin should always be tested for allergies by applying a small amount of oil to the area before treatment.
4. Oils should not be used during pregnancy.

8 Your class project is to prepare a speech on the functions of humor in nursing situations for your peers. Following the presentation, you know the participants understood your message when they respond that humor

1. increases the social distance between persons and assists in putting people at ease.
2. facilitates learning.
3. holds in anger and aggression.
4. aggravates coping mechanisms.

9 In evaluating the effectiveness of guided imagery for a client with preoperative anxiety, which data indicates that this therapy is successful?

1. "I hope that I don't have dreams like that tonight."
2. "I couldn't concentrate very much with all I have to do today."
3. "I'll practice what I learned next week."
4. "I feel less anxious about the upcoming surgery."

10 The nurse is using progressive relaxation in a client who is under a lot of stress. What nursing actions must be instituted prior to the start of the session to protect the client's safety?

1. Assess the client's muscle strength.
2. Check to make sure the client is not on any sedatives.
3. Remember to position the body so it is totally supported to prevent falls.
4. Assess for any allergies.

11 The nurse taught the client's wife how to perform a back massage on the client. Which observation by the nurse indicates that the spouse understands how to give a back massage?

1. Client is in his pajamas lying in bed.
2. The spouse is rubbing his back with large, circular motions.
3. The spouse is using cold lotion when performing the massage.
4. The spouse massages the client's back for 3 to 5 minutes.

12 The nurse taught the client about meditation. Which statement by the client demonstrates a correct understanding?

1. "Meditation is a technique used to quiet the mind and focus on the future."
2. "Meditation involves a religious conviction."
3. "There is only one way to meditate."
4. "Meditation involves both relaxation and focus of attention."

13 The nurse is performing an imagery session with a group of clients. What instructions should the nurse give the clients?

1. "Try to concentrate on your breathing, letting go of all your stress."
2. "Imagine that your body is healing itself, and it is using all its energy to attain this goal."
3. "Contract the muscles of your arm and then relax."
4. "Listen to some music of your choice and let the music take you away."

14 A client is using aromatherapy to treat stress. Which assessment data indicates an allergic reaction in a client who has received an aromatherapy session?

1. Presence of a new rash
2. Increased skin turgor
3. Decreased pigmentation
4. Edema peripherally

15 The preoperative waiting area has soft instrumental music playing in the background. The client asks the nurse, "Why are they playing this type of music instead of tuning into a radio station?" The nurse explains that the purpose of using music therapy in the preoperative client is that it

1. produces a hypermetabolic state.
2. helps reduce physiological stress, pain, anxiety, and isolation.
3. enhances the functions of the left hemisphere of the brain.
4. covers up the normal noises found in the hospital setting.

16 The client tells the nurse that when he walks, he develops a pain in his right leg. He describes the pain as cramping or burning in his muscles that subsides with rest. Based on these symptoms, the nurse supports the use of which of the following herbs?

1. Feverfew
2. Garlic
3. Ginkgo
4. Ginseng

17 A client is taking chlorpromazine (Thorazine). Based on metabolism of this prescribed medication, the nurse supports the concomitant use of which of the following herbs?

1. Valerian root
2. Ginger
3. Milk thistle
4. Hawthorn

18 Which of the following therapeutic changes in laboratory values would the nurse anticipate in the client taking garlic?

1. Increased platelet aggregation
2. Increased white blood cell count
3. Decreased serum cholesterol levels
4. Decreased serum glucose levels

19 The female client tells the nurse that she is planning a pregnancy soon. In providing client education related to the use of herbs during pregnancy, which of the following statements by the nurse is most appropriate?

1. "Most herbs are safe when taken as directed."
2. "Only herbs in the topical form are safe."
3. "Certain herbs are safe and effective when taken in lower doses."
4. "You should discuss the use of any herbs with your health care provider."

20 The client presents to the health care clinic with an abrasion to the left knee from a fall. After cleaning the abrasion, the nurse might support the use of which client-chosen herb as adjunct therapy to treat the abrasion?

1. Echinacea
2. Ginger
3. Valerian root
4. Feverfew

21 The client scheduled for arthroscopic surgery of the knee has been taking ginger for relief of arthritic pain preoperatively at home. The client asks the nurse about the use of ginger after surgery for continued relief of pain and also as a relief of postoperative nausea. In providing client education, the nurse explains that ginger

1. cannot be used safely postoperatively.
2. would not be effective in this situation.
3. may be repeated every 4 hours as needed.
4. may potentiate the effects of opioid medications.

22 In planning care for the client who is taking hawthorn, the nurse includes which of the following interventions?

1. Monitor blood glucose levels
2. Monitor blood pressure
3. Monitor white blood cell count
4. Monitor temperature

23 The client tells the nurse that a neighbor recommends the use of bilberry in treating simple diarrhea. The nurse supports the client's use of bilberry based on which of the following?

1. Anthocynanosides in the berry decrease peristalsis.
2. The berry contains pectin that acts as a soluble fiber.
3. Bilberry acts to counteract antimicrobial suppression of normal intestinal flora.
4. Action of the berry works to decrease bacterial or viral causes of diarrhea.

24 The nurse instructs the client taking St. John's wort that which of the following foods preferred by the client may be safely consumed while taking this herb?

1. Chocolate
2. Aged cheeses
3. Beer
4. Vanilla ice cream

25 Which of the following clients would benefit from the therapeutic effects of garlic? Select all that apply.

1. The client with decreased blood pressure
2. The client with liver disease
3. The client with coronary artery disease
4. The client with a bleeding disorder
5. The client with peripheral vascular disease

ANSWERS & RATIONALES

1 **Answer: 4** The client doesn't need prior experience to gain the benefits of imagery. The client with a 6 on a scale of 0 to 10 will benefit from the imagery session. Closing the eyes aids in establishing a state of internal awareness but is not necessary for an imagery session. The client could gaze at a fixed point 1 to 2 feet away instead of closing his or her eyes. When the client begins to trust the process, his or her eyes will get heavy and close. In clients with a history of organic

brain syndrome or psychosis, deep relaxation may exacerbate symptoms of psychosis. Other relaxation methods should be instituted.
Cognitive Level: Application **Client Need:** Physiological Integrity: Basic Care and Comfort **Integrated Process:** Nursing Process: Assessment **Content Area:** Fundamentals **Strategy:** To answer this question, the nurse needs to know what clients will benefit from imagery and what the contraindication is for this technique.

2 **Answer: 3, 4, 5** Music without words is recommended so that the client doesn't concentrate on the words. Music therapy needs to be at least 20 minutes in length to be effective. Music selections should be based on the type of music the client perceives as relaxing. The nurse should encourage the client to let the body respond to the music in any way it wishes, such as humming, relaxing muscles, or clapping. Analyzing the music will take away the focus from relaxing to thinking about the music. Any distracting thoughts should simply be let go, and the client should be instructed to concentrate on the music.
Cognitive Level: Application **Client Need:** Physiological Integrity: Basic Care and Comfort **Integrated Process:** Nursing Process: Implementation **Content Area:** Fundamentals **Strategy:** The answer to this question reflects the critical elements when using music therapy with a client.

3 **Answer: 2** The client needs to be involved in deciding which type of meditation to learn. The client's condition or schedule may prohibit the use of this holistic therapy. Meditation can be used in any facility and isn't restricted to outpatient settings. Anyone can learn how to meditate.
Cognitive Level: Application **Integrated Process:** Nursing Process: Assessment **Client Need:** Physiological Integrity: Basic Care and Comfort **Content Area:** Fundamentals **Strategy:** This question requires that you know when it is appropriate for the nurse to utilize meditation.

4 **Answer: 2, 3** Sympathetic nervous system is stimulated with humor therapy, leading to an increase in heart rate, respiratory rate, blood pressure, and oxygen saturation. The arousal state is followed by a relaxation state in which vital signs return to or below pre-laughter baseline. Research suggests that humor therapy increases IgA levels in the saliva, which helps prevent upper respiratory infections. Laughter decreasesstress hormones such as cortisol. Laughter increases T lymphocyte cells, thereby increasing the immune response. Temperature is not affected.
Cognitive Level: Analysis **Client Need:** Physiological Integrity: Basic Care and Comfort **Integrated Process:** Nursing Process: Implementation **Content Area:** Fundamentals **Strategy:** An understanding of the pathophysiological effects of humor on the body is needed in order to answer this question correctly.

5 **Answer: 3** The client needs to be in a comfortable position for relaxation to occur. Electromyogram sensors are applied to the forehead when using biofeedback to assess the physiological response to relaxation technique. The progressive relaxation response requires the client to contract and relax muscles to gain a deeper state of relaxation. Repeating a phrase or word silently helps the client turn off other thoughts and focus on a neutral, monotonous stimulus.
Cognitive Level: Application **Client Need:** Physiological Integrity: Basic Care and Comfort **Integrated Process:** Nursing Process: Implementation **Content Area:** Fundamentals **Strategy:** Knowledge of the process involved in performing progressive relaxation is needed to answer this question.

6 **Answer: 4** Massage stimulates circulation, thereby improving blood flow and preventing the formation of blood clots as well as decreasing muscle tension. Massage also stimulates the lymphatic system, enhancing lymphatic drainage. Massage causes the release of lactic acid that has accumulated during exercise.
Cognitive Level: Application **Client Need:** Physiological Integrity: Basic Care and Comfort **Integrated Process:** Nursing Process: Evaluation **Content Area:** Fundamentals **Strategy:** An understanding of the pathophysiological effects of massage on the body is needed to answer this question.

7 **Answer: 3** Essential oils are distilled from flowers, roots, bark, leaves, wood, resins, citrus rinds, and more; the quality of essential oils varies. Many oils should be kept out of the sunlight and heat. Essential oils can be toxic and produce an allergic reaction in some individuals. Some essential oils are unsafe during pregnancy, so it is critical to contact the primary care provider prior to trying aromatherapy to determine which oils are safe and which are toxic.
Cognitive Level: Analysis **Client Need:** Physiological Integrity: Basic Care and Comfort **Integrated Process:** Nursing Process: Implementation **Content Area:** Fundamentals **Strategy:** The core issue of the question is that essential oils can cause an allergic reaction in the client.

8 **Answer: 2** Humor decreases the social distance between persons, putting them at ease. Humor reduces the presenter's anxiety and gains the audience's attention, which facilitates learning. Humor helps individuals act out impulses in a safe, nonthreatening environment, thus releasing anger and aggression. Humor diminishes anxiety and fear, reducing tension and enabling the client to confront and deal with the situation.
Cognitive Level: Application **Integrated Process:** Nursing Process: Implementation **Client Need:** Physiological Integrity: Basic Care and Comfort **Content Area:** Fundamentals **Strategy:** An understanding of the benefits of humor therapy is needed to answer the question correctly.

9 **Answer: 4** The first statement indicates that the imagery session increases the client's anxiety level. The second statement indicates that the client did not focus well during the session, which prevents total relaxation. The third statement indicates the therapy was unsuccessful because guided imagery needs to be practiced daily to obtain the desired effect. The fourth statement indicates that the client's anxiety is decreased, which is the overall outcome of guided imagery therapy.
Cognitive Level: Analysis **Integrated Process:** Nursing Process: Evaluation **Client Need:** Physiological Integrity: Basic Care and Comfort **Content Area:** Fundamentals **Strategy:** Understanding that the purpose of imagery is to help the client relax will help you choose the correct answer.

10 **Answer: 3** It is not necessary to assess muscle strength prior to the relaxation therapy. It is not necessary to assess for the

use of sedatives because this therapy will cause relaxation. It is essential to have the body supported as the muscles begin to relax. The client could obtain injury if he or she falls as muscle tension dissolves. It is not pertinent to know the client's allergies before performing progressive relaxation.
Cognitive Level: Application **Integrated Process:** Nursing Process: Implementation **Client Need:** Physiological Integrity: Basic Care and Comfort **Content Area:** Fundamentals **Strategy:** The core issue of the question is the knowledge that a client can become so relaxed during the progressive relaxation session that falling is a risk if his or her body is not supported.

11 **Answer: 4** The skin being massaged needs to be exposed. Massaging the back requires long strokes along the spine with small circular strokes peripherally. Warmed lotion helps enhance relaxation. Massages should last 3 to 5 minutes and be given in an unhurried manner.
Cognitive Level: Analysis **Integrated Process:** Nursing Process: Evaluation **Client Need:** Physiological Integrity: Basic Care and Comfort **Content Area:** Fundamentals **Strategy:** Knowing the steps in giving a back massage will help you answer this question.

12 **Answer: 4** Meditation involves focusing on the present moment and not on the future. Although meditation was viewed as a religious practice, religious conviction is not required for meditation. Many types of meditation exist, and the techniques differ. All types of meditation involve relaxation and focused attention.
Cognitive Level: Analysis **Integrated Process:** Nursing Process: Evaluation **Client Need:** Physiological Integrity: Basic Care and Comfort **Content Area:** Fundamentals **Strategy:** In order to answer this question correctly, you need to know the definition of meditation, the types of meditation, and how it is utilized.

13 **Answer: 2** You would give the instructions in option 1 to a client who wants to meditate. Imagery involves visualization to assist in healing. An image often used in imagery is the healing of an ill area of the body. Other images that can be used include destroying certain foreign substances (e.g., cancer cells) or connecting with a higher level of consciousness. The instructions in option 3 are appropriate for progressive relaxation exercises. Listening to music is not essential for the use of imagery.
Cognitive Level: Application **Client Need:** Physiological Integrity: Basic Care and Comfort **Integrated Process:** Nursing Process: Implementation **Content Area:** Fundamentals **Strategy:** To answer this question, the nurse must know the difference between imagery and other therapies like meditation, progressive relaxation, and music therapy.

14 **Answer: 1** Dermatitis or eczema is a common allergic reaction to topical aromatherapy. Aromatherapy will not affect skin turgor. Aromatherapy will not change the pigmentation of the skin involved. Edema is not a side effect of aromatherapy.
Cognitive Level: Analysis **Client Need:** Physiological Integrity: Basic Care and Comfort **Integrated Process:** Nursing Process: Evaluation **Content Area:** Fundamentals **Strategy:** The question requires that the nurse know what to look for when a client has an allergic reaction to essential oils.

15 **Answer: 2** Music therapy causes a hypometabolic state that stimulates the parasympathetic system and causes a relaxation response. Music therapy does help reduce the stress and anxiety of the preoperative client. Music therapy stimulates the right hemisphere of the brain where creativity resides. A radio station or soft music can be used to cover up the normal noises found in the hospital setting.
Cognitive Level: Application **Client Need:** Physiological Integrity: Basic Care and Comfort **Integrated Process:** Implementation **Content Area:** Fundamentals **Strategy:** Knowledge of the physiological effects of music is needed to answer this question correctly.

16 **Answer: 3** All of the symptoms described suggest intermittent claudication. Ginkgo is the only herb effective for this condition because its anticoagulant properties will enhance blood flow to the extremities. All the other options are herbs that will not be effective with this painful condition of the calf caused by reduced peripheral circulation.
Cognitive Level: Analysis **Client Need:** Physiological Integrity: Pharmacological and Parenteral Therapies **Integrated Process:** Nursing Process: Planning **Content Area:** Pharmacology **Strategy:** The core issue of the question is the effect of gingko in reducing blood coagulation. Use this knowledge and the process of elimination to determine the correct option.

17 **Answer: 3** Chlorpromazine (Thorazine), a phenothiazine, is metabolized in the liver. Milk thistle, the liver herb, is known to reduce risk of hepatotoxicity caused by phenothiazines. The other options do not have this beneficial effect.
Cognitive Level: Analysis **Client Need:** Physiological Integrity: Pharmacological and Parenteral Therapies **Integrated Process:** Nursing Process: Planning **Content Area:** Pharmacology **Strategy:** The core issue of this question is recognition that milk thistle has a beneficial effect on the liver. Use this knowledge and the process of elimination to determine the correct option.

18 **Answer: 3** Garlic is used most widely to reduce total serum cholesterol and triglyceride levels. Option 1 is incorrect because garlic would reduce, not increase, platelet aggregation, thus leading to bleeding tendencies. Although garlic has been shown to boost immunity, it has not demonstrated effects on the white blood cell count, making option 2 incorrect. Option 4 is incorrect because there is no known relationship between garlic and serum glucose levels.
Cognitive Level: Application **Client Need:** Physiological Integrity: Pharmacological and Parenteral Therapies **Integrated Process:** Nursing Process: Analysis **Content Area:** Pharmacology **Strategy:** The core issue of the question is the use of garlic as an aid in reducing cholesterol and triglycerides levels. Use this knowledge and the process of elimination to determine the correct option.

19 **Answer: 4** The use of any herb should be discussed with the health care provider, particularly in pregnancy and lactation. Most herbs are contraindicated at this time, regardless of the form and even when taken as directed or in lower doses. (Although some sources recommend ginger for morning sickness, other sources claim safety during pregnancy is unknown. Black cohosh has been known to promote labor and should be avoided until birth is imminent.)
Cognitive Level: Analysis **Client Need:** Physiological Integrity: Pharmacological and Parenteral Therapies **Integrated Process:** Teaching and Learning **Content Area:** Pharmacology **Strategy:** The core issue of the question is that many herbs have

unknown or adverse effects on the developing fetus and are therefore used cautiously or avoided during pregnancy. Use this knowledge and the process of elimination to determine the correct option.

20 **Answer: 1** Echinacea is effective when used topically to promote wound healing. It is also used internally to boost the immune system, particularly in the prevention and adjunct treatment of colds and influenza. The other options do not have this beneficial effect.
Cognitive Level: Application **Client Need:** Physiological Integrity: Pharmacological and Parenteral Therapies **Integrated Process:** Nursing Process: Planning **Content Area:** Pharmacology **Strategy:** The core issue of the question is the use of echinacea in wound healing and immune system enhancement. Note the correlation between these properties and the skin injury of the client. Use this knowledge and the process of elimination to determine the correct option.

21 **Answer: 1** Ginger is known to inhibit thromboxane production. The inhibition of this prostaglandin reduces platelet aggregation, increasing the risk of bleeding in the postoperative client. Option 2 is incorrect because ginger would be effective in this situation but is unsafe. Option 3 is incorrect; although it is a true statement, it addresses dosing but not safety when used postoperatively. There is no data to support ginger as potentiating the effects of opioid medications (option 4).
Cognitive Level: Analysis **Client Need:** Physiological Integrity: Pharmacological and Parenteral Therapies **Integrated Process:** Teaching and Learning **Content Area:** Pharmacology **Strategy:** The core issue of the question is the risk of bleeding associated with the use of ginger. Note the association of that property of this herb and the word *postoperative* in the stem of the question. Use this knowledge and the process of elimination to determine the correct option.

22 **Answer: 2** The nurse should monitor blood pressure in the client taking hawthorn, which is known to decrease peripheral vascular resistance, thus decreasing blood pressure. There is no evidence that hawthorn has an effect on any of the other options.
Cognitive Level: Application **Client Need:** Physiological Integrity: Pharmacological and Parenteral Therapies **Integrated Process:** Nursing Process: Planning **Content Area:** Pharmacology **Strategy:** The core issue of the question is the effect of hawthorn on hemodynamics, such as lowering blood pressure and decreasing vascular resistance. Use this knowledge and the process of elimination to determine the correct option.

23 **Answer: 2** One of the principle active ingredients of bilberry is pectin, a soluble fiber that decreases diarrhea. The other options do not contain soluble pectin, and therefore they would be of no use in controlling simple diarrhea.
Cognitive Level: Analysis **Client Need:** Physiological Integrity: Pharmacological and Parenteral Therapies **Integrated Process:** Nursing Process: Implementation **Content Area:** Pharmacology **Strategy:** The core issue of this question is recognition that bilberry contains pectin and that pectin is used to control diarrhea. Use this knowledge and the process of elimination to determine the correct option.

24 **Answer: 4** The psychotherapeutic effects of St. John's wort are not well understood. The herb is thought to work by inhibition of serotonin reuptake, but it may have a slight inhibition of monoamine oxidase (MAO). It is therefore important for the nurse to instruct the client that it is safe to eat ice cream while taking St. John's wort. The other options are incorrect because they contain tyramine, which, when consumed with MAO inhibition, may lead to severe hypertension.
Cognitive Level: Analysis **Client Need:** Physiological Integrity: Pharmacological and Parenteral Therapies **Integrated Process:** Nursing Process: Implementation **Content Area:** Pharmacology **Strategy:** The core issue of the question is the risk of interactive effects of foods containing tyramine with the MAO inhibitor effect of St. John's wort. Use this knowledge and the process of elimination to determine the correct option.

25 **Answer: 3, 5** The client with coronary artery disease or peripheral vascular disease would benefit most from use of garlic because of its ability to lower cholesterol and triglyceride levels. Garlic is not helpful in treating low blood pressure or liver disease (options 1 and 2). Because it inhibits platelet aggregation, the use of garlic by clients with a bleeding disorder could be hazardous (option 4).
Cognitive Level: Analysis **Client Need:** Physiological Integrity: Pharmacological and Parenteral Therapies **Integrated Process:** Nursing Process: Analysis **Content Area:** Pharmacology **Strategy:** The core issue of the question is the use of garlic as an aid in reducing cholesterol and triglycerides as serum lipids. Use this knowledge and the process of elimination to determine the correct option.

ANSWERS & RATIONALES

Key Terms to Review

clinical aromatherapy p. 473
complementary therapy p. 471
imagery p. 472
meditation p. 472
music therapy p. 472

References

Adams, M., Josephson, D., & Holland, L. (2005). *Pharmacology for nurses: A pathophysiologic approach.* Upper Saddle River, NJ: Pearson Education.

Fontaine, K. L. (2005). *Complementary and alternative therapies for nursing practice.* (2nd ed.). Upper Saddle River, NJ: Pearson Education.

Harkreader, H., & Hogan, M. (2004). *Fundamentals in nursing: Caring and clinical judgment* (2nd ed.). St. Louis, MO: Elsevier.

Kozier, B., Erb, G., Berman, A., & Snyder, S. (2004). *Fundamentals of nursing: Concepts, process, and practice* (7th ed.). Upper Saddle River, NJ: Pearson Education.

Lehne, R. (2004). *Pharmacology for nursing care* (5th ed.). St. Louis, MO: Mosby.

McKenny, L., Tessier, E., & Hogan, M. (2006). *Mosby's pharmacology in nursing* (22nd ed.). St. Louis, MO: Elsevier Mosby.

Wilson, B., Shannon, M., & Stang, C. (2005). *Nurse's Drug Guide 2005.* Upper Saddle, NJ: Prentice Hall.

30 Dosage Calculation and Medication Administration

Test Yourself

Are you ready for the NCLEX-RN® or course exams? Use the practice tests on the companion CD-ROM to check.

In this chapter

Cross reference

Other chapters relevant to this content area are

Pediatric Dosage Calculation and Medication Administration	Chapter 31
Intravenous Therapy	Chapter 32

I. GENERAL PRINCIPLES OF MEDICATION ADMINISTRATION

A. Medication names

1. **Generic name:** a name that reflects chemical family of a drug and does not change according to manufacturer; an example is hydromorphone
2. **Brand name** or **trade name:** a proprietary name given to a generic drug by its manufacturer, resulting in various names for same drug; for example, Dilaudid is the trade name for the generic drug hydromorphone

B. Medication order components

1. Include drug name, dose, route, frequency, and special parameters, such as blood pressure (BP) or pulse, for administering or withholding dose; each order must be dated and timed
2. Medication order must include name of client and must be signed by prescriber
3. ! Call prescriber immediately if order is difficult to read or for any other questions about order; do not administer a medication that has an unclear order
4. ! Under law, nurses are responsible for their own actions (e.g., if a medication order is written incorrectly, the nurse who administers the incorrect order is also responsible for the error)
5. Telephone orders written by nurses are done as agency policy allows, must include all elements noted above, and must be cosigned by prescriber as soon as possible and within time frame of agency policy (usually 24 hours)
6. Verbal orders are generally discouraged and are usually used during emergency or near emergency situations; these orders are written as soon as possible and appropriately signed

C. **Essential concepts of pharmacology**

1. **Pharmacokinetics:** study of how body absorbs, distributes, metabolizes, and excretes medication (four processes)
2. **Absorption:** process by which a drug moves from administration site into bloodstream; drugs are absorbed through gastrointestinal (GI) tract, respiratory tract, or skin, and absorption depends upon correct drug form or preparation being administered by correct route
3. **Distribution:** movement of drug from site of absorption to site of action; depends upon vascularity for speed of onset and upon chemical and physical drug properties to attract drug to a certain area of body where it will exert its effect
4. **Metabolism:** conversion of a drug by enzymatic action of liver into a less active substance that is easily excreted through renal or biliary systems; can be affected by a variety of factors, including disease states
5. **Excretion:** elimination of drug and metabolites from body, primarily through kidneys but also through feces, respiration, perspiration, saliva, and breast milk
6. Prescriber determines frequency of drug dosing according to drug's **half-life,** the time it takes for total amount of drug to diminish by one-half; the drug's half-life provides information about its accumulation in body with repeated doses

D. **Principles and process of medication administration**

1. Determine completeness and accuracy of order
2. ! Check client allergies to ordered medication and to any of its ingredients
3. Assess client condition related to why medication is being ordered
4. ! Check ordered medication against other ordered medications for interactions; be aware of **side effects, adverse effects,** and **toxic effects**
5. ! Calculate dose properly, using any conversions needed (see next section)
6. Do not use any medication that has exceeded its expiration date
7. Label all drawn up or reconstituted medications with drug name, dose, date, time, and initials
8. Discard any partially used single-dose containers; label multiuse vials with date, time, and initials when opened or apply expiration date stickers used by some agencies (many expire 30 days after initial use; see product literature and agency policy)
9. ! Complete the six rights when administering medications: right drug, right dose, right route, right time, right client, and right documentation (date, time, initials and/or signature, site if parenteral, any parameters such as BP, pulse, or blood glucose)
10. ! Address any concerns client has about medication; do not administer a medication that client questions until order and dose are rechecked
11. Complete client teaching related to medication while administering dose

II. MEASUREMENT AND CONVERSION SYSTEMS

A. **Medication measurement systems**

1. **Metric system:** a decimal system of measurement based upon units of ten; gram is a unit of weight, and liter is a unit of liquid volume
2. **Apothecary system:** oldest system of pharmacologic measurement, expressed in roman numerals and special symbols; a unit of liquid measure is a minim, and unit for weight is a grain
3. Household: a less accurate system of measurement based upon drops, teaspoons, tablespoons, cups, and glasses

B. **Conversions**

1. When a medication order is written in one system and medication label utilizes another system, one system must be converted to equivalent measure in the other
2. See Table 30–1 ■ for approximate weight equivalents and Table 30–2 ■ for volume equivalents of various systems
3. When converting within the metric system, move decimal point 3 places to right to convert from a larger unit of measure to a smaller unit of measure (e.g., 2.5 grams converts to 2500 milligrams) and 3 places to left to convert from a

Table 30–1

Approximate Weight Equivalents

Metric System	Apothecary System
1 milligram (mg)	1/60 grain
60 mg	1 grain
1000 mg = 1 gram	15 grains
1000 grams or 1 kilogram	2.2 lb (pounds)

Table 30–2

Approximate Volume Equivalents

Metric	Apothecary	Household
0.06 mL (milliliter)	1 m (minim)	1 gtt (drop)
1 mL	15 m	15 gtt
5 mL	60 m = 1 dram	60 gtt = 1 tsp (teaspoon)
15 mL	4 dram	3 tsp = 1 tbsp (tablespoon)
30 mL	1 ounce	2 tbsp
240 mL	8 ounces	1 cup
500 mL	16 ounces	1 pint
1000 mL	2 pints	1 quart
4000 mL	4 quarts	1 gallon

smaller unit of measure to a larger unit of measure (e.g., 3000 milliliters converts to 3 liters)

4. All conversions must be done before dosage can be calculated

III. DOSAGE CALCULATIONS

A. **Medications are prescribed in a specific amount or weight per volume;** for instance, if a single tablet has 100 mg of medication, the volume of that tablet is 1; a medication that comes in 80 mg per 2 mL of liquid has a volume of 2

B. **A few liquid medications are prescribed by volume alone** because they are available in only one strength, such as a dose of 30 mL of a liquid antacid

C. **Common formulas for calculating medications** are ratio and proportion, "desired over have," and dimensional analysis (see Box 30–1)

Memory Aid

No single drug calculation formula is better than any other. Choose one that works for you and use it consistently.

D. **When giving liquid medications for injection,** round amounts greater than 1 mL to the nearest tenth (0.1) to coincide with calibrations on syringe (see next section)

E. **When giving liquid medications for injection,** round amounts less than 1 mL to the nearest hundredth (0.01) to coincide with calibrations on syringe (see next section)

F. **Rules for rounding generally require carrying out decimals to one place further than needed** and then rounding back only once at very end of calculation

IV. ORAL MEDICATIONS

A. **Tablets may be divided into partial dosages** (e.g., half or quarter dose) only when scored (marked in half with indented line)

B. **Extended-release and enteric-coated medications**

! 1. Do not break or crush enteric-coated medications, which are designed for release and absorption in small intestine

! 2. As a rule, do not break or crush extended-release medications; some scored formulations can be broken without affecting release mechanism; some mixed-

Box 30-1

Calculating Medication Dosages

Formula 1 "Desired over Have"

$$\frac{\text{Dose ordered (desired)}}{\text{Dose on hand (have)}} \times \text{Amount available (quantity)} = \text{amount to give}$$

Example: Lasix 60 mg IV is ordered and medication is labeled as 80 mg per 2 mL.

$$\frac{60\text{ mg}}{80\text{ mg}} \times 2\text{ mL} = 1.5\text{ mL}$$

Formula 2 Ratio and Proportion

Dose ordered is to (:) dose on hand as (::) x quantity is to (:) quantity available

Multiply the two outer values by the inner value and x to solve.

Example: Lasix 60 mg IV is ordered and medication is labeled as 80 mg per 2 mL.

$60\text{ mg} : 80\text{ mg} :: x : 2$

$80x = 120;\ x = 1.5\text{ mL}$

Formula 3 Dimensional Analysis

Utilizes a set of rules to set up problems for solving.

Rule 1: Multiplying one side of an equation by a conversion factor will not change the value of the equation.

Rule 2: Set up the problem in fractions called factors so that all labels cancel from the numerator and denominator except the label desired in the answer.

Example: Lasix 60 mg IV is ordered and medication is labeled as 80 mg per 2 mL.

$$\text{mL} = \frac{2\text{ mL}}{80\text{ mg}} \times 60\text{ mg}$$

$$\text{mL} = \frac{120}{80} = 1.5$$

release capsules can be opened and contents sprinkled on food; read product literature carefully

3. Abbreviations used in brand names identifying drugs as extended-release include CR (controlled release), CRT (controlled-release tablet), LA (long acting), SA (sustained action), SR (sustained release), TR (time release), and XL or XR (extended length or release)

C. Liquid doses

1. Use medicine cup to pour liquid volumes of 5 mL or greater; hold cup at eye level and measure to the middle of the meniscus
2. Use syringe with needle removed to draw up liquid volumes less than 5 mL
3. If a calibrated dropper is supplied with medication, it may be used

V. ENTERAL MEDICATIONS

A. Place client in semi-Fowler's position

B. Determine correct tube placement

1. It may not be possible to reliably determine placement of small-bore enteral tubes by any technique other than radiography, which is most reliable
2. Nasogastric tube: aspirate stomach contents and check pH of 4 or less, or auscultate air insufflation; secretions should be greenish tan to clear
3. Nasointestinal tubes: aspirate stomach contents and check pH higher than 6; duodenal secretions should be deep yellow
4. Percutaneous endoscopic gastrostomy (PEG) and percutaneous endoscopic jejunostomy (PEJ) tubes do not require placement verification prior to each medication administration

C. Flush enteral tube with approximately 30 mL water prior to administering medication

D. Administer medication in solution or elixir forms when available; crush tablets to a fine powder and mix in warm water to make a solution or suspension; do not mix medications—administer each medication separately; flush well between medications

E. If client is receiving enteral feeding, ensure compatibility of medication and feeding; if they are not, compatible, turn off tube feeding for 30 to 60 minutes before and after medication administration

F. Flush enteral tube with approximately 30 mL of water following each medication

G. If enteral tube is connected to suction, disconnect from suction for at least 30 minutes after administering medication

H. Maintain client in semi-Fowler's position for at least 30 minutes following administration of medication

VI. INJECTIONS

A. See Box 30–2 for withdrawing medications from a vial

B. See Box 30–3 for withdrawing medications from an ampule

C. Maintain sterility while assembling syringe and needle; select appropriate size needle and syringe based on volume and type of medication, desired site, client's size, and viscosity of medication

D. See Table 30–3 ■ for a summary of syringes, needles, and uses; see Figure 30–1 ■ for examples of 3 mL, insulin, and tuberculin syringes, with illustration of various calibrations

E. Using anatomical landmarks, select site of injection appropriate for type of injection and medication (e.g., intramuscular, intradermal, or subcutaneous); see Box 30–4 (p. 494) for a summary of injection sites

F. Wash hands and put on gloves

G. Cleanse area with alcohol swab and wait for it to dry

H. Inject medication

I. Discard syringe and needle into a sharps container

J. Specific information appropriate to injection sites

1. **Intradermal (ID):** gently pull skin taut; do not aspirate; inject medication slowly and observe for wheal formation and blanching at site
2. **Subcutaneous (SubQ):** grasp subcutaneous tissue; hold syringe like a dart (between thumb and forefinger) and insert needle; release subcutaneous tissue; aspirate (except with heparin or insulin) and inject medication slowly if no blood appears (if blood returns, withdraw needle, discard, and prepare a new injection); with insulin administration, rotate injection sites systematically to minimize tissue damage (**lipodystrophy,** atrophy, or hypertrophy of subcutaneous tissue), which affects absorption
3. **Intramuscular (IM):** hold syringe like a dart; spread skin taught or grasp skin in geriatric client; use quick, darting motion to insert needle; aspirate and inject medication slowly unless blood returns (if blood returns, withdraw needle, discard, and prepare new injection); Z-track technique prevents "tracking" and is used to administer medications irritating to subcutaneous tissue (e.g., hydroxyzine)—pull skin approximately 1 inch laterally away from injection site, inject medication, withdraw needle, then release tissue

Box 30–2

Withdrawing Medications from a Vial

1. Remove vial cap.
2. Cleanse rubber top of vial with alcohol.
3. Tighten needle on syringe or use needleless syringe.
4. Fill plunger with amount of air equal to amount of solution to be withdrawn.
5. Inject air into vacant area of vial, keeping needle above surface of medication.
6. Invert vial, touching only syringe barrel and plunger tip. Withdraw medication.
7. While syringe remains attached to vial, expel any air bubbles from syringe by tapping side of syringe sharply.
8. Recheck amount of medication in syringe.
9. Remove syringe from vial and recap needle, if appropriate, using scoop technique.

Box 30–3

Withdrawing Medications from an Ampule

1. Tap neck of ampule to move solution to body of ampule.
2. Using a pad, break ampule away from you.
3. Use a filter needle to withdraw solution. Solution can be withdrawn from either an upright or inverted position—insert needle, without touching sides of neck, with bevel down and touching bottom of ampule (it is not necessary to add air).
4. Return ampule to upright position.
5. Tap barrel below bubbles to dislodge air in syringe.
6. Eject air with syringe in upright position.
7. Recheck amount of medication in syringe.
8. Remove filter needle and replace with appropriate needle.

Table 30–3 Summary of Syringes, Needles, and Uses

Use/Purpose	Site	Maximum Volume	Syringe	Needle Size	Needle Angle
Insulin Slow absorption to produce a sustained effect	Abdomen, lateral and posterior aspects of upper arm or thigh, scapular area, upper ventrodorsal gluteal areas	1 mL	Insulin—calibrated on 100 unit scale	Non-removable ⅜ in. 29 gauge	45° or 90°
Intradermal or intracutaneous Antigens and skin testing Slow absorption	Inner aspect of fore-arm or scapular area, upper chest, medial thigh	0.10 mL	1 mL tuberculin syringe	⅜ in. 25–27 gauge	10–15° just under the epidermis; bevel of the needle up
Subcutaneous Absorbed slowly for sustained effect	Abdomen, lateral and posterior aspects of upper arm or thigh, scapular area of back, upper ventro-dorsal gluteal areas	1.0 mL	0.5–3 mL syringe	⅜–⅝ in. 25 gauge	⅝ in.– 45° when 1 in. of tissue can be grasped ⅜ in.–90° when 2 in. of tissue can be grasped
Intramuscular Promotes rapid absorption *Ventrogluteal*—preferred site for adults *Vastus lateralis*—preferred site for children < 7 months of age	Ventrogluteal, dorso-gluteal, vastus lateralis, deltoid	*Adult deltoid* 0.5–1 mL *Adult gluteus medius* 1–4 mL	1–5 mL syringe	*Deltoid* ⅝ –1 in. 23–25 gauge *Vastus lateralis, ventrogluteal, and dorsogluteal* 1½ in.	90°

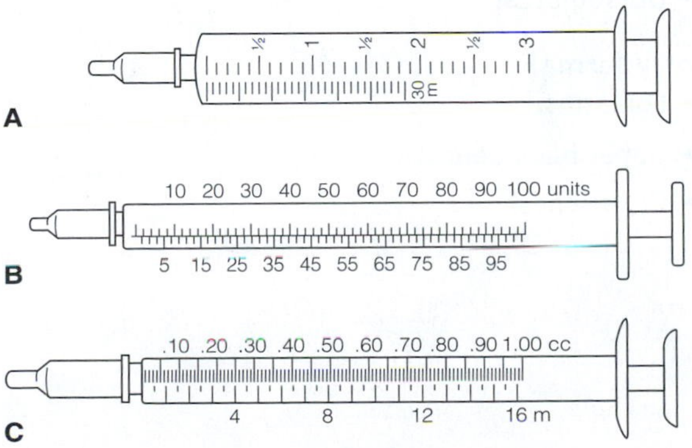

Figure 30–1

Three kinds of syringes for injection, (A) 3 mL hypodermic syringe is calibrated in tenths (0.1) milliliters and minims. (B) Insulin syringe is calibrated in 100 units for use with U100 insulin. (C) Tuberculin syringe is calibrated in tenths and hundredths (0.01) of an mL and in minims.

Box 30-4

Summary of Injection Sites

Intramuscular

Ventrogluteal

- Place client in side-lying position
- Use right hand for left anterior hip and left hand for right anterior hip
- Place palm over greater trochanter and point index finger toward client's anterior-superior iliac spine; spread out index finger from other three fingers to form a V area
- Inject at a 90-degree angle within V area

Dorsogluteal

- Place client either in prone position with toes pointed inward or in side-lying position with upper knee flexed and in front of lower leg
- Draw imaginary line between greater trochanter and postero-superior spine (prominence) of iliac crest
- Inject at 90-degree angle lateral and superior to imaginary line

Vastus Lateralis

- Place client in supine position
- Inject at a 90-degree angle using anterior-lateral middle third of thigh between greater trochanter and lateral femoral condyle

Deltoid

- Palpate lower edge of acromion and midpoint of lateral aspect of arm. Inject at 90-degree angle 2 inches below acromion process within triangle between boundaries
- Alternate method—place four fingers across deltoid muscle with first finger on acromion process; site is three finger breadths below acromion process

Z-Track Injection

- An alternative method of intramuscular injection designed to reduce seepage of medication into subcutaneous tissues
- Prior to injection, skin is displaced, needle is inserted at 90-degree angle while skin remains displaced; once needle is removed, skin is allowed to return to neutral position, thus eliminating an intact needle tract
- This method is used for medications that are irritating to subcutaneous tissues

Subcutaneous

Most Common Sites

- Lateral posterior aspect of upper arms
- Anterior thighs
- Lower quadrants of abdomen (outside 2-inch radius of umbilicus): preferred site for heparin

Other Sites

- Scapular areas
- Dorsogluteal

Intradermal

- Forearms
- Upper back beneath scapula
- Upper chest

VII. INTRAVENOUS (IV) MEDICATIONS

A. **Mixtures of medications within large volumes of IV fluids help to maintain constant therapeutic blood levels of medication;** examples are potassium (e.g., 20 mEq added to 1 liter of IV solution) or heparin (25,000 units added to 250 mL solution)

B. **To add medication to an IV solution,** prepare medication from a vial or ampule and draw into syringe

C. **To add medication to a new IV container**
1. Clean injection port with alcohol swab and allow to dry for 30 seconds
2. Remove needle cap from syringe, insert needle through center of injection port, and inject medication into IV solution
3. Mix medication and solution by gently rotating bag
4. Complete and attach medication label to IV solution; include name and dose of medication, date and time, and nurse's initials
5. Proceed with setting up IV for administration

D. **To add medication to an existing infusion**
1. Ensure that there is sufficient IV solution in container to properly dilute medication
2. Proceed as with adding a medication to a new IV container

E. **Injection by IV *bolus* or IV push**
1. A bolus, or IV push, is a direct injection of a medication intravenously
2. Used to obtain rapid serum concentrations when medications cannot be diluted, or for administration of emergency drugs
3. With PRN adaptor or heparin/saline lock device: when no solutions are running
   a. Prepare syringe with medication and two syringes with flush solution, usually normal saline, according to agency policy, and label all syringes
   b. Wash hands and put on gloves
   c. Instill normal saline to flush IV access device according to agency policy
   d. Cleanse infusion port with alcohol swab and let dry for 30 seconds
   e. Remove needle from syringe and attach syringe with medication to needleless port access device
   f. Administer medication following recommended IV push rate

Memory Aid

Look up in a drug handbook or other standard reference the infusion rate of IV push medications. They vary in length, but most should be given over 1 minute or longer.

   g. Flush IV access device again per agency policy
4. IV push medication through port of infusing IV line
   a. Draw up medication as ordered
   b. Pinch off IV tubing or shut off IV pump before injecting medication
   c. Inject medication over appropriate time frame through port in IV tubing close to client and remove syringe
   d. Resume IV infusion
5. Piggyback infusion without interrupting existing IV
   a. ! Ensure compatibility of piggyback medication with any other currently infusing IV solutions and any ingredients (such as potassium) or currently infusing medications; if incompatible, discontinue primary infusion temporarily if safe to do so or start a second IV line; set up secondary set following procedure for setting up an IV
   b. Hang existing infusion set lower than piggyback secondary set
   c. Cleanse uppermost infusion port with alcohol swab and let dry for 30 seconds
   d. Connect secondary set to primary set using needleless access device above existing IV roller clamp
   e. Maintain existing IV roller clamp position and regulate piggyback rate using roller clamp on secondary tubing or programming secondary rate and volume into infusion pump; piggyback solution will infuse first, and existing IV will resume at original rate when complete

f. When intermittent solution is in a syringe pump, connect syringe to secondary access port on pump; follow protocols for specific pump for administering intermittent medication as either a continuous infusion or an infusion that interrupts existing IV

VIII. TOPICAL MEDICATIONS

A. Medications applied to skin

! **1.** Put on gloves to prevent absorption of medication through fingertips
2. Remove prior applications remaining on client's skin unless otherwise specified
3. Remove ointments and creams from their containers and apply to skin with tongue depressors in thin layers unless otherwise specified
4. For transdermal patch or premeasured paper, read package insert for application directions
a. Remove previously applied patch or paper and cleanse skin
b. Record date and time of application and initials directly onto transdermal patch, and remove protective covering
c. Place prescribed amount of medication directly on premeasured paper and apply immediately; secure paper with tape
! **d.** Alternate application areas to prevent skin irritation and apply to clean, dry, intact, and hairless skin

B. Nasal medications

1. Apply gloves after washing hands
2. Ask client to blow nose and tilt client's head back
3. Occlude one nostril with gloved finger and have client inhale through nose while squeezing medication bottle if nasal spray is being used; client may self-medicate if able
4. Alternatively, fill dropper with prescribed amount of medication, place dropper just inside nares and instill correct number of drops, if bottle with dropper is being used
5. Wipe excess medication with tissue
6. Repeat with other nostril if appropriate
! **7.** Instruct client not to sneeze or blow nose and to keep head tilted back for 5 minutes until medication is absorbed

C. Optic medications

1. Ophthalmic drops
a. Tilt client's head slightly backward and ask client to look up
b. Supply tissue so that client can wipe off excess medication
c. Hold eyedropper ½ to ¾ inch above eyeball
d. Expose lower conjunctival sac by pulling down on cheek, creating a "cup"
! **e.** Drop prescribed number of drops into center of lower conjunctival sac while applying pressure to inner canthus to reduce systemic absorption of medication
f. Instruct client to close eyelids and move eyes; gently massage closed lid
g. Remove excess medication with tissue

2. Ophthalmic ointment
a. Supply tissue so that client can wipe off excess medication
b. Put on gloves
c. Gently separate client's eyelids with two fingers, grasping lower lid immediately below lashes; exert pressure downward over bony prominence of cheek to form a trough
d. Instruct client to look upward
! **e.** Apply eye medication along inside edge of entire lower eyelid, from inner canthus to outer canthus
f. Instruct client to close eyelids and move eyes to spread ointment under lids and over eye surface
g. Remove excess medication with tissue
h. Instruct client that vision may be blurred temporarily following administration of an ointment

D. Otic (ear) medications

1. Position client on side with ear to be treated facing up
2. Fill medication dropper with prescribed amount of medication
3. Put on gloves
4. Straighten ear canal; for an infant or young child, pull pinna of ear gently downward and backward; in an adult, pull pinna gently upward and backward
5. Instill medication drops, holding medication slightly above ear
6. Insert cotton loosely into ear canal, if ordered
7. Instruct client to remain on side for 5 to 10 minutes

E. Vaginal medications

1. Position client in dorsal recumbent or Sims' position
2. Perform hand hygiene and put on gloves
3. Suppository: remove foil wrapper and insert suppository into applicator
4. Cream: attach medication tube to applicator and squeeze tube to fill applicator with prescribed dose; remove tube
5. Insert applicator into vaginal canal 3 to 4 inches, push plunger until all medication is released, and remove applicator
6. Instruct client to lie quietly for 15 minutes until suppository is absorbed; vaginal medications may be ordered at bedtime to aid retention
7. Wash applicator and return to appropriate storage area

F. Rectal medications

1. Place client in Sims' (left lateral) position
2. Perform hand hygiene and put on gloves
3. Remove foil wrapper from suppository
4. Apply small amount of water-soluble lubricant to suppository
5. With index finger, insert suppository flat end first approximately 10 cm or 4 inches in adults beyond internal sphincter to ensure retention (studies indicate that inserting flat end first promotes better retention than inserting tapered end first)
6. Instruct client to lie quietly for 15 minutes while medication is absorbed

IX. INHALATION MEDICATIONS

A. Metered-dose inhaled (MDI) medication

1. Shake canister before each puff to mix medication and propellant
2. Instruct client to
   - a. Hold inhaler 2 inches away from mouth
   - b. Exhale through pursed lips
   - c. Depress inhalation device, inhaling slowly and deeply through mouth
   - d. Hold breath for 10 seconds and slowly exhale through pursed lips
   - e. Wait 2 to 5 minutes (as drug literature recommends) between puffs
3. Clean device according to manufacturer's instructions

B. Spacer with MDI

1. Insert MDI mouthpiece into spacer
2. Remove mouthpiece cover from spacer
3. Shake MDI with spacer
4. Hold MDI and spacer with drug canister upright
5. Instruct client to inhale, exhale slowly through pursed lips, then close lips around spacer mouthpiece
6. Activate MDI canister by pushing it further down into plastic adapter while client inhales slowly and deeply
7. Instruct client to hold breath for 10 seconds, then exhale and relax
8. Wipe mouthpiece after use
9. Remove rubber end of spacer, rinse with warm water, and dry thoroughly

PRACTICE TEST

Check Your NCLEX-RN® Exam I.Q.

You are ready for testing on this content if you can

- Assess the medication schedule of a client.
- Calculate medication dosages with accuracy.
- Reconstitute or mix medications appropriately.
- Verify dosage calculations before administering medications.
- Identify proper procedures for medication administration.
- Utilize the "six rights" of medication administration.
- Dispose of unused medications properly.

PRACTICE TEST

1 The nurse is administering an intradermal tuberculin skin test to a client. The client comments that this "shot" is different than other shots in the past. The nurse explains that because the medication goes into the dermal tissue, the angle for intradermal injections is

1. 10 to 15 degrees.
2. 30 to 40 degrees.
3. 45 degrees.
4. 90 degrees.

2 The nurse is preparing to administer a watery (less viscous) intramuscular injection into the deltoid muscle of a 160-pound male. What is the preferred needle size for the medication, muscle, and weight of the client?

1. 1.5 inch, 20 gauge
2. 1 inch, 20 gauge
3. 1.5 inch, 25 gauge
4. 1 inch, 25 gauge

3 A nurse giving an intramuscular injection places the heel of the hand on the client's greater trochanter, with the fingers pointing toward the client's head. The nurse places the index finger on the client's anterior-superior iliac spine, while the middle finger is stretched dorsally, palpating the iliac crest. After giving the injection in the triangle formed, the nurse documents the injection as being given in which intramuscular injection site?

1. Vastus lateralis
2. Ventrogluteal
3. Dorsogluteal
4. Rectus femoris

4 In teaching a mother to administer eardrops to her 4-month-old infant, the most important concept for the nurse to include is to do which of the following?

1. Wear gloves when administering the eardrops.
2. Avoid contaminating the bottle by not touching the nozzle to the ear.
3. Turn the baby on its back after administration because of the risk of SIDS.
4. Pull the pinna gently downward and backward.

5 A client is postoperative with an IV in place. The client is taking a soft diet and, when asked, rates the pain as 6 on a scale of 1 to 10. The following order is noted in the client's chart: morphine sulfate 6 to 8 mg q 4 hr prn for pain. Considering the client's pain level and noting that no route was ordered, the nurse should do which of the following?

1. Administer the dose IM because the client is on a soft diet and this is a safe IM dose.
2. Recognizing this to be a safe IV dose, administer the dose IV until clarification is received from the physician.
3. Withhold the dose and contact the physician for clarification of the order.
4. Withhold the dose until a route is ordered by the physician, but administer Tylenol™ from stock supplies since these are available over the counter.

6 The physician asks the nurse to take a telephone order for acetaminophen (Tylenol) 500 mg by mouth q 4 hr prn for a temperature elevation higher than 100 degrees F. What should be the nurse's response?

1. Explain to the physician that nurses are not permitted to write orders.
2. Record the order with "telephone order" from physician and the nurse's signature, and remind the physician to cosign it within the next 24 hours.
3. Record the order and sign the physician's name first, followed by the nurse's signature.
4. Ask the physician to restate the telephone order with another nurse witnessing and record the order with both the witness and the nurse's name.

7 The nurse is administering a medication to a client with a history of renal impairment. The medication is known to be excreted through the kidneys. To monitor the client for adverse reactions, the nurse would monitor which of the following?

1. Serum blood urea nitrogen (BUN) and creatinine
2. Color and odor of the urine
3. Urine sugar and acetone levels
4. Serum hemoglobin

8 A client has a continuously running peripheral intravenous (IV) infusion. The physician orders the addition of an antibiotic as a piggyback infusion 4 times a day. In order to administer the antibiotic safely, the nurse should do which of the following?

1. Start a new IV access to administer the antibiotic so that there will not be compatibility issues.
2. Start a new IV access to eliminate the problem of too much volume for one site.
3. Increase the flow rate of the continuous infusion to facilitate the administration of the antibiotic.
4. Check to see if the antibiotic is compatible with the continuous infusion.

9 The nurse is preparing to administer an oral medication to a client. Upon entering the client's room, the nurse finds that the client's condition has changed and the client is now vomiting, has diarrhea, is confused, and has a fever. What should the nurse do next?

1. Administer the medication IM.
2. Wait 2 hours and give the medication if vomiting subsides.
3. Withhold the medication and call the physician.
4. Omit this dose of medication.

10 A nurse has prepared an IM injection for a preoperative client. Suddenly, another client becomes entangled in an IV tubing and yells for help. The nurse rushes to assist. The surgery orderly is waiting for the preoperative client, so the nurse asks a second nurse to give the injection to the preoperative client. Which of the following is the best response by the second nurse?

1. Help the second client so the nurse can give the preoperative client the injection.
2. Give the client the preoperative medication.
3. Prepare a new syringe for the preoperative client.
4. Explain to the nurse that no other nurse can administer the already prepared medication.

11 The client is in the bathroom. When the nurse enters the room to give medications, the client asks the nurse to leave the pills on the bedside table. What is the best nursing action?

1. Leave the medication on the bedside table.
2. Wait in the room until the client comes out of the bathroom.
3. Go into the bathroom and give the client the pills.
4. Tell the client you will return in a little while with the medication.

12 The client has an order for dexamethasone (Decadron) 6 mg IV push stat. Available is a vial of dexamethasone with a concentration of 4 mg/mL. How many mL does the nurse draw into the syringe to administer the dose?

Provide an answer in the box below.

13 The client has an order for cefotaxime (Claforan) 1 gram IV q6h. The reconstituted vial in the client's medication drawer is labeled with a concentration of 95 mg/mL. How many milliliters of solution should be added to the IV bag for the intermittent infusion?

Provide an answer in the box below.

14 The client has an order for glyburide (DiaBeta) 1.25 mg before breakfast and dinner. Available are 2.5 mg tablets. How many tablets should the nurse plan to administer?

Provide an answer in the box below.

15 The client has an order for lorazepam (Ativan) 0.5 mg IV q6h PRN for agitation. Available is a vial containing 2mg/mL. How many mL of solution should the nurse draw up for injection?

Provide an answer in the box below.

16 A client has a temperature of 101.2°F. There is an order for acetaminophen (Tylenol) 650 mg PO for fever, and 325 mg tablets are available. How many tablets should the nurse give?

Provide an answer in the box below.

17 A client has an order for cefazolin (Ancef) 2 grams IVPB. Available are vials filled with powder containing 1 gram of cefazolin. The instructions state to "dilute each 1 gram with 10 mL of sterile water." After reconstituting the medication, how many total milliliters of solution should be drawn up to prepare the dose?

Provide an answer in the box below.

18 A client has an order for a dose of digoxin (Lanoxin) 0.25 mg IV push. Available is a vial containing 0.125 mg/mL. How many milliliters should the nurse draw up to administer the dose?

Provide an answer in the box below.

19 The client has an order to receive methylprednisolone (SoluMedrol) 120 mg IVPB q6h. Available is a solution containing 40 mg/mL. How many milliliters of medication should be added to the IV piggyback solution?

Provide an answer in the box below.

20 The client has an order to receive 40 mg prednisone (Deltasone) by mouth daily. Available are 10 mg tablets. How many tablets should the nurse prepare to give?

Provide an answer in the box below.

ANSWERS & RATIONALES

1 **Answer: 1** For an intradermal injection, the needle enters the skin at a 10- to 15-degree angle and the medication forms a bleb under the epidermis. The other angles would permit the medication to be deposited too deeply into either subcutaneous or muscle tissue, depending on needle length and size of client.

Cognitive Level: Application **Client Need:** Physiological Integrity: Pharmacological and Parenteral Therapies **Integrated Process:** Teaching and Learning **Content Area:** Fundamentals **Strategy:** The core issue is depth of penetration of medication utilizing correct needle angle. Choose the option that has the smallest angle, which will keep the injection from going too deeply.

2 **Answer: 4** Several factors indicate the size and length of the needle to be used: the muscle, the type of solution, the amount of adipose tissue covering the muscle, and the age of the client. A smaller needle such as a 23- to 25-gauge needle 1-inch long is commonly used for the deltoid muscle. More viscous solutions require a larger gauge (e.g., 20 gauge). The other answers are less appropriate because of incorrect needle length or gauge.
Cognitive Level: Application **Client Need:** Physiological Integrity: Pharmacological and Parenteral Therapies **Integrated Process:** Nursing Process: Implementation **Content Area:** Fundamentals **Strategy:** The critical concepts in the question are that the deltoid muscle allows the use of a shorter needle and a watery solution allows the use of a smaller gauge needle. Use the process of elimination to choose the option that combines these concepts.

3 **Answer: 2** The ventrogluteal site is in the gluteus medius muscle with the greater trochanter, the anterior-superior iliac spine, and the iliac crest as the landmarks. The vastus lateralis and the rectus femoris are located on the thigh, and the dorsogluteal is located on the buttocks, making the other options incorrect.
Cognitive Level: Application **Client Need:** Physiological Integrity: Pharmacological and Parenteral Therapies **Integrated Process:** Communication and Documentation **Content Area:** Fundamentals **Strategy:** Use the process of elimination. Basic knowledge of injection sites and landmarks is necessary to answer this question. Choose the option that matches the description given in the question.

4 **Answer: 4** Pulling the ear pinna down and back straightens the ear canal, allowing the drops to enter the ear. Not touching the dropper to the ear is a point of aseptic concern but has slightly lesser priority than correct instillation procedure. The infant should remain on the side for approximately 5 to 10 minutes after instillation and then placed on the back. It is unnecessary to wear gloves.
Cognitive Level: Analysis **Client Need:** Physiological Integrity: Pharmacological and Parenteral Therapies **Integrated Process:** Nursing Process: Analysis **Content Area:** Fundamentals **Strategy:** The critical words in the question are *most important.* This tells you that more than option may be partially or totally correct and that you must choose correctly. With this in mind, choose the option that indicates correct application technique.

5 **Answer: 3** The essential parts of a drug that must be present in order to implement the order are name of the drug, date and time the order was written, dosage, route, frequency, and signature of the person writing the order. Nurses may not independently administer a medication without all of the essential parts or determine a route based upon the client's condition. Administering Tylenol without a medical order constitutes practicing medicine without a license. In hospitalized clients, an order must be present for any medication to be given.
Cognitive Level: Application **Client Need:** Physiological Integrity: Pharmacological and Parenteral Therapies **Integrated Process:** Nursing Process: Implementation **Content Area:** Fundamentals **Strategy:** The core issue of the question is knowledge that medication cannot be given with an incomplete order. Eliminate options 1 and 2 because they do not specify a route in the original order, and eliminate option 4 because it gives a medication without an order.

6 **Answer: 2** A nurse can take a telephone order from a physician. When the nurse documents the order, "telephone order" and the physician's name must be written on the order and the physician must cosign the order, usually within 24 hours. The other answers are incorrect. Option 1 is a false statement, option 3 fails to note that it is a telephone order, and option 4 is unnecessary.
Cognitive Level: Application **Client Need:** Physiological Integrity: Pharmacological and Parenteral Therapies **Integrated Process:** Communication and Documentation **Content Area:** Fundamentals **Strategy:** The core issue of the question is knowledge of how to properly record a telephone order. The wording of the question tells you that only one option is correct. Use the process of elimination and basic nursing knowledge to make a selection.

7 **Answer: 1** Blood levels of two metabolically produced substances, urea and creatinine, are routinely used to evaluate renal function. Both are normally eliminated by the kidneys and are measured as serum BUN and creatinine. The color and odor of the urine are general observations (option 2). Sugar and acetone in urine are found in diabetes mellitus with ketoacidosis (option 3). Serum hemoglobin (option 4) is a measure of the red blood cell count but does not reflect kidney function.
Cognitive Level: Application **Client Need:** Physiological Integrity: Pharmacological and Parenteral Therapies **Integrated Process:** Nursing Process: Evaluation **Content Area:** Fundamentals **Strategy:** The core issue of the question is knowledge of what to assess to determine kidney function as an indicator of clearance of medications. Use the process of elimination and basic nursing knowledge to make a selection.

8 **Answer: 4** Before making a decision about how to infuse the antibiotic, the nurse should check compatibility of the antibiotic with the continuous IV solution. If the drug and the infusion were compatible, they would run together through the same line. If the drug and infusion were incompatible, the nurse would stop the infusion during the period of antibiotic administration and flush the line carefully before and after the antibiotic. It is always inadvisable to start a second IV site unless absolutely necessary. Increasing the IV flow rate constitutes changing a medical order, and does not address the issue of compatibility.
Cognitive Level: Application **Client Need:** Physiological Integrity: Pharmacological and Parenteral Therapies **Integrated Process:** Nursing Process: Implementation **Content Area:** Fundamentals **Strategy:** The core issue of the question is the need to check compatibility of medications and IV solutions as a beginning point to decision-making. Eliminate each of the incorrect options because they do not begin with compatibility checks (options 1 and 2) or are incorrect nursing actions (option 3).

9 **Answer: 3** The correct action should be to withhold the medication and call the physician. Nurses cannot independently change the route of a medication. Oral medications should not be administered to clients who are vomiting, which could

interfere with the ability to absorb the medication and possibly initiate further vomiting. The nurse should not just omit the dose without notifying the physician of the client's change in condition.
Cognitive Level: Application **Client Need:** Physiological Integrity: Pharmacological and Parenteral Therapies **Integrated Process:** Nursing Process: Implementation **Content Area:** Fundamentals **Strategy:** Use the process of elimination and general measures for administering medications safely to make a selection. The wording of the question tells you that there is only one correct answer.

10 **Answer: 1** The nurse who prepares the medication must be the nurse to give the medication. It would be prudent for the second nurse to assist the second client so that the first nurse may continue medication administration. Option 2 is incorrect. Option 3 is acceptable but requires destruction of the original medication, which is an added expense. Option 4 is appropriate but does not resolve the issue of the preoperative client.
Cognitive Level: Analysis **Client Need:** Physiological Integrity: Pharmacological and Parenteral Therapies **Integrated Process:** Nursing Process: Implementation **Content Area:** Fundamentals **Strategy:** Use the process of elimination. The core issue of the question is the principle that nurses may not administer medications prepared by another nurse. The wording of the questions tells you there is only one correct answer.

11 **Answer: 4** Medications should not be left at the bedside, with certain exceptions that are ordered in advance (e.g., nitroglycerin and cough syrup). The other answers are not prudent nursing actions because they either fail to ensure that the medication is taken (option 1), waste the nurse's time (option 2), or invade the client's privacy unnecessarily (option 3).
Cognitive Level: Application **Client Need:** Physiological Integrity: Pharmacological and Parenteral Therapies **Integrated Process:** Nursing Process: Implementation **Content Area:** Fundamentals **Strategy:** Use the process of elimination. There is one correct answer utilizing basic principles of medication administration.

12 **Answer: 1.5** Use the following formula to solve the problem:

$$\frac{\text{amount desired}}{\text{amount on hand}} \times \text{quantity}$$

Thus,

$$\frac{6}{4} \times 1 = 1.5$$

Cognitive Level: Application **Client Need:** Physiological Integrity: Pharmacological and Parenteral Therapies **Integrated Process:** Nursing Process: Implementation **Content Area:** Fundamentals **Strategy:** Use knowledge of basic pharmacological math to set up the question. Check your work carefully and double check placement of decimals for accuracy.

13 **Answer: 10.5** One gram is equal to 1000 mg. Use the following formula as one way to set up the problem:

$$\frac{1000\text{ mg (dose desired)}}{95\text{ mg (available)}} = \frac{x\text{(unknown)}}{1\text{ mL (quantity)}}$$

Cross–multiply 95 by x and 1000 by 1 to yield $95x = 1000$. Divide 1000 by 95 to yield 10.52 or 10.5 mL.
Cognitive Level: Application **Client Need:** Physiological Integrity: Pharmacological and Parenteral Therapies **Integrated Process:** Nursing Process: Implementation **Content Area:** Fundamentals **Strategy:** Use knowledge of basic pharmacological math to set up the question. Check your work carefully and double check placement of decimals for accuracy.

14 **Answer: 0.5** The following is one way to set up the calculation:

$$\frac{1.25\text{ mg (dose desired)}}{2.5\text{ mg (available)}} = \frac{x\text{(unknown)}}{1\text{ tablet (quantity)}}$$

Cross–multiply 2.5 by x and 1.25 by 1 to yield $2.5x = 1.25$. Divide 1.25 by 2.5 to yield 0.5 tablet.

Cognitive Level: Application **Client Need:** Physiological Integrity: Pharmacological and Parenteral Therapies **Integrated Process:** Nursing Process: Implementation **Content Area:** Fundamentals **Strategy:** Use knowledge of basic pharmacological math procedures to set up the question. Check your work carefully and double check placement of decimals for accuracy.

15 **Answer: 0.25** The following is one way to set up the calculation:

$$\frac{0.5\text{ mg (dose desired)}}{2.0\text{ mg (available)}} = \frac{x\text{(unknown)}}{1\text{ mL (quantity)}}$$

Cross–multiply 2.0 by x and 0.5 by 1 to yield $2x = 0.5$. Divide 0.5 by 2 to yield 0.25 mL.

Cognitive Level: Application **Client Need:** Physiological Integrity: Pharmacological and Parenteral Therapies **Integrated Process:** Nursing Process: Implementation **Content Area:** Fundamentals **Strategy:** Use knowledge of basic pharmacological math procedures to set up the question. Check your work carefully and double check placement of decimals for accuracy.

16 **Answer: 2** The following is one way to set up the calculation:

$$\frac{650\text{ mg (dose desired)}}{325\text{ mg (available)}} = \frac{x\text{(unknown)}}{1\text{ tablet (quantity)}}$$

Cross–multiply 325 by x and multiply 650 by 1 to yield $325x = 650$. Divide 650 by 325 to yield 2 tablets.

Cognitive Level: Application **Client Need:** Physiological Integrity: Pharmacological and Parenteral Therapies **Integrated Process:** Nursing Process: Implementation **Content Area:** Fundamentals **Strategy:** Use knowledge of basic pharmacological math procedures to set up the question. Check your work carefully.

17 **Answer: 20** Since the dose is 2 grams and each vial contains 1 gram, the nurse needs to use two vials. The nurse then adds 10 mL of sterile water to each vial of powder based on the direction to "add 10 mL of sterile water per 1 gram of medication." Once both vials are reconstituted, the concentration of each solution is 1 gram/10 mL. The nurse then must draw up the contents of both vials, making the total volume 20 mL.
Cognitive Level: Application **Client Need:** Physiological Integrity: Pharmacological and Parenteral Therapies **Integrated Process:** Nursing Process: Implementation **Content Area:** Fundamentals **Strategy:** Use knowledge of basic pharmacological math procedures to set up the question. Check your work carefully.

18 **Answer: 2** The following is one way to set up the calculation:

$$\frac{0.250\text{ mg (dose desired)}}{0.125\text{ mg (available)}} = \frac{x\text{(unknown)}}{1\text{ mL (quantity)}}$$

Cross–multiply 0.125 by x and 0.25 by 1 to yield $0.125x = 0.25$. Divide 0.25 by 0.125 to yield 2.0 mL.

Cognitive Level: Application **Client Need:** Physiological Integrity: Pharmacological and Parenteral Therapies **Integrated Process:** Nursing Process: Implementation **Content Area:** Fundamentals **Strategy:** Use knowledge of basic pharmacological math to set up the question. Check your work carefully and double check placement of decimals for accuracy.

19 **Answer: 3** The following is one way to set up the calculation:

$$\frac{120\text{ mg (dose desired)}}{40\text{ mg (available)}} = \frac{x\text{(unknown)}}{1\text{ mL (quantity)}}$$

Cross–multiply 40 by x and 120 by 1 to yield $40x = 120$. Divide 120 by 40 to yield 3.0 mL.

Cognitive Level: Application **Client Need:** Physiological Integrity: Pharmacological and Parenteral Therapies **Integrated Process:** Nursing Process: Implementation **Content Area:** Fundamentals **Strategy:** Use knowledge of basic pharmacological math procedures to set up the question. Check your work carefully for accuracy.

20 **Answer: 4** The following is one way to set up the calculation:

$$\frac{40\text{ mg (dose desired)}}{10\text{ mg (available)}} = \frac{x\text{(unknown)}}{1\text{ tablet (quantity)}}$$

Cross–multiply 10 by x and 40 by 1 to yield $10x = 40$. Divide 40 by 10 to yield 4 tablets.

Cognitive Level: Application **Client Need:** Physiological Integrity: Pharmacological and Parenteral Therapies **Integrated Process:** Nursing Process: Implementation **Content Area:** Fundamentals **Strategy:** Use knowledge of basic pharmacological math to set up the question. Check your work carefully for accuracy.

Key Terms to Review

absorption p. 489
adverse effects p. 489
apothecary system p. 489
bolus p. 495
brand name p. 488
distribution p. 489
excretion p. 489
generic name p. 488
half-life p. 489
inhalation p. 497
intradermal (ID) p. 492
intramuscular (IM) p. 492
intravenous p. 495
lipodystrophy p. 492
metabolism p. 489
metric system p. 489
ophthalmic p. 496
pharmacokinetics p. 489
side effects p. 489
subcutaneous (SubQ) p. 492
topical p. 496
toxic effects p. 489
trade name p. 488

References

Harkreader, H., & Hogan, M. (2004). *Fundamentals of nursing: Caring and clinical judgment* (2nd ed.). St. Louis, MO: Elsevier Science.

Kozier, B., Erb, G., Berman, A., & Snyder, S. (2004). *Fundamentals of nursing: Concepts, process, and practice* (7th ed.). Upper Saddle River, NJ: Pearson Education.

Pickar, G. (2004). *Dosage calculations* (7th ed.). Clifton Park, NY: Delmar Learning.

Smith, R., Duell, D., & Martin, B. (2004). *Clinical nursing skills: Basic to advanced skills* (6th ed.). Upper Saddle River, NJ: Prentice Hall.

31 Pediatric Dosage Calculation and Medication Administration

Test Yourself

Are you ready for the NCLEX-RN® or course exams? Use the practice tests on the companion CD-ROM to check.

In this chapter

Cross reference

Other chapters relevant to this content area are

I. DOSAGE CALCULATION USING BODY WEIGHT

A. **Consists of two steps:**
   1. Calculate body weight (often in kilograms)
   2. Calculate actual drug dosage

B. **Converting body weight between pounds and kilograms: see Box 31–1**

C. **Calculating pediatric drug dosages: see Box 31–2**
   1. Drugs are often ordered in mg/kg/day (total daily dose) or mg/kg/dose (actual single dose or divided daily dose)
   2. Occasionally a pediatric drug may be ordered in mg/pounds/day
   3. Most pediatric drugs are given in divided doses rather than a single daily dose
   4. ! It is critical to check ordered dose against safe dosage range to ensure that dose is within recommended range
   5. ! Question an order for a drug that does not fall within safe dosage range

II. DOSAGE CALCULATION USING BODY SURFACE AREA (BSA)

A. ***Body surface area* is a measurement of the surface area of the body;** it may be a more important factor than weight for calculating precise medication dosages for infants and children in selected circumstances

B. **A pediatric client's BSA can be estimated using a *nomogram* such as the one shown in Figure 31–1 ■**; a nomogram is a chart that contains graphs for height, BSA, and weight.

C. **Use simple multiplication** when dose is ordered based on either milligrams or micrograms of drug per meters squared (m^2) (Box 31–3)

D. **Use a formula** to calculate a pediatric drug dose when dosage is specified only for adults (see Box 31–3, p. 506)

Box 31-1

Converting Body Weight Between Pounds and Kilograms

Recall that 2.2 pounds (lb) = 1 kilogram (kg).

To convert from pounds to kilograms, divide the pounds by 2.2.

To convert from kilograms to pounds, multiply the kilograms by 2.2.

Express either pounds or kilograms to the nearest tenth (e.g., 20.6 kg or 45.3 lb).

Box 31-2

Calculating Pediatric Drug Dosages Using Body Weight

Calculating a Single Pediatric Dose by Body Weight

1. Multiply the child's weight in kilograms by the dosage ordered per kilogram. Example: A pediatrician orders a dose of 15 mg of a drug per kilogram of body weight (15 mg/kg).

$$20 \text{ kg weight} \times \frac{15 \text{ mg of drug}}{1 \text{ kg}}$$
$$= 300 \text{ mg of drug should be given as the dose}$$

2. Calculate the volume (tablets, solution) using a standard pharmaceutical math calculation (such as "desired over have multiplied by quantity" or ratio and proportion; see Chapter 30)

Calculating a Single Pediatric Dose from a Total Daily Dose Using Body Weight

1. Multiply the child's weight in kilograms by the daily dosage ordered per kilogram. Example: A pediatrician orders a dose of 45 mg of a drug per kilogram of body weight per day (45 mg/kg/day).

$$20 \text{ kg weight} \times \frac{45 \text{ mg of drug per day}}{1 \text{ kg}}$$
$$= 900 \text{ mg of drug should be given per day}$$

2. Divide the total daily dose by the number of doses per day to calculate the single dose.
Example (continued from above): 900 mg of drug per day divided by 3 doses per day = 300 mg per dose.

III. ORAL MEDICATIONS

A. **Children under 5 years old** often have difficulty swallowing tablets and capsules

B. **Most medications for pediatric use** are available in both solid dose forms (pill, tablet) and liquid forms (suspension, elixir, syrup)

C. **If a pill or tablet must be administered** to a child who cannot swallow it easily, dose may need to be crushed

! D. **Do not crush** enteric coated medications or time released or extended release medications

E. **If oral medications are crushed,** disguise taste by mixing with a small amount of flavored substance such as applesauce or juice

! F. **Check child's mouth** to ensure that oral pills or tablets are swallowed if given whole

G. **Pour liquid medications using a syringe or calibrated medicine cup or dropper,** especially if volumes are 5 mL or less

H. **Measure medication dose accurately**

! I. **Mix suspensions well before pouring** and administer immediately so dose does not precipitate out of suspension

J. **If it is necessary to disguise taste of a liquid dose,** mix in 30 mL or less of a flavored liquid such as juice

K. **Wear clean gloves when administering medications** to avoid coming in contact with child's saliva

! L. **To administer dose to an infant,** place small amounts of liquid along inside of mouth slowly and allow time for infant to swallow before giving more (to prevent aspiration and reduce likelihood of baby spitting out dose)

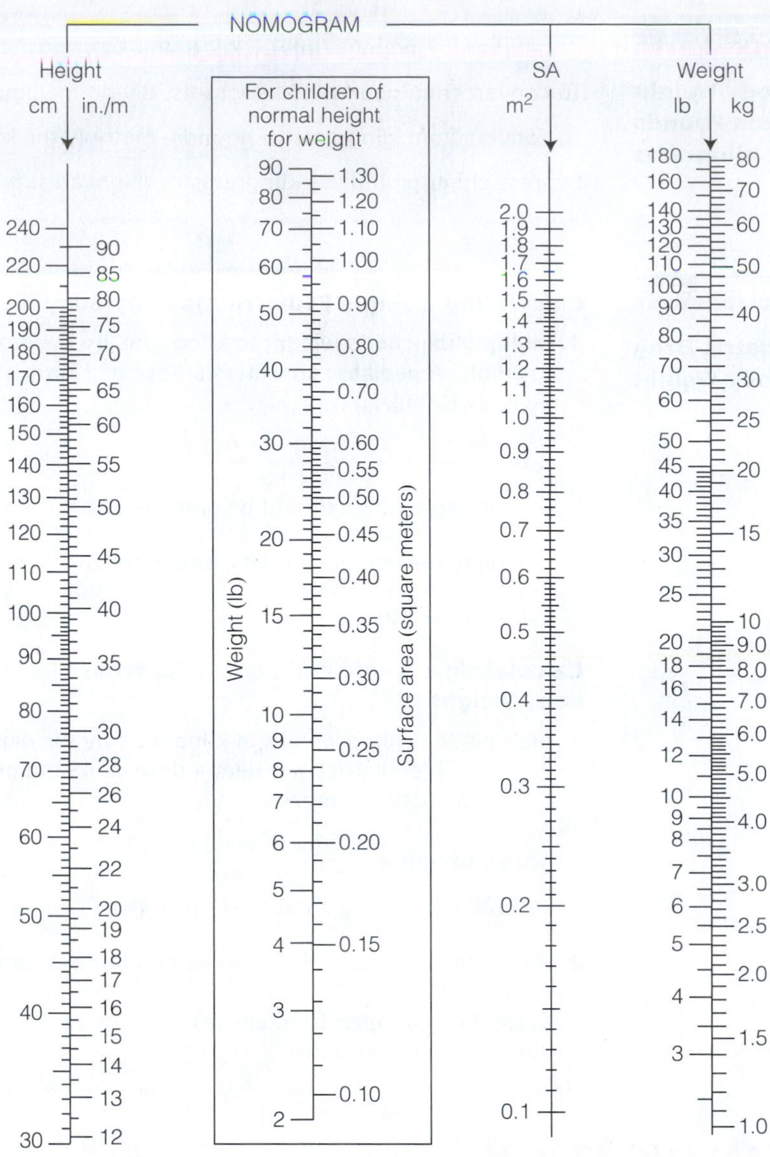

Figure 31–1

West nomogram for infants and children. Obtain child's height and weight and note those points on the nomogram. Draw a connecting line between these two points; the point where the line intersects the BSA column indicates the body surface area in square meters (m^2).

Source: Ball, J., & Bindler, R. (2006). *Child health nursing: Partnering with children & families.* Upper Saddle River, NJ: Prentice Hall, p. 1535.

Box 31–3

Calculating Pediatric Drug Dosages Using Body Surface Area

Calculating a Single Pediatric Dose Ordered by Body Surface Area

1. Multiply the recommended dosage (in milligrams or micrograms per m^2) by the body surface area (m^2).
   Example: 2.5 (mg per m^2) × 0.8 (m^2) = 2.0 mg dose
2. Calculate the volume (tablets, solution) using a standard pharmaceutical math calculation (such as "desired over have multiplied by quantity" or ratio and proportion; see Chapter 30).

Calculating a Single Pediatric Dose From an Adult Dose Using Body Surface Area

1. Divide the body surface area of the child (m^2) by 1.73 (m^2) and then multiply it by the adult dose.
   Example:
   $$\frac{0.8 \text{ m}^2}{1.73 \text{ m}^2} \times 25 \text{ mg (adult dose)} = 11.56 \text{ mg (child's dose)}$$
2. Calculate the volume (tablets, solution) using a standard pharmaceutical math calculation (such as "desired over have multiplied by quantity" or ratio and proportion; see Chapter 30).

M. **To administer dose to a small child,** sit child sideways in own lap or in parent/caregiver's lap; place child's closest arm under adult's arm and behind back; gently hold child's other arm near elbow, use dominant hand to give dose

IV. INJECTIONS

A. Subcutaneous (SubQ)

1. Site depends on age; for older children, use same sites as adults, but newborns, infants, and toddlers often require use of dorsum of upper arm or anterior thigh
2. Syringe size and needle length also depend on size of child, but infants and children often require 25- to 26-gauge needles that are ⅜- to ⅝-inch long
3. ! Medication volumes are typically not more than 0.5 mL for infant and 2 mL for large child; calculate doses to nearest hundredth and measure using a tuberculin syringe if less than 1 mL
4. Inject SubQ medications at 45-degree angle
5. Infants and toddlers need minimal to brief explanations but must be held securely for medication injection, as outlined previously in oral medication section
6. Preschoolers and young school-aged children often understand reason for injection and benefit from simple explanations, distraction, and praise for their cooperation; restraint is on an as-needed basis
7. ! Principles of administration not discussed in this section are same as for adult, including guidelines for aspiration before injecting and massaging site after administration (see Chapter 30)

B. Intramuscular

1. General principles are same as for SubQ injections; variations are presented here
   a. Site depends on age of child, amount of muscle mass, and volume of medication to be injected
   b. ! Typical volumes per single injection site are up to 0.5 mL for young infant, up to 1 mL for older infant or small children, and up to 2 mL in older (large) child
   c. ! Preferred injection site for infants is vastus lateralis muscle (middle third of anterior-lateral aspect of thigh)
   d. Dorsogluteal site can be used after child has been walking for 1 year, but it is not ideal for children under 5 years because these muscles are poorly developed
   e. Injection sites for older children and adolescents are same as for adult and include vastus lateralis, deltoid, and ventrogluteal muscles

V. INTRAVENOUS MEDICATIONS

A. ! **Always ensure that two mixed medications are compatible** and that medications and IV solutions are compatible

B. **Calculation of IV flow rates is often unnecessary due to use of pumps;** however, formula for calculation is same as for adults (volume multiplied by drop factor and divided by time in minutes; see Chapter 30)

C. **Principles for administration of IV medications to children** are same as for adults but with special considerations

1. For infants and children, place IV medications along with diluent in an IV administration set with a volume control chamber (such as a Soluset, Buretrol, Metriset); these sets have a small drop factor (60 drops/mL)
2. Take special care to ensure that tubing contains no air to prevent air injection into child's vein and subsequent air embolus
3. ! Use an electronic controller or pump to regulate IV fluids and intermittent IV medications
4. When setting pump or controller, calculate volume of added medications into total volume (e.g., set 55 mL as volume to be infused if IV bag has 50 mL and 5 mL of medication has been added)
5. For intermittent medication infusions, select a port close to child (ensures medication is delivered at proper time; with slowly running IVs, medication could take some time to travel from distal port to child's vein)
6. ! Check on IV medication and site several times during administration to ensure that client is not experiencing side effects and that IV is patent with no infiltration

PRACTICE TEST

VI. PEDIATRIC CONSIDERATIONS FOR OTHER ROUTES

A. Ophthalmic

1. Young children fear anything being placed in eyes; communicate in a manner to reduce anxiety and promote cooperation during procedure
2. Take care to maintain sterility in a child who is less than cooperative
3. Apply ointment or drops as for adults and close eyelids to prevent leakage
4. ! Encourage child not to squeeze eyes shut and have child lie quietly for 30 seconds

B. Otic

1. Use sterile technique if tympanic membrane is ruptured and draining
2. ! For children under 3, pull pinna straight back and slightly downward to straighten ear canal
3. ! For older children, pull pinna back and upward as for an adult

C. Nasal

1. Saline drops are commonly given to infants with nasal congestion
2. Because nasal medications drain into back of throat, they may cause tickling, bad taste, and occasional difficulty breathing
3. ! Check child for choking or vomiting after instillation of drops
4. Keep child in same position for 5 minutes after administration to allow medication to contact nasal mucosa

D. Aerosol: as per adults

E. Rectal

1. If suppository needs to be cut in half, do so lengthwise
2. Obtain assistance if needed to keep child in side-lying position (or prone in parent's lap if small enough)
3. ! After lubricating, insert gently into rectum just beyond internal sphincter
4. Hold buttocks together until urge to expel medication has passed (5 to 10 minutes)

Check Your NCLEX–RN® Exam I.Q. *You are ready for testing on this content if you can*

- Calculate pediatric medication dosages with accuracy.
- Verify dosage calculations before administering medications.
- Apply principles of medication administration to pediatric clients.

PRACTICE TEST

1 A 4-month-old client has an order for D_5 ½ NS IV to run at a rate of 40 mL/hr. While the unlicensed assistive person (UAP) is obtaining an IV infusion pump, the nurse sets the drip rate at which of the following, using a Soluset with microdrip tubing that has a drop factor of 60 gtts/mL?

Provide an answer in the box below. Round to the appropriate whole number (integer).

[ ] drops/minute

2 A 3½-month-old infant has an order for acetaminophen (Tylenol) suspension 45 mg po q4h prn. The product label lists a concentration of 500mg/5mL. After determining that the dosage is safe, how many mL should the nurse administer?

Provide an answer in the box below. Round to the nearest hundredth.

[ ] mL

3 A 4-year-old client's medication order reads, cefotaxime (Claforan) 1380 mg IV every 8 hours. The client weighs 13.8 kg. Which of the following nursing actions is appropriate if the safe dosage range for a child from 1 month to 12 years of age is listed as 100–200 mg/kg/day given in divided doses?

1. Give the dose as scheduled and document it appropriately.
2. Question the order for the excessively high dose.
3. Administer the slightly high dose but give it at half the recommended rate.
4. Withhold the dose and question the prescriber, since it is below the recommended range.

4 A 6-year-old client who weighs 18 kg is scheduled to receive a dose of vancomycin (Vancocin) 240 mg IV ordered every 6 hours. The safe dose range for a child is listed as 40mg/kg/day divided every 6 hours. What is the best nursing action?

1. Question the dosage of the order.
2. Question the frequency of the order.
3. Administer the dose, being sure to use an infusion pump.
4. Give the dose over at least 60 to 90 minutes to avoid adverse effects.

5 A 5-year-old client has an order for baclofen (Lioresal) ½ 10 mg tab po three times per day. The safe dose range for a 2- to 7-year-old child is 10 to 15 mg/day in divided doses. Which of the following nursing actions is most appropriate?

1. Question the total daily dose ordered.
2. Question the single dose ordered.
3. Refuse to give the dose because the child's weight is not factored into the dose.
4. Administer the dose as ordered.

6 A 3-year-old client has an order for 120 mg acetaminophen (Tylenol) every 4 to 6 hours prn for pain. The maximum total dose is 2.6 grams/day for a child of 2 to 3 years. How many times during a 24-hour period could the nurse legally administer the medication to this child?

Provide an answer in the box below using a whole number.

7 The client has an order for cefotaxime (Claforan) 1180 mg IV q6h. The reconstituted medication vial is labeled as having a concentration of 95 mg/mL. How many mL of solution should the nurse draw up to add to the bag of IV solution that will be used for the intermittent infusion?

Provide an answer in the box below. Round to the nearest tenth.

mL

8 The 6-year-old client has an order for fexofenadine (Allegra) ½ 60 mg tab po twice daily. The nurse calculates the child's total daily dose as how many mg?

Provide an answer in the box below. Round to the nearest tenth.

mg

9 The nurse is reviewing insulin administration techniques with a 13-year-old client with uncontrolled diabetes. The nurse evaluates that the client is using proper procedure after noting that the client does which of the following during self-injection?

1. Aspirates before injection but does not massage the site following injection
2. Uses a 45-degree injection angle and aspirates before injection
3. Uses a 90-degree angle and massages the site following injection
4. Uses a 90-degree injection angle and does not massage the site following injection

10 A 15-year-old client admitted with dehydration has an order for a bolus infusion of normal saline (NS) 500 mL IV over 1 hour. An infusion device is available that counts the number of drops per minute delivered. The IV tubing has a drop factor of 10 drops/mL. If the bolus is to infuse on time, the nurse should set the drip rate to how many drops per minute?

Provide an answer in the box below, rounding to the nearest whole number.

drops/min

11 A 6-year-old postoperative client has a medication order for cefazolin (Ancef) 500 mg IV every 6 hours. The client weighs 44 pounds. The safe dose range of cefazolin for a child is 25 to 100 mg/kg/day in three to four divided doses. What is the total daily dose that this client will receive in mg/kg/day?

Provide an answer in the box below, using a whole number.

mg/kg/day

12 A child who sustained a head injury has an order for mannitol (Osmitrol) 20 grams. Available is a bag of 20% solution that contains 20 grams mannitol in 100 mL volume. The medication may be administered over 30 to 90 minutes. If the nurse wishes to infuse the medication over 90 minutes, at how many mL/hour should the infusion pump be set if the pediatric infusion pump can be set to include tenths of a milliliter?

Provide an answer in the box below, rounding to the nearest tenth.

mL/hr

PRACTICE TEST

13 A client has a medication order for ceftazidime (Fortaz) 250 mg IV every 8 hours. The client weighs 55 pounds. The safe dose range of ceftazidime for a child is 30 to 50 mg/kg/day in three divided doses. What is the total daily dose ordered for this client in mg/kg/day?

Provide an answer in the box below, rounding to the nearest whole number.

______ mg/kg/day

14 A child has an order to receive an NS bolus 400 mL IV. If the nurse wishes to infuse this volume over 90 minutes, at what mL/hour should the infusion pump be set?

Provide an answer in the box below, rounding to the nearest whole number.

______ mL/hr

15 The nurse is about to administer a dose of acetaminophen (Tylenol) 200 mg via the NG tube to a child. Available is a suspension with a concentration of 80 mg per 5 mL. How many mL should the nurse administer to give the dose?

Provide an answer in the box below, rounding to the nearest tenth.

______ mL

ANSWERS & RATIONALES

1 **Answer: 40 drops/minute** Use the following formula to calculate the rate of IV solutions:

$$\frac{\text{Volume} \times \text{drop factor}}{\text{Time (in minutes)}}$$

Set up the problem as follows:

$$\frac{40 \times 60}{60}$$

Multiply 40 by 60 to yield 2400 and divide 2400 by 60 (or cancel out the 60's) to yield 40 drops/minute.
Cognitive Level: Application **Client Need:** Physiological Integrity: Pharmacological and Parenteral Therapies **Integrated Process:** Nursing Process: Implementation **Content Area:** Pharmacology **Strategy:** Use knowledge of basic IV calculation to set up the question. Calculate the problem carefully and double check your answer for accuracy.

2 **Answer: 0.45 mL** The problem can be set up using the following formula:

$$\frac{45 \text{ mg (dose desired)}}{500 \text{ mg (available)}} = \frac{x \text{ (unknown)}}{5 \text{ mL (quantity)}}$$

Multiply 500 by x and multiply 45 by 5 to yield $500x = 225$. Divide 225 by 500 to yield 0.45 mL.
Cognitive Level: Application **Client Need:** Physiological Integrity: Pharmacological and Parenteral Therapies **Integrated Process:** Nursing Process: Implementation **Content Area:** Pharmacology **Strategy:** Use knowledge of basic dosage calculation to set up the question. Calculate the problem carefully and double check your answer for accuracy.

3 **Answer: 2** First calculate the daily dose of the medication by dividing the number of mg (1380) by the client's weight in kg (13.8) to yield a single dose of 100 mg/kg. Because there are three doses ordered during a 24-hour period, multiply 100 by 3 to yield 300 mg/kg/day. Since the dose range is 100 to 200 mg/kg/day, the nurse should question the order for the excessively high dose as a safe nursing action.
Cognitive Level: Analysis **Client Need:** Physiological Integrity: Pharmacological and Parenteral Therapies **Integrated Process:** Nursing Process: Implementation **Content Area:** Pharmacology **Strategy:** Use knowledge of basic pediatric dosage calculation to set up the question. Calculate the problem carefully and double check your answer for accuracy. Recall that any dose that falls outside the safe dosage range needs to be questioned.

4 **Answer: 1** First calculate the total daily dose by dividing 240 mg by 18 kg to yield a single dose of 14.44 mg/kg. Multiply the single dose by 4 doses (every 6 hours) to yield a daily total dose of 57.76 mg/kg/day. Since this exceeds the safe total daily dose of 40 mg/kg/day, the nurse should question the order.
Cognitive Level: Analysis **Client Need:** Physiological Integrity: Pharmacological and Parenteral Therapies **Integrated Process:** Nursing Process: Implementation **Content Area:** Pharmacology **Strategy:** Use knowledge of basic pediatric dosage calculation to set up the question. Calculate the problem carefully and double check your answer for accuracy. Recall that any dose that falls outside the safe dosage range needs to be questioned.

5 **Answer: 4** The dose can be administered as ordered. The order for ½ of a 10 mg tab means that the child is receiving 5 mg per dose. If there are 3 doses per day, then the total daily dose is 15 mg, which is within the safe dosage range.
Cognitive Level: Analysis **Client Need:** Physiological Integrity: Pharmacological and Parenteral Therapies **Integrated Process:** Nursing Process: Implementation **Content Area:** Pharmacology **Strategy:** Use knowledge of basic pediatric dosage calculation to set up the question. Calculate the problem carefully and double check your answer for accuracy. Recall that any dose that falls within the safe dosage range may be administered.

6 **Answer: 6** Convert 2.6 grams to 2600 mg. Since a single dose is only 120 mg, the client could theoretically receive this dose 21 times (2600 divided by 120 = 21.66) within a 24-hour period without exceeding the top of the dosage range.

However, since the medication is ordered only every 4 to 6 hours, the nurse can legally administer the medication only 6 times maximum (every 4 hours).
Cognitive Level: Analysis **Client Need:** Physiological Integrity: Pharmacological and Parenteral Therapies **Integrated Process:** Nursing Process: Planning **Content Area:** Pharmacology
Strategy: Use knowledge of basic math calculations to determine your answer. If the drug can be given no more frequently than every 4 hours, it cannot exceed 6 doses, since 24 divided by 4 is 6.

7 **Answer: 12.4** The following formula illustrates one way to set up the problem:

$$\frac{1180 \text{ mg (dose desired)}}{95 \text{ mg (available)}} = \frac{x \text{ (unknown)}}{1 \text{ mL (quantity)}}$$

Multiply 95 by x and multiply 1180 by 1 to yield $95x = 1180$. Divide 1180 by 95 to yield 12.421 or 12.4 mL after rounding down to the nearest tenth.
Cognitive Level: Analysis **Client Need:** Physiological Integrity: Pharmacological and Parenteral Therapies **Integrated Process:** Nursing Process: Implementation **Content Area:** Pharmacology
Strategy: Use knowledge of basic dosage calculation procedures to set up the question. Calculate the problem carefully and double check your answer for accuracy.

8 **Answer: 60** One half of a 60 mg tablet is 30 mg. Because the dose is ordered twice a day, the total daily dose is 30 multiplied by 2, or 60 mg.
Cognitive Level: Analysis **Client Need:** Physiological Integrity: Pharmacological and Parenteral Therapies **Integrated Process:** Nursing Process: Implementation **Content Area:** Pharmacology
Strategy: Use knowledge of basic math calculation to set up the problem. Calculate carefully and double check your answer for accuracy.

9 **Answer: 4** Correct administration technique is to use a 90-degree angle (insulin syringes have a short ½-inch needle), avoiding aspiration before injection (to avoid tissue complications over time), and avoiding massaging the area after injection (which would enhance quicker absorption of the dose).
Cognitive Level: Analysis **Client Need:** Physiological Integrity: Pharmacological and Parenteral Therapies **Integrated Process:** Nursing Process: Evaluation **Content Area:** Pharmacology
Strategy: The core issue of the question is knowledge of subcutaneous injection techniques. Use the process of elimination and nursing knowledge to answer the question. To help eliminate incorrect answers, recall that insulin and heparin should not be massaged and that a 90-degree angle is used for injection.

10 **Answer: 83** Since the infusion device delivers fluid in drops/min, the nurse must calculate the number at which to set the machine. The formula to use is:

$$\frac{\text{Volume} \times \text{drop factor}}{\text{Time in minutes}}$$

Thus, the problem should be set up as follows:

$$\frac{500 \times 10}{60}$$

Multiply 500 by 10 to yield 5000 and divide it by 60 to obtain a flow rate of 83.33 gtts/min, which rounds down to 83 drops/minute.
Cognitive Level: Analysis **Client Need:** Physiological Integrity: Pharmacological and Parenteral Therapies **Integrated Process:** Nursing Process: Implementation **Content Area:** Pharmacology
Strategy: Use knowledge of basic IV calculation to set up the question. Calculate the problem carefully and double check your answer for accuracy.

11 **Answer: 100** First convert the child's weight to kg by dividing 44 by 2.2 to yield a weight of 20 kg. Then calculate the daily dose of the medication by dividing the number of mg (500) by the client's weight in kg (20) to yield a single dose of 25 mg/kg. Because there are four doses (every 6 hours) ordered during a 24-hour period, multiply 25 by 4 to yield a total daily dose of 100 mg/kg/day.
Cognitive Level: Analysis **Client Need:** Physiological Integrity: Pharmacological and Parenteral Therapies **Integrated Process:** Nursing Process: Implementation **Content Area:** Pharmacology
Strategy: Use knowledge of basic dosage calculation to set up the question. Calculate the problem carefully and double check your answer for accuracy.

12 **Answer: 66.7** Since the infusion pump delivers fluid in mL/hour, the nurse needs to calculate the equivalent hourly rate when infusing the 100 mL over 90 minutes. The problem can be set up as follows to cancel out the labels and end up with mL/hour:

$$\frac{100 \text{ mL (volume)}}{90 \text{ mins (time)}} \times \frac{60 \text{ mins}}{1 \text{ hour}} = \text{answer in mL/hour}$$

Multiply 1000 by 60 to yield 6000 and divide it by 90 (90 × 1) to obtain an equivalent hourly flow rate of 66.66 or 66.7 mL/hr. This answer also makes common sense because if the medication were infusing over 90 minutes, then two thirds of it would infuse in 1 hour; 66.7 mL is two thirds of 100 mL.
Cognitive Level: Analysis **Client Need:** Physiological Integrity: Pharmacological and Parenteral Therapies **Integrated Process:** Nursing Process: Implementation **Content Area:** Pharmacology
Strategy: Use knowledge of basic math calculation to set up the question. Read the question carefully, noting that the time needs to convert from minutes to hours in order to have the correct labeling. Calculate the problem carefully and double check your answer for accuracy.

13 **Answer: 30** First convert the child's weight to kg by dividing 55 by 2.2 to yield a weight of 25 kg. Then calculate the daily dose of the medication by dividing the number of mg (250) by the client's weight in kg (25) to yield a single dose of 10 mg/kg. Because there are 3 doses (every 8 hours) ordered during a 24-hour period, multiply 10 by 3 to yield a total daily dose of 30 mg/kg/day.
Cognitive Level: Analysis **Client Need:** Physiological Integrity: Pharmacological and Parenteral Therapies **Integrated Process:** Nursing Process: Implementation **Content Area:** Pharmacology
Strategy: Use knowledge of basic pediatric dosage calculation to set up the question. Calculate the problem carefully and double check your answer for accuracy.

14 **Answer: 267** Since the infusion pump delivers fluid in mL/hour, the nurse must calculate the equivalent hourly rate when infusing the 400 mL over 90 minutes. The problem can be set up as follows to cancel out the labels and end up with mL/hour:

$$\frac{400\text{ mL (volume)}}{90\text{ mins (time)}} \times \frac{60\text{ mins}}{1\text{ hour}} = \text{answer in mL/hour}$$

Multiply 400 by 60 to yield 24000 and divide it by 90 (90 × 1) to obtain an equivalent hourly flow rate of 266.66 or 267 mL/hr. **Cognitive Level:** Analysis **Client Need:** Physiological Integrity: Pharmacological and Parenteral Therapies **Integrated Process:** Nursing Process: Implementation **Content Area:** Pharmacology **Strategy:** Use knowledge of basic math calculation to set up the question. Read the question carefully, noting that the time needs to convert from minutes to hours in order to have the correct labeling. Calculate the problem carefully and double check your answer for accuracy.

15 **Answer: 12.5** The problem can be set up using ratio and proportion as follows:

$$\frac{200\text{ mg (dose desired)}}{80\text{ mg (available)}} = \frac{x\text{ (unknown)}}{5\text{ mL (quantity)}}$$

Multiply 80 by x and multiply 200 by 5 to yield $80x = 1000$. Divide 1000 by 80 to yield 12.5 mL. **Cognitive Level:** Analysis **Client Need:** Physiological Integrity: Pharmacological and Parenteral Therapies **Integrated Process:** Nursing Process: Implementation **Content Area:** Pharmacology **Strategy:** Use knowledge of basic pediatric dosage calculation to set up the question. Calculate the problem carefully and double check your answer for accuracy.

Key Terms to Review

body surface area (BSA) p. 504 **nomogram** p. 504

References

Kee, J., & Marshall, S. (2004). *Clinical calculations: With applications to general and specialty areas* (5th ed.). Philadelphia: Saunders.

Olson, J., Giangrasso, A., & Shrimpton, D. (2004). *Medical dosage calculations* (8th ed.). Upper Saddle River, NJ: Pearson Education.

Pickar, G. (2004). *Dosage calculations* (7th ed.). Clifton Park, NY: Delmar Learning.

Smith, R., Duell, D., & Martin, B. (2004). *Clinical nursing skills: Basic to advanced skills* (6th ed.). Upper Saddle River, NJ: Prentice Hall.

ANSWERS & RATIONALES

Intravenous Therapy

32

In this chapter

Test Yourself

Are you ready for the NCLEX-RN® or course exams? Use the practice tests on the companion CD-ROM to check.

Cross reference

Other chapters relevant to this content area are

Blood and Blood Component Therapy	Chapter 33
Fluid and Electrolyte Imbalances	Chapter 54

I. OVERVIEW OF INTRAVENOUS (IV) THERAPY

A. Indications

1. Provides fluid and electrolyte replacement for clients unable to take oral nourishment (such as with NPO status for diagnostic or surgical procedures or with problems related to swallowing or GI tract)
2. Provides a route for peripheral parenteral nutrition (PPN) or total parenteral nutrition (TPN) for clients with increased caloric needs, such as those with severe burns or other health problems leading to increased caloric needs above what can be taken orally
3. IV route can be used to give medications that would be destroyed by GI tract, are too irritating to be given by another route, to avoid discomfort of frequent intramuscular (IM) injections, or to maintain a constant blood level of a medication
4. In life-threatening situations, it provides rapid access for administration of medications and fluids directly into bloodstream, ensuring prompt onset of action and most complete absorption

B. Types of fluids provided by IV route

1. Hydrating solutions (see Table 32–1 ■)
2. Total parenteral nutrition (TPN); see Chapter 34

C. Equipment needed for IV therapy

1. Catheters and needles
   - **a.** Over-the-needle catheters: 16- to 26-gauge plastic catheter fits over a needle that pierces skin and vein; once in vein, needle is withdrawn and discarded, leaving catheter in place; available in a variety of lengths and gauges; use smallest length and gauge of catheter that is appropriate
   - **b.** Winged needle or butterfly: steel needle with plastic flaps (wings) attached to shaft to facilitate venipuncture; commonly used for obtaining some blood samples or for short-term therapy
   - **c.** These devices come in protected needle styles designed to protect nurse from accidental needlesticks and blood exposure

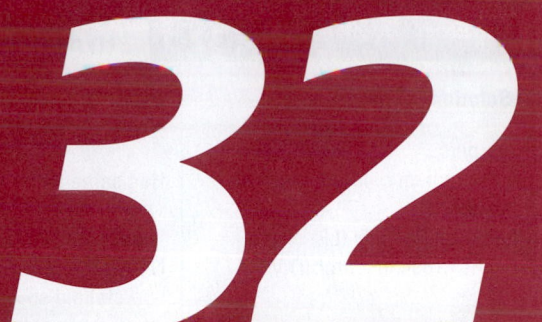

Table 32–1 Hydrating Solutions

Solution	Uses	Nursing Implications
Isotonic 0.9% sodium chloride (normal saline) Lactated Ringer's (LR) 5% dextrose in water (D_5W)	Has same concentration of solutes as plasma, therefore remains in the vascular compartment, expanding vascular volume Normal saline and lactated Ringer's are crystalloid solutions, increase fluid volume in both intravascular and interstitial space with minimal fluid volume expansion Normal saline is the only solution that may be administered with blood products 5% dextrose in water (D_5W) is isotonic on initial administration but provides free water when metabolized, expanding intracellular and extracellular fluid volumes	Assess for signs of hypervolemia • Bounding pulse • Shortness of breath • Distended neck veins Assess for signs of hypovolemia • Urine output < 30 mL/hr • Weak, thready pulse • Subnormal temperature • Flat neck veins
Hypotonic 0.45% sodium chloride (½ normal saline) 0.33% sodium chloride (⅓ normal saline)	Has lesser concentration of solutes than plasma, therefore treats cellular dehydration through fluid shifting out of the vascular compartment into cells; promotes elimination by kidneys	Do not administer to clients at risk for third-space fluid shift or sequestration of extracellular fluid in a body space (resulting in circulatory volume loss and the potential for organ failure or increased intracranial pressure)
Hypertonic 5% dextrose in normal saline (D_5NS) 5% dextrose in 0.45% sodium chloride (D_5 ½NS) 5% dextrose in lactated Ringer's (D_5LR) 10% dextrose in water ($D_{10}W$) 20% dextrose in water ($D_{20}W$) 50% dextrose in water ($D_{50}W$)	Has higher concentration of solutes than plasma, therefore causing fluid to shift from the cells into the vascular compartment, expanding vascular volume 10% dextrose—stand-by solution for clients receiving TPN 50% dextrose—used for hypoglycemia	Do not administer to clients with kidney or heart disease or clients who are dehydrated; monitor for signs of hypervolemia
Volume Expanders (colloid solutions) Albumin 5% (Albumin-5, Buminate 5%) Albumin 25% (Albumin-25, Buminate 25%) Dextran 40 (Gentran 40) Hetastarch (Hespan [HESI]) Plasma protein fraction (Plasmanate, PlasmaPlex, Plasmatein, Protenate)	Colloid solutions contain substances that cannot diffuse through capillary walls, resulting in increased plasma volume and increased osmotic pressure, causing fluids to move into the vascular compartment; used to treat hypovolemic shock	Establish baseline vital signs, lung and heart sounds, and central venous pressure; repeat per agency protocols Administer with a large-gauge (18–19 gauge) needle Monitor intake and output Monitor for signs of hypervolemia
Nutrient 5% dextrose (D_5W) 5% dextrose in 0.45% sodium chloride	Contain some form of carbohydrate (e.g., dextrose, glucose, or levulose) and water D_5 W provides 170 calories per liter	Useful in preventing dehydration but does not provide sufficient calories to promote wound healing, weight gain, or normal growth in children
Electrolyte 0.9% sodium chloride Ringer's solution (contains sodium, chloride, potassium, and calcium) 5% dextrose in 0.45% sodium chloride	Saline and electrolytes restore vascular volume and replace electrolytes Lactated Ringer's is also an alkalinizing solution that treats metabolic acidosis 5% dextrose in 0.45% sodium chloride is an acidifying solution to treat metabolic alkalosis	Monitor fluid and electrolytes Monitor arterial blood gases Monitor intake and output

2. Infusion pumps and electronic delivery devices (EDDs)
   a. Deliver fluids by exerting positive pressure on tubing or on fluid to maintain fluid flow despite increased venous resistance
   b. Regulate rate at preset limits and have alarms that are triggered when fluid level is low, air is in line, or an occlusion is present
   c. Should be utilized when volume must be carefully controlled
3. Regulators, controllers, and mechanical infusion devices
   a. Devices designed to aid in monitoring IV flow rates
   b. Regulators are in-line devices in which flow rate is set by a dial instead of relying on gravity flow drip counting
   c. Controllers sense drops that flow from bag of fluid into drip chamber
   d. Mechanical infusion devices include elastomeric balloon and spring-coil piston devices, which are disposable devices that control speed of infusion by size of tubing; frequently used with home infusions to simplify administration of medications
   e. All of these devices are convenience devices and are not to be used when flow rate must be carefully administered
4. Tubing: may be vented or nonvented
   a. Vented tubing is used with glass bottles; nonvented tubing is used with plastic bags
   b. When infusions flow by gravity, drip chamber of tubing determines size of drop
   c. Drip chambers commonly are rated at 10, 12, 15, or 20 drops per mL; pediatric sets usually are rated at 60 drops per mL
5. Filters: devices that may be part of infusion set or may be an addition to infusion line; filters remove contaminants such as air, bacteria, or particulate matter; not all medications or solutions can or must be filtered
   ! a. TPN requires a filter change every 24 hours when the tubing is changed
   ! b. Some medications, such as phenytoin (Dilantin) and pantoprazole (Protonix), require a filter change with each medication administration
   ! c. A filter must be used whenever blood is transfused; many blood administration sets are manufactured with an in-line filter, but nurse must be sure one is utilized
   d. To prime a filter, point filter downward so proximal half fills with fluid first, then invert to complete priming filter

II. TYPES OF INTRAVENOUS INFUSIONS

A. Peripheral infusion

1. IV device with an internal tip that terminates in a peripheral vein
2. In adults, internal tip lies between fingertips and shoulder
3. Some fluids and medications cannot be administered by peripheral line because of characteristics of fluids
4. Peripheral devices are usually rotated every 3 to 4 days, according to current agency policy and evidence-based research

B. Central infusion

1. IV device with an internal tip that lies in central venous system; these can include such catheters as central venous catheter (CVC) or peripherally inserted central catheter (PICC line)
2. Most commonly end at superior vena cava
3. These devices can remain in place for long periods of time
4. Any fluid or medication that can be administered in venous circulation can be administered by central lines
5. ! Most central lines require sterile dressings to reduce risk of contamination; agency policy and type of dressing determine frequency of dressing changes

C. Continuous infusion: an uninterrupted infusion that runs 24 hours a day

D. Intermittent infusion

1. An infusion designed for clients who do not require IV fluid replacement therapy but require an IV access

2. A saline lock or prn adapter is fitted to end of peripheral venous access device providing a connection for intermittent solution or medication administration
3. These devices require a saline flush at least once every 8 hours and before and after medication administration
4. Some central lines require saline flush be followed by an instillation of heparin flush (10 units/mL or 100 units/mL solutions) to maintain the device

III. PROCEDURES AND SKILLS FOR INTRAVENOUS THERAPY

A. Preparing for IV therapy

1. Verify allergies, such as latex
2. Gather equipment (IV catheter, tourniquet, alcohol and betadine cleansing wipes, sterile tape, gauze or semipermeable transparent membrane dressing materials, IV fluids and appropriate tubing, filter if indicated, pump and regulator device if desired or necessary, and gloves)
3. Wash hands
4. Verify type and amount of solution with physician's order, note expiration date
5. Prepare equipment
   - **a.** Obtain needleless adapter to connect to venous access device if device does not include one
   - **b.** Remove outer wrappers from tubing, connect tubing and filter device, and close tubing roller clamp
   - ! **c.** Remove outer wrapper around IV bag; inspect bag for leaks (small amount of condensation is normal), tears, discoloration, cloudiness, or particulate matter; discard bag if any of these conditions are present
   - **d.** Hang IV bag on pole
   - **e.** Using aseptic technique, remove port cap on IV bag and plastic protector from IV tubing spike (end with drip chamber) and insert spike into IV bag
   - **f.** Squeeze drip chamber until it is partially full
   - **g.** Remove protective cap on tubing if it is not an air-vented cap, open roller clamp on tubing to prime tubing and filter; invert and tap Y injection sites to remove air during priming, replace protective tubing cap
   - **h.** If solution to be hung is in a glass bottle (such as to administer medications that would absorb into plastic IV bag), use vented tubing, or solution will not infuse

B. Inserting an IV line

1. Follow agency policy when starting and maintaining an IV
2. ! Wear gloves for protection from blood-borne pathogens
3. Prepare client for infusion, explain procedure, and obtain client's permission for procedure
4. Identify appropriate vein for cannulation
   - **a.** In adults, peripheral IVs are inserted between fingers and shoulders depending on age
   - **b.** Peripheral IVs in children can also include scalp and leg veins
   - **c.** Avoid sites where veins are sclerotic, inflamed, or subject to decreased blood flow (as is common in adults following a stroke or mastectomy on that side)
5. Use tourniquet to distend vessel
   - ! **a.** Verify absence of latex allergy before applying
   - **b.** In absence of a tourniquet, a blood pressure cuff may be used
   - **c.** Some geriatric clients may be accessed without a tourniquet
   - **d.** Place tourniquet 4 to 6 inches above proposed site tightly enough to obstruct venous circulation but not arterial circulation (use light tapping, gravity, and/or topical heat application to aid vein distention)
6. Prepare skin; typical procedure is to clean site with alcohol followed by povidone-iodine; cleanse skin in a circular manner starting at inside and moving outward, to remove bacteria from insertion site; cleansing agent must be allowed to dry on skin for up to 2 minutes
7. Introduce needle at a 10- to 30-degree angle with bevel up; once blood return occurs, advance catheter until hub is in contact with insertion site
8. Release tourniquet and remove needle from catheter

9. Tape catheter to reduce accidental removal; apply tape in two directions, as common in the H or chevron styles, to reduce risk of accidental removal
10. Connect catheter to IV tubing and apply sterile dressing to insertion site; a label on side of insertion site identifies length and gauge of catheter, date and time of insertion, and nurse's initials
11. Apply date sticker to tubing
12. Initiate prescribed flow rate: gravity flow tubing is regulated by drops per minute, and drops delivered per mL of solution vary with different brands and types of infusion sets (drop drip factor) from 10 to 20 drops/mL; microdrip sets are always 60 drops/mL; to administer 1000 mL in 8 hours with a drip factor of 15 drops/mL, calculate as follows:

$$\frac{\text{Total infusion volume} \times \text{drop factor}}{\text{Total time of infusion in minutes}} = \text{drops/minute}$$

$$\frac{1000 \text{ mL} \times 15}{8 \times 60 \text{ min (480 min)}} = 31.25 \text{ drops/min (31 drops/minute)}$$

13. Dispose of sharps in rigid sharps disposal container
14. Document date, time, solution, amount, infusion device, rate, site location, and condition of site and dressing

C. Maintaining an IV infusion

1. Ensure that correct solution is infusing
2. Check rate of flow every hour or more frequently as per policy for selected situations
3. Inspect patency of IV tubing and needle
4. Maintain solution container 3 feet above IV site for gravity infusion devices; keep bag higher than IV pump when using this device
5. Inspect tubing for kinks or obstructions; ensure that it is not dangling below IV site
6. Check for blood return by lowering solution container below IV site and observe for blood return, or use a sterile syringe to withdraw fluid from port nearest venipuncture site, causing blood to flow into tubing
7. Splint a joint if IV site is positional (movement of extremity impedes flow of solution)
8. Ensure tight connections to prevent leakage
9. Discontinue solution and remove IV access device if there is no blood return and acceptable drip rate cannot be established
10. ! Inspect insertion site for fluid infiltration (IV access device becomes dislodged from vessel, causing fluid to flow into interstitial tissues and other complications); see Table 32–2 ■ for list of complications and associated nursing care
11. Instruct client to notify the nurse of any of the following conditions:
    a. Flow rate changes or solution stops dripping
    b. Solution container is nearly empty
    c. There is blood in IV tubing or at insertion site
    d. There is discomfort or swelling at insertion site
12. At least every 8 hours, document solution, amount, infusion device, rate, site location, and condition of site and dressing

IV. CENTRAL VENOUS ACCESS DEVICES (CVADs)

A. A CVAD enters a central vein that empties into superior vena cava; placement can occur in numerous settings but all placements must be verified by x-ray

1. Percutaneous (nontunneled) catheter: a single or multiple lumen catheters are inserted by physician at client's bedside
2. Tunneled catheter
    a. Terminates in central venous system
    b. Remainder of catheter passes through a subcutaneous tract and exits on chest wall or abdomen

Table 32-2 Complications of IV Therapy

Complication	Nursing Implications
Infection (catheter related) (sepsis)—common occurrence with TPN solutions that have high glucose concentration that invites bacteria; characterized by fever, chills, erythema, or drainage at insertion site, elevated white blood count, and possibly septic shock	Use strict aseptic technique when working with IVs. Change IV solutions at least every 24 hours. Change IV tubing and dressings per agency protocols (TPN tubing every day). When discontinuing central lines, remove tip of catheter and apply an occlusive dressing. Monitor site for 48 hours; the catheter tip may be sent to lab for culture if sepsis is suspected.
Air embolism—air is introduced into the IV line during catheter insertion, tubing change, or administration of solutions and medications; characterized by respiratory distress, chest pain, dyspnea, hypotension, and weak and rapid pulse	When changing tubing or reflux valves on CVADs without Groshong valves or catheters, instruct the client to perform the Valsalva maneuver (forcefully exhale with glottis, nose, and mouth closed). Ensure all catheter connections are tight. Ensure all connections on central lines are luer lock, not slip lock. During insertion of a percutaneous central venous catheter, position the client in head down position with head turned in opposite direction of insertion site. If an air embolism is suspected: • Clamp the catheter. • Position the client in left Trendelenburg's position. • Administer oxygen and contact the physician.
Hypersensitivity reaction—sensitivity to the medication; characterized by flushing, itching, and urticaria	Check client allergies prior to administering medications. Stop the infusion. Notify the physician. Monitor vital signs.
Circulatory overload—also called speed shock; fluids administered faster than the circulation can accommodate; characterized by cough, dyspnea, crackles, distended neck veins, tachycardia, hypertension, S_3 heart sounds, and cardiac rhythm	Use IV pumps or controllers to regulate the infusion rate. Do not "catch up" with IV solutions. Carefully monitor fluid volumes with administration of multiple concurrent IV solutions or medications. Check the client's IV infusion rates at least hourly per agency protocols. Avoid selecting an IV container with a larger volume than the volume ordered. Monitor the client's vital signs, intake and output, breath and heart sounds. For signs and symptoms of fluid volume overload: • Slow or stop the infusion rate per order. • Place the client in high Fowler's position. • Administer oxygen and diuretics per order. • Notify the physician.
Infiltration—localized swelling, coolness, pallor, and discomfort at the IV site	Stop the IV and remove the venous access device. Apply a warm compress to the site of the infiltration and elevate the extremity on a pillow. Restart the infusion at another site.
Phlebitis—inflammation of a vein; characterized by warmth, swelling, red streak at vein site, pain along the course of the vein, and localized warmth	Inspect and palpate the IV site at least every 8 hours for redness; if phlebitis is detected, discontinue the infusion and remove the venous access device. A medical order is not required to remove and replace a peripheral catheter that shows symptoms of phlebitis. Apply warm compresses to the venipuncture site. Select a large vein when administering irritating solutions or medications. Dilute irritating medications (e.g., promethazine [Phenergan]) and administer over prescribed amount of time on an infusion pump; if client complains of pain at the insertion site, further dilute the medication and slow the flow rate.
Hypoglycemia—decreased blood glucose level related to TPN being abruptly discontinued or due to excessive insulin administration; characterized by blood glucose less than 70 mg/dL, hunger, diaphoresis, weakness and anxiety	Monitor blood glucose per agency protocols (at least every day). Gradually decrease infusion when discontinuing TPN. Have 10% dextrose available as stand-by (medical order required for prn use).
Hyperglycemia—increased blood glucose related to TPN administration or administration of excessive dextrose solutions to diabetic clients; characterized by blood glucose greater than 200 mg/dL, excessive thirst, fatigue, restlessness, confusion, weakness, and diuresis	Monitor blood glucose per agency protocols (at least every day). Check medications affecting blood glucose levels (e.g., steroids). Begin infusion at a slow rate (40 mL/hr) and gradually increase. Do not "catch up" if infusion rate falls behind.

c. A Dacron cuff on catheter triggers scar formation that prevents ascending tract infection
d. This catheter does not require a sterile dressing once subcutaneous tract has healed

3. PICC
   a. Inserted into basilic or cephalic vein just above or below antecubital space of right arm by a physician or specially trained IV therapy nurse
   b. Used for longer term inpatient or outpatient therapy
   c. Although insertion site is in periphery, catheter terminates in superior vena cava
4. Implantable venous access devices or ports
   a. Surgically implanted into small subcutaneous pocket, usually on upper chest using local anesthesia
   b. Port is attached to catheter that terminates in central venous system
   c. Most subcutaneous ports are accessed with a Huber needle to preserve life of port's septum
5. Peripheral access system (PAS) ports are similar to a subcutaneous port except port itself is implanted in antecubital area

B. Internal tips: internal tip of catheter comes in two versions

1. Open-tipped: end of catheter opens directly into bloodstream; if flushing techniques are not performed correctly, blood can back up into catheter causing catheter occlusion; there are two open-tipped catheters; they must be flushed with saline followed by heparin flush solution to maintain patency when not in use
   a. Hickman: adult form of open-tipped catheter
   b. Broviac: pediatric version, which usually means smaller lumen size
2. Closed-tip catheter or Groshong: has a valve on its internal tip that prevents backflow of blood; Groshong catheters are routinely flushed with double volumes of saline but do not require instillation of heparin flush solution; advantages of Groshong catheter:
   a. Decreased risk of air emboli or bleeding
   b. Elimination of heparin flush
   c. Elimination of catheter clamping
   d. Reduced flushing protocols between use

C. Lumens: central catheters may have a single, double, triple, or quadruple lumen; each lumen corresponds to a separate catheter and has a separate exit point

1. Multiple lumens allow for administration of incompatible drugs
2. Blood drawn from one lumen will not be contaminated by drugs administered through another lumen of catheter
3. Each lumen is treated as a separate catheter and is flushed according to agency policy

D. Indications for use of CVC

1. Long-term IV therapy
2. Obtaining frequent blood specimens
3. Central venous pressure (CVP) monitoring
4. Administration of TPN and medications that are irritating to veins, thus requiring a high-flow vein for rapid dilution
5. Sclerosed peripheral veins
6. Limited peripheral venous access

E. Nursing care

! 1. Special precautions must be taken with all central venous devices to ensure asepsis and catheter patency; refer again to Table 32–2 for complications
2. Site care: subclavian, jugular, and PICC sites
   a. Require air occlusive dressings: dressings should be changed when soiled or loose
   ! b. Follow agency protocol for frequency of dressing changes—usually every 2 to 7 days; gauze dressings must be changed at least every 48 hours; semipermeable transparent membrane dressings may remain in place for up to 1 week
   c. Follow agency protocols for cleaning solutions and types of dressings; isopropyl alcohol followed by povidone-iodine are commonly used to clean insertion site

d. Using surgical asepsis and a mask, clean area 2 inches in diameter around site using alcohol swab; use a circular motion starting at center and work outward; allow to dry, clean with povidone-iodine; allow to dry, then apply air occlusive dressing over entire insertion site

! e. Assess site for redness, swelling, tenderness, or drainage, and compare length of external portion of catheter with its documented length to assess for displacement

f. Document date, condition of site, and dressing

3. Site care: implantable devices

a. Follow agency protocols for cleaning solutions and types of dressings; isopropyl alcohol and povidone-iodine are commonly used to clean insertion site

b. Before accessing port, using aseptic technique, clean an area 2 inches in diameter around the port with an alcohol swab, using a circular motion starting at center and working outward; allow alcohol to dry before cleaning with povidone-iodine; allow to dry before accessing

! c. Assess site for redness, swelling, tenderness, or drainage

d. Access site with an appropriate primed needle, usually a Huber needle; assess for patency by aspirating blood and then flushing according to policy

e. Apply a sterile dressing

4. Catheter care and flushing

a. Each lumen of catheter should be flushed according to agency policy; frequency of flush varies among catheters and may be as often as once a shift; subcutaneous ports that are not in use may not require flushing more often than once a month

b. Volume of flush solution should be at least twice the internal volume of catheter; closed-tip catheters (Groshong) should have flushing volume doubled

c. Flush solution is usually saline; some medications are incompatible with saline, and D_5W may be substituted

d. For closed-tip catheters, saline flush is followed by a heparin flush; volume should approximate internal volume of catheter

! e. Syringes smaller than 10 mL should not be used for flushing because they may contribute to catheter rupture

! f. Have client bear down (Valsalva maneuver) during tubing change and/or ensure catheter is clamped during tubing change; exception is Groshong catheter because of one-way valve

g. Blood draws: use distal lumen if possible; discard appropriate amount of blood prior to obtaining sample; following blood aspiration, flush line with a double volume of saline prior to instillation of weak heparin solution (if appropriate); change injection cap following a blood draw

5. Client teaching: provide clients with these instructions:

a. Do not allow anyone to take a blood pressure on arm with a PICC line or PAS port

b. Wear a Medic-Alert bracelet if device will be implanted for a long time

c. PICC and non-implanted CVADs: no activity restriction is necessary; do not immerse site in water

d. Implanted CVADs: no restriction of activities is necessary; there are no restrictions regarding bathing or swimming when device is not accessed

V. INTRAVENOUS MEDICATION ADMINISTRATION

A. **Mixtures of medications within large volumes of IV fluids** provide and maintain a constant, well-diluted level of a medication in bloodstream

B. **To add medication to an IV solution,** prepare medication from a vial or ampule and draw into a syringe

C. **To add medication to a new IV container**

1. Clean injection port with an alcohol swab and allow to dry for 30 seconds
2. Remove needle cap from syringe, insert needle through center of injection port, and inject medication into IV solution
3. Mix medication and solution by gently rotating bag

4. Complete and attach a medication label to IV solution, with name and dose of medication, date and time, and nurse's initials
5. Proceed with setting up IV for administration

D. To add medication to an existing infusion

1. Ensure that there is enough IV solution in container to properly dilute medication
2. Proceed as with adding a medication to a new IV container

E. Injection by *bolus* or push method

1. Direct injection of a medication intravenously (push) is used to obtain rapid serum concentrations, when medications cannot be diluted, or for administration of emergency drugs
2. With prn adaptor when no solutions are running
   a. Prepare medication, draw up into a syringe, and label syringe so that it will not be confused with syringe containing normal saline irrigating solution
   b. Wash hands and put on gloves
   c. Flush IV access device per agency policy
   d. Cleanse infusion port with an alcohol swab and let it dry for 30 seconds
   e. Remove needle from syringe and attach syringe with medication to needleless port access device
   ! f. Administer medication following recommended IV push rate
   g. Flush IV access device per agency policy

F. Tandem infusion

1. An intermittent method of administering medications to an existing IV (not frequently used)
2. Ensure that existing IV solution and intermittent infusion are compatible and client's condition, vein, and gauge of access device can tolerate volume of fluid
3. Medication will be administered in a second bag of fluid, usually 50 to 100 mL, by secondary line into Y port of a continuously running infusion; attach a needleless adapter to tubing of secondary set
4. Cleanse infusion port of continuous infusion line Y port with an alcohol swab and let it dry for 30 seconds
5. Hang secondary infusion and existing infusion at same level
6. Maintain existing IV rate and regulate piggyback rate using roller clamp on secondary tubing; primary and secondary solutions will run concurrently at their respective rates

G. Piggyback infusion

1. To administer intermittent infusion without disconnecting existing IV
   a. Set up secondary set following procedure for setting up an IV
   b. Hang existing infusion set lower than piggyback secondary set
   c. Cleanse uppermost infusion port with an alcohol swab and let it dry for 30 seconds
   d. Connect secondary set to primary set using a needleless access device placed above existing IV roller clamp
   e. Maintain existing IV roller clamp position, and regulate piggyback rate using roller clamp on secondary tubing; piggyback solution will infuse first, and when complete, existing IV will resume at original rate
2. To administer an intermittent infusion using an infusion pump that is regulating existing IV:
   a. When intermittent solution is in an IV bag, set up secondary administration set following procedure for setting up an IV; connect infusion tubing to secondary access port on pump; follow protocols for specific pump for administering intermittent medication as either a continuous infusion or an infusion interrupting existing IV
   b. When intermittent solution is in a syringe, connect syringe to secondary access port on pump; follow protocols for specific pump for administering intermittent medication as either a continuous infusion or an infusion interrupting existing IV

VI. SPECIAL CONSIDERATIONS IN IV THERAPY

A. **IV lines increase risk of bacteremia and sepsis** by breaking skin as a line of defense

B. **Various preparations (such as Emla cream or intradermal lidocaine) may be used to numb site before IV insertion,** but these are considered to be drugs and must be ordered by a physician

C. **Solutions and medications administered by IV route** act within seconds to minutes and cannot be retrieved once infused or injected

D. **It is a critical nursing responsibility to ensure that medications and IV solutions are compatible before administration;** this includes any additives (such as potassium) to an IV line, not only primary solution and intermittent medication

E. **The young and old are at greater risk of circulatory overload** as a speed-related complication of IV infusion

F. **Clients who have cardiac, renal, respiratory, or liver disease** may also be at greater risk of circulatory overload as a speed-related complication of IV infusion

! G. **Certain IV additives should be avoided in specific disease states**

1. Clients with diabetes mellitus should not receive dextrose
2. Clients with heart failure or otherwise at risk for excess fluid volume should not receive sodium in IV fluids; if sodium-containing solutions are necessary, they should be infused cautiously and with use of an IV pump
3. Clients with liver disease should not receive lactated Ringer's because of possible lack of ability to convert lactate to bicarbonate
4. Clients with renal failure should not receive potassium additives in IV solutions because they cannot excrete it

VII. DISCONTINUING AN IV

A. Indications

1. Client is able to take fluids orally
2. IV medication is no longer needed
3. Access route for emergency fluid and medication administration is no longer needed

B. Procedure

1. Gather equipment: (2 × 2 gauze, clean gloves, and tape)
2. Explain procedure to client
3. Turn off IV infusion
4. Apply gloves and loosen dressing and tape by peeling edges back; stabilize catheter to prevent vein injury
5. Fold sterile gauze in half or quarters and hold steadily over insertion site while withdrawing IV catheter flush to skin; apply pressure when catheter is completely removed from vein
6. ! Hold pressure for 2 minutes or until bleeding stops; assess site for bleeding, redness, or hematoma formation; apply clean gauze and tape in place
7. Inspect catheter tip to be sure it is intact
8. ! Document procedure and volume of IV fluid infused
9. Recheck site in 15 minutes for redness, swelling, or hematoma formation

Check Your NCLEX-RN® Exam I.Q.

You are ready for testing on this content if you can

- Utilize nursing knowledge and skills in the care of a client receiving IV therapy via a peripheral or central vein.
- Assess and monitor a client receiving IV therapy, including an infusion pump.
- Initiate, maintain, and discontinue a client's IV using appropriate technique.
- Document accurately a peripheral or central IV infusion.
- Monitor a client for complications of IV therapy.
- Provide care to a client with a central venous access device.
- Provide client teaching about IV therapy.

PRACTICE TEST

1 A client has a continuously running peripheral infusion. The physician orders an antibiotic as a piggyback infusion 4 times a day. In order to administer the antibiotic, the nurse should do which of the following?

1. Start a new IV access to administer the antibiotic so that there will not be compatibility issues.
2. Start a new IV access to eliminate the problem of too much volume for one site.
3. Increase the flow rate of the continuous infusion to facilitate the administration of the antibiotic.
4. Check to see if the antibiotic is compatible with the continuous infusion.

2 The family of a home infusion client calls the home health nurse one night to report that the electronic infusion pump is alarming. The nurse anticipates that the infusion pump alarm could be caused by which of the following?

1. The client's pulse and blood pressure falling
2. The client experiencing a reaction to the medication
3. The infusion is complete or there is an occlusion
4. An incompatibility with the medications

3 The home health nurse is monitoring a client who performs self-care of a central line. The nurse observes the client doing all of the following activities. Which activity indicates the need for further education?

1. Flushing the central line with a 3 mL syringe
2. Cleaning the needleless injection cap with alcohol before accessing
3. Using sterile gloves to change the central line dressing
4. Wearing a mask while changing the central line dressing

4 The client has a tunneled Groshong catheter for intermittent medication administration. After administering the medication, the nurse prepares to do which of the following?

1. Clamp the catheter.
2. Flush the catheter with saline, then heparin.
3. Flush the catheter with saline.
4. Ask the client to perform the Valsalva maneuver when the medication IV tubing is disconnected.

5 The client has a percutaneous jugular central venous line that is capped and used for intermittent infusions. After administering the medication, the best method to maintain patency is to do which of the following?

1. Flush the line first with 3–5 mL of normal saline, then with 1–3 mL of heparinized normal saline.
2. Flush the line with 3–5 mL of normal saline.
3. Flush the line with 3–5 mL of heparinized normal saline.
4. Flush the line first with 3–5 mL of heparin, then with 1–3 mL of normal saline.

6 The nurse is caring for a client with a Hickman central line. While changing the central line dressing, the nurse notes that the injection cap (heplock adapter) is of the slip lock variety instead of a luer lock device. The nurse recognizes that this adapter puts the client at risk for which of the following complications?

1. Sepsis
2. Occlusion
3. Phlebitis
4. Air embolism

7 The client is to receive vancomycin (Vancocin), an intravenous medication. To prevent adverse reactions from rapid infusion, the nurse would plan to administer this drug using which of the following methods?

1. By gravity
2. With a regulator
3. By electronic infusion pump
4. In an elastomeric pump

8 The physician is going to order a hypotonic intravenous solution for a client with cellular dehydration. The nurse would expect which of the following fluids to be administered?

1. 0.9% normal saline
2. 5% dextrose in normal saline
3. Lactated Ringer's solution
4. 0.45% sodium chloride

PRACTICE TEST

9 The nurse is caring for several clients with central venous catheters. While changing the tubing on the central lines, the nurse would not need to instruct the client to perform a Valsalva maneuver when the client has which of the following catheters?

1. Groshong catheter
2. Single-lumen catheter
3. Percutaneous catheter
4. Accessed subcutaneous venous port

10 The client is receiving 5% dextrose in 0.45% normal saline. The physician has ordered the client receive one unit of packed cells. Prior to hanging the blood, the nurse will prime the blood tubing with which of the following solutions?

1. 5% dextrose
2. Lactated Ringer's
3. 0.9% sodium chloride
4. 5% dextrose in 0.45% sodium chloride

11 While assessing a client's intravenous (IV) line, the nurse notes that the area is swollen, cool, pale, and causes the client discomfort. The nurse documents which of the following complications of IV therapy?

1. Infiltration
2. Phlebitis
3. Infection
4. Air embolism

12 The client is receiving 5% dextrose and 0.45% sodium chloride intravenously and is complaining of pain at the IV site. The nurse assesses the site and notes erythema and edema. Which of the following would be the appropriate nursing action?

1. Slow the infusion rate.
2. Discontinue the IV and apply a warm compress to the IV site.
3. Apply antibiotic ointment to the IV site.
4. Gently pull back the IV access device to reposition within the vein.

13 The nurse is starting a new peripheral intravenous (IV) line in a client. The client reports a latex allergy. The nurse has a typical IV start kit. Because of the latex allergy, the nurse should take which of the following actions?

1. Utilize a new tourniquet for this client.
2. Utilize a blood pressure cuff to distend the vein.
3. Avoid putting povidone iodine on the skin.
4. Suggest an alternative therapy to a peripheral intravenous line.

14 The nurse is inserting an intravenous (IV) line into a client. After piercing the skin and entering the vein, the nurse would refrain from advancing the catheter if which of the following were noted?

1. Blood backflow into the IV catheter
2. Mild resistance with advancement
3. No reports of client discomfort
4. The IV catheter was inserted bevel side up

15 The nurse is inserting a peripheral intravenous (IV) line. Place the following steps in order to perform this procedure correctly.

1. _____ Apply tourniquet.
2. _____ Insert catheter at 5 to 15 degree angle through skin
3. _____ Select vein
4. _____ Attach tubing primed with IV solution
5. _____ Gather equipment

ANSWERS & RATIONALES

1 **Answer: 4** Before making a decision about how to infuse the antibiotic, the nurse should check compatibility of the antibiotic with the continuous IV solution. If the drug and the infusion were compatible, they would be run at the same time. If the drug and infusion were incompatible, the nurse would stop the infusion during the period of antibiotic administration and flush the line carefully before and after the antibiotic. It is often inadvisable to start a second IV site unless absolutely necessary. The other answers are incorrect. **Cognitive Level:** Application **Client Need:** Physiological Integrity: Pharmacological and Parenteral Therapies **Integrated Process:** Nursing Process: Implementation **Content Area:** Fundamentals **Strategy:** The core issue of the question is the knowledge that it is critical to check for compatibilities when infusing IV solutions through the same line. Use this knowledge and the process of elimination to make a selection.

2 **Answer: 3** Alarms sound on electronic infusion devices when the infusion is complete, there is an occlusion, air is in the line, the battery is low, or the cassette is improperly loaded. The other answers are incorrect reasons for an alarm. **Cognitive Level:** Analysis **Client Need:** Physiological Integrity: Pharmacological and Parenteral Therapies **Integrated Process:** Nursing Process: Analysis **Content Area:** Fundamentals **Strategy:** The core issue of this question is the ability to interpret the

ANSWERS & RATIONALES

significance of an alarm on an infusion pump. Use knowledge of pump function in general and the process of elimination to make a selection.

3 **Answer: 1** All catheters should be flushed with syringes with barrels of 10 mLs or larger. The smaller the barrel size, the greater the pressure that comes from the tip. Smaller syringes could damage the catheter. All other activities are done correctly.
Cognitive Level: Analysis **Client Need:** Physiological Integrity: Pharmacological and Parenteral Therapies **Integrated Process:** Nursing Process: Evaluation **Content Area:** Fundamentals **Strategy:** The wording of the question tells you the correct option is an incorrect statement. Use knowledge of IV catheter flush protocols and the process of elimination to make a selection.

4 **Answer: 3** Groshong catheters have a three-way pressure-sensitive valve that restricts air from entering the venous system and prevents backflow of blood; therefore, the catheter should not be clamped and the client does not need to perform the Valsalva maneuver. The catheter is designed so that only saline is used to flush. The other answers are incorrect actions for catheter maintenance.
Cognitive Level: Application **Client Need:** Physiological Integrity: Pharmacological and Parenteral Therapies **Integrated Process:** Nursing Process: Implementation **Content Area:** Fundamentals **Strategy:** The core issue of the question is knowledge of proper management and care of Groshong catheters. Use this knowledge and the process of elimination to make a selection.

5 **Answer: 1** Although it is not necessary to flush peripheral capped access devices with heparinized normal saline (100 or 10 units per 1 mL of normal saline), central venous access devices that are not Groshong catheters are flushed per agency protocols with heparinized normal saline. When medications are administered, the access device is first flushed with normal saline, then with heparinized normal saline. Heparin is incompatible with many medications, and for this reason, normal saline is used prior to the administration of heparinized saline that maintains patency of the catheter. The other answers are incorrect procedure.
Cognitive Level: Application **Client Need:** Physiological Integrity: Pharmacological and Parenteral Therapies **Integrated Process:** Nursing Process: Implementation **Content Area:** Fundamentals **Strategy:** The core issue of the question is knowledge of proper management and care of central venous catheters. Use this knowledge and the process of elimination to make a selection.

6 **Answer: 4** One of the complications of IV therapy is air embolism—introduction of air into the vein. Air embolism can be prevented by using luer lock devices on all attachments. The other responses are unrelated to this connection.
Cognitive Level: Analysis **Client Need:** Physiological Integrity: Pharmacological and Parenteral Therapies **Integrated Process:** Nursing Process: Analysis **Content Area:** Fundamentals **Strategy:** The core issue of the question is the ability of the nurse to detect situations that could lead to complications of IV therapy. Use knowledge of these risks to aid in making a selection.

7 **Answer: 3** The device that provides the most accurate infusion rate is the electronic infusion pump. The other devices are less accurate and less controllable.
Cognitive Level: Analysis **Client Need:** Physiological Integrity: Pharmacological and Parenteral Therapies **Integrated Process:** Nursing Process: Planning **Content Area:** Fundamentals **Strategy:** The core issue of the question is the best method to prevent speed-related adverse reactions from a drug infused by IV. Use knowledge of IV infusion devices and the process of elimination to make a selection.

8 **Answer: 4** 0.45% sodium chloride (½ normal saline) is a hypotonic solution that draws fluid from the vascular compartment into the cells. Normal saline and lactated Ringer's are isotonic solutions, while 5% dextrose in normal saline is a hypertonic solution until the glucose is metabolized, then it is isotonic.
Cognitive Level: Application **Client Need:** Physiological Integrity: Pharmacological and Parenteral Therapies **Integrated Process:** Nursing Process: Planning **Content Area:** Fundamentals **Strategy:** The core issue of the question is knowledge of the tonicity of various intravenous solutions. Use this knowledge and the process of elimination to make a selection.

9 **Answer: 1** The Groshong catheter is designed with a three-way pressure-sensitive valve that restricts air from entering the venous system and prevents backflow of blood. The other options do not have this protection.
Cognitive Level: Application **Client Need:** Physiological Integrity: Pharmacological and Parenteral Therapies **Integrated Process:** Nursing Process: Implementation **Content Area:** Fundamentals **Strategy:** The core issue of the question is knowledge of various central venous catheters and which one poses the least risk of air embolism requiring Valsalva maneuver. Use this knowledge and the process of elimination to make a selection.

10 **Answer: 3** 0.9% sodium chloride (normal saline) is the only solution that can be administered with blood or blood products. Other solutions may cause the blood cells to clump or cause clotting. The other options are incorrect.
Cognitive Level: Application **Client Need:** Physiological Integrity: Pharmacological and Parenteral Therapies **Integrated Process:** Nursing Process: Implementation **Content Area:** Fundamentals **Strategy:** The core issue of the question is the knowledge that only normal saline is compatible with any blood product. Use this knowledge and the process of elimination to make a selection.

11 **Answer: 1** Infiltration is leakage of fluids into the surrounding tissues, resulting in edema around the insertion site, blanching, and coolness of skin around the site. The other options would not have these manifestations.
Cognitive Level: Analysis **Client Need:** Physiological Integrity: Pharmacological and Parenteral Therapies **Integrated Process:** Communication and Documentation **Content Area:** Fundamentals **Strategy:** The core issue of the question is the ability to accurately interpret an IV complication. Use knowledge of various IV complications and the process of elimination to make a selection.

12 **Answer: 2** Continuing the infusion at that site would only increase the phlebitis. The IV is discontinued and restarted at a

ANSWERS & RATIONALES

new site. Applying a warm compress to an area of phlebitis dilates the vessel, improving circulation, and reduces the resistance to blood flow from within the vein reducing the pain. The other options are incorrect.

Cognitive Level: Application **Client Need:** Physiological Integrity: Pharmacological and Parenteral Therapies **Integrated Process:** Nursing Process: Implementation **Content Area:** Fundamentals **Strategy:** The core issue of the question is the ability to accurately interpret an IV complication. Use knowledge of various IV complications and the process of elimination to make a selection.

13 **Answer: 2** Tourniquets are made of latex. A blood pressure cuff can be used as an alternative method of vein distention. A new tourniquet may not resolve the latex issue. The other responses do not address the latex issue.

Cognitive Level: Analysis **Client Need:** Safe Effective Care Environment: Safety and Infection Control **Integrated Process:** Nursing Process: Planning **Content Area:** Fundamentals **Strategy:** The core issue of the question is providing for safety of the client who has a latex allergy. Use this knowledge and the process of elimination to make a selection.

14 **Answer: 2** The nurse would refrain from advancing the catheter if mild resistance is noted. The other data are normal. The IV should be inserted bevel side up. The client should not experience pain, and a backflow is normal on insertion, indicating that the vein has been pierced.

Cognitive Level: Application **Client Need:** Physiological Integrity: Pharmacological and Parenteral Therapies **Integrated Process:** Nursing Process: Implementation **Content Area:** Fundamentals **Strategy:** The core issue of the question is knowledge of normal IV insertion procedure. Use this knowledge and the process of elimination to make a selection.

15 **Answer: 5, 3, 1, 2, 4** The first step is to gather equipment. The nurse then selects a vein and cleanses the site. The nurse applies a tourniquet and inserts the catheter. Finally, the nurse attaches the primed tubing and regulates the drip rate. Additional steps are to release the tourniquet, continue to assess the site, apply a dressing, and document the procedure.

Cognitive Level: Analysis **Client Need:** Physiological Integrity: Pharmacological and Parenteral Therapies **Integrated Process:** Nursing Process: Implementation **Content Area:** Fundamentals **Strategy:** Use this knowledge and the process of elimination to make a selection.

Key Terms to Review

bolus p. 521

intravenous p. 513

References

Ball, J., & Bindler, R. (2006). *Child health nursing: Partnering with children and families.* Upper Saddle River, NJ: Pearson Education.

Black, J., & Hawks, J. (2005). *Medical surgical nursing: Clinical management for positive outcomes* (7th ed.). St. Louis, MO: Elsevier Science.

Harkreader, H., & Hogan, M. (2004). *Fundamentals of nursing: Caring and clinical judgment* (2nd ed.). St. Louis, MO: Elsevier Science.

Ignatavicius, D., & Workman, L. (2006). *Medical-surgical nursing: Critical thinking for collaborative care* (5th ed.). Philadelphia: W. B. Saunders.

Kozier, B., Erb, G., Berman, A., & Snyder, S. (2004). *Fundamentals of nursing: Concepts, process, and practice* (7th ed.). Upper Saddle River, NJ: Pearson Education.

LeMone, P., & Burke, K. (2004). *Medical surgical nursing: Critical thinking in client care* (3rd ed.). Upper Saddle River, NJ: Pearson Education.

Lewis, S., Heitkemper, M., & Dirksen, S. (2004). *Medical surgical nursing: Assessment and management of clinical problems* (6th ed.). St. Louis, MO: Elsevier Science.

Smeltzer, S., Bare, B., & Boyer, M. (2006). *Brunner & Suddarth's textbook of medical surgical nursing:* (11th ed.). Philadelphia: Lippincott Williams & Wilkins.

Smith, S., Duell, D., & Martin, B. (2004). *Clinical nursing skills: Basic to advanced skills* (6th ed.). Upper Saddle River, NJ: Pearson Education.

Blood and Blood Component Therapy 33

In this chapter

Test Yourself

Are you ready for the NCLEX-RN® or course exams? Use the practice tests on the companion CD-ROM to check.

Cross reference

Other chapters relevant to this content area are:

Intravenous Therapy Chapter 32

I. SOURCES OF BLOOD FOR TRANSFUSION

A. Anonymous donor

1. An anonymous individual who donates blood to a blood bank
2. Donors must be at least 17 years old
3. May donate one unit (pint) every 8 weeks (56 days)

B. *Designated donor*

1. A donor who has volunteered to donate for a client or has been selected by client; is often a relative who has compatible blood
2. Does not reduce risk for transmission of blood-borne infections
3. Client often has less anxiety about receiving blood products from a known donor

C. *Autologous donor*

1. Client donates own blood for future transfusion
2. ! Process begins 4 to 6 weeks before scheduled surgery or procedure and ends at least 3 days before transfusion date
3. ! May donate every 3 days as long as hemoglobin level is satisfactory (no less than 11 grams/dL); iron supplements may be ordered
4. Especially useful for clients who have a rare blood type, history of transfusion reactions, and to prevent transmission of blood-borne viral infections
5. ! Contraindicated in clients with acute infection (including bacteremia), leukemia, significant cardiovascular or cerebrovascular disease, hemoglobin less than 11 grams/dL, or hematocrit less than 33%

D. *Blood salvage*

1. A type of autologous donation in which blood is suctioned (often during or after surgery) from body cavities, joint spaces, or other enclosed areas; an example is chest tube drainage following cardiac surgery
2. Blood may be "washed" to remove cellular and tissue debris before reinfusion into client

Table 33–1

Blood Group Compatibility

Blood Group	Can be donor for:	Can be recipient of:
0	0, A, B, AB (universal donor)	0
A	A, AB	0, A
B	B, AB	0, B
AB	AB	0, A, B, AB (universal receiver)

II. COMPATIBILITY

A. ***Compatibility* testing consists of several specific tests** done to ensure that a client receives blood or a blood product that will not lead to transfusion reaction

! B. **Client's blood is typed to determine blood group (see Table 33–1 ■) and Rh type (positive or negative)**

C. **Antibody screening may also be done (e.g., order reads "type and screen")** to detect antibodies other than anti-A and anti-B; this is often ordered when client might need blood at some time in very near future

D. ***Cross-match* is ordered (e.g., order reads "type and cross-match") when a unit of blood is to be transfused to client;** donor red blood cells (RBCs) are added to recipient's serum and Coomb's serum; if no RBCs agglutinate, the cross-match is compatible

! E. **After a sample of client's blood is drawn for typing, a special identification bracelet, often called a blood bank bracelet, is placed on client's wrist;** this bracelet has a unique blood donor number that must be matched to blood identification tag on any unit of blood client receives

III. BLOOD COMPONENTS

A. **Whole blood**

1. Replaces intravascular blood volume and all blood products; contains red blood cells, plasma, plasma proteins, fresh platelets, and other clotting factors
2. May occasionally be used for rapid treatment of hypovolemic shock caused by hemorrhage; otherwise not commonly used today
3. Each unit (approximately 500 mL) contains RBCs, plasma, and plasma proteins (including clotting factors), all of which are lost during hemorrhage
4. Intended outcome is resolution of symptoms of hypovolemic shock caused by hemorrhage

B. **Red blood cells (RBCs)**

1. Used to replace erythrocytes lost because of anemia or actual blood loss; they increase oxygen-carrying capacity of blood
2. ! Often contain a volume of 250 mL, although can be supplied in bags containing up to 400 mL; check bag for actual volume
3. ! Each transfused unit should raise hemoglobin by 1 gram/dL and hematocrit by 2 to 3%; blood sample should be drawn at 4 to 6 hours posttransfusion (not earlier) to evaluate effectiveness
4. Intended outcome is that client has increased RBC count and that symptoms of anemia (such as fatigue) resolve

C. **Fresh frozen plasma (FFP)**

1. Contains clotting factors and aids in volume expansion (though volume expansion is not primary purpose for use); RBCs and platelets have been removed
2. Requires ABO and Rh compatibility testing prior to use
3. A unit of FFP is often 200 to 250 mL in volume, but actual volume is labeled on the bag
4. ! Infuse as rapidly as possible and within 6 hours of thawing; this preserves viability of clotting factors as well as reducing risk of septicemia
5. Intended outcome is return to normal of coagulation studies, such as partial thromboplastin time and prothrombin time

D. **Platelets**

1. Play an important role in blood coagulation, homeostasis, and blood thrombus formation; used to treat thrombocytopenia or dysfunctional platelets

2. A transfusion of platelets can range from a volume of 50 to 70 mL or as high as 200 to 400 mL, depending on client condition and need; actual volume is noted on bag
3. Infuse as rapidly as possible immediately after obtaining from blood bank
4. Intended outcome is improved platelet counts at 1 hour and 24 hours posttranfusion

E. Albumin

1. Expands blood volume by providing plasma proteins that cannot diffuse through capillary walls
2. Increased osmotic pressure in blood vessels causing interstitial fluids to move back into vascular compartment
3. Used to treat hypovolemic shock
4. A bottle of albumin 25 grams/100 mL provides albumin content equal to that found in 500 mL of blood
5. Intended outcome is improved serum albumin level and resolution of hypovolemic shock and/or severe edema

F. Cryoprecipitate

1. Replaces various clotting factors found in blood, such as factor VIII, factor XIII, fibronectin, and fibrinogen; concentrates of factor VIII and IX are also available
2. Is prepared from fresh frozen plasma and must be used immediately upon thawing
3. Intended outcome is improved blood clotting times and/or serum fibrinogen level

IV. ADMINISTRATION OF BLOOD PRODUCTS

A. Safe administration of blood products is a vital concern to client and nurse

B. For proper procedure for administering blood, see Box 33–1

C. Additional safety concerns

1. Blood products will be released from blood bank only to personnel specified in agency policy
2. All agencies have very specific procedures related to blood product procurement and use
3. Do not store blood in any unit refrigerator; blood can be stored only in designated blood bank refrigerators
4. Do not add any medications or any solution other than normal saline to blood or blood products
5. Infuse blood product according to recommended timeframe, which may vary with type of blood product being given
6. To reduce risk of septicemia, change blood administration set every 4 hours or with each unit of blood
7. A filter is used for every blood transfusion; this is standardly built into blood administration tubing, but nurse should check to see that one is present

V. COMPLICATIONS

A. *Transfusion reaction*

1. Types of reaction are hypersensitivity, hemolytic, febrile, and bacterial reactions
2. Prescreen clients for risk by asking whether they have ever had a transfusion, a reaction to it, and what the symptoms were
3. Assessment: see Table 33–2 ■
4. Delayed reaction can occur days to months after a transfusion and manifests with increased temperature, decreased hematocrit and mild jaundice
5. Management
   a. Stop transfusion of blood or blood product
   b. Maintain IV access with infusion of normal saline (0.9% sodium chloride)
   c. Assess client and measure vital signs as often as every 5 minutes; do not leave client unattended
   d. Ensure that blood bank and physician are notified
   e. Provide supportive care and be ready to administer medications according to type of reaction; see Table 33–2 again
   f. Draw blood sample according to policy for culture, retyping, and/or hemoglobin and hematocrit level

Box 33–1

Procedure for Blood Administration

➤ Verify client consent and obtain baseline vital signs prior to initiating transfusion (some agencies require a physician's order to administer blood with a temperature elevation greater than 100°F).

➤ Ensure a suitable vein and appropriate gauge needle (18- or 20-gauge preferred; must be large enough to allow blood to infuse without damaging cells).

➤ Set up the blood infusion equipment:

- Obtain a Y-set with a blood filter; using aseptic technique, insert the spike into a container of 0.9% sodium chloride (normal saline) and prime the tubing. Ensure that the solution covers the filter and one third of the drip chamber above the filter. Back-prime the other Y leg with saline. Never use a solution containing dextrose because it will cause the blood to clump.
- Start the saline solution just prior to hanging the unit of blood.

➤ Obtain the correct blood component from the blood bank by checking the requisition form against the blood bag label with the lab technician. Verify client's name, identification number, blood type (A, B, AB, or O) and Rh group, blood donor number, and expiration date. Note any abnormal color, RBC clumping, gas bubbles, and extraneous material. Refuse to accept any blood product if date is expired or any abnormalities are noted.

➤ With another nurse, compare the client's identification bracelet against the tag on the unit of blood; ask the client to state and spell name, ask date of birth, and compare the name and identification number (located on the client's blood bank ID band), number on the blood bag label, and ABO group and Rh type on the blood bag label. If the information does not match exactly, notify the blood bank and do not administer the blood. Sign the appropriate form with the other nurse according to agency protocol.

➤ Immediately hang the blood—blood must be hung within 30 minutes of receipt from the blood bank:

- Wash hands and don gloves.
- Invert the blood bag gently several times to mix the cells with the plasma.
- Insert remaining Y-set spike into the blood bag.
- Open the upper clamp on the Y-set arm to the blood.
- Close the upper clamp below the IV saline solution and open the upper clamp below the blood bag to allow the blood to run into the saline-filled drip chamber.

➤ Begin transfusion at a slow rate of about 2 mL per minute; stay with the client and check vital signs every 5–15 minutes for the first 50–100 mL of blood transfused, monitoring for reactions: bacterial, allergic, or hemolytic.

➤ After the first 15 minutes, the rate of infusion is increased. An entire unit of blood must be administered within 4 hours, but often infuses in approximately 2 hours if the client can tolerate the speed and volume in that timeframe.

➤ Continue to monitor vital signs and lung sounds every hour until 1 hour after transfusion is complete.

➤ Document the procedure and client's reaction in the client's medical record.

g. Obtain urine specimen for hemoglobin measurement; observe voidings for hematuria

h. Return blood product bag, tubing, labels, and transfusion record to blood bank

B. Circulatory overload (formerly called speed shock)

1. Results from excessively rapid infusion of blood product beyond what client's circulatory system can tolerate

! 2. Assessment: signs of fluid overload

a. Tachycardia and bounding pulse

b. Hypertension

c. Distended neck veins

d. Crackles upon lung auscultation, dyspnea, and possibly cough

Table 33-2

Blood Transfusion Reactions

Type and cause	Assessment	Management
Hypersensitivity (antibodies in donor blood)	Fever Urticaria Anaphylactic shock	Airway management/oxygen Supportive care including treatment of shock state Diphenhydramine (Benadryl)
Febrile (nonspecific and most common)		Premedication with acetaminophen (Tylenol) or aspirin Airway management/oxygen Supportive care
Hemolytic (blood incompatibility)	Nausea and vomiting Lower back pain Tachycardia Hypotension Hematuria and decreased urine output	Airway management/oxygen Supportive care Diphenhydramine (Benadryl)
Bacterial (septicemia from contaminated blood product)	Fever and chills Tachycardia Hypotension/shock	Blood culture Antibiotic therapy Fluid resuscitation Vasopressors Corticosteroids

! 3. Management
   a. Slow infusion rate
   b. Elevate head of bed to upright with feet dependent
   c. Assess for cardiac dysrhythmias
   d. Notify physician
   e. Supportive care includes orders for oxygen and diuretics; morphine sulfate may be prescribed for vasodilating effect

C. Blood-borne infection (communicable disease)
1. Screening techniques and antibody testing of donor blood have greatly reduced this risk
2. Specific disease risks include hepatitis B and C, human immunodeficiency virus, Epstein-Barr virus, cytomegalovirus, human T-cell leukemia, and malaria

D. Electrolyte imbalances
1. Hyperkalemia
   a. Occurs when potassium is released from hemolyzed cells in stored blood
   b. Risk is greater to those with renal disease; therefore, these clients should receive fresh blood or blood that has not been stored very long
   c. Monitor serum potassium level and signs of hyperkalemia (see Chapter 54)
   ! d. Slow tranfusion rate, notify physician, and carefully assess cardiac status if signs of hyperkalemia occur
2. Hypocalcemia
   a. Occurs when calcium binds with citrate in banked blood and is excreted from body
   b. Clients receiving multiple transfusions are at greater risk
   c. Monitor serum calcium level and for signs of hypocalcemia (see Chapter 54)
   ! d. Slow tranfusion rate, notify physician, and carefully assess client status if signs of hypocalcemia occur (such as twitching of cheek, called Chvostek's sign)

E. Iron overload
1. Occurs only in those requiring repeated transfusions over time; is a delayed complication of transfusion
2. Assessment findings include nausea and vomiting, hypotension, and elevated iron level in blood
! 3. Management: administer desferoxamine (Desferal) subcutaneously or intravenously to clear iron via kidneys; teach client that urine will appear red during exretion of iron; monitor serum iron levels

PRACTICE TEST

Check Your NCLEX–RN® Exam I.Q. *You are ready for testing on this content if you can*

- Safely administer blood and blood products.
- Monitor a client during administration of blood and blood products.
- Complete proper documentation of blood and blood product therapy.
- Monitor the client's response to therapy with blood and blood products.

PRACTICE TEST

1 A nurse has obtained a unit of packed red blood cells (RBCs) from the blood bank. She and another nurse have confirmed that it is the correct blood for the patient. Immediately prior to starting the blood transfusion, the nurse should assess which of the following?

1. Vital signs
2. Skin color
3. Hemoglobin level
4. Creatinine clearance

2 A nurse is preparing to administer a unit of packed red blood cells (RBCs). When obtaining the necessary supplies, the nurse would obtain which of the following IV solutions to hang with the unit of blood?

1. Ringer's lactate
2. 5% dextrose in 0.9% sodium chloride
3. 5% dextrose in 0.45% sodium chloride
4. 0.9% sodium chloride

3 A nurse returns to evaluate a client who has been receiving a blood transfusion for the past 30 minutes. The client is observed to be dyspneic. Upon assessment, the nurse auscultates the presence of crackles in the lung bases and an apical heart rate of 110 beats per minute. The nurse suspects that the client is experiencing which of the following complications associated with blood transfusions?

1. Immune response to transfusion
2. Hypovolemia
3. Fluid overload
4. Polycythemia vera

4 A nurse determines that a client receiving a unit of packed red blood cells (RBCs) is experiencing a transfusion reaction. The nurse promptly stops the blood transfusion and does which of the following next?

1. Contact the physician
2. Obtain a white blood cell count
3. Run normal saline at keep vein open (KVO) rate
4. Infuse a normal saline bolus

5 A client arrives at the emergency department following a gunshot wound. The client is actively bleeding and has been taking warfarin (Coumadin) therapy. His prothrombin time is twice the desired amount. You expect that the physician will order a transfusion with which of the following blood products:

1. Fresh frozen plasma
2. Random donor platelets
3. Red blood cells
4. Crystalloids

6 An adult female client has a hemoglobin level of 9.2 grams/dL. A nurse interprets that this is most likely related to which of the following conditions?

1. Leukemia
2. Amenorrhea
3. Vitamin B_{12} deficiency anemia
4. Iron deficiency anemia

7 A nurse has received an order to transfuse a client with one unit of packed red blood cells (RBCs). In preparation for the infusion, the nurse selects the appropriate tubing for blood administration. The nurse is aware that the tubing is manufactured with which of the following?

1. A macrodrip chamber
2. An air vent
3. An in-line filter
4. Tinting that protects blood from exposure to light

8 A postoperative client is to receive a transfusion of platelets because of a critically low platelet count. The client requests information on the benefits of the transfusion. In response to the client's request, the nurse answers with which of the following statements?

1. Improvement of hemoglobin and hematocrit
2. Prevention of deep vein thrombosis
3. Decrease in bleeding from surgical site
4. Return of prothrombin time to expected range

9 The nurse has received an order to transfuse two units of packed red blood cells (RBCs) to a client over 2 hours each. The nurse notes after obtaining the first unit that it contains 350 mL. At what hourly rate would the nurse administer the infusion? Provide a numerical answer.

Answer: _____ mL/hour

10 A nurse has received a report on a client being admitted with anemia who requires a blood transfusion. The nurse will anticipate which of the following assessment findings? Select all that apply.

1. Tachycardia
2. Hypertension
3. Headache
4. Diaphoresis
5. Bounding peripheral pulses

11 A client is scheduled for elective surgery in 4 weeks. When the nurse in the surgeon's office initiates preoperative education, the client expresses concern regarding the potential need for a blood transfusion. The nurse's best response is which of the following:

1. "It is unlikely that you will lose that much blood during the surgery."
2. "Blood transfusions are safer now than in the past."
3. "Your family may be able to donate blood for you."
4. "You may want to consider an autologous blood transfusion."

12 A nurse is caring for an immunocompromised client with cancer. A nurse would consider implementing neutropenic precautions when the client's white blood cell (WBC) count is:

1. 10,500/mm^3
2. 7,650/mm^3
3. 6,000/mm^3
4. 2,000/mm^3

13 A client has experienced an adverse reaction shortly after a blood transfusion is initiated. The nurse documents the event according to hospital policy and does which of the following with the remainder of the blood that has not been transfused?

1. Discards the blood in the appropriate biohazard bag
2. Returns the blood to the blood bank
3. Sends the blood to the chemistry laboratory for analysis
4. Sends the blood to the infection control department

14 A client with a low hemoglobin and hematocrit is to receive a unit of packed red blood cells (RBCs). Prior to initiating the transfusion, the nurse determines that the client's temperature is 100.8°F orally. The most appropriate action for the nurse to take is which of the following?

1. Delay hanging the blood and notify the physician.
2. Begin the transfusion as prescribed.
3. Administer 650mg of acetaminophen (Tylenol) and begin the transfusion.
4. Administer an antihistamine and begin the transfusion.

15 A client presents to the emergency department following a motorcycle accident. The client is in hypovolemic shock. The health care provider has ordered plasma expansion. The nurse anticipates that the client will be transfused with which of the following blood products?

1. Packed red blood cells
2. Cryoprecipitate
3. Platelets
4. Albumin

16 A client has received a granulocyte transfusion. The nurse will assess which of the following labs to determine if the client has benefited from the transfusion?

1. Hemoglobin and hematocrit
2. Erythrocytes
3. White blood cells
4. Platelets

17 A client has experienced an adverse reaction to a blood transfusion. The client is found to have a pruritic rash and urticaria. The nurse anticipates that which of the following medications will be ordered for the client?

1. Diphenhydramine (Benadryl)
2. Acetaminophen (Tylenol)
3. Hydrocortisone cream
4. Acetylsalicylic acid (Aspirin)

ANSWERS & RATIONALES

1. **Answer: 1** Vital signs are taken immediately prior to beginning the transfusion. Because most blood transfusion reactions occur within 15 minutes of starting infusion, it is of great importance to establish the pre-infusion baseline immediately prior to beginning the transfusion. Skin color, hemoglobin levels, and renal function would be important considerations; however, it would not be essential that such assessments take place immediately prior to the start of the transfusion.
Cognitive Level: Application **Client Need:** Physiological Integrity: Pharmacological and Parenteral Therapies **Integrated Process:** Nursing Process: Assessment **Content Area:** Fundamentals **Strategy:** The question focuses on the action that should be taken *immediately* prior to beginning the transfusion.

2. **Answer: 4** Normal saline is the solution of choice when used as an adjunct to a transfusion. Ringer's lactate and dextrose solutions are contraindicated due to the potential for clotting and hemolysis.
Cognitive Level: Application **Client Need:** Physiological Integrity: Pharmacological and Parenteral Therapies **Integrated Process:** Nursing Process: Implementation **Content Area:** Fundamentals **Strategy:** The focus of the question is compatibility of blood with intravenous solutions. Use nursing knowledge and the process of elimination to make a selection.

3. **Answer: 3** Circulatory overload is a complication associated with rapid transfusion administration. Symptoms include bounding pulse, dyspnea, and crackles in the lungs. Crackles in the lungs would not be associated with an immune response, hypovolemia, or polycythemia vera.
Cognitive Level: Analysis **Client Need:** Physiological Integrity: Pharmacological and Parenteral Therapies **Integrated Process:** Nursing Process: Analysis **Content Area:** Fundamentals **Strategy:** The core issue of the question is the ability to recognize signs of circulatory overload. Use nursing knowledge and the process of elimination to make a selection.

4. **Answer: 3** The nurse is to stop the transfusion immediately and keep the IV line open with normal saline. The nurse would then notify the physician. A white blood cell count or a saline bolus may be ordered by the physician; however, these actions would not be independently initiated by the nurse without contacting the physician first.
Cognitive Level: Application **Client Need:** Physiological Integrity: Pharmacological and Parenteral Therapies **Integrated Process:** Nursing Process: Implementation **Content Area:** Fundamentals **Strategy:** The core issue of the question is the ability to take proper action when a transfusion reaction is suspected. Use nursing knowledge and the process of elimination to make a selection.

5. **Answer: 1** A transfusion of FFP is indicated for clients who are actively bleeding with a prothrombin time greater than 1.5 times normal. Platelets would be indicated for the client with thrombocytopenia. RBCs would be appropriate for the client with anemia. Crystalloids are given to help establish or maintain an adequate fluid and electrolyte balance.
Cognitive Level: Application **Client Need:** Physiological Integrity: Pharmacological and Parenteral Therapies **Integrated Process:** Nursing Process: Planning **Content Area:** Fundamentals **Strategy:** The core issue of the question is the ability to anticipate the need for fresh frozen plasma. Use nursing knowledge and the process of elimination to make a selection.

6. **Answer: 4** Iron deficiency anemia can result from blood loss and is common in menstruating women. Leukemia is reflected in the white blood cell count. Amenorrhea, the absence of menstruation, is unlikely to cause of iron deficiency anemia. Vitamin B_{12} deficiency anemia is often associated with dietary deficiency, such as experienced by vegetarians or those who avoid dairy products.
Cognitive Level: Analysis **Client Need:** Physiological Integrity: Pharmacological and Parenteral Therapies **Integrated Process:** Nursing Process: Analysis **Content Area:** Fundamentals **Strategy:** The core issue of the question is the ability to anticipate the needs of a client with iron deficiency anemia. Use nursing knowledge and the process of elimination to make a selection.

7. **Answer: 3** An in-line filter is required for the administration of blood. Tubing with a microdrip, an air vent, and tinting that protects the blood from light would not be indicated for blood administration.
Cognitive Level: Application **Client Need:** Physiological Integrity: Pharmacological and Parenteral Therapies **Integrated Process:** Nursing Process: Planning **Content Area:** Fundamentals **Strategy:** The core issue of the question is knowledge that an in-line filter is required for blood transfusion. Use nursing knowledge and the process of elimination to make a selection.

8. **Answer: 3** A transfusion of platelets is indicated for the client with active bleeding. A transfusion with packed RBCs would result in increased hemoglobin and hematocrit levels. Platelet administration is not associated with the prevention of deep vein thrombosis. The administration of platelets is not associated with the return of the prothrombin time to normal.
Cognitive Level: Analysis **Client Need:** Physiological Integrity: Pharmacological and Parenteral Therapies **Integrated Process:** Nursing Process: Implementation **Content Area:** Fundamentals **Strategy:** The core issue is knowledge of platelet transfusion therapy. Recall that platelets are critical for proper blood clotting to make a selection.

9. **Answer: 175 mL per hour** If a 350 mL unit of packed red blood cells is to infuse over 2 hours, the rate will be 175 mL per hour.
Cognitive Level: Application **Client Need:** Physiological Integrity: Pharmacological and Parenteral Therapies **Integrated Process:** Nursing Process: Implementation **Content Area:** Fundamentals **Strategy:** Use knowledge of pharmacological math to calculate the drip rate.

10. **Answer: 1, 3** Key features of anemia include coolness to touch, intolerance to cold, tachycardia, orthostatic hypotension, and headaches. Thus, hypertension, bounding pulses, and diaphoresis are not associated with anemia.
Cognitive Level: Application **Client Need:** Physiological Integrity: Pharmacological and Parenteral Therapies **Integrated Process:** Nursing Process: Assessment **Content Area:** Fundamentals **Strategy:** The core issue of the question is the ability to anticipate the needs of a client with moderately severe anemia.

Use nursing knowledge and the process of elimination to make a selection.

11 **Answer: 4** An autologous transfusion involves the collection of the client's blood prior to the anticipated need, thus compatibility is not problematic and the potential for contamination is eliminated. It would not be appropriate for the nurse to predict blood loss as a result of a surgical procedure. Further, stressing the safety of blood transfusions may elicit a false sense of comfort for the client. While the family may be able to donate blood, this would not be as potentially beneficial to the client as an autologous blood transfusion. Further, not all relatives share the same blood type.
Cognitive Level: Application **Client Need:** Physiological Integrity: Pharmacological and Parenteral Therapies **Integrated Process:** Nursing Process: Implementation **Content Area:** Fundamentals **Strategy:** The core issue of the question is knowledge of various types of transfusions. Use nursing knowledge and the process of elimination to make a selection.

12 **Answer: 4** The normal WBC count is between 5,000 and 10,000/mm^3. The nurse should consider implementing neutropenic precautions when the WBC count is at or below 2,000/mm^3.
Cognitive Level: Application **Client Need:** Physiological Integrity: Reduction of Risk Potential **Integrated Process:** Nursing Process: Implementation **Content Area:** Fundamentals **Strategy:** The core issue of the question is knowledge of white blood cell counts. Use nursing knowledge and the process of elimination to make a selection.

13 **Answer: 2** When a transfusion reaction has occurred, the nurse must return any remaining blood to the blood bank. If a reaction had not occurred, the nurse would dispose of the blood in an appropriate biohazard bag. It would not be appropriate for the nurse to send the blood to the laboratory or infection control department.
Cognitive Level: Application **Client Need:** Physiological Integrity: Pharmacological and Parenteral Therapies **Integrated Process:** Nursing Process: Implementation **Content Area:** Fundamentals **Strategy:** The core issue of the question is knowledge of critical actions to take when a transfusion reaction occurs. Use nursing knowledge and the process of elimination to make a selection.

14 **Answer: 1** Because the client is febrile, the nurse must notify the health care provider. The health care provider will determine if the client can tolerate the transfusion or if additional therapeutic intervention is warranted, which may include the administration of acetaminophen (Tylenol) or an antihistamine.
Cognitive Level: Application **Client Need:** Physiological Integrity: Pharmacological and Parenteral Therapies **Integrated Process:** Nursing Process: Implementation **Content Area:** Fundamentals **Strategy:** The core issue of the question is knowledge of critical actions to take when a client requiring a blood transfusion has an elevated temperature. Use nursing knowledge and the process of elimination to make a selection.

15 **Answer: 4** Albumin is used as a plasma expander and is used in the treatment of hypovolemic shock. Packed RBCs are indicated in the treatment of anemia. Platelets are indicated in the treatment of thrombocytopenia. Cryoprecipitate is administered to treat von Willebrand's disease and fibrinogen levels below 100 mg/dL.
Cognitive Level: Analysis **Client Need:** Physiological Integrity: Pharmacological and Parenteral Therapies **Integrated Process:** Nursing Process: Planning **Content Area:** Fundamentals **Strategy:** The core issue of the question is knowledge of the uses of various blood products. Use nursing knowledge and the process of elimination to make a selection.

16 **Answer: 3** Granulocyte transfusions are administered to neutropenic clients with infections for white blood cell replacement. Therefore, the white blood cell count would indicate the success of the treatment. The hemoglobin, hematocrit, erythrocytes, and platelet counts would not be appropriate for evaluating this therapy.
Cognitive Level: Application **Client Need:** Physiological Integrity: Pharmacological and Parenteral Therapies **Integrated Process:** Nursing Process: Evaluation **Content Area:** Fundamentals **Strategy:** The core issue of the question is knowledge of appropriate outcomes of blood component therapy. Use nursing knowledge and the process of elimination to make a selection.

17 **Answer: 1** Diphenhydramine (Benadryl) is administered for the treatment of anaphylaxis. Benadryl competes with the H_1 receptors on effector cells, thus blocking the effects of histamine. Tylenol and hydrocortisone would provide symptomatic relief from signs and symptoms of a transfusion reaction. Aspirin would not be indicated for treatment of a transfusion reaction.
Cognitive Level: Application **Client Need:** Physiological Integrity: Pharmacological and Parenteral Therapies **Integrated Process:** Nursing Process: Planning **Content Area:** Fundamentals **Strategy:** The core issue of the question is knowledge of appropriate treatments for transfusion reactions. Use nursing knowledge and the process of elimination to make a selection.

ANSWERS & RATIONALES

Key Terms to Review

autologous donor p. 527
blood salvage p. 527
compatibility p. 528
crossmatch p. 528
designated donor p. 527
transfusion reaction p. 529

References

Ignatavicius, D., & Workman, M. (2006). *Medical-surgical nursing: Critical thinking for collaborative care* (6th ed.). Philadelphia: Saunders.

Kozier, B., Erb, G., Berman, A., & Burke, K. (2004). *Fundamentals of nursing: Concepts, process, and practice* (7th ed.). Upper Saddle River, NJ: Pearson Education.

LeMone, P., & Burke, K. (2006). *Medical surgical nursing: Critical Thinking in Client Care* (4th ed.). Upper Saddle River, NJ: Pearson Education.

Smith, S., Duell, D., & Martin, B. (2004). *Clinical Nursing Skills: Basic to Advanced Skills* (6th ed.). Upper Saddle River, NJ: Pearson Education.

34 Total Parenteral Nutrition

Test Yourself

Are you ready for the NCLEX-RN® or course exams? Use the practice tests on the companion CD-ROM to check.

In this chapter

Cross reference

Other chapters relevant to this content area are

Meeting Nutritional Needs **Chapter 26**
Intravenous Therapy **Chapter 32**

I. BASIC CONCEPTS OF TOTAL PARENTERAL NUTRITION (TPN)

A. Overview

1. **Total parenteral nutrition (TPN)** is a form of nutrition provided intravenously when a client cannot take or tolerate oral or enteral feedings (see Box 34–1); may be utilized in home setting as well as hospital
2. TPN prevents catabolism of protein from muscle stores and fat from subcutaneous tissue
3. Composition of solution includes amino acids (3% to 15% calories), dextrose for carbohydrate (typically 25% of final concentration of solution providing 60% to 70% of calories), vitamins, minerals, trace elements (often twice weekly), electrolytes (according to individual need), and water
4. Lipids may be added to primary bag or infused as separate emulsion; provide up to 30% of calories and prevent or treat deficiency of fatty acids
5. Occasionally, regular insulin may be added to minimize blood glucose elevations in clients with diabetes mellitus, and heparin can be added to prevent clotting at tip according to individual need and agency protocol
6. Types of solutions
   a. TPN: formulas with amino acids and dextrose in a volume of 2 to 3 liters infused over 24 hours; intermittent infusion of 10% fat emulsion (Intralipid, 500 mL volume) may be given 1 to 3 times weekly
   b. Total nutrient admixture (TNA): also called 3-in-1 solution; contains amino acids, dextrose, and lipids; daily volume ordered to be given over 24 hours
   c. **Lipids** (fat emulsion): supplement TPN and provide fatty acids such as linoleic, linolenic, oleic, palmitic, and stearic acids

Box 34–1

Examples of Indications for TPN

Nonfunctional or poorly functioning GI tract (severe bowel inflammatory disease, malabsorption, severe GI side effects of chemotherapy or radiation therapy)

Conditions requiring bowel rest (extensive GI surgery, GI trauma, bowel obstruction)

High nutrient needs of client (burns, massive trauma, extensive wounds, malnutrition, cancer, acquired immunodeficiency syndrome)

B. Access sites

1. Peripheral line (used for **peripheral parenteral nutrition** or **PPN**)
   a. Peripheral veins are used for access
   b. Used for nutrient supplementation, not replacement
   c. Peripheral route often used for up to 7 days but should not exceed 2 weeks
   d. Maximal dextrose concentration is 10% to avoid irritation of blood vessel walls, phlebitis, and sclerosis
2. Central line (typical TPN)
   a. Utilizes catheter inserted percutaneously into a central vein (see Figure 34–1 ■); dextrose concentrations in solution are greater than 10%
   b. Triple lumen catheter common; 18-gauge middle lumen used for TPN infusion (other ports used for medication administration or IV blood draws according to agency policy); TPN administration through line limited to 4 weeks or less
   c. Peripherally inserted central catheter (PICC) line increasingly popular; catheter inserted into basilic or cephalic vein and advanced to superior vena cava; used when TPN needed for more than 4 weeks
   d. Single lumen catheters require secondary IV access site

Memory Aid

Do not administer or piggyback medications and blood into a line used for TPN. This will help to avoid incompatibilities and prevent infection.

II. NURSING MANAGEMENT

A. Assessment

1. Assess for pneumothorax (dyspnea, tachycardia, absent breath sounds on affected side, chest or shoulder pain) during catheter insertion; verify placement by x-ray following insertion
2. Assess insertion site each shift for patency and signs of infection (clear transparent dressing often used)
3. Monitor blood glucose as ordered (often every 6 hrs) to detect hyperglycemia

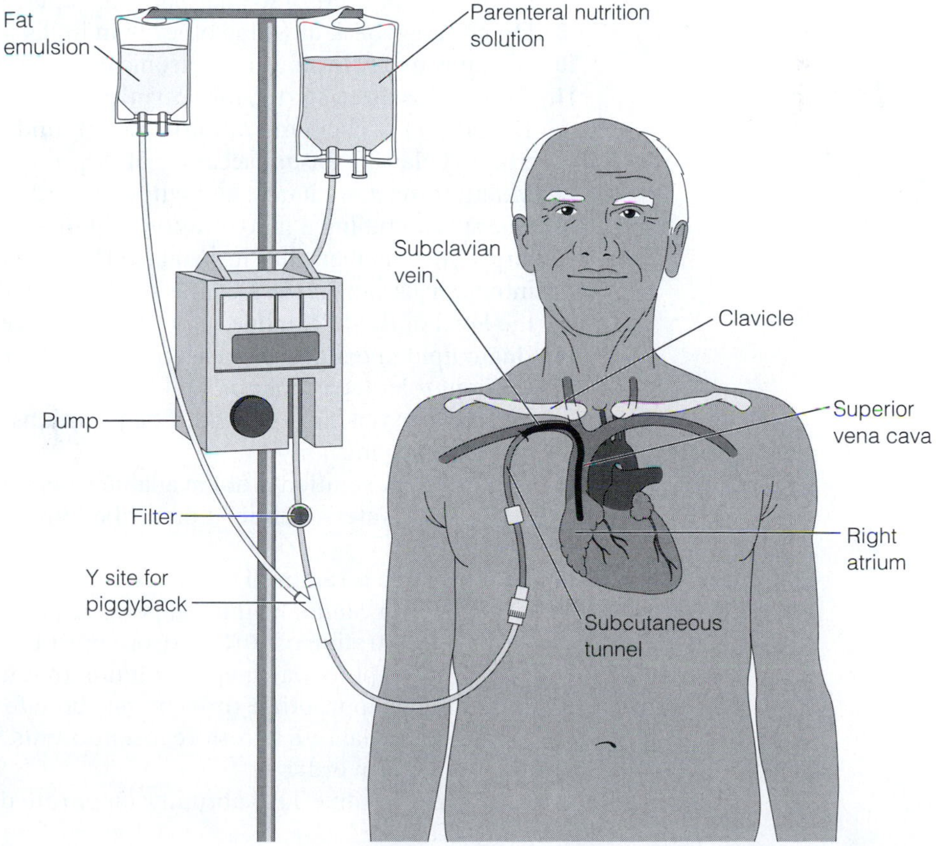

Figure 34–1

Total parenteral nutrition administered via right subclavian vein.

Source: LeMone, P., & Burke, K. (2003). Medical surgical nursing: Critical thinking in client care (3rd ed.). Upper Saddle River, NJ: Prentice Hall, p. 534.

4. Measure daily weight to determine fluid balance (1 liter = 1 kilogram) and nutritional weight gain (1–2 pounds per week) or weight maintenance, depending on individual client need
5. Monitor other laboratory results, such as serum electrolytes, total protein, prealbumin and albumin levels, blood urea nitrogen and creatinine (excess amino acid intake will cause increased levels), total lymphocyte count, and liver function test results (abnormally high values may indicate problems with glucose or protein metabolism, or excess lipids)

Memory Aid

In severely malnourished clients, watch for "refeeding syndrome," a precipitous drop in serum potassium, magnesium, and phosphate levels.

B. Planning and implementation

1. Client goals
   a. Maintains fluid and electrolyte balance
   b. Gains weight according to nutritional plan or maintains current weight and avoids loss of essential nutritional elements
   c. Remains free of complications of TPN therapy
2. Use strict aseptic technique if assisting with catheter insertion
3. Ensure that placement is correct before using catheter for any infusion
4. Keep TPN solution in refrigerator until 30 to 60 minutes prior to use to retard bacterial growth; change TPN bag and tubing every 24 hours to prevent infection
5. Administer TPN or PPN through IV tubing that has an inline filter to remove any crystals present in solution (0.22 micron filter without use of lipids; 1.2 micron filter or larger if lipids added)
6. Check every ingredient in TPN solution against physician's order; notify pharmacy and do not hang if any discrepancies are found; orders should be written daily
7. Do not add any other medication to the solution once distributed for use by pharmacy
8. Do not hang a solution that is cloudy, dark in color, has visible fat globules (if lipids present); return to pharmacy for replacement
9. Do not piggyback anything other than lipids into TPN line
10. Administer TPN using an electronic infusion device only
11. TPN rate is often started low (50 mL/hr) and gradually increased (often to 80 to 125 mL/hr) as client tolerates (based on fluid balance, blood glucose, and electrolyte balance); ensure accuracy of flow rate
12. Maintain accurate intake and output records every shift
13. Use special tubing if lipid infusion is hung separately; use 1.2 micron filter or larger (not smaller filter in standard IV tubing) to allow lipids to pass through into vein; use an electronic infusion device and piggyback into TPN line below the level of the TPN inline filter to ensure free flow
14. Begin lipid infusion at rate of 1 mL/minute, titrate upward as ordered according to client tolerance; monitor vital signs every 10 minutes for first half hour to detect adverse reactions (see III. Complications); measure serum lipids if ordered 4 hours post infusion
15. If a new TPN solution is not available when previous one has infused, hang 10% dextrose in water solution at prescribed rate to prevent hypoglycemia until TPN is available
16. If central line is removed because of dislodgement, sepsis, or leakage, the central TPN solution cannot be infused peripherally; a peripheral solution with a maximum concentration of 10% dextrose must be used
17. Do not attempt to "catch up" a solution that has fallen behind schedule for infusion; with an appropriate order, it may be safe to restart the rate at 10% higher than the original rate to restore lost nutrients, but this is highly individualized and requires an order
18. Do not discontinue TPN abruptly; taper rate down as ordered to prevent hypoglycemia

19. Change catheter dressing according to protocol
20. Collaborate on an ongoing basis with health care provider and dietitian to determine how well client is attaining goals of therapy

Memory Aid

Change a transparent central line dressing every 72 to 96 hours as per agency policy; change gauze dressing more frequently according to policy; change any dressing that is loose, wet, or soiled to prevent infection from contamination.

C. Client/family teaching

1. Includes intended purpose and effects of therapy and adverse effects that must be self-monitored
2. Home care skills
   a. How to self-administer TPN
   b. Technique for changing sterile dressing
   c. Clean hands before any contact with tubing or access area
   d. Do not allow caregivers with an infectious disease to work with catheter
   e. Monitor daily weight, and report more than 3 pounds per week gain (fluid overload/retention)
   f. Monitor blood glucose and report elevations
   g. Monitor catheter patency and report edema at catheter insertion site, jugular vein distention, and edema of affected arm (if applicable)
   h. Monitor for catheter displacement (leakage at insertion site, pain/discomfort during infusion)

! **D. Evaluation of outcomes**

1. Weight gain is satisfactory
2. Fluid and electrolytes are within normal limits
3. Client is free of complications of TPN therapy

III. COMPLICATIONS

! **A. Complications of TPN (see Table 34–1 ■)**

B. Adverse effects of lipids

1. See Box 34–2
2. If adverse reactions occur, discontinue lipid solution and notify prescriber; prepare to provide supportive measures according to symptoms

Table 34–1
Complications of Total Parenteral Nutrition

Complication	Client Manifestations	Nursing Management
Fluid overload (because of excess volume or hypertonicity)	Bounding pulse and increased BP, lung crackles, headache, jugular vein distention, excessive weight gain above goal	*Prevention:* always use electronic infusion device; do not "catch up" solutions that fall behind schedule; monitor I&O and weight daily *Intervention:* raise head of bed to alleviate respiratory symptoms; apply oxygen as ordered; carry out ordered therapies, such as diuretics, correctly
Air embolism (potentially fatal entry of air into catheter during insertion or tubing changes)	Rapid onset respiratory distress, dyspnea, apprehension, chest pain, rapid and weak pulse, low BP, churning heart murmur (hallmark sign)	*Prevention:* check catheter and tubing connections; have client use Valsalva maneuver during tubing and cap changes; place client in head-down position with head turned to opposite side (if tolerated) for cap and tubing changes to increase intrathoracic venous pressure *Intervention:* clamp catheter; place client in left Trendelenburg position (traps air in right ventricle away from pulmonic valve); notify physician; administer oxygen as prescribed

(continued)

Table 34-1 (cont.)

Complication	Client Manifestations	Nursing Management
Infection/sepsis (catheter-related; high-dextrose solution excellent medium for bacterial growth)	Fever and chills; redness, swelling, tenderness or drainage at insertion site; elevated WBC count; possible signs of septic shock	*Prevention:* use strict aseptic technique in all aspects of line management and site care; change solution every 12 to 24 hours as ordered and tubing every 24 hours according to agency protocol; change dressing according to protocol depending on dressing type (see text) *Intervention:* send tip of catheter for culture and sensitivity upon catheter removal; arrange for blood cultures to be drawn if ordered; administer antibiotics as ordered
Hyperglycemia (elevated blood glucose level from dextrose load in solution, infusion rate, or diabetes)	Glucose levels greater than 200 mg/dL, thirst, fatigue, confusion or restlessness, weakness and diuresis; coma when severe	*Prevention:* assess for history of glucose intolerance (e.g., diabetes); assess for use of medications that lead to hyperglycemia (e.g., corticosteroids); begin infusion at slow rate (often 40 to 60 mL/hr) and titrate upward over time as ordered; use infusion pump for TPN administration *Intervention:* monitor blood glucose levels q 6 hrs or as ordered; administer prescribed regular insulin "sliding scale" to keep blood glucose levels less than 200 mg/dL
Hypoglycemia (low blood glucose from abrupt termination of TPN or excess insulin)	Glucose level less than 70 mg/dL; weakness and shakiness, anxiety, diaphoresis, possible hunger	*Prevention:* use infusion pump for TPN administration; gradually decrease rate of infusion when discontinuing therapy; hang 10% dextrose in water solution for 1 to 2 hrs post-TPN as ordered *Intervention:* monitor blood glucose 1 hour after termination of TPN; administer source of glucose as needed

Box 34-2

Adverse Effects of Lipids

- Chills
- Fever and flushing
- Diaphoresis
- Chest and back pain
- Dyspnea and cyanosis
- Nausea and vomiting
- Headache
- Pressure over eyes
- Vertigo
- Thrombophlebitis
- Allergic reaction

Check Your NCLEX-RN® Exam I.Q.

You are ready for testing on this content if you can

- Identify various types of access for TPN therapy.
- Begin, maintain, and discontinue TPN therapy.
- Appropriately monitor TPN flow rate.
- Provide nursing care to the client receiving TPN therapy.
- Monitor for adverse effects or complications of TPN.
- Provide client/family teaching related to TPN.

PRACTICE TEST

1 While caring for a client receiving total parenteral nutrition (TPN), nursing responsibilities will include which of the following?

1. Covering elevated blood glucose levels with a sliding scale of regular insulin
2. Inspecting solution to ensure "layering" of contents is present
3. Adjusting rate of solution to client's output every shift
4. Changing injection caps on the intravenous tubing every shift

2 Clients suffering from profound malnutrition may experience the refeeding syndrome when first initiating total parenteral nutrition (TPN). To determine if this occurs, the nurse must do which of the following?

1. Monitor potassium, phosphorus, and magnesium levels closely.
2. Check blood glucose levels every 6 hours.
3. Assess client for hyperactive bowel sounds.
4. Assess client's level of consciousness every shift.

3 Which of the following conditions leads the nurse to conclude that a client's total parenteral nutrition (TPN) solution needs to be administered through a central venous catheter?

1. The client will be receiving fluids at a rate of 150 to 200 mL/hr.
2. The client will be receiving an infusion with a high caloric content.
3. The end concentration of dextrose in the solution will be 25%.
4. The use of a peripheral vein would require more frequent site changes.

4 A client recovering from multiple trauma is started on total parenteral nutrition (TPN) therapy. The nurse determines that which of the following is a major goal of this therapy?

1. Prevent a negative nitrogen balance in the client.
2. Maintain a high urine output.
3. Provide adequate hydration.
4. Ensure client receives needed trace minerals.

5 A 46-year-old male client has had a central venous catheter inserted in the subclavian vein recently so that he can be started on total parenteral nutrition (TPN) therapy. Which of the following assessment findings best indicates the client may have a pneumothorax?

1. Client complains of sharp chest pain.
2. Pulse oximetry is 90% on room air.
3. Catheter insertion site is red and swollen.
4. Radial pulse is rapid.

6 A 34-year-old female client recovering from severe weight loss secondary to Crohn's disease is being discharged and has received instructions on home parenteral nutrition. The nurse instructs the client to weigh herself weekly, suggesting the desired goal of therapy is

1. to maintain current weight.
2. a weight gain of 0.5 pound a week.
3. a weight gain of 2 pounds a week.
4. a monthly weight gain of 4 pounds.

7 Total parenteral nutrition (TPN) is being started on a client with malabsorption syndrome. Prior to starting the infusion, nursing responsibilities will include which of the following?

1. Calculating the nutrients needed for an individualized formula
2. Obtaining a baseline weight
3. Ensuring an EKG is done on client prior to starting infusion
4. Checking for allergies to wheat

8 Prior to hanging a total parenteral nutrition (TPN) solution, the nurse checks the content of the solution. Which of the following ingredients would the nurse expect to be included? Select all that apply.

1. Trace minerals
2. NPH insulin
3. Electrolytes
4. Diuretic
5. Multivitamin

9 A client is receiving an infusion of TPN at 83 mL/hr. The infusion is stopped for 4 hours while client is off the nursing unit. When the client returns, the standing order indicates the infusion should be restarted at a rate of 10% greater than the baseline rate. The infusion should be run at _____ mL/hour. Provide a numerical response.

PRACTICE TEST

10 The nurse is careful to ensure that when a client's total parenteral nutrition (TPN) infusion is discontinued, it is done gradually. The client questions why gradual tapering is necessary. The nurse responds that this measure will prevent which of the following?

1. Refeeding syndrome
2. Hypvolemia
3. Hyponatremia
4. Rebound hypoglycemia

11 The nurse is preparing to hang the next scheduled bag of total parenteral nutrition (TPN) solution. Prior to hanging the bag, the nurse does which of the following?

1. Irrigates the intravenous port with Heparin.
2. Removes solution from refrigerator 1 hour prior to hanging it.
3. Infuses 100 mL of normal saline to clear the intravenous line.
4. Has sterile gloves available to use when changing bags of solution.

12 A subclavian catheter has been inserted in a client who will be receiving total parenteral nutrition (TPN). Before beginning the infusion, it is most important for the nurse to do which of the following?

1. Obtain a baseline weight.
2. Confirm x-ray report of correct catheter placement.
3. Determine client is afebrile.
4. Check intake and output for the past 24 hours.

13 A client is receiving a continuous total parenteral nutrition (TPN) solution and is also on a regular diet while recovering from a multiple trauma. Which of the following nursing actions is of most importance when caring for this client?

1. Monitor blood glucose levels closely.
2. Assess urine output.
3. Encourage intake of high-protein foods.
4. Offer nutritional supplements at bedtime.

14 A client admitted with malnutrition has received total parenteral nutrition (TPN) for 2 weeks. To best evaluate the effectiveness of the treatment, the nurse should do which of the following?

1. Monitor recent blood glucose levels.
2. Check for recent weight gain.
3. Check prealbumin levels.
4. Evaluate skin turgor.

15 The nurse is assisting a student nurse in the preparation of a continuous infusion of total parenteral nutrition (TPN) solution. The nurse recognizes that which action by the student is unnecessary?

1. Dons sterile gloves when connecting tubing to the solution bag.
2. Attaches tubing that contains a micron filter to the solution bag.
3. Checks solution for evidence of layering and cracking.
4. Verifies orders are current for TPN.

ANSWERS & RATIONALES

ANSWERS & RATIONALES

1 **Answer: 1** TPN contains a 20% to 60% glucose solution, which often causes hyperglycemia and is routinely regulated by giving regular insulin. The solution should be clear and homogenous without layering or cracking. TPN solutions are infused at a steady rate. An alternative solution would be used to adjust fluids for urine output, NG losses, and so on. Injection caps are changed per institution protocol, usually every 72 hours. More frequent changes increase risk for bacterial contamination.
Cognitive Level: Application **Client Need:** Physiological Integrity: Pharmacological and Parenteral Therapies **Integrated Process:** Nursing Process: Implementation **Content Area:** Fundamentals
Strategy: The question asks for nursing responsibilities and the wording of the question indicates the correct option is also a true statement. Recall TPN solutions contain high concentrations of glucose. Systematically eliminate incorrect options, choosing option 1, which addresses the high glucose content.

2 **Answer: 1** Magnesium, potassium, and phosphate levels may drop because magnesium (needed for ATP synthesis) and phosphorus (a component of ATP) are utilized rapidly as the TPN solution is metabolized, and potassium is taken up intracellularly in energy metabolism. Blood sugars are checked frequently but are not related to the refeeding syndrome. Bowel sounds and level of consciousness would be part of a routine assessment but do not reflect refeeding syndrome.
Cognitive Level: Application **Client Need:** Physiological Integrity: Pharmacological and Parenteral Therapies **Integrated Process:** Nursing Process: Assessment **Content Area:** Fundamentals
Strategy: The question requires specific knowledge of the refeeding syndrome. Eliminate option 4 because it is unrelated to the other 3 options. Eliminate option 3 because TPN is often given to rest the bowel. Choose option 1 over 2 because it is more specific and blood sugars are specifically connected to hyperglycemia.

3 **Answer: 3** TPN solutions contain hypertonic glucose (20–70%), which would cause severe irritation and phlebitis to a peripheral vein. Central veins are much larger, and the solution becomes diluted quickly. A rate of 150 to 200 would

provide excessive fluid volume and calories. The infusion is of a high caloric content, but this fact does not explain why it must be given centrally. Peripheral sites do require more frequent changes, but frequency of changes does not influence the decision to use a central vein.
Cognitive Level: Application **Client Need:** Physiological Integrity: Pharmacological and Parenteral Therapies **Integrated Process:** Nursing Process: Analysis **Content Area:** Fundamentals **Strategy:** Recall the effect of osmolarity on blood vessels. Eliminate option 1 because it is an excessively high flow rate. Options 2 and 4 are correct statements but can be eliminated because they are not as specific. Option 3 gives a justification.

4 **Answer: 1** TPN provides a readily available source of carbohydrates, fats, and proteins in order to restore or maintain positive nitrogen balance. Recovery from multiple trauma utilizes protein and fat stores, leading to a negative nitrogen balance. TPN provides some hydration and helps to maintain urine output, but the primary purpose is to spare the body's own energy stores. Trace minerals are added to TPN solutions but are not the primary reason TPN solutions are used.
Cognitive Level: Application **Client Need:** Physiological Integrity: Pharmacological and Parenteral Therapies **Integrated Process:** Nursing Process: Planning **Content Area:** Fundamentals **Strategy:** A key word in the question is *major,* indicating some or all of the options may be correct, but one is considered more important. Recognize the major purpose of TPN is to provide calories and nutrition. Choose option 1 because it is more global and pertains to the nutritional needs.

5 **Answer: 1** Inspiration into a deflated lung produces sharp chest pain as resistance to airflow is met and is a sign of a pneumothorax. Oxygenation would decrease as ventilation capacity is decreased, but this effect could be attributed to many factors and is not the best indicator of a pneumothorax. A rapid pulse is also not a specific indicator of pneumothorax. A red and swollen insertion site is a sign of irritation or infection.
Cognitive Level: Analysis **Client Need:** Physiological Integrity: Pharmacological and Parenteral Therapies **Integrated Process:** Nursing Process: Assessment **Content Area:** Fundamentals **Strategy:** Note the question asks for the best answer, indicating one option is a better choice. Omit options 2 and 4 because they could be symptomatic of many respiratory and cardiovascular problems. Omit option 3 because it is the least related to a respiratory problem.

6 **Answer: 3** A 2-pound weekly gain is the ideal weight gain when TPN is given to restore nutritional balance and improve weight. It demonstrates the treatment is effective. Maintenance of weight would be a goal if weight gain were not desired. Weight gains of 0.5 to 1 pound a week are less than desirable.
Cognitive Level: Application **Client Need:** Physiological Integrity: Pharmacological and Parenteral Therapies **Integrated Process:** Teaching and Learning **Content Area:** Fundamentals **Strategy:** Key words in the question are *weekly* and *desired goal.* Also note the client is receiving the TPN to improve weight. Eliminate option 1 because a weight gain is desired. Eliminate option 4 because it is monthly; a weekly goal is desired. Choose option 3 over 2 because it gives an easily measurable weight (some scales do measure half pounds).

7 **Answer: 2** A baseline weight is needed to provide a foundation for clinical therapy and to assess response to treatment. The calculation of nutrients is done by a dietitian. It is not necessary to have a baseline EKG. Client should be assessed for allergies to eggs.
Cognitive Level: Application **Client Need:** Physiological Integrity: Pharmacological and Parenteral Therapies **Integrated Process:** Nursing Process: Implementation **Content Area:** Fundamentals **Strategy:** Recall the nurse's role in hanging TPN and the content of the solution. Eliminate option 1 because it is not the nurse's responsibility. Eliminate option 3 as unnecessary and option 4 as incorrect.

8 **Answer: 1, 3, 5** In addition to the base solution, TPN contains electrolytes, minerals, and multivitamins. Regular insulin may be added, but NPH cannot. If diuretics are needed because of underlying client condition, it would not be added to the TPN solution.
Cognitive Level: Application **Client Need:** Physiological Integrity: Pharmacological and Parenteral Therapies **Integrated Process:** Nursing Process: Planning **Content Area:** Fundamentals **Strategy:** Specific knowledge of the content of TPN is needed. Systematically eliminate ingredients that you recognize would not be appropriate.

9 **Answer: 91 mL/hour** If TPN infusion is interrupted, the nurse should not play "catch up," but TPN can be safely restarted at up to 10% of the baseline rate with an appropriate order to help replace nutrients missed.
Cognitive Level: Application **Client Need:** Physiological Integrity: Pharmacological and Parenteral Therapies **Integrated Process:** Nursing Process: Implementation **Content Area:** Fundamentals **Strategy:** Correctly calculate by multiplying the baseline rate of 83 by 10%. The exact calculation of 91.3 is rounded to the nearest tenth, making the correct answer 91 mL.
83 mL × 10%
83 mL × .10 = 8.3 mL
83 mL + 8.3 mL = 91.3 mL

10 **Answer: 4** TPN should be gradually discontinued over a 24 to 48 hour period to allow for adjustment in metabolic function and prevent a sudden drop in blood glucose. Refeeding syndrome occurs when TPN is first initiated. Hypovolemia and hyponatremia are not as significant a risk as hypoglycemia.
Cognitive Level: Analysis **Client Need:** Physiological Integrity: Pharmacological and Parenteral Therapies **Integrated Process:** Nursing Process: Analysis **Content Area:** Fundamentals **Strategy:** The question indicates the action should be done gradually, implying that abrupt withdrawal would have consequences. Consider each option in terms of what would occur if the solution were stopped suddenly. Eliminate option 1 because refeeding syndrome occurs at the beginning of TPN therapy.

11 **Answer: 2** It is recommended that TPN be brought to room temperature before infusing to prevent client discomfort and lowering of body temperature. It is not necessary to irrigate the IV line with heparin or saline. Bags should be changed using aseptic technique, but sterile gloves are not needed.
Cognitive Level: Application **Client Need:** Physiological Integrity: Pharmacological and Parenteral Therapies **Integrated Process:**

Nursing Process: Implementation **Content Area:** Fundamentals **Strategy:** Knowledge of nursing responsibilities related to TPN is necessary. Although protocols differ among institutions, the options are general and apply to basic principles. Eliminate option 4 because sterile technique is not used when changing IV bags.

12 **Answer: 2** Confirmation of correct catheter placement is essential before TPN is started to assure infusion will enter the superior vena cava. Confirming client is afebrile and obtaining a baseline weight are also important, but not of highest priorty. Intake and output should be monitored once TPN is started.
Cognitive Level: Analysis **Client Need:** Physiological Integrity: Pharmacological and Parenteral Therapies **Integrated Process:** Nursing Process: Planning **Content Area:** Fundamentals **Strategy:** The core concept in the question is identifying the action that must be taken before therapy can be started, and the key word is *most,* indicating all or some of the options are important, but one has a higher priority. Analyze each option and choose 2 because it is most critical.

13 **Answer: 1** The client is at greater risk for hyperglycemia because he or she is both receiving TPN and taking in additional calories on a regular diet. Assessing urine output, offering a nutritional supplement, and encouraging high-protein foods are all appropriate, but not of highest priority.
Cognitive Level: Analysis **Client Need:** Physiological Integrity: Pharmacological and Parenteral Therapies **Integrated Process:** Nursing Process: Implementation **Content Area:** Fundamentals **Strategy:** Recall TPN solutions contain a high caloric content and, combined with another source of calories, will increase risk of hyperglycemia for client. The key word in the stem is *most,* since all of the options are correct.

14 **Answer: 3** Prealbumin levels are the best indicators of protein stores and nitrogen balance, reflecting the client's nutritional status. Checking blood glucose levels assesses for hypoglycemia and hyperglycemia. Assessment of weight gain is indicated but is not the best indicator of nutritional status because fluid retention may influence the weight gain. Skin turgor is a measure of hydration status.
Cognitive Level: Analysis **Client Need:** Physiological Integrity: Pharmacological and Parenteral Therapies **Integrated Process:** Nursing Process: Evaluation **Content Area:** Fundamentals **Strategy:** The question asks that you evaluate effectiveness of treatment. A key word is *best,* indicating that some or all options are partially correct. Eliminate options 1 and 4 because they don't measure an outcome of treatment. Choose option 3 over 2 because it is a more specific measurement.

15 **Answer: 1** Aseptic technique is used when changing solution bags. Sterile gloves are not needed and would be contaminated as soon as the outside of the bag is touched. TPN requires use of a special micron filter. Solutions that are layered or cracked should not be used. The primary provider must order the content of TPN.
Cognitive Level: Analysis **Client Need:** Physiological Integrity: Pharmacological and Parenteral Therapies **Integrated Process:** Nursing Process: Analysis **Content Area:** Fundamentals **Strategy:** The word *unnecessary* is significant and indicates that three of the options are important or required for the task. Analyze each option for appropriateness to TPN therapy.

ANSWERS & RATIONALES

Key Terms to Review

lipids p. 536

peripheral parenteral nutrition (PPN) p. 539

total parenteral nutrition (TPN) p. 536

References

Abrams, A. (2004). *Clinical drug therapy: Rationales for nursing practice* (7th ed.). Philadelphia: Lippincott, Williams and Wilkins.

Ignatavicius, D., & Workman, M. (2006). *Medical-surgical nursing: Critical thinking for collaborative care* (5th ed.). Philadelphia: Saunders.

Kozier, B., Erb, G., Berman, A., & Burke, K. (2006). *Fundamentals of nursing: Concepts, process, and practice* (8th ed.). Upper Saddle River, NJ: Prentice Hall.

Lehne, R. (2004). *Pharmacology for nursing care* (5th ed.). St. Louis, MO: Mosby.

LeMone, P., & Burke, K. (2003). *Medical surgical nursing: Critical thinking in client care* (3rd ed.). Upper Saddle River, NJ: Prentice Hall.

Phipps, W., Monahan, F., Sands, J., Marek, J., & Neighbors, M. (2006). *Medical surgical nursing: Health and illness perspectives* (8th ed.). St. Louis: Mosby.

Smith, S., Duell, D., & Martin, B. (2004). *Clinical nursing skills: Basic to advanced skills* (6th ed.). Upper Saddle River, NJ: Pearson Education.

Maternal and Newborn Medications

35

In this chapter

Test Yourself

Are you ready for the NCLEX-RN® or course exams? Use the practice tests on the companion CD-ROM to check.

Cross reference

Other chapters relevant to this content area are

I. OXYTOCIN (PITOCIN)

A. Overview

1. Enhances uterine contractions in clients who are at term or provides stimulation of contractions with uterine inertia
2. Helps to induce labor in clients with maternal diabetes, preeclampsia, eclampsia, and erythroblastosis fetalis
3. Should be used only in carefully selected clients in labor after cervix has dilated and presentation of fetus has occurred

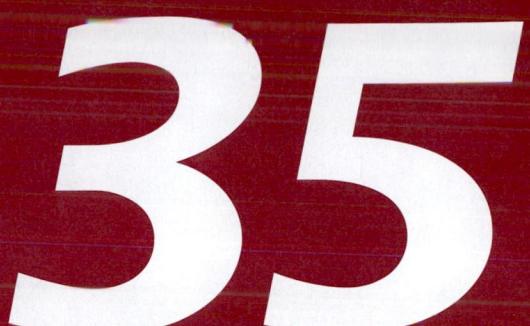

4. Stimulates letdown reflex in breast-feeding mother and relieves pain from breast engorgement
5. Controls postpartum hemorrhage and promotes postpartum uterine involution

B. Administration considerations

1. Dilute as ordered in IV solution and hang as a titratable IV drip, using an IV pump
2. Use normal saline as a primary line, with medication piggybacked at secondary port or stopcock
3. Monitor effects on contractions while titrating dosage
4. Nasal spray may be used to promote milk ejection
5. ! Keep magnesium sulfate on hand for use if needed to relax the myometrium
6. ! Do not confuse Pitocin (oxytocin) with Pitressin (vasopressin)

C. Side/adverse effects

1. Maternal: rare and with IV use, causes increased pain with contractions from increased uterine motility; also hypersensitivity, cardiac dysrhythmias, hypotension, hypertension if given following use of vasopressors, water intoxication (hyponatremia and hypochloremia), nausea and vomiting
2. Fetal: rare, but could include intracranial hemorrhage, hypoxia, or asphyxia

D. Nursing considerations

1. Use flowsheet to record baseline maternal BP and other vital signs, weight, I & O, contractions (frequency, duration, strength), and fetal heart tones and rate
2. Continue to monitor maternal pulse and BP, fetal heart rate, contractions, and resting uterine tone every 15 minutes
3. Record time medication was initiated and any changes in dosage
4. ! Monitor for hypertonic contractions (less than 2 minutes apart, greater than 90 seconds in length, and about 50 mmHg in strength), and shut off IV drip if uterine hyperstimulation or nonreassuring fetal heart rate occurs; turn client onto left side, increase rate of normal saline IV, and apply oxygen via facemask as appropriate
5. Effects of drug will diminish 2 to 3 minutes after discontinuing medication
6. Watch for hypertensive crisis in clients also receiving local or regional anesthesia (caudal, spinal); signs include sudden onset of intense occipital headache, palpitations, hypertension, stiff neck, nausea and vomiting, fever and sweating, photophobia and dilated pupils, constricting chest pain, and bradycardia or tachycardia
7. ! Monitor I & O; report signs of water intoxication (drowsiness, headache, confusion, anuria, and weight gain); also report decreasing urine output with adequate intake
8. Keep emergency resuscitation equipment available

E. Client teaching

1. Purpose and effect of medication
2. Importance of reporting sudden, severe headache immediately

II. UTERINE RELAXANTS

A. Overview

1. Inhibit contractions and therefore arrest labor for at least 48 hours so that corticosteroids (betamethasone) can be given to facilitate fetal lung maturity
2. Used for cessation of contractions to allow intrauterine fetal resuscitation when uterine hyperstimulation is present
3. Used to delay delivery in preterm labor
4. Common medications (Table 35–1 ■)

B. Administration considerations

1. Start medication at lowest possible dose and increase as indicated until contractions cease
2. Be certain about recommended dose
3. If GI symptoms occur, advise client to take medication with food
4. Dilute IV terbutaline by adding each 5 mg to 1000 mL D_5W or NS to yield a concentration of 5 micrograms/mL
5. Infuse medication via microdrip using an infusion pump

Table 35–1

Common Uterine Relaxant Medications

Generic (Trade Name)	Notes
Terbutaline sulfate (Brethine)	Not FDA-approved for preterm labor but most commonly used medication
Ritodrine (Yutopar)	FDA-approved for preterm labor, increased incidence of pulmonary edema
Nifedipine (Procardia)	Not FDA-approved for preterm labor but commonly used; may cause oligohydramnios
Indomethacin (Indocin)	Not FDA-approved for preterm labor but used as third line; increased risk of fetal complications

C. Side/adverse effects

1. ! Beta-adrenergics: maternal and fetal tachycardia, palpitations, tremors, jitteriness and anxiety, pulmonary edema
2. May cause or exacerbate constipation
3. Nausea and vomiting
4. Nifedipine (Procardia) and indomethacin (Indocin) can cause oligohydramnios
5. Indomethacin (Indocin) can cause premature closure of ductus arteriosus, leading to fetal death

D. Nursing considerations

1. Beta-adrenergics: if client delivers after receiving uterine relaxant medications, be prepared with oxytocic if needed to treat postpartum hemorrhage
2. Monitor vital signs and I & O
3. Nifedipine (Procardia): avoid grapefruit juice during administration (interferes with effect)
4. Use indomethacin for a short period of time (2 to 3 days)
5. If mother uses terbutaline during pregnancy, monitor neonate for hypoglycemia

E. Client teaching

1. Possible side effects and coping strategies
2. Use and dose of oral medications and importance of taking them on time
3. ! Nifedipine (Procardia): encourage client to change position slowly due to possible orthostatic hypotension
4. How to self-monitor pulse
5. Importance of consulting physician prior to taking over-the-counter (OTC) medications

III. ERGOT ALKALOIDS

A. Overview

1. Used to control postpartum hemorrhage; should not be used before delivery of placenta
2. Cause clonic contractions of uterus
3. Produce arterial vasoconstriction and possible vasospasm of coronary arteries
4. Common medications (Box 35–1)

B. Administration considerations: causes rebound uterine relaxation

C. Side/adverse effects

1. ! Contraindicated in pregnancy or hypersensitivity to ergot, hypertension
2. Should be used cautiously in unstable angina and recent myocardial infarction
3. Significant increase in systolic and diastolic BP
4. Uterine cramping
5. Decreased milk production
6. ! **Ergotism** or overdose: nausea, vomiting, weakness, muscle pain, insensitivity to cold, paresthesia of extremities

Box 35–1

Ergot Alkaloids

Ergonovine (Ergotrate)

Methylergonovine (Methergine)

D. Nursing considerations

1. Closely monitor blood pressure after administration; if hypertension noted, withhold dose and notify prescriber
2. Monitor lochia after administation and uterine contractions (strength, duration, and frequency)
3. Assess and report as indicated hypertension, chest pain, ergotism, or hypersensitivity (shortness of breath, itching)
4. Administer analgesics as needed to control pain of uterine contractions caused by ergot

E. Client teaching

1. Indication for administration
2. Route of administration (oral, IM, possible IV in emergency) and possible side effects, such as cramping
3. Report increased blood loss, increased temperature, or foul-smelling lochia
4. Perform pad count to monitor bleeding
5. Do not smoke because of increased/additive vasoconstriction with ergonovine use

IV. PROSTAGLANDINS

A. Overview

1. **Prostaglandins** terminate pregnancy from 12th week through second trimester (Table 35–2 ■); can also be used to stimulate myometrium to promote delivery
2. Dinoprostone (Prepidil, Cervidil) has FDA approval only for cervical ripening prior to labor induction; available as a gel
3. Carboprost tromethamine (Hemabate) has FDA approval only for control of postpartum bleeding

B. Administration considerations

1. Client should remain in supine position for 20 to 30 minutes after administration of dinoprostone
2. Before dinoprostone, client should receive antiemetic and antidiarrheal medications

C. Side/adverse effects

1. Diarrhea, nausea, vomiting, possible increase in BP
2. Uterine cramping
3. Tension headache
4. Flushing, cardiac dysrhythmias
5. Hypertension
6. Uterine tetany may develop with prelabor or intrapartum administration
7. Uterine rupture
8. Contraindicated with acute pelvic inflammatory disease and history of pelvic surgery; use cautiously in hypertension and with history of asthma

D. Nursing considerations

1. Prenatal: follow manufacturer's instructions for placement of medication; client must remain recumbent for 20 to 30 minutes after administration and have fetal monitoring during this time
2. Postpartum: monitor lochia and BP, be prepared for client to develop diarrhea

E. Client teaching

1. Prenatal: report long or continuous contractions, as uterine tetany may develop; count fetal movement as an indicator of fetal well-being
2. Postpartum: prepare client for route of administration and possible side effects

Table 35–2
Common Prostaglandins

Category	Generic (Trade Name)	Route	Indications for Use
Prostaglandin E2	Dinoprostone (Prepidil, Cervidil)	Prepidil intracervical gel Cervidil vaginal insert	Ripening of cervix prior to induction of labor
Prostaglandin F2	Carboprost tromethamine (Hemabate)	Hemabate: IM	Postpartum hemorrhage

V. MAGNESIUM SULFATE

A. Overview

1. When given parenterally, acts as central nervous system (CNS) depressant and also depresses smooth, skeletal, and cardiac muscle function
2. Used to arrest preterm labor and to prevent or to treat seizures with preeclampsia and eclampsia

B. Administration considerations

1. Use in conjunction with beta-adrenergics increases risk of pulmonary edema
2. A 4-gram loading dose is often utilized, which must be given over 20 to 30 minutes via infusion pump

C. Side/adverse effects

1. Flushed warm feeling, drowsiness
2. ! Decreased or absent deep tendon reflexes
3. Decreased strength or absence of hand grasp
4. Fluid and electrolyte imbalance, hyponatremia
5. Nausea and vomiting
6. ! Respiratory depression leading to respiratory arrest
7. Contraindicated in fetal anomaly incompatible with life, pulmonary edema or CHF, anuria, renal failure, and organic CNS disease

D. Nursing considerations

1. ! Check patellar reflex prior to initial dose and any subsequent doses; depression of reflex could indicate risk for respiratory arrest
2. ! Monitor hand grasps and deep tendon reflexes hourly for signs of toxicity
3. Monitor vital signs every 30 to 60 minutes, especially respiratory rate (needs to be 16/min or greater for additional doses to be safe)
4. ! Call prescriber for respiratory depression if respirations less than 12/minute
5. ! Ensure that calcium gluconate (antidote) is available at bedside
6. ! IV infusion flow rate is generally adjusted to maintain urine flow of at least 30 to 50 mL/hour, monitor I & O carefully; be certain to use infusion pump
7. Monitor IV site closely to avoid extravasation
8. Monitor serum magnesium levels for target range of 4 to 7 mEq/L and call prescriber if greater than 7 mEq
9. Take accurate daily weight

E. Client teaching

1. Side effects of medication
2. Report signs of preeclampsia, including headache, epigastric pain, and visual disturbance
3. Report any signs of confusion

VI. ANALGESICS

A. Overview (Box 35–2)

1. Used to manage moderate to severe pain of labor
2. Common opioid agonist analgesic is meperidine (Demerol)
3. Common opioid agonist-antagonists are butorphanol tartrate (Stadol) and nalbuphine (Nubain)
4. Epidural or intrathecal opioid agents commonly include fentanyl (Sublimaze) and sufentanil (Sufenta)
5. ! Antidote to opioids is naloxone (Narcan)

B. Administration considerations

1. Do not administer in early labor because it could slow labor

Box 35–2

Analgesics During Labor

Opioid Agonists	Opioid Agonist-Antagonists
Meperidine (Demerol)	Butorphanol (Stadol)
Fentanyl (Sublimaze)	Nalbuphine (Nubain)
Sufentanil (Sufenta)	

2. Birth should occur more than 4 hours or less than 1 hour after dose of meperidine to minimize neonatal CNS depression
3. Agonist-antagonists provide adequate analgesia, less respiratory depression, less nausea and vomiting, but equal or greater sedation when compared to meperidine
4. ! Do not use agonist-antagonists for women with opioid dependence because antagonist activity could precipitate withdrawal (abstinence) symptoms in mother and neonate (irritability, hyperactive reflexes, tremors, seizures, yawning, sneezing, vomiting and diarrhea; and excessive crying in neonate)

C. Side/adverse effects

1. Meperidine, fentanyl, and sufentanil: nausea and vomiting, sedation, drowsiness or confusion, tachycardia or bradycardia, hypotension, dry mouth, urinary retention, pruritis, respiratory depression
2. Butorphanol or nalbuphine: confusion, sedation, nausea and vomiting, sweating; respiratory depression less likely to occur

D. Nursing considerations

1. Meperidine, fentanyl, and sufentanil
   a. Monitor fetal heart rate and uterine contractions
   b. Assess for respiratory depression less than 12 breaths/minute
   c. ! Assess newborn for respiratory depression if born in 1 to 4 hours of dose
   d. Keep naloxone available as antidote
   e. Keep siderails raised for safety
   f. Supplement pain relief using nonpharmacologic methods, such as deep breathing, and imagery
2. Butorphanol or nalbuphine
   a. Similar to opioid analgesics
   b. Watch for withdrawal symptoms if administered to opioid-dependent women and neonates

E. Client teaching

1. Purpose and expected effects of medication
2. Use of nonpharmacological pain relief measures

VII. RH_0(D) IMMUNE GLOBULIN (RHOGAM)

A. Overview

1. Prevents anti-Rh_0(D) antibody formation (isoimmunization) in Rh-negative women
2. Used when there is potential or actual exposure to Rh-positive blood: pregnancy, labor and delivery, amniocentesis, chorionic villus sampling, termination of pregnancy, abdominal trauma, or transfusion

B. Administration considerations

1. ! Administer within 72 hours of potential or actual exposure to Rh-positive blood
2. ! Readminister with each subsequent possible or actual exposure
3. Do not administer if client has developed positive antibody titer to Rh antigen
4. ! In typical pregnancy, administer at 28 weeks gestation and within 72 hours of delivery
5. Do not administer to newborn infant

C. Side/adverse effects

1. Tenderness at injection site
2. Slight elevation in temperature
3. ! Contraindicated with hypersensitivity to human immunoglobulins and in Rh-positive women

D. Nursing considerations: administer as described previously

E. Client teaching: purpose and effects of medication and need for repeat injections with subsequent pregnancies

VIII. LUNG SURFACTANTS

A. Overview (Box 35–3)

1. **Surfactant** lowers surface tension on alveolar surfaces during respiration, which improves gas exchange

Box 35-3

Lung Surfactants

Beractant (Survanta)

Colfosceril palmitate (Exosurf)

2. Stabilizes alveoli against collapse at resting pressures
3. Prevents or treats respiratory distress syndrome (RDS) in premature infants

B. Administration considerations
1. Given by intratracheal route into endotracheal tube using #5 French catheter with end hole
2. Do not suction within 1 hour after dose unless significant airway obstruction occurs

C. Side/adverse effects
1. Oxygen desaturation
2. Transient bradycardia
3. Crackles and moist breath sounds occur transiently after dose; does not necessarily indicate suctioning is needed

D. Nursing considerations
1. Ensure proper endotracheal tube placement prior to dosing
2. Monitor heart rate, chest expansion, facial expression during administration
3. Monitor oxygen saturation and periodically assess arterial or transcutaneous oxygen and CO_2 levels

E. Client teaching: purpose and intended effects of medication to parents

IX. BETAMETHASONE (CELESTONE)

A. Overview
1. Synthetic glucocorticoid (corticosteroid)
2. Prevention of neonatal RDS as an unlabeled use
3. Enhances production of surfactant

B. Administration considerations
1. Administered to a client in preterm labor between 28 and 32 weeks gestation
2. Used if client and fetus can safely tolerate inhibition of labor for 48 hours
3. Administer as once-daily dose IM

C. Side/adverse effects
1. Contraindicated during lactation
2. Typically those of other corticosteroids, with risk of infection and delayed wound healing being notable

D. Nursing considerations
1. Monitor maternal vital signs and fetal well-being
2. Monitor for increased temperature and WBC as general indicators of infection

E. Client teaching: purpose and intended effects of medication to parents

X. PHYTONADIONE OR VITAMIN K_1 (AQUAMEPHYTON)

A. Overview
1. Fat-soluble vitamin that aids synthesis of clotting factors II, VII, IX, and X in immature newborn liver
2. Prevents and treats hemorrhagic disease of newborn until neonate has intestinal flora to absorb vitamin K from GI tract

B. Administration considerations
1. Give IM at time of delivery in vastus lateralis muscle of leg
2. Protect from light

C. Side/adverse effects: hyperbilirubinemia

D. Nursing considerations
1. Monitor for signs of bleeding, such as bruising at injection site or actual bleeding from umbilical cord
2. Assess for jaundice and monitor results of bilirubin levels to detect hyperbilirubinemia

E. Client teaching: purpose and intended effects of medication to parents

PRACTICE TEST

XI. NEONATAL EYE PROPHYLAXIS

A. **Overview**

1. Mandated by law for prophylaxis against *Neisseria gonorrhoeae* and *Chlamydia trachomatis*, which could be transmitted to neonate during birth
2. Common agents include erythromycin ophthalmic ointment and tetracycline ophthalmic ointment or solution
3. Previously silver nitrate (1%) solution used, but this practice is outdated because of irritating effects on eyes and insufficient prophylaxis against chlamydia infection

B. **Administration considerations**

!

1. Apply up to but within 1 hour of delivery (allow time for eye contact that promotes parent–infant bonding)
2. Cleanse eyes before application of dose
3. Administer 0.5 to 1 cm ribbon of ointment into each conjunctival sac
4. Do not rinse eyes following dose
5. Use a new tube of ointment for each neonate

C. **Side/adverse effects:** blurring of vision possible after application of ointment

D. **Nursing considerations:** as noted previously

E. **Client teaching:** purpose and intended effects of medication to parents

Check Your NCLEX-RN® Exam I.Q.

You are ready for testing on this content if you can

- Apply knowledge of expected actions and effects of maternal and newborn medications to client care.
- Correctly administer maternal and newborn medications to clients.
- Assess for side effects and adverse effects of maternal and newborn medications.
- Take appropriate action if a client has an unexpected response to a maternal or newborn medication.
- Monitor a client for expected outcomes or effects of treatment with maternal or newborn medications.

PRACTICE TEST

1 The nurse should anticipate that which of the following would be included in the therapeutic plan of care for a postpartum client with subinvolution?

1. Oral methylergonovine maleate (Methergine)
2. Oxytocin (Pitocin) IV infusion for 8 hours
3. Oral fluids to 3000 mL per day
4. Blood replacement

2 The nurse interprets that in which postpartum client would methylergonovine maleate (Methergine) be contraindicated?

1. A client with a blood pressure of 120/60
2. A client with a heart rate of 60
3. A client with a blood pressure of 140/100
4. A client with a respiratory rate of 12

3 A postpartum client has an epidural catheter in place following delivery of an infant via cesarean section. The nurse determines that which of the following medications is a priority to have on hand for use if needed?

1. Meperidine hydrochloride (Demerol)
2. Betamethasone (Celestone)
3. Carboprost (Hemabate)
4. Naloxone (Narcan)

4 The nurse is monitoring a client in labor who is receiving oxytocin (Pitocin) as a continuous infusion to augment labor. Which of the following observations of the client would indicate to the nurse that the infusion needs to be stopped?

1. Contractions lasting 120 seconds
2. Maternal blood pressure increase from 124/82 to 130/86
3. Early fetal heart rate decelerations on the fetal monitor
4. Squeezing eyes shut during each contraction

5 The nurse is evaluating the status of a pregnant client receiving magnesium sulfate. The nurse concludes that the medication is having the intended effect if which of the following is noted?

1. BP has stabilized at 128/76
2. Serum magnesium level reaches 2.2 mEq/L
3. Contractions are steady at a frequency of every 4 minutes
4. There is absence of seizure activity

6 The nurse notes that the client is Rh-negative and her baby is Rh-positive. Which maternal laboratory result would be important to interpret next in determining if the client is a candidate for RhoGAM?

1. Hemoglobin level
2. Direct Coomb's test
3. Indirect Coomb's test
4. Bilirubin level

7 In addition to routine assessment and care, nursing care of the client who is receiving terbutaline (Brethine) to prevent premature labor should include assessing which of the following as an indicator of adverse drug effects?

1. Oral temperature every 2 hours
2. Fetal heart tones every 30 minutes
3. Breath sounds every 4 hours
4. Deep tendon reflexes every 4 hours

8 A client in premature labor is scheduled to receive a dose of betamethasone (Celestone). In teaching the client about this medication, the nurse would explain that the purpose of the medication is to do which of the following?

1. Stop uterine contractions
2. Prevent infection
3. Hasten fetal lung maturity
4. Prevent cervical dilatation

9 The nurse is preparing to administer an intramuscular injection of phytonadione (AquaMEPHYTON) to a healthy newborn. Which of the following is the best explanation for the nurse to give the neonate's mother?

1. "This medication will treat hemorrhagic disease of the newborn."
2. "This medication supplies vitamin K, which the newborn cannot produce in the first 5 to 8 days of life."
3. "This medication is a multivitamin that has many effects, including helping to produce prothrombin in the blood."
4. "This medication is also known as vitamin K, and it is a water-soluble vitamin that is deficient in newborns."

10 The nurse caring for a newborn 30 minutes after birth would do which of the following when preparing to give a prescribed dose of ophthalmic erythromycin?

1. Withhold the dose for 2 hours to allow for parent–infant bonding.
2. Administer the dose into each lower conjunctival sac.
3. Irrigate the eyes after the dose to flush out microorganisms.
4. Use a tube of ointment from a previous birth that has only been open 2 hours.

11 A female client comes for her 24-week prenatal visit. The nurse midwife tells her, "Your blood tests reveal that you do not show immunity to the German measles." Which notation will the nurse include in the plan of care for the client? "Client will need:

1. Rh immune globulin at the next visit."
2. Rh immune globulin within 2 days of delivery."
3. Rubella vaccine at the next visit."
4. Rubella vaccine after delivery on the day of discharge."

12 A client who is breast feeding her newborn is to be discharged from the postpartum unit. She has been found to have no immunity to rubella and has orders to receive rubella vaccine on the day of discharge. What is the most important instruction for the nurse to include in the discharge plan?

1. Practice contraception and avoid conception for at least 2 to 3 months.
2. Discontinue breast feeding to prevent the infant from becoming infected with the rubella virus.
3. Avoid contact with women who are pregnant or who suspect they may be pregnant.
4. Have the infant screened for active rubella virus at the 2-month checkup.

PRACTICE TEST

13 A primigravida with blood type A-negative is at 28 weeks' gestation. Today her physician has ordered a RhoGAM injection. Which statement by the client demonstrates that more teaching is needed related to this therapy?

1. "I'm getting this shot so that my baby won't develop antibodies against my blood, right?"
2. "I understand that if my baby is Rh-positive I'll be getting another one of these injections."
3. "This shot will prevent me from becoming sensitized to Rh-positive blood."
4. "This shot should help to protect me in future pregnancies if this baby is Rh-positive, like my husband."

14 Aerosol therapy is an important part of the therapy for a pregnant woman with an exacerbation of asthma. Which of the following factors is most important for the nurse to consider in delivering aerosol medication?

1. It is used instead of postural drainage.
2. The particles of moisture produced must be large enough to dilate the bronchioles.
3. The aerosol delivers medication to the lower respiratory tract.
4. Unlike with many pulmonary diseases, medications administered through aerosol therapy are contraindicated in pregnancy.

15 The nurse explains to a new nurse orientee that phytonadione (AquaMEPHYTON) needs to be administered to the neonate for which of the following reasons?

1. It prevents gonorrhea, and it is a state law.
2. It inhibits the production of prothrombin by the liver.
3. The neonate lacks the intestinal flora for vitamin K production.
4. The neonate cannot synthesize phytonadione.

16 A pregnant client is receiving magnesium sulfate. The nurse evaluates which of the following as a sign of excessive blood levels of the drug?

1. Development of seizures
2. Disappearance of the knee-jerk reflex
3. Increase in respiratory rate
4. Increase in blood pressure

17 After receiving magnesium sulfate, a client develops signs of toxicity. The nurse should be prepared to administer which of the following?

1. Oxygen
2. Epinephrine
3. Potassium chloride
4. Calcium gluconate

18 Before administering IV magnesium sulfate therapy to a client with pregnancy-induced hypertension, the nurse would assess which of the following parameters that have highest priority?

1. Urinary glucose, acetone, and specific gravity
2. Temperature, blood pressure, and respirations
3. Urinary output, respirations, and patellar reflexes
4. Level of consciousness, funduscopic appearance, and knee reflex

19 During the administration of magnesium sulfate to the client with preeclampsia, the nurse would observe for which of the following toxic effects of the drug?

1. Dry pale skin
2. Hyporeflexia
3. Agitation
4. Increased respirations

20 A client in active labor is to have an epidural block. While this is being administered, the nursing action that takes priority is which of the following?

1. Checking the uterine contractions for an increase in strength
2. Positioning the mother flat in bed to avoid postspinal headache
3. Telling the mother she will feel the need to void more frequently
4. Monitoring the maternal blood pressure for possible hypotension

21 While a client is receiving magnesium sulfate for severe preeclampsia, the nurse would carry out which of the following appropriate nursing interventions? Select all that apply.

1. Limit fluid intake to 1000 mL/24 hours.
2. Prepare for the possibility of a precipitate delivery.
3. Restrict visitors and keep the room darkened and quiet.
4. Obtain calcium gluconate for use as an antagonist if necessary.
5. Assess for patellar reflexes.

ANSWERS & RATIONALES

1 **Answer: 1** Methergine provides long-sustained contraction of the uterus. It is commonly used to treat late postpartum hemorrhage (subinvolution). Oxytocin (option 2) and prostaglandin are more frequently used to treat early postpartum hemorrhage caused by uterine atony. When blood products are used (option 4), they are generally ordered for early postpartum hemorrhage. Increased fluid intake (option 3) is a general, helpful measure for any client who has lost body fluid volume, but it is not a specific therapy.
Cognitive Level: Application **Client Need:** Physiological Integrity: Pharmacological and Parenteral Therapies **Integrated Process:** Nursing Process: Planning **Content Area:** Maternal Newborn **Strategy:** Specific knowledge of ergonovine maleate (Methergine) is needed to answer this question. Use medication knowledge and the process of elimination to make your selection.

2 **Answer: 3** Methergine has a side effect of raising the blood pressure. A woman with hypertension or pregnancy-induced hypertension would not be a good candidate for use of Methergine. An alternative would be necessary. The client in option 1 has a normal blood pressure, which is not a contraindication. A pulse of 60 (option 2) or respiratory rate of 12 (option 4) are not contraindications to use of Methergine.
Cognitive Level: Analysis **Client Need:** Physiological Integrity: Pharmacological and Parenteral Therapies **Integrated Process:** Nursing Process: Planning **Content Area:** Pharmacology **Strategy:** Specific knowledge of ergonovine maleate (Methergine) is needed to answer this question. Use nursing knowledge and the process of elimination to make your selection.

3 **Answer: 4** Naloxone is the antidote to the opioid analgesics that are used with epidural analgesia. If respiratory depression occurs, this medication needs to be readily available for use. Meperidine is an opioid analgesic but is not used for epidural analgesia. Betamethasone is a glucocorticoid used to enhance fetal lung maturity before premature delivery. Carboprost is an abortifacient.
Cognitive Level: Analysis **Client Need:** Physiological Integrity: Pharmacological and Parenteral Therapies **Integrated Process:** Nursing Process: Planning **Content Area:** Pharmacology **Strategy:** The core issue of the question is a priority medication to have on hand during epidural analgesia. Use the process of elimination to select the antidote needed for respiratory depression, a priority adverse effect of epidural analgesia.

4 **Answer: 1** Contractions lasting longer than 90 seconds indicate uterine hyperstimulation, which is a reason to stop the oxytocin infusion. The increase in blood pressure is not of concern. Early decelerations of fetal heart rate do not indicate fetal distress; rather, they are a reassuring sign. Squeezing eyes shut during contractions could have variable meanings, including coping with the contraction, and needs to be correlated with other client data for proper interpretation.
Cognitive Level: Analysis **Client Need:** Physiological Integrity: Pharmacological and Parenteral Therapies **Integrated Process:** Nursing Process: Assessment **Content Area:** Pharmacology **Strategy:** The core issue of the question is knowledge of adverse effects of oxytocin and how to recognize them in the woman in labor. Use the process of elimination and knowledge of adverse drug effects and uterine hyperstimulation to make a selection.

5 **Answer: 4** The danger of preeclampsia is that it can progress to eclampsia, characterized by seizure activity. Magnesium sulfate is given to prevent seizures. It is not given to stabilize BP, although it can cause a transient decline in BP. It is not given to regulate magnesium level or uterine contractions.
Cognitive Level: Analysis **Client Need:** Physiological Integrity: Pharmacological and Parenteral Therapies **Integrated Process:** Nursing Process: Evaluation **Content Area:** Pharmacology **Strategy:** The core issue of the question is the action of magnesium sulfate in a client with preeclampsia. Use drug knowledge and the process of elimination to make a selection.

6 **Answer: 3** An indirect Coomb's test assesses for the presence of Rh antibodies in the maternal blood. Direct Coomb's test and bilirubin tests are conducted on the newborn. Hemoglobin is not a determinant for the administration of RhoGAM.
Cognitive Level: Analysis **Client Need:** Physiological Integrity: Pharmacological and Parenteral Therapies **Integrated Process:** Nursing Process: Analysis **Content Area:** Pharmacology **Strategy:** The core issue of the question is the laboratory indicator that signals the need for administration of Rhogam. Specific knowledge of this drug is needed to answer this question. Use the process of elimination.

7 **Answer: 3** Terbutaline, a beta-adrenergic agent, has many maternal and fetal side effects, including tachycardia, cardiac arryhthmias, and pulmonary edema. In addition to taking routine vital signs, the nurse should assess for pulmonary edema. The frequency of assessment of fetal heart tones and oral temperature depends on the intensity and length of the drug therapy as well as surrounding circumstances. Deep-tendon reflex assessment is not indicated.
Cognitive Level: Application **Client Need:** Physiological Integrity: Pharmacological and Parenteral Therapies **Integrated Process:** Nursing Process: Assessment **Content Area:** Pharmacology **Strategy:** Use the process of elimination. The core issue of the question is knowledge that terbutaline is a beta-adrenergic drug that can lead to adverse effects, including pulmonary edema. Use the ABCs to help focus on breathing and respiratory assessment.

8 **Answer: 3** Corticosteroids such as betamethasone have been shown to enhance fetal lung maturity and prevent respiratory distress. Betamethasone does not stop labor or cervical changes. A side effect is increased risk of infection.
Cognitive Level: Application **Client Need:** Physiological Integrity: Pharmacological and Parenteral Therapies **Integrated Process:** Nursing Process: Implementation **Content Area:** Pharmacology **Strategy:** Specific medication knowledge is needed to answer the question. Recall that a drug ending in *-sone* is likely to be a steroid, and this hastens lung maturity in the fetus at risk for premature delivery.

9 **Answer: 2** The best explanation is the one that explains the use of phytonadione. The medication is given to supply vitamin K, which the newborn cannot produce in the early days of life because of lack of intestinal flora needed to synthesize it. Although phytonadione does treat hemorrhagic disease of the newborn, its use in the healthy infant is prophylactic. The medication is not water soluble, nor is it a multivitamin.
Cognitive Level: Analysis **Client Need:** Physiological Integrity: Pharmacological and Parenteral Therapies **Integrated Process:** Communication and Documentation **Content Area:** Pharmacology **Strategy:** Note the critical word *best* in the stem of the question, which tells you that more than one or all answers may be factually correct. Note also the critical word *healthy,* which eliminates option 1. Eliminate options 3 and 4 because they contain inaccurate information.

10 **Answer: 2** The nurse would give the ophthalmic dose by applying a 0.5 to 1 cm ribbon of ointment into each lower conjunctival sac. The dose can be delayed up to an hour after birth, but not 2 hours. The eyes are not cleansed or irrigated after the dose, and a new tube is used for each newborn.
Cognitive Level: Application **Client Need:** Physiological Integrity: Pharmacological and Parenteral Therapies **Integrated Process:** Nursing Process: Implementation **Content Area:** Pharmacology **Strategy:** Use the process of elimination, keeping in mind principles of aseptic technique and standard procedure for administration of eye medications.

11 **Answer: 4** German measles is also termed rubella. Pregnant women are tested at their first prenatal visit for immunity to rubella. If the client is found to be nonimmune, immunization will be given after delivery, before discharge.
Cognitive Level: Application **Client Need:** Physiological Integrity: Pharmacological and Parenteral Therapies **Integrated Process:** Communication and Documentation **Content Area:** Pharmacology **Strategy:** Look for key differences in the answers. Here we have rubella and Rh isoimmunization, both of which are tested during pregnancy. Rh isoimmunization is prevented by giving RhoGAM at 28 weeks and again after delivery if the baby is found to be Rh-positive, Coomb's-negative. Rubella vaccine is not given during pregnancy.

12 **Answer: 1** The rubella vaccine is prepared with a live virus; therefore, it is not appropriate to administer during pregnancy. Clients are counseled to avoid pregnancy for 3 months after immunization.
Cognitive Level: Analysis **Client Need:** Physiological Integrity: Pharmacological and Parenteral Therapies **Integrated Process:** Nursing Process: Planning **Content Area:** Pharmacology **Strategy:** Knowledge of immunizations is critical to planning care for clients. Rubella vaccine is a live virus vaccine, and therefore pregnancy should be avoided while immunity is formed.

13 **Answer: 1** This client statement indicates that she does not understand the fundamental indications for treatment of this potential blood incompatibility. If an Rh-negative client is carrying an Rh-positive infant, the potential for mixing of fetal blood into the maternal system could occur at midpregnancy and again at delivery of the placenta. If the infant is found to be Rh-positive, the client will be given RhoGAM within 72 hours of delivery to block any antigen-antibody formation.
Cognitive Level: Analysis **Client Need:** Physiological Integrity: Pharmacological and Parenteral Therapies **Integrated Process:** Nursing Process: Evaluation **Content Area:** Pharmacology **Strategy:** Mapping out the case management of a client with Rh-negative blood is helpful in choosing potential interventions throughout pregnancy.

14 **Answer: 3** Aerosol medications are delivered via a liquid mist, which delivers medication to the lower respiratory tract. Postural drainage would be done if indicated. The droplets need to be small, not large. Drugs are always administered during pregnancy after evaluating both the benefit to the mother and the risks to the fetus.
Cognitive Level: Application **Client Need:** Physiological Integrity: Pharmacological and Parenteral Therapies **Integrated Process:** Nursing Process: Planning **Content Area:** Pharmacology **Strategy:** Remember the underlying principle of respiratory care entails postural drainage, mist oxygen that delivers medication to the lower respiratory, as well as oral medications to decrease viscous secretions. The pregnant client actually breathes in more volume than the nonpregnant client. The nurse would be wise to monitor the fetal effects of the medications given to the mother; in this case, beta-adrenergic agents cause fetal tachycardia.

15 **Answer: 3** The neonate intestinal tract is sterile at birth. Colonization of bacteria in the gut necessary for vitamin K synthesis takes approximately a week to occur. The other options listed contain incorrect rationales.
Cognitive Level: Application **Client Need:** Physiological Integrity: Pharmacological and Parenteral Therapies **Integrated Process:** Communication and Documentation **Content Area:** Pharmacology **Strategy:** Vitamin K is critical to normal clotting; careful attention to the subtle differences in the available answers will support better scores.

16 **Answer: 2** Magnesium sulfate is a CNS depressant; therefore, disappearance of the patellar or knee jerk reflex would indicate serious CNS depression. The other options do not indicate adverse effects of the medication.
Cognitive Level: Analysis **Client Need:** Physiological Integrity: Pharmacological and Parenteral Therapies **Integrated Process:** Nursing Process: Evaluation **Content Area:** Pharmacology **Strategy:** Remember your CNS assessments and the patellar reflex being a specific indicator of CNS integrity. In a client receiving magnesium sulfate, you would expect the patellar reflex to be diminished but not absent.

17 **Answer: 4** The antidote for magnesium sulfate is calcium gluconate. The other drugs listed are not.
Cognitive Level: Application **Client Need:** Physiological Integrity: Pharmacological and Parenteral Therapies **Integrated Process:** Nursing Process: Implementation **Content Area:** Pharmacology **Strategy:** Calcium gluconate is an antidote for excessive magnesium sulfate, and safe practice indicates that this drug should be available at the bedside.

18 **Answer: 3** Excretion of magnesium sulfate is primarily accomplished through the renal system. Critical assessments prior to administration of the drug would be focused on the body's ability to excrete the medication and the status of the CNS. Both assessments should be within normal limits, or the prescribing health care provider should be notified.

Cognitive Level: Analysis **Client Need:** Physiological Integrity: Pharmacological and Parenteral Therapies **Integrated Process:** Nursing Process: Assessment **Content Area:** Pharmacology **Strategy:** The key to correctly answering this question is to focus on indications for stopping the drug; if these signs are present prior to administration, they must be reported to the prescriber.

19 **Answer: 2** Magnesium sulfate is an anticonvulsant medication given to pregnant women with preeclampsia to diminish the risk of convulsions. The drug is a CNS depressant and therefore acts to reduce CNS activity. CNS activity should not be absent.

Cognitive Level: Application **Client Need:** Physiological Integrity: Pharmacological and Parenteral Therapies **Integrated Process:** Nursing Process: Implementation **Content Area:** Pharmacology **Strategy:** Remember CNS depressants should diminish reflex activity, not stop it altogether, or the client will cease respiratory and cardiac function.

20 **Answer: 4** Epidural medications cause vasodilatation, which can lead to hypotension. This is the primary risk factor the nurse needs to monitor after placement. Other considerations can be considered once the client's ABCs are stable.

Cognitive Level: Analysis **Client Need:** Physiological Integrity: Pharmacological and Parenteral Therapies **Integrated Process:** Nursing Process: Implementation **Content Area:** Pharmacology **Strategy:** Remember that many local anesthetics cause vasodilatation.

21 **Answer: 3, 4, 5** The most critical incident that could occur in a client receiving magnesium sulfate is toxic CNS depression, which could affect respiratory and cardiac function. Therefore, the antidote should be available at the bedside. The nurse should assess for patellar reflexes to detect excessive dosing. It is also important to keep the room quiet. It is not necessary to prepare for precipitous birth (option 2) or severely limit fluid intake (option 1).

Cognitive Level: Analysis **Client Need:** Physiological Integrity: Pharmacological and Parenteral Therapies **Integrated Process:** Nursing Process: Implementation **Content Area:** Pharmacology **Strategy:** The critical word in the stem of the question is *appropriate,* which tells you that the correct options are also correct interventions. Use knowledge of magnesium sulfate and the process of elimination to make a selection.

Key Terms to Review

ergotism p. 547 **prostaglandins** p. 548 **surfactant** p. 550

References

Abrams, A. (2004). *Clinical drug therapy: Rationales for nursing practice* (7th ed.). Philadelphia: Lippincott Williams & Wilkins.

Adams, M., Josephson, D., & Holland, L. (2005). *Pharmacology for nurses: A pathophysiologic approach.* Upper Saddle River, NJ: Pearson Education.

Deglin, J. H., & Vallerand, A. H. (2006). *Davis's drug guide for nurses* (10th ed.). Philadelphia: F. A. Davis.

Lehne, R. (2004). *Pharmacology for nursing care* (5th ed.). Philadelphia: Saunders.

Lowdermilk, D., & Perry, S. (2004). *Maternity and women's health care* (8th ed.). St. Louis: Elsevier Science, 220–265.

McKenry, L., Tessier, E., & Hogan, M. (2006). *Mosby's pharmacology in nursing* (22nd ed.). St. Louis: Elsevier Science.

Olds, S. B., London, M. L., & Davidson, M. (2004). *Maternal-newborn nursing & women's health care* (7th ed.). Upper Saddle River, NJ: Prentice Hall.

Wilson, B., Shannon, M., & Stang, C. (2006). *Prentice Hall nurse's drug guide 2006.* Upper Saddle River, NJ: Pearson Education.

36 Psychiatric Medications

Test Yourself

Are you ready for the NCLEX-RN® or course exams? Use the practice tests on the companion CD-ROM to check.

In this chapter

Cross reference

Other chapters relevant to this content area are

Mental Health Disorders	Chapter 22
Dependency and Addiction	Chapter 23
Crisis Intervention and Suicide	Chapter 24

I. GENERAL GUIDELINES FOR PSYCHIATRIC MEDICATIONS *(SEE BOX 36–1)*

II. ANTIPSYCHOTICS

A. Phenothiazines

1. Are **neuroleptics** (drugs used to treat psychosis); also called typical (traditional) antipsychotic agents (Box 36–2)
2. Assist in improving thought processes and positive symptoms in schizophrenia and other psychoses; are less effective in treating negative symptoms
3. Typical antipsychotics are predominantly dopamine **antagonists** (DA), which block postsynaptic D_2 receptors in several DA tracts in brain
4. Selected agents are also used as antiemetics and antihistamines; chlorpromazine is also used for intractable hiccups
5. **Tolerance** to antipsychotic medications is very uncommon; they are the most toxic drugs used in psychiatry
6. ! Medication effects can usually be seen in 1 to 2 days, but substantial improvement usually takes 2 to 4 weeks and full effects may not occur for several months
7. Initially, a thorough baseline evaluation is needed, including laboratory tests such as white blood cell (WBC) count and electrocardiogram (ECG)
8. Side/adverse effects
   a. Gynecomastia, galactorrhea, amenorrhea (occasionally), and weight gain
   b. Sedation and orthostatic hypotension
   c. ! **Anticholinergic effects** (dry mouth, blurred vision, urinary retention, photophobia, constipation, tachycardia)
   d. ! **Akathisia** (an uncontrollable need to move)
   e. ! **Parkinsonism** (a set of symptoms that resembles Parkinson's disease)

Box 36–1

General Guidelines for Psychiatric Medications

Administration Principles

1. Assess current medications (including OTC drugs and herbal products) and history of any allergies to identify potential risks to client.
2. Administer doses on time to maintain therapeutic blood levels.
3. Do not break or allow client to chew sustained release or enteric–coated preparations.
4. Many drugs cause CNS depression, so monitor client for adverse effects and maintain a safe environment.
5. Provide both verbal and written instructions to client, and provide phone number to call if questions arise or problems occur.
6. When risk of suicide is of concern, do not allow access to large quantities of medication; ensure that doses are swallowed and not "cheeked."

Client Teaching

1. Understand medication actions, side/adverse effects, signs of toxicity, importance of follow-up with prescriber and complying with follow-up laboratory tests, and how to self–administer.
2. Do not take any OTC or herbal preparations without first consulting prescriber.
3. Take exactly as prescribed and do not miss or double doses.
4. Report adverse or toxic effects promptly.
5. Many drugs used for psychiatric/mental health problems cause CNS depression; do not drive, use hazardous equipment, or engage in other activities requiring alertness until effects on individual client are known.
6. Do not drink alcohol or take other OTC medications that cause drowsiness to avoid interactive effects
7. Do not discontinue without consulting with prescriber

f. **Agranulocytosis** is rare, marked by a severe deficit or lack of granulocytic WBCs (neutrophils, basophils, eosinophils)

! g. **Neuroleptic malignant syndrome (NMS),** characterized by catatonia, rigidity, stupor, unstable blood pressure, hyperthermia, profuse sweating, dyspnea, and incontinence; treated with bromocriptine (Parlodel) and dantrolene (Dantrium) if usual treatment for hyperthermia is ineffective; the drug must be changed

Box 36–2

Typical and Atypical Antipsychotic Drugs

Typical Antipsychotics

Phenothiazine: aliphatic
Chlorpromazine (Thorazine)
Triflupromazine (Vesprin)

Phenothiazine: piperidine
Mesoridazine (Serentil)
Thioridazine (Mellaril)

Phenothiazine: piperazine
Acetophenazine (Tindal)
Fluphenazine (Prolixin)
Perphenazine (Trilafon)
Trifluoperazine (Stelazine)

Thioxanthene
Thiothixene (Navane)

Butyrophenone
Haloperidol (Haldol)

Dihydroindolone
Molindone (Moban)

Dibenzepin
Loxapine (Loxitane)

Atypical Antipsychotics

Dibenzodiazepine
Clozapine (Clozaril)
Olanzapine (Zyprexa)
Quetiapine (Seroquel)

Benzisoxazole
Risperidone (Risperdal)
Ziprasidone (Geodon)

Novel Antipsychotic

Aripiprazole (Abilify)

! h. **Tardive dyskinesia:** (inability to perform voluntary movement; "tardive" indicates late onset); a serious side effect of antipsychotic agents
! i. Overdoses are not usually fatal; treatment is supportive (e.g., gastric lavage to empty the stomach); can cause severe central nervous system (CNS) depression (somnolence to coma, hypotension), **extrapyramidal side effects** or ESPEs (parkinsonism, dystonia, akathisia, tardive dyskinesia) and restlessness or agitation, seizures, hyperthermia, increased anticholinergic symptoms, and dysrhythmias
j. Low-potency drugs are more likely to cause sedation and hypotension, while high-potency drugs cause more EPSEs

9. Nursing considerations
! a. Observe client taking medication in an inpatient setting to ensure medications are swallowed and not "cheeked"
b. Monitor vital signs and urine output
! c. Monitor and manage EPSEs, as appropriate (see Table 36–1 ■)
! d. Consider long-acting depot injections such as haloperidol and fluphenazine for long-term therapy of schizophrenia; this form of treatment usually reduces the rate of relapse
! e. Monitor results of periodic WBC counts and other laboratory studies

Table 36–1
Extrapyramidal Side Effects (EPSE)

Side Effects	Nursing Interventions
Peripheral Nervous System Effects	
Constipation	Increase fluid intake, encourage high dietary fiber intake, provide laxatives as necessary.
Dry mouth	Advise client to use sugarless hard candy or gum and to take sips of water frequently.
Nasal congestion	Suggest OTC nasal decongestants that are safe for use with antipsychotic agents.
Blurred vision	Ask client to avoid dangerous tasks. This symptom will usually last only a short time at the beginning of treatment. Eye drops should be used for the short-term need.
Mydriasis	Advise client to report any eye pain immediately.
Photophobia	Advise client to wear sunglasses when in sunlight.
Orthostatic hypotension	Advise client to get out of chair or bed slowly, to sit before standing, and to rise slowly. Observe to see if change to another antipsychotic is advisable.
Tachycardia	This is usually a reflex response to hypotension. When intervention for hypotension is effective, reflex tachycardia usually decreases. With clozapine, withhold the dose if pulse rate is over 140.
Urinary retention	Encourage client to void when urge is present and to void frequently. Catheterize for residual urine. Client should closely monitor output. Older men with benign prostatic hyperplasia are particularly susceptible to urinary retention.
Urinary hesitation	Provide privacy; encourage client to take the time to void, run water in sink, or pour warm water over perineum.
Sedation	Help client to get up, get dressed, and begin the day early.
Weight gain	Advise client to maintain appropriate diet.
Agranulocytosis	Monitor WBC counts weekly. There is a high incidence of agranulocytosis for clients who are taking clozapine. If the WBC is less than 3500 cells/mm^3 prior to therapy, no treatment should begin. After treatment has begun, a WBC under 3000 cells/mm^3 and a granulocyte count of under 1500 cells/mm^3 indicate that treatment should be interrupted to monitor for infection. If WBC is under 2000 cells/mm^3 and granulocyte count is less than 1000 cells/mm^3, halt therapy and do not begin treatment with the drug again. If infection develops, antibiotics should be prescribed.

Table 36–1 (*cont.*)

Side Effects	Nursing Interventions
Central Nervous System Effects	
Akathisia	Usually develops within the first 2 months. Client experiences an uncontrollable need to move; occurs most often with high-potency antipsychotics. Treatment is usually with beta-blockers, benzodiazepines, and anticholinergic drugs. The antipsychotic agent should be changed to a lower potency agent. It is important to distinguish between akathisia and exacerbation of psychosis. If akathisia is confused with anxiety or psychotic agitation, it is likely that antipsychotic dosage would be increased, thereby making akathisia more intense.
Dystonias	Acute: Usually occur early in treatment and are dangerous and severe. Oculogyric crisis or torticollis are the most common occurrences. Treatment includes antiparkinson drug or antihistamine immediately; offer reassurance. Obtain an order for IM administration when client begins treatment with antipsychotics, or if in acute state of dystonia, call physician immediately. For less acute dystonias, notify the physician when an order for an antiparkinson drug is warranted.
Drug-induced parkinsonism	A chronic disease characterized by a fine, slowly spreading tremor, muscular weakness and rigidity, and a peculiar gait induced by some antipsychotic medications. Assess for three major symptoms: tremors, rigidity, and bradykinesia. Report to physician immediately. Antiparkinson drugs will be indicated.
Tardive dyskinesia (TD)	Develops in 15% to 20% of clients during long-term therapy. The risk is related to duration of treatment and dosage size. For many clients, symptoms are irreversible. Assess for signs using the Abnormal Involuntary Movement Scale (AIMS). Anticholinergic agents will worsen TD, so use is contraindicated.
Neuroleptic malignant syndrome	This is a fatal side effect of antipsychotic medications. Routinely take client's temperature and encourage adequate water intake. Also routinely assess for rigidity, tremor, and similar symptoms.
Seizures	Occur in approximately 1% of clients taking antipsychotic medications. Clozapine causes an even higher rate, up to 5% of clients taking 600–900 mg/day. For dosages of clozapine greater than 600 mg/day, an EEG should be performed. If a seizure occurs, it may be necessary to discontinue clozapine.

10. Client teaching
- **a.** Take medication as prescribed; the major relapse factor for clients with schizophrenia is discontinuing medications
- **b.** Take oral doses with food, milk, or a full glass of water to decrease gastric irritation
- **c.** Dilute most concentrates in 120 mL of distilled or acidified tap water or fruit juice just before use; avoid skin contact with liquid to prevent contact dermatitis
- ! **d.** Use sunscreen and protective clothing such as long sleeves, pants, and hats when outdoors to prevent photosensitivity

Memory Aid

Many drugs cause photosensitivity as a side effect; when protection from the sun is an option, consider carefully whether this could be the correct answer.

- ! **e.** Expect observable response after 7 to 10 days, but full effects take 3 to 6 weeks
- ! **f.** Expect urine color to change from yellow to pinkish to red-brown; this is an expected change and is not harmful
- ! **g.** Change position slowly to avoid orthostatic hypotension
- **h.** Report fever, malaise, and other signs of infection such as sore throat; these may indicate agranulocytosis

i. Follow-up laboratory studies are needed to monitor WBC count and liver function
j. Avoid sudden withdrawal of drug, which may result in return of psychotic symptoms
k. Learn about other medications that may be prescribed to treat ESPEs (see Box 36–3)

B. Atypical antipsychotic drugs

1. Exert both dopamine receptor subtype 2 (D_2) and serotonin receptor subtype 2 ($5HT_2$) receptor-blocking action (are DA and 5HT antagonists)
2. Blockage of serotonin receptors is thought to liberate dopamine in cortex and may explain some reduction in negative symptoms
3. Atypical agents cause few or no EPSEs
4. ! Used to treat positive and negative symptoms of schizophrenia and other mental illnesses with psychotic features and to treat mood symptoms, hostility, violence, suicidal behavior, and cognitive impairment seen in schizophrenia

Memory Aid

Remember that typical drugs are effective against the positive symptoms of schizophrenia, while atypical antipsychotics are effective against both positive and negative symptoms.

5. Are especially useful for clients experiencing first psychotic episode and who have not responded well to typical antipsychotics or have suffered dose-limiting side effects from traditional neuroleptics
6. Refer back to Box 36–2 for listing of drugs in this category; clozapine (Clozaril), risperidone (Risperdal), and olanzapine (Zyprexa)
7. Side/adverse effects
   a. ! Clozapine (Clozaril): agranulocytosis, requiring weekly blood analysis and a limit of not more than a 1-week supply of prescription to enforce compliance with weekly labwork; NMS and seizures are also of concern

Memory Aid

Remember that clozapine begins with *c* and associate that with *CBC* to help you remember that white blood cell counts can drop with this medication, requiring close monitoring.

   b. Risperidone (Risperdal): orthostatic hypotension, insomnia, agitation, headache, anxiety, rhinitis, NMS
   c. Olanzapine (Zyprexa): few incidents of EPSEs, but NMS and seizures are possible
   d. Seizure incidence for clients taking clozapine is 3%; maximum dose should not exceed 900 mg/day
   e. ! See Table 36–2 ■ for common side effects of the atypical antipsychotics
8. Nursing considerations
   a. Clozapine is usually given 1 to 2 times daily and should not exceed 900 mg/day
   b. Risperidone is usually administered PO in 1 to 2 daily doses; for debilitated or elderly clients or for those with renal or hepatic impairment, dosage should be reduced

Box 36–3

Medications Used to Treat Extrapyramidal Side Effects

Anticholinergic

➤ Benztropine (Cogentin)

➤ Trihexyphenidyl (Artane)

Antihistamine

➤ Diphenhydramine (Benadryl)

Dopamine Agonist

➤ Amantadine (Symmetrel)

Table 36–2

Common Side Effects of Atypical Antipsychotics

	Clozapine	Risperidone	Olanzapine
Extrapyramidal	None	+	+
Cardiac	+++	++	+
Sedation	++++	++	+
Anticholinergic	++++	+	++
Weight gain	+++	++	++++

Occurrence: + = least, ++++ = greatest

c. Olanzapine is usually administered PO as well; dosage should not exceed 15 mg/day; for debilitated or nonsmoking female clients older than 65 years, therapy should be initiated at 5 mg/day

! d. Because of the risk of fatal agranulocytosis, clozapine is reserved for clients with severe schizophrenia who have not responded to traditional antipsychotic drugs

9. Client teaching: as per Box 36–1

III. ANTIDEPRESSANTS

A. Tricyclic antidepressants (TCAs)

1. TCAs block monoamine reuptake, elevate mood, increase activity and alertness, decrease client's preoccupation with morbidity, improve appetite, and regulate sleep patterns
! 2. Therapeutic effect occurs in 1 to 3 weeks; maximum response is achieved in 6 to 8 weeks
3. Other uses include treatment of chronic insomnia, attention-deficit/hyperactivity disorder (ADHD) and panic disorder
4. Common medications are listed in Table 36–3 ■
   a. TCAs are equally effective; major differences are in side effects; for example, doxepin has sedative effects and is more useful in clients with insomnia
   b. Elderly clients and those with glaucoma, constipation, or prostatic hyperplasia can be especially sensitive to anticholinergic effects of TCAs; therefore, a TCA such as desipramine with weak anticholinergic effects would be more appropriate with such clients
5. Administration considerations
   a. Dosing with TCAs is individualized and based on clinical response or plasma drug levels (must be above 225 ng/ml for antidepressant effects to occur)
   b. TCAs have long half-lives, so may be taken daily in a single dose
   ! c. Once-a-day dosing at bedtime has advantages: is more easily incorporated into daily routine, promotes sleep (sedative effect), and reduces intensity of daytime side effects
   d. For clients at risk for suicide, do not allow access to large quantity of medication; keep hospitalized until the risk of suicide has been ruled out
6. Significant drug interactions
   ! a. TCAs taken with a monoamine oxidase inhibitor (MAOI) can lead to severe hypertension from excessive adrenergic stimulation of the heart and blood vessels
   b. TCAs potentiate responses to direct-acting sympathomimetics (e.g., epinephrine and norepinephrine) because TCAs block uptake of these drugs into adrenergic terminals, prolonging their presence in the synaptic space
   c. TCAs decrease responses to indirect-acting sympathomimetics (e.g., ephedrine and amphetamine) because TCAs block uptake of these agents into adrenergic nerves, preventing them from reaching their site of action in nerve terminal
   ! d. TCAs exert anticholinergic actions of their own; therefore, they intensify effects of other medications with anticholinergic actions (antihistamines and OTC sleep aids); avoid these products while taking TCAs

Table 36-3

Medications Commonly Used to Treat Depression

Drug Class and Name: Generic (Trade)	Nursing Responsibilities
Tricyclic Antidepressants (TCAs)	
Amitriptyline (Elavil) Clomipramine (Anafranil) Desipramine (Norpramin) Doxepin (Sinequan) Imipramine (Tofranil) Trimipramine (Surmontil) Nortriptyline (Pamelor) Protriptyline (Vivactil)	• Educate client early about potential side effects • Inform client that side effects will diminish with time and, if needed, management alternatives can be implemented • Advise client that response will take some time and continued use is essential • Inform client that first-time treatment for major depression should continue for 6 to 12 months • Warn client of a possible significant weight gain • Monitor for improvement; if no change or minimum change after 2 to 4 weeks, it may be necessary to change medication
Second-Generation Tetracyclics	
Amoxapine (Asendin) Maprotiline (Ludiomil) Mirtazepine (Remeron)	• General considerations are same as for tricyclics.
Selective Serotonin Reuptake Inhibitors (SSRIs)	
Citalopram (Celexa) Escitalopram (Lexapro) Fluoxetine (Prozac) Fluvoxamine (Luvox) Paroxetine (Paxil) Sertraline (Zoloft)	• Inform client to take medication as prescribed; abrupt discontinuation of drug is contraindicated • Continuously monitor client for side/adverse effects, particularly in area of sexual dysfunction; client may be reluctant to discuss
Monoamine Oxidase Inhibitors (MAOIs)	
Phenelzine (Nardil) Tranylcypromine (Parnate)	• Educate client concerning a tyramine-restricted diet. • Caution client about side effects and adverse effects of MAOIs. • Educate client about careful use of OTC or other prescription medications and be sure client understands seriousness of effects. • Monitor efficacy of drugs and continuously re-educate client to avoid abruptly discontinuing medication or not taking medications as prescribed.
Atypical Antidepressants	
Bupropion (Wellbutrin) Trazodone (Desyrel) Nefazodone (Serzone) Venlafaxine (Effexor)	• Instruct client about adverse or side effect of medication, especially seizure risks at higher drug doses. • Instruct client concerning importance of taking this and all medication as prescribed. • Instruct client to take medication as prescribed and monitor for any adverse or side effects. • Instruct client to report any signs of sexual dysfunction, especially priapism, immediately.

e. CNS depression caused by TCAs adds to CNS depression caused by other drugs; avoid use of CNS depressants, including alcohol, antihistamines, opioids, and barbiturates

7. Side/adverse effects
   - a. ! Most common are orthostatic hypotension, sedation, and anticholinergic effects
   - b. Most serious one is cardiac toxicity; clients over age 40 and those with heart disease should have baseline ECG and then every 6 months
   - c. ! Adverse effects of each drug are more fully described in Table 36–4 ■
8. Nursing considerations
   - a. Advise clients of potential side effects and that therapeutic response will take some weeks to establish; clients and families often become impatient when client is experiencing medication side effects while still having original symptoms

Table 36–4

Most Common Adverse Effects from Antidepressant Medications

Effect	Manifestations
Orthostatic hypotension	Major decrease in blood pressure with body position changes
Anticholinergic	Blockade of muscarinic cholinergic receptors, which produces dry mouth, blurred vision, photophobia, constipation, urinary hesitancy, tachycardia
Sedation	Sleepiness and difficulty maintaining arousal are common responses to TCAs, caused by blockade of histamine receptors in CNS
Cardiac toxicity	TCAs can adversely affect heart's function by decreasing vagal influence (secondary to muscarinic blockade) and acting directly on bundle of His to slow conduction
Seizures	Lower seizure threshold
Hypomania	Mild mania can occur
Sexual dysfunction	Anorgasm, delayed ejaculation, decreased libido
Hypertensive crisis from dietary tyramine	Although MAOIs normally produce hypotension, can also cause severe hypertension if client eats tyramine-rich foods

b. Refer back to Table 36–3 for nursing responsibilities with TCAs, and see Table 36–4 for manifestations of common adverse effects

9. Client teaching

a. Side effects diminish with time and symptoms will lessen as medication regime is followed

b. Encourage client and family to utilize other available therapies as well

c. Refer back to Box 36–1 and Tables 36–3 and 36–4 for specific points to include in teaching

B. MAOIs

1. Because of potentially fatal food and drug interactions, MAOIs are not a first choice to treat depression unless client has atypical depression

2. Monoamine oxidase (MAO) is an enzyme present in liver, intestinal wall, and terminals of monoamine-containing neurons; it converts monoamine transmitters (norepinephrine, serotonin, and dopamine) into inactive products; in liver and intestine, MAO inactivates tyramine and other biogenic amines in food

3. MAOIs decrease amount of MAO in liver that breaks down amino acids tyramine and tryptophan

4. MAOIs have been used with some success to treat bulimia, obsessive-compulsive disorder, and panic disorder

5. Common medications: refer again to Table 36–3

6. Contraindications: clients over age 60 or those with pheochromocytoma, congestive heart failure, liver disease, severe renal impairment, cerebrovascular defect, cardiovascular disease, or hypertension

7. Significant drug interactions

! **a.** Taking SSRIs with MAOIs can cause **serotonin syndrome** (agitation, sweating, confusion, fever, hyperreflexia, tachycardia, hypotension, muscle rigidity, ataxia); avoid this combination

! **b.** Antihypertensive drugs potentiate hypotensive effects of MAOIs

c. Meperidine can produce hyperthermia in clients taking MAOIs and should be avoided

! **8.** Significant food interactions

a. Dietary tyramine, some other dietary constituents, and indirect-acting sympathomimetics (e.g., amphetamine, methylphenidate, ephedrine, cocaine) can precipitate a hypertensive crisis in clients taking MAOIs

b. See Box 36–4 for lists of foods to avoid and to use cautiously while taking an MAOI

! **9.** Side/adverse effects

a. Orthostatic hypotension

Box 36-4

Foods to Avoid with Monoamine Oxidase Inhibitors

Foods to Avoid

- All cheeses except those noted below
- Meats and fish: aged/cured
- Fruits and vegetables: broad bean pods, tofu, soybean extracts
- Alcohol: draft beer
- Other: sauerkraut, soy sauce, yeast extracts, soups (especially miso), and any non-fresh foods
- Drugs: other antidepressant drugs, nasal and sinus decongestants, allergy, hay fever and asthma remedies, narcotics (especially meperidine), epinephrine, stimulants, cocaine, amphetamines

Consume with Caution

- Cheeses: mozzarella, cottage, ricotta, cream, processed
- Meats and fish: beef and chicken liver, meats, herring
- Fruits and vegetables: raspberries, bananas, small amounts only of avocado, spinach
- Alcohol: wine
- Other: monosodium glutamate, pizza, small amounts only of chocolate, caffeine, nuts, dairy products
- Drugs: insulin, oral antidiabetics, oral anticoagulants, thiazide diuretics, anticholinergic agents, muscle relaxants

b. Edema, weight gain
c. Complaints of insomnia, anxiety, agitation, hypomania, and even mania
d. Sexual dysfunction

10. Nursing considerations
a. Assess client for ability to adhere to strict dietary regime
! **b.** Consult with primary physician about changes in vital signs to avoid potentially fatal hypertensive crisis

11. Client teaching
a. Teach symptoms of orthostatic hypotension and to avoid injury by rising from bed or chair slowly
! **b.** Provide dietary teaching to avoid hypertensive crisis (include written list of foods to avoid)

C. SSRIs

1. Block reuptake of serotonin and intensify transmission at serotonergic synapses; effects are often seen after 1 to 3 weeks and are equivalent to those produced from TCAs
2. SSRIs have the same efficacy as TCAs, exhibit fewer side effects than either TCAs or MAOIs, and have shorter time between initial dose and beginning of reduced signs and symptoms of depression
3. All SSRIs are effective in treatment of obsessive-compulsive disorder (OCD), panic disorder, and bulimia nervosa
4. Common medications (refer again to Table 36–3)
5. Administration considerations
a. Most SSRIs should not be prescribed for clients with a hypersensitivity to drug or severe hepatic or renal disease
! **b.** Lowered drug doses or longer dosing interval may be needed with impaired hepatic function, multiple drug therapy, or elderly clients
! **c.** To prevent serotonin syndrome SSRIs should not be administered with MAOIs
d. If a client is on an MAOI and is transferred to fluoxetine, at least 5 weeks should elapse before beginning the fluoxetine; to transfer from fluoxetine to MAOIs, at least 2 weeks should elapse before beginning MAOI

e. In a client taking fluoxetine and warfarin, monitor warfarin level closely because fluoxetine is highly bound to plasma proteins and may displace other highly bound drugs such as warfarin

! f. Monitor complete blood count (CBC), differential, and bleeding time periodically for signs of leukopenia, anemia, or thrombocytopenia or for increased bleeding time

6. Side/adverse effects

! a. Common initial side effects include nausea, drowsiness, dizziness, headache, sweating, anxiety, insomnia, anorexia, and nervousness; are generally milder and better tolerated than TCAs

b. Sexual dysfunction is experienced by 20% to 40% of clients, and must be discussed with client

7. Nursing considerations

a. Monitor mood changes; notify physician if client demonstrates an increase in anxiety, nervousness, or insomnia

! b. Assess for suicidal tendencies, especially during early drug therapy when client begins to have increased energy and has sufficient energy to act on suicidal thoughts

! c. Restrict amount of drug available to client to prevent overdose

d. Monitor appetite, nutritional intake, and weight

8. Client teaching: as per Box 36–1 and notify health care professional if a rash occurs, which may indicate hypersensitivity

D. Other antidepressants

1. Bupropion (Wellbutrin)

a. Similar in structure to amphetamines and can suppress appetite; does not have cardiotoxic, anticholinergic, and antiadrenergic side effects, so can be used more readily with elderly clients; can also be used for smoking cessation

b. Blocks reuptake of dopamine while having only minimal reuptake effects on norepinephrine

2. Trazodone (Desyrel)

a. Second-line agent for depression; often used in combination with another antidepressant; often prescribed to treat insomnia because of pronounced sedative effect

b. Alters effects of serotonin in CNS; antidepressant action may develop only over several weeks

3. Administration considerations

a. Bupropion can cause dose-related seizures

b. Dosage should be reduced in elderly or those with severe hepatic or renal disease

4. Side/adverse effects

a. Most common side effects of bupropion are agitation and insomnia

b. Common side effects of trazodone are sedation, orthostatic hypotension, nausea, and vomiting; in contrast to tricyclic agents, it lacks anticholinergic actions and is not cardiotoxic; it may cause priapism (sustained erection)

c. Major adverse effect of bupropion is seizure activity

d. Adverse effects of trazodone frequently include CNS changes

5. Nursing considerations

a. Assess individuals with a history of bipolar disorder taking bupropion for symptoms of mania

b. Monitor BP and pulse rate before and during initial therapy with trazodone; clients with pre-existing cardiac disease should have ECG monitored before and periodically during therapy to detect dysrhythmias

! c. Assess mental status and mood changes frequently; assess for suicidal tendencies, especially during early therapy; restrict amount of drug available to client

d. Give bupropion with food to decrease GI side effects; give trazodone immediately after meals to minimize side effects (nausea, dizziness) and allow for maximum absorption

6. Client teaching: as per Box 36–1

IV. ANTIMANIA MEDICATIONS

A. Lithium

1. The drug of choice for controlling manic episodes in bipolar disorder and for long-term prophylaxis against recurrent mania and depression
2. Alters many neurotransmitter functions, possibly correcting an ion exchange abnormality or normalizing neurotransmission of norepinephrine, serotonin, dopamine, and acetylcholine
3. Common medications (see Box 36-5)
4. Administration considerations
   a. Precise dosing is based on serum lithium levels
   ! b. Antimania effects are usually seen in 5 to 7 days after initial doses, but full effect does not usually occur for 2 to 3 weeks
   c. For many clients using lithium, adjunctive therapy with a benzodiazepine can provide the sedation clients need
   ! d. Contraindicated with sensitivity to drug; use cautiously in debilitated, dehydrated, or elderly clients; those with cardiac, renal, or thyroid disease; those with diabetes mellitus
   e. Should be used only where therapy (including blood levels) may be closely monitored (every 1 to 2 months and as needed based on client behaviors)
   ! f. Large changes in sodium intake may alter renal elimination of lithium; increasing sodium intake will increase renal excretion; conditions leading to loss of sodium (such as dehydration, sweating, diuretics, diarrhea) may lead to toxicity
   ! g. Therapeutic level and the toxic levels are very close; therapeutic range is 0.8 to 1.4 mEq/L, while the toxic dose is 1.5 mEq/L or greater
   h. It is essential to monitor serum lithium levels frequently because of danger of lithium toxicity
5. Side/adverse effects
   a. Fatigue, headache, lethargy
   b. Abdominal pain, anorexia, bloating, diarrhea, nausea, dry mouth, metallic taste in mouth
   c. Polyuria, glycosuria, nephrogenic diabetes insipidus, and renal toxicity
   d. Also reported are weight gain, muscle weakness, hyperirritability, rigidity, and tremors
   e. Toxic effects classified as mild, moderate, or severe
   ! f. Mild toxicity (1.5 mEq/L) is accompanied by mild CNS changes: lethargy, decreased concentration, slight muscle weakness, coarse hand tremors, and mild ataxia
   ! g. Moderate toxicity (1.5–2.5 mEq/L) is accompanied by GI symptoms (nausea, vomiting, severe diarrhea), blurred vision and tinnitus, muscle tremors/twitching, slurred speech, and worsening ataxia and incoordination
   ! h. Severe toxicity (higher than 2.5 mEq/L) is accompanied by nystagmus, hyperreflexia, impaired level of consciousness (LOC), hallucinations, muscle twitching/fasciculations, seizures, or renal shutdown; coma and death may result
6. Nursing considerations
   a. Assess mood, ideation, and behaviors frequently; initiate suicide precautions if indicated
   ! b. Monitor intake and output ratios; report significant changes in totals
   ! c. Unless contraindicated, provide fluid intake of at least 2000 to 3000 mL/day
   d. Monitor weight at least every 3 months

Box 36-5

Commonly Used Mood-Stabilizing Drugs

Lithium carbonate (Eskalith, Lithobid, lithium citrate, etc.)

Carbamazepine (Tegretol)

Valproic acid (Valproate, Depakote, Divalproex, others)

e. Assess client for signs and symptoms of lithium toxicity (vomiting, diarrhea, slurred speech, decreased coordination, drowsiness, muscle weakness, or twitching); if these occur, report before administration of the next dose

7. Client teaching
   a. Take medication even if feeling well; take a missed dose as soon as remembered unless within 2 hours of next dose (6 hours if extended release)
   b. May cause dizziness or drowsiness: avoid driving, operating heavy machinery, and other activities requiring alertness until response to medication is known
   c. Low sodium levels may lead to toxicity: drink 2000 to 3000 mL fluid each day and eat a diet with consistent and moderate sodium intake
   d. Avoid excessive amounts of coffee, tea, and cola (because of their diuretic effect); avoid activities that cause excess sodium loss; notify health care professional of fever, vomiting, and diarrhea, which also cause sodium loss
   e. Weight gain may occur: follow principles of a low-calorie diet
   f. Consult with health care professional before taking any OTC medications, before use of contraception, or if pregnancy is suspected
   g. For clients with cardiovascular disease or over 40 years of age: understand need for ECG evaluation before and periodically during therapy; report any irregular pulse, difficulty breathing, or fainting

B. Other antimania medications

1. A variety of anticonvulsant drugs demonstrate beneficial effects in bipolar disorder when lithium is ineffective, although they are not FDA approved for this use
2. Carbamazepine (Tegretol) and valproic acid (e.g., Valproate Depakote) have acute antimanic and long-term mood-stabilizing effects in bipolar disorder; are better than lithium in treating mixed or dysphoric bipolar states and in clients who are rapid cyclers
3. Carbamazepine's mechanism for stabilizing mood is unknown
4. Valproic acid seems to alter gamma-aminobutyric acid (GABA) mediated neurotransmission to exert mood-stabilizing effects
5. Contraindications
   a. Carbamazepine: hypersensitivity or bone marrow depression; pregnancy unless potential benefits outweigh fetal risks; use cautiously in clients with cardiac or hepatic disease, prostatic hyperplasia, or increased intraocular pressure
   b. Valproic acid: hypersensitivity or hepatic impairment; avoid use with products containing tartrazine; use cautiously with bleeding disorders, liver disease, organic brain disease, bone marrow depression, renal impairment, and in children (increased risk of hepatotoxicity); safe use in pregnancy not established
6. Side/adverse effects
   a. Carbamazepine: sedation, GI disturbance, tremor, ataxia, leukopenia, or agranulocytosis, aplastic anemia, thrombocytopenia, chills, fever, lymphadenopathy, and hepatotoxicity
   b. Valproic acid: sedation, confusion, dizziness, headache, nausea, vomiting, ataxia, paresthesias, tremor, hepatotoxicity, hair loss, and nausea (reduce nausea by using delayed-release tablets or by applying "sprinkle" formulation to food)
7. Nursing considerations
   a. Assess frequently for seizure activity when taking carbamazepine and assess for facial pain because of possibility of trigeminal neuralgia
   b. Perform liver function tests, urinalysis, and BUN routinely, and measure serum ionized calcium levels at least every 6 months or if seizure frequency increases
   c. Implement seizure precautions as indicated; administer medication with food to minimize gastric irritation; tablets may be crushed if client has difficulty swallowing—except for extended-release tablets
   d. Check results of routine CBC and serum iron weekly during the first 2 months and yearly thereafter for potentially fatal blood cell abnormalities; drug should be discontinued if bone marrow depression occurs

8. Client teaching
   a. Take carbamazepine around the clock, exactly as directed; drug dose should be tapered to prevent seizures
   b. Immediately report fever, sore throat, mouth ulcers, easy bruising, petechiae, unusual bleeding, abdominal pain, chills, rash, pale stools, dark urine, or jaundice
   c. Use sunscreen and protective clothing to prevent photosensitivity reactions with carbamazepine
   d. For female clients: use a nonhormonal form of contraception while taking carbamazepine
   e. Carry information, such as a Medic-Alert tag/bracelet, describing disease and medication regimen at all times
   f. Understand the importance of follow-up laboratory tests, eye examinations, and ECGs
   g. For valproic acid, be sure to take medication exactly as directed; abrupt withdrawal may lead to seizures in a susceptible client

V. SEDATIVE-HYPNOTIC AND ANXIOLYTIC MEDICATIONS

A. Benzodiazepines (BZs)

1. BZs are powerful potentiators (receptor agonists) of inhibitory neurotransmitter GABA
2. BZ molecules and GABA bind to each other at GABA receptor sites, resulting in *inhibition* of neurotransmission that results in a clinical decrease in anxiety level
3. **Metabolites** (the result of biotransformation of a drug) are pharmacologically active, so drug effects persist long after parent drug is gone from plasma
4. Major indications for use of BZs are anxiety, insomnia (sedative-hypnotic effect), and seizure disorders
5. Other uses include alcohol withdrawal, skeletal muscle relaxation, substance-induced (except for amphetamines) and psychotic agitation in emergency departments or in other crisis situations
6. Common medications are listed in Box 36–6

Memory Aid

Remember that a drug that ends with the suffix *-zepam* is a benzodiazepine.

7. Administration considerations
   a. BZs should be started at low doses and gradually increased to achieve desired clinical response; rapid onset of clinical action occurs once an appropriate dose is achieved
   b. For treatment of anxiety, BZs are usually dosed at bedtime or twice daily, only occasionally are 3 doses/day required
   c. Treatment for insomnia should be no longer than 7 to 10 days to avoid rebound insomnia; sleep hygiene techniques should also be used to establish regular sleep pattern
   d. BZs are contraindicated with drug sensitivity or during pregnancy or lactation (cross blood–brain barrier and enter breast milk with ease and develop quickly to toxic levels)
   e. BZs should not be used with clients who have pre-existing CNS depression, severe uncontrolled pain, or narrow-angle glaucoma
   f. Because hepatic metabolism is the primary mechanism for drug disposition, drugs that interfere with liver metabolism (e.g., alcohol) dangerously compound BZ effects
8. Side/adverse effects
   a. Hypotension
   b. Dry mouth, ataxia, dizziness, drowsiness, nausea
   c. Withdrawal symptoms (increased anxiety, flulike symptoms, tremors)

Box 36-6

Sedative-Hypnotic and Anxiolytic Medications*

Barbiturates

Amobarbital (Amytal)

Butabarbital (Butisol)

Pentobarbital (Nembutal)

Phenobarbital (Luminal)

Secobarbital (Seconal)

Benzodiazepines

Alprazolam (Xanax)

Chlordiazepoxide (Librium)

Clonazepam (Klonopin)

Clorazepate (Tranxene)

Diazepam (Valium)

Estazolam (ProSom)

Flurazepam (Dalmane)

Lorazepam (Ativan)

Midazolam (Versed)

Triazolam (Halcion)

Oxazepam (Serax)

Temazepam (Restoril)

Nonbarbiturate/Nondiazepines

Buspirone (Buspar)

Zolpidem (Ambien)

Benzodiazepine Antagonist

Flumazenil (Romazicon)

* Drug class and name: Generic (Trade)

9. Nursing considerations
   a. Assess degree and manifestation of anxiety before client begins therapy
   b. Assess client for drowsiness, light-headedness, and dizziness periodically during treatment; these usually disappear as therapy progresses
   c. Monitor blood pressure, pulse, and respirations, and provide supportive care as indicated
   d. Prolonged therapy may lead to psychological or physical dependence; risk is greater with larger doses of the medication; restrict amount of drug available to client
10. Client teaching
    a. As per Box 36–1
    b. If a dose is missed, take within 1 hour or skip dose and return to regular schedule
    c. If medication is less effective after a few weeks, check with prescriber; do not increase dose
    d. Abrupt withdrawal of medication may cause sweating, vomiting, muscle cramps, tremors, and convulsions

B. Benzodiazepine antagonist

1. Flumazenil (Romazicon) is a BZ antagonist that selectively blocks BZ receptors but does not block adrenergic or cholinergic receptors
2. Can reverse *sedative* effects of BZs but may not reverse BZ-induced *respiratory depression*
3. Because it does not stimulate CNS and does not block other receptors, it can be given for suspected BZ overdose and to reverse effects of BZs following general anesthesia
4. Works within 30 to 60 seconds of IV administration
5. Contraindicated with hypersensitivity; if receiving BZs for life-threatening medical problems, including status epilepticus or increased intracranial pressure; and for clients with serious TCA overdose
6. Side effects: minor side effects include dizziness, agitation, confusion, nausea, vomiting, hiccups, paresthesia, rigors, and shivering; principle adverse effect is seizures, which occur most often in clients with epilepsy or physical dependence on BZs
7. Nursing considerations
   a. Assess LOC and respiratory status before and throughout therapy
   b. Establish that client has patent airway before administration

c. Institute seizure precautions
d. For suspected DZ overdose: if no effects are seen after giving flumazenil, consider other causes of decreased LOC (alcohol, barbiturates, opioid analgesics)
e. Observe client for at least 2 hours after giving last dose for appearance of resedation; hypoventilation may occur

8. Client teaching
   a. Inform family that client may appear alert at time of discharge but sedative effects of BZ may reoccur; instruct client to avoid driving or other activities requiring alertness for at least 24 hours after discharge
   b. Instruct client not to take *any* alcohol or nonprescription drugs for at least 18 to 24 hours after discharge
   c. Client should resume usual activities only when no residual effects of BZs remain

C. Barbiturates

1. Cause relatively nonselective depression of CNS function and are prototypes of the general CNS depressants; used for daytime sedation, induction of sleep, suppression of seizures, and general anesthesia
2. Can cause tolerance and dependence, have a high abuse potential, and are subject to multiple drug interactions; are powerful respiratory depressants
3. Common medications (see again Box 36–4)
4. Administration considerations
   a. Avoid intramuscular (IM) route; barbiturate solutions are highly alkaline and can cause pain and necrosis when injected IM
   b. As dosage is increased, response progresses from *sedation* to *sleep* to *general anesthesia*
   c. At hypnotic doses, barbiturates may reduce BP and heart rate; by contrast, toxic doses can cause profound hypotension and shock (from direct depressant effects on both myocardium and vascular smooth muscle)
   d. Tolerance to sedative and hypnotic effects and to other effects that underlie barbiturate abuse develops with repeated drug use
5. Side/adverse effects
   a. Barbiturates have long half-lives and can produce residual effects (hangover) when taken to treat insomnia; can manifest as sedation, impaired judgment, and reduced motor skills
   b. Paradoxical excitement (especially the elderly and debilitated); the mechanism of this response is not known
   c. Barbiturates can intensify sensitivity to pain and may cause pain directly; their use has produced muscle pain, joint pain, and pain along nerves
   d. Acute barbiturate overdose produces a classic triad of symptoms: *respiratory depression, coma,* and *pinpoint pupils,* frequently accompanied by *hypotension* and *hypothermia*
6. Nursing considerations
   a. Monitor respiratory status, pulse, and blood pressure frequently
   b. Prolonged therapy may lead to psychological or physical dependence; restrict amount of drug available, especially if client is depressed, suicidal, or has a history of addiction
   c. Always monitor client for safety, alertness, and need for help with ambulation or self-care
7. Client teaching
   a. As per Box 36–1
   b. For female clients using oral contraceptives: use an additional nonhormonal contraceptive during therapy

D. Other sedative-hypnotics and anxiolytics

1. Buspirone: used to manage anxiety; binds to serotonin and dopamine receptors and increases norepinephrine metabolism in brain
2. Buspirone's major advantages are that it is nonsedative, has no abuse potential, and does not enhance CNS depression caused by BZs, alcohol, barbiturates, and related drugs; major disadvantage is delayed onset of anxiolytic effects

3. Zolpidem is used for short-term treatment of insomnia; produces CNS depression by binding to GABA receptors; it has no analgesic properties but produces sedation and induction of sleep
4. Administration considerations
   a. Buspirone undergoes extensive first-pass metabolism in the liver; giving it with food delays absorption but enhances bioavailability (by reducing first-pass metabolism)
   b. Zolpidem is rapidly absorbed following oral administration and is usually given just before bedtime because of its rapid onset of action
5. Side effects
   a. Buspirone is generally well tolerated; the most common reactions are dizziness, nausea, headache, nervousness, lightheadedness, and excitement
   b. Zolpidem has a side effect profile like that of the BZs; daytime drowsiness and dizziness are most common, but occur in only about 1% to 2% of clients
6. Nursing considerations
   ! a. Assess degree and manifestations of anxiety before and periodically throughout therapy with buspirone
   b. Buspirone does not appear to cause physical or psychological dependence or tolerance; however, assess clients with a history of drug abuse for tolerance or dependence, and restrict amount of drug available to these clients
   ! c. Clients changing from other antianxiety agents should receive gradually decreasing doses; buspirone will not prevent withdrawal symptoms
   ! d. With zolpidem, there may be a potential for physical or psychological dependence if used longer than 7 to 10 days; limit the amount of drug available to the client
   e. For clients taking zolpidem, assess alertness at time of peak effect; notify prescriber if desired sedation does not occur
   f. Assess client who has pain and medicate as needed; untreated pain decreases sedative effects of zolpidem
7. Client teaching
   a. As per Box 36–1
   ! b. With buspirone, report any chronic abnormal movements such as **dystonia** (muscle rigidity), motor restlessness, involuntary movements of facial or cervical muscles, or if pregnancy is suspected
   ! c. With zolpidem, go to bed immediately after taking dose because of rapid onset of action

VI. SUBSTANCE MISUSE

A. Alcohol abuse and disulfiram (Antabuse) therapy

1. Alcohol is a CNS depressant that causes general (relatively nonselective) depression of CNS function, primarily by enhancing GABA
2. Effect of alcohol on CNS is dose-dependent; low dosage primarily affects cortical brain function (thought processes, self-restraint, motor function); as dosage increases, CNS depression deepens, reflexes diminish greatly, and level of consciousness (LOC) is impaired
3. Management of withdrawal (outpatient versus inpatient) depends on degree of alcohol dependence
4. Most medical treatment for withdrawal includes use of BZs—chlordiazepoxide (Librium), diazepam (Valium) and lorazepam (Ativan); a regime of atenolol (a beta-adrenergic blocking agent) used in conjunction with BZs decreases amount of BZs necessary for safe detoxification
5. Disulfiram inhibits enzyme *alcohol dehydrogenase,* which catalyzes a major step in breakdown of alcohol
6. ! When enzyme is inhibited and an individual drinks alcohol, blood concentrations of toxic metabolite *acetaldehyde* increase significantly, producing unpleasant symptoms of flushing, tachycardia, nausea, vomiting, and hypotension
7. Administration considerations
   a. Disulfiram is used only with highly selected individuals in good physical health

b. At least 12 hours should elapse from time of last alcohol intake and initial disulfiram dose
c. Relatively long half-life of disulfiram ensures that several days must elapse between stopping the medication and safely drinking alcohol; this probably decreases impulsive relapse

8. Adverse effects/toxicity: acetaldehyde syndrome (from ingesting alcohol and disulfiram) is manifested by marked respiratory depression, cardiovascular collapse, cardiac dysrhythmias, myocardial infarction, acute congestive heart failure, convulsions, and death
9. Nursing considerations
   a. Simultaneous use with alcohol can precipitate acetaldehyde syndrome
   b. Effects of disulfiram may persist for about 2 weeks after last dose; alcohol must not be consumed until this interval has passed
10. Client teaching
   a. Avoid all forms of alcohol, including alcohol in sauces, cough and cold syrups, aftershave lotions, colognes, and liniments
   b. Adhere to all forms of self-help groups, both individual and group therapies, while using disulfiram therapy to establish a recovery program

B. Opioids

1. Opioids (e.g., morphine, heroin) are major drugs of abuse and are usually Schedule II substances
2. Opioid toxicity produces a classic triad of symptoms: respiratory depression, coma, and pinpoint pupils
3. Naloxone (Narcan), an opioid antagonist, rapidly reverses all signs of opioid poisoning
4. Naloxone dosage must be titrated carefully; too much naloxone causes client to swing from intoxicated state to one of withdrawal
5. Because of short half-life, naloxone must be given every few hours until opioid has dropped to a nontoxic level
6. Nalmefene (Revex), a long-acting opioid antagonist, is an alternative to naloxone; because of its long half-life, nalmefene does not require repeated dosing; however, if dose is excessive in an opioid-dependent person, it will lead to prolonged withdrawal
7. Methadone, a long acting oral opioid, is commonly used to ease opioid withdrawal and prevent abstinence syndrome; once stabilized on methadone, withdrawal is accomplished by administering it in gradually smaller doses
8. With methadone withdrawal, abstinence syndrome is mild, with symptoms resembling those of moderate influenza; entire process of methadone substitution and withdrawal takes about 10 days
9. Objective of maintenance methadone therapy is to avoid withdrawal and need to procure illicit drugs; methadone maintenance is most effective in conjunction with nondrug measures directed at altering patterns of drug use

C. Cocaine

1. Cocaine, extracted from coca plant, is a fine, white, odorless powder; it passes blood–brain barrier readily and causes an instantaneous high; when administered IV (mainlining), it is rapidly metabolized by liver, so "rush" does not last long
2. Cocaine exerts both CNS and peripheral nervous system (PNS) effects because it blocks norepinephrine and dopamine reuptake into presynaptic neurons; it depletes these neurotransmitters
3. Cocaine is highly addictive and produces mild physical withdrawal but severe psychological withdrawal
4. Treatment is aimed at restoring depleted neurotransmitters; three approaches include use of amino acid catecholamine precursors (such as tyrosine and phenylalanine), TCAs, and dopamine agonist bromocriptine

D. Cannabis (marijuana/hashish)

1. Marijuana is derived from the Indian hemp plant *Cannabis sativa;* major psychoactive substance is delta-9-tetrahydrocannabinol (THC), an oily chemical with high lipid solubility

2. Marijuana produces 3 principal subjective effects: euphoria, sedation, and hallucinations
3. Common effects of low-dose THC include euphoria and relaxation; an increased sensitivity to visual and auditory stimuli; enhanced sense of touch, taste, and smell; increased appetite and a more intense appreciation of flavor of food; distortion of time (times seems to move more slowly)
4. Cannabinoids are sometimes used to treat nausea and vomiting (more effectively than traditional antiemetics) as severe side effects of cancer chemotherapy; THC has been approved for stimulating appetite in clients with AIDS

Check Your NCLEX-RN® Exam I.Q. *You are ready for testing on this content if you can*

- Apply knowledge of expected actions and effects of psychiatric medications to client care.
- Correctly administer psychiatric medications to clients.
- Assess for side effects and adverse effects of psychiatric medications.
- Take appropriate action if a client has an unexpected response to a psychiatric medication.
- Monitor a client for expected outcomes or effects of treatment with psychiatric medications.

PRACTICE TEST

1 The client is reporting vague dread; she is pacing and hyperventilating. Her jaw is clenched, and she is wringing her hands. The nurse concludes that this client is in need of which of the following types of medications?

1. A barbiturate
2. An anxiolytic
3. An antipsychotic
4. A CNS stimulant

2 The client is taking zolpidem (Ambien). What would be a priority nursing diagnosis for this client?

1. Self-care deficit
2. Risk for violence
3. Disturbed sleep pattern
4. Deficient fluid volume

3 The nurse determines that the client understands the effects of flurazepam (Dalmane) ordered at a dose of 30 mg by which of the following client statements?

1. "After I take my medication at bedtime, I should be able to watch the boxing match or late night TV show, then go to bed and sleep."
2. "Once I take my medicine, I should be able to go to bed and read, and I will fall asleep within 1 hour."
3. "I will take my medicine, go to bed, and go to sleep."
4. "I will take my medicine, make my lunch for tomorrow, take my shower, and get my clothes ready for work tomorrow, and then go to bed."

4 The nurse conducting medication teaching with a client explains that a safe effective dose of clozapine (Clozaril) is established by weekly

1. physical exam by a psychiatrist.
2. hematological monitoring.
3. follow-up visits with a physician.
4. urinalysis.

5 A client is taking sertraline (Zoloft). The nurse explains to the client that how much time will pass before the onset of the medication occurs?

1. 5 to 7 days
2. 1 to 4 weeks
3. 4 to 6 weeks
4. 4 to 8 weeks

PRACTICE TEST

6 The visiting nurse is evaluating for client safety. The client is taking phenelzine (Nardil). A priority of the nurse's teaching includes which of the following?

1. Limiting daily intake of salt
2. Encouraging a fluid intake of at least 2000 mL
3. Encouraging the client to have scheduled blood tests on time
4. Eliminating foods containing tyramine

7 The client is diaphoretic, disoriented, has a temperature of 100°F., has insomnia, and is complaining of feeling anxious and unable to sit still. The nurse suspects this client may

1. be withdrawing from alcohol or CNS depressants.
2. be demonstrating flu symptoms.
3. be withdrawing from an antipsychotic medication.
4. have abruptly discontinued lithium carbonate.

8 Immediately after taking alprazolam (Xanax) the client says, "I know I shouldn't feel this guilty, but I don't want to take medicine that makes me feel this way." What would be the most appropriate response by the nurse?

1. "Are you worried about what people will say because you are taking this medicine?"
2. "Once the medication begins to work, you'll feel differently about taking it."
3. "Can we talk about how you're feeling about taking Xanax?"
4. "It will be better for your long-term mental health if you don't worry about what other people think."

9 The client is taking carbamazepine (Tegretol) for treatment of mania. The client is instructed to come to the laboratory weekly for monitoring of which of the following?

1. Neuroleptic malignant syndrome
2. Agranulocytosis
3. Thrombocytopenia
4. Anemia

10 A client with schizophrenia has been taking haloperidol (Haldol) for 3 weeks with good effect. Today, he comes to group but is complaining that he feels like his legs are on fire. He is moving continuously and states, "I can't sit here anymore." The nurse documents and reports that the client is experiencing which of the following medication side effects?

1. Anticholinergic effects
2. Gustatory hallucinations
3. Akathisia
4. Oculogyric crisis

11 The nurse concludes the client understands the desired effects and major side effects of trazodone (Desyrel) when he makes which of the following statements?

1. "I know I will be able to get up and go downstairs to the bathroom during the night as long as I leave a nightlight on."
2. "I am drinking more fluids now that I am taking this medication so it will work the way it is supposed to."
3. "This medicine should help me sleep without my having to worry about becoming addicted to it, and if I have a problem with priapism, I will notify my doctor immediately."
4. "I will feel more energetic after 3 or 4 weeks of taking this medication, and I understand I must take it only as prescribed so that I will not become addicted to it."

12 The client is hospitalized because of a suicide attempt while in a manic phase. The client has now been taking chlordiazepoxide (Librium) for 2 days. Which of the following is the most important safety measure for the nurse to implement with this client?

1. Frequently remind the client to remain visible to the nurses at all times.
2. Elicit the client's promise to tell someone if feeling suicidal.
3. Make a contract for safety.
4. Enforce the client's promise to eat all meals in the dining room.

13 If an overdose of benzodiazepines is suspected, the nurse obtains which of the following medications to reverse that drug's effects as ordered?

1. Diazepam (Valium)
2. Triazolam (Halcion)
3. Fluvoxamine (Luvox)
4. Flumazenil (Romazicon)

14 The nurse is making a plan of care for a client who is prescribed fluphenazine (Prolixin) 1 mg daily at bedtime. The nurse will include which of the following to monitor for side effects of the medication?

1. Frequently remind client to move slowly when getting out of bed or rising from a chair.
2. Assess for dizziness or lightheadedness frequently during the day.
3. Make sugarless hard candy, gum, and water available during the day.
4. Monitor frequently for confusion.

15 The client expresses an increase in appetite, a desire to participate in group today, and a request to have her mother come to visit later in the week. The client has been in the inpatient locked unit on suicide precautions for 5 days and is taking imipramine (Tofranil). The nurse does not make major changes to the nursing care plan at this time for which of the following reasons?

1. It is not safe after only 5 days to address too many changes at once. It is better to make gradual changes once the medication is more effective.
2. Imipramine (Tofranil) is beginning to make the client feel less suicidal.
3. After a suicide attempt, the likelihood of another attempt is rare, so it is better to let the client make adjustments, and then the nurse can change the care plan.
4. The client is less likely to attempt suicide again if there is no change in the care plan or expectations of her.

16 The client is receiving thioridazine (Mellaril) 100 mg TID. Today he comes to the clinic with the chief complaint of feeling like his mouth is "always dry." The nurse concludes this side effect is related to which of the following?

1. High anticholinergic effects of thioridazine
2. Extrapyramidal side effects (EPSE)
3. Weight loss effect of the medication
4. Neuroleptic malignant syndrome (NMS) side effect

17 A client asks the nurse if it is true that marijuana is not just a street drug but has legitimate uses, as he read in a magazine article. The nurse replies that marijuana does have therapeutic uses, such as the ability to

1. stimulate appetite.
2. stimulate clients to become more organized and motivated.
3. help clients to reduce stress.
4. act as an antibacterial agent.

18 The nursing diagnosis is "Anxiety related to recent attack and robbery in apartment evidenced by episodes of immobilizing apprehension." A short-term anxiolytic has been prescribed. What is the primary nursing priority for this client?

1. Help client learn alternative responses to the anxiety.
2. Promote involvement of family/client in group or community support activities.
3. Provide for physical safety.
4. Assist with desensitization to phobic place (apartment).

19 The client is admitted to the inpatient unit with a diagnosis of paranoid schizophrenia. He is prescribed risperidone (Risperdal). After 5 days of treatment, the client reports feeling dizzy. The nurse explains to the client that this is associated with

1. the desired effect of sedation.
2. the side effect of loss of appetite.
3. the anticholinergic side effects prominent with this agent.
4. the side effect of orthostatic hypotension.

20 Which of the following is the highest priority for the client after withdrawing from alcohol and beginning use of disulfiram (Antabuse)?

1. Social reintegration
2. Learning about the disease process
3. Remaining abstinent
4. Remaining in the rehabilitation unit

ANSWERS & RATIONALES

1 **Answer: 2** This client is suffering from anxiety. The correct answer is an anxiolytic. Option 1 is a sedative-hypnotic, which would not be prescribed. The client is not suffering from psychosis or hallucinations, so option 3 is inappropriate. Option 4 is be inappropriate for the signs and symptoms described.
Cognitive Level: Analysis **Client Need:** Physiological Integrity: Pharmacological and Parenteral Therapies **Integrated Process:** Nursing Process: Analysis **Content Area:** Pharmacology **Strategy:** This question requires you to interpret the client's symptoms as being representative of anxiety and to choose the drug category that is effective against it. Focus on the client manifestations to eliminate each of the incorrect options.

2 **Answer: 3** Zolpidem (Ambien) is a sedative-hypnotic medication used to treat insomnia. Therefore, disturbed sleep pattern is the appropriate priority nursing diagnosis. There is not enough information in the question to determine whether self-care deficit, risk for violence, or deficient fluid volume would be pertinent for the client.
Cognitive Level: Analysis **Client Need:** Physiological Integrity: Pharmacological and Parenteral Therapies **Integrated Process:** Nursing Process: Analysis **Content Area:** Pharmacology **Strategy:** First recall that zolpidem is a sedative-hypnotic medication. Next associate its use as a bedtime sleep aid to make the appropriate selection.

3 **Answer: 2** The medication normally works within 30 minutes to 1 hour after administration, making option 2 correct. Option 1 is incorrect because the client should not be watching stimulating shows on television before trying to fall asleep. Option 3 is incorrect because the medication will not work instantly. Option 4 is incorrect because the client should not take a sedative and then stay active for 30 minutes to 1 hour after taking medication.
Cognitive Level: Analysis **Client Need:** Physiological Integrity: Pharmacological and Parenteral Therapies **Integrated Process:** Nursing Process: Evaluation **Content Area:** Pharmacology **Strategy:** The word *understands* in the stem of the question tells you the correct answer is also a true statement. Recall that the medication is used to enhance sleep, and utilize principles of good sleep hygiene to eliminate each of the incorrect options.

4 **Answer: 2** In order to safely monitor clozapine, a weekly blood test is mandatory. If the client does not have the hematologic exam, the medication is not given for the following week. This is to monitor for agranulocytosis, the drug's major adverse effect. A full physical exam (option 1) and urinalysis (option 3) are unnecessary. Follow-up visits (option 3) are done periodically but may not be needed weekly with the physician.
Cognitive Level: Application **Client Need:** Physiological Integrity: Pharmacological and Parenteral Therapies **Integrated Process:** Nursing Process: Assessment **Content Area:** Pharmacology **Strategy:** The core issue of the question is knowledge of possible adverse effects of clozapine. Recall that the drug may cause bone marrow depression and agranulocytosis to choose the correct monitoring technique.

5 **Answer: 2** Sertraline is an antidepressant of the SSRI type. These agents work within 1 to 4 weeks. Option 1 is an insufficient amount of time, while options 3 and 4 are excessive as well as similar.
Cognitive Level: Application **Client Need:** Physiological Integrity: Pharmacological and Parenteral Therapies **Integrated Process:** Nursing Process: Implementation **Content Area:** Pharmacology **Strategy:** Specific knowledge of the time frame in which SSRIs exert an effect is needed to answer this question. Use medication knowledge and the process of elimination to make a selection.

6 **Answer: 4** With an MAOI such as phenelzine, the client must eliminate foods that contain tyramine. Intake of tyramine-containing foods could lead to severe hypertension and other complications. All of the other considerations are not major teaching considerations for MAOIs.
Cognitive Level: Application **Client Need:** Physiological Integrity: Pharmacological and Parenteral Therapies **Integrated Process:** Teaching/Learning **Content Area:** Pharmacology **Strategy:** The core issue of the question is knowledge that phenelzine is an MAOI. From there, recall that foods high in tyramine need to be avoided to make the correct selection.

7 **Answer: 1** These symptoms are the commonly seen symptoms of withdrawal from alcohol or other CNS depressants. Option 2 is incorrect because there would usually not be complaints of disorientation or insomnia with flu-like symptoms. Individuals do not usually have withdrawal symptoms from antipsychotic medications (option 3), nor are these the signs of lithium carbonate discontinuation (option 4).
Cognitive Level: Analysis **Client Need:** Physiological Integrity: Pharmacological and Parenteral Therapies **Integrated Process:** Nursing Process: Analysis **Content Area:** Pharmacology **Strategy:** Clients withdrawing from a substance are likely to experience the opposite effects of the original drug. With this in mind, review the client's symptoms and note that they represent excitation of the CNS. With this in mind, you can then deduce that the original substance was some type of CNS depressant, leading you to option 1.

8 **Answer: 3** In the correct response, the nurse acknowledges the client's feelings and asks the client to discuss the feelings and thoughts. In options 1, 2, and 4, the nurse is not acknowledging the client's feelings or thoughts. An open and trusting nurse–client relationship helps support the client in decisions related to medication therapy.
Cognitive Level: Application **Client Need:** Physiological Integrity: Pharmacological and Parenteral Therapies **Integrated Process:** Communication and Documentation **Content Area:** Pharmacology **Strategy:** The correct answer to the question is one that is the most therapeutic response by the nurse. Use knowledge of communication techniques and the process of elimination to make a selection.

9 **Answer: 2** The most serious side effect of carbamazepine is agranulocytosis (low WBC count). Neuroleptic malignant syndrome is not common with carbamazepine, nor is there a

need for weekly monitoring for low platelet count (option 3) or anemia (option 4) while taking carbamazepine.
Cognitive Level: Application **Client Need:** Physiological Integrity: Pharmacological and Parenteral Therapies **Integrated Process:** Nursing Process: Implementation **Content Area:** Pharmacology **Strategy:** The core issue of the question is that an adverse effect of carbamazepine is agranulocytosis. With this in mind, eliminate each of the incorrect responses that does not address this concern.

10 **Answer: 3** Akathisia is an inability to sit. This is the most common extrapyramidal side effect of haloperidol. The side effect described in option 1 would include dry mouth, urinary hesitance, constipation, mydriasis, tachycardia, and diminished lacrimation. Option 2, gustatory hallucination, is tasting something that is not present, while option 4 is a painful twisting and turning of the head and neck.
Cognitive Level: Analysis **Client Need:** Physiological Integrity: Pharmacological and Parenteral Therapies **Integrated Process:** Nursing Process: Assessment **Content Area:** Pharmacology **Strategy:** The core issue of the question is correct identification of side effects of haloperidol. First eliminate options 2 and 4 because *gustatory* refers to taste and *oculo-* refers to eyes. Choose option 3 over option 1 because the word *akathisia* is consistent with the client's presentation, while the word *anticholinergic* is not.

11 **Answer: 3** Trazadone is an atypical antidepressant that is used more for insomnia than for depression. Abuse potential is minimal, so option 4 is incorrect. Option 1, for safety reasons, is not a good practice when taking trazodone as a sleep aid, and option 2 is incorrect because taking more fluids will not increase the effectiveness of the medication.
Cognitive Level: Analysis **Client Need:** Physiological Integrity: Pharmacological and Parenteral Therapies **Integrated Process:** Nursing Process: Evaluation **Content Area:** Pharmacology **Strategy:** First recall that the use of trazodone is often as a sleep aid. With this in mind, eliminate each of the incorrect responses because they are not consistent with knowledge of its use for this purpose.

12 **Answer: 3** The client needs to make an agreement with the nurse to remain safe or report to the nurse if not feeling safe. Option 4 does not keep the client safe for 24 hours, only during meals. The agreement in option 1 is too vague and does not give specific responsibility either to the nurse or to the client. The promise in option 2 is also vague and does not make the client accountable to the health care professionals.
Cognitive Level: Application **Client Need:** Physiological Integrity: Pharmacological and Parenteral Therapies **Integrated Process:** Nursing Process: Implementation **Content Area:** Pharmacology **Strategy:** Note that the question contains a key phrase: *most important safety measure.* This tells you that more than one option might be partially or totally correct and that you must prioritize. Keep in mind that medication therapy alone is not sufficient in treating this client. Choose option 3 over the others because it is the most inclusive of the client's safety needs.

13 **Answer: 4** Flumazenil is the only drug available that acts as an antagonist to the benzodiazepines. Options 1 and 2 are benzodiazepines themselves, while option 3 is a selective serotonin reuptake inhibitor (SSRI) type of antidepressant.
Cognitive Level: Application **Client Need:** Physiological Integrity: Pharmacological and Parenteral Therapies **Integrated Process:** Nursing Process: Planning **Content Area:** Pharmacology **Strategy:** Specific knowledge of the antidote to benzodiazepines is needed to answer this question. It may help to remember that the antidote to benzodiazepines is a generic drug name that contains the letters *ze* and is not a benzodiazepene itself.

14 **Answer: 3** Dry mouth occurs from the anticholinergic effects seen with fluphenazine. Options 1 and 2 are incorrect because orthostatic hypotension is not a major side effect of fluphenazine. Confusion (option 4) is not a side effect of this agent.
Cognitive Level: Application **Client Need:** Physiological Integrity: Pharmacological and Parenteral Therapies **Integrated Process:** Nursing Process: Planning **Content Area:** Pharmacology **Strategy:** First eliminate options 1 and 2 because they are similar in referring to orthostatic hypotension. Choose option 3 over option 4 because it addresses anticholinergic effects of the drug, which are of concern.

15 **Answer: 1** Option 1 is the accurate response to the situation. Option 2 is incorrect because imipramine is very slow to become effective—2 to 6 weeks, not 5 days—and as the client begins to "feel better," it is not appropriate to make major changes, especially after a suicide attempt. Options 3 and 4 are not true, but gradual change and monitoring for changes in mood and behavior are still very critical for this client.
Cognitive Level: Analysis **Client Need:** Physiological Integrity: Pharmacological and Parenteral Therapies **Integrated Process:** Nursing Process: Planning **Content Area:** Pharmacology **Strategy:** To answer this question correctly, recall that antidepressants generally take more than 5 days for full effect. With this in mind, realize that the client is still a safety risk, and choose the option that keeps the client safest while medication therapy is progressing.

16 **Answer: 1** With thioridazine, the anticholinergic side effects of dry mouth, constipation, urinary retention, and blurred vision are usually high. Dry mouth is not associated with extrapyramidal side effects (option 2) or neuroleptic malignant syndrome (option 4). There is usually a weight gain, not a weight loss, as a side effect of thioridazine (option 3).
Cognitive Level: Analysis **Client Need:** Physiological Integrity: Pharmacological and Parenteral Therapies **Integrated Process:** Nursing Process: Analysis **Content Area:** Pharmacology **Strategy:** Specific knowledge of the intended effects and side effects of this medication is needed to answer the question. Use the process of elimination to make your selection.

17 **Answer: 1** Marijuana has been used for individuals with AIDS to increase their appetite. Marijuana does not increase organization and motivation (option 2), reduce stress (option 3), or have antibacterial properties (option 4).
Cognitive Level: Application **Client Need:** Physiological Integrity: Pharmacological and Parenteral Therapies **Integrated Process:** Nursing Process: Implementation **Content Area:** Pharmacology **Strategy:** The core issue of the question is legitimate uses for marijuana. To aid in making the correct selection, keep in mind that an effect of the drug is to stimulate appetite.

18 **Answer: 3** Although options 1, 2, and 4 are all appropriate nursing interventions, the need for physical safety is the

primary nursing priority for this client at this time. The others can be addressed once physical safety is established.
Cognitive Level: Analysis **Client Need:** Physiological Integrity: Pharmacological and Parenteral Therapies **Integrated Process:** Nursing Process: Planning **Content Area:** Pharmacology **Strategy:** Note that the drug prescribed is an anxiolytic. Next, relate the cause of the anxiety to the need for the medication. From there, choose option 3 over the others because it targets the best concern of the client and is congruent with the need for the medication.

19 **Answer: 4** Risperidone has very few side effects; they include orthostatic hypotension (option 4) and insomnia, agitation, headache, anxiety, and rhinitis. Options 1, 2, and 3 are incorrect conclusions about the causes of the client's dizziness.
Cognitive Level: Analysis **Client Need:** Physiological Integrity: Pharmacological and Parenteral Therapies **Integrated Process:** Nursing Process: Evaluation **Content Area:** Pharmacology **Strategy:** The core issue of this question is recognition of dizziness as a sign of orthostatic hypotension. With this concept in mind, eliminate each of the other options because they do not relate to this concern.

20 **Answer: 3** The principle of remaining abstinent is one of the three most important goals of treatment for alcoholism. It is also critical when taking disulfiram in order to avoid adverse effects from the interaction of the medication and alcohol. The other two goals of treatment are amelioration of concurrent psychiatric conditions and long-term prevention of relapse. Options 1, 2, and 4 are important components, but without option 3, the others could not occur, and they do not directly correlate with disulfiram therapy.
Cognitive Level: Application **Client Need:** Physiological Integrity: Pharmacological and Parenteral Therapies **Integrated Process:** Nursing Process: Planning **Content Area:** Pharmacology **Strategy:** The core issue of the question is the interactive effect of disulfiram and alcohol. With this in mind, eliminate each of the incorrect options because they do not address this critical concern.

ANSWERS & RATIONALES

Key Terms to Review

agranulocytosis p. 559
akathisia p. 558
antagonists p. 558
anticholinergic effects p. 558
dystonia p. 573
extrapyramidal side effects (EPSE) p. 560
metabolite p. 570
neuroleptic malignant syndrome (NMS) p. 559
neuroleptics p. 558
parkinsonism p. 558
serotonin syndrome p. 565
tardive dyskinesia (TD) p. 560
tolerance p. 558

References

Abrams, A. (2004). *Clinical drug therapy: Rationales for nursing practice* (7th ed.). Philadelphia: Lippincott Williams & Wilkins, pp. 124–182, 236–250.

Adams, M., Josephson, D., & Holland, L. (2005). *Pharmacology for nurses: A pathophysiologic approach.* Upper Saddle River, NJ: Pearson Education, pp. 108–118, 143–154, 172–207.

American Psychiatric Association. (2000). *Diagnostic and statistical manual of mental disorders, Fourth Edition, Text Revision* (DSM-IV-TR). Washington, DC: American Psychiatric Association.

Deglin, J. H. & Vallerand, A. H. (2006). *Davis's drug guide for nurses* (10th ed.). Philadelphia: F. A. Davis.

Laraia, M. (2004). Psychopharmacology. In G. Stuart & M. Laraia (Eds.), *Principles and practices of psychiatric nursing* (8th ed.). St. Louis, MO: Mosby, pp. 572–607.

Lehne, R. (2004). *Pharmacology for nursing care* (5th ed.). Philadelphia: W. B. Saunders, pp. 279–390, 666–672.

McKenry, L., Tessier., E. & Hogan, M. (2006). *Mosby's pharmacology in nursing.* (22nd ed.). St. Louis, MO: Elsevier Mosby, pp. 309–330, 378–413.

Wilson, B., Shannon, M., & Stang, C. (2005). *Prentice Hall nurse's drug guide 2005.* Upper Saddle River, NJ: Pearson Education.

Respiratory Medications

37

In this chapter

Test Yourself

Are you ready for the NCLEX-RN® or course exams? Use the practice tests on the companion CD-ROM to check.

Cross reference

Other chapters relevant to this content area are

Dosage Calculation and Medication Administration Chapter 30
Immunological and Anti-Infective Medications Chapter 46
Respiratory Disorders Chapter 56

I. GENERAL GUIDELINES FOR RESPIRATORY MEDICATIONS *(SEE BOX 37–1)*

II. BRONCHODILATORS

A. Beta-agonists (sympathomimetics)

1. Sympathetic nervous system (SNS) **adrenergic agonists** raise intracellular levels of cAMP (cyclic adenosine monophosphate) to dilate constricted bronchi and bronchioles by relaxing smooth muscle
2. Used during an **acute asthma attack,** characterized by bronchospasm with shortness of breath and wheezing, for quick airway dilation and relief of bronchospasm; used also for emphysema and acute and chronic bronchitis
3. **Sympathomimetics** can have beta$_1$ or beta$_2$ activity; beta$_1$ adrenergic receptors increase heart rate and force of myocardial contraction
4. Beta-adrenergic agents can be classified as **catecholamines** released from adrenal medulla in response to SNS stimulation or **noncatecholamines,** which are not released by SNS; all beta-adrenergic agents stimulate beta$_2$ receptors; catecholamines affect both alpha and beta receptors and cause cardiovascular effects
5. Selective beta$_2$ agonists are preferred for bronchial smooth muscle dilation because they produce fewer cardiac side effects
6. In contrast, alpha-adrenergic stimulants can act as a decongestant for allergic rhinitis caused by constriction of nasal cavity blood vessels

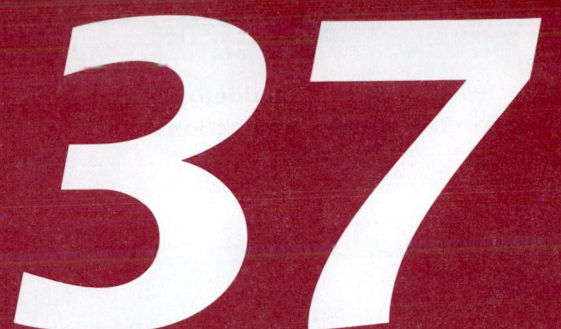

Box 37–1

General Guidelines for Respiratory Medications

Administration Principles

1. Assess current medications (including OTC drugs and herbal products) and history of allergies to identify any potential risks to client.
2. Administer doses on time to maintain therapeutic blood levels.
3. Do not break, crush or allow client to chew sustained release or enteric coated preparations.
4. Many drugs cause CNS depression so monitor client for adverse effects and maintain a safe environment.
5. Provide both verbal and written instructions to client, and provide phone number to call if questions arise or problems occur.

Client Teaching

1. Understand medication actions, side effects, signs of toxicity, importance of follow-up with prescriber and complying with follow-up laboratory tests, and how to self-administer.
2. Do not take any OTC drugs or herbal products without first consulting prescriber.
3. Take exactly as prescribed and do not miss or double doses.
4. Report adverse effects promptly.
5. Do not discontinue drug without consulting prescriber.
6. Do not drink alcohol while taking prescription medications.

7. Common medications are listed in Box 37–2

Memory Aid

If a medication ends in *-terol* or *-terenol*, it is a sympathomimetic type of bronchodilator.

8. Administration considerations
   a. ! Adverse effects may occur with albuterol, bitolterol, levalbuterol, and pirbuterol if used too frequently because they lose $beta_2$–specific actions at larger doses ($beta_1$ receptors are stimulated, leading to elevated heart rate [HR], nausea, anxiety, palpitations, and tremors)
   b. Epinephrine, ephedrine, and ethylnorepinephrine can be used as nasal decongestants because they are alpha-adrenergic stimulants
   c. ! Use with caution in young children and monitor for tremors, restlessness, hallucinations, dizziness, palpitations, tachycardia, and gastrointestinal (GI) difficulties
   d. Epinephrine is given subcutaneously for bronchoconstriction; effects are usually seen in 5 minutes and may last up to 4 hours

Box 37–2

Common Bronchodilators

Beta Agonists/Sympathomimetics

Albuterol (Proventil)

Bitolterol mesylate (Tornalate)

Epinephrine (Adrenalin, Bronkaid, Primatene) (alpha and beta agonist)

Formoterol fumarate (Foradil)

Isoetharine hydrochloride (Bronkosol, Bronkometer)

Isoproterenol (Isuprel)

Levalbuterol hydrochloride (Xopenex)

Metaproterenol sulfate (Alupent)

Pirabuterol acetate (Maxair)

Salmeterol (Serevent)

Terbutaline sulfate (Brethine)

Methylxanthines

Aminophylline (Truphylline)

Theophylline (Theo-Dur, others)

Anticholinergic

Ipratropium bromide (Atrovent, Combivent)

Tiotropium (Spiriva Handi Haler)

e. Salmeterol is not used in an acute asthma attack because of slow onset of action (20 minutes); do not dose more often than every 12 hours because of the 12-hour duration of action
f. Contraindicated with hypersensitivity to sympathomimetics or with tachydysrhythmias
g. Use with caution in clients with cardiovascular disease because of potential for increasing myocardial oxygen demand
h. Use with caution in clients with hypertension, diabetes mellitus, seizures, and hypothyroidism
i. Children under 12 should not use inhalations of albuterol, bitolterol, metaproterenol, and terbutaline
j. Concurrent use of monoamine oxidase inhibitors (MAOIs) may lead to hypertensive crisis

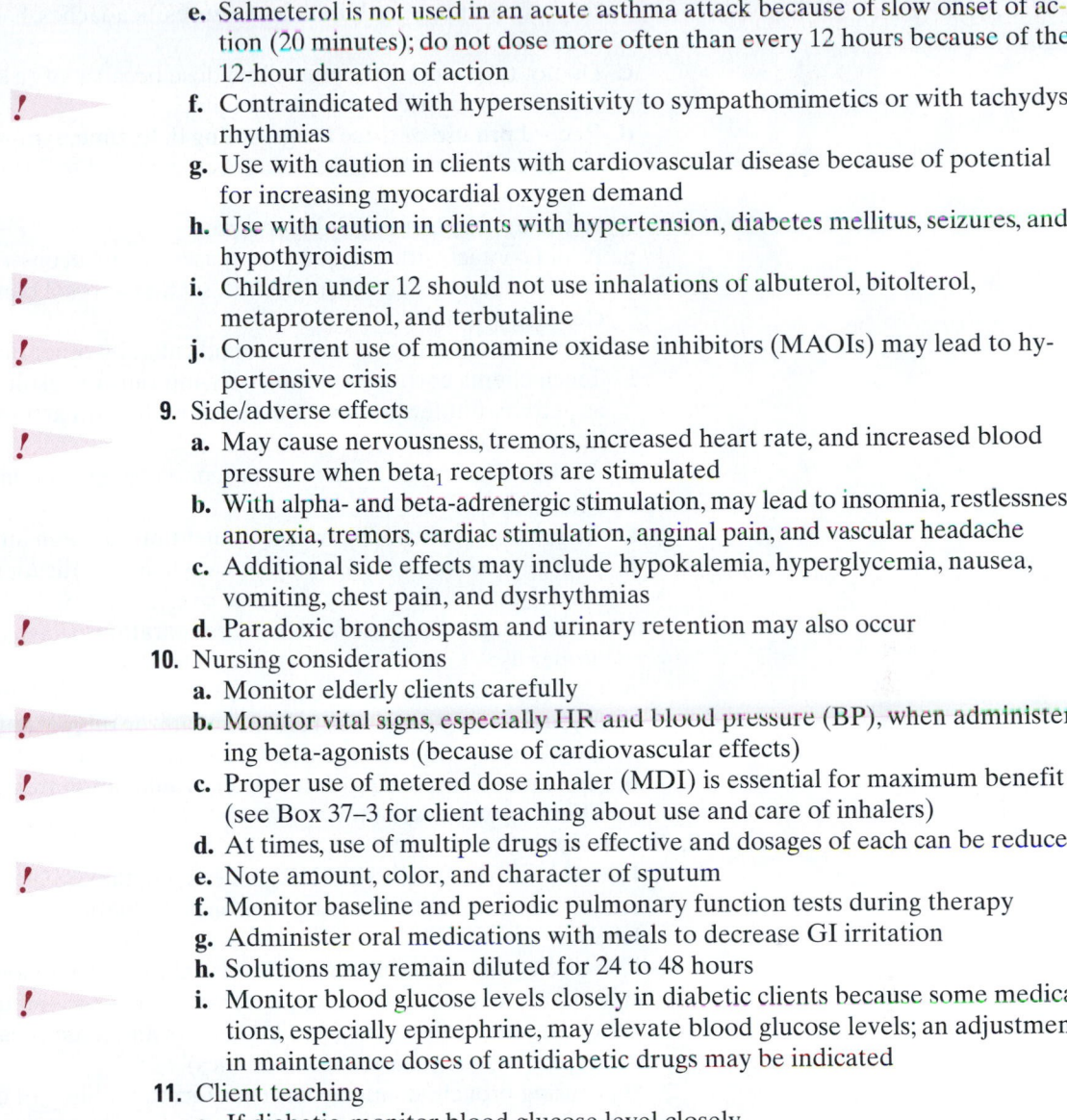

9. Side/adverse effects
a. May cause nervousness, tremors, increased heart rate, and increased blood pressure when $beta_1$ receptors are stimulated
b. With alpha- and beta-adrenergic stimulation, may lead to insomnia, restlessness, anorexia, tremors, cardiac stimulation, anginal pain, and vascular headache
c. Additional side effects may include hypokalemia, hyperglycemia, nausea, vomiting, chest pain, and dysrhythmias
d. Paradoxic bronchospasm and urinary retention may also occur

10. Nursing considerations
a. Monitor elderly clients carefully
b. Monitor vital signs, especially HR and blood pressure (BP), when administering beta-agonists (because of cardiovascular effects)
c. Proper use of metered dose inhaler (MDI) is essential for maximum benefit (see Box 37–3 for client teaching about use and care of inhalers)
d. At times, use of multiple drugs is effective and dosages of each can be reduced
e. Note amount, color, and character of sputum
f. Monitor baseline and periodic pulmonary function tests during therapy
g. Administer oral medications with meals to decrease GI irritation
h. Solutions may remain diluted for 24 to 48 hours
i. Monitor blood glucose levels closely in diabetic clients because some medications, especially epinephrine, may elevate blood glucose levels; an adjustment in maintenance doses of antidiabetic drugs may be indicated

11. Client teaching
a. If diabetic, monitor blood glucose level closely

Box 37–3

Client Education About the Use and Care of Metered Dose Inhalers

- Insert medication firmly into inhaler
- Remove cap and hold inhaler upright
- Shake inhaler for 3 to 5 seconds to ensure even mixing of medication in propellant
- Tilt head back slightly and hold inhaler upright
- Position inhaler 1 to 2 inches away from open mouth or attach it to spacer/holding chamber; if a medicine chamber is used, seal lips around mouthpiece
- Press on inhaler while beginning to breathe in slowly through mouth
- Breathe in slowly and deeply for 3 to 5 seconds
- Hold breath for 8 to 10 seconds as able to allow medication to move down into airways
- Wait 1 to 3 minutes per product directions before next inhalation if another is ordered
- Rinse mouth with water and blow nose
- Use mild soap and water to clean mouthpiece; allow to air dry
- Store inhaler at room temperature

b. Report chest pain, palpitations, seizures, headaches, hallucinations, or blurred vision to physician
c. Do not take more than prescribed dose because of risk for hypertension, tachycardia, dysrhythmias, and angina
d. Record prn use of these drugs, noting date, time, symptoms, and effectiveness
e. Wait 1 to 3 minutes (some references suggest 3 to 5 minutes) between inhalations of aerosol medications
f. Avoid eye contact with inhaler spray
g. Avoid contact with allergen that causes bronchoconstriction and avoid contact with smoke and other irritants, such as aerosol hair spray, perfumes, and cleaning products
h. Increase fluid intake if not contraindicated by other diseases
i. Teach clients early recognition of symptoms of respiratory difficulty (such as activity intolerance and waking at night with asthma symptoms) for early intervention
j. Avoid caffeine, which may increase nervousness and insomnia from bronchodilating drugs
k. An inhaled bronchodilator is treatment of choice in an acute asthma attack
l. Nervousness and tremors may occur when a medication is newly administered, but they frequently decrease over time
m. Understand proper use of inhaled preparations (have client demonstrate proper use)
n. Understand care of nebulizer and/or inhaler: wash daily in warm water and dry; use white vinegar to rinse the nebulizer tubing; read and follow manufacturer's instructions about use, storage, and cleaning of equipment
o. Anticipated response to a nebulizer or inhalation treatment is absence of wheezing and dyspnea

B. *Xanthines*

1. Inhibit phosphodiesterase (PDE), an enzyme that breaks down and thereby increases levels of cAMP, leading to bronchial dilation due to smooth muscle relaxation
2. Can also increase catecholamine levels, inhibit calcium ion movement into smooth muscle, inhibit prostaglandin synthesis, and inhibit release of bronchoconstrictive substances from leukocytes and **mast cells** (which contain histamine, prostaglandins, and thromboxanes)
3. By causing bronchodilation, xanthines increase ability of cilia to clear mucus from airways
4. Used to treat bronchoconstriction associated with COPD (diseases such as chronic bronchitis, asthma, and emphysema) and other chronic respiratory disorders
5. Have a slow onset of action and therefore are used to prevent rather than treat asthma attacks; can be used during an asthma attack if it is mild to moderate
6. Can be used as an additional treatment in pulmonary edema by decreasing vascular permeability and paroxysmal nocturnal dyspnea (PND)
7. Used in treatment of **status asthmaticus,** a bout of severe asthma that cannot be controlled with typical medications (use IV theophylline if client has not responded to the faster-acting beta agonist)
8. Common medications are listed in Box 37–2

Memory Aid

If a medication ends in *-phylline*, it is a xanthine type of bronchodilator.

9. Administration considerations
   a. Administer cautiously to elderly because of risk for increased sensitivity
   b. Carefully monitor serum drug levels and therapeutic response to avoid potential toxicity; therapeutic range of theophylline is 10 to 20 mcg/mL

Memory Aid

Remember 10–20 as the therapeutic serum range for aminophylline.

c. Xanthines exhibit a direct stimulating effect on CNS, which may be enhanced in children

! d. Use cautiously in clients with cardiovascular disorders

e. Theophylline dosages should be based on lean body weight because it does not enter the adipose tissue

f. Theophylline can enter breast milk and cross placenta

! g. Aminophylline is administered slowly by the intravenous route because of potential for cardiovascular collapse

h. Dosages are often started low and titrated up as needed for relief of symptoms

i. Children and adults who smoke cigarettes metabolize these medications more quickly and therefore may need higher doses for therapeutic effects

j. Theophylline levels may be increased in liver disease, congestive heart failure (CHF), and acute viral infections because of impaired biotransformation

k. Avoid with known hypersensitivity to xanthines; tachydysrhythmias; hyperthyroidism (exacerbates disease); history of seizure disorders unless unresponsive to other drugs (can cause seizures); peptic ulcer disease or other GI disorders, including acute gastritis, because of increased gastric acid secretion

! l. Avoid drinks and foods with caffeine, which have an additive effect with xanthines

! **10.** Side/adverse effects

a. Nausea, vomiting, anorexia, and gastroesophageal reflux during sleep

b. Sinus tachycardia, chest pain, palpitations, and ventricular dysrhythmias

c. Hyperglycemia and transient increased urination

d. Tremors, dizziness, hallucinations, restlessness, agitation, headache, and insomnia

11. Nursing considerations

! a. Assess for toxicity; note symptoms of restlessness, insomnia, irritability, tremors, nausea, and vomiting

! b. Because restlessness is also a symptom of hypoxia, assess client for hypoxia if restlessness occurs

c. Refrigerate suppository forms

! d. Children may exhibit hyperactive behavior with administration of theophylline because of CNS stimulation

12. Client teaching

a. As per Box 37–1; refrigerate suppository forms

b. Notify prescriber if suppositories cause rectal burning, itching, or irritation

! c. Notify prescriber if palpitations, nausea, vomiting, weakness, dizziness, chest pain, or convulsions occur

d. Comply with monitoring blood levels periodically

! e. Avoid use of caffeine, which could lead to an additive effect with xanthines

! f. Avoid contact with allergens if possible; avoid contact with smoke and other respiratory irritants such as aerosol hair spray, perfumes, and cleaning products

g. Increase fluid intake if no contraindication because of other disease process

h. Take medications even when there are no symptoms of asthma

i. Take medications with food if GI symptoms develop

III. INHALED CORTICOSTEROIDS

A. Overview

1. Exact mechanism of action is unknown; may stabilize cell membranes to decrease release of bronchoconstricting substances such as **histamine**
2. Cell membranes of **neutrophils** (white blood cells or WBCs that respond to inflammation) are stabilized so inflammatory substances are not released, leading to decreased inflammation, mucosal edema, and secretions, and reduced bronchoconstriction
3. May have a role in increasing responsiveness of bronchial smooth muscle to beta-agonist drugs
4. Appear to help inhibit movement of fluid and protein into tissues as well as inhibit production of prostaglandins, **leukotrienes** (substances released after

exposure to an allergen), and **interleukins** (plasma proteins that increase during inflammatory process)
5. Promote mobilization of mucus by increasing mucociliary action
6. Used in chronic asthma to decrease inflammation and therefore decrease airway obstruction, and are used prophylactically, not during acute attack
7. Used to treat bronchospastic disorders when bronchodilators are not completely effective
8. Used to treat chronic bronchitis, chronic obstructive pulmonary disease (COPD), and cystic fibrosis
9. Common inhalation medications are listed in Box 37–4; oral corticosteroids such as prednisone (Deltasone) and methylprednisolone (Depo-Medrol) may also be used

Memory Aid

Many corticosteroids contain *-cort* or *-sone* in either the generic or trade name.

B. Administration considerations

1. ! Proper technique is essential when administering medications by inhalation route
2. Beclomethasone has greater anti-inflammatory action and causes fewer side effects than dexamethasone
3. ! If client is also taking a systemic corticosteroid, that dose may need to be decreased with addition of inhaled corticosteroids
4. Beclomethasone, flunisolide, and fluticasone are available as nasal solutions for treatment of allergic rhinitis
5. Monitor for impaired bone growth in children receiving inhaled corticosteroids
6. ! Contraindicted with known allergy, psychosis, fungal infection, acquired immunodeficiency syndrome (AIDS), tuberculosis, idiopathic thrombocytopenia, and in children under age 2 years
7. Use cautiously in clients with diabetes, glaucoma, osteoporosis, ulcers, renal disease, congestive heart failure (CHF), myasthenia gravis, seizure disorders, inflammatory bowel disease, hypertension, thromboembolic disorders, esophagitis, and infections (due to potential for suppressed immune system)
8. ! Because of possible decreased response to skin test antigens, postpone skin testing if possible until after corticosteroid therapy

C. Side/adverse effects

1. Pharyngeal irritation, sore throat, and **rhinitis** (inflammation of nasal mucous membranes)
2. Coughing or dry mouth
3. Oral fungal infections
4. Increased susceptibility to infection, dermatologic effects, and osteoporosis
5. Diarrhea, nausea, vomiting, and stomach upset
6. Headache, fever, dizziness, angioedema, rash, urticaria, and paradoxical bronchospasm
7. Menstrual disturbances
8. Palpitations
9. Adrenocortical insufficiency, fluid and electrolyte disturbances, nervous system effects, and endocrine effects if absorbed systemically

Box 37–4

Inhaled Corticosteroid Medications

Beclomethasone dipropionate (Beclovent, others)

Budesonide (Pulmicort Turbohaler)

Flunisolide (AeroBid-M)

Fluticasone propionate (Flovent)

Triamcinolone acetonide (Azmacort)

D. Nursing considerations

1. Assess sputum color and viscosity for signs of infection
2. Pediatric clients may need a healthcare provider's order to keep an inhaler with them at school

E. Client teaching

1. As per Box 37–1
2. Keep equipment clean and in working order per manufacturer's guidelines
3. Rinse mouth after use of inhalation devices such as **inhaler** or **nebulizer**
4. Do not abruptly stop taking this medication; taper dose slowly over a 2-week period under direction of the prescriber
5. Wear a bracelet or necklace to identify self as a steroid user
6. Learn symptoms of steroid use, including moon face, acne, increased fat pads, increased edema; notify prescriber if these symptoms arise
7. Report signs of decreased amounts of steroid levels, including nausea, dyspnea, joint pain, weakness, and fatigue
8. Report weight gain of more than 5 pounds per week
9. Avoid contact with allergen responsible for producing allergic response if possible
10. Recognize early signs of respiratory difficulty so treatment can begin promptly
11. Take drug at approximately same time each day for maximal effectiveness
12. Use inhaled corticosteroids as maintenance drugs; they are ineffective in acute bronchospasm

IV. INHALED MAST CELL STABILIZERS

A. Overview

1. Stabilize mast cells to prevent release of bronchoconstrictive and inflammatory substances when stimulated by allergen; therefore, inflammation is limited
2. Used to prevent and treat inflammation of airways, and decrease mucosal edema, mucous secretions, and bronchoconstriction
3. Used for prophylaxis of acute asthma attacks
4. Used to prevent and treat allergic rhinitis
5. Common medications
   a. Cromolyn (Intal) is oral spray or nebulizer solution for oral inhalation; Nasalcrom is nasal spray form of cromolyn
   b. Nedocromil (Tilade): given by inhalation

B. Administration considerations

1. Bronchodilator and corticosteroid doses may be decreased with use of these drugs
2. Use with caution in clients with impaired hepatic or renal function; lower dosages may be required
3. Administer using proper inhalation technique
4. Nasal solution is used to prevent and treat allergic rhinitis
5. It may take 3 weeks of daily dosing to see therapeutic effects
6. Do not use in clients with acute bronchospasm, status asthmaticus, or hypersensitivity to drug

C. Side/adverse effects

1. Headache
2. Nasal irritation and sneezing
3. Dry mouth and unpleasant taste
4. Cough and irritation of throat and trachea, bronchospasm
5. Erythema, rash, urticaria

D. Nursing considerations

1. Use cautiously in clients with coronary artery disease (CAD) and/or dysrhythmias, which may be aggravated by propellants in aerosols
2. Pulmonary function testing may be ordered prior to therapy

E. Client teaching

1. As per Box 37–1
2. Use inhaler properly to ensure maximal effectiveness of medication; use spacer as appropriate
3. Record frequency and severity of asthma attacks

4. Allow 2 to 4 weeks for full medication effectiveness
5. Rinse mouth after taking medication to avoid dry mouth
6. Do not take during an acute attack because symptoms may be aggravated
7. Optimally, take bronchodilator 20 to 30 minutes prior to taking cromolyn; see individual product literature; always wait a minimum of 3 to 5 minutes between inhalations

V. LEUKOTRIENE MODIFIERS

A. Overview

1. Leukotrienes are substances released during an allergic response; they cause inflammation, bronchoconstriction, and mucus production that leads to coughing, sneezing, and shortness of breath
2. Leukotriene modifiers or inhibitors work by blocking action of leukotrienes
3. Prevent bronchoconstriction by inhibiting smooth muscle contraction of bronchial airways
4. Provide relief of inflammatory symptoms of asthma
5. Used for prophylaxis and chronic treatment of asthma in adults and children over 12; they are not used in managing an acute asthma attack
6. Common medications are listed in Box 37–5

Memory Aid

If a medication ends in *-lukast*, it is a leukotriene modifier.

B. Administration considerations

1. Leukotriene modifiers are used in adults and children 12 and over
2. Therapeutic effects may take up to a week
3. They have localized effects in lungs
4. They are used alone or in combination with corticosteroids
5. Montelukast and zafirlukast are taken orally, metabolized in liver, and excreted in feces
6. Zileuton is metabolized by liver and excreted in urine
7. Monitor hepatic aminotransferase enzymes when administering zileuton; discontinue if levels elevate to five times normal or if liver dysfunction develops
8. Zileuton is contraindicated in clients with liver disease and elevated transaminase (three times the norm), and all are contraindicated with hypersensitivity to drug

C. Side/adverse effects

1. Headaches may occur with all drugs
2. Zileuton may also cause dyspepsia, nausea, dizziness, insomnia, and hepatotoxicity
3. Zafirlukast may cause nausea and diarrhea
4. Monitor clients over age 55 for infection

D. Nursing considerations

1. Be sure drug is prescribed for chronic, not acute, treatment of asthma
2. Monitor liver function tests
3. Monitor liver enzymes during zileuton therapy and discontinue drug if elevated to five times normal value or if liver dysfunction develops

E. Client teaching

1. As per Box 37–1; expect drugs to take a week before therapeutic effects are seen
2. Follow-up liver function studies may be needed
3. Drugs prevent some symptoms of asthma but are not intended for use in acute attacks
4. Avoid contact with specific allergen if possible

Box 37–5

Leukotriene Modifiers

Zileuton (Zyflo)

Zafirlukast (Accolate)

Montelukast (Singulair)

5. Increase fluid intake if not contraindicated because of other disease processes
6. Take zafirlukast 1 hour before or 2 hours after meals
7. Montelukast and zileuton may be taken with or without food

VI. ANTIHISTAMINES

A. Overview

1. **Antihistamines** are used to treat allergies, allergic rhinitis (hay fever), allergic conjunctivitis, allergic contact dermatitis, vertigo, motion sickness, insomnia, allergic reactions, cough, and sneezing and runny nose from common cold
2. Compete with histamine for receptor sites and thereby block action of histamine following its release; work best early in response because they do not displace histamine from receptors
3. Cause bronchial smooth muscle relaxation and reduce bronchial, salivary, gastric, nasal, and **lacrimal** (tear) secretions
4. Reduce itching (urticaria) and are used to treat anaphylactic shock
5. Can be used to prevent or treat allergic reactions to medications
6. Common medications are listed in Box 37–6

B. Administration considerations

1. ! Treat symptoms but not the cause of a problem
2. Should not be used for treatment of acute asthma attack or lower respiratory disorder
3. Most antihistamines are tolerated better when taken with meals
4. Brompheniramine, chlorpheniramine, and diphenhydramine are available OTC
5. Hydroxyzine is effective with pruritis
6. Azelastine is topically applied to nasal mucosa and action peaks in 2 to 3 hours; it does not tend to cause drowsiness but does leave an unpleasant taste in mouth
7. ! Antihistamines may be used as premedication before administering blood products to decrease risk of allergic reactions
8. Oral antihistamines act in 15 to 60 minutes and last 4 to 6 hours; sustained-release medications last 8 to 12 hours
9. Use a rapid acting agent with an acute allergic reaction
10. Longer-acting agents give more consistent relief with chronic allergic conditions
11. Should be used cautiously with history of increased intraocular pressure, cardiac or renal disease, hypertension, bronchial asthma, stenosing peptic ulcer disease, prostatic hyperplasia, convulsive disorders, or during pregnancy
12. ! Can mask positive skin test results; discontinue use for 3 days (72 hours) before allergy skin testing

C. Side/adverse effects

1. ! Drowsiness is main side effect; however, children can experience paradoxical excitement

Box 37–6

Antihistamines

Second-Generation or Nonsedating Antihistamines

loratadine (Claritin)
cetirizine (Zyrtec)
fexofenadine (Allegra)
astemizole (Hismanal)

First-Generation or Traditional Antihistamines

diphenhydramine (Benadryl)
brompheniramine (Dimetane)
chlorpheniramine (Chlor-Trimeton)
dimenhydrinate (Dramamine)
doxylamine (Unisom)
meclizine (Antivert or Bonine)
azatadine (Optimine)
phenindamine (Nolahist)
tripelennamine (PBZ)
azelastine (Astelin)
clemastine (Tavist)
cyproheptadine (Periactin)
dexchlorpheniramine (Polaramine)
hydroxyzine (Vistaril, Atarax)
promethazine (Phenergan)

2. **Anticholinergic** side effects include dry mouth and nose, changes in vision, difficulty urinating, and constipation
3. Sedation from drowsiness to deep sleep, dizziness, syncope, muscular weakness, unsteady gait, paradoxical excitement (especially in older adults), restlessness, insomnia, and nervousness
4. Anorexia, nausea, vomiting, diarrhea, constipation, and jaundice
5. Urinary retention, impotence, vertigo, visual disturbances, blurred vision, tinnitus, hypotension, syncope, and headache
6. Agranulocytosis, hemolytic anemia, leukopenia, thrombocytopenia, and pancytopenia

D. Nursing considerations

1. Cetirizine, loratadine, and fexofenadine may be used in children over age of 6
2. Help client determine precipitating factors and symptoms of allergic reactions
3. Assess for drowsiness and dizziness, especially during first few days of therapy
4. Encourage fluid intake of 2000 to 3000 mL/day to loosen secretions unless contraindicated by another condition
5. Give antihistamines prior to contact with allergen if possible
6. Administer at bedtime to reduce side effect of drowsiness
7. Administer intramuscular antihistamines deep into large muscles
8. Intravenous injection should be over a few minutes

E. Client teaching

1. As per Box 37–1; take with meals to decrease stomach upset
2. Avoid contact with allergen responsible for reaction if possible; if unable, take medication prior to exposure
3. Do not take more than one medication at a time
4. Contact physician if excessive sedation, confusion, or hypotension occur
5. Use hard, sugarless candy to relieve dry mouth
6. Antihistamines may dry and thicken respiratory tract secretions and make them difficult to expectorate: increase fluid intake
7. Take loratadine on an empty stomach to increase absorption
8. Avoid prolonged exposure to sunlight because of potential for sunburn
9. Take medication at bedtime to reduce drowsiness, which should become less significant after repeated doses
10. Do not take antihistamines for 72 hours prior to allergen skin testing to reduce likelihood of false negative results

VII. MEDICATIONS TO CONTROL BRONCHIAL SECRETIONS

A. Nasal *decongestants*

1. Decongestants relieve nasal stuffiness by shrinking swollen nasal mucous membranes
2. Adrenergic agents (sympathomimetics) cause vasoconstriction, decreasing blood flow to nasal mucosa and thereby reducing swelling
3. Nasal steroids suppress inflammatory response
4. Used to relieve nasal congestion and nasal discharge caused by acute or chronic rhinitis (common cold), sinusitis, hay fever, and other allergies
5. May be used to decrease local blood flow prior to nasal surgery or as an aid to visualizing nasal mucosa during diagnostic exams
6. Common medications are listed in Box 37–7

Memory Aid

A medication that ends in *-zoline* is a nasal decongestant, although not all nasal decongestants end in *-zoline*.

7. Administration considerations
   a. Can be used topically (with sprays or drops) or orally
   b. Sustained use of topical drugs (longer than 3 days or in excessive amounts) can cause rebound congestion; therefore, oral agents should be used if needed for longer than 3 days

Box 37-7

Medications that Control Bronchial Secretions

Nasal Decongestants

Phenylephrine (Neo-Synephrine)

Pseudoephedrine (Sudafed)

Ephedrine (Vicks Vatronol)

Naphazoline (Privine)

Oxymetazoline (Afrin)

Tetrahydrozoline (Tyzine)

Xylometazoline (Otrivin)

Expectorants

Guaifenesin (Robitussin)

Potassium iodide (Pima syrup)

Terpin hydrate elixir

Antitussives

Nonopioid type

Benzonatate (Tessalon Perles)

Dextromethorphan (Robitussin DM, others)

Opioid type

Dimetane-DC

Tussar SF

Novahistine DH

Robitussin AC

Mucolytics

Sodium chloride solution by nebulization

Acetylcysteine (Mucomyst) (nebulizer)

Dornase alfa (rhDNAse; Pulmozyme—a proteolytic enzyme for clients with cystic fibrosis only)

c. Topical drugs are potent decongestants with prompt onset of action
d. Topical drugs are preferred if client has cardiovascular disease because of decreased risk of cardiovascular side effects

8. Side/adverse effects
   a. Local nasal mucosal irritation and dryness
   b. Rebound congestion is common
   c. Nervousness, insomnia, palpitations, and tremor (with systemic absorption) are rare
9. Nursing considerations
   a. Assess client for other medical history to determine risk for side effects; older adults with significant cardiac disease should avoid nasal decongestants because of high risk for hypertension, dysrhythmias, nervousness, and insomnia
   b. For administration of nose drops, have client lie down or sit with neck hyperextended
   c. Wash medication droppers after each use to prevent contamination
   d. Client should sit and squeeze nasal spray container once and avoid touching nares with spray dispenser; tip of dispenser should be rinsed after each use
   e. Observe client for intended decrease in nasal congestion
   f. Assess for tachycardia, hypertension and cardiac dysrhythmias; also observe for rebound nasal congestion, chronic rhinitis, and ulceration of the nasal mucosa
10. Client teaching
    a. As per Box 37–1; avoid use of caffeine while taking this medication because it can cause nervousness, tremors, and insomnia
    b. Avoid smoking because it increases secretions and decreases ciliary action
    c. Avoid exposure to crowds to minimize spread of disease
    d. Increase fluid intake to 2000 to 3000 mL/day unless contraindicated by another medical condition
    e. Nasal congestion in infants can decrease ability to suck effectively: apply nasal solution prior to feeding to increase infant's ability to feed
    f. Avoid eating or drinking for 30 minutes after medication administration
    g. Practice good hand washing
    h. Rinse droppers and spray bottles after each use to avoid contamination

B. *Expectorants*

1. Expectorants increase fluid flow in respiratory tract and reduce viscosity of secretions to aid in their removal by cough reflex and ciliary action

2. Used to relieve nonproductive cough associated with common cold, bronchitis, laryngitis, and influenza; they also thin secretions
3. Common medications are listed in see Box 37–7
4. Administration considerations
   a. Use with caution in elderly or debilitated clients
   b. Use with caution in clients with asthma and respiratory insufficiency
   c. Not used as commonly as in past because of questionable effectiveness
5. Side/adverse effects
   a. Nausea, vomiting, and gastric irritation
   b. Rash, dizziness and headache
6. Nursing considerations: as per Box 37–1
7. Client teaching
   a. As per Box 37–1
   b. Report a fever or cough to physician if it lasts longer than a week
   c. Increase fluid intake if not contraindicated by other disease processes
   d. Avoid smoking because it increases secretions and decreases ciliary action
   e. Avoid drinking fluids for 30 minutes after taking this medication
   f. Take iodide preparations with fruit juice or milk to decrease bitter taste

C. ***Antitussives***

1. **Opioid** (narcotic) and nonopioid antitussives suppress cough reflex by directly affecting cough center; nonopioid antitussives do so without CNS suppression
2. Peripherally acting agents (glycerin, ammonium chloride) have local anesthetic effects to decrease irritation of pharyngeal mucosa; they are available in gargles, lozenges, and syrups; lozenges increase saliva flow and therefore suppress cough
3. Used to stop a nonproductive cough or a dry, hacking, nonproductive cough that interferes with rest and sleep
4. Common medications are listed in Box 37–7
5. Administration considerations
   a. Potential exists for addiction and CNS and respiratory depression with opioid antitussives
   b. Most are given in a liquid form or as oral tablets; syrup form may soothe irritated mucosa in pharynx
   c. Dextromethorphan is preferred over codeine because it provides desired effect without use of opioids; is available in many OTC products and does not require a prescription
   d. Dextromethorphan is contraindicated with asthma, emphysema, chronic headaches, or hypersensitivity
   e. Codeine preparations are contraindicated with respiratory depression, increased intracranial pressure, severe liver or renal disease, hypothyroidism, adrenal insufficiency, or seizure disorders
6. Side/adverse effects
   a. Dizziness, headache, drowsiness or sedation, nausea, vomiting, constipation, pruritus, nasal congestion, dry mouth, blurred vision, and sweating
   b. Dependence and respiratory depression with codeine
   c. Dry mouth, palpitations, thickened respiratory mucus, anorexia, urinary retention or frequency, diarrhea, photosensitivity, and dysuria with nonopioids
   d. Nasal congestion and burning of the eyes with benzonatate
7. Nursing considerations
   a. Assess for inability to cough effectively from excessive cough suppression
   b. Observe for listed side effects and potential drug dependence
   c. Cough may be a useful diagnostic tool and protective measure for client; therefore, use antitussives cautiously for irritating, nonproductive, and ineffective cough
8. Client teaching
   a. As per Box 37–1
   b. Notify physician if cough lasts longer than a week or if persistent headache, fever, or rash occur

c. Do not drink liquids for 30 to 35 minutes after taking a chewable tablet or a lozenge
d. Avoid smoking because it increases secretions and decreases ciliary action
e. For excessive respiratory secretions, understand benefits of coughing, deep breathing, and ambulation
! f. Liquefy secretions with increased oral intake up to 2000 to 3000 mL/day unless contraindicated

D. *Mucolytics*

1. Mucolytics are administered by inhalation to liquefy (thin) mucus in respiratory tract and aid in removal of viscous secretions
2. Used with sinusitis and common cold
3. An oral form of acetylcysteine (Mucomyst) can be used to treat acetaminophen overdose
4. Common medications are listed in Box 37–7
5. Administration considerations
   a. No longer commonly used because of questionable effectiveness
   ! b. These drugs are nebulized using a face mask or a mouth piece; can be instilled into a tracheostomy
   c. Acetylcysteine is effective 1 minute after inhalation or immediately after direct instillation; maximal effect is in 5 to 10 minutes
   ! d. Activated charcoal limits effectiveness of acetylcysteine when used as antidote to acetaminophen overdose
6. Side/adverse effects
   a. Oral irritation and sore throat
   b. Cough and bronchospasm
   c. Nausea and vomiting, headaches
7. Nursing considerations
   ! a. May cause bronchospasm and are usually given with bronchodilators
   b. Suction client if cough is ineffective
   c. Rinse mouth after therapy to decrease oropharyngeal irritation
   ! d. Discard unused medication after 4 days
8. Client teaching
   a. As per Box 37–1
   ! b. Increase fluid intake unless contraindicated by other disease processes
   c. Avoid smoking because it increases secretions and decreases ciliary action

VIII. OXYGEN

A. Indications

1. **Hypoxia,** deficiency of oxygen (O_2) in cells and tissues, and **hypoxemia,** deficiency of O_2 in arterial blood
2. Conditions associated with decreased arterial oxygen (PO_2) levels (pulmonary edema), decreased cardiac output (myocardial infarction), decreased blood oxygen–carrying capacity (anemia), increased O_2 demand (sepsis, sustained fever), and others

B. Types of delivery systems

1. Nasal cannula (nasal prongs): most common form of O_2 delivery
   a. Two prongs go into nostrils and tubing attaches to oxygen source and flowmeter
   b. Client can eat and talk with a nasal cannula
   ! c. Oxygen can be administered at a rate ranging from 1 L/min to 6 L/min
   d. Dryness of mucous membranes can occur
2. Nasal catheter: inserted into throat through a nostril, change to other nostril every 8 hours; not used frequently because of client discomfort; gastric distention sometimes occurs
3. Oxymizer: a nasal cannula with a reservoir that can deliver higher concentrations of O_2 (approximately twice the amount) than a regular cannula without use of a mask

4. Face mask: a mask that fits over the client's mouth and nose
   a. Simple face mask: flow rate is 5 to 10 L/min with O_2 delivery capabilities of 40% to 60%
   b. Partial rebreather mask: consists of a face mask with a reservoir bag; some exhaled air goes into reservoir bag and is mixed with 100% O_2 for next inhalation; permits conservation of O_2 and can deliver 70% to 90% O_2 at rates of 6 to 15 L/min
   c. Nonrebreather mask: delivers highest concentration of O_2 by mask; no exhaled air goes into reservoir bag; reservoir bag contains O_2, which client breathes in with inspiration; exhaled air goes out through side vents and can deliver 60% to 100% O_2 at flow rates of 6 to 15 L/min
   d. Venturi mask: percentage of O_2 is adjusted by a dial at end of mask; amount of air pulled into system varies with needed amount of O_2 and gives precise oxygen concentrations

C. Oxygen toxicity

1. Lung tissue can be damaged from prolonged exposure to high O_2 concentrations
2. Exact amount of O_2 and length of time required to cause O_2 toxicity varies depending on degree of underlying lung disease; some sources say lung damage can occur with O_2 delivery of greater than 50% for more than 24 to 48 hours
3. **Atelectasis,** or alveolar collapse, can result with O_2 administration at rates of 60% for more than 36 hours or 90% for more than 6 hours
4. Adult respiratory distress syndrome (ARDS) can result from breathing 80% to 100% oxygen for more than 24 hours
5. Symptoms of O_2 toxicity begin as a nonproductive cough, substernal chest pain, GI upset, and dyspnea; as it worsens, client develops decreased vital capacity, lung compliance, and hypoxemia; atelectasis, pulmonary edema, and pulmonary hemorrhage can result if not reversed
6. Oxygen should be weaned as soon as possible and according to client's oxygen saturation (SaO_2) level

D. Nursing considerations

1. Oxygen therapy can be anxiety-provoking; provide sufficient explanation and allow client to express anxieties
2. Flow rate is measured in liters per minute; it is a measure of O_2 delivered but is not completely accurate because there is loss of O_2 content with leaking and mixing with room air
3. Oxygen analyzers are available to measure percentage of O_2 client inhales; this is recommended every 4 hours
4. Clients with COPD should not receive O_2 at high percentages because higher levels of O_2 in bloodstream can cause hypoventilation; a COPD client's drive to breathe is from low levels of O_2 tension; a client with COPD can usually tolerate a rate of up to 2 L/min by nasal cannula
5. Check O_2 delivery system frequently to ensure proper functioning
6. Oxygen should be humidified when client is receiving rates higher than 2 L/min
7. A face mask should fit client's face to avoid unnecessary leakage; if mask is too snug, skin irritation can occur
8. Masks can be replaced with a nasal cannula during mealtime with a physician's order
9. The reservoir bag on a partial rebreather should deflate slightly with inspiration
10. Provide reassurance if client becomes claustrophobic
11. Flaps on side of nonrebreather mask should be open during exhalation and closed during inhalation
12. Monitor SaO_2 with pulse oximeter during oxygen administration; with physician order, O_2 may be titrated to achieve desired SaO_2 level
13. Assess for signs of hypoxia and respiratory distress; also assess for changes in vital signs and color changes
14. Monitor arterial blood gases (ABGs) per physician order
15. Normal arterial O_2 levels decrease with age
16. Provide oral care for comfort because of potential drying of mucous membranes
17. Identify clients at high risk for developing O_2 toxicity

E. Client teaching

1. Expect noise with the flow of O_2
2. ! Avoid open flames with O_2 administration because it is flammable
3. ! Ensure there are no frayed electrical cords near O_2 so there is no chance of a spark causing combustion
4. ! Do not smoke when O_2 therapy is being utilized
5. Expect delivery to cause dryness of mouth and nasal mucosa
6. ! Remove O_2 when using an electric razor
7. Continue O_2 therapy at home as prescribed by physician
8. ! Keep O_2 tank in the holder and away from direct sunlight to reduce effects of heat
9. Understand signs of hypoxia and report them to physician

Check Your NCLEX-RN® Exam I.Q.

You are ready for testing on this content if you can

- Apply knowledge of expected actions and effects of respiratory medications to client care.
- Correctly administer respiratory medications to clients.
- Assess for side effects and adverse effects of respiratory medications.
- Take appropriate action if a client has an unexpected response to a respiratory medication.
- Monitor a client for expected outcomes or effects of treatment with respiratory medications.

PRACTICE TEST

1 A client with congestive heart failure is taking digoxin (Lanoxin) and furosemide (Lasix). A new diagnosis of acute bronchitis is made, and albuterol (Proventil) via inhalation is started. The nurse concludes that this client is at risk for which of the following complications?

1. Hyperkalemia
2. Hypernatremia
3. Hypocalcemia
4. Hypokalemia

2 A client with asthma has started to take a beta-adrenergic agent. The client also takes a monoamine oxidase inhibitor (MAOI). The nurse assesses the client for which of the following complications?

1. Hypotension
2. Hypertension
3. Tachycardia
4. Bradycardia

3 A diabetic client admitted to the emergency department with acute bronchospasm is given epinephrine (Bronkaid). The nurse should assess the client for which side effect of this medication?

1. Blood glucose level 156 mg/dL
2. Blood glucose level 77 mg/dL
3. Potassium level 5.4 mEq/L
4. Potassium level 3.1 mEq/L

4 The nurse is teaching a client with chronic obstructive pulmonary disease (COPD) how to administer multiple medications by inhalation. Which statement by the client indicates an understanding of the instruction?

1. "If my symptoms get worse I can double my dosage."
2. "I will wait at least 1 minute between use of my different inhalers."
3. "I can take any of the over-the-counter medications I need for my symptoms."
4. "I cannot rinse my inhaler equipment because it is not supposed to get wet."

5 A client complains that a newly prescribed beta-adrenergic agent is causing nervousness and tremors. Which statement by the nurse is effective?

1. "Sometimes those symptoms occur when first taking the medication but decrease over time."
2. "Stop taking the medicine because those symptoms will only get worse."
3. "Drinking coffee or tea will help decrease the symptoms."
4. "Those symptoms indicate a worsening disease process and should be reported to the physician."

PRACTICE TEST

6. The nurse is teaching the client about home administration of theophylline (Theo-Dur). Which statement by the nurse is reflective of appropriate teaching?

1. "Sustained-release forms can be crushed so they are easier to swallow."
2. "If a dose is omitted, take a double dose the next time."
3. "Only take the medication when acute symptoms occur."
4. "Take the medication with food if gastrointestinal symptoms occur."

7. A client who takes theophylline (Theo-Dur) complains of restlessness. Which is the most appropriate action for the nurse to take first?

1. Assess the client for hypoxia.
2. Explain this is a toxic reaction and call the physician.
3. Assess the client for other signs and symptoms of theophylline toxicity.
4. Call the physician to obtain an order for a theophylline level.

8. The client asks the nurse why the physician ordered beclomethasone (Beclovent) for his chronic obstructive pulmonary disease (COPD). Which statement by the nurse is most appropriate?

1. "Beclovent prevents airway dilation."
2. "Beclovent decreases inflammation and makes it easier to breathe."
3. "Beclovent suppresses the immune response."
4. "Beclovent decreases responsiveness to medications that dilate the airway."

9. The nurse is teaching a client about cromolyn (Intal). Which of the following statements should the nurse make about the mechanism of action of this medication?

1. "Cromolyn relaxes bronchial smooth muscle to assist with bronchodilation."
2. "Cromolyn limits inflammation and therefore bronchoconstriction with exposure to an allergen."
3. "Cromolyn helps to liquefy secretions to promote expectoration."
4. "Cromolyn promotes bronchoconstriction of overly dilated airways."

10. The nurse is assessing the client who takes cromolyn (Intal). Which symptom indicates to the nurse that the client is experiencing a potential side effect?

1. Vomiting
2. Moist mucous membranes
3. Tachycardia
4. Headache

11. A client beginning medication therapy with montelukast (Singulair) asks the nurse how the medication is helping his symptoms. Which is the best response?

1. "Singulair decreases inflammation and mucus secretion."
2. "Singulair increases mucus secretion and bronchodilation."
3. "Singulair prevents smooth muscle contraction by nervous system stimulation."
4. "Singulair increases the inflammatory response and mucus secretion."

12. The client asks the nurse about self-care related to newly ordered zafirlukast (Accolate). The nurse responds by telling the client that

1. renal function tests should be monitored.
2. liver function tests should be monitored.
3. fluid intake should be decreased.
4. the medication should be taken with meals.

13. A client asks the nurse if there is a benefit to taking second-generation antihistamines instead of first-generation antihistamines. The nurse replies that second-generation drugs cause less

1. nausea.
2. anxiety.
3. drowsiness.
4. euphoria.

14. A client asks the nurse about drug interactions with diphenhydramine (Benadryl). The nurse informs the client that which of the following will increase the effects of Benadryl?

1. Alcohol
2. Nicotine
3. Caffeine
4. Central nervous system stimulants

15 The nurse is teaching the client proper technique for administration of nasal sprays. Which explanation should the nurse use in order to provide accurate information?

1. "Lie down and instill the nasal spray, squeezing the bottle twice for each application."
2. "Sit and squeeze the nasal spray once as you inhale while holding your finger over the other nostril."
3. "Be careful not to rinse the tip of the spray bottle after use, or you will contaminate the medication."
4. "Lean your head back and administer two applications to each nostril for each dose to be sure some of the medication is instilled."

16 The nurse is developing a teaching plan for a client using nasal decongestant. The nurse should include which of the following instructions in the teaching plan?

1. "Be sure to stay on the medication for at least 7 days."
2. "Decrease fluid intake to 16 ounces/day to decrease nasal secretions."
3. "Avoid eating or drinking for 30 minutes after medication administration."
4. "Smoking decreases secretions and increases ciliary action."

17 The nurse is preparing to teach the client important information related to self-administration of guaifenesin (Robitussin). Which of the following should be included in the teaching plan?

1. Side effects include nausea, vomiting, and rash.
2. Report a cough to the physician if it lasts longer than 2 weeks.
3. Take the medication with meals.
4. If medication is not effective, double the dose.

18 The nurse is assessing a client for side effects of an opioid antitussive. Of the following, what is the most significant side effect assessed?

1. Dry cracked lips
2. Complaints of blurred vision
3. Inability to stay awake
4. Respirations of 10/min

19 Which of the following statements by a client taking a mucolytic agent indicates a need for further teaching?

1. "I will drink at least 2 to 3 liters of fluid each day."
2. "I will avoid smoking."
3. "I will rinse my mouth after I take my medicine."
4. "I can keep the medicine for a week before discarding what I do not use."

20 The nurse has an order to administer 50% oxygen to a client with pulmonary edema. The nurse would select which of the following oxygen administration systems that allows that percentage of oxygen to be delivered?

1. Nasal cannula
2. Nonrebreather mask
3. Partial rebreather mask
4. Venturi mask

ANSWERS & RATIONALES

1 **Answer: 4** Risk of hypokalemia is worsened by the concurrent use of a potassium-wasting diuretic (Lasix) and a beta-agonist (albuterol) medication. Furthermore, the risk of cardiac glycoside toxicity is worse in the presence of hypokalemia. Hyperkalemia (option 1), hypernatremia (option 2), and hypocalcemia (option 3) are not concerns with this drug regimen.
Cognitive Level: Analysis **Client Need:** Physiological Integrity: Pharmacological and Parenteral Therapies **Integrated Process:** Nursing Process: Analysis **Content Area:** Pharmacology **Strategy:** The core issue of this question is the effects of taking a potassium-losing diuretic with other cardiac or respiratory medications, which helps you to focus on hypokalemia. Note also that options 1 and 4 are opposite, so there is a greater chance that one of these may be the correct answer.

2 **Answer: 2** Concurrent use of an MAOI and a beta-agonist may lead to hypertensive crisis. The beta-agonist may lead to tachycardia (option 3), but since no specific agent is listed, the nurse should consider the potential interaction of the MAOI and the beta-agonist first. Hypotension (option 1) and bradycardia (option 4) are not of concern with this combination of medications.
Cognitive Level: Analysis **Client Need:** Physiological Integrity: Pharmacological and Parenteral Therapies **Integrated Process:** Nursing Process: Assessment **Content Area:** Pharmacology **Strategy:** The core issue of the question is interactive effects of

beta-agonists and MAOIs. Use the process of elimination and recall that an agonist type of drug enhances the action of a system, in this case the beta-adrenergic system. Then recall that these effects include increased pulse and blood pressure. Note also that two of these options are opposites, making it more likely that one of them is the correct answer.

3 **Answer: 1** Epinephrine is a beta-adrenergic agent used to dilate bronchial airways. It can cause an increased blood glucose level, which is especially an issue for a client with diabetes mellitus. Diabetic clients should be instructed to monitor blood glucose levels because an adjustment in maintenance doses of hypoglycemic agents may be indicated. Option 2, 3, and 4 are unrelated to effects of the medication on diabetic clients.
Cognitive Level: Analysis **Client Need:** Physiological Integrity: Pharmacological and Parenteral Therapies **Integrated Process:** Nursing Process: Assessment **Content Area:** Pharmacology **Strategy:** The core issue of the question is knowledge that beta-adrenergic medications stimulate the sympathetic nervous system and that one of the end effects of the stimulation is increased blood glucose. Correlate this knowledge with the client in the question, who has diabetes, to make a correct selection relative to hyperglycemia.

4 **Answer: 2** The client should wait at least 1 minute between inhalations. Dosages should be taken exactly as prescribed (option 1). The OTC products should not be added without consulting the physician (option 3). Inhaler equipment should be rinsed and dried daily to keep it clean (option 4).
Cognitive Level: Application **Client Need:** Physiological Integrity: Pharmacological and Parenteral Therapies **Integrated Process:** Nursing Process: Evaluation **Content Area:** Pharmacology **Strategy:** The core issue of the question is correct administration procedure for inhaled medications. The wording of the question tells you the correct answer is an option phrased as a true statement.

5 **Answer: 1** Nervousness and tremors may be experienced when medication is newly administered and frequently decrease over the time. Clients should not terminate medication use without consulting the prescriber (option 2). Caffeine would exacerbate the problem (option 3). The symptoms are likely related to the medication and not to the disease process (option 4).
Cognitive Level: Analysis **Client Need:** Physiological Integrity: Pharmacological and Parenteral Therapies **Integrated Process:** Communication and Documentation **Content Area:** Pharmacology **Strategy:** The wording of the question indicates the correct answer is also a true statement. Eliminate option 2 because this is not advice a nurse would give, and choose option 1 over 3 and 4 because it is the true statement.

6 **Answer: 4** Taking the medication with food can decrease GI symptoms. Sustained-release forms should not be crushed or chewed because doing so irritates the gastric mucosa and changes the absorption of the medication (option 1). Medications should be taken as prescribed without omissions or doubled doses (option 2). Medications should be taken at all times, not just when symptomatic (option 3). Prophylaxis is the goal, not acute treatment.
Cognitive Level: Application **Client Need:** Physiological Integrity: Pharmacological and Parenteral Therapies **Integrated Process:** Teaching and Learning **Content Area:** Pharmacology **Strategy:** The core issue of the question is general medication knowledge and instructions for use of theophylline. Eliminate options 1 and 2 first because they are not consistent with general principles of self-administration. Choose option 4 over 3 because the medication is not for prn use.

7 **Answer: 1** Restlessness is a sign of theophylline toxicity but often is a first indicator of hypoxia. The first and best action is to assess for hypoxia. After ruling it out, the other actions should be taken: assessing for other signs and symptoms of toxicity, obtaining an order for the blood level, and explaining toxicity to the client.
Cognitive Level: Analysis **Client Need:** Physiological Integrity: Pharmacological and Parenteral Therapies **Integrated Process:** Nursing Process: Planning **Content Area:** Pharmacology **Strategy:** The question contains the word *first,* which indicates that more than one option may be technically correct but that one is better than the others. Choose option 1 over options 2, 3, and 4 because all the incorrect options refer to the theme of toxicity. If options are very similar, none of them can be correct.

8 **Answer: 2** Beclovent is an inhaled corticosteroid that is thought to decrease inflammation and dilate the airway. The exact mechanism of action is unknown. Beclovent, as is true of any other corticosteroid, does suppress the immune response, but this is not the rationale for administration of the medication (option 3). Inhaled corticosteroids are thought to increase responsiveness of bronchial smooth muscle to beta-agonist drugs (option 4).
Cognitive Level: Application **Client Need:** Physiological Integrity: Pharmacological and Parenteral Therapies **Integrated Process:** Teaching and Learning **Content Area:** Pharmacology **Strategy:** The wording of the question tells you the correct answer is also a true statement. Use medication knowledge and the process of elimination to make a selection.

9 **Answer: 2** Cromolyn is a nonsteroidal agent that stabilizes mast cells so bronchoconstrictive and inflammatory substances are not released when stimulated with an allergen. It is used to treat inflammation of the airway. It does not cause bronchoconstriction (option 4) and is not a bronchodilator (option 1) or expectorant (option 3).
Cognitive Level: Application **Client Need:** Physiological Integrity: Pharmacological and Parenteral Therapies **Integrated Process:** Teaching and Learning **Content Area:** Pharmacology **Strategy:** The wording of the question tells you the correct answer is also a true statement. Use medication knowledge and the process of elimination to make a selection.

10 **Answer: 4** Side effects of cromolyn include dry mouth, irritated throat, cough, unpleasant taste, and headaches. Side effects do not include vomiting (option 1) or tachycardia (option 3). Moist mucous membranes (option 2) is a normal finding.
Cognitive Level: Application **Client Need:** Physiological Integrity: Pharmacological and Parenteral Therapies **Integrated Process:** Nursing Process: Assessment **Content Area:** Pharmacology **Strategy:** Specific medication knowledge is

needed to answer this question. Use the process of elimination to make a selection.

11 **Answer: 1** Leukotrienes are released when a client is exposed to an allergen. Leukotrienes cause inflammation, bronchoconstriction, and mucus production. Leukotriene modifiers such as montelukast block the action of leukotrienes and therefore decrease mucous secretion and reduce inflammation, which prevents bronchoconstriction.
Cognitive Level: Application **Client Need:** Physiological Integrity: Pharmacological and Parenteral Therapies **Integrated Process:** Teaching and Learning **Content Area:** Pharmacology **Strategy:** Specific medication knowledge is needed to answer this question. Use the process of elimination to make a selection.

12 **Answer: 2** Liver function tests should be monitored with leukotriene modifiers because of the potential for liver dysfunction with this type of medication. Renal studies are unnecessary (option 1) in relation to this medication. Fluid intake should be increased (option 3), unless contraindicated by another condition, in order to thin secretions and assist in their mobilization. The medication should be taken 1 hour before or 2 hours after meals (option 4).
Cognitive Level: Application **Client Need:** Physiological Integrity: Pharmacological and Parenteral Therapies **Integrated Process:** Teaching and Learning **Content Area:** Pharmacology **Strategy:** Recall that metabolism and excretion of many drugs occurs in either the hepatic or renal systems. This provides a clue that either option 1 or 2 is correct. Choose option 2 over option 1 by associating the letter *l* in leukotrienes with the letter *l* for liver.

13 **Answer: 3** Second-generation antihistamines cause less sedation than first-generation medications, so the client experiences less drowsiness. They are selective for peripheral H_1 histamine receptors and do not cross the blood–brain barrier. Nausea (option 1), anxiety (option 2), and euphoria (option 4) are unrelated as comparison points between first- and second-generation antihistamines.
Cognitive Level: Application **Client Need:** Physiological Integrity: Pharmacological and Parenteral Therapies **Integrated Process:** Teaching and Learning **Content Area:** Pharmacology **Strategy:** Recall that second-generation drugs generally have some type of improvement over first-generation drugs. In this case, since antihistamines often cause drowsiness, it is easy to reason that this side effect would be decreased in second-generation medications in this category.

14 **Answer: 1** The effects of first-generation antihistamines are increased with alcohol, tricyclic antidepressants, antianxiety agents, antipsychotic agents, opioid analgesics, sedative hypnotics, and monoamine oxidase inhibitors. Nicotine (option 2), caffeine (option 3), and CNS stimulants (option 4) would not have an additive effect.
Cognitive Level: Analysis **Client Need:** Physiological Integrity: Pharmacological and Parenteral Therapies **Integrated Process:** Teaching and Learning **Content Area:** Pharmacology **Strategy:** Recall first that first-generation antihistamines cause drowsiness, and look for an option that would have an additive effect. Since alcohol is a CNS depressant, it is the correct choice for this question; the others represent agents that stimulate the CNS.

15 **Answer: 2** The proper application of nasal spray decongestants is with the client sitting and squeezing the bottle once, holding a finger over the other nostril, and inhaling. Administering more than one squeeze application (options 1 and 4) would increase the dose. The applicator should be rinsed after each use to prevent contamination (option 3).
Cognitive Level: Application **Client Need:** Physiological Integrity: Pharmacological and Parenteral Therapies **Integrated Process:** Teaching and Learning **Content Area:** Pharmacology **Strategy:** A key word in the question is *accurate.* The core issue of the question is the instruction that is a true statement. Use the process of elimination and knowledge of basic medication administration procedures to make a selection.

16 **Answer: 3** Avoidance of eating or drinking for 30 minutes after medication administration allows the medication time to work. Nasal spray decongestants should not be taken for longer than 3 days because they can cause rebound congestion (option 1). Fluid intake should be increased to 2 to 3 L/day to liquefy secretions, not decreased (option 2). Smoking should be avoided because it increases secretions and decreases ciliary action (option 4).
Cognitive Level: Application **Client Need:** Physiological Integrity: Pharmacological and Parenteral Therapies **Integrated Process:** Teaching and Learning **Content Area:** Pharmacology **Strategy:** The wording of the question tells you the correct answer is also a true statement. Eliminate options 2 and 4 first as least likely to be true. Choose option 3 over option 1 knowing the side effects of decongestants.

17 **Answer: 1** It is important to teach clients side effects of medications. The side effects of expectorants include nausea, vomiting, gastric irritation, and rash. If a cough lasts longer than a week (option 2), it should be reported to the physician. The client should avoid eating or drinking for 30 minutes after medication administration to allow the medication to work (option 3). The medication should be taken as directed, and doses should not be doubled (option 4).
Cognitive Level: Application **Client Need:** Physiological Integrity: Pharmacological and Parenteral Therapies **Integrated Process:** Nursing Process: Planning **Content Area:** Pharmacology **Strategy:** Use the process of elimination and general medication knowledge to answer the question. Eliminate option 2 because the time frame is excessive and option 4 because it is not standard medication teaching. Choose option 1 over option 3 because it is a true statement and because option 3 may hinder medication absorption.

18 **Answer: 4** All of the symptoms listed are potential side effects of opioid antitussives. The most significant side effect is respiratory depression, evidenced by a respiratory rate of 10, when normal is 12 to 20 breaths/minute.
Cognitive Level: Analysis **Client Need:** Physiological Integrity: Pharmacological and Parenteral Therapies **Integrated Process:** Nursing Process: Assessment **Content Area:** Pharmacology **Strategy:** The key words *most significant* tell you that more than one option may be technically correct and that you must select the most important option. Use the ABCs (airway, breathing, and circulation) to make your selection.

19 **Answer: 4** Unused medication should be discarded after 4 days, not 7. Avoidance of smoking is necessary because

smoking increases secretions and decreases ciliary action (option 2). Increasing fluids assists with thinning secretions (option 1). Rinsing the mouth after administration decreases oropharyngeal irritation (option 3).
Cognitive Level: Application **Client Need:** Physiological Integrity: Pharmacological and Parenteral Therapies **Integrated Process:** Nursing Process: Evaluation **Content Area:** Pharmacology
Strategy: The phrase *further teaching* tells you the correct answer is an incorrect or false statement. Eliminate option 1 first because this is an important principle to follow and then option 3 because this is a general medication administration principle. Choose option 4 over 2 because smoking cessation is always recommended.

20 **Answer: 4** The Venturi mask has a dial to set the percentage of oxygen and can administer 50% oxygen. The nonrebreather mask (option 2) administers 60% to 100% oxygen. The partial rebreather mask (option 3) administers 70% to 90% oxygen. The nasal cannula (option 1) can administer up to 6 L/min, which is approximately 44% oxygen.
Cognitive Level: Application **Client Need:** Physiological Integrity: Pharmacological and Parenteral Therapies **Integrated Process:** Nursing Process: Implementation **Content Area:** Pharmacology
Strategy: Specific knowledge of the various concepts related to oxygen therapy is needed to answer this question. Use the process of elimination to make a selection, and remember that Venturi masks deliver precise oxygen concentrations.

Key Terms to Review

acute asthma attack p. 581
adrenergic agonist p. 581
anticholinergic p. 590
antihistamine p. 589
antitussive p. 592
atelectasis p. 594
catecholamine p. 581
decongestant p. 590
expectorant p. 591
histamine p. 585
hypoxemia p. 593
hypoxia p. 593
inhaler p. 587
interleukin p. 586
lacrimal p. 589
leukotrienes p. 585
mast cell p. 584
mucolytic p. 593
nebulizer p. 587
neutrophils p. 585
noncatecholamine p. 581
opioid p. 592
rhinitis p. 586
status asthmaticus p. 584
sympathomimetic p. 581
xanthines p. 584

References

Abrams, A. (2004). *Clinical drug therapy: Rationales for nursing practice* (7th ed.). Philadelphia: Lippincott, Williams & Wilkins.
Deglin, J., & Vallerand, A. (2006). *Davis's drug guide for nurses* (10th ed.). Philadelphia: F. A. Davis.
Kozier, B., Erb, G., Berman, A., & Burke, K. (2006). *Fundamentals of nursing: Concepts, process, and practice* (7th ed.). Upper Saddle River, NJ: Prentice-Hall.
Lehne, R. (2004). *Pharmacology for nursing care* (5th ed.). St. Louis, MO: Mosby.
LeMone, P., & Burke, K. (2007). *Medical surgical nursing: Critical thinking in client care* (4th ed.). Upper Saddle River, NJ: Prentice-Hall.
McKenry, L., Tessier, E., & Hogan, M. (2006). *Mosby's pharmacology in nursing* (22nd ed.). St. Louis, MO: Elsevier Mosby.
Smeltzer, S., & Bare, B. (2006). *Textbook of medical-surgical nursing* (11th ed.). Philadelphia: Lippincott, William & Wilkins.

Cardiovascular Medications

38

In this chapter

Test Yourself

Are you ready for the NCLEX-RN® or course exams? Use the practice tests on the companion CD-ROM to check.

Cross reference

Other chapters relevant to this content area are

Dosage Calculation and Medication Administration	Chapter 30
Cardiovascular Disorders	Chapter 57

I. GENERAL GUIDELINES FOR CARDIOVASCULAR MEDICATIONS *(SEE BOX 38–1)*

II. NITRATES AND NITRITES

A. **Increase oxygenated blood flow to myocardium** by dilating coronary and systemic blood vessels (BVs)

B. **Dilation of systemic vascular bed** leads to pooling of blood in peripheral BVs and reduced ***preload*** (volume in left ventricle just prior to contraction) and ***afterload*** (resistance to blood being ejected by left ventricle) and myocardial oxygen (O2) demand

C. **Common medications are listed in Box 38–2**

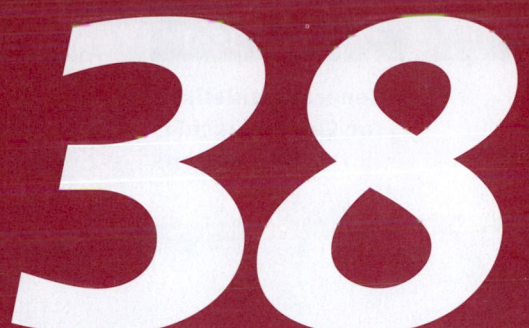

Box 38–1

General Guidelines for Cardiovascular Medications

Administration Principles

1. Assess current medications (including OTC drugs and herbal products) and history of allergies to identify any potential risks to client.
2. Administer doses on time to maintain therapeutic blood levels.
3. Do not break or allow client to chew sustained release or enteric coated preparations.
4. Many antihypertensive and vasodilating drugs cause orthostatic hypotension and dizziness, so assist client to arise slowly from lying to sitting, and from sitting to standing positions; provide a safe environment to decrease injury in case of falls.
5. Provide both verbal and written instructions to client, and provide phone number to call if questions arise or problems occur.

Client Teaching

1. Understand medication actions, side effects, signs of toxicity, importance of follow-up with prescriber and complying with follow-up laboratory tests, and how to self-administer.
2. Do not take any OTC drugs or herbal products without first consulting prescriber.
3. Take exactly as prescribed and do not miss or double doses.
4. Report adverse effects promptly.
5. Do not discontinue drug without consulting prescriber.
6. Do not drink alcohol while taking prescription medications.
7. Take measures described above to reduce risk of injury from orthostatic hypotension; avoid use hot baths and hot tubs and limit amount of time spent out of doors in hot weather to minimize risk of orthostatic blood pressure changes.

Memory Aid

Remember that drugs that are nitrates have the letters *nitro-* or *nitr-* in them.

D. Administration considerations

1. Ensure client's oral mucous membranes are moist when taking sublingual (SL) nitroglycerin (NTG) tablets
2. For a hospitalized client, keep NTG tablets at bedside with a physician order if policy allows; instruct client to report all chest pain episodes; count tablets daily if kept at bedside
3. Administer intravenous (IV) NTG as a continuous or intermittent infusion (not IV push) using an infusion pump
4. ! IV NTG must be diluted in 5% dextrose or 0.9% sodium chloride (normal saline) solution, mixed in glass bottles and infused only through manufacturer-supplied IV tubing; regular polyvinylchloride IV tubing can absorb 40% to 80% of NTG
5. Nitroglycerin IV drips are often **titrated** (dose adjusted according to a predetermined parameter, such as chest pain)
6. ! Monitor blood pressure (BP) and heart rate (HR) every 15 minutes when using IV form of NTG and titrating medication; be prepared to treat hypotension by decreasing or stopping NTG infusion
7. ! Use gloves or an applicator to spread NTG paste or ointment evenly and avoid absorption of medication into nurse's skin

Box 38–2

Nitrates and Nitrites

Nitroglycerin (Nitrostat, Nitro-Tab, Nitrogard, Nitro-Bid, Nitrol, Nitrodur, Transderm-Nitro, Tridil, others)

Isosorbide mononitrate (Ismo, Monoket, Imdur)

Isosorbide dinitrate (Isordil)

8. Rotate location of NTG paste or patch to reduce skin irritation and enhance absorption; place on hairless areas and avoid scar tissue or lesions; appropriate areas include chest, upper abdomen, anterior thigh, or upper arm
9. NTG dosing regimen should allow for an 8- to 10-hour nitrate-free period to prevent development of tolerance; NTG patch should be applied in morning and removed at bedtime
10. Do not administer any nitrate to a client who has hypersensitivity to nitrates, is hypotensive, has severe bradycardia or tachycardia, or has used erectile dysfunction medications such as sildenafil (Viagra) within 24 hours (causes profound hypotension)

E. Side/adverse effects

1. Headache (50%), postural or orthostatic hypotension, flushing, blurred vision, dry mouth
2. Weakness, dizziness, vertigo, and faintness
3. Severe postural hypotension
4. Nausea, vomiting, fecal and urinary incontinence, abdominal pain

F. Nursing considerations

1. Ensure that client is sitting or lying down when taking NTG to prevent dizziness or fainting
2. Allow SL tablet to dissolve naturally under tongue; if mouth is dry, instruct client to take a sip of water before placing tablet under tongue
3. Give client no more than 3 tablets total, one every 5 minutes; notify physician or emergency services if pain is unrelieved after third dose
4. Remove paste or patch each day at designated time before applying next dose
5. Store ointment in a cool, dry place with cap attached tightly
6. Monitor BP and HR frequently during medication titration (this may be as often as every 5 to 10 minutes)
7. Check infusion concentration carefully because many different dilutions are possible

G. Client teaching

1. As per Box 38–1; all forms of NTG might cause dizziness and headache; rest for at least 15 minutes after taking SL medication to avoid dizziness
2. Report to health care provider if symptoms become worse or increase in frequency
3. Sit down next to a phone when taking sublingual (SL) NTG tablets in case it becomes necessary to call for help
4. If pain persists after three NTG tablets (or sprays) at 5-minute intervals, notify physician because persistent pain could indicate an impending myocardial infarction (MI)
5. NTG degrades in heat, light, or moisture; store medication in original container in a cool, dry place
6. Replace NTG tablets every 3 to 6 months after opening; each tablet should produce a slight stinging or tingling sensation when placed under tongue if fresh
7. Write down emergency numbers and place them next to phone with home address and exact directions
8. Take a SL or spray NTG before an event that might cause angina, such as stair climbing, exercise, or sexual intercourse
9. Keep a written record for physician of times, dates, amount of medication required for relief of each attack, and possible precipitating factors
10. Shake aerosol spray well prior to use
11. If wearing an NTG patch or paste and experiencing an anginal attack, an NTG tablet may be taken SL following safety measures outlined above
12. Swimming or bathing with an NTG patch in place is acceptable
13. Frequent and prolonged use of NTG may reduce efficacy, requiring a medication adjustment

III. BETA-ADRENERGIC BLOCKERS

A. Block $beta_1$ adrenergic receptors are found chiefly in cardiac muscle, and in higher doses, they may cause blocking of $beta_2$ adrenergic receptors in airways, leading to increased airway resistance, especially in clients with asthma or chronic obstructive pulmonary disease (COPD)

Memory Aid

Use the number to remember the organs affected by beta-adrenergic receptors. Remember β_1—you have 1 heart, and β_2—you have 2 lungs.

B. Used therapeutically to manage hypertension, angina pectoris, acute MI, and supraventricular tachycardia

! **C. Block cardiac effects of beta-adrenergic stimulation, resulting in the following:**

1. Reductions in HR, myocardial **irritability** (cardiac muscle response to a variety of external stimuli such as hypoxia), and force of contraction
2. A negative **inotropic** (force of contraction) and **chronotropic** (heart rate) effect
3. Depression of **automaticity** (heart's ability to initiate impulses on its own without external stimulation) of sinus node
4. Reduction in atrioventricular (AV) node and intraventricular **dromotropic** (conduction velocity) effect

D. Also useful in controlling panic attacks and stage fright in some clients

E. Common medications are listed in Box 38–3

Memory Aid

Recognize beta-adrenergic blockers because they end in *-olol* or *-lol.*

F. Administration considerations

1. Assess client before, during, and after the initial dose
2. ! Monitor BP, apical pulse, and cardiac rhythm frequently during initial administration; if given orally, assess client 30 minutes before and 60 minutes after initial dose
3. Prior to next dose, reassess BP, HR, and cardiac rhythm
4. Give medication at consistent times with or without meals; recommended before meals and at bedtime
5. ! Beta-adrenergic blockers, when used concurrently with calcium channel blockers (see section to follow), may increase adverse response, including bradycardia and hypotension
6. Tablets may be crushed as needed (prn) before administration and taken with fluid of choice
7. ! Do not discontinue therapy abruptly; dosage is reduced gradually over 1 to 2 weeks, observe client for paradoxical reactions such as hypertension and tachycardia
8. ! Contraindicated with first-degree heart block (PR interval greater than 0.2 second), heart failure, bradycardia, shock, significant aortic or mitral valve disease, hyperactive airway syndrome (asthma or bronchospasm), severe seasonal allergies (allergic rhinitis during pollen season), concurrent use of psychotropic that augments adrenergic system or within 2 weeks of an monoamine oxidase inhibitor (MAOI)
9. Use cautiously in client before and after major surgery, in client with renal or hepatic impairment, diabetes mellitus, myasthenia gravis, or Wolff-Parkinson-White (WPW) syndrome, and systemic allergies to insect stings

Box 38–3

Common Beta-Adrenergic Blocker Medications

Atenolol (Tenormin)	Nadolol (Corgard)
Betaxolol (Kerlone)	Propranolol (Inderal)
Bisoprolol (Zebeta)	Propranolol long-acting (Inderal LA)
Metoprolol (Lopressor)	Timolol (Blocadren)
Metoprolol extended release (Toprol XL)	

G. Side/adverse effects

1. Dizziness, sleep disturbances, depression, confusion, agitation, or psychosis
2. Hypotension, bradycardia, heart block, acute heart failure, and peripheral paresthesias resembling Raynaud's phenomenon
3. Laryngospasm or bronchospasm
4. Dry eyes with a gritty sensation, blurred vision, tinnitus, or hearing loss
5. Dry mouth, nausea, vomiting, heartburn, diarrhea, constipation, abdominal cramps, and flatulence
6. Agranulocytosis, hypoglycemia, hyperglycemia and hypocalcemia in clients with hyperthyroidism

H. Nursing considerations

1. Take apical pulse and BP before administering; evaluate for fluid volume overload as sign of heart failure
2. Monitor intake and output (I & O) and daily weight
3. Withhold medication if HR is less than 60 beats per minute (bpm) or if systolic BP is less than 90 mmHg
4. Assess client for history of asthma, allergies, or COPD; realize beta-blockers may lead to bronchospasm in clients with no previously documented history of pulmonary disease
5. Assess HR, BP, and respiratory status carefully during periods of dosage adjustment; maintain effective communication with prescriber
6. Adverse reactions occur most frequently after IV dose and with oral doses in elderly and those with impaired renal function
7. Restrict dietary sodium as ordered to prevent fluid volume overload; check with prescriber regarding sodium restriction or concurrent use of a diuretic
8. Fasting longer than 12 hours may induce hypoglycemia, which is worsened by beta-blocker therapy because signs are masked
9. Review results of periodic renal, hepatic, cardiac, and hematologic studies
10. Beta-blockers may induce false-negative test results in exercise tolerance electrocardiogram (ECG)
11. Beta-blockers may increase or decrease blood glucose levels of diabetic clients

I. Client teaching

1. How to check pulse and BP and their desired ranges, how to record daily measurements, and when to call prescriber
2. Abrupt withdrawal can lead to severe paradoxical or rebound reactions, including sweating, tremulousness, severe headache, malaise, palpitations, hypertension, MI, and life-threatening heart rhythm disturbances
3. Establish a routine for taking medication and strive to comply with plan for results; write out a daily schedule for medication
4. Notify physician if any dizziness or lightheadedness occurs; avoid driving or operating machinery until these symptoms are relieved
5. Stop smoking because smoking might offset desired outcomes of controlled HR, BP, and prevention of angina; smoking also increases hepatic metabolism of beta-blocker medication, leading to unpredictable or diminished drug effects
6. Avoid OTC medications and herbal supplements without consulting physician
7. Inform all health care providers, including ophthalmologist or optometrist of medication; beta-blockers may lower intraocular pressure
8. As per Box 38–1; reduce salt intake while taking medication

IV. CALCIUM CHANNEL BLOCKERS

A. These are class IV antiarrhythmic drugs that inhibit calcium ion influx through slow channels into cells of myocardial and arterial smooth muscle (both cardiac and peripheral blood vessels)

1. Intracellular calcium remains below levels needed to stimulate cell
2. Dilate coronary arteries and arterioles and prevent coronary artery spasm
3. Increase myocardial O_2 delivery to prevent angina
4. Slow conduction through the sinoatrial (SA) node and AV node, lowering heart rate and decreasing strength of cardiac contraction (negative inotropic effect)

5. Decrease automaticity and **conductivity** (amount of force and pressure to pump blood out of ventricles) by blocking flow of calcium into cell
6. Decrease systemic vascular resistance (SVR) and thus afterload by dilating peripheral arteriols
7. Reduce arterial BP (antihypertensive effect) and HR

B. **Used for vasospastic angina (Prinzmetal's variant or angina at rest), chronic stable (classic and activity-induced) angina, and essential hypertension;** IV form is useful in atrial fibrillation, atrial flutter, and supraventricular tachycardia

C. **Common medications are listed in Box 38–4**

Memory Aid

Recognize many calcium channel blockers by noting the suffix *-dipine.* This is not true for all, however; exceptions are verapamil and diltiazem.

D. **Administration considerations**
1. Administer oral diltiazem before meals and at bedtime and oral verapamil with food to reduce gastric irritation
2. Evaluate BP and ECG before initiation of therapy
3. Monitor for headache; an analgesic may be required
4. Give IV forms of verapamil and diltiazem using infusion pump and carefully following package directions
5. ! Withhold dose if BP is less than 90/60
6. Contraindicated with known hypersensitivity to drug, sick sinus syndrome (without artificial pacemaker), second- or third-degree heart blocks
7. Does not alter serum calcium levels

E. **Adverse effects and toxicity**
1. Headache, dizziness, nervousness, insomnia, confusion, tremor, and gait disturbance
2. ! Postural hypotension, heart block and profound bradycardia, heart failure, possible syncope, palpitations, and fluid volume overload
3. Nausea, vomiting, constipation, and impaired taste
4. Skin rash

F. **Nursing considerations**
1. Evaluate BP and ECG prior to initiating treatment and monitor closely during medication adjustment; monitor for headache
2. Monitor hepatic and renal lab test results
3. May induce hyperglycemia; monitor diabetic clients closely

G. **Client teaching**
1. ! Take radial pulse before each dose (especially verapamil); report an irregular pulse or if slower than identified parameter (such as 50 or 60)
2. ! Change position slowly to prevent postural hypotension
3. Avoid driving if dizziness or faintness is noted; report these symptoms immediately
4. ! Report gradual weight gain and evidence of edema; may indicate onset of CHF
5. ! As per Box 38–1; avoid grapefruit and grapefruit juice when taking verapamil
6. Stop smoking

Box 38–4

Common Calcium Channel Blockers

Diltiazem extended release (Cardizem CD or LA, Dilacor XR, Tiazac)

Verapamil (Calan, Isoptin)

Amlodipine (Norvasc)

Felodipine (Plendil)

Isradipine (Dynacirc CR)

Nicardipine sustained release (Cardene SR)

Nifedipine long-acting (Adalat CC, Procardia XL)

Nisoldipine (Sular)

V. ANGIOTENSIN-CONVERTING ENZYME (ACE) INHIBITORS

A. **Inhibit renin-angiotensin-aldosterone mechanism** by blocking conversion of angiotensin I to angiotensin II and prevent peripheral vasoconstriction

! B. **Used to treat hypertension;** preferred for hypertensive clients with diabetic nephropathy

C. **Common medications are listed in Box 38–5**

Memory Aid

Generic names of ACE inhibitors can be recognized because they end in *-pril.*

D. **Administration considerations**
1. Discontinue with prescriber supervision if pregnancy is detected
2. Give moexipril and captopril on empty stomach due to decreased absorption with food
3. Contraindicated with hypersensitivity to ACE inhibitors
4. Avoid use with potassium supplements and potassium-sparing diuretics

E. **Side/adverse effects**
1. Headache, dizziness, anxiety, fatigue, insomnia, nervousness
2. ! Hypotension and palpitations
3. Nausea, vomiting, abdominal pain, constipation
4. ! Persistent dry nonproductive cough, dyspnea
5. Rash, arthralgia, impotence, and dysgeusia (altered taste)
6. ! Angioedema, leukopenia, agranulocytosis, pancytopenia, thrombocytopenia
7. Cerebrovascular accident (CVA), MI, and hypertensive crisis

F. **Nursing considerations**
1. Administer 1 hour before meals to increase absorption; tablets may be crushed
2. Do not administer to pregnant or lactating women
3. ! Monitor labs for increased potassium, liver enzymes, bilirubin, BUN and creatinine, and decreased sodium levels and WBC count
4. ! Take BP before giving dose and monitor regularly
5. ! Monitor for rashes or hives and for peripheral edema
6. If the client has renal disease, monitor urine protein on a regular basis by dipstick method
7. Discontinue diuretics 2 to 3 days before ACE inhibitor therapy

G. **Client teaching**
1. Report peripheral edema, signs of infection, facial swelling, loss of taste, or difficulty breathing
2. As per Box 38–1; do not skip doses or stop taking drug; it may cause serious rebound increase in BP
3. ! Persistent, dry cough is a side effect and does not indicate respiratory disease or infection
4. Take antacids 2 hours before or after dose of fosinopril and captopril
5. ! Avoid potassium-containing salt substitutes
6. Monitor for bruising, petechiae, or bleeding with captopril
7. Taste of food may be diminished during the first month of therapy
8. Take captopril 20 minutes to 1 hour before a meal

Box 38–5

Common ACE Inhibitors

Benazepril (Lotensin)	Moexipril (Univasc)
Captopril (Capoten)	Perindopril (Aceon)
Enalapril (Vasotec)	Quinapril (Accupril)
Fosinopril (Monopril)	Ramipril (Altace)
Lisinopril (Prinivil, Zestril)	Trandolapril (Mavik)

VI. ANGIOTENSIN II RECEPTOR BLOCKERS (ARBS)

A. Act as antagonists at angiotensin II receptor of vascular smooth muscle, blocking vasoconstriction and aldosterone-secreting effects and lowering BP

B. Common medications are listed in Box 38–6

Memory Aid

ARBs are easily recognized because they end in the suffix *-sartan*.

C. Administration considerations

1. Discontinue immediately if pregnancy is detected
2. Use cautiously in clients with renal or hepatic disease

D. Side/adverse effects

1. Hypotension and dizziness, tachycardia or bradycardia
2. Cough, GI upset, insomnia, nasal congestion, and myalgia
3. Neutropenia and hyperkalemia

E. Nursing considerations

1. Monitor client taking diuretics for additive hypotension
2. Regularly assess renal function, potassium level, and WBC with differential
3. Do not administer to pregnant or lactating women
4. Monitor BP and apical pulse regularly

F. Client teaching

1. As per Box 38–1; do not discontinue medication abruptly
2. Avoid salt substitutes because of potassium content
3. Notify physician immediately if pregnancy is suspected
4. Use alternate birth control methods
5. Maintain adequate hydration

VII. DIRECT-ACTING VASODILATORS

A. Potent antihypertensive agents that act directly on arterial smooth muscles

B. Produce peripheral vasodilation, resulting in lowered arterial BP, increased HR, and increased cardiac output (CO)

C. Some may also be used as an adjunct in treating heart failure or to treat Raynaud's disease by increasing blood flow to extremities

D. Common medications are listed in Box 38–7

E. Administration considerations

1. Take oral forms with food to increase bioavailability
2. IV hydralazine may be given undiluted via direct IV push at a rate of 10 mg/min
3. IV sodium nitroprusside is diluted to 50 mg in 250 mL D_5W (200 mcg/mL); infuse cautiously through an IV pump; when mixed, it appears orange and must be covered in a foil pouch to avoid exposure to light during infusion
4. Do not mix with other IV solutions
5. Discontinue all vasodilators slowly to avoid paradoxical hypertensive effects
6. Store medication in light-resistant container
7. Monitor HR and BP closely during administration to prevent sudden hypotension
8. Contraindicated in compensatory hypertension (arteriovenous shunt or coarctation of aorta), inadequate cerebral perfusion leading to a decreased cerebral perfusion pressure (CPP), or hypovolemia
9. During administration of sodium nitroprusside, monitor serum thiocyanate levels with prolonged IV infusion or in clients with impaired renal function

Box 38–6

Common Angiotensin II Receptor Blockers (ARBs)

Candesartan (Atacand)	Olmesartan (Benicar)
Eprosartan (Tevetan)	Telmisartan (Micardis)
Irbesartan (Avapro)	Valsartan (Diovan)
Losartan (Cozaar)	

Box 38–7

Direct-Acting Vasodilators

Diazoxide (Hyperstat)
Hydralazine (Apresoline)
Minoxidil (Loniten)
Nitroprusside (Nipride)
Trimethaphan camsylate (Arfonad)

F. Side/adverse effects

1. Headache, dizziness, tremors, apprehension, and muscle twitching
2. Angina, palpitations, tachycardia or bradycardia, flushing, paradoxical pressor response (sudden elevation in BP), ECG changes, profound hypotension, shock, and dysrhythmias
3. Systemic lupus erythematosus (SLE)–like syndrome (with hydralazine), edema
4. Anorexia, nausea, vomiting, constipation or diarrhea, abdominal pain, and paralytic ileus
5. Difficulty urinating and glomerulonephritis
6. Decreased hematocrit and hemoglobin, anemia, agranulocytosis (rare)
7. Rash, irritation at IV site, urticaria, pruritus, fever, chills, arthralgia, eosinophilia, and cholangitis; excessive hair growth with minoxidil
8. With sodium nitroprusside, thiocyanate toxicity, is noted by profound hypotension, tinnitus, fatigue, pink skin color, metabolic acidosis, and loss of consciousness

G. Nursing considerations

1. Assess carefully baseline vital signs including HR, cardiac rhythm, ECG, and neurological status
2. When administering IV vasodilators:
   a. Establish a large, stable IV site for infusions because they are irritating to tissue; administer with an IV infusion pump
   b. Monitor BP every 5 to 15 minutes with an automatic external BP machine or arterial line during initial infusion and medication adjustment
   c. Monitor I & O
   d. If hypotension occurs, decrease infusion and monitor client closely; if sudden, severe hypotension occurs, discontinue medication; maintain airway, breathing and circulation (ABCs); establish IV site; contact physician, and initiate emergency protocols as necessary
3. Obtain baseline vital signs and check BP, heart rate, and cardiac rhythm before each dose when administering orally

H. Client teaching

1. How to self-monitor pulse and BP
2. Possibility of headache and palpitations within 2 to 4 hours after first PO dose
3. As per Box 38–1; write down questions to ask provider on each follow-up visit
4. Stop smoking as this negates positive effects of medication
5. Monitor weight daily and report edema
6. Avoid hot tubs and hot baths that might induce profound vasodilation and hypotension

VIII. ANTI-ALPHA ADRENERGIC BLOCKERS (CENTRAL AND PERIPHERAL)

A. Centrally acting sympatholytics

1. Stimulate $alpha_2$ receptors in CNS to inhibit sympathetic cardio-accelerator and vasoconstrictor centers
2. Decrease sympathetic outflow from CNS, resulting in decreased arterial pressure

B. Peripheral anti-adrenergics

1. Deplete catecholamine stores in peripheral nervous system (PNS) and perhaps in CNS
2. Decrease total peripheral resistance, HR and CO

C. Common medications are listed in Box 38–8

D. Administration considerations

1. Do not discontinue abruptly; may result in rebound hypertension

Box 38-8

Alpha$_1$ and Alpha$_2$ Blockers

Alpha$_1$ blockers

Doxazosin (Cardura)

Prazosin (Minipress)

Terazosin (Hytrin)

Alpha$_2$ blockers

Clonidine (Catapres)

Clonidine patch (Catapres-TTS)

Methyldopa (Aldomet)

Reserpine (generic)

Guanabenz (Wytensin)

Guanfacine (generic)

Guanadrel (Hylorel)

2. Guanabenz: allow 1 to 2 weeks before adjusting dose
3. Guanfacine: administer at bedtime to decrease daytime somnolence; allow 3 to 4 weeks before adjusting dose
4. Methyldopa: allow 2 days for maximum response before adjusting dose
5. Contraindicated in hypersensitivity, active hepatitis or cirrhosis, co-administration with MAOIs (methyldopa), heart failure (methyldopa), history of mental depression, active peptic ulcer disease, ulcerative colitis, asthma, and bronchitis (reserpine)

E. Side/adverse effects

1. Sedation, headache, weakness, dizziness, and decreased mental acuity
2. Involuntary choreoathetoid movements, parkinsonism, depression, nightmares
3. Bradycardia, orthostatic hypotension, aggravation of angina, edema
4. GI disturbance, rash, gynecomastia, galactorrhea, amenorrhea, impotence, dry mouth, weight gain
5. Myocarditis, hemolytic anemia, thrombocytopenia
6. Hepatic necrosis
7. Severe rebound hypertension

F. Nursing considerations

1. Administer orally; tablets may be crushed and do not need to be given with food unless GI upset occurs
2. IV methyldopa should be given over 30 to 60 minutes; do not give subcutaneously or IM
3. ! Transdermal systems (Clonidine) are applied to dry, hairless areas of the skin of chest or upper arm; assess areas for rash
4. ! Monitor labs for elevated aspartate aminotransferase (AST), alanine aminotransferase (ALT), alkaline phosphatase, bilirubin, BUN, creatinine, potassium, sodium, and uric acid
5. May prolong prothrombin times
6. ! Obtain baseline BP and apical pulse, and monitor weight regularly
7. ! Assess client for peripheral edema
8. Dry mouth may contribute to development of dental caries, periodontal disease, oral candidiasis, and discomfort

G. Client teaching

1. As per Box 38–1
2. ! Possible need for sodium restriction and weight reduction; report weight gain of more than 5 lb per week
3. Relieve dry mouth by sipping water or chewing sugarless gum
4. Treat nausea by eating unsalted crackers, noncola beverages, or dry toast
5. Report mental acuity changes to health care provider

6. Some drugs cause urine to become darker
7. Do not drive a car or perform hazardous activities if drowsiness occurs
8. Take medication as prescribed; do not stop abruptly to avoid rebound hypertension

IX. CARDIAC GLYCOSIDES

A. **Used primarily to treat heart failure** but also used to treat atrial ***dysrhythmia*** (abnormality in electrical activity of heart)
B. **Increase *contractility* (force of contraction) and efficiency of myocardial contraction**
C. **Is a positive inotrope that increases force of myocardial contraction**
D. **Is a negative dromotrope that decreases conduction velocity through AV node**
E. **Common medications: digoxin (Lanoxin) and digitoxin (Crystodigin)**
F. **Administration considerations**
   1. May be given with or without food
   2. Tablet may be crushed and mixed with fluid or food as desired; pediatric elixir is also available
   3. IV push digoxin may be administered undiluted or diluted in 4 mL of sterile water, 5% dextrose, or NS; administer each direct IV dose over 5 minutes; client may receive a loading dose (digitalization) to achieve adequate serum drug levels
   4. Never administer digoxin IM because it would cause tissue irritation and great variation in bioavailability
   5. Infiltration into subcutaneous tissue can cause local irritation and tissue sloughing
   6. Contraindicated in clients with known hypersensitivity to digitalis or digoxin toxicity
   7. Full digitalizing dose should not be given if client has received digoxin during previous week
   8. Use cautiously with following conditions: renal insufficiency, hypokalemia, advanced heart disease, acute MI, heart block, cor pulmonale, hypothyroidism, and lung disease
   9. Use cautiously in pregnant or nursing mothers, children, premature infants, and elderly clients
G. **Side/adverse effects**
   1. Fatigue, muscle weakness, headache, facial neuralgia, depression, paresthesias, hallucinations, confusion, drowsiness, agitation, dizziness, and malaise
   2. Dysrhythmias, hypotension, A-V heart block, and diaphoresis
   3. Anorexia, nausea, vomiting, diarrhea, and dysphagia
   4. Visual disturbances (blurred, green or yellow vision, photophobia, or halo effect)
   5. Digoxin toxicity may be unrecognized because it may present same early manifestations as a flu, such as anorexia, nausea, vomiting, diarrhea, visual disturbances
H. **Nursing considerations**
   1. Obtain baseline data and perform ongoing physical assessments, including neurological status, HR, BP, and cardiac rhythm
   2. Check baseline serum digoxin level prior to initiating digoxin therapy
      a. Blood level is 0 if client has not taken digoxin before
      b. Therapeutic levels are 0.5 to 2.0 ng/mL (ranges vary slightly among texts)
      c. Toxic levels are greater than 2 ng/mL
   3. Assess baseline and ongoing serum electrolytes, creatinine clearance, magnesium, and calcium
   4. Monitor elderly clients taking digoxin and a diuretic to treat CHF or atrial fibrillation for digoxin toxicity
   5. Take apical pulse for 1 full minute prior to administering digoxin, noting rate, rhythm, and quality; if any changes are noted, withhold medication and notify prescriber; an ECG will likely be ordered
   6. Withhold dose of medication if client has symptoms of digoxin toxicity (anorexia, nausea, vomiting, diarrhea, or visual disturbances)
   7. In children, early signs of toxicity include cardiac dysrhythmias; children rarely demonstrate anorexia, nausea, vomiting, diarrhea, or visual disturbances
   8. Advise client to eat foods high in potassium, such as oranges, bananas, fruit juices, vegetables, and potatoes if taking loop diuretics

9. Monitor I & O and daily weight, especially in clients with impaired renal failure; auscultate breath sounds for crackles
10. Antidote: digoxin immune Fab (Digibind) is used in extreme toxicity
11. Assess extremities for edema as indicator of fluid volume overload
12. Concurrent antibiotic-digoxin therapy can precipitate toxicity because of altering of intestinal flora
13. Monitor client closely when changing from one drug form to another; often a dose adjustment is required (if tablet form is replaced by elixir, potential for toxicity increases)

I. **Client teaching**
1. As per Box 38–1
2. Check pulse for 1 full minute prior to taking dose; contact physician before taking dose if pulse is below 60 bpm or above 110 or if skipped beats are present
3. Suspect toxicity with nausea, vomiting, anorexia, diarrhea, or visual disturbances such as halos or green or yellow vision
4. Withhold next dose if digoxin toxicity is suspected, and contact physician immediately
5. Weigh self daily with same clothes and at same time; report weight gain greater than 2 lb/day
6. Take digoxin as ordered; do not to skip or add additional dose if experiencing chest discomfort (a common report from clients admitted with digoxin toxicity is that they take digoxin as a "heart pill" when experiencing chest pain)
7. Insist on receiving original brand of digoxin ordered by physician to avoid errors in dosing

X. ANTIDYSRHYTHMICS

A. **Class I-A (fast sodium channel blockers)**
1. Used to treat both atrial and ventricular dysrhythmias; prevent recurrence of premature ventricular contractions (PVCs) and ventricular tachycardia (VT) that are not severe enough to require cardioversion
2. Depress myocardial contractility and excitability and prolong **refractory period** (making cells able to respond only to strong stimulus)
3. Reduce rate of spontaneous diastolic depolarization in pacemaker cells, thereby suppressing ectopic focal activity
4. Disopyramide shortens sinus node recovery time and increases atrial and ventricular effective refractory period
5. Quinidine is classified as a chemical cardioversion agent used to convert atrial fibrillation to normal sinus rhythm
6. Common medications are listed in Box 38–9

Box 38–9

Common Antidysrhythmic Drugs

Group I-A drugs
Disopyramide (Norpace)
Procainamide (Pronestyl)
Quinidine (Quinaglute)

Group I-B drugs
Lidocaine (Xylocaine)
Tocainide (Tonocard)
Mexiletine (Mexitil)

Group I-C drugs
Flecainide (Tambocor)
Propafenone (Rhythmol)

Group I drugs (A, B, C)
Moricizine (Ethmozine)

Group II drugs
Beta-adrenergic blockers

Group III drugs
Bretylium (Bretylol)
Amiodarone (Cordarone)
Dofetilide (Corvert)
Sotalol (Betapace)

Group IV drugs
Calcium channel blockers

7. Administration considerations
   a. Give first dose of disopyramide 6 to 12 hours after last quinidine dose and 3 to 6 hours after last procainamide dose
   b. Do not administer controlled-release capsules as loading dose when a rapid control is required or when creatinine clearance is less than 40 mL/min
   c. Do not crush or open controlled-release capsules (may deliver potentially toxic dose of medication)
   d. Start controlled-release form of capsule 6 hours after last dose of conventional capsule when switching from a conventional to controlled-release form
   e. Contraindicated in cardiogenic shock, second- or third-degree heart block, severe heart failure, and hypotension
   f. Use caution when administering disopyramide in the presence of delayed cardiac conduction, hepatic or renal impairment, benign prostatic hypertrophy, myasthenia gravis, and angle-closure (narrow-angle) glaucoma
   g. Assess blood glucose levels and serum potassium levels because hyperkalemia worsens toxic effects; correct hypokalemia and other electrolyte imbalances before initiating therapy
   h. Follow ECG results closely; notify physician of conduction delays (prolonged QT interval, widening of the QRS greater than 25%), HR less than 60 or greater than 120, unusual change in pulse rate, rhythm, or quality
8. Adverse effects/toxicity
   a. Blurred vision, dizziness, headache, fatigue, muscle weakness, convulsions, paresthesias, nervousness, acute psychosis, and peripheral neuropathy
   b. Hypotension, chest pain, edema, dyspnea, syncope, bradycardia, tachycardia, increased dysrhythmias, CHF, cardiogenic shock, and heart block
   c. Nausea and vomiting, epigastric and abdominal pain, jaundice, dry mouth, constipation
   d. Urinary retention, frequency, urgency, and renal insufficiency
   e. Pruritis, urticaria, rash, photosensitivity, and laryngospasm
   f. Drying of nose, throat, and bronchial secretions
   g. Uterine contraction during pregnancy, precipitation of myasthenia gravis, agranulocytosis (decreased granulocytes), and thrombocytopenia
9. Nursing considerations
   a. Check apical pulse before administering the medication
   b. Monitor ECG and report any changes to physician immediately
   c. Monitor BP, especially during dosage adjustment and if receiving high doses of medication
   d. Monitor I & O especially in elderly clients and those with impaired renal function, prostatic hypertrophy, and urinary retention/hesitancy
   e. Monitor lab results as appropriate
   f. Assess for peripheral neuritis
10. Client teaching
    a. Weigh self daily and report gain of more than 2 to 4 lb/week
    b. Assess ankles and tibia daily for edema
    c. As per Box 38–1; avoid prolonged standing, and lie down if feeling lightheaded; avoid driving and other hazardous activities if dizzy or lightheaded
    d. Be sure to avoid use of nasal decongestants without contacting physician
    e. Avoid exposure to sunlight or ultraviolet radiation
    f. Notify all other health care providers of medication and have regular eye exams for glaucoma

B. Class I-B

1. Decrease refractory period and elevate electrical stimulation threshold of ventricle during diastole
2. Suppress automaticity in the bundle of His–Purkinje system
3. Treat or prevent ventricular dysrhythmias
4. Common medications are listed in Box 38–9

5. Administration considerations
   a. Bolus dose of lidocaine may be given undiluted IVP at a rate of 25 to 50 mg/min; be sure to use lidocaine manufactured specifically for IV use
   b. Add 1 gram lidocaine to 250 to 500 mL of D_5W for infusion; flow rate should not be more than 4 mg/mL
   c. Use microdrip tubing and infusion pump for an infusion
   d. Discontinue IV infusion as soon as client's basic cardiac rhythm stabilizes
   e. Correct hypokalemia prior to initiating tocainide
   f. Contraindicated in hypersenstivity to amide-type anesthetics, Stokes-Adams syndrome, untreated sinus bradycardia, and severe SA, AV, and intraventricular heart block
   g. Use cautiously with hepatic or renal disease, heart failure, hypovolemia or shock, myasthenia gravis, debilitated clients or elderly, and family history of malignant hyperthermia
6. Side/adverse effects
   a. Drowsiness or restlessness, confusion, disorientation, irritability, apprehension, euphoria, wild excitement, numbness of lips or tongue and other paresthesias, chest heaviness, and difficulty speaking
   b. Dyspnea and difficulty swallowing, muscular twitching, tremors, psychosis, convulsions and respiratory depression with high doses
   c. Hypotension, lightheadedness, bradycardia, heart block, cardiovascular collapse, and cardiac arrest
   d. Tinnitus and decreased hearing
   e. Severe blurred vision, double vision, and impaired color perception
   f. Anorexia, nausea, vomiting, and excessive perspiration
   g. Urticaria, rash, edema, and anaphylactoid reactions
7. Nursing considerations
   a. Assess ECG for changes including prolonged PR interval, widened QRS, aggravation of dysrhythmias, and heart block
   b. Monitor BP frequently
   c. Assess CNS status at baseline and frequently during infusions
   d. Administer via infusion pump and observe rate carefully
   e. Auscultate breath sounds for crackles and monitor respiratory rate
   f. Assess results of serum drug levels and creatinine levels
8. Client teaching: as per Box 38–1; notify physician if adverse effects occur; see previous section

C. Class I-C

1. Decrease automaticity and conductivity through AV node and ventricles
2. Used to treat life-threatening ventricular dysrhythmias
3. Common medications are listed in Box 38–9
4. Administration considerations
   a. Medications are available in oral forms
   b. Do not increase dosages more frequently than every 4 days, especially with elderly clients or those with previous extensive myocardial damage
   c. Dosage reduction should be considered in severe liver dysfunction and with significant widening of QRS complex
   d. Contraindicated with drug hypersensitivity, severe degrees of heart block or intraventricular block, cardiogenic shock, or hepatic failure
5. Side/adverse effects
   a. Headache, dizziness, prolonged lightheadedness, unsteadiness, paresthesias, fatigue, and fever
   b. Worsening dysrhythmias, chest pain, CHF, edema, and dyspnea
   c. Prolonged blurred vision and spots before eyes
   d. Nausea, constipation, and changes in taste perception
6. Nursing considerations
   a. Assess laboratory data and treat hypokalemia/hyperkalemia before initiating therapy

b. Monitor ECG rhythm for adverse changes; client may need Holter monitoring for ambulatory assessment
c. Determine threshold levels of pacemaker before initiating medication and at regular intervals thereafter

7. Client teaching: as per Box 38–1 and report any visual changes

D. Class II (beta-blockers): see previous section

E. Class III (potassium channel blockers)

1. Prolong repolarization and refractory period
2. Decrease intraventricular conduction
3. Used to treat ventricular tachycardia (VT) and ventricular fibrillation (VF)
4. May also be used to treat supraventricular tachycardias
5. Common medication: amiodarone (Cordarone, Pacerone)
6. Administration considerations
   a. Gastroenteritis symptoms may occur with high oral dose therapy and loading dose
   b. May be given by IV route
   c. Contraindicated with hypersensitivity to amiodarone, cardiogenic shock, severe sinus bradycardia or heart block, and hepatic disease
   d. Use cautiously in hyper- or hypothyroidism, heart failure, electrolyte imbalance, preexisting pulmonary disease, cardiac surgery, and sensitivity to iodine
7. Side/adverse effects
   a. Peripheral neuropathy, muscle wasting, weakness, fatigue, abnormal gait, dyskinesia, dizziness, paresthesias, and headache
   b. Bradycardia, hypotension, sinus arrest, cardiogenic shock, CHF, worsening dysrhythmias, and heart block
   c. Corneal microdeposits, blurred vision, optic neuritis, optic neuropathy, permanent blindness, corneal degeneration, macular degeneration, and photosensitivity
   d. Alveolitis, pneumonitis, and interstitial pulmonary fibrosis
   e. Slate-blue pigmentation to skin and rash; reverses slowly after drug is discontinued
   f. Anorexia, nausea, vomiting, and constipation
   g. Angioedema, hyperthyroidism or hypothyroidism, and hepatotoxicity
8. Nursing considerations
   a. Monitor BP during IV infusion and titrate to prevent hypotension and bradycardia
   b. Monitor client continually due to unusually long half-life of the medication (10 to 55 days)
   c. Check laboratory and other reports for liver, lung, thyroid, GI, and neurological dysfunction
   d. Baseline and regular ophthalmic examinations with a slit-lamp are recommended throughout therapy
   e. Report adverse reactions promptly
   f. Be alert to signs of pulmonary toxicity: dyspnea, fatigue, cough, pleuritic pain, or fever; auscultate breath sounds for adventitious sounds
   g. Monitor client for CNS changes, which generally develop within a week after amiodarone therapy begins; muscle weakness and tremors are a potential safety risk
   h. Observe client already receiving other antiarrhythmic therapy for adverse effects, especially heart block and worsening dysrhythmias
9. Client teaching
   a. As per Box 38–1; monitor pulse daily and report HR less than 60 bpm
   b. Have regular ophthalmic examinations every 6 months to 1 year
   c. Photophobia may be eased by wearing darkened glasses, but some clients should avoid daylight entirely
   d. Erythema and pruritus may develop when exposed to ultraviolet radiation; avoid sunlight, tanning beds, and sunlamps
   e. Wear protective clothing and a barrier-type sunblock to avoid exposure to sun (zinc-oxide or titanium-oxide preparations)

f. Blue-gray skin pigmentation (found after 1 year) may slowly disappear after medication is stopped

F. Class IV (calcium channel blockers): see previous section

G. Miscellaneous antidysrhythmic: Adenosine (Adenocard, Adenoscan)

1. Slows conduction through the SA and AV nodes
2. Interrupts the reentry pathways through the AV node
3. Depresses left ventricular function (very temporary)
4. Treats supraventricular dysrhythmias
5. Administration considerations
   a. Rapid IV bolus: administer directly into vein over 1 to 2 seconds and follow with a rapid normal saline flush
   b. Solution contains no preservatives so it must be clear; discard any unused portion
   c. Expect sudden slowing of the HR or even asystole for a brief period of time; do not repeat dose if high grade AV heart block develops after first dose
   d. Store at room temperature to avoid crystallization; if crystals appear, dissolve by warming to room temperature
   e. Contraindicated in severe heart block, sick sinus syndrome (without a pacemaker), atrial fibrillation or atrial flutter, VT
   f. Use cautiously with asthma, pregnancy, hepatic failure, and renal failure
6. Side/adverse effects
   a. During conversion to sinus rhythm, many dysrhythmias can occur
   b. Facial flushing, transient dyspnea, or hypotension
7. Nursing considerations
   a. Monitor ECG continuously
   b. Monitor HR and BP every 15 minutes after administration until stable
   c. Monitor carefully for bronchospasm, especially in clients with asthma
8. Client teaching: monitoring will be done during the medication administration, and transient facial flushing may occur

XI. ANTIHYPOTENSIVES (SYMPATHOMIMETICS)

A. Mimic fight-or-flight response of sympathetic nervous system (SNS), selectively stimulating alpha-adrenergic and beta-adrenergic receptors

B. Stimulation of alpha-adrenergic receptors results in vasoconstriction and increased systemic BP

C. Stimulation of beta-adrenergic receptors increases force and rate of myocardial contraction

D. Used to treat shock

E. Common medications are listed in Box 38–10

F. Administration considerations

1. Drug must be diluted before administration
2. Client should be attended constantly during drug administration
3. Contraindicated in uncorrected arrhythmias, mesenteric or peripheral vascular thrombosis, profound hypoxia, hypercapnia, hypotension due to blood volume deficit
4. Use with caution in those receiving MAOIs or imipramine-type antidepressants

G. Side/adverse effects

1. Anxiety, weakness, dizziness, tremor, restlessness
2. Bradycardia, tachycardia, palpitations
3. Nausea and vomiting, flushing, diaphoresis, sloughing upon extravasation
4. Azotemia, shortness of breath, and bronchospasm
5. Severe hypertension, anaphylaxis
6. Arrhythmias, cardiac arrest, ventricular tachycardia

Box 38–10

Antihypotensives (Sympathomimetics)

Norepinephrine (Levophed)	Dobutamine (Dobutrex)
Metaraminol (Aramine)	Isoproterenol (Isuprel)
Dopamine (Intropin)	

7. Seizures, asthmatic episodes

H. Nursing considerations

1. Reevaluate if 3 to 5 treatments in 6 to 12 hours provide minimal to no relief
2. Carefully monitor vital signs, ECG, and I & O
3. Monitor for rebound hypertension
4. Constant infusion pump prevents sudden infusion of excessive amounts of drugs
5. Correct blood volume depletion first
6. Monitor infusion site frequently; client should be attended constantly during administration
7. Antidote for extravasation: phentolamine mesylate (Regitine) diluted in normal saline injected at site of IV infiltration
8. Protect solution from light
9. Sympathomimetics are incompatible with sodium bicarbonate

I. Client teaching

1. Report adverse reactions and side effects immediately
2. Vital signs will be monitored frequently
3. Report anginal pain while on dobutamine

XII. ANTICOAGULANTS

A. Oral medication; sodium warfarin (Coumadin and its derivatives)

1. Oral **anticoagulants** prevent or delay blood coagulation and are used both to treat and prevent thromboembolic disorders in clients at risk
2. Oral anticoagulants such as warfarin prevent conversion of vitamin K, thereby decreasing its production in liver and subsequently reducing several clotting factors (II, VII, IX, and X)
3. Vitamin K plays an active role in **extrinsic pathway** (a pathway that forms fibrin and acts within seconds) in **clotting cascade** (a coagulation pathway)
4. Coumadin is bound to plasma proteins, most notably albumin; is metabolized in liver
5. Used to treat deep vein thrombosis (DVT), pulmonary embolism (PE), acute MI, heart valve replacement (bioprosthetic and mechanical), atrial fibrillation, and antiphospholipid syndrome
6. Administration considerations
   a. Warfarin is given orally at a usual dose of 1 to 15 mg daily
   b. Requires close monitoring because of a narrow therapeutic range, frequent need for dose adjustments, and high risk for food and drug interactions that can lead to either ineffective therapy or toxicity
   c. Full anticoagulant effect is not seen until after approximately 1 week's duration; therefore, drug may be started while client is still on heparin therapy and overlap while heparin is tapered
   d. **Prothrombin time (PT),** a diagnostic blood test used to measure extrinsic clotting response, and **international normalized ratio (INR),** a standard reference range for reporting PT levels, are both used to monitor client response and determine ongoing dose
   e. Desired range of PT and INR vary based on indication for use; PT levels are usually maintained at 1.5 to 2.5 times control value; INR levels range from a usual 2.0 to 3.0 range to a higher level of 3.0 to 4.5 range for mechanical cardiac valve replacement
   f. Coumadin is usually given in evening following careful attention to laboratory test results from earlier in day
   g. Duration of therapy can range from several months to lifelong depending on specific client need
   h. Refer to specific hospital protocol and physician's order for dose adjustments and monitoring of client's PT and INR levels
   i. Vitamin K is antidote for warfarin (Coumadin)
   j. Foods high in vitamin K such as liver, cheese, egg yolk, leafy vegetables (broccoli, cabbage, spinach, and kale) and oils (peanut, corn, olive, or

soybean) should be avoided or used sparingly during therapy; refer to dietitian for teaching

k. Contraindicated in pregnancy (although may be given if needed during lactation), hemorrhage or bleeding tendencies, clients with malignant hypertension, and those with history of allergic reaction)

7. Side/adverse effects
   a. Bleeding is the major adverse effect and is usually seen at higher dosage levels; also thrombocytopenia may occur
   b. Nausea, diarrhea, intestinal obstruction, anorexia, abdominal cramping
   c. Rash, urticaria, and purple toe syndrome (due to decreased perfusion from release of microemboli)
   d. Increased serum transaminase levels, hepatitis, jaundice
   e. Burning sensation in feet
   f. Transient hair loss
8. Nursing considerations
   a. Monitor baseline and ongoing PT and INR; report high or low abnormal values (ineffective therapy versus toxicity)
   b. Review drug and dietary history for potential drug and food interactions; be sure to include nutritional and herbal supplements
   c. Institute bleeding precautions (see Box 38–11)
   d. If client experiences adverse effects or toxicity, stop (withhold) Coumadin therapy; depending on INR or client manifestations, administration of phytonadione (vitamin K) may be indicated
   e. For significant bleeding, physician may order transfusion of fresh frozen plasma (FFP) or prothrombin concentrate
9. Client education
   a. Bleeding precautions (Box 38–11)
   b. As per Box 38–1, stressing need for frequent (weekly to monthly) follow-up blood tests to ensure safe therapy
   c. Point-of-care (POC) testing is available for self-monitoring PT and INR; physician may establish a home protocol to help manage care and necessary dosage adjustments
   d. Take dose on a daily basis; do not stop medication unless physician orders a dose to be withheld (pending PT and INR results) or client experiences a bleeding episode
   e. Use a soft toothbrush and an electric razor to minimize even mild trauma that could lead to bleeding
   f. Avoid intake of foods high in vitamin K (see previous section)

B. Heparin and related medications

1. Heparin plays an active role in the **intrinsic pathway** (pathway in which fibrin formation occurs) in clotting cascade; inhibits conversion of fibrinogen to fibrin, prevents formation of a fibrin clot, and inhibits thrombin

Box 38–11

Bleeding Precautions for Clients Taking Anticoagulant and Fibrinolytic (Thrombolytic) Drugs

1. Use a soft toothbrush and ensure gentle mouth care to minimize even mild trauma that could lead to bleeding.
2. Use an electric razor rather than a straight razor for shaving.
3. Use work gloves, do not go barefoot, and take other ordinary precautions as appropriate to avoid minor trauma to skin.
4. Observe for and report to prescriber evidence of bleeding, including bleeding gums, epistaxis (nosebleed), ecchymosis (bruising), petechiae, tarry stools, hematuria, hematemesis.
5. Notify health care providers, including dentists, about use of medications that cause bleeding, especially prior to any procedures or surgery.
6. Avoid use of OTC drugs that could increase risk of bleeding, such as acetylsalicylic acid (ASA or aspirin), non-steroidal anti-inflammatory drugs (NSAIDs).

2. Molecular weight of heparin varies depending on whether drug is unfractionated heparin (UFH) or **low molecular weight heparin (LMWH)**
3. Has immediate effect and is treatment of choice for DVT, PE, and embolism resulting from atrial fibrillation
4. Also used as a prophylaxis for clients at risk for developing thrombi following surgery
5. Also used in a weak concentration as a flush solution to maintain access and prevent thrombus formation in vascular access devices
6. LMWH is a newer class of heparin molecule consisting of heparin fragments, with enoxaprin (Lovenox) being most commonly used
7. Heparin (Liquaemin) sodium is most commonly used anticoagulant for treatment and prevention of recurrent thromboembolic episodes
8. Refer to Box 38–12 for a list of heparin anticoagulants
9. Administration considerations
   a. Heparin can be administered IV or subcutaneously
   b. LMWH has a higher bioavailability when compared to standard UFH
   c. **Activated partial thromboplastin time (APTT)** is used to monitor heparin therapy; results are trended over time to determine client response and therapeutic effect
   d. Low-dose UFH therapy: used as a prophylactic treatment for DVT; dosage ranges from 5,000 units subcutaneously every 8 to 12 hours or 3 doses in the immediate postoperative period depending on physician protocol; enoxaparin or Lovenox (an LMWH) comes in prefilled syringes ready for individual use
   e. High-dose UFH therapy achieves a therapeutic APTT; normal APTT value is 25 to 40 seconds, and therapeutic values are often 1.5 to 2.0 times control
   f. Use an infusion pump for IV administration; use a dedicated infusion line because of its incompatibility profile
   g. Be sure to carefully identify strength on product label; several concentrations of IV heparin are available; some are used only as flushes for IV lines
   h. **Protamine sulfate** is antidote that reverses action of heparin; dosage depends on amount of heparin given and time period following its administration; however, do not give more than 50 mg in a 10-minute period; protamine sulfate is administered IVP
   i. Hypersensitivity or allergic reactions can be seen in clients receiving heparin, so epinephrine 1:1000 should be readily available if a reaction develops
   j. Contraindicated with uncontrolled bleeding, known hypersensitivity, and thrombocytopenia
   k. Should not be given with aspirin (acetylsalicylic acid, or ASA) and nonsteroidal anti-inflammatory drugs (NSAIDs), which increase risk of bleeding
10. Side/adverse effects
    a. Hemorrhage, hematuria, epistaxis, bleeding gums
    b. Thrombocytopenia **heparin-induced platelet aggregation (HITT),** a more serious form of thrombocytopenia with platelet count less than 100,000/mm^3; also called white clot syndrome; can be fatal if not treated aggressively; begins 3 to 12 days following start of heparin therapy
    c. Clients who are on long-term heparin therapy (longer than 6 months) are prone to develop osteoporosis
11. Nursing considerations
    a. Monitor client's baseline labs according to heparin protocol (specifically APTT); commonly measured q 6 hours; when level is critically high, infusion may be stopped for 1 or more hours and APTT measured in 2 to 3 hours

Box 38–12

Heparins		
	Heparin (Liquaemin)	Danaparoid (Orgaran)
	Ardeparin (Normiflo)	Enoxaprin (Lovenox)
	Dalteparin (Fragmin)	Tinazaparin (Innohep)

b. Obtain daily weight for client on weight-based heparin protocol
! c. Institute bleeding precautions, hemocult all stools, and evaluate pertinent labs
d. Verify with pharmacy or another RN the correct dosage of heparin before administering or adjusting the heparin infusion
! e. Evaluate dosage for safety and therapeutic range based on normal adult dosage range of 20,000 to 40,000 units/24 hr; heparin is usually infused in units per hour
! f. Have antidote available (protamine sulfate)
! g. Subcutaneous administration of heparin requires rotation of sites; *do not aspirate or rub injection site*
! h. When administering heparin subcutaneously, inject into abdomen using a small (5/8-inch, 25- to 27-gauge) needle at a *90-degree angle*

12. Client teaching
    a. Heparin administration if used after discharge
    b. Frequent blood work monitoring is required to ensure effective anticoagulation
    ! c. As per Box 38–1 and Box 38–11

XIII. ANTIPLATELET AGENTS

A. Prevent or disrupt aggregation of platelets needed to form a clot

B. Often used as adjunctive therapy to other anticoagulant medications such as warfarin (Coumadin)

C. Used as both preventive and treatment measures for clients with history of MI, stroke, and cardiac surgery

D. Inhibit or block certain enzyme pathways to prevent clot formation

E. Common medications

1. ASA: most common antiplatelet medication; also has other therapeutic properties such as analgesic, anti-inflammatory, and antipyretic action
2. Ticlopidine (Ticlid): can be used by clients who cannot take aspirin
3. Dipyridamole (Persantine): used for antiplatelet effect and in cardiac stress testing
4. Clopidrogrel bisulfate (Plavix) is used as a form of secondary prevention for clients who have had MI, stroke, and peripheral arterial disease
5. Abciximab (ReoPro) is a fragment of a specific monoclonal antibody, called a Fab
6. Common antiplatelet medications are listed in Box 38–13

F. Administration considerations

1. ASA is administered in dosages ranging from 81 to 325 mg/day (baby ASA to adult strength); it can also be given as an enteric-coated preparation to minimize GI upset
2. Dipyridamole (Persantine) has a better profile when used with clients who have prosthetic mechanical heart valves; is contraindicated in pregnant or lactating clients
3. Ticlopidine (Ticlid) has been used effectively as a preventive measure in clients at risk for MI
4. Abciximab (ReoPro) is administered via the parenteral route, and client can receive a bolus dose as well as a constant infusion
5. ! ASA is contraindicated with known hypersensitivity to salicylates, bleeding disorders, asthma, or GI bleeding; do not give to pediatric clients because of risk for developing Reye syndrome
6. Antiplatelet agents are generally contraindicated in presence of conditions that increase risk of bleeding

Box 38–13

Antiplatelet Medications

Abciximab (ReoPro)	Eptifibatide (Integrilin)
Aspirin (many names)	Ticlopidine (Ticlid)
Clopidrogrel bisulfate (Plavix)	Tirofiban (Aggrastat)
Dipyridamole (Persantine)	

G. Side/adverse effects
1. ASA: blood dyscrasias, hemorrhage, GI symptoms, increased bleeding tendencies, hemorrhage, nausea and vomiting, dizziness, confusion, tinnitus, and ototoxicity
2. Persantine: GI complaints, nausea and vomiting, CNS alterations, headache, and dizziness
3. Ticlopidine: serious blood dyscrasias such as agranulocytosis and neutropenia; GI symptoms, such as nausea, vomiting, and jaundice
4. Clopidrogrel: flulike symptoms, chest pain, edema, and hypertension
5. Abciximab: allergic reaction
6. In general: bruising, hematuria, tarry stools

H. Nursing considerations
1. Perform baseline hematological labs on admission; monitor coagulation studies periodically
2. Monitor vital signs and for bleeding
3. Antiplatelet agents should be stopped at least 7 days prior to a planned surgery
4. Older adult clients may require closer monitoring to avoid toxicity because tinnitus and ototoxicity may be harder to assess if baseline hearing is already diminished
5. Life span concerns: children, pregnant women, and lactating women should not take antiplatelet medications

I. Client teaching
1. As per Box 38–1; carry a Medic-Alert bracelet
2. Monitor for and report side effects related to bleeding; may use bleeding precautions (Box 38–11) on advice of health care provider
3. Communication between client and health care team members is critical
4. Adults should not use aspirin for self-medication of pain for more than 5 days without consulting a physician
5. Maintain adequate fluid intake to prevent salicylate crystalluria
6. Prolonged use of ASA can lead to iron-deficiency anemia (especially important for females of childbearing age)

XIV. FIBRINOLYTICS

A. **Substances that dissolve or break down a thrombus or blood clot** to reestablish blood flow and increase perfusion to an ischemic area (also called ***thrombolytics***)
B. **Activate *fibrinolytic system* that breaks down thrombus or blood clot**
C. **Conversion of plasminogen to plasmin helps break down clot** by digesting fibrin and degrading fibrinogen and other procoagulant proteins into soluble fragments
D. **Indicated for clients at risk for developing thrombus with resultant ischemia,** such as acute MI, arterial thrombosis, DVT, pulmonary embolism, and occlusion of catheters or shunts
E. **Primarily used in emergency and critical care settings**
F. **Common medications are listed in see Box 38–14**

Memory Aid

Remember that the suffix *-ase* often indicates a fibrinolytic/thrombolytic drug.

G. Administration considerations
1. Record baseline vital signs and obtain baseline coagulation studies
2. Give IV according to specific protocols; monitor IV sites for signs of infiltration and/or phlebitis; change IV site to opposite extremity if any problems are noted with IV
3. Place client on cardiac monitor during administration
4. Antidote to streptokinase or urokinase is aminocaproic acid (Amicar)

Box 38–14

Fibrinolytics

Alteplase (Activase)	Streptokinase (Kabikinase, Streptase)
Anistreplase (Eminase)	Tenecteplase (TNKase)
Reteplase (Retavase)	Urokinase (Abbokinase Open-Cath)

5. Contraindicated in clients who are actively bleeding or have a recent history of CVA, severe uncontrolled hypertension, recent trauma, neoplasm, or are pregnant

H. Side/adverse effects (dose-related)

1. Hemorrhage
2. Hypersensitivity reactions
3. Nausea, vomiting, and hypotension
4. Cardiac dysrhythmias; reperfusion dysrhythmias may pose further problems for acutely ill client

I. Nursing considerations

1. Monitor coagulation studies and continue to assess client during therapy
2. Monitor for vital sign changes, because drug may cause variations in pulse, BP, and temperature
3. Maintain adequate IV site for medication administration; observe closely for infiltration
4. Institute bleeding precautions and limit invasive procedures and injections to reduce risk of bleeding
5. If bleeding occurs, medication should be stopped; fresh frozen plasma (FFP) and packed red blood cells (PRBCs) may be ordered
6. Monitor client closely for development of dysrhythmias
7. Maintain aseptic technique to prevent infection
8. Provide adequate nutrition and rest to support client

J. Client teaching

1. Treatment methods and medication administration; measurable signs of clinical response may not occur for 6 to 8 hours after therapy is started
2. Bleeding precautions as per Box 38–11
3. Lifestyle changes may be needed to prevent further abnormal clotting
4. Discontinue medication if bleeding occurs and notify physician

XV. ANTIHYPERLIPIDEMICS

A. HMG-CoenzymeA reductase inhibitors

1. Also called *statins;* reduce LDL cholesterol levels in clients for whom diet therapy has not been effective
2. Also have an a dose-dependent effect on HDL cholesterol; lipoprotein levels are not affected by use of statins
3. Common medications are listed in Box 38–15

Memory Aid

The suffix *-statin* indicates the cholesterol-lowering drugs known as HMG CoenzymeA reductase inhibitors.

4. Usually administered at night to increase the effectiveness because cholesterol synthesis normally occurs during evening hours
5. Contraindicated in clients with active liver disease, abnormal serum transaminase levels, and during pregnancy and lactation
6. Monitor for elevation of liver function tests
7. Side/adverse effects
   a. GI upset, dyspepsia, flatulence, pain and myalgias
   b. Headache, rash, dizziness, sinusitis
8. Nursing considerations
   a. Monitor lipid levels within 2 to 4 weeks after initiation of therapy
   b. May be given without regard to food

Box 38–15

HMG-Coenzyme A Reductase Inhibitors ("Statins")

Atorvastatin (Lipitor)	Pravastatin (Pravachol)
Fluvastatin (Lescol)	Rosuvastatin (Crestor)
Lovastatin (Mevacor)	Simvastatin (Zocor)

9. Client education
   a. Take dose with evening meal to coincide with body's timing of cholesterol production
   b. Required lab monitoring for compliance and client response
   c. Report immediately any unexplained muscle pain, tenderness, yellowing of skin or eyes, or loss of appetite (liver toxicity)
   d. Avoid or minimize alcohol intake

B. Bile acid sequestrants

1. Work in GI tract to bind with bile acids; liver cells respond by sending cholesterol to maintain bile acid synthesis, lowering plasma levels of LDL cholesterol
2. Indicated for use with elevated cholesterol levels with or without high triglyceride levels
3. Common medications: cholestyramine (Questran) and colestipol (Colestid)
   a. Colestipol is available as a tablet or powder, given in 2 to 4 doses before meals and at bedtime
   b. Cholestyramine is available as a powder, given 2 to 4 times daily before meals and at bedtime
4. Administration considerations
   a. Do not crush, chew, or cut colestipol tablets; they should be given with adequate fluids
   b. Mix powdered drug forms at bedside to prevent overthickening and esophageal obstruction; they may be plain or have orange flavoring; cholestyramine powder contains phenylalanine and should not be used in clients with phenylketonuria (PKU)
   c. Administer bile acids alone to avoid binding with other medications; give other drugs 1 to 2 hours before or 4 to 6 hours after bile acid administration
   d. Mix contents of one packet with at least 120 to 180 mL of water or other preferred liquid; dissolve before administration because drug is irritating to mucous membranes
5. Side/adverse effects
   a. Abdominal pain, bloating, reflux, constipation, steatorrhea, and hemorrhoids
   b. Associated fat-soluble vitamin deficiencies (A, D, K) and decreased erythrocyte folate levels
   c. Rash irritations of skin, tongue, and perianal areas
   d. Hypoprothrombinemia
6. Nursing considerations
   a. Not often used as first-line therapy because of poor compliance
   b. Vitamin deficiencies may require supplementation, if not discontinuation of bile acids, to restore normal levels
   c. Hemorrhoids and/or constipation may require intervention to provide client comfort
   d. If client develops GI complaints, dosage reduction may be needed to maintain client compliance
   e. Serum cholesterol levels are reduced within 24 to 48 hours after initiation of therapy
   f. Assess baseline cholesterol and triglyceride levels; continue to trend results to determine client response
   g. Decreased levels of LDL cholesterol should be seen within 1 month of therapy
   h. Long-term use of cholestyramine can increase bleeding tendency
7. Client teaching
   a. Proper administration and scheduling of medication to maximize effect
   b. Be alert for signs and symptoms indicating side effects of these agents
   c. Follow-up serum cholesterol levels are necessary
   d. Increase high-bulk diet with adequate fluid intake; report constipation immediately

C. Fibric acid derivatives

1. Act on very low lipid–density lipoproteins (VLDL) and chlyomicrons to reduce triglyceride levels

2. HDL cholesterol levels are increased but increase is not primary effect; there is also a variable effect on LDL levels
3. Indicated for use with elevated triglyceride levels and elevated cholesterol levels resistant to dietary management
4. Common medications are listed in Box 38–16
5. Administration considerations
   a. Usually given in divided doses, 30 minutes prior to morning and evening meals
   b. Contraindicated in clients with gallbladder disease, renal problems, liver or biliary cirrhosis, and in pregnant or lactating women
6. Side/adverse effects
   a. Abdominal or epigastric pain
   b. Jaundice, blurred vision, headache, and depression
   c. Rash, dermatitis, pruritus with gemfibrozil
   d. Back pain, muscle cramps, myalgia, and swollen joints
   e. Client may develop gallbladder disease and acute appendicitis
   f. Eosinophilia and/or hypokalemia
7. Nursing considerations
   a. Obtain baseline lipid levels, monitor periodically
   b. If there is no response to therapy or if liver function tests are persistently abnormal after 3 months, then therapy should be discontinued
   c. Hypokalemia may be seen in response to therapy
   d. Decreased hemoglobin, hematocrit, and WBC count may be seen with the use of gemfibrozil
   e. Monitor client for potential side effects and adverse effects
   f. Monitor closely for right upper quadrant (RUQ) abdominal pain or vomiting
8. Client teaching
   a. Need for periodic lab work to evaluate response
   b. Immediately report unexplained bleeding or any serious side effects such as acute appendicitis or gallbladder disease
   c. Restrict fat and alcohol intake

D. Nicotinic acid (niacin, vitamin B_3)

1. Water-soluble vitamin that lowers most lipoprotein levels (total cholesterol, LDL, triglyceride, and lipoproteins) and increases HDL levels
2. Indications for use are high cholesterol levels and as adjunctive therapy when dietary management is ineffective
3. Causes peripheral vasodilation and can be used for clients with peripheral vascular disease
4. Pellagra (dermatitis, diarrhea, and dementia) is a clinical deficiency state associated with niacin deficiency
5. Dosage for lowering cholesterol is higher (greater than 3 grams/day) than normal vitamin dose (500 mg/day in adults)
6. Administration considerations
   a. Tablets should be taken whole; do not crush or divide the pill
   b. Can be taken with meals to prevent GI upset
   c. Flushing is a common side effect of niacin caused by its vasodilator properties; it subsides usually after an hour
   d. Oral nicotinic acid should be taken with cold water
   e. Contraindicated with liver disease and/or unexplained elevated serum transaminases and with active peptic ulcer disease
   f. Contraindicated in clients with severe hypotension
   g. Leads to increases in blood glucose, uric acid, and serum transaminase levels

Box 38–16

Fibric Acid Derivatives

- Clofibrate (Abitrate, Atromid-S)
- Fenofibrate (Tricor)
- Gemfibrozil (Lopid)

7. Side/adverse effects
    a. Flushing, postural hypotension, vasovagal attacks
    b. Pruritus, increased sebaceous gland activity
    c. Dyspepsia, epigastric pain, and nausea
    d. Dark-colored urine
    e. Megadose therapy has been associated with liver damage, hyperglycemia, hyperuricemia, and cardiac dysrhythmias
8. Nursing considerations
    a. Dosing of nicotinic acid varies depending on whether prescribed to reduce cholesterol levels or merely as a vitamin supplement; be aware of specific dosing levels
    b. Expect side effect of flushing when administering medication
    c. Evaluate client for food sources high in niacin (dairy, meats, tuna, and egg) and assess dietary intake
9. Client teaching
    a. Change position slowly to avoid sudden BP drop
    b. Avoid direct exposure to sunlight
    c. Flushing in face, neck, and ears may occur within 2 hours after oral ingestion and immediately after IV administration and may last several hours; alcohol and niacin cause increased flushing
    d. Follow-up lab work will be done periodically to determine response to therapy
    e. Do not self-medicate with additional sources of niacin, which can lead to overdose

XVI. HEMOSTATICS

A. Systemic hemostatics

1. Systemic **hemostatics** are substances that inhibit bleeding after an injury to maintain hematologic balance
2. Common medications
    a. Aminocaproic acid (Amicar) and tranexamic acid (Cyklokapron) both impede **fibrinolysis**
    b. Aminocaproic acid is used to treat hyperfibrinolysis-induced hemorrhage after surgery and for hematologic disorders such as aplastic anemia, hepatic cirrhosis, and some neoplastic disease states; it is also an antidote to thrombolytic drugs
    c. Tranexamic acid is used 1 day before and 2 to 8 days after dental or other surgery in clients with hemophilia
    d. Phytonadione, vitamin K_1 (Aquamephyton), is antidote to warfarin and is fat-soluble; used to reverse excess effects of oral anticoagulants
    e. Menadiol sodium diphosphate, vitamin K_4 (Synkayvite), is a water-soluble compound
    f. Vitamin K is also used as mandatory treatment to prevent hemorrhagic disease of newborn
3. Nursing considerations
    a. Assess client's baseline labs for renal and liver function
    b. Monitor PT levels and response to therapy for vitamin K administration
    c. Monitor client's coagulation profile as antifibrinolytics can cause a **hypercoagulation** or rapid coagulation of blood
    d. Rotate injection sites for administration of vitamin K; assess client for signs of local irritation
    e. Monitor client closely for signs of hypersensitivity and development of allergic reactions
    f. Monitor client closely during administration of parenteral infusion because of potential for volume overload and adverse reactions
    g. Use an infusion pump for IV administration
4. Client teaching
    a. Dietary sources of vitamin K
    b. Periodic PT levels will be drawn to monitor response to therapy

c. Monitor for signs and symptoms of bleeding
d. Use of yogurt and buttermilk products in diet can help restore normal intestinal flora that aid in synthesis of vitamin K; clients who are on antibiotic therapy or who have intestinal problems may benefit from this supportive therapy
e. Report difficulty urinating or reddish brown urine (caused by myoglobinuria) while taking aminocaproic acid
f. Report chest pain, arm or leg pain, or difficulty breathing

B. Local absorbable hemostatic agents

1. Utilized to stop or inhibit bleeding at a specific site
2. Common medications: gelatin products, oxidized cellulose, thrombin, and epinephrine are all examples of topical hemostatic agents
3. Administration considerations
   a. Available in pads, powder, sponge, film, and liquid forms and are applied to local bleeding site to stop bleeding for 24–48 hours or more
   b. Irrigation with normal saline may be necessary to prevent further tissue destruction as topical is removed
   c. If product is a sponge or film, it may be completely reabsorbed into body
4. Nursing considerations
   a. Assess local site for signs of hypersensitivity, and document findings; antihistamine such as diphenhydramine (Benadryl) may be given to either prevent or treat allergic reaction
   ! b. Remove topical hemostatics as indicated by product guidelines; irrigate site with normal saline if necessary to prevent further tissue destruction with removal; document site assessment
   c. Clotting factor replacement therapy (see Chapter 33)

XVII. MEDICATIONS TO TREAT ANEMIA

A. Iron salts

1. Iron is an essential trace element that participates in oxygen transport, tissue respiration, and enzyme reactions
2. Iron is stored as ferritin; ferritin levels reflect visceral stores of iron that are available to body; transferrin levels reflect how iron is transported in body
3. Common medications are listed in Box 38–17
4. Administration considerations
   ! a. Oral iron is given with meals to decrease gastric upset
   ! b. Iron dextran is administered by Z-track technique to minimize discomfort, prevent tissue discoloration, and ensure absorption
   c. There is risk of anaphylaxis following iron dextran administration; a test dose may be ordered to determine client response
   d. Monitor client for intake of dietary sources of iron to avoid potential overdosing and toxicity
   ! e. Liquid (elixir) iron is administered by straw to avoid discoloration of tooth enamel
   f. Contraindicated in clients with ulcerative colitis, peptic ulcer disease, cirrhosis, and hemolytic anemia
   g. Contraindicated in clients with iron overload syndromes (hemosiderosis and hemochromatosis)
   ! h. Vitamin C can increase the absorption of oral iron medications
5. Side/adverse effects
   a. Upset stomach, nausea and vomiting, diarrhea, and constipation
   ! b. Dark and tarry stools
   c. Discoloration of skin and pain upon injection

Box 38–17

Iron Salts		
	Ferrous fumarate (Femiron, Fumerin)	Ferrous sulfate (Feosol)
	Ferrous gluconate (Fergon)	Iron dextran injection (DexFerrum)

d. **Pica** (ingestion of nonfood items) can interfere with iron levels in body and cause individuals to become anemic; pregnant women are the group most likely to be affected
e. Iron can accumulate in body, leading to potentially toxic levels
f. Chelation therapy should be instituted to remove iron from body; additional supportive measures include airway maintenance, correction of acidosis, and administration of IV fluids

6. Nursing considerations
   a. Monitor client for expected side effects, such as tarry stools
   b. Since anemia is often a symptom of a disease, assess client for underlying cause
   c. If client does not show a clinical response to iron therapy, notify physician
   d. Refer to dietitian as needed for instruction on foods rich in iron
   e. Evaluate client for pica if there is a high index of suspicion
   f. ! Monitor client's reticulocyte count, which will increase if RBC production is increasing
   g. ! If client's hemoglobin and hematocrit levels do not rise following iron therapy, additional testing may be required to determine type of anemia
7. Client education
   a. Proper self-administration of oral iron medications
   b. ! Importance of adequate food sources to maintain iron levels; these include lean meats, liver, egg yolks, dried beans, green vegetables (e.g., spinach)
   c. ! Expected changes in characteristics of stool (black, tarry)

B. Vitamin B_{12} (cyanocobalamin)

1. Vitamin B_{12} is a water-soluble vitamin utilized in body as part of many coenzyme reactions during process of metabolism of carbohydrate, protein, and fat
2. ! Vitamin B_{12} is found primarily in foods of animal origin (liver, meat, shellfish, and dairy food items)
3. Deficiency of vitamin B_{12} affects neurological, hematological, and GI systems
4. Vitamin B_{12} is considered to be an extrinsic factor, whereas intrinsic factor is released by parietal cells in stomach
5. ! Clients with GI surgeries that result in partial or complete removal and/or anastomosis of stomach and stop release of intrinsic factor will require weekly and then monthly injections of vitamin B_{12} for life; a nasal form is now available as well
6. **Pernicious anemia** is classification given to anemia that results from vitamin B_{12} deficiency
7. Vitamin B_{12} deficiency is classified as a megaloblastic macrocytic anemia
8. Atrophic gastritis is associated with vitamin B_{12} deficiency
9. Because B-complex vitamins work together, it is likely that more than one deficiency exists

Check Your NCLEX-RN® Exam I.Q.

You are ready for testing on this content if you can

- Apply knowledge of expected actions and effects of cardiovascular medications to client care.
- Correctly administer cardiovascular medications to clients.
- Assess for side effects and adverse effects of cardiovascular medications.
- Take appropriate action if a client has an unexpected response to a cardiovascular medication.
- Monitor a client for expected outcomes or effects of treatment with cardiovascular medications.

PRACTICE TEST

PRACTICE TEST

1. A client has an order to begin an IV nitroglycerin (Nitrostat) drip. The nurse prepares this medication by mixing the medication
   1. in a solution that is covered by a plastic bag.
   2. in a solution that is in a glass bottle.
   3. every 2 hours because it is unstable.
   4. under a laminar flow hood.

2. A client with angina pectoris received nitroglycerin tablets sublingually for chest pain. The client dislikes the medication because it causes headache. The nurse makes which of the following interpretations about the client's statement?
   1. This is a common but unhealthy response to the medication.
   2. This is a common response that will diminish as tolerance to the medication develops.
   3. This is a response caused by cerebral hypoxia induced by the medication.
   4. This is an adverse reaction that must be reported to the physician immediately.

3. A client who has just been diagnosed with hypertension also smokes and has diabetes mellitus. The nurse would question an order for which of the following antihypertensive medications?
   1. Diltiazem (Cardizem)
   2. Propranolol (Inderal)
   3. Prazosin (Minipress)
   4. Furosemide (Lasix)

4. Diltiazem (Cardizem) is prescribed for a client with chronic, stable angina. The clinic nurse determines that the client needs additional medication information if the client makes which of the following statements?
   1. "I will call the physician if shortness of breath occurs."
   2. "I will rise slowly when getting out of bed in the morning."
   3. "I will take medications after meals."
   4. "I will avoid activities requiring mental alertness until my body is adjusted to the medication."

5. The nurse has given medication instructions to the client receiving nicardipine (Cardene) for angina. The nurse would reinforce the teaching if the client makes which of the following statements?
   1. "I will keep track of angina episodes and report them if they increase."
   2. "I will ignore edema or weight gain as an expected side effect of the medication."
   3. "I will report a pulse rate of less than 50 beats per minute."
   4. "I will take missed dose as soon as remembered unless it is almost time for the next dose."

6. A client with hypertension has been given a prescription to treat the disorder. The nurse would explain that cough and loss of taste are side effects if which of the following antihypertensive agents is prescribed?
   1. Lisinopril (Prinivil)
   2. Propranolol (Inderal)
   3. Diltiazem (Cardizem)
   4. Furosemide (Lasix)

7. The physician prescribes losartan (Cozaar) for a client with hypertension. The nurse carrying out the order explains to the client that this medication promotes vasodilation by
   1. preventing calcium from going into the cells.
   2. promoting epinephrine and norepinephrine.
   3. promoting release of aldosterone.
   4. inhibiting conversion of a substance that would cause vasoconstriction.

8. The client with hypertension states he monitors his blood pressure daily. His medications include verapamil (Calan SR) 240 mg daily and hydrochlorothiazide (HCTZ) 12.5 mg daily. He states that if his BP reading is less than 140 systolic, he skips his dose for the day. What would be the most appropriate response by the nurse?
   1. "As long as the systolic is less than 140, it is okay to skip the dose."
   2. "You should not skip doses unless instructed by the ordering physician."
   3. "Maybe you won't even need your BP medications in a few more months."
   4. "Your doctor may want to stop the HCTZ and have you take only the Calan."

9 Adenosine (Adenocard) is to be administered to a client in the emergency room. Before preparing the medication, the nurse ensures that which of the following priority pieces of equipment is operational?

1. A pulse oximetry machine
2. An IV infusion pump
3. A cardiac monitor
4. An endotracheal tube

10 The home health nurse would be most concerned that a client is developing digoxin toxicity after noting which of the following during a routine visit?

1. Palpitations, elevated blood pressure, and shortness of breath
2. Anorexia, nausea, and reports of yellow vision
3. Chest pain, fatigue, and decreased blood pressure
4. Taste alterations, dry mouth, and constipation

11 A client with myocardial infarction is experiencing new, multiform, premature ventricular contractions (PVCs). The nurse checks the medication cart to ensure that which of the following medications is available for immediate use?

1. Digoxin (Lanoxin)
2. Metoprolol (Lopressor)
3. Verapamil (Isoptin)
4. Lidocaine (Xylocaine)

12 The nurse is preparing to administer amiodarone (Cordarone) IV. The nurse should assure that which of the following is in use at this time?

1. Oxygen therapy
2. Noninvasive blood pressure monitoring
3. Continuous cardiac monitoring
4. Oxygen saturation monitoring

13 Which medication does the nurse anticipate will be used for a pregnant client who requires anticoagulation therapy?

1. Low molecular weight heparin (LMWH)
2. Epoetin (Procrit)
3. Heparin (Liquaemin)
4. Enoxaparin (Lovenox)

14 The nurse would include in a teaching plan that a client taking warfarin (Coumadin) for atrial fibrillation will need to remain on drug therapy for what period of time?

1. Six months
2. Two to three months
3. Indefinite or long-term
4. One year

15 A client is placed on ticlopidine (Ticlid) following a stroke. What follow-up blood work is indicated in managing the client?

1. Frequent CBC monitoring to evaluate for blood dyscrasias
2. Monthly PT and INR levels to evaluate for clotting problems
3. ABGs to evaluate respiratory status
4. Serum chemistries to monitor for potential electrolyte imbalances

16 A client is undergoing percutaneous transluminal coronary angioplasty (PTCA) and requires an antiplatelet agent. The nurse prepares to administer which drug for this type of client immediately following the procedure?

1. Heparin (Liquaemin)
2. Abciximab (ReoPro)
3. Clopidrogrel bisulfate (Plavix)
4. Aspirin (ASA)

17 A client is receiving thrombolytic therapy. The nurse monitors the client for what potential problem?

1. Headache
2. Fever
3. Hematuria
4. Bone pain

18 The nurse would assess a client who is receiving thrombolytic therapy for which of the following?

1. Dry mouth
2. Decreased urine output
3. Decreased clotting times
4. Cardiac dysrhythmias

PRACTICE TEST

19 Which of the following would a nurse monitor for in a client taking folic acid (Folvite)?

1. Dark yellow urine
2. Dark green or black stools
3. Temperature elevations
4. Increased pulse rate

20 Which of the following measures should the nurse utilize when administering ferrous sulfate (Feosol) elixir?

1. Mix medication with milk to decrease GI effects.
2. Administer oral medication without food.
3. Administer medication through a straw.
4. Mix medication with carbonated beverages to minimize gastric upset.

21 A client has an order to receive 5,000 units of heparin subcutaneously. Available is a vial labeled Heparin 10,000 units per mL. How many mLs of heparin solution should the nurse administer?

Provide a numerical answer.

____

ANSWERS & RATIONALES

1 **Answer: 2** Intravenous nitroglycerin (NTG) must be prepared in only glass bottles and infused via the manufacturer-provided tubing. The polyvinyl chloride in regular tubing will adsorb (leech out) the nitroglycerin. NTG is stable in a glass bottle for 24 hours and does not require laminar flow ventilation.
Cognitive Level: Application **Client Need:** Physiological Integrity: Pharmacological and Parenteral Therapies **Integrated Process:** Nursing Process: Implementation **Content Area:** Pharmacology **Strategy:** The core issue of the question is knowledge that nitroglycerin adsorbs into plastic, making it necessary to use a glass bottle and special IV tubing from the manufacturer. Use nursing knowledge related to pharmacology and the process of elimination to make a selection.

2 **Answer: 2** Headache is a common side effect (not adverse reaction) related to the vasodilation properties of nitroglycerin. The incidence of headache decreases over time as the client develops tolerance to the medication. The client should be encouraged to continue its use as needed and to take acetaminophen or aspirin for headache, according to the preference of the physician.
Cognitive Level: Analysis **Client Need:** Physiological Integrity: Pharmacological and Parenteral Therapies **Integrated Process:** Nursing Process: Analysis **Content Area:** Pharmacology **Strategy:** The core issue of the question is knowledge of common adverse effects of nitroglycerin therapy. Use nursing knowledge related to pharmacology and the process of elimination to make a selection.

3 **Answer: 2** Adverse effects of beta-adrenergic blockers such as propranolol include their potential to cause bronchospasm and to mask hypoglycemia attacks. Therefore, the clients who are at risk for these conditions should not utilize beta-blockers as antihypertensive medications. Calcium channel blockers, alpha-blockers, and diuretics do not directly affect these conditions.
Cognitive Level: Application **Client Need:** Physiological Integrity: Pharmacological and Parenteral Therapies **Integrated Process:** Nursing Process: Implementation **Content Area:** Pharmacology **Strategy:** The core issue of the question is knowledge of contraindications for beta-adrenergic blockers such as propranolol. Use nursing knowledge related to pharmacology and the process of elimination to make a selection.

4 **Answer: 3** Diltiazem (Cardizem) is a calcium channel blocker. It is usually administered before meals and at bedtime to increase the absorption of the medication. Postural hypotension may occur, so the client must be instructed to rise slowly to avoid dizziness and falling. The medication may cause a decrease in mental alertness until the body adjusts and the proper dosage is established. The client should notify the physician if he or she develops shortness of breath, irregular heartbeat, pronounced dizziness, nausea, or constipation.
Cognitive Level: Analysis **Client Need:** Physiological Integrity: Pharmacological and Parenteral Therapies **Integrated Process:** Nursing Process: Evaluation **Content Area:** Pharmacology **Strategy:** The wording of the question tells you that the correct answer is an incorrect statement. Recall information about calcium channel blockers and use the process of elimination to make a selection.

5 **Answer: 2** Nicardipine (Cardene) is a calcium channel blocker. Weight gain and edema are potential signs of heart failure and must be reported to the physician. The client taking this medication should keep track of angina episodes and report an increase in the episodes or a change in the pattern. The client may take a missed dose of medication if not too close to the next dose; otherwise, the dose should be omitted. The client should be taught to check his or her pulse, note the rate, and report if the heart rate is less than 50 beats per minute.
Cognitive Level: Analysis **Client Need:** Physiological Integrity: Pharmacological and Parenteral Therapies **Integrated Process:** Nursing Process: Evaluation **Content Area:** Pharmacology **Strategy:** The core issue of the question is knowledge of teaching points regarding calcium channel blockers such as nicardipine. The wording of the question tells you that the

correct answer is an incorrect statement. Use nursing knowledge related to pharmacology and the process of elimination to make a selection.

6 **Answer: 1** Cough and loss of taste are common side effects of angiotensin-converting enzyme (ACE) inhibitors such as lisinopril. They disappear with discontinuance of the medication. The medications listed in the other options do not produce cough or change taste perception.
Cognitive Level: Analysis **Client Need:** Physiological Integrity: Pharmacological and Parenteral Therapies **Integrated Process:** Teaching and Learning **Content Area:** Pharmacology **Strategy:** The core issue of the question is knowledge that ACE inhibitors lead to cough and loss of taste perception. From there, you must be able to identify which drug is an ACE inhibitor. Recall that these drugs end in *-pril* to help make a selection.

7 **Answer: 4** Losartan is an angiotensin II antagonist that inhibits the conversion of angiotensin I to angiotensin II. Because angiotensin II is a powerful vasoconstrictor, this inhibition results in vasodilation and normalizing blood pressure. The client should be assessed for dizziness, cough, and diarrhea while taking this medication.
Cognitive Level: Application **Client Need:** Physiological Integrity: Pharmacological and Parenteral Therapies **Integrated Process:** Teaching and Learning **Content Area:** Pharmacology **Strategy:** The core issue of the question is knowledge of the mechanism of action of angiotensin receptor blockers. To reach the correct answer, it is necessary to recognize that the drug is in this class. Use nursing knowledge related to pharmacology and the process of elimination to make a selection.

8 **Answer: 2** Lack of adherence to pharmacologic treatment strategies prevents the client from establishing good control of the disease and ultimately places him or her at risk for developing long-term complications of hypertension. Noncompliance with the therapeutic program is a significant problem in people with hypertension. The client should not skip doses of medications without consulting the physician.
Cognitive Level: Application **Client Need:** Physiological Integrity: Pharmacological and Parenteral Therapies **Integrated Process:** Communication and Documentation **Content Area:** Pharmacology **Strategy:** The core issue of the question is knowledge that antihypertensive medications need to be taken as scheduled without missing or skipping doses. Use nursing knowledge related to pharmacology and the process of elimination to make a selection.

9 **Answer: 3** Adenosine (Adenocard) is an antidysrhythmic used in the treatment of paroxysmal supraventricular tachycardia (SVT). Cardiac performance must be assessed before and throughout treatment by cardiac monitoring. An endotracheal tube may be used if an emergency necessitates mechanical ventilation, but the tube itself is a rather isolated item. An IV pump may be needed but is not a priority because this medication is administered rapidly by IV push. A pulse oximetry machine may be helpful in assessing oxygenation but is not a priority item.
Cognitive Level: Analysis **Client Need:** Physiological Integrity: Pharmacological and Parenteral Therapies **Integrated Process:** Nursing Process: Planning **Content Area:** Pharmacology **Strategy:** The core issue of the question is the most important piece of equipment needed to monitor a client receiving adenosine. Recall that this drug is an antidysrhythmic to help choose the cardiac monitor as the appropriate answer.

10 **Answer: 2** Anorexia, nausea, and yellow vision are signs of digoxin toxicity. Other signs include other visual disturbances, vomiting, and diarrhea. The clusters of other symptoms listed do not fit the profile of digoxin toxicity.
Cognitive Level: Analysis **Client Need:** Physiological Integrity: Pharmacological and Parenteral Therapies **Integrated Process:** Nursing Process: Assessment **Content Area:** Pharmacology **Strategy:** The core issue of the question is knowledge of early signs of digoxin toxicity. Recall that early signs are usually more subtle than later signs. Use nursing knowledge related to pharmacology and the process of elimination to make a selection.

11 **Answer: 4** Lidocaine is a class-I antidysrhythmic used to treat ventricular dysrhythmias. Other medications that might be ordered include procainamide, amiodarone, or magnesium sulfate. The other medications would not be used as a primary treatment of ventricular dysrhythmias because they are a cardiac glycoside (option 1), a beta-blocker (option 2), and a calcium channel blocker (option 3).
Cognitive Level: Application **Client Need:** Physiological Integrity: Pharmacological and Parenteral Therapies **Integrated Process:** Nursing Process: Planning **Content Area:** Pharmacology **Strategy:** The core issue of the question is knowledge of first-line treatment for PVCs. Use nursing knowledge related to pharmacology and the process of elimination to make a selection.

12 **Answer: 3** Amiodarone is a class III antiarrhythmic used to treat life-threatening ventricular dysrhythmias that do not respond to the first-line drugs (like lidocaine). The client should have continuous EKG monitoring, and the medication should be infused through an IV pump. Oxygen therapy may be needed but is unrelated to this medication. Options 2 and 4 are not critical during administration of this medication, although they are generally useful adjuncts.
Cognitive Level: Application **Client Need:** Physiological Integrity: Pharmacological and Parenteral Therapies **Integrated Process:** Nursing Process: Implementation **Content Area:** Pharmacology **Strategy:** The core issue of the question is knowledge of what parameter needs to be monitored carefully during amiodarone therapy. Eliminate options 1 and 4 (oxygen and oxygen saturation monitor) because they are similar. Recall that the drug is an antidysrhythmic agent to make the final selection.

13 **Answer: 3** Heparin is the drug of choice in pregnancy. Low molecular weight heparins, of which enoxaparin is an example, are not recommended for use during pregnancy (options 1 and 4). Epoetin alfa (Procrit) is a colony-stimulating growth factor and is not used for anticoagulation (option 2).
Cognitive Level: Application **Client Need:** Physiological Integrity: Pharmacological and Parenteral Therapies **Integrated Process:** Nursing Process: Planning **Content Area:** Pharmacology **Strategy:** The core issue of the question is knowledge of the anticoagulant that is safe to use during pregnancy. Use nursing knowledge related to pharmacology and the process of elimination to make a selection.

14 **Answer: 3** Clients who have atrial fibrillation are at risk to develop emboli. Therapy with Coumadin is considered to be ongoing in nature in order to prevent such an occurrence. The other time frames are too short to achieve a preventative goal. In addition, the likelihood of emboli formation does not significantly diminish unless the client is anticoagulated on a long-term basis.
Cognitive Level: Application **Client Need:** Physiological Integrity: Pharmacological and Parenteral Therapies **Integrated Process:** Nursing Process: Planning **Content Area:** Pharmacology **Strategy:** The core issue of the question is knowledge that treatment for prevention of blood clot formation from atrial fibrillation is indefinite. Use nursing knowledge related to pharmacology and the process of elimination to make a selection.

15 **Answer: 1** A client taking ticlopidine should be monitored for potential blood dyscrasias that can occur with this drug. Monthly PT and INR levels are not indicated as follow-up for this medication but are used in conjunction with Coumadin therapy (option 2). ABGs are not indicated in the management of clients who are taking ticlopidine (option 3) There are no reported electrolyte imbalances with the use of this medication (option 4).
Cognitive Level: Application **Client Need:** Physiological Integrity: Pharmacological and Parenteral Therapies **Integrated Process:** Nursing Process: Planning **Content Area:** Pharmacology **Strategy:** The core issue of the question is knowledge of adverse effects of ticlopidine that can be detected using laboratory monitoring. Use nursing knowledge related to pharmacology and the process of elimination to make a selection.

16 **Answer: 2** ReoPro is often given IV following this type of procedure to help prevent possible reocclusion of the coronary artery that has been treated. It can be administered in conjunction with weight-based heparin therapy, but heparin is an anticoagulant agent (option 1). Plavix and ASA are examples of antiplatelet agents that are given orally and are not utilized in this particular acute-care setting (options 3 and 4). However, ASA can be given later as follow-up to the procedure to prevent possible complications related to vessel occlusion.
Cognitive Level: Application **Client Need:** Physiological Integrity: Pharmacological and Parenteral Therapies **Integrated Process:** Nursing Process: Planning **Content Area:** Pharmacology **Strategy:** The core issue of the question is knowledge of drugs that have antiplatelet properties and that can be used IV following interventional cardiology procedures such as PTCA. Use nursing knowledge related to pharmacology and the process of elimination to make a selection.

17 **Answer: 3** Clients taking thrombolytic therapy should be monitored closely for the possibility of hemorrhage because therapy increases the risk of bleeding. Monitoring includes evaluating the skin for bruising and gums and venipuncture sites for bleeding, and testing stool and urine for occult or obvious blood. Headache, fever, and bone pain are not directly related to thrombolytic therapy (options 1, 2, and 4).
Cognitive Level: Application **Client Need:** Physiological Integrity: Pharmacological and Parenteral Therapies **Integrated Process:** Nursing Process: Assessment **Content Area:** Pharmacology **Strategy:** The core issue of the question is knowledge that thrombolytics can lead to bleeding. With this in mind, recall the various ways that bleeding can manifest in a client taking drugs that interfere with clotting. Use nursing knowledge related to pharmacology and the process of elimination to make a selection.

18 **Answer: 4** The use of thrombolytic agents can cause cardiac irritation and lead to development of dysrhythmias that can be life threatening. The nurse must be aware of the serious likelihood that treatment can cause further cardiac compromise. Dry mouth, decreased urine output, and decreased clotting times (options 1, 2, and 3) are not seen with thrombolytic therapy.
Cognitive Level: Application **Client Need:** Physiological Integrity: Pharmacological and Parenteral Therapies **Integrated Process:** Nursing Process: Assessment **Content Area:** Pharmacology **Strategy:** The core issue of the question is knowledge that thrombolytic drugs can cause reperfusion dysrhythmias as a result of clot lysis. Use nursing knowledge related to pharmacology and the process of elimination to make a selection.

19 **Answer: 1** Folic acid (in large doses) can cause the urine to become discolored and turn to a darker yellow color. Dark green or black stools are more commonly associated with iron therapy (option 2). Temperature elevations and changes in pulse rate are not associated with folic acid (options 3 and 4).
Cognitive Level: Application **Client Need:** Physiological Integrity: Pharmacological and Parenteral Therapies **Integrated Process:** Nursing Process: Evaluation **Content Area:** Pharmacology **Strategy:** The core issue of the question is knowledge of expected side effects of folic acid. Recall that B complex vitamins may turn the urine a darker yellow as an aid to answering the question. Use nursing knowledge related to pharmacology and the process of elimination to make a selection.

20 **Answer: 3** Liquid iron preparations can cause staining of teeth. It is important for the nurse to be aware of proper administration methods, which includes drinking the mixture through a straw. Mixing medication with milk and carbonated beverages will decrease its absorption (options 1 and 4). The medication is usually taken with food to minimize GI upset (option 2).
Cognitive Level: Application **Client Need:** Physiological Integrity: Pharmacological and Parenteral Therapies **Integrated Process:** Nursing Process: Implementation **Content Area:** Pharmacology **Strategy:** The core issue of the question is knowing that liquid iron stains the teeth. With this in mind, select the option that prevents the liquid from being absorbed through tooth enamel. Keeping in mind other administration principles helps you to eliminate the incorrect options.

21 **Answer: 0.5 mL** To calculate the dose, divide the desired dose (5,000) by the dose on hand (10,000 units) and multiply that by the quantity (1 mL). The result is 0.5 mL.
Cognitive Level: Application **Client Need:** Physiological Integrity: Pharmacological and Parenteral Therapies **Integrated Process:** Nursing Process: Implementation **Content Area:** Pharmacology **Strategy:** The core issue of the question is the ability to calculate a drug dose. If necessary, memorize this basic formula for use in solving many medication questions.

Key Terms to Review

activated partial thromboplastin time (APTT) p. 619
afterload p. 601
anticoagulants p. 617
automaticity p. 604
chronotropic p. 604
clotting cascade p. 617
conductivity p. 606
contractility p. 611
dromotropic p. 604
dysrhythmia p. 611
extrinsic pathway p. 617
fibrinolysis p. 625
fibrinolytic system p. 621
hemostatics p. 625
heparin-induced platelet aggregation (HITT) p. 619
hypercoagulation p. 625
inotropic p. 604
international normalized ratio (INR) p. 617
intrinsic pathway p. 618
irritability p. 604
low molecular weight heparin (LMWH) p. 619
pernicious anemia p. 627
pica p. 627
preload p. 601
protamine sulfate p. 619
prothrombin time (PT) p. 617
refractory period p. 612
thrombolytics p. 621
titrate p. 602

References

Abrams, A. (2004). *Clinical drug therapy: Rationales for nursing practice* (7th ed.). Philadelphia: Lippincott Williams & Wilkins.

Adams, M., Josephson, D., & Holland, L. (2005). *Pharmacology for nurses: A pathophysiologic approach.* Upper Saddle River, NJ: Pearson Education.

American Psychiatric Association. (2000). *Diagnostic and statistical manual of mental disorders, Fourth Edition, Text Revision* (DSM-IV-TR). Washington, DC: American Psychiatric Association.

Deglin, J. H., & Vallerand, A. H. (2006). *Davis's drug guide for nurses* (10th ed.). Philadelphia: F. A. Davis.

Laraia, M. (2004). Psychopharmacology. In G. Stuart & M. Laraia (Eds.), *Principles and practice of psychiatric nursing* (8th ed.). St. Louis: Mosby.

Lehne, R. (2004). *Pharmacology for nursing care* (5th ed.). Philadelphia: W. B. Saunders.

McKenry, L., Tessier, E., & Hogan, M. (2006). *Mosby's pharmacology in nursing* (22nd ed.). St. Louis: Elsevier Science.

Wilson, B., Shannon, M., & Stang, C. (2006). *Prentice Hall nurse's drug guide 2006.* Upper Saddle River, NJ: Pearson Education.

39 Neurological and Musculoskeletal Medications

Test Yourself

Are you ready for the NCLEX-RN® or course exams? Use the practice tests on the companion CD-ROM to check.

In this chapter

Cross reference

Other chapters relevant to this content area are

Dosage Calculation and Medication Administration	Chapter 30
Psychiatric Medications	Chapter 36
Neurological Disorders	Chapter 58
Musculoskeletal Disorders	Chapter 62

I. GENERAL GUIDELINES FOR NEUROLOGICAL AND MUSCULOSKELETAL MEDICATIONS *(SEE BOX 39–1)*

II. ANALGESICS

A. Opioids

1. Used for symptomatic relief of severe acute and chronic pain
2. Produce effects by binding to opioid receptors throughout CNS and peripheral tissues
3. Considered controlled substances by FDA
4. Cross blood–brain and placental barriers and also into breast milk
5. Common medications are listed in Table 39–1 ■
6. Administration considerations
   - **a.** ! Use caution because of possibility of dependence
   - **b.** Determine client's pattern of use if long term; be aware that some opioids are used as street drugs
   - **c.** May increase intracranial pressure (ICP)
   - **d.** Closely monitor clients with severe heart, liver, or kidney disease or respiratory or seizure disorders
   - **e.** Decrease dosages for elderly or debilitated clients
   - **f.** ! Additional CNS depression can occur if used with barbiturates, other narcotics, hypnotics, antipsychotics, or alcohol

Box 39-1

General Guidelines for Neuromuscular Medications

Administration Principles

1. Assess current medications (including OTC drugs and herbal products) and history of allergies to identify any potential risks to client.
2. Administer doses on time to maintain therapeutic blood levels.
3. Do not break, crush, or allow client to chew sustained release or enteric coated preparations.
4. Many drugs cause CNS depression so monitor client for adverse effects and maintain a safe environment.
5. Provide both verbal and written instructions to client, and provide phone number to call if questions arise or problems occur.

Client Teaching

1. Understand medication actions, side effects, signs of toxicity, importance of follow-up with prescriber and complying with follow-up laboratory tests, and how to self-administer.
2. Do not take any OTC drugs or herbal products without first consulting prescriber.
3. Take exactly as prescribed and do not miss or double doses.
4. Report adverse effects promptly.
5. Do not discontinue drug without consulting prescriber.
6. Do not drink alcohol while taking prescription medications.

7. Side/adverse effects
   a. Nausea and vomiting, anorexia
   b. Sedation, respiratory or circulatory depression

Memory Aid

Remember that opioid analgesics are CNS depressants; watch for sedation as an early sign and respiratory rate decrease as a later sign of CNS depression.

   c. Constipation, gastrointestinal (GI) cramps, urinary retention, oliguria
   d. Pruritis, light-headedness, dizziness, increased ICP
8. Nursing considerations
   a. Assess pain type, intensity (pain scale), and location prior to administration
   b. Assess respiratory rate, depth, and rhythm; if less than 12, withhold medication
   c. Assess for CNS changes, including changes in level of consciousness (LOC); monitor vital signs (VS) regularly
   d. Assess for allergic reaction such as rash or urticaria

Table 39–1

Common Opioid Analgesics

Type	Generic/Trade Names
Pure agonists (no ceiling effect, increase in analgesia with increase in dose)	Codeine (Paveral) Dihydrocodeine, hydrocodone bitartrate (Vicodin) Oxycodone (Oxycontin) Propoxyphene (Darvon) Morphine sulfate (generic, Duramorph) Fentanyl citrate (Duragesic) Oxymorphone (Numorphan) Hydromorphone hydrochloride (Dilaudid) Meperidine (Demerol) Methadone hydrochloride (Dolophine) Levorphanal tartrate (Levo-dromoran)
Mixed agonists-antagonists (have ceiling effect)	Pentazocine hydrochloride (Talwin) Butorphanol tartrate (Stadol) Dezocine (Dalgan) Nalbuphine hydrochloride (Nubain)

e. Administer opiates for pain and antiemetics for nausea and vomiting
f. Evaluate therapeutic response and maintain comfort

! 9. Client teaching
a. As per Box 39–1; avoid other CNS depressants while using opioids
b. Use caution in ambulation, and avoid smoking, driving, and strenuous activities without assistance until drug response is known
c. Report any CNS changes, allergic reactions, or shortness of breath
d. If using medication on a long-term basis, be aware of withdrawal symptoms, including nausea, vomiting, cramps, fever, faintness, and anorexia

B. Opioid antagonists

1. Include naloxone (Narcan) and naltrexone (ReVia)
2. Compete with opioids at opiate receptor sites, blocking opioid effects
! 3. Reverse respiratory depression induced by overdose of opioids, pentazocine, and propoxyphene
4. Onset of effect is 1 to 2 minutes, duration is 45 minutes; assess client because CNS depression could recur when drug wears off
5. Side/adverse effects
! a. Reversal of analgesia
b. Increased or decreased blood pressure (BP), tachycardia, hyperpnea
c. Tremors, drowsiness, nervousness, convulsions
d. Nausea and vomiting
e. Ventricular tachycardia and fibrillation
f. Pulmonary edema
6. Nursing considerations
! a. Assess VS every 3 to 5 minutes, and cardiac status (tachycardia, hypertension)
b. Assess arterial blood gases (ABGs) and respiratory function (rate, rhythm)
c. Monitor electrocardiogram (ECG)
! d. Administer only with resuscitative equipment nearby
e. Evaluate therapeutic response, LOC, and need for reversal of respiratory depression

C. Nonopioids

1. Acetylsalicylic acid (ASA), or aspirin
a. Inhibits prostaglandins involved in production of inflammation, pain, and fever
b. Blocks pain impulses in CNS and provides relief of mild to moderate pain
c. Antipyretic action results from vasodilation of peripheral vessels
d. Powerfully inhibits platelet aggregation
! e. Assess for allergy to salicylates prior to administration
f. Decrease gastric irritation by administering with full glass of water, milk, food, or antacid, or by using an enteric coated preparation
! g. Side/adverse effects include visual changes, tinnitus, hepatotoxicity, allergic reactions and bleeding, instruct client to report these
h. Instruct client not to combine with other OTC medications that also contain ASA and avoid alcohol ingestion to decrease risk of GI bleeding
! i. Warn client that this medication should not be given to children or teens with flulike or chickenpox symptoms (can lead to Reye syndrome, characterized by encephalopathy and fatty liver degeneration)
2. Acetaminophen (Tylenol)
a. Used for mild to moderate pain or fever, especially when ASA or nonsteroidal anti-inflammatory drugs (NSAIDs) are not tolerated; blocks pain impulses peripherally
b. Antipyretic action occurs by inhibiting prostaglandins in CNS, resulting in peripheral vasodilation, sweating, and dissipation of heat
! c. Do not use if allergic to acetaminophen or phenacetin
d. Avoid use in clients with anemia or hepatic diseases, including alcoholism, malnutrition, or thrombocytopenia
! e. May cause **hepatotoxicity** at doses greater than 4 grams/day with chronic use; assess for dark urine, clay-colored stools, yellowing of skin or sclera, itching, abdominal pain, fever, and diarrhea, especially if on long-term therapy

f. Be prepared to administer acetylcysteine (Mucomyst) as antidote for acetaminophen poisoning
g. Evaluate client for therapeutic response, such as decreased pain or fever

3. NSAIDs
a. Decrease prostaglandin synthesis by inhibiting an enzyme needed for biosynthesis
b. Used to treat mild to moderate pain, osteoarthritis, rheumatoid arthritis, and dysmenorrhea
c. Common medications are listed in Box 39–2
d. Decrease gastric irritation by administering with full glass of water or milk or with food
e. Administer at least 30 minutes prior to physical therapy or planned activity to minimize discomfort
f. Contraindicated with asthma, severe renal or hepatic disease, GI bleeding, bleeding disorders, peptic ulcer disease, anemia, or while taking anticoagulant therapy
g. Instruct client to report blurred vision, ringing or roaring in ears; may indicate toxicity
h. Evaluate for therapeutic response, including decreased pain, stiffness in joints, decreased swelling in joints, ability to move more easily; may take up to 1 month

D. Medications to treat headaches

1. Aimed at prevention with prophylactic therapy and acute symptomatic treatment during attack
a. Ergot preparations for migraine headaches are alpha-adrenergic agonists or antagonists that cause vasoconstriction or vasodilation, depending on state of vessel; they also block uptake of serotonin by platelets that can cause precipitous decline of serotonin, leading to migraine attack
b. Prophylaxis for migraine headaches includes beta-adrenergic blockers, serotonin antagonists, and antiepileptics
c. Mild analgesics and muscle relaxants are first-line medications for tension-type headaches; antidepressants may be used with counseling; ASA, acetaminophen, and ibuprofen are used for pain; amitriptyline (Elavil) is helpful for muscle contraction pain
d. Preventative therapies for cluster headaches may include high-dose calcium channel blockers, lithium, methysergide, or corticosteroids

2. Common medications are listed in Box 39–3

3. Administration considerations
a. For abortive treatment medications, take early in headache to be effective
b. Start with dosage that was effective on last headache at beginning of this headache
c. Contraindicated with hypersensitivity to ergot alkaloids, pregnancy, cardiovascular disease, coronary artery disease, hypertension, sepsis, or severe pruritus

4. Nursing considerations
a. Planning for care must begin with careful history, including past treatments that were effective

Box 39–2

Common Nonsteroidal Anti-Inflammatory Agents

Celecoxib (Celebrex)	Ketoprofen (Actron)
Diclofenac sodium (Voltaren)	Ketorolac (Toradol)
Etodolac (Lodine)	Mefenemic acid (Ponstel)
Fenoprofen calcium (Nalfon)	Nabumetone (Relafen)
Flurbiprofen sodium (Ansaid)	Naproxen (Naprosyn)
Ibuprofen (Advil, others)	Piroxicam (Feldene)
Indomethacin (Indocin)	Sulindac (Clinoril)

Box 39-3

Medications Used to Treat Headaches

Ergotamine tartrate (Ergostat)

Dihydroergotamine mesylate (Migranal)

Sumatriptan (Imitrex)

b. Assess for medication-specific side effects as well as efficacy of treatment
c. Provide a quiet and low-light environment
d. Obtain an accurate dietary history to determine if onset of headache is associated with ingestion of certain foods
e. Avoid prolonged medication use
f. Beware of ergotamine rebound or an increase in frequency and duration of headache

5. Client teaching
   a. Identify triggers for headaches and how to ameliorate them
   b. Keep a headache diary
   c. Use stress reduction, stress management, lifestyle changes, including diet, to minimize headaches
   d. Do not eat, drink, or smoke while tablet is dissolving (if using sublingual tablet)
   e. Avoid prolonged exposure to cold weather (may increase adverse reactions to medication)
   f. Do not increase dose without consulting physician
   g. Use comfort measures during attack, such as lying in darkened, quiet room with cold compresses applied to head

III. ANTIEPILEPTICS

A. Hydantoins

1. Inhibit spread of seizure activity in motor cortex
2. Used in general **tonic-clonic seizures** (grand mal seizures), **status epilepticus seizures** (seizures that last longer than 4 minutes), and **psychomotor seizures** (complex focal seizures)
3. Common medications are listed in Table 39–2 ■
4. Administration considerations
   a. Fosphenytoin should only be given IV for status epilepticus in emergency department or critical care area; monitor respiratory rate, BP, and ECG
   b. Do not interchange chewable phenytoin products with capsules
   c. Phenytoin readily binds with protein, so do not give with gastric feedings, which inhibit uptake
   d. Carbamazepine given via nasogastric (NG) tube should be mixed with D_5W or NS and flushed with at least 100 mL solution afterwards
   e. Do not crush tablets or capsules of valproate sodium; take whole
   f. Contraindicated with hypersensitivity, pregnancy, bradycardia, SA and AV node block, Stokes-Adams syndrome, hepatic failure

Table 39–2

Antiepileptics

Type	Generic (Trade) names
Hydantoins	Fosphenytoin sodium (Cerebyx) Phenytoin (Dilantin)
Barbiturate	Phenobarbital sodium (Luminal)
Succinimide	Ethosuximide (Zarontin)
Benzodiazepines	Diazepam (Valium) Lorazepam (Ativan) Clonazepam (Klonopin)
Other	Carbamazepine (Tegretol) Valproate sodium (Depakote)

5. Side/adverse effects
   a. Drowsiness, dizziness, insomnia, **paresthesias** (abnormal sensations), depression, suicidal tendencies, aggression, headache, confusion, slurred speech
   b. **Nystagmus** (involuntary oscillation of eye), **diplopia** (double vision), blurred vision
   c. Nausea, vomiting, constipation, anorexia, weight loss, hepatitis, jaundice, **gingival hyperplasia** (increased growth of gum tissue)
   d. Urine discoloration
   e. Agranulocytosis, leukopenia, aplastic anemia, thrombocytopenia, megaloblastic anemia
   f. Rash, hirsutism, lupus erythematosus, **Stevens-Johnson syndrome** (an acute inflammatory disorder of the skin)
   g. Toxicity: bone marrow suppression, nausea, vomiting, ataxia, diplopia, cardiovascular collapse, slurred speech, confusion
6. Nursing considerations
   a. Assess for seizure activity, including type, location, duration, and character; provide seizure precautions
   b. Assess mental status for changes in mood, sensorium, affect, and memory (short and long term)
   c. Assess respiratory status for depression, rate, depth, and character of respirations
   d. Assess for blood dyscrasias, fever, sore throat, bruising, rash, and jaundice
   e. Evaluate client for therapeutic responses such as decreases in severity of seizures and decreased ventricular dysrhythmias
   f. Monitor results of periodic serum drug levels to ensure they are in therapeutic range

Memory Aid

Therapeutic serum theophylline levels are 10 to 20 mg/dL. Memorize this value because it is an important one to know in practice and in test situations.

7. Client teaching
   a. As per Box 39–1; carry Medic-Alert bracelet stating medication use
   b. Urine may turn pink
   c. Perform proper brushing of teeth with soft toothbrush and proper flossing to prevent gingival hyperplasia
   d. Do not change brands of medication once seizure activity has stabilized; bioavailability differs among formulations

B. Barbiturates

1. Decrease impulse transmission to cerebral cortex
2. Can be used in all forms of **epilepsy,** a chronic disorder characterized by recurring seizures
3. Common medications are listed in Table 39–2
4. Administration considerations
   a. Administer by intramuscular (IM) injection into large muscle mass to prevent tissue sloughing
   b. Use less than 5 mL/site
   c. When ordered IV, give slowly (after dilution) at a rate of 65 mg or less per minute
5. Contraindicated with hypersensitivity, pregnancy, porphyria, and liver disease
6. Side/adverse effects
   a. Paradoxical excitement (elderly), drowsiness, lethargy, hangover headache, flushing, hallucinations
   b. Nausea, vomiting, diarrhea, constipation
   c. Rash, urticaria, local pain or swelling or necrosis, Stevens-Johnson syndrome, angioedema, thrombophlebitis
7. Nursing considerations
   a. Assess mental status for changes in mood, sensorium, affect, and memory (long and short term)

b. Assess for respiratory depression
c. Assess for blood dyscrasias, fever, sore throat, bruising, rash, and jaundice
! d. Assess for seizure activity, including type, duration, and precipitating factors
e. Obtain routine blood studies and liver function tests during long-term treatment
f. Evaluate client for therapeutic responses such as decreased seizures or increased sedation

8. Client teaching
! a. As per Box 39–1; avoid use of other CNS depressants; carry Medic-Alert bracelet stating medication use
! b. Avoid hazardous activities until stabilized on drug; drowsiness may occur
c. Therapeutic effects may not be seen for 2 to 3 weeks

C. Succinimides

1. Inhibit spike and wave formation in absence seizures (petit mal); decrease amplitude, frequency, duration, and spread of discharges in minor motor seizures, partial seizures, and tonic-clonic seizures
2. Common medications are listed in Table 39–2
3. Administration considerations: give with food or milk to decrease GI symptoms; contraindicated with hypersensitivity
4. Side/adverse effects
! a. Drowsiness, dizziness, fatigue, euphoria, lethargy
b. Nausea, vomiting, heartburn, anorexia
! c. Pink urine
d. Urticaria, pruritic erythema, Stevens-Johnson syndrome
e. Myopia, blurred vision
f. Agranulocytosis, aplastic anemia, thrombocytopenia, leukocytosis, eosinophilia, pancytopenia
! g. Toxicity: bone marrow depression, nausea, vomiting, ataxia, diplopia, and cardiovascular collapse
5. Nursing considerations
a. Assess mental status for changes in mood, sensorium, affect, and behavior
! b. Monitor renal studies, including urinalysis, blood urea nitrogen (BUN), and creatinine
! c. Monitor blood studies, including complete blood cell count (CBC), hematocrit (Hct), hemoglobin (Hgb), and reticulocyte counts every week for 4 weeks
d. Monitor hepatic studies including aspartate aminotransferase (AST), alanine aminotransferase (ALT), and bilirubin
e. Assess for eye problems; may need regular ophthalmic exams
f. Assess for allergic reactions such as red, raised rash or exfoliative dermatitis
! g. Assess for blood dyscrasias, fever, sore throat, bruising, rash, or jaundice
6. Client teaching
a. As per Box 39–1; carry ID card or Medic-Alert bracelet with medication, client's name, physician's name, and phone number
! b. Avoid driving and other activities that require alertness; avoid alcohol ingestion and other CNS depressants because they may increase sedation
! c. Continue regular dental checkups to identify gingival hyperplasia

D. Benzodiazepines

1. Enhance inhibitory neurotransmitter gamma-aminobutyric acid (GABA) to decrease anxiety and as an adjunct for seizure activity
2. Used to treat delirium tremens
3. Common medications are listed in Table 39–2
4. Administration considerations
a. Give with food or milk to reduce GI symptoms; IV injection should be given into large vein
! b. Can lead to dependency; monitor client's use
5. Contraindicated with hypersensitivity, acute narrow-angle glaucoma or psychosis, children younger than 6 months, liver disease (clonazepam), or during lactation (diazepam)

6. Side/adverse effects
   a. Dizziness, drowsiness, confusion, headache, fatigue, blurred vision
   b. Orthostatic hypotension, ECG changes, tachycardia, respiratory depression
   c. Constipation, dry mouth, rash, itching, neutropenia
7. Nursing considerations
   a. Assess BP (lying, standing), pulse; if systolic BP drops 20 mmHg, withhold drug, notify physician because of orthostatic hypotension
   b. Assess hepatic and renal function (AST, ALT, bilirubin, creatinine, high density lipoprotein), alkaline phosphatase
   c. Assess mental status for changes in mood, sensorium, affect, memory (long and short term)
   d. Assess respiratory status for depression, rate, rhythm, depth
   e. Assess for seizure activity, including type, duration, and precipitating factors
   f. Evaluate client for therapeutic responses such as reduced or absent seizure activity, anxiety
8. Client teaching: As per Box 39–1; avoid other CNS depressants, including alcohol; avoid hazardous activities until stabilized on drug; drowsiness may occur

E. Other antiepileptics

1. Carbamazepine (Tegretol)
   a. Inhibits nerve impulses by limiting influx of sodium ions across cell membrane in motor cortex
   b. Used in tonic-clonic, complex-partial, and mixed seizures
   c. Give oral forms with food or milk to reduce GI symptoms
   d. When administered via NG tube, must be mixed with D_5W or NS and flushed with at least 100 mL solution afterwards
   e. Contraindicated with hypersensitivity to carbamazepine or tricyclic antidepressants (TCAs), bone marrow depression, and concomitant use of MAOIs
   f. Side/adverse effects are many and include drowsiness, dizziness, confusion, nausea, constipation, diarrhea, vomiting, tinnitis, dry mouth, blurred vision, nystagmus, thrombocytopenia, agranulocytosis, neutropenia, paralysis, worsening of seizures, Stevens-Johnson syndrome, and possible fatal reaction with MAOIs
   g. Assess for seizure activity, including type, duration, and precipitating factors
   h. Monitor blood, hepatic, and renal studies including RBC, Hct, Hgb, reticulocyte count, AST, ALT, bilirubin, urinalysis, BUN, creatinine
   i. Assess mental status for changes in mood, sensorium, affect, and memory (long and short term)
   j. Assess for eye problems; may need regular ophthalmic exams
   k. Assess for blood dyscrasias, fever, sore throat, bruising, rash, or jaundice
   l. Evaluate client for therapeutic response such as decreased or absent seizure activity
   m. Perform client teaching as in Box 39–1; instruct client to avoid other CNS depressants and activities that cause additive drowsiness
   n. Inform client that urine may turn pink to brown
2. Valproate sodium
   a. Increases levels of gamma-aminobutyric acid (GABA) in brain, which decreases seizure activity
   b. Used in simple (petit mal), complex (petit mal), absence, or mixed seizures; manic episodes associated with bipolar disorder and migraine headaches
   c. Do not crush tablets or capsules; take them whole; may give with food or milk to decrease GI symptoms
   d. Contraindicated with hypersensitivity, during pregnancy, and with hepatic disease
   e. Side/adverse effects include sedation, drowsiness, nausea, vomiting, constipation, diarrhea, thrombocytopenia, leukopenia, lymphocytosis, hepatic failure, pancreatitis, toxic hepatitis
   f. Assess for seizure activity, including type, duration, and precipitating factors
   g. Monitor blood, hepatic, and renal function
   h. Assess mental status for changes in mood, sensorium, affect, and memory (long and short term)

i. Assess respiratory status for depression, (rate, rhythm, and depth)
j. Evaluate client for therapeutic response, such as decreased seizure activity
! k. Provide client teaching as per Box 39–1; inform client that physical dependency may result from extended use
! l. Advise client to report visual disturbances, rash, diarrhea, light-colored stools, jaundice, or protracted vomiting to provider

IV. CENTRAL NERVOUS SYSTEM (CNS) STIMULANTS

A. Anorexiants

1. Most act similarly to amphetamines, as indirect sympathomimetic amines with alpha- and beta-adrenergic activity
2. Used for **narcolepsy** (inability to stay awake during day), **attention deficit disorder** (ADD), **attention deficit/hyperactivity disorder** (ADHD), and in short-term adjunct to control obesity
3. Common medications are listed in Table 39–3 ■
4. Administration considerations
   ! a. Anorexiant effects are temporary
   b. To avoid insomnia, take 6 hours prior to bedtime
   ! c. Do not abruptly discontinue medication
5. Contraindicated with hypersensitivity, angle-closure glaucoma, advanced cardiac disease, hyperthyroidism, agitated states, history of drug abuse, and children under 12 years
6. Side/adverse effects
   a. Restlessness, insomnia, decrease in seizure threshold in epilepsy
   ! b. Palpitations and tachycardia
   c. Dysmenorrhea
! 7. Nursing considerations
   a. Assess BP and pulse during treatment
   b. Current dosage of antihypertensives and antidiabetics may need to be adjusted
   c. Evaluate client for therapeutic response such as decrease in weight over time
! 8. Client teaching
   a. As per Box 39–1; discuss all medications currently taken (including OTC) with provider; serious or even fatal interactions can occur
   b. Avoid driving or other hazardous activities until reaction to medication is determined

B. Amphetamines

1. Increase release of norepinephrine and dopamine in cerebral cortex to reticular activating system
2. Used in treating narcolepsy, exogenous obesity, ADD
3. Common medications are listed in Table 39–3
4. Administration considerations
   ! a. Give first dose on awakening and last dose no closer than 6 hours before bedtime
   b. Administer on empty stomach 30 to 60 minutes before meal
5. Contraindicated with hypersensitivity, hyperthyroidism, hypertension, glaucoma, severe arteriosclerosis, drug abuse, cardiovascular disease, anxiety, and lactation
! 6. Side/adverse effects
   a. Hyperactivity, insomnia, restlessness, talkativeness

Table 39–3
Central Nervous System (Adrenergic) Stimulants

Type	Generic (Trade) Names	Use
Anorexiants	Benzphetamine hydrochloride (Didrex)	Weight loss
	Diethylpropion hydrochloride (Propion)	Weight loss
	Sibutramine hydrochloride monohydrate (Meridia)	Weight loss
Amphetamines	Amphetamine sulfate (Adderall)	Narcolepsy, weight loss
	Methylphenidate hydrochloride (Ritalin)	Narcolepsy, ADD
	Dextroamphetamine sulfate (Dexadrine)	Narcolepsy, ADD
	Pemoline (Cylert)	ADD

b. Dry mouth, nausea, vomiting
c. Impotence, change in libido
d. Palpitations, tachycardia

7. Nursing considerations
   a. Assess vital signs, especially BP, since anorexiants may reverse antihypertensive medication action
   b. Monitor CBC, urinalysis, and in diabetics, blood glucose levels; changes in insulin may be required
   c. Assess mental status for mood, sensorium, and affect; stimulation, insomnia, or aggressiveness may occur
   d. Assess for withdrawal symptoms: headache, nausea, vomiting, muscle pain, weakness
   e. Evaluate client for therapeutic responses such as decreased activity in ADHD, absence of sleeping during day in narcolepsy, decrease in weight
8. Client teaching
   a. As per Box 39–1
   b. Understand the importance of rest
   c. Avoid or decrease caffeine consumption (coffee, tea, cola, chocolate), which may increase irritability or stimulation

C. Medications to treat narcolepsy and ADHD

1. Increase release of norepinephrine and dopamine in cerebral cortex to reticular-activating system
2. Administer medication at least 6 hours before bedtime
3. Common medications are listed in Table 39–3
4. Contraindicated with hypersensitivity, anxiety, history of Tourette's syndrome, children under 6 years, and glaucoma
5. Increased stimulation and increased amine effect occurs with caffeine
6. Side/adverse effects
   a. Hyperactivity, insomnia, restlessness, and talkativeness
   b. Dry mouth, palpitations and tachycardia
   c. Rash, thrombocytopenic purpura, exfoliative dermatitis
   d. Uremia, leukopenia or anemia
7. Nursing considerations
   a. Assess vital signs, especially BP, since reversal of antihypertensive drug effects may occur
   b. Monitor CBC, urinalysis, and in diabetics, monitor closely blood glucose levels; changes in insulin may be required
   c. Assess mental status for changes in mood, sensorium, and affect; stimulation, insomnia, and aggressiveness may occur
   d. Assess for withdrawal symptoms: headache, nausea, vomiting, muscle pain, weakness
   e. Assess client for changes in appetite, sleep, speech patterns
   f. Assess client for increased attention span and decreased hyperactivity
   g. Evaluate client for therapeutic responses such as decreased activity in ADHD, absence of sleeping during day in narcolepsy, or decrease in weight
8. Client education
   a. As per Box 39–1
   b. Avoid or decrease caffeine consumption (coffee, tea, cola, chocolate), which may increase irritability or stimulation

Memory Aid

Foods or beverages containing caffeine or theobromine (coffee, tea, cola, chocolate), which are CNS stimulants, are often contraindicated with medications that affect the CNS.

   c. Avoid hazardous activities until stabilized on drug; drowsiness may occur
   d. Seizure threshold is decreased in clients with seizure disorders

V. MEDICATIONS TO TREAT PARKINSON'S DISEASE

A. Anticholinergics

1. Block or compete at central acetylcholine receptor sites in the autonomic nervous system
2. Used to decrease involuntary movements in parkinsonism
3. Common medications are listed in Table 39–4 ■
4. Administration considerations
   a. Parenteral dose of trihexyphenidyl is given with client in recumbent position to prevent postural hypotension
   b. Oral form of trihexyphenidyl is given with or after food to prevent GI upset; may give with fluids other than water
   c. Parenteral dose of benztropine is given slowly; keep client at rest at least 1 hour after administering medication and monitor vital signs
   ! d. Monitor dosage of medication very carefully; even slight overdose can lead to toxicity
5. Contraindicated for clients with narrow-angle glaucoma, myasthenia gravis, or GI obstruction
6. Side/adverse effects
   a. Dry mouth, constipation, paralytic ileus
   b. Urinary retention or hesitancy
   c. Headache or dizziness
7. ! Nursing considerations
   a. Monitor intake and output (I & O); retention may cause decreased urinary output
   b. Assess client for urinary hesitancy and retention; palpate bladder if retention occurs
   c. Assess client for constipation; increase fluids, bulk, and exercise to counteract constipation
   d. If tolerance occurs during long-term therapy, dose may need to be increased or changed
   e. Assess mental status for affect, mood, CNS depression, worsening of mental symptoms during early therapy
   f. Evaluate client for therapeutic responses such as decreased tremors, secretions, absence of nausea and vomiting
8. ! Client education: as per Box 39–1; avoid driving, other hazardous activities or use of OTC cough and preparations with alcohol or antihistamines; drowsiness may occur

B. Medications affecting amount of dopamine in brain

1. Include amantadine, levodopa, dopamine agonists, and MAO type B inhibitors (see Table 39–4)
   a. Amantadine (an antiviral) promotes the synthesis and release of dopamine
   b. L-dopa is the immediate, natural precursor of dopamine
   c. Dopamine agonists (DA) directly stimulate specific subclasses of dopamine receptors

Table 39–4
Medications Used to Treat Parkinson's Disease

Type of Medication	Generic (Trade) Names
Anticholinergics	Trihexyphenidyl hydrochloride (Artane) Benztropine mesylate (Cogentin)
Antiviral	Amantadine hydrochloride (Symmetrel)
Levodopa	In combination as Sinemet (L-dopa and Carbidopa)
Dopamine agonists	Bromocriptine mesylate (Parlodel) Pergolide (Permax)
Monoamine oxidase B inhibitor	Selegiline hydrochloride (Eldepryl)

d. MAO type B inhibitors (MAOBI) increase dopamine activity by an incompletely understood mechanism
e. DAs and MAOBIs are used to enhance the effects of L-dopa
f. All increase availability of dopamine, which reduces symptoms of Parkinson's disease

2. Administration considerations
   a. Administer medication after meals for better absorption and to decrease GI symptoms
   b. Give levodopa and selegiline with a low-protein snack or meal
3. Contraindicated with hypersensitivity, narrow-angle glaucoma, and undiagnosed skin lesions
4. Significant food interactions
   a. Decreased levodopa and selegiline absorption with high-protein foods
   b. With selegiline, tyramine-containing foods may increase hypertensive reactions
5. Side/adverse effects
   a. Nausea, vomiting, dry mouth, and constipation
   b. Dizziness, headache, and depression
   c. Cough
   d. Cardiac dysrhythmias and orthostatic hypotension
   e. Sleep disturbance, "on-off" phenomenon
   f. Amantadine: convulsions, congestive heart failure (CHF), leukopenia
   g. Levodopa: hemolytic anemia, leukopenia, agranulocytosis
   h. DAs: convulsions, shock
   i. MAOBIs: tachycardia or sinus bradycardia
   j. Levodopa toxicity: mental or personality changes, increased twitching, grimacing, tongue protrusion
6. Nursing considerations
   a. Assess BP and respirations
   b. Assess mental status for affect, mood, behavioral changes, depression; complete a suicide assessment
   c. Monitor for involuntary movement, akinesia, tremors, staggering gait, muscle rigidity, and drooling
   d. Evaluate client for therapeutic responses such as a decrease in akathisia and increased mood
7. Client education
   a. Change positions slowly to prevent orthostatic hypotension
   b. Report side effects such as twitching and eye spasm; may indicate overdose
   c. As per Box 39–1; never discontinue drugs abruptly because this may precipitate parkinsonian crisis
   d. Do not take medication with foods high in protein

VI. MEDICATIONS TO TREAT ALZHEIMER'S DISEASE

A. **Action and use:** cholinesterase inhibitors elevate acetylcholine concentrations in cerebral cortex by slowing degradation of acetylcholine released in cholinergic neurons; memantine is an N–methyl–O–aspartate receptor antagonist

B. **Common medications are listed in Box 39–4**

C. **Administration considerations**
   1. Administer medication between meals; may be given with meal to reduce GI symptoms
   2. Adjust dosage to response no more frequently than every 6 weeks

D. **Contraindications:** hypersensitivity to drug or development of jaundice when taking drug

Box 39–4

Medications Used to Treat Alzheimer's Disease

- Donepezil hydrochloride (Aricept)
- Galantamine (Razadyne)
- Memantine (Namenda)
- Rivastigmine (Exelon)
- Tacrine (Cognex)

E. Side/adverse effects

1. Insomnia, headache, dizziness, confusion, ataxia, anxiety, depression, hostility, and abnormal thinking
2. Nausea, vomiting, diarrhea, abdominal pain, and constipation
3. Urinary frequency and incontinence
4. Rhinitis or cough; rash
5. Seizures or hepatotoxicity

F. Nursing considerations

1. Assess BP for hypotension or hypertension
2. Assess mental status for affect, mood, behavioral changes, depression, hallucinations, confusion; complete a suicide assessment
3. Assess GI status for nausea, vomiting, anorexia, constipation, or abdominal pain
4. Assess client for urinary frequency and incontinence
5. Monitor liver function tests frequently
6. Evaluate client for therapeutic responses such as decrease in confusion, improved mood

G. Client teaching

1. Report side effects such as twitching, nausea, vomiting, sweating; they might indicate overdose
2. As per Box 39–1; drug may be taken with food to decrease GI upset
3. Medication is not a cure; it only relieves symptoms

VII. MEDICATIONS TO TREAT MYASTHENIA GRAVIS

A. Actions and use

1. Inhibit breakdown of acetylcholine at myoneural junction
2. Used to treat muscle weakness associated with myasthenia gravis
3. Edrophonium (Tensilon) is used to diagnose myasthenia gravis

B. Common medications are listed in Box 39–5

C. Administration considerations

1. Administer prior to mealtimes for optimal absorption
2. Administer medications on time to prevent muscle weakness from impairing ability to chew food and swallow medications

D. Use of edrophonium (Tensilon) as diagnostic aid

1. Tensilon test consists of giving a dose by IV injection
2. Aids in diagnosis of myasthenia gravis in an undiagnosed client or myasthenic crisis (undermedication) in a diagnosed client; positive findings noted when muscle tone improves within 30 to 60 seconds following dose, and improved muscle strength lasts 4 to 5 minutes (positive Tensilon test)
3. Diagnosis of cholinergic crisis (often caused by overmedication) in a diagnosed client is made when muscle strength does not improve after Tensilon injection, and symptoms may worsen (negative Tensilon test)
4. Keep atropine sulfate on hand as antidote

E. Contraindications: bowel obstruction or conditions characterized by decreased GI motility, or urinary tract obstruction

F. Side/adverse effects

1. Increased bronchial secretions
2. Nausea, vomiting, diarrhea
3. Sweating and drooling
4. Urge to urinate
5. Pinpoint pupils and eye watering

Box 39–5

Medications Used to Treat Myasthenia Gravis

- Edrophonium chloride (Tensilon, Enlon)
- Neostigmine bromide (Prostigmin Bromide)
- Pyridostigmine bromide (Mestinon)
- Ambenonium chloride (Mytelase)

G. Nursing considerations

1. Keep atropine sulfate on hand as antidote
2. Keep equipment for respiratory support on hand; muscles of head, neck, and respiratory system are affected before muscles in the lower body
3. Administer medications on time to prevent onset of myasthenic symptoms
4. Observe client for weakness; if it begins 1 hour after drug administration, overdose or cholinergic crisis may be occurring; if it begins 3 or more hours after dose, myasthenic crisis (undermedication) may be occurring
5. Observe for subtle changes in speech and facial expression, ptosis, and decreased ability to swallow as indicators that additional medication is needed
6. Assess general neuromuscular strength, including gait and reflexes
7. Monitor vital signs, especially respirations, pulse, and BP

H. Client teaching

1. As per Box 39–1; report side effects such as twitching, nausea, vomiting, sweating; they might indicate overdose
2. Do not increase or abruptly decrease dose; serious consequences may result
3. Medication is not a cure; it only relieves symptoms

VIII. CENTRALLY ACTING SKELETAL MUSCLE RELAXANTS

A. Medications for spasticity

1. Decrease synaptic responses at neurotransmitters to decrease frequency, severity of **spasms** (involuntary contractions of large muscles), and pain in musculoskeletal conditions)
2. Used to reduce spasticity after spinal cord injuries, strokes, and in cerebral palsy and multiple sclerosis
3. Common medications are listed in Box 39–6
4. Contraindicated in hypersensitivity, compromised pulmonary function, active hepatic disease, impaired myocardial function
5. Side/adverse effects
   a. Dizziness, weakness, fatigue, drowsiness, disorientation, seizures
   b. Nausea, vomiting
   c. Eosinophilia, hepatic injury
6. Nursing considerations
   a. Monitor BP, weight, blood glucose level, and hepatic function
   b. Assess for increased seizure activity; drugs decrease seizure threshold
   c. Monitor I & O; check for urinary frequency, retention, or hesitancy
   d. Monitor electroencephalogram (EEG) in epileptic clients due to poor seizure control
   e. Assess for allergic reactions, fever, rash, or respiratory distress
   f. Monitor for severe weakness or numbness in extremities
   g. Monitor for CNS depression, dizziness, drowsiness, or psychiatric symptoms
   h. Monitor hepatic function (AST, ALT) and renal function (BUN, creatinine, CBC)
   i. Evaluate client for therapeutic responses such as decrease in pain and spasticity
7. Client teaching
   a. As per Box 39–1; do not discontinue medication quickly; hallucinations, spasticity, tachycardia will occur; it should be tapered off gradually by provider
   b. Notify provider of abdominal pain, jaundiced sclera, clay-colored stools, or change in color of urine
   c. Do not break, crush, or chew capsules

Box 39–6

Skeletal Muscle Relaxants

Baclofen (Lioresal)	Cyclobenzaprine hydrochloride (Flexeril)
Dantrolene sodium (Dantrium)	Methocarbamol (Robaxin)
Carisoprodol (Soma)	

B. Medications used for spasms

1. Depress multisynaptic pathways in the spinal cord, causing skeletal muscle relaxation and/or sedation
2. Used for adjunct relief of spasms
3. Common medications are listed in Box 39–6
4. Contraindicated in hypersensitivity, children under 12, intermittent porphyria, acute recovery phase of myocardial infarction (MI), heart block, CHF, and thyroid disease
5. Side/adverse effects
   - a. Dizziness, weakness, drowsiness, seizures
   - b. Nausea
   - c. Erythema multiforme
   - d. Angioedema, anaphylaxis
   - e. Dysrhythmias
6. Nursing considerations
   - a. Periodically monitor results of blood studies (including CBC, WBC with differentials) and liver studies (including AST, ALT, alkaline phosphatase)
   - b. During and after injection, assess for CNS effects, rash, conjunctivitis, and nasal congestion
   - c. Monitor results of EEG in clients with seizures
   - d. Assess for allergic reactions, including idiosyncratic reaction, anaphylaxis, rash, fever, and respiratory distress
   - e. Assess for severe weakness or numbness in extremities
   - f. Assess for CNS depression, dizziness, drowsiness, and psychiatric symptoms
   - g. Monitor for psychological dependency, increased need for drug, and increased pain
   - h. Evaluate client for therapeutic responses such as decreased pain, spasm, and spasticity
7. Client teaching
   - a. As per Box 39–1; do not discontinue medication abruptly; insomnia, nausea, headache, spasticity, tachycardia will occur
   - b. Avoid hazardous activities if drowsiness or dizziness occurs

Check Your NCLEX–RN® Exam I.Q. *You are ready for testing on this content if you can*

- Apply knowledge of expected actions and effects of neurological and musculoskeletal medications to client care.
- Correctly administer neurological and musculoskeletal medications to clients.
- Assess for side effects and adverse effects of neurological and musculoskeletal medications.
- Take appropriate action if a client has an unexpected response to a neurological or musculoskeletal medication.
- Monitor a client for expected outcomes or effects of treatment with neurological and musculoskeletal medications.

PRACTICE TEST

1 A client who is receiving phenytoin (Dilantin) to control seizures indicates an understanding of medication by making which of the following statements?

1. "I need to take more of my Dilantin when I am having a stressful day."
2. "I will be able to stop taking this medicine in about a year."
3. "I will probably need to take this medicine all my life."
4. "I will never have another seizure if I take this medicine."

2 A client with a history of seizures is admitted with a partial occlusion of the left common carotid artery. The client has taken phenytoin (Dilantin) for 10 years. When planning care for this client, it is most important that the nurse does which of the following?

1. Obtains a history of seizure incidence
2. Places an airway, suction, and restraints at the bedside
3. Asks the client to remove any dentures
4. Observes the client for increased restlessness and agitation

3 A client with a history of seizures is scheduled for an arteriogram at 10:00 a.m. and is to have nothing by mouth before the test. The client is scheduled to receive phenytoin (Dilantin) at 9:00 a.m. The nurse should take which of the following actions?

1. Omit the 9:00 a.m. dose.
2. Give the same dosage of the drug rectally.
3. Ask the physician if the drug can be given IV.
4. Administer the drug with 30 mL of water at 9:00 a.m.

4 The nurse is assessing a client with Parkinson's disease to determine effectiveness of medication therapy. The nurse would determine that the medication is not working optimally if the client is demonstrating which of the following characteristics?

1. A flattened affect
2. Tonic-clonic seizures
3. Decreased intelligence
4. Changes in pain tolerance

5 The client with Parkinson's disease asks the nurse, "How will levodopa treat this disease?" The nurse would incorporate into a response that levodopa does which of the following?

1. Improves myelination of neurons
2. Increases acetylcholine production
3. Replaces dopamine in the brain cells
4. Causes regeneration of injured thalamic cells

6 A female client taking medications for seizures has been placed on warfarin (Coumadin) for thrombophlebitis. After the weekly prothrombin time, the client contacts the office to see if there will be a dosage change. The client also mentions that she is out of her barbiturate sleeping pill. She states that she will wait until her next appointment to get a refill. The nurse instructs her to come for the refill immediately for which of the following reasons?

1. She may develop withdrawal symptoms.
2. Absence of sleep may precipitate seizures.
3. Discontinuance of the drug may affect the prothrombin level.
4. Control of seizures is dependent on the combined action of phenytoin (Dilantin) and the sleeping medication.

7 A client is brought to the emergency department in the midst of a persistent tonic-clonic seizure. Diazepam (Valium) is administered intravenously. The nurse anticipates that the effects of diazepam will be to decrease central neuronal activity and

1. slow cardiac contractions.
2. relax peripheral muscles.
3. dilate the tracheobronchial structures.
4. provide amnesia of the seizure episode.

8 The nurse would assess for which of the following as symptoms of morphine overdose in a client receiving patient-controlled analgesia?

1. Slow pulse, slow respirations, sedation
2. Slow respirations, dilated pupils, restlessness
3. Profuse sweating, pinpoint pupils, deep sleep
4. Slow respirations, constricted pupils, sedation

9 Levodopa is prescribed for a client with Parkinson's disease. Which of the following would the nurse include in the teaching plan for the client about levodopa?

1. It is poorly absorbed if given with meals.
2. It must be monitored by weekly laboratory tests.
3. It causes an initial euphoria followed by depression.
4. It may cause a side effect of orthostatic hypotension.

10 When caring for the client who is receiving phenytoin (Dilantin), the nurse emphasizes meticulous oral hygiene to the client, stating that phenytoin has which of the following effects on oral tissue?

1. It causes hyperplasia of the gums.
2. It increases alkalinity of the oral secretions.
3. It irritates gingival tissue and destroys tooth enamel.
4. It increases plaque and bacterial growth at the gum lines.

11 The physician prescribes phenobarbital sodium (Luminal) for a client who has had a tonic-clonic seizure. The nurse concludes that the client understands the side effects of phenobarbital when the client states, "I should call the doctor if I develop

1. loss of appetite or persistent fatigue."
2. dizziness when I stand up or anal itching."
3. diarrhea or a rash on the upper part of my body."
4. decreased tolerance to common foods or constipation."

PRACTICE TEST

12 The nurse administering methylphenidate (Ritalin) is monitoring the client for symptoms associated with this medication. Which of the following is not a manifestation that the nurse would assess for?

1. Insomnia
2. Fever
3. Rash
4. Palpitations

13 The physician prescribes phenytoin (Dilantin) for a client to control tonic-clonic seizures. The nurse explains in simple terms to the client that the expected effect of the drug is to do which of the following?

1. Produce an antispasmodic action on the muscles
2. Prevent depression of the central nervous system
3. Control nerve impulses originating in the motor cortex
4. Alter the permeability of the cell membrane to potassium

14 The nurse is providing information to a client taking benztropine (Cogentin), an anticholinergic given for Parkinson's disease. Which of the following statements made by the client would indicate that more instruction is needed regarding this medication?

1. "I may crush the tablets to make them easier to take."
2. "I should avoid driving until I know how this medication will affect me."
3. "I can take OTC cough or cold pills that have alcohol in them."
4. "I should never discontinue the medication abruptly."

15 The nurse is providing discharge instructions to a client with Alzheimer's disease and his family after completing medication teaching. Because medication therapy will not reverse symptoms that have developed, which of the following should be included in this discussion?

1. Keep the client in his or her own home, regardless of circumstances.
2. Provide supervision to protect the client from becoming injured, humiliated, or lost.
3. Attend a 12-step program with a home-care agency.
4. Resist using adaptive-assistive equipment.

16 Which of the following would be the most important nursing diagnosis for the client newly diagnosed with Alzheimer's disease who is just beginning medication therapy?

1. Altered fluid and electrolytes
2. Pain
3. Disturbed sleep pattern
4. Disturbed thought processes

17 The nurse would include which of the following items in an assessment of the client with Alzheimer's disease who is receiving tacrine (Cognex)?

1. Blood pressure (BP), mental status, and gastrointestinal (GI) status
2. Hemoglobin (Hgb), white blood cells (WBCs), and liver function tests
3. Hgb, red blood cells (RBCs), and mental status
4. BP, electrolytes, and edema in legs

18 The client has migraine headaches. The provider has prescribed amitriptyline hydrochloride (Elavil) as prophylaxis for the headaches. What over-the-counter (OTC) medication may intensify the actions of Elavil that the nurse must alert the client about?

1. Acetaminophen (Tylenol)
2. Aspirin (ASA)
3. Nonsteroidal anti-inflammatory drugs (NSAIDs)
4. Cimetidine (Tagamet HB)

19 When administering anticholinergic medications for Parkinson's disease, the nurse would be least concerned with assessing the client for which of the following?

1. Dry mouth
2. Constipation
3. Fever
4. Urinary retention or hesitancy

20 The client receiving phenytoin (Dilantin) asks the nurse why the doctor has prescribed folic acid with this medication. The nurse's response would be based on which of the following statements about folic acid?

1. It improves absorption of iron from foods.
2. Its content in common foods is inadequate.
3. It prevents the neuropathy caused by phenytoin.
4. Its absorption from foods is inhibited by phenytoin.

ANSWERS & RATIONALES

1 **Answer: 3** Clients with seizure disorders rarely are able to stop taking the anticonvulsants. The last option is incorrect because of the word *never*. The first two options are incorrect statements. Extra doses are not taken related to stress, and there is no way to know at this time whether medication therapy could be terminated near the 1-year mark.
Cognitive Level: Analysis **Client Need:** Physiological Integrity: Pharmacological and Parenteral Therapies **Integrated Process:** Nursing Process: Evaluation **Content Area:** Pharmacology **Strategy:** The wording of the question tells you that the correct answer is also a true statement. Use the process of elimination and medication knowledge to make a selection.

2 **Answer: 1** Phenytoin (Dilantin) is an anticonvulsant most effective in controlling tonic-clonic seizures. Data collection before planning nursing care for a client with a seizure disorder should always include a history of seizure incidence. Option 4 may be a prodromal phase in some clients, but a history of incidence is more important data. Removal of dentures may be indicated during a seizure, but not at this time. Placing an airway or restraining a patient during a seizure could cause harm.
Cognitive Level: Analysis **Client Need:** Physiological Integrity: Pharmacological and Parenteral Therapies **Integrated Process:** Nursing Process: Planning **Content Area:** Pharmacology **Strategy:** The words *most important* in the stem of the question tell you that more than one or perhaps all options may be correct and that you must choose the best option. Use medication knowledge as well as knowledge of how to manage a client during a seizure to eliminate each of the incorrect options.

3 **Answer: 3** The therapeutic blood levels of the anticonvulsant need to be maintained. The nurse should question the physician about alternate routes of administration. Omission of a dose is not prudent, nor is changing the route without a physician order.
Cognitive Level: Application **Client Need:** Physiological Integrity: Pharmacological and Parenteral Therapies **Integrated Process:** Nursing Process: Implementation **Content Area:** Pharmacology **Strategy:** The core issue of the question is how to maintain the client in a seizure-free state while NPO. Analyze each of the options to determine the method that will best protect the client from seizure activity.

4 **Answer: 1** Destruction of the neurons of the basal ganglia in Parkinson's disease results in decreased muscle tone. This gives the face a masklike appearance and causes a monotone speech pattern that can be interpreted as flat. If medication therapy was ineffective, the client would still exhibit symptoms of the disorder, such as flattened affect. The other options do not apply to this disease.
Cognitive Level: Application **Client Need:** Physiological Integrity: Pharmacological and Parenteral Therapies **Integrated Process:** Nursing Process: Assessment **Content Area:** Pharmacology **Strategy:** The core issue of the question is the symptom that should be abolished by medication therapy. Use medication knowledge and the process of elimination to make a selection.

5 **Answer: 3** Levodopa is the precursor of dopamine. It is converted to dopamine in the brain cells until needed as a neurotransmitter. Improved neural myelination, acetylcholine production, and regeneration of injured cells cannot be attributed to levodopa.
Cognitive Level: Application **Client Need:** Physiological Integrity: Pharmacological and Parenteral Therapies **Integrated Process:** Communication and Documentation **Content Area:** Pharmacology **Strategy:** The wording of the question tells you that the correct option is also a true statement. Use medication knowledge and the process of elimination to make a selection.

6 **Answer: 3** Barbiturates decrease the body's response to warfarin (Coumadin). As a result, there is less suppression of prothrombin; when inhibition caused by barbiturates disappears, hemorrhage could result. Withdrawal symptoms are not a priority concern if the client just takes the barbiturate for sleep (option 1). Absence of sleep is not likely to result in seizure activity (option 2). The control of seizure activity is not dependent on combined use of phenytoin and the barbiturate sleep aid (option 4).
Cognitive Level: Application **Client Need:** Physiological Integrity: Pharmacological and Parenteral Therapies **Integrated Process:** Nursing Process: Implementation **Content Area:** Pharmacology **Strategy:** The word *mainly* in the stem of the question tells you that more than one or perhaps all options may be partially or totally correct and that you must choose the most important option. The core issue of the question is knowledge of the interactive effects of barbiturates and warfarin.

7 **Answer: 2** Diazepam is a benzodiazepene tranquilizer and an anticonvulsant used to relax smooth muscles during seizures. Diazepam does not slow cardiac contractions (option 1), dilate tracheobronchial structures (option 3), or provide amnesia of seizure activity (option 4).
Cognitive Level: Application **Client Need:** Physiological Integrity: Pharmacological and Parenteral Therapies **Integrated Process:** Nursing Process: Analysis **Content Area:** Pharmacology **Strategy:** The wording of the question tells you that the correct option is also a true effect of the medication. Use medication knowledge and the process of elimination to make a selection.

8 **Answer: 4** Morphine is a CNS depressant. Its major adverse effect is respiratory depression. It can also lead to lethargy, pupillary constriction, and depressed reflexes. Morphine does not slow the pulse rate (option 1), although it could lower blood pressure. It does not cause restlessness (option 2) or profuse sweating (option 3).
Cognitive Level: Application **Client Need:** Physiological Integrity: Pharmacological and Parenteral Therapies **Integrated Process:** Nursing Process: Evaluation **Content Area:** Pharmacology **Strategy:** The wording of the question tells you that the correct option is also a true effect of the medication. Use medication knowledge and the process of elimination to make a selection.

9 **Answer: 4** Levodopa is the precursor of dopamine. It reduces sympathetic outflow by limiting vasoconstriction, which may result in orthostatic hypotension. The medication should be administered with food to minimize gastric irritation (option 1). It is not monitored by weekly laboratory tests (option 2), nor does it cause initial euphoria followed by depression (option 3).
Cognitive Level: Application **Client Need:** Physiological Integrity: Pharmacological and Parenteral Therapies **Integrated Process:** Nursing Process: Planning **Content Area:** Pharmacology **Strategy:** The wording of the question tells you that the correct option is also a true statement that would be included in client teaching. Use medication knowledge and the process of elimination to make a selection.

10 **Answer: 1** Gingival hyperplasia is an adverse effect of long-term phenytoin (Dilantin) therapy. Maintaining therapeutic blood levels and meticulous oral hygiene, including regular check-ups with a dentist, can decrease the incidence of hyperplasia. It does not alkalinize oral secretions (option 2), destroy tooth enamel (option 3), or increase plaque and bacterial growth at gum lines (option 4).
Cognitive Level: Application **Client Need:** Physiological Integrity: Pharmacological and Parenteral Therapies **Integrated Process:** Nursing Process: Implementation **Content Area:** Pharmacology **Strategy:** The wording of the question tells you that the correct option is also a true statement that would be included in client teaching. Use medication knowledge and the process of elimination to make a selection.

11 **Answer: 1** Phenobarbital depresses the CNS, particularly the motor cortex, producing side effects such as lethargy, loss of appetite, depression, and vertigo. The other side effects listed for phenobarbital do not include anal itching or dizziness upon standing (option 2), diarrhea or upper body rash (option 3), or decreased tolerance to common foods and constipation (option 4).
Cognitive Level: Application **Client Need:** Physiological Integrity: Pharmacological and Parenteral Therapies **Integrated Process:** Nursing Process: Evaluation **Content Area:** Pharmacology **Strategy:** The wording of the question tells you that the correct option is also a true statement about medication therapy. Use medication knowledge and the process of elimination to make a selection.

12 **Answer: 2** Fever is not a side effect of methylphenidate. Insomnia (option 1), rash (option 3), and palpitations (option 4) are possible side effects of methylphenidate.
Cognitive Level: Application **Client Need:** Physiological Integrity: Pharmacological and Parenteral Therapies **Integrated Process:** Nursing Process: Assessment **Content Area:** Pharmacology **Strategy:** Note that the stem of the question contains the word *not,* which indicates that the correct option is an incorrect item. Use knowledge of side/adverse medication effects to make a selection.

13 **Answer: 3** The primary action is to reduce voltage, frequency, and spread of electrical discharges within the motor cortex, resulting in inhibition of seizure activity. The drug does not act directly on muscles (option 1), prevent CNS depression (option 2), or change permeability of cell membranes (option 4).
Cognitive Level: Application **Client Need:** Physiological Integrity: Pharmacological and Parenteral Therapies **Integrated Process:** Teaching and Learning **Content Area:** Pharmacology **Strategy:** The wording of the question tells you that the correct option is also a true statement. Use medication knowledge and the process of elimination to make a selection.

14 **Answer: 3** OTC medications with alcohol (another CNS depressant) should be avoided unless specifically directed by the provider. The other statements would indicate understanding of the medication teaching.
Cognitive Level: Analysis **Client Need:** Physiological Integrity: Pharmacological and Parenteral Therapies **Integrated Process:** Nursing Process: Evaluation **Content Area:** Pharmacology **Strategy:** Note that the question contains the words *more instruction,* which indicates that the correct answer is an option that represents incorrect information. Use medication knowledge and the process of elimination to make a selection.

15 **Answer: 2** The Alzheimer's client and family will need much support. Medication therapy will delay progression of symptoms but will not effect a cure. The primary concern is for the safety of the client, so constant supervision is necessary. The other options are incorrect approaches.
Cognitive Level: Application **Client Need:** Physiological Integrity: Pharmacological and Parenteral Therapies **Integrated Process:** Nursing Process: Evaluation **Content Area:** Pharmacology **Strategy:** The wording of the question tells you that the correct answer is an option that is a priority teaching measure. To make your selection recall the nature of the disorder and that medication therapy will not reverse symptoms.

16 **Answer: 4** The disturbance in thought processes is the primary nursing diagnosis. Effective medication therapy will reduce the progression of symptoms of the dementia. A disturbance in sleep pattern (option 3) may become important later, but initially the thought process is most significant. Altered fluid and electrolytes (option 1) is not a nursing diagnosis, while pain (option 2) is not applicable given the information in the question.
Cognitive Level: Analysis **Client Need:** Physiological Integrity: Pharmacological and Parenteral Therapies **Integrated Process:** Nursing Process: Analysis **Content Area:** Pharmacology **Strategy:** Note the key word *primary* in the stem of the question, which tells you that you need to prioritize your answer. Use knowledge of the key effects of medication therapy and the process of elimination to make a selection.

17 **Answer: 1** Tacrine (Cognex) increases the available acetylcholine in the brain; therefore, the parasympathetic system is stimulated. Blood pressure, mental status, and GI status would be affected. Hemoglobin, red and white blood cell count, liver function, electrocyte balance, and edema in legs do not relate to this medication.
Cognitive Level: Application **Client Need:** Physiological Integrity: Pharmacological and Parenteral Therapies **Integrated Process:** Nursing Process: Assessment **Content Area:** Pharmacology **Strategy:** The wording of the question tells you that the correct option is also a true statement that would be included in client teaching. Use medication knowledge and the process of elimination to make a selection.

18 **Answer: 4** Tagamet may increase the levels of Elavil in the blood, causing seizures, tachycardia, hypertension, or toxicity. Acetaminophen (option 1), aspirin (option 2), and NSAIDs (option 3) do not have that effect.
Cognitive Level: Application **Client Need:** Physiological Integrity: Pharmacological and Parenteral Therapies **Integrated Process:** Nursing Process: Planning **Content Area:** Pharmacology **Strategy:** Options that are similar are not likely to be correct. All of the incorrect options relate to analgesia and so must be eliminated.

19 **Answer: 3** Dry mouth, constipation, and urinary retention or hesitancy are all possible side effects of anticholinergic medications. Fever is not a side effect of anticholinergic medications.
Cognitive Level: Analysis **Client Need:** Physiological Integrity: Pharmacological and Parenteral Therapies **Integrated Process:** Nursing Process: Assessment **Content Area:** Pharmacology **Strategy:** The key words in the stem of the question are *least concerned.* This tells you that the correct answer is an option that is not characteristic of this medication. Use medication knowledge and the process of elimination to make a selection.

20 **Answer: 4** Phenytoin inhibits folic acid absorption and potentiates effects of folic acid antagonists. Folic acid is helpful in correcting some anemias that can result from phenytoin administration. The other options are incorrect statements.
Cognitive Level: Application **Client Need:** Physiological Integrity: Pharmacological and Parenteral Therapies **Integrated Process:** Nursing Process: Analysis **Content Area:** Pharmacology **Strategy:** The wording of the question tells you that the correct answer is also the option that contains correct information. Use knowledge of the key side effects of medication therapy and the process of elimination to make a selection.

Key Terms to Review

attention deficit disorder p. 642
attention deficit/hyperactivity disorder p. 642
diplopia p. 639
epilepsy p. 639
gingival hyperplasia p. 639
hepatotoxicity p. 636
narcolepsy p. 642
nystagmus p. 639
paresthesias p. 639
psychomotor seizures p. 638
spasms p. 647
spasticity p. 647
status epilepticus p. 638
Stevens-Johnson syndrome p. 639
tonic-clonic seizures p. 638

References

Abrams, A. (2004). *Clinical drug therapy: Rationales for nursing practice* (7th ed.). Philadelphia: Lippincott Williams & Wilkins.

Adams, M., Josephson, D., & Holland, L. (2005). *Pharmacology for nurses: A pathophysiologic approach.* Upper Saddle River, NJ: Pearson Education.

American Psychiatric Association. (2000). *Diagnostic and statistical manual of mental disorders, Fourth Edition, Text Revision* (DSM-IV-TR). Washington, DC: American Psychiatric Association.

Deglin, J. H., & Vallerand, A. H. (2006). *Davis's drug guide for nurses* (10th ed.). Philadelphia: F. A. Davis.

Lehne, R. (2004). *Pharmacology for nursing care* (5th ed.). Philadelphia: W. B. Saunders.

McKenry, L., Tessier, E., & Hogan, M. (2006). *Mosby's pharmacology in nursing* (22nd ed.). St. Louis, MO: Elsevier Science.

Wilson, B., Shannon, M., & Stang, C. (2006). *Prentice Hall nurse's drug guide 2006.* Upper Saddle River, NJ: Pearson Education.

40 Renal Medications

Test Yourself

Are you ready for the NCLEX-RN® or course exams? Use the practice tests on the companion CD-ROM to check.

In this chapter

Cross reference

Other chapters relevant to this content area are

Age-Related Care of Older Adults	Chapter 18
Dosage Calculation and Medication Administration	Chapter 30
Renal and Genitourinary Disorders	Chapter 59

I. DIURETICS

A. Loop diuretics

1. **Diuretics** (agents that increase amount of urine excreted) inhibit electrolyte reabsorption in thick ascending loop of Henle, promoting excretion of sodium, water, chloride, and potassium
2. Mechanism of action involves renal vasodilation, to provide a temporary increase in glomerular filtration rate (GFR) and decrease in peripheral vascular resistance
3. Loop diuretics are more potent than thiazide diuretics, causing rapid diuresis and reducing vascular fluid volume, cardiac output, and blood pressure (BP)
4. Used in clients with low GFR and hypertensive emergencies
5. Also used in clients with edema, pulmonary edema, congestive heart failure (CHF), chronic renal failure (CRF), and hepatic cirrhosis
6. May be used as treatment in drug overdose to increase renal elimination
7. Common medications (Box 40–1)
8. Administration considerations
   - a. Take early in day to avoid nocturia
   - b. Give IV doses slowly over 1 to 2 minutes; rapid injection may cause hypotension
   - c. For IV infusion, dilute in 5% dextrose in water, 0.9% NaCl, or lactated Ringer's; use infusion fluids within 24 hours

Box 40–1

Common Loop Diuretics

Bumetanide (Bumex)	Furosemide (Lasix)
Ethacrynic acid (Edecrin)	Toresemide (Demedex)

! **d.** Administer IV furosemide (Lasix) slowly (20 mg/minute or less), as hearing loss can occur if injected rapidly

Memory Aid

Remember that loop diuretics such as furosemide (Lasix) can cause ototoxicity, so be sure to assess hearing and avoid exceeding recommended injection rates.

9. Side/adverse effects

! **a.** Contraindicated with **anuria** (urine output less than 400 mL daily), electrolyte depletion

b. CNS: dizziness, headache, orthostatic hypotension, weakness

c. GI: nausea, vomiting, abdominal pain, elevated lipids with decreased high-density lipoprotein (HDL), pancreatitis, anorexia, constipation

d. GU: excessive urination, nocturia, urinary bladder spasms

! **e.** Photosensitivity, sulfonamide allergy, and ototoxicity (tinnitus, hearing impairment, deafness, vertigo, and sense of fullness in ears)

f. Skin: dermatitis, urticaria, pruritis, and muscle spasm

g. Severe watery diarrhea is a side effect of ethacrynic acid (Edecrin)

h. Electrolyte imbalances: hyponatremia, hypochloremia, hypokalemia, hypomagnesemia, hypocalcemia, and hypouricemia

i. Thrombocytopenia, systemic vasculitis, interstitial nephritis, thrombophlebitis, agranulocytosis, and aplastic anemia

10. Nursing considerations

! **a.** Monitor vital signs for hypotension and tachycardia

! **b.** Monitor serum electrolytes (especially potassium, as well as sodium and calcium) and uric acid levels

! **c.** Monitor and record body weight at regular intervals at same time of day and with same scale

d. Monitor intake and output (I & O)

e. Assess indicators of dehydration: thirst, poor skin turgor, coated tongue

f. Assess for inadequate tissue perfusion and weakness, decreased muscle strength, restlessness, anxiety and agitation

g. Monitor hemoglobin and hematocrit, which may become increased due to hemoconcentration

h. Monitor for blood dyscrasias, liver, or kidney damage

11. Client education

! **a.** Eat food high in potassium to prevent hypokalemia (such as bananas, cantaloupe)

! **b.** Restrict sodium intake; do not use salt substitutes if taking potassium supplement

c. Avoid dehydration by avoiding beverages with alcohol or caffeine and replacing fluids during exercise or hot weather

d. Avoid exposure to intense heat as with baths, showers, and electric blankets

e. Take small, frequent amounts of ice chips or clear liquids if vomiting

f. During episodes of diarrhea, replace fluids with fruit juice or bouillon

g. Diuretics increase amount and frequency of urination; therefore, take medication in morning (daily) and afternoon (twice-daily dosing) to avoid nighttime urination (nocturia)

h. Photosensitivity can occur while taking a loop diuretic

! **i.** Change position slowly to avoid dizziness and **orthostatic hypotension** (a fall of more than 10 to 15 mmHg of systolic blood pressure (SBP) or a fall of more than 10 mmHg of diastolic blood pressure (DBP) and a 10% to 20% increase in heart rate)

j. Weigh self daily and report sudden weight gains or losses

! **k.** Report ringing in ears immediately; this indicates ototoxicity

l. Loop diuretics should not be used while breast feeding

B. Thiazide diuretics

1. Increase urinary excretion of sodium and water by inhibiting sodium reabsorption in cortical diluting tubule of kidney

2. Hypotensive effect may be caused by direct arteriolar vasodilation and decreased total peripheral resistance
3. Used for edema and hypertension (SBP above 140 mmHg and DBP above 90 mmHg)
4. Not effective for immediate diuresis
5. Common medications (Box 40–2)
6. Administration considerations
   a. Give medication early in the day to avoid nocturia
   b. Thiazide diuretics are ineffective if creatinine clearance level is less than 30mL/min
   c. Allow 2 to 4 weeks for maximum antihypertensive effect
   d. Metolazone (Zaroxylin) is not recommended in children because safety has not been established
7. Side/adverse effects
   a. Dizziness, vertigo, headache, and weakness
   b. Dehydration, orthostatic hypotension, nausea and vomiting, abdominal pain, diarrhea, constipation, and frequent urination
   c. Dermatitis and rash
   d. Electrolyte imbalance, impaired glucose tolerance, jaundice, muscle cramps, photosensitivity, impotence, and hyperuricemia
   e. Contraindicated with hypersensitivity to thiazide diuretics or sulfonamide derivatives, anuria, severely impaired renal or hepatic function, pregnancy or lactation
   f. Renal failure, aplastic anemia, agranulocytosis, thrombocytopenia, and anaphylactic reaction
8. Nursing considerations
   a. Monitor vital signs for hypotension and tachycardia
   b. Monitor serum electrolytes (especially potassium), calcium, and uric acid levels
   c. Monitor and record body weight at regular intervals at same time of day and on same scale
   d. Monitor I & O
   e. Assess indicators of dehydration: thirst, poor skin turgor, coated tongue
   f. Assess for inadequate tissue perfusion and weakness, decreased muscle strength, restlessness, anxiety and agitation
9. Client education
   a. Eat foods high in potassium to prevent hypokalemia
   b. Restrict sodium intake; instruct client not to use salt substitutes if taking a potassium supplement
   c. Avoid dehydration by avoiding alcohol and caffeine-containing beverages and replacing fluids during exercise or hot weather
   d. Avoid exposure to intense heat as with baths, showers, and electric blankets

Box 40–2

Common Thiazide Diuretics

Short Acting

Chlorothiazide (Diuril, Microzide)

Hydrochlorothiazide (Esidrix, HCTZ)

Intermediate Acting

Bendroflumethiazide (Naturetin)

Benzthiazide (Exna)

Hydroflumethiazide (Diucardin)

Metolazone (Zaroxylin)

Quinethazone (Hydromox)

Long Acting

Chlorthalidone (Hygroton, Thalitone)

Indapamide (Lozol)

Methyclothiazide (Enduron)

Polythiazide (Minizide, Renese)

Trichlormethiazide (Diurese)

e. Take small, frequent amounts of ice chips or clear liquids if vomiting
f. During episodes of diarrhea, replace fluids with fruit juice or bouillion
g. Diuretics increase amount and frequency of urination; therefore, take medication in morning and afternoon to avoid nocturia
h. Change position slowly to avoid dizziness and orthostatic hypotension
i. Weigh self daily and report sudden weight gains or losses
j. Diabetic clients should check blood glucose as recommmended

C. Potassium-sparing diuretics

1. Act directly on distal convoluted tubule to increase sodium excretion and decrease potassium secretion
2. Used for hypertension and edema associated with heart failure
3. Spironolactone is also used for cirrhosis of liver, primary hyperaldosteronism, hirsutism, and premenstrual syndrome
4. Common medications (Box 40–3)
5. Administration considerations
   a. Take with food or milk
   b. Avoid salt substitutes, which are high in potassium
   c. Avoid excessive ingestion of foods high in potassium
   d. When administering spironolactone to children, crush tablet and mix in flavored syrup as oral suspension
6. Side/adverse effects
   a. CNS: headache, weakness, dizziness, and orthostatic hypotension
   b. GI: nausea, vomiting, diarrhea, and constipation
   c. Impotence, muscle cramps, urticaria, gynecomastia, and breast soreness
   d. Dry mouth, photosensitivity, transient elevated blood urea nitrogen (BUN) and creatinine
   e. Aplastic anemia and thrombocytopenia
   f. Hyperkalemia (potassium greater than 5.1 mEq/L)
   g. Contraindicated with serum potassium levels greater than 5.5 mEq/mL, concurrent use with other potassium-sparing diuretics, fluid and electrolyte imbalances, anuria, acute and chronic renal insufficiency, diabetic nephropathy, hypersensitivity, and impaired hepatic function
7. Nursing considerations
   a. Monitor vital signs
   b. Monitor urine output
   c. Discontinue potassium supplements
   d. Observe closely elderly and debilitated clients for drug-induced diuresis and hyperkalemia
   e. Monitor for dehydration and electrolyte imbalance
   f. Monitor periodic serum electrolytes such as BUN and creatinine
8. Client education
   a. Take medication with food to avoid GI upset except with triamterene
   b. Avoid consumption of large quantities of foods high in potassium
   c. Report any mental confusion or lethargy immediately
   d. Monitor for signs and symptoms of hyperkalemia such as nausea, diarrhea, abdominal cramps, and tachycardia followed by bradycardia
   e. Side effects usually disappear after the drug is discontinued, but gynecomastia may persist
   f. With spironolactone, maximal diuresis may not occur until day 3 of therapy and diuresis may continue 2 to 3 days after the drug is stopped
   g. Triamterene may turn urine blue
   h. Avoid salt substitutes because they contain potassium
   i. Avoid exposure to direct sunlight to prevent photosensitivity reaction

Box 40–3

Common Potassium-Sparing Diuretics

Amiloride (Midamor)
Spironolactone (Aldactone)
Triamterene (Dyrenium)

Box 40–4

Common Carbonic Anhydrase Inhibitors

Acetazolamide (Diamox)

Dichlorphenamide (Daranide)

Methazolamide (Neptazane)

D. Carbonic anhydrase inhibitors

1. Achieve noncompetitive reversible inhibition of enzyme carbonic anhydrase, which promotes excretion of bicarbonate, sodium, potassium, and water
2. Used to treat edema caused by CHF, to decrease intraocular pressure in open-angle glaucoma, and to treat epilepsy and metabolic alkalosis
3. Common medications (Box 40–4)
4. Administration considerations
   a. Increasing dose does not appear to increase diuresis
   b. Do not administer with high-dose aspirin
   c. Intramuscular administration is not recommended
5. Side/adverse effects
   a. Confusion, drowsiness, and paresthesias
   b. Hearing dysfunction, GI upset, polyuria, and transient myopia
   c. Electrolyte imbalance, fever, rash, renal calculus, and photosensitivity
   d. Metabolic acidosis
   e. Anaphylaxis
   f. Bone marrow depression
   g. Thrombocytopenia purpura, hemolytic anemia, leukopenia, pancytopenia, and agranulocytosis
   h. Severe reactions to sulfonamides, including Stevens-Johnson syndrome, toxic epidermal necrolysis, fulminant hepatic necrosis, coma, and death
   i. Contraindicated in narrow-angle or acute glaucoma, any situation with decreased sodium and/or potassium levels, marked kidney or liver dysfunction; use cautiously with chronic obstructive pulmonary disease (COPD)
6. Nursing considerations
   a. Monitor for signs and symptoms of dehydration
   b. Assess for alterations in skin integrity
   c. Assess for edema
   d. Assess vital signs, daily weight, and I & O
   e. Assess cardiovascular and respiratory status
   f. Assess changes in level of consciousness and activity level
   g. Assess dietary intake for foods high in salt
   h. Maintain fluid restriction as ordered
7. Client education
   a. Do not take aspirin or aspirin-containing medications
   b. Report symptoms of anorexia, lethargy, or tachypnea
   c. Use caution while driving or performing tasks that require alertness, coordination, or physical dexterity because they can cause drowsiness
   d. Monitor for signs of renal calculi
   e. Follow-up with scheduled lab tests is important
   f. Weigh self daily at same time of day and report any acute weight gain or loss (more than 2–3 pounds per day)
   g. Avoid foods and beverages containing high amounts of sodium

E. Osmotic diuretics

1. Increase osmotic pressure of glomerular filtrate in proximal tubule and loop of Henle inhibiting reabsorption of water and electrolytes, thus promoting diuresis
2. Used to prevent and manage acute renal failure (ARF) and oliguria
3. Used to decrease intracranial or intraocular pressure
4. Mannitol is used with chemotherapy to induce diuresis
5. Common medications (Box 40–5)
6. Administration considerations
   a. Medications are administered IV by slow infusion

Box 40–5

Common Osmotic Diuretics

Mannitol (Osmitrol)

Urea (Ureaphil)

b. Urea turns to ammonia if left standing
c. Do not infuse with blood or blood products
d. Mannitol crystallizes at low temperatures

7. Side/adverse effects
    a. Headache, syncope, and hypotension
    b. Nausea, vomiting, dry mouth, urine retention, electrolyte imbalance, and urticaria
    c. Seizures
    d. Thrombophlebitis
    e. CHF
    f. Cardiovascular collapse
    g. Contraindicated with severely impaired renal function, marked dehydration, breast feeding, hepatic failure, active intracranial bleed, anuria, severe pulmonary congestion, and severe CHF
8. Nursing considerations
    a. Maintain adequate hydration
    b. Monitor fluid and electrolyte balance
    c. Monitor BUN
    d. Indwelling catheter should be used in comatose clients for accurate I & O
    e. Monitor I & O and vital signs hourly while on Mannitol
    f. Daily weight
    g. Monitor renal function, fluid balance, serum and urinary sodium and potassium levels
    h. Assess for signs of decreasing intracranial pressure if appropriate
    i. Monitor lung and heart sounds for signs of pulmonary edema
9. Client education
    a. Monitor weight
    b. Report immediately pain in chest or legs, shortness of breath, or apnea
    c. Change position slowly to prevent dizziness or orthostatic hypotension
    d. Drink only fluids ordered if on a fluid restriction also
    e. Use sugarless hard candies to reduce dry mouth

II. URINARY ANTI-INFECTIVES

A. Overview

1. Act as **bacteriostatic** (inhibition of the growth of bacterial without destruction) and **bactericidal** (destroying bacteria) agents
2. Act as disinfectants within urinary tract
3. Used to treat urinary tract infections
4. Common medications (Box 40–6)

B. Administration considerations

1. May take with food or milk to decrease GI upset
2. Check renal and hepatic function before administering
3. Oral suspension of nitrofurantoin may stain teeth; instruct client to rinse mouth following dose
4. Complete full course of therapy to prevent reinfection or overgrowth of resistant organisms

Box 40–6

Common Urinary Tract Anti-Infectives

Methenamine (Hiprex, Mandelamine)	Sulfamethizole (Thiosulfil Forte)
Nalidixic acid (NegGram)	Sulfamethoxazole (Gantanol)
Nitrofurantoin (Macrodantin)	Sulfisoxazole (Gantrisin)
Trimethoprim (Proloprim)	Trimethoprim/sulfamethoxazole (Bactrim)

C. Side/adverse effects

1. Drowsiness, weakness, headache, dizziness
2. Sensitivity to light, blurred vision
3. GI distress, pruritis, rash, arthralgia
4. Seizures, increased intracranial pressure
5. Leukopenia, thrombocytopenia, angioedema
6. Contraindicated with hypersensitivity, megaloblastic anemia and folate deficiency, renal insufficiency, severe hepatic insufficiency, severe dehydration, anuria, oliguria, and seizure disorder

D. Nursing considerations

1. Drugs work best if client is well (but not overly) hydrated
2. Administer with meals to decrease GI distress
3. Monitor renal and liver function
4. Check urine pH before administration because some drugs work best in acidic urine
5. Cranberry juice or vitamin C may be added to acidify urine
6. Monitor CNS side effects
7. Ingestion of large amount of fluid while taking methenamide will reduce antibacterial effects by diluting medication and raising urinary pH

E. Client education

1. Long-term therapy is common even if feeling fine
2. Drink at least 8 glasses of water daily
3. Take medications with meals to decrease GI distress
4. Avoid alkalizing fluids such as milk, fruit juices, or sodium bicarbonate
5. Notify physician of any new medications
6. Use sunscreen and avoid excessive exposure to sunlight
7. Notify physician of any CNS side effects
8. Nitrofurantoin may discolor urine brown; this is not harmful and will disappear after drug is discontinued

III. URINARY ANTISPASMODICS

A. Overview

1. Relax smooth muscles of the urinary tract
2. Decrease bladder muscle spasms
3. Used to manage disorders of lower urinary tract associated with hypermotility: dysuria, urgency, nocturia, suprapubic pain, frequency, and incontinence
4. Common medications (Box 40–7)

B. Administration considerations: administer 1 hour before antacids or antidiarrheals

C. Side/adverse effects

1. Headache, insomnia, drowsiness, dizziness, confusion, excitement, palpitations
2. Blurred vision
3. Dry mouth, GI distress, urinary hesitancy, urine retention, urticaria
4. Leukopenia
5. Contraindicated in glaucoma, obstructive breathing, obstructive GI disease, severe ulcerative colitis, and myasthenia gravis, hypersensitivity to anticholinergics, paralytic ileus, unstable cardiovascular status, urinary tract obstruction

D. Nursing considerations

1. Monitor effect of medication
2. Monitor for CNS manifestations
3. Monitor I & O

Box 40–7

Common Antispasmodic Medications

Hyoscyamine (Cystospaz)	Oxybutynin chloride (Ditropan)
Tolterodine tartrate (Detrol)	Flavoxate (Urispas)

E. Client education

1. Drowsiness and blurred vision may occur; use caution with driving or operating machinery
2. Use hard, sugarless candy for dry mouth
3. Avoid alcohol, which increases drowsiness
4. Swallow pill whole and do not chew or crush
5. The shell of medication may appear in stool
6. Inform client of side effects and to report them to the provider

IV. URINARY ANALGESIC

A. Overview

1. Has a local anesthetic effect on urinary tract mucosa
2. Used to relieve pain with urinary tract infections or irritation
3. Does not have any antimicrobial properties
4. Common medication: phenazopyridine (Pyridium)

B. Administration considerations

1. Drug colors body fluids red or orange and may stain fabrics
2. May be used with antibiotics and should be discontinued after 2 days of antibiotic use

C. Side/adverse effects

1. Headache and vertigo
2. Nausea and GI distress
3. Anaphylaxis
4. Methemoglobinemia
5. Contraindicated in renal and hepatic failure

D. Nursing considerations

1. Assess for presence of urinary tract infection (UTI)
2. Assess urinary function and output
3. Monitor I & O
4. Monitor sclera for yellow tinge
5. Ensure renal function before administering
6. Use only as an analgesic

E. Client education

1. Maintain good hygiene to prevent UTI
2. Possible side effects
3. Drug discolors urine red or orange and may stain clothing or soft contact lenses
4. Do not double dose if a dose is missed
5. Take medication with food to decrease GI distress
6. Increase fluid intake
7. May be needed for only 24 to 48 hours once antibiotic therapy is begun for UTI
8. Notify provider if yellowing of the eyes occurs
9. Report symptoms that worsen or do not resolve

V. CHOLINERGIC AGENT

A. Overview

1. Direct-acting cholinergic agent is indicated for use with neurogenic bladder and urinary retention from nonobstructive causes
2. Contracts detrusor muscle of urinary bladder, which increases bladder tone and ability to initiate micturition (voiding)
3. Common medication: bethanechol chloride (Urecholine)

B. Administration considerations

1. Give oral dose on empty stomach to reduce nausea and vomiting (1 hour before or 2 hours after meals)
2. Alternate route is subcutaneous; do not give by IM or IV route to avoid life-threatening symptoms of cholinergic stimulation
3. Keep atropine sulfate available as an antidote

C. Side/adverse effects

1. Headache and malaise

2. Flushing and increased sweating
3. Hypotension with dizziness and faintness
4. Blurred vision and lacrimation
5. Nausea, vomiting, diarrhea, and abdominal cramps
6. Urgency with urination or defecation
7. Dyspnea or acute asthmatic attack
8. Contraindications of cholinergic drugs include mechanical obstruction of GI or urinary tracts, peptic ulcer disease, COPD, bradycardia, parkinsonism, hypotension, and A-V blocks

D. Nursing considerations

1. Monitor for 1 hour after subcutaneous dose for early signs of overdosage: salivation, sweating, flushing, abdominal cramps, and nausea
2. Use atropine as ordered for antidote
3. Monitor I & O to determine effectiveness
4. Monitor client's ambulation as needed according to response to drug

E. Client education

1. Change postions slowly, especially from lying to standing
2. Do not stand in place for long periods, and lie down at first sign of faintness
3. Use caution in activities to maintain safety because of risk of blurred vision

VI. DOPAMINE IN RENAL FAILURE

A. Action and use

1. Primary focus of pharmacologic management of renal failure is to restore and maintain renal perfusion and to eliminate drugs that are directly nephrotoxic
2. Dopaminergic receptors cause vasodilation in the renal, mesenteric, coronary, and intracerebral vascular beds
3. Used to increase urine flow

B. Dosage: dopamine (Intropin) 2 to 5 mcg/kg/min to increase renal perfusion; may increase to 50 mcg/kg/min IV to raise blood pressure

C. Administration considerations

1. Use an IV infusion device to control rate of flow
2. Administered into a large vein to prevent possibility of extravasation
3. Correct hypovolemia before initiation of dopamine therapy
4. Decrease dose as soon as hemodynamic condition is stabilized
5. Do not mix with other medications
6. Discard solution after 24 hours and replace with new solution

D. Side/adverse effects

1. Headache, tachycardia, angina, palpitations, hypotension, bradycardia, vasoconstriction, widening of QRS complex on electrocardiogram
2. Nausea and vomiting, piloerection, azotemia
3. Anaphylaxis
4. Asthmatic episodes
5. Severe hypertension
6. Contraindicated in uncorrected tachydysrhythmias, pheochromocytoma, or ventricular fibrillation; use cautiously with occlusive vascular disease, cold injuries, diabetic endarteritis, and arterial embolism

E. Nursing considerations

1. Carefully monitor I & O
2. Assess infusion site frequently for extravasation; possibly use phentolamine mesylate (Regitine) diluted in normal saline and injected into site of extravasation as an antidote
3. Monitor vital signs, cardiac output, and EKG frequently
4. Monitor for side effects

F. Client education

1. Purpose and effects of medication
2. Report side effects

VII. HEMATOPOIETIC GROWTH FACTOR

A. Action and use

1. Used to stimulate red blood cell (RBC) production
2. Reverses anemia associated with CRF, HIV infection, and chemotherapy used to treat nonmyeloid malignancies

B. Common medication: epoetin (Epogen, Procrit) dosed 3 times/wk

C. Administration considerations

1. Do not shake solution
2. Use only one dose per vial, and do not reenter vial
3. Inspect solution for particulate matter prior to use
4. IV administration: epoetin may be given undiluted by direct IV as a bolus dose or during hemodialysis
5. Rotate injection sites if given subcutaneously to minimize irritation

D. Side/adverse effects

1. Hypertension
2. Headache, seizure
3. Iron deficiency, sweating
4. Thrombocytosis, clotting of AV fistula
5. Bone pain, arthralgias
6. Contraindicated in uncontrolled hypertension, known hypersensitivity to mammalian cell-derived products, and albumin

E. Nursing considerations

1. Evaluate serum ferritin and transferrin levels prior to beginning therapy
2. Blood pressure may rise during early therapy as the Hct increases; notify physician of a rapid rise in Hct greater than 4 points in 2 weeks
3. Do not give with any other drug solution
4. Initial effects can be seen within 1 to 2 weeks
5. Hct reaches satisfactory levels (30% to 36%) in 2 to 3 months
6. Monitor for hypertensive encephalopathy in clients with CRF during period of increasing Hct
7. Client may require additional heparin during dialysis to prevent clotting of the vascular access

F. Client education

1. Self-monitor vital signs, especially BP
2. Headache is a common adverse effect; it should be reported if severe
3. Avoid driving and other hazardous activity because of possible seizure, especially during first 90 days of therapy
4. Keep all follow-up appointments

VIII. MEDICATIONS TO PREVENT ORGAN REJECTION

A. Cyclosporine (Neoral)

1. An immunosuppressant that acts on T lymphocytes to suppress production of interleukin-2, gamma interferon, and other cytokines
2. Used to prevent rejection of allogenic kidney transplant
3. Oral administration is preferred
4. Blood levels should be monitored frequently
5. Administer prednisone concurrently
6. Instruct client to monitor for signs of infection
7. Avoid drinking grapefruit juice, which can raise cyclosporine levels, thus increasing risk of toxicity
8. Mix concentrated medication solution with milk, chocolate milk, or orange juice just before administration
9. Place oral liquid into a glass (not plastic or Styrofoam cup) using calibrated pipette; stir well and drink immediately; rinse glass with diluent and drink it also to ensure complete dose is obtained
10. Side effects: nausea and vomiting, hypertension, tremor, hirsutism, depression, and anaphylactic shock

B. Tacrolimus (Prograf)

1. An immunosuppressant that is used concurrently with glucocorticoids
2. Increases risk of infection
3. Increases risk of development of lymphomas
4. Key toxicity is to kidney, but other adverse effects include neurotoxicity, hypertension, hyperkalemia, hyperglycemia, and GI effects

C. Azathioprine (Imuran)

1. Cytotoxic medication that suppresses cell-mediated and humoral immunity
2. Used with cyclosporine to help suppress transplant rejection; other uses include rheumatoid arthritis and other autoimmune disorders
3. Can cause neutropenia and thrombocytopenia secondary to bone marrow depression
4. Other adverse effects: nausea, vomiting, and secondary infection

D. Mycophenolate mofetil (CellCept)

1. A cytotoxic medication used in conjunction with cyclosporine and glucocorticoids
2. Is associated with increased risk of secondary infection and various malignancies
3. Adverse effects include GI (vomiting, diarrhea), neutropenia, sepsis, hypertension, fever, rash, and abdominal pain
4. Contraindicated for use during pregnancy

E. Prednisone (Deltasone), a glucocorticoid; see Chapter 42

F. Muromonab-CD3 (Orthoclone OKT3)

1. Antibody used to prevent acute allograft rejection of kidney transplants
2. Side effects: nausea and vomiting, chest pain, dyspnea, fever, and chills

G. Daclizumab (Zenapax)

1. Antibody used to prevent acute kidney rejection
2. Used in conjunction with glucocorticoids and cyclosporine
3. Give by IV route; first dose should be within 24 hours before surgery
4. Do not administer to client with allergy to protein (contraindication)
5. Side effects are many and include GI symptoms, chest pain, shortness of breath, edema, joint pain, and delayed wound healing

H. Basiliximab (Simulect)

1. Similar to daclizumab, but first dose is administered within 2 hours of transplant
2. Side effects are the same as for daclizumab and also CNS symptoms such as headache, dizziness, tremors, and insomnia

I. Client teaching for immunosuppressants to prevent organ rejection

1. Take medications as directed
2. Monitor temperature and other indicators of infection; report these to health care provider
3. Avoid crowds and being in company of people with communicable infections
4. Keep all appointments for follow-up care

Check Your NCLEX-RN® Exam I.Q. *You are ready for testing on this content if you can*

- Apply knowledge of expected actions and effects of renal medications to client care.
- Correctly administer renal medications to clients.
- Assess for side effects and adverse effects of renal medications.
- Take appropriate action if a client has an unexpected response to a renal medication.
- Monitor a client for expected outcomes or effects of treatment with renal medications.

PRACTICE TEST

1 A client is taking nalidixic acid (NegGram) for treatment of a urinary problem. The nurse explains to the client that the medication is best described as which of the following?

1. An antispasmodic
2. A uricosuric
3. An anti-infective
4. An analgesic

VIII. MUCOSAL PROTECTIVE AGENTS

A. Overview

1. Misoprostol (Cytotec) inhibits gastric secretion, protects gastric mucosa by increasing bicarbonate and mucus production, and decreases pepsin levels; is used to prevent gastric ulcers and has investigional use with duodenal ulcers
2. Sucralfate (Carafate) protects ulcer site from gastric acid by forming an adherent coating with albumin and fibrinogen; it absorbs pepsin, decreasing its activity; is used for short-term treatment of duodenal ulcers with continued maintenance treatment at lower doses; investigational use for gastric ulcers

B. Common medications: misoprostol (Cytotec), sucralfate (Carafate)

C. Administration considerations

1. Sucralfate should be taken 1 hour before meals and bedtime or 2 hours after meals
2. Sucralfate should be taken 2 hours after medications and not within 2 hours of antacids
3. Misoprostol should be taken with food

D. Contraindications

1. Misoprostol is contraindicated in clients who are allergic to prostaglandins, or who are pregnant or lactating
2. Use cautiously with clients with renal impairment and/or older than 64 years
3. Safety has not been established for children under age 18
4. Misoprostol may cause miscarriage with serious bleeding
5. No known contraindications with sucralfate, but safety in children and during lactation is not fully established

E. Side/adverse effects

1. Dizziness, headache, constipation, diarrhea, nausea, vomiting, flatulence, dry mouth, and rash
2. Misoprostol may cause spotting, cramping, dysmenorrhea, menstrual disorders, and postmenopausal bleeding
3. Angioedema
4. Respiratory difficulty, laryngospasm
5. Seizures

F. Nursing considerations

1. Assess effect of medication on GI symptoms and monitor side effects
2. Assess for pregnancy
3. Monitor concurrent medications
4. Assess respiratory status, swallowing, or change in gag reflex

G. Client teaching

1. Avoid gastric irritants such as caffeine, alcohol, smoking, and spicy foods
2. As per Box 41–1; report side effects to health care provider for possible dosage change
3. Follow contraceptive practices while on misoprostol
4. Report any abnormal vaginal bleeding
5. Do not take misoprostol if pregnant; discontinue use if pregnancy occurs or is suspected
6. Avoid pregnancy at least 1 month or 1 menstrual cycle after stopping medication
7. Increase fluids and fiber to decrease constipation
8. Follow instructions for antacid use to decrease interaction
9. Report immediately any difficulty swallowing or breathing

IX. ANTACIDS

A. Overview

1. Gastric acid–neutralizing agent
2. Used for symptomatic relief of hyperacidity associated with GI disorders
3. Used as antiflatulent to alleviate symptoms of gas and bloating

B. Common medications are listed in Box 41–8

C. Administration considerations: take at least 2 hours apart from other drugs where a drug interaction may occur

Box 41-8

Antacids	
	Aluminum carbonate (Basaljel)
	Aluminum hydroxide (Amphojel)
	Calcium carbonate (Tums, Dicarbisol)
	Dihydroxyaluminum sodium carbonate (Rolaids)
	Magnesium trisilicate (Gaviscon)
	Magnesium hydroxide and aluminum hydroxide (Maalox)
	Magnesium hydroxide, aluminum hydroxide, and simethicone (Mylanta, others)

D. Contraindications

1. Safety has not been established for use of antacids by lactating women
2. Magnesium hydroxide is contraindicated with abdominal pain, nausea, vomiting, diarrhea, severe renal dysfunction, fecal impaction, rectal bleeding, colostomy, ileostomy
3. Aluminum carbonate antacids: prolonged use of high doses with low serum phosphate
4. Calcium carbonate antacids: hypercalcemia and hypercalciuria, severe renal disease, renal calculi, GI hemorrhage or obstruction, dehydration
5. Dihydroxyaluminum sodium carbonate: aluminum sensitivity, severe renal disease, dehydration, clients on sodium-restricted diets

E. Side/adverse effects

1. Antacids increase gastric pH, and may bind with other drugs, decreasing their absorption and effectiveness; separate their administration from other drugs by 1–2 hours or as recommended by drug literature
2. Prolonged use of antacids may alter aluminum, calcium, sodium, and phosphate levels
3. Belching, constipation, flatulence, diarrhea, and gastric distention
4. Hypophosphatemia (anorexia, malaise, tremors, muscle weakness)
5. Aluminum toxicity (dementia) may occur with repeated dosing of aluminum-based products
6. Hypercalcemia and metabolic alkalosis may occur with antacids containing calcium carbonate
7. Use of antacids containing sodium carbonate may worsen hypertension and risk for heart failure from increased sodium intake
8. ! Aluminum-containing antacids can cause constipation, while magnesium-containing antacids tend to cause diarrhea

! **F. Nursing considerations**

1. Shake suspension well
2. Flush NG tube with water after administration
3. Observe for signs and symptoms of altered phosphate levels: anorexia, muscle weakness, and malaise
4. Liquid preparations act more quickly than tablets; follow liquid dose with 4 ounces of water to speed effectiveness

! **G. Client teaching**

1. Understand methods to avoid constipation; drink plenty of fluids
2. Take as directed; do not exceed maximum dose
3. Keep out of reach of children
4. Antacids may interact with certain medications; notify health care provider of any prescribed medications
5. Do not use without medical advice if diagnosed with kidney disease

X. TREATMENT REGIMENS FOR *HELICOBACTER PYLORI*

A. Overview

1. Antisecretory and antimicrobial action against most strains of *Helicobacter pylori* (*H. pylori*)

Box 41–9

Treatment Regimens for *Helicobacter pylori*

Lansoprazole, amoxicillin, clarithromycin (Prevpak) (currently most effective)

Bismuth subsalicylate, metronidazole, tetracycline (Helidac)

Omeprazole, clarithromycin (Prilosec/Biaxin)

Ranitidine, bismuth citrate, clarithromycin (Titrec/Biaxin)

Lansoprazole, amoxicillin (Prevacid/Amoxil)

2. Used to eradicate *H. pylori* infection and to reduce risk of duodenal ulcer recurrence

B. Common medication combinations are listed in Box 41–9

C. Administration considerations

1. Swallow all pills whole except bismuth, which should be chewed and not swallowed whole
2. If dose is missed, continue with normal dosage regimen; do not double dose
3. Do not administer it client has allergy to any component of therapy
4. Pregnant women should not take regimens containing clarithromycin

D. Side/adverse effects

1. Rash, nausea, vomiting, diarrhea, abnormal taste, abdominal pain, dyspepsia
2. Headache, photosensitivity
3. Transient CNS reactions such as anxiety, behavior changes, tinnitus, and vertigo
4. Ventricular dysrhythmias

E. Nursing considerations

1. Note signs and symptoms, onset, and duration of symptoms
2. Document allergy status
3. Determine pregnancy status; do not adminster bismuth subsalicylate to children because of risk of Reye syndrome
4. Document previous therapies used; document confirmation of infection

F. Client teaching

1. Understand importance of compliance
2. Avoid gastric irritants such as smoking, alcohol, and caffeine
3. Practice stress reduction techniques
4. Report side effects or continued symptoms to health care provider
5. Bismuth-containing preparations may cause darkening of tongue and stool
6. Review drug packaging (some preparations are prepackaged)
7. Do not double dose if dose is missed
8. Use additional contraceptive measures because antibiotics can decrease birth control pill effectiveness
9. Avoid prolonged exposure to sun

XI. GALLSTONE-DISSOLVING AGENT

A. Urosodiol (Actigall)

1. Used to dissolve gallbladder stones smaller than 20 mm
2. Absorbed in small bowel, secreted into hepatic bile ducts, and expelled into duodenum in response to eating
3. Natural occurring bile acid that inhibits hepatic synthesis and secretion of cholesterol

B. Administration considerations: use beyond 24 months has not been established

C. Contraindications

1. Clients who have calcified cholesterol stones, radiopaque stones, or radiolucent bile pigment stones
2. Excretion in breast milk is not known: use with caution
3. Avoid in clients with acute cholecystitis, biliary obstruction, pancreatitis, allergy to bile acids, and chronic liver disease

D. Side/adverse effects

1. Nausea, vomiting, abdominal pain, constipation, diarrhea, rash
2. Headache, fatigue, anxiety, sweating
3. Thinning of hair, arthralgia

E. Nursing considerations

1. If no dissolution of partial stone is observed in 12 months, drug will probably not be effective
2. Gallbladder ultrasound should be done every 6 months during first year of therapy
3. Document indications and length of therapy
4. Determine pregnancy status

F. Client teaching

1. Avoid antacid use with drug unless prescribed
2. Therapy may take up to 24 months, and stones may recur
3. Report any side effects to health care provider
4. Be aware that birth control pills may decrease drug effect
5. Understand importance of follow-up visits and diagnostic tests

XII. PANCREATIC ENZYME REPLACEMENT

A. Pancrelipase

1. Enzyme (lipase, amylase, and protease) replacement therapy for cystic fibrosis, chronic pancreatitis, ductal obstructions, or pancreatic insufficiency
2. Various formulations available with trade names of Creon 5, Ku-Zyme, Pancrease, and Viokase

B. Administration considerations

1. Swallow tablets/capsules whole; do not crush or chew
2. If swallowing is difficult, open capsules and give contents in applesauce or pudding to swallow without chewing
3. Take medications with meals; do not give with antacids or iron

C. Contraindications: hypersensitivity to pork protein or enzymes, or with acute pancreatitis

D. Side/adverse effects

1. Nausea, diarrhea, or abdominal cramps
2. Hyperuricemia

E. Nursing considerations

1. Monitor for side effects and monitor steatorrhea: it should diminish with appropriate dose of medication
2. Assess and monitor to maintain good nutritional status
3. Document allergies
4. Assess swallowing ability or difficulty
5. Monitor uric acid levels

F. Client teaching

1. Understand dietary interventions; consult with dietitian for counseling and meal planning
2. Take before or with meals with plenty of water
3. Report any side effects to health care provider

Check Your NCLEX-RN® Exam I.Q.

You are ready for testing on this content if you can

- Apply knowledge of expected actions and effects of gastrointestinal medications to client care.
- Correctly administer gastrointestinal medications to clients.
- Assess for side effects and adverse effects of gastrointestinal medications.
- Take appropriate action if a client has an unexpected response to a gastrointestinal medication.
- Monitor a client for expected outcomes or effects of treatment with gastrointestinal medications.

PRACTICE TEST

1 A 60-year-old client has been prescribed rabeprazole (Aciphex) for symptoms of gastroesophageal reflux disease (GERD). He has trouble swallowing pills. What alternate medication could be used for this client?

1. Omeprazole (Prilosec)
2. Pantoprazole (Protonix)
3. Lansoprazole (Prevacid)
4. There is no substitute for Aciphex

PRACTICE TEST

2. A nurse is teaching a female client newly diagnosed with *Helicobacter pylori* infection. The nurse expects that which of the following medications will not be used after learning the client is pregnant?

1. Metronidazole (Flagyl)
2. Amoxicillin (Amoxil)
3. Clarithromycin (Biaxin)
4. Ciprofloxacin (Cipro)

3. A client is taking bismuth for diarrhea. For which of the following side effects unique to this medication would a nurse monitor?

1. Darkening of the tongue
2. Dyspepsia
3. Abdominal pain
4. Diarrhea

4. A client's breath urease test is positive for *Helicobacter pylori* organisms. The nurse anticipates that which of the following medications will be ordered to eradicate this infection most effectively?

1. Antacids and amoxicillin
2. Omeprazole, ranitidine, and amoxicillin
3. Combination of proton pump inhibitor, amoxicillin, and clarithromycin
4. Clarithromycin and bismuth salicylate

5. The nurse would interpret that which of the following medications is ordered at a safe and effective dosage range for an adult client who is experiencing nausea and vomiting?

1. Promethazine (Phenergan) 25 mg every 4 to 6 hours prn
2. Prochlorperazine (Compazine) 200 mg every 6 hours
3. Metoclopramide (Reglan) 30 mg ac and HS
4. Trimethobenzamide hydrochloride (Tigan) 20 mg tid prn

6. A client is receiving omeprazole (Prilosec) for esophageal reflux. The nurse makes it a priority to monitor the results of which of the following laboratory studies?

1. Blood urea nitrogen (BUN)
2. Uric acid
3. Liver enzymes
4. White blood cell (WBC) count

7. When caring for a client with onset of severe nausea, the nurse telephones the health care provider for an order for which of the following emetics that has the fastest onset of action?

1. Oral promethazine (Phenergan)
2. Scopolamine transdermal (Transderm-Scop)
3. Oral metoclopramide (Reglan)
4. Haloperidol (Haldol)

8. A client has been diagnosed with severe erosive esophagitis. The nurse developing a medication teaching plan would be sure to include information about which of the following most appropriate medications to treat the disorder?

1. Sucralfate (Carafate)
2. Omeprazole (Prilosec)
3. Nizatidine (Axid)
4. Amoxicillin (Amoxil)

9. A client has been advised to take an antacid to neutralize gastric acid and thereby decrease the pain of gastric irritation. What antacid-related administration issues should be discussed with the client?

1. To chew tablets and follow with 4 ounces of water
2. To take the dose of antacid within 2 hours of any other prescribed medication
3. To take the antacids on a regular basis for up to 6 weeks
4. To take them after the onset of episodes of gastric irritation

10. A client who has a history of glaucoma is diagnosed with a gastrointestinal disorder. The nurse would consult with the physician after noting a medication order for which of the following medications that should be used very cautiously, if at all, for this client?

1. Dicyclomine (Bentyl)
2. Omeprazole (Prilosec)
3. Metoclopramide (Reglan)
4. Magnesium hydroxide (Milk of Magnesia)

11. A client who needs to take a histamine H_2 antagonist also has a history of several health problems. The nurse explains to this client that which histamine antagonist should be avoided because it has the greatest number of drug interactions?

1. Famotidine (Pepcid)
2. Ranitidine (Zantac)
3. Nizatidine (Axid)
4. Cimetidine (Tagamet)

PRACTICE TEST

12 A client newly diagnosed with a gastric ulcer has been prescribed sucralfate (Carafate). The nurse explains that this medication will have which of the following beneficial effects for the client?

1. It will reduce GI spasms.
2. It will protect the eroded ulcer surface from stomach acid.
3. It will help relieve nausea and vomiting.
4. It will act as an anticholinergic.

13 A client with chronic pancreatitis has been prescribed pancrelipase (Pancrease). The nurse who is teaching the client about this medication would include that pancrelipase increases digestion of what foods?

1. Proteins and starches
2. Proteins and fats
3. Starches and fats
4. Vitamins and starches

14 A female client reports having diarrhea for the past 24 hours. She took loperamide (Imodium) all day yesterday per dosage instructions without relief. Today, she has a temperature of 102°F, excessive thirst, and severe abdominal cramping. What is the highest priority action for the nurse at this time?

1. Obtain a further history of digestive disorders
2. Discuss dietary factors that may be causing the diarrhea
3. Suggest acetaminophen (Tylenol) for fever and pain
4. Notify the health care provider

15 A parent of a 2-year-old child asks the nurse why bismuth subsalicylate (Pepto-Bismol) should not be used for diarrhea in children under 3 years old. The nurse should include which of the following rationales in a response?

1. It has an offensive taste that children do not like.
2. It could lead to development of Reye syndrome because of its salicylate content.
3. It has a higher than recommended lead content.
4. It can cause darkening of the tongue, which is frightening for children of that age.

16 The nurse is giving follow-up instructions to a client with irritable bowel syndrome (IBS). The nurse provides information about which medication that would be beneficial to treat both the diarrhea and constipation associated with IBS?

1. Methylcellulose (Citrucel)
2. Docusate sodium (Colace)
3. Dicyclomine (Bentyl)
4. Bisacodyl (Dulcolax)

17 A 26-year-old female client comes to the clinic for an annual health examination. She has been taking misoprostol (Cytotec) for several years following a gastric ulcer. She is getting married next month. What is the priority nursing intervention for this client?

1. Discuss whether or not to continue taking her oral contraceptive.
2. Discuss family planning.
3. Ask the client about the need for sexually transmitted disease (STD) counseling.
4. Explain risks of using misoprostol during pregnancy.

18 An 82-year-old female who has had compensated congestive heart failure for years comes to the ambulatory care center for a quarterly routine health examination. At this time she reports increased fatigue, weakness, and dizziness, although physical examination findings are normal. Laboratory results include a normal CBC, sodium 123 mEq/L, and potassium 3.5 mEq/L. Her medications include Lasix 20 mg daily, K-Dur 10 mEq daily, Lanoxin 0.125 mg daily, and prn bisacodyl (Dulcolax) suppository. What information would be helpful to evaluate the cause of the client's hyponatremia?

1. How frequently the client uses the bisacodyl suppository
2. Whether the client has skipped digoxin doses in the last week
3. Whether the client has taken excess doses of K-Dur
4. How frequently the client eats salty foods in restaurants

19 The nurse would recommend which type of laxative as the best choice for a client with constipation and a history of coronary artery disease and congestive heart failure?

1. A bulk-forming laxative
2. A saline laxative
3. A stimulant laxative
4. PRN enemas

20 The client comes to the office to get a refill of the prescription dicyclomine hydrochloride (Bentyl). She tells the nurse she is leaving the next day for a vacation to Florida. What education should the nurse provide this client?

1. "You do not need to be so concerned about taking the medication on vacation because you probably won't be able to watch your diet very well anyway."
2. "This medication may make you more sensitive to high temperatures, which could lead to dizziness."
3. "You probably should discontinue the medication until you return home because alcohol can increase the drug's effects on the central nervous system."
4. "While you are away, you should take antacids with this medication to decrease any symptoms of GERD."

ANSWERS & RATIONALES

1 **Answer: 3** Omeprazole, pantoprazole, and rabeprazole must be swallowed whole. Lansoprazole and esomeprazole capsules may be opened and sprinkled on applesauce or dissolved in 40 mL of juice.
Cognitive Level: Application **Client Need:** Physiological Integrity: Pharmacological and Parenteral Therapies **Integrated Process:** Nursing Process: Planning **Content Area:** Pharmacology **Strategy:** The core issue of the question is knowledge of the formulations of various proton pump inhibitors. Use medication knowledge and the process of elimination to make a selection.

2 **Answer: 4** Ciprofloxacin is not recommended for *Helicobacter pylori* infection during pregnancy. The other medications can be used after consulting with the physician.
Cognitive Level: Application **Client Need:** Physiological Integrity: Pharmacological and Parenteral Therapies **Integrated Process:** Nursing Process: Assessment **Content Area:** Pharmacology **Strategy:** The core issue of the question is knowledge of what medications are safe for use in pregnancy for a client with *Helicobacter pylori* infection. Use medication knowledge and the process of elimination to make a selection.

3 **Answer: 1** Bismuth-containing preparations, such as Pepto-Bismol, can cause all the listed side effects, but transient darkening of the tongue and stool is a specific side effect to bismuth.
Cognitive Level: Application **Client Need:** Physiological Integrity: Pharmacological and Parenteral Therapies **Integrated Process:** Nursing Process: Assessment **Content Area:** Pharmacology **Strategy:** The critical word in the stem of this question is *unique.* This means that the answer is one that does not occur with other drugs that the client is receiving. Use specific medication knowledge and the process of elimination to make a selection.

4 **Answer: 3** The highest rate of eradication of *Helicobacter pylori* infection is by using a proton pump inhibitor and two antibiotics (usually clarithromycin and amoxicillin or metronidazole). The combinations of medications in options 1, 2, and 4 do not provide for this level of effectiveness.
Cognitive Level: Application **Client Need:** Physiological Integrity: Pharmacological and Parenteral Therapies **Integrated Process:** Nursing Process: Analysis **Content Area:** Pharmacology **Strategy:** The core issue of the question is knowledge of what medications are commonly used in treating *Helicobacter pylori* infection. Use medication knowledge and the process of elimination to make a selection.

5 **Answer: 1** Promethazine is usually given 25 mg every 4 to 6 hours prn. Dosing may start at 12.5 mg every 4 to 6 hours prn depending on client status; however, 25 mg is the usual dose. Normal doses of the other medications are as follows: prochlorperazine 5 to 10 mg tid–qid; metoclopramide 10 mg 30 minutes AC and HS; and trimethobenzamide hydrochloride 250 mg tid–qid prn.
Cognitive Level: Application **Client Need:** Physiological Integrity: Pharmacological and Parenteral Therapies **Integrated Process:** Nursing Process: Analysis **Content Area:** Pharmacology **Strategy:** The core issue of the question is knowledge of the dosing schedule for various antiemetics. Use medication knowledge and the process of elimination to make a selection.

6 **Answer: 3** Omeprazole can cause an increase in liver enzyme levels (AST, ALT, alkaline phosphatase, and bilirubin), leading to adverse reactions of liver necrosis and hepatic failure. For this reason the nurse should monitor these lab values as they become available. Monitoring of BUN, uric acid, and WBC count have a lesser priority and are monitored only as indicated based on an individual client's identified health need.
Cognitive Level: Application **Client Need:** Physiological Integrity: Pharmacological and Parenteral Therapies **Integrated Process:** Nursing Process: Planning **Content Area:** Pharmacology **Strategy:** The core issue of the question is knowledge of the laboratory values that could be affected by administration of omeprazole. With this group of medications, it is necessary to remember the liver. Use medication knowledge and the process of elimination to make a selection.

7 **Answer: 2** All the medications listed are antiemetic agents, but transdermal scopolamine has the fastest onset of action. For this reason, it is most effective in providing relief from nausea for a prolonged period of time.
Cognitive Level: Application **Client Need:** Physiological Integrity: Pharmacological and Parenteral Therapies **Integrated Process:** Nursing Process: Implementation **Content Area:** Pharmacology **Strategy:** The core issue of the question is knowledge of onset of action of various antiemetics. Recall that transdermal systems begin to absorb into the skin immediately after application, while oral doses take various amounts of time to absorb through the GI tract. Use medication knowledge and the process of elimination to make a selection.

8 **Answer: 2** Because of their antisecretory effect, proton pump inhibitors such as omeprazole are the drugs of choice for

moderate to severe erosive esophagitis. The course of therapy is usually 4 to 8 weeks. The other medications may be helpful for certain clients; however, proton pump inhibitors are the medication classification of choice.
Cognitive Level: Application **Client Need:** Physiological Integrity: Pharmacological and Parenteral Therapies **Integrated Process:** Nursing Process: Planning **Content Area:** Pharmacology **Strategy:** The core issue of the question is knowledge of the various GI medications that are useful in treating digestive system health problems. Recall that disorders that end in *itis* involve inflammation, so the correct answer is one that reduces inflammation either by its own action or by inhibiting other irritants, such as gastric acid. Use medication knowledge of omeprazole as a proton pump inhibitor to make a selection.

9 **Answer: 1** Antacids should be chewed well and followed with 4 ounces of water for optimal effect. They should be taken regularly after meals, but the client should allow at least 2 hours between taking the antacid and any other oral medication. Antacids should not be taken longer than 2 weeks without further evaluation. They can be taken before gastric upset occurs for better symptom control.
Cognitive Level: Application **Client Need:** Physiological Integrity: Pharmacological and Parenteral Therapies **Integrated Process:** Nursing Process: Planning **Content Area:** Pharmacology **Strategy:** The core issue of the question is knowledge of medication administration procedures for antacids. Recall that antacids are more effective when given with fluid to help disperse medication in the stomach. Use medication knowledge and the process of elimination to make a selection.

10 **Answer: 1** Clients with glaucoma should not take anticholinergic agents such as dicyclomine because the medication affects pupillary dilatation and therefore indirectly affects the outflow of aqueous humor. The other medications listed do not pose this problem to the client.
Cognitive Level: Analysis **Client Need:** Physiological Integrity: Pharmacological and Parenteral Therapies **Integrated Process:** Nursing Process: Planning **Content Area:** Pharmacology **Strategy:** The core issue of the question is knowledge of medications that are contraindicated with glaucoma. Specific medication knowledge is needed to answer the question. Use medication knowledge and the process of elimination to make a selection.

11 **Answer: 4** Cimetidine decreases metabolism of beta blockers, phenytoin, procainamide, quinidine, benzodiazepines, metronidazole, tricyclic antidepressants, and warfarin, leading to increased risk of drug toxicity. Ranitidine, famotidine, and nizatidine are histamine blockers that are newer than cimetidine and have fewer side effects.
Cognitive Level: Application **Client Need:** Physiological Integrity: Pharmacological and Parenteral Therapies **Integrated Process:** Nursing Process: Implementation **Content Area:** Pharmacology **Strategy:** The core issue of the question is knowledge of histamine antagonists that are highest in side or adverse effects. Specific medication knowledge is needed to answer the question. Use medication knowledge and the process of elimination to make a selection.

12 **Answer: 2** Sucralfate forms an adhesive barrier on the surface of the gastric mucosa, protecting it from gastric acid. It does not reduce spasms, relieve nausea or vomiting, or act as an anticholinergic.
Cognitive Level: Application **Client Need:** Physiological Integrity: Pharmacological and Parenteral Therapies **Integrated Process:** Nursing Process: Implementation **Content Area:** Pharmacology **Strategy:** The core issue of the question is knowledge of the mechanism of action of sucralfate (Carafate). Specific medication knowledge is needed to answer the question. Use this knowledge and the process of elimination to make a selection.

13 **Answer: 3** Pancrease, a pancreatic enzyme replacement, increases digestion of starches and fats and thereby decreases the incidence of steatorrhea (fatty, frothy, foul-smelling stools). Each of the other options is only partially correct.
Cognitive Level: Application **Client Need:** Physiological Integrity: Pharmacological and Parenteral Therapies **Integrated Process:** Teaching/Learning **Content Area:** Pharmacology **Strategy:** The core issue of the question is knowledge of the mechanism of action of pancrease. Specific medication knowledge is needed to answer the question. Use this knowledge and the process of elimination to make a selection.

14 **Answer: 4** Associated symptoms of fever, abdominal pain, and dehydration symptoms may suggest pathological diarrhea. The health care provider should be contacted for further evaluation. The other actions listed do not provide for the current physiological needs of the client.
Cognitive Level: Analysis **Client Need:** Physiological Integrity: Pharmacological and Parenteral Therapies **Integrated Process:** Nursing Process: Implementation **Content Area:** Pharmacology **Strategy:** The stem of the question contains the critical words *highest priority.* This tells you that more than one or all of the options may be partially or totally correct. Use general nursing knowledge about diarrhea associated with fever and the process of elimination to make a selection.

15 **Answer: 2** Bismuth subsalicylate contains small amounts of naturally occurring lead, but Reye syndrome is a theorized complication of salicylate use in young children. Taste and darkening of the tongue are not the issue being addressed in this question.
Cognitive Level: Application **Client Need:** Physiological Integrity: Pharmacological and Parenteral Therapies **Integrated Process:** Nursing Process: Implementation **Content Area:** Pharmacology **Strategy:** Note the critical word *salicylate* in the stem of the question. Immediately associate this word with *aspirin,* which is contraindicated for use in children because of the risk of developing Reye syndrome.

16 **Answer: 1** Methylcellulose is a bulk-forming cellulose that absorbs intestinal fluids. This action helps prevent constipation and reduce or eliminate diarrhea. Bisacodyl and docusate sodium are laxatives, while dicyclomine is an antispasmodic.
Cognitive Level: Application **Client Need:** Physiological Integrity: Pharmacological and Parenteral Therapies **Integrated Process:** Nursing Process: Analysis **Content Area:** Pharmacology **Strategy:** The core issue of the question is knowledge of a medication that relieves both constipation and diarrhea. With this in mind, you need to select a medication that regulates the

bowel. Use medication knowledge and the process of elimination to make a selection.

17 **Answer: 4** A serious adverse effect of misoprostol (Cytotec) is that a pregnant woman who takes medication may experience a miscarriage. Misoprostol should be discontinued at least 1 month before pregnancy occurs. Options 1 and 2 have lower priority, and option 3 may or may not be necessary for this client.
Cognitive Level: Application **Client Need:** Physiological Integrity: Pharmacological and Parenteral Therapies **Integrated Process:** Nursing Process: Implementation **Content Area:** Pharmacology **Strategy:** The core issue of the question is associated risks of taking misoprostol during pregnancy. Eliminate options 1 and 3 first because they do not relate to misoprostol. Then choose option 4 over option 2 because it is more specific to the medication.

18 **Answer: 1** Bisacodyl is a stimulant laxative that my cause fluid and electrolyte imbalance. This can have additive effects because the diuretic use would also contribute to this finding. For this reason, the nurse should assess the use of the laxative. The other options suggest items that would not help determine the cause of the client's current symptoms.
Cognitive Level: Analysis **Client Need:** Physiological Integrity: Pharmacological and Parenteral Therapies **Integrated Process:** Nursing Process: Analysis **Content Area:** Pharmacology **Strategy:** Note that the question contains the critical word *hyponatremia.* With this in mind, evaluate each option in terms of its relevance to the low sodium value. Eliminate each of the incorrect options because they would not cause the electrolyte imbalance stated in the question.

19 **Answer: 1** Bulk-forming laxatives, such as methylcellulose, absorb intestinal fluid, increasing stool volume, stimulating peristalsis, and decreasing straining on defecation. This type of laxative is the best choice for a client with a history of heart disease complicated by heart failure. The laxatives in the other options are more likely to cause straining at stool for the client and are therefore less helpful for the client's overall status.
Cognitive Level: Application **Client Need:** Physiological Integrity: Pharmacological and Parenteral Therapies **Integrated Process:** Nursing Process: Assessment **Content Area:** Pharmacology **Strategy:** The critical words in the stem of the question are *best choice.* This tells you that more than one option may be partially or totally correct, but one option is better than the others. Keeping in mind that the client has heart disease, use the process of elimination to choose the bulk-forming laxative as least likely to cause strain on the heart.

20 **Answer: 2** Dicyclomine HCl is an antispasmodic drug. Peripheral side effects include hot, flushed, dry skin; hyperthermia; and intolerance to high temperatures manifested by dizziness. The client should be advised to drink extra fluids (nonalcoholic) if exposed to high temperatures to reduce this occurrence.
Cognitive Level: Analysis **Client Need:** Physiological Integrity: Pharmacological and Parenteral Therapies **Integrated Process:** Nursing Process: Planning **Content Area:** Pharmacology **Strategy:** The core issue of the question is adverse effects of dicyclomine. A clue in the question is the reference to Florida, which suggests that option 2 (high temperature) is the correct option.

Key Terms to Review

antacid p. 679
anticholinergic p. 670
antispasmodic p. 670
cathartic p. 674
emesis p. 677
H_2 antagonist p. 679
Helicobacter pylori p. 679
laxative p. 673
proton pump inhibitor p. 680
surfactant p. 675

References

Abrams, A. (2004). *Clinical drug therapy: Rationales for nursing practice* (7th ed.). Philadelphia: Lippincott Williams & Wilkins.

Adams, M., Josephson, D., & Holland, L. (2005). *Pharmacology for nurses: A pathophysiologic approach.* Upper Saddle River, NJ: Pearson Education.

Deglin, J. H., & Vallerand, A. H. (2006). *Davis's drug guide for nurses* (10th ed.). Philadelphia: F. A. Davis.

Lehne, R. (2004). *Pharmacology for nursing care* (5th ed.). Philadelphia: W. B. Saunders.

McKenry, L., Tossier, E. & Hogan, M. (2006). *Mosby's pharmacology in nursing.* (22nd ed.). St. Louis: Elsevier Science.

Wilson, B., Shannon, M., & Stang, C. (2006). *Prentice Hall nurse's drug guide 2006.* Upper Saddle River, NJ: Pearson Education.

ANSWERS & RATIONALES

42 Endocrine Medications

Test Yourself	
Are you ready for the NCLEX-RN® or course exams? Use the practice tests on the companion CD-ROM to check.	

In this chapter

Cross Reference

Other chapters relevant to this content area are

Dosage Calculation and Medication Administration **Chapter 30**
Endocrine Disorders **Chapter 61**

I. GENERAL GUIDELINES FOR ENDOCRINE MEDICATIONS *(SEE BOX 42–1)*

II. MEDICATIONS AFFECTING THE PITUITARY GLAND

A. Growth hormone (GH)

1. Regulates growth of organs and tissues, specifically length of long bones; is approved for use in children to treat growth hormone deficiency or inadequate growth hormone secretion only
2. Common medications are listed in Table 42–1 ■
3. Administration considerations
   a. Is only given parenterally—intramuscularly (IM) or subcutaneously; oral route is inactivated by digestive enzymes
   b. Reconsititute packaged powder with 1 to 5 mL of approved diluent; mixture must be clear, not cloudy, and must not contain any undissolved particles; label date of reconstitution and discard refrigerated drug according to manufacturer's directions
   c. Rotate IM sites and use appropriate needle length to inject into muscle layer
   d. ! Contraindicated to stimulate growth in children who are short unrelated to growth hormone deficiency; during or after closure of epiphyseal plates in long bones; or with secondary intracranial tumors
   e. Use cautiously with diabetes or family history of same, hypothyroidism, or concurrent or previous use of thyroid or hormones in males before puberty
   f. Use of thyroid hormone, anabolic steroids, androgens, or estrogens may hasten closure of epiphyseal plates of long bones
4. Side/adverse effects
   a. Metabolic: glucose intolerance, adrenocorticotropic hormone (ACTH) deficiency, or hypothyroidism

Box 42–1

General Guidelines for Endocrine Medications

Administration Principles

1. Assess current medications (including OTC drugs and herbal products) and history of allergies to identify any potential risks to client.
2. Administer doses on time to maintain therapeutic blood levels.
3. Do not break or allow client to chew sustained release or enteric coated preparations.
4. Provide both verbal and written instructions to client, and provide phone number to call if questions arise or problems occur.

Client Teaching

1. Understand medication actions, side effects, signs of toxicity, importance of follow-up with prescriber and complying with follow-up laboratory tests and how to self-administer.
2. Do not take any OTC drugs or herbal products without first consulting prescriber.
3. Take exactly as prescribed and do not miss or double doses.
4. Report adverse effects promptly.
5. Do not discontinue drug without consulting prescriber.
6. Do not drink alcohol while taking prescription medications.

! **b.** Renal: **hypercalciuria** (excess calcium excretion in urine) during first 2 to 3 months of treatment; risk of renal calculi with complaints of flank pain, colic, gastrointestinal (GI) upset, urinary frequency, chills, fever, and hematuria
c. Other: recurrent intracranial tumor growth or presence of GH antibodies
d. Local allergic reaction: pain and edema at injection site
! **e.** Systemic allergic reaction: peripheral edema, headache, myalgia, and weakness
f. Excess dosage: diabetes mellitus, atherosclerosis, enlarged organs, hypertension, and features related to acromegaly

5. Nursing considerations
   a. Make sure there is documentation of growth rate for at least 6 to 12 months prior to initiating treatment
   b. Assess client for any adverse drug effects or toxicities
   c. Make sure annual bone age assessments are performed, especially for clients undergoing thyroid, androgen, or estrogen replacement therapy
6. Client teaching
   a. As per Box 42–1, advise parents or caregivers about need for regular bone age assessments
   ! **b.** A 3- to 5-inch growth rate is expected in first year and less in second year, with normal growth rate subsequent years; subcutaneous fat diminishes during treatment but will return later
   c. Teach client/caregiver to document monthly height and weight measurements and to report any less-than-expected growth to physician
   ! **d.** Teach signs and symptoms of slipped femoral epiphysis (hip or knee pain and limp) and to notify physician of same

Table 42–1

Growth Hormone Drugs

Generic (Trade) Name	Notes
Bromocriptine (Parlodel)	Suppresses growth hormone levels.
Ocreotide (Sandostatin)	Suppresses intestinal peptide hormones, insulin, glucagons, and growth hormone.
Sermorelin (Geref)	Stimulates release of growth hormone from intact pituitaries.
Somatrem (Protropin)	Used as replacement therapy.
Somatropin (Humatrope, Nutropin)	Used as replacement therapy.

e. Treatment is discontinued when adequate adult height is reached, epiphyseal plates fuse, or client fails to respond to GH

B. Antidiuretic hormone (ADH)

1. Promotes reabsorption of water; vasopressor effect due to constriction of smooth muscle; increases aggregation of platelets
! 2. Is a pituitary hormone for replacement therapy for clients with diabetes insipidus (DI); also for use in hemophilia A, von Willebrand's disease type 1
3. Common medications are listed in Box 42–2
4. Administration considerations

Memory Aid

Medications that are pituitary hormone replacements usually end with the suffix *-pressin*.

a. Give by intranasal, subcutaneous, IV, IM, or intra-arterial route according to order and preparation
b. Infusion pump is needed for IV or intra-arterial routes
! c. Contraindicated with coronary artery or vascular disease; vasoconstriction causes blood pressure elevation
d. Monitor serum osmolality and plasma osmolality if given to treat diabetes insipidus
e. Monitor Factor VIII coagulation level if given for hemostasis

5. Side/adverse effects
a. Drowsiness, headache, lethargy, nasal congestion and irritation; rhinitis
b. Abdominal cramps, nausea, heartburn, pain in vulva
c. Elevated BP
! d. IV route may cause anaphylaxis
e. Overdose may produce symptoms of water intoxication

6. Nursing considerations
a. Give initial dose in evening and increase amount until uninterrupted sleep is noted
! b. Check vital signs (BP and pulse) before giving by IV and subcutaneous routes
c. Assess for mental status changes such as disorientation, lethargy, and behavioral changes related to fluid overload
! d. Measure daily intake and output (I & O) to monitor water retention and sodium depletion; assess edema in extremities
! e. Weigh daily to monitor water retention
! f. For nasal spray, make sure nasal mucosa is intact by inspecting nares prior to dose
g. Store nasal spray at room temperature; all other solutions need refrigeration

7. Client teaching
a. Follow proper technique for nasal instillation (tube inserted into nostril to instill)
b. As per Box 42–1; especially avoid over-the-counter (OTC) medicines containing epinephrine that can decrease drug's action
c. Wear Medic-Alert identification
d. May take missed dose up to one hour before next dose
! e. Report any nasal congestion or upper respiratory tract infection

III. MEDICATIONS AFFECTING THE ADRENAL GLANDS

A. Mineralocorticoids

1. A **mineralocorticoid** is a steroid hormone that acts on kidneys to retain sodium and water and release potassium

Box 42–2

Drugs to Treat Diabetes Insipidus

Desmopressin (DDAVP, Stimate)

Lypressin (Diapid)

Vasopressin (Pitressin)

Table 42–2

Drugs for Adrenal Replacement Therapy (Mineralocorticoids)

Generic (Trade) Name	Notes
Cortisone (Cortone)	Has both mineralocorticoid and glucocorticoid action.
Fludrocortisone (Florinef)	Has strong mineralocorticoid action; used with glucocorticoid for replacement therapy.
Hydrocortisone (Cortef)	Has both mineralocorticoid and glucocorticoid action.

2. Synthesis is regulated by renin-angiotensin system
3. Replacement therapy is required with adrenal gland failure or hypofunction
4. Common medications are listed in Table 42–2 ■

Memory Aid

Medications that replace hormones from the adrenal cortex (either glucocorticoid or mineralocorticoid) often have the syllable *cort* somewhere in the name.

5. Administration considerations
   a. Fludrocortisone acetate is drug of choice for mineralocorticoid activity
   b. Contraindicated with hypersensitivity to glucocorticoids; idiopathic thrombocytopenic purpura (ITP); acute glomerulonephritis; viral/bacterial skin infections or infections not being treated with antibiotics; amebiasis; Cushing's syndrome; vaccinations/immunologic procedures
   c. Monitor serum electrolyte levels because drug's hypokalemic effect may potentiate action of other drugs and hypernatremia can result if given with high sodium drugs
6. Side/adverse effects
   a. Sodium and fluid retention
   b. Nausea
   c. Acne
   d. Impaired wound healing
   e. Thromboembolism
   f. Aggravation or masking of infection
   g. Anaphylactoid reactions are rare but may occur in clients hypersensitive to glucocorticoids
7. Nursing considerations
   a. Used with glucocorticoids for replacement therapy
   b. Monitor serum electrolyte levels
   c. Monitor weight and I & O and report weight gain of 5 lb per week
   d. Monitor/record BP daily and more frequently during periods of dosage adjustment
   e. Check for signs of overdosage related to hypercorticism (psychosis, excess weight gain, edema, congestive heart failure [CHF], increased appetite, severe insomnia, and elevated BP)
   f. Check for signs of underdosage: weight loss, poor appetite, nausea, vomiting, diarrhea, muscular weakness, increased fatigue, and low BP
8. Client teaching
   a. Report signs of low potassium associated with high sodium (muscle weakness, paresthesias, circumoral numbness, fatigue, anorexia, nausea, depression, delirium, diminished reflexes, polyuria, irregular heart rate, CHF, ileus)
   b. Eat foods high in potassium if so advised
   c. Salt intake regulates drug's effect: report signs of edema
   d. Weigh daily and report consistent weight gain
   e. Report any infections, trauma, or unexpected stress, which may warrant an order for increased medication dosage
   f. Wear/carry medical identification alert including drug use and prescriber's name

B. Glucocorticoids

1. A glucocorticoid is a steroid hormone with metabolic effects on carbohydrate, protein and fat metabolism, and anti-inflammatory and immunosuppressive activity
2. Synthesis is regulated by pituitary gland via negative feedback effect; may regulate metabolism of skeletal and connective tissues
3. Used in acute **adrenal insufficiency** (inability of adrenal glands to produce sufficient adrenocortical hormones) caused by trauma or thrombosis; chronic primary adrenal insufficiency (**Addison's disease**); and secondary adrenal insufficiency (diseased or destroyed adenohypophysis with inadequate production of ACTH)
4. Many miscellaneous uses
   a. Allergic conditions (asthma, angioedema, transfusion reactions, and serum sickness)
   b. Dermatological conditions, such as dermatitis and pemphigus
   c. Inflammatory GI disorders, such as Crohn's disease and ulcerative proctitis
   d. Hematologic disorders, such as autoimmune hemolytic anemia and thrombocytopenia
   e. Joint inflammation, bursitis
   f. With antineoplastic agents in leukemias and lymphomas
   g. Ophthalmic diseases, such as allergic conjunctivitis, chorioretinitis, iritis, iridocyclitis, and keratitis
   h. Rheumatic disease (acute inflammatory states of arthritis and systemic lupus erythematosus)
5. Common medications are listed in Table 42–3 ■
6. Administration considerations
   a. Routes of administration for systemic use to treat inflammatory conditions include IV, IM, and PO
   b. Routes of administration for nonsystemic use include inhalation, nasal, ophthalmic, otic, and topical
   c. Contraindicated with systemic fungal infections and known hypersensitivity
   d. Monitor CBC and differential, serum electrolytes, and blood glucose
   e. With long-term therapy, monitor hypothalamic-pituitary-adrenal (HPA) axis function to check adrenal function
7. Side/adverse effects
   a. Few side effects if high doses are given for only a few days
   b. Higher doses and prolonged therapy may alter metabolism of tissues and organs, leading to muscle wasting and increased fat tissue deposits in trunk and face; changes in behavior and personality may also occur
   c. Prolonged therapy may suppress growth in children and lead to osteoporosis in adults; impaired glucose tolerance and frank diabetes mellitus may also result

Table 42–3

Drugs for Adrenal Replacement Therapy (Glucocorticoids)

Generic (Trade) Name	Notes
Betamethasone (Celestone)	Has little or no mineralocorticoid action.
Cortisone (Cortone)	Has both mineralocorticoid and glucocorticoid action.
Dexamethasone (Decadron)	Has little or no mineralocorticoid action.
Hydrocortisone (Cortef)	Has both mineralocorticoid and glucocorticoid action.
Methylprednisolone (Medrol)	Has little mineralocorticoid action.
Prednisolone (Delta-Cortef)	Has both mineralocorticoid and glucocorticoid action.
Prednisone (Deltasone)	Has little mineralocorticoid action.
Triamcinolone (Aristacort, Kenacort)	Must be used with mineralocorticoid; has little or no mineralocorticoid action.

d. Prolonged therapy can suppress the HPA axis; **adrenal crisis** (acute, life-threatening state of profound adrenocortical insufficiency) may result if drug is abruptly withdrawn
e. Toxicity may include anaphylactoid reactions, hypertriglyceridemia, peptic ulcers, acute pancreatitis, aseptic necrosis of bone, cataracts, glaucoma, hypertension, and opportunistic infections

8. Nursing considerations
   - ! a. Check vital signs, BP, lung sounds, weight (including any history of gain or loss), nausea and vomiting, and signs of dependent edema
   - b. Conduct mental status exam and assess for signs of depression, withdrawal, insomnia, and anorexia
   - ! c. Check skin for striae, thinning, bruising, change in color, change in hair growth, and acne
   - d. In children on prolonged therapy, monitor height and growth pattern
   - e. Advise regular ophthalmic examinations with long-term therapy
   - ! f. Check stool for occult blood periodically; GI bleeding could result
   - ! g. With prolonged therapy, move and reposition immobilized clients carefully and limit use of adhesive tape on skin
9. Client teaching
   - ! a. As per Box 42–1; take oral doses with meals
   - b. If ordered every other day, take any missed dose as soon as remembered if on same day; if remembered next day, then take dose and readjust schedule to be every other day; do not double up missed doses
   - ! c. It may be advisable to lose weight, limit sodium intake, and increase potassium intake if excessive weight gain occurs
   - ! d. If diabetic, carefully monitor for increased blood glucose levels
   - ! e. Report any blood in stool or black tarry stools, mood changes or insomnia, vision changes or headache, weight gain of more than 5 lb per week, irregular menses or pregnancy, irregular heart rate, excessive fatigue, severe abdominal pain, serious injury, or infection
   - f. Avoid strenuous activities if skin is fragile and bruises easily
   - g. With long-term therapy, take prescribed doses every day and do not discontinue medication without notifying physician; do not increase or decrease dose on own; tapering of dose is necessary
   - h. Avoid immunizations during therapy and for 3 months after; avoid contact with anyone with measles or chicken pox or anyone receiving oral polio vaccine
   - i. Avoid skin testing during therapy
   - j. Wear specific medical identification during therapy
   - ! k. With long-term therapy, report any fever, cough, sore throat, malaise, and unhealed injuries; avoid contact with anyone with active infection

C. Adrenocorticotropic hormone (ACTH)

1. Directly stimulates adrenal cortex to synthesize adrenal steroids
2. ! Used in diagnosing adrenal disorders such as Addison's disease and secondary adrenal insufficiency caused by pituitary dysfunction
3. Used in treatment of adrenocorticoid-responsive diseases, such as multiple sclerosis
4. ! Limited use in treatment of adrenal insufficiency; corticosteroids used instead
5. Common medications are listed in Box 42–3
6. Administration considerations
   - a. Give IV, IM, PO, or subcutaneously according to manufacturer's instructions
   - b. Contraindicated with ocular herpes simplex, recent surgery, disorders such as CHF, scleroderma, osteoporosis, systemic fungoid infections, hypertension,

Box 42–3

Drugs Used in Diagnosis and Treatment of Adrenal Gland Disorders

Corticotropin (Acthar)
Cosyntropin (Cortrosyn)
Metyrapone (Metopirone)

sensitivity to porcine proteins, or conditions related to adrenocortical insufficiency or hyperfunction

7. Side/adverse effects
   a. Nausea and vomiting, dizziness, drowsiness, or light-headedness
   b. Hypersensitivity including urticaria, pruritus, dizziness, vomiting, and anaphylactic shock
   c. Cataracts or glaucoma; peptic ulcer with perforation; hirsutism and amenorrhea
   d. Sodium and water retention, potassium and calcium loss, and hyperglycemia
   e. Acne, impaired wound healing, fragile skin, petechiae, ecchymosis
   f. **Osteoporosis** (abnormal loss of bone density), decreased muscle mass, **cushingoid state** (having the appearance and facies characteristic of Cushing's disease), activation of latent tuberculosis or diabetes mellitus, vertebral compression fractures
8. Nursing considerations
   a. Individualized dosage and gradual dosage changes should be made only after apparent full effect from drug is seen
   b. Shake bottle well before injecting into deep gluteal muscle; observe closely for 15 minutes after dose for hypersensitivity reactions; prolonged treatment may increase risk of hypersensitivity
   c. Monitor vital signs and BP and assess for dizziness, fever, flushing, rash, and urticaria
   d. Monitor plasma or urinary cortisol levels and serum electrolytes
   e. Be aware that agents may suppress signs and symptoms of chronic disease; new infections may appear during treatment
   f. At high dosage levels, drug must be gradually tapered
   g. Carefully monitor growth and development in children
9. Client teaching
   a. As per Box 42–1; take oral doses with food, milk, or meals
   b. If ordered, follow low-salt or high-potassium diet
   c. If dizziness, drowsiness, or light-headedness occur, avoid driving or operating hazardous equipment

IV. MEDICATIONS AFFECTING THE THYROID GLAND

A. Thyroid hormones

1. Are replacement therapy for **hypothyroidism** (decreased activity of thyroid gland with a variety of specific causes); have same action as naturally produced thyroid hormones in body
2. Used to diagnose and treat thyroid deficiency and **myxedema** (most severe form of hypothyroidism characterized by swelling of face, feet, and periorbital tissues; may lead to coma and death), and to control goiter or thyroid carcinoma
3. Common medications are listed in Table 42–4 ■
4. Administration considerations

Table 42–4

Drugs for Diagnosing and Treating Thyroid Disorders or Replacement Therapy

Generic (Trade) Name	Notes
Levothyroxine (Levothroid, Levoxyl, Synthroid)	Chemically pure form of T_4 and preferred therapy for hypothythroidism. Given IV for myxedema coma.
Liothyronine (Cytomel)	Chemically pure form of T_3; for adult hypothyroidism; not used for cretinism since T_3 does not cross blood–brain barrier as well as T_4 does.
Liotrix (Thyrolar, Euthroid)	Chemically pure T_4 and T_3 in 4:1 ratio; used for hypothyroidism.
Thyroid (Thyrar)	Crude thyroid gland preparation containing variable amounts of T_3 and T_4. Dosage difficult to adjust and maintain.
Protirelin	Identical to natural hypothalamic hormone. Used in diagnosis.
Thyrotropin	Natural TSH extracted from animals. Used to differentiate primary hypothyroidism from secondary.

a. May be given IV, IM, PO, or subcutaneously
b. Contraindicated in thyrotoxicosis, acute myocardial infarction (MI) and cardiovascular disease, morphologic hypogonadism, nephrosis, and uncorrected hypoadrenalism
c. Use cautiously with angina pectoris; hypertension; elderly with cardiac disease; renal insufficiency; pregnancy; concurrent use of **catecholamines** (drugs that mimic effects of the sympathetic nervous system); diabetes mellitus; **hyperthyroidism** (hyperactivity of the thyroid gland), and malabsorption states
d. Note results of significant laboratory studies: serum T_4, free thyroxine, T_3 uptake, serum T_3, serum thyroid-stimulating hormone (TSH), protirelin test, thyroid uptake of radioiodine, TSH test, and thyroid suppression test

5. Side/adverse effects
a. Weight gain, vomiting, and tachycardia
b. Angina pectoris, coronary occlusion, or stroke in elderly or predisposed clients
c. Relative adrenal insufficiency in clients with inadequate pituitary function related to secondary hypothyroidism and secondary adrenal insufficiency; adrenal crisis
d. Overdosage causing signs of hyperthyroidism related to thyroid storm with shock and coma; thyrotoxicosis with CHF, angina, cardiac dysrhythmias, and shock
e. Reactions to thioamides include fever, itching, and skin rash; blood dyscrasias and peripheral neuropathy; pain and swelling of joints or lupus-like syndrome; dizziness; or alterations in taste
f. Overdosage of thioamides causes hypothyroidism

6. Nursing considerations
a. Assess vital signs, BP, weight and history of weight change, normal diet, energy level, mood, subjective feeling, and response to temperature
b. In children, check height
c. Monitor thyroid function test results and blood glucose levels
d. Start older adults on lower doses of thyroid hormones and increase dose by small increments; assess for symptoms of stress that could lead to angina or stroke

7. Client teaching
a. As per Box 42–1; learn how to monitor pulse, weight, and height; wear medical alert identification
b. With hormone replacement, adhere to dosage schedule and intervals; therapy is life-long; do not change brand of thyroid medication without prescriber approval because of differences in bioavailability
c. Immediately report any chest pain or other signs of aggravated cardiovascular disease
d. With juvenile hypothyroidism therapy, dramatic weight loss and catch-up growth can occur
e. Understand side effects and related treatment if changes in insulin or anticoagulants are needed
f. With radioactive iodine, most clients become hypothyroid and require replacement thyroid hormones; periodic thyroid evaluation is needed

B. Antithyroid medications

1. Used to treat hyperthyroidism and **Graves' disease** (pronounced hyperthyroidism often associated with enlarged thyroid gland and exophthalmos; also called thyrotoxicosis)
2. Common medications are listed in Table 42–5 ■
3. Administration considerations
a. Given PO; administer drug according to manufacturer's instructions
b. Contraindicated with previous allergic or other severe reactions to thioamides
c. Impaired hepatic function may require reduced doses
d. Monitor results of significant laboratory studies: serum T_4, serum T_3, free T_4, free T_3, T_3 resin uptake, serum thyroid uptake of radioiodine, and thyroid suppression test

Table 42-5

Drugs Used to Treat Hyperthyroidism and Graves' Disease

Generic (Trade) Name	Notes
Thioamides	
Methimazole (Tapazole)	Inhibits thyroid hormone synthesis but not release.
Propylthiouracil (generic)	Inhibits thyroid hormone synthesis but not release; in peripheral tissues inhibits conversion of T_4 to T_3.
Beta-Adrenergic Blocker	
Propranolol (Inderal)	Does not lower T_4 and T_3 release from thyroid.
Iodine	
Potassium iodide (Pima)	Has direct action on thyroid and used for short-term inhibition of thyroid hormone synthesis.
^{131}I as NaI (Iodotope)	Radioisotope concentrated in thyroid. Releases radiation and destroys tissue.

4. Side/adverse effects
   a. Fever, itching, and skin rash
   b. Blood dyscrasias and peripheral neuropathy
   c. Pain and swelling of joints or lupus-like syndrome
   d. Dizziness and alteration in taste
   e. Overdosage results in hypothyroidism
   f. Rare instances of agranulocytosis
5. Nursing considerations
   a. Assess for tingling of fingers and toes
   b. Monitor weight and check for hair loss and skin changes
   c. Check CBC, differential count, and thyroid and liver function tests
   d. Dilute oral iodine solutions well in milk, juice, or other beverage
   e. Assess for metallic taste in mouth, sneezing, edematous thyroid, vomiting, and bloody diarrhea
6. Client teaching
   a. As per Box 42–1; wear medical identification tag/bracelet
   b. Side effects may not appear for days or weeks after treatment begins
   c. Report any fever, chills, sore throat, and unusual bleeding/bruising
   d. Take medication at same time of day and with meals or snack; space additional daily doses throughout day

V. MEDICATIONS AFFECTING THE PARATHYROID GLANDS

A. Medications to treat hypocalcemia

1. Consist of calcium supplements that replace calcium to supply body's metabolic needs, help maintain bone strength, and prevent calcium loss from bones
2. Used to treat mild hypocalcemia and for supplementation of dietary calcium
3. Additional use as antacid
4. Common medications are listed in Box 42–4
5. Administration considerations
   a. Given orally, dosage differs among different oral calcium salts
   b. Must be taken with large glass of water and with or after meals for better absorption

Box 42-4

Calcium Salts Used to Treat Mild Calcium Deficiency

Calcium acetate (PhosLo)	Calcium glubionate (Neo-Calglucon)
Calcium chloride (generic)	Calcium gluconate (Kalcinate)
Calcium carbonate (Tums, others)	Calcium lactate (Cal-Lac)
Calcium citrate (Cal-Citrate 250)	Tricalcium phosphate (Posture)

Memory Aid

Most drugs that directly or indirectly affect calcium levels will have *calci* or *calc* somewhere in the generic or trade name.

c. When used as antacid, should be taken 1 hour after meals and at bedtime
d. Contraindications: hypercalcemia, renal calculi, and hypophosphatemia
e. Foods such as spinach, Swiss chard, beets, bran, and whole grains may reduce calcium absorption
f. Monitor results of periodic calcium levels for effectiveness

6. Side/adverse effects
   a. Constipation and flatulence
   b. Hypercalcemia may occur if frequent or high doses are used
   c. May also occur in clients receiving calcium as part of renal dysfunction therapy
7. Nursing considerations
   a. Take 1 to 1½ hours after meals
   b. Space additional daily doses throughout the day
   c. Note number and consistency of stools; for constipation, a laxative or stool softener may be ordered
   d. With prolonged therapy, monitor weekly serum and urine calcium levels
   e. Observe for signs of hypercalcemia if client is receiving frequent or high doses
   f. Monitor for acid rebound if used repeatedly as an antacid for more than 1 to 2 weeks
8. Client teaching
   a. Understand signs of hypercalcemia and report any nausea, vomiting, constipation, frequent urination, lethargy, or depression
   b. Do not take with cereals or other foods high in oxalates that form insoluble, nonabsorbable compounds with calcium
   c. If used as antacid, understand potential dangers of repeated use for more than 2 weeks

B. Vitamin D

1. Vitamin D, needed for proper absorption of calcium, is a fat-soluble vitamin that can accumulate in body
2. Used to control hypocalcemia or vitamin D deficiency
3. Used in treatment of rickets, **osteomalacia** (abnormal loss of calcification of lamellar bone matrix, resulting in bone softening and fracture), and **hypoparathyroidism** (insufficient secretion by parathyroid glands caused by primary parathyroid dysfunction or abnormal serum calcium level)
4. Common medications are listed in Box 42–5
5. Administration considerations
   a. Give PO or IM
   b. Adequate calcium is needed for optimal response to treatment
   c. Contraindicated with hypercalcemia or vitamin D toxicity and malabsorption syndrome
6. Side/adverse effects
   a. Hypercalcemia from overuse (ataxia, fatigue, irritability, seizures, somnolence, tinnitus, hypertension, GI tract distress or constipation, and hypotonia in infants)
   b. Vitamin D hypercalcemia may lead to dysrhythmias in clients taking digoxin
   c. Hypervitaminosis D caused by large therapeutic doses may lead to hypercalcemia, hypercalciuria, bone decalcification, and calcium deposits in soft tissues

Box 42–5

Drugs Used to Treat Vitamin D Deficiency

Calcifediol (Calderol)
Calcitrol (Calcijex, Rocaltrol)
Dihydrotachysterol (Hytakerol)
Ergocalciferol (Calciferol, Drisdol)
Paricalcitol (Zemplar)

7. Nursing considerations
   a. Assess for any CNS problems
   b. Monitor BP, pulse, and I & O
   c. Monitor BUN, serum creatinine levels, serum calcium and phosphorus levels, serum alkaline phosphatase and urinalysis
   d. If vitamin D toxicity occurs, make sure client stops drug immediately, drinks large amounts of fluid, and eats a low-calcium diet
8. Client teaching
   a. Make sure oral dose is swallowed intact without crushing or chewing tablet
   b. As per Box 42–1; consult prescriber before taking any OTC medications containing calcium, phosphorus, or vitamin D, and excessive vitamin D containing substances
   c. Do not drive or use heavy equipment if fatigue, somnolence, vertigo, or weakness develop
   d. Avoid magnesium-containing antacids

C. Medications to treat hypercalcemia

1. Promote urinary excretion of calcium
2. Decrease mobilization of calcium from bone
3. Decrease intestinal absorption of calcium
4. Form complexes with free calcium in blood
5. Used in emergency treatment of hypercalcemia and to control hypercalcemia resulting from malignancies of the bone
6. Common medications are listed in Table 42–6 ■
7. Administration considerations
   a. May be given IM, IV, PO, or subcutaneously
   b. Give IM doses at bedtime to minimize effects of flushing following injection
   c. In emergency situations, dilute IV dose before administration to prevent extravasation; infuse over prescribed period of time
   d. Contraindicated with known hypersensitivity and impaired renal function
   e. Significant drug interactions occur with antacids, mineral supplements, calcium salts, and vitamin D
   f. Decreased effects of digitalis occur when serum calcium is reduced
8. Side/adverse effects
   a. Nausea, vomiting, diarrhea, and dyspepsia with oral route
   b. Facial flushing and occasional inflammatory reaction at injection site
   c. Transient influenza-like symptoms with IV route
   d. Nasal dryness and irritation with intranasal spray
   e. Allergic reactions with calcitonin salmon
   f. IV administration may cause venous irritation, thrombophlebitis, and nephrotoxicity

Table 42–6
Drugs Used to Treat Hypercalcemia

Trade (Generic) Name	Notes
Calcitonin (Miacalcin)	Inhibits bone resorption.
Cinacalcet (Sensipar)	Decreases parathyroid hormone secretion by increasing parathyroid sensitivity to extracellular calcium.
Edetate disodium (Disotate, Endrate)	Strong chelating agent; used on short-term basis to remove excess calcium.
Etidronate (Didronel)	Inhibits bone resorption (biphosphonate).
Gallium nitrate (Ganite)	Used for hypercalcemia caused by cancer.
Pamidronate (Aredia)	Acts directly on bone by slowing bone reabsorption and lowering release of calcium (biphosphonate). Also used for Paget's disease.
Plicamycin (Mithramycin)	Cytotoxic antibiotic that inhibits malignancy-associated bone resorption.
Zoledronic acid (Zometa)	Inhibits bone resorption (biphosphonate).

g. Varying effects of hypocalcemia
h. Toxicity with higher doses causes more severe GI distress, such as esophagitis, severe nephrotoxicity, and severe hypocalcemia

9. Nursing considerations
   a. Assess for hypercalcemia and hypocalcemia
   b. Monitor weight and I & O if vomiting and diarrhea occur
   c. Monitor serum electrolytes, serum alkaline phosphatase, serum creatinine, BUN, liver function tests, CBC with differential, and urinalysis
   d. Monitor vital signs and assess for dysrhythmias with IV infusion
10. Client teaching
   a. Understand and demonstrate subcutaneous self-injection
   b. Do not discontinue therapy without notifying MD
   c. Taking dose in evening may lessen flushing
   d. Take PO doses on empty stomach
   e. Wear medical alert identification if on long-term therapy
   f. Review low-calcium and low-vitamin-D diet (decrease in dairy products, for example)
   g. Take sufficient fluid intake (at least 6 to 8 glasses of water per day and possibly more if not contraindicated by other health problems)

D. Medications to treat osteoporosis and *Paget's disease*

1. Reduce calcium release from bone, slow bone resorption and remodeling, and prevent high serum calcium concentrations
2. Used long-term for Paget's disease (a nonmetabolic disease of bone) and postmenopausal osteoporosis (abnormal loss of bone density)
3. Also used to treat heterotropic ossification after spinal cord injury and hip replacement
4. Common medications are listed in Box 42–6
5. Administration considerations
   a. Is given IM, PO, IV, subcutaneously and intranasally; intranasal spray is given once daily in alternate nostrils
   b. Contraindicated with known hypersensitivity or esophageal disorders
   c. Interacts with antacids, mineral supplements, calcium salts, vitamin D, and calcium-rich dairy products
6. Side/adverse effects
   a. Nausea, vomiting, diarrhea, and dyspepsia with oral route
   b. Facial flushing and occasional inflammatory reaction at injection site
   c. Transient influenza-like symptoms with IV route
   d. Muscle spasms; leukopenia with chills, fever, or sore throat
   e. Nasal dryness and irritation with intranasal spray
   f. Allergic reactions with calcitonin salmon
   g. IV administration may cause venous irritation, thrombophlebitis, and nephrotoxicity
   h. Varying effects of hypocalcemia
   i. Toxicity with higher doses causes more severe hypocalcemia, GI distress such as severe esophagitis with ulceration, and severe nephrotoxicity
7. Nursing considerations
   a. Assess for hypercalcemia and hypocalcemia
   b. Monitor weight and I & O if vomiting and diarrhea occur
   c. Monitor serum electrolytes, serum alkaline phosphatase, calcium and phosphorus, and 24-hour urinary hydroxyproline
   d. Monitor bone pain in clients with Paget's disease

Box 42–6

Drugs to Treat Osteoporosis and Paget's disease

Calcitonin human (Cibacalcin) or Calcitonin salmon (Calcimar, Miacalcin)

Etidronate (Didronel)

Pamidronate (Fosamax)

e. Check results of baseline values of bone mineral density (BMD) in hip, vertebrae, and forearm, and obtain periodic BMD values

8. Client teaching
   a. As per Box 42–1; understand and demonstrate how to self-administer subcutaneous injection and to rotate sites
   b. Taking doses in evening may lessen flushing
   c. Take PO doses on empty stomach and remain upright for 30 minutes after taking
   d. Recognize signs of esophagitis; withhold drug and notify prescriber if difficulty swallowing or worsening heartburn occur
   e. Wear Medic-Alert identification if on long-term therapy
   f. Review low calcium and low vitamin D diet
   g. Take in sufficient fluid
   h. Understand activation and use of metered dose pump for nasal spray use

VI. MEDICATIONS USED TO TREAT DIABETES MELLITUS

A. Insulin

1. Restores cells' ability to use glucose as an energy source and corrects **hyperglycemia** (higher than normal circulating glucose levels)
2. Corrects many associated metabolic derangements
3. Used to treat both type 1 and type 2 diabetes mellitus and diabetic ketoacidosis
4. Also lowers plasma potassium levels and is used as emergency treatment of hyperkalemia
5. Types of insulin are listed in Table 42–7 ■

Table 42–7

Types of Insulin Preparations

Insulin Type	Trade Name	Action	Notes
Lispro Glulisine	Humalog Apidra	**Onset:** 5 min **Peak:** 0.5–1 hr **Duration:** 2–4 hr	Rapid-acting; modified human type
Aspart	Novolog	**Onset:** 0.5 hr **Peak:** 1–3 hr **Duration:** 3–5 hr	Short-acting
Regular	Regular Iletin I Regular Iletin II Regular Purified Pork Insulin Humulin R Novolin R Velosulin BR	**Onset:** 0.5–1 hr **Peak:** 2–4 hr **Duration:** 5–7 hr	Short-acting; may be beef/pork, pork, or human insulin type
NPH (Isophane) Insulin	NPH Iletin I Pork NPH Iletin II NPH purified (N) Humulin N Novolin N	**Onset:** 1–2 hr **Peak:** 6–12 hr **Duration:** 18–24 hr	Intermediate-acting; may be beef/pork, pork, or human insulin type
Lente Insulin	Lente Iletin I Lente Iletin II (pork) Lente (L) Purified Pork Humulin L Novolin L	**Onset:** 1–2 hr **Peak:** 6–12 hr **Duration:** 18–24 hr	Intermediate-acting; may be beef/pork, pork, or human insulin type
Ultralente Insulin	Humulin U Ultralente Novolin L	**Onset:** 4–6 hr **Peak:** 16–18 hr **Duration:** 20–36 hr	Long-acting; human insulin type
NPH/Regular Mixture (70–30%)	Humulin 70/30 Novolin 70/30	**Onset:** 0.5–1 hr **Peak:** 4–8 hr **Duration:** 24 hr	Combination isophane insulin suspension and regular Insulin

6. Administration considerations
   a. Given only by injection (subcutaneous IM, IV); only regular insulin may be given IV; inactivated by digestive enzymes if given orally
   b. All insulins (except lispro and regular) are mixed in suspension so particles must be dispersed before insulin is drawn up into syringe
   c. Injection sites include upper arms, thighs, abdomen, and infrascapular area
   d. One general location is used at one time to maintain consistent absorption rates although sites within each general location are used only once each month
   e. Only mix insulins that are compatible with one another and use according to manufacturer's guidelines
   f. Store unopened vials in refrigerator; opened vials can remain at room temperature for up to one month; label vial with date and time opened and/or due to expire according to agency policy
   g. Alternate methods of delivery include jet injectors, pen injectors, portable insulin pumps, implantable pumps, and intranasal insulin
   h. Dosage must be monitored and linked with insulin needs
   i. Conventional therapy: short-acting and intermediate-acting insulin is given twice a day on a fixed regimen
   j. Intensified therapy: long-acting insulin taken in the evening and a fast-acting insulin given before meals according to blood glucose levels
   k. Continuous subQ insulin infusion: a portable infusion pump is connected to a catheter and infuses regular insulin at a steady rate
   l. Contraindicated with previous allergic response to local or systemic use of drug
   m. Concurrent use of beta-adrenergic blocking agents could delay response of insulin-related hypoglycemia and mask signs triggered by sympathetic nervous system (tachycardia and palpitations)
7. Side/adverse effects
   a. Hypoglycemic reactions when blood glucose levels drop below 50 mg/dL (headache, confusion, drowsiness, and fatigue)
   b. Coma related to inadequate dosage caused by uncontrolled diabetes with high blood glucose levels and ketoacidosis or hyperosmolar coma
   c. Coma related to insulin overdosage caused by inadequate food intake, excessive exercise, or excessive insulin administration
8. Complications
   a. Presence of insulin antibodies that can lead to insulin resistance
   b. **Lipodystrophy** (abnormal deposition of subcutaneous fat at injection sites)
   c. Local allergic reaction related to a contaminant in insulin preparation
   d. Systemic allergic reaction related to insulin itself and not to any contaminant
9. Nursing considerations
   a. Assess vital signs, weight, condition of skin and nails, serum and urine glucose levels, glycosylated hemoglobin (and electrolyte and arterial blood gas levels) when appropriate
   b. Assess for long-term complications related to acceleration of atherosclerosis (hypertension, heart disease, stroke); retinopathy leading to possible blindness; nephropathy leading to possible renal failure; neuropathy leading to lower limb ulcerations and amputation, impotence, and gastroparesis
   c. Consult with physician regarding insulin management when there is insufficient food intake or when client is NPO for surgery
   d. Adhere to agency policy regarding insulin administration
   e. Monitor results of random blood glucose, fasting blood glucose, glucose tolerance test, **glycosylated hemoglobin** A_{1c} (represents average blood glucose over past several weeks), urinary glucose and ketones, and serum electrolytes
10. Client teaching
   a. Participate in individualized teaching plan about insulin management
   b. Understand all aspects of insulin administration, including syringe use, mixing of insulins, stability of mixture, injection technique and sites
   c. Do not switch type or source of insulin or brand of syringe and avoid taking any new drug before notifying prescriber

d. Understand and be sure family understands signs and symptoms of hyperglycemia and hypoglycemia
e. Learn how to test blood glucose levels
f. Follow dietary restrictions and weight control measures; consult dietitian
g. Exercise regularly
h. Understand foot care and related aspects of personal hygiene
i. Learn sick-day management of diabetes and insulin administration (continue to eat and take liquids as able, check blood glucose, maintain insulin schedule, and call prescriber if blood glucose is higher than 250 mg/dL)
j. Obtain and wear a Medic-Alert tag or bracelet
k. Avoid smoking; avoid drinking alcoholic beverages unless approved by physician, since this can lead to hypoglycemia without proper food intake
l. Consult with physician before conceiving (if female)
m. Contact local home care agency and American Diabetic Association for additional follow-up and access to community-based resources

B. Oral antidiabetic (hypoglycemic) agents—sulfonylureas

1. Stimulate release of insulin from pancreatic islets
2. Used as an adjunct to nondrug therapy to reduce blood glucose levels in type 2 diabetes mellitus
3. Common medications are listed in Box 42–7
4. Administration considerations
   a. Dose is given orally 1 to 3 times a day
   b. Different agents possess different durations of action
   c. May be used alone or in combination with insulin
   d. Contraindicated during pregnancy, in women who are nursing/lactating, or in clients allergic to sulfa or urea

Memory Aid

The classification name *sulfonylurea* provides the clue as to what allergies to look for as contraindications for use. Break the word into component parts. The syllable *sulf* can trigger an assessment of sulfa allergy, while *urea* should trigger an assessment of allergy to urea.

   e. Beta-adrenergic blocking agents can suppress insulin release and delay response to hypoglycemia
5. Side/adverse effects
   a. GI tract distress
   b. Neurologic symptoms such as dizziness, drowsiness, or headache
   c. Alcohol may cause a disulfiram-like reaction: flushing, palpitations, and nausea
   d. Allergy noted by skin reaction
   e. **Hypoglycemia** related to drug overdosage, drug interactions, altered drug metabolism, or inadequate food intake, or because of renal or hepatic dysfunction
6. Nursing considerations
   a. Assess vital signs, weight, condition of skin and nails, serum and urine glucose levels, glycosylated hemoglobin, and electrolyte and arterial blood gas levels when appropriate
   b. Assess for long-term complications of diabetes as noted in previous section regarding nursing considerations with insulin

Box 42–7

Oral Antidiabetics/Hypoglycemics (Sulfonylureas)

First-Generation Agents	Second-Generation Agents
Acetohexamide (Dymelor)	Glipizide standard (Glucotrol)
Chlorpropamide (Diabinese)	Glipizide sustained release (Glucotrol XL)
Tolbutamide (Orinase)	Glyburide Nonmicronized (Diabeta, Micronase)
Tolazamide (Tolinase)	Glyburide Micronized (Glynase, PresTab)
	Glimepiride (Amaryl)

c. Consult with physician regarding management when client has insufficient food intake or is NPO for surgery

7. Client teaching
   a. Participate in individualized teaching plan based on previous knowledge, educational level, motivation to learn, and cultural considerations
   b. Understand all aspects of drug therapy; take with food if GI upset
   c. Take medication even if not feeling well
   d. Take dose with first daily meal and take any missed dose as soon as remembered unless time for next dose; do not double up doses
   e. Understand and be sure family understands signs and symptoms of hypoglycemia; notify physician if symptoms occur
   f. Learn how to test blood glucose levels
   g. Follow dietary restrictions and weight control measures; consult dietitian (very helpful for developing effective meal and weight management plans)
   h. Engage in regular aerobic exercise appropriate to health and abilities
   i. Understand foot care and related aspects of personal hygiene
   j. Understand sick-day management of diabetes and PRN insulin administration
   k. Obtain and wear Medic-Alert tag or bracelet
   l. Avoid smoking or drinking alcoholic beverages
   m. Consult with physician before conceiving (females); discontinue drug during pregnancy and lactation (may need insulin)
   n. Contact local home care agency and American Diabetic Association for additional follow-up and access to community-based resources

C. Oral antidiabetics (hypoglycemic) agents—nonsulfonylureas

1. Biguanides lower blood glucose by decreasing production of glucose by liver
2. Alpha-glucosidase inhibitors delay absorption of dietary carbohydrates and reduce blood glucose
3. Thiazolidinediones or "glitazones" reduce blood glucose by reducing glucose resistance and inhibiting gluconeogenesis in liver
4. All decrease blood glucose levels after meals in clients with type 2 diabetes mellitus not controlled by diet modification and exercise
5. Common medications are listed in Box 42–8
6. Administration considerations
   a. Given orally 1 to 3 times a day
   b. Biguanides are used alone or in combination with a sulfonylurea
   c. Alpha-glucose inhibitors are used alone or in combination with insulin or a sulfonylurea
   d. Contraindicated in renal insufficiency or other kidney disease
   e. Thiazolidinedione should be used cautiously in clients with liver disease; may cause liver damage
   f. Biguanides and alpha-glucosidase inhibitors should not be taken together because of significant GI distress
   g. Alcohol may increase risk of hypoglycemia or lactic acidosis

Box 42–8

Oral Antidiabetics/ Hypoglycemics (Nonsulfonylureas)

Biguanide

Metformin (Glucophage)

Meglitinides

Nateglinide (Starlix)

Repaglinide (Prandin)

Alpha-glucosidase Inhibitors

Acarbose (Precose)

Miglitol (Glyset)

Thiazolidinediones

Pioglitazone (Actos)

Rosiglitazone (Advandia)

Combination Drugs

Glipizide/metformin (Metaglip)

Glyburide/metformin (Glucovance)

Rosiglitazone/metformin (Avandamet)

7. Side/adverse effects
   a. Biguanides may cause decreased appetite, nausea, and diarrhea that usually subside over time; increased absorption of vitamin B_{12} and folic acid may occur
   b. Biguanides with hypoglycemia and lactic acidosis result in a mortality rate of 50%
   c. Alpha-glucosidase inhibitors cause flatulence, cramps, abdominal distension, borborygmus, and diarrhea; also may decrease absorption of iron, leading to anemia
   d. Alpha-glucosidase inhibitors may lead to hypoglycemia if given with insulin or a sulfonylurea
8. Nursing considerations
   a. Assess vital signs, weight, condition of skin and nails, serum and urine glucose levels, glycosylated hemoglobin, and electrolyte and arterial blood gas levels when appropriate
   b. Assess renal function and liver function studies
   c. Assess for early signs of lactic acidosis
   d. Assess for long-term complications of diabetes mellitus
   e. Consult with physician regarding management when client has insufficient food intake or is NPO for surgery
9. Client teaching
   a. Understand all aspects of diabetic management as outlined in previous client education section for sulfonylureas
   b. Understand early signs of hypoglycemia and lactic acidosis (hyperventilation, myalgia, malaise, unusual somnolence) and notify physician immediately if symptoms occur

D. Glucose-elevating medication—glucagon (Glucagen)

1. Promotes breakdown of glycogen, reduces glycogen synthesis, and stimulates synthesis of glucose
2. Used for emergency treatment of severe hypoglycemia in clients who are unconscious, unable to swallow, or receiving insulin shock therapy
3. Administration considerations
   a. Reconstitute according to manufacturer's directions
   b. Give IM, subcutaneously or by direct IVP; flush IV line with 5% dextrose instead of sodium chloride (NaCl) solution; incompatible with NaCl solutions or additives
   c. Incompatible in syringe with any other medication
   d. Contraindicated with hypersensitivity to glucagon or protein compounds
   e. Use cautiously in insulinoma and pheochromocytoma
4. Side/adverse effects: nausea and vomiting, hypersensitivity reactions, hyperglycemia and hypokalemia
5. Nursing considerations
   a. Client usually responds/awakens within 5 to 20 minutes after administration
   b. Give IV glucose if no response to glucagon
   c. After client awakens and is able to swallow, give PO carbohydrate
   d. After recovery, assess for persistent headache, nausea, and weakness
6. Client teaching
   a. Learn how to test blood glucose levels
   b. Be sure responsible family member knows how to administer subcutaneous or IM dose to treat hypoglycemic reactions
   c. Notify physician immediately after reaction to discover cause

Check Your NCLEX-RN® Exam I.Q.

You are ready for testing on this content if you can

- Apply knowledge of expected actions and effects of endocrine medications to client care.
- Correctly administer endocrine medications to clients.
- Assess for side effects and adverse effects of endocrine medications.
- Take appropriate action if a client has an unexpected response to an endocrine medication.
- Monitor a client for expected outcomes or effects of treatment with endocrine medications.

PRACTICE TEST

1 A young child who has been taking growth hormone (Somatropin) for 1 month is complaining of flank pain, colic, and GI symptoms. The nurse concludes this client is at increased risk for which of the following adverse effects that are more likely to occur during the first few months of treatment?

1. Acute glomerulonephritis
2. Renal calculi
3. Bowel obstruction
4. Duodenal ulcer

2 A client with coronary artery disease and hypertension was recently diagnosed with diabetes insipidus. The nurse concludes that treatment with antidiuretic hormone (ADH) is contraindicated for this client for which of the following reasons?

1. Fluid overload and elevated BP may occur.
2. Volume depletion and decreased blood pressure may occur.
3. Overstimulation and agitation may occur.
4. Hypercalciuria and renal calculi may occur.

3 A client with cardiovascular disease has been recently diagnosed with hypothyroidism, and levothyroxine (Levoxyl) has been prescribed. Which of the following signs and symptoms related to this medication are most important for the client to report to the physician?

1. Increased urine output
2. Chest pain
3. Increase in appetite
4. Loose stools

4 A client with a history of cardiac disease is exhibiting severe symptoms of hypothyroidism and is started on medication therapy with levothyroxine (Synthroid). The nurse anticipates that which of the following principles will be followed for initiation of drug therapy?

1. The client will be started with the highest dose possible, and the dose will then be titrated according to the client's response.
2. The client will be started with the highest dose possible and will be given a beta blocker to prevent any incidences of tachycardia.
3. The client will be started with as low a dose as possible, and the dose will gradually be increased over a period of weeks.
4. The client will receive a fixed dose calculated according to the client's weight; this dose will not be adjusted unless necessary.

5 A client with acute adrenal insufficiency (adrenal crisis) is admitted to the hospital. The nurse monitors for resolution of which of the following manifestations to determine that drug therapy with cortisone (Cortone) has been effective?

1. Hyperexcitability and restlessness
2. Increased appetite and weight gain
3. Vitiligo and hyperpigmentation
4. Hypertension and hypernatremia

6 The nurse is assessing the laboratory data of a client diagnosed with Cushing's syndrome. The nurse would expect to note which of the following laboratory values prior to initiation of drug therapy?

1. Elevated plasma cortisol level
2. Decreased blood glucose level
3. Decreased white blood cell count
4. Decreased sodium level

7 The nurse is caring for a client who has just been diagnosed with Graves' disease. Client education needs to include which of the following?

1. Atropine-like medication
2. Thyroid hormone replacement therapy
3. A low-calorie diet
4. Propylthiouracil (PTU)

8 A client with Graves' disease related to hyperthyroidism has been taking medication therapy as prescribed. Which of the following findings noted on cardiac assessment indicates to the nurse that the client has not had a sufficient response to medication therapy?

1. Decreased systolic blood pressure
2. Narrow pulse pressure
3. Bradycardia
4. Tachycardia

PRACTICE TEST

9. The nurse is caring for a client who has been recently diagnosed with hypoparathyroidism. To determine the effectiveness of medication therapy with calcitrol (Rocaltrol), the nurse assesses laboratory findings to see whether which of the following has occurred?

1. Hypercalcemia is resolving
2. Hypocalcemia is resolving
3. Hypermagnesemia is resolving
4. Vitamin D levels are decreasing

10. A client with type 2 diabetes mellitus has been prescribed pioglitazone (Actos). Which one of the following tests does the nurse anticipate will be done before drug therapy is initiated with this medication?

1. Liver function tests
2. Thyroid function tests
3. Respiratory function tests
4. Pituitary function tests

11. A client newly diagnosed with adrenal insufficiency is to begin therapy with fludrocortisone (Florinef). The nurse explains to the client in simple terms that this medication will do which of the following?

1. Decrease resorption of sodium by decreasing hydrogen and potassium excretion in the distal tubule
2. Increase resorption of sodium by increasing hydrogen and potassium excretion in the distal tubule
3. Decrease inflammation by suppressing migration of leukocytes and modifying the body's immune response to many stimuli
4. Increase inflammation by stimulating the production of leukocytes and enhancing the body's immune response to many stimuli

12. A homebound client with type 2 diabetes mellitus calls the nurse to report nausea and flulike symptoms for 2 days. What advice should the nurse give the client?

1. "Be sure to check your blood glucose level in the morning on a daily basis."
2. "Only take half of your regular dose of insulin and oral hypoglycemic agent."
3. "Limit fluid intake and eat only when you feel hungry."
4. "Test your urine for ketones if your blood glucose is greater than 240 mg/dL."

13. A client has been just diagnosed with hypothyroidism. The client also takes sodium warfarin (Coumadin). Before giving any thyroid replacement hormone, the nurse checks the results of what laboratory value that should be drawn?

1. Complete blood count (CBC)
2. Prothrombin time (PT) or international normalized ratio (INR)
3. Activated partial thromboplastin time (APTT)
4. Warfarin (Coumadin) level

14. A client who has osteoporosis has been receiving calcium supplements on a long-term basis. The physician has ordered the client to start taking digoxin (Lanoxin). What type of drug interaction would the home care nurse assess for in future visits?

1. Hypocalcemia
2. Hyperkalemia
3. Digoxin toxicity
4. Hypermagnesemia

15. The nurse who is working in a women's health clinic has several clients to see during the day. Which of these clients does the nurse anticipate will need medication teaching for calcium supplementation to treat primary osteoporosis?

1. A premenopausal client
2. An overweight client
3. An African American client
4. A Caucasian client

16. A client with osteoporosis has been prescribed hormone replacement therapy (HRT) in addition to calcium supplements. The nurse teaches the client that progesterone is given along with estrogen in this therapy to decrease occurrence of what condition?

1. Vaginitis
2. Endometrial or breast cancer
3. Benign breast tumors
4. Ovarian cysts

17 A client newly diagnosed with diabetes mellitus has begun taking insulin. The client asks the nurse about alcohol consumption. What should the nurse tell the client?

1. "Moderate to high alcohol consumption without food can cause your blood glucose level to go down too low."
2. "Moderate to high alcohol consumption without food can cause your blood glucose level to rise too high."
3. "Consumption of alcohol has no effect on your blood glucose as long as you don't eat while drinking."
4. "As long as you only drink beer and wine and not hard liquor then there should be no effect from the alcohol."

18 The nurse is instructing the newly diagnosed diabetic client how to mix regular insulin and NPH insulin. What should the nurse tell the client?

1. Shake the bottle of intermediate insulin before withdrawing the amount.
2. Withdraw the longer-acting insulin first.
3. Withdraw the shorter-acting insulin first.
4. Never inject air into the bottles before withdrawing.

19 Metformin (Glucophage) has been prescribed for a client newly diagnosed with type 2 diabetes mellitus. The nurse evaluates that the client understood medication teaching when the client states that this medication does which of the following?

1. Decreases sensitivity of peripheral tissue to insulin
2. Stimulates glucose production in the liver
3. Treats unstable type 2 diabetes mellitus
4. Decreases production of glucose by the liver

20 The physician has prescribed vitamin D for a client. The client asks the nurse what the medication is for. Which of the following is the best response by the nurse?

1. "Vitamin D decreases intestinal absorption of calcium and phosphorus and decreases their mobilization from bone."
2. "Vitamin D helps regulate calcium and phosphorus balance."
3. "Vitamin D helps the kidneys rid the body of excess calcium and phosphorus."
4. "Vitamin D decreases blood levels of calcium and phosphorus."

ANSWERS & RATIONALES

1 **Answer: 2** Adverse/side effects during the first 2 to 3 months of treatment with growth hormone include hypercalciuria with resultant renal calculi. The client is not at increased risk for acute glomerulonephritis, bowel obstruction, or duodenal ulcer (options 1, 3, and 4).
Cognitive Level: Analysis **Client Need:** Physiological Integrity: Pharmacological and Parenteral Therapies **Integrated Process:** Nursing Process: Analysis **Content Area:** Pharmacology **Strategy:** Note the key words in the question are *first few months.* This tells you the adverse effect occurs soon after medication therapy begins. Use medication knowledge and the process of elimination to make a selection.

2 **Answer: 1** Clients with coronary artery insufficiency and hypertensive cardiovascular disease who take ADH are at increased risk for developing fluid overload and edema. Option 2 is the opposite of what would occur. Options 3 and 4 are not related to this client's situation.
Cognitive Level: Analysis **Client Need:** Physiological Integrity: Pharmacological and Parenteral Therapies **Integrated Process:** Nursing Process: Analysis **Content Area:** Pharmacology **Strategy:** Note that options 1 and 2 are opposite, which may be a clue that one of them is correct. Recall that ADH causes fluid retention to link this information with the associated risks for a client with cardiac disease.

3 **Answer: 2** Clients with known cardiovascular disease who are prescribed thyroid hormone replacement therapy may develop chest pain that could lead to myocardial infarction. For this reason it is the most important manifestation for the client to report. The other manifestations, if they occurred in this client, would have a lesser priority.
Cognitive Level: Analysis **Client Need:** Physiological Integrity: Pharmacological and Parenteral Therapies **Integrated Process:** Nursing Process: Planning **Content Area:** Pharmacology **Strategy:** The critical words in the stem of the question are *most important,* which tells you that more than one answer may be correct and that you must prioritize your answer. Use the ABCs (airway, breathing, and circulation) to select the answer most important to a client with cardiac disease (which affects circulation).

4 **Answer: 3** Clients with severe symptoms of hypothyroidism and a history of cardiac disease must be started on the lowest dose possible of hormone therapy and have the dose gradually increased in order to prevent onset of severe hypertension, heart failure, and myocardial infarction (MI). The other options could put the client at risk for chest pain and subsequent MI.
Cognitive Level: Analysis **Client Need:** Physiological Integrity: Pharmacological and Parenteral Therapies **Integrated Process:**

Nursing Process: Planning **Content Area:** Pharmacology **Strategy:** The core issue of the question is knowledge of the principles of beginning a medication that stimulates metabolism in a client with heart disease. Use knowledge of pathophysiology to select the option that causes the least stress on the heart during initiation of therapy.

5 **Answer: 3** Clients with acute adrenal insufficiency will complain of musculoskeletal symptoms of weakness and fatigue; GI complaints of anorexia, nausea and vomiting, and weight loss; integumentary symptoms of vitiligo and hyperpigmentation; and cardiovascular symptoms related to anemia, hypotension, hyponatremia, hyperkalemia, and hypercalcemia. The manifestations in options 1, 2, and 4 are opposite those seen with adrenal insufficiency and are therefore incorrect.
Cognitive Level: Analysis **Client Need:** Physiological Integrity: Pharmacological and Parenteral Therapies **Integrated Process:** Nursing Process: Evaluation **Content Area:** Pharmacology **Strategy:** The wording of the question tells you that the core issue is knowledge of signs and symptoms of adrenal insufficiency that should respond to drug therapy. Use nursing knowledge and the process of elimination to make a selection.

6 **Answer: 1** Clients with Cushing's syndrome or hypercortisolism have elevated levels of cortisol, low ACTH levels, increased blood glucose levels, elevated white blood cell counts, elevated lymphocyte counts, increased sodium levels, decreased serum calcium levels, and decreased serum potassium levels. Drug therapy will reduce serum cortisol levels when given as directed. The laboratory trends noted in options 2, 3, and 4 are opposite what would be expected in Cushing's syndrome.
Cognitive Level: Application **Client Need:** Physiological Integrity: Pharmacological and Parenteral Therapies **Integrated Process:** Nursing Process: Assessment **Content Area:** Pharmacology **Strategy:** The core issue of the question is knowledge of laboratory values that are expected to change once drug therapy is initiated for Cushing's syndrome. Use nursing knowledge and the process of elimination to make a selection.

7 **Answer: 4** Graves' disease is caused by elevated levels of thyroid hormone. Clients experience tachycardia, nervousness, insomnia, increased heat production, and weight loss. Medication therapy with an agent such as propylthiouracil will help control the disorder. Option 1 is irrelevant, while option 2 is indicated for hypothyroidism. A client with this disorder needs a high-calorie diet, not a low-calorie one (option 3).
Cognitive Level: Analysis **Client Need:** Physiological Integrity: Pharmacological and Parenteral Therapies **Integrated Process:** Nursing Process: Planning **Content Area:** Pharmacology **Strategy:** The core issue of the question is the type of medication therapy that will be effective in treating hyperthyroidism or Graves' disease. Use nursing knowledge and the process of elimination to make a selection.

8 **Answer: 4** Cardiac problems related to Graves' disease and hyperthyroidism include increased systolic blood pressure, a widened pulse pressure, tachycardia, and other dysrhythmias. Appropriate control of the disorder with medication therapy would prevent these manifestations from occurring.
Cognitive Level: Application **Client Need:** Physiological Integrity: Pharmacological and Parenteral Therapies **Integrated Process:** Nursing Process: Assessment **Content Area:** Pharmacology **Strategy:** The core issue of the question is knowledge of what symptoms should resolve once medication therapy for Graves' disease has begun. Recall that Graves' disease represents a hypermetabolic state, and then eliminate each option that does not correlate with excess metabolic activity.

9 **Answer: 2** Management of hypoparathyroidism is aimed at correcting hypocalcemia, vitamin D deficiency, and hypomagnesemia. Options 1 and 4 are incorrect because they are the opposite of effective treatment of hypoparathyroidism, while option 3 is an unrelated finding.
Cognitive Level: Application **Client Need:** Physiological Integrity: Pharmacological and Parenteral Therapies **Integrated Process:** Nursing Process: Analysis **Content Area:** Pharmacology **Strategy:** The core issue of the question is knowledge of abnormal laboratory values that should resolve with effective medication therapy for hypoparathyroidism. Use knowledge of medication actions to eliminate each of the incorrect options. Options 1 and 2 are opposite, which is a clue that one of them is likely to be the correct answer.

10 **Answer: 1** Actos is a thiazolidinedione type of oral antidiabetic agent; its action enhances insulin action and promotes glucose utilization in peripheral tissues. This drug improves sensitivity to insulin in muscle and fat tissue and inhibits glucogenesis. Because of the potential for liver damage, clients taking drugs in this class must have liver function studies done before therapy is begun and periodically thereafter.
Cognitive Level: Application **Client Need:** Physiological Integrity: Pharmacological and Parenteral Therapies **Integrated Process:** Nursing Process: Planning **Content Area:** Pharmacology **Strategy:** The core issue of this question is knowledge of the adverse effects of thiazolidinedione antidiabetic agents. Recall as a general strategy that many drug classes have adverse effects on the liver. Use medication knowledge and the process of elimination to make a selection.

11 **Answer: 2** Adrenocortical replacement therapy medications are divided into mineralocorticoids and glucocorticoids. Mineralcorticoids such as fludrocortisone increase resorption of sodium by increasing hydrogen and potassium excretion in the distal tubule. Glucocorticoids decrease inflammation by suppressing leukocyte migration and modifying the body's immune response. The statements in the remaining options do not reflect these actions.
Cognitive Level: Application **Client Need:** Physiological Integrity: Pharmacological and Parenteral Therapies **Integrated Process:** Teaching and Learning **Content Area:** Pharmacology **Strategy:** Specific medication knowledge about the effects of mineralocorticoid drug therapy is needed to answer this question. Use medication knowledge and the process of elimination to make a selection.

12 **Answer: 4** If anorexia, nausea, or vomiting are present, sick-day diabetic management care requires clients to check their blood glucose level every 4 to 6 hours. Clients should not eliminate or adjust their doses of insulin or oral hypoglycemics. They also should drink 8 to 12 ounces of sugar-free liquids as tolerated every hour to prevent dehydration. Meals should be eaten at regular times, and they should consume foods and liquids that are more easily tolerated. To

prevent diabetic ketoacidosis, this client must regularly check urine ketone levels if the blood glucose level is greater than 240 mg/dL.

Cognitive Level: Application **Client Need:** Physiological Integrity: Pharmacological and Parenteral Therapies **Integrated Process:** Nursing Process: Implementation **Content Area:** Pharmacology **Strategy:** The core issue of the question is knowledge of how to manage medication therapy during illness. With this in mind, choose the option that does not decrease the drug dose (since blood glucose rises during illness) and provides for safe and effective treatment (calling the physician when the level is excessive).

13 **Answer: 2** Thyroid hormones increase the effects of anticoagulants. Assessment of PT or INR will determine if the anticoagulant dosage must be decreased. The nurse also assesses the client for evidence of bruising or bleeding. A CBC could detect anemia caused by bleeding as a complication of excessive warfarin therapy. APTT measures the effectiveness of heparin. Coumadin levels are not drawn.

Cognitive Level: Application **Client Need:** Physiological Integrity: Pharmacological and Parenteral Therapies **Integrated Process:** Nursing Process: Assessment **Content Area:** Pharmacology **Strategy:** The core issue of the question is understanding of interactive effects of thyroid hormones and anticoagulants such as warfarin. Use knowledge of both medications and associated laboratory values to make a selection.

14 **Answer: 3** Hypercalcemia, hypomagnesemia, and digitalis toxicity may result when calcium supplements interact with digoxin. Clients must be instructed to take these two drugs at separate times of the day. Also, antacids must not be taken with digoxin. Hyperkalemia is not a concern with calcium supplementation.

Cognitive Level: Analysis **Client Need:** Physiological Integrity: Pharmacological and Parenteral Therapies **Integrated Process:** Nursing Process: Assessment **Content Area:** Pharmacology **Strategy:** The core issue of the question is knowledge of the effects of calcium supplements in a client who also takes digoxin. Use knowledge of medication interactions and the process of elimination to make a selection.

15 **Answer: 4** Primary osteoporosis most often occurs in postmenopausal women who are thin and lean-built. It is more prevalent in Caucasian and Asian women.

Cognitive Level: Analysis **Client Need:** Physiological Integrity: Pharmacological and Parenteral Therapies **Integrated Process:** Nursing Process: Analysis **Content Area:** Pharmacology **Strategy:** The core issue of the question is knowledge of the clients at risk for osteoporosis and amenable to therapy with calcium supplementation. Use general nursing knowledge and the process of elimination to make a selection.

16 **Answer: 2** Progesterone frequently is given along with estrogen as part of HRT to minimize the occurrence of endometrial or breast cancer. The other options do not relate to this medication.

Cognitive Level: Application **Client Need:** Physiological Integrity: Pharmacological and Parenteral Therapies **Integrated Process:** Teaching/Learning **Content Area:** Pharmacology **Strategy:** The core issue of the question is knowledge of the adverse effects of HRT that is given in addition to calcium supplementation for prevention or treatment of osteoporosis. Use knowledge of adverse drug effects and the process of elimination to make a selection.

17 **Answer: 1** If diabetes if well controlled, blood glucose levels are not affected by mild consumption of alcohol. Male clients taking insulin may ingest two alcoholic beverages daily and female clients may ingest one alcoholic beverage with, or in addition to, the regular meal plan. Because of the risk of alcohol-induced hypoglycemia, diabetic clients must ingest alcohol only with or shortly after meals. In all cases, the client should confer with the prescribing physician and dietitian to determine whether alcohol should be utilized as part of the overall caloric intake.

Cognitive Level: Application **Client Need:** Physiological Integrity: Pharmacological and Parenteral Therapies **Integrated Process:** Communication and Documentation **Content Area:** Pharmacology **Strategy:** The core issue of the question is knowledge of how alcohol can affect blood glucose levels in a client taking insulin. Use knowledge of interactive effects of medications and alcohol to make a selection.

18 **Answer: 3** The following statements are commonly used to teach clients how to combine insulins in one syringe: Gently roll the bottle of intermediate insulin to mix because vigorous shaking creates bubbles, leading to an inaccurate dose. Air must be injected into each bottle before withdrawing. Withdrawing the shorter-acting insulin first prevents the longer-acting insulin from mixing in the bottle with the shorter-acting insulin.

Cognitive Level: Application **Client Need:** Physiological Integrity: Pharmacological and Parenteral Therapies **Integrated Process:** Teaching/Learning **Content Area:** Pharmacology **Strategy:** The core issue of the question is proper technique for drawing up mixed insulins. Choose the option that does not contaminate the shorter-acting insulin with the longer-acting one, which would necessitate discarding the contaminated vial.

19 **Answer: 4** Metformin is given to clients with stable type 2 diabetes mellitus to inhibit glucose production by the liver and increase sensitivity of peripheral tissue to insulin. The other three options contain factually incorrect statements.

Cognitive Level: Analysis **Client Need:** Physiological Integrity: Pharmacological and Parenteral Therapies **Integrated Process:** Nursing Process: Evaluation **Content Area:** Pharmacology **Strategy:** The core issue of the question is knowledge of the actions of metformin on reducing blood glucose. Use medication knowledge and the process of elimination to make a selection.

20 **Answer: 2** Vitamin D regulates calcium and phosphorus levels by increasing blood levels, increasing intestinal absorption and mobilization from bone, and reducing renal excretion of both elements. The statements in the other options are the opposites of the actions of vitamin D.

Cognitive Level: Application **Client Need:** Physiological Integrity: Pharmacological and Parenteral Therapies **Integrated Process:** Teaching/Learning **Content Area:** Pharmacology **Strategy:** The core issue of the question is knowledge of the effects of vitamin D. Use medication knowledge and the process of elimination to make a selection.

Key Terms to Review

Addison's disease p. 694
adrenal crisis p. 695
adrenal insufficiency p. 694
catecholamine p. 697
cushingoid state p. 696
glucocorticoid p. 694
glycosylated hemoglobin p. 703
Graves' disease p. 697
hypercalciuria p. 691
hyperglycemia p. 702
hyperthyroidism p. 697
hypoglycemia p. 704
hypoparathyroidism p. 699
hypothyroidism p. 696
lipodystrophy p. 703
mineralocorticoid p. 692
myxedema p. 696
osteomalacia p. 699
osteoporosis p. 696
Paget's disease p. 701

References

Abrams, A. (2004). *Clinical drug therapy: Rationales for nursing practice* (7th ed.). Philadelphia: Lippincott; Williams & Wilkins.

Adams, M., Josephson, D., & Holland, L. (2005). *Pharmacology for nurses: A pathophysiologic approach.* Upper Saddle River, NJ: Pearson Education.

Deglin, J. H., & Vallerand, A. H. (2006). *Davis's drug guide for nurses* (10th ed.). Philadelphia: F. A. Davis.

Lehne, R. (2004). *Pharmacology for nursing care* (5th ed.). Philadelphia: W. B. Saunders.

McKenry, L., Tessier, E. & Hogan, M. (2006). *Mosby's pharmacology in nursing.* (22nd ed.). St. Louis: Elsevier Science.

Wilson, B., Shannon, M., & Stang, C. (2006). *Prentice Hall nurse's drug guide 2006.* Upper Saddle River, NJ: Pearson Education.

Integumentary Medications 43

In this chapter

Cross reference

Other chapters relevant to this content area are

Dosage Calculation and Medication Administration	Chapter 30
Integumentary Disorders	Chapter 63

Test Yourself

Are you ready for the NCLEX-RN® or course exams? Use the practice tests on the companion CD-ROM to check.

I. GENERAL AGENTS

A. Soaps

1. Deodorant soaps (e.g., Dial™, Lever 2000™, Safeguard™) are relatively harsh soaps that contain triclosan or triclocarban as topical antibacterial agents; are useful in decreasing body odor, preventing bacterial spread, and assisting in treatment of cutaneous infections
2. True soaps (i.e., Ivory™) mechanically remove bacteria and remove sebum and environmental dirt
3. Synthetic detergent bars (i.e., Dove™, Neutrogena™, Tone™) are generally milder and comprise a group of products known as beauty bars
4. Allergic sensitization can occur to fragrances, dyes, antibacterial agents, or other additives in soaps
5. Medicated shampoos (with ingredients such as selenium sulfide 1%, may be used for dandruff, seborrheic dermatitis, or **psoriasis**—a chronic skin disorder characterized by periodic exacerbations of erythematous papules and plaques covered by prominent, thick, silvery-white scales)
6. Nursing considerations
   a. Assess any skin symptom, beginning with a history
   b. Monitor for local adverse effects/irritation from use of selected soap(s) and/or shampoo(s)
   c. Read product literature carefully because some shampoos are not recommended for small children

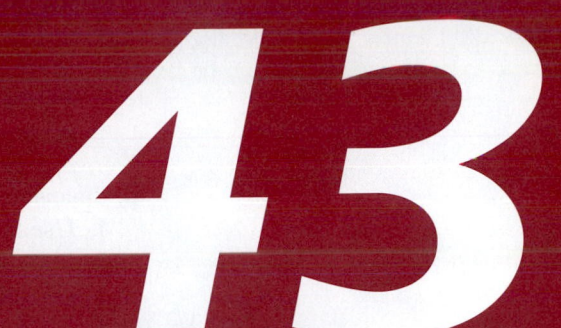

7. Client teaching
   a. Soaps can be irritating to people with dry skin, especially in winter with low humidity
   b. Apply a moisturizing preparation after bathing if dry skin is a problem
   c. Learn proper use of any prescribed shampoo

B. Cleansers

1. Used for preoperative cleansing of skin, treatment of wounds or abrasions
2. May be bacteriostatic or bactericidal depending on agent
3. Common preparations are listed in Table 43–1 ■
4. Nursing considerations
   a. Assess any skin symptom, beginning with a history
   b. Monitor for local irritation and/or drying as an adverse effect of these topical preparations
5. Client teaching
   a. Learn proper use of any prescribed cleanser
   b. If wounds or abrasions are present, understand inflammatory process and wound healing process

C. *Lotions*

1. Lotions historically were "shake lotions" or suspensions of a **powder** (finely divided solid drug or mixture of drugs) in water; powder would remain on skin as water evaporated to produce a drying effect
2. Today other types of liquid emulsions of thin, uniform consistency are also called lotions
3. Common preparations include calamine lotion (Calamox) zinc stearate, and others; may contain calamine, zinc oxide, glycerin bentonite magma, calcium hydroxide, and other ingedients
4. Nursing considerations
   a. Shake lotion before application to place powder in suspension
   b. Monitor for local and systemic adverse effects
5. Client teaching
   a. Learn proper use of any prescribed lotion
   b. Some preparations of calamine lotion also contain diphenhydramine (Benadryl), which can cause drowsiness; use cautiously until their effects are known

Table 43–1

Cleansers

Agent	Use
Povidone-iodine (Betadine, Betagen, Aerodine, Iodex, others)	Bactericidal
Iodine (iodine topical, iodine tincture)	Cleansing action
Benzalkonium chloride (Benza, Zephiran)	Bacteriostatic; can support growth of certain pseudomonas species; is inactivated by soap; do not cover with an occlusive dressing
Alcohol	Bactericidal; is not as effective as povidone-iodine
Hydrogen peroxide	Germicidal; has mechanical effectiveness; do not use after epithelium is formed because it will continue to debride newly growing cells
Chlorhexidine gluconate (Hibiclens, Dyna-Hex, Exidine, Hibistat, Peridex)	Cleansing action
Hexachlorophene (Phisohex, Septisol)	Cleansing action
Oxychlorosene sodium (Clorpactin XCB, Clorpactin WCS-90)	Cleansing action
Sodium hypochlorite (Dakin's)	Cleansing action

Box 43–1

Emollients

Aquaphor	Lac-Hydrin lotion 12% (prescription only)
Cetaphil lotion	Lubriderm lotions and oil
Curel moisturizing lotion	Moisturel lotion
Dermasil lotion	Neutrogena emulsion
Eucerin crème or lotion	Penecare lotion
Keri lotion	White petrolatum
Lac-Hydrin cream or lotion	

D. *Emollients*

1. Emollients are occlusive agents that make skin soft and pliable by increasing hydration of and filling gaps in stratum corneum created by dry, contracted skin cells
2. Include silicone oils, propylene glycol, isopropyl palmitate, and octyl stearate
3. Can also function as skin protectants if they soothe **pruritus** (intense itching) due to exposed, traumatized nerve endings
4. Moisturizers are intended to mimic function of sebum on skin, based on mechanisms of occlusion and humectancy
5. Occlusion function employs petrolatum, lanolin, cocoa butter, or mineral oil to prevent evaporation of water from skin
6. Humectancy function employs substances that attract moisture to skin, (e.g., glycerin, sorbitol, propylene glycol)
7. Common preparations are listed in Box 43–1
8. Nursing considerations
   a. Assess any skin symptom, beginning with a history
   b. Unless otherwise directed by product instructions, apply to skin after bathing while skin is slightly moist
9. Client teaching: proper use of any prescribed emollient

E. Protectants

1. Designed to protect skin from wetness or prevent and treat diaper rash, prickly heat, and/or chafing
2. Common preparations are listed in Box 43–2
3. Nursing considerations: assess any skin symptom, beginning with a history; monitor skin for desired effect
4. Client teaching
   a. Powders should be kept away from face to avoid inhalation
   b. Some preparations should not be used on broken skin
   c. If diaper rash or skin irritation worsens or does not improve within 7 days of beginning self-care, consult health care provider

F. Soaks and wet dressings

1. Acute lesions that are oozing, weeping, and crusting generally respond best to medication in aqueous, drying preparations
2. Scaling chronic lesions generally respond best to medication in moisturizing, lubricating preparations
3. Open soaks are applied for 20 minutes, 3 times a day
4. Closed soaks use a water-impermeable substance (occlusion) over a wet soak; this method causes heat retention, which is excellent for debridement but may lead to maceration; are applied for 1 to 2 hours 2 to 3 times a day
5. Continuous closed soaks are left in place for 24 hours to treat thick crusts; it is important to rewet dressing 4 to 5 times a day
6. Common preparations are listed in Table 43–2 ■
7. Nursing considerations: assess any skin symptom, beginning with a history, and monitor for achievement of intended effects
8. Client teaching: proper procedure for type of soak recommended or prescribed

Box 43-2

Protectants

A & D Ointment (lanolin, petrolatum, others)

A & D Medicated Diaper Rash Ointment (white petrolatum, zinc oxide, cod liver oil, light mineral oil, others)

Balmex Ointment (zinc oxide, balsam Peru, beeswax, mineral oil, others)

Caldesene Medicated Powder or Ointment (powder: calcium undecylenate; ointment: white petrolatum, zinc oxide, others)

Clocream Skin Protectant Cream (each ounce contains vitamins A and D equivalent to 1 ounce of cod liver oil, many others)

Desitin Cornstarch Baby Powder (zinc oxide 10% with cornstarch, others)

Desitin Ointment (zinc oxide 40% with cod liver oil in a petrolatum-lanolin base, others)

G. Rubs and liniments

1. Are OTC preparations for temporary relief of minor aches and pains of muscles and joints associated with strains, bruises, sprains, sports injuries, simple backache, and arthritis
2. Common preparations: BenGay™, Aspercreme™, capsaicin (Capsin™) with active ingredient from cayenne peppers; others
3. Nursing considerations: assess symptom for which agent is to be used and monitor for achievement of intended effects
4. Client teaching
   a. Clean skin of all other **ointments** (water in oil emulsions), **creams** (more complex preparations of oil in water than ointments), sprays, or liniments before applying product
   b. Apply to affected areas not more than 3 to 4 times daily
   c. Some products have specific directions (e.g., BenGay should not be used with heating pad or tight bandage)

II. PROTECTIVE AGENTS

A. Overview

1. This discussion is limited to sunscreen preparations and protective dressings
2. For other preparations that can be defined as offering protection, see previous section on *protectants*

B. Sunscreen preparations

1. Can help to prevent skin cancer
2. Chemical sunscreens absorb ultraviolet radiation in spectrum of ultraviolet (UV) light most responsible for sunburns
3. Chemical absorbers formulated against ultraviolet B (UVB) rays include cinnamates, *p*-aminobenzoic acid (PABA) and PABA esters, or salicylates
4. Chemical absorbers formulated against ultraviolet A (UVA) rays include benzophenones

Table 43-2

Soaks and Wet Dressings

Agent	Use
Burow's Solution (Bluboro Powder, Boropak Powder, Domeboro, Pedi-Boro Soak Paks): 5% aluminum acetate solution, 1 Domeboro tablet or packet to 1 pint of tap water	Acts as astringent to decrease exudation by precipitation of protein
Acetic Acid 0.1–1% solution: ½-cup white vinegar to 1 quart water	May be helpful for wound infected with *Pseudomonas* organisms
Potassium Permanganate: 1:4,000–1:16,000 solution	Formerly considered to be useful for fungal infections, but use has decreased because of staining property
Salt solution: 1 tbsp. of salt to 1 quart of water	Wetting action

5. Physical sunscreens reflect or scatter light to prevent skin penetration
6. Physical sunscreens contain ingredients such as titanium dioxide, zinc oxide, talc
7. ! Effectiveness of a sunscreen is indicated by its sun protection factor (SPF); a SPF of 15 means product offers 15 times greater protection than the use of no sunscreen; SPFs range from 4 to 60 in various products
8. A water-resistant sunscreen should continue to function after 40 minutes in water; a waterproof sunscreen withstands 80 minutes
9. Nursing considerations: assess skin for degree of burn if not used effectively
10. ! Client teaching
    a. If tendency to sunburn easily, use products with SPF of 15 or greater
    b. Avoid contact between products and eyes; follow product directions

C. Protective dressings

1. Includes occlusive biosynthetic dressings for certain wound therapies
2. For example, DuoDERM, as a hydrocolloid dressing hydrates wound surface; wound fluid interacts with wafer of preparation and melts it, forming a moist, jellylike substance that keeps wound moist and promotes healing
3. Common dressings are listed in Table 43–3 ■
4. Nursing considerations
    a. Assess any skin wound, beginning with a history
    b. ! Inspect dressing at least daily for leaks, dislodgment, wrinkling, or odor
    c. ! Change dressing when it becomes dislodged, leaks, or develops an odor
    d. ! If wound has substantial drainage, dressing might need changing every 24 to 48 hours but generally is left in place for 3 to 7 days
    e. When changing dressing, leave residue that is difficult to remove; it will wear off in time; attempts to remove can irritate surrounding skin
5. Client teaching: proper use of any prescribed occlusive biosynthetic dressing

III. ANTIPRURITICS

A. Overview

1. Medications that stop intense itching of pruritis
2. Pruritus brings more clients to the health care provider than any other dermatological symptom
3. Pruritus has a multitude of causes, and treatment must be tailored to specific cause
4. Types include winter pruritus, senior pruritus, lichen simplex chronicus, external otitis, pruritus ani (e.g., pinworm infestation in children), and genital pruritus
5. Antipruritic therapy for some types of pruritis might include topical corticosteroids to decrease inflammation and/or methods to promote skin hydration
6. Antipruritic therapy may also require use of a systemic antihistamine

Table 43–3

Common Protective Wound Dressings

Dressing	Transmits Oxygen	Transmits Water Vapor	Excludes Bacteria	Absorbs Fluids	Transparent	Adhesive
Bioclusive	+	+	–	–	+	+
DuoDERM	–	–	+	+	–	+
Geliperm	+	+	+	+	+	+
Intrasite	–	–	+	+	–	+
Op-site	+	+	+	–	+	+
Replicare	–	–	+	–	–	+
Tegasorb	–	–	+	+	–	+
Tegaderm	+	+	?	–	+	+
Vigilon	+	–	–	+	+	–
Zenoderm	+	+	+	+	+	+

+ has the stated action; – does not have the stated action; ? may or may not have the stated action

Box 43–3

Antipruritic Agents

Lotion or Cream

Aveeno Anti-itch Lotion or Cream

Aveeno Moisturing Lotion or Cream

Eucerin Crème or Lotion

Sarna Topical Lotion (camphor, menthol, and phenol)

Zonalon Cream

Hydrating Baths

Aveeno (colloidal oatmeal)

Aveeno Oil (colloidal oatmeal, mineral oil, glyceryl stearate, etc.)

Systemic H_1 Blockers or Combination

Hydroxyzine hydrochloride (Atarax)

Hydroxyzine pamoate (Vistaril)

Chlorpheniramine (Chlor-Trimeton)

Cyproheptadine hydrochloride (Periactin)

Unsafe

Benzocaine and other *-caine* derivatives

Antihistamines such as astemizole (Hismanal)

B. Common medications are listed in Box 43–3

C. Nursing considerations

1. Medications may be topical or oral
2. Take a history of systemic symptoms and any associated skin symptoms
3. ! Monitor for local and systemic adverse effects of any topical preparation
4. ! Monitor for anticholinergic adverse reactions if systemic antihistamines of anticholinergic type are used

! **D. Client teaching**

1. Limit bathing to once or twice a week; use only mild soaps, and use soap in a sparing manner
2. Understand negative effect of scratching and need to interrupt any itch-and-scratch cycle
3. Maintain cool environment, especially in bedroom for sleep

IV. ANTI-INFECTIVES

A. Antibacterials

1. Certain topical antibiotics inhibit growth of *Propionibacterium acnes* and reduce inflammatory lesions of acne
2. Topical antibacterial therapy may be useful for prophylaxis of infections in wounds and injuries
3. Common medications are listed in Table 43–4 ■
4. ! Nursing considerations
   a. Assess any skin symptom, beginning with a history
   b. Assess for hypersensitivity to any ingredient in product to be used
   c. Monitor for skin irritation and superinfection
5. ! Client teaching
   a. Wash hands before using any topical antibacterial agent; may wear gloves
   b. Generally, apply products sparingly and gently to affected area
   c. With some, a dressing should be applied; with others, it should not: follow prescriber instructions
   d. Report worsening of condition or lack of healing

Table 43–4

Antibacterial Agents

Medication	Source	Mechanism of Action	Notes
Bacitracin (Baciguent Topical)	*Bacillus subtilis*	Cell wall inhibitor	Effective against Gram-positive staphylococci and streptococci; used with impetigo, furunculosis, pyodermas
Bacitracin, polymyxin B, neosporin (Mycitracin Topical, Neomixin Topical, Neosporin Topical, Triple Antibiotic Topical)	*Bacillus subtilis, Streptomyces fradiae*	Cell wall inhibitor, 30S ribosome inhibition	Available as ointment to treat secondarily infected skin problems
Chloramphenicol (Chloromycetin)	*Streptococcus venezuelae* or synthetic	50S ribosome inhibition	Used infrequently because dose related bone marrow suppression has occurred following topical exposure
Clindamycin phosphate (Cleocin T, Clinda-Derm Topical Solution)	Semisynthetic	Binding to 50S ribosome and suppression of bacterial protein synthesis	Available as vaginal cream or suppositories, gel, solution, lotion; primarily for treatment of acne
Erythromycin and benzoyl peroxide (Benzamycin)			Gel for acne vulgaris
Gentamicin sulfate (G-myticin Topical)	Fermentation product from *Micromonospora purpura*	Interferes with bacterial protein synthesis	Cream or ointment used following ear surgery to provide prophylaxis against otitis externa due to *Pseudomonas aeruginosa*
Meclocycline sulfosalicylate (Meclan Topical)	Semisynthetic	30S ribosome inhibition	Gram positive and negative; cream to be applied generously but contact with eyes, nose, and mouth to be avoided; do not cover; may stain fabric
Metronidazole (MetroGel)		Unknown but may be due to antibiotic, antioxidant, and anti-inflammatory properties	Available as gel, topical treatment of rosacea
Mupirocin (Bactroban)	*Pseudomonas fluorescens*	tRNA synthetase inhibitor	Topical treatment of impetigo caused by Gram-positives such as *Staphylococcus aureus,* beta-*hemolytic Streptococcus,* and *S. pyogenes*
Neomycin (Mycifradin Sulfate Topical)	*Streptomyces fradiae*	30S ribosome inhibition	Gram negative; cream or ointment used for prophylaxis against infection in abrasions, cuts, burns, but can cause allergic contact dermatitis
Tetracycline (Achromycin Topical, Topicycline Topical)	Semisynthetic	30S ribosome inhibition	Gram positive and negative

B. Antivirals

1. Used to treat cutaneous **herpes simplex** (an acute viral disease marked by groups of skin vesicles, often on borders of lips, nares, or genitals) or herpes zoster
2. With some infections an oral agent instead of a topical agent may be needed
3. Common medication: acyclovir 5% ointment (Zovirax)

Memory Aid

Antiviral agents often can be recognized on sight because they contain *vir* in the beginning, middle, or end of the name.

! 4. Nursing considerations: assess skin symptoms (beginning with a history) and monitor for local adverse effects of topical product, such as mild pain, burning, stinging

! 5. Client teaching
   a. Wash hands before use and apply gloves or finger cot when applying product to avoid autoinnoculation of other body sites
   b. Apply as soon as symptoms of herpes lesions begins
   c. Apply sparingly and gently to affected area
   d. Wear loose clothing and keep area clean and dry
   e. Avoid sexual activity when skin lesions are present

C. Antifungals

1. Topical agents can be used in clients with limited disease and if infection is limited to glabrous (smooth, hairless) skin
2. Clients with extensive disease and infection of hair and nails are best treated with systemic therapy

! 3. Advantages of topical use over systemic use: absence of serious adverse reactions or drug interactions, OTC availability of some preparations, ability to localize treatment to affected sites, no need to monitor laboratory tests

4. New drugs have caused decrease in use of keratolytics and **antiseptics** (chemical agents that inhibit growth of microorganisms but do not necessarily kill them) used in past
5. Common medications
   a. Topical agents are listed in Box 43–4
   b. Oral agents include fluconazole (Diflucan), griseofulvin (Fulvicin, Grispeg), itraconazole (Sporanox), ketoconazole (Nizoral), and terbinafine (Lamisil)

Memory Aid

Antifungal agents are easy to recognize on sight because they generally end with the suffix *-azole*.

6. Nursing considerations
   a. Assess any skin symptom, beginning with a history
   b. Assess for predisposing factors, such as trauma, general health, suppressed immune status, hygiene practices, and exposure to infectious agent
   ! c. Monitor for local adverse effects of topical preparations (irritation, burning, or stinging)
   ! d. Monitor for skin sensitization, noted by increased redness, swelling, weeping, or any burning or itching that were not present before treatment began
   e. Systemic effects of topical products are negligible, since absorption rates generally are only 3% to 6%

! 7. Client teaching
   a. Use products as directed for full course of therapy (may be prolonged); apply liberally to clean and dry skin
   b. Leave exposed to air; do not apply protective dressing unless specifically ordered
   c. Wear shower shoes or thongs in public or communal showers and locker rooms (with **tinea pedis** or athlete's foot)
   d. Avoid going barefoot, and wear footwear of natural fibers (leather shoes, cotton or wool socks) to prevent tinea pedis; change socks daily

Box 43–4

Topical Antifungals

Medication

Allylamines

Naftifine hydrochloride (Naftin): cream gel

Terbinafine (Lamisal): cream

Imidazoles

Clotrimazole (Lotrimin, Mycelex): cream, solution, lotion, vaginal tablets, or cream

Econazole nitrate (Spectazole): cream

Ketoconazole (Nizoral): cream, shampoo

Miconazole nitrate (Monistat): cream, powder, spray, vaginal suppository, vaginal cream

Oxiconazole (Oxistat): cream, lotion

Sulfonazole nitrate (Exelderm): cream, solution

Miscellaneous

Ciclopirox olamine (Loprox): cream, lotion

Triacetin (Fungoid; includes triacetin, sodium propionate, benzalkonium chloride, cetylpyridium chloride, & chloroxylenol): solution, cream

Undecenoic acid, undecylenic acid (Desenex)

Nystatin (Mycostatin, Nilstat): cream, ointment, powder, vaginal tablet

Tolnaftate (Tinactin): cream, solution, spray, liquid, spray powder; (Aftate) gel, powder, spray liquid

e. To avoid other fungal infections, practice adequate hygiene by keeping affected areas clean, dry, and well ventilated (loose clothing), and use powders (with or without antifungal ingredients) to keep skin dry and prevent maceration

D. Antiparasitics

1. Used to treat infestations such as **scabies** (parasitic infestation caused by *Sarcoptes scabiei* mite) or **pediculosis** (parasitic infestation caused by lice); may involve hair (tinea capitus), body (tinea corporis), or pubic area (tinea pubis)
2. Recurrence of scabies is generally related to reinfection from incomplete treatment rather than resistance of mite
3. Crotamiton can be used in clients with scabies and pediculosis capitis who are ragweed-sensitive
4. Common medications are listed in Table 43–5 ■
5. Nursing considerations
   a. Assess any skin symptom, beginning with a history
   b. Monitor for local adverse effects, including irritation, pruritis, burning, or stinging
   ! c. Monitor for systemic effect of dizziness with lindane because it affects nervous system; avoid use in infants, children, and clients with known seizure disorders because of risk of convulsions

Table 43–5

Antiparasitics

Agent	Uses
Crotamiton (Eurax cream, lotion)	Scabies
Malathion (Ovide lotion)	Pediculosis capitis and their ova
Permethrin (Elimite cream, Nix liquid)	Pediculosis capitis, scabies
Pyrethrin, piperonyl butoxide (liquid, Rid shampoo)	Pediculosis capitis, pediculosis corporis, pediculosis pubis
Lindane (Kwell cream, lotion, shampoo)	Pediculosis capitis, pediculosis pubis, scabies

6. Client teaching: scabies
   a. Apply thin layer to dry skin from neck down and rub in thoroughly over entire body
   b. Permethrin and lindane: leave on 8 to 12 hours, remove thoroughly with washing
   c. Crotamiton: apply again after 24 hours, remove with washing 48 hours after initial application
7. Client teaching: pediculosis capitis
   a. Lindane lotion: apply lotion to dry hair, rub in thoroughly, leave on 12 hours, remove thoroughly
   b. Lindane shampoo: apply shampoo to dry hair, lather with small amount water, work into hair for 4 minutes, rinse thoroughly
   c. Second treatment in 7 to 10 days may be needed with malathion, RID

V. CORTICOSTEROIDS

A. Overview

1. Topical or systemic corticosteroids may be used with skin disorders; clinical effectiveness relates to four properties
   a. Vasoconstriction: decreases erythema
   b. Antiproliferative effects: inhibits DNA synthesis and mitosis
   c. Immunosuppression: mechanism poorly understood
   d. Anti-inflammatory effects: inhibits formation of prostaglandins
2. Responsiveness to topical corticosteroids varies: highly responsive diseases include psoriasis, atopic dermatitis in children, seborrheic dermatitis, intertrigo
3. Penetration of preparation varies according to skin site
4. Increased incidence of adverse reactions can occur when using these products on thin skin, on elderly or pediatric clients, or under occlusive dressing
5. Adverse effects more common in higher potency preparations
6. Local adverse reactions include atrophy, hypopigmentation, striae
7. Topical corticosteroids can cause systemic adverse reactions, including suppression of adrenal function
8. Low-potency agents are best used for diffuse eruptions, those involving the face or occluded areas such as axilla or groin, and chronic dermatoses
9. Medium-potency agents are appropriate for acute flare-ups of chronic dermatoses and acute self-limited eruptions where they can be used for periods of 14 to 21 days
10. High-potency agents are best used for acute localized eruptions for a short time of 7 to 14 days
11. High-potency agents should be avoided on areas susceptible to increased penetration and adverse reactions, such as face, intertriginous areas, perineum
12. A twice-a-day application is usually sufficient; more frequent application does not appear to improve response
13. Abrupt discontinuation of mid- or high-potency corticosteroids may result in rebound flare-up of disorder

Memory Aid

A corticosteroid drug often can be recognized because it ends in the suffix *-sone* or *-one*. As an alternative, it may contain *cort* in the beginning, middle, or end of the drug name.

B. Common medications are listed in Table 43–6 ■

C. Nursing considerations

1. Assess any skin symptom, beginning with a history
2. Generally, corticosteroids are applied sparingly and gently in a thin film to affected area
3. At times, preparation should be rubbed in thoroughly
4. Monitor for local adverse effects, which include acneiform skin eruptions, dryness, itching, burning, allergic contact dermatitis, hypopigmentation, and overgrowth of bacteria/fungi/viruses

Table 43-6 Corticosteroids

Potency Class	Generic Name	Brand Name
Lowest potency	Alclometasone 0.05% cream, ointment	Aclovate
	Desonide 0.05% cream, ointment, lotion	Desowen, Tridesilon
	Dexamethasone 0.04% aerosol	Decaspray
	Hydrocortisone 1% cream	Ala-Cort, Cort-Dome, Der-miCort, Hi-Cor-1.0, Hycort, Penecort, Synacort
	Hydrocortisone 1% lotion	Acticort 100, Cetacort, Cortizone-10, Dermacort, LactiCare-HC
	Hydrocortisone 1% ointment	Cortizone-10, Hycort, HydroSKIN, Hydro-Tex, Tegrin-HC
	Hydrocortisone 2.5% cream, ointment	
	Methylprednisolone acetate 0.25% ointment	Medrol
	Methylprednisolone acetate 1% ointment	Medrol
Low potency	Betamethasone valerate 0.025% cream	Valisone
	Clocortolone 0.1% cream	Cloderm
	Fluocinolone acetonide 0.01% cream, solution	Synalar
	Flurandrenolide 0.025% cream, ointment	Cordran
	Hydrocortisone valerate 0.2% cream	Westcort
	Triamcinolone acetonide 0.025% cream, ointment	Kenalog
Intermediate potency	Betamethasone benzoate 0.025% cream, gel, lotion	Uticort
	Betamethasone valerate 0.1% cream, ointment, lotion	Valisone
	Desoximetasone 0.05% cream, ointment	Topicort LP
	Fluocinolone acetonide 0.025% cream	Cutivate
	Halcinonide 0.025% cream, ointment	Halog
	Mometasone furoate 0.1% cream, ointment, lotion	Elocon
	Triamcinolone acetonide 0.1% cream, ointment	Kenalog
High potency	Amcinonide 0.1% cream, ointment	Cyclocort
	Betamethasone dipropionate 0.05% cream, ointment, lotion	Diprosone
	Desoximetasone 0.25% cream, ointment	Topicort
	Flucinolone 0.2% cream	Synalar HP
	Flucinolone 0.05% cream, ointment	Lidex
	Halcinonide 0.1% cream, ointment,solution	Halog
	Triamcinolone acetonide 0.5% cream, ointment	Kenalog
Very high potency	Augmented betamethasone dipropionate 0.05% ointment	Diprolene
	Clobetasol propionate 0.05% cream, ointment	Temovate
	Diflorasone 0.05% gel, ointment	Fluorone, Maxiflor, Psorcon
	Halobetasol propionate 0.05% cream, ointment	Ultravate

! 5. Monitor for systemic adverse effects, which are more likely to include hirsutism (usually of the face), moon facies, alopecia (scalp area), and immunosuppression

! 6. These drugs, especially those of higher potency, should be tapered and not discontinued abruptly

! **D. Client teaching**

1. Use exactly as directed; do not overuse
2. Do not apply to open wounds or weeping areas
3. Before using, wash and dry area gently
4. Report worsening of condition, signs of infection, or lack of healing

VI. KERATOLYTICS

A. Overview

1. Reduce thickness of hyperkeratotic stratum corneum and keratinocyte adhesion (remove or soften horny layer of skin)
2. Used to treat disorders of keratinization (e.g., forms of ichthyosis that generally have genetic component); some are used to treat certain warts
3. Concentration necessary for keratolytic action differs among available agents

B. Common medications are listed in Table 43–7 ■

C. Nursing considerations

1. Assess any skin symptom, beginning with a history
2. Monitor for local adverse effects of topical preparations

D. Client teaching

1. Understand purpose, use, side effects, and anticipated length of treatment
2. Use as directed; method will vary somewhat depending on condition for which it is used

VII. ACNE MEDICATIONS

A. Overview

1. Generally, a staged approach is used
2. Mild **acne** (noninflammatory and inflammatory lesions often on face, chest, back) with some comedones or few inflammatory lesions) is treated with topical agents such as salicylic acid, azelaic acid, benzoyl peroxide, and topical antibiotics
3. Moderate acne consisting of *comedones* (blackheads) and **papules** (small, circumscribed, superficial, solid elevations of the skin) can be managed by gradually increasing strength of topical tretinoin
4. Severe acne consisting of inflammatory papules and nodulocystic disease requires systemic antibiotics and isotretinoin (Accutane)
5. Choice of vehicle for topical preparation depends on whether client has dry or oily skin
6. Local adverse reactions to some topical preparations include erythema, burning or stinging, excessive dryness, and increased susceptibility to sunburn
7. Most clients develop tolerance to local side effects within 3 to 4 weeks

B. Common medications are listed in Table 43–8 ■

C. Nursing considerations

1. Assess skin lesions as baseline and periodically to evaluate effectiveness of therapy
2. Monitor for local adverse effects of topical preparations, such as excessive drying, erythema, and hypersensitivity
3. Monitor for systemic adverse effects as particular to individual product

D. Client teaching

1. Understand purpose, use, side effects, and anticipated length of treatment

Table 43–7

Keratolytics

Agent	Uses
Salicylic acid	Warts, psoriasis, lichen simplex or chronicus, tinea of feet or palms when peeling desired, seborrheic dermatitis
Resorcinol monoacetate (Resorcinol)	Acne vulgaris, rosacea, seborrheic dermatitis, psoriasis
Urea	Black hairy tongue, removal of nails affected by fungal infection or psoriasis
Sulfur (sulfur, precipitated)	Tinea of any area of body, acne vulgaris, rosacea, seborrheic dermatitis, pyodermas, psoriasis
Alpha-hydroxy acids (lactic, glycolic, glucuronic, pyruvic acids)	Ichthyosis, hyperkeratotic eczema, photoaging, acne, citric, hyperpigmentation
Propylene glycol	Ichthyosis

Table 43-8
Acne Medications

Medication	Action or Use	Preparation
Adapalene (Differin)	Retinoid	Alcohol-free gel, cream; solution with alcohol
Benzoyl peroxide (Benzac)	Antibacterial, keratolytic; antibacterial activity against *Propionibacterium acnes*	Gel, wash
Benzoyl peroxide (Benzagel)	Antibacterial, keratolytic	Gel, wash
Benzoyl peroxide, erythromycin (Benzamycin)	Antibacterial, keratolytic; contains erythromycin and benzoyl peroxide	Gel
Azelaic acid (Azelex)	Antibacterial, keratolytic; competitively inhibits tyrosinase, antimicrobial against *Propionibacterium acnes,* inhibits comedone formation; may take 4 weeks until beneficial effect observed	Cream
Clindamycin (Cleocin T)	Antibacterial	Solution, pads, lotion, gel
Erythromycin (Emgel, Erycette, T-Stat)	Anti-inflammatory, antibacterial; Emgel is gel, Erycette is swabs, T-Stat is solution, pads	
Sodium sulfacetamide (Klaron)	Antibacterial	Lotion
Tazarotene (Tazorac)	Retinoid	Aqueous gel
Tetracycline (Monodox, Sumycin, Doryx, Vibramycin)	Antibacterial	Capsules
Tretinoin (Retin-A)	Retinoic acid derivative; increases mitotic activity and turnover of follicular epithelial cells; loosens keratin debris; promotes drainage of preexisting comedones; inhibits formation of new comedones; maximal results take up to 6 weeks; maintenance therapy may be necessary	Gel, liquid, aqueous gel, cream
Tretinoin (Avita)	Retinoid	Cream, gel
Isotretinoin (Accutane)	Retinoic acid derivative	Capsules

2. Treatment is designed to control, not cure; therefore, periodic breakouts (especially premenstrual flares) may still occur
3. With topical preparation, wash and dry skin; massage thin film gently into affected areas twice daily
4. Avoid getting product into eyes, mouth, and mucous membranes; wash hands after use
5. With certain preparations, minimize exposure to sun and UV light
6. Isotretinoin (Accutane) is a teratogen; females of child-bearing age must strictly avoid becoming pregnant; they should have negative pregnancy test within 2 weeks before starting therapy and monthly during therapy
7. Avoid excess vitamin A intake with isotretinoin (Accutane), which is a vitamin A metabolite

VIII. BURN MEDICATIONS

A. Overview

1. Goals of therapy are to decrease inflammation, prevent infection, relieve pain, and promote healing
2. Topical agents are used to prevent infection in burn wounds, which could rapidly lead to sepsis

B. Common medications are listed in Table 43–9 ■

C. Nursing considerations

1. ! Apply agents under sterile conditions once or twice daily to a thickness of approximately 1/16-inch to clean and debrided wound
2. If hospitalized, client may undergo hydrotherapy (bathing in whirlpool) to aid debridement prior to application
3. ! Premedicate client with analgesic whenever possible 30 minutes prior to burn wound cleansing
4. Wound may be covered or left open
5. ! Monitor for adverse effects as outlined in Table 43–9
6. ! Watch for signs of infection and monitor WBC count in clients receiving silver sulfadiazine because of leukopenic effect

D. Client teaching

1. Understand purpose, use, side effects, and anticipated length of treatment
2. Use as directed if using preparation as an outpatient

Table 43–9
Burn Medications

Medication	Use	Notes
Mafenide (Sulfamylon)	Bacteriostatic against *Pseudomonas aeruginosa* and *Clostridia*	Adverse reactions include pain, burning, or stinging at application site for first 20–30 minutes after application With impaired renal function, high blood levels of agent may lead to metabolic acidosis; watch for compensatory respiratory alkalosis
Silver sulfadiazine (Silvadene, Thermazene, SSD Cream)	Silver is toxic to bacteria; prevents replication of *S. aureus, E. coli, Klebsiella, P. aeruginosa, P. mirabilis, Enterobacter, C. albicans*	Application is generally painless Watch for adverse reactions, including leukopenia, skin necrosis, erythema multiforme, skin discoloration, rashes Up to 10% may be absorbed; hazardous to use in clients with G6PD deficiency
Nitrofurazone (Furacin)	Adjunctive therapy when bacterial resistance to other agents occurs	Use cautiously in clients with impaired renal function; polyethylene glycol in preparation can be absorbed through denuded skin and may not be excreted normally by compromised kidney Watch for rash, itching, dermatitis, bacterial or fungal superinfection, and allergic reaction at site Drug darkens on exposure to light, but does not affect potency

Table 43-10

Debriding Preparations

Agent	Action	Notes
Collagenase (Santyl)	Digests collagen; active at pH 6–8, takes 10–14 days	Active at pH 6–8, such enzymes tend to be inactivated by extremes of pH; also inactivated by hydrogen peroxide, heavy metals like silver, detergents, iodine, nitrofurazone, and hexachlorophene
Sutilains (Travase)	Digests necrotic soft tissues by proteolytic action	Same as for Collagenase
Fibrinolysin and deoxyribonuclease (Elase)	Deoxyribonuclease attacks DNA; fibrinolysin attacks fibrin of blood clots and fibrinous exudates	Hypersensitivity reactions can occur; serious adverse reactions have been reported when using ointment preparation containing chloramphenicol
Papain and urea (Panafil White)	Ointment source is papaya	Chlorophyll derivatives control wound odor
Papain, urea, and chlorophyllin copper complex (Panafil)	Source is papaya	Same as for papain and urea
Trypsin, Balsam Peru, castor oil (Granulex)	Source of trypsin is bovine pancreas	Balsam Peru is capillary bed stimulant used to improve circulation; castor oil used to reduce premature epithelial cornification

IX. DEBRIDING MEDICATIONS

A. Overview

1. Debriding agents remove dirt, damaged tissue, and cellular debris from wound to prevent infection and promote healing
2. Effectiveness in removing necrotic tissue, clotted blood, purulent exudates, or fibrinous accumulations has been questioned
   a. Appear most effective when wound base has collagen that must be removed before epithelialization can proceed
   b. Specific indications may vary (e.g., collagenase is indicated for stage 3 and 4 pressure ulcers)

B. Common medications are listed in Table 43-10 ■

Memory Aid

Some enzymes that are used to debride wounds end in the suffix *-ase*. This may help you to choose an appropriate product at least some of the time.

C. Nursing considerations: assess skin problem before use and monitor progress in wound healing

D. Client teaching: understand purpose, use, and side effects of medications, and anticipated length of treatment

Check Your NCLEX-RN® Exam I.Q.

You are ready for testing on this content if you can

- Apply knowledge of expected actions and effects of integumentary medications to client care.
- Correctly administer integumentary medications to clients.
- Assess for side effects and adverse effects of integumentary medications.
- Take appropriate action if a client has an unexpected response to an integumentary medication.
- Monitor a client for expected outcomes or effects of treatment with integumentary medications.

PRACTICE TEST

PRACTICE TEST

1 The nurse explains to a client that a product containing which of the following ingredients would be the most useful agent to treat photoaging of the skin?

1. Propylene glycol
2. Salicylic acid
3. Alpha-hydroxy acids
4. Resorcinol

2 The nurse would include which of the following pieces of information when explaining the skin emollient Dermasil to a client?

1. It requires shaking before each use.
2. It has a drying effect on the skin when the water evaporates.
3. It includes a corticosteroid component.
4. It is of use when skin is dry.

3 What instructions should the nurse give the client who is receiving tretinoin (Retin-A)?

1. Apply the preparation in the morning.
2. Use gloves and apply a thick layer four times a day.
3. Avoid products containing vitamin C.
4. Apply to dry skin, 30 minutes after washing.

4 The nurse anticipates that mafenide (Sulfamylon) would be ordered for use if it is known that a client's burn is infected with which of the following organisms?

1. *Pseudomonas aeruginosa*
2. Tubercle bacillus
3. Methicillin-resistant *Staphylococcus aureus*
4. *Candida albicans*

5 A female client who is using salicylic acid to treat psoriasis asks how long she will have to use this drug. Which of the following would be the best response by the nurse?

1. "Response is rapid, and the drug will not be needed after 3 months of therapy."
2. "Drugs often do not produce prolonged remission, and maintenance therapy often is needed."
3. "Each situation is so individual it is not possible to answer the question accurately."
4. "The dermatologist caring for you is the best resource for such a question."

6 The nurse would recommend that a client with excessive dandruff use a medicated shampoo that contains which of the following active ingredients?

1. Silver sulfadiazine
2. Selenium sulfide
3. Corticosteroid
4. Lindane

7 It is winter and the client has extremely dry skin. Which type of preparation should the nurse recommend first?

1. Regular use of same soap, such as Dial
2. Shake lotion
3. Emollient or emollient-containing lotion
4. Antipruritic lotion

8 Which of the following client disorders might require the use of acyclovir (Zovirax)?

1. Herpes simplex viruses
2. Chronic dermatitis
3. Pseudofolliculitis
4. Candidiasis

9 A child has scraped his finger on a sharp spot on a shower door edge. The mother would like to use a topical antibiotic to prevent infection. Which agent would the pediatric telephone consultation nurse recommend?

1. Bacitracin (Baciguent Topical)
2. Malathion (Ovide Lotion)
3. Ketoconazole (Nizoral)
4. Mafenide (Sulfamylon)

10 The elderly client is being treated for a pressure ulcer. The nurse would anticipate use of which of the following types of agents to topically debride this ulcer?

1. Hydrocolloid dressing
2. Antibiotic-impregnated gauze packing
3. Allylamine
4. Enzyme

11 The nurse is preparing to do tracheostomy care and notes that the client's tracheostomy has encrusted debris around the tube. The nurse should dilute which of the following antiseptic solutions to half strength to most effectively clean the skin around the tracheostomy?

1. Iodine
2. Hydrogen peroxide
3. Chlorhexidine
4. Isopropyl alcohol

12 The physician's order sheet calls for topical application of the proteolytic enzyme Elase. The nurse carries out this order by applying this product to which of the following areas on the client?

1. External ear canal
2. Rectal area
3. Dry skin on feet
4. Sacral pressure ulcer

13 The nurse explains to a client who seeks treatment for a wart that which of the following types of products will be effective in removing this growth?

1. Astringent
2. Antiseptic
3. Keratinolytic
4. Proteolytic

14 The nurse would be most careful when using a topical drug for a client in which of the following age groups because of increased risk of toxicity?

1. Middle-aged adult
2. Older adult
3. Child
4. Adolescent

15 Which of the following types of dermatological products would the nurse recommend as having the most benefit for a client with acne?

1. Drying agent
2. Steroid
3. Emollient
4. Lubricant

16 The nurse would evaluate for which of the following effects in a client who has been using hydrocortisone 1% cream (Ala-Cort) as a topical agent?

1. Moisturizing
2. Drying
3. Antimicrobial
4. Anti-inflammatory

17 A client with psoriasis needs to apply a lubricating lotion to a psoriatic placque. The nurse plans to teach the client to use which of the following types of substances?

1. Emollient
2. Antiseptic
3. Alcohol
4. Astringent

18 The nurse prepares to apply which of the following ordered types of antiseptics to a client with a burn wound once the area has been cleansed with sterile saline?

1. Copper-containing
2. Silver-containing
3. Biguanide
4. Acetic acid

19 The nurse anticipates that a wound infection that is resistant to treatment with several antiseptics will most likely respond to treatment with which of the following antiseptics?

1. Hydrogen peroxide
2. Phenol derivative
3. Isopropyl alcohol
4. Dakin's solution

20 The nurse is choosing a protective wound dressing for a client. Which of the following products should be used when selecting a dressing that is permeable to oxygen?

1. Tegaderm
2. DuoDERM
3. Replicare
4. Tegasorb

ANSWERS & RATIONALES

1 **Answer: 3** Alpha-hydroxy acids are useful keratinolytics that help reduce the effects of photoaging. Propylene glycol is used to treat ichthyosis. Salicylic acid and resorcinol are keratinolytics that are used to treat a variety of other skin disorders.
Cognitive Level: Application **Client Need:** Physiological Integrity: Pharmacological and Parenteral Therapies **Integrated Process:** Nursing Process: Implementation **Content Area:** Pharmacology **Strategy:** The core issue of the question is knowledge of products that assist the skin to appear younger and resist the aging effects of light. Use knowledge of these ordinary products and the process of elimination to make a selection.

2 **Answer: 4** Emollients contain petrolatum, oils, propylene glycol, or other substances and make the skin soft and pliable by increasing hydration of the stratum corneum. They do not dry the skin (option 2) or contain corticosteroids (option 3). Option 1 is not always necessary.
Cognitive Level: Application **Client Need:** Physiological Integrity: Pharmacological and Parenteral Therapies **Integrated Process:** Nursing Process: Implementation **Content Area:** Pharmacology **Strategy:** The core issue of the question is general knowledge of integumentary products that are emollients. Use knowledge of these ordinary products and the process of elimination to make a selection.

3 **Answer: 4** Tretinoin is a retinoic acid derivative that needs to be applied once daily in a thin layer before retiring. The area to be treated should be washed at least 30 minutes before applying. Increased intake of vitamin A, not vitamin C, needs to be avoided.
Cognitive Level: Application **Client Need:** Physiological Integrity: Pharmacological and Parenteral Therapies **Integrated Process:** Nursing Process: Implementation **Content Area:** Pharmacology **Strategy:** The core issue of the question is knowledge of proper use of tretinoin. Use medication knowledge and the process of elimination to make a selection.

4 **Answer: 1** Mafenide is useful in treatment of partial- and full-thickness burns to prevent septicemia caused by organisms such as *Pseudomonas aeruginosa.* Mafenide does not have a defined use with the other infectious organisms mentioned.
Cognitive Level: Application **Client Need:** Physiological Integrity: Pharmacological and Parenteral Therapies **Integrated Process:** Nursing Process: Planning **Content Area:** Pharmacology **Strategy:** The core issue of the question is knowledge of the uses of mafenide in a client with burn injury. Use medication knowledge and the process of elimination to make a selection.

5 **Answer: 2** There is no cure for psoriasis. Psoriasis is notoriously chronic and recurrent. The cause is unknown. Each situation is individual, and the dermatologist who knows the client's situation the longest is a good resource, but nevertheless the best answer for most clients is that the disease is recurrent and therapy will need to be continued.
Cognitive Level: Application **Client Need:** Physiological Integrity: Pharmacological and Parenteral Therapies **Integrated Process:** Nursing Process: Implementation **Content Area:** Pharmacology **Strategy:** The core issue of the question is general knowledge about medications used to treat psoriasis. Use medication knowledge and the process of elimination to make a selection.

6 **Answer: 2** A 1% lotion of selenium sulfide is used to relieve the itching and flaking of the scalp associated with dandruff. A shampoo with lindane 1% (Kwell) would be used for pediculosis capitis. Corticosteroids have many uses, but dandruff is not one of them. Silver sulfadiazine is a cream used in the prevention and treatment of infection in partial- and full-thickness burns.
Cognitive Level: Analysis **Client Need:** Physiological Integrity: Pharmacological and Parenteral Therapies **Integrated Process:** Nursing Process: Planning **Content Area:** Pharmacology **Strategy:** The core issue of the question is general knowledge about medications used to treat dandruff. Use medication knowledge and the process of elimination to make a selection.

7 **Answer: 3** Dry skin may occur in otherwise healthy skin and is usually worse in winter, when forced-air heating reduces humidity inside many dwellings. Excessive washing with harsh soaps (such as Dial) strips stratum corneum of its natural lipids and exacerbates dry skin. No shake lotion is made specifically for management of dry skin. Itching may occur with dry skin, but before an antipruritic lotion is used, an emollient lotion or emollient should be tried. Emollient lotions are dilute dispersions of emulsified lipids in water. These provide smooth application and the most rapid hydration if applied to dry skin, but they do not provide a protective effect on the lipid barrier. Emollients (e.g., petrolatum) are occlusive agents that make the skin soft and pliable by increasing hydration of the stratum corneum.
Cognitive Level: Analysis **Client Need:** Physiological Integrity: Pharmacological and Parenteral Therapies **Integrated Process:** Nursing Process: Planning **Content Area:** Pharmacology **Strategy:** The core issue of the question is general knowledge about products used to treat dry skin. Use product knowledge and the process of elimination to make a selection.

8 **Answer: 1** Acyclovir is an antiviral agent that is useful in the treatment of herpes simplex viruses. The other conditions would require therapy with an antiinfective, but not of the antiviral type.
Cognitive Level: Application **Client Need:** Physiological Integrity: Pharmacological and Parenteral Therapies **Integrated Process:** Nursing Process: Implementation **Content Area:** Pharmacology **Strategy:** The core issue of the question is knowledge of the uses of acyclovir in a client with herpes infection. Use medication knowledge and the process of elimination to make a selection. Remember that an antiviral medication often contains *vir* somewhere in the name.

9 **Answer: 1** Bacitracin is a topical antibiotic that is bactericidal against Gram-positive cocci and bacilli, including staphylococci and streptococci. These organisms might cause infection in a skin wound. Malathion (option 2) is an antiparasitic agent for pediculosis. Ketoconazole (option 3) is an antifungal agent. Mafenide (option 4) is an agent used for burns.

Cognitive Level: Application **Client Need:** Physiological Integrity: Pharmacological and Parenteral Therapies **Integrated Process:** Nursing Process: Implementation **Content Area:** Pharmacology **Strategy:** The core issue of the question is knowledge of the types of medications used for various skin conditions. Use medication knowledge and the process of elimination to make a selection. Remember that cuts or open wounds often heal effectively when topical antibiotics are used to prevent infection at the site.

10 **Answer: 4** Ulcers with necrotic material should be debrided, either by sharp debridement (e.g., using scalpel) or chemical debridement (e.g., wound cleanser such as an enzyme). An example of such a preparation is collagenase (Santyl), which is inactivated by metal salts, hexachlorophene, or acidic solutions. Hydrocolloid dressings can be helpful with uninfected wounds with fibrinous bases. Topical antibiotics will not help remove necrotic material. Allylamines are selected for fungal infections.
Cognitive Level: Application **Client Need:** Physiological Integrity: Pharmacological and Parenteral Therapies **Integrated Process:** Nursing Process: Planning **Content Area:** Pharmacology **Strategy:** The core issue of the question is the type of topical agent to use when debridement is needed. Use medication knowledge and the process of elimination to make a selection. Enzymes often end in *ase,* which makes them easy to recognize on sight.

11 **Answer: 2** Hydrogen peroxide is an oxidizing antiseptic that can be used to clean wounds or tracheostomy tubes. Options 1 and 3 as cleaning agents do not have the bubbling action of hydrogen peroxide. Mafenide is an antimicrobial used to treat burn injury.
Cognitive Level: Application **Client Need:** Physiological Integrity: Pharmacological and Parenteral Therapies **Integrated Process:** Nursing Process: Implementation **Content Area:** Pharmacology **Strategy:** The core issue of the question is knowledge of the type of skin cleansing agent used for tracheostomy. Use knowledge of these agents and the process of elimination to make a selection.

12 **Answer: 4** Proteolytic enzymes such as Elase ointment can be used to chemically debride tissue. These areas commonly include venous stasis ulcers, burn wounds, and pressure ulcers. The areas listed in the other options are not appropriate for treatment with proteolytic enzymes.
Cognitive Level: Application **Client Need:** Physiological Integrity: Pharmacological and Parenteral Therapies **Integrated Process:** Nursing Process: Implementation **Content Area:** Pharmacology **Strategy:** The core issue of the question is knowledge of the debriding agents appropriate for use at various skin sites. Use knowledge of these agents and the process of elimination to make a selection.

13 **Answer: 3** A keratinolytic agent such as salicyclic acid is used to treat warts. Keratinolytics are also used to treat corns, calluses, and other keratin-containing skin lesions. Astringents cause topical vasoconstriction. Antiseptics inhibit bacterial growth. Proteolytic enzymes are used to debride tissue.
Cognitive Level: Application **Client Need:** Physiological Integrity: Pharmacological and Parenteral Therapies **Integrated Process:** Nursing Process: Implementation **Content Area:** Pharmacology **Strategy:** The core issue of the question is what type of medication is effective in treating warts. Begin to answer by reasoning that treatment of a wart includes breaking it down for removal. Next note the suffix *-lytic* in the correct option, which means "to break down."

14 **Answer: 3** Children have an increased risk of systemic toxicity from topically applied drugs because of the greater ratio of surface area to weight. The other responses are incorrect because they have similar body surface area to weight ratios.
Cognitive Level: Application **Client Need:** Physiological Integrity: Pharmacological and Parenteral Therapies **Integrated Process:** Nursing Process: Analysis **Content Area:** Pharmacology **Strategy:** The core issue of this question is that age group that is most at risk because of their skin characteristics when topical drugs are used. Recall that the greater the area involved, the greater risk of absorption and toxic effects. Finally, recall that infants and children have a greater skin surface to weight ratio than an adult of any age.

15 **Answer: 1** Acne can be successfully treated with the use of drying agents. Steroids would be of no benefit for this problem. Emollients and lubricants are moisturizers that may worsen the condition.
Cognitive Level: Application **Client Need:** Physiological Integrity: Pharmacological and Parenteral Therapies **Integrated Process:** Nursing Process: Planning **Content Area:** Pharmacology **Strategy:** The core issue of the question is what type of medication is effective in treating acne. Since this condition is characterized by inflammation and drainage, consider that an agent that has a drying effect would be opposite to the characteristics of the condition and help reduce symptoms.

16 **Answer: 4** Corticosteroids such as hydrocortisone are anti-inflammatory drugs. They do not exert antimicrobial action, and in fact, they can increase risk of infection by suppressing the inflammatory response. Corticosteroids are not moisturizing or drying agents.
Cognitive Level: Application **Client Need:** Physiological Integrity: Pharmacological and Parenteral Therapies **Integrated Process:** Nursing Process: Evaluation **Content Area:** Pharmacology **Strategy:** The core issue of the question is knowledge of the intended effects of corticosteroids as anti-inflammatory agents. Use this information and the process of elimination to make a selection.

17 **Answer: 1** Psoriatic plaques need to be lubricated so that they are easier to loosen and remove. Emollients and lubricants are fatty or oily substances that can be used for this purpose because they keep skin soft and prevent water evaporation. The other products listed are harsher and some may have a drying effect.
Cognitive Level: Application **Client Need:** Physiological Integrity: Pharmacological and Parenteral Therapies **Integrated Process:** Nursing Process: Planning **Content Area:** Pharmacology **Strategy:** Note the word *lubricating* in the stem of the question. This tells you that regardless of the client's health problem, the agent is one that must have a moisturizing effect on the skin. Use the process of elimination and knowledge of the categories of skin products to make a selection.

18 **Answer: 2** Silver sulfadiazine is a metallic type of antiseptic that is widely used on burns. The silver in the solution is

toxic to bacteria and prevents them from reproducing. The agents in options 3 and 4 would not be beneficial. Option 1 is a fictitious solution.

Cognitive Level: Application **Client Need:** Physiological Integrity: Pharmacological and Parenteral Therapies **Integrated Process:** Nursing Process: Planning **Content Area:** Pharmacology **Strategy:** The core issue of the question is the type of agent that would be effective in preventing microbial growth in a client with burn injury. Use knowledge of topical antimicrobial agents and the process of elimination to make a selection.

19 **Answer: 4** A chlorine preparation such as Dakin's solution is used for infected wounds when other treatments are ineffective. They are useful because they also dissolve necrotic materials and blood clots; however, a disadvantage is that they delay blood clotting, which may later interfere with wound healing. Options 1, 2, and 3 are not helpful in treating infections resistant to several antiseptics.

Cognitive Level: Application **Client Need:** Physiological Integrity: Pharmacological and Parenteral Therapies **Integrated Process:** Nursing Process: Analysis **Content Area:** Pharmacology **Strategy:** The core issue of the question is knowledge of antiseptics that are useful in treating problems involving the skin. Use this knowledge and the process of elimination to make a selection.

20 **Answer: 1** Tegaderm is a protective dressing that is permeable to oxygen. The other products listed do not have this advantage. DuoDERM and Tegasorb are absorbent products that exclude bacteria and adhere to the site. Replicare excludes bacteria.

Cognitive Level: Application **Client Need:** Physiological Integrity: Pharmacological and Parenteral Therapies **Integrated Process:** Nursing Process: Planning **Content Area:** Pharmacology **Strategy:** The core issue of the question is the type of dressing that is permeable to oxygen. The wording of the question tells you that only one answer is correct. Use the process of elimination and knowledge of wound care products to make a selection.

Key Terms to Review

acne p. 724
antiseptics p. 720
creams p. 716
emollients p. 715
herpes simplex p. 720
lotions p. 714
ointments p. 716
papules p. 724
pediculosis p. 721
powder p. 714
pruritus p. 715
psoriasis p. 713
scabies p. 721
tinea pedis p. 720

References

Abrams, A. (2004). *Clinical drug therapy: Rationales for nursing practice* (7th ed.). Philadelphia: Lippincott; Williams & Wilkins.

Adams, M., Josephson, D., & Holland, L. (2005). *Pharmacology for nurses: A pathophysiologic approach.* Upper Saddle River, NJ: Pearson Education.

Deglin, J. H. & Vallerand, A. H. (2006). *Davis's drug guide for nurses* (10th ed.). Philadelphia: F. A. Davis.

Lehne, R. (2004). *Pharmacology for nursing care* (5th ed.). Philadelphia: W. B. Saunders.

McKenry, L., Tessier, E. & Hogan, M. (2006). *Mosby's pharmacology in nursing.* (22nd ed.). St. Louis: Elsevier Science.

Wilson, B., Shannon, M., & Stang, C. (2006). *Prentice Hall nurse's drug guide 2006.* Upper Saddle River, NJ: Pearson Education.

Eye and Ear Medications

44

In this chapter

Test Yourself

Are you ready for the NCLEX-RN® or course exams? Use the practice tests on the companion CD-ROM to check.

Cross reference

Other chapters relevant to this content area are:

Dosage Calculation and Medication Administration Chapter 30
Eye and Ear Disorders Chapter 64

I. GENERAL GUIDELINES FOR EYE AND EAR MEDICATIONS *(SEE BOX 44–1)*

Box 44–1

General Guidelines for Eye and Ear Medications

Administration Principles

1. Assess current medications (including OTC drugs and herbal products) and history of allergies to identify any potential risks to client.
2. Administer doses on time.
3. Do not break or allow client to chew sustained release or enteric coated preparations; apply eyedrops or eye ointments or ear drops using proper technique.
4. Provide both verbal and written instructions to client, and provide phone number to call if questions arise or problems occur.

Client Teaching

1. Understand medication actions, side effects, signs of toxicity, importance of follow-up with prescriber and complying with follow-up laboratory tests, and how to self-administer.
2. Do not take any OTC drugs or herbal products without first consulting prescriber.
3. Take exactly as prescribed and do not miss or double doses.
4. Report adverse effects promptly.
5. Do not discontinue drug without consulting prescriber.
6. Do not drink alcohol while taking prescription medications.
7. Take care to maintain a safe environment in the presence of vision or hearing impairment.

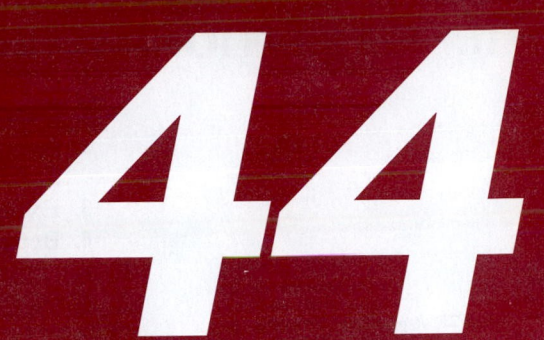

II. MEDICATIONS TO TREAT GLAUCOMA

A. Beta-blockers (beta-adrenergic antagonists)

1. Decrease production of **aqueous humor** (fluid formed by ciliary body in eye)
2. Reduce **intraocular pressure** (IOP; pressure within eye) in **open-angle glaucoma** (a change in appearance of optic disk resulting in visual loss)
3. Exact mechanism of action is unknown
4. Beta-blockers are the most commonly used class of drugs in management of chronic, primary open-angle glaucoma
5. Common medications are listed in Box 44–2

Memory Aid

Remember that a beta-blocking drug can be recognized easily because it ends with the suffix -olol or lol.

6. Administration considerations
   a. Available in ophthalmic solutions and suspensions
   b. Drugs cross placenta, enter breast milk
   ! c. Use nasolacrimal occlusion (press on inner canthus of eye) to minimize **systemic absorption** (entry of drug into body and circulating fluids)
   ! d. Use cautiously in clients with renal failure, diabetes, asthma, and chronic obstructive pulmonary disease (COPD)
   ! e. Administer with caution to clients receiving cardiovascular agents such as antihypertensives and antiarrhythmics
   f. May mask symptoms of hyperthyroidism
   g. Drug may be beta$_1$ selective (cardiac), beta$_2$ selective (pulmonary), or both beta$_1$ and beta$_2$ selective
   h. Because it is beta$_1$ selective, betaxolol (Betoptic) is usually the drug of choice for clients with pulmonary disease
7. Contraindicated in hypersensitivity, sinus bradycardia or second- or third-degree heart block, cardiogenic shock or congestive heart failure (CHF)
8. ! Adverse cardiovascular effects may occur when beta-adrenergic blockers are used in combination with other cardiovascular agents such as antihypertensives and antidysrhythmics
9. Side/adverse effects
   ! a. Primarily local reactions: eye irritation, burning, stinging
   ! b. Systemic adverse cardiovascular effects include bradycardia or tachycardia, CHF, dysrhythmias, hypotension, and edema of lower extremities
   ! c. Systemic adverse respiratory effects include wheezing, cough, exacerbation of asthma, and bronchospasm
   d. Systemic adverse central nervous system (CNS) effects include weakness, ataxia, confusion, and depression
   e. Systemic adverse gastrointestinal (GI) effects include nausea and vomiting
10. Nursing considerations
    ! a. Obtain baseline vital signs, neurologic status, vision and intraocular pressure data
    b. Assess for cardiovascular disease, renal failure, diabetes, lactation, or thyrotoxicosis
    c. Assess for signs and symptoms of hypersensitivity such as burning, itching, redness, and swelling occurring after medication administration
    ! d. Refer to Box 44–3 for administration of ophthalmic medications
11. Client teaching
    ! a. As per Box 44–1; beta-blocking agents may mask symptoms of hypoglycemia

Box 44–2

Beta-Adrenergic Blocking Agents for Ophthalmic Use

Betaxolol (Betoptic)	Metipranolol (OptiPranolol)
Carteolol (Ocupress)	Timolol (Timoptic)
Levobunolol (Betagan)	

Box 44–3

Administration of Ophthalmic Medications

Instillation of Eyedrops

- Wash hands
- Cleanse exudates from eye(s) if necessary
- Tilt client's head toward side of affected eye
- Gently pull lower eyelid down and have client look up (this forms a "sac")
- Instill drops in sac formed by lower lid, *not* onto eye
- Unless specifically indicated otherwise, apply gentle pressure for 30 seconds to 1 minute over inner canthus next to nose. This prevents absorption through tear duct and drainage of medication
- Unless specifically indicated otherwise, client should close eye(s) gently. Avoid squeezing eye(s) tightly as this forces medication out

Instillation of Eye Ointment

- Follow same procedure for instillation of eyedrops except that ointment is expressed directly into conjunctival sac from inner canthus to outer canthus
- Unless specifically indicated otherwise, client should close eye(s) and gently massage eye(s) to distribute medication

Note: To avoid contamination and risk of infection, do not touch dropper or tube to eye, eyelashes, or any other surface. Remove contact lenses before instilling ophthalmic medications.

b. Inform health care provider if surgery is being considered; gradual withdrawal of beta-blocking agent 48 hours before surgery may be required (withdrawal is controversial)
c. Have routine eye examinations and measurement of IOP
d. Do not stop medication unless instructed to do so by the health care provider
! e. Report symptoms of breathing difficulty, swelling of extremities, slow heart rate
! f. Wear dark glasses and avoid bright light if photophobia is present

B. Adrenergic medications (adrenergic agonists)

1. Decrease production of aqueous humor and decrease IOP
2. Used to manage open-angle glaucoma (often in combination with other drugs), glaucoma secondary to **uveitis** (intraocular inflammatory disorder), to produce **mydriasis** (pupil dilation) for ocular examination, and to produce local hemostasis during eye surgery to control bleeding
3. Common medications are listed in Box 44–4
4. Administration considerations
   a. If epinephrine hydrochloride (Epifrin, Glaucon) is used in conjunction with miotics, instill miotic first
   b. Drugs cross placenta, enter breast milk
   c. Do not administer ophthalmic solution that contains precipitates or has turned brown
5. ! Contraindicated in hypersensitivity to epinephrine and phenylephrine and for treatment of narrow-angle (angle-closure) glaucoma or abraded cornea, because pupil dilation further restricts ocular fluid outflow, precipitating an acute attack of glaucoma

Box 44–4

Adrenergic Agonist Agents for Ophthalmic Use

Apraclonidine (Iopidone), antiglaucoma

Brimonidine tartrate (Alphagan), antiglaucoma

Dipivefrin (Propine), antiglaucoma

Epinephrine hydrochloride (Epifrin, Glaucon), antiglaucoma

Hydroxyamphetamine (Paredrine), mydriatic

Phenylephrine (Neo-Synephrine), mydriatic

6. Side/adverse effects
   a. Local reactions include eye pain and stinging on initial instillation
   b. CNS side effects include headache, blurred vision, brow ache, photophobia, and difficulty with night vision
   c. Rebound **miosis** (constriction of pupils) may occur with phenylephrine
   d. Elderly clients with cardiac disease may experience BP elevations with phenylephrine
   e. Systemic adverse effects are unusual but may occur especially in clients with cardiovascular disease; symptoms include confusion, tachycardia, hypertension, diaphoresis, and tremors
7. Nursing considerations
   a. Obtain history of allergies or hypersensitivity to specific agents
   b. Obtain baseline vital signs, vision and intraocular pressure data
   c. Assess cardiac, respiratory, and renal function routinely
8. Client teaching
   a. Drugs may discolor contact lenses
   b. Do not blink for at least 30 seconds after instilling medication
   c. Report a decrease in visual acuity, floating spots, sensitivity to light, eye redness, or headache to health care provider

C. Cholinergic agents (miotics, cholinesterase inhibitors)

1. Increase outflow of aqueous humor, decrease resistance to aqueous flow in open-angle and angle-closure glaucoma
2. Produce miosis before ophthalmic examination or after ophthalmic surgery
3. Generally used for clients who fail to respond to first-line agents (beta-blockers)
4. Common medications are listed in Box 44–5
5. Administration considerations
   a. Drug crosses placenta, enters breast milk
   b. Do not administer ophthalmic solution that contains precipitates or has turned brown
   c. Pilocarpine can be stored at room temperature
   d. Contraindicated in acute iritis or conditions in which pupillary constriction is not desirable
   e. Concurrent use with beta-adrenergic blocking agents may increase risk of cardiovascular reactions
6. Side/adverse effects
   a. Visual blurring, myopia, irritation, brow pain, and headache
   b. Systemic reactions include abdominal pain, bronchoconstriction, diarrhea, hypotension, nausea, vomiting, diuresis, diaphoresis, exacerbation of asthma
   c. Toxic effects produce ataxia, confusion, seizures, coma, respiratory failure, hypotension, and death
   d. Prolonged use of cholinergics may lead to retinal detachments, obstruction of tear drainage, and cataracts
   e. Acute toxicity is reversible by IV administration of atropine, an anticholinergic agent that acts as antidote
7. Nursing considerations
   a. Obtain baseline vital signs, neurologic status, vision, and IOP data
   b. Assess for cardiovascular disease, renal failure, diabetes, lactation, or thyrotoxicosis

Box 44–5

Cholinergic Agents for Ophthalmic Use

Carbachol (Carboptic)

Demecarium bromide (Humorsol)

Echothiophate iodide (Phospholine Iodide)

Physostigmine sulfate (Eserine sulfate)

Pilocarpine (Isopto Carpine, Pilocar, others)

Pilocarpine ocular therapeutic system (Ocusert Pilo-20, Ocusert Pilo-40)

c. Assess for signs and symptoms of hypersensitivity such as burning, itching, redness, and swelling occurring after medication administration

8. Client teaching: miosis may cause difficulty adjusting quickly to changes in lighting; use proper administration technique

D. Carbonic anhydrase inhibitors (CAIs)

1. Are nonbacteriostatic sulfonamides that lower IOP by decreasing aqueous humor production
2. Oral CAIs are used to treat open-angle, secondary, and angle-closure glaucoma
3. Ophthalmic CAIs are used to treat open-angle glaucoma and ocular hypertension
4. ! Commonly used preoperatively in intraocular surgery
5. Common medications are listed in Table 44–1 ■

Memory Aid

Carbonic anhydrase inhibitors can often be recognized because many of them end with the suffix -zolamide.

6. Administration considerations
   a. ! Oral acetazolamide (Diamox) is administered for maintenance
   b. ! IV route is used preoperatively or to rapidly reduce increased IOP
   c. Give oral form with food or milk to decrease GI side effects
   d. May crush tablets and suspend in liquid
   e. Do not use alcohol or glycerin in administration of drug
   f. To minimize nocturia, schedule doses early in day
   g. Administer with caution to clients with adrenocortical insufficiency
   h. ! Contraindicated with hypersensitivity to antibacterial sulfonamides, chronic noncongestive angle-closure glaucoma, hyponatremia, hypokalemia, or other electrolyte imbalances, or hepatic or renal dysfunction
7. Side/adverse effects
   a. Oral agents: anorexia, diarrhea, diuresis, nausea, vomiting, lethargy, weakness, weight loss, metallic bitter taste, and paresthesia of fingers, hands, and toes
   b. ! Topical agents: topical allergic reaction, photosensitivity, superficial **keratitis** (inflammation of the cornea)
   c. ! Stevens-Johnson syndrome and bone marrow depression with acetazolamide (Diamox)
   d. Acidosis
   e. ! Blood dyscrasias
   f. Hypokalemia
8. Nursing considerations
   a. Potential exacerbation of renal stones; monitor renal function
   b. ! Monitor for fluid volume depletion related to diuresis; monitor intake and output (I & O), skin turgor, mucous membranes, and weight
   c. ! Monitor urinalysis, complete blood cell count (CBC), electrolytes
9. ! Client teaching
   a. Unless contraindicated, eat diet high in potassium and low in sodium
   b. Unless contraindicated, increase fluid intake to at least 2 liters per day to decrease risk of renal stones
   c. Report changes in urine color, rashes, fever

Table 44–1 Carbonic Anhydrase Inhibitors

Drug Name	Route
Acetazolamide (Diamox)	Oral, IV
Brinzolamide (Azopt)	Ophthalmic
Dichlorphenamide (Daranide)	Oral
Dorzolamide (Trusopt)	Ophthalmic
Methazolamide (Neptazane)	Oral

E. Sympathomimetic agents

1. Lower IOP by decreasing aqueous humor production and increasing its outflow; used to manage open-angle glaucoma
2. Common medications (ophthalmic): dipivefrin (Propine) and epinephrine
3. Administration considerations
   a. Administer with caution to clients with cardiovascular disease, hypertension, asthma, diabetes mellitus, hyperthyroidism, and parkinsonism
   b. Onset of action for epinephrine is 1 hour; peak effect occurs in 4 to 8 hours
   c. Onset of action for dipivefrin (Propine) is 30 minutes; peak effect in 1 hour
   d. Assess for sensitivity to sulfites
   e. Avoid concurrent use with monoamine oxidase inhibitors (MAOIs)
   f. Contraindicated with **narrow-angle glaucoma** (increased IOP from impaired rate of aqueous humor flow) or predisposition to narrow-angle glaucoma
4. Side/adverse effects
   a. Local: brow pain, burning, eye irritation, headache, watering eyes, stinging, **photophobia**
   b. Systemic: hypertension, diaphoresis, tachycardia, palpitation, tremors, light-headedness
5. Nursing considerations
   a. Assess vital signs; obtain baseline IOP and vision data
   b. Maintain pressure on lacrimal sac for 1 to 2 minutes after instillation of drug to minimize systemic absorption
   c. Obtain heart rate and BP periodically to detect systemic effects
6. Client teaching
   a. Prolonged use of epinephrine may result in pigment deposits in the conjunctiva
   b. Discuss use of contact lenses with prescriber; use may or may not be permitted
   c. Report symptoms of increased heart rate, heart palpitations, or elevated BP to health care provider

F. Prostaglandin agonists

1. Increases aqueous humor outflow
2. Used to manage open-angle glaucoma and ocular hypertension
3. Common medications are listed in Box 44–6

Memory Aid

Prostaglandin agonists can often be recognized because many of them end with the suffix *-prost*.

4. Administration considerations
   a. Administer 5 minutes apart from other antiglaucoma ophthalmic medications
   b. If pilocarpine (Isopto Carpine) is included in drug regimen, it should be administered 1 hour after prostaglandin agonist
   c. May be used in conjunction with other agents to lower IOP
5. Contraindications: hypersensitivity to latanoprost or benzalkonium
6. Side/adverse effects
   a. Blurred vision, photophobia, burning, stinging, and itching
   b. Longer, thicker, darker eyelashes
   c. Conjunctival hyperemia
   d. Increasing iris pigmentation
7. Nursing considerations
   a. Assess for hypersensitivity to latanoprost or benzalkonium chloride
   b. Assess for burning, itching, stinging after initial administration of medication
8. Client teaching
   a. Drug may cause an increase in iris pigmentation

Box 44–6

Prostaglandin Agonists

Bimatoprost (Lumigan)	Travaprost (Travatan)
Latanoprost (Xalatan)	Unoprostone isopropyl (Rescula)

b. Do not exceed once-a-day dose
c. Remove contact lenses before use and for 15 minutes after instillation of medication
d. Report symptoms of burning, itching, stinging after administration to prescriber

III. MYDRIATICS AND CYCLOPLEGICS

A. Anticholinergics

1. Produce mydriasis (pupil dilation) and/or **cycloplegia** (paralysis of ciliary muscle)
2. Used to treat ocular pain secondary to inflammatory disorders such as uveitis and keratitis or for relaxation of ciliary muscle to improve measurement of refractive errors
3. ! Used preoperatively and postoperatively for intraocular surgery
4. Common medications are listed in Box 44–7
5. Administration considerations
   a. ! Use with caution in clients with primary glaucoma or predisposition to angle-closure glaucoma
   b. Apply ointment several hours before vision examination
   c. ! Compress lacrimal duct during administration and for 2 to 3 minutes after
   d. Contraindicated with severe systemic reactions to atropine or hypersensitivity to anticholinergic drugs
6. Side/adverse effects
   a. Local: blurred vision, photophobia, allergic lid reactions
   b. ! Systemic: confusion, delirium, drowsiness, dry mouth, flushing, and tachycardia
   c. ! Acute glaucoma can be precipitated by pupillary dilation; if not recognized and treated, acute glaucoma can result in blindness
   d. Dry mouth and tachycardia may be symptoms of scopolamine toxicity
7. Nursing considerations
   a. Obtain baseline IOP and vision status data
   b. Combination drugs produce greater mydriasis
   c. Systemic side effects are more pronounced in infants and children with blond hair and blue eyes
   d. ! Monitor for tachycardia, confusion, slurred speech, dry mouth, dry skin, weakness, drowsiness
8. Client teaching
   a. Mydriasis may last from 3 days (scopolamine) to 12 days (atropine)
   b. Blurred vision may occur
   c. ! Wear dark sunglasses and avoid bright light for photophobia
   d. ! IOP and vision should be monitored over course of therapy
   e. Withhold medication if experiencing tachycardia or dry mouth (symptoms of toxicity)
   f. ! Use sugarless hard candy to relieve dry mouth
   g. Report symptoms of tachycardia and dry mouth to health care provider

B. Adrenergics: refer to previous section on medications to treat glaucoma

Box 44–7

Mydriatic and Cycloplegic Agents for Ophthalmic Use

- Atropine sulfate
- Cyclopentolate hydrochloride (Cyclogyl)
- Homatropine hydrobromide
- Scopolamine hydrobromide
- Tropicamide (Mydriacyl)
- Cyclopentolate and phenylephrine (Cyclomydril)
- Scopolamine and phenylephrine (Murocoll-2)
- Torpicamide and hydroxyamphetamine (Paremyd)

IV. ANTI-INFLAMMATORY AND ANTI-INFECTIVE EYE MEDICATIONS

A. NSAIDs

1. Flurbiprofen (Ocufen) and suprofen (Profenal) are used to inhibit intraoperative miosis
2. Diclofenac (Voltaren) is used to treat postoperative inflammation after cataract extractions
3. Ketorolac (Acular) is used to treat conjunctivitis and seasonal allergic ophthalmic pruritis
4. Common medications are listed in Box 44–8
5. Administration considerations
   a. Systemic effect may be produced if absorbed
   b. NSAIDs may cause increased bleeding; therefore, clients with increased bleeding tendencies should be monitored closely and have periodic CBC and coagulation studies done
   c. Contraindicated with sensitivity to aspirin or phenylacetic acid derivatives or to systemic NSAIDs
6. Side/adverse effects
   a. Local: transient burning or stinging on application, itching, allergic reaction, pain, and redness
   b. Systemic toxicity: bleeding
7. Nursing considerations: assess for bleeding and for hypersensitivity symptoms (burning, itching, redness, and swelling occurring after administration of medication)
8. Client teaching: NSAIDs may potentiate bleeding in clients with known bleeding tendencies

B. Antibacterial, antifungal, and antiviral agents

1. Antibacterial agents are used to manage bacterial infections such as conjunctivitis, blepharitis, keratitis, uveitis, and hordeolum (sty)
2. Antifungal agents are used to manage fungal blepharitis, conjunctivitis, and keratitis
3. Antiviral agents are used to manage herpes simplex virus keratitis and herpes simplex virus keratoconjunctivitis
4. Common medications are listed in Box 44–9
5. Administration considerations
   a. If indicated, obtain culture specimen from eye(s) before administering first dose of medication
   b. Remove exudates from eyes before administering medication
   c. Contraindicated with hypersensitivity to drug
   d. Ophthalmic anesthetics should not be administered within 30 minutes of sulfonamides (sulfacetamide sodium); sulfonamides are incompatible with thimerosol and silver preparations
6. Side/adverse effects
   a. Local: dermatitis, itching, stinging, swelling
   b. Systemic: chloramphenicol (Chloroptic) may cause blood dyscrasias
   c. Stevens-Johnson syndrome, systemic lupus erythematosus (SLE) with sulfacetamide sodium
7. Nursing considerations
   a. Monitor infected eye(s) for pain, drainage, redness, swelling
   b. Monitor for unusual bleeding or bruising with chloramphenicol

Box 44–8

Nonsteroidal Anti-Inflammatory Agents for Ophthalmic Use

Diclofenac (Voltaren)
Flurbiprofen (Ocufen)
Ketorolac (Acular)
Suprofen (Profenal)

Box 44–9

Antibacterial, Antifungal, and Antiviral Agents for Ophthalmic Use

Antibacterial

Bacitracin (Baciguent)

Chloramphenicol (Chloroptic)

Ciprofloxacin ophthalmic solution (Ciloxan)

Erythromycin (Ilotycin ophthalmic ointment)

Gentamicin sulfate (Garamycin)

Norfloxacin ophthalmic solution (Chibroxin)

Ofloxacin (Ocuflox)

Polymyxin B sulfate

Sulfacetamide sodium (Bleph-10 Liquifilm, Isopto Cetamide, Sodium Sulamyd)

Sulfisoxazole diolamine (Gantrisin)

Tobramycin (Tobrex solution and ointment)

Antiviral

Idoxuridine (Stoxil, Herplex)

Trifluridine (Viroptic)

Vidarabine (Vira-A)

Antifungal

Natamycin (Natacyn)

c. Store idoxuridine (Stoxil, Herplex) and trifluridine (Viroptic) in cool place or refrigerator

! 8. Client teaching: inform prescriber of photosensitivity, redness, swelling, increased drainage, pain, or if no improvement seen within a few days

C. Corticosteroids

1. Indicated for management of allergic and inflammatory ophthalmic disorders of conjunctiva, cornea, and anterior segment of eye
2. Common medications are listed in Box 44–10
3. Administration considerations
   - ! a. Corticosteroids should be used for short-term treatment only
   - b. Use with caution in clients with cataracts and chronic open-angle glaucoma
4. ! Contraindicated with hypersensitivity and corneal abrasion; may mask hypersensitivity reactions to other drugs
5. Side/adverse effects
   - a. Local: stinging after application
   - ! b. Toxicity: visual disturbances, headache, and eye pain
6. ! Nursing considerations
   - a. May mask symptoms of infection and hypersensitivity reactions
   - b. May increase susceptibility to infection

Box 44–10

Common Corticosteroid Agents for Ophthalmic Use

Dexamethasone (Maxidex, Decadron)

Fluorometholone (FML S.O.P., FML)

Hydrocortisone (Cortamed)

Medrysone (HMS Liquifilm)

Prednisolone (Pred-Forte)

7. Client teaching
   a. Avoid use of contact lenses during and for prescribed time after use of corticosteroid therapy
   b. As per Box 44–1, have eye(s) examined for progress

V. ANESTHETIC EYE MEDICATIONS

A. Action and use

1. Prevent initiation and transmission of nerve impulses
2. Prevent pain during procedures such as **tonometry** (measurement of IOP, used to detect glaucoma), subconjunctival injections, removal of foreign bodies, and removal of sutures

B. Common medications

1. Proparacaine hydrochloride (Ophthetic, Ophthaine)
2. Tetracaine hydrochloride (Pontocaine)

C. Administration considerations

1. Rapid onset within 20 seconds, and duration is 15 to 20 minutes
2. Tetracaine hydrochloride can cause systemic toxicity

D. Contraindications: hypersensitivity

E. Side/adverse effects

1. Proparacaine (Ophthaine, Ophthetic) causes allergic contact dermatitis, cycloplegia, conjunctival congestion, delayed corneal healing
2. CNS excitation symptoms: blurred vision, dizziness, nervousness, restlessness, trembling
3. CNS depression (follows CNS excitation): dyspnea, drowsiness, dysrhythmias

F. Nursing considerations

1. To protect cornea, apply eye patch until blink reflex has returned
2. Assess for hypersensitivity symptoms such as burning, itching, stinging

G. Client teaching: do not touch or rub the eye until anesthesia has worn off

VI. AUDITORY MEDICATIONS

A. Antibiotics for ear

1. Used to manage infections of external ear (external auditory canal surface)
2. Chloramphenicol (Chloromycetin Otic) is used to treat infections caused by such organisms as *Enterobacter aerogenes, Escherichia coli, Haemophilus influenzae, Pseudomonas aeruginosa,* and other organisms
3. Common medications
   a. Chloramphenicol (Chloromycetin Otic): 2 or 3 drops instilled in ear canal every 6 to 8 hours
   b. Gentamicin sulfate otic solution (Garamycin): 3 or 4 drops instilled in ear canal 3 times daily
   c. Note: otic preparation of gentamicin sulfate has not been approved by the Food and Drug Administration (FDA); prescribers in United States use *ophthalmic* preparation for otic infections
4. Administration considerations
   a. Unless contraindicated, warm ear drops by running medication bottle under warm water, immersing bottle in a cup of warm water, or holding bottle in hand or pocket for 30 minutes prior to administration
   b. Assess client's baseline hearing status, and presence of ear drainage, earache, erythema, pain, and **vertigo** (dizziness)
   c. Assess that ear canal is clear and not impacted with *cerumen* (earwax) before medication administration
   d. Assess for intact tympanic membrane
   e. Contraindicated in hypersensitivity and perforation of tympanic membrane
5. Side/adverse effects
   a. Local: burning, rash, redness, swelling, blurred vision
   b. Systemic: hypersensitivity reaction
   c. Rare occurrence of systemic hematologic toxicity
6. Nursing considerations

Box 44–11

Administration of Otic Medications

For instillation of eardrops in older children and adults

- Assess the ear canal for cerumen or edema
- Tilt client's head toward the unaffected side
- Gently pull the pinna of the ear up and back
- Instill the eardrops—*do not* insert dropper into the ear canal
- Gently massage the area anterior to the ear to facilitate entry of the drops into the ear canal

For instillation of eardrops in children 3 years and younger

- Assess the ear canal for cerumen or edema
- Tilt client's head toward the unaffected side
- Gently pull the pinna of the ear slightly down and back
- Instill the eardrops—*do not* insert dropper into the ear canal
- Gently massage the area anterior to the ear to facilitate entry of the drops into the ear canal

! a. Assess for local adverse effects
b. Discontinue use if hypersensitivity reaction occurs
c. Monitor auditory canal for drainage and pain
d. Monitor for hearing disturbances

7. Client teaching
   a. Inform prescriber of increased pain, drainage, or no improvement in symptoms within a few days of treatment
   ! b. Refer to Box 44–11 for instillation of otic medications

B. Corticosteroids

1. Used for anti-inflammatory, antipruritic, or antiallergenic effects; may be given with antibacterial or antifungal agents
2. Common medications are listed in Box 44–12
3. Administration considerations
   a. Assess client's hearing status and presence of ear drainage, earache, erythema, pain, and vertigo
   b. Assess that ear canal is clear and not impacted with cerumen before medication administration
   c. Assess for intact tympanic membrane
   d. May be given in combination with antibiotics to treat infections of external ear canal or mastoid cavity
   e. Contraindicated in hypersensitivity to sulfites or perforation of tympanic membrane
4. ! Side/adverse effects: corticosteroids may mask infection or exacerbate an existing infection
5. ! Nursing considerations: assess for hypersensitivity after administration of medication

Box 44–12

Corticosteroid Agents for Otic Use

Betamethasone (generic)
Hydrocortisone (Cortamed)
Dexamethasone (Decadron)
Hydrocortisone with acetic acid (VoSol HC, Acetasol HC)
Hydrocortisone with alcohol (EarSol-HC)
Hydrocortisone with acetic acid and benzethonium (AA-HC Otic)

PRACTICE TEST

Box 44–13

Common OTC Agents for Otic Use

- Boric acid and isopropyl alcohol (Auro–Dri Ear Drops)
- Carbamide peroxide (Auro Ear Drops)
- Carbamide peroxide and glycerin (Dent's Ear Wax Drops, E.R.O. Ear drops, Ear Wax Removal System)
- Hydrocortisone, propylene glycol, alcohol, benzyl benzoate (Earsol-HC Drops)
- Isopropyl alcohol (Aurocaine 2)
- Isopropyl alcohol in glycerin (Swim-Ear Drops)

6. Client teaching
   a. Hearing should be monitored during duration of treatment
   b. Inform prescriber of new onset of ear drainage, heat, fever, odor, or pain, or if no improvement is seen within a few days of treatment

C. Other medications (over-the-counter medications)

1. Acetic acid (alcohol, glycerin, or propylene glycol) is used after swimming or bathing to restore normal acid pH to the ear canal
2. Glycerin, mineral oil, and olive oil are used as emollients to relieve itching and burning in ear
3. Propylene glycol enhances antibacterial effects and acidity of acetic acid
4. Carbamide peroxide is an antibacterial agent used to help remove accumulated cerumen
5. Common medications are listed in Box 44–13
6. General considerations: generally considered safe and effective; contraindicated with hypersensitivity
7. Client teaching
   a. Seek evaluation by prescriber if symptoms do not improve within several days
   b. Inform prescriber if adverse reactions occur or if symptoms worsen

D. Medications that cause ototoxicity

1. Analgesics: aspirin and other salicylates, NSAIDs
2. Antibiotics; aminoglycosides, clarithromycin, erythromycin, vancomycin
3. Antineoplastic agents: cisplatin, mechlorethamine
4. Loop diuretics: bumetanide (Bumex), ethacrynic acid (Edecrin), furosemide (Lasix)

Check Your NCLEX–RN® Exam I.Q.

You are ready for testing on this content if you can

- Apply knowledge of expected actions and effects of eye and ear medications to client care.
- Correctly administer eye and ear medications to clients.
- Assess for side effects and adverse effects of eye and ear medications.
- Take appropriate action if a client has an unexpected response to an eye or ear medication.
- Monitor a client for expected outcomes or effects of treatment with eye and ear medications.

PRACTICE TEST

1 A client being treated for glaucoma complains of photophobia. The nurse's teaching instructions include which of the following?

1. Discontinue use of the medication.
2. Wipe eyes with tissue immediately after instillation of eye drops.
3. Wear dark glasses when outside or when around bright lights.
4. Special glasses are necessary while being treated for glaucoma.

PRACTICE TEST

2 Which of the following statements by the client demonstrates an understanding of client education regarding pilocarpine (Isopto Carpine)?

1. "I will see better at night."
2. "I may have trouble adjusting to darkness."
3. "I should not have any trouble adjusting to changes from light to dark."
4. "I will not use the medication if I plan to drive."

3 The nurse is providing care to a client taking methazolamide (Neptazane), a carbonic anhydrase inhibitor for glaucoma. The plan of care includes monitoring for which of the following electrolyte imbalances?

1. Hyperkalemia and hypernatremia
2. Hypokalemia and hyponatremia
3. Hyperkalemia and hyponatremia
4. Hypokalemia and hypernatremia

4 Which of the following statements by a client who has a prescription for otic chloramphenicol (Chloromycetin) indicates a need for further instructions?

1. "I will inform my doctor of increased ear pain."
2. "I will inform my doctor if my ear infection has not improved within 7 days."
3. "I will inform my doctor if I have an increase in drainage from my ear."
4. "I will inform my doctor if I experience any hearing disturbances."

5 A client is receiving pilocarpine (Isopto Carpine) for the treatment of glaucoma. Which of the following symptoms experienced by the client does the nurse attribute to systemic absorption?

1. Diaphoresis
2. Constipation
3. Tachycardia
4. Hypertension

6 A client is receiving cyclopentolate and phenylephrine (Cyclomydril) before an ocular examination. The nurse would explain the purpose of the medication as which of the following?

1. To constrict the pupil
2. To dilate the pupil
3. To provide anesthesia
4. To provide a prophylactic antibiotic

7 Which of the following symptoms described by a client would lead the nurse to suspect a systemic side effect of atropine ophthalmic solution?

1. Tachycardia
2. Bradycardia
3. Salivation
4. Diaphoresis

8 Which of the following statements demonstrates the client's understanding of proper administration of ophthalmic solutions?

1. "I will not use any medication if it has turned brown."
2. "I will not use my medication if it is clear in color."
3. "I will use a cotton swab to apply my medication."
4. "I will not use any medication that is more than 1 month old."

9 When teaching a client about side effects of medications, for which of the following over-the-counter medications would the nurse discuss ototoxicity?

1. Salicylates (aspirin)
2. Vitamin C
3. Diphenhydramine (Benadryl)
4. Vitamin A

10 During a follow-up visit at the clinician's office, a client states: "I insert the ear dropper deep into my ear so the medication doesn't run back out." The nurse's response and priority teaching to the client is based on which of the following?

1. The client's ear canal is likely obstructed with cerumen.
2. The client is using the appropriate technique for administering an otic solution.
3. The client should lie on the same side as the affected ear for 5 minutes to allow medication to flow into the ear.
4. The medication dropper or any other item should not be inserted into the ear canal.

11 Which of the following actions observed by the nurse demonstrates appropriate technique by a client self-administering an ophthalmic medication?

1. The client waits 5 minutes between instillation of two different ophthalmic solutions.
2. The client administers ophthalmic ointment immediately after administering ophthalmic solution.
3. The client administers the second ophthalmic solution immediately after administering the first ophthalmic solution.
4. The client administers ophthalmic solution immediately after administering ophthalmic ointment.

12 The nurse is observing a client give a return demonstration of the administration of eye drops. Which of the following actions taken by the client indicates a need for further teaching?

1. The client pulls the lower lid of the eye down, forming a sac.
2. The client instills the medication into the conjunctival sac.
3. The client cleanses the eyelid with cotton balls moistened with warm tap water.
4. The client cleanses the eye from inner canthus to outer canthus.

13 A client with open-angle glaucoma is receiving timolol (Timoptic) for treatment. When assessing the client's response to the medication, the nurse expects therapeutic effects to be the result of which of the following?

1. A decrease in the outflow of aqueous humor
2. An increase in the outflow of aqueous humor
3. A decrease in aqueous humor production
4. An increase in aqueous humor production

14 The nurse is providing information on safety measures to a family of an elderly client being treated with carbachol (Carboptic), an ophthalmic cholinesterase inhibitor. The safety measures implemented are related to which of the following?

1. The client will experience difficulty in making quick changes in illumination because of miosis.
2. The client will experience difficulty in making quick changes in illumination because of mydriasis.
3. The client will experience a side effect of constipation.
4. The client will experience a side effect of hypertension.

15 The nurse is developing a plan of care for a client receiving a carbonic anhydrase inhibitor for treatment of glaucoma. The nurse identifies that the client is at risk for which nursing diagnosis?

1. Excess fluid volume
2. Deficient fluid volume
3. Electrolyte imbalance: hyperkalemia
4. Electrolyte imbalance: hypocalcemia

16 A client who just self-administered the first dose of vidarabine (Vira-A) calls the clinic and reports eye redness and swelling not present before treatment began. The nurse instructs the client to take which of the following actions?

1. No action is necessary because these are normal signs and symptoms of the medication.
2. Discontinue use of the medication and return to clinic immediately for evaluation.
3. If redness continues after 3 days, return to the clinic for evaluation.
4. Discontinue use of the medication and return to clinic at the next scheduled appointment.

17 Which of the following statements made by a client being treated with ophthalmic trifluridine (Viroptic) indicates an understanding of the medication instructions?

1. "I will stop the medication once healing has occurred."
2. "I will administer the treatment for 7 days."
3. "I will store the medication in a warm place."
4. "I will continue the medication for 5 to 7 days after healing has occurred."

18 The parent of a 2-year-old child exhibits correct administration technique for otic solutions when doing which of the following in a return demonstration?

1. The parent pulls the child's pinna down and back before administering the medication.
2. The parent pulls the child's pinna up and back before administering the medication.
3. The parent places the dropper into the child's ear canal before administering the medication.
4. The parent tilts the head of the child towards the affected side before administering the medication.

19 A client in the rural health clinic complains of frequent urination during the night. Upon evaluation, the nurse suspects that which of the following actions by the client taking acetazolamide (Diamox) is likely the cause of the nocturia?

1. The client takes oral Diamox every morning.
2. The client consumes 2,000 mL of fluid per day.
3. The client takes oral Diamox before supper.
4. The client takes oral Diamox with juice.

20 The nurse is orienting a newly hired nurse to the outpatient ophthalmic clinic. The nurse concludes that the orientee understands instructions for administering ophthalmic anesthetics for tonometry after observing which of the following actions?

1. The orientee administers proparacaine hydrochloride (Ophthaine) 15 minutes before the scheduled tonometry.
2. The orientee administers Ophthaine immediately before the scheduled tonometry.
3. The orientee administers Ophthaine 5 minutes before the scheduled tonometry.
4. The orientee administers Ophthaine after the tonometry is completed.

ANSWERS & RATIONALES

1 **Answer: 3** Clients experiencing photophobia are instructed to wear dark sunglasses and to avoid bright lights. Not enough information is provided to warrant discontinuing the medication. Eyes should not be wiped with tissue immediately after instillation of drops, and no special glasses are required.
Cognitive Level: Application **Client Need:** Physiological Integrity: Pharmacological and Parenteral Therapies **Integrated Process:** Teaching and Learning **Content Area:** Pharmacology **Strategy:** The wording of the question tells you the correct answer is also a true statement. Focus on the word *photophobia* and use the process of elimination to choose the answer that shields the eyes from light.

2 **Answer: 2** Difficulty in adjusting quickly to changes in illumination occurs as a result of miosis, an effect of pilocarpine. The client will experience more difficulty seeing at night (option 1). Driving is not contraindicated (option 4); however, nighttime driving may not be possible because of the miosis.
Cognitive Level: Analysis **Client Need:** Physiological Integrity: Pharmacological and Parenteral Therapies **Integrated Process:** Nursing Process: Evaluation **Content Area:** Pharmacology **Strategy:** The wording of the question tells you the correct answer is also a true statement. Specific knowledge of the important teaching points related to pilocarpine is needed to answer the question. Use this knowledge and the process of elimination to make a selection.

3 **Answer: 4** The diuretic effects of methazolamide may lead to electrolyte disturbances of hypokalemia and hypernatremia. Options 1, 2, and 3 are either partially or totally incorrect.
Cognitive Level: Analysis **Client Need:** Physiological Integrity: Pharmacological and Parenteral Therapies **Integrated Process:** Nursing Process: Planning **Content Area:** Pharmacology **Strategy:** The core issue of the question is knowledge of electrolyte disturbances for which the client is at risk during therapy with methazolamide. Recall that the medication has a diuretic effect and reason that potassium may be lost while sodium is retained. Use this knowledge and the process of elimination to make a selection.

4 **Answer: 2** Improvement of the infection should be noticed within a few days of beginning the antibiotic therapy. Superinfections are known to occur with this medication; therefore, 7 days is too long to seek further evaluation and treatment. Options 1, 3, and 4 are correct actions by the client experiencing any ear infection or disorder.
Cognitive Level: Analysis **Client Need:** Physiological Integrity: Pharmacological and Parenteral Therapies **Integrated Process:** Nursing Process: Evaluation **Content Area:** Pharmacology **Strategy:** The wording of the question tells you that the correct answer is an incorrect option. Use the process of elimination and selection the option that represents incorrect factual information.

5 **Answer: 1** Symptoms of systemic absorption of pilocarpine include diaphoresis, diarrhea, bradycardia, and hypotension. Options 2, 3, and 4 are incorrect because they are opposites of actual signs of systemic absorption.
Cognitive Level: Application **Client Need:** Physiological Integrity: Pharmacological and Parenteral Therapies **Integrated Process:** Nursing Process: Analysis **Content Area:** Pharmacology **Strategy:** The core issue of the question is recognition of signs of systemic absorption of pilocarpine. Specific knowledge of systemic effects of this medication is needed to answer the question. Use this knowledge and the process of elimination to make a selection.

6 **Answer: 2** Cyclomydril and other mydriatics are applied topically to produce mydriasis (dilated pupil) to facilitate ocular examination. Options 1, 3, and 4 are incorrect because they do not constrict the pupil, provide anesthesia, or prevent infection, respectively.
Cognitive Level: Application **Client Need:** Physiological Integrity: Pharmacological and Parenteral Therapies **Integrated Process:** Nursing Process: Implementation **Content Area:** Pharmacology **Strategy:** The core issue of the question is knowledge of the intended effects of Cyclomydril. Note that the name of the drug contains the letters *myd,* which is also the beginning of the word *myd*riasis (meaning to dilate the pupils). Using simple word association will sometimes assist in making the correct selection.

7 **Answer: 1** Systemic side effects of ophthalmic atropine include tachycardia, confusion, dry mouth, drowsiness, and slurred speech. Options 2 and 3 are opposites of known systemic side effects, while option 4 (diaphoresis) is unrelated. **Cognitive Level:** Application **Client Need:** Physiological Integrity: Pharmacological and Parenteral Therapies **Integrated Process:** Nursing Process: Analysis **Content Area:** Pharmacology **Strategy:** The core issue of the question is knowledge of side/adverse effects of atropine. Recall that when used for cardiac reasons, the medication speeds up heart rate. With this in mind, eliminate each of the incorrect responses and choose tachycardia as the correct answer.

8 **Answer: 1** Ophthalmic solution that has darkened or become cloudy should be discarded. Most solutions are clear (option 2). Swabs should not be used to apply medication (option 3), and the medications generally have a shelf life of 3 months (option 4).
Cognitive Level: Analysis **Client Need:** Physiological Integrity: Pharmacological and Parenteral Therapies **Integrated Process:** Nursing Process: Evaluation **Content Area:** Pharmacology **Strategy:** The wording of the question tells you the correct option is also a correct statement. The core issue of the question is safe self-administration of ophthalmic medications. Use nursing knowledge and the process of elimination to answer the question.

9 **Answer: 1** Salicylates may cause tinnitus, vertigo, and hearing loss if ingested in high doses. Vitamin C (option 2), diphenhydramine (option 3), and vitamin A (option 4) do not present this concern.
Cognitive Level: Application **Client Need:** Physiological Integrity: Pharmacological and Parenteral Therapies **Integrated Process:** Nursing Process: Implementation **Content Area:** Pharmacology **Strategy:** The core issue of the question is an understanding of the types of drugs that can cause ototoxicity. Use nursing knowledge and the process of elimination to make a selection.

10 **Answer: 4** Inserting objects into the ear canal, including medication droppers, may perforate the tympanic membrane. Though the ear canal may be obstructed with cerumen (option 1), there are other reasons, such as inappropriate instillation technique, for the medication to not flow into the ear canal (option 2). The client is instructed to lie on the unaffected side, not the affected side (option 3), to allow flow of medication into the ear.
Cognitive Level: Analysis **Client Need:** Physiological Integrity: Pharmacological and Parenteral Therapies **Integrated Process:** Nursing Process: Planning **Content Area:** Pharmacology **Strategy:** The core issue of the question is an understanding of the procedure for safe self-administration of an otic medication. Use nursing knowledge and the process of elimination to make a selection.

11 **Answer: 1** The recommended wait time between administrations of two ophthalmic solutions is 5 minutes. If an ophthalmic ointment is instilled, the waiting time is 10 minutes between the ointment and the next medication.
Cognitive Level: Application **Client Need:** Physiological Integrity: Pharmacological and Parenteral Therapies **Integrated Process:** Nursing Process: Evaluation **Content Area:** Pharmacology **Strategy:** The core issue of the question is an understanding of the procedure for safe self-administration of an ophthalmic medication. Use nursing knowledge and the process of elimination to make a selection.

12 **Answer: 3** The eye is cleansed with sterile irrigating solution or sterile normal saline to decrease risk of contamination. Options 1, 2, and 4 represent appropriate techniques demonstrated by the client.
Cognitive Level: Analysis **Client Need:** Physiological Integrity: Pharmacological and Parenteral Therapies **Integrated Process:** Nursing Process: Evaluation **Content Area:** Pharmacology **Strategy:** The wording of the question tells you that the correct option is an incorrect statement. Analyze each option to decide if it is a true or false statement and make the selection that represents false information.

13 **Answer: 3** Timolol is a beta-adrenergic blocker that decreases the production of aqueous humor, thereby decreasing intraocular pressure. Sympathomimetics also decrease aqueous humor production. Prostaglandins increase the outflow of aqueous humor to decrease intraocular pressure.
Cognitive Level: Analysis **Client Need:** Physiological Integrity: Pharmacological and Parenteral Therapies **Integrated Process:** Nursing Process: Evaluation **Content Area:** Pharmacology **Strategy:** Note that the drug name ends in *olol* and reason that the medication is a beta-blocking agent. With this in mind, recall the actions of beta-blocker medications in the eye. Use nursing knowledge and the process of elimination to make a selection.

14 **Answer: 1** Carbachol causes miosis (pupil constriction), making quick changes in illumination difficult. Nighttime is particularly hazardous for the elderly client. The client and family are instructed on methods, such as lighting hallways and bathrooms at night, to reduce the potential for injury. Mydriasis (option 2) is not a concern. Systemic side effects of carbachol include diarrhea (option 3) and hypotension (option 4).
Cognitive Level: Application **Client Need:** Physiological Integrity: Pharmacological and Parenteral Therapies **Integrated Process:** Nursing Process: Implementation **Content Area:** Pharmacology **Strategy:** Note that options 1 and 2 are opposites. When two options are opposite, consider the possibility that one of them is the correct answer. In this case, note that the client is elderly and is not in a situation (such as an eye exam) when the pupils would be dilated. With this in mind, choose option 1 over 2.

15 **Answer: 2** Carbonic anhydrase inhibitors produce increased urinary elimination and subsequent increased excretion of potassium. Clients are monitored for fluid volume deficit (not excess as in option 1) and hypokalemia (options 3 and 4). Assess electrolytes, intake and output, daily weights, mucous membranes, and skin turgor.
Cognitive Level: Analysis **Client Need:** Physiological Integrity: Pharmacological and Parenteral Therapies **Integrated Process:** Nursing Process: Planning **Content Area:** Pharmacology **Strategy:** The core issue of the question is knowledge of what to monitor regarding side effects of carbonic anhydrase inhibitors. Use medication knowledge and the process of elimination to make a selection. Note

also that options 1 and 2 are opposites, which suggests that one of them may be correct.

16 **Answer: 2** Redness and swelling are signs of hypersensitivity to vidarabine. The medication should be discontinued, and the client should return to the clinic immediately for evaluation. Options 1, 2, and 4 are incorrect because they place the client at risk.
Cognitive Level: Analysis **Client Need:** Physiological Integrity: Pharmacological and Parenteral Therapies **Integrated Process:** Nursing Process: Implementation **Content Area:** Pharmacology
Strategy: Note that the question contains key information about adverse effects that began after the first dose of the medication. When symptoms suddenly appear as in this question, consider the possibility of a hypersensitivity reaction and choose an option accordingly.

17 **Answer: 4** Viroptic, used in the treatment of viral infections such as herpes, is administered for an additional 5 to 7 days after healing has occurred. Ophthalmic medications are stored in a cool, dry place (option 3), and some are recommended for refrigeration (check label for instructions). Options 1 and 2 are incorrect because their timeframes are too limited.
Cognitive Level: Analysis **Client Need:** Physiological Integrity: Pharmacological and Parenteral Therapies **Integrated Process:** Nursing Process: Evaluation **Content Area:** Pharmacology
Strategy: The core issue of the question is knowledge of appropriate information about Viroptic as an ophthalmic medication. Use nursing knowledge and the process of elimination to make a selection.

18 **Answer: 1** The child's pinna is pulled down and back for administration of otic solutions. The pinna in the adult is pulled up and back. Droppers should never be inserted into the ear canal, and the head is tilted toward the unaffected side.
Cognitive Level: Analysis **Client Need:** Physiological Integrity: Pharmacological and Parenteral Therapies **Integrated Process:** Nursing Process: Evaluation **Content Area:** Pharmacology
Strategy: One quick way to remember the direction for pulling the pinna is to associate the direction with the height of the person. Since an adult is taller, pull the pinna up and back, while in a child who is shorter, pull the pinna down and back.

19 **Answer: 3** Acetazolamide, a carbonic anhydrase inhibitor, causes diuresis. The nurse should instruct the client to take the medication early in the day to avoid nocturia. Clients receiving acetazolamide are encouraged to consume at least 2,000 mL of fluid per day to avoid fluid volume depletion, and acetazolamide may be taken with juice or food to minimize gastrointestinal irritation.
Cognitive Level: Analysis **Client Need:** Physiological Integrity: Pharmacological and Parenteral Therapies **Integrated Process:** Nursing Process: Evaluation **Content Area:** Pharmacology
Strategy: The core issue of the question is recognition of and client teaching to prevent nocturia, a side effect of carbonic anhydrase inhibitors. Use medication knowledge and general principles for timing the administration of diuretics to answer the question.

20 **Answer: 2** Proparacaine is administered to prevent pain during procedures such as tonometry and removal of foreign bodies. The medication has a rapid onset within 20 seconds and duration of 15 to 20 minutes. Options 1, 3, and 4 are incorrect actions taken by the nurse because of the timeframes identified.
Cognitive Level: Analysis **Client Need:** Physiological Integrity: Pharmacological and Parenteral Therapies **Integrated Process:** Nursing Process: Evaluation **Content Area:** Pharmacology
Strategy: Note that the name of the drug ends in *-caine* to help remember that this drug has an anesthetic action. With this in mind, choose the option that best protects an eye that has no sensation, which in this case is the option that utilizes the medication just prior to the exam.

Key Terms to Review

aqueous humor p. 734
cycloplegia p. 739
intraocular pressure p. 734
keratitis p. 737
miosis p. 736
mydriasis p. 735
narrow-angle glaucoma p. 738
open-angle glaucoma p. 734
photophobia p. 738
systemic absorption p. 734
tonometry p. 742
uveitis p. 735
vertigo p. 742

References

Abrams, A. (2004). *Clinical drug therapy: Rationales for nursing practice* (7th ed.). Philadelphia: Lippincott Williams & Wilkins.

Adams, M., Josephson, D., & Holland, L. (2005). *Pharmacology for nurses: A pathophysiologic approach.* Upper Saddle River, NJ: Pearson Education.

Deglin, J. H., & Vallerand, A. H. (2006). *Davis's drug guide for nurses* (10th ed.). Philadelphia: F. A. Davis.

Lehne, R. (2004). *Pharmacology for nursing care* (5th ed.). Philadelphia: W. B. Saunders.

McKenry, L., Tessier, E. & Hogan, M. (2006). *Mosby's pharmacology in nursing.* (22nd ed.). St. Louis: Elsevier Science.

Wilson, B., Shannon, M., & Stang, C. (2006). *Prentice Hall nurse's drug guide 2006.* Upper Saddle River, NJ: Pearson Education.

45 Antineoplastic Medications

Test Yourself

Are you ready for the NCLEX-RN® or course exams? Use the practice tests on the companion CD-ROM to check.

In this chapter

Cross reference

Other chapters relevant to this content area are:

Dosage Calculation and Medication Administration	Chapter 30
Oncological Disorders	Chapter 66

I. ALKYLATING AGENTS

A. Overview

1. Interfere with DNA replication through cross-linking of DNA strands, DNA strand breaking, and abnormal base pairing proteins
2. Most agents are **cell cycle nonspecific,** which means that they exhibit a cytotoxic effect regardless of cell cycle stage
3. ! Major toxicities occur in hematopoietic, gastrointestinal (GI) and reproductive systems

B. Common medications are listed in Box 45–1

Box 45–1

Common Alkylating Agents

Altretamine (Hexalen)	Ifosfamide/mesna (Ifex/Mesnex)
Busulfan (Myleran)	Mechlorethamine (Mustargen)
Carboplatin (Paraplatin)	Melphalan (Alkeran)
Chlorambucil (Leukeran)	Oxaliplatin (Eloxatin)
Cisplatin (Platinol)	Procarbazine (Matulane)
Cyclophosphamide (Cytoxan)	Temozolomide (Temodar)
Dacarbazine (DTIC-Dome)	Thiotepa (Thioplex)
Estramustine (Emcyt)	

C. Administration considerations

1. Cyclophosphamide (Cytoxan)
   - **a.** Administer PO (per os, or orally) on an empty stomach; if nausea and vomiting are severe, it may be taken with food; antiemetic agent should be given before administering drug
   - **b.** Should be administered by intravenous piggyback (IVPB) over 60 to 90 minutes
2. Busulfan (Myleran)
   - **a.** Should be taken as directed at same time every day
   - **b.** Taking drug on an empty stomach may minimize nausea and vomiting
   - **c.** Store drug tightly capped in light-resistant container
3. Cisplatin (Platinol)
   - **a.** Provide hydration with 1 to 2 liters of IV fluid before and after administration
   - **b.** Administer parenteral antiemetic agent 30 minutes before cisplatin therapy is instituted and give it on a scheduled basis throughout day and night as long as necessary
4. Carboplatin (Paraplatin)
   - **a.** Do not use needles or IV sets containing aluminum
   - **b.** Premedication with an antiemetic 30 minutes before and on a scheduled basis thereafter is generally recommended
   - **c.** Dosage should not be repeated until neutrophil count is at least 2,000/mm^3
   - **d.** Store unopened vials at room temperature, protect from light
5. Mechlorethamine (Mustargen, a nitrogen mustard)
   - **a.** Potent **vesicant** (causes severe skin and tissue necrosis if medication extravasates from vein)
   - **b.** Should be administered through side-arm portal of a freely running IV to avoid extravasation
   - **c.** If drug should extravasate, subcutaneous and intradermal injection with isotonic sodium thiosulfate and application of ice compresses may reduce local irritation
   - **d.** Short **nadir** period (6–8 days), which is lowest point to which blood counts will drop after chemotherapy administration

D. Contraindications

1. Cyclophosphamide (Cytoxan): childbearing age, serious infections including chicken pox and herpes zoster, immunosuppression, pregnancy (category C), and nursing mothers
2. Busulfan (Myleran): therapy-resistant chronic lymphocytic leukemia, blast crisis of chronic myelogenous leukemia, bone marrow depression, pregnancy (category D), and nursing mothers
3. Cisplatin (Platinol): history of sensitivity to cisplatin or other platinum-containing compounds, impaired renal function and/or hearing, history of gout or urate renal stones; safe use in pregnancy (category D) and nursing women not established
4. Carboplatin (Paraplatin): history of severe reactions to carboplatin or cisplatin, severe bone marrow depression, impaired renal function, pregnancy (category D), and with other nephrotoxic drugs
5. Ifosfamide (Ifex): severe bone marrow suppression or known hypersensitivity to ifosfamide, cautious use in clients with impaired renal function, prior radiation therapy, prior cytotoxic agents, or pregnancy (category D) and nursing mothers
6. Mechlorethamine (nitrogen mustard; Mustargen): **myelosuppression** (a decrease in blood counts usually related to chemotherapy), infectious granuloma, known infectious diseases, including herpes zoster, pregnancy (category D), and lactation

E. Significant assessment parameters

1. Cyclophosphamide (Cytoxan)
   - **a.** Determine total differential leukocyte count, platelet count, and hematocrit initially and at least every 2 weeks thereafter
   - **b.** Obtain baseline and periodic determinations of liver and kidney function in addition to serum electrolytes
   - **c.** Microscopic urine examinations are recommended after large doses

2. Busulfan (Myleran)
   a. Determine total differential leukocyte count, platelet count, and hematocrit initially and at least every 2 weeks thereafter
   b. There may be abrupt onset hematological toxicity; recovery from busulfan-induced **pancytopenia** (a decrease in all blood cell components) may take from 1 month to 2 years
   c. Ovarian suppression, amenorrhea, and menopausal symptoms are common
3. Cisplatin (Platinol)
   a. Pretreatment electrocardiogram (ECG) is indicated because of possible myocarditis or focal irritation
   b. Monitor urine output and specific gravity for 4 consecutive hours before therapy and for 24 hours after therapy; report less than 100 mL/hr output or specific gravity greater than 1.030; a urine output of less than 75 mL/hr necessitates medical intervention
   c. Audiometric testing should be performed before initial dose
   d. Anaphylactic reactions may occur within minutes of drug administration
   e. Blood urea nitrogen (BUN), serum uric acid, serum creatinine, and urinary creatinine clearance should be assessed before initiating therapy and every subsequent course of therapy
   f. Nephrotoxicity usually occurs within 2 weeks after drug administration and becomes more severe and prolonged with repeated courses
   g. Suspect ototoxicity if client manifests tinnitus or difficulty hearing in high-frequency range
   h. Assess BP, mental status, pupils, and optic fundi every hour during therapy because hydration increases danger of elevated intracranial pressure
   i. Monitor and report abnormal bowel patterns because constipation may be an early sign of neurotoxicity
4. Carboplatin (Paraplatin)
   a. Allergic reaction can occur within first 15 minutes of administration; monitor closely for signs of anaphylaxis during first 15 minutes of infusion
   b. Frequently monitor peripheral blood counts; nadir usually occurs at day 21
   c. Periodically monitor kidney function and creatinine clearance, although it has less renal toxicity than cisplatin
   d. Monitor for peripheral neuropathy, ototoxicity, and visual disturbances, although they occur less frequently than with cisplatin
   e. Monitor clients on diuretic therapy closely because carboplatin may also decrease serum sodium, potassium, calcium, and magnesium levels
5. Ifosfamide (Ifex)
   a. Monitor complete blood count (CBC) with differential before each dose; hold ifosfamide if WBC is below $2000/mm^3$ or platelet count is below $50{,}000/mm^3$
   b. Monitor urine before and during each dose for microscopic hematuria
   c. Hydrate with at least 3000 mL of fluid daily to reduce risk of **hemorrhagic cystitis** (excessive bleeding from bladder due to chemical irritation)

F. Side effects/toxicity

1. Cyclophosphamide (Cytoxan)
   a. Cardiotoxicity, acute cardiomegaly with high dose; prior radiation therapy and prior anthracycline therapy increases risk
   b. Hemorrhagic cystitis (occasionally chronic and severe)
   c. Metallic taste on administration

Memory Aid

Notice that the words cyclophosphamide, Cytoxan, and cystitis all begin with *cy*. Use these letters to associate this drug with hemorrhagic cystitis of the bladder.

   d. Acute myelosuppression
   e. **Acral erythema** (palmar redness) and sloughing of skin on palms of hands and soles of feet

f. Diffuse hyperpigmentation
g. Gonadal dysfunction
h. Nausea and vomiting

2. Busulfan (Myleran)
a. Myelosuppression
! b. Severe nausea and vomiting, mucositis
c. Pulmonary fibrosis, sometimes called *busulfan lung*

Memory Aid

Notice that busulfan begins with *b*, which can help you to think of blue and pulmonary complications of therapy with busulfan. Look at the trade name Myleran, which begins with *my*, to help remember that it also causes myelosuppression.

d. Hepatic dysfunction leading to veno-occlusive disease
e. Diffuse hyperpigmentation; development of bullae
f. Chronic **alopecia:** partial or complete hair loss usually on the scalp

3. Cisplatin (Platinol)
a. Renal and hepatic toxicity
! b. Eighth cranial nerve damage because of ototoxicity
c. Myelosuppression
d. Peripheral neuropathy; neurotoxicity
e. Intense nausea and vomiting
f. Metallic taste on administration

4. Carboplatin (Paraplatin)
! a. Myelosuppression with pronounced thrombocytopenia
b. Severe nausea and vomiting
c. Hepatotoxicity and ototoxicity, mild nephrotoxicity

5. Ifosfamide (Ifex)
! a. Hemorrhagic cystitis, occasionally chronic and severe
! b. Neutopenia and thrombocytopenia
c. Nausea and vomiting
d. Hepatic dysfunction
e. Nephrotoxicity
f. Somnolence, confusion, and hallucinations

G. Client and family education

1. Cyclophosphamide (Cytoxan)
a. Because of mutagenic potential, employ adequate contraception during and for at least 4 months after termination of drug therapy
! b. Void frequently and maintain hydration with oral fluids to at least 3000 mL/24 hours

2. Cisplatin (Platinol)
! a. Continue maintenance of adequate hydration with oral fluids to at least 3000 mL/24 hours; report reduced urinary output, anorexia, nausea and vomiting uncontrolled by antiemetics, fluid retention, and weight gain
b. Keep vestibular stimulation to a minimum to avoid dizziness or falling
! c. Tingling, numbness, tremors of extremities, loss of position sense and taste, and constipation are early warning signs of neurotoxicity

3. Carboplatin (Paraplatin)
! a. Give special attention to strategies to prevent nausea
! b. There is potential for infection and hemorrhage related to bone marrow suppression
c. Report paresthesias, visual disturbances, or symptoms of ototoxicity (hearing loss/tinnitis)

4. Ifosfamide (Ifex)
! a. Void frequently and maintain hydration
b. Susceptibility to infection will increase
c. Report any unusual bleeding or bruising

5. Procarbazine (Mutalane)
   a. Avoid foods high in tyramine (e.g., beer, wine, cheese, brewer's yeast, chicken livers, and bananas) while taking procarbazine; may lead to hypertension and possible intracranial hemorrage
   b. Disulfiram-like reaction can occur if client consumes alcohol and procarbazine

II. ANTIMETABOLITES

A. Overview

1. Inhibit protein synthesis, substitute erroneous metabolites or structural analogues during DNA synthesis, and inhibit DNA synthesis
2. Most agents are **cell cycle–specific,** exhibiting cytotoxic effect during a specific phase of cell cycle, such as S phase
3. Most toxicity occurs in hematopoietic and GI systems
4. Used to treat leukemia, solid tumors, and lymphoma

B. Common medications are listed in Box 45–2

C. Administration considerations

1. Rotate IV sites every 48 hours to decrease hyperpigmentation
2. Determine whether dosage ordered is standard or high dose and obtain appropriate rescue therapy before administration (i.e., methotrexate with leucovorin)
3. Dosage of mercaptopurine should be reduced by 75% if given concurrently with allopurinol (Zyloprim); however, no dosage reduction is required when giving thioguanine
4. Fludarabine (Fludara) should be given as a 30-minute infusion

D. Contraindications

1. Myelosuppression
2. Pregnancy (category D) and nursing women
3. Concurrent administration of hepatotoxic drugs and hematopoietic depressants
4. Cautious use in following situations
   a. Clients with major surgery during previous month
   b. Previous use of alkylating agents
   c. History of high-dose pelvic irradiation
   d. Preexisting bone marrow impairment
   e. Men and women during childbearing years
   f. Hepatic or renal impairment

E. Significant assessment parameters

1. Assess baseline CBC, WBC differential, and platelet count prior to administration
2. Assess for signs and symptoms of infection or bleeding

F. Side effects/toxicity

1. General toxicities for this drug group include myelosuppression, nausea and vomiting, mucosal inflammation or stomatitis, photosensitivity with or without hyperpigmentation, and diarrhea (most commonly associated with antimetabolites)
2. Fluorouracil (5-FU): specific side effects/toxicity
   a. Cardiotoxicity resembling acute myocardial infarction (MI), angina, cardiogenic shock
   b. Photosensitivity and hyperpigmentation
   c. Cerebellar toxicity
3. Cytarabine (Ara-C): specific side effects/toxicity
   a. Maculopapular rash, with or without fever

Box 45–2

Common Antimetabolites

Capecitabine (Xeloda)	Gemcitabine (Gemzar)
Cladribine (Leustatin)	Mercaptopurine (Purinethol)
Cytarabine (Ara-C, Cytosar-U)	Methotrexate (Folex)
Floxuridine (FUDR)	Pemetrexed (Alimta)
Fludarabine (Fludara)	Pentostatin (Nipent)
Fluorouracil (5-FU, Adrucil)	Thioguanine (generic only)

b. Cytarabine syndrome (rash with or without fever, myalgia, bone pain, malaise)
c. Chemical conjunctivitis
d. Acute neurotoxicity: cerebellar toxicity; clients over 50 years of age at highest risk
e. Hepatotoxicity
f. Acral erythema

G. Client and family education

1. Teach importance of self-care measures to avoid infection and bleeding
   a. Avoid large crowds
   b. Avoid proximity to people with infections
   c. Avoid over-the-counter (OTC) aspirin-containing medications
2. Assess condition of oral cavity, maintain scheduled mouth care, and report development of stomatitis to healthcare professional
3. Maintain a low residue diet after discharge and report excessive diarrhea (more than 3 loose stools in 24 hours) to prescriber
4. Darkening of veins, mucous membranes, and fingernails may occur
5. Photosensitivity precautions should be followed year round
   a. Use sunscreen with a sun protection factor (SPF) of at least 15
   b. Avoid sun exposure between 10 a.m. and 2 p.m.
   c. Wear long sleeves and a large brimmed hat

III. ANTITUMOR ANTIBIOTICS

A. Overview

1. Interfere with nucleic acid synthesis and function, inhibit ribonucleic acid (RNA) synthesis, and inhibit DNA synthesis
2. Most agents are cell cycle–nonspecific
3. Major toxicities occur in hematopoietic, GI, reproductive, and cardiac systems (cumulative doses)

B. Common medications are listed in Box 45–3

C. Administration considerations

1. Most antitumor antibiotics are severe vesicants except for bleomycin (see signs and symptoms of extravasation in Table 45–1 ■ and antidotes for vesicant drugs in Table 45–2 ■)
2. Administer slowly by IV push (IVP) via side-arm portal of a freely flowing IV
3. Maintain clear visualization of injection site during administration
4. IV catheter should have an excellent blood return, be recently placed, and not more than 48 hours old before administering vesicant therapy
5. Avoid use of antecubital veins, in dorsum of hand, or in wrist, where extravasation could damage underlying tendons and nerves
6. Avoid venous access in extremity with compromised venous or lymphatic drainage

D. Contraindications

1. Doxorubicin (Adriamycin): myelosuppression, impaired cardiac function, obstructive jaundice, impaired hepatic or renal function, safe use in pregnancy not established
2. Bleomycin (Blenoxane): history of hypersensitivity or idiosyncrasy to bleomycin; pregnancy (category D) and women of childbearing age; cautious use with compromised hepatic, renal, or pulmonary function; previous cytotoxic drug or radiation therapy

Box 45–3

Anti-Tumor Antibiotics

Bleomycin (Blenoxane)	Idarubicin (Idamycin)
Dactinomycin (Cosmegen)	Mitomycin (Mutamycin)
Daunorubicin (Cerubidine)	Mitoxantrone (Novantrone)
Doxorubicin (Adriamycin)	Plicamycin (Mithracin)
Epirubicin (Ellence)	

Table 45–1

Signs and Symptoms of Extravasation

Assessment Parameter	Immediate Manifestations	Delayed Manifestations
Pain	Severe pain or burning that lasts minutes to hours and eventually subsides; usually occurs around needle site while drug is being given	Up to 48 hours
Redness	Blotchy redness around the needle site; not always present at time of extravasation	Later occurrence
Ulceration	Develops insidiously; usually occurs 48 to 96 hours later	Later occurrence
Swelling	Severe swelling; usually occurs immediately	Up to 48 hours
Blood return	Inability to obtain a blood return	Good blood return during administration
Other	Change in quality of infusion	Local tingling and sensory deficits

3. Plicamycin (Mithramycin): bleeding and coagulation disorders, myelosuppression, electrolyte imbalance (especially hypocalcemia), pregnancy (category C); cautious use in clients with prior abdominal or mediastinal radiation
4. Mitoxantrone (Novantrone): hypersensitivity, myelosuppression, pregnancy (category D) and lactation, cautious use in impaired cardiac, renal, or hepatic function
5. Mitomycin (Mutamycin): hypersensitivity to Mutamycin, pregnancy (category D) and lactation, thrombocytopenia, and coagulation disorders

E. Significant assessment parameters

1. Doxorubicin (Adriamycin)
   - **a.** Assess hepatic, renal, hematopoietic, and cardiac function prior to administration and at regular intervals thereafter
   - **b.** Begin a flowchart to establish baseline data, including temperature, pulse, respiration, BP, body weight, laboratory values, intake and output (I & O) ratio and pattern, and cardiac ejection fraction
   - ! **c.** Give prompt attention to complaints of stinging or burning sensation at injection site
   - ! **d.** Be alert to and report early signs of cardiotoxicity and hepatic dysfunction

Memory Aid

Notice that doxorubicin contains the letters *rub.* Think of ruby and red when you see this name to help you think of the heart and cardiotoxicity.

   - **e.** Stomatitis is greatest at 2 weeks following therapy, begins with burning sensation
   - **f.** Nadir usually occurs 10 to 14 days after administration
   - ! **g.** Radiation recall, erythema that develops in previously irradiated field, is common
2. Bleomycin (Blenoxane)

Table 45–2

Antidotes for Vesicant Therapy

Chemotherapeutic Drug	Antidote
Nitrogen mustard (Mustargen), Cisplatin (Platinol)	Thiosulfate
Dactinomycin (Cosmegen)	Apply ice and elevate; heat may enhance tissue damage
Doxorubicin (Adriamycin)	Cold pack with circulating ice water first 24 to 48 hours
Vinblastine (Velban), Vincristine (Oncovin), Vinorelbine (Navelbine)	Hyaluronidase; apply warm pack for first 24 to 48 hours
Paclitaxel (Taxol)	Hyaluronidase; apply ice for first 24 hours

a. Inject test dose of 2 units or less deeply into muscle to assess anaphylactic response before IV administration
b. Assess vital signs; a febrile reaction is relatively common
c. Bone marrow toxicity is rare
d. Pulmonary toxicity occurs in about 10% of clients, most usually in clients over 70 years of age and when cumulative dose reaches 400 units

Memory Aid

Notice that bleomycin (Blenoxane) begin with *bl*, which can help you to think of blue and pulmonary toxicity from chemotherapy with this agent.

e. Radiation recall is common
3. Plicamycin (Mithramycin)
a. Assess bowel function to prevent high impaction
b. Assess liver, hematological, and renal function before and periodically throughout therapy
c. Thrombocytopenia is common and is frequently evidenced by a single or persistent episode of epistaxis or hematemesis
4. Mitoxantrone (Novantrone)
a. Assess IV insertion site; transient blue discoloration may occur
b. Assess cardiac function throughout course of therapy; report signs and symptoms of CHF
c. Assess uric acid levels and initiate hypo-uricemic therapy before antileukemia therapy
5. Mitomycin (Mutamycin)
a. Assess serum creatinine because drug is rarely given if greater than 1.7 mg/dL
b. Assess platelet count, PT, and bleeding times
c. Assess I & O ratio and pattern, dysuria, hematuria, and oliguria; maintain hydration because drug is nephrotoxic
d. Is incompatible with dextrose-containing solutions

F. Side effects/toxicity

1. Anthracycline(s), which end in –rubicin
a. Vesicant: flare reaction is common and may be difficult to distinguish from an extravasation
b. Cardiotoxicity leading to degenerative cardiomyopathy occurs over time
c. Lifetime dosage is 450 to 550 mg/m^2
d. Prior radiation therapy to chest wall may predispose client to enhanced cardiotoxicity
e. Alopecia
f. Severe mucositis, stomatitis
g. Hyperpigmentation of nail beds and dermal creases
h. Acute myelosuppression
2. Bleomycin (Blenoxane)
a. Pulmonary toxicity that is dose- and age-related
b. Anaphylactic reaction may occur
c. Mild febrile reaction commonly occurs
d. Diffuse alopecia, hyperpigmentation of skin, vesiculation, acne, thickening of skin and nailbeds
3. Plicamycin (Mithramycin)
a. Vesicant
b. Depression of platelet count, usually severe; thrombocytopenia may be of rapid onset and occur at any time during the therapy
c. Hypocalcemia (because it is often given to treat hypercalcemia)
4. Mitoxantrone (Novantrone)
a. Is an **irritant:** a drug capable of causing pain and inflammation at administration site if extravasation occurs
b. Sclera and urine may turn blue to blue-green
c. Potent myelosuppression

d. Increased cardiotoxicity with cumulative dose higher than 180 mg/m^2

5. Mitomycin (Mutamycin)
   - ! a. Vesicant; has unique ability to produce ulceration at distal sites
   - b. Myelosuppression is delayed and cumulative initial nadir is 4 to 6 weeks
   - ! c. Nephrotoxic; can cause hemolytic uremia syndrome

G. Client and family education

1. Anthracycline agents
   - ! a. Alopecia, which may also involve eyelashes, eyebrows, beard/mustache, and pubic and axillary hair; regrowth of hair usually begins 2 to 3 months after completion of administration
   - ! b. Urine may turn red
2. Mitoxantrone (Novantrone)
   - ! a. Blue-green urine is common for 24 hours after drug therapy and sclera may also take on a bluish color
   - b. Stomatitis and mucositis may occur within one week of therapy

IV. PLANT EXTRACTS

A. Overview

1. Arrest or inhibit mitosis
2. Most agents are cell cycle–specific, M-phase
3. Major toxicities occur in the hematopoietic, integumentary, neurologic, and reproductive systems; also, hypersensitivity reactions may occur

B. Common medications are listed in Box 45–4

C. Administration considerations

1. Etoposide (VP-16): administer by slow IVPB over 60 to 90 minutes to avoid hypotension
2. Paclitaxel (Taxol)
   - a. Do not use equipment or devices containing polyvinyl chloride (PVC)
   - b. Tissue necrosis occurs with extravasation
   - c. Administer via nitroglycerine tubing with an in-line filter of 0.22 micron or less
   - ! d. Requires strict premedication (preferably with dexamethasone, diphenhydramine, and either cimetidine or ranitidine) per protocol order set before administration to prevent anaphylaxis
3. Vincristine (Oncovin)
   - a. Vesicant: administer into side-arm portal of freely flowing IV
   - ! b. Hyaluronidase is antidote if extravasation occurs; also apply moderate heat to disperse drug and minimize sloughing

D. Contraindications

1. Etoposide (VP-16): severe bone marrow depression, severe hepatic or renal impairment, existing or recent viral infection or bacterial infection, safe use in pregnancy (category D) and nursing mothers not established
2. Paclitaxel (Taxol): hypersensitivity to paclitaxel, baseline neutropenia of less than 1500 cells/mm^3, cautious use in presence of cardiac arrhythmias and impaired liver function, pregnancy (category X)
3. Vincristine (Oncovin): obstructive jaundice, demyelinating neurological diseases; preexisting neuromuscular disease, pregnancy (category D)

Box 45–4

Plant Extracts and Miscellaneous Agents

Vinca Alkaloids

Vinblastine (Velban)

Vincristine (Oncovin)

Vinorelbine (Navelbine)

Taxanes

Docetaxel (Taxotere)

Paclitaxel (Taxol)

Topoisomerase Inhibitors (miscellaneous agents)

Etoposide (Vepesid)

Teniposide (Vumon)

Irinotecan hydrochloride (Camptosar)

Topotecan hydrochloride (Hycamtin)

E. Significant assessment parameters

1. Etoposide (VP-16)
   a. Assess IV site before and after infusion; extravasation can cause thrombophlebitis and necrosis
   b. Be prepared to treat an anaphylactic reaction
   c. Monitor vital signs during and after infusion; if hypotension occurs, stop infusion
   d. Assess CBC, WBC and differential, and hepatic and renal function before administration and periodically during treatment
2. Paclitaxel (Taxol)
   a. Monitor for hypersensitivity during first and second administrations of drug; immediately discontinue if angioedema and generalized urticaria develop
   b. Monitor vital signs frequently; bradycardia occurs in 12% of clients who receive drug
   c. Assess for peripheral neuropathy
3. Vincristine (Oncovin)
   a. Assess for leukopenia, which occurs in a significant number of clients
   b. Assess hand grasps and deep tendon reflexes; depression of Achilles reflex is earliest sign of neuropathy

F. Side effects/toxicity

1. Etoposide (VP-16)
   a. Severe mucositis
   b. Acral erythema and sloughing of the skin on palms and soles
   c. Myelosuppression
   d. Severe blood fluctuations
   e. Fever and chills during infusion
2. Paclitaxel (Taxol)
   a. Transient bradycardia
   b. Peripheral neuropathy
   c. Neutropenia, thrombocytopenia
   d. Hypersensitivity reaction including hypotension, bronchospasm, urticaria, and angioedema
   e. Alopecia
3. Vincristine
   a. Neurotoxicity, loss of sensation on the soles of the feet and the fingertips
   b. Depression of the Achilles reflex is the earliest sign of neuropathy
   c. Paralytic ileus

G. Client and family education

1. Etoposide (VP-16)
   a. Inform about possible adverse effects (blood dyscrasias, alopecia, and carcinogenesis)
   b. Make position changes slowly, particularly from a recumbent position
   c. Inspect mouth daily for ulcerations and bleeding and avoid obvious irritants
2. Paclitaxel (Taxol)
   a. Report dyspnea, chest pain, palpitations, or angioedema
   b. Stress need for periodic laboratory testing
   c. There is high probability of developing alopecia
3. Vincristine
   a. Maintain a prophylactic regimen against constipation and paralytic ileus
   b. Report a change in bowel habits
   c. Alopecia is most common side effect; is reversible after treatment is complete

V. NITROSOUREAS

A. Overview

1. Interfere with DNA replication and repair
2. Not cross-resistant to alkylating agents
3. Most agents are cell cycle–nonspecific
4. Most agents cross the blood–brain barrier
5. Major toxicities occur in hematopoietic and GI systems

Box 45-5

Nitrosoureas

Carmustine (BCNU)	Streptozocin (Zanosar)
Lomustine (CeeNu)	

B. Common medications are listed in Box 45-5

C. Administration considerations

1. Carmustine (BiCNU)
   a. Administer over 1 to 2 hours by slow IV infusion with constant monitoring if given peripherally
   b. Vesicant: if possible, avoid starting IV in dorsum of hand, wrist, or antecubital veins because extravasation may cause damage to underlying tissues
2. Lomustine (CeeNU): should be taken on an empty stomach to avoid nausea
3. Streptozocin (Zanosar)
   a. Vesicant: administer via side arm portal of a freely flowing IV
   b. ! Administer antiemetic routinely before dose and Q 4 to 6 hours after for first 24 hours

D. Contraindications

1. Carmustine (BiCNU): history of pulmonary function impairment, decreased platelets, leukocytes, or erythrocytes; safe use during pregnancy (category D) not established
2. Lomustine (CeeNU): decreased platelets, leukocytes, or erythrocytes; safe use during pregnancy (category D) not established
3. Streptozocin (Zanosar): hepatic and renal dysfunction; safe use during pregnancy (category C) not established

E. Significant assessment parameters

1. Carmustine (BiCNU)
   a. ! Persistent nausea and vomiting may occur 2 hours after drug administration and persist up to 6 hours; prior administration of an antiemetic will help
   b. Blood counts should be monitored prior to beginning course of therapy and weekly for at least 6 weeks after last dose
   c. Assess results of pulmonary function studies prior to therapy and periodically thereafter
   d. ! Symptoms of lung toxicity should be reported to physician: cough, dyspnea, fever
   e. Be alert to hepatic and renal insufficiency
2. Lomustine (CeeNU): blood counts should be monitored prior to therapy and weekly for at least 6 weeks after last dose; liver and kidney function tests should also be performed
3. Streptozocin (Zanosar)
   a. Assess for early evidence of renal dysfunction with hypophosphatemia, mild proteinuria, and changes in I & O pattern
   b. Monitor CBC prior to therapy and weekly during therapy
   c. Do liver function studies prior to each dose

F. Side effects/toxicity

1. Carmustine (BiCNU)
   a. Severe nausea and vomiting
   b. Ocular infarctions, retinal hemorrhage, suffusion of the conjunctiva
   c. Delayed myelosuppression
   d. Pulmonary infiltration or fibrosis
2. Lomustine (CeeNU)
   a. Delayed myelosuppression
   b. Severe nausea and vomiting
3. Streptozocin (Zanosar)
   a. Nausea and vomiting
   b. Mild to moderate myelosuppression, can be severe in 10% to 20% of clients
   c. Insulin shock due to effect on the pancreatic beta cells
   d. Nephrotoxicity

G. Client and family education

1. Myelosuppression is severe and may be cumulative; teach neutropenic precautions and symptoms of sepsis
2. Teach signs and symptoms of hypoglycemia when administering streptozocin
3. Teach signs and symptoms of pulmonary toxicity when administering carmustine

VI. HORMONES AND HORMONE MODULATORS

A. Overview

1. Corticosteroids: lyse lymphoid malignancies and have indirect effect on malignant cells
2. Estrogens: suppress testosterone production in males and alter response of breast cancers to prolactin
3. Progestins: promote palliation and tumor cell regression; exact mechanism of action unknown
4. Antiestrogens: compete with estrogens for binding with estrogen receptor sites on malignant cells
5. Androgens: hormone therapy that has palliative use in metastatic/advanced carcinoma of breast; used if surgery and irradiation inappropriate; otherwise, tamoxifen (Nolvadex) is drug of choice for this purpose
6. Antiandrogens: inhibit binding of androgens at androgen receptor sites in target tissues; indicated for use in metastatic/advanced prostate cancer

B. Common medications are listed in Box 45–6

C. Administration considerations

1. Corticosteroids
   a. Oral forms should be administered with meals and may be crushed
   b. IV form should be given slowly by IVPB to prevent vaginal and anal burning
2. Estrogens
   a. Give orally immediately after solid food
   b. An exception is estramustine (Emcyt), a combination estrogen and nitrogen mustard compound; this must be taken with water an hour before meals and requires that no milk, dairy products, or calcium-containing products be used concurrently

Box 45–6

Hormones and Hormone Modulators

Corticosteroids

Prednisone (Deltasone)

Dexamethasone (Decadron)

Hydrocortisone (SoluCortef)

Methylprednisolone (SoluMedrol)

Estrogens

Chlorotrianisene (TACE)

Diethylstilbestrol (DES)

Ethinyl estradiol (Estinyl)

Polyestradiol (Estradurin)

Estramustine (Emcyt)

Antiestrogens

Tamoxifen (Nolvadex)

Toremifene (Fareston)

Anastrozole (Arimedex)

Fulvestrant (Faslodex)

Progestins

Medroxyprogesterone acetate (Depo-Provera)

Megestrol acetate (Megace)

Leuprolide (Lupron)—a Gn-RH agonist

Antiandrogens (androgen receptor blockers)

Bicalutamide (Casodex)

Flutamide (Eulexin)

Nilutamide (Nilandron)

Goserelin (Zoladex)—a Gn-RH agonist

Androgens

Testosterone (generic)

Testolactone (Teslac)

Fluoxymesterone (Halotestin)

3. Progestins: give orally without regard to meals
4. Estrogen antagonists: give orally; dosage may be decreased if side effects are severe
5. Androgens and antiandrogens: give orally

D. Contraindications

1. Corticosteroids: systemic infections, ucerative colitis, diverticulitis, active or latent peptic ulcer disease; safe use in pregnancy (category C) and nursing mothers not established
2. Estrogens: known or suspected pregnancy, estrogen-dependent neoplasms, history of thromboembolic disorders
3. Progestins: severe arrhythmias if taking a calcium-channel blocker; psychiatric depression, pregnancy (category C); cautious use in lactation
4. Antiestrogens: first trimester of pregnancy (category C)

E. Significant assessment parameters

1. Corticosteroids
   a. Establish baseline and continuing data on blood pressure, I & O, weight, and sleep patterns
   b. Measure 2-hour postprandial blood glucose, serum potassium, and serum calcium prior to therapy and at regular intervals thereafter
   c. Watch for changes in mood, emotional stability, and sleep patterns
2. Estrogens
   a. Spotting or breakthrough bleeding may occur
   b. Severe hypercalcemia may occur
3. Progestin
   a. Assess weight periodically
   b. Assess for allergic reactions, rash, urticaria, anaphylaxis, tachypnea
4. Antiestrogens: assess CBC, including platelet count, periodically
5. Androgens: monitor serum calcium levels; hypercalcemia can result, requiring temporary termination of drug therapy and administration of large volumes of IV fluid
6. Antiandrogens: monitor liver function studies periodically to detect rare complication of hepatitis

F. Side effects/toxicity

1. Corticosteroids
   a. Euphoria, headache, insomnia, psychosis
   b. Edema
   c. Muscle weakness, delayed wound healing, osteoporosis, spontaneous fractures
   d. Hyperglycemia
2. Estrogens: thromboembolic disorders, nausea
3. Progestins
   a. Vaginal bleeding and breast tenderness
   b. Abdominal pain, nausea, and vomiting
   c. Increased appetite and weight gain
4. Antiestrogens
   a. Thrombosis
   b. About 25% of clients experience nausea and vomiting
   c. Hot flashes, weight gain, changes in menstrual cycle, leaking from breasts
5. Androgens
   a. Virilization, including clitoral enlargement, increases in facial and body hair, deepened voice, increased libido, and male-pattern baldness
   b. Hypercalcemia
6. Anti-androgens
   a. Gynecomastia
   b. GI disturbances (nausea, vomiting, constipation, diarrhea)
   c. Hepatitis

G. Client and family teachings: for all drug groups, teach clients about adverse effects and when to report them

VII. OTHER ANTINEOPLASTICS

A. Overview

1. Asparaginase (Elspar) depletes extracellular supply of asparagine, an amino acid essential to DNA synthesis
2. Hydroxyurea (Hydrea) blocks incorporation of thymidine into DNA and may damage already formed DNA molecules

B. Common medications: asparaginase (also called L-asparaginase) and hydroxyurea

C. Administration considerations

1. Asparaginase (Elspar)
   a. Administer intradermal (ID) skin test before initial dose because of potential for anaphylaxis; a negative skin test does not preclude possibility of allergic reaction
   b. Fiberlike particles may develop in vial after reconstitution; use a 5-micron filter to remove particles (will not affect potency)
2. Hydroxyurea: capsule may be opened and mixed with water if client has difficulty swallowing

D. Contraindications

1. Asparaginase (Elspar): history of or existing pancreatitis; safe use during pregnancy (category C) and nursing mothers is not established
2. Hydroxyurea: pregnancy (category D)

E. Significant assessment parameters

1. Asparaginase (Elspar)
   a. Prepare for anaphylaxis and have personnel, emergency medications, oxygen, and airway equipment readily available
   ! b. During administration, monitor vital signs and be alert for hypersensitivity or anaphylactic reaction, which usually occurs 30 to 60 minutes after medication administration
   c. Assess laboratory values prior to treatment and routinely thereafter, including CBC, amylase, serum calcium, coagulation factors, hepatic and renal function studies, and ammonia and uric acid levels
2. Hydroxyurea (Hydrea)
   a. Determine status of kidney, liver, and bone marrow function before and periodically during therapy
   ! b. Monitor I & O and increase fluid intake, especially in clients with high serum uric acid levels

F. Side effects/toxicity

1. Asparaginase (Elspar)
   a. Severe anaphylaxis is possible; crash cart should be readily available
   b. Severe nausea and vomiting
   c. Potential for bleeding because of reduced clotting factors, decreased circulating platelets, and decreased fibrinogen levels
2. Hydroxyurea (Hydrea)
   a. Bone marrow suppression
   b. Stomatitis
   c. Maculopapular rash
   d. Hyperuricemia

VIII. SAFE HANDLING OF CHEMOTHERAPEUTIC AGENTS

A. Drug preparation and administration

! 1. All individuals preparing and administering cytotoxic drugs should be specially trained in safety procedures for handling them and comply with agency, government, and professional practice standards
2. Chemotherapy doses are generally individualized according to body weight (in kg) or body surface area (in m^2)
3. Most chemotherapy protocol order sets consist of short, intermittent, high-dose courses of medications (often in combination) to maximize cancer-cell kill while allowing healthy cells time to heal and recover

4. Chemotherapy drugs should be prepared for use in an air-vented space, such as a clean-air workstation or biohazard cabinet; access to this area should be limited
5. Wear a disposable, leak-proof gown, surgical latex gloves, a mask, and eye protection when preparing chemotherapeutic agents
6. Do not prepare or administer IV chemotherapy if pregnant because of possible risk to fetus

B. Safe handling of antineoplastic agents and spill management

1. Use leak-proof, puncture-resistant containers to dispose of all antineoplastic drug preparation equipment; double-bag and identify container with a biohazard label
2. To avoid leaking medication from them, do not separate needle from syringe or break needles
3. If drug accidentally touches a nurse or client, wash area well with soap and water; immediately remove any contaminated clothing; copiously flush eyes if involved while keeping eyelids open
4. Double-glove to clean a drug spill, washing hands before and after
5. For powdered medications, wear a mask and eye protection as well
6. Place spilled substance in a plastic bag; wipe remaining area with a damp cloth and place the cloth in same bag; place this bag into another plastic bag (double-bag) and label it as biohazardous
7. All materials used for drug preparation and administration must be disposed of by incineration

C. Disposal of client's body fluids

1. Handle cautiously all body substances, such as blood, urine, vomitus, stool, and others; carefully follow standard precautions and other procedures as designated by agency policy
2. Wear gloves when in contact with all body substances; carefully dispose of them in toilet; clean containers carefully and thoroughly

IX. NURSING MANAGEMENT OF TREATMENT SIDE EFFECTS

A. Neutropenia

1. Neutropenia is an absolute neutrophil count of 1,500/mm^3 or less
2. Lowest point in WBC count reached after chemotherapy (nadir) most commonly occurs 7 to 14 days following chemotherapy administration
3. Fever of more than 38° C or 100.4° F is most reliable and often only sign of infection in clients with neutropenia
4. Management
    a. Avoid exposure to fresh fruits, vegetables, flowers, and live plants; people recently vaccinated with live organisms or viruses; or pet excreta including fish tanks and aquariums
    b. Teach people who come in contact with client to wash hands prior to touching client
    c. Encourage client to practice good personal hygiene
    d. Prevent trauma to skin and mucous membranes
    e. Culture urine, peripheral blood, all lumens of central venous catheters (CVCs) and suspected sources of infection; obtain chest x-ray (CXR); administer antibiotics as ordered for empiric therapy
    f. Institute neutropenic precautions for hospitalized clients whose absolute neutrophil count drops as described, using previously described measures
    g. Administer filgrastim (Neupogen), a granulocyte colony-stimulating factor that increases production of neutrophils, either IV or subcutaneously as ordered; client may complain of bone pain 1 to 3 days before blood count increases, which may be controlled with nonopioid analgesics
5. Client and family education
    a. Report temperature greater than 38° C or 100.4° F, shaking chills, dysuria, dyspnea, sputum production, or pain
    b. Meticulous hygiene is important to prevent infection
    c. Avoid contact with people who have contagious illness

d. Teach self-administration of granulocyte colony-stimulating factor (G-CSF) for neutropenia or granulocyte/macrophage colony-stimulating factor (GM-CSF) for treatment of blood-forming organ cancers as ordered

B. Thrombocytopenia

1. Bone marrow suppression decreases platelet production
2. Circulating platelets diminish gradually because platelet life span is only 10 days
3. Chemotherapy drugs accelerate platelet destruction
4. Assessment
a. Platelet count below 50,000/mm^3; risk significantly increases when platelet count falls below 20,000/mm^3
b. Petechiae, bruising, and hemorrhage
c. Neurological changes, which may indicate intracranial bleeding
d. Hypotension and tachycardia
5. Management
a. Institute bleeding precautions (refer to Chapter 38)
b. Decrease activity to prevent falls and maintain a safe environment
c. Discourage heavy lifting and Valsalva maneuver, which may increase risk of intracranial bleeding
d. Encourage client to eat a high-fiber diet and drink adequate liquids
e. Avoid using nail clippers; use a nail file instead
f. Avoid using vaginal douches, rectal suppositories, or enemas
g. Use water-soluble lubricant for sexual intercourse
h. Avoid intercourse when platelet count is below 50,000/mm^3
i. Instruct menstruating women to monitor pad count and amount of saturation; tampon use should be avoided
j. Encourage client to blow nose gently or wipe nose instead
k. Avoid administration of aspirin or aspirin-containing products as well as NSAIDs
l. Apply pressure for 5 to 10 minutes following venipuncture, bone marrow biopsy, or other invasive procedures; platelet transfusion prior to procedure may be indicated
6. Client and family education
a. Notify physician of symptoms of bleeding
b. Test urine and stool for occult blood
c. Implement other safety recommendations for daily management as above

C. Nausea and vomiting

1. **Anticipatory nausea**: a conditioned response resulting from repeated association of chemotherapy-induced nausea and vomiting and stimulus from environment
2. Acute nausea: occurs 0 to 24 hours after chemotherapy administration
3. Delayed nausea: persistent vomiting lasting 1 to 4 days after chemotherapy administration
4. Assessment parameters
a. Women have higher incidence than men
b. Younger clients experience more nausea than older clients
c. A history of motion sickness can predispose some to experience chemotherapy-induced nausea
d. Dehydration may accelerate nausea and vomiting
5. Administer antiemetics to cover emetogenic period; these may include (but are not limited to) ondansetron (Zofran) and metoclopramide (Reglan), a prokinetic GI stimulant
6. Provide additional antiemetics to manage breakthrough nausea
7. Dexamethasone may be most effective agent in preventing anticipatory nausea/vomiting
8. Client and family education
a. Eat small frequent meals and avoid fatty or spicy foods
b. Notify prescriber if vomiting persists for 24 or more hours and client is unable to take oral hydration
c. Maintain antiemetic schedule for 48 to 72 hours to avoid delayed nausea

D. Diarrhea

1. Chemotherapy affects rapidly dividing cells of villae and microvillae in GI mucosa
2. Combined chemotherapy and radiation therapy to pelvis can lead to added cellular destruction
3. Monitor number of stools, amount, and consistency
4. Replace fluid and electrolytes, including potassium
5. Administer antidiarrheal medication to reduce peristalsis and stool frequency and volume
6. Client and family education
   a. Consume low-residue, high-protein, high-calorie diet to promote bowel rest
   b. Eliminate irritating foods, such as alcohol, coffee, cold liquids, popcorn, and raw fruits and vegetables
   c. Drink 6 to 8 glasses of water per 24-hour period
   d. Implement liquid diet if diarrhea is severe
   e. Avoid milk products and chocolate
   f. Decrease activity when diarrhea is severe to provide rest and decrease peristalsis
   g. Clean rectal area with mild soap and water after each bowel movement and apply moisture barrier
   h. Take warm sitz baths for comfort

E. Stomatitis

1. Epithelial cells of oral mucosa are destroyed, causing inflammatory response and denudation of oral mucosa
2. Initial presentation: burning sensation with no physical changes in oral mucosa, sensitivity to heat and cold, and sensitivity to salty and spicy foods
3. Promote well-balanced intake, including protein intake of greater than 1 gram/kg of body weight
4. Promote consistent, thorough oral hygiene after each meal and before sleep
5. Administer antifungal/antiviral medication for prophylaxis as directed
6. Client and family education
   a. Use consistent oral hygiene
   b. Avoid using lemon/glycerin swabs, hydrogen peroxide, and products containing alcohol, which promote dryness and irritation

F. Constipation

1. Neurotoxic effects of chemotherapy can decrease peristalsis or cause paralytic ileus
2. Assess patterns of elimination including amount and frequency
3. Assess usual fiber and fluid intake
4. Determine laxative and cathartic use, including frequency and amounts taken
5. Initiate bowel maintenance program for clients receiving neurotoxic chemotherapeutic agents or those at high risk for constipation
6. Recognize complications associated with constipation, such as fecal impaction
7. Client and family education
   a. Drink warm liquids to stimulate bowel movement
   b. Increase fiber intake to increase peristalsis and stool bulk
   c. Drink at least 8 glasses of water per day
   d. Exercise regularly
   e. Develop a regular bowel program, avoiding use of laxatives if possible

G. Alopecia

1. Cells responsible for hair growth have a high mitotic rate and are affected to some degree by most chemotherapeutic agents
2. Hair loss begins approximately 2 weeks after drug administration and continues until 3 to 5 months after last chemotherapy treatment is completed
3. Devices to decrease circulation to scalp are contraindicated because they can also promote micrometastasis
4. Provide emotional support to client who is experiencing body image change
5. Client and family education
   a. Rationale and expected timeframe of hair loss and regrowth

b. Provide gentle hair care, avoiding permanent waves, coloring, peroxide, electric rollers, and curling irons until regrowth has been reestablished long enough for two haircuts
c. Hair prosthesis (wig)
d. Emotional support strategies to cope with changing body image

H. Cardiotoxicity

1. May occur within 24 hours to up to 4 to 5 weeks after drug administration; is self-limiting; warrants immediate drug discontinuation
2. Higher doses over a shorter period of time increase its incidence
3. Baseline ejection fraction should be assessed before administration of cardiotoxic agents
4. Characteristics of cardiotoxicity include a variety of EKG changes, premature ventricular contractions, bradycardia, angina, hypotension, atypical chest pain, cardiomegaly, pulmonary congestion, and ventricular tachycardia
5. Cardiotoxicity may manifest more commonly as cardiomyopathy leading to heart failure and less commonly as hemorrhagic myocardial necrosis
6. Maintain ongoing documentation of client's cumulative dose
7. Cardioprotective iron chelating agents (e.g., dexrazoxane) may be administered to prevent cardiotoxicity in clients who have received 75% of their lifetime dosage
8. Client and family education
   a. Cardiotoxicity is an expected side effect of some chemotherapy medications
   b. Recognize signs and symptoms of CHF and report them to prescriber as directed
   c. Chronic cardiotoxicity is dose-related and possibly irreversible

I. Pulmonary toxicity

1. Lung tissue is sensitive to toxic effects of chemotherapy, causing direct damage to alveoli and capillary endothelium
2. Dyspnea is cardinal symptom
3. Deteriorating creatinine clearance (renal dysfunction) is an important predictor for pulmonary pneumonitis
4. High oxygen concentrations can enhance pulmonary toxicity of bleomycin
5. Risk of pulmonary toxicity increases significantly after age 70
6. Monitor pulmonary function studies as indicated
7. Client education
   a. Recognize and report symptoms associated with pulmonary toxicity (e.g., dyspnea, chest pain, shallow breathing, chest wall discomfort)
   b. Use pursed-lipped breathing and use a small fan to decrease symptoms of dyspnea
   c. Use opioid analgesic as prescribed to decrease fear of air hunger
   d. Be aware of safety issues related to oxygen administration
   e. Explore with client and family their wishes for intubation and resuscitation; breast-feeding should be discontinued

J. Hemorrhagic cystitis

1. Bladder mucosal irritation and inflammation results from contact with acrolein, a metabolic by-product of cyclophosphamide and ifosfamide
2. Prior radiation therapy to pelvis or bladder increases risk
3. It presents with dysuria, frequency, burning upon urination, and hematuria
4. A chemoprotectant agent (mesna) may be given to bind to acrolein in bladder, inactivating it and allowing excretion from bladder
5. Client education
   a. Hemorrhagic cystitis is possible side effect of cyclophosphamide (Cytoxan) and ifosfamide (Ifex) therapy
   b. Report signs and symptoms of hemorrhagic cystitis
   c. Void frequently and take medication early in day
   d. Drink at least 6 to 8 glasses of fluid daily and to empty bladder at least every 4 to 6 hours

K. Hepatotoxicity

1. It is caused by direct toxic effect on liver when drugs are metabolized

2. Prior liver infection, tumor involvement in liver, advanced age, total bilirubin higher than 2 mg/100 dL, or cirrhosis increase incidence
3. Clinical manifestations include jaundice, ascities, fatigue, anorexia, nausea, hyperpigmentation, upper right quadrant pain, hepatomegaly, and changes in urine and stool
4. Avoid hepatotoxic drugs if liver function tests are abnormal
5. Client and family education
   a. Avoid alcohol-containing beverages
   b. Hepatotoxicity is possible adverse effect of some chemotherapeutic agents
   c. Instruct client about signs and symptoms of liver failure

L. Nephrotoxicity

1. It is caused by direct damage to glomeruli, renal blood vessels, different parts of nephron, and/or precipitation of metabolites in acid environment of urine; leads to obstructive nephropathy
2. Advancing age, preexisting renal disease, poor nutritional status, and administration of other nephrotoxic agents predispose client to nephrotoxicity
3. It is manifested by increasing serum creatinine, declining creatinine clearance, hypomagnesemia, proteinuria, and hematuria
4. Continuation of nephrotoxic agents should be reviewed if BUN is higher than 22 mg/dL and/or creatinine is higher than 2 mg/dL
5. Institute hydration of 3000 mL/day to prevent or minimize renal damage
6. Induce diuresis with mannitol (Osmitrol) or furosemide (Lasix) when administering cisplatin
7. Administer allopurinol (Zyloprim) to decrease uric acid production from high tumor-cell kill (e.g., leukemia, lymphoma, small cell lung cancer)
8. Maintain alkalinization of urine with sodium bicarbonate to a pH level greater than 8 to prevent renal damage when giving high-dose methotrexate (Folex)
9. Avoid administration of aspirin and NSAIDs
10. Client and family education
    a. Nephrotoxicity is possible side effect of selected chemotherapeutic agents
    b. It is important to comply with measures to prevent nephrotoxicity, such as collecting 12- or 24-hour urine for creatinine clearance, increasing fluid intake, complying with instructions to alkalinize urine, and completing leucovorin rescue and/or allopurinol (Zyloprim) therapy

M. Neurotoxicity

1. Caused by direct toxicity on nervous system, metabolic encephalopathy, or intracranial hemorrhage related to chemotherapy-induced coagulopathy
2. Risk factors
   a. Administration of agents that cross blood–brain barrier
   b. Specified chemotherapeutic agents, especially cumulative doses of vinca alkaloids
   c. Concurrent radiation therapy to brain
   d. Incidence increases with age
   e. Impaired renal function
3. Assess for fine motor losses, numbness, tingling, gait disturbance, constipation, and change in mentation, which are early warning signs
4. Use measures outlined in Table 45–3 ■ for collaborative management of neurotoxicity
5. Client and family education
   a. Neurotoxicity is a possible side effect of some chemotherapy agents
   b. Recognize and report to prescriber early warning signs

N. Sexual and reproductive dysfunction

1. Infertility occurs in men primarily through depletion of germinal epithelium that lines seminiferous tubules
2. Women experience reproductive dysfunction primarily as a result of hormonal alterations or direct effects that cause ovarian fibrosis and follicular destruction
3. Chemotherapy compromises fertility by exerting cytotoxic effects on gametogenesis; degree is related to therapeutic agent and duration of treatment

Table 45-3 Neurotoxicity

Area Affected	Assessment	Collaborative Management
Cerebrum	Confusion, memory loss, and level of consciousness	1. Use positive support and encouragement 2. Maintain a consistent schedule
Sensory	Decreased deep tendon reflexes, numbness, decreased sensation, jaw pain, paresthesia of hands or feet	1. Avoid extreme temperatures 2. Use assistive devices as required 3. Use opioids, antidepressants, and anticonvulsants for neuropathic pain
Autonomic	Abdominal pain, constipation, ileus, bladder atony	1. Recommend a high-fiber diet 2. Increase fluid intake 3. Administer stool softeners and laxatives as required 4. Initiate a bowel management program 30 minutes after meals 5. Monitor for bladder infection with urinary retention
Auditory	Assess for tinnitis, hearing loss	1. Report auditory changes 2. Reduce or discontinue chemotherapy

4. Approximately 40% to 100% of clients experience some sexual dysfunction following treatment; it is frequently underreported because it often is not assessed by health care personnel
5. ! Males should be encouraged to bank sperm before starting treatment
6. Although expensive (and not always successful), females should be informed of opportunities to bank oocytes or cryopreserve embryos
7. Water-based lubricants or estrogen supplements may help to decrease vaginal dryness
8. Client education and counseling
   a. Provide an unbiased, sexually neutral environment that promotes open discussion
   b. Identify whether sexual issues pose a problem for client and/or partner
   c. Explain implications of treatments on sexuality
   d. ! Provide information related to contraception
   e. ! Discourage pregnancy during treatment
   f. Advise the client of possible long-term side effects on reproductive function
   g. ! Encourage communication between client and significant other

Check Your NCLEX-RN® Exam I.Q.

You are ready for testing on this content if you can

- Apply knowledge of expected actions and effects of antineoplastic medications to client care.
- Correctly describe administration of antineoplastic medications to clients.
- Assess for side effects and adverse effects of antineoplastic medications.
- Take appropriate action if a client has an unexpected response to an antineoplastic medication.
- Monitor a client for expected outcomes or effects of treatment with antineoplastic medications.

PRACTICE TEST

1 The nurse instructs the client receiving chemotherapy to avoid which of the following reduce the risks associated with thrombocytopenia?

1. Being near individuals with upper respiratory infection
2. Keeping fresh flowers and plants in the home
3. Shaving with an electric razor
4. Trimming nails with a nail clipper

PRACTICE TEST

2 A newly registered nurse asks the nurse preceptor what qualifications are needed in order to administer chemotherapy agents. The nurse preceptor should reply that a requirement is to

1. hold a bachelor's degree in nursing.
2. be certified by an approved chemotherapy administration program.
3. be certified as an oncology nurse.
4. have at least 1 year of clinical experience after graduation.

3 During an intravenous (IV) push administration of doxorubicin peripherally into client's left forearm, the nurse becomes unable to obtain a blood return. The client has no complaints of discomfort at the site, and no swelling is noted. The nurse should take which of the following actions?

1. Remove the IV catheter and restart it at another site.
2. Flush the IV with saline to ensure no extravasation has occurred.
3. Reposition the needle in hopes of obtaining a blood return.
4. Since the client has no complaint of pain, continue the administration.

4 The nurse should become concerned about which of the following risks to a client receiving chemotherapy who had prolonged diarrhea at home without adequate management?

1. Malnutrition
2. Increased gastric motility
3. Insidious weight gain and jaundice
4. Renal failure

5 The nurse would apply which of the following clinical labels to nausea and vomiting experienced by a client 24 hours after chemotherapeutic drug administration with cisplatin (Platinol)?

1. Delayed nausea and vomiting
2. Retching
3. Acute nausea and vomiting
4. Anticipatory nausea and vomiting

6 The client is receiving chemotherapy with fluorouracil (5-FU) and concurrent radiation therapy to the abdomen for colon cancer. The client is at greatest risk for developing which of the following adverse effects?

1. Peripheral neuropathy
2. Alopecia
3. Thrombocytopenia
4. Diarrhea

7 The nurse would assess for pulmonary toxicity in a client receiving which of the following chemotherapeutic agents?

1. Doxorubicin (Adriamycin)
2. Vincristine (Oncovin)
3. Cyclophosphamide (Cytoxan)
4. Bleomycin (Blenoxane)

8 A client receiving cyclophosphamide (Cytoxan) as treatment for cancer experiences painful urination, dysuria, suprapubic pain, and blood in the urine. The nurse determines that these classic signs are compatible with which of the following problems?

1. Thrombocytopenia
2. Hemorrhagic cystitis
3. Renal dysfunction
4. Urinary tract infection

9 What major risk factors influencing gonad toxicity would a nurse assess for in a client who is receiving chemotherapy drugs?

1. Renal function, specific agents, and blood levels of chemotherapeutic drugs
2. Gender, age, and specific agents
3. Renal function, blood levels of drugs, and age
4. Age, blood levels of drugs, and gender

10 The nurse suspects that a client receiving chemotherapy with which of the following classes of drugs is most likely to be at risk for developing a second malignancy?

1. Antimetabolite
2. Taxane
3. Alkylating agent
4. Vinca alkaloid

11. The nurse caring for a client receiving chemotherapy incorporates which of the following practices into the routine for the day's work shift?
    1. Determine if dosage reductions should be made based on the client's laboratory values.
    2. Dispense the drugs that are part of the treatment regimen for the client.
    3. Encourage the client to consider alternative nonpharmaceutical treatment options.
    4. Educate the client about how to manage treatment side effects to maintain dose intensity.

12. Which of the following is the most appropriate nursing diagnosis for a client who has experienced ototoxicity as a result of chemotherapy administration?
    1. Chronic pain related to side effects of chemotherapy
    2. Anxiety related to potential or actual sensory loss secondary to chemotherapy
    3. Risk for ineffective tissue perfusion related to decrease in cerebral blood flow
    4. Risk for impaired skin integrity related to decreased cerebral blood flow

13. A client who is 90 years old is exhibiting altered mental status after chemotherapy with a neurotoxic agent. Which of the following statements provides the most appropriate reality orientation when the client first awakens in the morning?
    1. "Do you remember who I am or what day it is? Would you like to write it down so you can refer to it later?"
    2. "Did you sleep well? Which gown would you prefer to wear today, the pink or the blue?"
    3. "Today is Tuesday, and we will be having pancakes and sausage for breakfast."
    4. "This is your second day in St. Elizabeth's hospital. My name is Susan, and I will be your nurse for today."

14. In teaching the client receiving a continuous fluorouracil (5-FU) infusion, the nurse should instruct the client about the importance of an oral care protocol, including which of the following statements?
    1. "Assess the inside of your mouth weekly."
    2. "Remove white patches with your toothbrush and apply a lanolin-based jelly."
    3. "Eat a low-residue, semi-soft diet to prevent stomatitis."
    4. "Call your doctor if white patches appear on your tongue or mouth."

15. The nurse is developing a plan of care for a client who will receive chemotherapy with a neurotoxic agent. The nurse plans to implement client and family education regarding these side effects at which of the following appropriate times?
    1. When the client requests it
    2. Before the treatment begins
    3. When the symptoms occur
    4. When the physician requests client education

16. Which of the following is an important intervention in a client receiving chemotherapy who has an absolute granulocyte count (AGC) of less than 500/mm^3?
    1. Assess the client's rectal temperature every 4 hours.
    2. Administer broad-spectrum antibiotics according to physician orders.
    3. Encourage intake of fresh fruits to increase potassium level.
    4. Avoid bathing for 2 days to reduce risk of skin irritation.

17. Which of the following nursing interventions should be the highest priority of the oncology nurse to decrease nausea in a client receiving chemotherapy?
    1. Avoid oral nutrition 24 hours before chemotherapy administration.
    2. Encourage the client to eat salty snacks, such as potato chips.
    3. Encourage the client to avoid fatty or spicy foods.
    4. Administer an antiemetic each time vomiting is experienced.

18. The nurse would explain to a client receiving which of the following chemotherapeutic agents that the drug may cause a metallic taste during administration and lead to taste changes?
    1. Etoposide (VP-16)
    2. Cyclophosphamide (Cytoxan)
    3. Doxorubicin (Adriamycin)
    4. Prednisone (Deltasone)

19 The nurse would assess the client receiving bleomycin (Blenoxane) as treatment for cancer for which of the following cardinal symptoms of pulmonary toxicity?

1. Absent breath sounds in upper lobes
2. Generalized fatigue
3. Dyspnea on exertion and at rest
4. Respiratory acidosis on arterial blood gases

20 The oncology nurse assesses a client receiving chemotherapy for which of the following most well-known and common chronic cardiac toxicity?

1. Cardiomyopathy
2. Asymptomatic bradycardia
3. Hemorrhagic myocardial necrosis
4. Coronary artery spasm

ANSWERS & RATIONALES

1 **Answer: 4** A client with thrombocytopenia should avoid activities that could result in injury and bleeding. For this reason, the client should avoid trimming the nails with a nail clipper and should use a nail file instead. Option 3 indicates the safe method for shaving; straight razors should be avoided, but electric razors are acceptable. Not all clients with thrombocytopenia also experience concurrent leukopenia. Options 1 and 2 should be avoided to minimize risk of infection or when the client's white blood cell count is low.
Cognitive Level: Application **Client Need:** Physiological Integrity: Pharmacological and Parenteral Therapies **Integrated Process:** Nursing Process: Planning **Content Area:** Pharmacology **Strategy:** The core issue of the question is safety measures for chemotherapy-induced thrombocytopenia. The wording of the question tells you that the correct option is a true statement or selection. Use nursing knowledge and the process of elimination to make a selection.

2 **Answer: 2** Upon graduation, the registered nurse has attained adequate knowledge to manage standard clinical problems. Before accepting an assignment to administer chemotherapy, the nurse should receive additional education on the management of treatment side effects, pharmacology, administration principles, and safe handling. Although a bachelor's degree and 1 year of clinical experience may be helpful, they are not required to safely administer chemotherapy. Certification in oncology nursing does not imply skill or knowledge of chemotherapy administration procedures.
Cognitive Level: Application **Client Need:** Physiological Integrity: Pharmacological and Parenteral Therapies **Integrated Process:** Communication and Documentation **Content Area:** Pharmacology **Strategy:** The core issue of the question is prerequisite qualifications to administering chemotherapy. Make your selection based on knowledge that this is a specialized skill requiring additional certification.

3 **Answer: 2** It is not uncommon to lose a blood return during IV administration of a vesicant. Repositioning the IV will only ensure infiltration due to manipulation. Restarting the IV is no assurance that the blood return will not be lost again. Clients can experience extravasation without pain, but not without swelling. With no evidence of swelling or pain, it is safe to flush with 20 to 30 c mL of saline to ensure an extravasation has not occurred.
Cognitive Level: Application **Client Need:** Physiological Integrity: Pharmacological and Parenteral Therapies **Integrated Process:** Nursing Process: Implementation **Content Area:** Pharmacology **Strategy:** The core issue of the question is safe nursing practice relative to administration of IV medications that are chemotherapeutic agents. Choose the option that is safest in avoiding harm to the client if the line is infiltrated after losing a blood return. Eliminate options 3 and 4 first because they are potentially dangerous. Choose option 2 over 1 because option 1 may be unnecessary and excessive at this point.

4 **Answer: 1** Prolonged diarrhea without adequate management will cause dehydration, nutritional malabsorption, and circulatory collapse. Option 2 may accompany diarrhea but is not a resulting clinical problem. Options 3 and 4 do not result from untreated diarrhea.
Cognitive Level: Analysis **Client Need:** Physiological Integrity: Pharmacological and Parenteral Therapies **Integrated Process:** Nursing Process: Analysis **Content Area:** Pharmacology **Strategy:** The core issue of the question is knowledge of complications of side effects from chemotherapeutic agents. Recall that nausea and vomiting deplete both fluid volume and nutrients. Make the selection that is consistent with one of these, which is option 1.

5 **Answer: 1** Delayed nausea may occur 24 to 48 hours after chemotherapy administration, primarily due to the ongoing effect that the metabolites exert on the CNS or GI tract. Despite effective antiemetic regimens, 93% of clients receiving cisplatin experience delayed nausea. Anticipatory nausea occurs in approximately 25% of clients because of the classic conditioning response from prior therapy. Acute nausea occurs 1 to 2 hours after chemotherapy administration.
Cognitive Level: Analysis **Client Need:** Physiological Integrity: Pharmacological and Parenteral Therapies **Integrated Process:** Nursing Process: Analysis **Content Area:** Pharmacology **Strategy:** The critical words in the stem of the question are *24 hours after.* From there, evaluate each option in terms of timeframe. Eliminate options 2 and 3 because they are focused on present time, and eliminate option 4 because it is future-oriented related to the chemotherapy administration.

6 **Answer: 4** Both 5-FU and radiation therapy to the abdomen can cause diarrhea. Alopecia is uncommon with 5-FU and only occurs with irradiation to the skull. Some myelosuppression could result but is not the greatest risk. Peripheral neuropathy is not related to either therapy.

Cognitive Level: Analysis **Client Need:** Physiological Integrity: Pharmacological and Parenteral Therapies **Integrated Process:** Nursing Process: Analysis **Content Area:** Pharmacology **Strategy:** Note the stem of the question contains the critical words *highest risk*. This tells you that more than one or all options are correct and that you must prioritize your answer. Choose the option that is a lower GI symptom, which is the area that both chemotherapy and radiation therapy will target.

7 **Answer: 4** Pulmonary toxicity is a dose- and age-related toxic effect of bleomycin. Cardiotoxicity is a toxic effect of doxorubicin. Vincristine causes neurotoxicity. Cytoxan can cause hemorrhagic cystitis.
Cognitive Level: Analysis **Client Need:** Physiological Integrity: Pharmacological and Parenteral Therapies **Integrated Process:** Nursing Process: Assessment **Content Area:** Pharmacology **Strategy:** The core issue of the question is knowledge of toxicity caused by bleomycin. If you associate the *bl* in bleomycin with the color blue for cyanosis, this may help you to recall that this drug causes pulmonary toxicity.

8 **Answer: 2** Although painful urination, dysuria, suprapubic pain, and blood-tinged urine may occur when a client experiences a urinary tract infection, in the oncology client receiving Cytoxan or Ifex, the cause is usually chemically induced. A decreased platelet count may cause blood in the urine but rarely causes the other symptoms. Renal dysfunction unusually causes anuria.
Cognitive Level: Analysis **Client Need:** Physiological Integrity: Pharmacological and Parenteral Therapies **Integrated Process:** Nursing Process: Analysis **Content Area:** Pharmacology **Strategy:** The core issue of the question is knowledge of toxicity caused by cyclophosphamide. If you associate the *cy* in cyclophosphamide or Cytoxan with the beginning of the word *cystitis,* this may help you to recall that this drug can lead to hemorrhagic cystitis as a toxic effect of the drug.

9 **Answer: 2** The likelihood that chemotherapy will affect a client's fertility depends in part on the client's gender and age and the specific agent. Since chemotherapy affects rapidly dividing cells, men are more affected than women. Women over 30 are less likely to regain ovarian function because they have fewer oocytes.
Cognitive Level: Analysis **Client Need:** Physiological Integrity: Pharmacological and Parenteral Therapies **Integrated Process:** Nursing Process: Assessment **Content Area:** Pharmacology **Strategy:** The critical word in the stem of the question is *gonad.* From there, eliminate the options that refer to renal function (options 1 and 3). Choose option 2 over 4 because not all agents have the same degree of gonadal toxicity.

10 **Answer: 3** One of the most serious consequences of cancer is that the treatment intended to cure the client may contribute to the occurrence of a second malignancy. The alkylating agents, nitrosoureas, and procarbazine are the agents most likely to cause chemotherapy-related malignancies.
Cognitive Level: Analysis **Client Need:** Physiological Integrity: Pharmacological and Parenteral Therapies **Integrated Process:** Nursing Process: Analysis **Content Area:** Pharmacology **Strategy:** The core issue of the question is knowledge of chemotherapeutic agents that cause added risk for future malignancy. Specific knowledge of the drug classes is needed to answer the question. Use this knowledge and the process of elimination to make a selection.

11 **Answer: 4** Educating clients to manage treatment side effects so that their treatment programs can remain on course is an essential function of nursing. Although the nurse should review laboratory values before administering chemotherapy, it is the physician's responsibility to make dose reductions. Only a pharmacist can dispense medications. It is inappropriate to influence the client's decision making related to alternative treatment options.
Cognitive Level: Application **Client Need:** Physiological Integrity: Pharmacological and Parenteral Therapies **Integrated Process:** Nursing Process: Analysis **Content Area:** Pharmacology **Strategy:** The core issue of the question is knowledge of the nurse's role related to chemotherapy that is prescribed for a client. Use general nursing knowledge and the process of elimination to make a selection.

12 **Answer: 2** Since many chemotherapeutic agents can cause ototoxicity, continued administration may cause irreparable hearing loss. Clients may become anxious when their hearing is compromised. The hearing loss is not related to cerebral blood flow, and there is no pain related with the condition. Hearing deficits are unrelated to skin integrity.
Cognitive Level: Application **Client Need:** Physiological Integrity: Pharmacological and Parenteral Therapies **Integrated Process:** Nursing Process: Analysis **Content Area:** Pharmacology **Strategy:** The core issue of the question is the ability to translate the label ototoxicity into a working nursing diagnosis that can be used to guide nursing care. Use general nursing knowledge and the process of elimination to make a selection.

13 **Answer: 4** The nurse should be specific when addressing a confused/disoriented client. In options 1 and 2, questions about the environment and the need to make choices may be too challenging and may decrease the client's self-esteem. Option 3 provides irrelevant information.
Cognitive Level: Application **Client Need:** Physiological Integrity: Pharmacological and Parenteral Therapies **Integrated Process:** Communication and Documentation **Content Area:** Pharmacology **Strategy:** The core issue of the question is communication techniques that will be most effective in a client who has experienced confusion secondary to neurotoxicity. Use knowledge of general communication techniques and the process of elimination to make a selection.

14 **Answer: 4** The client should assess the oral cavity daily (not weekly) when receiving chemotherapy. A low-residue, semi-soft diet does not prevent stomatitis but may decrease diarrhea. White patches on the mouth or tongue should be reported to the physician so that an antifungal agent (Nystatin) can be prescribed. The patches should not be manually removed because doing so will cause bleeding of the mucous membranes.
Cognitive Level: Application **Client Need:** Physiological Integrity: Pharmacological and Parenteral Therapies **Integrated Process:** Teaching and Learning **Content Area:** Pharmacology **Strategy:** The core issue of the question is knowledge of oral assessment protocols for a client receiving chemotherapy. Use knowledge of the signs and symptoms of stomatitis and fungal infection to choose option 4 over the others, which do not allow for appropriate recognition (option 1) or treatment (options 2 and 3).

15 Answer: 2 Client education is a nursing intervention and does not require a physician's order. Although the nurse should assess client readiness, education related to chemotherapeutic agents should occur before the treatment is administered rather than when the symptoms develop. If the client does not want to receive education, then the nurse should educate the caregiver.
Cognitive Level: Application **Client Need:** Physiological Integrity: Pharmacological and Parenteral Therapies **Integrated Process:** Teaching and Learning **Content Area:** Pharmacology **Strategy:** The core issue of the question is appropriate timing of client and family teaching related to adverse effects of chemotherapy. Recall that a principle of client education is to conduct teaching about a problem beforehand whenever possible. This will easily help you to choose option 2 over the others.

16 Answer: 2 Broad-spectrum antibiotics may be ordered for a client according to individual client circumstances when the client is notably neutropenic and at great risk of infection. A rectal temperature should not be performed on a neutropenic client. The neutropenic client should avoid fresh fruits and vegetables. A daily bath will remove pathogens from the skin and decrease their potential for causing infection.
Cognitive Level: Application **Client Need:** Physiological Integrity: Pharmacological and Parenteral Therapies **Integrated Process:** Nursing Process: Implementation **Content Area:** Pharmacology **Strategy:** The core issue of the question is recognition that the client is neutropenic and selection of an appropriate action. Eliminate options 3 and 4 first because they increase the risk of infection. Then choose option 2 over 1 because it focuses on infection instead of possible bleeding as the risk.

17 Answer: 3 Avoiding fatty, spicy foods will often decrease nausea related to chemotherapy. Avoiding nutrition before treatments should be discouraged and has little to no benefit. Salty foods may help, but potato chips are also high in fat. Antiemetics should be administered on a scheduled basis, not after vomiting has already occurred.
Cognitive Level: Application **Client Need:** Physiological Integrity: Pharmacological and Parenteral Therapies **Integrated Process:** Nursing Process: Implementation **Content Area:** Pharmacology **Strategy:** The core issue of the question is knowledge of methods to reduce nausea and vomiting in a client receiving chemotherapy. Recall that fatty and spicy foods can aggravate nausea to help you make the appropriate selection. Note also that options 2 and 3 are opposite in terms of dietary fat, which is a clue that one of them may be the correct answer.

18 Answer: 2 A common complaint of clients receiving nitrogen mustard, cisplatin, and cyclophosphamide is of a metallic taste. Some clients become so sensitized to this taste that they become nauseated in anticipation of their administration. Sucking on peppermints during administration may help. None of the other drugs listed are known to cause this problem.
Cognitive Level: Analysis **Client Need:** Physiological Integrity: Pharmacological and Parenteral Therapies **Integrated Process:** Nursing Process: Analysis **Content Area:** Pharmacology **Strategy:** The core issue of this question is knowledge of chemotherapeutic agents that cause metallic taste as a side effect of therapy. Specific medication knowledge is needed to answer this question. Use the process of elimination to make a selection. You might be able to partially remember this by realizing that Cytoxan and tongue both have the letters *to.*

19 Answer: 3 The cardinal sign of pulmonary toxicity is dyspnea, which may be present both on exertion and at rest. The client may also have generalized fatigue and respiratory acidosis, but these are not cardinal signs. A client does not have absence of breath sounds in upper lobes with pulmonary toxicity.
Cognitive Level: Analysis **Client Need:** Physiological Integrity: Pharmacological and Parenteral Therapies **Integrated Process:** Nursing Process: Assessment **Content Area:** Pharmacology **Strategy:** The core issue of the question is recognition of manifestations of pulmonary toxicity in a client receiving chemotherapy for cancer. The critical word *cardinal* tells you that more than one or all options may be partially or totally correct, and you must prioritize your answer. Recall that a classic sign of respiratory distress or pulmonary toxicity would be dyspnea to help you to prioritize this answer over the others.

20 Answer: 1 Cardiomyopathy occurs in 40% of clients receiving anthracycline chemotherapy agents. While other cardiac problems can occur, cardiomyopathy is by far the most common.
Cognitive Level: Analysis **Client Need:** Physiological Integrity: Pharmacological and Parenteral Therapies **Integrated Process:** Nursing Process: Assessment **Content Area:** Pharmacology **Strategy:** The critical words in the stem of the question are *most common.* This tells you that more than one option may be partially or totally correct and that you must prioritize your answer. Use medication knowledge and the process of elimination to make a selection.

Key Terms to Review

acral erythema p. 752
alopecia p. 753
anticipatory nausea p. 765
cell cycle–nonspecific p. 750
cell cycle–specific p. 754
hemorrhagic cystitis p. 752
irritant p. 757
myelosuppression p. 751
nadir p. 751
pancytopenia p. 752
radiation recall p. 756
vesicant p. 751

References

Abrams, A. (2004). *Clinical drug therapy: Rationales for nursing practice* (7th ed.). Philadelphia: Lippincott Williams & Wilkins.

Adams, M., Josephson, D., & Holland, L. (2005). *Pharmacology for nurses: A pathophysiologic approach.* Upper Saddle River, NJ: Pearson Education.

Deglin, J. H., & Vallerand, A. H. (2006). *Davis's drug guide for nurses* (10th ed.). Philadelphia: F. A. Davis.

Lehne, R. (2004). *Pharmacology for nursing care* (5th ed.). Philadelphia: W. B. Saunders.

McKenry, L., Tessier, E., & Hogan, M. (2006). *Mosby's pharmacology in nursing.* (22nd ed.). St. Louis, MO: Elsevier Science.

Wilson, B., Shannon, M., & Stang, C. (2006). *Prentice Hall nurse's drug guide 2006.* Upper Saddle River, NJ: Pearson Education.

Immunological and Anti-infective Medications

46

In this chapter

Test Yourself

Are you ready for the NCLEX-RN® or course exams? Use the practice tests on the companion CD-ROM to check.

Cross reference

Other chapters relevant to this content area are

Dosage Calculation and Medication Administration Chapter 30
Immunological Disorders Chapter 67
Communicable or Infectious Diseases Chapter 68

I. IMMUNOMODULATORS

A. Description

1. Immunomodulators can either suppress or enhance immune response
2. Depending on intended immune response, client is administered either an immune stimulant or an **immunosuppressant,** which suppresses body's response to an **antigen** (a substance that stimulates production of antibodies)
3. Can be used to stimulate platelet production to prevent severe thrombocytopenia (abnormally low platelet count) caused by platelet destruction
4. Increase development of bone marrow, which is adversely affected by administration of chemotherapy agents used after bone marrow transplantation or to treat cancer

B. *Colony-stimulating factors*

1. Action and use
   a. Glycoproteins that increase production of white blood cells that enhance cellular immunity (immunity of host affecting body cells)
   b. Are described as granulocyte colony-stimulating factors (G-CSF) or macrophage and granulocyte colony stimulating factors (GM-CSF)

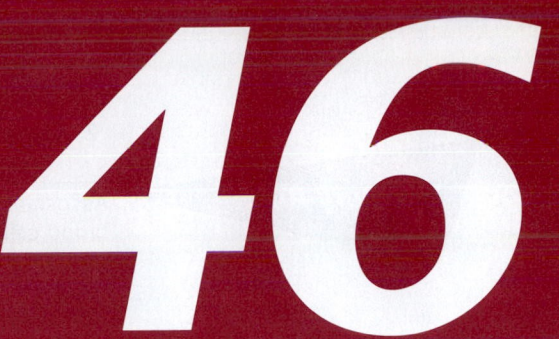

c. Reduce **neutropenia** (abnormally low neutrophil count) and decrease incidence of infection; they assist in mobilization of stem cells, allowing for stem cell collection

2. Common medications are listed and described in Table 46–1 ■

Memory Aid

Associate the *E* in epoetin alfa with the *E* in erythrocyte to recall that it stimulates red blood cell growth. Use the same strategy to associate *Neu*pogen with *neu*trophil count (WBC).

3. Administration considerations
   a. Sargramostim (Leukine: reconstitute with sterile water; avoid shaking vial during reconstitution; use for 21 days after bone marrow transplantation and, in clients with acute myelogenous leukemia, around either day 11 following chemotherapy dose or 4 days after chemotherapy induction
   b. ! Epoetin alfa (Erythropoetin): goal of administration in clients with acquired immunodeficiency syndrome (AIDS) receiving zidovudine therapy should be to maintain hematocrit (Hct) at 30% to 33% (maximum 36%); usually given 3 times per week
   c. ! Filgrastim (Neupogen): do not give during or 24 hrs after a dose of cytotoxic chemotherapy; dosage may be titrated depending on neutrophil count, stop drug if absolute neutrophil count (ANC) exceeds 10,000/mm^3
4. ! Contraindications
   a. Sargramostim: pregnancy, hypersensitivity to yeast products or *E. coli;* leukemic myeloblasts in the bone marrow; use cautiously with hepatic or renal insufficiency and lactation
   b. Epoetin alfa: uncontrolled hypertension, pregnancy, and hypersensitivity to albumin
   c. Filgrastim: pregnancy, hypersensitivity to *E. coli* products
5. Side/adverse effects
   a. Nausea, vomiting, anorexia, constipation, diarrhea
   b. Headache, stomatitis, edema, rash, mucositis, generalized pain, bone pain
   c. Supraventricular dysrhythmias, tachycardia
   d. Renal or hepatic dysfunction, dyspnea, seizures, porphyria
   e. Report neutrophil count of 20,000/mm^3 to physician
   f. Adult respiratory distress syndrome (ARDS), pleural effusion
   g. Myocardial infarction (MI), gastrointestinal (GI) hemorrhage, thrombus formation
6. Nursing considerations for sargramostim (Leukine)
   a. Assess CBC and platelet count before administration and 2 times per week during medication administration
   b. Assess renal and hepatic function
   c. Assess for excessive myeloid blasts in bone marrow
   d. Do not administer during pregnancy; use cautiously during lactation
   e. Dilute with normal saline and store in the refrigerator; administer only one dose per vial

Table 46–1
Common Immunostimulant Medications

Generic/Trade Names	Actions
Sargramostim (Leukine)	Increases the production of granulocytes and macrophages before and after bone marrow transplantation, so labeled as a GM-CSF
Epoetin alfa (Epogen)	Increases the RBC count in clients with chronic renal failure, cancer, or human immunodeficiency virus; is actually a hematological, not an immunological, colony stimulating factor, but is used in clients who have immunodeficiency
Filgrastim (Neupogen) Pegfilgrastim (Neulasta)	Increases neutrophil (granulocyte) production in cancer clients to prevent infection, so labeled as a G-CSF

! 7. Nursing considerations for epoetin alfa (Epogen)
   a. Assess blood pressure (BP) prior to administration and regularly during therapy; hypertension may occur if hematocrit level rises rapidly
   b. Epoetin alfa should be used cautiously during lactation
   c. The client should eat foods rich in iron and possibly take an iron supplement to increase effectiveness of therapy on RBC formation
   d. Assess Homan's sign periodically to detect thrombus development with increased RBC counts
   e. Administer cautiously with lactation
   f. Do not shake solution after it has been reconstituted
   g. Assess Hct to determine if it has risen 4 points in 2 weeks; a rapid elevation of 4 points may lead to hypertension and seizures

! 8. Nursing considerations for filgrastim (Neupogen)
   a. Assess results of CBC, differential, and platelet count before administration and 2 times per week during therapy
   b. Do not administer 24 hours before or after chemotherapy
   c. Assess for hypersensitivity to *E. coli* products
   d. Filgrastim is pregnancy category C; use cautiously with lactation
   e. Administer only one dose per vial, and discard after 24 hours; store medication in the refrigerator
   f. Reconstitute in dextrose 5%, and avoid shaking the bottle to prevent damage to the protein
   g. Avoid exposure to infection because client's lowered white cell count indicates increased risk of infection

9. Client education for sargramostim (Leukine)
   a. Avoid exposure to infection and be aware of signs and symptoms of infection
   b. Report difficulty breathing and fever
   c. CBC and platelet counts must be done periodically
   d. Address body image with client because of alopecia

10. Client education for epoetin alfa (Epogen)
   a. Administration of medication at home with home dialysis; action, side effects, and nursing implications associated with epoetin alfa administration
   b. Signs and symptoms of clot formation
   c. Self-monitor BP
   d. Eat a diet high in iron and take iron supplement if ordered

11. Client education for filgrastim (Neupogen)
   a. Report pain in the joints and bones
   b. Maintain good hygiene and avoid exposure to crowds because of susceptibility of infection

C. Cell-stimulating medications

1. Action and use
   a. Interleukins are biologic response modifiers that prevent thrombocytopenia and stimulate platelet production
   b. In the helper T cells, cellular immunity is increased along with number of lymphocytes
   c. Interleukins are a group of proteins, produced by lymphocytes, that have antitumor activity, causing cells to change to a nonproliferative type
   d. Aldesleukin (Proleukin) is used to treat renal carcinoma and prevents severe thrombocytopenia
   e. Levamisole (Ergamisol) increases immune response by increasing activity of B cells, T cells, and macrophages; it is used in combination with fluorouracil to treat Duke's stage C colon cancer
   f. Oprelvekin (Neumega) is used following chemotherapy that causes **myelosuppression** chemotherapy (suppressed bone marrow function in manufacture of blood cells); it increases thrombocyte and megakaryocyte production to prevent and treat thrombocytopenia in clients receiving chemotherapy

2. Common medications are listed in Table 46–2 ■

Table 46–2

Common Cell-Stimulating Medications

Generic/Trade Names	Actions
Aldesleukin (Proleukin)	Increases lymphocytes, platelets, and tumor necrosis factor
Levamisole (Ergamisol)	Increases B cell activity and antibody formation by increasing monocyte and macrophage action
Oprelvekin (Neumega)	Increases thrombocyte and megakaryocyte production, thus preventing thrombocytopenia

3. Administration considerations
   a. Aldesleukin (Proleukin): because of seriousness of side effects, this medication is given in a hospital that has an intensive care unit with medical specialists available; after 14 doses, a waiting period ensues, followed by another 14 doses
   b. Levamisole (Ergamisol): drug therapy should begin 7 to 30 days after bowel resection surgery; maintenance dose is 50 mg every 8 hours for 3 days with fluorouracil
   c. Oprelvekin (Neumega): administration can be continued for 21 days or until platelet count is greater than 100,000 cells/mm^3; reconstitute in an isotonic solution; do not agitate; administer within 3 hours of reconstitution
4. Side/adverse effects
   a. Aldesleukin: cardiac dyshythmias, fluid retention, lethargy, myalgia
   b. Levamisole: flulike symptoms, bone marrow depression, GI upset
   c. Oprelvekin: cardiac dysrhythmias, fluid retention
5. Nursing considerations
   a. Assess CBC, differential, and platelet count
   b. Assess heart rate, BP, respirations, and lung sounds
   c. Maintain fluid and electrolyte balance, particularly during flulike symptoms
   d. Provide good hygiene practices
6. Client and family education
   a. Home medication administration
   b. Assessment of fluid retention and irregular heart rate
   c. Measures to assist in preventing infection
   d. Care and management of flulike symptoms

D. Immunosuppressants

1. Action and use
   a. Immunosuppressants inhibit inflammatory response and block immune response to an antigen
   b. Inhibit T cells and block production of antibodies by B cells
   c. ! Prevent rejection of organs that have been transplanted
2. ! Common medications are listed in Table 46–3 ■
3. Administration considerations
   a. Azathioprine (Imuran): reaches the peak blood concentration in 1 to 2 hours and duration of action is 10 hours
   b. Cyclosporine (Sandimmune): reaches its peak level in 4 to 5 hours after administration and duration of action is 20 to 54 hours
   c. Basiliximab (Simulect): administered IV 24 hours after transplant, then 4 days after transplant
   d. Daclizumab (Zenapax): administered IV 24 hours after transplant for total of 5 doses
   e. Muromonab CD3 (Orthoclone OKT 3): therapy should begin as soon as rejection is identified
   f. Mycophenolate (CellCept): renal transplant clients receive 1 gram 2 times per day; therapy should begin 72 hours after transplant
   g. Tacrolimus (Prograf): administered 6 hours after transplant
4. Side/adverse effects
   a. ! Increased risk for infection; hypertension; acne
   b. Hepatotoxicity and/or renal toxicity

Table 46–3 Common Immunosuppressant Medications

Generic/Trade Names	Actions
Azathioprine (Imuran)	Prevents rejection in renal transplants; administered for life after the transplant
Basiliximab (Simulect)	Prevents acute renal transplant rejection; must be given in combination with cyclosporine and a glucocorticoid
Daclizumab (Zenapax)	Prevents renal transplant rejection
Cyclosporine (Sandimmune)	Prevents rejection in solid organ transplant
Muromonab CD3 (Orthoclone OKT3)	Suppresses T cells to prevent renal transplant rejection
Mycophenolate (CellCept)	Prevents rejection in renal, liver, and cardiac transplants
Sirolimus (Rapamune)	Prevents rejection in kidney transplant
Tacrolimus (Protopic, Prograf)	Prevents rejection in solid organ transplant, primarily liver transplant

c. Flulike symptoms and/or headache, diarrhea, nausea, and/or vomiting
d. Contraindicated with allergy to drug, or during pregnancy, or lactation

5. Nursing considerations
   a. Assess for signs and symptoms of infection
   b. Provide supportive care for flulike symptoms
   c. Complete serum laboratory tests as ordered, such as CBC, platelet count, BUN, creatinine, and hepatic function tests
   d. Assess nutritional status; encourage well-balanced meals with small, frequent feedings
6. Client education: need for lab studies, prevention of infection, and all aspects of medication administration, including action, side effects, and nursing implications

II. MEDICATIONS TO TREAT MULTIPLE SCLEROSIS (MS)

A. Action and use

1. Goal is to decrease inflammation, suppress immune system to prevent nerve tissue destruction, and decrease fatigue and ataxia
2. A wide variety of medications are used to treat multiple sclerosis; they include beta-adrenergic blockers, corticosteroids, anti-inflammatory agents, and interferon

B. Common medications are listed in Table 46–4 ■

C. Administration considerations

1. Beta 1b (Betaseron) should be discontinued in 6 months if disease does not enter remission
2. These medications should be administered cautiously with hepatic or renal insufficiency and when client has been diagnosed with a neoplasm
3. Contraindicated in pregnancy, lactation, and hypersensitivity to drug

D. Side/adverse effects

1. Azathioprine (Imuran): increased risk of infection, renal or hepatic insufficiency; leukopenia and thrombocytopenia
2. Beta 1a (Avonex): anorexia, nausea, vomiting, dizziness, and flulike symptoms
3. Beta 1b (Betaseron): anorexia, confusion, dizziness, flulike symptoms, and photosensitivity
4. Cyclophosphamide (Cytoxan): anorexia, nausea, vomiting, or hemorrhagic cystitis
5. Cyclosporine (Sandimmune): hepatotoxicity, hirsutism, and renal toxicity
6. Glatiramer acetate (Copaxone): anxiety, diarrhea, flulike symptoms, hypertonia, and pain at the injection site
7. Medications used to treat symptoms of multiple sclerosis have been noted to increase pulmonary edema leading to chest pain and shortness of breath

Table 46–4

Common Medications to Treat Multiple Sclerosis

Generic/Trade Names	Actions
Azathioprine (Imuran)	Decreases the severity of symptoms and the progress of the disease process
Interferon Beta 1a (Avonex)	Reduces the severity of acute exacerbations; decreases demyelination in the brain tissue; can be used for long-term treatment
Interferon Beta 1b (Betaseron)	Reduces the severity of acute exacerbations, decreases demyelination in the brain tissue; can be used for long-term treatment
Cyclophosphamide (Cytoxan)	Reduces the rate and progression of disease by interfering with replication of susceptible cells
Cyclosporine (Sandimmune)	Reduces severity of acute exacerbations
Glatiramer acetate (Copaxone)	Prevents destruction of brain and nerve tissue; used for long-term treatment
Methylprednisolone (Medrol) followed by tapered oral prednisone (PredPak)	Reduces severity of acute exacerbations

E. Nursing considerations

1. Assess client for signs and symptoms of pulmonary edema, chest pain, and shortness of breath
2. Assess laboratory tests as ordered by physician
3. Provide comfort measures when client experiences flulike symptoms
4. Assess injection sites for inflammation and pain

F. Client education

1. Side effects of medication and need for periodic laboratory studies
2. Report any side effects to prescriber
3. Supportive care of flulike symptoms, including adequate fluid intake, rest, and use of acetaminophen for relief of pain and fever
4. Signs and symptoms of pulmonary edema

III. MEDICATIONS TO TREAT MYASTHENIA GRAVIS

A. Action and use

1. Goal of anticholinesterase medications is to treat symptoms of myasthenia gravis
2. Increase concentration of acetylcholine at neuromuscular junction
3. Increase nerve impulses and strength

! **B. Common medications are listed in Table 46–5** ■

C. Administration considerations

! 1. Edrophonium (Tensilon): single dose is for diagnostic purposes only; may be repeated once to aid in uncertain diagnosis

Table 46–5

Common Medications to Treat Myasthenia Gravis

Generic/Trade Names	Actions
Ambenonium (Mytelase)	Long-acting medication to treat myasthenia gravis
Edrophonium (Tensilon)	Used for diagnostic purposes; clients who exhibit temporary relief of symptoms with injected dose have decreased acetylcholine in neuromuscular junction (myasthenia gravis)
Neostigmine (Prostigmin)	Has a duration of action of 2–4 hours, and it increases acetylcholine concentration, facilitating neuromuscular function
Physostigmine (Antilirium)	Anticholinesterase agent that crosses blood–brain barrier; used as an antidote for anticholinergic poisoning and to treat glaucoma
Pyridostigmine (Mestinon)	Increases acetylcholine concentration facilitating neuromuscular function; taken every 3–6 hours

2. Neostigmine (Prostigmin): can be administered subcutaneously during an acute exacerbation of myasthenia gravis
3. Physostigmine (Antilirium): IV administration should be no faster than 1 mg per minute
4. Pyridostigmine (Reganol, Mestinol): a timed-release preparation can be administered at bedtime; can also be administered IM during acute exacerbation
5. Contraindicated in pregnancy and lactation, bradycardia, intestinal or urinary obstruction
6. Use cautiously in clients with asthma, heart disease, Parkinson's disease, and seizure disorders

D. Side/adverse effects

! 1. Bradycardia, hypotension, or cardiac arrest
2. Increased gastric secretions, nausea and vomiting, diarrhea
3. Increased urinary urgency
4. Involuntary incontinence of stool
! 5. Severe cholinergic reactions include excessive salivation, sphincter relaxation, diarrhea, and vomiting

E. Nursing considerations

! 1. Assess respiratory and general muscle strength, including swallowing and heart rate prior to administration
2. Administer with meals to enhance absorption and decrease GI irritation
! 3. Administer on time to prevent difficulty with respirations and swallowing caused by undermedication or late medication administration
4. Administer IV preparations slowly to prevent cholinergic reaction
! 5. Have atropine available as antidote to counteract cholinergic reaction
6. Assess client's response to medication and ability to perform activities of daily living

F. Client education

1. All aspects of medication administration, side effects; take with food to decrease GI irritation
2. Coordination of medication administration with activities of daily living
3. Overmedication will result in cholinergic reaction
4. Assessment of apical pulse

IV. MEDICATIONS TO TREAT RHEUMATOID ARTHRITIS

A. Action and use

1. Early stage rheumatoid arthritis is managed with NSAIDs
2. Later stages are treated with disease-modifying antirheumatic drugs (DMARDs)
3. These medications decrease erythrocyte sedimentation rate (ESR), thus reducing inflammation, stiffness, swelling, and pain
4. Gold salts or gold compounds decrease prostaglandin activity that contributes to joint destruction

! **B. Common medications are listed in Table 46–6 ■**

C. Administration considerations

1. Gold sodium thiomalate (Aurolate) should be injected into intragluteal muscle
! 2. Never administer medications to clients who have a known allergy to animal products
3. Contraindicated with pregnancy, lactation, liver disease, renal disease
4. Penicillamine is contraindicated with a known hypersensitivity to penicillin
! 5. Gold salts are contraindicated with systemic lupus erythematosus or blood dyscrasias; inject gold preparations into gluteal muscle
6. Inject etanercept into abdomen, thigh, or upper arm subcutaneously

D. Side/adverse effects

1. Alopecia, itching, and rash
2. Colitis and diarrhea, stomatitis and black furry tongue
3. Dizziness, hepatotoxicity, pericarditis, pulmonary edema
4. Thrombosis, Stevens-Johnson syndrome
5. Death

Table 46–6

Common Medications to Treat Rheumatoid Arthritis

Generic/Trade Names	Actions
Auranofin (Ridaura)	Decreases rheumatoid factor and immunoglobulins to suppress arthritic symptoms
Aurothioglucose (Solganal)	Inhibits phagocytosis and lysosomal enzyme activity to decrease rheumatoid factor and decrease inflammation
Etanercept (Enbrel)	Tumor necrosis factor from Chinese hamsters that reacts with active lymphocytes to reduce signs and symptoms of rheumatoid arthritis
Gold sodium thiomalate (Myochrysine)	Suppresses the activity produced by prostaglandins, which contributes to joint destruction
Hylan G-F 20 (Synvisc)	Lubricating hylan obtained from chicken combs that is injected into arthritic joint to provide lubrication
Leflunomide (Arava)	Produces anti-inflammatory process by blocking enzyme DHODH
Methotrexate (Amethopterin)	Inhibits DNA synthesis and folic acid reductase to reduce inflammation
Penicillamine (Depen)	Lowers IgM rheumatoid factor
Sodium hyaluronate (Hyalgan)	Lubricating hylan injected into joint to provide cushioning

E. Nursing considerations

1. Avoid antacid use for at least 2 hours following medication administration
2. ! Assess for bone marrow suppression, pulmonary fibrosis, and GI ulceration/bleeding with methotrexate
3. Protect from exposure to sunlight
4. ! Check for proteinuria and hematuria before giving initial dose and during therapy with gold drugs
5. Observe client for signs of allergic reaction for 30 minutes after gold injection for first 2 doses
6. Assess for signs of infection with etanercept

F. Client education

1. Protect self from infection when taking etanercept
2. Use good oral hygiene to protect from stomatitis
3. If taking gold preparations, report signs of gold toxicity, including metallic taste and pruritus
4. Monitor for and report bruising, petechiae, bleeding gums, or blood in stool
5. Monitor blood glucose and report elevations
6. All aspects of medication administration, including side effects, action, use, and contraindications

V. MEDICATIONS TO TREAT SYSTEMIC LUPUS ERYTHEMATOSUS (SLE)

A. Action and use

1. Cytotoxic drugs or purine analogs are used along with NSAIDs, and corticosteroids to treat symptoms of SLE
2. Provide immunosuppressive action to treat autoimmune diseases

! **B. Common medications are listed in Table 46–7** ■

Table 46–7

Common Medications to Treat Systemic Lupus Erythematosus

Generic/Trade Names	Actions
Azathioprine (Imuran)	Decreases the severity of symptoms and disease process
Methotrexate (Amethopterin)	Inhibits DNA synthesis and folic acid reductase to reduce inflammation

C. Administration considerations: do not administer with agents known to be hepatotoxic, or during pregnancy or lactation

D. Side/adverse effects

1. Alopecia, itching or rash
2. Diarrhea or colitis, stomatitis or black furry tongue
3. Dizziness
4. Leukopenia or thrombocytopenia
5. Hepatotoxicity, pericarditis, or pulmonary edema
6. Stevens-Johnson Syndrome
7. Death

E. Nursing considerations: assess for side effects of medications, pulmonary edema and shortness of breath, and ordered laboratory tests

F. Client education

1. Protect self from infection
2. Use good oral hygiene to protect from stomatitis
3. Monitor blood glucose level and report elevations
4. Learn all aspects of medication administration, including side effects, actions, use, and contraindications
5. Learn signs and symptoms of pulmonary edema and report such signs to provider

VI. ANTIBIOTICS

A. Aminoglycosides

1. Action and use
   a. **Bactericidal:** aminoglycosides kill bacteria cells
   b. Effective against aerobic Gram-negative infections
   c. Used to sterilize bowel prior to surgery
   d. Used to destroy urease-producing bacteria to prevent absorption of ammonia in hepatic encephalopathy
   e. Toxicity limits use to serious Gram-negative infections and specific conditions involving Gram-positive cocci
   f. Used in infections caused by *Acinetobacter, Citrobacter, E. coli, Klebsiella pneumoniae, proteus, pseudomonas, Providencia, Salmonella, Serratia,* and *staphylococcus* organisms; also active against protozoal infections
2. Common medications are listed in Box 46–1

Memory Aid

Recognize an aminoglycoside by the suffix *-mycin*. Note that not all drugs that end in *-mycin* are aminoglycosides, but all aminoglycosides end in *-mycin*.

3. Administration considerations
   a. IV route preferred for optimal distribution to tissues
   b. Used intramuscularly (IM) as well
   c. Oral route: poorly absorbed, so effective orally only to decrease bacteria in bowel before surgery or to prevent absorption of ammonia in hepatic encephalopathy
   d. Intrathecal or intraventricular injection: can be used to counteract poor penetration of cerebral spinal fluid (CSF) by other routes
   e. Periocular instillations: because of poor penetration of eye fluids, direct instillations are used

Box 46–1

Aminoglycosides

Amikacin (Amikin)	Netilmicin (Netromycin)
Gentamicin (Garamycin)	Paromomycin (Humatin)
Kanamycin (Kantrex)	Streptomycin (generic)
Neomycin (Mycifradin)	Tobramycin (Nebcin)

f. Contraindicated with allergy to aminoglycosides; preexisting renal disease; if receiving renal toxic agents such as amphotericin B (Fungizone), vancomycin (Vancocin), or loop diuretics such as furosemide (Lasix); in myasthenia gravis; and cautious use in pregnancy and lactation

4. Significant laboratory studies
   a. **Peak drug level:** blood specimen drawn 30 minutes after completion of IV infusion of aminoglycoside to determine that toxic levels do not occur; dose may need to be decreased if peak too high
   b. **Trough drug level:** blood specimen drawn immediately prior to starting next IV infusion of aminoglycoside to assure that therapeutic drug levels are maintained between administrations; if drug level is too low, an increase in dose and/or dosing frequency may be indicated
   c. WBC count to monitor effectiveness of drug therapy; counts decrease as infection resolves
   d. Serum creatinine and blood urea nitrogen (BUN) to monitor renal function; expected BUN to creatinine ratio is 20:1 or 15:1 depending on laboratory criteria; creatinine is most specific test for renal function; if creatinine level rises 3 to 4 days into treatment, renal damage has occurred
5. Side/adverse effects
   a. Headache, paresthesias, skin rash, fever
   b. Nephrotoxicity and ototoxicity are two common toxicities associated with aminoglycosides
   c. Nephrotoxicity: increased risk factors include advancing age (with associated declining renal function), hypotension, dehydration, preexisting renal disease, and coadministration of other nephrotoxic drugs
   d. Ototoxicity: may be irreversible; auditory impairment and vestibular damage; possible damage to 8th cranial nerve
   e. Risk is increased with nephrotoxic drugs, prolonged treatment with aminoglycosides, impaired renal function, and other ototoxic drugs, such as furosemide (Lasix), vancomycin (Vancocin), amphotericin B, and certain antineoplastic agents
   f. Neuromuscular blockade: secondary to inhibition of acetylcholine release; may be seen in clients with myasthenia gravis or those receiving neuromuscular blockers such as pancuronium bromide (Pavulon) or succinylcholine (Anectine); use calcium salts to reverse blockade
   g. **Candidiasis** superinfection: secondary infection usually of skin and mucous membranes caused by *Candida albicans;* appears as discrete white plaques that are not easily removed
   h. **Pseudomembranous colitis** superinfection secondary infection of bowel, usually caused by *Clostridium difficile;* manifested by 4 to 6 watery stools per day with blood and/or mucus, abdominal pain, and fever; antibiotic is discontinued and vancomycin (Vancocin) PO or Flagyl IV or PO is prescribed
6. Nursing considerations
   a. See Box 46–2 for general nursing considerations with antibiotic therapy
   b. **Empiric therapy** (based on probable offending organism) is usually begun before test results available because of seriousness of infection
   c. Monitor peak and trough aminoglycoside levels
   d. Monitor for nephrotoxicity: monitor serum creatinine, BUN, urine creatinine clearance and urinalysis (urinary casts and proteinuria)
   e. Make certain the client is not taking other nephrotoxic drugs
   f. Keep accurate record of intake and output (I & O)
   g. Monitor for ototoxicity: assess for dizziness, lightheadedness, tinnitus, fullness in ears, and hearing loss; monitor vestibular integrity with Romberg's test
   h. Maintain fluid hydration to protect the kidneys; intake should be 2,500 to 3,000 mL/day unless contraindicated by other conditions
   i. Provide small, frequent, nutritious meals with high-quality proteins; drugs that may be taken with food may be associated with decreased GI upset

Box 46–2

General Nursing Considerations for Antibiotic Therapy and Other Anti-infectives

- Collect appropriate specimen for culture and sensitivity (C&S), whenever possible, prior to initiation of antibiotic therapy to ensure proper drug selection. Empiric therapy may be started so that infection can be treated promptly.
- Assess client's medication profile (including OTC and herbal products) for agents that may cause drug interactions.
- Assess for allergy prior to administration and withhold dose and notify prescriber for documented hypersensitivity reaction (such as hives, urticaria, stridor, dyspnea, and anaphylaxis).
- Administer doses on time to maintain therapeutic blood levels; when an IV antibiotic is scheduled at same time as another IV medication (e.g. ranitidine [Zantac]); give IV antibiotic first to assist in maintaining standardized times and keep drug level within therapeutic range.
- Assess for, document, and report adverse effects of prescribed antibiotic.
- Monitor for superinfection.
  - Candidiasis: vaginal yeast infection or oral thrush; is treated with appropriate anti-infective agent.
  - Pseudomembranous colitis: 4 to 6 or more watery stools per day, accompanied by blood and mucus in stools, abdominal cramps, and fever; usually caused by overgrowth of *clostridium difficile;* is treated with oral or IV metronidazole (Flagyl) or oral vancomycin; place client on contact precautions; original antibiotic is discontinued and another is selected.
- Maintain adequate fluid hydration and increase fluids if indicated (up to 3 liters daily) depending on antibiotic class.
- Ensure that client takes full course of antibiotic therapy for full beneficial effects, even if signs of infection resolve; otherwise, microorganism re-growth and drug resistance can occur.
- Observe for evidence that infection is resolving with symptom improvement within 48 to 72 hours of beginning therapy (decreased temperature, WBC count, and local signs of infection); report to prescriber if infection is not resolving and prepare to do additional cultures as ordered.

7. Client education

   ! **a.** See general teaching points for antibiotic therapy (Box 46–3)

   b. Keep liquid drug refrigerated if so recommended

   c. Take oral drug with food if not contraindicated to reduce risk of GI upset

   d. Eat small, frequent meals with at least 6 to 8 glasses of fluid a day

B. Cephalosporins

1. Action and use

   a. Structurally and chemically related to penicillins; practically identical to penicillin in mechanism of action, drug actions, therapeutic effects, side and adverse effects, and drug interactions; **cross-sensitivity** may occur between penicillins and cephalosporins, meaning that allergy to one class may indicate hypersensitivity to the other in some clients

   b. Four generations of cephalosporins exist with various uses but generally include Gram-negative organisms and anaerobes; fourth generation has increased activity against Gram-positive cocci and Gram-negative bacilli

   c. Usually bactericidal

   d. Used to treat sexually transmitted infections (STIs); respiratory infections such as bronchitis, pharyngitis, otitis media, sinusitis, and pneumonia; urinary tract infections (UTIs); skin and tissue infections; and Lyme disease

   e. Used prophylactically and therapeutically in orthopedic disorders; cefazolin (Ancef) is drug of choice to prevent or treat bone infections associated with orthopedic surgery

   f. Used for endocarditis prophylaxis prior to surgery for clients with history of rheumatic heart disease

Box 46–3

General Client Teaching Points for Antibiotic Therapy

- ➤ Know drug, dose, purpose, route, and schedule of drug regimen.
- ➤ Take at evenly spaced intervals around the clock without disrupting sleep to maintain serum levels.
- ➤ Take with food, if not contraindicated, to minimize GI upset.
- ➤ If medication must be taken on empty stomach, take 1 hour before or 2 hours after a meal.
- ➤ Ensure adequate fluid intake of 2,000 to 3,000 mL fluid intake daily if not contraindicated by heart failure, kidney disease, or other condition.
- ➤ If using a liquid preparation, use calibrated measuring device rather than household measurement (kitchen teaspoons can vary by 2 to 10 mL).
- ➤ Know side and adverse effects of drug and which ones require notification of prescriber.
- ➤ Report sore throat or white patches in mouth, watery stools more often than 4 to 6 times per day, or severe nausea or vomiting, indicating possible superinfection with pseudomembranous colitis or *candida* (candidiasis).
- ➤ Before taking any over-the-counter (OTC) drugs, check efficacy and possible adverse reactions with prescriber.
- ➤ Take full course of therapy as ordered; do not discontinue drug on own even if feeling better and symptoms have resolved; do not “save” medication for future illnesses.
- ➤ Do not take drugs with expired date; discard any drug that is not used (full course of therapy should be taken).
- ➤ Report to prescriber if symptoms aren’t resolving or not feeling better after 48 to 72 hours.

g. Important to reserve use for appropriate clinical infections because bacterial resistance is increasing

h. Most cephalosporins are excreted through urine; exceptions are cefoperazone (Cefobid) and ceftriaxone (Rocephin), which are excreted in bile

! **2.** Common medications are listed in Box 46–4

Memory Aid

Recognize a cephalosporin by the by the prefix or root *cef-* or *ceph-*.

3. Administration considerations

a. Well absorbed from GI tract; do not readily enter CSF except for cefuroxime; third-generation drugs readily enter CSF in presence of meningeal inflammation

b. Check renal function prior to and during therapy; renal impairment significantly extends drug half-life; use extreme caution if creatine clearance is less than 50 mL/min

c. Crosses placenta

d. Separate oral administration of antacids, H_2 receptor antagonists, iron supplements, and foods fortified with iron by 2 hours before and after oral administration of cephalosporins

e. Intramuscular administration is painful and irritating; administer deep IM into large muscle; avoid repeated IM injections; IV is preferred parenteral route

f. Shake suspensions to disperse or dissolve particles of drug immediately before measurement

g. Continue drug administration for at least 10 days to decrease risk of rheumatic fever in beta-hemolytic streptococcal bacterial infections such as strep throat; also, acute glomerulonephritis can become a sequela of this infection if treatment is inadequate

Box 46-4

Cephalosporins

First-generation cephalosporins
- cefadroxil (Duricef)
- cefazolin (Ancef)
- cephalexin (Keflex)
- cephapirin (Cefadyl)
- cephradine (Velosef)

Second-generation cephalosporins
- cefaclor (Ceclor)
- cefmetazole (Zefazone)
- cefonicid (Monocid)
- cefprozil (Cefzil)
- cefotetan (Cefotan)
- cefoxitin (Mefoxin)
- cefuroxime axetil (Ceftin)
- cefuroxime sodium (Zinacef)
- loracarbef (Lorabid)

Third-generation cephalosporins
- cefdinir (Omnicef)
- cefditoren (Spectracef)
- cefixime (Suprax)
- cefoperazone (Cefobid)
- cefotaxime (Claforan)
- cefpodoxime proxetil (Vantin)
- ceftazidime (Fortaz)
- ceftibuten (Cedax)
- ceftizoxime (Cefizox)
- ceftriaxone (Rocephin)

Fourth-generation cephalosporins
- cefipime (Maxipime)

h. Contraindications include cross-sensitivity with penicillins; not recommended for those who have had a type I (anaphylactic) reaction to penicillin
i. Hepatotoxicity with cefoperazone and ceftriaxone
j. Caution in pregnancy and lactation

4. Side/adverse effects
a. Central nervous system (CNS): lethargy, hallucinations, anxiety, depression, twitching, convulsions, coma
b. GI: nausea, vomiting, mild diarrhea, abdominal cramps or distress, elevated liver function tests such as aspartate aminotransferase (AST) and alanine aminotransferase (ALT), abdominal pain, colitis
! **c.** Hematologic: anemia, increased bleeding time, bone marrow depression, granulocytopenia
d. Metabolic: hyperkalemia, hypokalemia, alkalosis
e. Other: taste alteration, sore mouth; dark, discolored, or sore tongue; hives, pruritis, rash, edema
f. Hypersensitivity occurs in 5% to 16% of clients
! **g.** Cross-sensitivity with penicillins
h. Serum-sickness–like illness: usually follows second course of treatment and is noted by erythema multiforme and other skin rashes, arthralgia, and fever; treated with antihistamines and corticosteroids
i. Seizure activity: especially in renal impairment; discontinue cephalosporin to resolve activity
j. In renal impairment, cancer, impaired vitamin K synthesis, malnutrition, low vitamin K stores, there is increased risk for coagulation disturbances with parenteral administration
! **k.** Pseudomembranous colitis
! **l.** Use of ethanol with some cephalosporins such as cefoperazone and cefotetan can cause disulfiram-like reaction during therapy and up to 72 hours after drug is discontinued; can occur within 30 minutes of alcohol ingestion; manifestations include weakness, pulsating headache, and abdominal cramps

5. Nursing considerations
a. As per Box 46–2

b. Monitor injection sites for induration and tenderness; provide warm compresses and gentle massage to injection sites if painful or swollen; if phlebitis or redness at IV site develops, remove IV device and restart IV
c. Monitor for renal toxicity: check serum creatinine, BUN, urine creatinine clearance; keep accurate I & O
d. Monitor for unusual lethargy beginning after drug started; provide safety measures, including adequate lighting, use of side rails, and assistance with ambulation to protect client if CNS effects occur
e. For client with diabetes mellitus, use blood glucose monitoring; false-positive urine glucose can occur with copper sulfate technique (Clinitest)
f. Offer small, frequent meals with quality protein as tolerated
g. Provide frequent oral care; offer ice chips or sugarless candy if stomatitis and sore mouth occur
h. Monitor for increased bleeding if taking anticoagulants
i. Monitor for hemolytic anemia (rare): check RBCs with indices, tiredness or weakness, yellow skin or eyes; to observe for icterus in dark-skinned clients, check the hard palate

6. Client education
a. As per Box 46–3
b. Take safety precautions, including changing position slowly and avoiding driving and hazardous tasks, if CNS effects occur
c. Drink fluids and maintain nutrition, especially protein, to ensure adequate protein for drug binding and efficacy of action
d. Shake suspensions well to dispense or dissolve particles of drug immediately before measurement; use a measuring device for liquid/suspension and not a kitchen teaspoon (may vary from 2 to 10 mL/teaspoon)
e. Report manifestations of hypersensitivity to health care provider: difficulty breathing, severe rash, hives, severe headache, dizziness or weakness, aching joints
f. Report side effects to the prescriber: anorexia, epigastric pain, nausea/vomiting indicating biliary sludge or pseudolithiasis if on ceftriaxone; discontinue drug and manifestations will resolve
g. Refrain from alcohol during therapy and for 72 hours after drug is discontinued to avoid disulfiram-like reaction

C. Fluoroquinolones

1. Action and use
a. Newer class of broad-spectrum bactericidal antibiotics
b. Used against Gram-negative and selected Gram-positive organisms; used in various bacterial infections: lower respiratory tract infections, sinusitis, bone and joint infections, infectious diarrhea, UTIs, skin and soft tissue infections, intra-abdominal infections, and STIs
c. Many oral formulations are as effective as parenteral forms

2. Common medications are listed in Box 46–5

Memory Aid Recognize a fluoroquinolone by the suffix *-oxacin*.

3. Administration considerations
a. Administer around the clock, evenly spaced, and do not interrupt sleep, if possible, to maintain therapeutic blood level
b. Oral drug is tolerated better with food
c. Use cautiously in clients with renal dysfunction, including those with advanced age, children, pregnant or lactating women, and those with history of seizures
d. Elimination of caffeine is decreased with ciprofloxacin (Cipro), enoxacin (Penetrex), and norfloxacin (Noroxin)

4. Side/adverse effects
a. Headache, dizziness, fatigue, lethargy, insomnia, depression, restlessness, confusion, and convulsions

Box 46–5

Fluoroquinolones

First Generation
Cinoxacin (Cinobac)
Nalidixic acid (NegGram)

Second Generation
Ciprofloxacin (Cipro)
Enoxacin (Penetrex)
Lomefloxacin (Maxaquin)
Norfloxacin (Noroxin)
Ofloxacin (Floxin)

Third Generation
Gatifloxacin (Tequin)
Levofloxacin (Levaquin)
Sparfloxacin (Zagam)

Fourth Generation
Gemifloxacin (Factive)
Moxifloxacin (Avelox)
Trovafloxacin (Trovan)

b. Nausea, vomiting, diarrhea, constipation, flatulence, epigastric distress, oral candidiasis, dysphagia, pseudomembranous colitis, and elevated liver function tests, such as ALT, AST, bilirubin, and alkaline phosphatase
c. Rash, pruritus, urticaria, photosensitivity, flushing
d. Fever, chills, piloerection, blurred vision, tinnitus
e. Hypersensitivity reaction

5. Nursing considerations
a. As per Box 46–2
b. Separate drug from oral antacids, iron and zinc salts, or sucralfate by 2 hours
! c. Monitor PT, INR, and manifestations of increased bleeding or bruising if also on oral anticoagulants
d. Monitor renal function
e. Provide more frequent meals with complete or complementary proteins to better ensure adequate albumin levels for drug efficacy
f. Monitor for increased CNS irritability if client has history of epilepsy, ethanol abuse, or is concurrently taking theophylline
g. Maintain hydration with 3 L fluid/day, if not contraindicated

6. Client education
a. As per Box 46–3
b. Take safety precautions including changing position slowly and avoiding driving and hazardous tasks if CNS effects occur
! c. Drink fluids and maintain nutrition, especially protein, to provide adequate protein for drug-binding and drug efficacy
d. Report difficulty breathing, severe headache, dizziness, or weakness to health care provider
e. Baseline electrocardiogram may be necessary if client receives sparfloxacin or moxifloxacin
! f. Wear sunglasses, long-sleeves and long-legged garments, and hat to protect from direct sunlight; sunscreen or sunblock may not prevent photosensitivity reaction; avoid ultraviolet lights, tanning beds, and direct sunlight

D. Macrolides and lincosamides

1. Action and use
a. **Bacteriostatic** (inhibiting the growth of bacteria) but can be bactericidal in high doses with some bacteria
b. Highly protein-bound
c. Action is similar to other antibiotics
d. Used in upper and lower respiratory tract infections, skin and soft tissue infections caused by *Streptococcus* or *Haemophilus* organisms
e. Used to treat syphilis, gonorrhea, chlamydia, Lyme disease, and *mycoplasma, listeria,* and *corynebacterium* infections
f. Clarithromycin (Biaxin) is used with omeprazole (Prilosec) to treat *Helicobacter pylori* associated with peptic ulcers

g. Lincosamides may be bactericidal and bacteriostatic; used to treat chronic bone infections, genitourinary (GU) infections, intra abdominal infections, pneumonia, and streptococcal or staphylococcal septicemia

2. Common medications are listed in Box 46–6
3. Administration considerations
   a. If erythromycin form has bitter taste, give with juice or applesauce; give with food to reduce GI irritating effects
   b. Give clindamycin (Cleocin) and lincomycin (Lincocin) with at least 8 ounces of fluid or on an empty stomach
   c. If clindamycin (Cleocin) is given IV, do not give by intravenous push (IVP) method; instead, give by IV infusion
   d. Zithromax: longer half-life with less frequent dosing, shorter term of therapy, and fewer or less intense GI side effects than others (may contribute to better compliance)
   e. Contraindicated with hypersensitivity, ulcerative colitis/enteritis (lincosamides), and children under 1 year (lincosamides)
   f. Use caution with liver or renal dysfunction, GI disorders, the elderly, and pregnant or lactating women
4. Side/adverse effects
   a. Stimulation of smooth muscle and GI motility results in diarrhea (may be used therapeutically as a GI stimulant to facilitate passage of intestinal tube or to prevent gastroesophageal reflux)
   b. Palpitations and chest pain
   c. Headache, dizziness, vertigo, lethargy, somnolence, confusion, hearing loss usually preceded by tinnitus
   d. Stomatitis, flatulence, epigastric distress, anorexia, nausea, vomiting, abnormal taste (clarithromycin/Biaxin)
   e. Jaundice, rash, pruritis, urticaria
   f. Thrombophlebitis at peripheral IV site
   g. Toxicities: hepatotoxicity, nephrotoxicity, and ototoxicity (erythromycin)
   h. Superinfections such as pseudomembranous colitis, candidiasis
5. Nursing considerations
   a. Collect data such as age, hypersensitivity to drugs, hepatic and renal function; also check cardiac status if appropriate for prescribed drug
   b. As per Box 46–2
   c. Assess GI function and elimination pattern
   d. Observe for bleeding if taking oral anticoagulants
   e. Observe for superinfections
   f. Monitor ALT, AST, bilirubin, and alkaline phosphatase as indicated for hepatic dysfunction prior to and during therapy
   g. Monitor serum creatinine, BUN, creatinine clearance, I & O as appropriate for development of renal dysfunction
   h. Assess baseline hearing and monitor for hearing loss; arrange for discontinuation of drug if hearing loss occurs
   i. Hydrate with at least 2,000 to 2,400 mL/day if not contraindicated
6. Client education
   a. As per Box 46–3
   b. Include protein in diet because these drugs are highly protein bound and require protein for therapeutic efficacy

Box 46–6

Macrolides and Lincosamides

Azithromycin (Zithromax)	Troleandomycin (Tao)
Clarithromycin (Biaxin)	Clindamycin (Cleocin)
Dirithromycin (Dynabac)	Lincomycin (Lincocin)
Erythromycin (Erythrocin)	Telithromycin (Ketek)

E. Penicillins (beta-lactams) and penicillinase-resistants

1. Action and use
   - **a.** Derived from fungus or mold evidenced on bread or fruit
   - **b.** Similarities exist among penicillins, cephalosporins, monobactams, carbapenems, and beta-lactamase inhibitors; they share many of the same actions and uses; cross-sensitivity is possible
   - **c.** Most effective against Gram-positive organisms; less effective against Gram-negative ones
   - **d.** Used to treat infections caused by meningococci, pneumococci, streptococci, treponema pallidum, staphylococci such as in upper respiratory infections, pneumonia, STIs such as syphilis but not gonorrhea, wound infections, and urinary tract infections
   - **e.** Used prophylactically against endocarditis for oral, GI, pulmonary procedures when bacteria may enter circulation; usually amoxicillin (Amoxil) or ampicillin (Omnipen) are used
   - **f.** Used in beta-hemolytic streptococci Group A infections associated with rheumatic fever or acute glomerulonephritis, such as pharyngitis (V-Cillin) often used with PO route preferred
   - **g.** Increasing resistance developing, especially in facility-acquired or nosocomial infections
2. Common medications are listed in Box 46–7

Memory Aid

Recognize a penicillin by the suffix *-cillin.*

3. Administration considerations
   - **a.** Oral dosing needs to be 3 to 4 times greater than parenteral dose because of hepatic first-pass effect and instability of penicillin in acid environment of stomach
   - **b.** For serious systemic infections, parenteral route is recommended
   - **c.** Absorption erratic from IM route; limit due to irritability of tissue; IM injection should be slow and steady over 12 to 15 seconds to minimize discomfort and prevent needle obstruction, especially with thick preparations
   - **d.** Nafcillin (Unipen): IV extravasation can cause necrosis; avoid IM or, if not possible, inject by Z-track method
   - **e.** Contraindicated with hypersensitivity reaction and anaphylaxis, serum sickness, exfoliative dermatitis, blood dyscrasias
   - **f.** Penicillin G procaine or benzathine not to be given IV: lethal
   - **g.** Most likely drug category to cause allergic reactions
   - **h.** Use caution in anemia, thrombocytopenia, bone marrow depression, and concurrently with anticoagulants because some penicillins cause increased bleeding
4. Side/adverse effects
   - **a.** ! Most common allergic responses are skin rash, urticaria, pruritis, angioedema; a maculopapular, pruritic rash that is like measles with ampicillin or

Box 46–7

Penicillins (Beta-Lactams) and Penicillinase-Resistants

Amoxicillin (Amoxil)	Carbenicillin (Geopen)
Amoxicillin/clavulanate (Augmentin)	Mezlocillin (Mezlin)
Ampicillin (Omnipen)	Cloxacillin (Apo-Cloxi)
Ampicillin/sulbactam (Unasyn)	Dicloxacillin (Dynapen)
Bacampicillin (Spectrobid)	Methicillin (Staphcillin)
Piperacillin (Pipracil)	Nafcillin (Unipen)
Piperacillin/tazobactam (Zosyn)	Oxacillin (Bactocil)
Ticarcillin (Ticar)	Penicillin G (Pentids)
Ticarcillin/clavulanate (Timentin)	Penicillin V (V-Cillin)

amoxocillin is not a true allergic reaction but develops after 7 to 10 days of therapy and may last several days after discontinuation of penicillin; is not a contraindication to give drug in the future

b. Most common adverse effects are GI, such as nausea, vomiting, diarrhea, epigastric distress, abdominal pain, colitis, elevated liver enzymes; also taste alteration, sore mouth, or dark, discolored, sore tongue

c. Anemia, bone marrow suppression, granulocytopenia, increased bleeding time

d. Lethargy, anxiety, depression, hallucinations, twitching, convulsions, coma

e. Hypokalemia or hyperkalemia, metabolic alkalosis

f. Type I hypersensitivity often fatal immediately if untreated within 2 to 30 minutes; noted by nausea, vomiting, urticaria, pruritis, severe dyspnea, stridor, tachycardia, hypotension, diaphoresis, vertigo, loss of consciousness/circulatory collapse

g. Serum sickness–like reaction: skin rash, arthralgia, fever

h. Exfoliative dermatitis: red, scaly skin

i. Blood dyscrasias: hemolytic anemia, neutropenia, leukopenia

5. Nursing considerations

a. As per Box 46–2

b. Monitor renal studies, liver enzymes, and electrolytes; many of the penicillins contain sodium salts that can result in hypokalemia

c. Monitor for adverse effects; may not be necessary to discontinue penicillin if mild diarrhea develops; give yogurt or buttermilk to restore normal flora; use absorbent antidiarrheal agents (Kaolin and Pectin/Kao-tin); avoid antiperistaltic agents that delay or prevent elimination of intestinal toxins

d. Provide good nutrition and hydration

e. Some penicillins cause false-positive results on urine glucose testing; use blood glucose monitoring

6. Client education

a. As per Box 46–3

b. Take oral drug on empty stomach; take 1 hour before meals or 2 hours after meals, except amoxicillin (which is not affected by food)

c. Chewable tablets must be crushed or chewed in order for the penicillin to be effectively absorbed

d. Shake suspensions to disperse particles prior to measurement; use a calibrated device to measure liquid because kitchen teaspoons may vary by 2 to 10 mL; most suspensions maintain potency for 14 days if refrigerated

e. Ensure antibiotic drops are used for correct route: oral, eye, ear

f. Take missed doses as soon as possible; do not take a double dose at the next administration time

g. Report rash, urticaria, pruritis, difficulty breathing

h. Take small, frequent meals with high-quality protein and drink 6 to 8 glasses or more of water per day if not contraindicated by other conditions

F. Sulfonamides

1. Action and use

a. First effective group of antibiotics (1935); bacteriostatic

b. Used to treat UTIs (especially caused by *Escherichia coli,* the most common cause of cystitis), *Chlamydia trachomatis* causing blindness, pneumonia, brain abscesses, mild to moderate ulcerative colitis, active Crohn's disease, and rheumatoid arthritis; pyrimethamine is only effective drug treatment for toxoplasmosis; drugs of choice for treatment of nocardiosis

c. Sulfacetamide (silver sulfadiazine) to prevent bacterial growth in burns and wounds

d. Cross-sensitivity possible with penicillins and cephalosporins

2. Common medications are listed in Box 46–8

Memory Aid Recognize a sulfonamide by the root *sulf* in the drug name.

Box 46-8	
Sulfonamides	Sulfisoxazole (Gantrisin)
	Sulfadiazine (Microsulfon)
	Sulfamethoxazole–Trimethoprim (Bactrim)
	Sulfasalazine (Azulfidine)

3. Administration considerations
   a. Fluid intake should be 3,000 to 4,000 mL/day to promote urinary output at least 1,500 mL/day to prevent crystalluria/stone formation; if not possible, may administer antacids or sodium bicarbonate to alkalinize urine; alkaline ash diet may be helpful, which includes fruit (except plums, prunes, and cranberries), vegetables, and milk
   b. Store in light-resistant, tightly closed container at room temperature
4. Contraindications
   a. History of hypersensitivity to sulfonamindes, salicylates, penicillins, cephalosporins
   b. In lactation and in children younger than 2 months unless used to treat congenital toxoplasmosis
   c. In porphyria, advanced or severe renal or hepatic dysfunction, or with intestinal and urinary blockage; use with caution in impaired renal or hepatic function, asthma, blood dyscrasias, or glucose-6-phosphate dehydrogenase (G6PD) deficiency
5. Side/adverse effects
   a. Rash common; most are urticaria and maculopapular
   b. Nausea, vomiting, diarrhea, abdominal pain, jaundice, stomatitis
   c. Headache, insomnia, drowsiness, depression, psychosis, photosensitivity
   ! d. Crystalluria
   e. Peripheral neuritis/neuropathy
   f. Tinnitus, hearing loss, vertigo, ataxia, seizures
   g. Hepatitis, pancreatitis
   h. Anemia, agranulocytosis, thrombocytopenia, leukopenia, eosinophilia, prothrombinemia
   ! i. Exfoliative dermatitis, Stevens-Johnson syndrome (an adverse reaction of skin that resembles appearance of second-degree burns)
   j. Serum sickness, drug fever
6. Nursing considerations
   a. As per Box 46–2
   b. Assess baseline laboratory findings for liver and renal function, and monitor during therapy
   ! c. Provide hydration to assure daily urinary output of 1,500 mL or more to prevent stone and crystal formations; alkalinize urine as indicated; keep accurate I & O record
   d. Provide for safety if neurotoxicities develop, such as ataxia or convulsions
   e. Provide small, frequent, nutritious meals with high-quality proteins; drugs that may be taken with food may decrease GI upset
7. Client education
   a. As per Box 46–3
   b. Take safety precautions if vertigo, ataxia, or seizures occur
   c. Avoid driving or performing hazardous tasks if drowsiness occurs
   d. Take with food, if not contraindicated, to minimize GI upset
   ! e. Eat small, frequent meals with at least 2,500 to 3,000 mL fluid intake a day
   f. Empty bladder frequently, at least every 2 hours while awake
   ! g. Report flank or suprapubic pain, increased dysuria, disruption of skin integrity to health care provider

G. Tetracyclines

1. Action and use
   a. Broad spectrum; bacteriostatic; can be bactericidal in high concentrations

b. Effective against most chlamydia, mycoplasmas, rickettsiae, cholera, and certain protozoa
c. Suppress *Proprionibacterium acnes* in treating acne; topical application may be as effective as oral preparation for acne; both forms may be used for severe acne
d. Used prophylactically for traveler's diarrhea
e. Used to treat Rocky Mountain Spotted Fever, **amebiasis** (a protozoan infection), brucellosis, shigellosis, cholera, tetanus, chronic bronchitis, Lyme disease
f. Used to treat syphilis and gonorrhea in clients with penicillin allergy
g. Used as a sclerosing agent for pleural and pericardial effusion, such as in metastasis of cancer; causes inflammation resulting in fibrosis, leaving scar tissue that does not allow fluid to accumulate
h. Used in *Helicobacter pylori* peptic ulcer disease, Q fever, Rickettsia pox, typhus, Mycoplasma pneumonia, epididymo-orchitis, pelvic inflammatory disease (PID)
i. Used with quinine for treatment of malaria
j. Anti-infective prophylaxis for rape victims
k. Treat syndrome of inappropriate antidiuretic hormone (SIADH) with demeclocyline (Declomycin) by inhibiting antidiuretic hormone (ADH)

2. Common medications (generic name ends in *-cycline;* see Box 46–9)

Memory Aid

Recognize a tetracycline by the suffix *-cycline* in the drug name.

3. Administration considerations
a. Avoid administering outdated drug: Fanconi-like syndrome with polyuria, polydipsia, nausea and vomiting, glycosuria, proteinuria, acidosis can occur; renal tubular dysfunction and lupus erythematosus–like syndrome have occurred and are attributed to preparations used beyond expiration date
b. Oral: give with full glass of water on empty stomach at least 1 hour before or 2 hours after meals; food, milk, and milk products decrease absorption by one-half
c. IM injection contains procaine, so assess for allergies to local anesthetics ending with *-caine*
d. Administer deep IM into large muscle such as the gluteus; alternate sites; not to be administered IV
e. If topical, clean area with soap and water, rinse and dry well prior to application
f. ! Tetracyclines bind to calcium, preventing normal bone growth and causing tooth hypoplasia in developing fetus or child younger than 8 years old; contraindicated during last half of pregnancy when tooth development occurs, from birth to 8 years of age, and in lactating women
g. Use caution with history of renal or liver dysfunction, allergy, asthma, hay fever, urticaria, or in myasthenia gravis

4. Side/adverse effects
a. Nausea, vomiting, diarrhea, epigastric distress, abdominal discomfort, flatulence, dry mouth, dysphagia, bulky or loose stools, steatorrhea
b. Headache, photosensitivity, increased intracranial pressure (rare)
c. Maculopapular rash, urticaria, exfoliative dermatitis, angioedema
d. Stinging/burning with topical application
e. Discoloration of developing teeth
f. Pigmentation of conjunctiva related to drug deposits
g. Discoloration and loosening of nails

Box 46–9

Tetracyclines

Demeclocycline (Declomycin)	Doxycycline (Vibramycin)
Oxytetracycline (Terramycin)	Minocycline (Minocin)
Tetracycline (Achromycin)	

h. Retrosternal pain
i. Elevated liver function tests and decreased cholesterol level
j. Drug fever, serum sickness, and anaphylaxis
k. Hepatotoxicity, pancreatitis, nephrotoxicity
l. Blood dyscrasias such as thrombocytopenia, hemolytic anemia
m. Fatty degeneration of liver results in jaundice, azotemia, increased nitrogen retention, hyperphosphatemia, and metabolic acidosis
n. Topicycline topical application can cause itching, wheezing, anaphylaxis in client with asthma allergies

5. Nursing considerations
a. As per Box 46–2
b. Assess for history of renal or liver problems and related laboratory results
c. Assess history of immunosuppression
d. Check CBC, including WBC, with differential, RBC indices, and platelet count
e. Monitor I & O
f. Check IM injection sites every day for induration, redness, edema

6. Client education
a. As per Box 46–3
b. Unstable with age and light exposure; store in tightly covered container in dry area, protected from light at room temperature
c. Report side effects, particularly severe diarrhea
d. Practice good oral care and hygiene
e. Avoid exposure to direct sunlight or ultraviolet light or tanning beds; wear hat, long sleeves, long-leg pants, and sunglasses outside during and for a few days after treatment; sunscreen or sunblock may not prevent erythema
f. If on long-term treatment, report onset of severe headache or visual disturbances that may indicate increased intracranial pressure (rare); requires discontinuation of tetracycline to prevent irreversible vision loss
g. Take oral doses with full glass of water on empty stomach (1 hour before or 2 hours after meal or dairy product) to promote absorption and decrease risk of esophagitis; report sudden dysphagia to health care provider
h. Topical form may stain clothing or cause affected skin to reflect yellow or green fluorescence under an ultraviolet or "black" light

H. Urinary tract antiseptics

1. Action and use; drugs that act against bacteria in urine (urinary tract infections) but have little or no systemic antibacterial effects
2. Common medications are listed in Box 46–10
3. Administration considerations
a. Use caution in clients with impaired renal and/or hepatic function
b. Use caution during lactation and pregnancy
c. Controversial if pH of urine has any effect on UTI
d. Alkaline ash diet may interfere with the required acidity of urine for antiseptic action; alkaline ash foods include fruits (except cranberries, prunes, plums), milk, vegetables
e. Acid ash foods that may or may not increase urine acidity include meat, cheese, eggs, whole grains, as well as cranberries, prunes, and plums
f. Fluids that may acidify urine and potentially facilitate drug action include cranberry and prune juice
4. Side/adverse effects (do not commonly occur):
a. Nausea, vomiting, anorexia, diarrhea, epigastric distress
b. Rash, pruritus, photosensitivity, photophobia, tinnitus, insomnia, headache, dizziness, drowsiness

Box 46–10
Urinary Tract Antiseptics

Cinoxacin (Cinobac)
Methenamine mandelate (Mandelamine)
Methenamine hippurate (Hiprex)
Nalidixic acid (NegGram)
Nitrofurantoin (Furadantin)

c. Low back pain, dysuria
d. Nitrofurantoin: urine may become brown

5. Nursing considerations
   a. As per Box 46–2; assess for previous renal or liver dysfunction
   b. Encourage at least 3,000 mL/day fluids, including cranberry juice, if not contraindicated by fluid restriction, diabetes mellitus, or other conditions
   c. Monitor urine pH at bedside with test strip as indicated
   d. Give medication with or after food to limit GI adverse effects
6. Client education
   a. As per Box 46–3
   b. Take with or after food to minimize GI distress
   c. Drink at least 3 liters of fluid a day, including cranberry and prune juice, unless contraindicated by other conditions
   d. Include acid ash foods in diet, such as cranberries, prunes, plums, cheese, eggs, meat, whole grains; limit or avoid alkaline ash foods, such as citrus fruits and juices, vegetables
   e. Do not take other medications unless approved by the prescriber; avoid drugs that may alkalinize the urine, such as antacids, Alka-Seltzer, sodium bicarbonate (baking soda)
   f. Nalidixic acid (NegGram) can cause photophobia; avoid bright sunlight, wear sunglasses, and report any visual disturbances; photosensitivity can also occur several weeks after drug is discontinued so avoid direct sunlight or ultraviolet light
   g. Nitrofurantoin may cause urine to be brown; may stain clothing
   h. Do not drive or perform hazardous tasks if drowsiness or dizziness occurs
   i. If diabetic, urine testing for glucose with Clinitest can yield a false-positive result; test blood glucose

I. Miscellaneous antibiotics are listed in Box 46–11

1. Quinupristin/dalfopristin (Synercid): used to treat bacteremia and life-threatening infections caused by vancomycin-resistant *Enterococcus faecium* (VREF); also complicated skin and skin structure infections caused by *Staphylococcus aureus,* including vancomycin-resistant strains, and *Streptococcus pyogenes*
   a. Administration considerations: IV use only, preferably via central line
   b. Side/adverse effects: arthralgias, myalgias (possibly severe); with peripheral IV administration, frequently pain, inflammation, edema, and thrombophlebitis
   c. Nursing considerations and client education: same as for other antibiotics
2. Vancomycin (Vancocin): bactericidal; parenteral antibiotic of choice for methicillin-resistant *Staphylococcus aureus* (MRSA) and other Gram-positive bacteria, yeast, and fungi; antibiotic-induced pseudomembranous colitis caused by *Clostridium difficile* and staphylococcal enterocolitis (oral drug form)
   a. Administration considerations: poorly absorbed from GI tract so indicated for local surface-infected areas of GI tract; IV dose should be through a central venous access device (CVAD) because of high risk for phlebitis; can cause necrosis if it extravasates
   b. Side/adverse effects: nausea, hypotension, flushing; pain and thrombophlebitis at injection site; ototoxicity, nephrotoxicity, temporary leukopenia;

Box 46–11

Miscellaneous Antibiotics

Generic/Trade Names

Monobacterium
Aztreonam (Azactam)

Carbapenems
Imipenem/Cilastatin (Primaxin)
Ertapenem (Invanz)
Meropenem (Merrem)

Streptogramin
Quinupristin/dalfopristin (Synercid)

Other
Vancomycin (Vancocin)

"red neck (or man) syndrome": too rapid IV infusion results in profound hypotension, erythematous rash on face, neck, upper chest, and arms

c. Nursing considerations: as for other antibiotics; give IV dose over 60 to 90 minutes to avoid hypotension and red neck syndrome

d. Client education: as for other antibiotics; also, if client is receiving IV therapy in home, ensure appropriate knowledge and ability to perform procedures correctly, including monitoring BP and heart rate

3. Imipenem/cilastatin (Primaxin), meropenem (Merrem), ertapenem (Invanz)

a. Classified as broad-spectrum carbapenems

b. May be used in serious infections of urinary tract, lower respiratory tract, bones, joints, skin and skin structures; intraabdominal, gynecologic, and mixed infections

c. Meropenem (Merrem) is used in bacterial meningitis because of its ability to enter CSF, especially if inflammation is present

d. Administration considerations: preparations are specific for IM or for IV use; do not interchange; give IM deep into gluteal muscle

e. Contraindicated with known hypersensitivities to components of drugs or penicillins or cephalosporins; also allergy to amide local anesthetics

f. Side/adverse effects: headache, dizziness, mental changes, somnolence, tremors, paresthesia, heartburn, nausea, vomiting, diarrhea, glossitis, rash, pruritis, urticaria, candidiasis, flushing, sweating, facial edema, fever, pain/phlebitis at injection site, drug fever, hyperkalemia, hyponatremia, polyuria, oliguria, weakness, arthralgias

g. Nursing considerations and client education: same as for other antibiotics; eat small, frequent meals with high-quality protein; drink at least 6 to 8 glasses of fluids a day

VII. ANTIMYCOBACTERIALS

A. Antituberculins

1. Action and use

a. Inhibit cell wall synthesis, protein synthesis, RNA synthesis

b. Effects limited primarily to *Mycobacterium tuberculosis* and then certain other mycobacterium strains

c. Prophylaxis or treatment of pulmonary tuberculosis and extrapulmonary tuberculosis in adults and children

d. Often used in combination with other antituberculin agents

e. Used to prevent or delay onset of *Mycobacterium avium* bacteremia in clients with advanced human immunodeficiency virus (HIV); in combination with other antituberculin antibiotic

f. Rifampin eradicates meningococci from nasopharynx of asymptomatic *Neisseria meningitides* carriers when there is increased risk for infection outbreaks in a community

g. Rifampin is used prophylactically with exposure to *Haemophilus influenzae* type B (HIB) infection

h. Antituberculins are used in combination to treat leprosy

i. Used to treat endocarditis with methicillin-resistant staphylococci, chronic prostatitis with staphylococcal organisms, and anti-infective-resistant pneumococci

j. Effective treatment requires compliance and therapy over months to years

2. Common medications are listed in Box 46–12

3. Administration considerations

a. Effectiveness depends on correct drug, correct combination therapy, adequate dosing, adequate duration of therapy, and compliance

b. Empiric treatment is initiated with isoniazid, rifampin, pyrazinamide, and ethambutol or streptomycin

c. Multicombination drug therapy decreases risk or rate of developing resistance to any single drug

d. Give isoniazid one 1 hour before meals on empty stomach

e. Give clofazimine (Lamprene) with meals

Box 46–12
Antituberculins

Capreomycin (Capostat sulfate)	Rifampin (Rifadin)
Clofazimine (Lamprene)	Streptomycin (also an aminoglycoside)
Ethambutol HCL (Myambutol)	Rifabutin (Mycobutin)
Ethionamide (Trecator-SC)	Cycloserine (Seromycin)
Isoniazid (INH)	Kanamycin (Kantrex)
Pyrazinamide (Tebrazid)	

f. Contraindications: hypersensitivity to drug, hepatic or renal damage, use caution in pregnancy unless risk is significant
g. Caution in renal or liver dysfunction, history of seizures, ethanol abuse
h. Caution in older clients, children, diabetics, those with gout or blood dyscrasias, and optic neuritis or defects

4. Side/adverse effects
a. Fairly well tolerated
b. Nausea, vomiting, anorexia, constipation, diarrhea, dyspepsia
c. Headache, dizziness, malaise, fever, chills, arthralgia, flulike symptoms, weakness
d. Skin rash, dry skin, peripheral paresis, photophobia, photosensitivity, vision changes
e. Dysrhythmias
f. Urinary retention (in males)
! g. Change in color to orange-red of excretions/secretions such as urine, tears, feces, perspiration (with rifampin and rifabutin)

Memory Aid

Remember the *R* for rifampin can indicate a *R*eddish orange discoloration to body fluids.

h. Electrolyte imbalances
i. Metallic taste with ethionamide (Trecator-SC)
j. Disulfiram-like effect with alcohol ingestion
k. Nephrotoxicity or hepatotoxicity, or ototoxicity

Memory Aid

Remember the *H* in INH can stand for *H*epatotoxicity as an adverse drug effect.

l. Hematologic disorders: agranulocytosis, thrombocytopenia, eosinophilia, anemia
m. Seizures, depression, confusion, ataxia, paresis, paresthesias, drowsiness

5. Nursing considerations
a. Follow same principles as for antibiotic therapy (Box 46–2)
b. Assess baseline and periodic liver and renal function, C & S results, CBC with WBC and differential, RBC indices, and platelet count
c. Assess for pregnancy
! d. Coadminister pyridoxine (vitamin B_6) and/or cyanocobalamin (vitamin B_{12})
! e. Encourage food high in B-complex vitamin (especially pyridoxine), such as meat (chicken, beef, and pork), liver, soybeans, baked potato with skin, raw avocado
f. Evaluate client compliance with full course of therapy to lessen risk of reinfection or development of drug resistance
g. Encourage good hydration and good nutrition with high-quality protein

6. Client education
a. As per Box 46–3
b. Take isoniazid (INH) 1 hour before meals
! c. Rifampin (Rifadin): may discolor urine, tears, saliva; may stain contact lens and undergarments
d. Keep follow-up appointments with health care provider and for tests

e. Use infection control measures to protect self and others
f. Avoid alcohol because of increased risk for hepatitis or disulfiram-like effect
g. Use alternative contraception during therapy and for at least 1 month after therapy is discontinued if using oral contraceptives
h. For dry skin, use emollients or oils

B. Leprostatics

1. Action and use
   a. Treat leprosy and some AIDS-related opportunistic infections
   b. Bacteriostatic against *Mycobacterium leprae, Pneumocystis carinii, Plasmodium, Mycobacterium tuberculosis:* dapsone (DDS)
   c. Bactericidal against *Mycobacterium leprae* and *Mycobacterium avium:* clofazimine (Lamprene)
2. Common medications are listed in Box 46–13
3. Administration considerations:
   a. Give clofazimine with food
   b. Contraindicated with hypersensitivity to DDS and possible sulfonamides
   c. Use cautiously in clients with hepatic disease or G6PD deficiency (an inherited type of hemolytic anemia associated with stress or certain drug interactions)
   d. Not established for safe use in pregnant and lactating clients
4. Side/adverse effects
   a. Skin pigmentation changes, as pink to brownish black color; may resolve in weeks to months
   b. Dry skin
   c. Nausea, vomiting, diarrhea, abdominal pain
   d. Headache, insomnia, malaise, paresthesias, nervousness, tinnitus, vertigo, vision changes
   e. Agranulocytosis
   f. Hepatotoxicity, phototoxicity
   g. Dose-related hemolysis (increased in G6PD deficiency)
   h. Methemoglobinemia may occur resulting in rhinitis, fatigue, difficulty breathing, cyanosis
   i. Male infertility with DDS
5. Nursing considerations
   a. As per Box 46–2
   b. Give clofazimine with food
   c. Monitor laboratory test for hemoglobin and reticulocyte count
6. Client education
   a. As per Box 46–3
   b. Take clofazimine with meals; skin discoloration may be pink to brownish black; resolves in months to years after drug is discontinued
   c. Ensure infection control measures are used
   d. Encourage hydration and good nutrition with complete or complementary proteins for tissue healing

VIII. ANTIVIRALS

A. Medications to treat herpes and cytomegalovirus

1. Action and use
   a. Virustatic; drugs convert to compound that is a counterfeit nucleotide; it is taken into viral cell where DNA chain is developing and terminates chain, resulting in cell death with help from host's immune system
   b. Drug has little effect on host cells; effective only during acute phase of infection, not during latent phase; virus must be in living cell to survive and replicate

Box 46–13

Leprostatics	Dapsone (DDS) Clofazimine (Lamprene)

c. Used to treat broad spectrum of diseases, including cold sores, viral encephalitis, shingles, and genital infection
d. Viruses include herpes simplex virus-1 (HSV-1) in oral herpes or herpes labialis, herpes simplex virus-2 (HSV-2) in genital herpes, herpes zoster in shingles, herpes varicella zoster virus (VZV) in chickenpox, and some Epstein-Barr viruses
e. Acyclovir (Zovirax) is drug of choice in herpes simplex encephalitis; genital herpes treatment is its most frequent use; used prophylactically with immunosuppressed seropositive clients before bone marrow transplantation and after other organ transplants; not found to be beneficial in treating those who are not immunosuppressed, although it may help prevent shedding of virus
f. Ganciclovir (DHPG) is approved to treat only cytomegalovirus (CMV) retinitis in immunosuppressed clients; has good intraocular penetration; foscarnet (Foscavir) is used to treat ganciclovir-resistant CMV retinitis; cidofovir (Vistide) is also given IV for CMV retinitis
g. Famciclovir (Famvir) is used to treat acute herpes zoster (shingles)
h. Trifluridine is a topical treatment for keratoconjunctivitis caused by herpes simplex
i. Valacyclovir (Valtrex), an improved oral form of acyclovir, is drug of choice for genital herpes;
j. Penciclovir (Denavir) is used to treat herpes infections; topical only; it is negligibly absorbed so is well tolerated and shortens pain and healing by one-half day
k. Cidofovir (Vistide) IV to treat CMV retinitis in client with AIDS

2. Common medications are listed in Box 46–14

Memory Aid

Recognize an antiviral drug by the root *vir* in the drug name.

3. Administration considerations
a. Hydrate client to decrease risk or extent of nephrotoxicity
b. Administer as soon as possible to improve effectiveness
c. Wear gloves for topical application to limit exposure to drug or lesions
d. Preferred central venous access for IV administrations
e. Foscarnet: precipitates with many drugs when used as IV administration; use with D_5W or NaCl solutions

4. Contraindicated with hypersensitivity to drug; use caution in preexisting hepatic or renal dysfunction, concurrent use of nephrotoxic drugs, and in pregnant and lactating women

5. Side/adverse effects
a. Anemia, headache, mood changes, seizures
b. Nausea, vomiting, diarrhea
c. Local irritation including phlebitis at IV site
d. Neutropenia; often dose-dependent because of bone marrow suppression
e. Fever, hypocalcemia, hypomagnesemia, hypokalemia, metabolic acidosis, dysrhythmias
f. Increased risk for CNS disturbances and fluid overload in clients with impaired hepatic or renal function

Box 46–14

Antivirals: Medications to Treat Herpes and Cytomegalovirus

Acyclovir (Zovirax)	Penciclovir (Denavir)
Cidofovir (Vistide)	Trifluridine (Viroptic)
Ganciclovir (DHPG)	Valacyclovir (Valtrex)
Famciclovir (Famvir)	Valganciclovir (Valcyte)
Foscarnet (Foscavir)	

g. Ocular hypotony
h. Additive neutropenia with zidovudine
i. Carcinogenic, embryotoxic, antiteratogenic in experimental animals
j. Infertility in males and females: ganciclovir
k. Nephrotoxicity or hepatoxicity
l. Thrombocytopenic purpura
m. Pancreatitis

6. Nursing considerations
   a. Check allergies, including allergy to antiviral agents
   b. Assess baseline data to monitor effectiveness of drug and side effects
   c. Assess for neutropenic infection if immunosuppressed
   d. Assess renal function: creatinine, BUN, creatinine clearance, I & O
   e. Check hepatic function: ALT, AST, alkaline phosphatase, bilirubin
   f. Collaborate with prescriber if dosage needs adjustment for hepatic or renal dysfunction
   g. Analyze findings of CBC with differential, CD4 count, platelet count to monitor bone marrow activity, and for effectiveness of drug therapy
   h. Preexisting CNS disturbances may be exacerbated; assess orientation and reflexes; implement safety measures if CNS disturbances exist
   i. Assess skin and lesions regularly
   j. Hydrate to decrease risk of nephrotoxicity (e.g., 2,000 to 3,000 mL/fluids per day) if not contraindicated by other conditions
   k. Monitor relief of infection and of pain
   l. Monitor platelets and evidence of petechiae or increased risk of bleeding
   m. Monitor electrolytes and fluid balance
   n. Monitor nutritional status, especially if GI side effects occur; ensure adequate protein intake
   o. Provide safety measures if CNS effects occur to protect from injury

7. Client education
   a. Similar principles as in antibiotic therapy (Box 46–2); importance of completing full course of therapy with evenly distributed dosing that does not interrupt sleep (to improve effectiveness and prevent drug resistance)
   b. Self-administration techniques if indicated
   c. Clinical manifestations to report: severe side effects; evidence of increased bleeding, edema, fatigue; severe rash, especially if accompanied by blisters, fever, and other indications of infection to avert serious complications
   d. Avoid sexual intercourse if genital herpes being treated
   e. Avoid tactile contact of lesions by self and others to avoid spreading infection to new sites
   f. Avoid hazardous tasks and driving if drowsiness, dizziness, seizure activity occurs
   g. Ensure client follows up with labs and appointments with health care provider
   h. Offer frequent, small, high-protein meals
   i. Encourage 2,000 to 3,000 mL/day intake
   j. Female clients should have annual Pap smear since there is increased risk of cervical cancer with genital herpes infection
   k. Antiviral agents do not cure herpes and CMV infections
   l. Notify health care provider if lesions do not heal or if they recur

B. Protease inhibitors

1. Most potent of antiviral agents; inhibit cell protein synthesis that interferes with viral replication
2. Not curative but slow progression of AIDS and prolongs life
3. Used prophylactically because viral replication peaks before clinical manifestations of infection emerge and antiviral efficacy is then more limited; virus relies on using resources within live host cell, and there is increased risk for toxicity to host cell
4. Used in AIDS and AIDS-related complex (ARC) to decrease viral load and opportunistic infections

Box 46–15

Antiviral Medications for HIV and AIDS: Protease Inhibitors

Amprenavir (Agenerase)	Lopinavir/ritonavir (Kaletra)
Atazanavir (Reyataz)	Nelfinavir (Viracept)
Fosamprenavir (Lexiva)	Ritonavir (Norvir)
Indinavir (Crixivan)	Saquinavir (Invirase)

5. Used in combination to decrease viral load, increase CD4 counts, and decrease incidence or rate of development of drug resistance
6. Common medications are listed in Box 46–15
7. Administration considerations
   a. Give saquinavir (Invirase) with high-fat meals or within 2 hours of full meal
   b. Give ritonavir (Norvir) with chocolate milk, nutritional supplement, or food (ritonavir is unpalatable)
   c. Indinavir (Crixivan) requires an acidic gastric environment for absorption, so it should be taken 1 hour before or 2 hours after a light, low-fat snack and client should drink 1.5 liters or more of fluid daily
   d. Contraindicated in pregnant or lactating women, children, and hypersensitivity to drug
8. Side/adverse effects
   a. Headache, fatigue, nausea, vomiting, diarrhea, abdominal discomfort, anemia, taste perversion, asthenia, circumoral paresthesia with ritonavir
   b. Reversible hyperbilirubinemia and nephrolithiasis with indinavir (Crixivan): 1.5 liters or more of fluid daily are needed to prevent nephrolithiasis
   c. Hepatotoxicity; reduce dose in liver dysfunction
9. Nursing considerations
   a. Similar principles as for antibiotic therapy (Box 46–2)
   b. Monitor for hepatotoxicity: ALT, AST, alkaline phosphatase, bilirubin; observe for nausea, vomiting, jaundice, upper right abdominal quadrant enlargement and tenderness
   c. Monitor for nephrotoxicity: creatinine, BUN, creatinine clearance, urinalysis; keep accurate I & O
   d. Monitor CBC for blood dyscrasias such as neutropenia, thrombocytopenia, or anemia, and for improvement as evidenced by increased T-cell count
   e. Monitor for side effects; if neutropenic, observe for occult signs of infection (e.g., low back, flank, or suprapubic pain), normal temperature or low-grade fever related to UTI
   f. Saquinavir (Invirase): take with high-fat foods or within 2 hours of full meal
   g. Ritonavir (Norvir): take with chocolate milk, nutritional supplement, or food to counteract unpleasant taste
   h. Indinavir (Crixivan): take 1 hour before or 2 hours after light, low-fat snack; drink more than 1500 mL/day of fluids
   i. Provide neutropenic care as appropriate
10. Client education
   a. Similar principles as for antibiotic therapy (Box 46–3)
   b. Ensure fluid intake of at least 1,500 mL/day
   c. Take with food: saquinavir (Invirase) (high-fat foods recommended) and ritonavir (unpalatable taste)
   d. Take 1 hour before or 2 hours after light, low-fat snack: indinavir
   e. Eat small, frequent meals with complete or complementary proteins
   f. Use neutropenic precautions

C. Reverse transcriptase inhibitors

1. Block viral reverse transcriptase; stops replication/growth; effectiveness diminishes over time
2. Used for all symptomatic HIV clients with a CD4 count less than 500/mm^3 and some with higher counts; possible prophylaxis for known occupational HIV exposure

3. Penetrates blood–brain barrier
4. AZT is used to prevent maternal transmission of HIV
5. A major advantage of nonnucleoside reverse transcriptase inhibitors (NNRTIs) is that they do not adversely affect development of blood cells
6. There is no cross-resistance between nucleoside reverse transcriptase inhibitors (NRTIs) and NNRTIs
7. Used in combination because resistant strains rapidly evolve if used as single-agent therapy
8. Common medications are listed in Box 46–16
9. Administration considerations
   a. Crush or chew buffered tablets that are chewable because drug has acid lability
   b. Food may slow absorption but does not affect total absorption
   c. May administer at bedtime for better tolerance of CNS adverse effects
   d. Contraindicated with concurrent use of drugs that cause peripheral neuropathy
10. Side/adverse effects
    a. Neurological side effects of insomnia, confusion, peripheral neuropathies (numbness and tingling of extremities), dizziness, anxiety, tremors or seizures
    b. Diarrhea, pancreatitis
    c. Hypermagnesemia
    d. Discolored fingernails, rash
    e. Myalgias, altered taste sensations, cough
    f. Anemia, leukopenia, thrombocytopenia with nucleosides
    g. Nevirapine (Viramune): severe hepatotoxicity and dermatologic effects such as Stevens-Johnson syndrome
11. Nursing considerations
    a. Similar principles as for other anti-infective drugs (Box 46–2)
    b. Monitor baseline and periodic renal and liver test results
    c. Ensure client takes complete course and all drugs included in the regimen to improve effectiveness and retard risk for resistant strains emerging
    d. Administer around the clock as needed to maintain therapeutic levels
    e. Stop administration if severe rash or other hypersensitivity reaction occurs
    f. Assess client for complications of HIV infection (e.g., opportunistic infections, cancer, neurologic disease)
    g. Monitor level of consciousness (LOC), strength, appropriateness of activity, short-term memory, ability to follow complex commands, reasoning and calculation abilities, and peripheral sensation
    h. Assess for compromised respiratory or cardiovascular status
    i. Provide safety measures to protect from injury if CNS adverse effects occur
    j. Assess nutritional intake and tolerance
    k. Monitor skin and mucous membranes frequently
    l. Monitor renal function with labs, I & O, daily weight; monitor for reduced symptoms of AIDS or ARC and for increase in CD4 count
12. Client education
    a. Similar principles as for other anti-infective therapy (Box 46–3)
    b. Caution about risks of dizziness or altered mentation; do not drive or perform hazardous tasks

Box 46–16

Antiviral Medications for HIV and AIDS: Reverse Transcriptase Inhibitors

Nucleoside Reverse Transcriptase Inhibitors

Abacavir sulfate (Ziagen)
Didanosine (DDI)
Lamivudine (Epivir)
Stavudine (Zerit)
Zalcitabine (Hivid)
Zidovudine (AZT, Retrovir)

Nonnucleoside Reverse Transcriptase Inhibitors

Nevirapine (Viramune)
Delavirdine (Rescriptor)
Efavirenz (Sustiva)

c. Avoid crowds and persons with infections
d. Hair loss possible with zidovudine (AZT)
e. Drug does not cure but helps manage infection; it reduces viral load, decreases risk for complications, and extends survival
f. Practice good hygiene and safe sex practices

D. Medications for influenza and respiratory viruses

1. Are virustatic; most of viral replication has occurred before symptoms appear; bacterial replication occurs as signs of infection emerge, so antibacterial agents are more effective against bacterial infections than antiviral agents are against viral infections, since drug therapy relies on viral replication for effectiveness
2. Amantadine (Symmetrel and rimantadine (Flumadine) are used prophylactically for influenza A; increased efficacy if initiated at time of exposure or at least within 48 hours
   a. Adjunctive therapy for temporary immunization of influenza A
   b. May limit severity of influenza symptoms and/or decrease length or duration
3. Administration considerations
   a. Initiate drug therapy as soon as possible to enhance effectiveness and prevent complications of infection
   b. Administer before flu season for prophylactic purpose
4. Side/adverse effects
   a. Most are transient and resolve quickly after drug discontinued
   b. Dizziness, lightheadedness, headache, palpitations, mood and mental changes, drowsiness, insomnia, irritability, nightmares
   c. Dyspnea, rash, peripheral edema
   d. Orthostatic hypotension, nausea, vomiting, mouth dryness, urinary retention
   e. Slurred speech, ataxia, convulsions
   ! f. Leukopenia
   g. Possible digitalis toxicity with concurrent digoxin therapy
   h. Possible teratogenic
5. Nursing considerations
   a. Similar principles as for other anti-infectives (Box 46–2)
   b. Assess hepatic and renal dysfunction
   c. Assess baseline neurological status (e.g., orientation, affect, coordination, reflexes)
   d. Initiate drug therapy as soon as possible after exposure
   e. Monitor for respiratory deterioration in infants
   f. Provide safety precautions if CNS adverse effects develop
   g. Keep accurate I & O; monitor for urinary retention
   h. Avoid commercial mouthwashes that may potentiate dryness of mouth; provide oral care with water or saline rinses
6. Client education
   a. As per other types of anti-infectives (Box 46–3)
   b. Change position slowly to minimize risks of orthostatic hypotension
   c. Report increased respiratory distress or severe adverse effects to health care provider
   d. If drowsiness, dizziness, lightheadedness, confusion, ataxia, or blurred vision occur, do not drive or perform hazardous tasks
   e. If dry mouth develops, rinse mouth with plain warm water or warm water with one teaspoon of salt; avoid commercial mouthrinses with alcohol content and hydrogen peroxide that increase dry mouth; hard sugarless candy may stimulate salivation
   f. Drink at least 6 to 8 glasses of fluids a day

Box 46–17

Medications for Influenza and Respiratory Viruses

Amantadine (Symmetrel)
Rimantadine (Flumadine)

Box 46–18 Locally Active Antiviral Agents		
	Idoxuridine (Herplex)	Trifluridine (Viroptic)
	Imiquimod (Aldara)	Vidarabine (Vira–A)
	Penciclovir (Denavir)	

E. Locally active antiviral agents

1. Action and use: not absorbed systemically
2. Common medications are listed in Box 46–18
   - **a.** Idoxuridine (Herplex): topical ophthalmic agent to treat herpes simplex keratitis
   - **b.** Imiquimod (Aldara): genital and perianal warts
   - **c.** Penciclovir (Denavir): herpes simplex 1 or herpes labialis; cold sores on face and lips; do not apply to mucous membranes
   - **d.** Fomivirsen (Vitravene): ophthalmic solution injected into eye to treat CMV retinitis in clients with AIDS
   - **e.** Trifluridine (Viroptic): ophthalmic agent to treat herpes simplex infection of the eye
   - **f.** Vidarabine (Vira-A): ophthalmic agent to treat herpes simplex infection of eye not responsive to idoxuridine (Herplex)
3. Administration considerations
   - **a.** Wash hands well before applying medication
   - ! **b.** Wear gloves or use cotton-tip applicator to apply to skin lesions, being cautious not to contaminate drug or other sites on skin
   - **c.** Ensure proper administration technique
   - **d.** Stop drug if severe local adverse effect or open lesions develop
4. Contraindications use: caution in known hypersensitivity, pregnancy, lactation
5. Side effects
   - **a.** Local burning, stinging, discomfort may occur at time of application but usually resolve without intervention
   - **b.** Temporary visual impairment possible with optic application
6. Adverse effects/toxicity: skin eruptions and hypersensitivity
7. Nursing considerations
   - **a.** See previous section on administration considerations
   - **b.** Monitor for comfort, safety, and compliance
8. Client education
   - **a.** Similar principles as for other anti-infectives (Box 46–3)
   - **b.** Does not cure but alleviates pain and discomfort and prevents extended damage to uninvolved tissue
   - **c.** Report severe local discomfort or reaction to health care provider

IX. ANTIFUNGALS

A. Systemic antifungals

1. Fungistatic or fungicidal depending on therapeutic serum levels and sensitivity to fungi
2. Treat candida infections, cryptococcus, blastomycosis, histoplasmosis, aspergillus fumigates, and **tinea** infections (a fungal infection caused by ringworm)
3. Increased permeability of cell membranes better enables other drugs to enter fungus cell
4. Common medications are listed in Box 46–19
5. Administration considerations
   - **a.** Administer carefully as ordered, especially IV dosages
   - **b.** Combination of antifungal agents may deter or retard drug resistance
   - **c.** May premedicate amphotericin with an antipyretic such as acetaminophen (Tylenol), an antihistamine such as diphenhydramine (Benadryl), an antiemetic, and meperidine (Demerol) to reduce severity of fever/chills response; heparin or hydrocortisone (Cortaid) added to the IV solution may reduce risk for thrombophlebitis at IV site

Box 46–19

Systemic Antifungal Medications

Amphotericin B (Fungizone)
Amphotericin B Liposomal Complex (Ambisome)
Amphotericin B Cholesteryl Sulfate Complex (Amphotec)
Clotrimazole (Mycelex troche)
Fluconazole (Diflucan)
Flucytosine (Ancobon)
Griseofulvin (Grifulvin V)
Itraconazole (Sporanox)
Ketoconazole (Nizoral)
Miconazole (Monistat)
Nystatin (Mycostatin)
Terbinafine (Lamisil)
Variconazole (V fend)

d. Give with amphoteracin B with heparin or hydrocortisone and over 4 to 6 hours to avert clinical manifestations of hypersensitivity or drug toxicity

! **e.** Hydrate with IV fluids usually 2 hours before and 2 hours after amphoteracin B administration to decrease risk for nephrotoxicity

f. To test for hypersensitivity to amphoteracin B prior to administration, deliver 1 mg/20 mL D_5W IV over 10 to 30 minutes; if test elicits hypersensitivity response, a lipid preparation such as amphotericin B liposomal complex (Ambisome) may be given to minimize the severe fever, shaking, and chills; premedicate as above

g. Mix amphoteracin B in D_5W only; precipitates form in any solution containing sodium chloride

h. Amphotericin B Liposomal Complex: shake gently to distribute drug particles; use 5-micrometer filter needle to inject agent into container of D_5W and thoroughly disperse drug throughout solution; redisperse drug in solution every 2 hours if infusion time extends beyond 2 hours; no in-line filter used

i. Contraindicated in hypersensitivity; use cautiously in pregnant and lactating clients, or those with renal impairment or severe bone marrow depression

6. Side/adverse effects
a. Thrombophlebitis with administration through peripheral vein
b. Fever, chills, shaking, headache
c. Anorexia, nausea, vomiting during or after administration; heartburn, diarrhea, flatulence
d. Myalgia, arthralgia, weakness, hypotension
e. Insomnia, vertigo, confusion
f. Taste acuity diminished or causes unpleasant taste; furry tongue with griseofulvin (Grifulvin V)
g. Photosensitivity, rash, pruritus, dry skin, urticaria
h. Hypokalemia or hypomagnesemia, especially with concurrent use of glucocorticosteroids or diuretics
i. Ketoconazole (Nizoral): sexual impotency, hair loss, and gynecomastia
j. Bone marrow depression resulting in neutropenia, thrombocytopenia, anemia
k. Ototoxicity and nephrotoxicity with amphotericin B preparations
l. Drug toxicity or hypersensitivity: fever, chills, shaking, piloerection, headache, anorexia, nausea and vomiting
m. Stevens-Johnson syndrome, **superinfections** (candidiasis, diarrhea)
n. Cardiovascular collapse with too rapid infusion

7. Nursing considerations
a. Similar principles as for other anti-infectives (Box 46–2); check for incompatibility of solutions as there are many
b. Assess for pregnancy, lactation, liver or renal dysfunction; monitor liver and renal laboratory studies throughout therapy
c. Monitor serum levels of antifungal agents
d. Monitor WBC for improvement and for early detection of developing neutropenia, thrombocytopenia, anemia
e. Give potassium supplements if hypokalemia occurs

f. Protect amphoteracin B from light, and monitor client's intake and output

8. Client education
   a. Similar principles as for other anti-infectives (Box 46–3); know length of therapy (e.g., Amphotericin B may be given over weeks or months)
   b. Report adverse effects such as burning at IV site, increased bleeding or bruising, evidence of superinfection
   c. Febrile reaction may decrease over time
   d. Fluid intake of 2,000 to 3,000 mL/day if not contraindicated by other conditions
   e. Eat small, frequent meals with high-quality protein
   f. Take oral agents with food to minimize GI distress

B. Topical antifungals

1. Action and use
   a. Local infections of skin and mucous membranes of oropharynx, vagina, or intestines caused by Candida species; infections of tinea pedis (athlete's foot), tinea cruris (in scrotal, crural, anal, and genital areas, called "jock itch"), tinea corporis (skin), tinea unguium or onychomycosis (nail fungus), tinea manus, tinea versicolor (infection of skin with yellow or beige brawny patches)
   b. Use vaginal tablets up to 6 weeks prior to delivery to prevent newborn thrush
2. Common medications are listed in Box 46–20
3. Administration considerations
   a. Oral tablets or lozenges/troches are not to be chewed or swallowed whole; swallow saliva as lozenge/troche dissolves slowly over 5 to 30 minutes; avoid food or drink during and for 30 minutes after administration
   b. For oral infections in client with dentures, remove dentures at bedtime; with oral suspension, remove dentures before each rinse or before each oral lozenge/troche
   c. ! For application to skin: wear latex gloves, cleanse area with tepid water (soap if prescribed), dry thoroughly (without application of heat), and apply antifungal to infected area sparingly; do not cover with an occlusive dressing or tight clothing; wash hands well after removing gloves
   d. For treatment of tinea pedis (athlete's foot), apply antifungal powder such as nystatin (Mycostatin) to inside of shoes and stockings
   e. For vulvovaginal use: insert one applicator full or one vaginal tablet into vagina at bedtime as instructed; continue therapy during menstruation
   f. Avoid contact of antifungal with eyes; with certain agents, avoid contact with mucous membranes
   g. ! Do not apply occlusive dressing unless prescribed; client to avoid restrictive clothing in areas of infection
   h. Store creams, vaginal application, and topical preparation at room temperature; if specified for vaginal tablets and troches, refrigerate but do not freeze
   i. Contraindicated with drug hypersensitivity
4. Side/adverse effects
   a. Topical: stinging, burning, erythema, edema, dry skin, vesication, pruritis, urticaria, desquamation, skin fissures
   b. Vaginal: slight burning, lower abdominal discomfort, bloating, erythema, itching, vaginal soreness during intercourse
   c. Oral troches or swish and swallow: nausea and vomiting
   d. Possible hepatotoxicity in client with liver impairment

Box 46–20

Topical Antifungal Medications

Amphotericin B (Fungizone)	Butenafine (Mentax)
Ketoconazole (Nizoral)	Edorazole nitrate (Spectazole)
Miconazole (Monistat)	Haloprogin (Halotex)
Nystatin (Mycostatin)	Terbinafine cream (Lamisil)
Clotrimazole (Mycelex)	

5. Nursing considerations
   a. Ensure complete course of therapy taken
   b. Observe for clinical signs of improvement
   c. Observe for clinical evidence of liver dysfunction, such as upper right quadrant tenderness, abdominal discomfort or bloating, lethargy, mentation changes, icterus, enlarged liver, elevated liver enzymes (ALT, AST, alkaline phosphatase, bilirubin)
   d. Stop application if severe burning or exacerbation of lesions occur and collaborate with prescriber
6. Client education
   a. Know drug name, purpose, dose, strength, how to apply, schedule of administration, length of therapy
   b. Observe for resolution of signs and symptoms within first week of therapy; some infections require 2 to 4 weeks of treatment; notify health care provider if condition worsens or no improvement is noted in 1 to 2 weeks
   c. Store in tightly covered container at room temperature; if vaginal tablet or suppository, store as recommended, usually in refrigerator or above 59 degrees F; avoid freezing or excess heat of all products
   d. If taken vaginally, refrain from sexual intercourse or have partner wear condom to avoid burning or irritation of penis or urethra
   e. ! Clothing and linens in contact with infectious sites should be washed after each treatment with soap and water; ointments may be removed from fabric with commercial cleaning products
   f. If severe burning, stinging, or eruptions occur, discontinue use and notify health care provider
   g. See previous administration considerations for specific information regarding types of applications

X. ANTIPROTOZOALS

A. Antimalarials

1. Action and use
   a. Therapeutic use to treat acute episodes or prophylaxis to prevent malarial infection
   b. Chloroquine treatment for **giardiasis** (a protozoan intestinal infection) and amebiasis outside the GI tract
   c. Quinacrine (Atabrine): treat dwarf tapeworm giardiasis and cestodiosis (infestation with tapeworms); pleural sclerosing agent to prevent recurrence of pneumothorax
2. Common medications are listed in Box 46–21
3. Administration considerations
   a. Separate drug from antacid administration by 4 hours before or after antacids

Box 46–21

Antiprotozoal Medications

Antimalarials	**Other Antiprotozoal Medications**
Chloroquine HCl (Aralen HCl)	Emetine HCl
Chloroquine phosphate (Aralen Phosphate)	Paromomycin (Humatin)
Hydroxychloroquine sulfate (Plaquenil Sulfate)	Pentamidine isoethionate (Pentam 300)
Mefloquine HCl (Lariam)	Lindane (Kwell)
Primaquine phosphate	Atovaquone (Mepron)
Pyrimethamine (Daraprim)	Iodoquinol (Dioquinol)
Quinacrine (Atabrine)	Metronidazole (Flagyl)
Quinine sulfate (Quinamm)	Primaquine phosphate

b. Take quinine sulfate with food to decrease GI distress and mask bitter taste; do not crush capsule
c. Quinacrine HCL (Atabrine): take after food with full glass of water, tea, or juice
d. Chloroquine HCL (Aralen HCL), hydroxychloroquine sulfate (Plaquenil Sulfate), and pyrimethamine (Daraprim): take with food to minimize GI distress
e. For prophylaxis, take as prescribed, such as same day every week when entering high-risk area and for 10 weeks after departing
f. Mefloquine HCL (Lariam): take with at least 8 ounces water; separate by at least 8 hours from ingestion of quinine or quinidine, an antidysrhythmic

4. Side/adverse effects
   a. Dizziness, vertigo, headache, visual impairment, angina
   b. Nausea, vomiting, diarrhea, gastric distress, abdominal cramps
   c. Confusion, apprehension, insomnia, nightmares, syncope, delirium
   d. Cutaneous flushing, pruritus, rash, paresthesia, dyspnea, weight loss, fatigue
   e. Quinacrine HCL: may cause reversible yellowing of skin or gray-blue hue to ears, nasal cartilage, and nail beds (not jaundice/cyanosis)
   f. Chloroquine HCL and hydroxychloroquine sulfate: alopecia, bleaching of scalp or hair (including eyebrows and body hair) and freckles; bluish black hue of skin or mucous membranes, rash, pruritis, photophobia
   g. Tinnitus, hearing loss
   h. Cardiotoxicity in clients with atrial fibrillation
   i. Leukopenia, thrombocytopenia, agranulocytosis, hypoprothrombinemia, hemolytic anemia
   j. Hypotension, tachypnea, tachycardia, hypothermia
   k. Convulsions, coma, cardiovascular collapse, blackwater fever (extensive intravascular hemolysis with renal failure), death
   l. Visual halos, blurring, inability to focus
5. Nursing considerations
   a. Similar principles as for other anti-infectives (Box 46–2)
   b. Assess hepatic and cardiac function at intervals
   c. Assess for electrolyte disturbances, blood disorders as anemia, thrombocytopenia
   d. If client is taking anticonvulsants, monitor drug levels of these agents
   e. Ensure regular ophthalmic exams, electcardiograms, and lab tests as ordered
   f. Assess for G6PD deficiency as indicated
   g. Assess for muscle weakness and depressed deep tendon reflexes periodically; assess for CNS side effects; collaborate with prescriber regarding discontinuation of agent
6. Client education
   a. Similar principles as for other anti-infectives (Box 46–3)
   b. If weekly, take on same day every week
   c. Do not drive or perform hazardous tasks if drowsiness, dizziness, vertigo, visual disturbances occur
   d. Report fever, sore throat, myalgias, visual disturbances, anxiety, mental changes, hallucinations
   e. Chloroquine HCl: sunglasses may decrease risk of photophobia or ocular changes; urine may become rusty yellow or brown

B. Other antiprotozoals

1. Action and use
   a. Amebic dysentery, hepatic amebiasis, or abscess
   b. Some are bacteriocidal as well as amebicidal, especially in GI tract
   c. Paromomycin (Humatin): bactericidal and amebicidal related to tape worms
   d. Destroy intestinal bacteria that form nitrogen to decrease ammonia in hepatic disease and coma
   e. Pentamidine isethionate (Pentem 300): treat *pneumocystis carinii* pneumonia, an opportunistic infection in client with AIDS
   f. Kills insects, parasites, and their ova, such as in head lice, body lice, and scabies
2. Common medications are listed in Box 46–21

3. Administration considerations
   a. Pentamidine isoethionate: decreased doses in renal dysfunction
   b. Rotate IM injection sites
   c. Administer atovaquone with high-fat meal (more than 23 grams fat) to increase absorption
   d. Use caution in pregnancy and lactation; contraindicted with hypersensitivity to drug or to iodine, iodoquinol (Dioquinol), or primaquin
4. Side/adverse effects
   a. Hypotension, tachycardia, dizziness, headache, syncope, dysrhythmias
   b. Flushing, pruritis, dyspnea
   c. Abdominal cramps, diarrhea, nausea, vomiting, epigastric distress, unpleasant taste
   d. Myalgia, precordial stiffness
   e. Tremors, restlessness
   f. Nephrotoxicity: mild, reversible
   g. Leukopenia, neutropenia, anemia, thrombocytopenia
   h. Hypoglycemia related to pancreatitis
   i. Large doses can cause abscess, cellulitis, or lesion in muscle in the GI tract, heart, liver, and kidneys
   j. Pain at injection site
   k. Lindane (Kwell) topical shampoo can cause CNS problems, such as convulsions, or eczematous eruptions
5. Nursing considerations
   a. Ensure complete course of therapy is taken for full benefit
   b. Assess skin for scabies, tracking, lesions, nits
   c. For scabies: warm (not hot) shower and apply topical Kwell, then rinse off after 24 hours
   d. For lice: massage Kwell into head or area infected; leave on for 5 minutes and shampoo out; do not get agent into eyes or on face; do not repeat in less than 1 week
6. Client education
   a. Know drug, dose, purpose, schedule, proper administration technique
   b. Take full course of therapy for best effect
   c. Report side or adverse effects to health care provider
   d. Wash clothes and linens after treatment to prevent reinfection
   e. Know clinical manifestations of infections to recognize and report

XI. ANTIHELMINTHICS

A. Action and use

1. Intestinal worms: *Ascaris lumbricoides, Trichostrongylus*
2. Pinworm: *Enterobius vermicularis*
3. Hook worms: *Ancytostoma duodenale, Necator americanus*

B. Common medications are listed in Box 46–22

C. Administration considerations

1. Mebendazole: may be chewed, swallowed whole, crushed, mixed with food
2. Pyrantel pamoate: may take with food
3. Thiabendazole: take after meals

D. Contraindications

1. Known hypersensitivity
2. Paromomycin: in intestinal obstruction
3. Piperazine citrate: in renal or hepatic impairment, convulsive disorders
4. Caution with other antihelminthics in clients with hepatic or renal dysfunction
5. Safety not established in pregnancy and lactation

Box 46–22
Antihelminthics

Mebendazole (Vermox)	Pyrantel pamoate (Antiminth)
Piperazine citrate (Antepar)	Thiabendazole (Mintezol)

E. Side/adverse effects
1. Nausea, vomiting, diarrhea, abdominal cramps, anorexia
2. Rash, urticaria, erythema multiforme, photosensitivity, purpura, lacrimation, rhinorrhea
3. Dizziness, drowsiness, vision changes
4. Fever, productive cough, anemia
5. Thiabendazole: urinary odor
6. Neurotoxicity: headache, vertigo, ataxia, tremors, jerking movements, muscle weakness, paresthesia, depressed reflexes, mental changes, abnormal ECG, seizures
7. Dose-related neutropenia; reversed with discontinuation of drug

F. Nursing considerations
1. Similar principles as for other anti-infectives (Box 46–2)
2. Assess laboratory findings for hepatic, renal, or blood disorders and to verify diagnosis
3. Collect stool specimen for ova and parasites (O & P) for baseline and follow-up to verify eradication of infectious agents

G. Client education
1. Similar principles as for other anti-infectives (Box 46–3)
2. Agents may be taken with or after food to minimize GI distress
3. Store drug at room temperature protected from light and heat
4. Do not repeat drug therapy for continued infection until one week after initial treatment
5. Practice personal hygiene to prevent transmission
6. Urine odor may occur with thiabendazole

Check Your NCLEX-RN® Exam I.Q.

You are ready for testing on this content if you can

- Apply knowledge of expected actions and effects of anti-infective and immunological medications to client care.
- Correctly describe administration of anti-infective and immunological medications to clients.
- Assess for side effects and adverse effects of anti-infective and immunological medications.
- Take appropriate action if a client has an unexpected response to an anti-infective or immunological medication.
- Monitor a client for expected outcomes or effects of treatment with anti-infective and immunological medications.

PRACTICE TEST

1 A client has a new order to receive vancomycin (Vancocin) to treat a systemic infection. The nurse anticipates the order would indicate which of the following routes to be best administered?

1. Peripheral venous access
2. Central venous access
3. Intramuscular
4. Oral

2 Gentamicin (Garamycin) therapy is to be initiated. Which of the following laboratory test results would indicate to the nurse that the client is manifesting a common adverse effect?

1. Elevated urine creatinine clearance
2. Increased prothrombin time (PT)
3. Increased serum creatinine
4. Hypokalemia

3 The nurse teaches the client who is taking isoniazid (INH) and experiencing paresthesia as a common side effect to include what food in the diet?

1. Liver
2. Peanuts
3. Whole milk
4. Raw apples

PRACTICE TEST

4 A client taking digoxin (Lanoxin) along with amphotericin B (Fungizone) may experience digitalis toxicity because of which of the following?

1. Hypokalemia
2. Antifungal attaching to receptors before digoxin
3. Increased plasma concentration of amphotericin B
4. Increased gastrointestinal absorption of digoxin and amphotericin B

5 A client is receiving levofloxacin (Levaquin) in addition to an oral anticoagulant. Which of the following treatments would the nurse anticipate administering if the client experiences an adverse drug effect as a result of this combination?

1. Albumin
2. Platelets
3. Protamine sulfate
4. Phytonadione (Vitamin K)

6 The nurse assesses a client taking doxycycline (Vibramycin) as being jaundiced and lethargic. What laboratory study would be most specific for the nurse to assess?

1. Bilirubin
2. Alkaline phosphatase (ALP)
3. Alanine aminotransferase (ALT or SGPT)
4. Aspartate aminotransferase (AST or SGOT)

7 A client taking ampicillin (Omnipen) develops a macular rash on the chest. The nurse should draw which of the following conclusions about this assessment finding?

1. This reaction is a Stevens-Johnson syndrome.
2. A minor rash usually precipitates the development of more severe reactions.
3. A minor rash requires notification of the prescriber but may be well tolerated and fade with continued treatment.
4. Hypersensitivity reactions requiring discontinuation of the antibiotic occur to some extent with many clients taking a penicillin agent.

8 The nurse teaches the client who is started on erythromycin (Erythrocin) as treatment for pneumonia to contact the health care provider for which of the following reasons?

1. Improvement of fever, cough, or respiratory effort is not observed in 48 to 72 hours
2. Client is taking fluids orally but continues to refuse to eat after 24 hours
3. Client develops anorexia and nausea within 24 hours
4. Fever fluctuates

9 A child with otitis media is taking trimethoprim-sulfamethoxazole (TMP-SMZ) as a suspension. The nurse provides what instruction to the mother?

1. Do not allow the child to drink water immediately after taking the medication.
2. The medication is to be taken on an empty stomach.
3. The medication must be kept refrigerated.
4. Use a calibrated measuring device.

10 A client receiving an anti-infective drug begins to wheeze. The nurse anticipates initial administration of what drug?

1. Epinephrine HCL (Adrenalin Chloride)
2. Methylprednisolone (Solu-Medrol)
3. Atropine sulfate (Atropine)
4. Dopamine HCL (Intropin)

11 The nurse would teach a client that alcohol taken in conjunction with which of the following ordered medications can cause a reaction causing flushing, dizziness, pounding headache, sweating, abdominal cramps, nausea, irritability, and low blood pressure?

1. Cefoxitan (Mefoxin)
2. Metronidazole (Flagyl)
3. Clindamycin (Cleocin)
4. Ampicillin (Omnipen)

12 The nurse assesses the client receiving cefotazime (Claforan) and notes three diarrhea stools in the past 24 hours, rectal itching, glossitis, and fever. The nurse concludes these adverse effects probably indicate which of the following?

1. Leukocytosis
2. Opportunistic infection
3. Bone marrow depression
4. Drug failure against original infective organism

13 What teaching or intervention is appropriate for a client taking an antibiotic that causes diarrhea secondary to elimination of normal intestinal flora?

1. Test stool for occult blood.
2. Include yogurt or buttermilk products in the diet.
3. Arrange for IV administration instead of oral route for the antibiotic.
4. Take antacids with oral antibiotic to slow absorption of antibiotic and reduce severity of the diarrhea.

14 A disulfiram-like reaction occurs in a client taking cefoperazone sodium (Cefobid). The nurse suspects this reaction is a drug interaction resulting from the client's ingestion of which of the following substances within the last few hours?

1. Caffeine in tea or coffee
2. Sulfamethoxazole (Gantonol) for a chronic urinary tract infection
3. Alcohol-containing cough syrup
4. Ampicillin (Omnipen), which has a cross-sensitivity to cephalosporins

15 The nurse evaluates for an adverse reaction to tobramycin sulfate (Tobrex) by conducting what assessment?

1. Capillary refill
2. Romberg's test
3. Chvostek's sign
4. Babzinski's reflex

16 What does the nurse teach an adult premenopausal client receiving griseofulvin microsize (Grisfulvin V) for a systemic antifungal condition?

1. If taking oral contraceptives, use an alternative form of contraception during and for 1 month after use of griseofulvin.
2. Keep a record of the number of absorbent products used daily to monitor for increased menstrual flow while taking griseofulvin.
3. Check blood pressure daily during treatment if taking oral contraceptive and griseofulvin because both can increase blood pressure.
4. Avoid taking calcium supplements concurrently with griseofulvin.

17 Because of the mechanisms of action of tetracycline, the client needs to have which of the following in order for the drug to be effective?

1. A competent client immune system
2. Concurrent administration of iron
3. Supplemental pyridoxine HCL (Vitamin B_6)
4. Weekly evaluation of the complete blood count

18 The nurse assesses for which lab result when a client is receiving long-term oral anticoagulation therapy and is also taking a Beta-lactam penicillin?

1. Decreased bleeding time
2. Increased thrombin time (TT)
3. Increased prothrombin time (PT)
4. Increased activated partial thromboplastin time (APPT)

19 During a routine screening, a client has a positive response to intradermal injection of purified protein derivative (PPD or Mantoux test). The nurse draws which of the following conclusions about this result?

1. The client is currently infectious.
2. The client has active tuberculosis.
3. The client has been exposed to the tubercle bacillus within the past 2 weeks.
4. The client has been infected with tuberculosis and has developed a cellular (T cell) response to the tubercle bacillus.

20 Appropriate teaching for a young adult female related to a new prescription for ampicillin (Omnipen) orally would include to do which of the following?

1. Observe for easy bruising.
2. Observe for clinical extrapyramidal tract manifestations.
3. Change positions slowly to avoid orthostatic hypotension.
4. If applicable, use an alternative to oral contraceptives during and for 1 month after therapy.

PRACTICE TEST

21 A female client is taking sargramostim (Leukine) following a bone marrow transplant. During an assessment, the client voices concern about her hair falling out. Based on this assessment, which of the following would be the priority nursing diagnosis?

1. Impaired skin integrity
2. Alopecia
3. Disturbed body image
4. Anxiety

22 A client receiving aldesleukin (Proleukin) begins to complain of a fever and pain. Which of the following is the priority nursing diagnostic statement for this client?

1. Risk for deficient fluid volume related to flulike symptoms
2. Ineffective airway clearance related to fever
3. Excess fluid volume related to flulike symptoms
4. Ineffective airway clearance related to increased pulmonary secretions

23 Clients receiving oprelvekin (Neumega) should be assessed frequently for signs and symptoms of which of the following?

1. Dehydration
2. Congestive heart failure (CHF)
3. Anxiety
4. Hyperuricemia

24 Based on the prescribed therapy of mycophenolate (Cell Cept), the nurse can expect the renal transplant client to receive the first dose at which of the following times?

1. In the postanesthesia recovery area
2. Within 1 hour of admission to intensive care
3. Seventy-two hours following the transplant
4. One week following the transplant

25 A 28-year-old male client is admitted to the emergency department with a 3-inch laceration over his left eye. The nurse should assess which of the following priority items related to the risk of infection before beginning drug therapy to prevent infection?

1. The client's temperature
2. The date of the client's last tetanus vaccine
3. If the client's blood pressure is decreased
4. Whether the client is taking corticosteroid medication

26 A pitbull dog has bitten a 28-year-old woman. Upon admission to the emergency room, the nurse will administer the prescribed antirabies serum (equine) into which of the following locations?

1. Intravenously
2. Intramuscularly into the right gluteal muscle
3. Into the animal bite
4. Z-track into the anterolateral thigh

27 In conducting client teaching about Beta 1b (Betaseron), the nurse would explain that the goal of the administration is which of the following?

1. Cure the client of multiple sclerosis.
2. Prevent signs and symptoms of anaphylaxis.
3. Destroy nerve tissue that is laden with plaque.
4. Decrease the demyelination in brain tissue.

28 To decrease renal insufficiency side effects in clients receiving cyclophosphamide (Sandimmune), the nurse should instruct the client to do which of the following?

1. Consume a diet high in fiber.
2. Have a creatinine level assessed weekly.
3. Drink 3,000 mL of fluid per day.
4. Administer hydrochlorothiazide (HCTZ) with cyclophosphamide.

29 To assess a client's baseline prior to the administration of azathioprine (Imuran), the nurse should put highest priority in evaluating which of the following laboratory test results?

1. Creatinine
2. Uric acid
3. PT and PTT
4. Red blood cell count

30 Azathioprine (Imuran) and allopurinol (Zyloprim) are administered to a client diagnosed with both multiple sclerosis and gout. It is important for the nurse to assess the results of which of the following laboratory tests in this client?

1. Creatinine
2. Uric acid
3. Blood glucose
4. Blood urea nitrogen (BUN)

31 A client is scheduled for diagnostic testing for myasthenia gravis. The nurse would prepare which of the following medications necessary for this testing?

1. Ambenonium (Mytelase)
2. Edrophonium (Tensilon)
3. Neostigmine (Prostigmin)
4. Physostigmine (Eserine)

32 Which of the following points should be included in a teaching plan for a client regarding medications to treat multiple sclerosis?

1. The signs and symptoms of pulmonary edema
2. The restriction of fluids
3. The requirement to remain restricted from crowds
4. The requirement to exercise to enhance muscle strength

33 A client has been exposed to hepatitis A. Which of the following client factors would be an indication for withholding administration of immune serum globulin to the client?

1. The client has received a hepatitis B vaccine.
2. The client has recently fallen and suffered a hip fracture.
3. The client has a history of a coagulation disorder.
4. The client is scheduled for foreign travel.

34 A client with Parkinson's disease is admitted to the emergency department with lethargy, hypotension, and weakened gait. The nurse should be prepared to administer which of the following medications?

1. Carbidopa (Lodosyn)
2. Levodopa (Dopar)
3. Atropine (generic)
4. Physostigmine (Eserine)

35 To prevent toxicity during IV administration of physostigmine (Eserine), the nurse should administer the medication:

1. retrograde.
2. through a central line.
3. concurrently with Parlodel.
4. no faster than 1 mg per minute.

ANSWERS & RATIONALES

1 **Answer: 2** Because vancomycin (Vancocin) can cause thrombophlebitis, this adverse effect is less likely to occur with central IV administration than with a peripheral IV administration (option 1). Dilution of the drug lessens irritation to the vein. Vancomycin is not absorbed in the GI tract, so oral route is used only to treat *Clostridium difficile* associated with antibiotic-induced pseudomembranous colitis (option 4). Intramuscular administration is contraindicated (option 3). **Cognitive Level:** Application **Client Need:** Physiological Integrity: Pharmacological and Parenteral Therapies **Integrated Process:** Nursing Process: Planning **Content Area:** Pharmacology **Strategy:** Focus on the critical word *systemic* in the stem of the question. Use this word and knowledge of safe administration of this drug to eliminate the incorrect options regarding best route.

2 **Answer: 3** Increased serum creatinine indicates renal dysfunction. Nephrotoxicity is a common adverse effect of aminoglycosides such as gentamicin. The urine creatinine clearance would be decreased in renal impairment (option 1). Coagulation disturbances and hypokalemia are not attributed to this class of antibiotic as a direct adverse reaction (options 2 and 4). **Cognitive Level:** Application **Client Need:** Physiological Integrity: Pharmacological and Parenteral Therapies **Integrated Process:** Nursing Process: Analysis **Content Area:** Pharmacology **Strategy:** Note the critical words *common adverse effect* in the stem. Recall that aminoglycosides often adversely affect the kidneys to narrow the options to 1 and 3. Note that 3 indicates renal impairment to select it over option 1.

3 **Answer: 1** Peripheral neuritis is the most common side effect of isoniazid (INH). Adding vitamin B_6 (pyridoxine) to the client's intake is the therapy to correct this side effect. The diet may be supplemented with vitamin B_6. Foods highest in vitamin B_6 include beef, liver, chicken, and pork including beef liver and chicken liver. Other foods listed are not high in pyridoxine. Foods other than meats that could be included are raw avocados, baked potato with skin, raw banana, figs, and soybeans. **Cognitive Level:** Application **Client Need:** Physiological Integrity: Pharmacological and Parenteral Therapies **Integrated Process:** Nursing Process: Implementation **Content Area:** Pharmacology **Strategy:** The core issue of the question is knowledge of what nutrient will reduce adverse drug effects of INH. Recall that vitamin B_6 will assist in this action and then choose the food that is highest in this vitamin.

4 **Answer: 1** Amphotericin-induced hypokalemia may potentiate toxicity of digoxin because hypokalemia is a primary cause for digitalis toxicity. Amphotericin B is available for only intravenous and topical routes. Antifungal agents and cardioglycosides do not compete for the same receptor sites. **Cognitive Level:** Comprehension **Client Need:** Physiological Integrity: Pharmacological and Parenteral Therapies **Integrated Process:** Nursing Process: Analysis **Content Area:** Pharmacology **Strategy:** The core issue of the question is knowledge of drug

interaction of digoxin and amphotericin B. Use specific nursing knowledge and the process of elimination to make a selection.

5 **Answer: 4** Eradication of the intestinal flora can occur during antibiotic therapy. Absorption of vitamin K from the intestines can be interrupted, and prolonged bleeding may result because of inadequate serum level of prothrombin (hypothrombinemia). Vitamin K is essential to the synthesis of prothrombin (factor II) by the liver. Appropriate therapy in this case is to administer phytonadione or menadiol sodium diphosphate (Synkayvite). Since intestinal absorption may not be optimal, parenteral route is preferred. In addition, the nurse must assess for and protect against increased bleeding.
Cognitive Level: Analysis **Client Need:** Physiological Integrity: Pharmacological and Parenteral Therapies **Integrated Process:** Nursing Process: Planning **Content Area:** Pharmacology **Strategy:** The core issue of the question is knowledge of drug interaction between levofloxacin and oral anticoagulants. Recall that vitamin K reverses bleeding to help narrow down the selection to a drug that reverses the effect of oral anticoagulant drugs.

6 **Answer: 3** ALT is specific for diagnosing and monitoring liver disease or impairment. Differential diagnosis of etiology of jaundice between hepatic dysfunction and hemolysis of red blood cells is indicated by the bilirubin. AST may help to diagnose or monitor clients with heart disease or disease of the liver.
Cognitive Level: Analysis **Client Need:** Physiological Integrity: Pharmacological and Parenteral Therapies **Integrated Process:** Nursing Process: Analysis **Content Area:** Pharmacology **Strategy:** The core issue of the question is the laboratory test that will help evaluate the presence of jaundice as an adverse effect of doxycycline. Use specific nursing knowledge and the process of elimination to make a selection.

7 **Answer: 3** A minor rash is the most common side effect of the penicillins and may be relatively insignificant. Its presence does not signify an allergic reaction and does not prohibit future administration of penicillin. However, the nurse closely monitors for further hypersensitivity reaction because other clinical manifestations may develop, such as fever, urticaria, chills, erythema, Stevens-Johnson syndrome, respiratory distress, and anaphylaxis. If itching occurs, an antihistamine as diphenhydramine (Benadryl) may be prescribed. All available antimicrobials are capable of stimulating an exaggerated immune response, but not all clients experience allergy with antibiotic therapy. Stevens-Johnson syndrome is a more serious aberration of the skin associated with antimicrobial adverse reactions; it resembles a second-degree burn in that necrolysis separates the epidermis from the dermis, causing blisters.
Cognitive Level: Analysis **Client Need:** Physiological Integrity: Pharmacological and Parenteral Therapies **Integrated Process:** Nursing Process: Analysis **Content Area:** Pharmacology **Strategy:** The core issue of the question is the significance of a rash that develops in a client taking ampicillin. Use specific nursing knowledge and the process of elimination to make a selection. Recall that not all drug rashes indicate hypersensitivity to aid in choosing the correct option.

8 **Answer: 1** Improvement in clinical manifestations of the infection should be noted within 48 to 72 hours. Otherwise, compliance with prescribed drug therapy should be assessed and adjustment of drug, dose, and/or administration frequency may be needed. Anorexia, nausea, and fluctuating febrile state may be common sequelae in systemic infections (options 3 and 4). The client's ability to take in fluids can temporarily sustain his or her nutritional status for a few days, particularly if dietary supplements are also included, which is appropriate for client education (option 2).
Cognitive Level: Application **Client Need:** Physiological Integrity: Pharmacological and Parenteral Therapies **Integrated Process:** Nursing Process: Implementation **Content Area:** Pharmacology **Strategy:** The core issue of the question is knowledge of unsatisfactory progress after beginning erythromycin and indicators that need to be reported to the prescriber. Use specific nursing knowledge and the process of elimination to make a selection.

9 **Answer: 4** The volume of a household teaspoon may vary by 2 to 10 mL, so a calibrated device is necessary for accurate dosing. The suspension is to be shaken to disperse the particles just prior to measurement. It is recommended that a glass of water be given with the medication and that adequate urinary output be maintained (option 1). The medication is stable at room temperature, but the taste may be more palatable if cold (option 3). Food does not interfere with absorption of the medication and may help to minimize gastrointestinal side effects (option 2).
Cognitive Level: Application **Client Need:** Physiological Integrity: Pharmacological and Parenteral Therapies **Integrated Process:** Nursing Process: Implementation **Content Area:** Pharmacology **Strategy:** The core issue of the question is the proper method of administration of trimethoprim-sulfamethoxazole to a child. Use specific nursing knowledge and the process of elimination to make a selection.

10 **Answer: 1** Epinephrine is the primary drug used when bronchoconstriction causes inadequate respiratory exchange, as in anaphylactic shock. Marked improvement in respiration occurs within a few minutes after subcutaneous administration of 0.1 to 0.5 mL of 1:1000 strength epinephrine. Corticosteroids may be given to minimize the inflammation and edema but are not the initial agent given (option 2). Atropine may minimize secretions but would not be given unless vagal-induced bradycardia or asystole occurs; then atropine may be given as an IV bolus rapidly before, during, or after cardiopulmonary arrest (option 3). Dopamine HCL, a catecholamine (as is epinephrine), may be given to increase blood pressure if shock develops (option 4).
Cognitive Level: Analysis **Client Need:** Physiological Integrity: Pharmacological and Parenteral Therapies **Integrated Process:** Nursing Process: Implementation **Content Area:** Pharmacology **Strategy:** The core issue of the question is knowledge of drugs that are used to treat hypersensitivity or anaphylactic reactions. Use specific nursing knowledge and the process of elimination to make a selection.

11 **Answer: 2** A disulfiram-like effect is associated with certain drugs, including metronidazole (Flagyl). Onset is usually within 15 to 30 minutes of ingestion of alcohol but can occur up to 72 hours after Flagyl has been discontinued. The reaction lasts approximately 20 to 30 minutes but can remain up to 24 hours.
Cognitive Level: Application **Client Need:** Physiological Integrity: Pharmacological and Parenteral Therapies **Integrated Process:** Nursing Process: Implementation **Content Area:** Pharmacology **Strategy:** The core issue of the question is knowledge of which drugs can cause a disulfiram-like reaction when used with alcohol. Use specific nursing knowledge and the process of elimination to make a selection.

12 **Answer: 2** Opportunistic infections or superinfections are manifested by these signs and symptoms. Common ones are vaginal and GI tract infections, including candidiasis and diarrhea. They often result from broad-spectrum antibiotic use that destroys bacteria in the normal flora, allowing the resistant pathogens to proliferate. Early recognition and intervention with administration of sensitive anti-infectives is important in controlling discomfort and the severity of the reaction. The other options represent incorrect conclusions about the data presented.
Cognitive Level: Analysis **Client Need:** Physiological Integrity: Pharmacological and Parenteral Therapies **Integrated Process:** Nursing Process: Analysis **Content Area:** Pharmacology **Strategy:** The core issue of the question is knowledge of adverse drug effects of cefotazime and their significance. Use specific nursing knowledge and the process of elimination to make a selection.

13 **Answer: 2** Yogurt and buttermilk products can decrease the diarrhea as well as add protein to the diet to provide albumin for drug binding. Blood or mucus in the stool with increased number of stools indicates the possibility of pseudomembranous colitis that should be reported to the health care provider. Antacids would interfere with the effectiveness of the antibiotic (option 4). The route of administration of antibiotics is not the cause for destruction of normal flora (option 3). Clients are not usually taught to test their stool for occult blood (option 1).
Cognitive Level: Application **Client Need:** Physiological Integrity: Pharmacological and Parenteral Therapies **Integrated Process:** Nursing Process: Implementation **Content Area:** Pharmacology **Strategy:** The core issue of the question is knowledge of client teaching points related to antibiotic therapy that has diarrhea as a side effect. Use specific nursing knowledge and the process of elimination to make a selection.

14 **Answer: 3** Disulfiram-like or antabuse-like reactions can occur when cephalosporins are taken with ingestion of alcohol during and up to 72 hours after discontinuation of the cephalosporin. Caffeine and the other medications listed would not cause this reaction.
Cognitive Level: Analysis **Client Need:** Physiological Integrity: Pharmacological and Parenteral Therapies **Integrated Process:** Nursing Process: Analysis **Content Area:** Pharmacology **Strategy:** The core issue of the question is knowledge of the causes of disulfiram-like drug reactions. Use specific nursing knowledge and the process of elimination to make a selection.

15 **Answer: 2** Vestibular ototoxicity as well as cochlear otoxicity can occur with administration of an aminoglycoside such as tobramycin. A positive Romberg's test indicates vertigo or loss of balance and may suggest a vestibular problem. Babinski's reflex present in the adult reflects a possible lesion in the corticospinal tract (option 4). Chvostek's sign is seen in tetany and hypocalcemia (option 3). One method of assessing peripheral circulation is to check the capillary refill (option 1).
Cognitive Level: Application **Client Need:** Physiological Integrity: Pharmacological and Parenteral Therapies **Integrated Process:** Nursing Process: Implementation **Content Area:** Pharmacology **Strategy:** The core issue of the question is knowledge of assessment techniques that will help determine whether ototoxicity is occurring in a client taking tobramycin. Use specific nursing knowledge and the process of elimination to make a selection.

16 **Answer: 1** Griseofulvin does not cause increased bleeding unless the client is also on anticoagulant therapy (option 2). The agent also has no known effect on blood pressure or known interaction with calcium intake (options 3 and 4). However, griseofulvin can interfere with the effectiveness of estrogen-containing oral contraceptives (option 1).
Cognitive Level: Application **Client Need:** Physiological Integrity: Pharmacological and Parenteral Therapies **Integrated Process:** Communication and Documentation **Content Area:** Pharmacology **Strategy:** The core issue of the question is knowledge of key teaching points regarding systemic griseofulvin. Use specific nursing knowledge and the process of elimination to make a selection.

17 **Answer: 1** Bacteriostatic agents inhibit or retard bacterial growth and replication, but they do not kill the entire bacteria. These agents depend on the host's defense mechanisms to complete elimination of the bacteria. Bactericidal agents actually kill and lyse the bacteria. Tetracyclines are bacteriostatic. Supplemental vitamin B_6 is indicated with isoniazid (INH) administration (option 3). Iron, as well as antacids and laxatives, food, and dairy products should be separated 1 hour before or 2 hours after administration of a tetracycline (option 2). These substances interfere with the absorption of tetracyclines. Option 4 is unnecessary.
Cognitive Level: Comprehension **Client Need:** Physiological Integrity: Pharmacological and Parenteral Therapies **Integrated Process:** Nursing Process: Analysis **Content Area:** Pharmacology **Strategy:** The core issue of the question is the mechanism of action of tetracycline and how it leads to eradication of infection. Use specific nursing knowledge and the process of elimination to make a selection.

18 **Answer: 3** The prothrombin time (PT) and the international normalization ratio (INR) values are standard tests to monitor warfarin (Coumadin) levels. The beta-lactam antibiotics may cause increased PT and INR. The bleeding time (option 1) evaluates the integrity of the vascular and platelet factors associated with stagnated blood. Thrombin time (option 2) evaluates the fibrinogen to fibrin conversion factor that can be used to gauge heparin effectiveness. However, the APPT (option 4) is currently used most often in regulating heparin therapy.

Cognitive Level: Analysis **Client Need:** Physiological Integrity: Pharmacological and Parenteral Therapies **Integrated Process:** Nursing Process: Analysis **Content Area:** Pharmacology **Strategy:** The core issue of the question is the expected change in laboratory results for a client taking a beta lactam penicillin and an oral anticoagulant. Use specific nursing knowledge and the process of elimination to make a selection.

19 **Answer: 4** The PPD injection stimulates a local inflammatory response at the injection site in the client who has been exposed to the tubercle bacillus in the past. The client develops a cellular response to tubercle bacillus at 3 to 10 weeks after infection. A positive PPD result does not indicated the client currently has active tuberculosis or is in an infectious state (options 1 and 2). Follow-up sputum tests for tubercle bacillus and/or chest films are done to clarify current status.
Cognitive Level: Analysis **Client Need:** Physiological Integrity: Pharmacological and Parenteral Therapies **Integrated Process:** Nursing Process: Analysis **Content Area:** Pharmacology **Strategy:** The core issue of the question is the significance of PPD test results. Use specific nursing knowledge and the process of elimination to make a selection.

20 **Answer: 4** Antibiotics, especially the aminopenicillins such as ampicillin, may decrease the effectiveness of oral contraceptives. The other clinical manifestations are not related to penicillin therapy.
Cognitive Level: Application **Client Need:** Physiological Integrity: Pharmacological and Parenteral Therapies **Integrated Process:** Nursing Process: Implementation **Content Area:** Pharmacology **Strategy:** The core issue of the question is client teaching that is needed for a client beginning drug therapy with ampicillin. Use specific nursing knowledge and the process of elimination to make a selection.

21 **Answer: 3** It is the responsibility of the nurse to address the client's body image related to alopecia. Option 1 does not apply. Option 2 is not a nursing diagnosis. Option 4 is a secondary diagnosis that could apply, but option 3 is more relevant to the side effect of the medication.
Cognitive Level: Analysis **Client Need:** Physiological Integrity: Pharmacological and Parenteral Therapies **Integrated Process:** Nursing Process: Analysis **Content Area:** Pharmacology **Strategy:** The core issue of the question is knowledge of how adverse drug effects of sargramostim can affect a client, necessitating formulation of a nursing diagnosis. Use specific nursing knowledge and the process of elimination to make a selection.

22 **Answer: 1** Potential flulike symptoms can occur with aldesleukin (Proleukin). For this reason, the nurse must provide for adequate fluid and electrolyte balance to prevent deficient fluid volume. Options 2 and 4 have lesser priority because they are not side effects (although they are usually general priority items), and option 3 is the opposite of the actual problem.
Cognitive Level: Analysis **Client Need:** Physiological Integrity: Pharmacological and Parenteral Therapies **Integrated Process:** Nursing Process: Analysis **Content Area:** Pharmacology **Strategy:** The core issue of the question is knowledge of how adverse drug effects of aldesleukin can affect a client, necessitating formulation of a nursing diagnosis. Use specific nursing knowledge and the process of elimination to make a selection.

23 **Answer: 2** Oprelvekin (Neumega) can cause cardiopulmonary insufficiency with irregular heart rate and fluid retention. Thus, it is a nursing priority to assess the client frequently for signs and symptoms of congestive heart failure. The other options do not address this priority concern.
Cognitive Level: Application **Client Need:** Physiological Integrity: Pharmacological and Parenteral Therapies **Integrated Process:** Nursing Process: Assessment **Content Area:** Pharmacology **Strategy:** The core issue of the question is knowledge of adverse drug effects of oprelvekin. Use specific nursing knowledge and the process of elimination to make a selection.

24 **Answer: 3** Mycophenalate (Cell Cept) is administered orally 72 hours after transplant. The time frames listed in each of the other options is incorrect.
Cognitive Level: Application **Client Need:** Physiological Integrity: Pharmacological and Parenteral Therapies **Integrated Process:** Nursing Process: Planning **Content Area:** Pharmacology **Strategy:** The core issue of the question is knowledge of time frames to begin drug therapy with mycophenolate following transplant. Use specific nursing knowledge and the process of elimination to make a selection.

25 **Answer: 2** It is recommended that every client have a tetanus vaccine every 10 years to prevent infection caused by tetanus. The primary opportunity for this assessment is following a laceration. Delayed wound healing is a possibility with corticosteroid therapy, but assessment of tetanus immunization status takes priority. Temperature and blood pressure measurement (options 1 and 3) do not address the risk of infection caused by trauma while the client is in the emergency room.
Cognitive Level: Application **Client Need:** Physiological Integrity: Pharmacological and Parenteral Therapies **Integrated Process:** Nursing Process: Assessment **Content Area:** Pharmacology **Strategy:** The critical words in the question are *laceration* and *emergency department.* Recall that the skin is the first line of defense against infection to choose option 2.

26 **Answer: 3** Antirabies serum, equine 55 U/Kg IM, can be applied to the animal bite wound. The medication does not need to be administered parenterally (options 1, 2, and 4).
Cognitive Level: Application **Client Need:** Physiological Integrity: Pharmacological and Parenteral Therapies **Integrated Process:** Nursing Process: Implementation **Content Area:** Pharmacology **Strategy:** The core issue of the question is knowledge of how to administer antirabies serum. Use specific nursing knowledge and the process of elimination to make a selection.

27 **Answer: 4** Beta 1b (Betaseron) reduces the severity of acute exacerbations of multiple sclerosis. The drug decreases the demyelination in brain tissue. The other responses do not accurately reflect the action of this medication.
Cognitive Level: Application **Client Need:** Physiological Integrity: Pharmacological and Parenteral Therapies **Integrated Process:** Nursing Process: Implementation **Content Area:** Pharmacology **Strategy:** The core issue of the question is knowledge of goals of drug therapy with interferon (Betaseron). Use specific nursing knowledge and the process of elimination to make a selection.

28 **Answer: 3** Adequate fluid intake greater than 2,000 to 3,000 mL per day allows for the kidneys to flush renal toxins and prevents renal insufficiency. Option 1 is a general measure to prevent constipation. Option 2 would be a monitoring function but would not prevent renal insufficiency from occurring. The nurse would not instruct the client to take additional medication that is not specifically part of the plan of care (option 4).
Cognitive Level: Application **Client Need:** Physiological Integrity: Pharmacological and Parenteral Therapies **Integrated Process:** Nursing Process: Implementation **Content Area:** Pharmacology **Strategy:** The core issue of the question is knowledge of measures to prevent the development of renal side effects with use of cyclophosphamide. Use specific nursing knowledge and the process of elimination to make a selection.

29 **Answer: 1** The most significant laboratory test to utilize prior to medication therapy with azathioprine is creatinine level because renal and hepatic function should be assessed. Option 2 is irrelevant, while options 3 and 4 evaluate blood clotting and components of the blood, respectively. Other risks of azathioprine would be increased white cell count (infection) and decreased platelet count.
Cognitive Level: Application **Client Need:** Physiological Integrity: Pharmacological and Parenteral Therapies **Integrated Process:** Nursing Process: Evaluation **Content Area:** Pharmacology **Strategy:** The core issue of the question is knowledge of adverse drug effects of azathioprine and which laboratory test to use as a baseline measure. Use specific nursing knowledge and the process of elimination to make a selection.

30 **Answer: 2** Azathioprine (Imuran) is administered to treat multiple sclerosis, and allopurinol (Zyloprim) is administered to treat symptoms of gout. When these two medications are administered together, the dose of azathioprine should be reduced. The uric acid level and client symptoms should be assessed to determine the control of gout.
Cognitive Level: Application **Client Need:** Physiological Integrity: Pharmacological and Parenteral Therapies **Integrated Process:** Nursing Process: Assessment **Content Area:** Pharmacology **Strategy:** The core issue of the question is knowledge of drug interactive effects of azathioprine and allopurinol. Use specific nursing knowledge and the process of elimination to make a selection.

31 **Answer: 2** Edrophonium (Tensilon) is used for diagnostic purposes. Clients who receive an injection of edrophonium and exhibit a temporary relief of symptoms are diagnosed with myasthenia gravis, which is characterized by a decrease in the concentration of acetylcholine in the neuromuscular junction. The medications listed in the other options are not used to diagnose myasthenia gravis.
Cognitive Level: Application **Client Need:** Physiological Integrity: Pharmacological and Parenteral Therapies **Integrated Process:** Nursing Process: Planning **Content Area:** Pharmacology **Strategy:** The core issue of the question is knowledge of medications used for diagnosis of myasthenia gravis. Use specific nursing knowledge and the process of elimination to make a selection.

32 **Answer: 1** Medications used to treat symptoms of multiple sclerosis have been noted to increase pulmonary edema, leading to chest pain and shortness of breath. Option 2 could increase risk of urinary tract infection. Option 3 is useful to avoid infection but does not specifically relate to medication teaching. Option 4 could increase fatigue if done to excess and lead to exacerbation of symptoms.
Cognitive Level: Application **Client Need:** Physiological Integrity: Pharmacological and Parenteral Therapies **Integrated Process:** Nursing Process: Implementation **Content Area:** Pharmacology **Strategy:** The core issue of the question is knowledge of essential teaching points for a client being treated with drug therapy for multiple sclerosis. Use specific nursing knowledge and the process of elimination to make a selection.

33 **Answer: 3** Immune serum globulin should not be administered to clients with a history of coagulation disorders. The other options do not represent contraindications to administration of this medication.
Cognitive Level: Application **Client Need:** Physiological Integrity: Pharmacological and Parenteral Therapies **Integrated Process:** Nursing Process: Assessment **Content Area:** Pharmacology **Strategy:** The core issue of the question is knowledge of safe administration of serum immune globulin. Use specific nursing knowledge and the process of elimination to make a selection.

34 **Answer: 4** Physostigmine (Eserine) is an anticholinesterase agent that crosses the blood–brain barrier. It is used as an agent to correct anticholinergic poisoning. The other medications listed do not have this effect.
Cognitive Level: Application **Client Need:** Physiological Integrity: Pharmacological and Parenteral Therapies **Integrated Process:** Nursing Process: Planning **Content Area:** Pharmacology **Strategy:** The core issue of the question is knowledge of drug therapy to reverse excessive effects of medications used to treat Parkinson's disease. Use specific nursing knowledge and the process of elimination to make a selection.

35 **Answer: 4** The intravenous administration of physostigmine (Eserine) should be no faster than 1 mg per minute to prevent toxic adverse reactions. The other options do not relate to toxicity of physostigmine.
Cognitive Level: Application **Client Need:** Physiological Integrity: Pharmacological and Parenteral Therapies **Integrated Process:** Nursing Process: Implementation **Content Area:** Pharmacology **Strategy:** The core issue of the question is knowledge of safe administration technique for physostigmine. Use specific nursing knowledge and the process of elimination to make a selection.

Key Terms to Review

amebiasis p. 794
antigen p. 775
bactericidal p. 783
bacteriostatic p. 789
candidiasis p. 784
colony-stimulating factors p. 775
cross-sensitivity p. 785
empiric therapy p. 784
giardiasis p. 808
immunosuppression p. 775
myelosuppression p. 777
neutropenia p. 776
peak drug level p. 784
pseudomembranous colitis p. 784
superinfection p. 806
tinea p. 805
trough drug level p. 784

References

Abrams, A. (2004). *Clinical drug therapy: Rationales for nursing practice* (7th ed.). Philadelphia: Lippincott Williams & Wilkins.

Adams, M., Josephson, D., & Holland, L. (2005). *Pharmacology for nurses: A pathophysiologic approach.* Upper Saddle River, NJ: Pearson Education.

Deglin, J. H., & Vallerand, A. H. (2006). *Davis's drug guide for nurses* (10th ed.). Philadelphia: F. A. Davis.

Lehne, R. (2004). *Pharmacology for nursing care* (5th ed.). Philadelphia: W. B. Saunders.

McKenry, L., Tessier, E., & Hogan, M. (2006). *Mosby's pharmacology in nursing.* (22nd ed.). St. Louis: Elsevier Science.

Wilson, B., Shannon, M., & Stang, C. (2006). *Prentice Hall nurse's drug guide 2006.* Upper Saddle River, NJ: Pearson Education.

Common Laboratory Tests

47

In this chapter

Test Yourself

Are you ready for the NCLEX-RN® or course exams? Use the practice tests on the companion CD-ROM to check.

Cross reference

Other chapters relevant to this content area are

Common Diagnostic Tests and Procedures	Chapter 48
Fluid and Electrolyte Imbalances	Chapter 54
Acid-Base Imbalances	Chapter 55

I. GENERAL PRINCIPLES OF SPECIMEN COLLECTION

A. Routine specimens

1. Usually collected in early morning before intake of food and fluids
2. Tests done in the fasting state require withholding food and fluids for 8 to 12 hours prior to test
3. Should be collected using standard precautions to protect caregiver from exposure to blood or other body fluids and using strict aseptic technique to protect client from infection
4. Label specimens with client name, date, exact time of collection, and type of specimen
5. Laboratory requisition slip should note client name, age, gender, room, physician, possible diagnosis, and test (or tests) being requested; record any factors that could interfere with results, such as foods or drugs

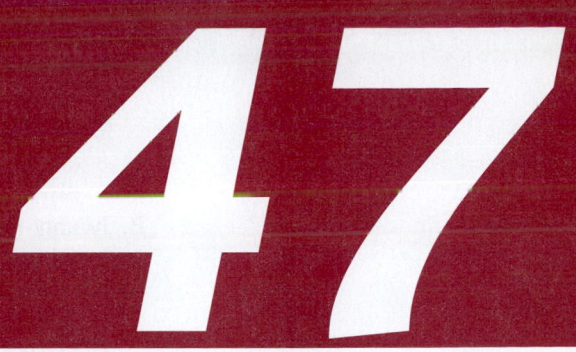

! 6. Avoid shaking blood specimens to avoid hemolysis
7. Send specimens promptly to lab
8. Values that fall within the laboratory reference range are considered normal
! 9. Critical (panic) values are abnormal results that could increase risk of harm to client; these are telephoned to nursing unit and must be reported to charge nurse and/or health care provider

! **B. Twenty-four-hour urine specimens**
1. Obtain a 24-hour specimen collection container from lab
2. Place container on ice, if indicated for test, and place 24-hour specimen collection sign above client bed, in bathroom, and on chart as a reminder not to discard urine
3. Have client void prior to test and discard this urine; save all urine for next 24 hours
4. Instruct client to void each time into container, such as a specimen hat, and avoid contaminating specimen with feces or toilet paper
5. Transfer voided specimen into collection device using standard precautions
6. At end of collection time, have client void and save this specimen
7. Label container with client's name, date, type of specimen, and exact time of collection (e.g., 12/29/06 07:00 to 12/30/06 07:00)

II. ARTERIAL BLOOD GASES *(See also Chapter 55)*

A. Analysis of serum pH, partial pressure of arterial oxygen (PaO_2), partial pressure of carbon dioxide ($PaCO_2$), bicarbonate (HCO_3^-), and base excess

B. See Table 47–1 ■ for normal reference ranges

C. See Chapter 55 for further discussion of arterial blood gases (ABGs)

III. SERUM ELECTROLYTES *(See also Chapter 54)*

A. Consist of cations sodium, potassium, calcium, and magnesium; and anions chloride and phosphorus

B. Standard reported values include sodium, potassium, chloride, bicarbonate; see Table 47–2 ■ for normal reference ranges

C. See Chapter 54 for further discussion of full range of electrolytes

IV. GLUCOSE STUDIES

A. Fasting blood glucose (FBG)
1. Glucose is an end product of carbohydrate digestion, glycogenolysis, and gluconeogenesis
2. It is primary fuel source of cellular energy, especially for brain, which is only fueled by glucose and oxygen
! 3. FBG is used to diagnose diabetes mellitus (type 1 or 2) and hypoglycemia; see Table 47–3 ■ for normal reference range
! 4. Client must fast for 8 to 12 hours prior to drawing lab sample, with no ingestion of foods, beverages, or medications (oral antidiabetics or insulin)

B. Random blood glucose
1. Measures blood glucose as above but in nonfasting state
2. May be checked using capillary blood as in fingerstick blood glucose measurements
! 3. See Table 47–3 for normal reference range

C. Two-hour postprandial blood glucose: measures serum glucose 2 hours after eating

D. Glucose tolerance test (GTT)
1. Used as a screening test for clients at risk of diabetes mellitus and as diagnostic aid

Table 47–1
Normal Arterial Blood Gases

Test	Normal Reference Range
Serum pH	7.35–7.45
Oxygen (PaO_2)	80–100 mmHg
Carbon dioxide ($PaCO_2$)	35–45 mmHg
Bicarbonate (HCO_3^-)	22–26 mEq/L
Base excess	+3 – −3

Table 47-2

Normal Serum Electrolytes

Test	Normal Reference Range
Sodium	35–145 mEq/L
Potassium	3.5–5.1 mEq/L
Chloride	98–107 mEq/L
Bicarbonate (venous)	23–29 mEq/L

2. Glucose levels should rise and fall in predictable amounts following ingestion of a specific glucose load (see Table 47–3); with diabetes mellitus, glucose levels peak at higher levels and fall more slowly than normal

!

3. Client teaching
   a. Eat high-carbohydrate (CHO) diet (200–300 grams daily) for 3 days prior to test (give client list of high-CHO foods as needed)
   b. Do not drink alcohol or coffee or smoke for 36 hours before test (eliminates alcohol, caffeine, and nicotine as interfering factors with test results)
   c. Fast for 10 to 16 hours before test as instructed by healthcare provider
   d. Do not take any oral antidiabetic medications or insulin prior to test
   e. Do not exercise vigorously for 8 hours before or after test; sit quietly during test
   f. Test consists of baseline glucose level, ingestion of oral or IV glucose load, and series of blood glucose samples
   g. Two-hour GTT takes about 3 hours to complete; abnormal results may require a longer (3 to 5 hours) GTT

E. Glycosylated hemoglobin A_{1c}

1. Measures glucose that binds irreversibly to hemoglobin for life of red blood cell (RBC lifespan is 120 days)

!

2. Indicates glycemic control over period of 3 to 5 weeks (takes into account continuous production and destruction of RBCs in body)
3. See Table 47–3 for interpretation of results
4. No fasting is required before test

V. COAGULATION STUDIES

A. Prothrombin time (PT) and international normalized ratio (INR)

1. Measures time needed for prothrombin (a vitamin-K–dependent glycoprotein) to form a fibrin clot via extrinsic clotting pathway
2. Commonly used to assess effectiveness of oral anticoagulant such as sodium warfarin (Coumadin) or to diagnose disseminated intravascular coagulopathy (DIC), vitamin K deficiency, or liver dysfunction

Table 47-3

Normal Adult Glucose Levels

Test	Normal Reference Range
Fasting blood glucose	70–110 mg/dL
Random (capillary) glucose	60–110 mg/dL
2-hour postprandial blood glucose	< 140 mg/dL
Oral glucose tolerance test (OGTT)	
Fasting baseline	70–110 mg/dL
30-minute sample	110–170 mg/dL
60-minute sample	120–170 mg/dL
90-minute sample	100–140 mg/dL
120-minute sample	70–120 mg/dL
Glycosylated hemoglobin A_{1c}	
Normal	3.5–6%
Good diabetic control	7.5% or lower
Fair diabetic control	7.6–8.9%
Poor diabetic control	9% or higher

3. Normal reference ranges vary slightly by lab (9.6–11.8 seconds for adult males and 9.5–11.3 seconds for adult females); normal level is control value plus or minus 2 seconds; therapeutic range for warfarin is 1.5 to 2 times the control value
4. INR is similar to PT but standardizes normal values across all lab systems; it also measures effectiveness of oral anticoagulation
5. Normal reference ranges are 2.0–3.0 for standard warfarin therapy and 3.0–4.5 for high-dose therapy
6. Draw baseline PT before beginning oral anticoagulation and repeat at specified intervals to monitor progress of therapy
7. Report abnormals or any values outside therapeutic ranges; low values indicate ineffective therapy and high values indicate risk for bleeding or hemorrhage
8. Teach client to limit green leafy vegetables in diet because they are rich in vitamin K and will decrease PT

B. Activated partial thromboplastin time (aPTT)

1. Measures time needed for recalcified, citrated plasma to clot after adding activated thromboplastin reagent
2. Commonly used to assess heparin therapy; can be used to screen for all clotting factor deficiencies except VII and XIII
3. Elevated in liver disease and DIC
4. Normal reference range is 20–35 seconds, and therapeutic range for heparin therapy is 1.5–2.5 times the control in seconds
5. Draw baseline aPTT before beginning heparin therapy and repeat at specified intervals to monitor progress of therapy
6. Do not draw lab sample from vein in same arm in which heparin is infusing
7. Report abnormals or any values outside therapeutic ranges; low values indicate ineffective therapy and high values indicate risk for bleeding or hemorrhage

C. Clotting time

1. Measures time required to complete all steps in clotting process
2. Normal reference range: 8–15 minutes
3. Results can be affected by anticoagulant therapy, high temperatures, and test tube agitation

VI. COMPLETE BLOOD COUNT

A. Hematocrit (Hct)

1. Measures proportion of RBCs in a volume of whole blood
2. Blood is centrifuged and proportions of **plasma** and solid components are measured and reported as a percentage
3. Can be falsely elevated when white blood cell (WBC) counts are markedly elevated (referred to as "buffy coat")
4. Can be falsely lowered with hemodilution (increased water component of blood)
5. Normal reference range for males is 40% to 50% and for females is 38% to 47%

B. Hemoglobin (Hgb)

1. Heme consists of red pigment porphyrin and iron and is capable of combining loosely with oxygen (O_2) and carbon dioxide (CO_2)
2. Globin is a complex protein that, can result in hemoglobinopathies when abnormal amino acid sequencing is present
3. Abnormal hemoglobinopathies include sickle cell disease and thallasemias; decreased hemoglobin commonly indicates anemia
4. Normally, Hgb and Hct levels parallel each other; Hct is usually 3 times higher than Hgb level
5. Normal reference range for males is 13.5–18 grams/dL and for females is 12–16 grams/dL

C. RBC count

1. RBCs are formed in bone marrow and removed by liver, spleen, and bone marrow
2. Life span of RBC is approximately 120 days
3. Carry hemoglobin molecules responsible for O_2 transport to tissues
4. Normal reference range: 4.0–5.5 million cells/microliter for adult females and 4.5–6.2 million cells/microliter for adult males
5. Abnormal values indicate anemia or blood dyscrasias

Table 47-4

White Blood Cell Differential Counts

Cells	Normal Adult Reference Range
Neutrophils (total) Segments (mature) Bands (immature)	50–70% or 2500–7000 cells/microliter 50–65% or 2500–6500 cells/microliter 0–5% or 0–500 cells/microliter
Eosinophils	1–3% or 100–300 cells/microliter
Basophils	0.4–1.0% or 40–100 cells/microliter
Lymphocytes	25–35% or 1700–3500 cells/microliter
Monocytes	4–6% or 200–600 cells/microliter

D. Platelet count

!

1. Normal reference range: 150,000 to 450,000 per cubic mm (mm^3)
2. When microtrauma occurs and damages blood vessels, platelets aggregate and adhere to altered surface to form hemostatic plug to initiate clot formation
3. Platelets produce prostaglandins, which also promote platelet adherence and aggregation
   - **a.** Aspirin is an antiplatelet drug that inhibits platelet aggregation
   - **b.** Aspirin is given to prevent platelet aggregation along walls of atherosclerotic lesions (and initiating clot formation that could occlude vessel)
4. Decreased levels occur with cancer chemotherapy from bone marrow suppression, idiopathic thrombocytopenic purpura (ITP), most leukemias, uremia, and some infections such as infectious mononucleosis
5. Normal platelet life span is about 10 days

E. WBC

1. Consist of agranulocytes (monocytes and lymphocytes; no stainable granules in nucleus) and granulocytes (neutrophils, eosinophils, and basophils)

!

2. Normal total WBC reference range: 5,000–10,000/mm^3
3. Normal WBC differential reference ranges: see Table 47-4 ■
4. Neutrophils function as immune system defenses against inflammation, tissue injury, and infection

!

   - **a.** A "shift to the left" indicates a greater number of neutrophils are immature (bands) because of need for more rapid production to combat inflammation or infection
   - **b.** A "shift to the right" indicates cells with excessive nuclear segments, seen with liver disease, megaloblastic and pernicious anemias, and Down syndrome
5. Eosinophils increase during allergic and parasitic conditions and decrease with higher levels of steroids
6. Basophils increase during healing process and decrease when steroid levels increase
7. Monocytes ("monos") are second line of defense against bacterial infection and foreign substances; they are macrophages that ingest larger particles and debris from cellular destruction; may also kill tumor cells—mechanism unclear
8. Lymphocytes ("lymphs") elevate during chronic and viral infections and lymphocytic leukemia; consist of B lymphocytes and T lymphocytes
   - **a.** B lymphocytes lie dormant in lymph nodes until stimulated by antigenic substance and provide for humoral immunity by transforming into plasma cells that secrete immunoglobulins; IgG is immunoglobulin responsible for antiviral, antitoxin, and antibacterial work
   - **b.** T lymphocytes mature in thymus, although they reside in lymph nodes, spleen, and other peripheral lymphoid tissue; are also stimulated when presented with an antigen that has been preprocessed by a macrophage; see immune studies section later in chapter for additional information on T cells

VII. CARDIOVASCULAR FUNCTION STUDIES

A. Serum lipids

1. Primary measurements include total cholesterol, low-density lipoproteins (LDLs), high-density lipoproteins (HDLs), and triglycerides

Table 47–5

Serum Lipid Levels

Type of Lipid	Normal Reference Range
Cholesterol (total)	< 200 mg/dL
LDL	< 130 mg/dL
HDL	30–70 mg/dL
Triglycerides	< 200 mg/dL

2. Normal reference ranges: see Table 47–5 ■
3. Elevated levels (except for HDLs) increase risk of heart disease, stroke, and peripheral vascular disease; high HDL levels seem to have cardioprotective function; elevated triglycerides indicate hyperlipidemia (possibly familial)
4. Teach client to avoid alcohol intake for 24 hours before test and avoid high-cholesterol foods the evening before blood is drawn
5. Client must fast (except water) for 12 to 14 hours prior to test

B. Creatine kinase (CK) or creatinine phosphokinase (CPK)

1. An enzyme found in large amounts in cardiac and skeletal muscle and in low amounts in brain tissue; enzyme is released from cells upon cell death
2. Enzyme can be fractionated into isoenzymes to identify tissue of origin; CK-MB is cardiac band; CK-MM is skeletal muscle band; CK-BB is brain tissue band
3. Normal reference range and pattern of elevation: see Table 47–6 ■
4. Avoid intake of alcohol 24 hours prior to test
5. Avoid injections, which could give false elevations to level
6. Instruct client to avoid excessive physical exertion if monitoring skeletal muscle band; make note of soft tissue injury or falls that could cause false elevations
7. Monitor results serially over 3 days if monitoring myocardial infarction (MI) and correlate with clinical picture

C. Lactic dehydrogenase (LDH)

1. An enzyme sometimes used to detect MI; elevates with myocardial cell death
2. Normal reference range and pattern of elevation: see Table 47–6
3. Considered diagnostic for MI when level of LDH_2 rises or "flips" above LDH_1
4. Monitor results serially over 3 days and correlate with clinical picture

D. Troponins

1. Regulatory proteins found in skeletal and cardiac muscle (striated muscle cells)
2. Released into bloodstream with myocardial cell death; early indicator of cardiac damage; myoglobin also rises (12–90 mcg/L normal); peaks in 8–12 hrs
3. Normal reference range and pattern of elevation: see Table 47–6
4. Monitor results serially over 3 days and correlate with clinical picture

Table 47–6

Cardiac Enzymes

Enzyme/Isoenzyme	Normal Reference Range	Pattern of Elevation and Decline
Creatine kinase (CK)	Males 55–170 units/L Females 30–135 units/L	Begins to rise 4–6 hours after myocardial or skeletal muscle damage
CK-MM	94–100%	Peaks at 18–24 hours
CK-MB	0–6%	Returns to normal within 3–4 days
CK-BB	0%	
Lactic dehydrogenase (LDH)	140–280 units/L	Begins to rise 24 hours after myocardial damage
LDH_1	14–26%	Peaks in 48–72 hours
LDH_2	29–39%	Returns to normal within 7–14 days
LDH_3	20–26%	
LDH_4	8–16%	
LDH_5	6–16%	
Cardiac Troponins		Rise within 3 hours of myocardial infarction
Troponin I	<0.1 to <1.0 ng/mL	
Troponin T	<0.2 to <1.0 ng/mL	Returns to normal in 5–9 days (I) or 10–14 days (T)

VIII. THYROID FUNCTION STUDIES

A. Thyroxine (T_4)

1. Major hormone secreted by thyroid gland
2. Aids in diagnosis of hypo- or hyperthyroidism with low or high levels respectively
3. Normal reference range: 4.5–11.5 mcg/mL T_4 or 1.0–2.3 ng/dL free T_4

B. Triiodothyronine (T_3)

1. A short-acting but potent thyroid hormone; present only in small amounts in blood
2. More useful for diagnosing hyperthyroidism than hypothyroidism
3. Normal reference range: 80–200 ng/dL

C. Thyroid-stimulating hormone (TSH)

1. A hormone secreted via negative feedback loop by anterior pituitary gland in response to decreased T_4
2. Used with results of T_4 level to differentiate between pituitary and thyroid dysfunction
   a. Decreased T_4 and normal or elevated TSH is consistent with thyroid disorder
   b. Decreased T_4 and decreased TSH is consistent with pituitary disorder
3. Normal reference range: 0.35–5.5 microinternational units/mL

D. No special preparation is needed for any thyroid test, but results can be affected by antithyroid drugs

IX. RENAL FUNCTION STUDIES

A. Blood urea nitrogen (BUN)

1. Formed in liver as end product of protein metabolism; consists of nitrogen portion of urea
2. Excreted via kidneys with only small amounts reabsorbed in renal tubules
3. ! Normal reference range is 8–22 mg/dL
4. ! Rises with reduced glomerular filtration rate, (GFR) increased dietary protein, increased catabolism (such as starvation), crush injuries, febrile illness, absorption of blood from intestines, and with hemoconcentration from dehydration
5. Decreases with overhydration, inadequate protein intake, or liver disease (because liver is not functioning to convert ammonia to urea)
6. ! Must be assessed concurrently with serum creatinine for true indication of renal status; if BUN and creatinine rise together, indicates renal insufficiency or failure

B. Serum creatinine

1. End product of creatine metabolism in muscles; is a specific indicator of GFR and renal status
2. ! Elevated levels commonly indicate renal insufficiency or failure
3. Teach client to avoid eating red meat for 24 hours prior to test and heavy exercise 8 hours prior in order to avoid falsely high values
4. Normal reference range is 0.6–1.3 mg/dL

X. URINALYSIS

A. Normal results: see Table 47–7 ■

B. Possible causes of abnormal results: see Table 47–8 ■

C. Nitrites

1. If present, nitrites suggest urinary tract infection (UTI)
2. Mechanism
   a. Dietary nitrates are excreted in urine
   b. When Gram-negative bacteria (such as common *E. coli*) are present in urine, these nitrates are converted to nitrites
   c. Test *suggests* a UTI with Gram-negative bacteria
   d. False-negatives can result if urine does not sit in bladder long enough for reaction to take place ($\geq$ 4 hours), if infection is caused by an organism that is not Gram-negative, or if dietary nitrate is absent

D. Leukocyte esterase

1. ! Simple test that may be done on a voided urine sample; positive result suggests UTI
2. Mechanism
   a. WBCs contain esterases that react with substances in urine

Table 47-7

Normal Urinalysis Findings

Component	Normal Finding
Color	ranges from pale yellow to amber
Clarity	clear when first excreted
Odor	faintly aromatic
Specific gravity	1.005–1.030
pH	4.6–6.0
Protein	trace to none
Glucose	none
Ketones	none
Sediment	0–3 RBCs, 0–4 WBCs; occasional cast; occasional renal epithelial cell

Table 47-8

Possible Causes of Abnormal Urinalysis Findings

Urinalysis	Significance of Abnormal Findings
Color	Pale: diabetes insipidus, drinking of excess free water Reddish: RBCs Burgundy: porphyria Orange: phenazopyridine HCl (Pyridium) or rifampin (Rifadin) Green: bile Black-brown: mercury poisoning Milky: pus, fat globules
Clarity	Cloudy: infection, phosphate precipitation from standing Turbid: spermatozoa, prostatic fluid
Odor	Sweet: acetonuria Strong: drugs, asparagus Ammonia: after standing for a time
Specific gravity	Decreased: diabetes insipidus, diuretics, excessive intake of free water Increased: diabetes mellitus, hypovolemia, liver disease, heart failure, SIADH, IV contrast medium
pH	Acid: acidosis, diabetes mellitus, fever, starvation, dehydration Alkaline: citrus, salicylate poisoning, sodium bicarbonate, urinary tract infection; urine becomes alkaline after standing because urea-splitting bacteria result in ammonia production
Protein	Transient: fever, stress 0.5 gm/day: chronic pyelonephritis 0.5–4 gm/day: multiple myeloma, diabetic nephropathy 5 gm/day: nephrotic syndrome, glomerulonephritis
Glucose	Present: diabetes mellitus
Ketones	Present: acidosis, diabetic ketoacidosis, starvation, or dieting (fat breakdown)
Sediments	Casts: clumps of material or cells that form in renal collecting tubule, assuming shape of tubule; are seen in various renal disease states Granular casts: acute tubular necrosis, glomerulonephritis, UTI, stress, renal transplant rejection Pus: glomerulonephritis RBC casts: glomerulonephritis WBCs: UTI RBCs or bleeding within glomeruli, transfusion reaction, malaria, hemolytic hemoglobin, anemia

b. More than 100,000 colonies of bacteria (per high-powered field) are needed before diagnosis of UTI is made

XI. LIVER FUNCTION STUDIES

A. Alanine aminotransferase (ALT) or serum glutamic pyruvic transaminase (SGPT)

1. An enzyme found primarily in liver cells but also found in small amounts in heart, kidney, and skeletal muscle
2. Normal reference range: 10–25 units/L
3. Rises as high as 200–400 units with hepatitis or liver damage from drugs and chemicals
4. ! Used to differentiate between jaundice from liver disease (often > 300 units/L) and causes outside liver (often < 300 units/L)
5. There is no food or fluid restriction before test

B. Aspartate aminotransferase (AST) or serum glutamic oxaloacetic transaminase (SGOT)

1. An enzyme found mainly in heart muscle and liver, with moderate amounts also found in skeletal muscle, kidneys, and pancreas
2. Normal reference range: 8–38 units/L
3. Rises with cellular injury and release of enzyme into circulation
4. Rises following MI in 6–10 hours, peaks in 24–48 hours, and returns to normal in 4–6 days; rarely used because not specific to myocardial tissue
5. ! With liver injury (hepatitis, necrosis), levels rise by 10 times or more and stay elevated longer; also rises with pancreatitis and musculoskeletal trauma, including injections
6. There is no food or fluid restriction before test

C. Bilirubin

1. A by-product of hemoglobin breakdown; produced also by liver, spleen, and bone marrow
2. Consists of total bilirubin, direct or conjugated bilirubin (excreted by GI tract), and indirect or unconjugated bilirubin (circulates protein-bound in blood)
3. Normal reference ranges
   a. Total: 0.1–1.2 mg/dL adults and 1–12 mg/dL newborn
   b. Direct: 0.1–0.3 mg/dL
   c. Indirect: calculated by subtracting direct from total bilirubin level
4. ! Levels are elevated with jaundice and liver disease
5. Draw infant blood sample from heel of foot
6. ! Protect specimen from sunlight and artificial light and avoid hemolysis
7. Alcohol and many drugs will increase levels; write medications given on lab requisition
8. Teach client to reduce intake of yellow vegetables (beans, carrots, sweet potatoes, squash) for 3–4 days before test and to fast for 4 hours prior to test

D. Ammonia

1. End product of nitrogen breakdown during protein metabolism
2. Metabolized by liver and excreted via kidneys
3. Normal reference range: 35–65 micrograms/dL
4. Elevated results indicate liver disease and could lead to encephalopathy (and hepatic coma)
5. ! Degree of elevation does not correlate directly with risk of developing hepatic coma
6. Teach client not to smoke for 24 hours prior to test and to fast (except for water) for 8–10 hours prior

XII. PANCREATIC ENZYMES

A. Amylase

1. Produced by pancreas and salivary glands for CHO digestion and excreted via kidneys
2. Normal reference range: 25–151 units/L
3. ! Increased with pancreatitis; elevation begins 3 to 6 hours after pain begins, peaks in 24 hours and returns to normal in 2 to 3 days

4. Many drugs affect results, so list them on lab requisition; false results can occur if measured within 72 hours of cholecystography with radiopaque dyes

B. Lipase

1. Produced by pancreas to break down fats and triglycerides into fatty acids and glycerol
2. Normal reference range: 10–140 units/L
3. Increased with pancreatic disorders; may rise as late as 24 to 36 hours after onset of disorder and return to normal as much as 14 days later

XIII. GASTROINTESTINAL (GI) FUNCTION STUDIES

A. Albumin

1. A plasma protein that maintains oncotic pressure (to prevent edema) and transports water-insoluble substances such as fatty acids, hormones, bilirubin, and drugs
2. Normal reference range: 3.4–5.0 grams/dL
3. May be decreased in malnourished states and monitored as an indicator of nutritional status

B. Alkaline phosphatase

1. Enzyme present in intestines, liver, bone, and placenta
2. Normal reference range: 4.5–1.3 King-Armstrong units/dL
3. Rises with periods of bone growth and with liver disease or bile duct obstruction
4. Results may be affected by hepatotoxic drugs administered during 12 hours prior to test
5. Fasting may be required for 12 hours prior to test

C. Total protein

1. Consists of circulating albumin and globulins in serum; serve many functions, including tissue growth and repair, pH buffering, enzymes, hormones, and coagulation factors
2. Normal reference range: 6.0–8.0 grams/dL
3. May be decreased with malnutrition, low-protein diet, GI disorders, severe liver disease, chronic renal failure, severe burns, or water intoxication
4. May be increased with dehydration (hemoconcentration), vomiting, diarrhea, and myeloma
5. Teach clients to avoid high-fat foods for 24 hours prior to test

D. Uric acid

1. By-product of purine metabolism that is elevated in gout and is affected by dietary intake and renal function
2. Normal reference range: 3.5–8.0 mg/dL adult males and 2.8-6.8 mg/dL females (results may vary among laboratories)
3. Excessive uric acid can lead to kidney stone formation with renal clearance
4. Teach client to avoid high-purine foods (liver, kidney, brain, heart, sweetbreads, scallops, sardines) for 24 hours prior to test; otherwise, no food or drink restriction
5. Write medications taken on lab requisition, since many drugs affect results

XIV. IMMUNE FUNCTION STUDIES

A. Human immunodeficiency virus (HIV) tests

1. Consist of enzyme-linked immunosorbent assay (ELISA), Western blot, and immunofluorescence assay (IFA)
2. ELISA is tested first, and if positive, test may be repeated using same blood sample; if positive again, Western blot or IFA is done; if second test is negative, client should be retested in 3 to 6 months
3. Positive IFA or Western blot confirms diagnosis of HIV

B. CD4 T cell counts

1. Function of T helper cells is primarily to help B cells and promote increased immunoglobulin production

2. Normal reference range: 500–1600 cells/microliter
3. CD4 counts decrease with HIV, increasing risk of client infection at levels of 200–499 cells/microliter and causing severe risk of infections when count is less than 200 cells/microliter

C. CD4 to CD8 ratio

1. CD8 or T suppressor cells are responsible for down-regulation of immune response or once an infection has been eradicated
2. Normal ratio of CD4 to CD8 cells is 2:1
3. With decrease in CD4 counts as HIV progresses to acquired immunodeficiency syndrome (AIDS) and client condition worsens, this ratio decreases

D. Viral load testing

1. Measures amounts of HIV viral RNA or other viral protein in blood
2. Values increase or decrease according to current level of infection

XV. THERAPEUTIC DRUG LEVELS

A. Measure amount of drug circulating in bloodstream, usually before scheduled daily dose of drug in question

B. If measurement is required before and after drug administration, referred to as peak and trough drug levels

1. Trough level is drawn when dose circulating in bloodstream is lowest (just prior to next dose)
2. Peak level is drawn when dose circulating in bloodstream is highest (approximately 30 minutes after drug has finished infusing and dose has equilibrated in bloodstream)

C. Drug levels need to remain within therapeutic range at all times

D. High drug levels could cause signs of toxicity; low levels could result in symptoms of original health problem (ineffective dose)

E. Teach client not to take daily dose before routine drug level is drawn

F. Alert prescriber immediately of abnormal levels so dosage adjustment can be made

G. See Table 47–9 for common therapeutic drug levels

Table 47–9
Common Therapeutic Drug Levels

Drug	Therapeutic Range
Acetaminophen (Tylenol)	10–20 mcg/mL
Amitriptyline (Elavil)	120–150 ng/mL
Carbamazepine (Tegretol)	5–12 mcg/mL
Digoxin (Lanoxin)	0.5–2.0 ngmL
Ethosuximide (Zarontin)	40–100 mcg/mL
Lidocaine (Xylocaine)	1.5–5.0 mcg/mL
Lithium (Lithobid)	0.5–1.3 mEq/L
Magnesium sulfate	4.0–7.0 mg/dL
Phenytoin (Dilantin)	10–20 mcg/mL
Procainamide (Pronestyl)	4–10 mcg/mL
Quinidine (Cardioquin)	2–5 mcg/mL
Salicylate	100–250 mcg/mL
Theophylline (Theo-Dur)	10–20 mcg/mL
Valproic acid (Depakene)	50–100 mcg/mL

PRACTICE TEST

Check your NCLEX-RN® Exam I.Q.

You are ready for testing on this content if you can

- Collect blood and body fluid specimens correctly for laboratory analysis.
- Perform client teaching about specimen collection for laboratory analysis.
- Identify normal and abnormal values for common laboratory tests.
- Correlate pathophysiology with results of laboratory tests.
- Make appropriate clinical decisions after reviewing laboratory test results, including notification of primary care provider.

PRACTICE TEST

1 The nurse is providing care to a client who underwent removal of a pituitary tumor. Eighteen hours after surgery, the urine output is markedly increased and the urine specific gravity is 1.002. The nurse expects to note which of the following corresponding findings when reviewing results of laboratory tests?

1. Serum sodium 148 mEq/L
2. Serum potassium 3.4 mEq/L
3. Serum osmolality 263 mosm/L
4. Hematocrit 29%

2 The nurse would be most concerned about which of the following laboratory values obtained for a client receiving furosemide (Lasix) therapy?

1. Blood urea nitrogen 20 mg/dL
2. Hematocrit 46%
3. Creatinine 1.1 mg/dL
4. Potassium 3.2 mEq/L

3 The nurse inserts a nasogastric tube, and it immediately drains 1000 mL of fluid. Which of the following electrolyte assessments is of greatest concern to the nurse at this time?

1. Sodium
2. Potassium
3. Chloride
4. CO_2 content

4 A client who was just admitted to the nursing unit has a uric acid level of 9.5 mg/dL. Which assessment would the nurse make initially?

1. "Do you have a history of gallbladder disease?"
2. "Do you drink large amounts of green tea?"
3. "Do you have a history of gout?"
4. "Have you been having any pains in the flank area?"

5 The nurse is caring for a client who received a renal transplant 24 hours previously. Which of the following trends in lab studies indicates to the nurse that the new kidney is functioning?

1. Hemoglobin 12%, increased from 11.8%
2. Serum creatinine 1.6 mg/dL, decreased from 1.9 mg/dL
3. Serum sodium 140 mEq/L, increased from 136 mEq/L
4. Serum phosphate 4.4 mg/dL, decreased from 4.8 mg/dL

6 The nurse is caring for a client who has just returned from the operating room. Blood loss was minimal, but the client was given large volumes of crystalloid fluid during the procedure. Which of the following laboratory test results suggests overhydration?

1. Sodium 147 mEq/L
2. Hemoglobin 14%
3. Hematocrit 33 %
4. Calcium level 8.8 mg/dL

7 A client is being evaluated for possible appendicitis. Which of the following results of laboratory tests suggests most strongly to the nurse the presence an acute bacterial infection?

1. Elevated neutrophils
2. Elevated erythrocytes
3. Elevated lymphocytes
4. Elevated platelets

8 The nurse is assigned to the care of a client who has been admitted with meningitis. A spinal tap has been performed. Which of the following cell types in the spinal fluid suggests that the client has become infected with viral meningitis?

1. Platelets
2. Neutrophils
3. Red blood cells
4. Lymphocytes

9 In caring for a female client who has a urinary tract infection with more than 100,000 colonies of *Escherichia coli* bacteria, which of the following would the nurse expect to see on the client's urinalysis report?

1. Negative nitrites
2. Positive leukocyte esterase
3. Positive potassium
4. Negative WBCs

10 The nurse is reviewing the results of follow-up laboratory studies on a client diagnosed with hyperlipidemia. Which of the following total cholesterol levels indicates to the nurse that the client has been compliant with diet and medication therapy?

1. 198 mg/dL
2. 174 mg/dL
3. 269 mg/dL
4. 214 mg/dL

11 A nurse notes the client's albumin level is 2.4 grams/dL. The nurse should plan to assess the client for which of the following at this time?

1. Fluid retention
2. Inelastic skin turgor
3. Hypoactive bowel sounds
4. Dry mucous membranes

12 A client is admitted with complaints of severe nausea and vomiting for several days. The nurse expects the client is at risk for experiencing which acid base imbalance?

1. Metabolic acidosis
2. Metabolic alkalosis
3. Respiratory acidosis
4. Respiratory alkalosis

13 Troponin levels are ordered on a client to confirm a myocardial infarction. When should the nurse plan to have blood drawn for this test?

1. Within 1 to 2 hours of onset of chest pain
2. Within the first 24 hours of onset of chest pain
3. Between 6 and 24 hours of onset of chest pain
4. Between 24 and 48 hours of onset of chest pain

14 The nurse would anticipate that a client with cirrhosis of the liver would have decreased levels of which of the following?

1. Albumin
2. Bilirubin
3. Ammonia
4. Prothrombin time

15 The nurse checks the prothrombin time on a client with aortic valve replacement who is receiving sodium warfarin (Coumadin). The client's level is 20 seconds; control is 13 seconds. The nurse should take which of the following actions?

1. Encourage client to eat foods high in vitamin K.
2. Administer the daily dose of Coumadin as ordered.
3. Monitor the client closely for signs of a deep vein thrombosis.
4. Withhold the next scheduled dose of Coumadin and notify the prescriber.

16 A client is being evaluated for hypothyroidism and has had blood drawn to determine TSH and T_4 levels. Which of the following would support the diagnosis?

1. An elevated TSH and elevated T_4 level
2. An elevated TSH and decreased T_4 level
3. A decreased TSH and elevated T_4 level
4. A decreased TSH and decreased T_4 level

17 A client is admitted with dehydration secondary to prolonged nausea and vomiting. Which of the following lab values would the nurse expect to see?

1. Sodium 138 mEq/dL
2. Potassium 4.2 mEq/dL
3. BUN 30 mg/dL
4. Hematocrit 40%

18 The nurse is establishing a plan of care for a client who has a hemoglobin level of 7.6 grams/dL. Which of the following does the nurse identify as a priority nursing diagnosis?

1. Activity intolerance
2. Constipation
3. Risk for deficient fluid volume
4. Imbalanced nutrition: less than body requirements

19 The nurse should assess for a Trousseau sign in the client with which of the following electrolyte abnormalities?

1. Hypokalemia
2. Hyponatremia
3. Hypochloremia
4. Hypocalcemia

20 The white blood cell (WBC) count of a client is 18,000 cells/microliter. The nurse attributes this value to which of the following health problems of this client?

1. Rheumatoid arthritis
2. History of alcoholism
3. Viral infection
4. Wound dehiscence

21 The nurse would assess the client for fever and other signs of infection if the client's white blood cell count was noted to be greater than how many cells/mm^3 on the laboratory report? Provide a numerical response.

Answer: _____ cells/mm^3

ANSWERS & RATIONALES

1 **Answer: 1** Diabetes insipidus is a complication for any client who has undergone removal of a pituitary tumor. Edema of the remaining pituitary gland may cause reduction in the release of antidiuretic hormone (ADH), resulting in movement of water from the glomerulus into the collecting tubules of the nephron. The client excretes large volumes of urine with a low specific gravity. As water is removed from the vascular compartment, the serum sodium becomes concentrated. Thus, the lab result indicates hypernatremia. The serum potassium, osmolality, and hematocrit would not be low (options 2, 3, and 4).
Cognitive Level: Analysis **Client Need:** Physiological Integrity: Reduction of Risk Potential **Integrated Process:** Nursing Process: Assessment **Content Area:** Adult Health: Endocrine and Metabolic **Strategy:** This question calls for specific knowledge of ADH and the alteration in ADH secretion that commonly occurs following surgery for removal of a pituitary tumor. Remember that ADH results in the movement of free water (that is, water without sodium) into the collecting tubules of the nephron, which results in large volumes of water being removed from the blood. The specific gravity (concentration) of the urine decreases. In addition, removal of water from the serum concentrates (and thereby elevates) the serum sodium. Recall also that hemoconcentration could also raise, not lower, other lab values.

2 **Answer: 4** Furosemide inhibits reabsorption of sodium, water, and potassium from the distal renal tubules and the loop of Henle, leading to a diuresis. The most common electrolyte disturbance associated with furosemide administration is hypokalemia. BUN and creatinine may be either elevated or lowered depending on a client's individualized response to therapy. Similarly, the hematocrit could rise or fall depending on the amount of fluid retained in the vascular compartment.
Cognitive Level: Analysis **Client Need:** Physiological Integrity: Reduction of Risk Potential **Integrated Process:** Nursing Process: Assessment **Content Area:** Adult Health: Renal and Genitourinary **Strategy:** This question calls for specific knowledge of the action of furosemide and that hypokalemia is a common side effect of furosemide therapy. Use nursing knowledge and the process of elimination to make a selection.

3 **Answer: 2** Hypokalemia is an almost universal complication of loss of gastric hydrochloric acid. In this scenario, loss of the hydrogen ions results in a metabolic alkalosis. In turn, compensation for this loss takes place in the nephron where hydrogen ions are retained. The nephron is obligated to excrete potassium, which may result in profound hypokalemia and require vigilant IV replacement. Other electrolytes may be affected, but not to the degree that potassium homeostasis is altered.
Cognitive Level: Application **Client Need:** Physiological Integrity: Reduction of Risk Potential **Integrated Process:** Nursing Process: Analysis **Content Area:** Adult Health: Gastrointestinal **Strategy:** This question calls for specific knowledge that loss of hydrochloric acid triggers the mechanism whereby the kidneys lose potassium. Use nursing knowledge and the process of elimination to make a selection.

4 **Answer: 3** Elevated uric acid levels are commonly seen with gout, and this is the initial question to ask the client. Uric acid does not rise with gallbladder disease and is not affected by green tea. Although the client could experience renal stones from precipitation of uric acid crystals (causing flank pain), this is not the initial question to ask since renal stones are a complication of gout.

Cognitive Level: Analysis **Client Need:** Physiological Integrity: Reduction of Risk Potential **Integrated Process:** Nursing Process: Assessment **Content Area:** Adult Health: Endocrine and Metabolic **Strategy:** Note that the stem of the question has the critical word *initially,* which tells you that more than one option may be technically correct but one is better than the others. Use nursing knowledge related to uric acid level and gout and the process of elimination to make a selection.

5 **Answer: 2** Serum creatinine is the best indicator of renal function. Often, decreases in serum creatinine are dramatic following renal transplantation. Regular monitoring of serum creatinine levels is imperative in assessing the function of the transplanted kidney. Hemoglobin levels may increase postoperatively because of blood transfusions. Serum phosphate may decrease long term as the kidney increases excretion of phosphates. However, this is not a reliable indicator of renal function. Serum sodium levels may fluctuate according to individual client's sodium–water balance. **Cognitive Level:** Analysis **Client Need:** Physiological Integrity: Reduction of Risk Potential **Integrated Process:** Nursing Process: Assessment **Content Area:** Adult Health: Renal and Genitourinary **Strategy:** This question calls for specific knowledge that creatinine is the best indicator of renal function. Use nursing knowledge and the process of elimination to make a selection.

6 **Answer: 3** The hematocrit is an indicator of the proportion occupied by the cells in a given volume of blood. The hematocrit may decrease when cell volume of the blood is decreased because of blood loss. In addition, the hematocrit may decrease when the liquid portion of the blood volume increases, as would be the case when large volumes of intravenous fluid are administered. Hemoglobin would not be increased in this client situation, nor would sodium and calcium balance be altered.
Cognitive Level: Analysis **Client Need:** Physiological Integrity: Reduction of Risk Potential **Integrated Process:** Nursing Process: Assessment **Content Area:** Adult Health: Endocrine and Metabolic **Strategy:** This question calls for specific knowledge that hematocrit may be reduced even if there is no blood loss. In this case, it is indicative of increased volume, most likely due to administration of intravenous fluids. Use nursing knowledge and the process of elimination to make a selection.

7 **Answer: 1** Neutrophils are responsible for destruction of bacterial invaders. In acute bacterial infections, such as appendicitis, the percentage of neutrophils (especially immature bands) in the complete blood count will increase. This presence of an increased number of bands in the CBC is known as a "shift to the left." Lymphocytes are responsible for destruction of viruses. Erythrocytes and platelets are not affected by infections.
Cognitive Level: Analysis **Client Need:** Physiological Integrity: Reduction of Risk Potential **Integrated Process:** Nursing Process: Assessment **Content Area:** Adult Health: Gastrointestinal **Strategy:** This question calls for specific knowledge that neutrophils are responsible for destruction of bacterial invaders and will be elevated in acute bacterial infections. Use nursing knowledge and the process of elimination to make a selection.

8 **Answer: 4** Lymphocytes are responsible for the destruction of viruses. Thus, the presence of lymphocytes in the cerebrospinal fluid (CSF) suggests that the meningitis is viral in etiology, which is significant because the infection is most commonly self-limiting and will not respond to antibiotic therapy (as would bacterial meningitis). The presence of neutrophils would suggest bacterial meningitis. Normally, CSF is free of all cell types.
Cognitive Level: Application **Client Need:** Physiological Integrity: Reduction of Risk Potential **Integrated Process:** Nursing Process: Analysis **Content Area:** Adult Health: Neurological **Strategy:** This question calls for specific knowledge that lymphocytes are responsible for destruction of viruses. Use nursing knowledge and the process of elimination to make a selection.

9 **Answer: 2** A positive leukocyte esterase suggests a urinary tract infection. Leukocytes (white blood cells) contain esterases that react with substances contained in urine. More than 100,000 colonies of bacteria (per high-powered field) are needed before the patient can be diagnosed with a UTI. Testing for the presence of leukocyte esterase may be done using a voided urine sample, which is simple compared to the need for a catheterized urine sample. Nitrites may be positive in this situation. White blood cells may be elevated. Potassium in the urine is unaffected and rarely measured.
Cognitive Level: Application **Client Need:** Physiological Integrity: Reduction of Risk Potential **Integrated Process:** Nursing Process: Analysis **Content Area:** Adult Health: Renal and Genitourinary **Strategy:** This question calls for specific knowledge that leukocyte esterase will be positive in a sample of urine infected with bacteria. Use nursing knowledge and the process of elimination to make a selection.

10 **Answer: 2** The goal for total serum cholesterol is to keep the value below 200 mg/dL. Although options 1 and 2 are within the normal range, the best outcome of therapy is the value that is the lower of the two.
Cognitive Level: Analysis **Client Need:** Physiological Integrity: Reduction of Risk Potential **Integrated Process:** Nursing Process: Assessment **Content Area:** Adult Health: Cardiovascular **Strategy:** The core issue of the question is knowledge of normal serum cholesterol levels. Use nursing knowledge and the process of elimination to make a selection.

11 **Answer: 1** Albumin is a protein responsible for increasing osmotic pressure and maintaining intravascular fluid volume. Low albumin levels result in a decrease in intravascular colloid osmotic pressure, which in turn allows fluid to move out of the blood vessel and into interstitial tissues. This condition will be assessed as fluid retention in the form of edema, crackles, and so on. Skin turgor will be elastic when fluid shifts into the interstitial spaces. Bowel sounds and mucous membranes would not be affected.
Cognitive Level: Analysis **Client Need:** Physiological Integrity: Reduction of Risk Potential **Integrated Process:** Nursing Process: Planning **Content Area:** Adult Health: Endocrine and Metabolic **Strategy:** Determine that this test result is an abnormal and low albumin level. Recall that albumin is

necessary for maintenance of fluid balance between body compartments. Systematically eliminate incorrect options.

12 **Answer: 2** The loss of stomach acids creates an imbalance leading to an excess of alkaline fluids in the body. The source of the loss is metabolic, not respiratory.
Cognitive Level: Application **Client Need:** Physiological Integrity: Reduction of Risk Potential **Integrated Process:** Nursing Process: Analysis **Content Area:** Adult Health: Endocrine and Metabolic **Strategy:** First, determine if the imbalance is metabolic or respiratory. Loss of GI fluids is a metabolic function, so options 3 and 4 can be eliminated. Next, determine if the imbalance is acid or base. Loss of body acids will lead to an excess of bicarbonate in the body.

13 **Answer: 3** Troponin is a specific marker for cardiac injury. Elevations in serum levels usually begin 4 to 6 hours after onset of symptoms and peak in 12 to 24 hours. Drawing the blood in the first 2 hours would be too soon, and waiting longer than 24 hours would miss the times for peak levels.
Cognitive Level: Application **Client Need:** Physiological Integrity: Reduction of Risk Potential **Integrated Process:** Nursing Process: Planning **Content Area:** Adult Health: Cardiovascular **Strategy:** The question calls for specific knowledge of troponin physiology. Recall the times for elevations following cardiac injury and choose the option closest. Choose option 3 over 2 because it is more specific.

14 **Answer: 1** In cirrhosis, the damaged liver is unable to properly metabolize amino acids and synthesize albumin, resulting in decreased serum concentrations. The damaged liver is unable to completely break down bilirubin, and serum levels are elevated. Ammonia is normally converted to urea; serum levels are increased with liver damage. Prothrombin times are increased when the liver is unable to synthesize clotting factors.
Cognitive Level: Application **Client Need:** Physiological Integrity: Reduction of Risk Potential **Integrated Process:** Nursing Process: Assessment **Content Area:** Adult Health: Gastrointestinal **Strategy:** This question tests knowledge of liver functions and cirrhosis. Recall the liver's function as related to each of the lab values and systematically eliminate incorrect options.

15 **Answer: 2** Prothrombin times should be 1.5 to 2 times the control when anticoagulation therapy is being given, indicating the Coumadin is effective. The level is in the therapeutic range, and the next dose should be given as scheduled. Encouraging the client to eat foods high in vitamin K would reduce effectiveness of the Coumadin. The client would be at risk for bleeding, not for deep vein thrombosis, when prothrombin times are prolonged.
Cognitive Level: Analysis **Client Need:** Physiological Integrity: Reduction of Risk Potential **Integrated Process:** Nursing Process: Implementation **Content Area:** Adult Health: Cardiovascular **Strategy:** First, determine if the level is abnormal. Recall that in order to be therapeutic, prothrombin times must be 1.5 to 2 times the control. Eliminate options 1 and 4 because they would be counterproductive to the purpose of the Coumadin therapy. Eliminate option 3 because the client is not at risk for this problem.

16 **Answer: 2** In hypothyroidism, the thyroid gland does not produce thyroxine (T_4) despite being stimulated by the pituitary gland (TSH, thyroid-stimulating hormone) to do so. Elevated TSH and T_4 levels are seen with secondary hyperthyroidism caused by excessive TSH production by the pituitary. A decreased TSH and elevated T_4 are seen with primary hyperthyroidism. Decreased TSH and T_4 levels are seen in hypothyroidism secondary to insufficient pituitary secretions.
Cognitive Level: Application **Client Need:** Physiological Integrity: Reduction of Risk Potential **Integrated Process:** Nursing Process: Assessment **Content Area:** Adult Health: Endocrine and Metabolic **Strategy:** The question requires knowledge of pituitary and thyroid hormone functions. Recall the negative feedback loop of the endocrine system. Eliminate options 1 and 4 because there is an increased T_4 level, which would not be seen with primary hypothyroidism.

17 **Answer: 3** Dehydration results in loss of fluids, causing a hemoconcentration of the BUN, which is elevated. Sodium would be elevated, not normal, with dehydration. The potassium level is normal and would most likely be lower because of losses from the vomiting. The hematocrit would also be elevated secondary to hemoconcentration.
Cognitive Level: Analysis **Client Need:** Physiological Integrity: Reduction of Risk Potential **Integrated Process:** Nursing Process: Assessment **Content Area:** Adult Health: Gastrointestinal **Strategy:** The question requires analysis of fluid losses on common lab values. Recall that vomiting will result in loss of sodium, potassium, and water. Eliminate options 1 and 2 because they are normal and you are looking for abnormal values. Eliminate option 4 because it is also normal and would be elevated with fluid losses.

18 **Answer: 1** Hemoglobin is the oxygen-carrying component of red blood cells. When levels are decreased the client will be fatigued and tire easily. Altered nutrition may be the cause of the low hemoglobin, but it is not of highest priority since intolerance to activity involves safety concerns. Constipation and risk for deficient fluid volume would not be as high in priority.
Cognitive Level: Analysis **Client Need:** Physiological Integrity: Reduction of Risk Potential **Integrated Process:** Nursing Process: Analysis **Content Area:** Adult Health: Hematological **Strategy:** The question asks to choose a priority, indicating all options may be partially or totally correct. Eliminate options 2 and 3 because they are not as high a priority. Choose option 1 over 4 because it addresses a problem related to the function of hemoglobin.

19 **Answer: 4** Hypocalcemia causes excitability of skeletal, cardiac, and smooth muscle tissues. Evidence of this is seen in the Trousseau sign, a carpopedal spasm. Hypokalemia, hyponatremia, and hypochloremia would not cause this sign.
Cognitive Level: Application **Client Need:** Physiological Integrity: Reduction of Risk Potential **Integrated Process:** Nursing Process: Assessment **Content Area:** Adult Health: Endocrine and Metabolic **Strategy:** Specific knowledge of the Trousseau sign is needed to answer this question. Recall this is a carpopedal spasm seen with low calcium and magnesium levels. Eliminate options 1, 2, and 4 because they would lead to muscle weakness, not neuromuscular excitability.

ANSWERS & RATIONALES

20 **Answer: 4** Tissue injury can cause an increase in WBCs. The WBC count could decrease with rheumatoid arthritis, alcoholism, and viral infections (options 1, 2, and 3).
Cognitive Level: Analysis **Client Need:** Physiological Integrity: Reduction of Risk Potential **Integrated Process:** Nursing Process: Assessment **Content Area:** Adult Health: Gastrointestinal **Strategy:** First, determine that the value is abnormal and that is it elevated. Recall conditions that elevate the white count, such as bacterial infections, stress, and tissue injury. Evaluate each option to eliminate conditions in which the white count is decreased. Choose option 4 because wound dehiscence is a type of tissue injury.

21 **Answer: 10,000** The normal range for the white blood cell count is 5,000 to 10,000/mm^3. For this reason, the nurse would be concerned about the risk of infection if the count exceeded 10,000.
Cognitive Level: Analysis **Client Need:** Physiological Integrity: Reduction of Risk Potential **Integrated Process:** Nursing Process: Assessment **Content Area:** Adult Health: Endocrine and Metabolic **Strategy:** The core issue of the question is knowledge of normal laboratory values. Use this knowledge to choose an answer. Since specific knowledge is needed to answer correctly, memorize this value if you found the question difficult.

Key Terms to Review

plasma p. 824

serum p. 822

References

Corbett, J. (2004). *Laboratory tests and diagnostic procedures with nursing diagnoses* (6th ed.). Upper Saddle River, NJ: Pearson Education.

Fischbach, F. (2004). *A manual of laboratory and diagnostic tests* (7th ed.). Philadelphia: Lippincott.

Kacmarek, R. (2005). *The essentials of respiratory care* (4th ed.). Philadelphia: Elsevier Mosby.

Leeuwen, A., Kranpitz, T., & Smith, L. (2006). *Davis's comprehensive handbook of laboratory and diagnostic tests with nursing implications* (2nd ed.). Philadelphia: F.A. Davis.

Malley, W. J. (2005). *Clinical blood gases* (2nd ed.). Philadelphia: Elsevier Saunders.

Smith, S., Duell, D., & Martin, B. (2004). *Clinical nursing skills: Basic to advanced skills* (6th ed.). Upper Saddle River, NJ: Pearson Education.

Wilkins, R. (2005). *Clinical assessment in respiratory care* (5th ed.). Philadelphia: Elsevier Mosby.

48 Common Diagnostic Tests and Procedures

Test Yourself

Are you ready for the NCLEX-RN® or course exams? Use the practice tests on the companion CD-ROM to check.

In this chapter

Cross Reference

Other chapters relevant to this content area are

Common Laboratory Tests **Chapter 47**

I. GENERAL DIAGNOSTIC TESTS

A. Client safety in diagnostic testing

1. Ensuring client safety is a requirement of the Joint Commission on Accreditation of Healthcare Organizations (JCAHO)
2. Client safety for any diagnostic test implies knowledge of the procedure, its risks and benefits, and pre- and post-care
3. Ensure that informed consent form is signed and witnessed, especially for invasive diagnostic tests involving penetration of tissues or blood vessels (contrast dye, radioisotopes)
4. ! Before beginning a diagnostic test, a *time out* or pause is called to double check that the right procedure is being carried out on the right client at the right site

B. Biopsy

1. Overview
   - a. Removal and examination of body tissue to detect malignancy or other disease process
   - b. Methods include aspiration by suction, brush method (scrapes cells using stiff bristles), excision by surgical cutting, needle aspiration, or punch biopsy (using punch-type instrument)
   - c. Common sites are bone marrow, breast, endometrium of uterus, kidney, colon, and liver
2. Preprocedure care
   - a. Take baseline vital signs
   - b. Explain that biopsy site will be anesthetized just prior to procedure

c. Explain that with needle biopsy client may be asked to take a breath and hold it
d. Keep client NPO for 6 hours prior to liver biopsy to decrease liver congestion

3. Postprocedure care
   a. Monitor vital signs as prescribed
   b. Apply pressure to site for 20 minutes (kidney) or place client on right side (liver) to reduce risk of bleeding; apply pressure dressing
   c. Observe for bleeding at site and instruct client to report bleeding
   d. Instruct client to rest and avoid heavy lifting for 24 hours or longer if indicated (liver, kidney)
   e. Increase fluid intake and teach client to report decreased urine output or burning on urination (kidney)
   f. Do not administer aspirin, anticoagulants (heparin or warfarin), or nonsteroidal anti-inflammatory drugs (NSAIDs) from immediately after biopsy until 2 weeks post-biopsy to prevent bleeding

C. Computed tomography (CT) scan

1. Overview
   a. Screens commonly for abscesses, infection, vascular disease, stroke, bone destruction, tumors, edema, lesions in head, liver, and kidney; soft tissue foreign bodies
   b. Common areas for scanning are head and brain, chest (thoracic), abdominal, spine, long bones, joints, and pelvis
   c. CT scanning may be done with or without contrast dye (most are without contrast)
   d. Produces narrow x-ray beam that examines body sections from many angles
   e. Protective shields must be worn by personnel and over client's reproductive area to prevent adverse effects of x-ray exposures
   f. Clients of child-bearing age should have urine pregnancy testing done
2. Preprocedure care
   a. Ensure informed consent when contrast is used
   b. Assess for allergy to eggs, iodine, or contrast media
   c. No food or fluid restriction if contrast dye is not used; with IV contrast studies, keep client NPO for 4 hours prior and assess kidney function for contrast clearance
   d. If client is allergic to contrast medium, hypoallergenic contrast may be used or client may be premedicated with prednisone, diphenhydramine (Benadryl), and ranitidine (Zantac)
   e. Ensure client has patent IV access
   f. Remove metal objects prior to scanning
   g. Teach client that machine is circular and makes series of "clicking" sounds, test is not painful, and takes usually about 15 minutes
   h. Teach client that contrast media may cause a warm, flushed feeling or salty, fishy, or metallic taste in mouth, and possibly nausea for 1 to 2 minutes
3. Postprocedure care
   a. Assess for delayed reaction to contrast dye if used (skin rash, urticaria, headache, vomiting, renal dysfunction) and increase fluid intake to clear contrast from kidneys
   b. Explain that client can resume usual diet and activity unless otherwise ordered

D. Fluoroscopy

1. Overview
   a. Views functions of organs in motion on fluorescent screen
   b. Often used with many diagnostic tests for visualization and guidance
   c. Common areas include thorax, abdomen, heart, and brain
   d. Room is darkened for visualization and those remaining in room should wear protective aprons to prevent exposure
2. Preprocedure care
   a. Explain that there is no discomfort with procedure
   b. Ask if client is pregnant or suspects pregnancy because procedure contraindicated during pregnancy; complete a pregnancy test if indicated

c. Barium sulfate is given to clients undergoing abdominal procedures
d. Teach client that x-ray personnel may give specific instructions during test

3. Postprocedure care
   a. Food and fluids permitted after abdominal and thorax fluoroscopy, but cardiac catheterization aftercare is performed following fluoroscopy of heart (see section later in chapter)
   b. Laxative is usually ordered post-fluoroscopy of abdomen

E. Magnetic resonance imaging (MRI)

1. Overview
   a. Produces images similar to CT scanning but does not use ionizing radiation, so client is free of hazards caused by exposure to x-rays
   b. Consists of magnet enclosed in large, doughnut-shaped cylinder; client is guided into cylinder until body part undergoing diagnosis is within magnetic field
   c. ! Implanted metal devices (pacemakers or wires, aneurysm or surgical clips, metal rods or screws in bones, some hearing aids, nerve stimulators) are contraindications to MRI
   d. Used to detect central nervous system lesions, vascular problems such as with blood flow or hemorrhage, cardiac perfusion problems, injury, edema, or tumors
2. Preprocedure care
   a. Obtain history related to implanted metal objects, which are contraindications for test
   b. ! Remove all jewelry and other objects containing metal (eyeglasses, hearing aids, hair pins, cosmetics that may have metallic fragments)
   c. Food and fluids are not restricted for adults, but children may be NPO for 4 hours
   d. ! IV access may be inserted for contrast (usually gadolinium is used—nonallergenic, but may affect calcium absorption for next 24 hours)
   e. Teach client that procedure involves lying on narrow table that will slide into machine; clients with claustrophobia may need sedation or use of open machine if available; test is painless
   f. ! Teach client that machine makes series of loud noises (clicks and thumps) but that earplugs are available and client can communicate with personnel via intercom; family member or friend may remain in room with client (no radiation)
   g. MRI machines have weight limits
3. Postprocedure care: none specific

F. Nuclear scan (also called radionuclide imaging or radioisotope scan)

1. Overview
   a. Scintillation camera records distribution of radioisotope in specific organ(s) under study after oral or IV administration or by inhalation, depending on area under study
   b. Common radioisotopes include technetium 99m (most common), iodine 123 and 125, thallium 201, xenon, indium 111 (for labeling white blood cells), and gallium citrate
2. Preprocedure care
   a. Keep NPO for nuclear scans of heart, GI tract and gallbladder, and thyroid; no restriction for bone, brain, kidney (keep well hydrated), liver and spleen, and lung
   b. ! Administer ordered blocking agent (Lugol's solution, potassium perchlorate) prior to radioiodine study except for thyroid scan
   c. Adhere to specific preparation protocols for administration of radioisotopes and waiting periods before scanning; ensure client arrives for appointment on time
   d. Teach client to avoid high-iodine foods and iodized salt for 3 days prior to thyroid scan
   e. ! Teach client that radionuclide leaves body in 6 to 24 hours and should not affect other people

f. Teach client that scans cause no discomfort, that client should lie still during procedure unless asked to change position, and that more than one imaging session may be needed (client may need to return for additional imaging at specified times)

g. Remove jewelry and other metal objects in area under study

3. Postprocedure care: none specific

G. Positron emission tomography (PET) scan

1. Overview

a. Most common purpose is to detect blood flow to brain and heart

b. Other uses include to differentiate between types of dementia, identify stages of cranial tumors, differentiate between benign and malignant lesions, and stage malignant lesions and disease

c. Measures concentrations of positron-emitting isotope after receiving a substance tagged with a radionuclide (radioactive glucose, rubidium 82, oxygen 15, nitrogen 13)

2. Preprocedure care

a. Ensure that client has patent IV access and measure vital signs

b. Teach client to follow instructions given during test, Velcro straps may be used to limit movement during test, and radiation from test is short-lived

3. Postprocedure care

a. Monitor vital signs; avoid postural hypotension by moving client slowly to upright position

b. Increase fluid intake to aid in clearing radioisotope via kidneys

H. Ultrasonography (sonogram)

1. Overview

a. Uses a probe (transducer) over skin surface or in body cavity to produce ultrasound beam that is reflected or echoed from tissues and can be captured by computer into scans, graphs, or audible sounds (Doppler)

b. Detects tissue abnormalities such as masses, cysts, edema, fluid, and stones; evaluates blood flow in arteries and veins

c. Can be used for many body tissues, including abdominal aorta, brain, breast, arteries and veins, gallbladder, heart, kidney, liver, pelvis including pregnant or nonpregnant uterus, pancreas, prostate, scrotum, spleen, thorax, and thyroid

2. Preprocedure care

a. Restrict food and fluids for 4 to 8 hours prior to tests of abdomen, abdominal aorta, gallbladder, liver, spleen, and pancreas

b. Have client eat fat-free meal on evening prior to abdominal, gallbladder, liver, pancreas, kidney, or liver sonogram

c. For pelvic and renal ultrasound (including obstetrics), client should drink 24 ounces water 1 hour prior to exam or three to four 8-ounce glasses of clear fluid 90 minutes prior to exam; teach client not to void until after test is completed

d. Instruct client that ultrasound gel is applied to skin surface of site being examined; probe is moved smoothly with light pressure over area

e. Teach client that test is usually painless and no radiation is involved

3. Postprocedure care: none specific

I. X-rays

1. Overview

a. Performed to detect abnormal size, structure, and shape of bone or body tissues

b. May be done as initial screening test

c. Common tests include chest, heart, abdominal (flat plate), KUB (kidneys, ureter, bladder), skull, and skeletal

d. Because of risk of radiation, protective garb is provided to client to wear over reproductive organs and to personnel as well; pregnant clients should avoid x-rays, especially during first trimester of pregnancy (perform urine pregnancy test prior to x-rays)

2. Preprocedure care

a. Food and fluids are generally not restricted unless it is anticipated that client may go to surgery following tests (such as to repair bone fractures)

! b. Remove hairpins, glasses, jewelry, and other metallic objects prior to test
c. Explain that more than one x-ray film may be needed and that client may need to wait while staff ensures that films are of good quality

3. Postprocedure care: none specific

II. RESPIRATORY DIAGNOSTIC TESTS

A. Bronchoscopy

1. Overview
   a. Allows for direct inspection or visualization of larynx, trachea, and bronchi using a metal or flexible fiberoptic bronchoscope
   b. Indicated to diagnose tracheobronchial tumor or bleeding site, remove foreign body or mucus plugs, or obtain secretions for cytologic examination or culture
   c. Client generally receives premedication and local anesthetic sprayed in throat and sometimes nose (if fiberoptic instrument used) before insertion of bronchoscope
2. Preprocedure care
   a. Ensure that informed consent form and complete preprocedure or preoperative checklist are completed
   ! b. Assess for allergies to drugs (especially analgesics, anesthetics, and antibiotics), food, and latex
   ! c. Have client void before giving premedication
   d. Remove dentures, contact lenses, and jewelry
   e. Obtain baseline vital signs; ensure admission vital signs also available for reference and comparison
   f. Instruct client to relax during test if using local anesthesia; general anesthesia may also be used; explain that throat may be sore after procedure but will resolve
! 3. Postprocedure care
   a. Monitor vital signs every 15 minutes for first hour, every 30 minutes for second hour, and then hourly until stable
   b. Keep head of bed elevated in semi-Fowler's position; if unconscious, lie client onto side with head slightly elevated to prevent aspiration
   c. Assess for and notify physician of respiratory distress (dyspnea, wheezing, apprehension, decreased breath sounds)
   ! d. Explain that coughing with minimal blood-tinged mucus may be expected; assess for and immediately report hemoptysis (coughing up of excessively bloody secretions)
   ! e. Do not give food or fluids until gag and swallow reflexes have returned (usually 2 to 8 hours postprocedure); offer ice chips and sips of water before giving food
   f. Offer throat lozenges to relieve sore throat once client is taking food and fluids
   g. Evaluate for and report complications after procedure, including laryngeal edema, bronchospasm, pneumothorax, cardiac dysrhythmias, and bleeding from biopsy site

B. Pulmonary function tests

1. Overview
   a. Detect pulmonary dysfunction, differentiate between obstructive and restrictive lung disease, evaluate response to drug therapy (such as bronchodilators or steroids), and obtain baseline parameters for planning pulmonary rehabilitation program
   b. Common pulmonary tests include vital capacity tests, lung volume studies, flow volume loop, diffusion capacity test, bronchial provocation studies, exercise studies, pulse oximetry, nutritional studies (indirect calorimetry), and body plethysmography
2. Preprocedure care
   a. Contact laboratory for specific restrictions, which can vary among labs
   ! b. Instruct client to avoid eating heavy meal prior to test and to avoid smoking for 4 to 6 hours before test

c. Record client's age, height, and weight for use in predicting normal range of results
d. Tell client to wear nonrestrictive clothing
e. Cancel test if client has active cold, fever, or is under influence of alcohol
f. Withhold medications that affect results, including sedatives and narcotics; check whether bronchodilators are allowed (they may be withheld beforehand and be given during test)
g. Help client practice breathing patterns for test, such as normal breathing, rapid breathing, forced deep inspiration, and forced deep expiration

3. Postprocedure care: none specific

C. Ventilation scan (pulmonary ventilation scan)

1. Overview
a. A nuclear scan of lungs in which client inhales mixture of air, oxygen, and radioactive gas
b. Often performed in conjunction with pulmonary perfusion scan to differentiate between ventilatory problem and vascular abnormality in lungs
c. Also done to detect lung cancer, sarcoidosis, or tuberculosis, and to determine hypoventilation caused by excessive smoking or chronic obstructive pulmonary disease (COPD)

2. Preprocedure care
a. There is no food or fluid restriction
b. Remove all jewelry and other metal objects from neck and chest area
c. Teach client that he or she will inhale radioactive gas and will be asked to take deep breath and hold it while single image of lung is taken; other images will be recorded during three phases of test: wash-in (gas builds up in lungs), equilibrium (steady state), and wash-out (gas is expelled while breathing room air)

3. Postprocedure care
a. Assess respiratory status and breath sounds; report changes in rate and difficulty breathing
b. Assess for and report chest pain, especially if pulmonary embolism is suspected as underlying problem being diagnosed

III. CARDIOVASCULAR DIAGNOSTIC TESTS

A. Angiography (angiogram)

1. Overview
a. Injection of contrast dye via catheter into femoral, brachial, subclavian, or carotid arteries to visualize blood vessels; also called arteriography
b. Used to detect aneurysms, thrombosis, emboli, space-occupying lesions, stenosis, and plaques, and to evaluate cerebral, pulmonary, and renal blood flow
c. Type is generally specified by prefacing *angiography* or *angiogram* with the name of the area under study, such as cerebral angiography or pulmonary angiogram; may also be used to evaluate extent of peripheral arterial disease

2. Preprocedure care
a. Keep client NPO for 8 to 12 hours prior to test
b. Shave access site
c. Discontinue anticoagulants, such as heparin, for specified time prior to test (e.g., 6 hours)
d. Record baseline vital signs
e. Assess for allergy to contrast dye
f. Have client void before procedure
g. Ensure that client has patent IV access before procedure and begin any ordered IV fluids at time specified; administer any ordered premedication
h. Give cleansing enema as ordered prior to renal angiography to enhance visualization; perform vascular studies before any barium studies are done
i. Explain that client will receive local anesthetic to site and must remain still during procedure

3. Postprocedure care
   - ! **a.** Apply pressure for up to 30 minutes or longer until bleeding has stopped; check injection site for bleeding, swelling, or hematoma with each set of vital signs
   - ! **b.** Monitor vital signs every 15 minutes for first hour, every 30 minutes for 2 hours, every hour for next 4 hours, or longer until stable, then routine per agency policy
   - ! **c.** Assess peripheral pulses in affected area (femoral and dorsalis pedis or radial) with vital signs and document and report diminished or absent pulses to physician
   - ! **d.** Note neurovascular status of affected extremity (color, temperature, motion, sensitivity) when assessing pulses and report abnormal findings (pale, cool, numbness, weakness)
   - **e.** Monitor body temperature every 4 hours for 24 to 48 hours as ordered
   - **f.** Maintain bedrest for 6 to 8 hours as ordered and restrict activities until following day
   - ! **g.** Apply sandbag, pressure device, cold compress, or ice bag to site as ordered to relieve edema or discomfort
   - ! **h.** Assess for delayed reaction to contrast media (tachycardia, dyspnea, skin rash, urticaria, falling blood pressure, and decreased urine output)
   - **i.** Teach client that coughing may be expected following pulmonary angiography
   - ! **j.** Assess for and report dysphagia and respiratory distress following cerebral angiography, and also for weakness or numbness in an extremity, confusion, slurred speech, or visual changes (may indicate transient ischemic attack or TIA)

B. Cardiac catheterization

1. Overview
   - **a.** Also known as cardiac angiography, angiocardiography, and coronary arteriography
   - **b.** May be performed as right-cardiac catheterization with access via femoral vein to diagnose tricuspid or pulmonic valve stenosis or regurgitation, pulmonary hypertension, and septal defects
   - **c.** May be performed as left-heart catheterization with access via brachial or femoral artery up through aorta to diagnose metal or aortic valve stenosis or regurgitation, coronary artery disease, left ventricular hypertrophy, and ventricular aneurysm
   - **d.** Left-sided catheterization is more commonly performed and uses principles of angiography outlined in previous section

! 2. Preprocedure care
   - **a.** Ensure that informed consent is signed and witnessed and ensure that provider has discussed possible risks with client and family
   - **b.** Restrict food and fluids for 8 hours before test or as per agency policy
   - **c.** Assess for allergy to contrast media and administer any ordered antihistamines and steroids on the evening before or on day of test
   - **d.** Withhold medications, including anticoagulants such as heparin, for 6 to 8 hours as ordered by physician
   - **e.** Cleanse and shave/prep insertion site on morning of procedure
   - **f.** Measure and record client's height and weight to calculate dye needed (1mL/kg body weight), and record baseline vital signs and peripheral pulses
   - **g.** Ensure client voids before administering any premedication (given 30 minutes to 1 hour prior)
   - **h.** Ensure client has patent IV access
   - ! **i.** Explain that client will be in cardiac cath room on a padded table; IV fluids will be administered; cardiac rhythm will be monitored; skin anesthetic will be applied to injection site; client may feel flushed or warm with dye injection and this will pass; client may be asked to cough or deep breathe during procedure; coughing can reduce nausea from dye and possible cardiac dysrhythmias

! 3. Postprocedure care
   a. Monitor vital signs (BP, pulse, respirations) every 15 minutes for an hour, every 30 minutes until stable, then every hour as ordered, and then every 4 hours; monitor temperature every 4 hours
   b. Assess catheter insertion site for bleeding or hematoma and change dressing as needed
   c. Assess peripheral pulses, neurovascular status of affected extremity, pain or discomfort
   d. Assess cardiac rhythm and report rate or rhythm abnormalities
   e. Assess for and report chest pain, chest heaviness, shortness of breath, and abdominal or groin pain
   f. Administer prescribed analgesics for comfort and antibiotics if ordered
   g. Instruct client to remain on bedrest for 8 to 12 hours or as indicated by agency policy
   h. Client may turn from side to side and head of bed may be elevated to no more than 30 degrees (some agencies have head flat or only 15 degrees elevation); affected leg must be kept straight for 8 to 12 hours; if arm used for access, it must be immobilized for 3 hours (smaller blood vessel)
   i. Increase fluid intake to aid contrast dye excretion unless contraindicated by heart failure or renal disease
   j. Assess for and report complications, including myocardial infarction, dysrhythmias, cardiac tamponade, and pulmonary or cerebral embolism

C. Echocardiography

1. Overview
   a. A noninvasive ultrasound test to identify abnormalities in heart size, structure, and function, and to diagnose valvular disease
   b. Handheld transducer is moved over chest in area of heart and other identified areas; sound waves are emitted and reflected back to produce images that appear on a video screen and are recorded on videotape and graph paper
   c. Several specific types of studies are available, including M-mode, two-dimensional, spectral Doppler, color Doppler, transesophageal, contrast, and stress echocardiography
2. Preprocedure care
   a. Measure and record baseline vital signs
   b. There is no food or fluid restriction and no medications need to be withheld unless ordered by physician; exceptions are transesophageal and stress echocardiography, which require NPO status 4 hours prior to test
   ! c. For transesophageal test, client will be given IV sedation
   ! d. For contrast test, an IV access line must be inserted
   e. Have client undress from waist up and wear hospital gown
   f. Explain procedure to client (outlined earlier in general ultrasound section)
   g. Explain that client will lie supine or on left side
3. Postprocedure care
   a. None for most tests
   b. Client is monitored during recovery for 1 to 2 hours following transesophageal test

D. Electrocardiography (electrocardiogram or ECG, EKG)

1. Overview
   a. Measures electrical activity of heart
   ! b. Detects cardiac dysrhythmias and electrolyte imbalance (hyperkalemia—tall peaked T wave)
   ! c. Electrodes are placed on extremities and chest (excess hair may be shaved in small spots) and electrical activity is recorded with each heartbeat
   d. Records cardiac waveforms or complexes in 12 leads: six limb leads (three bipolar: leads I, II, and III; three unipolar: leads aVR, aVL, and aVF), and six chest or precordial leads (V1 through V6)

! 2. Preprocedure care
   a. No food or fluid restriction is needed; no, consent form is required

b. Position client in supine position and expose arms and legs for lead placement
c. Clothing should be removed to waist, with females given a gown to wear
d. Note medications client is receiving, since some drugs (e.g., antidysrhythmics and beta-blockers) may alter readings
e. Instruct client to relax muscles and breathe normally during ECG, and that procedure does not cause pain or electric shock
f. Instruct client to state if chest pain is experienced during ECG

3. Postprocedure care: remove electrode paste or jelly if used and assist client to dress if needed

E. Holter monitoring

1. Overview
a. Evaluates heart rate and rhythm during normal activities over a 24-hour period; identifies cardiac dysrhythmias
b. Consists of a cassette tape and clock inside a 1-pound monitor that is worn by client
! c. Client keeps a diary to record timing of symptoms such as palpitations, chest pain, shortness of breath, syncope, vertigo, and usual daily activities (eating, exercise, sleep) for correlation with ECG readings

2. Preprocedure care
a. No food or fluid restriction is necessary
b. Clean and shave as necessary skin areas needed for electrode placement
c. Place five to seven electrodes on chest as per particular monitor
! d. Instruct client to avoid vigorous exercise or sweating, and not to shower, take a bath, or swim until electrodes are removed
e. Postprocedure care: none specific except to review items in diary with client for clarification if necessary

F. Stress/exercise tests

1. Overview
a. Include a variety of specific tests, such as treadmill exercise electrocardiography, exercise myocardial perfusion imaging test (thallium or technetium stress test), nuclear persantine (dipyridamole) stress test, and nuclear dobutamine stress test (investigational by FDA currently)
b. Used to screen for coronary artery disease, evaluate myocardial perfusion, differentiate between cardiac ischemia and infarct, develop cardiac rehabilitation program, evaluate cardiac status for work capability, and evaluate effectiveness of cardiac drug therapy
c. Electrodes are applied to chest; baseline vital signs are recorded and monitored periodically during test, and client exercises per age-based protocol on treadmill or bicycle (except for persantine test, prescribed for those who cannot tolerate exercise)

2. Preprocedure care
a. Maintain NPO status after midnight (persantine, dobutamine) or for 2 to 3 hours prior to test (others)
! b. Avoid alcohol, caffeine, and nicotine during NPO status
! c. Teach client to wear comfortable clothes (shorts or slacks with belt, sneakers or tennis shoes with socks, shirt with buttons in front for ECG electrodes)
! d. Instruct client to inform staff so that test can be stopped if client has dyspnea, severe fatigue, chest pain, rapid increase in pulse rate or blood pressure, life-threatening dysrhythmias, or palpitations
e. Make note of any medications, such as beta-blockers, that could interfere with test results

3. Postprocedure care
a. Return client to department for any follow-up testing
b. Record vital signs and ECG tracings at end of test and 5 to 10 minutes later
! c. Explain client can resume usual activity but may need to avoid strenuous activity or taking hot baths or showers posttest depending on procedure

G. Venography (venogram), also called phlebography

1. Overview
   a. A fluoroscopic and/or x-ray examination of deep leg veins following injection of contrast dye
   b. Detects deep vein thrombosis and congenital venous abnormalities, and aids in selecting vein for arterial bypass grafting
2. Preprocedure care
   a. NPO for 4 hours before test (some hospitals permit clear liquids)
   ! b. Assess for allergy to contrast media and prepare to use antihistamines or steroids if necessary
   c. Record baseline vital signs and have client void prior to procedure
   d. Explain that client will lie on radiographic table tilted at 40- to 60-degree angle, tourniquet is applied above ankle, and dye is injected into vein over 2 to 4 minutes
3. Postprocedure care
   a. Monitor vital signs until stable, then as per routine
   b. Assess peripheral pulses (femoral, popliteal, dorsalis pedis)
   ! c. Assess injection site for bleeding, hematoma, or infection (redness, edema, pain); document and report if any of these are found
   ! d. Elevate extremity as ordered; if deep vein thrombosis is found, expect client to have orders for bedrest, heparin, leg elevation, and warm moist compresses

IV. RENAL OR URINARY DIAGNOSTIC TESTS

A. Cystoscopy and cystography (cystogram)

1. Overview
   a. *Cystoscopy* is direct visualization of bladder wall and urethra using a cystoscope (tubular lighted telescopic lens), usually by urologist
   b. *Cystography* is instillation of contrast dye into bladder using a catheter
   c. Purposes are to detect and remove urinary calculi, determine cause of hematuria or urinary tract infections, and detect tumors or prostatic hyperplasia
2. Preprocedure care
   ! a. Ensure informed consent is signed and witnessed prior to giving any ordered premedication (usually 1 hour before test)
   ! b. Record baseline vital signs and urine characteristics (amount, color, odor, specific gravity)
   ! c. Assess for allergy to medications, food, and latex
   d. Explain to client that procedure will be done under local or general anesthesia; local anesthesia will be injected into urethra several minutes before cystoscope is inserted
   e. Complete preoperative or preprocedure checklist as per agency policy
3. Postprocedure care
   ! a. Monitor vital signs every 15 minutes for an hour, then possibly every half hour until stable
   ! b. Monitor urine output for 48 hours after cystoscopy; increase fluid intake if less than 200 mL in 8 hours; report low urine output to physician
   c. Apply heat to lower abdomen to relieve pain and muscle spasm as ordered; explain to client that some pressure or burning may be present after test
   ! d. Assess for and report gross hematuria; blood tinged urine may be expected
   e. Monitor for complications of cystoscopy, such as hemorrhage, bladder perforation, urinary retention, and infection
   ! f. Teach client that slight burning on urination is expected for 1 to 2 days after procedure; use analgesic if prescribed and avoid alcoholic beverages for 2 days after test (bladder irritant)

B. Intravenous pyelography (IVP)

1. Overview
   a. Also called excretory urography, because test visualizes entire urinary tract rather than just pelvis of kidney

b. Consists of injecting IV radiopaque contrast and taking series of x-rays at specified times (3, 5, 10, 15, and 20 minutes postinjection), and a final x-ray after client voids to visualize residual dye in bladder
c. Used to identify abnormal size, shape, and function of kidneys and detect renal calculi, tumors, and cysts

2. Preprocedure care
   a. Keep client NPO for 8 to 12 hours prior to test
   b. Administer laxative in evening before test and enema on morning of test as ordered
   c. Assess for allergy to contrast media; antihistamines or steroids may be ordered
   d. Record baseline vital signs and check blood urea nitrogen (BUN) lab result (test might be canceled if greater than 40 mg/dL [normal 8–22 mg/dL])
3. Postprocedure care
   a. Monitor vital signs and urine output
   b. Assess for and report delayed reaction to contrast dye (dyspnea, rash, flushing, urticaria, tachycardia, and others); prepare to treat with ordered antihistamines or steroids

C. Retrograde pyelography (retrograde pyelogram)

1. Overview
   a. May be performed after or in place of IVP and is usually done in conjunction with cystoscopy
   b. Consists of injecting contrast dye via catheter into ureters and renal pelvis to diagnose suspected nonfunctioning kidney, unlocated calculus, tumor, or renal stricture
   c. Not as frequently performed today
2. Preprocedure care
   a. NPO for 8 hours prior to test; some clients may be allowed water to avoid dehydration unless undergoing general anesthesia
   b. Administer laxative and/or cleansing enema as ordered
   c. Assess for allergy to contrast media; antihistamines or steroids may be ordered
   d. Record baseline vital signs
   e. Explain that client is placed in stirrups; there should be little to no pain for discomfort although pressure and urge to void may occur with insertion of cystoscope
3. Postprocedure care
   a. Monitor vitals signs as per protocol
   b. Observe for and report delayed reaction to contrast dye as noted under IVP
   c. Monitor urine output and report if less than 240 mL in 8 hours or if client does not void in 8 hours
   d. Assess for and report hematuria; explain to client that blood-tinged urine is common
   e. Provide ordered analgesics for pain or discomfort and report severe pain
   f. Observe for and report signs of infection (fever, chills, abdominal pain, tachycardia, and later hypotension)

V. NEUROLOGICAL DIAGNOSTIC TESTS

A. Electroencephalography (EEG)

1. Overview
   a. Measures electrical impulses produced by brain cells to detect seizure disorder, brain tumor, abscess, and intracranial hemorrhage, and to assist in determination of brain death
   b. Consists of applying electrodes to scalp and in specific positions, and recording brain activity on moving paper
   c. Procedure may be performed while client is awake, drowsy, asleep, undergoing stimuli (hyperventilation, flashes of bright light), or combinations of these
2. Preprocedure care
   a. Shampoo hair night before test and instruct client not to use oil or hair spray on hair

! b. Food and fluids are permitted and encouraged (hypoglycemia could affect results) but client may not have coffee, tea, cola, or alcohol before test
c. Do not administer sleep aids or other sedatives on night before test because they affect readings; check with physician regarding whether other medications should be administered or withheld (such as antiepileptic drugs)
d. Explain that procedure is painless and may be done with client lying down or seated in reclining chair
e. Explain electrode placement and that electric shock will not occur; alleviate any client fears including that machine cannot determine intelligence and cannot read client's mind
! f. Observe for and report seizure activity; note whether client is extremely anxious, restless, or upset

3. Postprocedure care
! a. Shampoo client's hair to remove paste or collodion; acetone may be used to remove paste
b. Allow client to resume normal activity unless client was sedated

B. Myelography (myelogram)

1. Overview
a. A fluoroscopic and radiologic exam of spinal subarachnoid space (spinal canal) using air or contrast agent (oil- or water-based)
b. Detects spinal lesions (herniated intervertebral disks, cysts or tumor in spinal column, or spinal nerve root injury)

2. Preprocedure care
! a. NPO for 4 to 8 hours prior to test; client may have light breakfast or clear liquids in morning if test is scheduled for afternoon
b. Administer cleansing enema if ordered to remove feces and gas to improve visualization
c. Administer ordered premedications such as sedative or narcotic analgesic and atropine
! d. Assess for allergy to contrast dye and record baseline vital signs
! e. Explain to client that spinal puncture will be performed and dye will be injected; table may be tilted as dye enters spinal column to enhance visualization of structures
f. Instruct client to tell physician of any discomfort (such as pain going down legs)

3. Postprocedure care
a. Monitor vital signs until stable, then per protocol
! b. Monitor urine output and notify physician if client does not void in 8 hours
! c. Position client properly: keep head of bed flat if oil-based contrast used and elevated to 60 degrees for 8 hours or longer if water-based contrast was used (to prevent irritation from residual dye; oil-based dye is aspirated out but some microdroplets could remain)
! d. Increase fluid intake to excrete dye via kidneys and to replace lost spinal fluid
e. Assess for signs of chemical or bacterial meningitis (severe headache, fever, chills, stiff neck, irritability, photophobia, and seizures)
f. Encourage use of good body mechanics

VI. MUSCULOSKELETAL DIAGNOSTIC TESTS

A. Arthroscopy

1. Overview
a. An endoscopic examination of interior joint (usually knee) using fiberoptic endoscope; usually preceded by arthrography (x-ray exam of joint using air, contrast media, or both)
b. Performed to diagnose meniscal, patellar, extrasynovial, and synovial problems
c. Also used to perform joint surgery

2. Preprocedure care
a. No food or fluid restriction if done using local anesthetic; NPO after midnight for spinal and general anesthesia
b. Assess involved skin area for lesion or infection; document and report if found

3. Postprocedure care
   a. Assess vital signs and local bleeding or swelling; report abnormal findings
   b. Apply covered ice bag to area if ordered
   c. Administer ordered analgesics for pain or discomfort
   d. Instruct client to rest joint for specified amount of time and avoid excessive use of joint for 2 to 3 days after procedure; minimize walking

B. Bone densitometry

1. Overview
   a. Detects early osteoporosis by determining density of bone mineral content
   b. Normal result is determined according to client age, gender, and height
   c. Most frequent population is postmenopausal women, who are at risk for greatest annual bone loss
2. Preprocedure care
   a. Food and fluids do not need to be restricted
   b. ! Teach client to remove all metal objects in area to be scanned and that test takes 30 to 60 minutes and is not painful
3. Postprocedure care: none

VII. GASTROINTESTINAL DIAGNOSTIC TESTS

A. Barium enema

1. Overview
   a. An x-ray examination of large intestine (colon) to detect polyps, tumor, diverticuli, intestinal stricture or obstruction, intussusception, or ulceration
   b. Consists of administering barium sulfate (alone as single contrast or with air as double contrast) via rectal tube into large intestine
   c. Filling process is monitored by fluoroscopy, and then x-rays are taken
   d. Indicated for clients who have lower abdominal pain or cramps; stool that contains blood, mucus, or pus; changes in bowel habits or stool characteristics
2. ! Preprocedure care
   a. Some institutions ask that clients eat low-residue diet for 2 to 3 days before test (tender meats, eggs, bread, clear soup, pureed bland fruits and vegetables, boiled milk, potatoes)
   b. Ensure that ordered abdominal x-rays, ultrasound studies, radionuclide studies and proctosigmoidoscopy are done prior to this test
   c. Withhold oral medications for 24 hours prior to test unless ordered by physician
   d. Provide, or instruct client to take, clear liquid diet for 18 to 24 hours before test and maintain water and clear liquid intake 24 hours prior to maintain hydration
   e. Administer laxatives (such as magnesium citrate) in late afternoon or early evening (4 to 8 pm) of day before test
   f. Administer cleansing enema or laxative suppository such as bisacodyl (Dulcolax) on evening before test as ordered
   g. Administer saline enemas in early morning of day of procedure until clear (maximum of three) is ordered
   h. Black coffee or tea is permitted up to 1 hour prior to test
3. Postprocedure care
   a. Instruct client to try to expel barium in bathroom or on bedpan immediately after test
   b. ! Increase fluid intake for hydration and prevent constipation from retained barium
   c. ! Administer ordered laxative or oil retention enema to expel barium; laxative may need to be repeated on day following test

B. Cholangiography

1. Overview
   a. May be done as IV, percutaneous, or T-tube cholangiography
   b. IV test examines biliary ducts to detect strictures, stones, or tumor, but gallbladder may not be well visualized
   c. Percutaneous test is indicated when biliary obstruction is indicated because contrast is injected directly into biliary tree

d. T-tube test may be done 7 to 8 hours after cholecystectomy to explore common bile duct for patency and determine if any gallstones are blocking duct after removal of gallbladder; dye is injected into T-shaped tube, which is placed into common bile duct during surgery to promote drainage

2. Preprocedure care
   a. NPO for 8 hours prior to test
   b. Take usual precautions regarding allergy to contrast media
   c. Provide laxative (evening before test) and cleansing enema (morning of test) as ordered; for T-tube test, only cleansing enema may be ordered
3. Postprocedure care
   a. Check vital signs as ordered and instruct client to remain in bed for 6 hours after percutaneous test
   b. T-tube may or may not be taken out after procedure
   c. Otherwise, no specific aftercare is indicated

C. Cholecystography (oral)

1. Overview
   a. An x-ray test to visualize stones in gallbladder or determine obstruction in cystic duct
   b. Oral contrast media is administered, dye concentrates in gallbladder in 12 to 14 hours
   c. Specific sequence of dietary instructions must be followed for best results
   d. Liver disease, inadequate client preparation, obstruction of cystic duct, and diarrhea (eliminates contrast agent) can interfere with results
2. Preprocedure care
   a. ! Assess allergy history; assess for signs of jaundice (yellow sclera, skin or serum bilirubin greater than 3 mg/dl); notify provider if found
   b. Provide fat-free diet for 24 hours before test (some agencies suggest high-fat meal at noon to empty gallbladder and low-fat meal in evening)
   c. ! Begin NPO status with sips of water after dinner the evening before test
   d. Administer radiopaque tablets 2 hours after dinner meal according to package directions with total of 240 mL (8 ounces) of water
   e. Saline enema may be ordered on morning of test in some agencies to clear GI tract
   f. Explain to client that fasting x-rays will be taken and then high-fat meal or fat-containing substances (Bilevac) will be given in x-ray department; follow-up x-rays will be done over next 1 to 2 hours to monitor gallbladder emptying
   g. Explain that test does not cause discomfort
   h. Explain that client should not become alarmed if test needs to be repeated but should remain on low-fat diet until test is repeated
3. Postprocedure care: none specific

D. Colonoscopy

1. Overview
   a. An endoscopic procedure that inspects large intestine (colon) using long, flexible fiberoptic tube (colonoscope)
   b. Tube is inserted anally and advanced through rectum, sigmoid colon, and large intestine to cecum, and air is used to insufflate area for better visualization
   c. Detects lower GI bleeding, polyps, diverticulitis, and benign or malignant lesions in colon
2. Preprocedure care
   a. Withhold medications that interfere with coagulation (aspirin, NSAIDs) and alcohol 1 week prior to test
   b. Explain that another person must be available to drive client home if performed on outpatient basis
   c. Follow preprocedure preparation to clear bowel of feces: usually GoLytely or Colyte solution or Fleet PhosphoSoda beginning on day prior to test
   d. Avoid soapsuds enemas, which could irritate wall of colon
   e. Record baseline vital signs

- **f.** Client will lie in Sims or left lateral position, will receive IV moderate sedation immediately prior to test, and will be asked to breathe deeply during insertion of colonoscope

3. Postprocedure care

- **a.** Monitor vital signs and report abnormal changes
- **b.** Do not administer anything by mouth following IV moderate sedation until gag and swallow reflexes have returned
- **c.** Assess for and report anal bleeding, abdominal distention, severe pain or abdominal cramps, or fever
- **d.** Maintain client safety post-sedation

E. Endoscopic retrograde cholangiopancreatography (ERCP)

1. Overview

- **a.** Examines biliary and pancreatic ducts endoscopically after injection of contrast medium into duodenal papilla
- **b.** Identifies causes of biliary obstruction (usually accompanied by jaundice), such as stricture, cyst, stones, or tumor
- **c.** May be done as follow-up study to ultrasound, CT scan, liver scan, or biliary tract x-rays

2. Preprocedure care

- **a.** Assess for allergies to contrast media
- **b.** Maintain NPO status for 8 hours prior to test
- **c.** Obtain baseline vital signs
- **d.** Ensure that informed consent is obtained and that client voids before premedication (mild sedative or narcotic and atropine, usually)
- **e.** Explain that local anesthetic is sprayed in throat to decrease gag reflex prior to insertion of endoscope

3. Postprocedure care

- **a.** Monitor vital signs including temperature (fever could indicate infection) and respiratory rate (respiratory status could be compromised from anesthetic spray in throat and/or endoscope)
- **b.** Ensure gag and swallow reflexes are present before offering food and fluids
- **c.** Provide warm saline gargles or lozenges to reduce sore throat caused by endoscope; may be needed for a few days
- **d.** Note and report presence of persistent abdominal pain, discomfort, or fullness

F. Esophagogastroduodenoscopy

1. Overview

- **a.** Also includes or is known as gastroscopy, esophagoscopy, esophagogastroscopy, duodenoscopy, endoscopy
- **b.** Directly visualizes esophagus, stomach, and duodenum with flexible fiberoptic endoscope
- **c.** Used to diagnose esophageal, gastric, or duodenal disease; diverticulosis or *H. pylori* infection; to obtain cytologic specimens; or to remove foreign bodies

2. Preprocedure care

- **a.** NPO status for 8 to 12 hours prior to test; if done as emergency and NPO status not possible, perform stomach lavage/suction to prevent aspiration
- **b.** Record baseline vital signs and have client void
- **c.** Administer any prescribed premedication; client's usual prescribed medications may often be taken at 6 a.m. on day of test; check with physician
- **d.** Give client hospital gown to wear and remove dentures, eyeglasses, and jewelry; note any loose teeth
- **e.** Explain that client may feel some pressure with insertion of scope, but that IV sedation and local anesthetic to throat will be used

3. Postprocedure care

- **a.** NPO for 2 to 4 hours after test as ordered; ensure that gag and swallow reflexes have returned before offering fluids or food
- **b.** Monitor vital signs
- **c.** Explain that "burping up air" or passing gas is expected because air is instilled during procedure to visualize area

d. Provide gargles, lozenges, or analgesics for throat discomfort, which is expected and caused by endoscope
e. Observe for possible complications, such as perforated GI tract; assess for and report epigastric, abdominal, or back pain; dyspnea; fever; tachycardia; and subcutaneous emphysema in neck

G. Gastric analysis

1. Overview
   a. Examines acidity of gastric secretions via nasogastric tube during basal state (without stimulation) and at peak or maximal secretion (with drug stimulation)
   b. Decreased levels indicate pernicious anemia, gastric malignancy, and atrophic gastritis
   c. Increased levels indicate peptic ulcer (duodenal) or Zollinger-Ellison syndrome
2. Basal gastric analysis
   a. NPO for 8 to 12 hours prior to test and restrict smoking for 8 hours
   b. Restrict selected drugs (antacids, steroids, cholinergics, and anticholinergics) and coffee and alcohol for at least 24 hours prior; note on test request form if not complied with
   c. Record baseline vital signs and remove loose dentures
   d. Insert nasogastric tube and obtain residual gastric specimen as well as four additional specimens 15 minutes apart
   e. Properly label specimens as basal secretions with client name, date, time, and specimen number
3. Stimulation test (a continuation of basal gastric analysis test)
   a. Administer gastric stimulant such as Histalog, histamine, or pentagastrin
   b. Obtain four to eight specimens 15 minutes apart depending on agent used
   c. Label specimens obtained after stimulation with client name, date, time, and specimen number
   d. Monitor vital signs postprocedure

H. Gastrointestinal (GI) series

1. Overview
   a. Also known as upper GI series, barium swallow, or small bowel series
   b. Consists of fluoroscopic and x-ray examinations of esophagus, stomach, and small intestine after ingestion of oral barium sulfate or water-soluble contrast such as Gastrografin
   c. Used to detect esophageal, gastric, or duodenal ulcer, polyps, tumors, hiatal hernia, foreign bodies, esophageal varices, or esophageal or small bowel strictures
2. Preprocedure care
   a. Low-residue diet may be ordered for 2 to 3 days prior to test
   b. Maintain NPO status with no smoking for 8 to 12 hours before test
   c. Withhold medications for 8 hours before test unless otherwise ordered; withhold narcotics and anticholinergics for 24 hours because they reduce gastric motility
   d. Administer laxatives as ordered on evening before test
   e. Explain that client swallows a chalk-flavored (chocolate or strawberry) barium meal or Gastrografin and x-rays are taken periodically over 1 to 2 or 4 to 6 hours depending on length of area to be visualized; follow-up film (post-GI series) at 24 hours may be ordered as well
3. Postprocedure care
   a. Check with radiology department that studies are completed before giving late breakfast or late lunch
   b. Administer ordered laxative following test to excrete barium
   c. Explain to client that stool will be light in color for some days after test and to notify physician if no bowel movement in 2 to 3 days

VIII. REPRODUCTIVE DIAGNOSTIC TESTS

A. Fetal nonstress test (NST)

1. Overview
   a. Evaluates fetal functioning and well-being in response to fetal movement

b. Is inexpensive, rapidly accomplished, lacks side effects, and helps identify at-risk fetuses for mothers with high-risk pregnancy conditions (such as diabetes and pregnancy-induced hypertension)
c. Monitors fetal heart rate (FHR) with fetal movement, which should accelerate 15 beats per minute for 15 seconds
d. If FHR does not increase within 20 minutes, can rub mother's abdomen or make loud noise nearby to stimulate fetal movement
e. If no increase in FHR after 40 minutes, test indicates a nonreactive fetus; normal is a reactive fetus

2. Preprocedure care
   a. Obtain informed consent and measure baseline vital signs and FHR
   b. Position mother in semi-Fowler or lateral position with roll or wedge under right hip to displace uterus to left slightly
   c. Instruct client to press pressure transducer when she feels fetus move so FHR acceleration can be monitored
3. Postprocedure care
   a. Encourage client to rest
   b. Provide general teaching that instructs client to report bleeding, continuous contractions, or lack of fetal movement
4. Nonreactive test may be followed up with contraction stress test
   a. Evaluates fetal functioning during spontaneous or induced uterine contractions
   b. May also be performed as routine test for selected high-risk mothers
   c. Uses nipple stimulation or oxytocin to stimulate uterine contraction
   d. Normal result is absence of late decelerations in FHR during three contractions; presence of late decelerations indicates condition that leads to placental dysfunction or insufficient blood supply

B. Hysteroscopy

1. Overview
   a. Visualizes uterine cavity and allows for endometrial biopsy or removal of uterine polyps
   b. Contraindicated with cervical or vaginal infection, pelvic inflammatory disease, purulent vaginal discharge, or if cervical surgery performed previously
   c. Risks to procedure include perforation of uterus and infection
2. Preprocedure care
   a. Obtain menstrual history because test should be done after menses but before ovulation
   b. Restrict food and fluids for 8 hours before test
   c. Have client void before test
   d. Explain that client will be in lithotomy position; hysteroscope will be inserted and carbon dioxide will be instilled to distend uterus for visualization
3. Postprocedure care
   a. Monitor vital signs
   b. Assess for excessive bleeding or discharge
   c. Explain that cramping may occur following test and mild analgesic will reduce discomfort; client should report severe discomfort or shortness of breath immediately
   d. Teach client to avoid sexual intercourse or douching for 2 weeks or as instructed by physician

C. Mammography

1. Overview
   a. X-ray examination of breasts to detect cysts or tumors
   b. Detects approximately 90% of breast malignancies
   c. Recommended annually for women over 40 years and every 2 years for women ages 35 to 40
2. Preprocedure care
   a. Food and fluids are not restricted prior to test

! b. Instruct client not to use ointment, powder, or deodorant on breasts or under arms on day of test; client will need to remove clothes to waist and wear a paper gown that opens in front
c. Explain that procedure will not cause pain but some discomfort may occur during breast compression during test
d. Explain that client will need to wait while films are developed, and reassure client that additional films are sometimes needed and not to be alarmed
3. Postprocedure care: none specific

D. Papanicolaou smear (pap smear)

1. Overview
a. A cytological test to detect precancerous lesions or cancerous cells of cervix
b. Also identifies viral, fungal, and parasitic conditions and evaluates response to chemotherapy or radiation therapy
2. Preprocedure care
a. Food and fluids are not restricted
! b. Client should not douche, insert vaginal medications, or have sexual intercourse for 24 hours before test
c. Obtain menstrual history, including any problems, and document whether or not client is taking any hormones or oral contraceptives
d. Ask client to remove all clothes; provide paper gown; breast examination is done after Pap smear is taken
e. Explain that client will lie on examining table in lithotomy position and speculum will be inserted into vagina to aid in specimen collection
3. Postprocedure care: none specific

IX. INTEGUMENTARY DIAGNOSTIC TESTS

A. Tuberculin skin test

1. Overview
a. Screens for tuberculosis
b. Tine test or Mono-Vacc test is multipuncture test that uses tines impregnated with purified protein derivative (PPD); used for mass screening and is read in 48 to 72 hours
! c. Mantoux test involves injection of PPD intradermally using a tuberculin (1 mL) syringe with a 25- to 27-gauge needle, and is read in 48 to 72 hours
2. Preprocedure care
a. Food and fluids are not restricted
! b. Assess whether client has tested positive to test before; test should only be performed if previous results were negative
c. Cleanse inner aspect of forearm with alcohol and let dry before injecting 0.1 mL of antigen intradermally
3. Postprocedure care
! a. Explain that client needs to return to have results read in 48 to 72 hours; a 72-hour reading is more accurate; client may be asked to return for reading at 72 hours if 48-hour result is questionable
! b. Explain that positive test does not always indicate active infectious disease but that organism is present in body in either an active or dormant state; follow-up x-ray and sputum cultures are indicated

B. Other skin tests

1. Include tests for blastomycosis, coccidioidomycosis, histoplasmosis, trichinosis, and toxoplasmosis
2. Procedures are similar to that described above for tuberculosis
! 3. For allergy skin tests, the area injected may be outlined with a marker and a diagram made of injection sites, especially if more than one antigen is planted concurrently; antihistamines are withheld 3 to 4 days prior to avoid false negatives

PRACTICE TEST

Check Your NCLEX-RN® Exam I.Q.

You are ready for testing on this content if you can

- Apply knowledge from foundational sciences to the care of clients undergoing diagnostic testing.
- Correlate client pathophysiology with specific nursing interventions needed before and after diagnostic testing.
- Assess a client appropriately before and after diagnostic testing.
- Compare the results of client assessments before and after diagnostic testing.
- Monitor the results of serial or periodic diagnostic tests.
- Reinforce client teaching about diagnostic tests.

PRACTICE TEST

1 A client is about to undergo skin biopsy to determine if a skin lesion is malignant. The client asks how much the biopsy will hurt. Which response by the nurse is best?

1. "We will give you a pain pill in just a moment that will minimize any pain during the biopsy."
2. "Luckily, this type of procedure does not cause any pain for most people."
3. "You may feel some discomfort while the local anesthetic is injected, but this will numb the area for the actual biopsy."
4. "This procedure does cause some pain, but you can manage any soreness afterward with over-the-counter medications such as acetaminophen (Tylenol)."

2 The client is about to undergo a computerized tomography (CT) scan of the head with contrast. Which of the following questions by the nurse is most important to ask while preparing the client for the test?

1. "Have you ever had a procedure like this before?"
2. "Do you have an allergy to iodine or shellfish?"
3. "Would you like something to drink before you go to the radiology department?"
4. "Have you voided in the bathroom in the last few hours?"

3 The client is scheduled for a magnetic resonance imaging (MRI) study of the spine. The outpatient nurse explains to the client that which of the following is an important part of preprocedure care?

1. "Do not eat or drink after midnight of the day before the test."
2. "Plan to have someone drive you home after the test."
3. "Expect to stay in the MRI department for an hour afterward for observation."
4. "Do not wear any metal, such as jewelry or hairclips."

4 A client will undergo a radionuclide scan of the thyroid. A nursing assistant asks what needs to be done to protect staff from any residual radiation following the scan. Which of the following is an appropriate response by the nurse?

1. "All caregivers and visitors need to stand 6 feet away from the client for 24 hours. I need to put a sign above the bed."
2. "Using standard precautions for handling body fluids will be sufficient to protect staff."
3. "I have arranged for the client to be moved to a private room for 48 hours after the test."
4. "The client will need to be on contact precautions. I will have the unit secretary call the central processing department for a cart with gowns and gloves."

5 A 17-year-old girl is brought to the emergency department for x-rays after twisting her ankle while playing basketball. Which of the following questions is most important for the nurse to ask the client before sending her to the radiology department?

1. "Do you experience claustrophobia when in small spaces?"
2. "Are you wearing any necklaces or other metal objects?"
3. "When was your last monthly period?"
4. "Have you ever had an x-ray before?"

6 A female client is returning to the nursing unit following a pelvic ultrasound. The nurse plans to do which of the following at this time for the client?

1. Make the client comfortable and ask if she needs anything.
2. Instruct the client to drink at least one quart of water over the next hour.
3. Explain that analgesic medication is available to relieve the expected cramping pain.
4. Tell the client that she will be able to eat in one hour.

7 A client who underwent bronchoscopy 4 hours ago is asking for something to drink to ease his sore throat. The nurse obtains some juice for the client after noting which of the following assessment data for the client?

1. Respiratory rate has ranged from 16 to 18.
2. Breath sounds are clear bilaterally.
3. The client has had no hemoptysis.
4. Gag and swallow reflexes have returned.

8 A client underwent angiography of the left leg. Which of the following data obtained during the current assessment is of greatest concern to the nurse?

1. Skin paler on left foot than right
2. Skin temperature cooler on left foot than right
3. Left dorsalis pedis pulse audible by Doppler, previously 2+
4. Band-aid at femoral access site has trace amount of dark red blood

9 The client who will undergo a cardiac catheterization says to the nurse, "I am nervous about having a cardiac catheterization. Can you tell me what to expect during this test?" Which of the following replies by the nurse is appropriate?

1. "The procedure will be done in the operating room to help ensure sterile conditions."
2. "The room will be brightly lit at all times."
3. "The insertion of the catheter in the femoral area will be one of the few painful moments of the procedure."
4. "The physician will ask you to lie still except to do specific things, such as cough or take a deep breath."

10 A client who is scheduled for a cardiac echocardiogram at 9 a.m. on the following morning asks the nurse if he will be able to eat breakfast before the test. Which of the following responses by the nurse is appropriate?

1. "Yes, we can arrange for your breakfast tray to arrive a half hour early so that you have time to eat before the test."
2. "Yes, but you will need to get up at 5 o'clock so that you will be without food or fluids for 4 hours before the test."
3. "Yes, but you can only drink clear liquids such as ginger ale, black tea, or apple juice, and you cannot eat solid food until after the test."
4. "No, you cannot eat or drink before the test, but you can have a full breakfast after the test."

11 A client has just received a Holter cardiac monitor to wear for the next 24 hours. The nurse determines that the client understands its use when the client makes which of the following statements?

1. "I should write in the diary what I am doing every half hour."
2. "I should only take a bath, not a shower, for the next 24 hours."
3. "I can continue with my usual activity and exercise pattern while wearing the monitor."
4. "I need to try to walk a total of 3 miles over the next 24 hours while wearing the monitor."

12 A client who underwent cystography 16 hours ago has a urinary output of 225 mL in the previous 8 hours. Which of the following actions should the nurse take as a priority at this time?

1. Measure the specific gravity of the urine.
2. Document the volume on the client's flowsheet.
3. Encourage the client to drink increased amounts of fluid.
4. Notify the physician.

13 The nurse has assigned a nursing assistant to a client who just returned to the nursing unit at 09:45 after electroencephalography. Which of the following directions should the nurse give the nursing assistant regarding care for the client?

1. "Do not give any food or fluids until lunchtime."
2. "Wash the client's hair at your earliest opportunity."
3. "Keep the client on bedrest for the remainder of the shift."
4. "Encourage the client to drink fluids to flush dye through the kidneys."

PRACTICE TEST

14 A client has just returned to the nursing unit following a myelogram, which was done to diagnose a herniated intervertebral disk. The medical record indicates a water-based contrast medium was used during the test. The nurse should assist the client to which of the following positions in bed after transferring from the stretcher?

1. Supine with head of bed elevated 60 degrees
2. Supine with head of bed elevated 15 degrees
3. Left side lying with head of bed flat
4. Any position of client choice, with head of bed elevated 30 degrees

15 A client has received discharge instructions after undergoing arthroscopy of the knee earlier in the day. The nurse concludes that the client understands self-care after discharge when the client makes which of the following statements?

1. "I should not expect to need pain medication following this procedure."
2. "I should apply warm, moist heat to my knee to maintain comfort."
3. "I should limit my activities, including walking, for 2 to 3 days."
4. "I should expect increased swelling and perhaps some bleeding in the knee area after going home."

16 A client with gastroesophageal reflux disease has just undergone esophagogastroscopy. Which of the following client data is the nurse's highest priority for continued monitoring?

1. Inability to swallow saliva
2. Temperature of 99.4 degrees oral
3. Client report of heartburn
4. Client report of sore throat

17 The nurse has given instructions to a client who will have a barium swallow in 3 days. The nurse determines that the client understands how to properly prepare for the test after the client makes which of the following statements?

1. "I should eat a low-fat meal for the next two days, and then have clear liquids the day before the test."
2. "I should stop taking all medication except antacids the day before the test."
3. "I should not eat or drink anything after midnight on the day of the test."
4. "I should eat a high-carbohydrate diet for the three days before the test."

18 The nurse is providing instructions to a client who is returning to home following colonoscopy. Which of the following statements would be appropriate for the nurse to include?

1. "You may drive in about 6 hours after all the medication given during the procedure has fully worn off."
2. "It is alright to eat and drink, but it is helpful to resume the diet gradually."
3. "You should call the doctor if you feel distended or begin passing gas."
4. "Bleeding from the rectum is expected after this procedure, but call the physician if it gets severe."

19 The nurse would give which instruction regarding preprocedure care to a woman who is scheduled for a mammogram?

1. "Drink liquids, but don't eat breakfast on the morning of the mammogram."
2. "Do not use any deodorant or lotions on the chest or underarms before the mammogram."
3. "Take a mild analgesic such as acetaminophen (Tylenol) before coming to the clinic for the mammogram."
4. "Plan a light schedule for the day of the mammogram so you can plan on getting some rest after the procedure."

20 The occupational health nurse has given an intradermal injection of purified protein derivative (PPD) to a client to screen for tuberculosis. After noting that the current day is Monday, the nurse instructs the client to return to have the result read on which of the following days?

1. Tuesday or Wednesday
2. Wednesday or Thursday
3. Thursday or Friday
4. Friday or the following Monday

21 A client will undergo basal gastric acid secretion analysis. The client is taking the following types of medications. Which of the following types of drugs should the nurse withhold prior to the test? Select all that apply.

1. Anticholinergic
2. Cardiac glycoside
3. Antacid
4. Diuretic
5. Steroid

ANSWERS & RATIONALES

1 **Answer: 3** The area is anesthetized using a local anesthetic before skin biopsy, so the client should only feel discomfort while the anesthetic is administered. Analgesics are not given before the procedure (option 1), and the procedure is not pain-free (option 2). The client may take medication such as acetaminophen following the procedure (option 4), but this does not address the client's question about pain during the procedure.
Cognitive Level: Analysis **Client Need:** Physiological Integrity: Reduction of Risk Potential **Integrated Process:** Communication and Documentation **Content Area:** Adult Health: Integumentary **Strategy:** The core issue of the question is pain during a skin biopsy procedure. Eliminate option 4 because it does not address the client's concern. Use knowledge that local anesthesia is used during the procedure to make your selection.

2 **Answer: 2** Because a contrast agent will be used for the test, it is most important for the nurse to ask about an allergy to iodine or shellfish. While it is good to know if the client has had a similar test for anxiety reduction, it is not the priority. The client should not have anything to eat or drink for 4 hours prior to the test. It is generally helpful for the client to void before leaving the unit to avoid having to do so during the test, but this is also a lower priority item than assessing for allergy.
Cognitive Level: Analysis **Client Need:** Physiological Integrity: Reduction of Risk Potential **Integrated Process:** Nursing Process: Assessment **Content Area:** Adult Health: Neurological **Strategy:** The core issue of the question is knowledge that a client who is allergic to iodine or shellfish is likely to have an allergic reaction to iodinated contrast media. Eliminate options 1 and 4 as least important, and then eliminate option 3 because fluids are not allowed prior to CT scans with contrast.

3 **Answer: 4** Because the MRI scanner uses magnets, the client cannot wear any metal, and clients who have implanted metal may be ineligible for this study. The client does not need to withhold food or fluids before the test. The client does not need to remain in the department for additional observation after the test and can drive himself or herself home.
Cognitive Level: Application **Client Need:** Physiological Integrity: Reduction of Risk Potential **Integrated Process:** Communication and Documentation **Content Area:** Adult Health: Musculoskeletal **Strategy:** The core issue of the question is knowledge that metal cannot be worn in the vicinity of an MRI scanner because of the magnetic field. Use nursing knowledge about this test and the process of elimination to make a selection.

4 **Answer: 2** The amount of residual radioactivity following radionuclide scanning is very small and poses no risk to visitors or staff. Using standard precautions in handling blood or body fluids is sufficient for protection. It is unnecessary to stand 6 feet away from the client, use a private room, or place the client on contact precautions.
Cognitive Level: Application **Client Need:** Physiological Integrity: Reduction of Risk Potential **Integrated Process:** Communication and Documentation **Content Area:** Adult Health: Endocrine and Metabolic **Strategy:** The core issue of the question is knowledge that the amount of radioactivity following radionuclide imaging is very small. With this in mind, eliminate each of the incorrect options, which contain excessive and unnecessary steps for protection of staff.

5 **Answer: 3** The most important question is to determine whether the client could be pregnant, since x-rays are contraindicated during pregnancy, especially during the first trimester. The second question in importance would be asking about whether the client is wearing any metal, but possible pregnancy is a priority. It is helpful, but not of highest priority, to know if the client has had an x-ray before to alleviate concerns. Asking about fear of small or closed spaces would be important for MRI machines and possibly for CT scanning machines.
Cognitive Level: Analysis **Client Need:** Physiological Integrity: Reduction of Risk Potential **Integrated Process:** Nursing Process: Assessment **Content Area:** Adult Health: Musculoskeletal **Strategy:** The core issue of the question is knowledge that x-rays are contraindicated during pregnancy. Note the critical words *most important* in the question, which tells you that more than one option may be correct, and you must prioritize your answer. Use general knowledge of x-rays and the process of elimination to make a selection.

6 **Answer: 1** There is no special aftercare following pelvic ultrasound. For this reason, the nurse should make the client comfortable and ask if she needs anything before leaving the room. The client does not need to drink fluids, should not have cramping pains, and does not need to wait an hour before eating.
Cognitive Level: Application **Client Need:** Physiological Integrity: Reduction of Risk Potential **Integrated Process:** Nursing Process: Planning **Content Area:** Adult Health: Renal and Genitourinary **Strategy:** The core issue of the question is knowledge that there is no special aftercare following ultrasound as a diagnostic test. Use nursing knowledge and the process of elimination to make a selection.

7 **Answer: 4** Before offering food or fluids to a client following bronchoscopy, it is essential to ensure that gag and swallow reflexes have returned. A local anesthetic is used to numb the throat to ease passage of the bronchoscope, and if protective reflexes have not returned, the client could aspirate. The other client data is also normal but would not indicate whether the client can safely swallow.
Cognitive Level: Analysis **Client Need:** Physiological Integrity: Reduction of Risk Potential **Integrated Process:** Nursing Process: Assessment **Content Area:** Adult Health: Respiratory **Strategy:** The core issue of the question is knowledge that gag and swallow reflexes need to be present before offering clients food or beverages to prevent aspiration. Think of gag

and swallow reflexes as a possible priority concern whenever a client has had a procedure ending in *-oscopy*. Otherwise, use nursing knowledge of this key principle and the process of elimination to make a selection.

8 **Answer: 3** The assessment finding that should be of greatest concern to the nurse is the adverse change in the distal pulse on the leg that underwent angiography. Skin that is paler and cooler is also of concern, but the reason for these adverse changes is the reduced circulation to the leg, which is in turn caused by the decreased pulse. A bandage that has a small amount of old blood is expected and is not of concern at this time.

Cognitive Level: Analysis **Client Need:** Physiological Integrity: Reduction of Risk Potential **Integrated Process:** Nursing Process: Analysis **Content Area:** Adult Health: Cardiovascular **Strategy:** The core issue of the question is the most serious adverse change in the neurovascular status of a client who underwent angiography. The critical words in the stem of the question are *greatest concern,* which indicates that more than one piece of data may be abnormal. Use nursing knowledge about adverse circulatory changes and the process of elimination to make a selection.

9 **Answer: 4** The client is asked to lie still except for specific requests, such as to cough or deep breathe to aid in catheter movement or to terminate cardiac dysrhythmias caused by irritation of the catheter. The procedure is done in a special cardiac catheterization room in the radiology department, not in the operating room. The lights in the room may be dimmed at times so catheter movement can be visualized on a fluoroscopy screen. The catheter insertion site is anesthetized with a local anesthetic, so the client should feel pressure but not pain.

Cognitive Level: Application **Client Need:** Physiological Integrity: Reduction of Risk Potential **Integrated Process:** Teaching and Learning **Content Area:** Adult Health: Cardiovascular **Strategy:** The core issue of the question is knowledge of typical events during a cardiac catheterization. Knowledge of these factors helps alleviate client fears. Use nursing knowledge and the process of elimination to make a selection.

10 **Answer: 1** There is no restriction of food or fluids prior to a cardiac (or any) echocardiogram. This test uses sound waves emitted from and reflected back to a transducer, and it is noninvasive. Options 2 through 4 are all variations of an incorrect response.

Cognitive Level: Analysis **Client Need:** Physiological Integrity: Reduction of Risk Potential **Integrated Process:** Teaching and Learning **Content Area:** Adult Health: Cardiovascular **Strategy:** The core issue of the question is knowledge of client preparation for echocardiography. Recall that this is a noninvasive test to eliminate option 4, and then use nursing knowledge and the process of elimination to make a selection.

11 **Answer: 3** The client should go about his or her usual daily activities and exercise pattern while wearing the monitor and should record activities and any symptoms experienced in the diary. The client does not need to make diary entries every 30 minutes, but as needed to provide an overview of activity so that it can be correlated with any cardiac abnormalities on the time-stamped electrocardiogram being recorded. The client should not take a bath or a shower while wearing the device, which has electrical circuitry. The client does not need to walk a total of 3 miles during the 24-hour period.

Cognitive Level: Analysis **Client Need:** Physiological Integrity: Reduction of Risk Potential **Integrated Process:** Nursing Process: Evaluation **Content Area:** Adult Health: Cardiovascular **Strategy:** The core issue of the question is knowledge of proper use of a Holter monitor. The wording of the question tells you that only one option is a correct statement. Use nursing knowledge and the process of elimination to make a selection.

12 **Answer: 3** The client has 15 mL less than the expected minimum urine output of 240 mL in 8 hours. The first step by the nurse would be to assess the client's fluid intake and encourage the client to drink increased fluids. Although it is not incorrect to measure specific gravity, the nurse could expect the value to be high if the urine output volume was low because of poor intake. Documenting the value is insufficient because further nursing action is warranted. The nurse should call the physician if the reduced output continues after increasing the client's fluid intake.

Cognitive Level: Analysis **Client Need:** Physiological Integrity: Reduction of Risk Potential **Integrated Process:** Nursing Process: Implementation **Content Area:** Adult Health: Renal and Genitourinary **Strategy:** The critical words in the question are *at this time,* which tell you that more than one option may be plausible but there is a sequence of nursing actions appropriate to the situation. Recall that when urine output is low, an early measure is to offer increased fluids. Use this nursing knowledge and the process of elimination to make a selection.

13 **Answer: 2** The nursing assistant should wash the client's hair to remove the paste or colloidon that was used to secure the electrodes to the head for the diagnostic test. The client should be able to eat and drink and can resume usual activity unless otherwise ordered. There is no dye used in this diagnostic test.

Cognitive Level: Application **Client Need:** Physiological Integrity: Reduction of Risk Potential **Integrated Process:** Nursing Process: Implementation **Content Area:** Adult Health: Neurological **Strategy:** Use nursing knowledge and the process of elimination to make a selection.

14 **Answer: 1** Following myelogram with water-based contrast, the head of bed needs to be elevated to 60 degrees to reduce the risk of meningeal irritation from any residual contrast in the spinal fluid. If an oil-based contrast was used, the head of the bed would need to remain flat. The other options indicate incorrect responses because the head of bed is too low to prevent headache from meningeal irritation as a complication of the procedure.

Cognitive Level: Application **Client Need:** Physiological Integrity: Reduction of Risk Potential **Integrated Process:** Nursing Process: Implementation **Content Area:** Adult Health: Neurological **Strategy:** The core issue of the question is knowledge of correct head position following myelogram using water-based contrast. Use nursing knowledge and the process of elimination to make a selection.

15 **Answer: 3** The client should limit joint movement, including walking, for 2 to 3 days after arthroscopy. Analgesics are often needed to manage pain, and the client should be instructed about what to use and how often to take it. The physician may order ice to control swelling, but not heat, which would aggravate swelling. Increased swelling and bleeding after discharge should be reported because these are abnormal findings and could indicate a complication of the procedure.
Cognitive Level: Analysis **Client Need:** Physiological Integrity: Reduction of Risk Potential **Integrated Process:** Nursing Process: Evaluation **Content Area:** Adult Health: Musculoskeletal **Strategy:** The core issue of the question is knowledge of measures to prevent complications and aid healing after arthroscopy. The wording of the question indicates that only one answer is a correct statement. Use nursing knowledge about care following arthroscopy and the process of elimination to make a selection.

16 **Answer: 1** Because the throat is anesthetized so the client can tolerate the endoscope, the client's gag and swallow reflexes are temporarily lost during any upper endoscopy procedure, such as esophagogastroscopy. The nurse's priority is to monitor for return of these protective airway reflexes. While mildly elevated temperature and reports of heartburn and sore throat also bear continued monitoring, they are of lesser priority than concerns related to the client's airway.
Cognitive Level: Analysis **Client Need:** Physiological Integrity: Reduction of Risk Potential **Integrated Process:** Nursing Process: Assessment **Content Area:** Adult Health: Gastrointestinal **Strategy:** Use the ABCs—airway, breathing, and circulation—to answer the question. Options that involve the airway are frequently the highest priority items. Use nursing knowledge and the process of elimination to make a selection.

17 **Answer: 3** The client should not eat or drink anything for 8 to 12 hours before the test, and so the client should not eat or drink anything after midnight. Oral medications are usually withheld before the procedure as well.
Cognitive Level: Analysis **Client Need:** Physiological Integrity: Reduction of Risk Potential **Integrated Process:** Nursing Process: Evaluation **Content Area:** Adult Health: Gastrointestinal **Strategy:** The core issue of the question is knowledge of dietary preparation before a barium swallow or upper GI series. Use ordinary logic to determine that the GI organs would be difficult to visualize if they contained food or fluid. Use nursing knowledge and the process of elimination to make a selection.

18 **Answer: 2** The diet may be resumed after colonoscopy, but the client usually tolerates it better if it is resumed gradually. The client should not drive for about 24 hours until all medications have fully worn off. It is normal to pass gas and feel bloated because of the carbon dioxide used to insufflate the colon to visualize the area. It is abnormal for bleeding to be present, and the client should notify the physician if it occurs.
Cognitive Level: Analysis **Client Need:** Physiological Integrity: Reduction of Risk Potential **Integrated Process:** Teaching and Learning **Content Area:** Adult Health: Gastrointestinal **Strategy:** The core issue of the question is knowledge of self-care following colonoscopy. Use nursing knowledge and the process of elimination to make a selection.

19 **Answer: 2** The client should avoid using any skin products, such as lotions or deodorant, on the skin of the breast or underarm prior to mammogram. The client may eat and drink as usual. Although the procedure may cause some women discomfort with compression of the breast, it is not necessary to premedicate with analgesics. There is no activity restriction following the test.
Cognitive Level: Application **Client Need:** Physiological Integrity: Reduction of Risk Potential **Integrated Process:** Teaching and Learning **Content Area:** Adult Health: Integumentary **Strategy:** The core issue of the question is knowledge that skin products should be avoided to prevent possible skin damage prior to a radiographic procedure such as a mammogram. The wording of the question tells you that only one option is a correct statement. Use nursing knowledge and the process of elimination to make a selection.

20 **Answer: 2** A Mantoux test (or PPD test) to screen for tuberculosis should be read in 48 to 72 hours. If the test was planted on Monday, the result must be read in 2 to 3 days, which is Wednesday or Thursday. The other options are either partially (options 1 and 3) or completely incorrect (option 4).
Cognitive Level: Application **Client Need:** Physiological Integrity: Reduction of Risk Potential **Integrated Process:** Nursing Process: Implementation **Content Area:** Adult Health: Respiratory **Strategy:** The core issue of the question is knowledge of specific timeframes for reading a PPD test. Remember, when there is more than one part to an option, the entire option must be correct in order for that option to be the correct answer. Use nursing knowledge and the process of elimination to make a selection.

21 **Answer: 1, 3, 5** Selected drugs (antacids, steroids, cholinergics, and anticholinergics) and coffee and alcohol should be restricted for at least 24 hours prior to test; note on test request form if client has not complied with restrictions. There is no reason to withhold a cardiac glycoside or a diuretic because these medications would not affect the test results.
Cognitive Level: Application **Client Need:** Physiological Integrity: Reduction of Risk Potential **Integrated Process:** Nursing Process: Implementation **Content Area:** Adult Health: Gastrointestinal **Strategy:** The core issue of the question is knowledge of drugs that could interfere with basal gastric acid testing and analysis. The wording of the question tells you that more than one may be correct; you must have the necessary knowledge to make your selections. Use nursing knowledge and the process of elimination.

Key Terms to Review

computed tomography (CT) scan p. 839
magnetic resonance imaging (MRI) p. 840
nuclear scan p. 840
ultrasonography p. 841
x-ray p. 841

References

Corbett, J. (2004). *Laboratory tests and diagnostic procedures with nursing diagnoses* (6th ed.). Upper Saddle River, NJ: Pearson Education.

Fischbach, F. (2004). *A manual of laboratory & diagnostic tests* (7th ed.). Philadelphia: Lippincott.

Kacmarek, R. (2005). *The essentials of respiratory care* (4th ed.). Philadelphia: Elsevier Mosby.

Leeuwen, A., Kranpitz, T., & Smith, L. (2006). *Davis's comprehensive handbook of laboratory and diagnostic tests with nursing implications* (2nd ed.). Philadelphia: F. A. Davis.

Smith, S., Duell, D., & Martin, B. (2004). *Clinical nursing skills: Basic to advanced skills* (6th ed.). Upper Saddle River, NJ: Pearson Education.

Wilkins, R. (2005). *Clinical assessment in respiratory care* (5th ed.). Philadelphia: Elsevier Mosby.

Perioperative Care

49

In this chapter

Test Yourself

Are you ready for the NCLEX-RN® or course exams? Use the practice tests on the companion CD-ROM to check.

Cross reference

Other chapters relevant to this content area are

Preventing and Controlling Infection Chapter 8
Maintaining Function of Drainage and Wound Tubes Chapter 28
Blood and Blood Component Therapy Chapter 33

I. OVERVIEW OF PERIOPERATIVE NURSING

!

A. Perioperative phases

1. **Preoperative phase** begins with determination that surgery is necessary and ends with transport of client to operating room (OR); general nursing activities include the following:
   - **a.** Client identification
   - **b.** Client assessment
   - **c.** Identifying potential or actual health problems
   - **d.** Beginning postoperative teaching about self-care
2. **Intraoperative phase** (surgical period) begins when client is transferred to operating table and ends when client is admitted to postanesthesia care unit (PACU); general nursing activities include:
   - **a.** Preparing client for induction of anesthesia
   - **b.** Maintaining homeostasis and asepsis throughout procedure
   - **c.** Assisting surgeon and team as needed by providing an aseptic, hazard-free environment and necessary supplies in a timely manner
3. **Postoperative phase** begins with client's admission to PACU and ends with a follow-up evaluation in either the clinical setting or home; general nursing activities include:
   - **a.** Assessing for physical adaptation following anesthesia and surgical intervention
   - **b.** Assisting in orienting client back to consciousness

c. Providing continuity of information between nursing units about client progress and adaptation following procedure

B. Summary of nursing responsibilities during preoperative period

1. Interview: current health status, allergies, medication currently taking, previous surgical experiences, mental status, understanding of the surgical procedure and anesthesia, smoking habit, alcohol and drug use, coping strategies, social resources, and cultural considerations
2. Arranging for preadmission testing, consultations, and education related to management of recovery from surgery and anesthesia
   a. Scheduling appropriate ordered laboratory tests, electrocardiogram, X-rays
   b. Ensuring reports are available on chart
   c. Reporting to surgeon or anesthesiologist any pertinent abnormalities
   d. Asking client if arrangements for autologous or directed blood donation (family/friends) have been made; if so, attach pertinent lab requisitions
3. ! Day of surgery: after appropriate identification of client, nurse verifies completion of paperwork and secures valuables; if procedure is being performed on an outpatient basis, transportation home is verified; nurse then proceeds to:
   a. Determine client's cognitive understanding of procedure and obtain signed **informed consent** form; ensure consent is obtained before administering premedication with sedative effects; some agencies have client mark limb that will be operated on, if appropriate
   b. Perform a physical assessment
   c. Implement preoperative teaching for postoperative care
   d. Physical preparation: skin preparation, vital signs, antiembolism stockings, catheterization, and starting an IV infusion
   e. Complete preoperative checklist; note client status and pertinent recent lab results; assist client to remove clothing, jewelry, and other articles, and to don hospital gown
   f. If client refuses to remove wedding band, tape in place and notify operating room personnel; leave eyeglasses in place if consistent with hospital policy; keep hearing aid(s) in place; remove dentures

C. Summary of nursing responsibilities during intraoperative period

1. Administer IV infusions and medications as needed
2. ! Provide safe, effective care
   a. Position client to ensure functional alignment and exposure of surgical site
   b. Apply grounding device
   c. Provide emotional and physical support if awake
   d. Account for all equipment and supplies
   e. Maintain aseptic environment
   f. Perform physiologic monitoring
   g. Assess fluid loss or gain
   h. Monitor cardiac, respiratory, and neurological status
   i. Monitor client response to preoperative medications
3. Nursing roles during the intraoperative period (the period of surgery)
   a. Circulating nurse assists scrub nurses and surgeons; sterile scrubbing and gloving not necessary
   b. Scrub nurses assist surgeons; maintain sterile gowns, gloves, shoe covers; wear eye protection and caps
   c. Circulating nurse and scrub nurse account for used sponges, needles, and instruments during and after the case

D. Summary of nursing responsibilities during postoperative period

1. Immediate care
   a. Assess the effects of anesthetic agents and surgical procedure
   b. Monitor vital functions
   c. Provide comfort and pain relief
2. ! Ongoing care
   a. Assess for client adaptation to effects of surgery
   b. Provide pain management

c. Position client appropriately
d. Promote use of the incentive spirometry
e. Assist with postoperative exercises
f. Maintain hydration
g. Promote urinary elimination
h. Maintain suction to devices as needed
i. Provide wound care
j. Continue client teaching and discharge planning

II. PURPOSES AND TYPES OF SURGERY AND ANESTHESIA

!

A. Purposes

1. Diagnostic or exploratory: establishes a diagnosis, such as a breast biopsy
2. Curative: removes pathological cause, such as removal of cancer
3. Ablative: removes a diseased body part, such as tonsils for tonsillitis
4. Reconstructive: restores function or appearance, such as cleft lip repair
5. **Palliative:** relieves or reduces pain or symptoms of a disease, such as removal of sensory nerves for intractable pain

B. General classification of surgery

1. Major (higher risk) versus minor (lower risk)
a. Major: may include prolonged intraoperative period, a large loss of blood, involvement of a vital organ, or postoperative complications; examples are lung surgery, colectomy
b. Minor: usually associated with few complications, may be described as "one-day surgery" or outpatient surgery; examples are cyst removal, ingrown toenails

!

2. Urgency classification
a. Emergent: performed immediately to save a person's life, limb, or organ, such as testicular torsion
b. Urgent: requires prompt attention, usually within 24 hours, such as reduction of a broken bone
c. Required: necessary for client's well-being, usually within weeks to months, such as cholecystectomy, if not acute
d. Elective: surgery is necessary but condition is not imminently life-threatening; surgery will improve the client's life, such as plastic surgery
e. Optional: based on client preference, such as gastric stapling

C. Administration of *anesthesia* (partial or complete loss of sensation)

1. Anesthetic agents are drugs used to effect a partial or complete loss of pain sensation; client may be conscious or unconscious

!

2. **Conscious sedation** (or moderate sedation)
a. An anesthesia state involving minimal depression of level of consciousness (LOC), allowing client to respond to verbal and physical stimuli; client maintains a patent airway while pain threshold is raised; examples are with burn dressings, balloon angioplasty
b. Uses IV narcotics and anti-anxiety agents

!

3. **Regional anesthesia:** loss of sensation in one part of body
a. Local: injected in a specific area for minor surgical procedures, such as lidocaine for suturing a small wound
b. Nerve block: anesthetic agent is injected into and around a nerve or group of nerves, such as a pudendal block used to numb the perineum for an episiotomy in childbirth
c. Epidural block: anesthetic agent injected into epidural space to anesthetize larger areas, such as in vaginal childbirth; client is awake and aware of surroundings but feels no pain
d. Spinal anesthesia: anesthesia is injected through a lumbar puncture into the subarachnoid space, such as for hernia repairs or cesarean section deliveries; client is conscious but has no sensation or movement of lower extremities up to a specific area

!

4. General anesthesia
a. Anesthesia that involves loss of all sensation and consciousness

b. It is usually administered by IV infusion or by inhalation of gases
c. Examples of use: major surgery, exploratory laparotomy

D. Stages of general anesthesia

1. Stage I: beginning of anesthesia; client is drowsy and dizzy; pain sensation is depressed
2. Stage II: excitement stage
   a. Client demonstrates irregular breathing and involuntary motor movements
   b. It is important to avoid stimulating client, which can trigger vomiting, holding the breath, and increased activity
   c. Ensure client safety by proper use of safety straps
3. Stage III
   a. Stage of anesthesia appropriate for surgical procedures
   b. Client demonstrates skeletal muscle relaxation, constricted pupils, and absence of eyelid reflex
4. Stage IV
   a. Medullary depression
   b. Pupils are fixed and dilated, respirations are weak, and pulse is rapid and thready
   c. The client is near death

E. Preanesthesia classification of client's physical condition

1. Anesthesiologist reviews client's medical history as well as current findings related to diagnosis, medication use, allergies, and drug reactions
2. Client is then assigned a risk category for surgery, from I (healthiest) to VI (brain dead; organs being donated) or E for emergency surgery

F. Anesthetic agents may be administered by either inhalation or IV routes

1. Inhalation anesthetic agents are inhaled in gaseous forms
   a. Administered by mask or by endotracheal tube
   b. Induction is usually rapid
   c. Drugs are eliminated by respiratory system
   d. With normal lung function, recovery rate is predictable
2. IV anesthesia
   a. Administered alone or in combination with inhalation anesthesia
   b. Rapid onset of unconsciousness
   c. Metabolized primarily by liver and excreted by kidneys
   d. Reversal agents may be required to stop drug's effects

III. COMPONENTS OF PREOPERATIVE ASSESSMENT

A. Client's history

1. Medical history: current and past
   ! a. Family history of malignant hyperthermia
   b. Current health status including any chronic disease that might affect the client's response to surgery and anesthesia
   c. Past medical illnesses and treatments; previous surgical experiences including complications that occurred with any previous surgical or anesthesia experience (such as malignant hyperthermia)
   d. Report of severe anxiety associated with surgery
2. ! Medication use: all current medications, including prescription, over-the-counter, and herbal or other agents
3. ! Allergies
   a. Food or medication
   b. Environmental: latex allergies, tape, soap, and antiseptic agents
4. Tobacco use: may indicate potential problems of the respiratory tract
   a. Type of product
   b. Amount and frequency
   c. When possible, urge client to stop smoking 6 to 8 weeks prior to major surgery
5. Alcohol and controlled substance use
   a. Type of product
   b. Amount and frequency
   c. Potential for problems with withdrawal

6. Psychosocial and economic factors
   a. Occupation and financial concerns
   b. Support systems
   c. Spiritual needs
   d. Cultural beliefs
   e. Coping mechanisms used in the past
   f. Fear and anxiety related to procedure, such as changes in body image, pain, or grieving a loss of body part

B. Physical assessment

1. Assessment of factors that will affect client's response to surgery or anesthesia
2. General assessments
   a. Overall appearance, gestures, facial expression
   b. Height and weight (obesity increases risk)
   c. Vital signs (hypertension increases risk)
3. Head and neck
   a. Oral mucous membranes reveal hydration status
   b. Identify loose teeth, dentures, and orthodontia work
   c. Inspect soft palate, nasal sinuses, cervical lymph nodes
   d. Note presence of jugular venous distention
4. Integumentary
   a. Evaluate skin over entire body
   b. ! Note any areas where skin is thin, dry, or has poor turgor or breakdown
5. Chest and lungs
   a. ! Auscultate for adventitious breath sounds
   b. Note degree of chest expansion, presence of cough, upper airway congestion, and/or obstructed nasal passages
6. ! Cardiovascular system
   a. Assess apical rate and rhythm
   b. Check color and temperature of extremities
   c. Note presence of pacemaker, A-V fistula or graft
7. Gastrointestinal (GI) system
   a. Distinguish between obesity and distention of abdomen
   b. Assess baseline bowel sounds and elimination patterns
   c. Note gag reflex and history of nausea/vomiting postoperatively
   d. ! Validate NPO (nothing by mouth) status when applicable; anesthetics are known to depress GI functioning; clients are usually NPO for 6 to 8 hours prior to surgery to reduce the risk of vomiting and aspiration
8. Genitourinary and reproductive system
   a. Determine alterations in urinary elimination, color, appearance, and usual amount of urine output
   b. Note presence of abnormal vaginal discharge, uterine bleeding in women
   c. Pregnancy status
9. Neurological and mobility status
   a. Determine baseline LOC
   b. ! Note presence of sensory or perceptual deficits
   c. Assess range of motion and ability to perform activities of daily living

C. Diagnostic screening

1. Laboratory tests are done prior to surgery to screen for existing abnormalities and to use as a baseline for future assessments
2. Additional tests may be ordered related to specific condition
3. ! Nurse should verify that test results are present prior to surgery
4. ! Abnormal findings may need to be corrected prior to surgery
5. See Table 49–1 ■ for routine preoperative screening tests

IV. INFORMED CONSENT

A. Description

1. Written permission obtained from client prior to any invasive procedure or one that has potentially serious side effects or complications

Table 49–1
Routine Preoperative Screening Tests

Test	Purpose for Assessment
Urinalysis	Urine composition and possible abnormal components
Chest x-ray	Respiratory status and heart size
Electrocardiogram	Preexisting cardiac disease or rhythm abnormalities
Complete blood count (CBC)	Red blood cells, hemoglobin, and hematocrit for oxygen-carrying capacity of blood White blood cells as indicator of immune function (infection)
Blood typing and cross-matching	Blood transfusion, ABO and Rh matching
Serum electrolytes (Na^+, K^+, Ca^{++}, Mg^{++}, Cl^-, $HCO3^-$)	Electrolyte balance
Fasting blood glucose	Detection or control of diabetes mellitus
Blood urea nitrogen (BUN) and creatinine	Renal function
ALT, AST, LDH, bilirubin	Liver function
Serum albumin and total protein	Nutritional status

2. Client has right to accept or reject procedure after receiving explanation
3. Informed consent includes providing client with information about the following:
   a. Nature and purpose of a treatment or procedure
   b. Expected outcomes and probabilities of success, material risks, benefits and consequences of treatment
   c. Alternatives to procedure and supporting information
   d. Effect of doing without the procedure or treatment, including effect on prognosis

B. Three elements of informed consent

1. It is given voluntarily
2. It is given by an individual with the capacity and competence to understand what the procedure involves
   a. Adults have legal authority to make decisions for themselves
   b. If client is a minor, parent or legal guardian has right to provide consent
   c. Many states recognize emancipated minors who can provide consent for themselves
   d. Many states allow minors to provide consent for treatment in cases related to venereal disease, pregnancy, abortion, and contraception
   e. Legal power of attorney for health care allows another individual to make decisions should client become incapacitated
3. Sufficient information must be provided to client to allow for an informed decision
   a. Health care workers must communicate in a way the client can understand
   b. An interpreter may be needed to ensure adequate communication
4. In emergencies, when informed consent cannot be obtained from client or next of kin, consent is implied by law; specific information about the emergency situation and the reason informed consent was not obtained must be documented in medical record

C. Nurse's role with informed consent

1. Informed consent is part of physician–client relationship
2. Because nurse does not perform surgery or procedures, informed consent is not part of nursing responsibility; nurse can reinforce physician explanations
3. Physician has obligation to obtain consent
4. Nurse's role is to serve as witness to the following:
   a. Authority on consent form is authentic
   b. Client has capacity to make informed consent
   c. Client has authority to consent
   d. Consent is being given voluntarily

V. DEVELOPMENTAL CONSIDERATIONS OF INDIVIDUALS HAVING SURGERY

! **A. Children and adolescents**

1. Take care with all children and adolescents while explaining procedures because they may misinterpret meaning
2. Infancy: surgery and separation from parents may interfere with bonding; children of this age have no understanding of the process but are aware of adult emotions; no explanations about procedures are required for a child, but parents will need complete preparation
3. Toddler: children of this age may suffer from separation anxiety; their security lies in the presence of their caregivers; when caregivers are not present, child may suffer; immediately prior to a procedure, give toddler a brief, simple explanation
4. Preschoolers: often view illness as a punishment for bad behavior; have an inadequate understanding of cause–effect and thus misinterpret relationships; explanations continue to be simple and in close proximity to time of procedure; play therapy may be beneficial in aiding preschooler to express feelings
5. School-aged children: better able to withstand separation from parents and are accustomed to dealing with adults other than family; children of this age fear pain and mutilation; more complete, yet age-appropriate instructions are required, and may benefit from pictures, dolls, and videos
6. Adolescents: concerns are separation from peers and body image/physical attractiveness; protect child's privacy

B. Adults

1. Fear of the unknown and separation from support systems
2. Dependence and loss of control
3. Disruption in career goals, family living patterns, and financial worries
4. Concern over disability and/or death

VI. PHYSICAL PREPARATION OF INDIVIDUALS HAVING SURGERY

A. Preparing for anesthesia

1. Anesthetic needs and risks are assessed by anesthesiologist
2. Type of anesthetic along with method of administration, risks, and recovery is explained

B. Preparing the skin

1. Purpose: cleansing and removing transient microbes from skin
2. Includes the following components:
   a. Cleansing: begins with morning shower or bath; surgical site is then cleansed with an antimicrobial agent immediately prior to surgical procedure
   b. Hair removal from surgical site: may be ordered to further reduce microbial growth; care must be taken to maintain intact skin (clip but don't shave)

C. Preparing the GI tract

! 1. NPO prior to OR in order to
   a. Reduce risk of vomiting or aspiration
   b. Prevent contamination of operative site from fecal material
   c. Reduce postoperative nausea, vomiting, gastric distention, or bowel obstruction
2. Colon cleansing may be ordered for surgical procedures involving GI tract; this reduces contamination of surgical field; postoperative constipation may be prevented; cleansing may occur using
   a. Enemas
   b. Laxatives
   c. Oral antibiotics

D. Preparation on the day of surgery

! 1. Routine care for most outpatient as well as hospitalized clients
   a. Consent form is signed
   b. Preoperative medications are given
   c. Emotional support to client and family is provided
   d. Preoperative teaching is completed, including postoperative routine

2. General care
   a. Vital signs are recorded for baseline information
   b. Dentures, bridgework (or both) are removed; loose teeth are noted on chart
   c. Hospital gown is put on without undergarments in most cases (for children and minor procedures, there may be exceptions)
   d. Bladder is emptied
   e. Cosmetics and nail polish is removed
   f. Jewelry is removed per agency policy and is placed in secure area for safekeeping; if client does not want to remove wedding band, it can be taped in place; in certain situations, removal of wedding band may be required because of risk of postoperative edema
   g. Hearing aids are left in place and are noted on preoperative checklist
   h. Eyeglasses, contact lenses, and other prostheses are removed
   i. Antiembolism stockings may be ordered; these stockings promote return circulation from legs

E. Preoperative medications

1. May be ordered at a scheduled time or "on call" to OR
2. Purposes
   a. Sedate or tranquilize
   b. Decrease respiratory tract secretions
   c. Provide analgesia
   d. Reduce nausea and prevent vomiting
   e. Reduce gastric acid
3. Classifications of preoperative medication
   a. Barbiturates are used for sedation and as narcotic enhancer; major side effects are CNS depression, respiratory depression
   b. Benzodiazepines are used to reduce anxiety and as a medication enhancer; major side effect is CNS depression
   c. Narcotic or opioid analgesics are used to reduce dosages needed of anesthetics; major side effect is CNS depression
   d. Anticholinergics are used to reduce secretion of body fluids such as saliva; major side effect is GI system depression
   e. Antinausea agents are used to reduce probability of emesis and aspiration; major side effect is respiratory depression
   f. Antacid, H_2-receptor blockers are used to reduce gastric acidity and reflux; major side effect is rebound acidity
   g. Prophylactic anti-infectives are used to reduce risk of infection; major side effect is resistance to antibiotics; hypersensitivity is always a concern if first dose

VII. INTRAOPERATIVE FACTORS AFFECTING POSTOPERATIVE PHASE

A. Principles of perioperative asepsis

1. General
   a. Keep sterile supplies dry and unopened
   b. Check package sterilization expiration date to verify sterility
   c. Maintain general cleanliness in surgical suite
   d. Maintain **surgical asepsis** (activities designed to keep sites free of microorganisms) throughout procedure (see Box 49–1)
2. Personnel with signs of illness should not report to work
3. **Surgical scrub,** a specific handwashing technique used by operating room personnel designed to reduce microorganisms on hands and arms, is done for length of time designated by hospital policy
   a. A sensor-controlled or knee- or foot-operated faucet allows water to be turned on and off without use of hands
   b. Remove all rings and watches
   c. Use liquid soaps to prevent spread of microorganisms
   d. Keep fingernails short and well-trimmed; clean fingernails with a nail stick under running water; artificial nails pose risk of infection and are prohibited

Box 49-1

Principles of Surgical Asepsis

All objects within a sterile field must remain sterile at all times.

Sterile objects are no longer sterile when they are touched by unsterile objects.

Objects that are below the nurse's waist level or out of the nurse's vision are considered unsterile.

Sterile objects lose their sterility with prolonged exposure to airborne microorganisms.

Fluids always flow in the direction of gravity.

Moisture that wicks or passes through a sterile object draws microorganisms through it from above or below by capillary action (also called strikethrough).

A one-inch margin at any edge of a sterile field is considered unsterile.

The skin can never be sterilized and is therefore unsterile.

Maintaining surgical asepsis requires conscientiousness, alertness, and honesty.

Adapted from Kozier, B., Erb, G., Berman, A., & Snyder, S. (2004). *Fundamentals of nursing: Concepts, process, and practice* (7th ed.). Upper Saddle River, NJ: Pearson Education, 655–656.

e. Hold hands higher than elbows throughout procedure so that run-off goes to elbows; this allows cleanest area to be the hands
f. A scrub brush facilitates removal of microorganisms; clean all areas of skin on hands and arms in sequence, starting at hands and ending at elbows
g. After rinsing, dry hands with sterile towels, drying first one arm from hand to elbow, then using a second towel to dry second hand

! **4.** Maintaining a **sterile field** (a microoganism-free area)
a. Create a sterile field using sterile drapes
b. Use sterile field to place sterile supplies where they will be available during procedure
c. Drape equipment prior to use
d. Keep drapes dry and out of contact with nonsterile objects
e. Utilize sterile technique while adding or removing supplies from sterile fields

! **5.** Sterile supplies and solutions
a. Check expiration dates for sterility
b. Don't use solutions that were opened prior to current use
c. "Lip" solutions after initial use by pouring a small amount of liquid out of bottle into a waste container to cleanse bottle lip

B. Potential environmental health hazards during intraoperative period

1. Injuries caused by equipment
a. Laser tools used for a surgical procedure can cause burns
b. Improperly grounded cautery devices can cause burns
c. Ensure proper grounding for electrical equipment and check equipment prior to beginning surgical procedure

! **2.** Latex allergy affects many people, both clients and hospital personnel
a. Clients with spina bifida and those who have had multiple surgical procedures are at greatest risk
b. Exposure can occur percutaneously, mucosally, parenterally, and via inhalation
c. Symptoms can vary from contact dermatitis to anaphylaxis
d. Symptoms in an anesthetized client would include flushing, facial swelling, urticaria, bronchospasm, hypotension, and cardiac arrest
e. Be aware of equipment that contains latex, including tourniquets, Ambu bags, balloon catheters, surgical gowns, boots, and drapes

! **3.** Exposure to blood and body fluids
a. A concern for client and staff alike
b. Use goggles and fluid-protectant shields; gloves worn for extended period can leak and should be changed periodically
c. Use caution with sharps

C. Potential intraoperative complications

1. Nausea and vomiting: ensure that client is NPO for prescribed time period
2. Hypoxia and respiratory complications
   a. Loss of pharyngeal and cough reflexes may lead to aspiration of secretions or vomitus
   b. Respiratory depression can occur from anesthetic agents
   c. Respiratory muscles become weakened or paralyzed by neuromuscular agents
   d. Positioning can negatively affect lung expansion
   e. Tissue perfusion is monitored by anesthesiologist
   f. Use of a pulse oximeter assists with monitoring oxygenation
3. Hypothermia
   a. Related to OR temperature and exposure of internal organs
   b. Minimized by preventing exposure of nonsurgical body parts, use of head covering and blankets, warmed IV fluids and anesthetic agents
4. ! Malignant hyperthermia
   a. Excessive heat production related to stress, trauma, infection; may be attributed to anesthetic agent; seen more commonly in males; there is a tendency toward development if inherited as an autosomal-dominant trait
   b. Symptoms include rapid rise in body temperature, tachycardia and tachypnea, and respiratory and metabolic acidosis
   c. Skin initially appears flushed, then becomes mottled and cyanotic
   d. Treatment includes administering 100% oxygen, cooling blankets and ice packs, cool IV fluids, and stomach irrigation
   e. Can be fatal
5. Paresthesia and impaired skin integrity related to positioning
6. Excessive fluid and blood loss

VIII. POSTOPERATIVE NURSING CARE

A. Assessments in immediate period following surgery in PACU (see Box 49–2)

1. Confirm client's identity
2. Receive report from surgical nurse: surgical procedure, anesthesia, drugs and intravenous fluids administered, and estimated blood loss
3. Note location, types, and conditions of catheters, **drains,** or packs; drains are tubes inserted into wounds to allow the removal of excessive **serosanguineous** (fluid composed of serum and blood) or **purulent** (containing pus) material from wound

B. Nursing management in PACU

1. ! Maintain a patent airway: priority nursing concern
   a. May be impaired by continued effects of anesthesic drugs, relaxation of the tongue, oropharyngeal secretions, or vomitus
   b. Position client on side unless contraindicated
   c. Monitor respiratory rate (should be 10–30 breaths/minute)
   d. Assess breath sounds for crackles (fluid) or rhonchi (secretions) and suction as necessary
   e. Wheezing or stridor may signal broncho- or laryngospasm; assess carefully and maintain airway; notify surgeon or anesthesiologist immediately
   f. Assess for return of cough, gag, and swallow reflexes
2. ! Maintain cardiovascular stability
   a. Client is typically on a cardiac and respiratory monitor
   b. Monitor vital signs according to hospital policy (often every 15 minutes) until stable and then every 30 minutes until PACU discharge
   c. Report changes in vital signs immediately; small but persistent trends are early signs that client's condition is deteriorating
   d. Apply pneumatic boots or antiembolism stockings as ordered to promote circulation in lower extremities
3. Assess for hypotension or shock
   a. May be related to fluid or blood loss or as a reaction to drugs
   b. Symptoms include restlessness, desreased urine output, cool moist skin, pallor followed by cyanosis, and dropping BP with increasing pulse

Box 49–2

Clinical Assessment in the Postanesthetic Phase

- Adequacy of airway
- Oxygen saturation
- Adequacy of ventilation
  - Respiratory rate, rhythm, and depth
  - Use of accessory muscles
  - Breath sounds
- Cardiovascular status
  - Heart rate and rhythm
  - Peripheral pulse amplitude and equality
  - Blood pressure
  - Capillary filling
- Level of consciousness
  - Not responding
  - Arousable with verbal simuli
  - Fully awake
  - Oriented to time, person, and place
- Presence of protective reflexes (e.g., gag, cough)
- Activity, ability to move extremities
- Skin color (pink, pale, dusky, blotchy, cyanotic, jaundiced)
- Fluid status
  - Intake and output
  - Status of IV infusions (type of fluid, rate, amount in container, patency of tubing)
  - Signs of dehydration or fluid overload
- Condition of operative site
  - Status of dressing
  - Drainage (amount, type, and color)
- Patency, character, and amount of drainage from catheters, tubes, and drains
- Discomfort (i.e., pain: type, location, and severity), nausea, vomiting
- Safety (e.g., necessity for side rails, call bell within reach)

Source: Kozier, B., Erb, G., Berman, A., & Snyder, S. (2004). *Fundamentals of Nursing: Concepts, Process, and Practice* (7th ed.). Upper Saddle River, NJ: Pearson Education, 913.

c. Monitor and maintain IV infusion flow rates to prevent hypovolemia as a cause of shock

! **4.** Assess for hemorrhage

a. Monitor dressings and drains for amount of discharge; observe appearance and amount of urine (concentrated and decreased volume with hypovolemia); observe for distention of body tissues

b. A client with excessive blood loss may require a transfusion; ensure blood product and type are correct (see Chapter 33)

5. Assess for hypertension and dysrhythmias

6. Relieve pain and anxiety

a. Pain can negatively affect vital signs and recovery

b. Assess location and cause of pain

c. Administer analgesics (often opioids by IV) as ordered

d. Observe effectiveness of analgesics

7. Neurological status
   a. Assess LOC with vital signs and prn
   b. Frequently attempt to arouse client until fully awake
   c. Orient to environment when awake
   d. Maintain quiet environment during recovery period from anesthesia
8. Temperature
   a. Measure temperature
   b. Apply warm blankets or Bear hugger to keep client warm if hypothermic from cool operating room and exposure during surgery
9. Integumentary
   a. Monitor status of incision if visible; otherwise, monitor status of incisional dressing
   b. Assess for skin redness or breakdown because of surgical positioning or burns from cautery or grounding pad; report and complete incident report if found

C. Discharge criteria from PACU

1. Vital signs are stable and spontaneous respirations have returned
2. Gag reflex is present
3. Client is easily arousable
4. Additional client discharge criteria from ambulatory surgical unit:
   a. Is alert and oriented
   b. Has no respiratory distress
   c. Is able to cough, swallow, and walk
   d. Is free of vomiting
   e. Has voided (may not be required in minor procedures per some agency policies)
   f. Has mild or minimal pain
   g. Has minimal, if any, bleeding from incisional area
   h. Has responsible adult to drive client home

D. Nursing management on clinical unit

1. Immediate nursing interventions
   a. Assess breathing and apply oxygen if prescribed
   b. Check vital signs and skin warmth, moisture, color
   c. Assess surgical site and wound drains; the partial or total rupture of a sutured wound is termed **dehiscence;** dehiscence may be preceded by sudden straining as occurs during coughing (see also section on complications that follows)
   d. Note and document wound **exudate** (fluid and cells that accumulate in a wound); exudate varies in appearance: **serous** (like serum—watery and clear), purulent (thick and contains pus; may be blue, green, or yellow tinged), **sanguineous** (bloody and may be dark red or bright red depending on freshness of blood)
   e. Connect tubes to drain devices or suction
   f. Perform pain assessment and utilize appropriate pain relief interventions
   g. Position client properly using support devices as necessary
   h. Monitor IV fluids and infusion pumps
   i. Monitor urine output hourly or less frequently as ordered; hourly urine output should be 30 mL or more
   j. Bladder distention is possible for up to 24 hours following spinal anesthesia; spontaneous voiding should occur within 6 to 8 hours postoperatively; if unable to void, catheterization may be ordered and repeated as necessary
2. Ongoing nursing interventions
   a. Encourage deep breathing and coughing exercises every 2 hours while awake to prevent atelectasis and pneumonia; encourage client to sit up in bed and place hands one on top of the other directly on wound (splint incision) to reduce discomfort of coughing
   b. Teach and encourage leg exercises, use of support stockings or sequential compression device
   c. Keep call light, emesis basin, ice chips, bedpan, urinal within reach
   d. Communicate with family and significant others
   e. Monitor for infection by noting wound characteristics, temperature, and WBC test results

f. Teach self-care according to surgical procedure and client and family needs
g. Encourage activity as tolerated
! h. Promote GI status: provide diet and fluids once bowel sounds return; begin with clear liquids and advance to full liquids, soft and regular as tolerated (no nausea, vomiting, abdominal distention) and ordered; encourage early ambulation to promote bowel function
! i. Continue to monitor voiding and compare to intake; diuresis from mobilization of fluids given during surgery can occur by second postoperative day
j. Provide wound care as ordered (monitor incision, change dressing as ordered); document findings
! k. Provide for adequate pain management using patient-controlled analgesia or other opioids; assess pain at least every 4 hours; assess effectiveness of pharmacological and nonpharmacological (e.g., music, distraction, massage) measures
! l. Participate in discharge planning according to client needs: ensure client understands diet, activity, medications, and when to call surgeon for complications; schedule follow-up care; ensure that home care or other support services are in place (see Box 49–3)

Box 49–3

Common Postsurgical Discharge Instructions

Diet

Drink at least 6 to 8 glasses of fluid daily unless otherwise ordered (water is beneficial)

Adhere to any diet restrictions (provide individualized instruction according to diet)

Make sure meals are well balanced and high in vitamin C and protein to aid in wound healing

Activity

Maintain activity restriction if ordered by surgeon

Resume activities gradually (all clients)

Avoid heavy lifting for 6 weeks after major surgery

Avoid lifting more than 10 pounds or performing activities involving pushing or pulling with an abdominal incision

Often may return to work in 6 to 8 weeks (depending on surgery and client status preoperatively)

Medications

Continue to take pain medication as needed; follow directions on prescription bottle

Take other medications as ordered (teach specifics regarding medication action, dose, how to take, and side or adverse effects to watch for and report)

Wound Care

Take care of incision and/or change dressing as taught (specific information is individualized to client and surgery; provide 1 to 2 days of dressing materials or according to hospital policy)

Cover incision with plastic wrap before showering (if allowed)

Sutures or staples are often removed in surgeon's office 7 to 14 days postoperatively

Steri-Strips will fall off by themselves (if used instead of sutures or if applied for support when sutures are removed before discharge)

Follow-up Care

Contact surgeon if signs of complications occur (fever, signs of wound infection, increased pain, other signs specific to surgery)

It is important to keep follow-up appointments to aid in continued recovery from surgery

Table 49–2

Postoperative Complications

Respiratory	Hypoxia Atelectasis and possible pneumonia Aspiration Pulmonary embolism
Cardiovascular	Hemorrhage Shock Thrombophlebitis
GI	Paralytic ileus Constipation
GU	Urinary retention Urinary tract infection (with indwelling catheter)
Wound-related	Infection Dehiscence (abdominal wound) Evisceration (abdominal wound)

IX. POSTOPERATIVE COMPLICATIONS *(See Table 49–2 ■)*

A. Respiratory

1. Hypoxia (inadequate arterial oxygenation)
   - **a.** Assess for restlessness as early sign, decreasing oxygen saturation levels (by pulse oximetry), increasing dyspnea, tachycardia, rising BP, possible diaphoresis and cyanosis (late sign)
   - **b.** Prevent with use of deep breathing and coughing, incentive spirometry, turning and repositioning every 2 hours, and early ambulation
   - **c.** Provide oxygen as ordered and provide ongoing monitoring
2. Atelectasis and pneumonia
   - **a.** Atelectasis: alveolar collapse with retained mucus; often occurs within 1 to 2 days postoperatively; is most common complication
   - **b.** Pneumonia: alveolar inflammation caused by infection, aspiration, or immobility leading to atelectasis; often develops 3 to 5 days postoperatively
   - **c.** Assess for signs of hypoxia, dyspnea, crackles over affected area, fever, chest pain, and productive cough
   - **d.** Perform regular respiratory assessments, including breath sounds and oxygen saturation
   - **e.** Encourage deep breathing, coughing, incentive spirometry, frequent repositioning, and ambulation; suction client if needed to mobilize secretions
   - **f.** Implement ordered interventions such as antibiotic therapy, chest physiotherapy (CPT), and oxygen

B. Pulmonary embolism

1. Occurs when an embolus obstructs a pulmonary artery and blocks blood flow to one or more lung segments; usually occurs after surgery as a complication of thrombophlebitis (see next section)
2. Signs include sudden pain in chest (often sharp), although occasionally described as upper abdominal pain; dypsnea with possible air hunger, tachycardia, hypotension, and pallor deteriorating to cyanosis; declining oxygen saturation readings
3. Sit client up in bed as much as tolerated; assess vital signs and notify physician; be prepared for emergency interventions including resuscitation if needed

C. Hemorrhage and shock

1. Occurs when there is rapid and large blood loss; hemorrhage can lead to shock state
2. Signs include restlessness, deteriorating LOC, rapid and weakening pulse, decreasing BP, increasing respirations, pale diaphoretic skin, and decreasing urine output
3. If bleeding is external, provide manual pressure over site after applying gloves
4. Notify surgeon
5. Provide oxygen, fluid resuscitation, and blood or blood products as ordered

6. Place client in modified Trendelenburg position (legs elevated to low Fowler's but thorax flat) to support BP; if client had spinal anesthesia, elevate legs on only one pillow so spinal anesthetic does not affect diaphragm and breathing
7. Prepare client for return to OR if necessary
8. Treatment of hemorrhage usually helps resolve shock, but prepare to use vasopressors as adjunct therapy
9. Monitor for return of stable vital signs, urine output, and LOC as signs that shock has resolved

D. Thromblophlebitis

1. Occurs when clot formation and inflammation are present in a vein, usually in the leg
2. Best prevention is use of pneumatic boots (for intermittent pulsatile pressure to mimic leg muscle action on veins) or antiembolism stockings, postoperative ankle/leg exercises or passive range of motion every 2 hours, adequate fluid inake (1.5 to 2 liters daily at least), and early ambulation
3. Signs include pain at site (usually cramping or aching), possible vein inflammation (may be visible if superficial, but is often deep), enlarged calf on affected side, unilateral edema, positive Homan's sign (non-specific), and increased temperature
4. Elevate leg 30 degrees without allowing pressure on popliteal space (avoid knee gatch); keep on bedrest as ordered until risk of pulmonary embolus passes
5. Administer anticoagulation (heparin or warfarin sodium) as prescribed; enoxaprin (Lovenox) may be ordered for prevention in high-risk clients
6. When client is allowed out of bed, do not let client dangle legs at bedside, sit or stand for prolonged periods, or cross knees or ankles (all impair venous return)

E. Paralytic ileus

1. Occurs when bowel motility does not return following anesthesia; may be affected also by manipulation of bowel during abdominal surgery
2. Signs include absent bowel sounds, increasing abdominal distention, lack of flatus or bowel movement, and nausea and vomiting
3. Maintain NPO status until return of bowel sounds
4. Maintain patency of nasogastric tube if present; if not, one may be ordered to be inserted and placed to low wall suction to provide gastric decompression
5. Administer IV fluids or total parenteral nutrition until gut motility returns
6. Monitor intake and output and document accurately
7. Encourage ambulation to stimulate bowel
8. Administer GI stimulants, histamine-2 receptor blockers, or gastric pump inhibitors as ordered

F. Constipation

1. Defined as inadequate or infrequent passage of stool; is cause for concern if client cannot have a bowel movement within 48 hours of surgery
2. Signs include increasing abdominal distention and possible discomfort, lack of bowel movement, and possibly anorexia and nausea
3. Increase fluid intake to as much as 3 liters per day unless contraindicated
4. Increase intake of fiber in diet if solid diet is allowed and appropriate
5. Encourage and assist with frequent ambulation if able to be out of bed
6. Administer ordered stool softeners and laxatives
7. Provide for privacy during elimination and allow sufficient time
8. Monitor and document frequency and characteristics of stool; also teach assistive personnel the importance of monitoring; use a stool chart if necessary

G. Urinary retention

1. Occurs when urine collects in bladder because of loss of tone from anesthetic agents and opioid analgesics; is evident within 6 to 8 hours postoperatively
2. Signs include inability to void, increasing bladder distention, drumlike sound on bladder percussion, increasing volume of urine noted via bladder scanner, lower abdominal discomfort, possible restlessness, disphoresis, increasing BP
3. Provide privacy and upright position for voiding (on bedpan, commode, or in bathroom); may assist male clients to stand for more natural position for voiding

4. Run water in sink or pour water over perineum to stimulate urge to void
5. Obtain order for straight catheterization when noninvasive measures are ineffective; some surgeons will order catheter to remain inserted if drainage exceeds a certain volume; use Foley catheter kit instead of straight catheter kit if order is written in this manner; ensure sterile technique to prevent urinary tract infection
6. Continue to monitor subsequent ability to void following straight catheterization until regular voiding pattern resumes and risk of retention has passed

H. Wound infection

1. Occurs because of improper aseptic technique in perioperative period or because of wound contamination preoperatively
2. Signs include warmth, redness, and tenderness at incision site; possible edematous suture line with taut sutures, elevated temperature and white blood cell count, possible malaise and chills
3. Monitor temperature; assess status of incision with dressing changes (report any adverse changes)
4. Maintain function of any surgical drains and use aseptic technique while handling them
5. Administer ordered prophylactic or therapeutic anti-infective therapy (antibiotics); give medications on time to maintain therapeutic blood levels

I. Wound dehiscence and evisceration

1. Dehiscence: separation of incisional wound edges that often occurs 6 to 8 days postoperatively; occurs more frequently in clients with abdominal wounds or poor wound healing or who are obese
2. Signs of dehiscence include separating wound edges with visible underlying tissue; drainage may be increased
3. Evisceration: protrusion of internal structures or organs through an area of dehiscence; is an emergency situation that generally requires additional surgery to repair
4. Signs of evisceration include appearance of bowel or other abdominal tissue through wound, new or increased serosanguinous fluid drainage from wound, and possible client reports of a "popping" sensation after an event that raises intra-abdominal pressure (coughing, sneezing, turning in bed)
5. Assist client to lie down
6. Position client in low Fowler's with knees bent to remove tension from abdominal suture line
7. Place sterile saline-moistened dressings on wound
8. Notify surgeon immediately after taking actions to safeguard client
9. Administer antiemetics as ordered to avoid further stress on incision from vomiting
10. Administer antibiotics as ordered and prepare client with evisceration for return to surgery
11. Teach measures to prevent recurrence, such as splinting when moving, coughing, or sneezing

Check Your NCLEX-RN® Exam I.Q.

You are ready for testing on this content if you can

- Determine a client's readiness for surgery.
- Prepare a client for surgery.
- Monitor a client before, during, and after surgery.
- Provide preoperative, intraoperative, and postoperative care to a client.
- Assess a client's response to recovery from various types of anesthesia.
- Provide client education about preoperative and postoperative care.
- Assess a client's response to a surgical procedure.
- Evaluate effectiveness of interventions designed to prevent postoperative complications.

PRACTICE TEST

1 The nurse has taught the client to perform deep breathing and coughing exercises. The nurse determines that the client needs more teaching when the client is observed doing which of the following activities?

1. Sitting upright before performing deep breathing and coughing exercises
2. Taking deep breaths before attempting to cough
3. Placing both hands vertically and lightly on either side of the incision
4. Using a pillow for splinting during coughing

2 A toddler is being prepared for a surgical procedure. This is the child's first experience with surgery. The child's mother expresses concern about the child's psychological adaptation to the surgery. While planning for postoperative care, the nurse recognizes that which of the following is likely to be the child's greatest concern?

1. Anticipated pain
2. Body image changes
3. Communication difficulties
4. Separation from parents

3 A female client is being prepared for surgery. When the nurse asks the client to remove her wedding ring, the client refuses. Which of the following would be the most appropriate response by the nurse?

1. Encourage the client to use soapy water to remove the ring if it is tight.
2. Explain that the hospital cannot be responsible for jewelry worn during surgery.
3. Notify the surgeon's office that the surgeon must see the client in the preoperative holding area.
4. Tape the ring in place before the client is transported to the preoperative holding area.

4 The nurse is caring for clients in the preanesthesia room. The nurse notes one client, who is an older adult, has an increased surgical risk based on which of the following factors?

1. Decreased kidney function leading to potential fluid and electrolyte imbalances
2. Increased hunger sensations leading to postoperative complications from hyperacidity
3. Inability to comprehend the seriousness of surgical interventions leading to noncompliance
4. Poor cardiovascular status leading to decreased pain sensation

5 A client who takes numerous medications is being prepared for surgery. The nurse reviewing the client medication list is most concerned about which medication that increases surgical risk?

1. An antidysrhythmic
2. A sedative-hypnotic
3. A corticosteroid
4. An oral hypoglycemic

6 The following clients are in the preanesthesia holding room. The nurse determines that the client undergoing which procedure is having the most serious or major surgery?

1. Tonsillectomy
2. Biopsy of the breast
3. Arthroscopy
4. Nephrectomy

7 All of the following clients will be having surgery this morning. The nurse concludes that which client is most likely to be at higher surgical risk?

1. A client who has dementia
2. A client who is culturally different than the medical personnel
3. A client who has mild anxiety
4. A client who has had previous surgeries

8 The nurse is preparing a client for surgery. Prior to completing the skin preparation, the nurse assesses the surgical site for which of the following?

1. Presence of pustules or abrasions
2. Absence of hair growth
3. Presence of lanugo
4. Absence of pulsation

PRACTICE TEST

9 The nurse asks the client about previous surgeries. The client asks the nurse why this information is important. The nurse would explain that previous surgeries can do which of the following?

1. Interfere with the absorption of anesthetic agents
2. Affect the ability of the client to comprehend the instructions prior to surgery
3. Affect the central nervous system
4. Alter the client's responses to surgery

10 A client who is scheduled for an outpatient surgical procedure arrives at the hospital. During the preoperative assessment, the nurse smells alcohol on the client's breath. The nurse reports this finding to the surgeon, prior to completing the preoperative assessment, after drawing which conclusion about the significance of this finding?

1. Alcohol can affect the client's response to anesthesia and surgery.
2. Alcohol can increase the risk for respiratory complications.
3. Use of sedatives and hypnotics prior to surgery can decrease the alcohol effects.
4. Physiological and psychological responses are slowed down by recent alcohol intake.

11 The staff nurse is questioning the preoperative client's vision and hearing. A family member asks the nurse why these questions are important prior to surgery. What information should the nurse provide as the primary reason for seeking this information?

1. "This will help us determine the need for additional resources after discharge postoperatively."
2. "This will help assess the risk of accidents in the home after surgery, which could affect the surgical outcome."
3. "This helps identify any unanticipated needs prior to beginning the surgery."
4. "This will help us to individualize how we provide preoperative and postoperative teaching."

12 A client is admitted for surgery. During the preoperative assessment, the nurse learns the client is taking warfarin sodium (Coumadin). When planning postoperative care for this client, the nurse would include monitoring for which of the following?

1. Delirium tremens
2. Respiratory depression
3. Bleeding or oozing at the surgical wound
4. Hypovolemia

13 While planning postoperative care for an obese client prior to surgery, the nurse would develop which nursing diagnosis specific to the effect obesity has on postsurgical recovery?

1. Risk for ineffective tissue perfusion (cardiopulmonary)
2. Excess fluid volume
3. Risk for impaired skin integrity (pressure ulcers)
4. Ineffective thermoregulation

14 The postsurgical unit nurse is implementing measures to prevent thrombophlebitis. Which of the following is the priority action by the nurse?

1. Apply ordered antiembolic stockings
2. Reinforce importance of smoking cessation
3. Assess the legs with each set of vital signs
4. Teach the client to report Homan's sign

15 A client has been admitted for surgery for resection of nerve roots. The client, observing the written comment that the surgery is palliative, asks what this means. The nurse would offer which of the following explanations?

1. The surgery schedule is overbooked, so the client's surgery may be delayed.
2. The surgeon is against performing the surgery.
3. The exact surgical procedure has not been decided.
4. The procedure will be done to relieve pain but will not cure the problem.

16 The physician progress note indicated a plan to let a client's wound heal by tertiary intention. The nurse determines that healing has occurred when which of the following is observed?

1. Wound is smaller but irregular.
2. Very little scarring has occurred.
3. Tissue loss prevents edges from approximating.
4. A wide scar is present over the area of wound closure.

17 A postoperative client is observed to have moderate wound drainage that has a greenish tinge. The nurse should take which of the following actions next?

1. Document the expected findings.
2. Check for bleeding at the base of the wound.
3. Take pulse and blood pressure and compare to previous readings.
4. Note latest temperature and white blood cell (WBC) count.

18 A client experiences wound dehiscence when coughing. After assisting the client to a low Fowler's position with legs slightly elevated, what is the next best action?

1. Push the internal organs back into the abdominal opening.
2. Cover the wound with a moist hydrocolloid dressing.
3. Cover the wound with a sterile, saline-moistened dressing.
4. Use Steri-Strips to hold the wound together.

19 A client is scheduled for surgery and has been placed on NPO status. The client complains of thirst and hunger and asks for breakfast. The nurse would explain that which of the following is the purpose of NPO status?

1. To make anesthesia induction easier
2. To avoid the risk of aspiration
3. To prevent excessive bleeding
4. To allow the wound to heal faster

20 The nurse is teaching a client about wound care in preparation for discharge. How should the nurse evaluate the effectiveness of home care teaching on wound care? Select all that apply.

1. Give a paper-and-pencil quiz.
2. Have the caregiver or client demonstrate the procedure.
3. Have the client or caregiver explain the procedure.
4. Have the client or caregiver critique a video on the procedure.
5. Ask the client detailed questions while demonstrating the procedure.

ANSWERS & RATIONALES

1 **Answer: 3** Placing the hands *directly on* the incision during coughing will diminish the discomfort associated with coughing. Each of the other options indicates correct procedure on the part of the client.
Cognitive Level: Application **Client Need:** Physiological Integrity: Reduction of Risk Potential **Integrated Process:** Nursing Process: Evaluation **Content Area:** Fundamentals **Strategy:** The words *needs more teaching* in the stem of the question tells you that the incorrect client statement is the correct option. Use knowledge of nursing fundamentals to make a selection.

2 **Answer: 4** The child fears separation from parents. The child has no previous experiences to compare to this experience, so he or she will not anticipate pain. The child cannot anticipate any changes in his or her body and does not worry about communication.
Cognitive Level: Application **Client Need:** Physiological Integrity: Reduction of Risk Potential **Integrated Process:** Nursing Process: Planning **Content Area:** Fundamentals **Strategy:** The critical word *greatest* in the stem of the question provides a clue that more than one option could be partially true. Use knowledge of growth and development to make a selection, recalling that toddlers fear separation from parents.

3 **Answer: 4** Taping a wedding band in place is acceptable for the client who does not wish to remove it unless there is danger the finger may swell during or after surgery. The other options are incorrect because option 1 assumes the ring is tight and that the client wishes to remove it. Option 3 is a false statement, while option 2 creates unnecessary fear during a time when anxiety is likely to be already enhanced.
Cognitive Level: Application **Client Need:** Nursing Process: Implementation **Integrated Process:** Physiological Integrity: Reduction of Risk Potential **Content Area:** Fundamentals **Strategy:** Identify the core issue of the question, which is the method of safeguarding client property during surgery. Choose the option that meets the needs of the client and protects both the hospital and the client's property.

4 **Answer: 1** Option 1 is correct because with increased age, there is a greater likelihood that the kidneys start to degenerate. All the other options are incorrect: hunger does not necessarily cause hyperacidity, comprehension is not altered in all older adults, and cardiovascular problems do not necessarily diminish pain sensations.
Cognitive Level: Analysis **Client Need:** Physiological Integrity: Reduction of Risk Potential **Integrated Process:** Nursing Process: Analysis **Content Area:** Fundamentals **Strategy:** For questions that ask you to choose one client over others, determine which client description indicates the worst client status or highest risk for complications. In this case, note that fluid and electrolyte balance poses the most risk in the intraoperative period, which is the core issue of the question.

5 **Answer: 3** Corticosteroids may lead to weight gain because of salt and water retention and may also delay wound healing. An antidysrhythmic helps to regulate the cardiac rhythm (option 1). A sedative-hypnotic may interfere with the uptake of the anesthetics but does not affect healing (option 2). An oral hypoglycemic agent is used for diabetes, but the medication itself does not pose added risk to the client during surgery (option 4).
Cognitive Level: Analysis **Client Need:** Physiological Integrity: Reduction of Risk Potential **Integrated Process:** Nursing Process: Assessment **Content Area:** Fundamentals **Strategy:** To answer this question, recall the actions and adverse effects of each drug class listed. Use the process of elimination, focusing on the risk to the client during an actual surgical procedure, to make your selection.

6 **Answer: 4** Nephrectomy is a major type of surgery because the kidney is a major vital organ, loss of blood is more likely to be greater than with the other mentioned surgeries, and there is more likelihood of complications. Options 1, 2, and 3 are all examples of minor surgery because they do not involve a high degree of risk.
Cognitive Level: Analysis **Client Need:** Physiological Integrity: Reduction of Risk Potential **Integrated Process:** Nursing

Process: Analysis **Content Area:** Fundamentals **Strategy:** The core issue of the question is the degree of surgical risk associated with each surgical procedure. Use the process of elimination, focusing on the nature of each surgical procedure and the seriousness of each one.

7 **Answer: 1** Dementia affects the person's understanding of the proposed surgery and ability to cooperate with the perioperative care; it also affects the medications given. Cultural differences should not pose a risk unless the client's beliefs are contrary to the proposed measures. Mild anxiety will not create a risk, and previous surgeries may be helpful for the client to draw on previous experiences.
Cognitive Level: Analysis **Client Need:** Physiological Integrity: Reduction of Risk Potential **Integrated Process:** Nursing Process: Assessment **Content Area:** Fundamentals **Strategy:** The core issue of the question is the degree of surgical risk associated with each client circumstance. Use the process of elimination, recalling that physiological issues take precedence over psychosocial ones and that previous surgery may or may not be relevant to the current surgery.

8 **Answer: 1** Abrasions, pustules, or other skin conditions have to be assessed and documented because they may interfere with wound healing or increase the risk of infection. Hair growth—lack of it or presence of lanugo or fine hair—will not interfere with the skin preparation. Pulsation is not always visible or available to assess depending upon the part of the body being operated on.
Cognitive Level: Application **Client Need:** Physiological Integrity: Reduction of Risk Potential **Integrated Process:** Nursing Process: Assessment **Content Area:** Fundamentals **Strategy:** The core issue of the question is knowledge of integumentary risks to a surgical procedure. Use the process of elimination, focusing on skin breaks or alterations as the option that interferes with the protective function of the skin.

9 **Answer: 4** Previous surgeries can reveal possible difficulties or problems with certain anesthetic agents but do not necessarily interfere with absorption of anesthetics (option 1), hinder comprehension of instructions (option 2), or affect the central nervous system (option 3). However, they may affect the physiological or psychological responses of the client to the planned surgery.
Cognitive Level: Application **Client Need:** Physiological Integrity: Reduction of Risk Potential **Integrated Process:** Nursing Process: Implementation **Content Area:** Fundamentals **Strategy:** Focus on the issue of the question, which is the need to gather assessment data that could put the client at risk during the surgical procedure. With this concept in mind, eliminate each of the other options that are false statements.

10 **Answer: 1** Alcohol affects the central nervous system and therefore the client's response to surgery and the anesthetic itself. Smoking, not alcohol (in small amounts), poses respiratory risks. Alcohol effects cannot be reduced by the use of sedatives or hypnotics. Past and recent intake of alcohol can impact responses which can be either slowed down or escalated.
Cognitive Level: Application **Client Need:** Physiological Integrity: Reduction of Risk Potential **Integrated Process:** Nursing Process: Analysis **Content Area:** Fundamentals **Strategy:** The core issue of the question is knowledge that alcohol has an interactive effect with anesthesia and possibly other medications used during surgery. Focus on the option that safeguards the client's physical status as the reason for notifying the surgeon.

11 **Answer: 4** The ability of the client to see and hear may affect the preoperative and postoperative teaching methods used. Social resources and accident prevention rely not only on the client's vision and hearing (options 1 and 2) but also on family supports and the client's physical and mental status. *Unexpected needs* is a very general term that can be applied not just to vision and hearing but also to any area of client functioning (option 3).
Cognitive Level: Application **Client Need:** Physiological Integrity: Reduction of Risk Potential **Integrated Process:** Teaching and Learning **Content Area:** Fundamentals **Strategy:** Eliminate options 1 and 2 because the postdischarge time frame makes these less relevant to the current situation. Choose option 4 over option 3 because it is more specific and applies to the situation of the client.

12 **Answer: 3** Anticoagulants inhibit clotting of the blood, putting the client at increased risk for bleeding postoperatively. Delirium tremens needs to be monitored for clients who had problems with alcohol use (option 1). Respiratory compromise may occur if clients take sedatives or hypnotics (option 2). If clients are taking diuretics or cardiovascular agents, fluid volume may be a problem (option 4).
Cognitive Level: Application **Client Need:** Physiological Integrity: Reduction of Risk Potential **Integrated Process:** Nursing Process: Planning **Content Area:** Fundamentals **Strategy:** The core issue of the question is knowledge that warfarin sodium is an anticoagulant and that this medication increases risk of bleeding unless stopped for a sufficient amount of time before surgery (approximately 7 days depending on client and surgery). With this in mind, eliminate options 1 and 2 first. Choose option 3 over 4 because there are other causes besides bleeding for hypovolemia, such as inadequate fluid replacement during surgery or the postoperative period.

13 **Answer: 1** Wound and cardiovascular complications are more common among clients who are obese. The heart is stressed from its workload, and the added stress of surgery may place the client at risk. The client has no risk for excess fluid volume (option 2), and decreasing fluid intake could complicate wound healing. Pressure ulcers occur more frequently in emaciated clients than in obese ones (option 3). The obese client has no problem with thermoregulation (option 4).
Cognitive Level: Application **Client Need:** Physiological Integrity: Reduction of Risk Potential **Integrated Process:** Nursing Process: Planning **Content Area:** Fundamentals **Strategy:** Recall that obesity leads to increased cardiovascular risks in general and that it can also be a risk factor for poor wound healing after surgery. Eliminate options 2 and 4 first as being least related to the core issue of the question, and choose option 1 over 3 as the priority risk.

14 **Answer: 1** Antiembolic stockings facilitate venous return from the lower extremities. Smoking may contribute to cardiovascular events, but cessation will not necessarily lessen the chance of thrombophlebitis in the immediate postsurgical period. Assessment of the leg will help with detection, but it will not prevent thrombophlebitis. Homan's sign is

pain on dorsiflexion of the leg, and this is also a means of detection, not prevention.
Cognitive Level: Application **Client Need:** Physiological Integrity: Reduction of Risk Potential **Integrated Process:** Teaching and Learning **Content Area:** Fundamentals **Strategy:** Focus on the critical word in the stem, *prevent.* Discriminate between options that address assessment versus prevention.

15 **Answer: 4** A surgical procedure that relieves symptoms of disease or pain but does not cure is described as palliative. The other options are incorrect explanations.
Cognitive Level: Application **Client Need:** Physiological Integrity: Reduction of Risk Potential **Integrated Process:** Teaching and Learning **Content Area:** Fundamentals **Strategy:** Use the process of elimination, selecting the answer that is an accurate description of the meaning of the term *palliative.*

16 **Answer: 4** A wide scar occurs in tertiary intention because the edges are not approximated, and they regenerate via granulation. Options 1 and 3 refer to secondary healing, while option 2 is characteristic of primary healing.
Cognitive Level: Analysis **Client Need:** Physiological Integrity: Reduction of Risk Potential **Integrated Process:** Nursing Process: Evaluation **Content Area:** Fundamentals **Strategy:** First recall the definition of the wound that heals by tertiary intention. Then visualize the appearance of the wound to make your selection.

17 **Answer: 4** Purulent drainage is made up of tissue debris, WBCs, and bacteria; it may be of different colors depending upon the type of bacteria, and it is thick in consistency. It often indicates wound infection. The next action by the nurse would be to gather additional data that could indicate infection, such as elevated temperature and WBC count. The nurse would document the findings at some point, but this is not the priority action. There is no reason to assess for bleeding within the wound or to measure pulse and BP.
Cognitive Level: Analysis **Client Need:** Physiological Integrity: Reduction of Risk Potential **Integrated Process:** Nursing Process: Assessment **Content Area:** Fundamentals **Strategy:** The critical word in the stem of the question is *next.* This means that the correct option is the one that contains a critical-thinking sequence based on the information presented. Correlate the word *purulent* with infection, and then choose the option that assesses for signs of infection.

18 **Answer: 3** Covering the wound with sterile, saline-moistened gauze keeps the wound moist and protects it from infection. Option 1 is incorrect; in wound dehiscence, the layers of the wound are disrupted, but there is no protrusion of vital organs. In addition, pushing back organs such as the intestines is extremely dangerous because it could cause strangulation. A hydrocolloid dressing is not indicated (option 2) because its absorptive properties are not needed. Option 4 would be ineffective and does not protect underlying tissue.
Cognitive Level: Application **Client Need:** Physiological Integrity: Reduction of Risk Potential **Integrated Process:** Nursing Process: Implementation **Content Area:** Fundamentals **Strategy:** The core issue of the question is nursing management of wound dehiscence. Recall that the priority sequence of actions is to remove the effects of gravity on the wound and then to protect the wound. Eliminate options 1 and 4 as ineffective, and then choose correctly based on knowledge of various types of wound dressings.

19 **Answer: 2** By keeping the stomach empty during surgery, the risk of vomiting and aspiration is decreased. The other options are unrelated to NPO status.
Cognitive Level: Application **Client Need:** Physiological Integrity: Reduction of Risk Potential **Integrated Process:** Nursing Process: Implementation **Content Area:** Fundamentals **Strategy:** Use knowledge of basic principles of preoperative care to make a selection. The wording of the question tells you that there is only one correct choice.

20 **Answer: 2, 3** Return demonstration is the best way to evaluate teaching of a procedure. Ideally, the teaching is done over a few days and is then evaluated. Having the client explain the procedure is also appropriate because it indicates that the client has the necessary knowledge to perform the procedure. Giving a paper-and-pencil quiz and critiquing a video would measure cognitive aspects of learning but are not realistic. Asking the client detailed questions during the procedure is not helpful because it detracts from learning.
Cognitive Level: Analysis **Client Need:** Physiological Integrity: Reduction of Risk Potential **Integrated Process:** Teaching and Learning **Content Area:** Fundamentals **Strategy:** Use fundamental principles of teaching and learning to answer the question, recalling that the best methods of evaluation involves knowledge and action on the part of the client, which can be determined by verbal explanation and return demonstration.

ANSWERS & RATIONALES

Terms to Remember

anesthesia p. 865
conscious sedation p. 865
dehiscence p. 874
drain p. 872
exudate p. 874
informed consent p. 864
intraoperative phase p. 863
palliative p. 865
postoperative phase p. 863
preoperative phase p. 863
purulent p. 872
regional anesthesia p. 865
sanguinous p. 874
serosanguinous p. 872
serous p. 874
sterile field p. 871
surgical asepsis p. 870
surgical scrub p. 870

References

Ball, J., & Bindler, R. (2004). *Pediatric nursing: Caring for children* (3rd ed.). Upper Saddle River, NJ: Pearson Education.

Harkreader, H. & Hogan, M. (2004). *Fundamentals of nursing: Caring and clinical judgement* (2nd ed.). St. Louis: Elsevier.

Kozier, B., Erb, G., Berman, A. J., & Burke, K. (2004). *Fundamentals of nursing: Concepts, process, and practice* (7th ed.). Upper Saddle River, NJ: Pearson Education.

LeMone P., & Burke, K. (2004). *Medical surgical nursing: Critical thinking in client care* (3rd ed.). Upper Saddle River, NJ: Pearson Education.

50 Complicated Antenatal Care

Test Yourself

Are you ready for the NCLEX-RN® or course exams? Use the practice tests on the companion CD-ROM to check.

In this chapter

Cross reference

Other chapters relevant to this content area are:

I. ASSESSMENT AND DIAGNOSTIC TESTING FOR HIGH-RISK PRENATAL CLIENT

A. **Identifying clients at risk**
   1. Begins with first prenatal visit and continues through puerperium
   2. Risk factors (physiological, psychological, sociodemographic, or environmental) may be associated with a negative pregnancy outcome

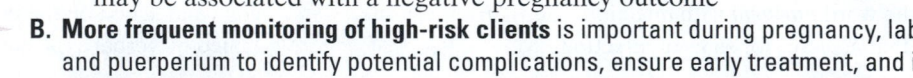

! B. **More frequent monitoring of high-risk clients** is important during pregnancy, labor, birth, and puerperium to identify potential complications, ensure early treatment, and improve maternal–fetal outcomes

C. **Ongoing care** consists of routine antenatal care plus special considerations as noted in following text

D. **Diagnostic tests**
   1. **Biophysical profile (BPP)**
      a. Overview: a method of assessing fetal well-being by determining scores on five criteria: fetal breathing movements, body movements, muscle tone, fetal heart rate (FHR), and amniotic fluid volume
      b. Total score ranges from 0 to 10; individual scores are 2 (normal) or 0 (abnormal)
      c. A total score of 8 to 10 is normal, 4 to 6 is possibly abnormal, and less than 4 may indicate a need for delivery
   2. **Doppler blood flow analysis**
      a. Overview: a noninvasive assessment of fetal blood flow across placenta
      b. Provides data about blood flow and resistance in placental circulation and is useful in detecting intrauterine growth restriction (IUGR)

c. Can be done as early as 15 weeks
d. Velocity waveforms from umbilical and uterine arteries are reported as systolic/diastolic (S/D) ratios
e. Persistently elevated ratios of greater than 3 after 30 weeks gestation are considered abnormal and have been associated with IUGR

3. Nonstress test (NST)

a. Overview: a screening test that assesses fetal well-being that analyzes response of FHR to fetal movement
b. Advantages: noninvasive, easily interpreted, and can be performed in outpatient setting at low cost; NST is a good indicator of fetal well-being
c. Disadvantages: high number of false-positive results caused by fetal sleep cycles, medications, and fetal immaturity; NST is not a good predictor of poor fetal outcomes
! d. Test procedure: semi-Fowler's position used; an ultrasound transducer and tocodynamometer record contractions and FHR; client may be asked to press a handheld button that graphs FHR when fetal movement is felt
e. Episodes of fetal movement can then be compared to changes in FHR; acoustical stimulation can be done if absence of fetal movement
! f. Findings: normal (reactive) if there are two or more accelerations of 15 beats per minute lasting for 15 seconds over a 20-minute period, normal baseline, and long-term variability of 10 or more beats per minute
! g. If these criteria are not met within 40 minutes, test is considered nonreassuring (nonreactive) and further testing is indicated

4. Contraction stress test (CST)

a. Overview: assesses ability of fetus to withstand stress of uterine contractions and evaluates placental capacity for O_2/CO_2 exchange; since contractions reduce blood flow to fetus, can predict a fetus that may not be able to tolerate stress of labor
b. Indications: factors that place fetus at risk for asphyxia such as IUGR, diabetes, postdates, nonreactive NST, and BPP score less than 6
c. Contraindications: third-trimester bleeding and previous cesarean birth with classical uterine incision; advantages of CST should be weighed against danger of preterm labor if this is a risk, such as with premature rupture of membranes or incompetent cervix
! d. Test procedure: explain procedure and obtain informed consent; electronic monitoring of contractions and FHR are begun; after obtaining baseline fetal heart tracing, contractions (if not spontaneous) are initiated with IV oxytocin or breast self-stimulation
! e. Findings: when at least three contractions of 40- to 60-second duration occur in a 10-minute time period, the FHR pattern is assessed; result is reassuring (negative) if no late decelerations occur; is not reassuring (positive) if late decelerations occur with at least two of three contractions; is suspicious (equivocal) if there is late deceleration with one of three contractions or contractions every 2 minutes for 10 minutes (hyperstimulation pattern)

5. Amniocentesis

a. Overview: used to assess fetal well-being and maturity; a needle is inserted through abdominal wall (see Figure 50–1 ■) to collect sample of amniotic fluid; can be done after 14 to 16 weeks gestation
b. Purpose: prenatal diagnosis of genetic disorders or congenital anomalies, assessment of pulmonary maturity, and diagnosis of fetal hemolytic disease
! c. Complications: in fewer than 1% of cases; possible maternal complications include hemorrhage, infection, labor, **abruptio placentae,** damage to intestines or bladder, and amniotic fluid leakage or embolism; possible fetal complications include death, hemorrhage, infection, and direct needle injury
d. Test procedure: explain procedure and obtain informed consent; if client is more than 20 weeks gestation, she should empty bladder and assume supine position; using sterile technique, physician inserts a needle through

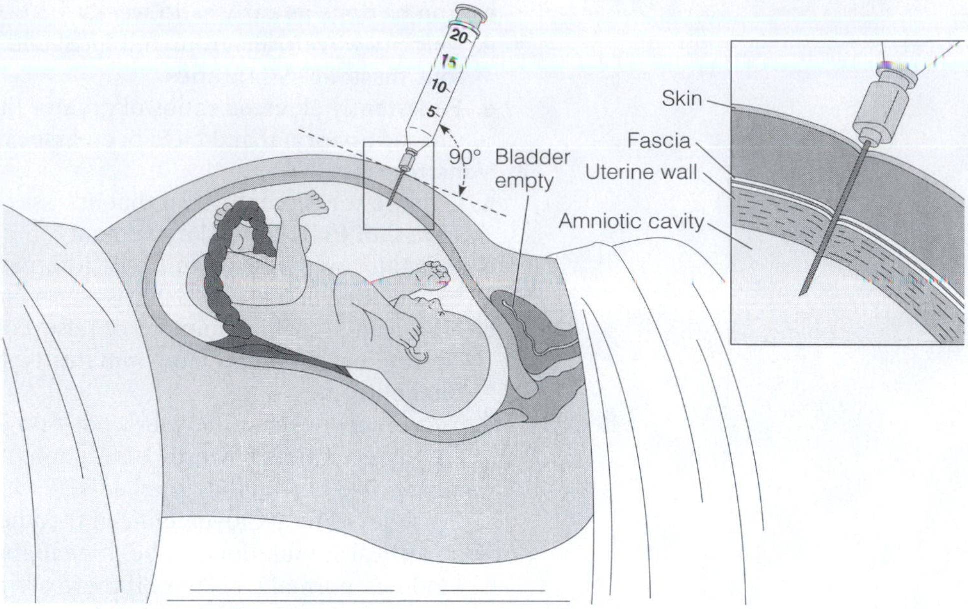

Figure 50–1

Amniocentesis.

abdomen into uterus; ultrasound assists in guiding needle; 15 to 20 mL of fluid are withdrawn

e. Monitor FHR and maternal vital signs throughout procedure and for 30 minutes postprocedure

f. Rh-negative clients should receive RhoGAM following procedure because of risk of isoimmunization from fetal blood

g. Follow-up: instruct client to contact physician for fluid loss, bleeding, fever, abdominal pain, increased or decreased fetal activity

h. Inform client that test results will be available in about 2 weeks

6. Lecithin to sphingomyelin (L/S) ratio

a. Obtained via amniocentesis to assess fetal lung maturity

b. Ratio of 2:1 or greater indicates probable lung maturity; contamination with meconium or blood may alter the results

7. Phosphatidylglycerol (PG)

a. Obtained via amniocentesis; is a phospholipid found in pulmonary surfactant

b. Presence in amniotic fluid indicates fetal lung maturity

8. Karyotype

a. Obtained via amniocentesis; analyzes chromosomes to determine gender and chromosomal aberrations

b. Gender identification is important in assessment of sex-linked diseases

c. Rh isoimmunization status and severity of hemolytic anemia can be assessed by measuring bilirubin pigment in amniotic fluid

d. Alpha-fetoprotein (AFP) levels, either increased or decreased, can indicate anatomic abnormalities; fetal blood contamination of amniotic fluid can alter AFP results

9. Chorionic villus sampling (CVS)

a. Involves collecting small specimen of tissue from fetal portion of placenta for fetal genetic studies

b. Specimen can be obtained either transcervically or transabdominally

c. Indications: over 35 years old (because of increased risk for Down syndrome), frequent spontaneous **abortions,** fetuses with chromosomal anomalies or other defects, or a client with a genetic defect

d. Advantages: earlier diagnosis and rapid return of results compared to amniocentesis; can be performed at 10 to 12 weeks gestation with results returned in 1 to 2 weeks

e. Test preparation: instruct client to come for procedure with full bladder; explain procedure and obtain informed consent; use lithotomy position

f. Test procedure: using sterile technique, physician visualizes cervix using ultrasound guidance, a suction cannula is used to collect specimen transvaginally or transabdominally (if necessary)
g. Rh-negative clients should receive RhoGAM postprocedure
h. Complications (rare): vaginal spotting or bleeding, miscarriage, rupture of membranes, and chorioamnionitis; limb anomalies if procedure done before 10 weeks gestation
i. Follow-up includes teaching client signs and symptoms of complications to report, stating when results will be available, and arranging genetic counseling as needed

II. PREGESTATIONAL CONDITIONS

A. Cardiac disease

1. Pregnancy increases workload on heart; cardiac output increases 30% to 50% by mid-pregnancy (cardiac workload greatest at 28 to 30 weeks gestation when blood volume peaks)
2. A compromised heart with inadequate cardiac capacity and decreased reserves may be unable to adapt to added requirements of pregnancy
3. Treatment options and outcome depend on degree of cardiac compromise
4. Clients with class I and II cardiac disease have potential for good pregnancy outcome, while class III or IV clients may have serious maternal or fetal compromise (Table 50–1 ■)
5. ! Nursing assessment: most common complication of heart disease during pregnancy is congestive heart failure (CHF)
   a. Edema of varying degree from pedal edema, pitting edema, generalized edema (anasarca), and pulmonary edema
   b. Dyspnea on exertion, increasing fatigue, dyspnea at rest, moist cough, basilar crackles, cyanosis of nail beds, circumoral cyanosis
   c. Tachycardia, irregular pulse, murmurs, chest pain
6. Collaborative management
   a. Monitor client and fetal well-being more frequently during pregnancy; changes in maternal vital signs or signs of fetal compromise may indicate inability to handle increasing demands on heart
   b. ! Teach adequate nutrition for pregnancy and provide prenatal vitamins and iron to prevent anemia; monitor for signs of infection
   c. ! Instruct client to avoid excessive weight gain and emotional stress, which place added stress on cardiac reserves
   d. Teach client to report signs of infection so treatment may begin early
   e. Diagnostic procedures may include auscultation, electrocardiogram, echocardiogram, and possible cardiac catheterization
   f. ! Prophylactic antibiotics are used for invasive procedures, including dental work and at time of birth, to prevent bacterial endocarditis; penicillin (PCN) is usually prescribed unless client is allergic
   g. Cardiac glycosides (Digitalis) may be used to increase myocardial contractility and slow heart rate for effective filling
   h. Antidysrhythmia agents may be used for cardiac dysrhythmias

Table 50–1

Classification of Functional Capacity for Clients with Cardiac Disease (NYHA 1979)

Classification	Functional Capacity
I	Uncompromised: No limitation on physical activity due to angina or symptoms of cardiac insufficiency
II	Slightly compromised: Normal activity causes fatigue, palpitation, dyspnea, or angina
III	Markedly compromised: May be comfortable at rest but less than usual activity causes fatigue, dyspnea, palpitations, or angina
IV	Severely compromised: Cannot perform any activity without increasing discomfort; may experience angina and cardiac insufficiency while at rest.

i. The diuretic furosemide (Lasix) may be used to decrease fluid excess; take care to ensure adequate circulating volume to maintain uteroplacental perfusion

! j. Heparin is considered safe for use in pregnancy if an anticoagulant is indicated (pregnancy category C); warfarin (Coumadin) is a pregnancy category X drug (Table 50–2 ■) and must be avoided

! k. Teach client to avoid exertion and to plan frequent rest periods

l. Provide adequate pain relief during labor to avoid excessive maternal stress

m. Vaginal delivery is preferred with epidural anesthesia, continuous maternal oxygen administration, and low-forceps delivery to decrease maternal straining

! n. Observe client carefully for complications from hemodynamic changes immediately after delivery

B. Diabetes mellitus

1. Description

a. A pancreatic endocrine disorder with major effects on carbohydrate (CHO) metabolism

b. Results from insufficient insulin production in beta cells of islets of Langerhans

c. Insulin facilitates movement of glucose from blood into cells for storage or energy

d. **Gestational diabetes** results when pancreas is unable to meet increased demands for insulin production during pregnancy

2. Effect of pregnancy on glucose metabolism

a. During first half of pregnancy, maternal hormones increase demand for insulin production to facilitate increased storage of glycogen in maternal tissue

! b. During last half of pregnancy, human placental lactogen (hPL) from placenta causes resistance to action of maternal insulin, increasing circulating glucose for fetal use and demand on maternal pancreas to produce more insulin

c. Fetus produces own insulin but obtains glucose from mother across placenta; amount of glucose available in maternal circulation stimulates fetal pancreas to produce insulin

3. Effects of diabetes on pregnancy and fetus relate to degree of blood glucose control within 70 to 120 mg/dL range and degree of vascular involvement

4. Complications are more common with type 1 diabetes mellitus and include

a. Polyhydraminos, preeclampsia, eclampsia, ketoacidosis and worsening retinopathy

b. Dystocia and stillbirth (usually after 36 weeks)

! c. Neonatal **macrosomia** (excessively large body), hypoglycemia, hyperbilirubinemia, delayed fetal lung maturity resulting in respiratory distress syn-

Table 50–2

FDA Pregnancy Categories for Prescription Drugs

Category	Risk to the Fetus	Examples of Drugs
A	Controlled studies in women do not demonstrate a risk to the fetus in the first trimester, and the possibility of fetal harm appears remote.	RDA dose of Vitamin C
B	Animal studies have not demonstrated fetal risk but there are no controlled studies in women, or animal studies show an adverse effect not confirmed in controlled studies in women in the first trimester.	Acetaminophen (Tylenol) Penicillins
C	Animal studies show adverse effects and there are no controlled studies in women, or studies in women and animals are not available. Drug should be given only if potential benefit justifies the potential risk to the fetus.	Zidovudine (Retrovir) Heparin
D	Positive evidence of fetal risk in humans, but the benefits to the mother may be acceptable despite the risk in certain situations.	Phenobarbitol (Luminol)
X	The risks to the fetus clearly outweigh any possible benefit to the mother. The drug is contraindicated in women who may become pregnant.	Warfarin (Coumadin) Diethylstilbestrol (DES)

drome (RDS), and increased incidence of congenital anomalies including neural tube defects (NTD)

5. Nursing assessment
   a. Risk factors: family history of diabetes, maternal obesity, previous large-for-gestational-age (LGA) infants, previous unexplained stillbirth
   b. Classic symptoms of diabetes mellitus include polyuria, polydipsia, and polyphagia
   c. Possible increasing frequency of urinary tract infections and vaginal candidiasis (yeast) infections caused by altered pH in reproductive tract
   d. Urine testing for ketones as part of routine prenatal care
   e. Diabetes screening should be done around 28 weeks gestation with a 50-gram oral glucose tolerance test (GTT); if blood glucose is greater than 140 mg/dL at 1 hour, a 3-hour 100-gram oral GTT is performed
   f. Long-term glucose control is estimated with glycosylated hemoglobin (HbA_{1c}), which measures the percent of hemoglobin with glucose bound to it (glycohemoglobin); levels depend on amount of circulating glucose in previous weeks (see Chapter 47)
6. Collaborative management
   a. Teach prescribed ADA diet regulation with no concentrated sweets
   b. Dietary regulation usually adequate, excessive weight gain should be avoided; caloric needs will increase as pregnancy progresses
   c. Medications: oral hypoglycemic medications are contraindicated during pregnancy; insulin (human) should be carefully regulated and adjusted as pregnancy progresses with up to a fourfold dose increase needed at term
   d. Instruct client in frequent blood glucose and urine ketone testing and to keep a diary of test results and activity levels
   e. Encourage regular nonstrenuous exercise such as walking for weight and blood glucose control
   f. Monitor fetal well-being: maternal AFP at 16 to 18 weeks, ultrasound for anomalies, amniotic fluid volume, and fetal size; fetal movement counts, weekly NST from 28 to 32 weeks, possible oxytocin challenge test (OCT), BPP, and amniocentesis for lung maturity; L/S ratio needs to be 1:3 (normal is 1:2); PG should be present
   g. Monitor client for development of complications: infection, preeclampsia, and diabetic ketoacidosis
   h. Prepare for possible induction of labor at 38 to 39 weeks for clients with type 1 diabetes mellitus to reduce risk for stillbirth caused by premature placental aging
   i. Insulin requirements drop dramatically after delivery of placenta and removal of hormonal influences; client may need no insulin or a very decreased dose; gestational diabetics generally may eat a regular diet

C. Substance abuse

1. Description and etiology
   a. As many as 10% of pregnant women use tobacco, alcohol, or other drugs, often in combination; clients using illegal drugs may delay seeking care for fear of prosecution; all pregnant women should be screened for substance abuse
   b. Substances frequently used are tobacco, alcohol, marijuana, cocaine, crack cocaine, MOMA (Ecstasy), and heroin; effects on pregnancy include spontaneous abortion, IUGR, preterm labor, placental abruption, stillbirth, neonatal addiction, and fetal alcohol syndrome (FAS)
2. Nursing assessment
   a. Establish trusting relationship with client by remaining open, matter-of-fact, and nonjudgmental; women seeking prenatal care are interested in improving and safeguarding their health and that of fetus
   b. Encourage client to describe all substances used, amounts, times and triggers to use, and any previous attempts to discontinue use
   c. Evaluate client's motivation, support systems, and personal strengths that may be elicited to change behaviors

3. Collaborative management
   a. Monitor client for complications: anemia, inadequate nutrition and weight gain, hypertension, preterm labor; random urine toxicology screens may be ordered
   b. Monitor fetal growth and well-being: fundal height, ultrasound, NST, BPP
   c. Teach client about potential negative effects of substances used on pregnancy and fetus/neonate
   d. Assist with referrals for client as indicated: smoking cessation classes, Alcoholics Anonymous, addiction counseling, psychological counseling, and possible hospitalization
   e. Reinforce teaching about nutrition and effects on fetal development; teach client danger signs of pregnancy including signs of preterm labor and abruption of placenta
   f. Support client's efforts to change negative behaviors
   g. Client may need to be followed by a perinatologist during pregnancy; an addicted neonate will require intensive care at birth
   h. Client should not go through "cold turkey" drug withdrawal during pregnancy; clients with heroin addiction may receive methadone hydrochloride (Dolophine)—a narcotic agonist analgesic that blocks more severe symptoms of heroin withdrawal

D. HIV/AIDS

1. Overview
   a. Human immunodeficiency virus (HIV) leads to acquired immunodeficiency syndrome (AIDS) over years of time
   b. HIV is transmitted through contact with infected blood and body secretions, usually during sexual contact or use of contaminated needles by IV drug users
   c. AIDS is characterized by decreased immunity and overwhelming opportunistic infection
   d. Pregnancy doesn't appear to change course of illness for mother; fetus may contract HIV transplacentally or through breast milk, but generally fetal infection is considered to occur during vaginal birth
   e. Current maternal treatment with antiretroviral drugs including zidovudine (AZT) orally during pregnancy and IV during labor and delivery has decreased neonatal transmission to less than 7% with vaginal birth and less than 1% with cesarean birth
   f. Maternal HIV antibodies cross placenta so all infants of HIV-positive mothers will test positive at birth and until maternal antibodies are depleted at between 15 to 18 months of age
2. Nursing assessment
   a. Antibodies to HIV are detected with ELISA test and results confirmed by Western blot test
   b. All pregnant women should be offered HIV testing because most clients are asymptomatic for 5 to 10 years before signs of opportunistic infection appear
3. Collaborative management
   a. Provide emotional support and reproductive counseling to client and family
   b. Evaluate client for other sexually transmitted diseases and hepatitis B
   c. Review lab results for signs of anemia, thrombocytopenia, leukopenia, and decreased CD-4 T-lymphocyte counts
   d. Monitor client for signs of opportunistic infection: fever, weight loss, fatigue, candidiasis, cough, skin lesions
   e. Administer prophylactic antiretroviral drugs as ordered during pregnancy and labor and delivery
   f. Monitor fetal growth and well-being
   g. Be meticulous in use of standard blood and body fluid precautions with all clients
   h. Protect fetus from maternal secretions by not using fetal scalp electrode or invasive devices during labor
   i. Wash infant's eyes and face at birth before administering prophylactic eye drops or ointment

j. Bathe entire newborn as soon as possible after delivery to remove all maternal secretions; delay any newborn injections or heel-sticks until after bath
k. Encourage mother to formula-feed infant to avoid transmission by breast milk

E. Rh-sensitization

1. Overview
   a. Rh-negative women who have Rh-positive embryo/fetus (from an Rh-positive father) may become sensitized to the Rh antigen with contact between maternal and fetal blood
   b. Other causes of Rh-sensitization might be blood transfusion of Rh-positive blood to an Rh-negative woman or fetomaternal blood contact during amniocentesis or other invasive procedure
   c. Sensitized Rh-negative women develop anti-Rh antibodies, which may cross placenta in subsequent Rh-positive pregnancies and attack and destroy fetal RBCs
   d. Fetal effects of Rh incompatibility and sensitization are progressively severe
2. Hemolysis of fetal erythrocytes leads to greatly increased immature RBC production, termed **erythroblastosis fetalis**
3. Continued RBC destruction and anemia results in jaundice and marked fetal edema known as **hydrops fetalis;** may lead to fetal CHF
4. Breakdown of RBCs releases bilirubin, causing jaundice; high levels of circulating bilirubin can cause **kernicterus,** a yellow staining of basal ganglia and brain, and may result in permanent neurological damage
5. Nursing assessment
   a. All pregnant women should be tested for blood group and Rh factor and should have routine antibody screening; note history of previous miscarriage, blood transfusions, or infants experiencing jaundice
   b. If client is Rh-negative, infant's father is tested to determine Rh status; an Rh-negative father and mother will only produce Rh-negative offspring who will not be affected by Rh-incompatibility
   c. An indirect **Coombs' test** on maternal blood determines whether Rh-negative client has developed antibodies to Rh antigen; serial antibody screening should continue throughout pregnancy; a direct Coombs' test on infant's blood after birth identifies maternal antibodies attached to fetal RBCs
6. Collaborative management
   a. Provide support and education to client and family; client should carry Rh-negative identification card and recognize that she may need medication (RhoGAM) with future reproductive events
   b. Unsensitized Rh-negative clients should be given 300 mcg of Rh-immune globulin (RhoGAM) IM at 28 weeks and also within 72 hours of delivery
   c. Antibodies in immune globulin bind with Rh antigens in maternal circulation; this provides passive immunity so mother will not become sensitized to Rh antigens and will not produce antibodies of her own
   d. RhoGAM is not given to mothers who are already sensitized and have antibodies (positive indirect Coombs' test)
   e. Rh-immune globulin is also given after abortion, **ectopic** pregnancy, amniocentesis, and any other situation that might result in maternal exposure to fetal Rh antigen
   f. Kleihauer-Betke test estimates amount of fetal blood in maternal circulation; used to determine dose of Rh-immune globulin when a larger fetal–maternal bleed is suspected
   g. Evaluate fetus for development of complications by serial ultrasound for amniotic fluid volume, fetal size, and development of edema or enlarged heart
   h. A sinusoidal electronic fetal monitoring pattern indicates severe fetal anemia; BPP may be used to identify a compromised fetus
   i. Amniocentesis or percutaneous umbilical cord blood sampling (PUBS) may be used to determine fetal Rh; both procedures carry risk of causing maternal exposure and sensitization, so RhoGAM should be given

j. An early delivery with phototherapy and exchange transfusions may be planned if fetus is developing anemia close to term
k. Intrauterine exchange transfusion may be performed for severely affected fetus until viability is reached

III. GESTATIONAL CONDITIONS

A. Hyperemesis gravidarum (pernicious vomiting of pregnancy)

1. Overview
   a. Extreme nausea and vomiting during first half of pregnancy associated with dehydration, weight loss, and electrolyte imbalances
   b. Emesis is much more severe than in common "morning sickness" of early pregnancy and occurs in only 0.1% of pregnancies
   c. Theories about etiology include psychological and physiological factors but actual cause remains unknown; condition is rare in developing countries
   d. High levels of hCG, as are found in **gestational trophoblastic disease** (hydatidiform mole, molar pregnancy), are associated with severe nausea and vomiting
   e. Fetus is at risk for abnormal development, IUGR, or death from lack of nutrition, hypoxia, and maternal ketoacidosis
2. Nursing assessment
   a. Intractable vomiting during first 20 weeks of pregnancy
   b. Dehydration with weight loss of greater than 5% of prepregnancy weight, poor skin turgor, dry mucous membranes, possible hypotension, tachycardia, and increased hematocrit and urine specific gravity
   c. Signs and symptoms of electrolyte or acid-base imbalance (acidosis): ketosis, confusion, drowsiness, muscle weakness, cramps, clumsiness, tremors, irregular heartbeat, decreased level of consciousness (LOC)
   d. Signs and symptoms of starvation: muscle wasting, ketonuria, jaundice, bleeding gums (vitamin deficiency)
3. Collaborative management
   a. Client may need hospitalization with IV fluid therapy with glucose, electrolytes, and vitamins to begin treatment and then continue at home once stabilized
   b. Monitor daily weight and measure intake and output (I & O); assess vital signs as appropriate, hydration, and nutritional status
   c. Administer antiemetic medications such as phenothiazines or antihistamines as ordered to control nausea and vomiting
   d. Encourage 6 small feedings/day after acute nausea and vomiting pass; salty foods and clear liquids such as lemonade and herbal teas are sometimes better tolerated at first
   e. Total parenteral nutrition (TPN) may be required in severe cases when client cannot tolerate oral feedings
   f. Monitor fetal growth with serial ultrasounds
   g. Provide emotional support; help client to identify healthy coping mechanisms and support systems she can rely on during pregnancy
   h. Refer for additional counseling and support as indicated

B. Ectopic pregnancy

1. Overview
   a. Implantation of fertilized ovum outside uterus; most common site is a fallopian tube narrowed by scarring or adhesions; other sites may include ovary or elsewhere in abdominal cavity
   b. Ascending infections, pelvic inflammatory disease (PID), use of IUD contraception, or tubal surgery are risk factors for tubal damage that may result in an ectopic pregnancy
2. Nursing assessment
   a. Interview reveals last normal menstrual period (LNMP) consistent with possible pregnancy and possible subjective symptoms of pregnancy such as breast tenderness and nausea
   b. Unilateral lower abdominal pain: may be slowly increasing or sudden and severe with abdominal rigidity and referred right shoulder pain

! c. Possible irregular vaginal bleeding or signs of hypovolemic shock if fallopian tube has ruptured; prioritize care accordingly
d. Laboratory tests: β-hCG confirms pregnancy
e. Ultrasound confirms an extrauterine pregnancy

3. Implementation and collaborative care
! a. Monitor BP, pulse, and respiration every 15 minutes or more frequently if indicated by client condition
b. Start an IV of ordered fluid with at least an 18-gauge needle in case blood products need to be given
! c. Provide oxygen as indicated for shock
d. Medicate for pain as ordered
e. Obtain laboratory tests: β-hCG, CBC, and blood group and type; type and cross-match if hemorrhage is suspected
f. Prepare client for surgery; if possible, pregnancy will be evacuated and tube preserved for future fertility if desired
g. Provide standard preoperative care and teaching; offer emotional support to client and family
! h. Provide general postoperative care; facilitate grieving; provide RhoGAM for Rh-negative mothers with an Rh-positive partner

C. Gestational trophoblastic disease (GTD; hydatidiform mole; molar pregnancy)

1. Overview
a. An abnormal growth of trophoblastic tissue including placenta and chorion
b. Is more common in Japan and Taiwan for unknown reasons
c. Characterized by abnormal development of placenta (with either complete or partial hydatiform mole)
d. Chorionic villi grow rapidly into fluid-filled, grapelike clusters; a complete mole develops from an empty ovum that contains no maternal genetic material; a partial mole may have an abnormal embryo that usually spontaneously aborts in first trimester
e. Abnormal development of chorion may result in choriocarcinoma, a rapidly growing malignant neoplasm
f. Twenty percent of women with complete molar pregnancy will develop malignant trophoblastic disease

2. Nursing assessment
a. Variable vaginal bleeding usually occurs during first trimester; may be brown, like prune juice, and may contain some grapelike vesicles
! b. Unusual uterine growth measured by fundal height; no fetal parts can be palpated and no FHR heard; "snowstorm" pattern seen on ultrasound
c. Abnormal labs include very high hCG levels and very low maternal AFP levels
! d. Complications include hyperemesis gravidarum (probably associated with high hCG levels) and severe hypertension that occurs during first half of pregnancy; others include hyperthyroidism and possible trophoblastic pulmonary embolism

3. Collaborative management
! a. Monitor client for signs of hemorrhage, hypertension, or other complications, including disseminated intravascular coagulopathy (DIC)
b. Prepare client and assist with suction uterine evacuation of molar pregnancy; hysterectomy may be chosen for clients who do not want to preserve fertility
c. Provide RhoGAM to appropriate clients (Rh-negative with Rh-positive partners) postprocedure
! d. Teach client about need for frequent follow-up care during next year to rule out development of cancer (choriocarcinoma)
e. Weekly hCG levels are done initially with other testing to rule out cancer; reinforce need for diligent follow-up care because 1 in 5 women develop cancer
! f. Client should not become pregnant for 1 year following molar pregnancy in case chemotherapy is indicated; provide contraceptive counseling
g. Provide emotional support for client and family who are grieving pregnancy loss and living with fear of developing a malignancy

D. Incompetent cervix

1. Overview
   - **a.** A painless cervical effacement and dilatation not associated with contractions that usually occurs in second trimester resulting in spontaneous abortion or very preterm birth
   - **b.** Maternal DES (diethylstilbestrol) exposure or congenital uterine anomalies may be associated with incompetent cervix
   - **c.** Other possible contributing factors are cervical inflammation or previous cervical trauma
2. Nursing assessment
   - **a.** Previous unexplained second-trimester pregnancy losses may indicate undiagnosed incompetent cervix
   - **b.** Cervical effacement and dilatation without contractions or pain; client may present for care completely dilated with bulging membranes
3. Collaborative management
   - **a.** Provide emotional support and grief support group referral for client with pregnancy loss from an incompetent cervix
   - **b.** Provide client teaching if client is managed on bedrest at home for a cervix just beginning to efface (shorten)
   - **c.** Provide teaching about cervical **cerclage** if this is treatment method chosen; cerclage is a technique of reinforcing closure of cervix with sutures during pregnancy
   - **d.** Monitor for signs of preterm labor or infection; client may be placed in Trendelenburg position and receive tocolytics; provide appropriate nursing assessments and care related to medication
   - **e.** Instruct client to return if contractions begin because suture must be removed before vaginal birth is accomplished

E. Spontaneous abortion

1. Overview
   - **a.** An unintended pregnancy loss before 20 weeks gestation; lay term is *miscarriage*
   - **b.** Most common cause of bleeding in first trimester; usually results from chromosomal abnormalities in embryo
   - **c.** Other causes may be teratogen exposure, inadequate implantation, and maternal endocrine disorders or chronic illness
   - **d.** Late spontaneous abortion may be result of incompetent cervix; classification of spontaneous abortion is presented in Box 50–1
2. Nursing assessment
   - **a.** Vaginal spotting or bleeding is common; client may pass clots and tissue
   - **b.** Pelvic cramping or dull backache is usually present
   - **c.** Falling hCG levels indicate death of embryo; ultrasound is used to identify gestational sac and note whether there is current cardiac movement

Box 50–1

Classification of Spontaneous Abortion

Terminology associated with spontaneous abortion helps to classify the clinical condition.

- Threatened abortion: The client experiences vaginal bleeding, but the cervix remains closed. There may be some mild cramping or backache.
- Inevitable abortion: The client experiences cramping and bleeding. The cervix dilates, and the membranes may rupture.
- Incomplete abortion: The client experiences bleeding, cramping, and expulsion of part of the products of conception. Tissue remains in the uterus, and the cervix is dilated. Hemorrhage is possible.
- Complete abortion: The client experiences bleeding, cramping, and expulsion of all the products of conception. The cervix is closed, and the uterus contracts.
- Missed abortion: The client experiences decreasing signs of pregnancy because the fetus has died in utero but has not been expelled. The client may be at risk for DIC if the products of conception are not removed.

3. Collaborative management
   - **a.** Instruct client with threatened abortion about bedrest at home and when to return if bleeding or cramping worsens
   - **b.** Assess amount of bleeding; instruct client to save all clots and tissue that may be passed for further examination
   - **c.** Monitor BP, pulse, and respirations frequently if bleeding is heavy; evaluate client for signs of impending shock
   - **d.** Initiate IV therapy with at least an 18-gauge needle as ordered
   - **e.** Assist with dilatation and curettage (D & C) as indicated for an incomplete abortion
   - **f.** Provide emotional support, without false hope, to client and family; never discount importance of even a very early pregnancy
   - **g.** Refer to pregnancy loss or grief support groups
   - **h.** Give RhoGAM to Rh-negative clients with Rh-positive partners within 72 hours of abortion

F. *Placenta previa*

1. Overview
   - **a.** Placenta is abnormally implanted near to or over internal cervical os; as cervix softens and begins to efface and dilate, placental sinuses are opened causing progressive hemorrhages
   - **b.** May be a low implantation near cervix, a partial previa covering part of os, or a complete placenta previa that covers entire internal cervical os
   - **c.** Incidence of placenta previa is higher with multiple gestation and multiparity
   - **d.** Delivery of client with complete previa is by cesarean section, usually with a classical uterine incision to avoid placenta
   - **e.** Vaginal birth may be possible with a low-lying placenta if fetal head is down to press against placenta and occlude sinuses
2. Nursing assessment
   - **a.** Episodic painless vaginal bleeding after 20th week of pregnancy without contractions; each successive bleeding episode is usually heavier than the last; profuse hemorrhage may occur as cervix dilates under placenta
   - **b.** Ultrasound identification of placental location
3. Collaborative management
   - **a.** Never perform vaginal exam on pregnant client presenting with painless vaginal bleeding because doing so may create profuse hemorrhage
   - **b.** Assist with double setup procedure if indicated: physician performs a careful vaginal exam in OR with equipment and staff ready to perform either a cesarean or a vaginal delivery depending on whether bleeding is caused by placenta previa or is increased bloody show of advanced labor
   - **c.** Maintain preterm clients on bedrest with bathroom privileges until fetal maturity is reached or until hemorrhage warrants immediate cesarean delivery
   - **d.** Monitor maternal vital signs to rule out ascending infection or shock
   - **e.** Assess blood loss by weighing peripads and bed pads that are bloody (1 gram = 1 mL)

Memory Aid

Remember when weighing small amounts of blood or other fluids that one gram equals one milliliter (1 gram = 1 mL); weigh the dry object (such as peripad) and subtract weight from that of wet object to obtain weight of blood or other fluids.

   - **f.** Monitor serial hemoglobin and hematocrit levels; obtain blood group and type, cross-match as needed
   - **g.** Perform continuous or intermittent fetal monitoring and other testing as indicated
   - **h.** Maintain IV access with at least an 18-gauge needle and provide replacement fluids as ordered
   - **i.** Provide emotional support to client on bedrest; facilitate family visits
   - **j.** Promote adequate nutrition with prenatal vitamins and iron to prevent maternal anemia

k. Provide routine preoperative and postoperative cesarean care if indicated; instruct client about location of uterine incision as it relates to future desire for a vaginal birth after cesarean (VBAC)

G. Abruptio placentae

1. Overview
   a. Premature separation of placenta away from uterine wall during pregnancy
   b. Placenta may separate only at margins, causing vaginal bleeding but perhaps little pain
   c. A central (concealed) abruption may not result in vaginal bleeding but does cause increasing uterine irritability and tenderness
   d. A complete (100%) separation from uterine wall leads to profuse hemorrhage
   e. Most common identified precipitating factors are maternal hypertension, cocaine abuse, and abdominal trauma
   f. Client is at increased risk of depleting clotting factors and developing DIC
2. Nursing assessment
   a. ! A painful, rigid, boardlike abdomen with vaginal bleeding is classic sign; abdomen may increase in size as bleeding continues; ultrasound confirms diagnosis
   b. A central abruption causes severe pain from bleeding behind placenta that distends uterine muscle but there may be little or no vaginal bleeding; uterus is very irritable and fetus shows consistent late decelerations
   c. ! Bleeding behind placenta is forced into myometrium and may result in a Couvelaire uterus, which becomes bluish-purple, extremely irritable, distended, and rigid; uterus does not contract efficiently after delivery, leading to postpartum hemorrhage
   d. Marginal placental abruption may present with more vaginal bleeding but less pain than a concealed abruption
   e. Fetal outcome depends on degree of placental separation and fetal maturity at delivery
3. Collaborative management
   a. Monitor maternal BP, pulse, and respiration for signs of impending shock
   b. ! Monitor fetus continuously for signs of distress: increased fetal movement, decreased FHR variability, changes in baseline FHR, late decelerations
   c. ! Assess client for bleeding, uterine activity, and abdominal pain; place on external fetal monitor to evaluate uterine irritability and fetal well-being; palpate uterine tone
   d. ! Measure client's abdominal girth at umbilicus for baseline size and repeat periodically to evaluate occult bleeding
   e. Review lab values to estimate blood loss (hemoglobin and hematocrit) and monitor for potential development of DIC (decreased platelets and fibrinogen; increased fibrin degradation products, PT, and PTT)
   f. Monitor client for signs of developing coagulation defects: unusual bleeding from injection sites, gums, development of petechiae
   g. Start and maintain IV fluids with at least an 18-gauge needle; monitor I & O; a Foley catheter may be inserted with expected urine output of 30 mL/hour or greater
   h. ! Provide oxygen as indicated at 8 to 12 L/min via snug-fitting face mask
   i. Carefully monitor client and fetus if vaginal delivery is attempted; prepare for emergency cesarean delivery if fetus develops distress
   j. Provide ongoing information and emotional support for client and family

H. Premature rupture of membranes

1. Overview
   a. Premature rupture of membranes refers to amniotic membrane rupture before labor begins; labor usually begins spontaneously within 24 hours of rupture
   b. Preterm rupture of membranes refers to membrane rupture prior to term gestation or before 38 weeks; risk factors include infection, incompetent cervix, and trauma
   c. Prolonged rupture of membranes refers to membranes ruptured more than 12 hours before birth; many caregivers will induce labor rather than risk prolonged rupture with possible ascending infection

2. Nursing assessment
   a. Gush of watery, clear, or meconium-stained fluid from vagina with continued leakage
   b. Amniotic fluid turns nitrazine paper blue, indicating an alkaline pH; urine is almost always acidic and doesn't change the yellow color of nitrazine paper
   c. Amniotic fluid shows characteristic ferning pattern on microscopic examination of a slide containing dried fluid; urine and vaginal secretions do not display ferning
   d. An unengaged fetus is at risk for prolapsed cord when membranes rupture
3. Collaborative management
   a. Assess FHR when membranes rupture to rule out prolapsed cord; note time, color, and amount of fluid; obtain a baseline maternal temperature
   b. Evaluate client's temperature every 2 hours; other vital signs may be routine
   c. Avoid vaginal exams to prevent introduction of microorganisms that may cause an ascending infection
   d. Monitor for development of uterine contractions and evaluate fetal well-being; decreased amniotic fluid may cause variable decelerations of FHR
   e. Monitor client for signs of **chorioamnionitis** (inflammation and infection of fetal membranes and amniotic fluid): elevated temperature, abdominal tenderness, increased WBCs and erythrocyte sedimentation rate
   f. Obtain vaginal culture for group B streptococcus as ordered
   g. Provide client teaching and reassurance that amniotic fluid is continuously produced and that there is no such thing as a "dry birth"
   h. Administer antibiotics if ordered; some caregivers prefer to wait and treat newborn

I. Pregnancy-induced hypertension

1. Overview
   a. A group of hypertensive disorders of unknown etiology that begin during pregnancy; other term used is *preeclampsia;* associated with vasospasm and vascular endothelial damage
   b. Is more common in young primigravidas, women over 35, multiple gestation, diabetes mellitus, and hydatidiform mole; client is at risk for CVA, DIC, renal failure, hepatic rupture, and hemorrhage
   c. Gestational hypertension is a high BP during pregnancy that resolves after delivery; it is not associated with proteinuria or edema
   d. Mild preeclampsia is characterized by BP higher than 140/90 after 20 weeks gestation, proteinuria of 1–2+ by dipstick
   e. Severe preeclampsia is characterized by a BP of 180/110 or higher and proteinuria 3^+ or greater
   f. Sudden onset of severe edema indicates a need for evaluation for preeclampsia or renal disease
   g. Eclampsia is the term for preeclampsia that has progressed to include maternal tonic-clonic seizures
   h. HELLP (hemolysis, elevated liver enzymes, and low platelet count) syndrome may be associated with PIH; the client is at risk for hemorrhage, pulmonary edema, and hepatic rupture
   i. Fetal complications include IUGR, fetal distress from hypoxia, and death

Memory Aid

Remember HELLP to recall a syndrome that is a complication of pregnancy-induced hypertension:
Hemolysis, **E**levated **L**iver enzymes and **L**ow **P**latelet count

2. Nursing assessment
   a. Symptoms usually develop during third trimester except in cases of gestational trophoblastic disease (hydatidiform mole); client is at risk for seizures and other complications up to 48 hours after delivery; see Table 50–3 ■
   b. Systemic responses: CNS irritability causes severe or continuous headache, hyperreflexia (greater than +2, baseline, or clonus), or visual disturbance

Table 50–3

Comparison of Mild and Severe Preeclampsia

	Mild Preeclampsia	Severe Preeclampsia
Blood pressure	140/90 or increase of 30/15 from baseline	Greater than 160/110
Proteinuria	Trace to +1	3+ to 4+ or more than 5 grams in a 24-hour urine specimen
Edema	Mild to moderate pretibial edema	Facial edema and pitting pretibial edema
Weight gain	2 to 2.5 pounds/week	Sudden large weight gain
Other	———	Possible signs of CNS irritation

(blurred vision, seeing spots or flashing lights); renal damage is indicated by oliguria (less than 30 mL/hr); portal hypertension may result in epigastric pain and may precede hepatic rupture

! **c.** Lab values: increased hematocrit (as fluid moves out of intravascular space), serum uric acid and BUN; increased liver enzymes (alanine aminotransferase [ALT] and aspartate aminotransferase [AST]); decreased RBCs and platelets as condition worsens

3. Collaborative management: the only cure for PIH is delivery; goal is to deliver healthy, viable infant while safeguarding mother's health

! **a.** Bedrest at home is indicated if preeclampsia is mild; hospitalization if severe until fetus is mature enough for delivery; bedrest on left side to facilitate uteroplacental perfusion

b. Maintain quiet, calm environment to decrease CNS stimulation; keep siderails up and padded for clients with severe preeclampsia who are at risk of progressing to seizures

! **c.** A high-protein diet without salt restriction is indicated; restricting salt intake may result in hypovolemia and fetal distress

! **d.** Implement frequent assessments (every 15 minutes to 1 to 4 hours as indicated by client condition) to include BP, pulse and respirations, edema, deep tendon reflexes, and clonus checks; assess client for headache, visual disturbances, and epigastric pain

e. Foley catheter is inserted to monitor renal function, record strict I & O; evaluate urine for protein; assess daily weight

f. Monitor fetal well-being by continuous electronic fetal monitoring, serial NSTs, BPP, or amniocentesis as indicated

! **g.** Administer magnesium sulfate as ordered for seizure prevention; monitor client for signs of magnesium toxicity (see also Chapter 34)

h. Prepare for induction or cesarean birth when fetus is mature or if maternal condition worsens

i. Provide teaching and support to client and family about condition and therapeutic interventions; clients with mild preeclampsia frequently do not feel ill and may have difficulty maintaining bedrest

j. Evaluate newborn for signs of depression related to magnesium sulfate

k. Continue to monitor client for complications; seizures may occur for 48 hours after delivery

Check Your NCLEX-RN® Exam I.Q.

You are ready for testing on this content if you can

- Implement nursing care for clients undergoing diagnostic testing.
- Determine whether the condition of a client undergoing diagnostic testing has changed from preprocedure to postprocedure.
- Position clients appropriately for diagnostic testing.
- Take action to prevent complications of diagnostic procedures.
- Implement nursing care for clients experiencing complications of pregnancy.
- Instruct clients who have a complication of pregnancy about ongoing care.

PRACTICE TEST

1 The client is a 37-year old gravida one at 38 weeks gestation. She was diagnosed with diabetes at age 17 and is scheduled for an amniocentesis. The nurse concludes that the procedure is probably being done to assess for the presence of which of the following?

1. Neural tube defects
2. Down syndrome
3. Effects of TORCH syndrome
4. Lung maturity

2 A client has been scheduled for an amniocentesis. Which of the following actions should the nurse plan to take in the care of this client?

1. Arrange for the client's admission to the hospital.
2. Arrange for access to an ultrasound machine for use during the procedure.
3. Assist the woman in assuming a supine position.
4. Arrange for administration of general anesthetic.

3 The client is scheduled to have an amniocentesis for assessment of lung maturity. She seems upset and says that she doesn't understand how this test could tell if a baby's lungs are mature. What is the best response by the nurse?

1. "There is no need for you to worry about that. Your doctor knows the procedure well."
2. "The fluid changes color as the fetal lungs mature. We assess the color to determine the lung maturity."
3. "A chemical called lecithin is made by the fetal lungs. The amount of it increases as gestation continues. It flows out into the amniotic fluid where we can measure it."
4. "The amount of bilirubin in the fluid increases as lung maturity increases. We measure the yellow color in the fluid to assess lung maturity."

4 The nurse would formulate which of the following as the highest priority nursing diagnosis for a client about to undergo an amniocentesis?

1. Imbalanced nutrition: less than body requirements related to NPO status
2. Risk for aspiration related to anesthesia
3. Anxiety related to concern for fetal well-being
4. Risk for deficient fluid volume related to removal of amniotic fluid

5 The nurse assesses that which of the following findings would be a contraindication for conducting a contraction stress test?

1. Intrauterine growth restriction
2. Diabetes mellitus
3. Pregnancy at 42 weeks gestation
4. Marginal abruptio placentae

6 A primigravida is hospitalized at 32 weeks gestation after a second hemorrhage from a complete placenta previa. The client appears subdued and sad after the physician informs her she will remain in the hospital until delivery. She says that she is worried about her husband, who will be at home alone much of the time. The nurse interprets the client's response as which of the following?

1. Anxiety
2. Denial
3. Immaturity
4. Ineffective coping

7 The nurse reviews the client's chart for results of which of the following diagnostic tests that will best indicate a diagnosis of erythroblastosis fetalis?

1. Amniocentesis
2. Biophysical profile
3. Indirect Coombs' test
4. Percutaneous umbilical blood sampling

8 The nurse caring for a client with a concealed abruptio placentae prepares to assess the client for which complication as a priority after delivery?

1. Retained placental fragments
2. Urinary tract infection
3. Uterine atony
4. Vaginal hematoma

PRACTICE TEST

9 A pregnant client who has class II heart disease has progressed throughout her pregnancy without complication and is admitted to the labor and delivery unit in active labor. The nurse anticipates administering which medication based on the client's history?

1. An antibiotic
2. An antihypertensive
3. A cardiac glycoside
4. A loop diuretic

10 A client with placenta previa reports that she has religious beliefs that prohibit receiving blood or blood products. The nurse provides client teaching and evaluates that the teaching has been effective if the client states:

1. "A judge will force me to accept a transfusion if I really need it."
2. "I may have to sign out of the hospital against medical advice (AMA)."
3. "I will meet with the dietician to increase the amount of iron in my diet."
4. "There is little chance that I will bleed heavily during this pregnancy."

11 The nurse would assess the pregnant client with a history of multiple sexual partners for which complication of pregnancy that is of greatest concern in this situation?

1. Ectopic pregnancy
2. Premature rupture of membranes
3. Pregnancy-induced hypertension
4. Rh-incompatibility

12 The nurse anticipates that a pregnant client with a history of which of the following might benefit from a scheduled cesarean birth to achieve an improved outcome for the infant?

1. Diabetes mellitus
2. Herpes simplex type II
3. Human immunodeficiency virus
4. Systemic lupus erythematosus

13 Which of the following short-term client outcomes would be most appropriate for a client admitted to the hospital with hyperemesis gravidarum and the nursing diagnosis of imbalanced nutrition: less than body requirements?

1. Assess hourly intake and output
2. Maintain present weight
3. Provide favorite foods
4. Verbalize risks to the fetus

14 A type 1 diabetic prenatal client asks the clinic nurse whether she will be able to breast-feed her baby. Which response by the nurse is most accurate?

1. "Breast-feeding is contraindicated for insulin-dependent moms."
2. "Certainly, breast-feeding will be beneficial for both of you."
3. "I think this is a good idea because it also prevents pregnancy."
4. "You will have a lot of difficulty maintaining a stable blood sugar."

15 A client is admitted with membranes that ruptured 4 hours ago and occasional mild contractions. The term fetus looks healthy on external monitoring. Which of the following is the priority in the nursing plan of care for this client?

1. Encourage ambulation
2. Monitor vital signs
3. Promote rest
4. Provide clear liquids

16 A prenatal client at 14 weeks gestation complains of continuous nausea and vomiting and a severe headache. The client has elevated blood pressure and the fundal height is 21 centimeters. Which diagnostic test does the nurse anticipate will be ordered to confirm a hydatidiform mole?

1. Biophysical profile
2. Human chorionic gonadotropin
3. Maternal serum alpha-fetoprotein
4. Sonography

17 An HIV-positive client in active labor with ruptured membranes is being transported to the hospital via ambulance. The labor and delivery nurse anticipates priority administration of which medication to this client?

1. Antibiotics
2. Immune globulin
3. Oxytocin (Pitocin)
4. Zidovudine (Retrovir)

18 A client who admits to crack cocaine use during her pregnancy asks the nurse not to inform the baby's father about the substance abuse. Which response by the nurse is most appropriate?

1. "You must be very worried about how he will react to that information."
2. "This is your pregnancy and your body, so I'll keep your information private."
3. "Your baby will probably not survive, so there is no need for him to know."
4. "Have you considered that he deserves to know what you may have done to his baby?"

19 A client experiencing profuse hemorrhage from placenta previa is being prepared for an emergency cesarean birth. The client exhibits signs of hypovolemia. The nurse makes it a priority to place the client into which of the following positions?

1. Knee-chest
2. Left lateral
3. Semi-Fowler's
4. Trendelenburg

20 Which of the following nursing diagnoses has the highest priority for a client with a missed abortion who has developed disseminated intravascular coagulopathy (DIC)?

1. Anticipatory grieving
2. High risk for deficient fluid volume
3. High risk for injury
4. Spiritual distress

21 A client with premature spontaneous rupture of membranes (SROM) at 33 weeks gestation is to be given betamethasone (Celestone) to increase fetal lung maturity. The nurse checks the client's record to ensure that the client does not have what disorder that would be a contraindication for this drug?

1. Diabetes mellitus
2. History of alcohol abuse
3. Incompetent cervix
4. Intrauterine growth restriction (IUGR)

22 The nurse concludes that a client is at risk for pregnancy-induced hypertension (PIH) when the vital signs taken today show that the blood pressure has increased during pregnancy from

1. 90/56 to 110/70.
2. 100/60 to 130/76.
3. 122/80 to 138/86.
4. 134/80 to 140/88.

23 A client who has experienced a spontaneous abortion at 8 weeks asks the nurse why this happened. The nurse provides accurate information by stating that the most common cause of "miscarriage" is

1. Chromosome abnormalities.
2. Environmental teratogens.
3. Excessive activity.
4. Substance abuse.

24 A client who received no prenatal care delivers a 9-pound 4-ounce baby boy who exhibits signs of respiratory distress. The nurse obtains a blood sample from the infant to assess for which of the following?

1. Hemolysis
2. Hyperbilirubinemia
3. Hypoglycemia
4. Sepsis

25 The nurse explains to a client who had a cervical cone biopsy several years ago that she is now at increased risk for which complication of pregnancy?

1. Abdominal pregnancy
2. Incompetent cervix
3. Gestational trophoblastic disease
4. Placenta previa

ANSWERS & RATIONALES

1 **Answer: 4** Amniocentesis for genetic testing is usually done early in the second trimester. This test, on a client who has diabetes and is at 38 weeks gestation, is probably being done to assess lung maturity in anticipation of delivery.

Cognitive Level: Analysis **Client Need:** Physiological Integrity: Physiological Adaptation **Integrated Process:** Nursing Process: Implementation **Content Area:** Maternal-Newborn **Strategy:** The critical words in the question are *38 weeks gestation.* Use knowledge of the timing of tests used to diagnose genetic defects to systematically eliminate the incorrect options. As an alternative, consider that lung maturity is a key concern as a pregnant client approaches the due date.

2 **Answer: 2** The test, completed on an outpatient basis, is done under guidance of ultrasound visualization. The test is done without anesthetic or with a local anesthetic. The client is positioned on her back with a wedge under her left hip to avoid hypotension from pressure of the uterus on the vena cava. **Cognitive Level:** Application **Client Need:** Physiological Integrity: Reduction of Risk Potential **Integrated Process:** Nursing Process: Planning **Content Area:** Maternal-Newborn **Strategy:** The wording of the question tells you that the correct answer is also a true statement about care for this client. Use knowledge of the procedure to eliminate options 1 and 4. Choose option 2 over 3 because the procedure is guided by ultrasound and option 3 does not address risk of pressure on the vena cava in the supine position.

3 **Answer: 3** The amount of lecithin increases as the fetal lungs mature. The ratio of lecithin to sphingomyelin is used to assess lung maturity; changes in color (options 2 and 4) are not. Option 1 is not a therapeutic response. **Cognitive Level:** Application **Client Need:** Physiological Integrity: Reduction of Risk Potential **Integrated Process:** Communication and Documentation **Content Area:** Maternal-Newborn **Strategy:** Recall that amniotic fluid is clear to eliminate options 2 and 4. Choose option 3 over 1 because option 1 is not a therapeutic response.

4 **Answer: 3** Most women view invasive antenatal testing with anxiety because of the reason for the test, the impending results, and concern about maternal and fetus complications. Because of the small amount of fluid removed, option 4 is unnecessary. Options 1 and 2 are completely incorrect. **Cognitive Level:** Analysis **Client Need:** Physiological Integrity: Reduction of Risk Potential **Integrated Process:** Nursing Process: Analysis **Content Area:** Maternal-Newborn **Strategy:** Use knowledge of the procedure to assist in eliminating incorrect options. Eliminate options 1 and 2 first because there is no need for NPO status and there is no anesthesia. Choose option 3 over 2 (it is a valid concern but a psychosocial issue rather than a physiological one) because the amount of fluid removed is very small.

5 **Answer: 4** Contractions elicited during the test could cause increased bleeding if an abruption is present. Intrauterine growth restriction, diabetes mellitus, and postterm pregnancy are all indications for completing a contraction stress test. **Cognitive Level:** Analysis **Client Need:** Physiological Integrity: Reduction of Risk Potential **Integrated Process:** Nursing Process: Assessment **Content Area:** Maternal-Newborn **Strategy:** Note the critical word *contraindication* in the stem of the question. This tells you that the correct answer is likely an item that could pose risk of harm to the fetus. From there, recall that abruptio placentae can lead to bleeding to help you choose correctly.

6 **Answer: 1** The client has stated that she is worried, which creates anxiety. The information presented does not represent denial or immaturity. There is insufficient data to determine whether the client's coping is effective or ineffective at this time. **Cognitive Level:** Analysis **Client Need:** Physiological Integrity: Physiological Adaptation **Integrated Process:** Communication and Documentation **Content Area:** Maternal-Newborn **Strategy:** Note that the client has appropriate nonverbal behavior (subdued and sad) and is able to articulate a concern (worried about husband). Consider that all of these are expected reactions to choose anxiety over each of the other options.

7 **Answer: 4** Percutaneous umbilical blood sampling (PUBS) obtains an actual sample of fetal blood for analysis. The other options provide information about fetal well-being but do not directly sample the fetal erythrocytes. **Cognitive Level:** Analysis **Client Need:** Physiological Integrity: Reduction of Risk Potential **Integrated Process:** Nursing Process: Analysis **Content Area:** Maternal-Newborn **Strategy:** Note the word *erythroblastosis* in the question and correlate that with erythrocyte or red blood cell. Eliminate options 1 and 2 first because they are not related to red blood cells. Then choose option 4 over 3 because it allows access to fetal cells, not maternal cells.

8 **Answer: 3** A concealed abruption may result in a Couvelaire uterus, which doesn't contract effectively after delivery, leading to uterine atony. The other complications may occur in any client. **Cognitive Level:** Analysis **Client Need:** Physiological Integrity: Physiological Adaptation **Integrated Process:** Nursing Process: Assessment **Content Area:** Maternal-Newborn **Strategy:** Specific knowledge of the risks of concealed abruptio placentae is needed to answer the question. Use nursing knowledge and the process of elimination to make your selection.

9 **Answer: 1** Prophylactic antibiotics are given during labor to prevent bacterial endocarditis. The other medications may need to be given based on additional assessment findings and may not be needed at all for a client with class II heart disease. **Cognitive Level:** Analysis **Client Need:** Physiological Integrity: Physiological Adaptation **Integrated Process:** Nursing Process: Planning **Content Area:** Maternal-Newborn **Strategy:** The core issue of the question is knowledge of the significance of class II heart disease during labor. Use nursing knowledge and the process of elimination to make your selection. Consider that antihypertensives, cardiac glycosides, and diuretics are used to manage symptoms, which are not present in the stem of the question. An antibiotic is the only drug listed that could prevent a new problem (infection).

10 **Answer: 3** The client is likely to lose some blood with a placenta previa. Increasing iron in her diet is a positive response that does not interfere with her religious beliefs. Option 1 is not a true statement. Option 2 does not address the client's need or right to care. **Cognitive Level:** Analysis **Client Need:** Physiological Integrity: Physiological Adaptation **Integrated Process:** Nursing Process: Evaluation **Content Area:** Maternal-Newborn **Strategy:** The core issue of this question is culturally competent care to reduce risk of complications. Eliminate option 1 because of the word *force,* and eliminate option 2 because of *against medical advice.* Choose option 3 over 4 because the client cannot predict the risk of bleeding during pregnancy.

11 **Answer: 1** The client with multiple partners is at high risk for sexually transmitted diseases and ascending infection that

may lead to blockage in the fallopian tubes. Ultimately, this process could lead to ectopic pregnancy. The other options do not address this particular pathophysiological concern.
Cognitive Level: Analysis **Client Need:** Physiological Integrity: Physiological Adaptation **Integrated Process:** Nursing Process: Assessment **Content Area:** Maternal-Newborn **Strategy:** Note the critical words *multiple sex partners* and *greatest concern* in the question. This tells you that the correct answer has a connection to risks associated with multiple sex partners. Use knowledge of complications of sexually transmitted infections to choose option 1 over the others.

12 **Answer: 3** The transmission of HIV is less than 1% if the infant is delivered by cesarean prior to membrane rupture. Only the client with active herpes lesions should be delivered by cesarean to prevent transmission of the virus during vaginal birth.
Cognitive Level: Application **Client Need:** Physiological Integrity: Physiological Adaptation **Integrated Process:** Nursing Process: Planning **Content Area:** Maternal-Newborn **Strategy:** The core issue of the question is knowledge of methods of transmitting infection from mother to newborn during the delivery process. Eliminate options 1 and 4 first because they do not address infection. Choose option 3 over 2 because there is greater risk of transmitting HIV during delivery, while only active herpes lesions transmit that virus.

13 **Answer: 2** A short-term outcome of maintained weight is appropriate while the client is being stabilized in the hospital. An outcome is the result of nursing care. Options 1 and 3 are nursing interventions. Option 4 does not address the nursing diagnosis.
Cognitive Level: Analysis **Client Need:** Physiological Integrity: Physiological Adaptation **Integrated Process:** Nursing Process: Planning **Content Area:** Maternal-Newborn **Strategy:** The critical words in the question are *client outcomes.* With this in mind, eliminate options 1 and 3 because they are interventions. Choose option 1 over 4 because it directly correlates with nutrition, which is the focus of the nursing diagnosis.

14 **Answer: 2** Breast-feeding should be encouraged because it benefits both the mother and her infant. It is not contraindicated for diabetic mothers (option 1), may or may not help prevent future pregnancy during lactation (option 3), and does not necessarily lead to loss of blood glucose control with careful management (option 4).
Cognitive Level: Application **Client Need:** Physiological Integrity: Physiological Adaptation **Integrated Process:** Nursing Process: Implementation **Content Area:** Maternal-Newborn **Strategy:** Note the key words *most accurate,* which tell you that the correct answer is the one that is a true statement, while the others are false to a greater or lesser degree. Eliminate options 1 and 4 first because of the words *contraindicated* and . . . *a lot of difficulty* . . . respectively. Then choose option 2 over 3 because option 3 may or may not be true depending on individual circumstances.

15 **Answer: 2** The client with premature ruptured membranes is at risk for developing an infection and should have her vital signs monitored every 2 hours, specifically temperature. The client may be on bedrest, not ambulating, following rupture of the membranes (option 1). Promoting rest (option 3) and providing clear liquids (option 4) are slightly lesser priorities for this client.
Cognitive Level: Analysis **Client Need:** Physiological Integrity: Physiological Adaptation **Integrated Process:** Nursing Process: Planning **Content Area:** Maternal-Newborn **Strategy:** The core issue of the question is knowledge of infection as the key risk following rupture of the membranes. Eliminate options that do not address this risk. Only option 2 addresses vital signs, which includes monitoring temperature as one way of detecting infection.

16 **Answer: 4** Ultrasound confirms the diagnosis of molar pregnancy that is indicated by the client's symptoms. The client will have high hCG levels and low maternal serum alphafetoprotein levels, but these are not conclusive for hydatidiform mole. Option 1 is inappropriate before the third trimester because it evaluates the fetus.
Cognitive Level: Application **Client Need:** Physiological Integrity: Reduction of Risk Potential **Integrated Process:** Nursing Process: Assessment **Content Area:** Maternal-Newborn **Strategy:** The core issue of the question is the best method to determine hydatidiform mole. Choose option 4 over all the others because it is the only one that provides for visualization of the reproductive structures and allows discrimination of true pregnancy from hydatidiform mole.

17 **Answer: 4** The rate of transmission of HIV to the newborn is decreased from 17% to less than 7% if the mother is given prophylactic zidovudine (Retrovir) orally during pregnancy and by IV during labor. There are no indications presented in the question for any of the other medications listed, although an antibiotic could be administered if the mother acquired an infection secondary to ruptured membranes.
Cognitive Level: Analysis **Client Need:** Physiological Integrity: Physiological Adaptation **Integrated Process:** Nursing Process: Planning **Content Area:** Maternal-Newborn **Strategy:** The core issue of the question is management of the HIV client in active labor with respect to preventing transmission of HIV to the newborn. With this in mind, eliminate options 2 and 3 first, which do not prevent or treat infection. Choose option 4 over 1 because it is an antiviral rather than antibacterial (note also the *vir* that indicates *virus* in the drug name Retrovir).

18 **Answer: 1** Option 1 is a therapeutic response to the client's concerns. The nurse should remain nonjudgmental when clients reveal information about substance abuse. Option 2 is nontherapeutic because it does not explore the client's concern. Option 3 is inaccurate, and option 4 is judgmental.
Cognitive Level: Application **Client Need:** Physiological Integrity: Physiological Adaptation **Integrated Process:** Communication and Documentation **Content Area:** Maternal-Newborn **Strategy:** The core issue of the question is a therapeutic response to a concern shared by the client. Eliminate each of the incorrect options systematically because they do not invite further sharing of information between client and nurse.

19 **Answer: 2** The left lateral position facilitates uteroplacental perfusion. Semi-Fowler's position would decrease maternal cerebral perfusion, Trendelenburg puts the weight of the gravid uterus against the maternal lungs, and knee-chest is unlikely to be maintained by a client in shock.
Cognitive Level: Analysis **Client Need:** Physiological Integrity: Physiological Adaptation **Integrated Process:** Nursing Process:

Implementation **Content Area:** Maternal-Newborn **Strategy:** The core issue of the question is how to maintain uteroplacental perfusion for the client in shock. With this in mind, choose the position that turns the client to the left side and takes pressure of the gravid uterus off the great vessels in the abdomen.

20 **Answer: 2** The client with DIC is at risk for hemorrhage, which takes priority over the non-life-threatening options 1 and 4. The client could experience bruising or other areas of local bleeding from the disorder, but hypovolemia from hemorrhage takes priority over risk for injury (option 3).
Cognitive Level: Analysis **Client Need:** Physiological Integrity: Physiological Adaptation **Integrated Process:** Nursing Process: Analysis **Content Area:** Maternal-Newborn **Strategy:** The issue of the question is knowledge of complications of DIC, specifically hemorrhage and loss of circulating volume. With this in mind, focus on physiologically based nursing diagnoses, and eliminate options 1 and 4. Choose option 2 because it addresses a greater and more specific physiological risk.

21 **Answer: 1** Glucocorticoids such as betamethasone are contraindicated for use in diabetic clients because they raise the blood glucose level even further. The other disorders are not contraindications for giving betamethasone.
Cognitive Level: Application **Client Need:** Physiological Integrity: Physiological Adaptation **Integrated Process:** Nursing Process: Assessment **Content Area:** Maternal-Newborn **Strategy:** The core issue of the question is knowledge of key side effects of betamethasone, which helps to select the client for whom it should not be used. Recall that the glucocorticoids often end in *sone* to help you recognize the drug as a glucocorticoid. Recall next the risk of elevating blood glucose levels to choose option 1 over the others.

22 **Answer: 2** An increase of 30 mmHg systolic and 15 mmHg diastolic on two occasions is diagnostic for PIH. The blood pressures in each of the other options do not meet the criteria for increase in either the systolic or the diastolic blood pressure reading.
Cognitive Level: Analysis **Client Need:** Physiological Integrity: Physiological Adaptation **Integrated Process:** Nursing Process: Assessment **Content Area:** Maternal-Newborn **Strategy:** Specific knowledge of the criteria for PIH is needed to answer this question. Use nursing knowledge and the process of elimination to make your selection. As an alternative, choose option 2 because it has the greatest degree of change in *both* systolic and diastolic measurements.

23 **Answer: 1** The majority of early abortions are related to abnormal chromosomes. The client may fear that she has caused the loss and should be provided with accurate information. The other responses are not accurate.
Cognitive Level: Application **Client Need:** Physiological Integrity: Physiological Adaptation **Integrated Process:** Communication and Documentation **Content Area:** Maternal-Newborn **Strategy:** Specific knowledge of the etiologies of spontaneous abortion is needed to answer the question. Use nursing knowledge and the process of elimination to make your selection.

24 **Answer: 3** An LGA infant who demonstrates respiratory immaturity may have a diabetic mother. The infant produces his own insulin during pregnancy and stores the excess glucose as fat to compensate for high maternal glucose loads. However, after delivery the infant is at high risk for hypoglycemia because excess maternal glucose is now absent from the infant's circulation.
Cognitive Level: Analysis **Client Need:** Physiological Integrity: Physiological Adaptation **Integrated Process:** Nursing Process: Assessment **Content Area:** Maternal-Newborn **Strategy:** The core issue of the question is prenatal risks for LGA infants and the consequences after delivery. Use nursing knowledge and the process of elimination to make your selection.

25 **Answer: 2** Cervical trauma and scarring may result in cervical incompetence during pregnancy. The other options are unrelated to cone biopsy.
Cognitive Level: Analysis **Client Need:** Physiological Integrity: Physiological Adaptation **Integrated Process:** Nursing Process: Teaching and Learning **Content Area:** Maternal-Newborn **Strategy:** Note the critical word *cervical* in the stem of the question and choose option 2 over the others because it also refers to the cervix.

Key Terms to Review

References

Condon, M. (2004). *Women's health: An integrated approach to wellness and illness.* Upper Saddle River, NJ: Pearson Education.

Kozier, B., Erb, G., Berman, A., & Snyder, S. (2004). *Fundamentals of nursing: Concepts, process, and practice* (7th ed.). Upper Saddle River, NJ: Pearson Educaton.

Lowdermilk, D., & Perry, S. (2004). *Maternity and women's health care* (8th ed.). St. Louis, MO: Elsevier Science.

Olds, S. B., London, M. L., & Davidson, M. (2004). *Maternal-newborn nursing & women's health care* (7th ed.). Upper Saddle River, NJ: Prentice-Hall.

Smith, S. F., Duell, D. J., & Martin, B. C. (2003). *Clinical nursing skills: Basic to advanced skills* (6th ed.). Upper Saddle River, NJ: Pearson Education.

Complicated Labor and Delivery Care

51

In this chapter

Cross reference

Other chapters relevant to this content area are

Reproduction, Family Planning, and Infertility	Chapter 9
Uncomplicated Antenatal Assessment and Care	Chapter 10
Uncomplicated Labor and Delivery	Chapter 11
Uncomplicated Postpartum Assessment and Care	Chapter 12
Uncomplicated Newborn Care	Chapter 13
Complicated Antenatal Care	Chapter 50
Complicated Postpartum Care	Chapter 52
Complicated Newborn Care	Chapter 53

Test Yourself

Are you ready for the NCLEX-RN® or course exams? Use the practice tests on the companion CD-ROM to check.

I. GENERAL NURSING CARE OF THE CLIENT

A. High-risk factors

1. May develop at any time during labor in client who has been otherwise healthy throughout pregnancy
2. Etiology may be related to fetus, pelvic bones and other pelvic structures, uterine contractions, or client's psychological state

B. Client response to onset of high-risk factors in labor

1. Stress, fear, and anxiety brought about by unexpected complications during labor may have profound effects on maternal and fetal outcomes
2. Maternal anxiety can increase tension, produce higher pain perception, and may make labor contractions less effective
3. Catecholamines released during stress produce vasoconstriction that may negatively affect uterine blood flow

C. Family members

1. May be overwhelmed with concern
2. May become less capable of providing needed emotional support for client

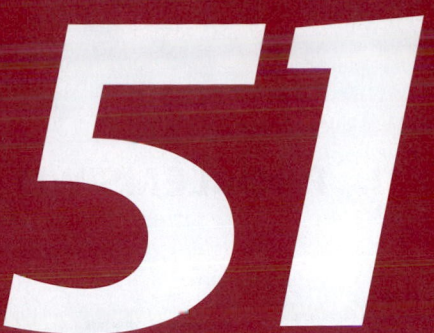

D. **Nursing care**
   1. Basic intrapartal care is still important
   2. Nursing care during complicated labor requires additional special knowledge and skill in assessment and care of mother and fetus

II. PROBLEMS WITH THE FETUS

A. **Fetal *malpositions***
   1. Ideal fetal position is flexed with occiput in right or left anterior quadrant of maternal pelvis
   2. Various types of malpositions are possible
   3. Occiput posterior (OP) position
      a. Right or left OP position occurs in about 25% of all term pregnancies but usually rotates to occiput anterior (OA) as labor progresses
      b. Failure to rotate is termed persistent occiput posterior
      ! c. Maternal risks include prolonged labor, potential for operative delivery, extension of episiotomy, or 3rd- or 4th-degree laceration of perineum
      ! d. Maternal symptoms include intense back pain in labor, dysfunctional labor pattern, prolonged active phase, secondary arrest of dilatation, and/or arrest of descent
   4. Occiput transverse (OT) position
      a. Incomplete rotation of OP position to OA results in fetal head being in horizontal or transverse position
      b. Persistent OT position occurs because of ineffective contractions or flattened bony pelvis
      c. If pelvic structure is adequate, vaginal delivery can be accomplished by stimulating contractions with oxytocin (Pitocin,) and use of forceps
   5. Collaborative management of fetal malpositions
      a. Key maternal assessments are pain and coping skills
      ! b. Encourage client to lie on side opposite from fetal back, which may help with rotation
      ! c. Knee-chest position or pelvic rocking may facilitate rotation
      ! d. Apply sacral counterpressure with heel of hand to relieve back pain
      e. Provide support and encouragement by keeping client and family informed of progress, prasing efforts to maintain control, and encouraging relaxation with contractions
      f. Anticipate forceps rotation and forceps-assisted birth or vacuum extraction
      g. Forceps: metal instruments applied to fetal head to provide traction or a means to rotate fetal head
      ! h. Risks of forceps use are fetal ecchymosis or edema of face, transient facial paralysis, maternal lacerations, or episiotomy extensions
      i. Vacuum extraction: a suction cup applied to fetal head to provide traction to shorten second stage of labor
      ! j. Risks of vacuum extraction are newborn cephalohematoma, retinal hemorrhage, and intracranial hemorrhage

B. **Fetal *malpresentations***
   1. Vertex malpresentations are caused by failure of fetus to assume a flexed attitude; include brow presentation, face presentation, and sincipital presentation
   2. With brow presentation, fetal forehead is presenting part; 50% convert to vertex or face presentation
   3. With face presentation, there is increased risk of prolonged labor and operative delivery
      a. Anticipate vaginal delivery if mother's pelvis is adequate and infant's chin (mentum) is in anterior position
      ! b. Anticipate cesarean delivery if mentum is posterior or signs of fetal distress occur
      ! c. Fetal monitor electrode should not be placed on presenting part (infant's face); requires external fetal heart rate (FHR) monitoring

d. Edema and bruising of face, eyes, and lips are common occurrences—clients should be prepared for this possibility before seeing infant for first time

4. With sincipital presentation (military attitude), larger diameter of fetal head is presented; labor progress is slowed with slower descent of fetal head

5. Breech presentations

a. Three types (see Figure 51–1 ■)

b. Maternal risks include prolonged labor (decreased pressure exerted by breech on cervix), premature rupture of membranes (risk of infection), cesarean or forceps delivery, trauma to birth canal during delivery (manipulation and forceps), and intrapartum or postpartum hemorrhage

c. Fetal risks include compressed or prolapsed umbilical cord, entrapment of fetal head in incompletely dilated cervix, aspiration and asphyxia at birth, and birth trauma from manipulation and forceps to free fetal head

d. Vaginal delivery of breech: fetal body may pass through an incompletely dilated cervix, entrapping the larger fetal head; head must be delivered quickly to avoid hypoxia; Piper (long handle) forceps may be applied to after-coming fetal head

e. **Cesarean section:** most breech presentations are delivered by cesarean section, or abdominal delivery

6. Shoulder presentation (transverse lie): acromium process is presenting part

a. Vaginal delivery is not considered possible in term infant; cesarean birth is preferred method of delivery

b. **External cephalic version:** manipulation of fetus through abdominal wall from breech or shoulder presentation to vertex presentation

c. Collaborative management during external cephalic version includes placing client on external fetal monitor, starting IV fluids, administering terbutaline (Brethine) via a piggybacked IV line to relax uterine muscle, closely monitoring FHR during version attempt, and discontinuing version if undue maternal or fetal distress occurs

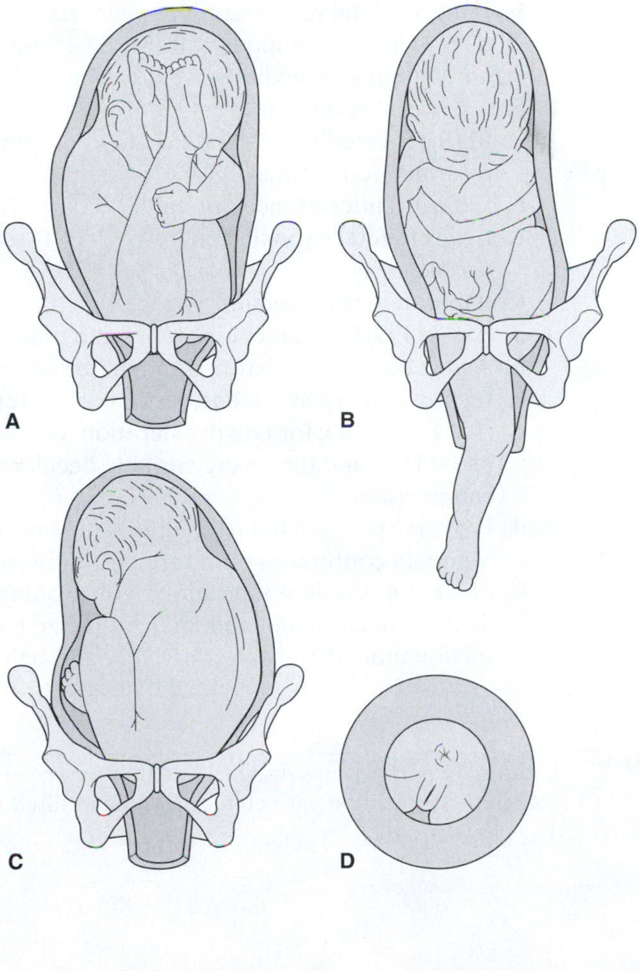

Figure 51–1

Breech presentation. *A.* Frank breech: sacrum is presenting part, knees extended. *B.* Incomplete (footling) breech: one or both feet presenting, increasing risk of umbilical cord prolapse. *C.* Complete breech: sacrum is presenting part, knees flexed, left sacral anterior position shown. *D.* On vaginal exam, nurse may feel anal sphincter; tissue of fetal buttocks feels soft.

7. Compound presentations: more than one part of fetus presents
   a. Most common type is a hand or arm prolapsing beside head
   b. Risk of cord compression and prolapse is increased
   c. Vaginal versus cesarean delivery depends on size of fetus, presence of fetal distress, and progress in labor
8. Collaborative management of clients with fetal malpresentations
   a. Leopold's maneuvers may help detect abnormal presentation
   b. Observe closely for abnormal labor patterns
   c. Monitor FHR and contractions continuously
   d. Provide client and family teaching
   e. Provide client support and encouragement
   f. Anticipate forceps-assisted birth
   g. Anticipate cesarean birth for incomplete breech or shoulder presentation
   h. Be prepared for childbirth emergencies such as neonatal resuscitation

C. Fetal distress: insufficient oxygen supply to meet demands of fetus

1. Causes include compression of umbilical cord and uteroplacental insufficiency (from placental abnormalities or maternal condition)
2. May be signaled by meconium-stained (green-tinged) amniotic fluid (excluding breech presentation)
3. Changes in FHR baseline
   a. Tachycardia (above 160): early sign of distress
   b. Bradycardia (below 110): late sign of distress
4. Decreased or absence of variability of heart rate
   a. Heart rate varies less than 2 to 5 beats per minute (bpm), causing a flattened appearance to the heart rate
   b. Indicates depression of the autonomic nervous system that controls heart rate
   c. Fetal sleep, sedation, and hypoxia may affect variability
5. Late deceleration pattern
   a. FHR slows following peak of contraction and slowly returns to baseline rate during resting phase
   b. Indicates fetal response to hypoxia from uteroplacental insufficiency
   c. Considered an omnious pattern regardless of depth of deceleration of FHR and requires immediate intervention
6. Severe variable deceleration pattern
   a. FHR repeatedly decelerates below 90 bpm for more than 60 seconds before returning to baseline
   b. Indicates interference of fetal blood flow from cord compression
   c. Leads to fetal hypoxia and low APGAR scores unless corrective steps are taken
7. Collaborative management
   a. Assess FHR baseline, variability, and pattern of periodic changes
   b. Assess contraction pattern and maternal response to labor
   c. Institute emergency measures to correct fetal hypoxia based on FHR pattern (see Box 51–1); for late deceleration, take steps to improve uteroplacental blood flow and for severe variable deceleration, take steps to relieve cord compression
   d. Provide appropriate information and emotional support to client and family
   e. Maintain continuous monitoring of FHR, uterine activity, and labor progress
   f. Prevent meconium aspiration by suctioning neonate's nasopharynx prior to delivery of chest and abdomen; visualize larynx and vocal cords with deep suction immediately after delivery and before first breath is taken

Memory Aid

To correctly perform nasotracheal suction on an infant, slightly hyperextend the head to a "sniffing" position with chin up and head tilted back slightly.

Box 51-1

Nursing Management of Fetal Distress

Late decelerations (uteroplacental insufficiency)
The goal is to improve maternal blood flow to the placenta

- Reposition the mother on her left side
- Administer O_2 by face mask at 8–10 L/min
- Increase IV fluids
- Discontinue oxytocin infusion if labor is being induced
- Notify the health care provider immediately

Severe variable decelerations or prolonged bradycardia (cord compression)
The goal is to relieve pressure on the umbilical cord

- Reposition the mother on either side
- If not corrected, reposition to opposite side
- Administer O_2 by face mask at 8–10 L/min
- Trendelenburg or knee-chest position if not corrected
- Perform vaginal examination and apply upward digital pressure on the presenting part to relieve pressure on the umbilical cord

g. **Amnioinfusion:** amniotic fluid may be replaced with warmed sterile saline through an intrauterine catheter using an infusion pump when signs of cord compression are present during labor; monitor FHR monitor continuously and discontinue infusion when signs of cord compression disappear

h. **Intrauterine resuscitation:** consists of administration of terbutaline (Brethine), a tocolytic agent, to stop uterine contractions and provide an opportunity for uteroplacental circulation to improve when fetal distress is present during first stage of labor; see Chapter 35 for discussion of medication

D. Prolapsed umbilical cord

1. Cause: fetus is not firmly engaged, allowing room for umbilical cord to move beyond (prolapse) or alongside presenting part (occult prolapse)
2. Contributing factors include rupture of membranes before engagement of presenting part, small fetus, breech presentation, multifetal pregnancy, and transverse lie (shoulder presentation)
3. Collaborative management
   a. Identify client at risk for prolapsed umbilical cord
   b. ! Place mother's hips higher than her head: knee-chest position or Trendelenburg position
   c. ! Perform sterile vaginal exam pushing fetal presenting part upward with fingers to relieve pressure on cord
   d. Administer O_2 by face mask at 8 to 10 L/min
   e. Maintain continuous electronic fetal monitoring
   f. Prepare for rapid delivery vaginally or by cesarean section
   g. ! If cord protrudes through vagina, determine that pulsation is present and wrap cord loosely with warm sterile saline soaked towel or dressing to prevent drying; do not allow dressing or towel to cool, which could cause spasms of umbilical cord vessels and decrease fetal oxygen

III. PROBLEMS WITH PELVIC STRUCTURES

A. Abnormal size or shape of pelvis

1. Contracted pelvic inlet: anterior–posterior diameter less than 10 centimeters (cm); transverse diameter less than 12 cm
   a. Makes engagement difficult
   b. Influences fetal position and presentation
2. Contracted midpelvic plane: interspinous diameter less than 9.5 cm
   a. Hampers internal rotation of fetal head
   b. Secondary arrest of dilatation or arrest of descent of fetal head occurs

3. Contracted pelvic outlet: interischial tuberous diameter less than 8 cm
4. **Trial of labor (TOL):** physician may allow labor to continue or may even stimulate labor with oxytocin when pelvic measurements are borderline to see if fetal head will descend, making vaginal delivery possible; if progressive changes in dilatation and station do not occur, a cesarean delivery is performed

B. ***Cephalopelvic disproportion (CPD)***
1. Fetal head is too large to pass through bony pelvis
2. Signs and symptoms: fetal head does not descend despite strong contractions
3. Maternal risks include prolonged labor, exhaustion, hemorrhage, and infection
4. Fetal risks include hypoxia and birth trauma
5. Cesarean birth is necessary

C. **Shoulder dystocia: an obstetric emergency resulting from difficulty or inability to deliver shoulders**
1. Fetal macrosomia increases risk of shoulder dystocia
2. Inability to deliver shoulders leads to fetal hypoxia and death
3. Maternal risks: lacerations and tears of birth canal and postpartum hemorrhage
4. Neonatal risks: hypoxia, fractures of clavicle, and injury to neck and head
5. Collaborative management
   a. Identify client at risk for shoulder dystocia: obesity, increased fundal height, history of macrosomia, maternal diabetes or gestational diabetes, prolonged second-stage labor
   b. Assist with positioning during delivery: use McRoberts maneuver, flexing thighs up onto abdomen to change angle of pelvis, increase pelvic diameters, and facilitate delivery of shoulders
   c. Assess for maternal and newborn injury following delivery

IV. PROBLEMS WITH UTERINE CONTRACTIONS

A. ***Induction of labor***
1. Methods consist of pharmacologic (see also Chapter 35) and nonpharmacologic measures to initiate contractions and cervical change
2. Cervical ripening with prostaglandins (PGE_2) gel or with laminaria (hydrophilic agent): when inserted into cervix, absorbs water from cervical mucus, expands, and dilates cervix
3. **Amniotomy** or artificial rupture of membranes (AROM)
   a. Auscultate FHR prior to and immediately after AROM to detect prolapse of umbilical cord or fetal distress
   b. Take maternal temperature every 1 to 2 hours following AROM to detect signs of infection

Memory Aid

Remember that *-otomy* means "cutting into"; amniotomy is thus artificial rupture of the amniotic membranes.

4. Misoprostol (Cytotec)
   a. A synthetic prostaglandin agent administered intravaginally and/or orally to stimulate onset of contractions
   b. Continuous monitoring of FHR, uterine activity, and maternal vital signs is essential
5. Oxytocin (Pitocin) administration (see also Chapter 35)
   a. Use **Bishop score** to assess maternal readiness for induction by determining dilatation, effacement, station, cervical consistency, and position of the cervix
   b. Begin external fetal monitoring and monitor FHR closely throughout induction
   c. Assess and record maternal vital signs, intake and output (I & O), and contraction frequency and intensity
   d. Always administer using IV infusion pump for safety; stop infusion immediately if contractions are closer than 2 minutes, last longer than 90 seconds, or for any indication of fetal distress

6. Absolute contraindications to induction of labor
   a. Placenta previa
   b. Transverse lie and other fetal malpresentations
   c. Prior classic uterine incision
   d. Pelvic structure abnormality
   e. Prolapsed umbilical cord
   f. Active genital herpes
   g. Invasive cervical cancer

B. ***Dystocia* or difficult labor**

1. **Hypertonic uterine dysfunction:** uncoordinated irregular contractions with decreased intensity and increased uterine resting tone
   a. Maternal risks are prolonged or nonprogressive labor, pain, and fatigue
   b. Fetal risks include hypoxia caused by decreased uteroplacental blood flow
   c. Medical treatment includes sedation aimed at stopping contractions, promoting rest, and allowing a normal labor pattern to develop
   ! d. Provide hydration, monitor I & O, and promote relaxation
2. Hypotonic uterine dysfunction: infrequent contractions with decreased intensity
   ! a. Maternal and fetal risks are related to nonprogressive labor (often associated with prolonged rupture of membranes) and frequent vaginal examinations leading to infection
   b. More commonly occurs in active phase of labor
   c. Medical treatment includes ruling out CPD and initiating **augmentation of labor,** or stimulation of contractions, with oxytocin
3. Abnormal progress in labor: a **labor graph,** or **Friedman curve,** identifies deviations from normal progress in labor by plotting cervical dilatation and descent of fetal head over time
   a. Prolonged latent phase: more than 20 hours for nulliparous client or more than 14 hours for multiparous client; may indicate CPD; may be caused by false labor; medical treatment is sedation and rest
   b. Protracted active phase: dilatation less than 1.2 cm per hour in nulliparous client or less than 1.5 cm per hour in multiparous client; may be caused by malposition; assess for CPD and fetal presentation and position
   c. Protracted descent: less than 1 cm per hour change in station in nulliparous client or less than 2 cm per hour in multiparous client; rule out CPD; assess contraction intensity and duration; labor may be augmented with oxytocin
   d. Secondary arrest of dilatation: cessation of dilatation for more than 2 hours in nulliparous client or more than 1 hour in multiparous client; rule out CPD and, if absent, augment labor with oxytocin
   e. Arrest of descent: no progress in fetal station for more than 1 hour; assess for CPD and, if absent, augment labor
4. Retraction rings
   a. Physiologic retraction ring is a boundary between upper and lower uterine segments that normally forms during labor; upper segment contracts and becomes thicker as muscle fibers shorten; lower segment distends and becomes thinner
   ! b. Bandl's ring: a pathological retraction ring that forms when labor is obstructed due to CPD or other complications; upper segment continues to thicken while lower segment continues to distend; risk of uterine rupture increases if contractions continue, so cesarean delivery is indicated
   c. Constriction ring: retraction ring forms and impedes fetal descent; relaxation of constriction ring with analgesics, anesthetics, or both allows vaginal delivery

C. ***Premature labor:* contractions occurring between 20 to 37 weeks gestation**

! 1. Client teaching for every woman about signs and symptoms of premature labor
   a. Contractions occurring every 10 minutes or less with or without pain
   b. Low abdominal cramping with or without diarrhea
   c. Intermittent sensation of pelvic pressure, urinary frequency
   d. Low backache (constant or intermittent)
   e. Increased vaginal discharge, may be pink-tinged
   f. Leaking amniotic fluid

2. Immediate actions to be taken by clients experiencing suspected premature labor
   a. Empty bladder
   b. Assume a side-lying position, left preferred
   c. Drink 3 to 4 cups of water
   d. Palpate abdomen for uterine contractions; if 10 minutes apart or closer, contact health care provider
   e. Rest for 30 minutes and slowly resume activity if symptoms disappear
   f. If symptoms do not subside within 1 hour, contact health care provider
3. Medical management
   a. Bedrest
   b. Continued monitoring of uterine activity and FHR
   c. Administer ordered **tocolytic agents,** drugs to stop contractions, if labor continues (see also Chapter 35), including ritodrine (Yutopar), terbutaline (Brethine), and magnesium sulfate
   d. Administration of betamethasone (Celestone) or dexamethasone to stimulate fetal lung maturity
4. Collaborative management
   a. Identify clients at risk for premature labor
   b. Provide client and family teaching regarding signs and management of premature labor
   c. Promote bedrest encouraging left lateral position
   d. Monitor uterine activity and FHR
   e. Administer tocolytics and monitor for adverse reactions
   f. Provide emotional support encouraging client and family to express feelings and concerns

D. ***Precipitate labor and birth:*** rapid labor (under 3 hours) resulting in precipitous (unattended or nurse attended) birth

1. Maternal risks: cervical, vaginal, or rectal lacerations and hemorrhage
2. Fetal risks: hypoxia (decreased perfusion to intervillous spaces), intracranial hemorrhage (rapid passage through the birth canal), and injury at birth
3. Collaborative management
   a. Identify client at risk for precipitous labor and birth
   b. Do not leave client; send someone or call for help
   c. Don sterile gloves if time allows
   d. Instruct client to pant or blow to decrease urge to push
   e. Support perineum with a sterile towel as crowning occurs
   f. Apply gentle pressure on fetal head to prevent rapid delivery; lacerations of perineum can occur and subdural or dural tears may occur with sudden expulsion of infant's head

Memory Aid

Remember to "protect the head" during a precipitous birth. Apply enough pressure to guide the descent and prevent rapid intracranial pressure changes within the infant's molded skull.

   g. After delivery of head, suction infant's mouth then nose with bulb syringe
   h. Check around infant's neck for possible tight umbilical cord; if present, cord must be clamped and cut before delivery

Memory Aid

Remember that the umbilical cord could choke the fetus and is dangerous. If, during delivery, the umbilical cord can't be loosened and slipped away from the infant's neck, two clamps should be applied to the cord and the cord should be cut between the clamps.

   i. Place hands on each side of infant's head and instruct client to push
   j. Gentle downward pressure facilitates birth of anterior shoulder
   k. Gentle upward traction facilitates birth of posterior shoulder
   l. Support infant's body with a towel during expulsion from birth canal

m. Suction and dry infant thoroughly
n. Place infant on mother's abdomen as soon as stable
o. Clamp and cut umbilical cord
p. Observe for signs of placental separation: gush of bright blood; lengthening of the cord
q. Gently pull cord while massaging fundus to deliver placenta
! r. Continue to massage fundus to prevent hemorrhage or put infant to breast
s. Inspect perineum for lacerations or tears

E. Uterine prolapse

1. Vigorous massage of fundus and pulling on umbilical cord to speed placental separation may cause prolapse of cervix and lower uterine segment through introitus
2. **Uterine inversion:** turning inside out of uterus
   a. Complete inversion: inverted uterus is visible outside introitus; is life-threatening because of severe hemorrhage and shock; uterus must be immediately replaced manually to stop blood loss
   b. Partial inversion: uterine fundus is partially inverted, impeding contraction and control of hemorrhage; is not visible but can be palpated; corrected by physician using a bimanual technique

F. ***Uterine rupture:*** tearing open or separation of uterine wall

1. Rare but serious complication, occurring in 1 in 1,500 to 2,000 births
2. Most common causes
   ! a. Separation of scar from previous classical cesarean
   b. Uterine trauma
   c. Intense uterine contractions
   d. Overstimulation of labor with oxytocin
   e. Difficult forceps-assisted birth
   f. External cephalic or internal version
3. Risk factors: multiparity, overdistension of uterus with multifetal pregnancy, malpresentation, or previous uterine surgery
4. Types
   a. Complete: extends through uterine wall into peritoneal cavity
   b. Incomplete: extends into peritoneum but not into peritoneal cavity; often due to partial separation of cesarean scar; may go unnoticed until repeat cesarean is performed
5. Collaborative management
   a. Attempt to prevent from occurring by identifying clients at risk and avoiding hyperstimulation of uterus during induction
   b. Assess for signs and symptoms that may be either silent or dramatic
   ! c. Assess for sudden, sharp, lower abdominal pain, tearing sensation, signs of shock, cessation of contractions, cessation of FHR
   d. Note that blood loss is often concealed and that fetal parts may be easily palpated through abdominal wall
! 6. Specific medical management depends on type of rupture
   a. Complete rupture requires management of shock, replacement of blood, and hysterectomy
   b. Incomplete rupture may require laparotomy, repair, and blood transfusion

V. PROBLEMS WITH MATERNAL PSYCHOLOGICAL STATUS

A. Factors influencing psyche of client in labor

1. Fear and anxiety
2. Perception of situation
3. Self-image
4. Preparation for childbirth
5. Support systems
6. Coping ability

B. Effects of fear and anxiety on labor progress

1. Epinephrine secreted in response to stress
2. Vascular changes divert blood from uterus to skeletal muscles

3. Oxygen and glucose supplies decrease with accumulation of lactic acid in uterine muscle
4. Higher perception of pain
5. Decrease in available energy supply to support effective contractions
6. Labor progress is slowed

C. Collaborative management

1. Assess client's past experiences with, preparation for, and expectations of labor and birth
2. ! Assess client's current coping behaviors and their effectiveness with current situation
3. Establish trusting relationship with client and family
4. ! Remain at bedside with client and family during labor
5. Encourage relaxation
6. Keep client and family informed about progress and procedures
7. ! Encourage positive coping behaviors and discourage negative ones
8. Promote self-image by praising efforts

VI. CESAREAN DELIVERY

A. Overview

1. Is delivery of infant by an abdominal incision
2. Purpose is to facilitate delivery to preserve health of mother and fetus
3. Number of cesarean births increased dramatically beginning in late 1970s and early 1980s
4. National goal of Healthy People 2010 is to reduce incidence from current rate (25% to 30%) to 15% of all deliveries
5. Major indications for cesarean delivery include dystocia or CPD, fetal distress, breech presentation, and previous cesarean birth

! **B. Maternal risks**

1. Aspiration or pulmonary embolism
2. Hemorrhage or infection
3. Injury to bowel or bladder
4. Thrombophlebitis

! **C. Fetal/neonatal risks**

1. Prematurity
2. Injury at birth
3. Respiratory problems caused by delayed absorption of fetal lung fluid

D. Surgical techniques

1. Skin incisions: vertical or Pfannenstiel's (transverse lower abdominal incision)
2. Uterine incisions
   a. Classical: through upper uterine segment
   b. Low cervical transverse: lower uterine segment
   c. Lower uterine segment vertical

E. Collaborative management

1. Determine reason for cesarean delivery
2. Assess client's understanding of indication, procedure, and implications for recovery from abdominal delivery
3. Assess whether cesarean birth was discussed in childbirth preparation classes
   a. Clients and families cope better if they have time to learn about cesarean birth
   b. Emergency cesarean birth increases anxiety and alters couple's expectations about childbirth
4. ! Preoperative care
   a. Assess NPO status (being NPO decreases risk of aspiration)
   b. Explain procedure so that client and family know what to expect
   c. Obtain client signature on consent form
   d. Perform abdominal prep
   e. Insert Foley catheter to prevent bladder trauma during surgery
   f. Start IV fluids using a large bore catheter

g. Administer an antacid either IV or PO to decrease risk of lung damage from aspirating acidic gastric contents during surgery
h. Administer antibiotics as ordered
i. Assist with positioning and administration of regional anesthesia if used

5. Intraoperative care
   a. Provide heated crib and supplies to receive newborn
   b. Provide immediate care to newborn or assist nursery personnel as needed
   c. Provide assistance to surgical team and immediate care for mother
6. Postoperative care
   a. Begin postanesthesia (recovery room) monitoring of vital signs, pulse oximetry, and cardiac monitoring; monitor vitals signs every 15 minutes for first hour and until stable
   b. Assess fundus for firmness and location (if boggy, massage until firm)
   c. Assess vaginal bleeding
   d. Assess abdominal dressing
   e. Assess catheter and urine output
   f. Turn, cough, and deep breathe hourly
   g. Assess for return of sensation post-anesthesia
   h. Administer medications for pain as needed
   i. Promote maternal–infant contact and bonding

F. ***Vaginal birth after cesarean (VBAC)***

1. Labor and vaginal birth after a previous cesarean is considered a safe option if indication for cesarean delivery is not likely to be repeated
2. Contraindications
   a. Previous classical incision into the uterus
   b. Large infant (over 4000 grams)
   c. Malpresentation
   d. Pelvic measurements inadequate
   e. Any fetal or placental problem that may require cesarean section
   f. Delivery in an alternative birth setting: access to a facility where emergency cesarean may be performed is necessary
3. Risks of VBAC
   a. Possible uterine rupture and hemorrhage: less likely to occur if previous uterine incision was in the lower uterine segment; risk of rupture is approximately 1%
   b. Failure of trial of labor, requiring a repeat cesarean
4. Benefits of VBAC
   a. Ability to experience labor and vaginal delivery, which is desired by some clients; success rates are approximately 70%
   b. Vaginal delivery is less costly than cesarean delivery with faster, easier recovery period and less risk of complications
   c. Does not preclude induction or augmentation of labor
5. Collaborative management
   a. Monitor uterine activity and progress in labor; identify deviations from normal progress in labor and report to physician (essential)
   b. Monitor FHR and response to contractions, identify and report indications of fetal distress quickly
   c. Provide teaching before onset of labor that early period of labor carries greatest risk of uterine rupture for VBAC clients
   d. Observe for indications of uterine rupture, including signs of shock or hemorrhage, report of "ripping or tearing" sensation or sharp uterine pain, abrupt cessation of contractions, abrupt onset of fetal distress, and more easily palpable fetus (lying outside uterus)
   e. Be alert and prepared for possible emergency cesarean delivery
   f. Provide support and encouragement for client attempting VBAC

PRACTICE TEST

Check Your NCLEX–RN® Exam I.Q. *You are ready for testing on this content if you can*

- Assess the client experiencing complications of labor and delivery.
- Provide care to the client experiencing complications of labor and delivery.
- Take action to prevent fetal distress during complications of labor and delivery.
- Evaluate client's response to interventions to treat complications of labor and delivery.
- Communicate effectively to increase client and family understanding of complications of labor and delivery.

PRACTICE TEST

1 The nurse caring for a high-risk client in labor observes the presence of variability of the fetal heart rate of 10 to 12 beats per minute as recorded by the internal fetal monitor. Which of the following conditions does the nurse suspect?

1. Fetal hypoxia
2. Fetal well-being
3. Umbilical cord compression
4. Uteroplacental insufficiency

2 The nurse locates fetal heart tones in the upper-right quadrant. This finding should cause suspicion that the fetus is in a(n)

1. Occiput posterior position.
2. Occiput transverse position.
3. Breech presentation.
4. Shoulder presentation.

3 A client's contractions have become less frequent and less intense in the past hour. Vaginal examination reveals 6 cm dilatation and 0 station, indicating there has been no change since the last examination over 2 hours ago. The nurse should take which of the following actions at this time?

1. Notify the physician of the last exam.
2. Continue to observe over the next hour for further progress.
3. Encourage the client to turn on her side and relax.
4. Anticipate the need for cesarean delivery.

4 A delivery of a client who has shoulder dystocia is best accomplished using the McRoberts maneuver. The nurse should have the client perform this maneuver by doing which of the following?

1. Flexing the thighs against the abdomen
2. Placing her legs in stirrups
3. Assuming a side-lying position for delivery
4. Sitting upright for delivery

5 The nurse explains to a client with premature labor that betamethasone (Celestone) is administered for which of the following purposes?

1. Stop uterine contractions.
2. Prevent infection.
3. Hasten fetal lung maturity.
4. Prevent cervical dilatation.

6 After teaching the client and her husband about premature labor, the nurse recognizes that the intervention was effective when the client states,

1. "I will call the office if I notice excessive fetal movement."
2. "I will come to the hospital if I have back pain."
3. "I will lie down and rest awhile if I notice watery vaginal discharge."
4. "I will call the office if I have abdominal cramps or pressure that does not go away after I drink 3 or 4 cups of liquid and rest for an hour."

7 The client is admitted in active labor with a breech presentation. Which of the following signs would indicate fetal distress?

1. Meconium-stained amniotic fluid
2. Fetal heart rate of 180 beats per minute
3. Mild variable decelerations
4. Increased fetal heart rate variability

8 A nulliparous client has not made any progress in cervical dilatation or station since she was 7 cm and 0 station over 2 hours ago. According to the labor graph, or Friedman curve, this represents

1. Prolonged deceleration phase.
2. Protracted active phase.
3. Arrest of descent.
4. Secondary arrest of dilatation.

9 The nurse explains to a client that the presence of a Bandl's ring, which the client overheard from the physician, will alter the client's plan of care because it is

1. A serious complication requiring cesarean section.
2. A constriction ring that may prolong labor.
3. The normal physiologic division between the upper and lower uterine segments.
4. An abnormal depression in the lower uterine segment.

10 The client in labor tells the nurse that she overheard the physician say she is having hypertonic uterine contractions. She is worried that this will harm the baby. The nurse explains that they could increase the risk of fetal distress because

1. Maternal exhaustion occurs, producing a build-up of lactic acids.
2. Umbilical cord compression occurs decreasing oxygen supply.
3. Increased uterine tone and frequent contractions interfere with blood flow from mother to fetus through the uterine arteries.
4. Placental separation may occur.

11 After the initial care following amniotomy, the nurse should include which of the following assessments every 2 hours?

1. Maternal blood pressure and pulse
2. Fetal movement
3. Color and consistency of amniotic fluid
4. Oral temperature

12 Which of the following conditions, if identified in the pregnant client's history, places her at increased risk for uterine inversion during the current labor and delivery?

1. Forceps delivery of the infant
2. Fundal pressure during delivery of the head and body
3. Precipitous birth of less than 3 hours duration
4. Traction on the umbilical cord and vigorous fundal massage in the third stage

13 Which of the following is the priority nursing goal in helping a client during a complicated labor?

1. Establish a trusting relationship
2. Ensure that the client knows what to expect
3. Prevent invasion of privacy
4. Prevent fear and anxiety

14 Late decelerations on the fetal monitor should cause the nurse to suspect which of the following conditions?

1. Head compression
2. Cord compression
3. Decreased uteroplacental blood flow
4. Close uterine contractions

15 A client asks what trial of labor means. Which of the following is the best response by the nurse?

1. "The doctor has decided to give you more time to make progress in labor before considering a cesarean delivery."
2. "You will be expected to make progress in the next hour or a cesarean will be done."
3. "Even though your pelvis is small, sometimes it is possible to deliver your baby vaginally."
4. "A cesarean delivery will be done because you have had a trial of labor and have not made much progress."

16 The nurse should suspect cephalopelvic disproportion after noting documentation about which of the following for a laboring client?

1. Pelvic outlet is less than 9 cm
2. Midpelvis is contracted
3. Fetal shoulders are too large to pass through the bony pelvis
4. Fetal head is too large to pass through the bony pelvis

17 The nurse explains to a pregnant client at 37 weeks gestation that a Bishop score is being completed to determine which of the following?

1. The client's readiness for labor
2. The fetus's readiness for labor
3. Progress during induction
4. Cervical changes in labor

18 Which of the following priority items should the nurse assess because of the potential impact on the laboring client's psychological status?

1. Attitude about parenting
2. Relationship with the client's own mother
3. Self-image
4. Beliefs about health

19 A client is experiencing contractions that occur every 3 to 4 minutes, of 35-second duration and mild intensity, during the active phase of labor. After making this assessment, the nurse suspects which of the following?

1. Hypertonic uterine dysfunction
2. Hypotonic uterine dysfunction
3. Normal uterine activity
4. Progressive labor pattern

20 In preparing the client in labor for vacuum extraction, it is important to teach her that the infant may initially have which of the following after delivery?

1. A large caput and bruising of the scalp
2. Red marks on the face
3. Edema of the face
4. Swelling of the eyes

ANSWERS & RATIONALES

1 **Answer: 2** Variability of fetal heart rate indicates fetal well-being. Loss of variability or decreased variability (less than 2 to 5 beats per minute) is associated with depression of the autonomic nervous system that regulates heart rate. Hypoxia can cause loss of variability of the FHR, as can maternal sedation and fetal sleep, though the latter two are less serious signs. The presence of variability is assessed by internal fetal monitoring, since there is less artifact that could be mistaken for variability of heart rate.
Cognitive Level: Analysis **Client Need:** Physiological Integrity: Physiological Adaptation **Integrated Process:** Nursing Process: Assessment **Content Area:** Maternal-Newborn **Strategy:** The core issue of the question is knowledge of the significance of variability in fetal heart rate. Recall that less or loss of variability may be a cause for concern, depending on the circumstance leading to it. Use nursing knowledge and the process of elimination to make your selection.

2 **Answer: 3** Fetal heart tones are heard loudest over the fetal back. In breech presentation, this tends to be above the umbilicus. Fetal heart tones are heard just below the midline of the umbilicus in shoulder presentation or transverse lie.
Cognitive Level: Analysis **Client Need:** Physiological Integrity: Physiological Adaptation **Integrated Process:** Nursing Process: Analysis **Content Area:** Maternal-Newborn **Strategy:** Specific knowledge related to fetal position and associated location of fetal heart sounds is needed to answer the question. Use nursing knowledge and the process of elimination to make your selection.

3 **Answer: 1** The nurse should suspect CPD because of the lack of progress since the last exam. The physician may assess the maternal pelvis by CT, MRI, or other means, or may stimulate contractions with oxytocin (Pitocin) opting for a trial of labor (TOL). Lack of progress may be caused by inadequate contractions and a vaginal delivery could be possible, so it is too early to anticipate cesarean delivery. Encouraging rest and continued observation will do nothing to resolve the problem.
Cognitive Level: Analysis **Client Need:** Physiological Integrity: Physiological Adaptation **Integrated Process:** Nursing Process: Implementation **Content Area:** Maternal-Newborn **Strategy:** The core issue of the question is recognition of lack of progress in labor and the nurse's decision-making ability once this is detected. Eliminate options 2 and 3 first because they do nothing to help labor progress again, and choose option 1 over 4 because there is not enough information yet to indicate that cesarean delivery is needed.

4 **Answer: 1** Flexing the thighs against the abdomen (McRoberts maneuver) increases the pelvic angle from symphysis pubis to sacrum and facilitates delivery by making the bony pelvis less restrictive.
Cognitive Level: Application **Client Need:** Physiological Integrity: Physiological Adaptation **Integrated Process:** Nursing Process: Implementation **Content Area:** Maternal-Newborn **Strategy:** Specific knowledge of McRoberts maneuver is needed to answer this question. Use nursing knowledge and the process of elimination to make your selection.

5 **Answer: 3** Corticosteroids such as betamethasone have been shown to enhance fetal lung maturity and prevent respiratory distress. Betamethasone does not stop labor or cervical changes. A side effect is increased risk of infection.
Cognitive Level: Application **Client Need:** Physiological Integrity: Pharmacological and Parenteral Therapies **Integrated Process:** Nursing Process: Implementation **Content Area:** Maternal-Newborn **Strategy:** Specific knowledge of the purpose of

betamethasone late in pregnancy is needed to answer this question. Use nursing knowledge and the process of elimination to make your selection.

6 **Answer: 4** Signs of premature labor may include abdominal cramping and pressure or persistent back pain. The client should be instructed to empty her bladder, lie down on her side, and drink 3 to 4 cups of water. If symptoms do not disappear within an hour, the health care provider should be notified. Unusual vaginal discharge should be reported sooner. Excessive fetal movement can sometimes indicate fetal distress but is not a sign of premature labor.
Cognitive Level: Analysis **Client Need:** Physiological Integrity: Physiological Adaptation **Integrated Process:** Teaching and Learning **Content Area:** Maternal-Newborn **Strategy:** The wording of the question tells you that the correct answer is an option that contains a true statement. Eliminate option 3 because this symptom should not be ignored and would not be relieved by rest. Eliminate option 1 because it does not have to do with labor, and eliminate option 2 because back pain may or may not indicate labor. Also, option 4 is very detailed and comprehensive, which is a clue that this is the correct choice.

7 **Answer: 2** Fetal heart rate greater than 160 beats per minutes is considered fetal tachycardia, an early sign of distress. Meconium passage often occurs in breech presentation because of pressure on the presenting part and is not an indication of fetal distress in this situation. Mild variable decelerations and increased variability are not indications of fetal distress and occur more frequently in breech presentations.
Cognitive Level: Analysis **Client Need:** Physiological Integrity: Physiological Adaptation **Integrated Process:** Nursing Process: Assessment **Content Area:** Maternal-Newborn **Strategy:** The core issue of this question is the ability to correlate knowledge of breech presentation with knowledge of fetal distress. Choose option 2 over the other options by recalling that the normal fetal heart rate (FHR) is 120 to 160 beats per minute. An FHR outside this range is generally a cause for concern regardless of the specific situation.

8 **Answer: 4** Dilatation has stopped (arrested) after considerable progress. Causes may be hypotonic uterine contractions, malposition, or cephalopelvic disproportion. The terms *prolonged* (option 1) and *protracted* (option 2) mean that progress occurs at a very slow rate. Arrest of descent (option 3) occurs when the station rather than cervical dilatation does not change.
Cognitive Level: Analysis **Client Need:** Physiological Integrity: Physiological Adaptation **Integrated Process:** Nursing Process: Assessment **Content Area:** Maternal-Newborn **Strategy:** Note the critical phrases *not made any progress* and *over 2 hours ago.* Correlate these phrases with the word *arrest* to eliminate options 1 and 2. Choose option 4 over 3 because dilatation has not changed and because the word *secondary* implies that labor was active at one time, which is true in this situation.

9 **Answer: 1** Bandl's ring forms when labor is obstructed. The upper uterine segment continues to thicken while the lower segment thins and retracts. If left untreated, uterine rupture can occur. Bandl's ring necessitates cesarean section.
Cognitive Level: Application **Client Need:** Physiological Integrity: Physiological Adaptation **Integrated Process:** Nursing Process: Implementation **Content Area:** Maternal-Newborn **Strategy:** Specific knowledge of Bandl's ring is needed to answer this question. Use nursing knowledge and the process of elimination to make your selection.

10 **Answer: 3** Frequent contractions and increased uterine muscle tone impede the blood flow through uterine arteries to the placenta. The incidence of umbilical cord compression is not increased, and hypertonic contractions are not necessarily associated with placental separation. While maternal exhaustion and lactic acid accumulation may occur over time, this does not immediately threaten fetal well-being.
Cognitive Level: Application **Client Need:** Physiological Integrity: Physiological Adaptation **Integrated Process:** Communication and Documentation **Content Area:** Maternal-Newborn **Strategy:** The core issue of the question is knowledge of how hypertonic uterine contractions affect the well-being of the fetus. Eliminate options 1 and 4 as least likely to happen, then eliminate option 2 because the cord may or may not be compressed depending on the position of the fetus.

11 **Answer: 4** The risk of infection is increased after rupture of membranes. Therefore, the nurse should assess for signs of infection, including fever, foul-smelling amniotic fluid, and tenderness. Blood pressure, pulse, and fetal movement are checked more often during active labor. Color and consistency of amniotic fluid is assessed immediately after rupture and each time the under pad is changed.
Cognitive Level: Application **Client Need:** Physiological Integrity: Physiological Adaptation **Integrated Process:** Nursing Process: Assessment **Content Area:** Maternal-Newborn **Strategy:** Recognize that the term *amniotomy* (*-otomy* means "cutting into") refers to artificial rupture of the membranes. Correlate this with increased risk for infection as a complication to choose option 4 as an indicator of infection.

12 **Answer: 4** Although not always preventable, uterine inversion can occur because of excessive traction on the umbilical cord during the third stage of labor with or without vigorous fundal massage to remove the placenta, especially if the placenta is implanted in the fundus. The other options are not associated with inversion.
Cognitive Level: Analysis **Client Need:** Physiological Integrity: Physiological Adaptation **Integrated Process:** Nursing Process: Analysis **Content Area:** Maternal Newborn **Strategy:** Specific knowledge of the etiology and risks of uterine inversion is needed to answer this question. Use nursing knowledge and the process of elimination to make your selection.

13 **Answer: 1** While all of the answers are appropriate goals, establishing a trusting relationship with the client and her family is a priority. In an emergency situation, the nurse may have little time to ensure that the client knows what to expect or to protect her privacy. It is not always possible to prevent fear and anxiety. A trusting relationship increases the likelihood of cooperation and compliance during a crisis.
Cognitive Level: Application **Client Need:** Psychosocial Integrity **Integrated Process:** Nursing Process: Planning **Content Area:**

Maternal-Newborn **Strategy:** Note the critical word *priority* in the question, which tells you all options may be partially or totally correct, and you must choose the most important one. A client experiencing a complicated labor is likely to experience both fear and lack of knowledge. Choose option 1 over the others because a trusting relationship is the foundation for assisting the client through the labor process and reducing fear and lack of knowledge.

14 **Answer: 3** Uteroplacental insufficiency (UPI) is believed to be the cause of late decelerations. The insufficiency or decreased uteroplacental blood flow leads to fetal hypoxia. Several factors, including maternal hypotension, anemia, vasoconstriction, uterine tetany, and dehydration, can be primary causes of UPI. Head compression (option 1) causes early deceleration, and cord compression (option 2) causes variable deceleration. Option 4 is incorrect because it may or may not lead to UPI and eventual late deceleration.
Cognitive Level: Analysis **Client Need:** Physiological Integrity: Physiological Adaptation **Integrated Process:** Nursing Process: Analysis **Content Area:** Maternal-Newborn **Strategy:** Specific knowledge of the significance of late decelerations is needed to answer this question. Use nursing knowledge and the process of elimination to make your selection.

15 **Answer: 1** A trial of labor means that the client will be followed closely and given more time to show progress before considering a cesarean. Options 2 and 3 make cesarean delivery seem inevitable and can increase the client's anxiety. Option 4 is incorrect because the client will be allowed to continue laboring as long as some progress is made.
Cognitive Level: Application **Client Need:** Physiological Integrity: Physiological Adaptation **Integrated Process:** Communication and Documentation **Content Area:** Maternal-Newborn **Strategy:** Eliminate option 4 because it provides knowledge to the client in retrospect, while nursing information is given in a current and timely manner whenever possible. Eliminate option 3 because it does not directly answer the client's question. Choose option 1 over option 2 because of the time frame and because there is an undercurrent of threat in the wording of the option.

16 **Answer: 4** Cephalopelvic disproportion (CPD) means that the fetal head is too large to pass through the bony pelvis. Options 1 and 2 refer to a smaller than normal pelvis but do not take into account the fetal head size. Option 3 refers to shoulder dystocia.
Cognitive Level: Analysis **Client Need:** Physiological Integrity: Physiological Adaptation **Integrated Process:** Nursing Process: Analysis **Content Area:** Maternal-Newborn **Strategy:** Specific knowledge of cephalopelvic disproportion is needed to answer this question. Use nursing knowledge and the process of elimination to make your selection.

17 **Answer: 1** The Bishop score, an assessment of the mother's physical readiness for labor, takes into account cervical dilatation, effacement, consistency, cervical position, and station before contractions begin. The higher the score, the more likely a client can be successfully induced.
Cognitive Level: Analysis **Client Need:** Physiological Integrity: Physiological Adaptation **Integrated Process:** Nursing Process: Implementation **Content Area:** Maternal-Newborn **Strategy:** Recall that a Bishop score focuses primarily on the mother rather than on the fetus, which eliminates option 2. Choose option 1 over options 3 and 4 because the stem indicates that the client is not yet in labor.

18 **Answer: 3** Self-image refers to how a client feels about herself. A positive self-image enables a client to deal with labor and delivery realistically, even in the event of complications. Research has shown that self-image impacts the laboring patient's psyche. Other options have not been identified as having a significant impact during labor.
Cognitive Level: Analysis **Client Need:** Psychosocial Integrity **Integrated Process:** Nursing Process: Assessment **Content Area:** Maternal-Newborn **Strategy:** Note that the focus of the question is on the client in active labor. With this in mind, choose option 3 because it is the only option that specifically relates to the client as it pertains to her current status.

19 **Answer: 2** Hypotonic uterine dysfunction occurs most often during the active phase. It is characterized by contractions that have become farther apart, less intense, and of shorter duration. Contractions are typically 2 to 3 minutes apart, strong, and last 45 to 60 seconds in the active phase of labor.
Cognitive Level: Analysis **Client Need:** Physiological Integrity: Physiological Adaptation **Integrated Process:** Nursing Process: Assessment **Content Area:** Maternal-Newborn **Strategy:** Note that the question contains the critical words *mild intensity* and *active phase.* Reasoning that active labor should be characterized by strong contractions, you would select option 2 because it contains the word *hypotonic.* Alternatively, eliminate options 3 and 4 because they are similar, and eliminate option 1 because the word *hypertonic* conveys the opposite of what the client in the question is experiencing.

20 **Answer: 1** Suction applied over the occiput commonly causes edema and bruising of the scalp. Although it may appear to be a deformity of the fetal head, the edema disappears in 2 to 3 days. Suction is not applied to the face (options 2, 3, and 4).
Cognitive Level: Application **Client Need:** Physiological Integrity: Physiological Adaptation **Integrated Process:** Nursing Process: Planning **Content Area:** Maternal-Newborn **Strategy:** Note the critical word *vacuum* in the stem of the question, and eliminate each of the incorrect options because they refer to a part of the face rather than to the occiput of the head.

Key Terms to Review

amnioinfusion p. 909
amniotomy p. 910
augmentation of labor p. 911
Bishop score p. 910
cephalopelvic disproportion (CPD) p. 910
cesarean section p. 97
dystocia p. 911
external cephalic version p. 907
hypertonic uterine dysfunction p. 911
hypotonic uterine dysfunction p. 911
induction of labor p. 910
intrauterine resuscitation p. 909
labor graph (Friedman's curve) p. 911
malpresentation p. 906
malposition p. 906
precipitate labor and birth p. 912
premature labor p. 911
tocolytic agents p. 912
trial of labor (TOL) p. 910
uterine inversion p. 913
uterine rupture p. 913
vaginal birth after cesarean (VBAC) p. 915

References

Condon, M. (2004). *Women's health: An integrated approach to wellness and illness.* Upper Saddle River, NJ: Pearson Education.

Lowdermilk, D., & Perry, S. (2004). *Maternity and women's health care* (8th ed.). St. Louis, MO: Elsevier Science.

Olds, S. B., London, M. L., & Davidson, M. (2004). *Maternal–newborn nursing & women's health care* (7th ed.). Upper Saddle River, NJ: Prentice Hall.

Davis, L. J., Okuboye, S., & Ferguson, S. L. (2000). Healthy people 2010: Examining a decade of maternal and infant health. *AWHONN Lifelines, 4*(3): 26–33.

52 Complicated Postpartum Care

Test Yourself

Are you ready for the NCLEX-RN® or course exams? Use the practice tests on the companion CD-ROM to check.

In this chapter

Cross reference

Other chapters relevant to this content area are

Reproduction, Family Planning, and Infertility	Chapter 9
Uncomplicated Antenatal Assessment and Care	Chapter 10
Uncomplicated Labor and Delivery	Chapter 11
Uncomplicated Postpartum Assessment and Care	Chapter 12
Uncomplicated Newborn Care	Chapter 13
Maternal and Newborn Medications	Chapter 34
Complicated Antenatal Care	Chapter 50
Complicated Labor and Delivery Care	Chapter 51
Complicated Newborn Care	Chapter 53

I. NURSING CARE OF THE HIGH-RISK POSTPARTUM CLIENT

! **A. Assessment**

1. Degree of homeostasis, amount of intrapartum blood loss, hematocrit, hemoglobin, and complete blood cell (CBC) count results
2. Vital signs: elevated temperature, blood pressure (BP), heart rate; low BP, symptoms of shock
3. Fundus: height, tone, and position
4. Lochia: amount, color, consistency, odor, and presence/size of clots (larger than quarter-size of concern)
5. Perineum: edema, ecchymosis, pain, hemorrhoids
6. Bladder: distension and displacement, ability to void
7. Bowel: constipation, distended abdomen, decreased or no bowel sounds (risk of ileus)
8. Breasts: cracked, bleeding, or blistered nipples; engorgement, red streaks, lumps, clogged milk ducts
9. Homan's sign (nonspecific), redness, tenderness, areas of heat in calves, severe abdominal or flank pain
10. Rest, activity tolerance
11. Bonding or attachment behaviors, maternal–infant interaction

B. Priority nursing diagnoses
1. Safe, effective care: risk for injury, risk for infection, deficient knowledge
2. Physiologic integrity: interrupted breast-feeding, deficient fluid volume, impaired gas exchange, fatigue, pain (perineal), imbalanced body temperature
3. Psychosocial integrity: fear, disturbed body image, ineffective coping, impaired adjustment
4. Health promotion/maintenance: self-care deficit, interrupted family processes, risk for impaired parent–infant attachment

C. Planning
1. Develop a nursing care plan that reflects knowledge of etiology, pathophysiology, and current clinical management for client experiencing a postpartum complication
2. The goal/expected outcome of care is that client will be free from undetected problems and will maintain physiological and psychosocial integrity

D. Implementation
1. Teach client normal adaptation
2. Observe for actual or potential problems in immediate postpartum period (first 2 hours after delivery) and continue into the later postpartum period
3. Administer treatment or medication as ordered
4. Educate client about signs of complications prior to discharge
5. Reinforce importance of keeping appointment for postpartum checkup
6. Provide client with telephone numbers to call to obtain answers to questions

II. POSTPARTUM HEMORRHAGE

A. Early-postpartum hemorrhage
1. Approximately one third of maternal deaths are related to postpartum hemorrhage
2. ! Definition: a blood loss greater than 500 mL in first 24 hours after vaginal delivery; may be greater with cesarean delivery
3. Predisposing factors: early postpartum hemorrhage occurs within first 24 hours of birth; at term, 600 mL/minute of blood perfuse pregnant uterus; most common causes are uterine atony (75%) and lacerations
4. **Uterine atony**
   a. ! Description: lack of uterine muscle tone; after birth, contraction of interlacing uterine muscles occludes open areas at site of placental attachment; absence of uterine contraction can cause significant blood loss
   b. ! Predisposing factors that overdistend uterus: delivery of a large infant, multiple gestation, hydramnios/polyhydramnios
   c. ! Predisposing factors that affect uterine contractility: multiparity, precipitous labor, dysfunctional or prolonged labor, prolonged third stage of labor, retained placental fragments
   d. Predisposing medications: general anesthesia, magnesium sulfate, oxytocin induction or augmentation of labor, tocolytics
   e. Predisposing maternal condition: low platelet count secondary to pregnancy-induced hypertension (PIH)
5. Lacerations
   a. Description: more common after operative obstetrics, a firm uterus with bright red blood or a steady stream or trickle of unclotted blood
   b. Types/locations: perineal, vaginal, cervical
   c. ! Predisposing factors: primiparous state, epidural anesthesia, precipitous childbirth, macrosomia, forceps or vacuum-assisted birth, mediolateral episiotomy
6. **Hematoma**
   a. Overview: a collection of blood, often vulvar or vaginal, that results from injury to a blood vessel during spontaneous delivery; in an assisted vaginal delivery, most common site is lateral wall in area of ischial spine
   b. ! Predisposing factors: prolonged pressure of fetal head on vaginal mucosa, operative delivery (forceps or vacuum extraction), prolonged second stage of labor, precipitous labor, macrosomia, pudendal anesthesia

7. **Disseminated intravascular coagulopathy (DIC)**
   a. Overview: complex disorder of clotting mechanisms in blood; consumption of clotting factors because of widespread clotting can lead to overwhelming and diffuse hemorrhage; oozing from puncture sites or development of petechiae may be initial clues of coagulopathy
   b. Predisposing factors: PIH, amniotic fluid embolism, sepsis, abruptio placentae, prolonged intrauterine fetal demise, excessive blood loss
8. Other causes of early postpartum hemorrhage: uterine rupture or uterine inversion

B. Late-postpartum hemorrhage
1. **Subinvolution:** failure of uterus to return to normal size after pregnancy
2. Late-postpartum hemorrhage occurs most often within 1 to 2 weeks after childbirth because of retention of placental tissue; blood loss may be excessive but usually poses less risk than immediate postpartum hemorrhage
3. Lochia often fails to progress from rubra to serosa to alba normally; lochia rubra that exists longer than 2 weeks is suggestive of subinvolution
4. Subinvolution is most commonly diagnosed at 4- to 6-week postpartum exam

C. Nursing assessment
1. Assess client's history and labor and delivery record for predisposing factors to postpartum hemorrhage
2. Assess vaginal bleeding after delivery every 10 to 15 minutes for 1 hour, then every 30 minutes for 1 hour until stable; more frequent assessments may be necessary depending upon client's condition
   a. Bleeding may be slow and continuous or rapid and profuse
   b. Blood may escape from vagina or pool in uterus and vagina, becoming evident as clots
   c. Bleeding from a laceration occurs in presence of a firm uterus and may be noted as a slow, steady trickle
   d. Large and numerous clots may occur
   e. Assist client to a side-lying position and check pad underneath frequently; blood may accumulate under client
   f. Weigh peri-pads to estimate blood loss if careful measurement is deemed necessary
3. Palpate fundus for firmness, assess for height in relation to umbilicus and position
4. Assess for signs of shock
5. Assess bladder for fullness and distension
6. Assess for pelvic pain or backache

D. Implementation
1. Remain with client
2. Massage boggy uterus gently but firmly, cupping uterus between two hands and avoiding overmassage
3. Administer uterine stimulants as prescribed to prevent or manage uterine atony and hemorrhage; these often include oxytocin (Pitocin) IV or IM, ergonovine maleate (Methergine) IM or PO (commonly used for subinvolution); or prostaglandin (Hemabate) IM; hypertension is a common adverse effect; see Chapter 35 for additional information
4. If bleeding is excessive, health care provider may perform bimanual massage
5. Monitor vital signs, intake and output (I & O), level of consciousness (LOC), fundal tone and placement, and amount of bleeding during episode of acute hemorrhage; elevate legs 15 to 30 degrees (modified Trendelenburg position)
6. Encourage frequent voiding to prevent bladder distension that contributes to uterine atony; a Foley catheter may be inserted or a bed pan may be used during postpartum hemorrhage
7. Replace fluids by IV and administer blood products as ordered
8. Assist with any preoperative preparation as necessary for surgical removal of placental fragments, ligation of bleeding vessel, suturing of laceration, or to correct more serious causes of bleeding, such as uterine rupture (see also Chapter 51)
9. Maintain asepsis
10. Ensure that surgical consent form is signed if necessary
11. Support significant other

III. POSTPARTUM INFECTIONS

A. Reproductive tract infections (see Table 52–1 ■)

1. Overview: any infection in reproductive system within 6 weeks of delivery; occurs after delivery in about 6% of births in United States
2. Predisposing factors: anemia, prolonged rupture of membranes, soft tissue trauma or hemorrhage, invasive procedures including internal fetal monitoring, multiple vaginal examinations, retention of placental fragments, chorioamnionitis, pre-existing bacterial vaginosis, manual removal of placenta, lapses in aseptic technique by staff, use of forceps or vacuum-extraction, and obesity
3. ! Cesarean delivery is single most significant risk, with infection occurring in 12% to 15% of cases
4. Localized infections of perineum, vulva, and vagina
   a. Local infection may extend through venous circulation, resulting in infectious thrombophlebitis or septicemia
   b. Local infection may extend through lymphatic vessels, resulting in **pelvic cellulitis/parametritis,** an infection involving connective tissue of broad ligament or connective tissue of all pelvic structures
   c. Can lead to **peritonitis,** an infection involving peritoneal cavity
5. **Endometritis or endomyometritis:** localized infection of uterine lining, usually beginning at the placental site; is a common complication after cesarean delivery; antibiotic prophylaxis at time of cord-clamping reduces incidence of postpartum endometritis in both elective and emergent cesarean sections
6. Bacterial causative agents are many and include *Escherichia coli, staphylococcus aureus, chlamydia trachomatis, beta-hemolytic streptococcus,* and others
7. Nursing assessment
   a. ! Temperature higher than 100.4°F on any 2 of first 10 days postpartum excluding first 24 hours
   b. ! Abnormal lochia: prolonged rubra phase, foul odor, scant or profuse in amount
   c. Tachycardia
   d. Delayed involution: fundal height does not descend as expected; uterus may feel larger and softer; pain or tenderness over uterus

Table 52–1 Summary of Specific Reproductive System Infections and Assessment Findings

Type of Infection	Assessment Findings
Metritis	Fever initially 101–102°F, (38.3–38.9°C); then jagged temperature elevations between 101 and 104°F (38.3 and 40°C) Uterine tenderness on palpation of fundus or on bimanual exam Grimacing, guarding, complaints of pain Prolonged or bothersome afterpains Subinvolution of uterus Positive bacteria culture of lochia
Parametrial cellulitis (parametritis)	Prolonged elevation of temperature to 102–104°F (38.9–40°C) with fluctuations Abdominal pain extending laterally; possible rebound tenderness Hypotension, subinvolution, chills Decreased bowel sounds, nausea, and vomiting
Peritonitis	Elevated temperature up to 105°F (40.5°C) Severe pain Paralytic ileus and abdominal rigidity; frequent vomiting with dehydration Possibly weak and thready pulse Rapid, shallow respirations Excessive thirst and marked anxiety
Septic pelvic thrombophlebitis	Elevation of temperature to 105°F (40.5°C); dramatic fluctuations (possible) over short periods Pain in flank or lower abdomen
Bacteremia and septic shock	Rapid elevation of temperature to 103–104°F (39.4–40°C) Profuse, foul-smelling lochia Symptoms of shock, including reduced urinary output

e. Pain, tenderness, or inflammation of perineum
f. Backache and chills
g. Malaise and fatigue
h. Abnormal laboratory results: increased sedimentation rate; leukocytosis—white blood cell (WBC) level of 14,000 to 16,000/mm^3 is not unusual during postpartum period; an increase in WBC level greater than 30% in a 6-hour period indicates infection

8. Implementation
   a. Administer antibiotics, analgesics, and antipyretics as ordered
   b. Promote comfort; change linen frequently
   c. Promote adequate nutrition and hydration (3000 to 4000 mL/day); monitor and record I & O
   d. Use aseptic technique and good handwashing; provide frequent perineal care and educate client in correct technique
   e. Assess vital signs; monitor laboratory results
   f. Assess fundus for involution and lochia; encourage semi-Fowler's position to facilitate drainage
   g. Promote adequate rest and sleep; allow family and friends to visit per client's wishes
   h. Encourage client to care for self first before taking care of baby; allow client to care for and feed infant per client's condition; provide client positive reinforcement

B. Wound infections

1. Description: infection of abdominal incision for cesarean delivery or episiotomy; infection rate following cesarean births is 4% to 12%, with highest rate occurring after emergency cesarean because of greater tissue trauma; culture of wound drainage frequently reveals mixed pathogens
2. Predisposing factors: obesity, diabetes mellitus, prolonged postpartum hospitalization, steroid therapy, immunosuppression
3. Nursing assessment
   a. REEDA assessment; see Box 52–1

Memory Aid

Use the mnemonic **REEDA!** See Box 52–1 to remember to assess episiotomies and wounds for **r**edness, **e**dema, **e**cchymosis, **d**ischarge, and **a**pproximation of wound edges.

   b. Generalized fever, localized tissue warmth
   c. Tenderness
4. Implementation
   a. Administer antibiotics, analgesics, and antipyretics as ordered
   b. Promote comfort, change linen frequently
   c. Promote adequate nutrition and hydration (3000 to 4000 mL/day); monitor and record I & O
   d. Use aseptic technique and good handwashing; provide frequent wound or perineal care; educate client in correct technique
   e. Assess vital signs; monitor laboratory results
   f. Assess incision or episiotomy site every 8 to 12 hours for signs of infection
   g. Promote adequate rest and sleep; allow family and friends to visit per client's wishes

Box 52–1

REEDA Assessment

Redness: erythema around wound

Edema: swelling of tissues

Ecchymosis: skin discoloration

Discharge: purulent drainage from incision site

Approximation of skin edges: gaping of the wound edges

h. Encourage client to care for self first before taking care of baby; allow client to care for and feed infant per client's condition; provide client positive reinforcement

C. **Breast infection (mastitis)**

1. Overview: an infection of breast connective tissue, primarily in women who are lactating; usual causative organisms are *Staphylococcus aureus, Escherichia coli, Streptococcus* species, and occasionally *Candida albicans*
2. Predisposing factors
   a. Traumatized tissue, fissured or cracked nipples
   b. Engorgement, milk stasis or poor drainage of milk, missed feedings
   c. Lowered maternal defenses caused by fatigue or stress
   d. Poor hygiene practices
   e. Tight clothing or poor support of pendulous breasts
3. ! Nursing assessment
   a. Breast consistency, nipple condition
   b. Warm, reddened, painful area
   c. Axillary lymph nodes enlarged or tender
   d. Flulike symptoms
   e. Generalized fever
4. Implementation
   a. Culture and sensitivity of breast milk may be ordered; note that infection usually is not transmitted to breast milk
   b. Administer antibiotics, analgesics, and antipyretics as ordered
   c. ! Promote comfort: a well-fitting, supportive bra is needed 24 hours a day
   d. Promote adequate nutrition, hydration, rest, and sleep
   e. ! Remind mother and staff to use good handwashing technique before handling breasts or assisting with breast-feeding; continue breast-feeding as advised by health care provider
   f. Assess vital signs as ordered
   g. ! Educate client regarding breast care, proper latch on, let-down reflex, necessity for frequent breast-feeding, signs of complications, and telephone numbers client can call with questions, provide client positive reinforcement
   h. ! Change position of infant for feeding to relieve pressure on same area of nipple; breast-feed frequently to prevent stasis of milk

D. **Urinary tract infections (UTI)**

1. Overview: occurs in 2% to 4% of postpartum women; infection can occur as **cystitis** (lower urinary tract infection) and often appears 2 to 3 days after birth, or as **pyelonephritis** (upper urinary tract infection); postdelivery urinary tract infections are usually caused by *E. coli* bacteria and generally occur soon after vaginal delivery
2. ! Predisposing factors
   a. Increased bladder capacity
   b. Decreased bladder sensitivity from stretching or trauma
   c. Possible inhibited neural control of bladder following use of general or regional anesthesia
   d. Contamination from catheterization
   e. Obesity
3. ! Nursing assessment
   a. Overdistension of bladder in early postpartum period
   b. Frequent urination of small amounts, burning, dysuria
   c. Hematuria
   d. Elevated temperature; low-grade temperature occurs with cystitis, higher fever occurs with pyelonephritis
   e. Flank pain (pyelonephritis)
   f. Costovertebral angle tenderness (pyelonephritis)
   g. Chills, nausea, vomiting (pyelonephritis)

4. Implementation
    a. Monitor bladder frequently during recovery period to institute preventative measures
    b. Culture and sensitivity of urine may be ordered prior to giving antibiotics
    c. Administer antibiotics as ordered; commonly sulfamethoxazole/trimethoprim (Bactrim), Macrodantin™
    d. Promote comfort; administer analgesic, antispasmodic, antipyretic medications
    e. Promote nutrition and hydration; increase oral fluids to 3000 to 4000 mL/day
    f. Assess vital signs as ordered
    g. Promote rest and sleep

IV. THROMBOEMBOLIC DISORDERS

A. Overview

1. Usually occur antepartally but are often considered a postpartum complication
2. When thrombus forms in response to inflammation in vein wall, it is called **thrombophlebitis;** in this type of thrombosis, the clot is more firmly attached and is less likely to result in an embolism
3. Thromboembolic disorders are more likely to occur after a cesarean birth

B. Contributing factors

1. Increased amounts of blood clotting factors in postpartum period
2. Postpartum thrombocytosis (increased quantity of circulating platelets and increased adhesiveness)
3. Release of thromboplastin substances from placental tissue and fetal membranes
4. Increased amounts of fibrinolysis inhibitors

C. Predisposing factors

1. Maternal factors such as obesity, increased maternal age, high parity, anemia, or hypothermia
2. Anesthesia or surgery resulting in vessel trauma or venous stasis, prolonged bedrest
3. Disorders such as heart disease, endometritis, varicosities or injury to leg, and history of deep vein thrombosis (DVT)

D. Types of thromboembolic disorders

1. Superficial thrombophlebitis (more common in the postpartum period)
2. DVT
    a. More frequently seen in women with a history of thrombosis
    b. Increased incidence in women with obstetric complications such as hydramnios, PIH, and operative birth
3. Septic pelvic thrombophlebitis
    a. Develops in conjunction with infections of reproductive tract
    b. More common in women with a cesarean birth
    c. DVT and septic pelvic thromboemboli predispose clients to pulmonary embolization

E. Nursing assessment

1. Superficial thrombophlebitis
    a. Symptoms become apparent about third or fourth postpartum day
    b. Tenderness is apparent in portion of vein
    c. Local heat and redness is present; may have low-grade fever
    d. Pulmonary embolism is extremely rare
2. Deep vein thrombosis
    a. Frequently occurs in women with history of thrombosis
    b. Characterized by edema of ankle and leg
    c. Initial low-grade fever followed by chills and high fever
    d. Pain located in lower leg or lower abdomen
    e. Homan's sign may or may not be positive, but pain results from calf pressure
    f. Peripheral pulses may or may not be decreased
    g. May result in pulmonary embolism; signs include dyspnea and chest pain, diagnosis may be verified by VQ (ventilation quotient) scan, blood gas studies, or x-ray

3. Septic pelvic thrombophlebitis
   a. Infection ascends upward along the venous system, and thrombophlebitis develops in uterine, ovarian, or hypogastric veins
   b. Usually unresponsive to antibiotics
   c. Characterized by abdominal or flank pain present with guarding
   d. Occurs on second to third postpartum day with fever and tachycardia
   e. Intermittent fever and chills may persist
   f. Pulmonary embolism may result; signs include dyspnea and chest pain, diagnosis may be verified by V/Q scan, blood gas studies, or x-ray

F. Implementation

1. Evaluate regarding need for support hose during labor and postpartum period
2. Encourage early ambulation following birth; women who have had a cesarean birth should perform regular leg exercises to promote venous return
3. If the diagnosis of DVT is made, monitor client for signs of pulmonary embolism
4. Monitor for signs of bleeding related to heparin or sodium warfarin (Coumadin) therapy, and keep protamine sulfate (antagonist for heparin) available; keep vitamin K available if receiving warfarin
5. Keep legs elevated and use warm, moist soaks if ordered
6. Obtain clotting times as ordered in client who is on anticoagulant therapy
7. Maintain bedrest as ordered; if client can get up, educate client to avoid standing or sitting for long periods of time; advise client against crossing legs
8. Review need for client to wear support stockings, if ordered, and to plan for rest periods with legs elevated
9. Promote increased fluid intake
10. Promote comfort
    a. Administer nonaspirin analgesic for pain
    b. Elevate extremities on pillow to decrease venous aching
    c. Promote adequate rest and sleep
11. Take serial measurements of both extremities daily to compare for any increase in swelling
12. Report to physician any heavy vaginal bleeding, generalized petechiae, bleeding from mucous membranes, hematuria, or oozing from venipuncture sites

V. POSTPARTUM PSYCHIATRIC DISORDERS

A. Overview

1. Various psychiatric problems may occur during postpartum period
2. *Adjustment reaction* with depressed mood is also known as postpartum, maternal, or baby blues; may be associated with rapid alteration in estrogen, progesterone, and prolactin levels after birth
   a. Is characterized by mild depression interspersed with happier feelings
   b. Typically occurs within a few days after baby's birth and is self-limiting, lasting from 1 to 10 days, more severe in primiparas
   c. New mothers feel overwhelmed, unable to cope, fatigued, anxious, irritable, and oversensitive; episodic tearfulness occurs without any reason
3. *Postpartum major mood disorder,* also known as postpartum depression
   a. Develops in about 8% to 26% of all postpartum women
   b. May occur anytime in first postpartum year, most often occurs around the fourth week
   c. Symptoms: sadness, frequent crying, insomnia, appetite change, difficulty concentrating and making decisions, feelings of worthlessness, obsessive thoughts of inadequacy as a person/parent, lack of interest in usual activities, lack of concern about personal appearance; possible irritability and hostility toward new baby
   d. Risk factors: primiparity, ambivalence about pregnancy, history of postpartum depression or bipolar illness, lack of social support or stable relationship with parents or partner, body image and eating disorders
   e. Treatment: medication, primarily selective serotonin reuptake inhibitors such as sertraline (Zoloft), paroxetine (Paxil), and fluoxetine (Prozac); only small

amounts of drug found in breast milk; individual or group psychotherapy, and practical assistance with child care and other demands of daily life

4. Postpartum psychosis
   a. Evident within the first 3 months postpartum
   b. Symptoms: agitation, hyperactivity, insomnia, mood lability, confusion, irrationality, difficulty remembering or concentrating, poor judgment, delusions, and hallucinations
   c. Risk factors: previous postpartum psychosis, history of bipolar disorder, prenatal stressors such as lack of support, obsessive personality, and a family history of mood disorder
   d. 10% to 25% recurrence rate in subsequent pregnancies
   e. Treatment: hospitalization, antipsychotic medications, sedatives, electroconvulsive therapy, removal of the infant, social support, and psychotherapy
5. *Postpartum onset panic disorder:* characterized by frightening panic attacks that include acute onset of anxiety, fear, rapid breathing, palpitations, and sense of doom

B. Nursing assessment

1. History of previous psychological problems
2. Adequacy of coping skills
3. Degree of self-esteem
4. Presence of mood swings, emotional distress, restlessness, irritability, guilt, extreme anxiety about the baby, anorexia, inability to complete activities of daily living, or trouble concentrating or expressing self

C. Implementation

1. Observe client with baby, by herself, and with family and friends
2. Recognize early signs of problems
3. Seek client referral to psychiatrist for evaluation of psychological status
4. Support positive parenting behaviors
5. Discuss client's plans for her baby and herself
6. Refer client to social services if indicated

Check Your NCLEX-RN® Exam I.Q. *You are ready for testing on this content if you can*

- Identify signs and symptoms of complications in the postpartum period.
- Implement nursing interventions to prevent postpartum complications or assist the client to recover from them.
- Perform client teaching about postpartum complications and their management.
- Evaluate the client and family response to therapy for postpartum complications.

PRACTICE TEST

1 The nurse determines that the postpartum client who is most at risk for postpartum hemorrhage is the client who delivered which of the following infants?

1. 5-pound 12-ounce infant
2. 6-pound infant after a 2-hour labor
3. 7-pound 6-ounce infant after a 9-hour labor
4. 8-pound infant after a 12-hour labor

2 The nurse is preparing for beginning-of-shift rounds on assigned postpartum clients. After reviewing the assignment, the nurse plans to assess for hematoma formation in which of the following clients who is at greatest risk for this postpartum complication?

1. A 17-year-old client who gave birth to a small-for-gestational-age infant
2. A 26-year-old client with gestational diabetes and forceps delivery of a large-for-gestational-age infant
3. A 35-year-old client having twins
4. A 40-year-old client having her first infant

3 The clinic nurse receives a telephone call from a 7-day postpartum client who states she is having increased vaginal bleeding and asks if it is serious and what could be causing it. The nurse suspects which of the following as the most common cause of this late-postpartum hemorrhage?

1. Uterine atony
2. Disseminated intravascular coagulation (DIC)
3. Retained placental fragments
4. Laceration

4 The postpartum nurse would utilize which of the following therapeutic measures to help prevent a urinary tract infection (UTI) in an assigned client who has just delivered an infant?

1. Promote bedrest for 12 hours postdelivery.
2. Discourage voiding until the bladder regains the sensation of being full.
3. Force fluids to at least 3000 mL per day.
4. Encourage the intake of orange, grapefruit, or apple juice.

5 A newly postpartum client is going into hypovolemic shock as a result of uterine inversion. Which initial order should the nurse expect to implement to restore fluid volume?

1. Administer oxygen at 3 to 4 L/min via nasal cannula.
2. Administer an oxytocic drug via IV.
3. Monitor heart rate every 5 minutes.
4. Increase the IV infusion rate.

6 A client delivered by vaginal birth after cesarean (VBAC). During postpartum recovery, she suddenly complains of severe pain in the abdomen and between her scapulae. She has a minimal amount of vaginal bleeding. The nurse's priority action should be to

1. Put the client in Trendelenburg.
2. Continue to assess for uterine atony.
3. Maintain the rate of IV fluids.
4. Notify the physician promptly.

7 The nurse interprets that which client would be classified as having early postpartum hemorrhage?

1. A client who had a blood loss of 350 mL in the first 24 hours after delivery
2. A client who had a blood loss of 700 mL in the first 48 hours after a cesarean delivery
3. A client with a greater than 500 mL blood loss in the first 24 hours postdelivery
4. A client with a blood loss of 500 mL in the first 48 hours postdelivery

8 To prevent early-postpartum hemorrhage in the woman who just had a cesarean birth, the recovery nurse should implement which of the following measures?

1. Maintain an IV rate of 125 mL/hr.
2. Assess the uterus for firmness every 15 minutes.
3. Assess abdominal dressing for drainage.
4. Monitor urinary output.

9 A client has been taking methylergonovine maleate (Methergine) for uterine subinvolution. It has not been effective in controlling late-postpartum hemorrhage. Which procedure does the clinic nurse anticipate will be ordered to correct the cause of this condition?

1. Dilatation and curettage
2. Laparotomy
3. Hysterotomy
4. Hysterectomy

10 The husband of a client who delivered 4 days ago calls the nurses' station stating that his wife is happy one minute and crying the next. He states, "She never was like this before the baby was born." The nurse's initial response should be to

1. Tell him to ignore the mood swings, they will go away.
2. Reassure him that this is normal in the postpartum period because of hormonal changes.
3. Advise him to contact a psychiatrist immediately; this is the first step in postpartum psychosis.
4. Instruct the husband in signs and symptoms of postpartum psychiatric disorders.

11 The postpartum nurse reviews the clinical assignment and determines that the client at greatest risk for early-postpartum hemorrhage is which of the following?

1. A client with an infant weighing 5 pounds 7 ounces
2. A client who is 17 years old
3. A client with endometritis
4. A client with uterine atony

PRACTICE TEST

12. While performing a postpartum assessment, the nurse notices the client's lochia is very heavy. Which of the following should be the nurse's first response?

1. Palpate and massage the uterus.
2. Elevate the head of the bed to Fowler's position.
3. Reevaluate in 10 minutes to see if the problem has corrected itself.
4. Place client in modified Trendelenburg position.

13. The postpartum nurse would use which of the following interventions as most effective in detecting the development of thrombophlebitis?

1. Monitoring the client's temperature
2. Assessing for Homan's sign
3. Asking the client if she has pain when the nurse massages her leg
4. Assessing for petechiae on the lower extremities

14. The nurse expects that the client's lochia and location of the uterine fundus on the second day after delivery would most likely be documented as which of the following?

1. Yellowish-white lochia with no clots and fundus three finger breadths below the umbilicus
2. Dark red lochia with small clots, fundus midline and two fingerbreadths below the umbilicus
3. Pinkish brown lochia with no clots, fundus midline and four fingerbreadths below the umbilicus
4. A large amount of bright red lochia with large clots, fundus midline and at the umbilicus

15. The clinic nurse working with women during the postpartum period would interpret that which of the following behaviors exhibited by a client is typical during this time?

1. The mother experiences feelings of depression as she assumes responsibility for her new baby.
2. The mother does not take care of herself but attends well to her infant.
3. The mother is receptive to learning about her baby and demonstrates bonding.
4. The mother does not sleep or eat well, but tries to take care of herself.

16. The nurse has been caring for a postpartum client diagnosed with a right labial hematoma. When planning care, the nurse should explain to the client that

1. A hot pack will be used to increase comfort and to decrease blood loss.
2. Witch hazel pads will be applied to reduce discomfort.
3. She needs to give informed consent for surgery to incise and drain the hematoma.
4. A cold pack will help to decrease bleeding and reduce the swelling.

17. A postpartum client develops thrombophlebitis in her right calf and is started on heparin therapy. Which of the following interventions would be most appropriate?

1. Encourage the client to ambulate to reduce lower extremity swelling.
2. Encourage the client to take salicylic acid (aspirin) for leg pain.
3. Instruct the client to remain on bedrest to reduce the possibility of embolism.
4. Inform the client that she will experience numbness in her leg for several months.

18. A postpartum client receiving heparin asks whether she can continue to breast-feed. Which of the following is the best advice for the nurse to give?

1. She should stop breast-feeding immediately.
2. She can continue to breast-feed but must assess the baby daily for ecchymotic spots.
3. Heparin will not affect the breast-feeding and requires no special precautions.
4. She should alternate breast- and bottle-feeding.

19 During a home visit, a postpartum client complains of a reddened, swollen, and tender breast 10 days after delivery. Based on this finding, the nurse would advise the client that

1. These symptoms suggest an inflammatory or infectious process and require immediate physician notification.
2. She should mention it to her physician at her 2-week checkup because it will be abnormal if it continues after 2 weeks.
3. This is normal breast engorgement and should subside within another week.
4. She has to stop breast-feeding immediately until the swelling and redness resolve on their own.

20 The postpartum nurse is caring for a client who developed disseminated intravascular coagulopathy (DIC) following a placenta previa. The nursing priority would be to

1. Assess Homan's sign hourly.
2. Frequently monitor her vaginal bleeding.
3. Administer antibiotics.
4. Monitor reflexes hourly.

21 The postpartum nurse is caring for a client with thrombophlebitis. The nurse monitors the client for which of the following symptoms of complications? Select all that apply.

1. Confusion
2. Sudden high fever
3. Dyspnea
4. Diaphoresis
5. Sudden onset of chills

ANSWERS & RATIONALES

1 **Answer: 2** A rapid labor and delivery may cause exhaustion of the uterine muscle and prevent contraction of the uterus after delivery, which controls the amount of bleeding. The infants in the other options either were not identified for length of labor (option 1) or were delivered after 9-hour and 12-hour labors (options 3 and 4).
Cognitive Level: Analysis **Client Need:** Physiological Integrity: Physiological Adaptation **Integrated Process:** Nursing Process: Analysis **Content Area:** Maternal-Newborn **Strategy:** First eliminate options that are similar (options 3 and 4) because they identify infants of similar size who were delivered within reasonably similar time frames. Choose option 2 over 1 because of the very short duration of labor.

2 **Answer: 2** A hematoma is a collection of blood in the pelvic tissue caused by damage to a vessel wall without laceration of the tissue. A gestational diabetic client is more prone to have a large baby that could cause tissue trauma during delivery. She had to be delivered with forceps, which is also another high-risk factor for developing a postpartum hematoma. Maternal age does not affect the development of a hematoma (options 1 and 4). The size of the newborn, rather than the number, determines risk for hematoma formation (option 3).
Cognitive Level: Analysis **Client Need:** Physiological Integrity: Physiological Adaptation **Integrated Process:** Nursing Process: Assessment **Content Area:** Maternal-Newborn **Strategy:** The core issue of the question is knowledge of fetal size at the time of delivery as a risk factor for hematoma formation. Eliminate option 1 first because of the infant's size; next eliminate option 3 because twins are more likely to be small than large. Choose option 2 over 4 because option 4 addresses age rather than size.

3 **Answer: 3** Late-postpartum hemorrhage occurs anytime after the first 24 hours postdelivery. The causes of early hemorrhage are uterine atony, DIC, hematomas, and lacerations. This leaves retained placental fragments as the cause for late-postpartum hemorrhage. The retained fragments undergo necrosis, forming fibrin deposits. These deposits form polyps, which eventually detach from the myometrium, causing hemorrhage.
Cognitive Level: Analysis **Client Need:** Physiological Integrity: Physiological Adaptation **Integrated Process:** Nursing Process: Analysis **Content Area:** Maternal-Newborn **Strategy:** Specific knowledge of how to discriminate etiology of early- and late-postpartum hemorrhage is needed to answer this question. Use nursing knowledge and the process of elimination to make your selection.

4 **Answer: 3** Adequate fluid intake (up to 3000 mL/day) prevents urinary stasis, dilutes urine, and flushes out waste products, all of which help to prevent UTI. Bedrest is of no value (option 1). The client should attempt to void every few hours rather than waiting to regain a sense of a full bladder (option 2). While intake of juices is healthy (option 4), it is the large volume of fluid consumed that aids in flushing out wastes.
Cognitive Level: Application **Client Need:** Physiological Integrity: Physiological Adaptation **Integrated Process:** Nursing Process: Implementation **Content Area:** Maternal-Newborn **Strategy:** The core issue of the question is knowing how to decrease risk for UTIs. Recall that increased fluid intake and intake of foods and beverages that yield acidic urine (cranberry juice, ascorbic acid in high doses) can decrease the risk. With this in mind, eliminate each of the incorrect options easily.

5 **Answer: 4** Increasing the rate of IV fluids is an effective initial measure necessary to replace lost fluid volume that occurs in uterine inversion caused by hemorrhage. Blood products may also be necessary but generally take some time to obtain from the blood bank. Oxygen would be given (option 1) also to increase perfusion to tissues but does not restore circulating volume. An oxytocic drug (option 2) will help to limit further bleeding but will not restore circulating volume. Monitoring pulse is an assessment and will not limit the condition (option 3); an intervention is needed in this situation.

Cognitive Level: Application **Client Need:** Physiological Integrity: Physiological Adaptation **Integrated Process:** Nursing Process: Planning **Content Area:** Maternal-Newborn **Strategy:** The core issue of the question is fluid volume replacement. Eliminate each of the incorrect options because they do not replace fluids, although they may be helpful in a specific way.

6 **Answer: 4** A common risk associated with VBAC is uterine rupture. Pain in the abdomen and between the scapulae may occur when the uterus ruptures, the hemorrhage is concealed, and blood accumulates under the diaphragm. This is an emergency and requires immediate medical intervention, which is initiated by calling the physician. The client may be put in modified Trendelenburg to manage shock, not Trendelenburg (option 1); uterine atony is not the problem (option 2); and IV fluids would be increased rather than maintained (option 3).

Cognitive Level: Application **Client Need:** Physiological Integrity: Physiological Adaptation **Integrated Process:** Nursing Process: Implementation **Content Area:** Maternal-Newborn **Strategy:** Note the core issue of the question is recognition of internal hemorrhage because of uterine rupture. Eliminate each of the incorrect options because they fail to provide effective treatment for this medical emergency.

7 **Answer: 3** The traditional definition of early postpartum hemorrhage after a vaginal birth is greater than 500 mL in the first 24 hours. With this in mind, each of the other options is incorrect.

Cognitive Level: Analysis **Client Need:** Physiological Integrity: Physiological Adaptation **Integrated Process:** Nursing Process: Assessment **Content Area:** Maternal-Newborn **Strategy:** The core issue of the question is an understanding of criteria for postpartum hemorrhage. Use nursing knowledge and the process of elimination to make your selection.

8 **Answer: 2** Maintaining contraction of the uterus is important in controlling bleeding from the placental site. Assessing the fundus every 15 minutes helps assure that this is taking place. Early detection of a boggy uterus can lead to actions that will prevent hemorrhage. While the other assessments may be appropriate for the client, they will not help to detect early-postpartum hemorrhage.

Cognitive Level: Application **Client Need:** Physiological Integrity: Physiological Adaptation **Integrated Process:** Nursing Process: Implementation **Content Area:** Maternal-Newborn **Strategy:** Note that the critical word in the question is *prevent.* Use the process of elimination to make a selection. Note that none of the incorrect options addresses the root cause of postpartum hemorrhage.

9 **Answer: 1** Late-postpartum hemorrhage most frequently occurs because of retained placental tissue. Dilatation and curettage is the vaginal procedure of choice to remove retained tissue from the uterus. The other procedures are abdominal surgeries and are not used to treat this condition.

Cognitive Level: Analysis **Client Need:** Physiological Integrity: Physiological Adaptation **Integrated Process:** Nursing Process: Planning **Content Area:** Maternal-Newborn **Strategy:** Consider first that the client is bleeding and determine the most likely cause, retained placental fragments. Then visualize each of the surgeries described and use the process of elimination and nursing knowledge to choose the one that will effectively treat the condition.

10 **Answer: 2** Before providing further instructions, explain that these are signs of postpartum blues, which is a normal process related to hormonal changes. Option 1 does not address the client's concern (in this case, the husband is the client). Option 3 is excessive, and option 4 is unnecessary and excessive.

Cognitive Level: Application **Client Need:** Psychosocial Integrity **Integrated Process:** Communication and Documentation **Content Area:** Maternal-Newborn **Strategy:** The core issue of the question is recognition and appropriate instruction regarding mood changes in the postpartum period. Use nursing knowledge and the process of elimination to make your selection.

11 **Answer: 4** Uterine atony accounts for 80% to 90% of all early (within first 24 hours) hemorrhage. Infants weighing between 5 and 7 pounds would not overdistend the uterus (option 1). The client's age (option 2) also does not increase the incidence of postpartum hemorrhage. Endometritis (option 3) could cause late-postpartum hemorrhage, not early hemorrhage.

Cognitive Level: Analysis **Client Need:** Physiological Integrity: Physiological Adaptation **Integrated Process:** Nursing Process: Analysis **Content Area:** Maternal-Newborn **Strategy:** First recall the causes of early postpartum hemorrhage, which may help you to easily select the correct option. Alternatively, eliminate option 3 first because it is a different postpartum complication, then option 1 because the baby is small, and finally option 2 because it is irrelevant.

12 **Answer: 1** Excessive bleeding must be evaluated and managed immediately to prevent excessive loss of blood and shock. Repositioning the client will do nothing. Waiting will only hurt the client. Bleeding should be assessed immediately.

Cognitive Level: Application **Client Need:** Physiological Integrity: Physiological Adaptation **Integrated Process:** Nursing Process: Implementation **Content Area:** Maternal-Newborn **Strategy:** The core issue of the question is knowledge of measures to reduce postpartum bleeding. With this in mind, eliminate option 3 first because it delays action. Choose option 1 over options 2 and 4 because positioning will not correct a boggy uterus.

13 **Answer: 2** Calf pain upon dorsiflexion of the foot indicates a positive Homan's sign, a sign of thrombophlebitis. If there is any question of thrombus formation, the legs, especially the calves, should not be massaged because doing so may dislodge a potential clot. Petechiae are not a clinical sign of thrombophlebitis.

Cognitive Level: Analysis **Client Need:** Physiological Integrity: Physiological Adaptation **Integrated Process:** Nursing Process: Assessment **Content Area:** Maternal-Newborn **Strategy:** Specific knowledge of assessment of thrombophlebitis is needed to answer this question. You can easily eliminate option 3 because legs should not be massaged and option 4 because the problem is not evidenced by bleeding into skin tissue. Choose option 2 over option 1 because it is a more specific sign than elevated temperature.

14 **Answer: 2** The fundus should be midline, two fingerbreadths below the umbilicus with dark red lochia, which may contain small clots. This explains lochia rubra. Option 1 explains lochia alba, which does not occur until about 10 days postpartum. Option 3 describes lochia serosa, which usually occurs between days 4 and 9 postpartum. Option 4 describes a complication of subinvolution.
Cognitive Level: Analysis **Client Need:** Physiological Integrity: Physiological Adaptation **Integrated Process:** Nursing Process: Assessment **Content Area:** Maternal-Newborn **Strategy:** Specific knowledge of changes in lochia during the postpartum period is needed to answer this question. Use nursing knowledge and the process of elimination to make your selection.

15 **Answer: 3** Option 3 indicates the mother is interacting with her infant and accepting responsibility for self-care and care of her infant. Options 1 and 2 indicate potential psychiatric problems, which require additional investigation. Option 4 requires investigation of why the mother is not eating well, which is important during the postpartum period.
Cognitive Level: Analysis **Client Need:** Psychosocial Integrity **Integrated Process:** Nursing Process: Assessment **Content Area:** Maternal-Newborn **Strategy:** The core issue of the question is healthy adaptation to life with a new infant. Choose the option that indicates the greatest resemblance to healthy behavior and adaptive coping.

16 **Answer: 4** Applying a cold pack will minimize swelling, bleeding, and discomfort. Labial hematomas do not necessarily need to be drained (option 3); they will usually resolve on their own. A hot pack is incorrect because it will increase engorgement at the site via vasodilation (option 1). Witch hazel will not decrease the swelling in the area (option 2).
Cognitive Level: Application **Client Need:** Physiological Integrity: Physiological Adaptation **Integrated Process:** Nursing Process: Implementation **Content Area:** Maternal-Newborn **Strategy:** The core issue of the question is knowledge of heat and cold applications to aid in reabsorption of hematoma. Use basic nursing knowledge and the process of elimination to make your selection.

17 **Answer: 3** Bedrest is recommended following a diagnosis of thrombophlebitis to help prevent an embolus. Clients receiving heparin therapy should avoid aspirin or nonsteroidal anti-inflammatory drugs because they will potentiate the action of heparin. Once the thrombophlebitis resolves, the client should not experience any residual effects.
Cognitive Level: Analysis **Client Need:** Physiological Integrity: Physiological Adaptation **Integrated Process:** Nursing Process: Implementation **Content Area:** Maternal-Newborn **Strategy:** The core issue of the question is knowledge of measures to prevent complications of thrombophlebitis. Note that options 1 and 3 are opposites, which means that one of them likely is correct. Use knowledge that activity can cause thrombi to yield emboli to choose option 3 over 1.

18 **Answer: 3** A woman can continue to breast-feed while on heparin. Heparin will not affect the breast-feeding and requires no special precautions. Heparin does not pass to the breast milk.
Cognitive Level: Application **Client Need:** Physiological Integrity: Physiological Adaptation **Integrated Process:** Nursing Process: Implementation **Content Area:** Maternal-Newborn **Strategy:** Specific knowledge of acceptable medication to use while breast-feeding is needed to answer this question. Use nursing knowledge and the process of elimination to make your selection.

19 **Answer: 1** These symptoms are suggestive of mastitis and require prompt attention by the client's physician. It is not therapeutic to wait for the symptoms to resolve on their own. Breast-feeding does not have to be stopped if mastitis is present.
Cognitive Level: Analysis **Client Need:** Physiological Integrity: Physiological Adaptation **Integrated Process:** Nursing Process: Assessment **Content Area:** Maternal-Newborn **Strategy:** The core issue of the question is recognition of mastitis and applying knowledge of appropriate intervention. Use nursing knowledge and the process of elimination to make your selection.

20 **Answer: 2** DIC is a disorder of widespread microvascular clotting that can then result in bleeding once clotting factors are consumed. Vaginal bleeding can be excessive if a coagulation disorder is present. Antibiotics will not affect a clotting disorder, DIC does not affect a client's reflexes, and Homan's sign is associated with thrombophlebitis, not DIC.
Cognitive Level: Analysis **Client Need:** Physiological Integrity: Physiological Adaptation **Integrated Process:** Nursing Process: Assessment **Content Area:** Maternal-Newborn **Strategy:** The core issue of the question is knowledge that DIC may be evidenced by bleeding once clotting factors have been consumed. When answering questions about DIC, look first for an option that addresses bleeding.

21 **Answer: 1, 3, 4** Symptoms of pulmonary embolus include sudden onset of dyspnea, chest pain, anxiety, diaphoresis, elevated pulse, and hypotension. Confusion can also occur because of decreased oxygenation to the brain resulting from loss of adequate gas exchange in the affected area of the lung. The client would not experience chills or fever; these are more indicative of infection.
Cognitive Level: Analysis **Client Need:** Physiological Integrity: Physiological Adaptation **Integrated Process:** Nursing Process: Assessment **Content Area:** Maternal-Newborn **Strategy:** Specific knowledge of manifestations of pulmonary embolism is needed to answer this question. Use nursing knowledge and the process of elimination to make your selection.

Key Words to Review

cystitis p. 927
disseminated intravascular coagulopathy p. 924
early-postpartum hemorrhage p. 923
endometritis/metritis p. 925
hematoma p. 923
late-postpartum hemorrhage p. 924
mastitis p. 927
pelvic cellulitis/parametritis p. 925
peritonitis p. 925
postpartum psychiatric disorders p. 929
pyelonephritis p. 927
subinvolution p. 924
thrombophlebitis p. 928
urinary tract infection p. 927
uterine atony p. 923

References

Ladewig, M., London, M., Moberly, S., & Olds, S. (2002). *Contemporary maternal newborn nursing care* (5th ed.). Upper Saddle River, NJ: Pearson Education.

Lowdermilk, D., & Perry, S. (2004). *Maternity and women's health care* (8th ed.). St. Louis, MO: Elsevier Science.

Mattson, S., & Smith, J. (2004). *Core curriculum for maternal newborn nursing* (3rd ed.). St. Louis, MO: Elsevier.

Olds, S. B., London, M. L., & Davidson, M. (2004). *Maternal-newborn nursing & women's health care* (7th ed.). Upper Saddle River, NJ: Pearson Education.

Complicated Newborn Care

53

In this chapter

Test Yourself

Are you ready for the NCLEX-RN® or course exams? Use the practice tests on the companion CD-ROM to check.

Cross reference

Other chapters relevant to this content area are

Reproduction, Family Planning, and Infertility	Chapter 9
Uncomplicated Antenatal Assessment and Care	Chapter 10
Uncomplicated Labor and Delivery	Chapter 11
Uncomplicated Postpartum Assessment and Care	Chapter 12
Uncomplicated Newborn Care	Chapter 13
Maternal and Newborn Medications	Chapter 34
Complicated Antenatal Care	Chapter 50
Complicated Labor and Delivery Care	Chapter 51
Complicated Postpartum Care	Chapter 52

I. GENERAL NURSING CARE OF THE HIGH-RISK NEWBORN

A. **Assessments that identify high-risk newborns**

1. Certain prenatal and intrapartal risk factors increase risk of neonatal complications after delivery
   a. Maternal preexisting diabetes or development of gestational diabetes during the pregnancy; a primary concern in infants of diabetic mothers (IDMs) is hypoglycemia after delivery
   b. Woman received opioid analgesics/anesthetics during labor, especially systemically and immediately before delivery; they cross placenta and can cause respiratory depression in neonate after delivery

c. Fetal asphyxia causes fetus to pass meconium into amniotic fluid, which could be aspirated during delivery; common causes include placental insufficiency, prolapsed cord, placental abruption, and placenta previa
d. Difficult or prolonged labor, which increases risk of birth trauma
e. Multiple gestation pregnancy
f. Preterm or postterm delivery
g. Life-threatening congenital anomalies
h. Maternal or neonatal infection
i. Small for gestational age (SGA) or large for gestational age (LGA)

! 2. Apgar scores: an Apgar score of less than 6 at 1 minute or 7 at 5 minutes indicates unsatisfactory transition to extrauterine life and requires careful monitoring

! 3. Changes in physical assessment are often vague, so thorough assessment is essential (see Box 53–1)

4. Gestational age
! a. Gestational age less than 37 weeks based on due date
b. Perform a quick assessment if due date unknown; follow up with a thorough gestational age assessment as soon as possible
c. Eyelids fused until 26 weeks gestation
d. Creases cover a third of soles of feet at 36 weeks gestation
e. Breast buds are absent until 37 weeks gestation
f. Ear cartilage has little recoil until 30 weeks gestation
g. Vernix covers body by 31 to 33 weeks gestation
h. Lanugo covers shoulders by 33 to 36 weeks gestation

B. General planning and implementation for all high-risk newborns

1. Constantly monitor infant for subtle changes in condition and intervene promptly when necessary

! 2. Decrease risk of nosocomial infections; provide each neonate with own supplies; handwashing is most important method of preventing infection

! 3. Conserve infant's energy and decrease physiologic stress by organizing care and minimizing interruptions; monitor each neonate for signs of stress

4. Provide appropriate stimulation for infant growth and development; high-risk neonates have same developmental needs as healthy neonate

5. Pulse oximeter; estimates arterial oxygen saturation through sensor placed on skin
a. Place sensor on palm of hand, sole of foot, or wrap around finger
! b. Assess skin integrity at sensor site every 4 hours and rotate site every 12 hours
! c. Pulse oximeter reading of 88% to 92% reflects safe clinical range

6. Arterial blood gas (ABG)
a. Direct measurement of amount of oxygen (O_2), carbon dioxide (CO_2), and select electrolytes in a sample of arterial blood by arterial puncture or from **umbilical arterial line (UAL)**
b. Compare oximeter reading at time of blood sample to correlate values
! c. Apply pressure to puncture site for 3 to 5 minutes if obtained by arterial puncture

Box 53–1

Critical Neonatal Assessment Indicators

The appearance of any of these signs in a neonate could indicate the presence of a serious complication:

- Respiratory: bradypnea or tachypnea, respiratory distress, weak or absent respiratory effort
- Cardiovascular: bradycardia or tachycardia, murmur
- Neuromuscular: lethargy, temperature instability, tremors, unusual behaviors such as lip-smacking
- Gastrointestinal: poor feeding tolerance, poor suck/swallow reflex
- Skin color: cyanosis (acrocyanosis is normal for the first 24 to 48 hours after delivery), jaundice (especially within the first 24 hours)
- Obvious major anomalies

7. Blood glucose monitoring (Dextrostick, Accucheck)
   a. Warm foot prior to obtaining blood sample to increase circulation
   b. Lance heel to obtain blood sample; heel is preferred site
8. Umbilical lines
   a. An umbilical arterial line (UAL) is inserted into an umbilical artery primarily to obtain ABG
   b. An **umbilical venous line (UVL)** is inserted into umbilical vein to give IV fluids and medications and to obtain blood for lab tests
   c. Assess all neonates with umbilical lines closely for blue discoloration or blanching on lower extremities or buttocks, which could indicate an embolus or vasospasm and may necessitate removal of line
   d. Assess closely for line placement, bleeding from umbilicus, or disconnected tubing; position infant in a side-lying or prone position for close monitoring
9. Oxygen administration
   a. Administered by **oxygen hood** (hood placed over infant's head), nasal cannula, **continuous positive airway pressure (CPAP)** (pressurized air), or endotracheal tube (ET)
   b. Warm and humidify O_2 prior to administration to decrease insensible fluid loss and heat loss
   c. Monitor amount of O_2 being administered and O_2 saturation and/or ABGs; administer minimum amount of O_2 to meet infant's O_2 needs to prevent complications
10. Gavage tubes
   a. Used to decompress stomach or administer formula, breast milk, or oral medications
   b. It is preferred to insert tube orally instead of nasally because infants are obligate nose-breathers
   c. A 5 Fr. or 8 Fr. tube is commonly used; measure tube from earlobe to nose and then to tip of xyphoid process; insert tube and secure placement
   d. Check placement of tube prior to administering any feeding or medication; administer feedings over 3 to 5 minutes to avoid dumping syndrome; offer a pacifier during feeding
11. Parenting the high-risk newborn
   a. Parents are initially in a state of shock and disbelief and may grieve loss of "perfect baby"
   b. Assess bonding
   c. Explain equipment and infant's condition
   d. Present positive, realistic attitude and establish trust
   e. Encourage parents to touch infant and perform care-taking activities as infant's condition allows
   f. Encourage parents to verbalize feelings
   g. Give Polaroid pictures of infant to parents prior to transfer to neonatal intensive care unit (NICU)
   h. Teach parents care of infant in preparation for discharge

II. PROBLEMS RELATED TO MATURITY

A. Prematurity

1. Description: infant born before completion of 37th week of pregnancy
   a. Prognosis and severity of complications related to level of maturity: the earlier infant is born, the greater chance of complications
   b. Earliest age of viability is 23 to 24 weeks gestation
   c. Major complications are related to **respiratory distress syndrome (RDS)**—a disorder caused by lack of surfactant—difficulty regulating body temperature, infection, and hemorrhage
   d. Generally ready for discharge near their due date
2. Etiology
   a. Maternal risk factors: age, smoking, poor nutrition, placental problems (placenta previa, placental abruption, preeclampsia/eclampsia), previous preterm delivery, incompetent cervix

b. Fetal risk factors: multiple gestation pregnancy, infection
c. Other risk factors: low socioeconomic status, environmental exposure to harmful substance

3. Respiratory assessment
a. Insufficient surfactant allows alveoli to collapse with each expiration
b. Inadequate number and maturity of alveoli makes adequate alveolar gas exchange difficult
c. Skeletal muscles weak so may not be able to reposition head and body to maintain patent airway
d. Signs of respiratory distress typically develop within 1 to 2 hours after delivery (see Box 53–2)

Memory Aid

Remember respiratory distress in a premature infant by the mnemonic SIN:
S Substernal retractions
I Inspiratory grunting
N Nasal flaring

e. Respiratory failure is most common cause of death in preterm infants within the first 72 hours of life

4. Respiratory interventions
a. Maintain respirations at 30 to 60/min, assess every 1 to 2 hours and prn (as needed)
b. Assess oxygenation and administer O_2 as ordered
c. Auscultate breath sounds
d. Monitor for signs of respiratory distress
e. Suction prn
f. Monitor O_2 saturation and/or ABGs

5. Assessment of thermoregulation
a. Lack of subcutaneous fat to insulate body and small muscle mass
b. Large body surface area in proportion to body weight, so more likely to lose heat quickly
c. Absent sweat or shiver mechanisms
d. Increased insensible fluid loss
e. Increased risk of hypothermia

6. Interventions to assist thermoregulation
a. Maintain **neutral thermal environment** (temperature that prevents heat loss) and prevent cold stress
b. Place infant under radiant warmer or in double-wall isolette
c. Warm equipment and linen before contact with infant
d. Generally, infant can be weaned to an open bassinet when temperature is stable and infant is gaining weight
e. Assess infant's temperature every 2 to 3 hours and prn

7. Low resistance to infection
a. Lack of immunoglobulins from mother (these usually cross placenta in third trimester)
b. Difficulty localizing infection and poor white blood cell (WBC) response
c. Increased risk of infection, so monitor carefully for signs of infection

Box 53–2

Signs of Neonatal Respiratory Distress

- Tachypnea
- Intercostal and/or subcostal retractions
- Nasal flaring
- Expiratory grunting
- Seesaw respiratory movements
- Diminished breath sounds
- PaO_2 less than 50 mm Hg
- PCO_2 above 60 mm Hg
- Increasing exhaustion
- Cyanosis (late finding)

8. Hepatic assessment
   a. Liver is immature at birth
   b. Increased risk of hyperbilirubinemia caused by difficulty in eliminating bilirubin released by normal breakdown of red blood cells (RBCs); monitor for jaundice
   c. Immature production of clotting factors resulting in increased risk of bleeding disorders
   d. Increased risk of hypoglycemia related to inadequate glucose stores
   e. Prolonged drug metabolism related to immature liver
9. Hematopoetic assessment: bruises easily related to fragile capillaries and prolonged prothrombin time
10. Gastrointestinal (GI) assessment
    a. ! Weak suck/swallow reflex until 33 to 34 weeks gestation and poor gag/cough reflexes increase risk of aspiration
    b. Increased risk of **necrotizing enterocolitis (NEC),** a neonatal disorder related to immature GI system and hypoxia
11. Feeding
    a. Feed according to abilities
    b. Assess tolerance of feedings
    c. ! Monitor suck/swallow reflex to assess the risk of aspiration; if poor, gavage feed as indicated
    d. ! Use "preemie" nipple if bottle feeding; burp frequently
    e. Assess for abdominal distention and emesis, which could indicate neonate is not tolerating feedings
    f. Monitor intake and output (I & O), daily weight; assess for dehydration
    g. Monitor for hypoglycemia
12. Renal assessment
    a. Unable to concentrate urine effectively, increasing the risk of dehydration
    b. Prolonged drug excretion time related to immature kidneys
13. Neuromuscular assessment
    a. Immature control of vital functions
    b. Increased risk of **intraventricular hemorrhage (IVH),** which is bleeding into ventricles of brain
    c. Increased risk of apnea
    d. Poor muscle tone and weak or absent reflexes
    e. Weak, feeble cry
14. Organize care to minimize stress
15. Provide skin care with special attention to cleanliness and careful positioning to prevent skin breakdown
16. Assess apical heart rate for 1 min every 1 to 2 hours
17. Monitor potential bleeding sites (umbilicus, injection sites)
18. Monitor overall growth and development; check daily weight, measure length and occipital frontal circumference (OFC) weekly
19. ! Monitor closely for medication side effects caused by decreased ability to metabolize and excrete medications

B. Potential complications related to prematurity

1. RDS, also known as hyaline membrane disease
   a. Usually appears during first 24 to 48 hours after birth and peaks around 72 hours
   b. Other predisposing factors include fetal hypoxia and postnatal hypothermia
   c. Protection against RDS can be achieved by administering prenatal betamethasone to mother to accelerate fetal lung maturity and artificial surfactant (Exosurf, Survanta) in infant's airway after delivery to keep alveoli from collapsing and causing atelectasis
2. **Bronchopulmonary dysplasia (BPD),** a chronic pulmonary disease requiring mechanical ventilation and high oxygen levels in first weeks of life
3. **Retinopathy of prematurity (ROP)**
   a. Etiology: prolonged exposure to high concentrations of O_2 causes hemorrhage within retina and leads to retinal detachment and loss of vision

!
b. Preventable with cautious administration of O_2; it is critical to administer minimum amount of O_2 needed to maintain a PaO_2 of 50 to 70 mm Hg
c. All premature infants who receive O_2 should be screened prior to discharge by an ophthalmologist

4. Intraventricular hemorrhage (IVH)
   a. Etiology: rupture of thin, fragile capillaries within ventricles of brain leading to increased intracranial pressure
   b. Prematurity and hypoxia are primary risk factors
   c. Assessment: neurological changes such as hypotonia and lethargy, bulging fontanels, increasing OFC, bradycardia, apnea
5. Necrotizing enterocolitis (NEC)
   a. Etiology: intestinal ischemia related to shunting of blood to brain and heart in response to fetal or neonatal distress
   b. Assessment: abdominal distention, poor feeding, vomiting, blood in stool
   c. Treatment involves nothing by mouth (NPO), IV fluids and antibiotics until intestines healed
6. Apnea and bradycardia
   a. Preterm neonates are at risk for apnea related to immature regulation of vital functions; if apnea is prolonged, eventually bradycardia occurs
   b. Infants almost always experience respiratory arrest before cardiac arrest; by supporting respiratory function, heart rate should return to normal range

   !
   c. If apnea occurs, first stimulate respirations with gentle tactile stimulation; if unsuccessful, reposition neonate, and finally, support respirations with a manual resuscitation bag if necessary

C. Postmaturity

1. Overview
   a. Born after completion of 42 weeks of pregnancy
   b. Problems caused by progressively less efficient actions of placenta
   c. At risk for birth injury related to dystocia
   d. Placental insufficiency may occur with an aging placenta that can no longer meet fetal needs; increases risk of fetal asphyxia that results in passage of meconium in utero and increased risk of **meconium aspiration syndrome (MAS),** inhalation of meconium into lungs
2. Nursing assessment
   a. Absence of vernix and minimal lanugo
   b. Dry, cracked skin related to metabolism of fat to meet energy needs in utero
   c. Hypoglycemia related to metabolism of glycogen to meet energy needs in utero
   d. Minimal subcutaneous fat
   e. Skin and cord yellow/green caused by meconium staining
   f. Long fingernails and often has scratches on face and trunk

!
3. Interventions: assess for presence of meconium at delivery, birth injuries, and hypoglycemia

III. PROBLEMS RELATED TO SIZE

A. Small for gestational age

1. Overview
   a. Defined as birth weight below 10th percentile (under 2500 grams or 5 pounds, 8 ounces)

Memory Aid

Remember that a low-birth-weight infant weighs 2500 grams (5 pounds 8 ounces) at birth or less.

!
   b. Etiology: placental insufficiency, infections, smoking, hypertension, malnutrition
2. Nursing assessment
   a. Skin: loose and dry, little fat or muscle mass
   b. Little scalp hair

c. Hypoglycemia
d. Weak cry
3. Interventions
a. Assess for presence of meconium during labor and delivery; thoroughly suction airway immediately after delivery if present
b. Assess temperature and provide neutral thermal environment
c. Assess for signs of hypoglycemia
d. Weigh daily and assess changes in weight
4. Outcomes: infant maintains stable temperature and blood glucose level and gains weight

B. Large for gestational age
1. Overview
a. Defined as birthweight above 90th percentile (over 4000 grams or 8 pounds 13 ounces)
b. Primary etiology: infant of diabetic mother (IDM)
2. Risks
a. Hyperbilirubinemia related to increased bilirubin released from damaged RBCs secondary to traumatic delivery
b. Birth injury: fractured clavicle, Erb-Duchenne paralysis secondary to shoulder dystocia
c. If preterm, risk for RDS
d. If postterm, risk for meconium aspiration
3. Nursing assessment
a. Macrosomia (large body size and high birthweight)
b. Signs of birth trauma related to cephalopelvic disproportion (CPD)
c. Hypoglycemia, especially in an IDM
4. Interventions: assess for signs of birth injury, and/or hypoglycemia

IV. PROBLEMS RELATED TO BIRTH TRAUMA

A. Facial paralysis
1. Etiology: temporary facial paralysis caused by pressure on facial nerve during delivery
2. Nursing assessment: face on affected side is unresponsive when neonate cries, eye remains open, forehead does not wrinkle
3. Self-resolves within hours or days of delivery; permanent paralysis is rare
4. Assess and support ability to feed orally

B. Erb-Duchenne paralysis
1. Definition: brachial paralysis of upper portion of arm
2. Etiology
a. Most common type of paralysis associated with difficult delivery
b. Paralysis is related to stretching or pulling head away from shoulder during difficult delivery
3. Nursing assessment
a. Flaccid arm with elbow extended and hand rotated inward
b. Moro reflex absent on affected side
c. Grasp reflex intact
4. Interventions
a. Intermittent immobilization
b. Brace, splint, or pin sleeve to mattress
c. Reposition every 2 to 3 hours
d. Delay range of motion until 10th day to prevent further damage

C. Fractures
1. Etiology
a. Clavicle is bone most frequently fractured during delivery
b. Other bones fractured during delivery are skull, humerus, and femur
c. CPD is often a predisposing factor
2. Nursing assessment (fractured clavicle): limited range of motion, crepitus over affected bone and absence of Moro reflex on affected side

3. Interventions (fractured clavicle)
   a. Instruct parents to handle affected arm gently
   b. Usually self-resolves

D. Asphyxia

1. Definition: inadequate tissue perfusion that fails to meet metabolic needs of tissues
2. Etiology
   a. Nonreassuring fetal heart rate (FHR) pattern during labor (late or variable decelerations, loss of variability, bradycardia), difficult delivery, prematurity, passage of meconium in utero
   b. Initial goal is to identify neonates at risk so resuscitation can begin immediately if necessary
3. Nursing assessment
   a. Fetal scalp pH during labor; 7.20 or less is considered ominous sign of fetal asphyxia
   b. Apgar score of 4 to 7 indicates need for stimulation; score less than 4 indicates need for resuscitation; resuscitative efforts should begin immediately if needed
   c. Passage of meconium prior to or during delivery
4. Interventions
   a. At delivery, hold neonate in head-down position and thoroughly suction mouth and nares
   b. Place neonate under prewarmed radiant warmer
   c. Stimulate respiratory effort by rubbing back and feet
   d. If respirations inadequate, place neonate in "sniffing" position; inflate neonate's lungs with positive pressure using bag and mask with 100% O_2 at rate of 40 to 60 breaths/min
   e. Once breathing established, check heart rate; if less than 60, or if 60 to 80 and not increasing, begin cardiac compressions; compress lower third of sternum with two fingertips or both thumbs at rate of 90 beats/min; use a 3:1 ratio of compressions to assisted ventilation; see also Chapter 69
   f. Administer as ordered resuscitative medications, primarily epinephrine, after 30 seconds of assisted ventilation and compressions if neonate's heart rate is not more than 80 beats/min
   g. Administer naloxone (Narcan) as ordered if mother received narcotics near time of delivery

V. GENERAL CARE OF THE NEONATE EXPERIENCING RESPIRATORY DISTRESS

A. Common causes of neonatal respiratory distress

1. RDS, typically in preterm infants
2. Meconium aspiration syndrome (MAS), typically in term and postterm infants
3. **Transient tachypnea of the newborn (TTN)** from delayed absorption of fluid in lungs from delivery; typically in term and postterm infants

B. Nursing assessment (see Box 53–2 again)

C. Interventions

1. Maintain neutral thermal environment due to increased O_2 demand if neonate is hypothermic
2. Administer warmed, humidified O_2 as ordered, generally attempting to keep O_2 saturation higher than 90% and PaO_2 between 50 and 70 mm Hg
3. Withhold oral feedings if respiratory rate is higher than 60 breaths/min because of increased risk of aspiration; notify health care provider
4. Position neonate side-lying or supine with neck slightly extended (sniffing position); arms at sides
5. Suction prn to maintain a patent airway
6. Monitor O_2 saturation and/or ABGs as ordered

D. Meconium aspiration syndrome

1. Definition: aspiration of meconium into tracheobronchial tree during first few breaths after delivery in a term neonate

2. Etiology
   a. Prenatal asphyxia causes increased fetal intestinal peristalsis, relaxed anal sphincter, and passage of meconium into amniotic fluid, which may be aspirated into lungs during first few breaths after delivery
   b. Meconium-stained fluid occurs in 8% to 13% of all pregnancies
   c. Meconium in lungs produces a ball-valve action (air is allowed in but cannot be exhaled) and is irritating to airway; as lungs become hyperinflated, pulmonary perfusion decreases, leading to increasing hypoxia
   d. Can lead to persistent pulmonary hypertension of the newborn (PPHN)
3. Nursing assessment
   a. May demonstrate signs of fetal distress during labor and delivery
   b. Apgar score less than 6 at 1 and 5 minutes
   c. ! Immediate signs of respiratory distress at delivery (cyanosis, tachypnea, retractions)
   d. Overdistended, barrel-shaped chest
   e. Diminished breath sounds
   f. Yellow staining of skin, nails, and umbilical cord
4. Interventions
   a. ! Suction baby's oropharynx then nasopharynx after neonate's head is born, and while shoulders and chest are still in birth canal, to remove as much meconium as possible before baby's first breath
   b. ! If meconium is thick in amniotic fluid, place neonate under radiant warmer, visualize glottis, and suction any meconium from trachea before stimulating respirations
   c. Administer O_2 to maintain adequate PO_2 and O_2 saturation
   d. Anticipate need for mechanical ventilation, high-frequency ventilation, or **extracorporeal membrane oxygenation (ECMO),** which is used for prolonged heart–lung bypass to allow lungs to heal
   e. Perform chest physiotherapy routinely

E. Transient tachypnea of the newborn

1. Etiology
   a. Failure to clear airway of excess lung fluid at delivery
   b. Primarily occurs in term infants, especially if delivered by cesarean because they have not experienced mechanical squeezing that occurs during vaginal delivery
2. Nursing assessment
   a. Expiratory grunting, nasal flaring, mild cyanosis
   b. ! Tachypnea by 6 hours of age, respiratory rate may climb to 100 to 140 breaths/min
3. Interventions
   a. Administer O_2 as needed to maintain PO_2 and O_2 saturation within normal limits
   b. Usually self-resolves within 72 hours

VI. CONGENITAL INFECTIONS

A. TORCH (see also Chapter 10)

1. Toxoplasmosis
   a. Overview: protozoan *Toxoplasma gondii;* contracted by mother's ingestion of raw or undercooked meat or contact with feces of infected cats; maternal–fetal transmission occurs during pregnancy
   b. Often results in spontaneous abortion if contracted during first trimester
   c. Severe neonatal disorders associated with congenital infection include convulsions, coma, microcephaly, and hydrocephalus
   d. ! Advise pregnant client to
      1) Practice good handwashing
      2) Avoid eating raw meat
      3) ! Avoid exposure to cat litter during pregnancy
      4) Have toxoplasma titer checked prenatally if cats live in the household
2. Other infections, usually hepatitis B (HBV)
   a. Transmitted from mother to neonate in about 90% of cases

b. Transmitted transplacentally and by contact with blood and body fluids
c. Associated with 32% increase in risk of preterm labor
d. Infected neonates may be symptom-free or have acute hepatitis, with a 75% mortality rate
e. Infants of mothers with positive HbsAg should receive hepatitis B immune globulin (HBIG) 0.5 mL IM within first 12 hours of life
f. Infants of mothers with positive HbsAg should also receive hepatitis B vaccine, with first dose within first 12 hours of life, second dose at 1 month, and third dose at 6 months
g. Centers for Disease Control (CDC) recommends all women be screened prenatally for HbsAg to determine newborns at risk

3. Rubella
   a. Overview: also called German measles; up to 20% of women of childbearing age are not rubella immune; a rubella titer of 1:8 or greater indicates immunity
   b. Eighty to ninety percent of fetuses exposed during first trimester will be affected by either spontaneous abortion or congenital anomalies
   c. Nursing assessment: clinical signs of congenital infections are congenital heart disease, **intrauterine growth restriction (IUGR)** or fetal undergrowth, and hearing loss
   d. Intervention: infants born with congenital rubella syndrome are infectious and should be isolated
4. Cytomegalovirus (CMV)
   a. Respiratory or sexual transmission; neonate can contract during delivery through an infected birth canal
   b. Most common cause of congenital viral infection (1% of all newborns); most (90% to 95%) are asymptomatic at birth; remaining 5% to 10% may experience hemolytic anemia and jaundice, hydrocephaly or microcephaly, pneumonitis, deafness, and fetal or neonatal death
   c. Disease is usually progressive through infancy and childhood
5. Herpes simplex virus (HSV)
   a. Overview: HSV type 1 or type 2
   b. Nursing assessment: maternal symptoms include vesicles on genitalia that are usually painful; fetal symptoms include fever or hypothermia, jaundice, seizures, poor feeding; 50% develop vesicular skin lesions
   c. There is no known cure
   d. Virus can be lethal to fetus and is transmitted during birth; cesarean delivery is indicated if mother has active lesions at time of delivery

B. Sexually transmitted infections, or STIs (see also Chapter 10)

1. Syphilis
   a. Overview: caused by *treponema palladium,* a spirochete, that crosses placenta after 16 weeks gestation and infects fetus; Langhans' layer in chorion prevents fetal infection early in pregnancy until this layer begins to atrophy between 16 and 18 weeks gestation
   b. There is no increased risk of anomalies, but spirochete may cause inflammatory and destructive changes in liver, spleen, kidneys, and bone marrow
   c. If syphilis is untreated during pregnancy, 25% will end in stillbirth and 40% to 50% of neonates will have symptomatic congenital syphilis
   d. Assessment: clients with syphilis have a positive rapid plasma reagin (RPR) test
2. Gonorrhea
   a. Causative organism is *Neisseria gonorrhea*
   b. Neonate can be exposed to organism during birth, which can result in sepsis or ophthalmia neonatorum, possibly leading to permanent blindness
   c. Penicillin is treatment of choice
   d. Eye prophylaxis with erythromycin (Ilotycin) ointment within 4 hours after birth decreases risk of ophthalmia neonatorum
3. Chlamydia
   a. Overview: most common sexually transmitted disease; caused by *Chlamydia trachomatis*

b. Can be transmitted to neonate during delivery and cause neonatal conjunctivitis and pneumonia
c. Eye prophylaxis with erythromycin ointment shortly after birth can prevent neonatal conjunctivitis; silver nitrate has been used prophylactically in past but is not effective against *Chlamydia trachomatis*

4. Candidiasis
   a. Overview: a neonatal oral yeast infection commonly called thrush; most commonly caused by vaginal *Candida albicans*
   b. Excessive yeast growth occurs more commonly in sick newborns and those receiving antibiotics or steroids
   c. Neonate may contract thrush during birth process or from contaminated hands or feeding equipment
   d. Nursing assessment: white patches on oral mucosa, gums, and tongue, which cannot be manually removed and may bleed when touched; occasional difficulty in swallowing
   e. Interventions: antifungal medications to affected area (feed sterile water prior to administration to rinse out milk); nystatin (Mycostatin) using medicine dropper or swab to mucosa, gums, and tongue after a feeding; Gentian violet swabbed over mucosa, gums, and tongue (avoid staining skin, clothes, and equipment)
5. HIV/AIDS
   a. Overview: transmission can occur across placenta during childbirth or through breastmilk or contaminated blood; transmission rate 20% to 30%; decreases by two thirds when zidovudine (AZT) given prenatally and intrapartally to mother, and to newborn after delivery
   b. It may take up to 15 months for infants to form their own antibodies against HIV
   c. For infants, average survival time between testing positive for HIV infection and death is 9 months, with a 70% to 80% mortality rate by 2 years of age
   d. HIV testing should be done at birth and 3 to 6 months of age
   e. Nursing assessment: typically asymptomatic at birth, failure to thrive with developmental delays, hepatomegaly and/or splenomegaly, lymphoid interstitial pneumonitis, recurrent infections, persistent thrush, chronic diarrhea
   f. Interventions: standard precautions; specific isolation not required; promote comfort; keep well nourished (bottle-feeding to prevent HIV transmission in breast milk); thorough cord care to prevent infection, prevent exposure to infections; provide all routine vaccines; (no live virus vaccines) give skin and mouth care; administer AZT as ordered

C. Sepsis

1. Overview: generalized infection that spreads rapidly through bloodstream; aided by immature neonatal immune system, inability to localize infection, and lack of IgM immunoglobulin (necessary to protect against bacteria and does not cross placenta)
2. Etiology
   a. Prolonged rupture of membranes
   b. Long, difficult labor
   c. Resuscitation and other invasive procedures
   d. Maternal infection
   e. Beta-hemolytic streptococcal vaginosis is most common cause of neonatal sepsis and meningitis; obtain cervical culture prior to delivery; if positive, antibiotics given during intrapartum period decrease risk of transmission
   f. Aspiration of amniotic fluid, formula, or mucus
   g. Nosocomial: caused by infected health care workers or equipment
3. Assessment
   a. Symptoms often vague initially
   b. Temperature instability, especially hypothermia
   c. Feeding intolerance as evidenced by decreased intake, abdominal distention, vomiting, poor sucking

d. Subtle behavior changes, "the infant just doesn't look right," lethargy, seizure activity, pallor
e. Progressive respiratory distress
f. Hyperbilirubinemia
g. Tachycardia initially, followed by periods of apnea and bradycardia

4. Interventions
   a. ! Obtain cultures (blood, urine, cerebral spinal fluid) before antibiotics are initiated
   b. Administer antibiotics as ordered
   c. After 72 hours of treatment, antibiotics may be discontinued if final culture reports are negative and symptoms have subsided; antibiotics are generally continued for 10 to 14 days if final culture reports are positive
   d. Observe for changes in vital signs and physical assessment

VII. COLD STRESS

A. Overview

1. Neonates produce body heat by nonshivering thermogenesis; this process requires increased O_2 and glucose consumption to burn brown fat
2. Subcutaneous fat acts as an insulator and helps conserve body heat
3. A flexed position decreases exposed surface area and conserves body heat
4. Can cause infant to develop hypoglycemia, hypoxemia, and acidosis

B. Etiology

1. Hypothermia because of large surface-area-to-mass ratio
2. ! Large amount of heat lost from head
3. All newborns are at risk for hypothermia, especially preterm and SGA infants

C. Interventions

1. Maintain neutral thermal environment
   a. Reduce or eliminate heat lost through drafts and contact with cold objects
   b. Postpone initial bath until temperature has stabilized
   c. Dry infant immediately after delivery and when bathing
2. Place newborn under servo-controlled warmer or on mother's abdomen immediately after delivery
3. Assess body temperature; keep axillary temperature 97.6° to 99.2°F
4. If axillary temperature is less than 97.6°F:
   a. Put hat on infant's head
   b. Wrap newborn with warm blankets
   c. Assess oxygenation status and assess for hypoglycemia
   d. ! Rewarm infant slowly to prevent hypotension and apnea
5. Chronic hypothermia could be an early sign of sepsis

VIII. HYPERBILIRUBINEMIA

A. Etiology

1. Bilirubin is formed by breakdown of hemoglobin from RBCs; direct (conjugated) is water-soluble and easier for body to eliminate, and indirect (unconjugated) is fat-soluble so it can more easily cross blood–brain barrier and is harder for body to eliminate
2. Before birth, unconjugated bilirubin is eliminated via placenta; after delivery, bilirubin converts from unconjugated to conjugated form in liver and is excreted via bile ducts into intestines; it can be reabsorbed from intestines if peristalsis slows
3. **Kernicterus** is a potential complication; bilirubin deposits in basal ganglia of brain and causes permanent impaired neurological function; bilirubin level, gestational age, condition, and poor fluid–caloric balance increase risk of kernicterus at low serum bilirubin levels

B. Physiologic jaundice

1. Healthy newborn has twice as much bilirubin as an adult related to higher concentration of circulating RBCs; immature liver has impaired ability to conjugate

bilirubin during transition from fetal to neonatal circulation; a shorter life span of fetal RBCs is also a factor

2. Factors that increase risk of physiologic jaundice
   a. Resolution of enclosed hemorrhage (cephalhematoma, large amount of bruising from difficult delivery)
   b. Infection
   c. Dehydration
   d. Sepsis
3. Physiologic jaundice usually begins after first 24 hours of life

C. Pathologic jaundice

1. Rh incompatibility (hemolytic anemia)
   a. RBCs from Rh-positive fetus enter Rh-negative maternal bloodstream late in pregnancy and after separation of placenta at delivery, causing maternal antibody formation, and destruction of fetal RBCs (erythroblastosis fetalis)
   b. In subsequent pregnancy with fetus of same blood type, maternal antibodies attack fetal RBCs, causing hemolysis and anemia
   c. RhoGAM prevents development of antibodies, but cannot reverse reaction once it occurs
   d. Hydrops fetalis is most severe hemolytic reaction, causing severe anemia, cardiac decompensation, edema, ascites, hypoxia, and possible fetal death
2. ABO blood type incompatibility (hemolytic anemia)
   a. Type O mother carries type A, B, or AB fetus
   b. Maternal antibodies cross placenta, enter and attack fetal RBCs, causing hemolysis and fetal anemia
   c. Reaction tends to be less severe than with Rh incompatibility
3. Pathologic jaundice begins within first 24 hours of life

D. Nursing assessment

1. Determine mother's blood type and Rh factor; if mother is Rh-negative or type O blood, determine infant's blood type and Rh factor
2. Evaluate results of Coombs' tests
   a. Indirect Coombs' determines presence of antibodies (sensitization) in maternal blood; a positive test indicates presence of antibodies
   b. Direct Coombs' determines presence of maternal Rh antibodies in fetal blood; cord blood is generally used; a positive test indicates presence of antibodies
3. Golden colored amniotic fluid indicates severe hemolytic disease
4. Assess for jaundice by gently pressing on sternum or forehead; in dark-skinned infants, assess sclera, palms of hands, soles of feet, nose, or palate

Memory Aid

Remember that natural light is best for assessing jaundice; apply slight pressure to blanche the forehead (preferred), tip of nose or gum line and watch for yellow discoloration when pressure is released.

5. Evaluate results of bilirubin levels
   a. Bilirubin can be assessed noninvasively with a bilimeter
   b. Total serum bilirubin levels higher than 13 to 15 mg/dL indicate hyperbilirubinemia
6. Enlarged liver and spleen
7. Anemia
8. Concentrated, dark urine

E. Interventions

1. Early and frequent feedings to stimulate peristalsis
2. **Phototherapy** (exposure of infant to bright light)
   a. Cover infant's closed eyes when under phototherapy light; remove eye covers every 2 hours during light therapy to assess for conjunctivitis and when not under phototherapy to promote bonding
   b. Undress infant to maximize amount of circulating blood exposed to phototherapy light; genitalia can be covered to prevent soiling

c. Change infant's position every 2 hours and assess for skin breakdown
d. Assess for loose green stools as bilirubin is excreted through intestines
e. Increase fluid intake to prevent dehydration
f. Assess temperature every 2 hours and monitor for hypothermia or hyperthermia
g. Monitor bilirubin levels

3. **Exchange transfusion**
a. Used to quickly decrease high bilirubin level by exchanging infant's circulating blood volume with donor blood; also removes anti-Rh antibodies and fetal cells coated with antibodies from infant's blood and corrects anemia
b. Only use Type O Rh-negative blood to decrease risk of transfusion reaction
c. Warm blood to room temperature to prevent cardiac arrest
d. Give calcium gluconate, as ordered, after each 100 mL
e. Assess vital signs before procedure, every 15 minutes during procedure and postprocedure
f. Record time, and amount of blood withdrawn, time and amount injected, medications given
g. Assess for dyspnea, listlessness, bleeding, cyanosis, bradycardia or arrythmias, hypoglycemia

IX. HYPOGLYCEMIA

A. Etiology

1. Definition: blood glucose lower than 30 to 35 mg/dL in a term newborn
2. Glucose levels are assessed with a heel-stick
3. Newborns at risk: IDM, SGA, premature, and infants experiencing cold stress, hypothermia, or delayed feedings
4. Poor prognosis if hypoglycemia is not treated
5. Blood glucose usually stabilizes within 48 to 72 hours

B. Nursing assessment

1. Tremors, jitteriness
2. Lethargy
3. Decreased muscle tone
4. Apnea
5. Anorexia

C. Interventions

1. Check blood glucose on all infants at risk by 1 hour of age (30 minutes if IDM) and any symptomatic newborn as ordered
2. Treat hypoglycemia by breast-feeding immediately or giving formula (avoid glucose water to prevent rebound hypoglycemia); do not feed a lethargic infant orally because of increased risk of aspiration; give lethargic infant dextrose via IV
3. If treated for hypoglycemia, reassess blood glucose level before next feeding

X. INFANT OF A DIABETIC MOTHER

A. Etiology

1. Hormones secreted during pregnancy (human placental lactogen, or HPL) increase maternal resistance to insulin, increasing insulin requirements; in diabetic clients, pancreas cannot secrete additional insulin and blood glucose levels increase
2. Maternal insulin cannot cross placenta but glucose can; fetal glucose levels rise; fetal pancreas secretes more insulin, which metabolizes additional glucose and acts as a growth hormone; increased insulin needs decrease surfactant production

B. Nursing assessment

1. LGA; birth trauma more likely
2. Maternal dystocia related to CPD
3. Enlarged internal organs: cardiomegaly, hepatomegaly, splenomegaly
4. Hypoglycemia
5. Hypocalcemia
6. Hyperbilirubinemia
7. RDS

! 8. False positive lecithin to sphingomyelin (L/S) ratio
9. Increased risk for congenital anomalies, particularly cardiac and spinal defects

C. Interventions

1. Assess for birth trauma
! 2. Assess blood glucose at 30 minutes and at 1, 2, 4, 6, 9, 12, and 24 hours after birth
3. Treat hypoglycemia per orders

XI. SUBSTANCE ABUSE

A. Fetal alcohol syndrome (FAS)

1. Etiology
   a. Alcohol crosses placenta and interferes with protein synthesis
   b. Increased risk of congenital anomalies, mental deficiency, intrauterine growth restriction (IUGR)
2. Nursing assessment
   a. Small for gestational age
   b. Facial features: epicanthal folds, maxillary hypoplasia, long and thin upper lip
   ! c. Irritable, hyperactive
   ! d. High-pitched cry
3. Interventions
   ! a. Reduce environmental stimuli
   ! b. Swaddle to increase feeling of security
   c. Administer sedatives as ordered to decrease side effects of withdrawal
   d. Maintain nutrition and hydration

B. Neonatal abstinence syndrome (NAS)

1. Etiology
   a. Repeated intrauterine absorption of drugs from maternal bloodstream causes fetal drug dependency
   b. Increased risk of spontaneous abortion, preterm labor, stillbirth
   c. Degree of drug withdrawal depends on type and duration of addiction and maternal drug levels at delivery
2. Nurisng assessment
   ! a. Hyperactivity, jitteriness
   b. Absence of "step" reflex and "head-righting" reflex
   c. Shrill, persistent crying
   d. Frequent yawning and sneezing; nasal stuffiness
   e. Respiratory distress
   f. Sweating
   ! g. Feeding difficulties (regurgitation, vomiting, and diarrhea), increased need for nonnutritive sucking
   h. Developmental delays
! 3. Interventions
   a. Position infant on side to facilitate drainage of mucus
   b. Suction prn to maintain patent airway
   c. Decrease environmental stimuli, swaddle for comfort

Memory Aid

Remember that infants are jittery during withdrawal. Create a soothing environment by keeping the room dark and quiet.

   d. Monitor I & O; measure daily weight
   e. Obtain meconium and/or urine for drug screening as ordered
   f. Administer medications as ordered: paregoric elixir to wean infant; chlorpromazine (Thorazine) and diazepam (Valium) to decrease hyperirritability (diazepam predisposes to hyperbilirubinemia and is contraindicated in jaundiced newborns); methadone; phenobarbital to decrease hyperirritability and hyperbilirubinemia
   g. Provide pacifier for nonnutritive sucking

PRACTICE TEST

Check Your NCLEX–RN® Exam I.Q.

You are ready for testing on this content if you can

- Identify signs and symptoms of neonatal complications after delivery.
- Implement nursing interventions to prevent neonatal complications or assist the client to recover from them.
- Teach mother about neonatal complications and their management.
- Evaluate the client and family response to therapy for neonatal complications.

PRACTICE TEST

1 The following neonates are admitted to the nursery. The nurse should withhold the scheduled initial feeding on which newborn?

1. A neonate with a sustained heart rate of 118 beats/min
2. A neonate with an axillary temperature of 97.5°F
3. A neonate with a sustained respiratory rate of 68 breaths/min
4. A neonate who is small for gestational age (SGA)

2 The nurse hears the parents of a 26-week-gestation newborn tell family members, "We'll be ready to bring the baby home in a few weeks." The most therapeutic response by the nurse is which of the following?

1. "I'm glad he's doing so well."
2. "He probably won't be ready to come home for a few months."
3. "A therapist could help you resolve your feelings of denial."
4. "Do you have the nursery ready yet?"

3 While observing the parents interact with their high-risk newborn, the nurse recognizes that teaching has been effective if the parents do which of the following?

1. Wear gloves every time they touch their baby.
2. Put family pictures in the isolette.
3. Bring a 2-year-old sibling to visit.
4. Turn off the cardiac monitor when at the newborn's bedside.

4 The nurse is developing a plan of care for an infant born at 28 weeks gestation. A realistic goal for this infant is that within 1 week the infant will

1. Drink from a bottle.
2. Recognize parents.
3. Maintain respiratory rate between 30 and 60 breaths/minute.
4. Maintain body temperature in a bassinet.

5 The nurse is making client assignments. Which baby could be appropriately assigned to an LPN/LVN?

1. An infant being admitted with hypoglycemia
2. An infant scheduled to receive blood this shift
3. A stable premature infant being fed every 2 hours
4. An infant with rising bilirubin levels

6 A newborn is receiving phototherapy for the treatment of hyperbilirubinemia. The nurse evaluates that teaching has been effective when the parents do which of the following?

1. Cover the infant with a blanket while under the bililights.
2. Stop breastfeeding because of the jaundice.
3. Limit the infant's formula intake due to loose green stools.
4. Cover the infant's eyes before placing under the bililight.

7 Which of the following would be most important to note as part of the initial assessment of a newborn's history?

1. Mother received meperidine (Demerol) 50 mg IV 20 minutes before delivery.
2. Mother reports drinking a glass of wine with dinner each night.
3. Mother's age is 14.
4. Mother's blood type is O negative.

8 The parents of a preterm neonate ask why their baby gets cold so easily. The nurse explains that preterm neonates

1. Are able to shiver to produce body heat.
2. Have minimal body fat to retain body heat.
3. Have blood vessels that are deep under the skin surface.
4. Lose heat faster because they lay in a fetal position.

9 While feeding an infant, the nurse notices white adherent patches on the infant's gums and buccal cavity. The nurse should take which of the following actions?

1. Document this normal finding.
2. Further evaluate for yeast infection.
3. Verify that vitamin K (Aqua-Mephyton) was given at delivery.
4. Assess for maternal history of herpes simplex.

10 Which of the following data would alert the nurse that the infant is experiencing dehydration?

1. Urine specific gravity 1.006
2. Urine volume 2 mL/kg/hr
3. Low serum sodium
4. Sunken anterior fontanel

11 A newborn male is admitted to the nursery 15 minutes after delivery. His skin is mottled and mucous membranes are blue; he is active and is wrapped in a blanket. The primary nursing assessment should be to assess which of the following?

1. Umbilical cord for bleeding
2. Infant's temperature
3. Visible deformities
4. Patent airway

12 Which nursing intervention is appropriate in the care of an infant with respiratory distress syndrome (RDS)?

1. Maintain a neutral thermal environment.
2. Perform a complete gestational age assessment.
3. Perform chest physiotherapy twice a day.
4. Suction meconium from airway as needed.

13 A 26-week-gestation neonate has received 80% to 100% oxygen via mechanical ventilation for 2 weeks and has received several blood transfusions for anemia. The nurse should plan for which of the following interventions?

1. Begin phototherapy.
2. Schedule eye exam by ophthalmologist prior to discharge.
3. Discontinue oxygen immediately.
4. Administer surfactant via the endotracheal tube.

14 The nurse is caring for an infant born to a mother who is HIV positive. Which sign in the newborn should be evaluated further?

1. Absence of tears
2. White bumps on nose
3. Enlarged liver
4. Fine, red rash over trunk

15 An infant of a diabetic mother (IDM) is admitted to the nursery. Which of the following is the priority nursing intervention at this time?

1. Clean the cord with alcohol.
2. Administer vitamin K (Aqua-Mephyton) intramuscularly.
3. Complete a gestational age assessment.
4. Assess the infant's blood glucose level.

16 A father asks how the bilirubin lights make the bilirubin level go down. The nurse's best reply is which of the following?

1. "The lights prevent more bilirubin from being released into your baby's body."
2. "Exposing the skin to the air helps get rid of the jaundice. The bililights really just keep the baby warm while this occurs."
3. "The bililights help convert the bilirubin to a form the baby can get rid of."
4. "The bililights release a substance in the body which attacks the bilirubin and destroys it."

17 The nurse assesses a 10-day old infant and obtains the following information: left arm limp and extended, left hand internally rotated, positive grasp reflex bilaterally, no response on left side to Moro reflex. What is the most appropriate nursing intervention for this infant?

1. Assess for congenital hip dysplasia
2. Turn infant to left side
3. Passive range of motion
4. Prepare supplies for a cast application

18 A neonatal nurse is attending a high-risk delivery and is told that the mother received morphine sulfate IV 30 minutes ago. The nurse should be prepared to give which of the following medications to the infant immediately after delivery?

1. Naloxone (Narcan)
2. Regular insulin
3. Double dose of vitamin K (Aqua-Mephyton)
4. Magnesium sulfate

19 Which of the following infants is at greatest risk for the nursing diagnosis of high risk for infection?

1. 38 weeks gestation, small for gestational age (SGA)
2. 39 weeks gestation, diagnosed with caput succedaneum
3. 38 weeks gestation, cesarean delivery for breech presentation
4. 41 weeks gestation, infant of a diabetic mother (IDM)

20 An infant with fetal alcohol syndrome is about to be discharged to home with foster parents. Place in order (without spaces or commas) the priority of the nurse in teaching the following topics to the foster parents.

1. Toy safety
2. Infection prevention
3. Feeding methods
4. Immunizations

ANSWERS & RATIONALES

1 **Answer: 3** Feeding a baby orally with a respiratory rate greater than 60 breaths/min increases the risk of aspiration. A heart rate of 118 is slightly below the normal range of 120 to 160 beats/min, but it is not a contraindication to feeding the infant. A hypothermic or SGA infant are both at risk for hypoglycemia and require a consistent source of glucose. **Cognitive Level:** Analysis **Client Need:** Physiological Integrity: Physiological Adaptation **Integrated Process:** Nursing Process: Analysis **Content Area:** Maternal-Newborn **Strategy:** Recall simply that breathing and swallowing cannot be done at the same time. This will help you to easily select the infant with an elevated respiratory rate as the one who is at risk if given feedings orally.

2 **Answer: 2** Families are often in a state of denial with the birth of a sick newborn. It is important for nurses to gently encourage the parents to be realistic. By agreeing with the parent's statement (option 1), the nurse is prolonging the state of denial and making it more difficult for the parents to see the situation realistically. Some parents do benefit from professional counseling, but nurses still need to provide support when working with families. It is not important if the nursery is ready yet (option 4) and this distracts from the real issues this family is facing at this time.
Cognitive Level: Application **Client Need:** Psychosocial Integrity **Integrated Process:** Communication and Documentation **Content Area:** Maternal-Newborn **Strategy:** Use knowledge of therapeutic communication techniques to answer the question. The correct response is one that provides factual information about the infant's status while respecting the parent's potentially vulnerable status.

3 **Answer: 2** The act of taping family pictures to the sides of the isolette promotes bonding and infant stimulation. Parents should wash their hands when they enter the unit but do not need to wear gloves when in contact with their infant. Young children often harbor organisms that could be transmitted to vulnerable newborns and should not have contact until the infant is moved out of the neonatal intensive care unit.
Cognitive Level: Analysis **Client Need:** Physiological Integrity: Physiological Adaptation **Integrated Process:** Nursing Process: Evaluation **Content Area:** Maternal-Newborn **Strategy:** The wording of the question tells you that the correct answer is an option that contains an appropriate action on the part of the parents. Use nursing knowledge and the process of elimination to make a selection.

4 **Answer: 3** A healthy respiratory rate for all newborns is 30 to 60 breaths/min. The other interventions are not timely for a 28-week-gestation infant at 1 week of age.
Cognitive Level: Application **Client Need:** Physiological Integrity: Physiological Adaptation **Integrated Process:** Nursing Process: Analysis **Content Area:** Maternal-Newborn **Strategy:** Specific knowledge of expected fetal development by gestational age is needed to answer this question. Use nursing knowledge and the process of elimination to make your selection.

5 **Answer: 3** An LPN/LVN is qualified to perform certain procedures and care for stable patients (option 3). An LPN/LVN is not qualified to admit a client, administer blood, or make nursing decisions based on changes in a client's assessment. The infants identified in the other options require assessment and care by a registered nurse.
Cognitive Level: Application **Client Need:** Safe Effective Care Environment: Management of Care **Integrated Process:** Nursing Process: Planning **Content Area:** Maternal-Newborn **Strategy:** Specific knowledge of scope of practice by RNs and LPNs/LVNs is needed to answer this question. Use this knowledge and the process of elimination to make your selection.

6 **Answer: 4** It is important to protect the infant's eyes from the bililight to prevent permanent damage. The infant should be unclothed to allow as much skin exposure to the bililight as possible. Breast-feeding is not contraindicated with hyperbilirubinemia. Loose green stools are a side effect of bilirubin excretion through the intestines.
Cognitive Level: Application **Client Need:** Physiological Integrity: Physiological Adaptation **Integrated Process:** Nursing Process: Evaluation **Content Area:** Maternal-Newborn **Strategy:** The core issue of the question is knowledge that the ultraviolet light used to treat jaundice can cause damage to the infant's retinas. Specific knowledge of treatment of jaundice is needed to answer this question. Use nursing knowledge and the process of elimination to make your selection.

7 **Answer: 1** Narcotics cross the placenta and, if given close to delivery, can cause respiratory depression in the newborn. The other three answers may warrant further investigation, but the priority at delivery is to establish and maintain an airway.

Cognitive Level: Analysis **Client Need:** Physiological Integrity: Physiological Adaptation **Integrated Process:** Nursing Process: Assessment **Content Area:** Maternal-Newborn **Strategy:** Note that critical words in the stem of the question are *most important.* This tells you that some or all of the options are correct, but you must select the priority option. Use nursing knowledge and the process of elimination to make your selection.

8 **Answer: 2** Preterm infants have minimal adipose tissue, so they lose heat more quickly through their skin. The skin is thin with blood vessels near the surface, which increases the amount of heat lost through their skin. Because they are weak and neurologically immature, they aren't able to lay in a tight fetal position, allowing exposure of a greater percentage of the body to the air, which causes heat loss. In general, infants are not able to shiver to produce body heat when they are cold.
Cognitive Level: Application **Client Need:** Physiological Integrity: Physiological Adaptation **Integrated Process:** Communication and Documentation **Content Area:** Maternal-Newborn **Strategy:** The wording of the question tells you that the correct option must be a true statement. Use knowledge about the physical characteristics of premature infants and the process of elimination to make your selection.

9 **Answer: 2** The primary sign of an oral yeast infection, or thrush, is the presence of white patches in the mouth that tend to bleed if they are touched. This is not a normal finding, and is unrelated to whether vitamin K was given at delivery, or maternal history of herpes simplex.
Cognitive Level: Application **Client Need:** Physiological Integrity: Physiological Adaptation **Integrated Process:** Nursing Process: Analysis **Content Area:** Maternal-Newborn **Strategy:** The core issue of the question is the significance of white patches in the infant's mouth. Eliminate option 1 because this is not a normal finding. Eliminate option 3 because vitamin K aids in blood clotting. Herpes simplex (cold sores) would present as vesicles, not white patches.

10 **Answer: 4** Signs of dehydration in an infant include dry mucous membranes, sunken fontanel, dry skin turgor. The other assessment data are expected findings in an infant.
Cognitive Level: Analysis **Client Need:** Physiological Integrity: Physiological Adaptation **Integrated Process:** Nursing Process: Analysis **Content Area:** Maternal-Newborn **Strategy:** Specific knowledge of manifestations of dehydration is needed to answer this question. Use nursing knowledge and the process of elimination to make your selection.

11 **Answer: 4** The highest priority after delivery is to maintain and support respiratory function. This infant is demonstrating initial signs of respiratory deficiency. Once this is done, the nurse may then check the umbilical cord for bleeding, measure temperature, and finally, check for visible deformities.
Cognitive Level: Analysis **Client Need:** Physiological Integrity: Physiological Adaptation **Integrated Process:** Nursing Process: Analysis **Content Area:** Maternal-Newborn **Strategy:** Follow the ABC's of resuscitation—airway, breathing, and circulation—to select the correct answer to this question. Airway and breathing are assessed before circulation (bleeding).

12 **Answer: 1** Infants use additional oxygen and glucose when faced with cold stress. Infants with RDS are already compromised, so it is important to keep environmental temperatures stable to minimize their oxygen and glucose requirements. A complete assessment could increase oxygenation requirements even further (option 2). Chest physiotherapy (option 3) may or may not be needed. There is no specific evidence in the question that meconium is present (option 4).
Cognitive Level: Analysis **Client Need:** Physiological Integrity: Physiological Adaptation **Integrated Process:** Nursing Process: Implementation **Content Area:** Maternal-Newborn **Strategy:** Note that the core issue of the question is care of an infant with respiratory distress. First eliminate option 2 because of the word *complete.* Choose option 1 over options 3 and 4 because there is no evidence in the question that these are needed.

13 **Answer: 2** This infant has been receiving high levels of oxygen for several weeks and is at risk for retinopathy of prematurity (ROP). All preterm infants who receive oxygen should have a thorough eye exam done by an ophthamologist prior to discharge. It is important to administer the minimum amount of oxygen to infants to decrease the risk that this condition will develop. Oxygen should be weaned and not withdrawn suddenly. Artificial surfactant may be administered within the first several days of life to decrease the risk of respiratory distress syndrome (RDS).
Cognitive Level: Application **Client Need:** Physiological Integrity: Physiological Adaptation **Integrated Process:** Nursing Process: Planning **Content Area:** Maternal-Newborn **Strategy:** The core issue of the question is knowledge of the effects of long-term oxygen therapy for a neonate. Use nursing knowledge and the process of elimination to make your selection.

14 **Answer: 3** Hepatosplenomegaly (enlarged liver and spleen) may be an early sign of HIV infection in an infant. All other assessment data are within normal limits.
Cognitive Level: Application **Client Need:** Physiological Integrity: Physiological Adaptation **Integrated Process:** Nursing Process: Analysis **Content Area:** Maternal-Newborn **Strategy:** The core issue of the question is discriminating normal from abnormal findings in a newborn born to a mother who is HIV positive. Use nursing knowledge and the process of elimination to make your selection.

15 **Answer: 4** An infant of a diabetic mother is at risk for hypoglycemia and should be monitored closely after delivery. All other interventions are important but are not the highest priority. Therefore, these can be completed once the blood glucose level has been measured and treated if necessary.
Cognitive Level: Application **Client Need:** Physiological Integrity: Physiological Adaptation **Integrated Process:** Nursing Process: Implementation **Content Area:** Maternal-Newborn **Strategy:** Note critical word *priority* in the stem of the question. This tells you that more than one or all options are technically correct, but you must decide which has the greatest importance at this time. Note the connection between the word *diabetic* in the stem and the word *glucose* in the correct option to help you make a selection.

16 **Answer: 3** Phototherapy assists the body in converting unconjugated bilirubin to conjugated bilirubin, which is water soluble and easier for the body to eliminate. The other statements do not reflect accurate explanations.
Cognitive Level: Application **Client Need:** Physiological Integrity: Physiological Adaptation **Integrated Process:** Communication

and Documentation **Content Area:** Maternal-Newborn **Strategy:** The core issue of the question is knowledge of how phototherapy assists in lowering the bilirubin levels of a jaundiced newborn. Use nursing knowledge and the process of elimination to make your selection.

17 **Answer: 3** This infant has signs of Erb-Duchenne paralysis. It is important to provide passive range of motion on the affected side to prevent muscle wasting. The infant should not be positioned on the affected side. Occasionally, a splint may be applied, but a cast is not indicated.
Cognitive Level: Analysis **Client Need:** Physiological Integrity: Physiological Adaptation **Integrated Process:** Nursing Process: Implementation **Content Area:** Maternal-Newborn **Strategy:** The core issue of this question is recognition of and appropriate intervention for an infant with Erb-Duchenne paralysis. Use nursing knowledge and the process of elimination to make your selection.

18 **Answer: 1** Narcotics cross the placenta and can cause respiratory depression in a neonate when given shortly before delivery. Naloxone (Narcan) is the drug of choice to reverse respiratory depression in the neonate caused by narcotics. Insulin would be given for hyperglycemia. Double doses of vitamin K are not given. Magnesium sulfate is given to the mother prevent eclampsia.
Cognitive Level: Application **Client Need:** Physiological Integrity: Pharmacological and Parenteral Therapies **Integrated Process:** Nursing Process: Planning **Content Area:** Maternal-Newborn **Strategy:** The core issue of the question is knowledge of adverse effects of morphine sulfate. Use nursing knowledge and the process of elimination to make your selection. The wording of the question tells you that there is only one correct option.

19 **Answer: 1** SGA infants often experience intrauterine growth restriction related to decreased blood flow to the placenta, which increases their risk for infection. In comparison, the infants in the other options are at less risk for infection.
Cognitive Level: Analysis **Client Need:** Physiological Integrity: Physiological Adaptation **Integrated Process:** Nursing Process: Analysis **Content Area:** Maternal-Newborn **Strategy:** The wording of the question tells you the correct answer is the infant who is at greatest risk for infection. Knowledge of the relative risk for infection in each of the neonates listed is needed to answer this question. Use nursing knowledge and the process of elimination to make your selection.

20 **Answer: 3241** Infants with fetal alcohol syndrome have an increased risk of feeding difficulties related to hyperactivity. Nutrition is a key concern for this infant for proper growth and development. Infection prevention is the next concern, since this will help to maintain healthy physiological condition. The immunization schedule has third priority because it is also related to prevention of communicable diseases and infection. Finally, although toy safety is important, it is the fourth priority because newborns are not developed sufficiently to play with toys.
Cognitive Level: Analysis **Client Need:** Physiological Integrity: Physiological Adaptation **Integrated Process:** Nursing Process: Planning **Content Area:** Maternal-Newborn **Strategy:** Use Maslow's hierarchy of needs to guide priority setting. Physiological needs come first, followed by safety needs, then psychosocial needs.

ANSWERS & RATIONALES

Key Terms to Review

bronchopulmonary dysplasia (BPD) p. 941
continuous positive airway pressure (CPAP) p. 939
exchange transfusion p. 950
extracorporeal membrane oxygenation (ECMO) p. 945
intrauterine growth restriction (IUGR) p. 946
intraventricular hemorrhage (IVH) p. 941
kernicterus p. 948
meconium aspiration syndrome (MAS) p. 942
necrotizing enterocolitis (NEC) p. 941
neutral thermal environment p. 940
oxygen hood p. 939
phototherapy p. 949
retinopathy of prematurity (ROP) p. 941
respiratory distress syndrome (RDS) p. 939
transient tachypnea of the newborn (TTN) p. 944
umbilical arterial line (UAL) p. 938
umbilical venous line (UVL) p. 939

References

Condon, M. (2004). *Women's health: An integrated approach to wellness and illness.* Upper Saddle River, NJ: Pearson Education.

Ladewig, P., London, M., & Davidson, M. (2006). *Contemporary maternal newborn nursing care* (6th ed.). Upper Saddle River, NJ: Pearson Education.

Lowdermilk, D., & Perry, S. (2004). *Maternity and women's health care* (8th ed.). St. Louis, MO: Elsevier Science.

Olds, S. B., London, M. L., & Davidson, M. (2004). *Maternal-newborn nursing and women's health care* (7th ed.). Upper Saddle River, NJ: Pearson Education.

Fluid and Electrolyte Imbalances

54

In this chapter

Cross reference

Other chapters relevant to this content area are

Meeting Nutritional Needs	Chapter 26
Common Laboratory Tests	Chapter 47

Test Yourself

Are you ready for the NCLEX-RN® or course exams? Use the practice tests on the companion CD-ROM to check.

I. CONCEPTS OF FLUID AND ELECTROLYTE BALANCE

A. Fluid transport

1. Body fluid compartments
   - **a.** Intracellular fluid (ICF): fluid within cells; two thirds of body fluid is ICF
   - **b.** Extracellular fluid (ECF): fluid outside of cells; made up of two components, interstitial fluid (fluid surrounding cells) and fluid within vascular space (blood vessels)
   - **c.** Fluid constantly moves among intracellular, interstitial, and vascular spaces to maintain body fluid balance
   - **d.** ICF is most stable and is fairly resistant to major fluid shifts
   - **e.** Vascular fluid is least stable; it is quickly lost or gained in response to fluid intake or losses
   - **f.** Interstitial fluid is reserve fluid, replacing fluid either in blood vessels or cells, depending on need

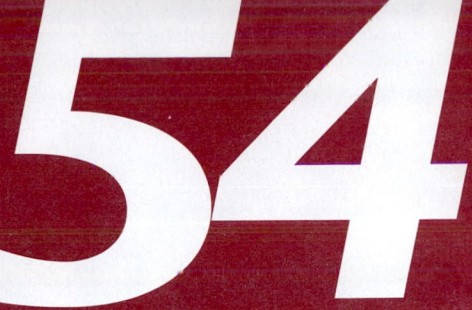

2. Osmosis
   a. Water moves through a semipermeable membrane (allows water and small particles, but not large particles, to easily pass through) from an area of lower concentration (fewer particles, more water) to an area of higher concentration (more particles, less water) until concentrations are equalized
   b. Osmosis is a major force in body fluid movement and intravenous (IV) fluid therapy; cell membranes and capillary membranes are semipermeable; water moves into and out of cells and capillaries by osmosis
3. Osmolality and osmotic pressure
   a. Osmolality and osmalarity refer to concentration of a solution, which creates its osmotic pressure (pulling power of a solution for water)
   b. Osmolality is concentration of solute (particles) measured per *kilogram* of water, while osmolarity is concentration of solute (particles) measured per *liter* of solution (solvent does not have to be water)
   c. Because body fluid solvent is water and one liter of water weighs one kilogram, the terms can be used interchangeably in discussing human fluids
   d. The higher the osmolality of a solution, the greater its pulling power for water
   e. Serum osmolality is concentration of particles (major particles are sodium and protein) in plasma: normal is 275 to 295 mOsm/L
   f. Isotonic: having same osmolality as normal plasma (see Table 54–1 ■ for examples of IV solutions that are isotonic; also see Chapter 32)
   g. **Hypotonic:** having a lower osmolality than normal plasma; water is pulled out of blood vessels into cells, resulting in decreased vascular volume and increased cell water (see Table 54–1 for examples of hypotonic IV solutions; also see Chapter 32)
   h. **Hypertonic:** having a higher osmolality than normal plasma; water is pulled from cells into blood vessels, resulting in increased vascular volume and decreased cell water (see Table 54–1 for examples of hypertonic IV solutions; also see Chapter 32)
4. Diffusion
   a. Particles move from an area of higher concentration (more particles, less water) to lower concentration (fewer particles, more water) until equalized
   b. Electrolytes (e.g., sodium, potassium, chloride, calcium, magnesium, and phosphate) are small particles that move easily through semipermeable membranes

Table 54–1

Tonicity of Typical IV Solutions

Tonicity	Examples of IV Solutions	Comments
Isotonic	Normal saline (NS; 0.9% NaCl) Ringer's solution Lactated Ringer's solution (LR) 5% dextrose in water (D_5W)	Same osmolality as normal plasma; no osmotic pressure difference is created, so fluids remain primarily in ECF; isotonic IV fluids replace ECF losses and expand vascular volume quickly D_5W is isotonic in bag but has hypotonic effect in body after dextrose is metabolized; two thirds of water goes to body cells
Hypotonic	0.45% sodium chloride (½ NS) 0.225% sodium chloride (¼ NS)	Provides free water and small amounts of sodium and chloride to cells
Hypertonic	5% dextrose in 0.45% sodium chloride (D_5 ½ NS) 5% dextrose in 0.225% sodium chloride (D_5 ¼ NS) 5% dextrose in 0.9% sodium chloride (D_5 NS) 3% sodium chloride (3% NaCl) 5% sodium chloride (5% NaCl) 10% dextrose 50% dextrose	D_5 ½ NS and D_5 ¼ NS are hypertonic in IV bag and provide dextrose and some water to cells D_5 NS is isotonic after dextrose is metabolized 3% and 5% NaCl: used to treat specific problems; administered in carefully controlled, limited doses to avoid vascular volume overload and cell dehydration; also used to pull excess fluid from cells and promote osmotic diuresis

c. Urea, glucose, and albumin are large particles that do not pass easily through semipermeable membranes

B. Capillary fluid movement

1. Hydrostatic pressure: pushing force of a fluid against walls of space it occupies; generated in blood vessels by heart's pumping action and varies within vascular system
2. Oncotic pressure (also called colloid osmotic pressure, or COP): pulling force exerted by colloids (such as albumin, other plasma proteins) that normally remain in bloodstream
3. Starling's Law of the capillaries
   a. Filtration (net fluid movement into or out of capillary) is determined by difference between forces favoring filtration and those opposing it (like a tug of war—pushing and pulling)
   b. Interstitial hydrostatic pressure (pushing water into capillary) and interstitial oncotic pressure (pulling water out of capillary) are very low and essentially equal, thus normally exerting little influence on fluid movement into or out of capillaries
   c. Capillary hydrostatic pressure (pushing water out of capillary) and capillary oncotic pressure (pulling water into capillary) are not equal, and fluid movement is seen in capillary bed

C. Chemical regulation of fluid and electrolyte balance

1. Antidiuretic hormone (ADH): a hormone synthesized by hypothalamus and secreted by posterior pituitary that regulates water (see also Chapter 61); is released and inhibited in a feedback loop
2. Aldosterone: hormone produced by adrenal gland that conserves sodium by causing renal retention of sodium and potassium excretion; water follows sodium because of osmosis, thus aldosterone has an indirect effect on water; is released and inhibited in a feedback loop as part of the renin-angiotensin-aldosterone (RAA) system
3. Glucocorticoid (cortisol): hormone produced and released by adrenal gland when body is stressed; promotes renal retention of sodium and water
4. Atrial natriuretic peptide (ANP): a cardiac hormone found in atria of heart and released when atria are stretched by high blood volume or high BP; ANP causes vasodilation by direct effects on blood vessels, suppresses RAA system, decreases ADH release, and increases glomerular filtration rate (GFR) in kidneys; these actions all promote fluid excretion
5. Thirst mechanism: occurs with fluid losses or increases in serum osmolality; stimulated by receptors in hypothalamus that can detect as little as 1 mOsm/L change in plasma concentration; stimulates ADH and aldosterone release, which promotes reabsorption of water; thirst is depressed in people over 60 years, including those who are healthy and those with debilitating illnesses
6. Fluid losses occur mainly via kidneys (approx. 1500 mL/day), but also via skin through diffusion (400 mL/day) and perspiration (100 mL), lungs via moisture in exhaled air (350 mL/day), and feces (150 mL/day); fluid losses that are not measureable are called insensible losses

II. DEFICIENT FLUID VOLUME (DEHYDRATION)

A. Overview

1. Occurs when fluid intake is inadequate for bodily needs; goal is to replace fluid and any necessary electrolytes and eliminate cause of deficit
2. Types of fluid loss: isotonic, hypotonic, hypertonic (see Table 54–2 ■)
   a. Isotonic dehydration involves equal losses of all fluid components and is most common type of fluid volume deficit
   b. Hypertonic dehydration involves greater losses of ECF volume than electrolytes, leading to an increased plasma osmolality; fluid shifting occurs as body tries to compensate to restore balance
   c. Hypotonic dehydration involves greater losses of electrolytes, leading to a decreased plasma osmolality; fluid shifting occurs as ECF volume decreases

Table 54–2

Comparison of Isotonic, Hypertonic, and Hypotonic Dehydration

Type of Dehydration	Description	Causes
Isotonic	Fluid and solute are lost in proportional or equal amounts; serum osmolality remains normal, and no osmotic force is created Intracellular water is not disturbed, and fluid losses are primarily ECF (especially vascular), which can quickly lead to shock Is primarily an ECF loss that requires ECF replacement, with emphasis on the vascular volume	Hemorrhage Gastrointestinal losses (mild nausea and vomiting, gastric suction, etc.) Fever, environmental heat, and diaphoresis Burns (especially large burns) Diuretics Third space fluid shifts (when fluid moves from vascular space into physiologically useless extracellular spaces, (becoming unavailable as reserve fluid or to transport nutrients)
Hypertonic	More water than solute (primarily sodium) is lost, creating a fluid volume deficit and a relative solute excess Solute (sodium or glucose more commonly) can also be gained in excess of water, creating a similar imbalance Serum osmolality is elevated, resulting in hypertonic ECF that pulls fluid into vessels from cells by osmosis and causes the cells to shrink and become dehydrated	Inadequate fluid intake (those unable to respond to thirst, nausea, anorexia, dysphagia) Severe or prolonged isotonic fluid losses (vomiting, watery diarrhea, diabetes insipidus) Increased solute intake (salt, sugar, protein) without proportional fluid increase, such as concentrated enteral feedings, hyperglycemia, excess salt or sugar ingestion, excess osmotic diuretic use)
Hypotonic	More solute than water is lost Fluid moves into cells, causing cellular swelling	Chronic illness Malnutrition Excess hypotonic fluid replacement)

3. Third spacing
   a. Occurs when fluid is deposited into extracellular body spaces that do not normally hold large amounts of fluid but in which fluids can accumulate; fluid is useless because it is not available as reserve fluid or to transport nutrients
   b. Common locations for third space fluid to accumulate include tissue spaces (edema), abdomen (ascites), pleural spaces (pleural effusion), and pericardial space (pericardial effusion); see Box 54–1 for causes of third spacing

Box 54–1

Causes of Third Spacing

Injury or inflammation (increases capillary permeability, allowing fluid, electrolytes, and proteins to leak from vessels)

Massive trauma

Crush injuries

Burns

Sepsis

Cancer

Intestinal obstruction

Abdominal surgery

Malnutrition or liver dysfunction (prevents liver from producing albumin, thus lowering capillary oncotic pressure)

Starvation

Cirrhosis

Chronic alcoholism

High vascular hydrostatic pressure (pushes abnormal volumes of fluid from vessels)

Heart failure

Renal failure

Other forms of vascular fluid overload

B. Nursing assessment

1. Presence of risk factors: age: (very young or old), acute or chronic illness, vigorous exercise or heat injuries, dysphagia, malnutrition, and medications (diuretics, chemotherapy agents that cause vomiting)
2. Thirst (an early sign), unreliable as an indicator in elderly and in children who cannot express needs
3. Low urine volume: less than 1 to 2 mL/kg/hour in children, 30 mL/hour (240 mL/8 hours) for adults
4. Concentrated, dark urine with specific gravity higher than 1.035 (normal 1.010 to 1.030); note that if diabetes insipidus is causing fluid loss, urine will be pale, dilute, and high in volume
5. Dry mucous membranes, dry tongue with longitudinal furrows in all ages, dry skin and decreased skin turgor (tenting, which occurs when skin in pinched gently and it takes time to return to normal—forming a "tent")
   a. Skin of older clients loses elasticity with aging, so tenting is not a reliable sign in elderly; test elderly skin on sternum, forehead, inner thigh, or top of hip bone rather than arms or legs
   b. Decreased tearing and dry conjunctiva
6. Sunken eyeballs; sunken or depressed anterior and possibly posterior fontanels in infants under 18 months old
7. Flat neck veins (with head of bed 30 to 45 degrees) and poor peripheral vein filling when hand is placed lower than heart (normally fill within 3 to 5 seconds)
8. Hypotension (late sign in infants and young children); may be postural or frank
   a. Complaints of weakness, dizziness, lightheadedness
   b. Syncope when rising from lying position
9. Tachycardia (early sign, especially in infants and young children); weak, thready pulse; cool extremities with delayed capillary refill
10. Tachypnea (usually without dyspnea)
11. Low-grade fever (higher fever can occur in severe dehydration)
12. Mental status changes (e.g., irritability, restlessness, lethargy, confusion, drowsiness)
    a. Often first signs noticed in elderly and also often cause alarm in parents of infants and small children
    b. Are a serious sign of significant fluid loss; if fluid loss is severe, client can progress to seizures and coma
13. Acute weight loss (an important sign in infants and young children)
    a. 1 liter (L) water = 1 kg (2.2 pounds)
    b. Monitoring weight is considered more accurate than monitoring intake and output (I & O) because of difficulty in keeping accurate records
14. Laboratory findings: normal or high hematocrit (Hct) and blood urea nitrogen (BUN), high urine specific gravity (>1.030) except in diabetes insipidus (<1.010); possible elevated serum osmolality (>300 mOsm/kg), hypernatremia over 150 mEq/L

C. Therapeutic management

1. Oral replacement therapies if deficit is mild, thirst is intact, and client can drink; during initial rehydration, avoid fluids with sugar or salts, which can worsen fluid loss, and caffeinated beverages, which have diuretic effect
2. Parenteral replacement therapies: IV fluid replacement depending on type of fluid loss (isotonic, hypertonic, hypotonic)
3. Monitor specific assessment parameters (vital signs, urine output, mental status, IV site, I & O, and daily weight)
4. Provide comfort measures such as mouth care and lip moisturizer; avoid giving client hard candy or chewing gum with sugar, which have drying effect
5. Provide measures to prevent fluid volume deficits and dehydration
   a. Provide additional plain water boluses periodically during enteral feedings
   b. Implement measures to control nausea, vomiting, diarrhea, and high fever because these conditions may cause further complications

c. Recognize acutely ill clients at risk for inadequate fluid intake and initiate measures to provide adequate fluids by the oral, enteral, or parenteral routes
6. Medication therapy as needed (antiemetics, antidiarrheals, ADH (vasopressin), antipyretics for fever

D. Client teaching

1. Awareness of predisposing or risk factors; contact physician if illness lasts more than 24 hours, if client is elderly or very young, or if client has a chronic illness (such as diabetes, heart disease, kidney or liver disease)
2. Measures to help prevent fluid deficit and dehydration (frequent fluid intake during day in hot weather even if not thirsty; avoid highly salty fluids and excess table salt; avoid caffeine)
3. Specific measures that treat underlying cause

III. EXCESS FLUID VOLUME (FLUID OVERLOAD)

A. Overview

1. A state in which rate of fluid intake or retention exceeds rate of fluid loss in body; goal is to restore fluid balance
2. Types of fluid volume excess (FVE)
   a. Isotonic fluid excess is caused by renal failure, heart failure, excess fluid intake, high corticosteroid levels, or high aldosterone levels
   b. Hypotonic fluid excess (water intoxication) is caused by repeated plain water enemas or repeated plain water NG tube or bladder irrigations, overuse or excessive speed of hypotonic IV fluid infusions, excessive plain water intake (such as in extreme dieting), syndrome of inappropriate ADH secretion (SIADH), or psychogenic polydipsia
   c. Hypertonic: caused by excessive salt intake

! **B. Nursing assessment**

1. Predisposing risk factors: age (very old or young), surgery, chronic illess (especially cardiac or renal failure), and medications such as long-term glucocorticoid therapy
2. Peripheral edema
3. Tense or bulging fontanels in children under 18 months old
4. High central venous pressure (CVP) with venous engorgement (distended neck veins with head of bed at 45 degrees or higher), delayed peripheral vein emptying, S_3 heart sound in adults, hepatomegaly and splenomegaly are signs of venous congestion
5. Signs of pulmonary edema because of increasing extravascular fluid retention
   a. Tachypnea and dyspnea, irritated cough (often early sign of fluid in alveoli)
   b. Hacking cough that eventually becomes moist and productive (clear to white sputum); a late sign of fluid in alveoli and larger airways
   c. Labored breathing (seen as intercostal and substernal retractions, nasal flaring, and expiratory grunting in infants)
   d. Wet lung sounds (moist crackles) on auscultation (first appear in bases bilaterally and progress upward as lung water increases)
   e. Decreased O_2 saturation due to inadequate or mismatched ventilation and perfusion as a result of FVE
   f. Cyanosis (a late sign of hypoxemia)
6. Vital signs (reflect normal or increased cardiac output): normal heart rate, full or bounding peripheral pulses, warm extremities, brisk capillary refill
7. Third space fluid accumulations may be present (ascites, pleural effusion, pericardial effusion)
8. Acute, rapid weight gain
9. Increased urine output that is dilute
10. A weight gain of 3 pounds or more can occur over 2 to 5 days
11. Hct and BUN are decreased because of hemodilution (plasma has more water than normal, thus is more dilute), possible significant decreases in serum osmolality (<275 mOsm/kg) or serum sodium (<125 mEq/L); chest x-ray may show pleural effusions

C. Therapeutic management

1. Restrict fluid intake (sometimes as low as 1,000–1,500 mL per 24-hour period) and restrict sodium (helps decrease water retention); keep IV access with saline lock instead of infusing IV fluids
2. Involve client in dividing fluid allowances over 24-hour period; plan for more fluids during meals and with oral medications
3. Promote excretion (diuretics, cardiac glycosides in heart failure to increase cardiac output and renal perfusion)
4. Increase protein intake in clients who are malnourished and have low serum proteins to increase capillary oncotic pressure (and pull fluid into blood vessels for excretion)
5. Monitor cardiac, and respiratory status
6. Monitor fluid I & O carefully, ice chips count as fluid intake (1 cup ice chips equals 1/2 cup water); improved urine output indicates response to therapy
7. Monitor daily weights (same time, same clothing, same scale); remember: a change of 2.2 lbs (1 kg) equals a 1 liter water loss or gain
8. Assess for peripheral edema (differentiate dependent, or stasis, edema from more generalized edema related to heart, kidney, or liver problems)
9. Observe for developing or worsening water intoxication (hypotonic fluid volume excess), often associated with neurological changes
10. Monitor for overcorrection, in which signs of fluid volume deficit begin to appear
11. Evaluate follow-up electrolytes, BUN, serum osmolarity for return to normal values
12. Use an infusion pump to help prevent inadvertent administration of excess fluid
13. Institute measures to prevent fluid volume excess: irrrigate NG tube and bladder with normal saline rather than plain water; avoid repeated plain tap water enemas; mix infant formula according to package directions; do not use a water bottle as a pacifier for infants

D. Client teaching

1. Risk factors for excess fluid volume
2. Weigh self (adult) daily and report a gain of more than 2 pounds per week
3. Elevate extremities and change position frequently if peripheral edema present
4. Dietary education: sodium-restricted diet and use of alternative seasonings (natural, sodium-free herbs and spices); clients taking potassium-sparing diuretics and/or ACE inhibitors (which cause potassium retention) should not use salt substitutes because most contain potassium; avoid adding salt while cooking or at table; assess sodium content by reading food/OTC drug labels

IV. HYPONATREMIA

A. Overview

1. **Hyponatremia** is a serum sodium (Na^+) level below 135 mEq/L (normal range 135–145 mEq/L)
2. Usually associated with **hypervolemia** (increased fluid volume), which can then be referred to as dilutional hyponatremia or **water intoxication** (excess fluid that dilutes serum Na^+); can also occur in euvolemia (normal volume) and **hypovolemia** (low volume) states (see Table 54–3 ■)
3. Predisposing conditions (see Box 54–2)

B. Nursing assessment

1. Common signs relate to shift of water into cells and sodium's role in nerve impulse transmission and muscle contraction
2. Cardiovascular: bounding pulse, tachycardia, hypotension (with decreased ECV), hypertension (with increased ECV)
3. Integument: pale, dry skin and dry mucous membranes (with decreased ECV); edema and weight gain (with increased ECV)
4. Renal: increased urine output with low specific gravity (<1.010)
5. Neuromuscular: lethargy, agitation, dizziness, weakness, headache, confusion, seizures
6. Gastrointestinal (GI): anorexia, vomiting, diarrhea, hyperactive bowel sounds, abdominal cramping

Table 54–3

Hyponatremia in Various Fluid Volume States

Euvolemic State	Hypervolemic State	Hypovolemic State
Description Decrease in fluids in both the intravascular and interstitial space	High-glucose states that pull water from cells, leading to cellular dehydration as seen in diabetic ketoacidosis (DKA)	Glucose in isotonic solutions is oxidized, leading to cellular swelling
Results in a normal serum osmolality Use of sodium-free solutions that dilute the ECF	Fluid loss from ECF is greater than solute loss, leading to increased serum osmolality	Loss of solute from ECF is greater than excess of water, resulting in a decreased serum osmolality
Clinical presentations SIADH, medications, hypothyroidism, psychiatric disorders	CHF, cirrhosis, nephrotic syndrome, and renal failure	GI fluid loss, diuretic therapy, osmotic diuresis, adrenal insufficiency, burns, and sweating, hypotonic dehydration
Treatment Water restriction, correction of underlying cause, treat SIADH with demeclocycline (unlabeled use), and increase dietary salt intake	Water restriction, treat existing disease states, loop diuretics such as furosemide (Lasix), and restrict dietary salt intake	NS to correct ECF deficits, increase dietary salt intake; hypertonic saline to raise Na level

7. Decreased blood urea nitrogen (BUN) and hematocrit (Hct)
8. Dietary: prolonged NPO status; excess infusion of nonelectrolyte solutions, causing free water accumulation

C. Therapeutic management

1. Focuses on restoring normal levels, preventing complications, and treating underlying problems
2. ! Encourage inclusion of high-sodium foods in diet (refer to Box 54–3 for Na^+ food sources)

Box 54–2

Causes of Hyponatremia

- Loss of sodium
- Renal losses through excretion, diuretic administration, and renal disease (salt-wasting nephropathy)
- GI losses through vomiting, diarrhea, suctioning, tap water enemas (TWE), GI surgery, and bulimia
- Skin losses through perspiration, environmental conditions, burns, and tissue destruction
- Conditions that increase extracellular water
- Hormone regulation response of ADH and aldosterone, leading to fluid shifting and water gain
- Disease states that add to increased volume, such as CHF, cirrhosis, and nephrotic syndrome
- Disease states such as psychiatric disorders that involve compulsive water drinking
- Disease states such as tumors, SIADH, and adrenal insufficiency that affect hormonal response, leading to increased secretion
- Hyperglycemic states such as diabetic ketoacidosis (DKA) that cause cellular dehydration
- Prolonged or excessive use of hypotonic fluid administration
- Conditions that lead to inadequate dietary intake of sodium
- Prolonged use of fluids without sodium replacement
- The presence of anorexia and other eating disorders

Box 54-3

Sodium Food Sources

The following foods are considered adequate sources of sodium:

- Processed food products (highest sources of sodium in the diet)
- Lunch meats
- Ham, bacon, and pork products (high sodium levels)
- Dill pickles, corned beef, and products that are "pickled" in brine solutions
- Potato chips and other snack foods
- Butter, cheese, and milk
- Condiments such as ketchup, mustard, soy sauce, relishes.
- Anchovies, mackerel, and other saltwater fish products

3. For hyponatremia with normal fluid volume (euvolemic) or hypertonic dehydration, use water restriction and treat underlying cause
4. For hyponatremia with hypovolemic volume, treat with normal saline (NS) or lactated Ringer's (LR) solution
5. Use isotonic saline for wound or other irrigations
6. Loop diuretics, salt and fluid restrictions, 3% saline infusions, and even dialysis may have to be utilized if clinical picture so dictates
7. Continue to monitor laboratory results; aim is to raise Na^+ level no more than 25 mEq/L in the first 48 hours with a rate not to exceed 1 to 2 mEq/L/hr
8. Keep accurate I & O records
9. ! Obtain daily weights; a weight loss of more than 0.5 pounds in 24 hours is considered to be caused by fluid loss
10. ! Monitor for resolution of manifestations of hyponatremia, including CNS changes such as confusion, lethargy, and seizures
11. ! Protect client from injury and maintain a safe environment if client experiences neurological changes due to hyponatremia
12. Medication therapy: salt tablets, loop diuretics, LR or 0.9% sodium chloride (isotonic dehydration) or 3% or 5% hypertonic saline (severe deficits)

D. Client teaching

1. Predisposing factors: age (elderly and very young), environmental conditions (heat and humidity)
2. Dietary education: high-sodium foods
3. Preventing a recurrence: observe for and report early signs and symptoms of hyponatremia such as abdominal cramps, muscle weakness, and nausea
4. Observe for changes in mental status, especially if client already has cardiac, renal, or endocrine problems that might exacerbate hyponatremia

V. HYPERNATREMIA

A. Overview

1. **Hypernatremia** is a serum Na^+ level greater than 145 mEq/L (normal range 135–145 mEq/L)
2. Sodium excess always exists in a **hyperosmolar** (osmotic pressure greater than normal plasma pressure) state
3. Sodium excess can exist in hypovolemic, euvolemic, and hypervolemic states (see Table 54-4 ■ for summary of this disorder)
4. Predisposing clinical conditions
   a. Disturbances in water regulation such as decreased intake, increased insensible loss, or watery diarrhea predispose to development of hypernatremia
   b. Water loss due to fever, hyperventilation, diuretic therapy, and burns tends to develop into hypernatremia
   c. Increased Na^+ intake either due to dietary intake or infusion of sodium-containing fluids
   d. Renal losses or disease or hormonal states such as Cushing's syndrome (increased cortisol production) or diabetes insipidus

Table 54-4

Hypernatremia in Various Fluid Volume States

Euvolemic State	Hypervolemic State	Hypovolemic State
Description Decrease in water that leads to elevation of serum sodium levels Does not present with contracted volume unless there is a severe water loss	Greater gain of sodium in relation to fluids, leading to elevation of serum sodium levels	Greater loss of water than sodium, leading to elevation of serum sodium levels
Clinical presentations Increased fluid loss via skin or lungs (hyperventilation)	Seen primarily with administration of hypertonic saline solutions or $NaHCO_3$ hyperaldosteronism or hypertonic dehydration	Renal losses with osmotic diuresis, insensible loss with sweating and/or fever, GI losses with diarrhea Young and elderly clients are most at risk
Treatment Free water replacement either orally or by fluid-hydrating solutions	Remove sodium source, administer diuretics, and replace water	NS to correct intravascular volume deficit, then hypotonic fluids can be used to restore Na level

e. Clients who experience near-drowning in salt water are at risk for developing hypernatremia

! **B. Nursing assessment**

1. Common signs are related to water shift from cells (cellular dehydration) into vascular space and sodium's role in nerve impulse transmission and muscle contraction
2. Cardiovascular: tachycardia, hypertension, decreased cardiac contractility
3. Integumental: dry and sticky mucous membranes; rough, dry tongue; flushed skin
4. Renal: thirst, increased urine output
5. Neuromuscular: twitching, tremor and hyperreflexia, agitation and CNS irritability, hallucinations, seizures, coma
6. GI: watery diarrhea, nausea, thirst
7. Risk factors: age (very young or old), OTC or prescribed medications, high-sodium diet or excessive use of salt as flavoring

! **C. Therapeutic management**

1. Focuses on restoring normal levels, preventing complications, and treating underlying problems
2. Decrease Na^+ intake depending on severity to 3 grams, 2 grams, 1 gram, or 500 mg/day
3. Refer client to a dietitian to evaluate dietary intake for hidden sources of Na^+
4. Maintain safe environment because of CNS irritability and risk of seizure activity; initiate seizure precautions
5. Assess I & O and daily weight
6. Medication therapy: loop diuretics (sodium excess), IV fluids as needed

D. Client teaching

1. Awareness of predisposing factors in elderly: limited mobility, multiple medication profile, and restricted access to fluids
2. Report recurrence of early signs of hypernatremia to health care provider
3. ! Dietary education
   a. Na^+ content of foods and sources of hidden Na^+
   b. Follow a low-sodium diet after discharge
   c. Read all labels for Na^+ content prior to ingestion
   d. Use herbs, lemon juice, spices, and vinegar instead of salt or salt substitutes to season foods
   e. Do not routinely salt food prior to tasting

VI. HYPOKALEMIA

A. Overview

1. **Hypokalemia** is a serum potassium (K^+) level below 3.5 mEq/L (normal range 3.5–5.1 mEq/L)
2. Has widespread effects on body, and if severe or not corrected quickly, death can result from cardiac and respiratory arrest
3. Predisposing factors
   - **a.** Increased secretion of aldosterone leading to excretion of K^+ from renal tubules (adrenal adenomas, cirrhosis, nephrosis, heart failure and hypertensive crisis, Cushing's syndrome, diabetes insipidus)
   - **b.** Excessive loss of K^+ by loop diuretics, thiazide diuretics, corticosteroids, cardiac glycosides, penicillins, amphotericin B, gentamicin, theophylline, cisplatin, and tocolytic agents
   - **c.** GI loss by vomiting, diarrhea, prolonged nasogastric suctioning, newly created ileostomy, villous adenoma on intestinal tract, laxative abuse, or enema administration
   - **d.** Heat induced diaphoresis
   - **e.** Renal disease affecting reabsorption of K^+ seen in diuretic phase of renal failure
   - **f.** Hemodialysis and peritoneal dialysis
   - **g.** Altered intake (K^+-restricted diets), NPO status without sufficient IV replacement therapy, starvation, malnutrition, alcoholism, anorexia, high glucose levels (leading to diuresis), large ingestion of black licorice (causes aldosterone effects)

B. Nursing assessment

1. Cardiovascular: variable pulse rate; weak, thready pulse; pedal pulses difficult to palpate; ECG changes (ST segment depression, flattened T wave, appearance of U wave, ventricular dysrhythmias, and heart block); digitalis toxicity is potentiated
2. Respiratory: decreased breath sounds; weak, shallow respirations; dyspnea
3. Renal: polyuria and nocturia, decreased specific gravity
4. Neuromuscular: anxiety, lethargy, depression, confusion, paresthesias, weakness, leg cramps
5. GI: nausea, diarrhea or constipation (from decreased peristalsis), polydipsia

C. Therapeutic management

1. Treatment focuses on restoring normal levels, preventing complications, and treating underlying problems
2. If client also has hypocalcemia and/or hypomagnesemia, all electrolyte levels must be corrected together
3. Check for signs of metabolic alkalosis (including irritability and paresthesias) because hypokalemia is present in alkalotic states
4. Monitor pertinent client assessment data for potential effects related to hypokalemia and for response to therapeutic treatment
   - **a.** Vital signs, especially BP (hypokalemia can lead to orthostatic hypotension) and respiratory rate, depth, and pattern
   - **b.** Serum electrolyte levels
   - **c.** ECG changes and heart rate and rhythm pattern
   - **d.** I & O and possibly daily weight
5. Monitor therapeutic serum drug levels for clients taking cardiac glycosides (digoxin) and serum K^+ levels for clients taking loop and thiazide diuretics
6. Protect client from injury and maintain a safe environment because client may experience weakness due to hypokalemia
7. Dietary interventions to promote normal K^+ levels
   - **a.** Encourage high-fiber diet and increased fluid intake, if not on fluid restriction, to prevent constipation
   - **b.** Provide adequate dietary sources of K^+; see Box 54–4 for good food sources of K^+

Box 54-4

Potassium Food Sources

The following foods are considered adequate sources of potassium:

- Vegetables such as spinach, broccoli, carrots, green beans, tomato juice, acorn squash, and potatoes
- Fruits such as bananas, cantaloupe, apricots, oranges, and raisins
- Milk, milk products, yogurt, and meat
- Legumes, nuts, and seeds
- Whole grains

8. Oral replacement therapy (note: K^+ supplements should never be given unless client has a urine output of at least 0.5 mL/kg/hour)
    a. Usual dose is 20 mEq; higher doses (up to 100 mEq in divided doses) may be given depending on client's baseline
    b. Medication can be given in either liquid or pill form
9. Administer parenteral K^+ carefully
    a. Verify additive K^+ in solution prior to hanging infusion
    b. Always use an infusion pump, paying attention to rate, intake, and output
    c. Do not exceed an infusion rate of 5 to 10 mEq/hr unless there is moderate hypokalemia
    d. Dilute K^+ in a solution that provides no more than 1 mEq/10 mL
    e. If more than 20 mEq/hr is given, use continuous ECG monitoring and check serum level every 4 to 6 hours until normal
    f. Monitor IV site closely because potassium chloride (KCl) is irritating to vessels and can lead to infiltration, phlebitis, and tissue necrosis; this threat to tissue integrity could cause sloughs that may require skin grafts
    g. Never administer K^+ by IV push or intramuscular routes because these methods can lead to fatal dysrhythmias
10. Diet therapy
    a. Foods high in K^+ include raisins, bananas, apricots, oranges, avocados, beans, beef, potatoes, tomatoes, cantaloupe, and spinach
    b. Avoid foods such as black licorice that, when eaten in large quantities, can cause hypokalemia

D. Client teaching

1. Report signs and symptoms of hypokalemia to physician
2. Take K^+ supplements with at least 4 ounces fluid or with food
3. Never crush or break K^+ tablets or capsules.
4. Dissolve powder form of K^+ in at least 4 ounces of water or other fluids (no carbonated beverages)
5. Take K^+ after meals to prevent GI upset
6. Do not use salt substitutes when taking K^+ supplements
7. Know signs and symptoms of hyperkalemia and report these to health care provider
8. Get regular serum K^+ levels drawn as per health care provider's recommendations

VII. HYPERKALEMIA

A. Overview

1. **Hyperkalemia** is a serum K^+ level greater than 5.1 mEq/L (normal range 3.5–5.1 mEq/L)
2. Actual hyperkalemia (K^+ level in the ECF is elevated)
    a. Excessive K^+ intake from K^+-rich food or medications, use of salt substitutes, or rapid infusion of K^+-containing IV solutions
    b. Decreased K^+ excretion due to adrenal insufficiency (Addison's disease), renal failure, K^+-sparing diuretics, or use of ACE inhibitors
3. Relative hyperkalemia (movement of K^+ from ICF to ECF leading to elevated serum K^+ levels without a true body increase of K^+)
    a. Excessive cellular release: massive cell damage, burns, hyperuricemia in tumor lysis syndrome, major surgeries, and hypercatabolism
    b. Pseudohyperkalemia: hemolysis of blood sample

c. Excessive transcellular shifting: metabolic acidosis, insulin deficiency, rapid increase in blood osmolality
d. Medication therapy: digoxin use, overdose of replacement therapy, administration of stored blood (hemolysis of RBCs in solution increases serum K^+), use of K^+-sparing diuretics
e. Addison's disease is associated with decreased aldosterone that leads to Na^+ depletion and K^+ retention

B. Nursing assessment

1. Cardiovascular: irregular, slow heart rate, decreased BP, ECG changes (narrow, peaked T waves, widened QRS complexes, prolonged PR intervals, flattened P waves, frequent ectopy, ventricular fibrillation, and ventricular standstill)
2. Respiratory: unaffected until levels are very high, leading to muscle weakness and paralysis and causing respiratory failure
3. Neuromuscular: muscle twitching (early) and cramps, irritability, anxiety; a late sign is ascending flaccid paralysis involving arms and legs
4. GI: hyperactive bowel sounds, diarrhea, nausea

C. Therapeutic management

1. Decrease K^+ intake: implement prescribed K^+ restrictions; do not administer K^+ supplements; refer client to dietitian to evaluate hidden dietary intake of K^+
2. Promote K^+ excretion: increase urinary output and monitor adequate renal function
3. Continued monitoring of client: serum K^+ levels; report abnormals; assess cardiac status, and signs and symptoms of hyperkalemia and metabolic acidosis
4. Whenever possible, determine and treat underlying cause to restore balance
5. Dialysis may be performed for intractable conditions to prevent development of potentially lethal problems or if client's clinical condition warrants immediate intervention
6. Monitor for response to therapeutic treatment
7. Sodium polystyrene sulfonate (Kayexalate), to reduce K^+ levels, can be given either orally or as an enema with an osmotic agent (sorbitol) to decrease possible constipation
8. Intravenous medications
   a. Calcium gluconate
   b. Regular insulin and dextrose (usually 50%) solution (shifts K^+ from ECF to ICF)
   c. Sodium bicarbonate
9. K^+-wasting diuretics (loop diuretics and thiazide and thiazide-like diuretics)

D. Client teaching

1. Recognize predisposing factors
2. Avoid foods that are high in K^+
3. Examine food labels and medication packages to determine K^+ content
4. Avoid salt substitutes

VIII. HYPOCALCEMIA

A. Overview

1. **Hypocalcemia:** abnormally low calcium (Ca^{++}) level (<8.5 mg/dL) or decreased availability of ionized Ca^{++}
2. Predisposing clinical conditions result from decreased physiologic availability of Ca^{++}, decreased Ca^{++} intake or absorption, or increased Ca^{++} excretion (see Box 54–5)
3. Other risk factors
   a. Postmenopausal women not taking estrogen
   b. Post-thyroidectomy or parathyroidectomy
   c. Family history of hereditary hypoparathyroidism
   d. History of Crohn's or small bowel dysfunction
   e. Increased incidence of fractures; osteoporosis and/or osteopenia
   f. Immobility
   g. Dietary patterns that lack adequate Ca^{++} and vitamin D sources
   h. Excessive use of dietary phosphorous supplements
   i. Eating disorders with laxative use as part of dietary pattern

Box 54-5

Clinical Conditions That Lead to Hypocalcemia

- Hypoparathyroidism
- Hypomagnesemia
- Alkalotic states
- Multiple blood transfusions
- Medications (loop diuretics, anticonvulsants, citrate-buffered blood products, phosphates, antineoplastic agents, radiographic contrast media, corticosteroids, biphosphonates, antacids, and heparin)
- Hypoalbuminemia
- Acute pancreatitis
- Hyperphosphatemia
- Vitamin D deficiency
- Malabsorptive states
- Renal disease
- Alcoholism
- Neonatal hypocalcemia
- Gram-negative sepsis
- Medullary thyroid carcinoma
- Burns

j. Lactose-intolerance unless alternative products are used
k. Dietary factors that limit absorption of Ca^{++} (oxalates such as spinach and rhubarb, phytates such as bran and whole grains, and tannins as in tea)

!

B. Nursing assessment

1. Cardiovascular: decreased BP; ECG changes include prolonged QT interval and lengthened ST segment; cardiac arrest can occur
2. Respiratory: laryngospasm can occur, leading to respiratory compromise and airway failure; respiratory arrest can occur
3. Renal: low serum calcium levels are associated with renal failure; other electrolyte disturbances are seen in conjunction with clinical manifestations of renal failure
4. Neuromuscular : paresthesias and tingling in hands and feet; muscle spasms of extremities and face; positive Chvostek's (twitching of cheek) and Trousseaus's sign (spasm of arm when BP cuff inflated); hyperactive reflexes and increased irritability and apprehension; mental status changes ranging from depression, memory impairment, delusion, and hallucinations, to convulsions
5. GI: possible hyperactive bowel sounds and diarrhea, intestinal cramps
6. Musculoskeletal: possible bone fractures due to demineralization; in children, chronic hypocalcemia may retard growth and cause rickets; can lead to osteomalacia and osteoporosis in adults
7. Other systems: development of cataracts; dry, brittle nails and dry hair; complaints of bone pain; increased bleeding or bruising, bone thinning, and fractures

!

C. Therapeutic management

1. Treatment focuses on restoring normal levels, preventing complications, and treating underlying problems
2. Replacement therapies
   a. Calcium gluconate (more common) or calcium chloride (less common; irritating to vein) by slow IV push in an emergency; may give slow IV infusion of calcium gluconate until tetany has been controlled or until calcium reaches 8 to 9 mg/dL
   b. Daily oral doses of elemental Ca^{++}, usually 1.0 to 3.0 grams/day
   c. Calcitriol, vitamin D supplements, or phosphorus-binding antacids based on need
   d. Thiazide diuretics may be used to decrease urinary excretion of calcium

3. Continue monitoring client (laboratory values and physical manifestations) for treatment effectivesss
   a. Continuous ECG monitoring, especially during calcium gluconate or calcium chloride administration
   b. Continually reassess neurologic, respiratory, and cardiac status
   c. Monitor clients receiving Ca^{++} replacement who are also on digitalis for enhanced digitalis effect—check pulse
4. Protect client from injury and maintain a safe environment
   a. Be knowledgeable about and prepared for emergencies that may result from hypocalcemia, such as tetany, seizures, laryngospasm, and respiratory and cardiac arrest
   b. Initiate seizure precautions and maintain a quiet environment
   c. Closely observe respiratory and airway status; have emergency tracheostomy kit available and IV calcium gluconate at bedside for postoperative thyroidectomy clients (may have inadvertent removal of parathyroid gland)
   d. Observe for signs of tetany in clients receiving multiple blood transfusions
   e. Observe for signs of bleeding or increased bruising
5. Monitor for possible hypercalcemia resulting from replacement therapy
6. Encourage foods high in Ca^{++}, such as dairy products

D. Client teaching

1. Predisposing factors
2. Paresthesias, tingling and numbness in extremities are early warning signs of tetany
3. Report onset of signs of tetany or seizures immediately to health care provider
4. Take oral replacements as prescribed
5. Avoid overuse of antacids and/or laxatives containing phosphorus
6. Increase intake of foods rich in Ca^{++} (dairy products) and protein
7. Vitamin D and protein are important to keep Ca^{++} within normal limits
8. Use appropriate substitutes for milk and dairy products if lactose intolerant
9. Avoid foods high in phosphorus
10. Limit foods that decrease absorption of Ca^{++} in diet

IX. HYPERCALCEMIA

A. Overview

1. **Hypercalcemia:** an abnormally elevated serum Ca^{++} level (>10.5 mg/dL); symptoms may not appear until serum Ca^{++} level is higher than 12 mg/dL
2. Predisposing clinical conditions (see Box 54–6)
3. Other risk factors
   a. Clients with cancer or known metastasis
   b. Clients with hyperparathyroidism
   c. Clients who are immobile due to clinical conditions or sedentary lifestyle
   d. Excessive dietary intake of Ca^{++}-rich foods
   e. Excessive intake of antacids for gastric distress

! B. Nursing assessment

1. Cardiovascular: hypertension, decreased ST segments and shortened QT interval on ECG, cardiac dysrhythmias such as heart block, and cardiac arrest
2. Neuromuscular: headache and confusion, subtle changes in personality to acute psychosis, fatigue, decreased deep tendon reflexes (DTRs); impaired memory and bizarre behavior, lethargy, or coma (seizures are rare)

Box 54–6

Clinical Conditions That Lead to Hypercalcemia

- Hyperparathyroidism
- Metastatic cancer
- Use of thiazide diuretics
- Sarcoidosis
- Immobility
- Hypophosphatemia
- Hyperthyroidism (thyrotoxicosis)
- Renal tubular acidosis
- Milk-alkali syndrome
- Familial hypocalciuric hypercalcemia
- Lithium therapy
- Vitamin D intoxication

3. GI: anorexia, nausea and vomiting; abdominal pain; constipation, hypotonic bowel sounds
4. Renal: polyuria and polydipsia due to altered renal function; decreased ability of kidneys to concentrate urine; renal colic from development of kidney stones due to high Ca^{++} levels; renal failure may occur
5. Musculoskeletal: pathologic bone fractures; bone thinning, deep bone pain

! **C. Therapeutic management**

1. Decrease Ca^{++} intake
   a. Limit milk and dairy products
   b. Eliminate use of calcium carbonate antacids until Ca^{++} levels return to normal
2. Promote calcium excretion
   a. Use loop diuretics, such as furosemide (Lasix) or ethacrynic acid (Edecrin), to promote increased urine output so that more Ca^{++} will be excreted
   b. Maintain hydration of 3,000 to 4,000 mL (3–4 L) of fluid/day; oral fluids should be high in acid-ash, such cranberry or prune juice
   c. Give 0.9% sodium chloride (NaCl) infusion of 300 to 500 mL/hr up to 6 liters as ordered until volume status restored, then 0.45% NaCl may be used; watch for fluid overload as a complication of therapy, especially with preexisting cardiac or respiratory disease
   d. Corticosteroids to decrease GI absorption of Ca^{++}: prednisone 20 to 50 mg po BID is usual dose or 40 to 100 mg daily in four divided doses; may take 5 to 10 days for Ca^{++} levels to fall
   e. Chronic management of hypercalcemia is effective only with parathroidectomy for primary hyperparathyroidism
3. Continued monitoring of client: strict I & O, daily weight, serum Ca^{++} and phosphorus levels, possible ECG monitoring
4. Treatment of hypercalcemic crisis
   a. Isotonic saline (0.9% NaCl) at 300 to 500 mL/hr initially and up to 6 liters until intravascular volume restored or calcium level is 8 to 9 mg/dL
   b. Biphosphonates, such as pamidronate (Aredia) IV to inhibit bone resorption; returns Ca^{++} to normal within 24 to 48 hours with effects lasting for weeks in most clients
   c. Plicamycin (Mithracin) IV to inhibit bone resorption specifically if hypercalcemia induced by metastasis
   d. Salmon calcitonin may temporarily lower Ca^{++} level by 1 to 3 mg/dL in clients with severe hypercalcemia
   e. Phosphorus IV to decrease Ca^{++} because of inverse relationship in emergency situations only
5. Dialysis: during oliguric/anuric stage, severe renal dysfunction can lead to life-threatening fluid and electrolyte imbalances
6. Prevent injuries and maintain safe environment
   a. Monitor for pathologic fractures in clients with long-term hypercalcemia
   b. Assist client with mobility to prevent injury and maintain safety

D. Client teaching

1. Predisposing factors associated with hypercalcemia
2. Take phosphorus agents or other medications as prescribed
3. Notify health care provider if flank pain develops (risk of kidney stones)
4. How to strain urine (check for kidney stones) if indicated
5. Notify health care professional if symptoms worsen
6. Avoid foods and OTC antacids that are high in Ca^{++}
7. Increase fluid intake to 2,000 to 3,000 mL in 24 hours, especially fluids high in acid-ash such as prune or cranberry juice
8. Increase dietary fiber and fluid to prevent constipation
9. Do not take large doses of vitamin D supplements

X. HYPOMAGNESEMIA

A. Overview

1. **Hypomagnesemia:** a serum magnesium (Mg^{++}) level that falls below 1.4 mEq/L (normal range 1.4–2.1 mEq/L)

2. Usually occurs with nutritional or metabolic abnormalities, altered absorption, increased renal loss, or redistribution of body magnesium
3. Predisposing clinical conditions
   a. Chronic alcoholism is most common cause
   b. Decreased dietary intake or prolonged IV therapy without Mg^{++} supplementation; in parenteral nutrition therapy, Mg^{++} moves into cells from bloodstream, leading to low serum Mg^{++} levels
   c. Decreased absorption: inflammatory bowel disease, small bowel resection (less surface available to absorb), GI cancer, chronic pancreatitis, or medications such as gentamicin (Garamycin, an aminoglycoside antibiotic) or cisplatin (Platinol, an antineoplastic agent)
   d. Increased intestinal (lower GI) losses: prolonged diarrhea, draining intestinal fistulas, and ileostomy
   e. Increased renal excretion: loop diuretic use, hyperaldosteronism that leads to volume expansion, diabetes that leads to osmotic diuresis
   f. Losses can also occur because of burns and debridement therapy

! **B. Nursing assessment**
1. Clinical manifestations usually appear when serum Mg^{++} level drops below 1 mEq/L
2. Respiratory: laryngeal stridor
3. Cardiovascular: supraventricular tachycardia, premature ventricular contractions and ventricular fibrillation, and increased susceptibility to digitalis toxicity (possibly enhanced by concurrent hypokalemia)
4. ECG changes: diminished voltage of P wave; broad, flat, or inverted T waves; depressed ST segments; prolonged QT interval; possible prominent U wave
5. Neuromuscular: mood changes, such as apathy, depression, and confusion; muscle twitching, tremors, hyperreactive reflexes
6. GI: nausea and vomiting, diarrhea, and anorexia (from concurrent hypokalemia)
7. Growth failure in children can occur
8. Severe deficiency can lead to convulsions, hallucinations, or tetany
9. Signs and symptoms are similar to hypokalemia or hypocalcemia (all are cations and may occur together); positive Chvostek's sign (twitching of cheek when stimulated) can occur

Memory Aid

Rember the *Ch* in *Ch*vostek and in *ch*eek to help remember how Chvostek's sign is manifested.

! **C. Therapeutic management**
1. Identify risk factors: malabsorption and/or GI dysfunction, renal disease, diabetes, alcohol intake, and medications such as diuretics
2. Monitor client with continuous IV fluid therapy without Mg^{++} replacement
3. Monitor client with hyperaldosteronism because volume expansion may result in decreased Mg^{++}
4. Monitor client taking a diuretic for increased renal excretion of Mg^{++}
5. Institute ECG monitoring and seizure precautions
6. Monitor for stridor and/or difficulty swallowing
7. Keep bed rails raised if client is confused; take other safety precautions as needed
8. Maintain accurate intake and output records
9. Monitor DTRs in clients receiving IV solutions containing Mg^{++}; depressed DTRs indicate a rebound elevated Mg^{++} level
10. Medication therapy
    a. Oral replacement therapy: Mg^{++}-containing antacids; magnesium oxide; use caution because oral administration may cause diarrhea, leading to decreased absorption
    b. Parenteral magnesium sulfate or magnesium chloride
    c. Ensure urine output of at least 30 mL/hr or 120 mL every 4 hours during therapy to avoid rebound hypermagnesemia if renal insufficiency is present

d. Monitor DTRs (such as patellar reflex) before each dose of parenteral Mg^{++}; if reflex is present, hypermagnesemia from previous doses has not occurred

11. Dietary therapy: for mild hypomagnesemia, encourage foods high in Mg^{++}, such as legumes, whole grain cereals, nuts, dark green vegetables, seafood, bananas, oranges, and chocolate

D. Client teaching

1. Predisposing factors
2. Increase intake of foods high in Mg^{++}
3. Increase intake of hard water or mineral water, which are high in Mg^{++}
4. Take 300 to 350 mg magnesium daily with an extra 150 mg for pregnant or lactating women

XI. HYPERMAGNESEMIA

A. Overview

1. **Hypermagnesemia:** serum Mg^{++} level greater than 2.1 mEq/L (normal range 1.4–2.1 mEq/L)
2. Predisposing factors
   a. Decreased renal excretion of Mg^{++}, such as with decreased urine output or renal failure
   b. Increased Mg^{++} intake, such as with overuse of Mg^{++}-containing antacids, cathartics, or enemas; total parenteral nutrition; or hemodialysis using hard water dialysate
3. Predisposing clinical conditions
   a. Untreated diabetic ketoacidosis (glucose carries cations across cell membranes)
   b. Adrenal insufficiency (Addison's disease): causes fluid and electrolyte shifts
   c. Mg^{++} treatment in preeclampsia of pregnancy
   d. Lithium ingestion
   e. Volume depletion

! **B. Nursing assessment**

1. Neuromuscular symptoms (most common): decreased DTRs and depressed neuromuscular activity; symptoms are similar to those seen in hyperkalemia
2. Cardiovascular: hypotension, bradycardia, bradyarrhythmias, flushing and sensation of warmth, possible cardiac arrest
3. ECG may show prolonged PR interval, widened QRS complex, and elevated T wave
4. CNS: somnolence, weakness and lethargy, respiratory depression, and coma

! **C. Therapeutic management**

1. Decrease Mg^{++} intake; withhold Mg^{++}-containing drugs (antacids) and enemas
2. Promote Mg^{++} excretion using diuretics (in stable renal function)
3. Provide rehydration to promote increased urinary output and Mg^{++} excretion
4. Emergency treatment includes IV calcium gluconate to antagonize effect of Mg^{++} and counteract cardiac and respiratory symptoms
5. Dialysis: in clients with renal failure, dialysis may be necessary for Mg^{++} removal; if hemodialysis is not feasible, peritoneal dialysis is an option
6. Monitor I & O
7. Identify risk factors such as antacid use, laxative use, diabetic instability, and renal failure
8. Promote client safety

D. Client teaching

1. Predisposing factors
2. Signs and symptoms of hypermagnesemia to report
3. Avoid foods high in mg^{++} such as legumes, whole-grain cereals, nuts, dark green vegetables, and cocoa

XII. HYPOCHLOREMIA

A. Overview

1. **Hypochloremia:** a serum chloride (Cl^-) level that falls below 95 mEq/L (normal range 95–108 mEq/L)

a. Decreases in Cl^-) usually are accompanied by decreases in Na^+ and K^+
b. A reduction in hydrochloric acid decreases Cl^-)
c. Chloride is excreted with cations during massive diuresis and when the bicarbonate level is elevated

2. Predisposing clinical conditions
a. Hyponatremia, metabolic alkalosis, hypokalemia, prolonged administration of D_5W IV therapy
b. Chronic respiratory acidosis
c. Chronic lung disease accompanied by high pCO_2 levels and bicarbonate levels that result in decreased serum Cl^-)
d. Diabetic ketoacidosis because of increased anion gap
e. Acute infections, although mechanism by which they lower serum Cl^-) is unclear
f. Vomiting (loss of HCl), GI suctioning, perspiration, diarrhea, and presence of fistulas
g. Metabolic stress conditions, such as severe burns, fever, heat and exhaustion states
h. Disease states such as Addison's disease, anorexia, salt-wasting renal nephropathy, SIADH, and hypervolemic states such as congestive heart failure (CHF) and cirrhosis
i. Various medications that promote electrolyte loss, have diuretic activity, or promote alkalosis

B. Nursing assessment
1. Neuromuscular: tremors and twitching
2. Respiratory: slow and shallow breathing
3. Cardiac: hypotension if severe Cl^- and ECF losses
4. Seldom a primary problem; usually associated with hyponatremia, hypokalemia, metabolic alkalosis or hypokalemic alkalosis

C. Therapeutic management
1. Administer oral salt tablets
2. Provide IV infusion of Cl^- (as NaCl or KCl) if levels are critical or if client is unable to tolerate oral administration
3. Monitor I & O because excess water administration can cause dilutional hypochloremia and hyponatremia
4. Monitor BP because a drop in BP can occur if hypochloremia is caused by ECF volume loss
5. Monitor ABG results if client's clinical presentation or underlying medical history suggests accompanying acid-base imbalance
6. Maintain safety precautions by keeping bed rails up and assisting client with ambulation if client presents with muscle tremors and/or decreased BP
7. Dietary therapy: foods high in Cl^-, such as salt, processed foods, canned vegetables, dates, bananas, cheese, spinach, milk, eggs, celery, crabs, fish, olives, and rye

D. Client teaching
1. Predisposing factors
2. Include in diet Na^+ and processed foods that are also high in Cl^-
3. Electrolyte replacement as well as fluid replacement is important if activity level is increased and client perspires excessively

XIII. HYPERCHLOREMIA

A. Overview
1. **Hyperchloremia:** a serum Cl^- level greater than 108 mEq/L (normal range 95–108 mEq/L)
2. Predisposing clinical conditions
a. Fluid and electrolyte imbalances such as hypernatremia and metabolic acidosis
b. Ingestion or administration of drugs that promote Cl^- retention, such as IV saline, certain diuretics, salicylate intoxication, corticosteroids, guanethidine, and phenylbutazone
c. Dehydration

d. Endocrine disturbances that result in diabetes insipidus and certain cases of hyperparathyroidism (seen in association with hypercalcemia)
e. Hyperaldosteronism (increased sodium and chloride reabsorption)
f. Renal changes that manifest as renal tubular acidosis or acute renal failure

B. Nursing assessment

1. Neuromuscular: weakness and lethargy; can progress to significant CNS damage
2. Respiratory: deep, rapid, vigorous breathing that can lead to unconsciousness (results from attempt to compensate for acidotic state due to loss of bicarbonate)
3. Cardiac: dysrhythmias due to retained Cl^- levels and accompanying acid-base disturbances
4. Increased aldosterone leads to greater reabsorption of both Na^+ and Cl^-
5. Fluid volume disturbances: dehydration, retention of salt and water due to drug administration, and a greater Na^+ loss than Cl^- loss
6. Increased Cl^- sweat levels are seen in diabetes insipidus, hypothyroidism, malnutrition, acute renal failure, and certain genetic disorders such as cystic fibrosis and glucose-6-phosphate-dehydrogenase (G6PD) deficiency
7. Associated electrolyte imbalances that usually occur with elevated Cl^- levels are elevated K^+ and Na^+ levels and decreased bicarbonate levels

C. Therapeutic management

1. Decrease Cl^- intake; withdraw all chloride-containing agents used as treatment measures
2. Promote Cl^- excretion by administering diuretics
3. Continue monitoring client, including acid-base, respiratory, and cardiac status
4. Administer appropriate IV therapy to restore fluid and electrolyte balance
5. Correct dehydration states with oral and parenteral fluids to restore serum Cl^- levels
6. Monitor vital signs and I & O parameters
7. Promote client safety
8. Parenteral administration: hypotonic solutions such as 0.45% NaCl or D_5W or IV diuretics

D. Client teaching

1. Predisposing factors
2. Avoid foods high in Cl^- and restrict processed foods (high in both Na^+ and Cl^-)
3. Maintain adequate hydration status

XIV. HYPOPHOSPHATEMIA

A. Overview

1. **Hypophosphatemia:** serum phosphorus level of less than 2.5 mg/dL (normal range 2.5–4.5 mg/dL)
2. May be associated with increased Ca^{++} levels (hypercalcemia)
3. Predisposing factors
   a. A complication of refeeding severely malnourished clients; has a high mortality rate
   b. Decreased intestinal absorption from vitamin D deficiency, malabsorption disorders, and starvation
   c. Prolonged use of aluminum- and Mg^{++}-containing antacids, which bind to phosphorus
   d. Severe vomiting and diarrhea; prolonged gastric suction
   e. Diabetic ketoacidosis
   f. Alcoholism and severe alcohol abuse (especially during withdrawal) related to poor nutritional intake, vomiting, diarrhea, and the use of antacids
   g. Poor dietary intake, malnutrition, hypomagnesemia
   h. Administering total parenteral nutrition (TPN) without adequate levels of phosphorus
   i. Increased renal excretion from hyperparathyroidism, hypomagnesemia, hypokalemia, thiazide diuretic therapy, the diuretic phase of acute tubular necrosis, renal tubular disorders, polyuria, and glycosuria from uncontrolled diabetic ketoacidosis

j. Respiratory alkalosis (may stimulate glycolysis, which enhances movement of phosphorus into cells)

B. Nursing assessment

1. Hematologic effects (anemia from the increased fragility of RBCs from low ATP levels), altered granulocyte functioning (immunosuppression), bruising and bleeding from platelet dysfunction and destruction
2. Neuromuscular: slurred speech, confusion, apprehension, seizures, coma, numbness and tingling of fingertips and around lips, muscle weakness, paresthesias, tremors, spasms, tetany
3. Cardiac: chest pain, dysrhythmias related to decreased oxygenation, heart failure and shock from decreased myocardial contractility
4. Respiratory: alkalosis from an increased rate/depth of breathing in response to hypoxemia; respiratory muscle fatigue leading to respiratory failure
5. GI: hypoactive bowel sounds, anorexia, dysphagia, vomiting, gastric atony and ileus related to reduced gastric motility

C. Therapeutic management

1. Administer phosphorus via oral supplements or IV replacement
2. Dissolve oral preparations in a full glass of water and administer after meals to minimize gastric irritation and laxative effect and to enhance palatability
3. Monitor IV infusion site for signs of infiltration, which may lead to tissue necrosis or sloughing
4. Avoid use of phosphorus-binding antacids
5. Assess clients for difficulty speaking; note weakening respiratory efforts; have appropriate size airway available
6. Assess serial hand grasps for increasing weakness
7. Investigate episodes of bleeding and/or bruising
8. Monitor for other associated fluid and electrolyte imbalances, especially in those with nausea, vomiting, and/or diarrhea
9. Assess orientation and neurologic status with each set of vital signs
10. Incorporate seizure precautions into care
11. Carefully monitor fluid I&O
12. Increase intake of foods high in phosphorus, such as red and organ (brain, liver, kidney) meats, fish, poultry, eggs, milk and milk products, legumes, whole grains, and nuts
13. Reduce dietary sources of oxalates (spinach and rhubarb) and phytates (bran and whole grains), which bind phosphates in GI tract and reduce absorption

D. Client teaching

1. Predisposing factors and signs and symptoms of hypophosphatemia
2. Avoiding phosphorus-binding antacids
3. Increase intake of foods high in phosphorus

XV. HYPERPHOSPHATEMIA

A. Overview

1. **Hyperphosphatemia:** serum phosphorus level of greater than 4.5 mg/dL (normal range 2.5–4.5 mg/dL)
2. Predisposing factors
   a. Acute and chronic renal failure
   b. Hypocalcemia from antacids, diuretic agents, steroids
   c. Chemotherapy for malignant tumors
   d. Hypoparathyroidism (primary or secondary), which causes a decrease in Ca^{++} and increased renal absorption of phosphorus
   e. Excessive intake of phosphorus or its supplements
   f. Vitamin D excess or increased GI absorption
   g. Massive transfusions because phosphorus can leak from cells during storage of blood
   h. Hyperthyroidism, hyperparathyroidism
   i. Large milk intake
   j. Overzealous administration of oral or IV phosphorus supplements

k. Rhabdomyolysis (breakdown of striated muscle), which releases cellular phosphorus

B. Nursing assessment

1. Most signs relate to the development of hypocalcemia or soft tissue calcification
2. Metastatic calcification includes oliguria, corneal haziness, conjunctivitis, irregular heart rate
3. ECG changes and conduction disturbance, tachycardia
4. Calcium phosphate deposits in nonosseous sites such as the kidney and heart
5. Numbness and tingling around the mouth and in the fingertips, muscle spasms, and tetany from the increased phosphorus and corresponding decreased Ca^{++}
6. Anorexia, nausea, vomiting

C. Therapeutic management

1. Restrict or eliminate phosphorus in diet, phosphorus-containing medications or enemas
2. Administer phosphate binding agents
3. Perform renal dialysis in clients with renal failure
4. Treat concurrent hypocalcemia
5. Monitor renal function carefully, particularly urine output, BUN, creatinine
6. Monitor I & O; keep clients well hydrated; pay particular attention to types of fluids being ingested (avoid carbonated beverages, which are high in phosphates)
7. Monitor for signs and symptoms of tetany, such as positive Trousseau's and Chvostek's signs

D. Client teaching

1. Purpose of phosphate binders; take them with or after meals to maximize effectiveness
2. Avoid OTC phosphorus medications such as laxatives, enemas, and vitamin-mineral supplements
3. Use bulk-building supplements or stool softeners to combat constipating effects of some phosphate-binders, especially those with an aluminum base
4. Avoid or limit foods high in phosphorus, as previously described, and avoid carbonated beverages, which have low nutrient value and are also high in phosphates

Check your NCLEX-RN® Exam I.Q.

You are ready for testing on this content if you can

- Describe the pathophysiology and etiology of fluid and electrolyte imbalances.
- Discuss expected assessment data and diagnostic test findings for fluid or electrolyte imbalance.
- Discuss therapeutic management of a client experiencing a fluid or electrolyte imbalance.
- Discuss nursing management of a client experiencing a fluid or electrolyte imbalance.
- Identify expected outcomes for the client experiencing a fluid or electrolyte imbalance.

PRACTICE TEST

1 A 10-month-old infant is admitted to the emergency department with a 102°F rectal temperature and a history of vomiting and diarrhea for the past 48 hours. What signs and symptoms should the nurse look for related to this client's likely fluid imbalance?

1. Bulging fontanels, tearless cry, and low urine output
2. Sunken eyes, lethargy, and dry, furrowed tongue
3. Weight loss, dilute urine, and peripheral edema
4. Dry skin, thready pulse, and neck vein distention

2 Which observation by the nurse is a reliable indicator that therapy for fluid volume excess is achieving the desired outcome?

1. Full, bounding peripheral pulses
2. Flat neck veins with head of bed elevated
3. Hand vein emptying longer than 20 seconds
4. S_3 heart sound clearly audible on auscultation

3 The nurse concludes that which of the following is a reliable sign that ascites fluid is being effectively mobilized in response to therapy?

1. Weight gain of 1 pound in 24 hours
2. Increase in urine output
3. Drop in blood pressure
4. Hand veins fill slowly

4 Which of the following should be included in an education program to prevent dehydration for a hiking club that is planning a 12-mile hike in the summer?

1. Take water and commercial sports drinks to sip often along the way
2. Drink large amounts of water, at least 16 ounces every hour, while hiking
3. Take salt tablets every 3 to 4 hours and drink plenty of water while in the heat
4. Stop every 4 hours along the way and drink a few ounces of water while resting

5 Which one of the following postoperative clients would be at risk for developing a sodium imbalance?

1. A client who has just had a tonsillectomy
2. A client who has a primary cesarean section for failure to progress in labor
3. A client who has a transurethral resection of the prostate (TURP)
4. A client who has a right knee arthroscopy

6 The nurse is caring for a client experiencing hyponatremia. As part of the care, the nurse will restrict which of the following items for this client?

1. Sports drinks such as Gatorade
2. Eggs and cheese products
3. Salt on the diet tray
4. Water

7 The nurse is caring for a client experiencing hypernatremia. The nurse concludes that it is important to administer which of the following to this client?

1. Cough suppressant to treat symptomatic cough
2. 3% saline solution
3. Water
4. Lactulose (Chronulac)

8 The community health nurse is assigned to a client who has been recently discharged from the hospital with resolving hypernatremia. During the initial assessment interview, what information would be of critical importance in determining a plan of care for this client?

1. The client lives on the second floor of an apartment building that has an elevator.
2. The client has a neighbor who picks up the mail each day and brings it to the apartment.
3. The client performs self-monitoring of blood glucose once a day.
4. The client uses Alka-Seltzer on a frequent basis for gastrointestinal complaints.

9 The nurse is caring for a client who has sustained partial and full thickness burns over 30% of his body. The nurse assesses for which of the following electrolyte imbalances, which occurs as electrolyte shifts from the intracellular fluid (ICF) to the extracellular fluid (ECF)?

1. Hyperkalemia
2. Hypokalemia
3. Hypervolemia
4. Hypercalcemia

10 The nurse concludes that a history of which of the following conditions places a client at risk for possible hypokalemia?

1. Chronic obstructive pulmonary disease (COPD)
2. Cirrhosis
3. Malignant melanoma
4. Chronic renal failure (CRF)

PRACTICE TEST

11 Which of the following orders should the nurse question regarding a client with severe hypokalemia?

1. Infuse 1,000 mL normal saline with 20 mEq-potassium chloride IV over 8 hours.
2. Give KCl 20 mEq PO daily after meals.
3. Infuse 1,000 mL normal saline with 40 mEq KCl at 200 mL/hour.
4. Give 20 mEq KCl/IV over 10 minutes.

12 Which of the following treatment options does the nurse anticipate will be appropriate for a client with a potassium level of 3.5 mEq/L?

1. Administration of Kayexalate per rectum
2. Use of salt substitutes in the diet
3. Administration of oral KCl
4. Continue to monitor and offer foods high in potassium

13 Which one of the following assessments should be included in a plan of care for a client who is at risk for developing hypocalcemia?

1. Monitor BUN and creatinine levels to determine renal dysfunction.
2. Monitor client for constipation.
3. Monitor serum albumin and magnesium levels.
4. Monitor for fluid volume excess related to intravenous saline therapy.

14 A client with hypocalcemia is taking supplemental vitamin D. The nurse explains the rationale for vitamin D is that

1. It directly opposes calcitonin.
2. It prevents renal disease in clients with hypocalcemia.
3. Calcium is absorbed in the intestines only under the influence of activated vitamin D.
4. The only way to obtain vitamin D is with oral supplementation.

15 Which of the following medications reported by a client during a nursing history could be associated with the development of hypocalcemia?

1. Phenytoin (Dilantin)
2. Calcium carbonate (TUMS)
3. Calcitriol
4. Hydrochlorothiazide (Hydro-Diuril)

16 The family of a client with hypercalcemia states that the client is "not acting like himself." The nurse focuses assessment on which of the following symptoms?

1. Personality change
2. Anxiety
3. Convulsions
4. Carpal spasms

17 The nurse who is assessing the client for signs of hypocalcemia would conclude that this electrolyte imbalance exists after noting which of the following?

1. Negative Chvostek's sign
2. Positive Trousseau's sign
3. Positive Kernig's sign
4. Hypoactive bowel sounds

18 The nurse would review a client's electrolyte levels to detect a possible increase in magnesium if the client had which of the following conditions?

1. Cushing's syndrome
2. Diabetes
3. Addison's disease
4. Splenomegaly

19 The nurse concludes that a client does not have an increased magnesium level based on which of the following findings?

1. Hypotension
2. Bradycardia
3. Supraventricular tachycardia (SVT)
4. Flushing and sweating

20 A client with renal failure is experiencing hypermagnesemia. The nurse explains that which of the following treatments will be used to most effectively decrease the magnesium level?

1. Dialysis
2. Diuretics
3. Fluid restriction
4. High volume IV fluids

21 The nurse reviews the laboratory test results for a client with preeclampsia, expecting to find which of the following values?

1. Sodium 148 mEq/L
2. Sodium 125 mEq/L
3. Magnesium 3.1 mEq/L
4. Magnesium 1.2 mEq/L

22 A client was admitted to the hospital with a weight gain of 30 pounds over the past month. Upon assessment, the client was noted to have a moon face and a "buffalo hump." On admission, lab results indicated decreased serum potassium and magnesium and elevated serum chloride and sodium levels. The nurse interprets that which of the following disorders is consistent with these manifestations?

1. Addison's disease
2. Cushing's syndrome
3. Burns
4. Syndrome of inappropriate ADH (SIADH)

23 A home health nurse is making a visit to an elderly client who has a history of heart failure (CHF). The client was prescribed diuretics twice a day and a low sodium diet. The nurse should be most concerned about which of the following laboratory results?

1. Na^+ 145 mEq/L
2. Cl^- 90 mEq/L
3. K^+ 4.2 mEq/L
4. HCO_3^- 27 mEq/L

24 Which of the following findings in a client's history would alert the nurse to assess for signs and symptoms of hypophosphatemia?

1. Withdrawal from alcohol
2. The oliguric phase of acute tubular necrosis
3. Short-term gastric suction
4. Occasional use of aluminum-containing antacids

25 Which of the following concurrent electrolyte imbalances should the nurse anticipate while assigned to the care of a client with hyperphosphatemia?

1. Potassium 2.8 mEq/L
2. Sodium 131 mEq/L
3. Calcium 6.8 mEq/L
4. Magnesium 3.4 mEq/L

26 The nurse would report to the charge nurse that an assigned client has hyperkalemia after noting that the serum potassium level drawn that morning was greater than how many mEq/L? Provide a numerical answer.

Answer: ______________________

PRACTICE TEST

ANSWERS & RATIONALES

ANSWERS & RATIONALES

1 **Answer: 2** The client's history suggests fluid volume deficit and dehydration. Sunken eyes, altered mental status and behavior, and dry, furrowed tongue are reliable signs of fluid volume deficit in infants. Bulging fontanels, peripheral edema, and neck vein distention are seen with fluid volume excess. **Cognitive Level:** Application **Client Need:** Physiological Integrity: Physiological Adaptation **Integrated Process:** Nursing Process: Assessment **Content Area:** Adult Health: Endocrine and Metabolic **Strategy:** The core issue of the question is the ability to correlate a clinical picture with risk for hypovolemia. Use nursing knowledge of signs of dehydration and the process of elimination to make a selection.

2 **Answer: 2** Venous congestion results from fluid volume excess and causes full, bounding pulses, delayed hand vein emptying, and S_3 heart sounds. Flat neck veins with head of bed elevated is an indicator of the absence of venous congestion. **Cognitive Level:** Application **Client Need:** Physiological Integrity: Physiological Adaptation **Integrated Process:** Nursing Process: Evaluation **Content Area:** Adult Health: Endocrine and Metabolic **Strategy:** The core issue of the question is knowledge of signs of fluid overload and normal findings. Use nursing knowledge and the process of elimination to make a selection.

3 **Answer: 2** Ascites is a form of third space fluid. Therapy is aimed at moving third space fluid back into the circulation where it can be eliminated by the kidneys. When this fluid is drawn back into the vascular space (leading to a rise in BP and venous pressure), the kidneys increase the urine output to eliminate the excess fluid. Loss of fluid results in loss of weight. **Cognitive Level:** Analysis **Client Need:** Physiological Integrity: Physiological Adaptation **Integrated Process:** Nursing Process: Evaluation **Content Area:** Adult Health: Endocrine and Metabolic **Strategy:** The core issue of the question is recognition of ascites as a third space fluid and knowledge of effective mobilization of that fluid. Recall that mobilized fluid must be eliminated via the kidneys to assist in making a selection.

4 **Answer: 1** Those who exercise in hot climates need to continuously replace both fluid and electrolyte losses. Sports drinks

provide carbohydrates, water, and electrolytes. Drinking large amounts of only water fails to replace electrolytes, which can lead to water intoxication. Salt tablets are no longer recommended because too much salt has a hypertonic effect, causes diuresis, and can actually worsen fluid loss.
Cognitive Level: Analysis **Client Need:** Physiological Integrity: Physiological Adaptation **Integrated Process:** Nursing Process: Implementation **Content Area:** Adult Health: Endocrine and Metabolic **Strategy:** The core issue of the question is knowledge of measures to prevent fluid and electrolyte imbalance during exercise. Use nursing knowledge and the process of elimination to make a selection.

5 **Answer: 3** A TURP procedure can place a client at risk for developing hyponatremia in the postoperative period due to increased fluid irrigation used during and after surgery. Clients with a TURP procedure have a CBI (continuous bladder irrigation) as a routine part of their postoperative care. The other options do not place a client at risk for development of sodium imbalances because they do not require lengthy fluid and dietary restrictions or excessive fluid irrigation.
Cognitive Level: Application **Client Need:** Physiological Integrity: Physiological Adaptation **Integrated Process:** Nursing Process: Analysis **Content Area:** Adult Health: Endocrine and Metabolic **Strategy:** The core issue of the question is knowledge that procedures and surgeries requiring the use of water for irrigation can lead to dilutional hyponatremia. Use nursing knowledge and the process of elimination to make a selection.

6 **Answer: 4** Hyponatremia can also be referred to as dilutional hyponatremia or water intoxication. Water restriction would be an important part of the treatment plan when caring for a client who has hyponatremia. The restriction of Gatorade (electrolyte-rich solution), eggs, cheese products, and salt on the diet tray are not indicated because the client is experiencing a sodium deficit.
Cognitive Level: Application **Client Need:** Physiological Integrity: Physiological Adaptation **Integrated Process:** Nursing Process: Implementation **Content Area:** Adult Health: Endocrine and Metabolic **Strategy:** The core issue of the question is effective treatment measures for hyponatremia. Use nursing knowledge and the process of elimination to make a selection.

7 **Answer: 3** Clients with hypernatremia are thirsty and need water replacement to balance the increased sodium levels. Cough medication and lactulose can further increase sodium levels and should not be administered unless there is sufficient clinical information to warrant their use. Three percent saline is a hypertonic solution that would also increase serum sodium levels and should not be given to this client.
Cognitive Level: Application **Client Need:** Physiological Integrity: Physiological Adaptation **Integrated Process:** Nursing Process: Implementation **Content Area:** Adult Health: Endocrine and Metabolic **Strategy:** The core issue of the question is knowledge of measures that effectively treat hypernatremia. Use nursing knowledge and the process of elimination to make a selection.

8 **Answer: 4** The frequent use of Alka-Seltzer can cause an increase in serum sodium levels. It is important during an initial assessment to obtain information about all medications (prescription and OTC) that a client is taking. Options 1 and 2 are incorrect because they do not relate to potential sodium imbalance. They are helpful in determining the client's support system and mobility status. Option 3 suggests that the client may have diabetes, but this does not relate to increases in serum sodium levels.
Cognitive Level: Application **Client Need:** Physiological Integrity: Physiological Adaptation **Integrated Process:** Nursing Process: Assessment **Content Area:** Adult Health: Endocrine and Metabolic **Strategy:** The core issue of the question is knowledge of factors that can lead to elevated serum sodium levels. Use nursing knowledge and the process of elimination to make a selection.

9 **Answer: 1** During periods of major trauma, potassium shifts from the ICF to the ECF because of cell death, leading to high serum levels of potassium. Hypokalemia is not seen in burn clients during the time of fluid shifting secondary to trauma. The client with burns is more likely to be hypovolemic and hypocalcemic at this point in time because there is fluid and electrolyte loss caused by altered capillary integrity.
Cognitive Level: Application **Client Need:** Physiological Integrity: Physiological Adaptation **Integrated Process:** Nursing Process: Assessment **Content Area:** Adult Health: Endocrine and Metabolic **Strategy:** The core issue of the question is knowledge that burn injury increases the risk of hyperkalemia. Use nursing knowledge and the process of elimination to make a selection.

10 **Answer: 2** In clients with cirrhosis, increased amounts of aldosterone are secreted, which leads to sodium retention and potassium excretion from the kidneys; these clients are likely to become hypokalemic. Clients with COPD, malignant melanoma, and CRF are likely to develop hyperkalemia due to retention of acids.
Cognitive Level: Analysis **Client Need:** Physiological Integrity: Physiological Adaptation **Integrated Process:** Nursing Process: Analysis **Content Area:** Adult Health: Endocrine and Metabolic **Strategy:** The core issue of the question is the ability to discriminate predisposing factors for hypokalemia from hyperkalemia. Use nursing knowledge and the process of elimination to make a selection.

11 **Answer: 4** Potassium is never given as a bolus when it is administered intravenously. All of the other orders are within a safe and therapeutic range. KCl should never be given rapidly or by IV push because serious arrhythmias or cardiac arrest can occur.
Cognitive Level: Analysis **Client Need:** Physiological Integrity: Pharmacological and Parenteral Therapies **Integrated Process:** Nursing Process: Planning **Content Area:** Adult Health: Endocrine and Metabolic **Strategy:** The core issue of the question is knowledge of safe and unsafe methods of administering potassium as replacement therapy. Use nursing knowledge and the process of elimination to make a selection.

12 **Answer: 4** A serum potassium level of 3.5 mEq/L is at the low end of the normal range. With a low normal level, it is better to continue to monitor the client and offer foods that are good sources of potassium. In the absence of additional medical history, it is not advisable to use additional treatment options at this point in time. Therefore, options 1 and 3 would not be indicated: they would be included for a client who is hypokalemic. The use of salt substitutes would require more background information because the client may have other conditions in which their use is not advisable.

Cognitive Level: Application **Client Need:** Physiological Integrity: Physiological Adaptation **Integrated Process:** Nursing Process: Planning **Content Area:** Adult Health: Endocrine and Metabolic **Strategy:** The core issue of the question is knowledge of treatment measures depending on the severity of hypokalemia. First recognize that this is a value at the low end of normal, and then select the mildest intervention of the choices provided.

13 **Answer: 3** A client who is at risk for developing hypocalcemia requires monitoring of serum albumin (provides information relative to physiologically available calcium) and magnesium levels (decreased magnesium levels are usually seen concurrently with low serum calcium levels). The other options reflect assessments that would be included for a client who would be at risk to develop hypercalcemia.
Cognitive Level: Application **Client Need:** Physiological Integrity: Physiological Adaptation **Integrated Process:** Nursing Process: Planning **Content Area:** Adult Health: Endocrine and Metabolic **Strategy:** The core issue of the question is the ability to choose assessments to detect hypocalcemia. Use nursing knowledge and the process of elimination to make a selection.

14 **Answer: 3** Calcium is absorbed in the intestines only under the influence of vitamin D, which is activated in the kidneys. Option 1 is incorrect because parathyroid hormone directly opposes calcitonin. Option 2 is incorrect because renal disease prevents activation of vitamin D, thereby reducing the body's ability to absorb calcium. Option 4 is incorrect: there are other ways to obtain vitamin D in the body (such exposure to sunlight).
Cognitive Level: Application **Client Need:** Physiological Integrity: Pharmacological and Parenteral Therapies **Integrated Process:** Nursing Process: Implementation **Content Area:** Adult Health: Endocrine and Metabolic **Strategy:** The core issue of the question is knowledge of the purpose and effects of vitamin D in a client with hypocalcemia. Use nursing knowledge and the process of elimination to make a selection.

15 **Answer: 1** Anticonvulsants such as phenytoin (Dilantin) alter vitamin D metabolism and lead to hypocalcemia. Options 2 and 3 represent calcium sources, and the inclusion of these in a treatment plan would lead to increased serum calcium levels. Option 4 is incorrect because thiazide diuretics can lead to calcium retention.
Cognitive Level: Application **Client Need:** Physiological Integrity: Physiological Adaptation **Integrated Process:** Nursing Process: Assessment **Content Area:** Adult Health: Endocrine and Metabolic **Strategy:** The core issue of the question is knowledge of medications that increase risk of hypocalcemia. Use nursing knowledge and the process of elimination to make a selection.

16 **Answer: 1** Clinical manifestations of hypercalcemia include personality changes. All other options are signs and symptoms of hypocalcemia.
Cognitive Level: Application **Client Need:** Physiological Integrity: Physiological Adaptation **Integrated Process:** Nursing Process: Assessment **Content Area:** Adult Health: Endocrine and Metabolic **Strategy:** The core issue of the question is knowledge of manifestations of hypercalcemia. Use nursing knowledge and the process of elimination to make a selection.

17 **Answer: 2** Clinical manifestations of hypocalcemia include a positive Trousseau's sign, which is an ischemia-induced carpopedal spasm. A positive Chvostek's sign is associated with hypocalcemia, while hypoactive bowel sounds are a sign of hypercalcemia. Kernig's sign is an indication of meningeal irritation.
Cognitive Level: Application **Client Need:** Physiological Integrity: Physiological Adaptation **Integrated Process:** Nursing Process: Assessment **Content Area:** Adult Health: Endocrine and Metabolic **Strategy:** The core issue of the question is knowledge of manifestations of hypocalcemia. Use nursing knowledge and the process of elimination to make a selection.

18 **Answer: 3** Addison's disease, known also as adrenal insufficiency, can cause increased magnesium levels resulting from volume depletion. Cushing's disease is hyperfunction of the adrenal gland. Diabetes could lead to low magnesium levels if osmotic diuresis is present from hyperglycemia. Splenomegaly is an unrelated finding.
Cognitive Level: Application **Client Need:** Physiological Integrity: Physiological Adaptation **Integrated Process:** Nursing Process: Assessment **Content Area:** Adult Health: Endocrine and Metabolic **Strategy:** The core issue of the question is knowledge of risk factors for hypermagnesemia. Use nursing knowledge and the process of elimination to make a selection.

19 **Answer: 3** SVT is seen with decreased magnesium levels, as are premature ventricular contractions and ventricular fibrillation. The other three options are findings with hypermagnesemia.
Cognitive Level: Analysis **Client Need:** Physiological Integrity: Physiological Adaptation **Integrated Process:** Nursing Process: Assessment **Content Area:** Adult Health: Endocrine and Metabolic **Strategy:** The core issue of the question is the ability to discriminate signs of hyper- and hypomagnesemia. Use nursing knowledge and the process of elimination to make a selection.

20 **Answer: 1** Either hemodialysis or peritoneal dialysis is used to remove excess magnesium in the client with renal failure. Diuretics will not be effective if the kidneys are not functional. Fluid restriction would be ineffective, and high-volume IV fluid replacement would be contraindicated in renal failure.
Cognitive Level: Application **Client Need:** Physiological Integrity: Physiological Adaptation **Integrated Process:** Nursing Process: Implementation **Content Area:** Adult Health: Endocrine and Metabolic **Strategy:** The core issue of the question is knowledge of effective therapies for increased magnesium levels. Note the critical words *renal failure,* which leads you to look for a treatment that does not involve functional kidneys. Use nursing knowledge and the process of elimination to make a selection.

21 **Answer: 4** Decreased magnesium level (option 4) may occur in toxemia of pregnancy, preeclampsia, and eclampsia, in turn causing convulsions (seizures). The other responses are incorrect because they are directed at sodium (options 1 and 2) or increased magnesium level (option 3).
Cognitive Level: Application **Client Need:** Physiological Integrity: Physiological Adaptation **Integrated Process:** Nursing Process: Assessment **Content Area:** Adult Health: Endocrine and Metabolic **Strategy:** The core issue of the question is knowledge of conditions that are consistent with decreased magnesium levels, and the ability to determine a reduced level. Use nursing knowledge and the process of elimination to make a selection.

22 **Answer: 2** Cushing's syndrome causes low potassium and magnesium levels and an increase in sodium and chloride levels. The moon face and buffalo hump are also symptoms of excess corticosteroids. Option 1 is incorrect because Addison's disease causes low sodium and increased magnesium and potassium. Option 3 is incorrect because burn states cause significant fluid and electrolyte disturbances (loss of sodium, chloride, and magnesium with alterations in potassium depending on stage of burn), but the presence of a moon face and buffalo hump is characteristic of Cushing's syndrome. Option 4 is incorrect because SIADH is associated with hyponatremia.
Cognitive Level: Analysis **Client Need:** Physiological Integrity: Physiological Adaptation **Integrated Process:** Nursing Process: Assessment **Content Area:** Adult Health: Endocrine and Metabolic **Strategy:** The core issue of the question is the ability to synthesize electrolyte results with a clinical picture in a client with Cushing's syndrome. Use nursing knowledge and the process of elimination to make a selection.

23 **Answer: 2** The home health nurse should be most concerned with the decreased chloride level because it can lead to complications such as dilutional hypochloremia. The client's history of CHF places the client in a higher risk category for fluid retention, electrolyte disturbances, and acid-base disorders. All of the other options reflect laboratory values that are within normal range and are reassuring.
Cognitive Level: Analysis **Client Need:** Physiological Integrity: Physiological Adaptation **Integrated Process:** Nursing Process: Assessment **Content Area:** Adult Health: Endocrine and Metabolic **Strategy:** The core issue of the question is the ability to determine abnormal electrolyte levels. Use nursing knowledge and the process of elimination to make a selection.

24 **Answer: 1** Poor nutritional intake, vomiting, diarrhea, and the overuse of antacid are related to alcoholism and alcohol abuse. These can lead to hypophosphatemia. During oliguria, the kidneys are unable to excrete phosphorus (option 2). Clients with prolonged (not short-term) gastric suction are more likely to experience hypophosphatemia (option 3). Prolonged or continuous use of aluminum-containing antacids (not occasional use) leads to hypophosphatemia (option 4).
Cognitive Level: Analysis **Client Need:** Physiological Integrity: Physiological Adaptation **Integrated Process:** Nursing Process: Assessment **Content Area:** Adult Health: Endocrine and Metabolic **Strategy:** The core issue of the question is knowledge of risk factors for hypophosphatemia. Use nursing knowledge and the process of elimination to make a selection.

25 **Answer: 3** Calcium and phosphorus have an inverse relationship in the body. For this reason, when phosphorus levels are high, calcium levels are low (option 3). The other responses do not address this relationship.
Cognitive Level: Analysis **Client Need:** Physiological Integrity: Physiological Adaptation **Integrated Process:** Nursing Process: Assessment **Content Area:** Adult Health: Endocrine and Metabolic **Strategy:** The core issue of the question is knowledge that hypocalcemia accompanies hypermagnesemia. To answer the question correctly, you must also be able to recognize abnormal laboratory values. Use nursing knowledge and the process of elimination to make a selection.

26 **Answer: 5.1** Hyperkalemia exists when the serum potassium level rises above the upper limit of normal, which is 5.1 mEq/L.
Cognitive Level: Analysis **Client Need:** Physiological Integrity: Physiological Adaptation **Integrated Process:** Nursing Process: Analysis **Content Area:** Adult Health: Endocrine and Metabolic **Strategy:** The core issue of the question is knowledge that hypocalcemia accompanies hypermagnesemia. To answer the question correctly, you must also be able to recognize abnormal laboratory values. Use nursing knowledge and the process of elimination to make a selection.

Key Terms to Review

hypercalcemia p. 971
hyperchloremia p. 975
hyperkalemia p. 968
hypermagnesemia p. 974
hypernatremia p. 965
hyperosmolar p. 965
hyperphosphatemia p. 977
hypertonic p. 958
hypervolemia p. 963
hypocalcemia p. 969
hypochloremia p. 974
hypokalemia p. 967
hypomagnesemia p. 974
hyponatremia p. 963
hypophosphatemia p. 976
hypotonic p. 958
hypovolemia p. 963
water intoxication p. 963

References

Black, J., & Hawks, J. (2005). *Medical surgical nursing: Clinical management for positive outcomes* (7th ed.). St. Louis: Elsevier Science.

Corbett, J. (2004). *Laboratory tests and diagnostic procedures with nursing diagnoses* (6th ed.). Upper Saddle River, NJ: Pearson Education.

Harkreader, H., & Hogan, M. (2004). *Fundamentals of nursing: Caring and clinical judgment* (2nd ed.). St. Louis: Elsevier Science.

Hockenberry, M., Wilson, D., Winkelstein, M., & Kline, N. (2003). *Nursing care of infants and children* (7th ed.). St. Louis: Mosby.

Ignatavicius, D., & Workman, L. (2006). *Medical-surgical nursing: Critical thinking for collaborative care* (5th ed.). Philadelphia: W. B. Saunders.

Kozier, B., Erb, G., Berman, A., & Snyder, S. (2004). *Fundamentals of nursing: Concepts, process, and practice* (7th ed.). Upper Saddle River, NJ: Pearson Education.

LeMone, P., & Burke, K. (2004). *Medical surgical nursing: Critical thinking in client care* (3rd ed.). Upper Saddle River, NJ: Pearson Education.

Lewis, S., Heitkemper, M., & Dirksen, S. (2004). *Medical surgical nursing: Assessment and management of clinical problems* (6th ed.). St. Louis: Elsevier Science.

Porth, C. (2004). *Pathophysiology: Concepts of altered health states* (7th ed.). Philadelphia: Lippincott Williams & Wilkins.

Acid-Base Imbalances

55

In this chapter

Test Yourself

Are you ready for the NCLEX-RN® or course exams? Use the practice tests on the companion CD-ROM to check.

Cross reference

Other chapters relevant to this content area are

Common Laboratory Tests Chapter 47
Fluid and Electrolyte Imbalances Chapter 54

I. NORMAL ACID-BASE BALANCE

A. Nature of acids and bases

1. An **acid** is a substance that releases a hydrogen (H^+) ion when dissolved in water
2. A **base** is a substance that will bind to an H^+ ion when dissolved in water
3. Weak acids do not completely separate in water; they only release some of H^+ ions
4. A weak base accepts H^+ ions less easily, but it is extremely valuable in preventing major alterations in **pH** of extracellular fluid (ECF)

B. Chemical buffer systems in body

1. A **buffer** prevents major changes in ECF by releasing or accepting H^+ ions
2. The major chemical buffers (found in blood) include bicarbonate–carbonic acid buffer system, phosphate buffer system, and protein buffer system
3. Chemical buffers are present in both intracellular fluid (ICF) and ECF
4. Buffers are found in all body tissues, including bone
5. Chemical buffers act within seconds to neutralize acids and bases and keep pH within narrow normal range of 7.35 to 7.45
6. Bicarbonate buffer system
   a. Consists of a water solution that contains a weak acid, carbonic acid (H_2CO_3), and a bicarbonate salt, usually sodium bicarbonate ($NaHCO_3$)
   b. Normally, body maintains pH by keeping ratio of bicarbonate (**HCO_3^-**) to H_2CO_3 at a proportion of 20:1; this ratio is changed if pH goes up or down
   c. Once compensation occurs, ratio becomes stable again
   d. The bicarbonate–carbonic acid buffer system is linked to both respiratory and renal systems
   e. H_2CO_3 is respiratory compensatory component; it can dissociate into carbon dioxide (CO_2) and water, with CO_2 being exhaled by lungs
   f. HCO_3^- is the primary renal compensatory component; it can be excreted by kidneys or retained with excretion of H^+ ions

g. This function is illustrated by the following equation:
$CO_2 + H_2O \leftrightarrow H_2CO_3 \leftrightarrow HCO_3^- + H^+$

7. The phosphate buffer system buffers both ICF and ECF to maintain a normal pH
8. The protein buffer system acts similarly to bicarbonate–carbonic acid buffer system because it releases or accepts H^+ readily and can exist as either an acid or a base; it is a major intracellular buffer
9. The hemoglobin-oxyhemoglobin buffer system helps to maintain pH within normal range in both arterial and venous blood, which have different amounts of CO_2

C. Physiologic buffers in body

1. Pulmonary regulation
   a. Lungs control the respiratory carbonic acid buffer system and compensate for acid-base disturbances that are primarily metabolic in nature (e.g., lactic acidosis that occurs with exercise)
   b. Under control of medulla oblongata, lungs increase or decrease respiratory rate and depth in response to amount of CO_2 in ECF
   c. Respiratory system is extremely sensitive to changes in pH and begins compensatory efforts within seconds to minutes but can become quickly exhausted and is not as efficient as renal compensation
   d. Older adults have reduced gas exchange during breathing and less alveolar membrane so CO_2 retention and increased H^+ ion concentrations may be a problem
2. Renal regulation
   a. Kidneys control the metabolic buffer $NaHCO_3^-$ by excreting an acidic urine or an alkaline urine
   b. This system works within several hours to days but is powerfully effective by eliminating either acids or bases as needed
   c. Kidneys control HCO_3^- in ECF by either reabsorbing or excreting H^+ ions; they also combine ammonia (NaH_3) with hydrochloric acid (HCl) to form ammonium (NH_4Cl), which is excreted by kidneys; approximately 50% of excess H^+ can be excreted by this mechanism
   d. Kidneys can also excrete weak acids into urine
   e. Body depends on kidneys to excrete acids from cellular metabolism; thus urine is normally acidic (average pH 6)
   f. Renal function decreases with age, so older adults do not excrete H^+ ions or synthesize HCO_3^- as efficiently, making their acid-base imbalances more difficult to correct, especially if other conditions such as pneumonia, fever, or infection occur
3. **Compensation** for an acid-base imbalance occurs when body uses regulatory mechanisms to return pH to normal by transforming acids and bases within body; pH becomes normal, but there are abnormal amounts of CO_2 and/or HCO_3^-
   a. A primary metabolic disturbance will cause respiratory compensation
   b. A primary respiratory disturbance will activate blood buffers and cause metabolic compensation by kidneys
   c. Complete compensation means that buffers have achieved homeostasis and pH is fully corrected
   d. Partial compensation means that buffers are working to restore homeostasis
   e. Decompensation refers to a worsening state of acid-base imbalance
4. Correction of acid-base imbalance occurs when lungs and/or kidneys eliminate offending substance(s) from body, and both CO_2 and HCO_3^- levels (not just pH) are returned to normal

D. Indicator measures of acid base status

1. pH: the negative logarithm of H^+ ion concentration in mEq per liter
   a. Actual concentration of H^+ ions is very small (less than 0.0001 mEq/liter); therefore, it has a negative logarithm
   b. Because pH is calculated as a negative value, there is an inverse relationship between pH and H^+ ion concentration; therefore, as H^+ ion concentration increases, pH decreases
   c. Normal pH in arterial blood is 7.35 to 7.45; in venous blood, it is 7.32 to 7.42

d. A pH less than 7.35 is labeled acidotic; acidosis has depressant effect on central nervous system (CNS)
e. A pH greater than 7.45 is labeled alkalotic; alkalosis has excitatory effect on CNS

Memory Aid

The pH is like the center of a seesaw; it wants to stay balanced.

2. **$PaCO_2$** (partial pressure of carbon dioxide): measurement of CO_2 pressure being exerted on plasma; is directly related to amount of CO_2 being produced
   a. $PaCO_2$ is regulated by lungs and indicates amount of H_2CO_3 that is available to act as a buffer
   b. $PaCO_2$ indicates whether condition is a respiratory disturbance
   c. Normal value of $PaCO_2$ is 35 to 45 mm Hg
   d. Values less than 35 mm Hg indicate alkalosis
   e. Values greater than 45 mm Hg indicate acidosis

Memory Aid

Carbon dioxide (CO_2) acts as an acid in the body. It is also the indicator of how the respiratory system is functioning.

3. HCO_3^- (bicarbonate): measurement of HCO_3^- in plasma and is directly related to attraction and release of H^+ ions from H_2CO_3
   a. HCO_3^- is regulated by kidneys and indicates body's ability to buffer H^+ ions (acid) by combining to form H_2CO_3
   b. HCO_3^- is the value that indicates whether there is a metabolic disturbance
   c. Normal value of HCO_3^- is 22 to 26 mEq/L
   d. Values less than 22 mEq/L indicate acidosis
   e. Value greater than 26 mEq/L indicate alkalosis

Memory Aid

Bicarbonate (HCO_3^-) acts as a base in the body. It is also the indicator of how the metabolic system is functioning.

4. **PaO_2** (partial pressure of oxygen): measures amount of pressure exerted by oxygen on plasma
   a. Range of normal values for PaO_2 is 80 to 100 mm Hg for adults under 60 years of age; for every year above 60, there is an expected decrease in PaO_2 of 1 mmHg
   b. If PaO_2 drops dramatically, then O_2 saturation also decreases greatly
5. **SaO_2**: percentage of hemoglobin saturated with O_2; since most O_2 is carried on hemoglobin, total O_2 concentration is measured using hemoglobin saturation (SaO_2)
   a. A relationship between PaO_2 and SaO_2 influences binding affinity and dissociation of oxygen and hemoglobin (called oxygen–hemoglobin dissociation curve)
   b. Acidosis causes a shift toward right on oxygen–hemoglobin dissociation curve that results in a decreased affinity; oxygen is more easily released to tissues
   c. Alkalosis causes a shift toward left on oxygen–hemoglobin dissociation curve that results in an increased affinity; oxygen is held more tightly and is less available to tissues
   d. Other factors that affect oxygen affinity include body temperature and transfusion of banked blood
6. Electrolyte interactions
   a. HCO_3^- is a direct reflection of renal system's ability to compensate for pH changes; a decreased HCO_3^- level is consistent with acidosis, and an increased HCO_3^- level is consistent with alkalosis

b. Base excess (BE) indicates amount of HCO_3^- available in ECF, and normal values range from −3.0 to +3.0 in adults; values above +3.0 indicate metabolic alkalosis, while values below −3.0 indicate metabolic acidosis
c. Serum anion gap (AG) (normal range 10 to 12mEq/L) calculates concentrations of anions (HCO_3^-, chloride [Cl^-], proteins, phosphates, and sulfates) and cations (sodium [Na^+], potassium [K^+], magnesium [Mg^{++}], calcium [Ca^{++}]) by using the following equation:
$Na^+ - [Cl^- + HCO_3^-]$
d. Increased AG of more than 12 mEq/L indicates metabolic acidosis (AG acidosis); however, a normal AG can exist with a metabolic acidosis (non-AG acidosis) when there is a decrease in HCO_3^- balanced by an increase in Cl^-
e. Decreased AG of less than 10 mEq/L can be seen with low albumin levels or in conditions in which there is an increase in unmeasured cations (multiple myeloma, lithium toxicity, or nephrotic syndrome)
f. Potassium (K^+) helps to maintain acid-base balance by exchanging for H^+ ions across cell membranes; in acidosis, K^+ comes out of cell and allows H^+ in to reduce circulating acids; in alkalosis, K^+ goes into cell and allows H^+ to come out to increase circulating acids
g. Chloride levels are used to evaluate clients who are at risk for metabolic alkalosis; this can help to determine cause of alkalosis and thus corrective treatment

E. Arterial blood gas (ABG) analysis (see Table 55–1 ■ for normal values)

! 1. Follow a systematic approach (see Figure 55–1 ■)
2. Interpret pH: a pH less than 7.35 indicates acidosis, while a pH greater than 7.45 indicates alkalosis
3. Identify primary cause—respiratory or metabolic
   a. Examine first $PaCO_2$ value and then HCO_3^- value
   b. If $PaCO_2$ is abnormal and direction of change in value is inversely related to direction of change in pH, then primary problem is respiratory
   c. If HCO_3^- is abnormal and direction of change in value is same as direction of change in pH, then problem is metabolic

Memory Aid

Interpret ABGs by looking first at the pH, then at the CO_2, then at the HCO_3^-. Determine first whether there is acidosis or alkalosis, then evaluate whether the imbalance is respiratory (CO_2) or metabolic (HCO_3^-) in origin. The cause will be the value that *matches* or correlates with the change in the direction of the pH.

4. Determine presence of compensation
   a. Determine if $PaCO_2$ and HCO_3^- are decreased or increased as body attempts to maintain ratio of HCO_3^- to H_2CO_3 at 20:1

Table 55–1

Normal Arterial Blood Gas Values

Serum Laboratory Value	Normal Reference Ranges: Adult	Child	Infant
pH (arterial)	7.35–7.45	7.37–7.43 (c) 7.35–7.41 (a)	7.36–7.42
PCO_2 (mmHg)	35–45	35–41 (c) 38–44 (a)	30–34
HCO_3^- (mEq/L)	22–26	18–25 (c) 23–25 (a)	17.2–23.6
PO_2 (mm Hg)	80–100	80–100	80–100
SaO_2 (%)	95–100	95–100	95–100
Anion Gap Base Excess	10–12 mEq/L +3 to −3 (+/− 2 mEq/L)	10–12 mEq/L +3 to −3 (+/− 2 mEq/L)	10–12 mEq/L +3 to −3 (+/− 2 mEq/L)

c, children; a, adolescents

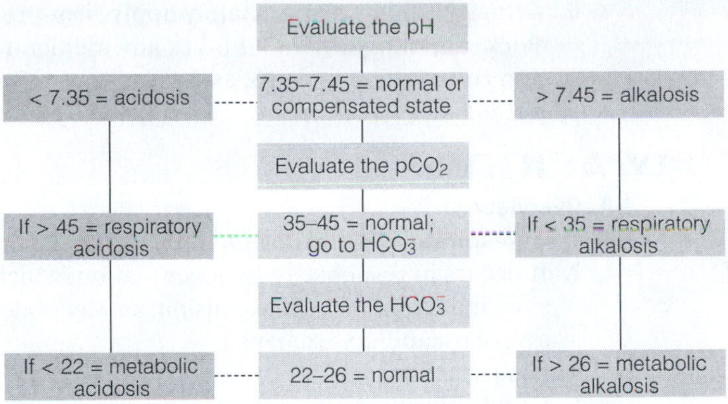

Figure 55–1

Interpreting ABGs: If CO_2 and HCO_3^- are both abnormal, look to see which one has a change that *matches* the change in the pH (CO_2 acts as an acid; HCO_3^- acts as a base). This match will be the primary imbalance, while the other system is compensating.

b. Partial compensation exists when pH remains abnormal but parameter that did not originally alter pH now changes (e.g., pH indicates an acidotic state and CO_2 is high, indicating respiratory origin, but HCO_3^- is also increased, indicating that body is utilizing buffer systems to bring pH back into line)

Memory Aid

The pH is like a seesaw. The CO_2 and the HCO_3 are like riders on the ends of the seesaw. When one side goes up, the other tries to go up to compensate. When one side goes down, the other side also tries to go down to compensate and bring the pH back toward normal.

c. Full or complete compensation occurs when buffer system is working effectively and brings pH back to a value of 7.35 to 7.45 (e.g., respiratory acidosis exists as indicated by an elevated $PaCO_2$; however, pH is normal and HCO_3^- is increased)

Memory Aid

If CO_2 and HCO_3^- are both abnormal, again look to see which one has a change that *matches* the direction of the change in the pH (e.g., CO_2 acts as an acid; HCO_3^- acts as a base). This match will be the primary imbalance, while the other system is compensating. If the pH is back in normal range, the value will be a number that is nearer to the side of the primary imbalance (e.g., 7.43 is nearer to alkalosis than acidosis, while 7.36 is nearer to acidosis than alkalosis). Remember that the body does not overcompensate!

F. Assisting with obtaining an ABG specimen

1. Determine site of specimen collection (radial or femoral artery, intra-arterial line) and obtain baseline vital signs
2. Perform Allen test prior to radial artery puncture
   - **a.** Apply simultaneous pressure to radial and ulnar arteries of affected hand
   - **b.** Ask client to repeatedly make a fist and open it; note that hand should blanch
   - **c.** Maintain pressure on radial artery and release pressure on ulnar artery; note color of hand
   - **d.** A return of normal pink color within 6 seconds indicates adequate collateral circulation from ulnar artery, making it safe to use radial artery for puncture; otherwise, site should not be used
3. Assist with specimen preparation by preparing heparinized syringe and placing ice in collection bag prior to blood draw; prepare specimen labels
4. Note on laboratory requisition any factors that could affect results, such as body temperature and O_2 or ventilator settings; also mentally note client's activity level in last 20 minutes
5. Explain procedure to client and provide emotional support during blood draw, which may be uncomfortable

6. After procedure, immediately apply firm pressure for a full 5 minutes by the clock, and longer if client takes any medications that interfere with coagulation (e.g., anticoagulants, aspirin); arrange for specimen to be sent immediately for analysis

II. RESPIRATORY ACIDOSIS

A. Overview

1. In **respiratory acidosis**, CO_2 is retained and pH is decreased (Table 55–2 ■)
2. It occurs in response to hypoventilation, which occurs with respiratory depression, inadequate chest expansion, airway obstruction, or interference with alveolar-capillary exchange

B. Nursing assessment

1. Cardiovascular
   - a. Hypotension
   - b. Delayed cardiac conduction that can lead to heart block, peaked T waves, prolonged PR intervals, and widened QRS complexes on cardiac rhythm strip
   - c. Peripheral vasodilation with thready, weak pulse
   - d. Tachycardia
   - e. Warm, flushed skin related to peripheral vasodilation as well as to impaired gas exchange
2. Respiratory
   - a. Dyspnea
   - b. May have hypoventilation with hypoxia
3. Central nervous system (CNS)
   - a. Headache
   - b. Muscle twitching or seizures
   - c. Altered mental status or decreased level of consciousness (LOC)

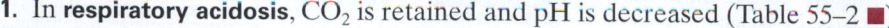

Table 55–2 Overview of Acid-Base Imbalances

Primary Abnormality	Compensation	Common Etiologies	Clinical Manifestations
Respiratory acidosis pH ↓ < 7.35 CO_2 ↑ > 45	HCO_3^- ↑ to raise pH	COPD, sedative or barbiturate overdose, chest wall abnormalities, pneumonia, atelectasis, respiratory muscle weakness, hypoventilation	Respiratory rate ↑ and shallow to attempt to blow off CO_2, hypotension, heart block, peaked T waves, prolonged PR interval, weak and thready pulse, tachycardia, warm and flushed skin, headache, papilledema, decreased level of consciousness, drowsiness, coma
Respiratory alkalosis pH ↑ > 7.45 CO_2 ↓ < 35	HCO_3^- ↓ to lower pH	Hyperventilation caused by hypoxia, fever, fear, pain, exercise, anxiety, or pulmonary embolus; mechanical ventilation, septicemia (respiratory center stimulation), brain injury, encephalitis, salicylate poisoning	↑ myocardial irritability, ↑ heart rate, ↑ sensitivity to digitalis preparations, dyspnea, chest tightness, dizziness, anxiety, panic, tetany, seizures, blurred vision
Metabolic acidosis pH ↓ < 7.35 HCO_3^- ↓ < 22	CO_2 ↓ to raise pH	DKA, lactic acidosis, starvation, severe diarrhea, renal tubule acidosis, renal failure, GI fistulas, shock	Hypotension, dysrhythmias, peripheral vasodilation, cold clammy skin, deep rapid respiratory pattern (Kussmaul respirations), drowsiness, headache, confusion, lethargy, weakness, coma, nausea and vomiting, diarrhea, abdominal pain
Metabolic alkalosis pH ↑ > 7.45 HCO_3^- ↑ < 26	CO_2 ↑ to lower pH	Severe vomiting, excessive nasogastric suctioning, diuretic therapy, hypokalemia, excess licorice intake, excessive $NaHCO_3$ use, excessive mineralocorticoids	↑ heart rate, dysrhythmias secondary to hypokalemia, hypotension, premature ventricular contractions, atrial tachycardia, hypoventilation, respiratory failure, dizziness, irritability, nervousness, confusion, tremors, muscle cramps, tetany, hyperreflexia, parasthesias in fingers and toes, seizures

   d. Papilledema
   e. Drowsiness that can progress to a coma
4. Diagnostic findings
   a. pH decreased below 7.35
   b. $PaCO_2$ elevated above 45 mm Hg
   c. Hyperkalemia
5. Compensation
   a. Increased rate and depth of respirations to blow off CO_2
   b. Kidneys eliminate H^+ ions and retain HCO_3^- (urine pH less than 6)
   c. HCO_3^- levels rise when body is compensating for acidosis

C. Collaborative management

1. Treatment is aimed at correcting underlying cause and improving ventilation
2. Implement pulmonary hygiene measures to clear respiratory tract of mucus and purulent drainage
3. Provide adequate fluid intake to liquefy secretions
4. If indicated, administer supplemental O_2 cautiously to a client with chronic respiratory acidosis
   a. Note that clients with chronic acidosis have compensated and are adjusted to living with higher $PaCO_2$ levels
   b. Remember CO_2 level is the mechanism that stimulates respiratory drive
   c. O_2 administration at higher levels can lead to a decreased ventilatory drive and can cause further hypoxia
   d. Low-flow oxygen is expected treatment
   e. Collaborate with physician and respiratory therapist to manage chronic respiratory disease
5. Mechanical ventilation may be required to improve respiratory status; CO_2 is decreased gradually to prevent alkalosis and seizures from occurring
6. Assess respiratory rate and depth
7. Position to facilitate maximum lung expansion (upright as tolerated)
8. Monitor client for complications and response to therapy
9. Take apical pulse and assess for tachycardia and irregularities; assess color of skin, nail beds, and mucous membranes
10. Assess LOC
11. Monitor ECG for dysrhythmias
12. Monitor results of ABGs and serum electrolytes, especially potassium
13. Administer medications as ordered
    a. Bronchodilators to decrease bronchospasm
    b. Antibiotics to treat infections in respiratory tract
    c. Respiratory agents to decrease viscosity of pulmonary secretions, such as acetylcystine (Mucomyst)
    d. Anticoagulants and thrombolytics to prevent or treat pulmonary emboli
    e. Medications are usually administered IV in acute situations and then changed to oral route as client's condition stabilizes
    f. Respiratory therapists often administer medications as part of treatment plan; they are often called on a prn (as needed) basis to assist clients during acute episodes
14. Provide good oral hygiene frequently
15. Provide adequate fluid intake
16. Keep side rails up, bed at lowest level, and call bell within client's reach
17. Maintain a calm, quiet environment
18. If client is confused, orient frequently to person, place, and time
19. Satisfactory outcomes include ABGs improved to client's baseline, decreased anxiety, improved breathing with less effort, freedom from injury, absence of cardiac dysrhythmias, improved LOC, and decreased rate but increased depth of respirations

D. Client education

1. Teach preventive measures to clients at risk
2. Teach deep breathing techniques

3. Teach signs and symptoms of infection to report to the health care provider
4. Report signs of infections, shortness of breath, fatigue, and increased pulse rate to health care provider

III. RESPIRATORY ALKALOSIS

A. Overview

1. In **respiratory alkalosis**, the pH is elevated and $PaCO_2$ is decreased (Table 55–2)
2. Occurs with hyperventilation and leads to a decreased level of CO_2; sometimes called an H_2CO_3 deficit
3. Other causes can include infection, excessive mechanical ventilation, and respiratory center stimulation from fever, salicylate intoxication, and trauma to CNS

B. Nursing assessment

1. Cardiovascular
   a. Increased myocardial irritability; palpitations
   b. Increased heart rate
   c. Increased sensitivity to digitalis
2. Respiratory
   a. Rapid, shallow breathing
   b. Chest tightness and palpitations
3. CNS
   a. Dizziness and light-headedness, blurred vision
   b. Difficulty concentrating
   c. Anxiety, panic
   d. Numbness and tingling in extremities
   e. Hyperactive reflexes
   f. Tetany and convulsions
4. Diagnostic findings
   a. High pH (over 7.45)
   b. Low $PaCO_2$ (under 35 mm Hg)
   c. Hypokalemia
   d. Hypocalcemia (as pH increases, calcium binding occurs in plasma and calcium levels decrease)
5. Compensation
   a. Kidneys conserve H^+ and excrete HCO_3^- (urine pH greater than 6)
   b. Low HCO_3^- indicates body is attempting to compensate

C. Collaborative management

1. Treat underlying cause
2. Assist client to breathe more slowly
3. If needed, have client rebreathe CO_2 by using a rebreather mask or a paper bag
4. Give oxygen therapy if client is hypoxic
5. Medicate as needed with antianxiety drugs to control anxiety or sedatives to control hyperventilation associated with anxiety
6. Provide support and reassurance
7. Monitor vital signs and ABGs
8. Protect from injury
9. Satisfactory outcomes include decreased respiratory rate, absence of numbness and tingling in extremities, return of ABGs to normal or client's baseline, and diminished anxiety; additionally, client remains free from injury

D. Client education

1. Teach client relaxation techniques
2. Encourage client to attend stress management classes as indicated
3. Teach parents to keep aspirin and other salicylates out of reach of children and to follow current poison control guidelines if exposure occurs

IV. METABOLIC ACIDOSIS

A. Overview

1. In **metabolic acidosis**, the pH decreases and HCO_3^- decreases (Table 55–2)
2. Occurs when there is a loss of HCO_3^- or when acids other than carbonic acid (H_2CO_3) accumulate in ECF

3. This condition rarely occurs spontaneously but rather is accompanied by other problems, such as gastrointestinal (GI) conditions (starvation, malnutrition, and chronic diarrhea), renal (kidney failure), diabetic ketoacidosis (DKA), hyperthyroidism, trauma, shock, increased exercise, severe infection, and fever

B. Nursing assessment

1. Cardiovascular
   a. Peripheral vasodilation and hypotension
   b. Dysrhythmias
   c. Cold, clammy skin
2. Respiratory: deep rapid pattern, Kussmaul respirations
3. CNS
   a. Drowsiness progressing to coma
   b. Headache
   c. Confusion, lethargy and weakness

Memory Aid

Acidosis of any origin tends to be a CNS depressant.

4. GI
   a. Nausea and vomiting, diarrhea
   b. Abdominal pain
5. Diagnostic findings
   a. pH less than 7.35
   b. HCO_3^- less than 22 mEq/L
   c. Hyperkalemia frequently seen
   d. ECG may show changes related to K^+ levels
   e. AG calculation increases
   f. BE decreases
6. Compensation
   a. Lungs eliminate CO_2; kidneys conserve HCO_3^-
   b. Urine pH less than 6
   c. $PaCO_2$ decreases when compensation is occurring

C. Collaborative management

1. Treatment is aimed at correcting underlying problem
2. Provide hydration to restore water, nutrients, and electrolytes
3. Administration of alkalotic IV solution (sodium bicarbonate or sodium lactate) may be indicated to correct acidosis
4. Mechanical ventilation is used only if other treatment modalities are ineffective
5. Monitor ABGs
6. Monitor I&O and measure daily weights
7. Assess vital signs, especially respiration for rate and depth
8. Assess LOC
9. Assess GI function
10. Monitor ECG for conduction problems
11. Monitor serum electrolytes
12. Protect from injury
13. Administer IV fluids and medications as ordered, based on underlying cause
    a. If cause is secondary to DKA, implement hydration with normal saline, regular insulin, and possibly potassium
    b. If diarrhea is cause, treat with hydration and antidiarrheal agents
    c. Administer $NaHCO_3$ cautiously and only when HCO_3^- levels are very low (below 16 to 18 mEq/L); can cause metabolic alkalosis and hypokalemia; titrate closely to avoid further acid-base imbalances
14. Satisfactory outcomes include that client is free from injury and has no dysrhythmias, ABGs return to normal, fluid volume deficits are corrected, LOC returns to normal, and GI upset is relieved

D. Client education

1. Teach clients to seek health care for prolonged diarrhea
2. Teach diabetic clients importance of preventing occurrences of DKA and how to manage DKA should it occur

V. METABOLIC ALKALOSIS

A. Overview

1. In **metabolic alkalosis**, there is an increased pH and increased HCO_3^- (see Table 55–2)
2. ! Occurs when there is a loss of H^+ ions (e.g., because of vomiting or nasogastric suctioning) or an increase in HCO_3^- level (such as with ingestion of bicarbonate-based antacids)

B. Nursing assessment

1. Cardiovascular
   a. ! Tachycardia and hypertension
   b. Dysrhythmias such as atrial tachycardia or premature ventricular contractions
2. ! Respiratory: hypoventilation and respiratory failure
3. CNS
   a. Dizziness
   b. ! Irritability, nervousness, or confusion
   c. Tremors or muscle cramps
   d. Hyperreflexia
   e. ! Paresthesias in fingers and toes
   f. ! Tetany and seizure activity

Memory Aid

Alkalosis of any origin tends to have an excitatory effect on the CNS.

4. GI
   a. Anorexia, nausea and vomiting
   b. Paralytic ileus if hypokalemia occurs
5. ! Diagnostic findings
   a. pH greater than 7.45
   b. HCO_3^- above 26 mEq/L
   c. Hypokalemia
   d. Hypocalcemia (as pH increases, Ca^{++} binding occurs and serum Ca^{++} levels decrease)
   e. Hyponatremia and hypochloremia
   f. Urine chloride levels reveal whether client is chloride responsive (under 10 mEq/L) or chloride resistant (over 10 mEq/L)
   g. BE increases
6. Compensation
   a. Lungs retain CO_2; kidneys conserve H^+ and excrete HCO_3^-
   b. $PaCO_2$ increases with compensation
   c. Urine pH greater than 6

C. Collaborative management

1. Treatment aimed at correcting underlying problem
2. Provide sufficient Cl^- to enhance renal absorption of Na^+ and excretion of HCO_3^-
3. Restore normal fluid balance
4. ! Assess LOC
5. ! Assess vital signs, especially respiratory rate and depth
6. Administer medication and IV fluids as ordered
   a. Normal saline-based IV fluid replacement
   b. Potassium supplementation if hypokalemic
   c. Histamine-2 receptor antagonists such as ranitidine (Zantac) or famotidine (Pepcid) to reduce secretion of H^+ ions and loss of H^+ ions from GI drainage
   d. If client is chloride responsive, then administer acetazolamide (Diamox) to increase renal bicarbonate excretion

e. If client is chloride resistant, then correct K^+ and Mg^{++} deficits with appropriate supplementation
7. Monitor I&O
8. ! Protect from injury
9. Monitor ECG for conduction abnormalities
10. Monitor results of ABGs and serum electrolytes
11. Satisfactory outcomes include that client is free from injury, ABGs return to normal, hypertension is corrected, electrolytes are restored to normal, cardiac conduction is normal, and client states ways to prevent reoccurrance

D. Client education
1. Teach clients to take antacids correctly to prevent excessive dosing
2. Teach signs and symptoms to report to health care provider for those at risk, especially older adults
3. Teach signs and symptoms of hypokalemia to report to health care provider

VI. MIXED ACID-BASE DISORDERS

A. Identification and treatment of primary disorder
1. A **mixed acid-base disorder** occurs when two or more independent acid-base disorders occur at same time
2. pH depends on type and severity of each simple disorder
3. Respiratory acidosis and alkalosis cannot occur concurrently; it is impossible to have hyperventilation and hypoventilation at same time
4. Treatment is aimed at correcting underlying cause of each disorder
5. When identifying acid-base imbalances, mathematical formulas can be used to assess degree of expected compensation
   a. These equations are usually used when there is an intermediate level of acid-base balance
   b. However, it is important to know that calculations will identify degree of compensatory changes
6. AG and urine pH values will also help determine which imbalance is occurring

B. Chronic and superimposed acid-base disturbances
1. Mixed metabolic acidosis and respiratory acidosis
   a. Clients with acute pulmonary edema
   b. Clients with cardiac arrest as a result of buildup of lactic acidosis and CO_2 retention due to inadequate ventilation
   c. ! pH values decrease and are more pronounced because of decreasing HCO_3^- level coupled with increasing CO_2 level
2. Mixed metabolic alkalosis and respiratory acidosis
   a. ! Clients with chronic obstructive pulmonary disease (COPD) and who have treatment with potassium-wasting diuretics, severe vomiting, or development of diarrhea
   b. Clients with COPD who have a quick improvement in ventilation
   c. pH values tend to become balanced because of an increase in both HCO_3^- and $PaCO_2$ values
3. Mixed metabolic acidosis with respiratory alkalosis
   a. Clients with a rapid correction of metabolic acidosis
   b. ! Clients with salicylate intoxication
   c. Clients with Gram-negative septicemia
   d. pH values tend to become balanced because of decreases in both HCO_3^- and $PaCO_2$
4. Mixed metabolic alkalosis and respiratory alkalosis
   a. Postoperative clients with severe hemorrhage
   b. Clients who have massive transfusions
   c. Clients with excessive nasogastric (NG) drainage
   d. pH values increase and are more pronounced because of increasing HCO_3^- coupled with decreasing CO_2 levels
5. Mixed metabolic acidosis and metabolic alkalosis
   a. ! Seen in clients with gastroenteritis, vomiting, and diarrhea

b. If imbalance is present in same proportion, there is usually no change in values (pH, HCO_3^-, and $PaCO_2$) even though there is volume depletion

6. Chronic and acute respiratory acidosis

! a. Chronic respiratory conditions with an acute condition superimposed can lead to increased $PaCO_2$ levels, causing further pulmonary dysfunction and leading to serious consequences that can compromise both treatment and expected response to treatment

b. Clients with both a chronic and a superimposed acute respiratory acid-base imbalance should be closely monitored by a pulmonologist

c. Respiratory therapist should be part of collaborative health care team plan during client's treatment

C. Diagnostic and laboratory findings

1. Increased $PaCO_2$ with decreased pH
   a. Respiratory acidosis
   b. Respiratory acidosis with incompletely compensating metabolic alkalosis
   c. Respiratory acidosis with coexisting metabolic acidosis
2. Increased $PaCO_2$ with increased pH
   a. Metabolic alkalosis with incomplete compensating respiratory acidosis
   b. Metabolic alkalosis with coexisting respiratory acidosis
3. Decreased $PaCO_2$ with decreased pH
   a. Metabolic acidosis with incomplete respiratory alkalosis
   b. Metabolic acidosis with coexisting respiratory alkalosis
4. Decreased $PaCO_2$ with increased pH
   a. Respiratory alkalosis
   b. Respiratory alkalosis with incomplete compensating metabolic acidosis
   c. Respiratory alkalosis with coexisting metabolic alkalosis
5. Normal pH values
   a. Increased $PaCO_2$ leads to respiratory acidosis with compensated metabolic alkalosis
   b. Decreased $PaCO_2$ leads to respiratory alkalosis with compensated metabolic acidosis
6. Changes in AG levels and $NaHCO_3^-$ levels
7. Abnormal serum electrolyte levels can reflect changes in acid-base balance
8. ECG results may show electrolyte disturbances
9. Chest x-ray (CXR) may show underlying cardiac or pulmonary disease
10. Hemoglobin and hematocrit levels can indicate O_2-carrying potential

D. Collaborative management

1. Treatment focuses on correcting underlying causes of disorder
2. Mixed disorders must be treated before acid-base balance can be restored
3. A collaborative team approach (including a pulmonologist, respiratory therapist, nurses, and dietitian) is needed to assist client in restoring acid-base balance, increasing activity tolerance, and improving physiological function
4. ! Monitor vital signs and LOC
5. Monitor ABGs, pulmonary function tests, pulse oximetry, and CXR
6. ! Protect from injury
7. Monitor ECG, hemoglobin and hematocrit levels, and serum electrolytes
8. Ensure adequate fluid intake
9. ! Implement therapeutic measures as ordered, such as O_2 therapy and medications to resolve underlying causes of imbalances
10. Satisfactory outcomes include that client remains free from injury, ABGs return to normal or baseline, cardiac conduction is normal; fluid balance and electrolyte levels are restored, LOC is improved, and client is able to report ways to prevent problem from reoccurring

E. Client education

1. Clients with chronic respiratory conditions should report exacerbations to health care provider

2. Clients who experience fluid losses through emesis or diarrhea are at increased risk for acid-base imbalance and should notify health care provider if condition is not self-limiting (lasts more than 2 or 3 days)
3. Clients with diabetes are at risk for acid-base imbalance due to alterations in glucose levels and should closely monitor serum glucose levels and use appropriate interventions to maintain normal levels
4. Clients who have renal problems are prone to develop acid-base imbalance due to alterations in electrolyte levels; closely monitor renal status to identify potential disturbances and allow for intervention

Check your NCLEX–RN® Exam I.Q.

You are ready for testing on this content if you can

- Use knowledge from the biological and physical sciences to assess acid-base status.
- Apply concepts of pathophysiology to acid-base imbalances.
- Identify signs and symptoms of acid-base imbalances.
- Describe interventions to treat acid-base imbalances.
- Evaluate the client's response to treatments for acid-base imbalances.

PRACTICE TEST

1 A client has been admitted for dehydration after fasting for 5 days. For which of the following acid-base imbalances would the nurse assess this client?

1. Metabolic acidosis
2. Metabolic alkalosis
3. Respiratory acidosis
4. Respiratory alkalosis

2 A client is admitted to the hospital after vomiting for 3 days. Which of the following ABG results would the nurse expect?

1. pH 7.30, $PaCO_2$ 50, HCO_3^- 27
2. pH 7.47, $PaCO_2$ 43, HCO_3^- 28
3. pH 7.34, $PaCO_2$ 50, HCO_3^- 28
4. pH 7.47, $PaCO_2$ 30, HCO_3^- 23

3 A client is admitted to the hospital with a diagnosis of respiratory acidosis secondary to overdose of barbiturates. Which of the following assessments would the nurse make?

1. Slow, shallow respirations
2. Tetany symptoms
3. Increased deep tendon reflexes
4. Palpitations

4 A client is admitted with a diagnosis of renal failure. Which of the following ABG results would the nurse expect to see with this client?

1. pH 7.49, $PaCO_2$ 36, HCO_3^- 30
2. pH 7.30, $PaCO_2$ 35, HCO_3^- 18
3. pH 7.31, $PaCO_2$ 50, HCO_3^- 23
4. pH 7.43, $PaCO_2$ 48, HCO_3^- 30

5 A client is admitted to the hospital with atelectasis and complaints of chest pain. Which of the following acid-base imbalances would the nurse assess this client for?

1. Respiratory alkalosis
2. Metabolic acidosis
3. Metabolic alkalosis
4. Respiratory acidosis

6 A client is admitted to the hospital with respiratory acidosis. Which of the following conditions most likely leads to the development of this state?

1. Severe diarrhea for several days
2. Diabetic ketoacidosis
3. Obesity
4. Diuretics

PRACTICE TEST

7 Which of the following signs and symptoms indicates that a client has metabolic acidosis?

1. Weight gain
2. Rapid, deep respirations
3. Melena
4. Decreased respiratory rate and depth

8 Which of the following medications should the nurse review first for its potential interaction in a client admitted to the hospital with alkalosis?

1. Warfarin (Coumadin)
2. Metformin (Glucophage)
3. Digoxin (Lanoxin)
4. Ibuprofen (Motrin)

9 A client is admitted to the hospital with complaints of sudden onset of severe abdominal pain. Which of the following values in the arterial blood gas would the nurse expect to see?

1. $PaCO_2$ 48
2. HCO_3^- 18
3. pH 7.32
4. SaO_2 90

10 A client is admitted to the hospital with an acid-base imbalance. ABG results are pH 7.33, $PaCO_2$ 49, HCO_3^- 28. The nurse interprets these results as which of the following?

1. Respiratory acidosis, uncompensated
2. Metabolic alkalosis, uncompensated
3. Respiratory acidosis, partially compensated
4. Metabolic acidosis, partially compensated

11 A client is admitted to the hospital with numerous complaints of muscle weakness and twitching. ABG results are pH 7.44, $PaCO_2$ 49, HCO_3^- 30. The nurse interprets these as which of the following?

1. Metabolic acidosis, uncompensated
2. Respiratory alkalosis, compensated
3. Respiratory alkalosis, uncompensated
4. Metabolic alkalosis, compensated

12 The nurse would suspect that a client who frequently uses which of the following is at risk for the development of metabolic alkalosis?

1. Calcium carbonate (Tums)
2. Ibuprofen (Motrin)
3. Acetylsalicylic acid (aspirin)
4. Acetaminophen (Tylenol)

13 The nurse is admitting a client who has metabolic alkalosis. The nurse plans to assess for signs and symptoms of which of the following electrolyte imbalances?

1. Hypernatremia
2. Hypochloremia
3. Hypermagnesemia
4. Hypocalcemia

14 A client's blood gas results are pH 7.48, $PaCO_2$ 30, HCO_3^- 23. How will the nurse interpret these results?

1. Respiratory alkalosis, compensated
2. Metabolic alkalosis, uncompensated
3. Respiratory alkalosis, uncompensated
4. Metabolic alkalosis, compensated

15 The nurse determines that a client with a nasogastric tube to low suction for 5 days is at risk for developing which acid-base imbalance?

1. Respiratory acidosis
2. Metabolic alkalosis
3. Metabolic acidosis
4. Respiratory alkalosis

16 The following ABG results are on the client's chart: pH 7.50, $PaCO_2$ 36, HCO_3^- 30. How will the nurse interpret these blood gas reports?

1. Metabolic alkalosis, partially compensated
2. Respiratory alkalosis, compensated
3. Metabolic alkalosis, uncompensated
4. Respiratory alkalosis, uncompensated

17 A client is admitted to the hospital. ABG results are pH 7.50, $PaCO_2$ 40, HCO_3^- 29. Which of the following questions should the nurse ask the client in order to help determine an etiology for this ABG result?

1. "Have you had diarrhea lately?"
2. "Do you have a history of COPD?"
3. "How long have you had nausea and vomiting?"
4. "Do you smoke?"

18 A client's blood gas results are pH 7.36, $PaCO_2$ 50, HCO_3^- 28. What do these results indicate to the nurse?

1. Respiratory acidosis, compensated
2. Metabolic acidosis, compensated
3. Metabolic acidosis, uncompensated
4. Respiratory acidosis, uncompensated

19 Which of the following statements by the client indicates that discharge teaching for respiratory alkalosis is understood?

1. "I will not take so many antacids anymore."
2. "I will take a stress management class."
3. "I will not take my Lasix without taking my potassium supplement."
4. "I will tell the doctor the next time I have diarrhea for so long."

20 A client is admitted with severe diarrhea. ABGs are pH 7.33, $PaCO_2$ 42, HCO_3^- 20. The nurse concludes this client has which of the following?

1. Metabolic acidosis, uncompensated
2. Respiratory acidosis, compensated
3. Metabolic acidosis, compensated
4. Respiratory acidosis, uncompensated

PRACTICE TEST

ANSWERS & RATIONALES

1 **Answer: 1** A prolonged fasting state can lead to dehydration. During fasting, the body reverts to cellular breakdown to maintain energy, and lactic and pyruvic acids build up in the body. This accumulation of acids leads to the development of metabolic acidosis. Options 2 and 4 are incorrect because alkalosis would not occur. Option 3 is incorrect because the primary disturbance is not respiratory.
Cognitive Level: Application **Client Need:** Physiological Integrity: Physiological Adaptation **Integrated Process:** Nursing Process: Assessment **Content Area:** Adult Health: Endocrine and Metabolic **Strategy:** Note the critical word *fasting* that indicates this is a metabolic rather than respiratory problem, which eliminates options 3 and 4. Choose option 1 over 2 because metabolic by-products are acidic in nature, not alkaline.

2 **Answer: 2** Vomiting leads to the loss of hydrochloric acid from gastric acids. Hydrogen ions must leave the blood to replace this acidity in the stomach. Option 2 reflects metabolic alkalosis—elevated pH and HCO_3^- and normal $PaCO_2$. Option 1 is incorrect because it reflects respiratory acidosis with partial compensation—decreased pH, elevated $PaCO_2$ and HCO_3^-. Option 3 is incorrect because it reflects a mixed acid-base imbalance—metabolic alkalosis with respiratory acidosis—normal pH and elevated $PaCO_2$ and HCO_3^-. Option 4 is incorrect because it reflects respiratory alkalosis—increased pH, decreased $PaCO_2$, and normal HCO_3^-.
Cognitive Level: Application **Client Need:** Physiological Integrity: Physiological Adaptation **Integrated Process:** Nursing Process: Assessment **Content Area:** Adult Health: Endocrine and Metabolic **Strategy:** Note the critical word *vomiting* and recall that stomach contents are rich in acid. Loss of acid would raise the pH (eliminating option 1 and 3) and lead to increased free circulating HCO_3^-, eliminating option 4.

3 **Answer: 1** Clients with respiratory acidosis from ingestion of barbiturates would have slow and shallow respirations, leading to hypoventilation. Palpitations are a subjective complaint reported by the client; the nurse cannot directly assess this symptom. In addition, palpitations are associated with respiratory alkalosis. Tetany symptoms and increased deep tendon reflexes are also associated with respiratory alkalosis.
Cognitive Level: Application **Client Need:** Physiological Integrity: Physiological Adaptation **Integrated Process:** Nursing Process: Assessment **Content Area:** Adult Health: Respiratory **Strategy:** The wording of the question guides you to look for objective data, which eliminates option 4. Also recall that barbiturates are CNS depressants, while options 2 and 3 indicate CNS excitation. For this reason, eliminate options 2 and 3, which leaves option 1 as the correct option.

4 **Answer: 2** Clients with renal failure have difficulty synthesizing HCO_3^- in the renal tubules secondary to the renal failure. These clients also retain K^+ and subsequently develop metabolic acidosis. Option 2 reflects uncompensated metabolic acidosis. Option 1 is incorrect because it reflects metabolic alkalosis—increased pH and HCO_3^- and normal $PaCO_2$. Option 3 is incorrect because it reflects respiratory acidosis—decreased pH, increased $PaCO_2$, and normal HCO_3^-. Option 4 is incorrect because it reflects a mixed acid-base imbalance—metabolic alkalosis with a respiratory acidosis—normal pH, increased $PaCO_2$ and HCO_3^-.
Cognitive Level: Application **Client Need:** Physiological Integrity: Physiological Adaptation **Integrated Process:** Nursing Process: Assessment **Content Area:** Adult Health: Endocrine and

ANSWERS & RATIONALES

Metabolic **Strategy:** First recognize renal failure as a metabolic condition in which there is an impaired ability to eliminate metabolic acids and wastes. With this in mind, eliminate options 1 and 4 because of an elevated pH and a normal pH, respectively. Then choose option 2 over 3 because the bicarbonate (indicating metabolic status) is lower in option 2.

5 **Answer: 4** A client with atelectasis has collapsed alveoli that retain CO_2, which can lead to respiratory acidosis. The client would most likely have hypoventilation as a respiratory pattern, which would further contribute to the development of respiratory acidosis. Options 1 and 3 are incorrect because the client would not be in an alkalotic state. Option 2 is incorrect because the primary disturbance is respiratory; clients with respiratory problems can report "chest pain." Further information would be needed to rule out cardiac problems. **Cognitive Level:** Application **Client Need:** Physiological Integrity: Physiological Adaptation **Integrated Process:** Nursing Process: Assessment **Content Area:** Adult Health: Respiratory **Strategy:** The critical word in the stem of the question is *atelectasis.* Recall that this term is associated with respiratory problems to eliminate options 2 and 3. Choose option 4 over option 1, recalling that CO_2 retention characterizes many respiratory conditions, leading to acidosis (since CO_2 acts as an acid in the body).

6 **Answer: 3** Obesity can lead to chest wall abnormalities and hypoventilation. Respiratory acidosis results from hypoventilation. Option 1 is incorrect because prolonged diarrhea likely leads to the development of metabolic acidosis. Option 2 is incorrect because DKA leads to the development of metabolic acidosis. Option 4 is incorrect because diuretic administration leads to the development of metabolic alkalosis. **Cognitive Level:** Analysis **Client Need:** Physiological Integrity: Physiological Adaptation **Integrated Process:** Nursing Process: Analysis **Content Area:** Adult Health: Respiratory **Strategy:** Note the term *acidosis* in both the stem of the question and in the correct option to help you choose option 2 correctly. Alternatively, eliminate options 1 and 4 because they are similar in that they both lead to fluid loss, and then eliminate option 3 as irrelevant.

7 **Answer: 2** Clients who have metabolic acidosis develop Kussmaul respirations (rapid and deep respirations). Weight gain and melena are not associated with the development of metabolic acidosis. Option 4 is incorrect because shallow breathing is associated with the development of metabolic alkalosis. **Cognitive Level:** Application **Client Need:** Physiological Integrity: Physiological Adaptation **Integrated Process:** Nursing Process: Analysis **Content Area:** Adult Health: Endocrine and Metabolic **Strategy:** The critical words in the stem of the question are *metabolic acidosis.* Recall that in metabolic abnormalities, the respiratory system helps to compensate; this will help to eliminate options 1 and 3. Choose option 2 over option 4 because it is the option that assists the body to "blow off" acid in the form of CO_2.

8 **Answer: 3** Alkalosis, especially respiratory, makes the client more sensitive to the effects of digoxin; toxicity can develop even at therapeutic levels. A serum digoxin level should be obtained and the client evaluated for potential digoxin toxicity; warfarin affects clotting factors; metformin may cause the development of lactic acidosis; and ibuprofen may cause gastric irritation. **Cognitive Level:** Application **Client Need:** Physiological Integrity: Physiological Adaptation **Integrated Process:** Nursing Process: Planning **Content Area:** Adult Health: Endocrine and Metabolic **Strategy:** Specific knowledge of medications that are affected by alkalosis is needed to answer this question. Use nursing knowledge and the process of elimination to make your selection.

9 **Answer: 2** Acute pain usually leads to hyperventilation, which causes CO_2 to be blown off, leading to an increased pH and decreased CO_2 level. If the client has not compensated, the bicarbonate level would be normal. If the client is compensating, then the bicarbonate level would decrease in an attempt to restore the pH. Option 1 is incorrect because it reflects only a slight elevation of $PaCO_2$; if the client is in severe pain, the level would likely be higher. Option 3 is incorrect because the pH is only slightly acidotic. Option 4 is incorrect because the oxygen saturation is within normal limits. **Cognitive Level:** Analysis **Client Need:** Physiological Integrity: Physiological Adaptation **Integrated Process:** Nursing Process: Assessment **Content Area:** Adult Health: Endocrine and Metabolic **Strategy:** Visualize a picture of the client in pain. This person is most likely to have an increased respiratory rate, which blows off carbon dioxide (eliminating option 1) and decreases the bicarbonate level as a compensatory mechanism. This will help you to easily choose option 2 as correct.

10 **Answer: 3** The pH is low, indicating acidosis; the $PaCO_2$ is elevated, indicating a respiratory basis; and the HCO_3^- is elevated, indicating that compensatory mechanisms are partially working. Option 1 is incorrect because compensation is taking place because of increased HCO_3^- level. Option 2 is incorrect because the client is not alkalotic. Option 4 is incorrect because the primary disturbance is respiratory. The change in the $PaCO_2$ level is greater than the change in the HCO_3^- level, which indicates a respiratory disturbance. **Cognitive Level:** Analysis **Client Need:** Physiological Integrity: Physiological Adaptation **Integrated Process:** Nursing Process: Analysis **Content Area:** Adult Health: Respiratory **Strategy:** First eliminate option 2 because it is an alkalosis and the client's pH of 7.33 indicates acidosis. Next note that both the CO_2 and HCO_3^- levels are abnormal, indicating that the body is attempting to compensate (eliminating option 1). Choose option 3 over 4 because the elevated CO_2 "matches" a respiratory acidosis, and the HCO_3^- (an alkaline substance), is rising to try to compensate.

11 **Answer: 4** The pH is just below the high limit and the HCO_3^- is elevated, indicating a metabolic problem. The $PaCO_2$ is elevated, indicating that compensation is taking place. Option 1 is incorrect because the client is not acidotic. Option 2 is incorrect because the CO_2 would be decreased rather than elevated. Option 3 is incorrect because the primary disturbance is metabolic and the CO_2 is elevated rather than decreased. **Cognitive Level:** Analysis **Client Need:** Physiological Integrity: Reduction of Risk Potential **Integrated Process:** Nursing Process: Analysis **Content Area:** Adult Health: Endocrine and Metabolic **Strategy:** Note that the pH is within normal range,

which indicates that the condition is compensated, thus eliminating options 1 and 3. Note that the high HCO_3^- is a metabolic indicator (not a respiratory one) and is consistant with a pH near the high end of normal to help you choose option 4 over 2.

12 **Answer: 1** Excessive use of oral antacids can lead to metabolic alkalosis. Use of ibuprofen and acetominophen is not associated with the development of metabolic alkalosis. Overdoses of aspirin can be associated with the development of respiratory alkalosis and eventually lead to metabolic acidosis.
Cognitive Level: Application **Client Need:** Physiological Integrity: Physiological Adaptation **Integrated Process:** Nursing Process: Assessment **Content Area:** Adult Health: Endocrine and Metabolic **Strategy:** Knowledge of medication side effects is needed to answer this question. First eliminate options 2 and 4 because they are similar (non-opioid analgesics). Then eliminate option 3 because acid would not lead to alkalosis. Alternatively, recall that calcium carbonate is an antacid, which in excess could lead to metabolic alkalosis.

13 **Answer: 4** Clinical manifestations of metabolic alkalosis are associated with the presence of tetany-like symptoms. Clients should be monitored for the presence of these symptoms because they usually correlate with low levels of calcium. Although it is important to assess all serum electrolyte values to obtain a comprehensive picture, the presence of hypocalcemia can cause the client to have significant clinical symptoms. Early monitoring and prompt intervention can result in restoration of balance.
Cognitive Level: Application **Client Need:** Physiological Integrity: Physiological Adaptation **Integrated Process:** Teaching/Learning **Content Area:** Adult Health: Endocrine and Metabolic **Strategy:** Specific knowledge of the association between metabolic alkalosis and various electrolytes is needed to answer this question. Use nursing knowledge and the process of elimination to make your selection.

14 **Answer: 3** The client's pH is high, indicating alkalosis. The $PaCO_2$ is abnormal, indicating a respiratory basis. The HCO_3^- is normal, indicating that compensation has not started. Option 1 is incorrect because the HCO_3^- level would decrease with compensation. Options 2 and 4 are incorrect because the primary disturbance is respiratory, as indicated by the decrease in the CO_2 parameter.
Cognitive Level: Analysis **Client Need:** Physiological Integrity: Reduction of Risk Potential **Integrated Process:** Nursing Process: Analysis **Content Area:** Adult Health: Respiratory **Strategy:** Note that the pH is high, so the condition is not compensated, eliminating options 1 and 4. Choose option 3 over 2 because a low CO_2 correlates with a high pH, whereas an HCO_3^- at the lower end of the normal range does not correlate with a high pH.

15 **Answer: 2** A client who has prolonged nasogastric suction is apt to have higher levels of bicarbonate because of hydrogen ion loss. Bicarbonate excess leads to a metabolic disturbance and the development of metabolic alkalosis. Options 1 and 3 are incorrect because the client will not experience acidosis. Option 4 is incorrect because the primary disturbance is caused by retained levels of bicarbonate in the body.
Cognitive Level: Application **Client Need:** Physiological Integrity: Physiological Adaptation **Integrated Process:** Nursing Process: Analysis **Content Area:** Adult Health: Endocrine and Metabolic **Strategy:** Eliminate options 1 and 4 first because impaction is a GI (metabolic) problem rather than a respiratory one. Choose option 2 over 3, recalling that pancreatic juices are rich in bicarbonate. A client who is impacted cannot eliminate bicarbonate in the stool, and thus it may be reabsorbed.

16 **Answer: 3** The pH indicates alkalosis; HCO_3^- is high, indicating a metabolic basis; and the $PaCO_2$ is normal, which indicates that compensation has not taken place. Option 1 is incorrect because with compensation the $PaCO_2$ level would be increased. Options 2 and 4 are incorrect because the primary disturbance is metabolic, as reflected by the increased bicarbonate level.
Cognitive Level: Analysis **Client Need:** Physiological Integrity: Reduction of Risk Potential **Integrated Process:** Nursing Process: Analysis **Content Area:** Adult Health: Endocrine and Metabolic **Strategy:** First note that the pH is high, and so the imbalance cannot be compensated (eliminating option 2). Then note that HCO_3^- is the abnormally high value (not CO_2), so the imbalance must be metabolic rather than respiratory (eliminating option 4). Choose option 3 over option 1 because the CO_2 (normally 35 to 45) has made no attempt to rise to compensate for the high HCO_3^-.

17 **Answer: 3** ABG results reflect elevated pH, indicating alkalosis; normal $PaCO_2$ and an increased HCO_3^-, indicating metabolic alkalosis. Vomiting is a common cause of this condition. The presence of diarrhea is associated with metabolic acidosis. COPD and smoking are associated with respiratory acidosis.
Cognitive Level: Analysis **Client Need:** Physiological Integrity: Physiological Adaptation **Integrated Process:** Nursing Process: Assessment **Content Area:** Adult Health: Endocrine and Metabolic **Strategy:** An ability to interpret ABGs and specific knowledge of manifestations of metabolic alkalosis are needed to answer this question. Use nursing knowledge and the process of elimination to make your selection.

18 **Answer: 1** The pH is just within normal range, so the blood gas results are either normal or compensated. However, the $PaCO_2$ is high, indicating a respiratory problem and thus the ABGs cannot be normal. The HCO_3^- is also high, which along with a normal pH indicates complete compensation. Options 2 and 3 are incorrect because the primary disturbance is respiratory, as reflected by the correlation between an elevated $PaCO_2$ and a pH toward the low end of normal. Option 4 is incorrect because the HCO_3^- level would be normal if there was no compensation taking place.
Cognitive Level: Analysis **Client Need:** Physiological Integrity: Reduction of Risk Potential **Integrated Process:** Nursing Process: Assessment **Content Area:** Adult Health: Respiratory **Strategy:** Because the pH is within normal range, eliminate options 3 and 4. Choose option 1 over 2 because the pH is near the acidic end of the range and the high CO2 correlates with acidosis, whereas the high HCO_3^- would correlate with an alkalosis.

19 **Answer: 2** Respiratory alkalosis is caused by hyperventilation. Stress and anxiety are two things that can cause hyperventilation. It is important for clients who are prone to develop respiratory alkalosis be aware of how to manage causative factors. Options 1 and 3 are incorrect because antacids and diuretics are associated with the development of metabolic alkalosis. Option 4 is incorrect because diarrhea is associated with the development of metabolic acidosis. **Cognitive Level:** Analysis **Client Need:** Physiological Integrity: Physiological Adaptation **Integrated Process:** Teaching and Learning **Content Area:** Adult Health: Respiratory **Strategy:** The critical word in the question is *respiratory.* Eliminate each of the incorrect options because they would correlate better with a metabolic condition than with a respiratory one. Alternatively, consider that a common cause of respiratory alkalosis is hyperventilation, which is often caused by anxiety and managed with stress management.

20 **Answer: 1** The pH and HCO_3^- are decreased, indicating metabolic acidosis. The $PaCO_2$ is normal, indicating that compensatory mechanisms have not started working. Options 2 and 4 are incorrect because the primary disturbance is metabolic, as indicated by the low bicarbonate level. Option 3 is incorrect because with compensation, a decrease in $PaCO_2$ to restore balance would be expected. **Cognitive Level:** Analysis **Client Need:** Physiological Integrity: Physiological Adaptation **Integrated Process:** Nursing Process: Analysis **Content Area:** Adult Health: Endocrine and Metabolic **Strategy:** First correlate diarrhea with a metabolic problem to eliminate options 2 and 4. Then note that the pH is not within normal limits to choose option 1 over option 3.

Key Terms to Review

acid p. 985
base p. 985
buffer p. 985
compensation p. 986
HCO_3^- p. 985
metabolic acidosis p. 992
metabolic alkalosis p. 994
mixed acid-base disorder p. 995
$PaCO_2$ p. 987
PaO_2 p. 987
pH p. 985
respiratory acidosis p. 990
respiratory alkalosis p. 992
SaO_2 p. 987

References

Harkreader, H., & Hogan, M. (2004). *Fundamentals of nursing: Caring and clinical judgment* (2nd ed.). St. Louis, MO: Elsevier Science.

Malich, M. (2004). Fluid, electrolyte, and acid-base imbalances. In S. M. Lewis, M. M. Heitkemper, & S. R. Dirksen (Eds.), *Medical-surgical nursing: Assessment and management of clinical problems.* St. Louis, MO: Mosby.

Kozier, B., Erb, G., Berman, A., & Snyder, S. (2004). *Fundamentals of nursing: Concepts, process, and practice* (7th ed.). Upper Saddle River, NJ: Pearson Education.

LeMone, P., & Burke, K. (2004). *Medical-surgical nursing: Critical thinking in client care* (3rd ed.). Upper Saddle River, NJ: Pearson Education.

Respiratory Disorders

56

In this chapter

Cross reference

Other chapters relevant to this content area are

Test Yourself

Are you ready for the NCLEX-RN® or course exams? Use the practice tests on the companion CD-ROM to check.

I. OVERVIEW OF ANATOMY AND PHYSIOLOGY

A. Respiratory system structures

1. Upper respiratory tract (conducting airways)
   a. Nose: filters, humidifies, and heats inspired air; nasal hairs trap airborne particles in mucus; olfactory nerve receptors allow for sense of smell
   b. Paranasal sinuses: air-filled cavities in frontal, maxillary, ethmoid, and sphenoid bones that contribute to mucus production and voice resonance
   c. Pharynx: nasopharynx, laryngopharynx, and oropharynx; adenoids in the nasopharynx and tonsils in oropharynx contain lymphatic tissue that contributes to immune function
   d. Larynx: contains vocal cords that vibrate to produce voice; epiglottis closes during swallowing to prevent passage of food into trachea
   e. Trachea: passageway between upper and lower respiratory tract; divides into right and left mainstem bronchi
2. Lower respiratory tract (conducting airways and gas exchange airways)
   a. Bronchi: right and left mainstem bronchi (conducting airways) lead into smaller bronchioles that eventually terminate in alveoli; right mainstem bronchus curves less sharply than left, making it a more common passage for aspirated gastric contents and dislocated endotracheal tubes
   b. **Alveoli**: air-filled sacs in lungs; oxygen (O_2) diffuses from alveoli (gas exchange airways) into blood across alveolar-capillary membrane (primary site of gas exchange); carbon dioxide (CO_2) diffuses back into alveoli; surfactant decreases surface tension
   c. Lungs: right lung has three lobes—upper, middle, and lower; left lung has two lobes—upper and lower; upper area is called the apex; lower area is called base
   d. Pleura: two-layer membrane covering lungs (visceral pleura) and thoracic cavity (parietal pleura); pleural fluid lubricates pleural layers and holds them together during inspiration and expiration
   e. Pleural cavity: air-filled space of thoracic cavity housing structures of lower respiratory tract
3. Accessory structures: contribute to the mechanics of breathing and/or provide support and protection
   a. Rib cage: 12 pairs of ribs and sternum
   b. Intercostal muscles: located between ribs
   c. Diaphragm: separates thoracic cavity from abdominal cavity; flattens (contracts) during inspiration via phrenic nerve to allow greater chest expansion

B. Respiratory system functions

1. Primary function is gas exchange; process of **respiration** (process of O_2 and CO_2 exchange) involves ventilation, perfusion, diffusion, and nervous system control
2. Ventilation: passage of gases between atmosphere and lungs during inspiration and expiration; adequacy is influenced by tissue properties, airway resistance, lung volumes and capacities, body position, and disease processes
   a. **Pulmonary ventilation:** total volume of gas exchange between atmosphere and lungs
   b. **Alveolar ventilation:** volume of air that undergoes gas exchange
   c. **Inspiration:** stimulation of phrenic nerve causes diaphragm to contract and increase diameter of thoracic cavity; intrapleural pressure becomes more negative; air moves from atmosphere to alveoli and pulmonary capillaries where gas exchange occurs
   d. **Expiration:** diaphragm relaxes and pushes upward; intrapulmonic pressure becomes higher than atmospheric pressure, allowing passive air flow from lung into atmosphere; smaller airways may collapse during expiration, particularly in supine position
   e. Intrapulmonary (intra-alveolar) pressure: equals atmospheric pressure (760 mmHg) when glottis is open and there is no air movement

f. Intrapleural pressure: negative pressure produced by opposite forces of elastic recoil between lungs and chest wall; normally negative intrapleural pressure prevents lung collapse
g. Intrathoracic pressure: generally has negative pressure that equals intrapleural pressure; with forced expiration against a closed glottis (Valsalva maneuver), it becomes positive
h. **Compliance:** elastic property of lung because of elastic and collagen fibers; higher compliance allows for easier lung distention; lower compliance (lung stiffness) makes distention more difficult
i. Elastic recoil: ability of lungs to return to original shape after air is expelled
j. Airway resistance: obstruction to airflow caused by conditions of respiratory system tissues (elastic recoil, compliance), changes in airway diameter (bronchoconstriction, mucus obstruction), and/or pressure differences between atmospheric air and intrapulmonary air
k. Lung volumes and capacities: volumes are normal individual quantities of air exchanged during specific period of breathing cycle; capacities are combined quantities of lung volumes during specific periods of breathing cycle (see Box 56–1)
l. Body position: gravity accounts for greater ventilation in dependent areas of lung; with upright body (sitting, standing) during inspiration, airflow has less resistance in reaching lung bases

3. **Perfusion:** blood flow through pulmonary capillary bed in pulmonary and bronchial circulation to respiratory system structures
   a. Pulmonary circulation: pulmonary artery carries deoxygenated (venous) blood from right ventricle, branches into pulmonary capillaries, and connects to alveoli; CO_2 is exchanged for O_2 at pulmonary capillary membranes; capillary membranes merge into pulmonary venules and pulmonary veins that carry oxygenated blood back to left atrium of heart
   b. Bronchial circulation: bronchial arteries branch from thoracic aorta to circulate blood to conducting airways and other respiratory tract tissues; bronchial blood does not circulate to alveoli and is not included in gas exchange
   c. Characteristics of respiratory system circulation: blood pressure (BP) and resistance to blood flow are lower in pulmonary blood vessels than systemic blood vessels
4. **Diffusion:** movement of air and O_2 from atmosphere into alveoli; O_2 crosses into pulmonary capillaries; CO_2 diffuses out of pulmonary capillaries into alveoli;
   a. Variables that influence gas exchange (see Table 56–1 ■)

Box 56–1

Lung Volumes and Capacities

- Tidal volume (V_T): total air volume inspired and expired during one breathing cycle.
- Inspiratory reserve volume (IRV): maximum air volume inspired with forced inspiration (i.e., movement of air from the atmosphere into the respiratory system) following normal inspiration.
- Expiratory reserve volume (ERV): air volume that can be expired with force following normal expiration.
- Residual volume (RV): air volume remaining in lungs following forced expiration.
- Total lung capacity (TLC): maximum capacity of air volume of the lungs. $TLC = IRV + V_T + ERV + RV$
- Inspiratory capacity (IC): maximum air volume that can be inhaled following a normal exhalation. $IC = V_T + IRV$
- Vital capacity (VC): maximum air volume that can be exhaled after a maximum inhalation. $VC = IRV + V_T + ERV$
- Functional residual capacity (FRC): residual air volume in lungs after a normal exhalation. $FRC = ERV + RV$

Table 56-1

Variables That Influence Gas Exchange

Variable	Example
Partial pressure of the gas	Supplemental oxygen increases partial pressure of inspired air
Surface area	Loss of lung tissue by surgery or disease decreases surface area available for gas exchange
Molecular weight and gas solubility	CO_2 is more soluble in the membranes and diffuses more quickly than oxygen
Thickness of membrane	Membrane is thickened by some disease processes, such as pneumonia, pulmonary edema; a thicker membrane impedes effective air exchange

b. Ventilation–perfusion relationship: adequate gas exchange requires alveolar ventilation of about 4 L/min balanced with alveolar capillary perfusion of about 5 L/min (see Figure 56–1 ■); normal ventilation-perfusion (V/Q) ratio: 4:5

5. Nervous system control of breathing: initiates within medulla oblongata (inspiration, expiration, and breathing pattern) and pons (rate and depth) of brainstem

a. Sensory inputs to brainstem that influence respiration: chemoreceptors (increased PCO_2 and/or decreased blood pH), stretch receptors (alveolar septa, bronchi, and bronchioles), proprioceptors (muscles and tendons of moveable joints), baroreceptors (aortic arch and carotid sinus), and external environment factors (cold, physical stress, air pollution, smoking, pain, infection, and fever)

b. Motor nerve impulses travel from brain stem via phrenic nerve to diaphragm and stimulate muscle contraction for breathing

II. DIAGNOSTIC TESTS AND ASSESSMENTS

A. Radiological studies

1. Chest x-ray: visualizes structures, fluid, and air in thoracic cavity; anterior–posterior and lateral views are most common; appropriate use of lead shielding reduces overall exposure to x-rays

2. Computed tomography (CT): provides a cross-sectional view of tissue; detects lesions not identified by x-ray; performed with or without contrast media (check allergies to iodine or seafood if contrast used)

3. Magnetic resonance imaging (MRI): computerized images similar to CT identify subtle changes in tissue structure; assess client to ensure metal sources are removed; clients with metal implants may be ineligible for MRI

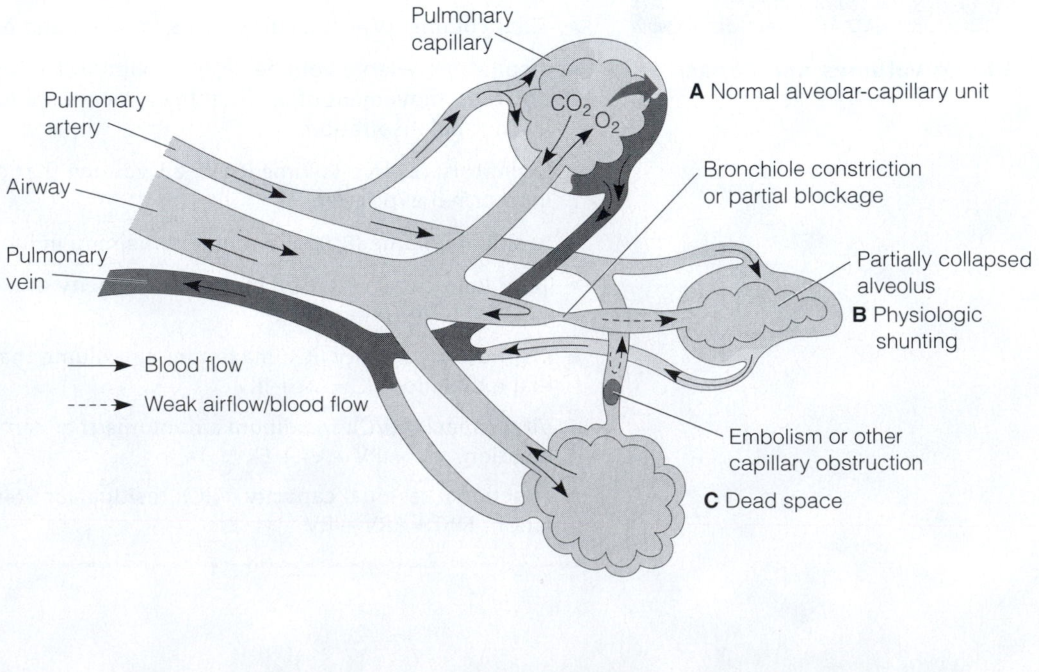

Figure 56-1

Ventilation perfusion relationships. A. Normal alveolar-capillary unit with an ideal match of ventilation and blood flow. Maximum gas exchange occurs between alveolar wall and blood. B. Physiologic shunting: a unit with adequate perfusion but inadequate ventilation. C. Dead space: a unit with adequate ventilation but inadequate perfusion. In the latter two cases, gas exchange is impaired.

4. Pulmonary angiogram: outlines pulmonary vasculature; radioactive contrast medium is injected through a central venous catheter into right side of heart and pulmonary artery; identifies tumors and circulation abnormalities (congenital, thromboembolism) demarcation; assess for iodine and/or seafood allergies
5. Ventilation–perfusion scan: radioactive isotope injected to identify areas of ventilation and perfusion within lungs; also called VQ (ventilation quotient) scan

B. Pulse oximetry

! 1. Monitors arterial or venous **oxygen saturation** ([percentage of O_2] bound to hemoglobin [Hgb] compared to volume that Hgb is capable of binding); normal is usually 95% or greater in a client with no lung disease; in clients with lung disease, target oxygen saturation is 90% or greater; may be measured intermittently (such as with vital signs or ambulation) or continuously
2. Uses a light spectroscopy probe attached to a finger, earlobe, or nose
! 3. Accuracy is lower with diminished peripheral perfusion, brightly lit environment, acrylic fingernails, and dark skin color

C. Pulmonary function test

1. Uses a spirometer to measure lung volumes and capacities during forced breathing techniques; identifies normal or abnormal pulmonary functions
2. Differentiates restrictive versus obstructive lung disease, and assesses effects of bronchodilator therapy; see also Chapter 48

D. Bronchoscopy (see Chapter 48)

E. Thoracentesis

1. Introduction of a needle into thoracic cavity for diagnostic and/or therapeutic reasons
2. Allows withdrawal of pleural fluid for laboratory analysis—microbiology, cytology—such as to determine if cancerous cells are present
3. Permits drainage of pleural effusion to relieve dyspnea

F. Laboratory

1. Arterial blood gases: blood specimen obtained by arterial puncture or drawn from arterial line; identifies oxygenation status, acid-base balance and compensatory mechanisms
   a. Results can indicate acidosis (pH <7.35) or alkalosis (pH >7.45) and may be of respiratory (CO_2) or metabolic (HCO_3^-) origin
   ! b. See Table 56–2 ■ for normal values and refer to Chapter 55 for additional information
2. Sputum analysis: specimen obtained for microbiology (Gram stain, culture and sensitivity) or cytology
   a. Sputum collection procedure: obtained by expectoration, suctioning, saline-induced from the airways, thoracentesis, lung needle biopsy, or transtracheal aspiration; for sputum collection from individuals who can cooperate, have client rinse mouth prior to attempting to obtain expectorated specimen
   ! b. Specimens for acid-fast bacilli (mycobacterium tuberculosis) may be collected on three different days; specimen collection following a long sleep period (early morning) is desirable because of greater concentration; if unable to obtain a sputum specimen for acid-fast bacilli, gastric specimen may be obtained because mycobacterium tuberculosis is not altered by acidic gastric contents
   ! c. Specimen processing: collect specimens in appropriate container and send to laboratory promptly

Table 56–2

Normal Arterial Blood Gas Values

Arterial Blood Gas Parameter	Normal Value
pH	7.35–7.45
PCO_2	35–45 mmHg
HCO_3^-	22–26 mEq/L
PO_2	80–100 mmHg

3. Skin testing: assesses for allergic reactions to specified antigens (type I hypersensitivity), exposure to tuberculosis-causing organisms (type IV hypersensitivity), or fungi
   a. Administer by intradermal route; circle injection site with a long-lasting marker; diagram forearm injection site on chart
   b. Measure area of induration (if present), *not* reddened area; read result 48 to 72 hrs after placement; an uncertain reading at 48 hrs may be reread at 72 hrs
   c. Positive result: individual has been exposed to antigen; does not mean that individual currently has active disease, only that there has been exposure/infection
   d. Induration of 5 mm or greater: indicates recent exposure to tuberculosis or possible HIV infection; chest x-ray findings with characteristic Ghon tubercles are likely healed and not active sites of infection
   e. Induration of 10 mm or greater: indicates typical finding of active tuberculosis infection in populations with chronic, complicating diseases such as diabetes, end-stage renal disease, gastrointestinal (GI) cancer; finding is compatible in high-risk populations such as intravenous (IV) drug users, homeless, and residents of high infection incidence areas
   f. Negative result: indicates no exposure; false-negative findings occur with suppression of cell-mediated immunity such as occurs with HIV infection
   g. When performing skin tests to assess for type I allergies, ensure that antihistamines, which could interfere with test results, are discontinued 72 hours prior to testing

III. COMMON NURSING TECHNIQUES AND PROCEDURES

A. Airway management: goal is to maintain patent airway

1. Head and jaw position
   a. Upper airway obstruction is often caused by loss of local muscle tone or a foreign object
   b. Open airway by head tilt and anterior chin lift maneuver
   c. In individuals with suspected neck injury, open airway by anterior chin displacement and/or jaw thrust; do *not* perform head tilt
   d. Perform Heimlich maneuver in individuals who are conscious with suspected foreign body obstruction of airway
2. Oropharyngeal airway: maintains airway patency by preventing posterior tongue displacement
   a. Oropharyngeal airway is intended only for unconscious individuals because of possible vomiting or laryngeal spasms
   b. Airway must be sized for each client
   c. Assess oral cavity for possible foreign body or vomitus
   d. Tongue blade may be needed to temporarily displace tongue during insertion
   e. Head and jaw position must be maintained independent of airway placement
3. Nasopharyngeal airway: maintains airway patency via nasal route in individual who is semiconscious or in whom placement of oropharyngeal airway is not feasible
   a. Airway must be sized for individual; an excessively long tube may pass into esophagus, causing stomach distention and inadequate ventilation
   b. Maintain head and jaw position even when an airway is in place
4. Endotracheal (ET) intubation: a long, cuffed ET tube is inserted with a laryngoscope by specially trained personnel for long-term airway management or connection to a mechanical ventilator; see Chapter 28
5. Tracheostomy: surgical placement of cuffed airway into trachea by specially trained personnel to assist in maintaining an effective airway in clients who cannot maintain an airway or require prolonged mechanical ventilation; see Chapter 28
6. Cricothyrotomy: emergency surgical opening of cricothyroid membrane to maintain patent airway when other methods fail or are not feasible
7. Techniques for airway clearance
   a. Oropharyngeal suctioning: nonsterile procedure to remove secretions from upper airway; alert individuals may be taught to do self-suctioning

b. Nasotracheal suctioning: sterile procedure to remove secretions from tracheal area; may be performed to obtain a sterile sputum specimen
c. Tracheobronchial suctioning: sterile procedure using individual suction catheters or in-line suction catheter for clearing secretions via ET tube
d. Ensure that catheter diameter is no more than two thirds of airway lumen
e. Limit suctioning to 10 seconds per catheter pass (5 in children) to reduce risk of inadequate oxygenation and cardiac dysrhythmias from hypoxia

B. Body positioning

1. Physiology: fluid shift theory
   a. Lung ventilation and perfusion are gravity-dependent
   b. Changes in body position from supine (0 degrees) to varying degrees of head elevation or lateral positioning activates reflexive cardiovascular changes that produce fluid shifts in lungs and chest blood vessels
2. Acute respiratory failure
   a. Elevate head at least 45 degrees to increase chest expansion
   b. Elevation also mobilizes fluid from chest into more dependent areas
3. Unilateral lung disease
   a. Position with unaffected lung in dependent position ("good lung down")
   b. Position by using gravity to promote ventilation–perfusion matching
4. Adult respiratory distress syndrome (ARDS)
   a. Prone positioning may be used for clients on maximal mechanical ventilation with unresponsive hypoxemia
   b. Prone position allows previously nondependent air-filled alveoli to become dependent, increasing perfusion to air-filled alveoli and possibly improving ventilation—perfusion matching
   c. Use caution to avoid unintentional dislodgment of ET tube during position changes

C. Oxygen (O_2) administration

1. Nasal cannula
   a. Typical O_2 flow of 1 to 6 L/min will provide O_2 concentrations of 24% to 44%
   b. For each 1 L of O_2 flow, O_2 concentration increases by about 4% (room air O_2 concentration is about 21%)
   c. Individuals with chronic obstructive pulmonary disease (COPD) should receive low flow oxygen, about 1 to 2 L/min, to prevent respiratory depression; these clients are used to high CO_2 levels and low O_2 levels, so increased O_2 (greater than 2 L/min) can cause a loss of respiratory drive
2. Face mask
   a. Provides O_2 concentration of 40% to 60%
   b. Exhaled CO_2 trapped by mask can be rebreathed
   c. Oxygen flow should be greater than 5 L/min to minimize rebreathing CO_2
3. Face mask with O_2 reservoir (partial rebreather)
   a. Constant flow of O_2 into attached reservoir bag attached to mask allows rebreathing of ⅓ of exhaled air along with O_2
   b. Typical O_2 flow of 6 to 10 L/min provides 60% to 90% O_2 concentration
4. A nonrebreather mask is used for clients who require higher O_2 concentrations; provides 95% to 100% O_2 with flow rate of 10 to 15 L/min
5. Venturi mask
   a. Delivers O_2 in precise concentrations of 24%, 28%, 35%, and 40%
   b. Used in individuals with COPD and chronic CO_2 retention

D. Pulmonary hygiene

1. Pursed lip breathing: client exhales through pursed lips, which slows exhalation and reduces airway collapse, thus enhancing respiration
2. Coughing
   a. Coughing adequate for airway clearance requires higher airway pressures
   b. Augmented coughing: caregiver places hand below xiphoid process and thrusts downward on abdomen as client ends inspiration
   c. Huff coughing: client attempts sequential coughing while saying "huff"; maneuver keeps glottis open during coughing; beneficial in clients with COPD

3. Chest physiotherapy (CPT)
   a. Mobilizes bronchial secretions into larger airways for removal by coughing or suctioning; useful for clients with more than 30 mL secretions per day, secretions with artificial airway, and/or atelectasis
   b. Percussion: client is positioned for maximal drainage from affected area; involves use of cupped hands alternately percussing indicated area; contraindicated with lung cancer, hemoptysis, and bronchospasm
   c. Vibration: pressure is applied with palm of hand or electrical vibrator over affected area of chest; may be used in some clients when percussion is contraindicated
   d. Postural drainage: uses gravity to mobilize bronchial secretions; nebulized bronchodilators may be administered prior to postural drainage; contraindicated about 1 hour before and within 3 hours after a meal to reduce risk of vomiting and/or aspiration (see Box 56–2)

E. Mechanical ventilation

1. Purpose: to assist with breathing and provide for adequate gas exchange using a ventilator attached to ET tube or tracheostomy tube
2. Types of ventilators
   a. Positive-pressure volume-cycled, which exerts a positive pressure on airway to deliver a predetemined volume of gas; this type of ventilator allows for pressure and time limits to be set and is the most common ventilator used
   b. Positive-pressure time-cycled ventilator, which exerts a positive pressure on airway, delivering a set volume of gas over a preset time
   c. Positive-pressure pressure-cycled ventilator, which exerts positive pressure on airway within pressure limits set to stop inspiration if that pressure is exceeded
   d. Positive-pressure jet ventilator, which exerts a positive pressure on airway and delivers small volumes of gas at a very high rate
   e. Negative-pressure ventilator, which exerts a negative pressure on external chest and does not require intubation; rarely used; an iron lung used for clients with polio is an example
3. Modes of ventilation
   a. Intermittent mandatory ventilation (IMV): delivers a preset tidal volume (V_T) at a preset rate despite client breathing spontaneously at his or her own rate and V_T
   b. Assist control ventilation (ACV): delivers a preset volume for every breath set on machine as well as those initiated by client; allows for hyperventilation which may or may not be beneficial to an individual client
   c. Controlled mandatory ventilation (CMV): delivers a preset volume at a preset rate and is most frequently utilized for those clients with no ventilatory effort; sometimes requires neuromuscular blockade in clients not tolerating ventilation
   d. Synchronized intermittent mandatory ventilation (SIMV): delivers a preset, mandatory volume synchronized to client's inspiratory effort; most common ventilation currently used

Box 56–2

Chest Physiotherapy (CPT)

- Client is dressed in a lightweight shirt.
- Percussion is performed with a cupped hand striking the chest over a portion of the lung; if done properly, a popping sound will be heard.
- Postural drainage facilitates removal of secretions that are loosened during percussion; for drainage, various head-down positions drain all lung segments.
- Positioning for bronchial drainage can be achieved by child standing on his head, hanging upside down on monkey bars, and other playground activities that are fun for the child.
- Avoid performing CPT immediately after eating.

4. Key ventilator settings
   a. Rate: number of breaths per minute delivered by ventilator; is a number that is combined with the mode often in clinical practice (e.g., SIMV of 6/min)
   b. FiO_2: fraction of inspired O_2 or O_2%; amount of O_2 in air inhaled via ventilator; is expressed as a decimal instead of a percentage (e.g., FiO_2 of .40 versus 40%)
   c. Tidal volume (V_T): amount of air delivered with each breath; often expressed in milliliters or liters (e.g., 700 mL or 0.7 L)
   d. PEEP: abbreviation for positive end-expiratory pressure; the amount of positive pressure set in system at end of exhalation; keeps alveoli open during exhalation to increase gas exchange; is expressed in terms of centimeters of pressure (e.g., 5 cm)
5. Indications: ineffective breathing pattern or hypoxia (e.g., dyspnea, cyanosis, altered mental status, absent breath sounds, tachycardia with no underlying cardiac disease); O_2 saturation levels under 80%, pH less than 7.35, $PaCO_2$ greater than 50 mmHg, V_T less than 5 mL/kg, or minute volumes less than 10 L/min
6. Nursing management
   a. Position client for maximum alveolar ventilation and comfort; maintain soft restraints to avoid accidental extubation
   b. Monitor for any changes in respiratory status or effort
   c. Maintain ventilator settings as ordered and remain knowledgeable about how to troubleshoot ventilator alarms (high pressure frequently indicates need for suctioning or kinking/compression of ET tube; low pressure indicates leak or disconnection); manually ventilate client if alarms sound without apparent cause
   d. Monitor arterial blood gases (ABGs) and maintain continuous O_2 saturation monitoring
   e. Complete a thorough physical assessment with emphasis on cardiac, neurological, and respiratory areas
   f. Administer antibiotics, neuromuscular blocking agents, and sedatives as ordered
   g. Maintain nasogastric suction to prevent aspiration
   h. Supply nutritional support as ordered
   i. Perform frequent oral care and suctioning to maintain airway patency
   j. Provide emotional support to client and family as well as alternative communication method
7. Potential complications: pneumothorax, GI stress ulcers, hypotension caused by decreased venous return from increased intrathoracic pressure, increased intracranial pressure, infection

F. Laryngectomy

1. Purpose: excision of larynx as treatment for cancer
2. Preoperative teaching: educate client and family about long-term implications, including loss of voice, swallowing difficulties, altered route for nutrition, and permanent tracheostomy
3. Postoperative care
   a. Maintain patent airway
   b. Provide pain management
   c. Provide appropriate nutritional support
   d. Teach client and family how to care for tracheostomy and feeding tube (if applicable)
   e. Provide access to communication devices, such as writing supplies, picture or word board, speaking tracheostomy valve
   f. Provide emotional support to client and family; make appropriate referrals

G. Respiratory isolation

1. The Occupational Safety and Health Administration (OSHA) mandates that employers provide protective materials to caregivers at risk for exposure to infectious substances
2. Standard precautions include handwashing, gloves, and protective face gear utilized with all clients independent of actual or potential risk for infection; use

these precautions with all clients whenever there is possible contact with blood, mucous membranes, nonintact skin, or parenteral devices

3. Droplet precautions (transmission-based precautions)
   a. In addition to standard precautions, persons should wear mask when near client who has known or suspected pathogen transmitted by droplet route
   b. Limit client transport within facility; when transport is necessary, place mask on client
   c. Limit contamination of equipment and/or environment
   d. Place client in private room or with a cohort (client with same diagnosis)
4. Airborne precautions: use same principles as droplet precautions but use fit-tested N95 respirator and place client in private room with negative air pressure; keep door closed (see also Chapter 8)

IV. NURSING MANAGEMENT OF CLIENT HAVING THORACIC SURGERY

A. Preoperative period

1. Reduce anxiety through preoperative teaching about procedure and postoperative course and care
2. Assess client's support systems and ability to care for self after surgery
3. Administer preoperative medications, such as antibiotics, opioid analgesics, and anti-anxiety agents, as ordered
4. Obtain baseline vital signs, oxygenation status, and cognitive status for comparison postoperatively

B. Postoperative period

1. Perform baseline assessments for vital signs, oxygenation status, and cognitive status as for all postoperative clients
2. Maintain patent airway
3. Position client for optimal ventilation and perfusion; note any specific surgeon's orders for positioning; be prepared to initiate respiratory support (intubation, emergency tracheostomy, mechanical ventilation) as needed
4. Provide standard care to client with a chest tube, if present; see also Chapter 28
5. Maintain sterility of operative dressing
6. Maintain client safety
7. Administer antibiotics, bronchodilators, corticosteroids, inhalation agents, or other medications as ordered
8. Administer analgesics as ordered; adequate pain management facilitates chest expansion and optimal ventilation
9. Assess for and report possible surgical complications to maintain oxygenation
   a. Change in level of consciousness (LOC) ranging from restlessness and agitation to lethargy or unresponsiveness
   b. Increase in respiratory rate, unequal chest expansion, decreased breath sounds, and/or use of accessory muscles for breathing
   c. Loss of water seal drainage in closed chest drainage system
   d. Greater than desired volume of chest drainage (75–100 mL drainage over 1 hour is an average acceptable upper limit); orders should specify volume of acceptable chest tube drainage; should decrease over first 24 hours
10. Teach client and family about postdischarge home care and follow-up
11. Refer to community health resources for assistance with postdischarge care if needed

C. Positioning client after lung surgery: orders should specify turning parameters for individual client

1. Lobectomy: positioning includes lying on back or turned to either side
2. Segmental resection: positioning includes lying on back and turned onto nonoperative side; positioning on operative side may place tension on sutures and promote bleeding
3. Pneumonectomy
   a. Positioning includes lying on back and turned toward operative side

b. Client may be turned temporarily and slightly toward nonoperative side but should not remain in this position
c. Positioning client with operative side in dependent position promotes desired consolidation of fluid in pleural space previously occupied by removed lung, prevents the remaining lung from shifting into operative side, and facilitates ventilation and perfusion
! d. Avoid complete lateral turning to either side, which changes pressure dynamics within chest and could lead to mediastinal shift

V. OBSTRUCTIVE PULMONARY DISEASES

A. Emphysema

1. Overview
   a. Progressive destruction of alveoli related to chronic inflammation
   b. Decreased surface area of respiratory bronchioles, alveoli, and alveolar ducts available for gas exchange
   c. Airway collapse due to loss of elasticity in respiratory system tissues
   d. A chronic form of obstructive pulmonary disease (COPD)
   e. Common symptom is difficulty with exhalation caused by airways obstructed by edema or excessive mucus production
   f. Lung hyperinflation causes alveolar air trapping and leads to frequent pulmonary infections
   g. Cigarette smoking is primary etiology associated with emphysema
   h. Contributing factors include chronic respiratory inflammation from air pollution or occupational substances such as coal, glass, and asbestos
   i. Diagnosis in young and middle-aged adults may be associated with hereditary deficiency of alpha-1-antitrypsin, an enzyme that prevents breakdown of lung tissue protein
   j. Air trapping in respiratory bronchioles, alveoli, and alveolar ducts leads to repeated infections and characteristic **barrel chest** appearance
   k. Work of breathing requires more energy and greater use of accessory muscles

! 2. Assessment
   a. "Pink puffer" is a classic clinical description characterized by barrel chest, pursed-lip breathing (caused by forced exhalation), obvious use of accessory muscles when breathing, and underweight appearance
   b. Exertional dyspnea progresses with advancing disease
   c. Persistent tachycardia is related to inadequate oxygenation
   d. Overall diminished breath sounds, and possible wheezes or crackles
   e. ABGs: slightly decreased PO_2; PCO_2 is not elevated until later stages
   f. Chest x-ray: hyperinflated lungs with a flattened diaphragm; heart size is normal or small
   g. Pulmonary function tests: low vital capacity and forced expiratory volume (FEV_1)

! 3. Therapeutic management
   a. Goals are to improve ventilation and promote patent airway by removing secretions
   b. Remove environmental pollutants and encourage smoking cessation
   c. Prescribed treatments include bronchodilator therapy, beta-adrenergic agonists, corticosteroid therapy, oxygen and nebulization therapy, chest physiotherapy, intermittent positive-pressure breathing (IPPB), possibly mechanical ventilation, and possible surgical procedures such as bullectomy, lung volume reduction surgery, or lung transplantation
   d. Provide education and referrals for clients with behaviors (such as smoking) that increase risk for COPD
   e. Refer clients to a structured pulmonary conditioning program and provide reinforcement as appropriate
   f. Teach clients to avoid pulmonary irritants
   g. Assist clients to develop appropriate nutritional plans to provide adequate calories

h. Administer supplemental low-flow O_2 as necessary; be prepared to initiate mechanical ventilatory support
i. Administer and teach clients about antibiotic therapy, bronchodilator therapy, and use of measured-dose (metered dose) inhalants
j. Position clients to optimize and maintain airway and effective breathing patterns, usually with head elevated according to comfort
k. Provide immunization against pneumonia and influenza
l. Ensure adequate but not excessive nutritional intake

4. Client education: smoking cessation, avoiding occupational or environmental pollutants, maintaining adequate nutrition with emphasis on higher calorie intake, energy conservation techniques

B. Chronic bronchitis

1. Overview
a. A disorder of chronic airway inflammation with a chronic productive cough lasting at least 3 months during 2 years; is a form of COPD
b. Cigarette smoking is primary etiology of chronic bronchitis
c. Contributing factors include chronic respiratory inflammation from air pollution or occupational substances such as coal, glass, and asbestos
d. Chronic inflammation of airways produces hyperplasia of mucous glands, resulting in excessive sputum production
e. Cilia disappear, and their airway clearance function is lost
f. Goblet cells develop in abnormal sites of terminal bronchioles, also increasing sputum production
g. Mucosal edema and increased production of thick mucus progressively obstructs airflow
h. Work of breathing increases with progressive airway obstruction
i. Repeated pulmonary infections result from increased sputum production with ineffective airway clearance
j. Polycythemia develops as a compensatory response to chronic hypoxemia

! 2. Assessment
a. Frequent cough, occurring during winter season, with foul-smelling sputum
b. Frequent pulmonary infections
c. Classic appearance of "blue bloater" includes tendency for obesity and bluish-red skin discoloration from cyanosis and polycythemia
d. Dyspnea and activity intolerance occurs as disease progresses
e. Increased anterior–posterior chest diameter
f. Elevated red blood cell count; hemoglobin and hematocrit elevated in later stages
g. Chest x-ray reveals enlarged heart, congested lung fields, and normal or flattened diaphragm
h. Pulmonary function indicates increased residual volume, decreased vital capacity, FEV_1, and FEV_1/FVC ratio

! 3. Therapeutic management
a. Includes measures previously described in section on emphysema
b. Provide education or referrals to clients with behaviors that increase the risk of developing COPD
c. Refer clients to a structured pulmonary conditioning program and provide reinforcement as appropriate
d. Teach clients how to avoid pulmonary irritants
e. Assist clients to develop appropriate nutritional plans that provide adequate calories but maintain ideal weight
f. Administer supplemental low-flow O_2 as necessary; be prepared to initiate mechanical ventilation
g. Surgical interventions include bullectomy, lung volume reduction surgery, and lung transplantation
h. Medication therapy includes immunization against pneumonia and influenza, antibiotics, possible bronchodilators (beta-adrenergic agonists, anticholiner-

gics such as ipratropium (Atrovent), long-acting theophylline (controversial use in COPD), corticosteroids (controversial use in COPD)

4. Client education: smoking cessation, avoiding occupational or environmental pollutants, nutritional therapies for adequate energy needs and weight management

C. Asthma

1. Overview
   - **a.** A form of COPD
   - **b.** Chronic inflammation of airways leads to intermittent obstruction
   - **c.** Severity and duration of symptoms are unpredictable
   - **d.** Progressive airway obstruction that is unresponsive to treatment can lead to status asthmaticus, an emergency condition
   - **e.** Intrinsic etiologies: uncertain causes; physical or psychological stress; exercise-induced
   - **f.** Extrinsic etiologies: antigen–antibody (allergic) reaction to specific irritants; common **triggers** (initiators) include air pollutants, sinusitis, cold and dry air, medications, food additives, hormonal influences, and gastroesophageal reflux
   - **g.** Characterized by widespread spasms of bronchial smooth muscle with airway edema
   - **h.** Excessive secretion of thick mucus contributes to airway obstruction
   - **i.** Lungs become hyperinflated and alveolar air trapping occurs
   - **j.** Gas exchange becomes impaired as **ventilation–perfusion mismatching** occurs

! 2. Assessment
   - **a.** Severe **dyspnea** (difficulty breathing)
   - **b.** Wheezing with expiration; intensity of wheezing is not related to severity of airway obstruction; clients with severe airway obstruction may not be able to move enough air to produce wheezing sound
   - **c.** Cough
   - **d.** Feelings of chest tightness
   - **e.** Prolonged expiration
   - **f.** Mild to greatly diminished breath sounds; may be related to **atelectasis** or narrowed airway lumens
   - **g.** Hyperresonant sound on percussion
   - **h.** Increased heart rate and blood pressure (BP)
   - **i.** Extreme restlessness, anxiety, agitation
   - **j.** **Tachypnea** (rapid respirations) with use of accessory muscles
   - **k.** Decreased PO_2, mild respiratory alkalosis during "attack"
   - **l.** Elevated eosinophil count
   - **m.** Increased residual volume, decreased vital capacity, decreased FEV_1 and peak expiratory flow rate (PEFR)

! 3. Therapeutic management
   - **a.** Acute episodes are managed with inhaled beta agonists, bronchodilators, anti-inflammatory agents, corticosteroids, and oxygen therapy; in severe cases, mechanical ventilation may be instituted
   - **b.** Chronic management: short-acting beta-agonist inhaler (mild symptoms occurring twice weekly or less, intermittent symptomatic relief) anti-inflammatory inhaler: used for mild symptoms occurring daily; corticosteroid inhaler: used for moderate symptoms occurring daily or more often; systemic corticosteroids (oral) can be used for severe symptoms occurring daily or more often
   - **c.** Assess respiratory and oxygenation status; administer supplemental O_2 as needed
   - **d.** Administer bronchodilators as prescribed
   - **e.** Observe characteristics of sputum
   - **f.** Identify, avoid, and remove precipitating factors
   - **g.** Teach client relaxation techniques during nonacute periods
   - **h.** Allergy desensitization therapy if appropriate
   - **i.** Be prepared to establish IV access
   - **j.** Be prepared to initiate mechanical ventilation if indicated

k. Diagnostic testing during nonacute period includes chest x-ray, pulmonary function studies, allergy skin testing, serum eosinophils, and IgE
l. Provide emotional support to client and family
m. If appropriate, allergy desensitization therapy

4. Client education
   a. Identify asthma triggers
   b. Teach client and family proper use of metered-dose inhaler
   c. Instruct client/family regarding the use of peak-flow meter for self-assessment of asthma status; goal is to remain in green zone (80–100% of personal best); use action plan for medications when PEFR is in yellow zone (50–80%); use action plan and seek health care when in red zone (less than 50%)
   d. Asthma symptoms requiring emergency intervention

VI. PLEURAL EFFUSION

A. Overview

1. Accumulation of fluid in pleural space that indicates underlying pulmonary disease or abnormality; a form of restrictive lung disease
2. Transudative pleural effusion: contains small amounts of protein and may be associated with increased hydrostatic pressure (heart failure) or decreased oncotic pressure from low albumin level (chronic renal or liver disease); fluid moves from capillaries into pleural space
3. Exudative pleural effusion: contains larger quantity of protein; results from increased capillary permeability and fluid shift out of capillaries associated with inflammatory processes such as pulmonary tumors, infection, or emboli
4. Empyema: pleural fluid containing pus associated with infectious processes such as pneumonia, lung abscess, and tuberculosis
5. Chylothorax: pulmonary lymph vessels disrupted by surgery or trauma can lead to abnormal accumulation of lymph fluid in pleural space; produces fat malabsorption from GI tract

! B. Assessment

1. Worsening dyspnea
2. Diminished or absent breath sounds on affected side
3. Dullness to percussion on affected side
4. Chest wall pain
5. Fever, persistent cough, night sweats, and weight loss with empyema
6. Visible on chest x-ray if greater than 250 mL fluid accumulates
7. Diagnostic thoracentesis: differentiates source of pleural fluid

! C. Therapeutic management

1. Goal is to treat underlying cause
2. Thoracentesis to drain pleural cavity
3. Antibiotic therapy
4. Surgical procedure may include decortication, or the separation of pleural membranes
5. Monitor respiratory and oxygenation status
6. Physician performs thoracentesis or thoracostomy if indicated
7. Provide supplemental O_2 if indicated
8. Provide adequate nutrition with focus on adequate protein intake
9. Medication therapy: analgesics, antipyretics; IV lipids if chylothorax present

D. Client education

1. Explain underlying cause of pleural effusion
2. Teach client/family to monitor for changes in respiratory and oxygenation status
3. Instruct about purpose of thoracentesis/thoracostomy

VII. PNEUMOTHORAX AND HEMOTHORAX

A. Overview

1. Pneumothorax: air accumulation in pleural space
   a. Spontaneous: rupture of air-filled bleb allows air to move between respiratory system and pleural space; collapse of involved tissue may seal leak with

minimal client symptoms; air leak may progress until pressure between thoracic cavity and atmosphere equalizes and client is symptomatic

b. Primary: spontaneous rupture of bleb in otherwise healthy individual; occurs more often in tall, slender males aged 20 to 40

c. Secondary: rupture of overly distended alveolus/alveoli; occurs in those with known COPD; severity of symptoms varies with size of pneumothorax

d. Tension: disruption of chest wall or lungs causes air accumulation in pleural space; pressure on mediastinum causes pressure on other lung and interrupts venous return to heart; is a medical emergency that requires emergency placement of chest tube to relieve increasing pressure in thoracic cavity and restore adequate cardiac output

e. Traumatic: disruption of pleura, bronchi, or lung tissue caused by blunt or penetrating trauma with air accumulation in pleural space

f. Iatrogenic: disruption of pleura, bronchi, or lung tissue during central venous line placement, lung biopsy, or thoracentesis produces unintentional air leak within respiratory system; clinical manifestations and treatment are same as for spontaneous pneumothorax

2. Hemothorax: blood accumulation in pleural space; clinical manifestations and treatment are same as for pneumothorax

B. Assessment

1. Dyspnea
2. Tracheal deviation toward unaffected side
3. Diminished breath sounds on affected side
4. Percussion dullness on affected side
5. Unequal chest expansion (reduced on affected side)
6. Crepitus over chest
7. Chest x-ray reveals pneumothorax
8. ABG shows decreased PO_2

C. Therapeutic management

1. In mild cases, no chest tube is required; if pneumothorax is significant, a chest tube is inserted and attached to water seal drainage
2. Spontaneous pneumothorax: in otherwise healthy client, may resolve without invasive treatment
3. If spontaneous pneumothorax occurs repeatedly, may require pleurodesis, an instillation of an agent (such as talc or tetracycline) in pleural spaces to allow pleura to adhere together; other procedures include partial pleurectomy, stapling, or laser pleurodesis for pleural sealing
4. Care of client with a chest tube: previously discussed in Chapter 28
5. Monitor respiratory and oxygenation status
6. Provide supplemental oxygen as indicated
7. Maintain infection control practices
8. Medication therapy: analgesics and antibiotics

D. Client education: purpose of chest tube, activity limitations, and pain management

VIII. ATELECTASIS

A. Overview

1. Incomplete expansion or collapse of the lung resulting from obstruction of airway by secretions or a foreign body
2. Collapsed alveoli
3. Common complication among postoperative or immobilized clients
4. Pulmonary secretions and/or exudates contribute to airway obstruction
5. Airway obstruction increases intra-alveolar pressure, causing alveolar collapse
6. Surface area available for gas exchange is decreased

B. Assessment

1. Low-grade fever
2. Breath sounds diminished or absent in affected area
3. Diminished rate and depth of respiration

4. Physical inactivity caused by immobility or pain
5. Diagnostic and laboratory test findings: chest x-ray reveals area of collapse

C. Therapeutic management

1. Primary goal is prevention of atelectasis
2. Chest physical therapy and general pulmonary hygiene measures
3. Intermittent positive pressure breathing treatments
4. Supplemental oxygen as indicated
5. Monitor respiratory and oxygenation status
6. Deep breathing and coughing exercises
7. Incentive spirometry
8. Frequent position change
9. Ambulation as soon as feasible with client condition
10. Maintain adequate hydration and nutrition
11. Medication therapy: analgesics and antipyretics

D. Client education: diaphragmatic and abdominal breathing techniques, and nonpharmacologic pain control measures

IX. PNEUMONIA

A. Overview

1. Acute inflammation of lung parenchyma (alveoli and respiratory bronchioles)
2. Classified as viral versus bacterial, community-acquired versus hospital-acquired, atypical, or pneumocystis
3. Causative agent can be infectious (bacteria, viruses, fungi, and other microbes) or noninfectious (aspirated or inhaled substances)
4. Most common organism for both community-acquired and hospital-acquired pneumonia is the Gram-positive bacteria *Streptococcus pneumoniae*
5. Other common organisms associated with community-acquired pneumonia include *Klebsiella pneumoniae, Pseudomonas aeruginosa, Escherichia coli, haemophilus influenzae,* and other influenzae viruses
6. Spread of microbes in alveoli activates inflammatory and immune response
7. Antigen–antibody response damages mucous membranes of bronchioles and alveoli resulting in edema
8. Microbe cellular debris and exudate fill alveoli and can impair gas exchange

B. Assessment

1. Viral
   - **a.** Fever: low-grade
   - **b.** Cough: nonproductive
   - **c.** White blood cell count: normal to low elevation
   - **d.** Chest x-ray: minimal changes evident
   - **e.** Clinical course: less severe than pneumonia of bacterial origin
2. Bacterial
   - **a.** Fever: high
   - **b.** Cough: productive
   - **c.** White blood cell count: high elevation
   - **d.** Chest x-ray: obvious infiltrates
   - **e.** Clinical course: more severe than pneumonia of viral origin

C. Therapeutic management

1. Antibiotic therapy, analgesics, antipyretics
2. Oxygen therapy to treat hypoxemia
3. Maintain patent airway; monitor respiratory and oxygenation status
4. Provide supplemental oxygen as indicated
5. Be prepared to initiate mechanical ventilatory support
6. Provide nutritional support and fluids (2 liters per 24 hours or greater if no contraindications) via appropriate route
7. Provide adequate opportunities for physical rest
8. For all hospitalized clients, take measures to prevent pneumonia
   - **a.** Identify clients at high risk for pneumonia
   - **b.** Maintain appropriate infection control measures

c. Maintain adequate nutrition
d. Initiate aspiration precautions for clients at risk (ex: stroke)
e. Encourage activity and mobility as soon as feasible

9. Medication therapy: antibiotics or other antimicrobials as indicated, analgesics, antipyretics

D. Client education

1. Immunization against influenza and pneumococcal pneumonia
2. Activity limitations and importance of rest
3. Effects and dosages of medications
4. Avoid pollutants and irritants such as smoke
5. Symptoms to report to health care provider (return of fever, worsening respiratory status)

X. PULMONARY TUBERCULOSIS

A. Overview

1. Lung infection caused by *Mycobacterium tuberculosis*
2. Any tissue can be infected, but often found in lungs
3. *M. tuberculosis* is an acid-fast, Gram-positive bacillus with transmission via airborne droplets
4. Infection usually results from frequent close contact with an infected individual
5. Inhaled bacilli inhabit respiratory bronchioles and alveoli
6. Bacilli travel through lymph circulation and may spread throughout body before cell-mediated immunity can contain its movement
7. Eventual activation of cell-mediated immunity produces a granuloma lesion
8. Liquified necrotic material from Ghon tubercle portion of granuloma lesion results in passage of infectious particles into major airways where they can be exhaled into air

! **B. Assessment**

1. Frequent cough with copious frothy pink sputum; nonproductive cough develops first as an early symptom (especially in early morning)
2. Night sweats
3. Anorexia
4. Weight loss
5. History may indicate recent exposure to infected individual
6. Positive tuberculin skin test (indicates exposure)
7. Appearance of characteristic Ghon tubercle on chest x-ray
8. Positive acid-fast bacillus sputum cultures (provides definitive diagnosis of infection)

! **C. Therapeutic management**

1. Monitor respiratory and oxygenation status
2. Provide adequate nutrition and hydration
3. Institute standard precautions (Centers for Disease Control [CDC] Tier 1) and airborne precautions (Tier 2, transmission-based precautions); see also Chapter 8
   a. Use a private room with negative air pressure that has 6 to 12 full air exchanges per hour and is vented to the outside or has its own air filtration system
   b. Wear specially fitted mask (N95 respirator) whenever entering client's room; fit-test the mask with each use
   c. Provide visitors with appropriate masks
   d. Wear gown and masks if client does not reliably cover mouth during coughing or sneezing to reduce risk of transmission to others
   e. Provide client with a surgical mask if it is necessary to bring client to another department; choose shortest and least busy route and alert that department ahead of time about client's status; schedule tests for least busy times of day
   f. Administer antimicrobial therapy as prescribed
   g. Provide supplemental oxygen as indicated
   h. Obtain periodic sputum cultures following onset of antimicrobial therapy
4. Medication therapy
   a. Antibiotic prophylaxis: for individuals exposed to clients with active disease; isoniazid (INH) is drug of choice for 6 months if no clinical evidence of disease

b. INH drug of choice for 12 months if abnormal chest x-ray or high-risk population such as with HIV or drug-induced immunosuppression
c. Active disease option 1 (CDC): INH, rifampin (Rifadin), pyrazinamide (Tebrazid), and ethambutol (Myambutol) or streptomycin given daily or two to three times weekly (if therapy verified); if cultures report sensitivity to rifampin or INH, ethambutol or streptomycin can be stopped; minimal 6 months of drug therapy; drug therapy continues for at least 3 months after first negative sputum culture obtained
d. Active disease option 2 (CDC): INH, rifampin, pyrazinamide, and ethambutol or streptomycin given daily for 2 weeks, then twice weekly for 6 weeks, then twice weekly INH and rifampin for 16 weeks
e. Active disease option 3 (CDC): INH, rifampin, pyrazinamide, and ethambutol or streptomycin three times weekly for 6 months
f. Active disease option 4 (CDC): active TB with HIV; option 1, 2, or 3 for minimum of 9 months and to continue for at least 6 months after first negative sputum culture

D. Client education

! 1. Infection control measures, including handwashing, coughing into tissues and disposing of them in a closed bag
2. No special precautions need to be taken with clothing, books, personal objects, or eating utensils because inanimate objects do not easily spread the bacteria
! 3. Teach client, family, and close contacts about mechanisms of transmission and antimicrobial therapy, including need to take medication for full course of therapy to prevent recurrence and/or development of drug-resistant organisms
4. Teach client about adverse effects of medications; see also Chapter 37
5. Maintain adequate nutrition for healing and provide rest periods to minimize fatigue

XI. PULMONARY EMBOLISM

A. Overview

1. Emboli lodge in pulmonary vasculature and impede blood flow through pulmonary capillaries
2. **Ventilation–perfusion mismatch**: a clinically significant imbalance between volume of air and volume of blood circulating to gas exchange area of lungs; leads to impaired gas exchange
3. Pulmonary embolism (PE) more commonly occurs in immobilized clients who develop deep vein thrombosis
4. Other sites of origin of emboli include veins in pelvis, or thrombi in right side of heart
5. Risk factors for PE include immobility, hypercoagulability, trauma to endothelial layer of blood vessels, and long bone fractures
6. Venous thrombus dislodges and circulates to pulmonary vasculature; fat emboli travel from site of long bone fractures and traumatized vessels
7. Emboli obstruct small to large areas of pulmonary vasculature, preventing adequate perfusion and gas exchange
8. A massive area of obstructed tissue leads to pulmonary infarction
9. Severe impairment of gas exchange can be rapidly fatal

! **B. Assessment**

1. Restlessness, anxiety, agitation
2. Vital signs: tachycardia, tachypnea, hypotension, fever
3. Chest pain
4. Hemoptysis
5. Mental status changes with possible decreasing level of consciousness (LOC)
6. Cyanosis
7. Recent history of thromboembolism and/or long bone fractures
8. Lung crackles upon auscultation
9. Atrial fibrillation
10. Chest x-ray may be normal

11. Pulmonary angiogram reveals pulmonary embolism
12. Ventilation–perfusion scan indicates areas of mismatch
13. Abnormal arterial blood gases (significantly low PaO_2)

C. Therapeutic management

1. Supplemental oxygen therapy; maintain patent airway
2. Be prepared to initiate mechanical ventilation
3. Maintain IV access and provide circulatory support as needed
4. Anticoagulant and/or thrombolytic therapy
5. Opioid analgesies and anti-anxiety agents as needed
6. Embolectomy
7. To prevent future pulmonary emboli, a vena cava filter may be inserted to trap emboli from a known source

D. Client education

1. Prevention of thromboembolism
2. Avoid immobility as much as feasible
3. Teach signs/symptoms of venous occlusion
4. Instruct client/family regarding anticoagulant therapy as indicated

XII. BRONCHOGENIC CARCINOMA

A. Overview

1. Lung cancer is leading cause of death from malignancy
2. Five-year survival rate is less than 15%
3. Greater than 90% of lung cancers originate in bronchus epithelium
4. Cigarette smoking is leading cause; cancer risk increases with length of smoking exposure
5. Contributing factors include inhaled environmental substances such as air pollution, arsenic, asbestos, iron, radon, and aromatic hydrocarbons
6. Some individuals have a genetic predisposition to bronchogenic carcinoma
7. Tumor growth commonly begins in bronchus then migrates to upper lobes of lungs
8. Nonspecific inflammatory cellular changes lead to excessive mucus production, desquamation, metaplasia of epithelium, and slow-growing bronchogenic carcinoma
9. Tumor types include small cell and non-small cell
10. Metastasis occurs by direct contact and transport in blood and lymph

B. Assessment

1. Symptom onset is often late in course of disease
2. Persistent cough with or without hemoptysis
3. Localized chest pain
4. Dyspnea
5. Unilateral wheeze upon auscultation
6. Swallowing difficulty
7. Anorexia and weight loss
8. Enlarged neck lymph nodes
9. Mass visible on chest x-ray
10. CT scan or MRI of chest may better differentiate mass
11. Sputum for cytology reveals tumor cells
12. Bronchoscopy for direct biopsy or washings for cytology reveal tumor cells

C. Therapeutic management

1. Surgical resection
   - a. Pneumonectomy: removal of entire lung
   - b. Lobectomy: removal of a lobe of lung
   - c. Segmentectomy (segmental resection): removal of a segment or segments of a lung
   - d. Wedge resection: dissection and removal of a defined area in lung
2. Chemotherapy
3. Radiation therapy
4. Laser therapy
5. Immunotherapy

6. Provide psychological support for client and family
7. Provide preoperative and postoperative care for client having surgery
8. Administer oxygen therapy as prescribed
9. Assist client with pain management
10. Position to optimize oxygenation (see previous discussion)
11. Provide care of chest tubes (see also Chapter 28)
12. Medication therapy: opioid analgesics and antiemetics

D. Client education: treatment plan, pain management, and assistance with coping skills

XIII. CANCER OF THE LARYNX

A. Description

1. Most laryngeal tumors are benign
2. Most common form of malignant laryngeal cancer is squamous cell carcinoma
3. Primary etiologies include long-term cigarette smoking and alcohol ingestion
4. Contributing factors include chronic laryngeal irritation caused by singing, air pollution, and environmental hazards
5. Tumor growth occurs in glottis, supraglottis, and subglottis; symptoms are specific to site of tumor
6. Chronic laryngeal irritation leads to precancerous lesions, leukoplakia, and erythroplakia
7. Carcinoma may develop at site of precancerous lesions
8. Most common site for laryngeal metastasis is lungs; larynx is, however, a rare site for metastasis of other tumors

! **B. Assessment**

1. Hoarseness and/or change in voice characteristics
2. Palpable jugular nodes
3. Pain when swallowing
4. Unexplained earache
5. Diagnostic test results: laryngeal biopsy findings, x-ray visualization, MRI or CT findings, barium swallow visualization

! **C. Therapeutic management**

1. Depends on stage of disease and general condition of client
   - **a.** Radiation therapy or brachytherapy (placement of a radioactive source next to tumor)
   - **b.** Chemotherapy
   - **c.** Laryngectomy
   - **d.** Radical neck dissection
2. Maintain patent airway (tracheostomy performed with laryngectomy)
3. Pain management
4. Provide adequate hydration and nutrition (temporary or permanent altered route for nutrition)
5. Provide alternate means for communication and plan for permanent means of communication (artificial larynx or esophageal speech)
6. Monitor respiratory and oxygenation status
7. Provide oxygen supplementation as indicated
8. Medication therapy: opioid analgesics and antipyretics

D. Client education

1. Smoking cessation
2. Changes in body image
3. Care of tracheostomy
4. Use of artificial larynx
5. Supraglottic swallowing for voice production (esophageal speech)
6. Nutritional access device if indicated
7. Pain management
8. Signs of tumor spread

XIV. THORACIC TRAUMA

A. Overview

1. Alteration of breathing mechanics and/or gas exchange caused by respiratory system trauma
2. Blunt trauma: injury to chest wall without disruption of pleura
   a. Rib fractures
   b. Flail chest
   c. Soft tissue rupture: diaphragm, trachea, bronchi, and major blood vessels
   d. Tension pneumothorax
   e. Contusion: lungs, heart
   f. Mechanism of injury commonly involves motor vehicle collisions, falls, and assaults
3. Penetrating trauma: injury involves disruption of pleura
   a. Internal wounds communicate with external atmosphere
   b. Open air-sucking wounds
   c. Pneumothorax and hemothorax
   d. Tissue wounds: heart, lungs, major blood vessels
   e. Mechanism of injury commonly involves firearms, motor vehicle collisions, falls, or assaults
4. Flail chest
   a. Multiple rib fractures in two or more places (separated from bony skeleton)
   b. Chest wall unstable with paradoxical chest expansion (flail segment moves inward with inhalation and outward with exhalation)
   c. Ventilation–perfusion mismatch
   d. Possible underlying lung injury
5. Rupture of diaphragm
   a. Abdominal contents dislocate upward into thoracic cavity
   b. Decrease in diaphragmatic control of breathing

! B. Assessment

1. Chest pain, may be severe such as with flail chest
2. Shallow breathing with splinting
3. Possible unequal chest expansion
4. Tachycardia, tachypnea, hypotension
5. Crepitus over chest
6. Chest x-ray findings show white opacifications
7. ABGs reveal hypoxemia

! C. Therapeutic management: same as pneumothorax and hemothorax

1. Ventilation support
2. Be prepared to initiate mechanical ventilation
3. Maintain IV access
4. Possible placement of chest tube with water seal drainage
5. Medication therapy: opioid analgesics, patient-controlled or epidural analgesia may be appropriate

D. Client education

1. Techniques for pulmonary hygiene
2. Pain management: patient-controlled analgesia may be appropriate
3. Prevention of thromboembolic phenomena
4. Measures to decrease anxiety

XV. CYSTIC FIBROSIS (CF)

A. Overview

1. Multisystem disorder of exocrine glands, leading to increased production of thick mucus in bronchioles, small intestines, and pancreatic and bile ducts
2. Increased viscosity of secretions obstructs small passageways of these organs and interferes with normal pulmonary and digestive functioning
3. Respiratory problems are most serious threat to life; thick, sticky secretions pool in bronchioles, cause atelectasis, and serve as a medium for bacterial growth

4. Pancreatic ducts become clogged with thick secretions and prevent pancreatic enzymes from reaching duodenum, impairing digestion and absorption
5. Small intestines, without aid of pancreatic enzymes, are unable to absorb fats and protein; thus, growth and puberty are retarded
6. Inherited as an autosomal-recessive trait; gene on chromosome 7 responsible for functioning of cystic fibrosis transmembrane regulator (CFTR) is defective; absence of CTFR as a chloride channel interferes with sodium-chloride (Na^+–Cl^-) transport, prohibiting movement of water across cell membranes
7. Usually diagnosed in infancy and early childhood; affects white children primarily; rarely seen in children of Asian of African descent; males and females are affected equally
8. Life expectancy has increased to median age of 30 years, but disease is terminal; death usually results from resistant pulmonary organisms and fibrosis and destruction of lung tissues

! **B. Assessment**

1. **Sweat test** (pilocarpine iontophoresis) analyzes Na^+ and Cl^- content in sweat; a chloride concentration greater than 60 meq/L is diagnostic of cystic fibrosis; parents often report that infants taste salty when kissed
2. 72-hour fecal fat analysis
3. Chest x-ray
4. Prior to delivery, prenatal DNA analysis of amniotic fluid shows intestinal alkaline phosphatase is reduced in a fetus with cystic fibrosis
5. History usually reveals frequent bouts of respiratory infections
6. Observe for any respiratory impairment (i.e., cough, presence and color of sputum, dyspnea, retractions) color of nailbeds and mucous membranes, O_2 saturation; auscultate breath sounds for equality, crackles, wheezes, or any increased effort during breathing; observe for clubbing of fingers and toes; **digital clubbing,** an indication of hypoxia, produces nails with increased rounding and a loss of normal angle at base of nail
7. Assess nutritional status by obtaining height and weight and plot on growth charts; skin turgor and mucous membranes reveal hydration status; record diet history and activity tolerance; signs of malabsorption include bulky, frothy, foul-smelling stools called steatorrhea and unusually protruberant abdomen and thin extremities; often first sign of CF is meconium ileus, where intestine is blocked with thick, tenacous secretions in newborn period and neonate is unable to pass first meconium stool

! **C. Therapeutic management**

1. Respiratory: ensure pulmonary hygiene is performed; auscultate breath sounds before and after treatments; encourage coughing and deep breathing exercises and physical activity as tolerated; administer prescribed antibiotics and bronchodilator(s)
2. Digestive: provide high-calorie (150% above normal recommendations), high-protein diet and snacks; give infants a predigested formula such as pregestimil or nutramigen; administer pancreatic enzymes with all meals and snacks; individualize to achieve stools as near normal as possible; administer fat-soluble vitamins; determine food preferences to encourage acceptance of diet; weigh daily; avoid pulmonary treatments immediately after meals to decrease risk of vomiting
3. Medications: antibiotics for treatment of pulmonary infection and purulent secretions, pancreatic enzymes for fat absorption, vitamin supplementation, mucolytics to decrease viscosity of sputum, bronchodilators to improve lung function; see Chapter 37 for overview of commonly ordered respiratory care medications

D. Child and family education

1. Avoid exposure to respiratory infections; report immediately any fever, increase in cough, or change in sputum
2. Chest percussion and postural drainage must be performed 3 to 4 times daily; noncompliance will result in increased hospitalizations and infections; see Box 56–2 for instructions on chest physiotherapy and postural drainage (p. 1010)

! 3. High-calorie, high-protein diet is essential; give pancreatic enzymes with all meals and snacks; may need extra salt in hot weather
4. Physical activity and exercise loosen secretions and promote lung expansion
5. Provide information on community resources, such as Cystic Fibrosis Foundation, American Lung Association; provide social service consults, home-health referrals with visiting nurses and respiratory therapists
6. Genetic counseling
7. Provide written information on medications, breathing exercises, chest physiotherapy, and postural drainage
8. Suggest clergy, mental health services, respite care, and families of other children with CF to assist with psychologic and emotional coping with chronic, progressive illness

XVI. BRONCHOPULMONARY DYSPLASIA (BPD)

A. Overview

1. A chronic obstructive pulmonary disorder occurring in infants as a sequela to prolonged O_2 therapy and mechanical ventilation
2. Premature infants with BPD have usually survived respiratory distress syndrome (RDS) at birth; term infants who develop BPD also generally had serious respiratory problems that required ventilatory assistance
3. High O_2 concentrations and mechanical ventilation damage bronchial epithelium and alveoli; thickened alveolar walls, scarring, and fibrosis lead to atelectasis, poor airway clearance of mucus, and poor gas exchange; chronic low oxygenation results in decreased lung compliance and altered function
4. Lung immaturity is a major contributor to occurrence of BPD, and improved survival rates of premature infants have increased incidence of BPD; as little as 3 days of positive pressure ventilation can increase an infant's risk of developing BPD
5. There may be a genetic predisposition; males have increased morbidity

! B. Assessment

1. Diagnosed by chest x-ray, which reveals lung changes and air trapping with or without hyperinflation
2. Blood gases reveal hypercapnia (increased CO_2) and respiratory acidosis
3. Respiratory observations include tachypnea (rapid respirations), tachycardia, increased work of breathing, retractions, wheezing, and barrel chest (rounding of chest caused by trapped air)
4. Pallor, activity intolerance, and poor feeding result from chronic hypoxia

! C. Therapeutic management

1. Infants with BPD are cared for in intensive care units and require an artificial airway; avoid pressure or trauma to ET tube and infant's airway
2. Suctioning, turning, and weighing is done carefully to ensure adequate O_2 saturation levels are maintained
3. Monitor respiratory status continuously; infant's condition can worsen in a short period of time
4. Monitor for fluid overload; infants are at increased risk for pulmonary edema; weigh daily; maintain strict I & O
5. Strict handwashing; avoid exposure to respiratory infections
6. Cluster nursing care to minimize O_2 requirements and caloric expenditure
7. Plan quiet stimulation and activities to foster normal infant development and parental bonding with extended and often repeated hospitalizations of infants with BPD
8. Medications
   a. Bronchodilators open airways and increase lung compliance
   b. Corticosteroids reduce airway edema and inflammation
   c. Diuretics remove excess fluid from lungs and help prevent pulmonary edema
   d. Antibiotics may be given prophylactically

D. Client and family education

1. Infants are discharged with multiple needs; assess family's understanding and ability to follow treatment regimen

2. Teach parents cardiopulmonary resuscitation (CPR), use of home monitoring equipment and O_2 therapy; infants are usually discharged with a tracheostomy when O_2 concentration requirements are low
3. Review infection control practices such as handwashing and avoidance of family members with respiratory infections; teach warning signs of illness
4. Teach safety precautions regarding O_2 therapy and tracheostomy care; see Box 56–3 for instructions on home tracheostomy care; before discharge, notify utility companies, emergency services, and telephone companies of a technology-dependent infant or child
5. Review basic care—feeding, bathing, playing, holding—with parents; allow parents an opportunity to care for child in hospital before discharge; after basic care is mastered, medical treatment plan is developed with assistance of parents
6. Make referrals to community agencies for supplies, medications, nutrition, parental support, and stimulation programs to foster growth and development

XVII. LARYNGOTRACHEOBRONCHITIS (LTB)

A. Overview

1. Viral infection that causes inflammation, edema, and narrowing of larynx, trachea, and bronchi; usually LTB is preceded by a recent upper respiratory infection (URI)
2. LTB is most common in infants and toddlers and affects boys more often than girls; is the most common of the croup syndromes

Box 56–3

Tracheostomy Home Care and Oxygen Therapy

Discharge instructions for a child with a tracheostomy should include the following:

- Keep small toys, talcum powder, plastic bibs and bedding, and any small particles away from child to decrease risk for aspiration or occlusion of trachea.
- Be sure child wears cloth bib loosely over tracheostomy when eating to prevent food particles from entering tube.
- Be careful when bathing to keep water from entering trachea; showers are not recommended.
- Cover tracheostomy loosely when outside in strong wind and cold to prevent tracheal spasms.
- Observe skin around tracheostomy daily for redness, breakdown, or any signs of infection.
- Change tracheostomy ties weekly; be sure to use nonfraying material; always have assistance to change ties.
- Clean area around tracheostomy daily with half-strength saline and hydrogen peroxide and cotton applicators.
- Suction tracheostomy tube when needed to remove secretions from the child's airway; use sterile gloves and limit suctioning to 5 seconds. Insert suction catheter only to the length of the tracheostomy tube and apply intermittent suction while withdrawing the catheter.
- Be sure child is allowed to rest between suctioning if catheter is passed more than once.
- Notify physician if tracheal secretions are increased or become purulent, or if child develops a fever.
- Keep written instructions available at all times.
- Keep emergency bag with extra suction catheters and tracheostomy tubes available.
- Notify utility companies and emergency medical services that child in the home requires emergency equipment.
- Do not allow smoking in the home of child with oxygen therapy.
- Keep oxygen tanks away from any heat source; keep a fire extinguisher nearby.

3. LTB is usually caused by parainfluenzae virus, influenzae A and B, respiratory syncytial virus (RSV), and mycoplasma pneumoniae
4. Inflammation and narrowing of airways cause inspiratory stridor and suprasternal retractions as child struggles to inhale air; increased production of thick secretions and edema further obstruct airway and cause hypoxia accumulation of carbon dioxide, and lead to respiratory acidosis and failure

B. Assessment

1. Onset is gradual after URI
2. Child awakens with low-grade fever, barking cough, and acute stridor; noisy breathing and use of accessory muscles increase
3. Child is agitated, restless, has a frightened appearance, sore throat, and rhinorrhea
4. Pulse oximetry is used to detect hypoxemia; anteroposterior (AP) and lateral upper airway x-rays are ordered

C. Therapeutic management

1. Monitor child's respiratory effort continuously to ensure a patent airway; observe for diminished breath sounds, circumoral cyanosis, diminishing noisy breathing, and drooling
2. Quiet respiratory effort is a sign of physical exhaustion and impending respiratory failure
3. Provide humidity and supplemental O_2; IV fluids prevent dehydration and help liquefy secretions
4. Assist child to assume upright position or any position of comfort; promote a calm, quiet environment; keep parents nearby to decrease child's stress and to lessen crying
5. Keep emergency intubation equipment available at bedside; readily respond to call bell or requests for assistance
6. Assess parental and child's anxiety level; provide emotional support
7. Medications
   a. Bronchodilators decrease mucosal constriction and laryngeal edema; nebulized racemic epinephrine has a rapid onset with improvement of symptoms, although relapse may occur within 2 hours
   b. Corticosteroids decrease inflammation and edema

D. Child and family education

1. Assess parental anxiety and ability to adhere to medical recommendations
2. Symptoms are usually worse at night and may recur for several nights; instruct parents that child can be cared for at home if able to take fluids by mouth and has no stridor at rest
3. Cool mist humidifier and parental presence can be initial treatment of crisis; comforting measures include cuddling, rocking, singing, and any calming measures until breathing becomes easier
4. Instruct parents to seek medical attention immediately if breathing becomes labored, child seems exhausted or very agitated, or if symptoms do not improve after cool air humidity treatment
5. Teach parents that LTB is a viral illness; avoid contact with large groups of people and practice infection control measures

XVIII. EPIGLOTTITIS

A. Overview

1. Inflammation and swelling of epiglottis, primarily affecting children ages 2 to 8
2. Epiglottis covers larynx during swallowing to prevent food from entering trachea
3. Bacteria, usually *Haemophilus influenzae,* cause epiglottis to become cherry red, swollen, and so edematous that it obstructs airway; secretions pool in pharynx and larynx above epiglottis; child has a sore throat and is unable to swallow; complete airway obstruction can occur within 2 to 6 hours
4. Onset is sudden in a previously healthy child; Hib vaccine has reduced incidence of epiglottitis, although causative organisms may also be streptococcus and staphylococcus

! **B. Assessments**

1. Child awakens with sudden onset of high fever (102°F), extremely sore throat, and pain on swallowing
2. Child is very anxious, restless, looks ill, and insists on sitting upright leaning on arms, with chin thrust out and mouth open (tripod position)
3. Dysphonia (muffled voice), dysphagia (difficulty swallowing), drooling of saliva, and distressed respiratory effort are classic signs
4. Edematous, cherry-red epiglottis is most reliable diagnostic sign
5. Examination of throat is contraindicated, however, unless emergency intubation equipment and trained personnel are available; physical manipulation of hypersensitive and irritated airway muscles may result in spasm and complete obstruction
6. Lateral neck x-ray confirms an enlarged epiglottis; portable x-rays are completed in examination room with child on parent's lap to minimize stress and maximize child's comfort and calm behavior
7. Complete blood count (CBC) and blood cultures are taken once child is intubated and stabilized

! **C. Therapeutic management**

1. Assess continuously for respiratory distress and decrease in respiratory effort; report changes in status
2. Never leave child unattended; support child in position of comfort; encourage parents to hug and cuddle their child
3. Keep ET and tracheotomy tubes and suction equipment at bedside; assist with emergency ventilation if needed before child is taken to operating room (OR) for airway insertion
4. Child is usually intubated for 24 hours; restraints may be necessary to prevent tube dislodgment, because swelling of epiglottis may prohibit reintubation
5. Provide support for child and family and alleviate anxiety; explain all procedures clearly and calmly
6. All invasive procedures, including starting an IV infusion, ABGs, and blood cultures are performed in OR
7. Keep child NPO; IV fluids provide hydration; administer antipyretics and antibiotics as prescribed
8. After extubation, monitor child closely in intensive care unit to ensure immediate assessment if respiratory effort is compromised
9. Medications
   a. Antibiotics treat bacterial infection (usually given for 7 to 10 days); child is discharged in about 3 days with oral antibiotics
   b. Antipyretics treat fever and manage pain of sore throat
   c. Corticosteroids may be given for 24 hours before extubation to decrease edema

D. Client and family education

1. Provide emotional support and explain all procedures calmly; encourage parents to cuddle and comfort child
2. Prepare child and parents for airway insertion in OR
3. Teach parents importance of completing antibiotic regimen after discharge; explain medications, how to administer, and any side effects to be expected
4. Discuss importance of Hib vaccine and reassure parents that recurrence of epiglottitis is uncommon

XIX. BRONCHIOLITIS

A. Overview

1. Inflammation of bronchioles with edema and excess accumulation of mucus; air trapping and atelectasis result from increased airway resistance because of small obstructed bronchioles
2. A major cause of hospitalization of high-risk infants
3. RSV is primary causative organism; virus is spread by contact with contaminated objects; RSV is not airborne but can live for several hours on nonporous surfaces

4. RSV bronchiolitis is most prevalent during first 2 years of life, with most occurrences in spring and winter; bronchiolitis usually begins with a mild URI; as disease progresses, gas exchange is compromised, hypoxemia results, and metabolic acidosis develops

B. Assessment

1. Clinical manifestations include worsening of URI with tachypnea, retractions, low-grade fever, anorexia, thick nasal secretions, and increasingly labored breathing; older infants may have a frequent, dry cough
2. Auscultation of lungs reveal wheezing or crackles
3. Nasopharyngeal washing to obtain respiratory secretions identifies causative virus; chest x-ray may be normal or indicate hyperinflation or nonspecific inflammation

C. Therapeutic management

1. Assess respiratory status hourly; provide humidified O_2 to ease respiratory effort; use pulse oximetry to assess O_2 saturation
2. Clear nasal passages with bulb syringe; elevate head of bed
3. Cluster nursing care to allow for rest; assess anxiety level of parents and provide support; maintain a calm environment
4. IV fluids may be needed if oral intake is compromised; monitor strict I & O; weigh daily to assess fluid loss
5. Maintain strict handwashing and contact precautions; caregivers should not care for other high-risk children
6. Medications: bronchodilators and steroids are sometimes used; prevention of bronchiolitis in high-risk children under age 2 may be achieved with use of palivizumab (Synagis) or IV RSV immunoglobulin

D. Child and family education

1. Explain disease process and provide support to lessen anxiety
2. Encourage parents to assist in care of infant; explain all procedures and treatments
3. Teach parents to use bulb syringe as needed to keep nasal passages clear
4. Teach parents to provide frequent oral fluids; notify physician if child demonstrates symptoms of dehydration, including crying without tears, sunken eyes, lethargy, or "acts sick"
5. Instruct parents to notify physician if child refuses to eat or breathing becomes worse
6. Instruct parents to use humidifier in child's bedroom
7. Teach parents to avoid smoking in child's vicinity
8. Teach parents to practice strict handwashing and keep child away from individuals with upper respiratory infections; RSV can reoccur

XX. FOREIGN BODY ASPIRATION

A. Overview

1. Inhalation of an object into respiratory tract, intentional or otherwise
2. Peak age for foreign body aspiration is children under 3 years; it is a leading cause of death in children under 1 year
3. Foreign bodies usually lodge in right main bronchus because it is shorter and wider than left; obstruction may be partial or complete and causes atelectasis, air trapping, and hyperinflation distal to site of obstruction
4. The type and shape of object, as well as small diameter of an infant's airway, determines severity of problem; round objects such as hot dogs, round candy, nuts, and grapes do not break apart and are more likely to occlude airway; latex balloons are particularly hazardous; objects with irregular shapes may irritate airway and partially obstruct airflow
5. Failure to remove a foreign object is usually fatal; a delay in removal may cause aspiration pneumonia

B. Assessment

1. Sudden coughing and gagging is first sign, and objects in upper airway may be expelled by coughing
2. Partial obstruction may cause symptoms of respiratory infection for days or even weeks; child may have hoarseness, croupy cough, wheezing, and dyspnea

PRACTICE TEST

3. If obstruction is complete, child will demonstrate stridor, cyanosis, difficulty swallowing and speaking
4. A child who cannot speak, is cyanotic, and collapses requires immediate attention for complete airway obstruction
5. Fluoroscopy and chest x-ray reveal foreign body in respiratory tract

! C. Therapeutic management

1. Assess respiratory status to determine severity of problem and degree of obstruction; continuously monitor and provide assistance if obstruction worsens
2. If total airway obstruction occurs, perform back blows and chest thrusts for infants and Heimlich maneuver in children older than 1 year
3. Keep NPO; foreign body is usually removed in surgery
4. Position for comfort and to optimize airway; provide emotional support to parents and child and alleviate anxiety
5. After removal of object, assess for additional obstruction that may result from laryngeal edema and tissue swelling
6. Medications: antibiotics may be administered if secondary infection is suspected, or if purulent secretions are present in airway, with or without signs of pneumonia

D. Child and family education

1. Teach parents about hazards of aspiration and importance of child-proofing home
2. Review age-appropriate foods and discuss most frequently aspirated objects: coins, hot dogs, balloons, nuts, popcorn, grapes, round candy, peanut butter
3. Discuss toy safety and avoidance of toys with small, removable parts; caution against allowing child to run and play with objects in his or her mouth
4. Teach parents CPR and techniques of chest thrusts, back blows, and abdominal thrusts

Check Your NCLEX-RN® Exam I.Q. *You are ready for testing on this content if you can*

- Identify basic structures and functions of the respiratory system.
- Describe the pathophysiology and etiology of common respiratory disorders.
- Discuss expected assessment data and diagnostic test findings for selected respiratory disorders.
- Discuss therapeutic management of a client experiencing a respiratory disorder.
- Discuss nursing management of a client experiencing a respiratory disorder.
- Identify expected outcomes for the client experiencing a respiratory disorder.

PRACTICE TEST

1 The nurse teaching health maintenance strategies for the client with COPD should include which of the following items?

1. Yearly influenza immunizations
2. Annual tuberculin skin test
3. Limitation of physical activity
4. Fluid restriction

2 The nurse who is explaining the pathophysiology of COPD to a client includes that alveolar destruction results in which of the following?

1. Decreased surface area for gas exchange
2. Increased dead space air
3. Pulmonary emboli
4. Chronic dilation of bronchioles

3 The nurse explains to a client and family that the development of COPD in a young adult is likely caused by which of the following?

1. Hereditary deficiency of alpha-1-antitrypsin
2. Onset of smoking during childhood
3. Heavy secondary smoke exposure during childhood
4. Use of smokeless tobacco during childhood

4 A client who develops acute respiratory distress syndrome (ARDS) is exhibiting hypoxemia unresponsive to oxygen therapy. In explaining the client's condition to the family, the nurse would incorporate which of the following concepts?

1. Blood is shunted past alveoli with no ventilation.
2. The individual has difficulty expelling air trapped in the alveoli.
3. There is excess surfactant production by the alveoli.
4. Thick secretions block the airways.

5 What intervention does the nurse identify as the priority for the client with a nursing diagnosis of ineffective airway clearance related to tumor mass?

1. Provide supplemental oxygen
2. Keep the head of the bed elevated
3. Teach the client coughing and deep breathing, and maintain hydration
4. Prepare the client for the possible insertion of a tracheostomy tube

6 When assisting with psychological issues for the client with lung cancer, which epidemiological factor should the nurse keep in mind?

1. Five-year survival rate for lung cancer is less than 15 percent.
2. Symptoms usually occur early during lung cancer progression.
3. Tumor growth usually begins in a bronchus, then migrates upward in the tissue.
4. Risk of lung cancer is associated with length of exposure to cigarette smoking.

7 The nurse administers which of the following medications as a part of pharmacological treatment aimed at prevention of pulmonary embolism?

1. Streptokinase
2. Aquamephyton (vitamin K)
3. Enoxaparin (Lovenox)
4. Protamine sulfate

8 In the client with respiratory distress, which finding by the nurse is most compatible with a worsening clinical state?

1. Increased respiratory rate
2. Tachycardia
3. Agitation
4. Cyanosis

9 For the hospitalized client, which factor would the nurse assess to be a symptom of pulmonary embolism?

1. Slow increase in heart rate and respiratory rate
2. Cyanosis of the upper torso
3. Abrupt onset of dyspnea and apprehension
4. Significant bilateral wheezing

10 A client underwent a thoracentesis a few hours earlier. Which finding should the nurse report immediately to the physician?

1. Oozing of blood from the puncture site
2. Crepitus
3. Diminished breath sounds on the affected side
4. Fever

11 The nurse who is assisting the client with obstructive pulmonary disease to learn effective breathing techniques would use which of the following statements to explain why dyspnea occurs?

1. "Decreased surfactant causes many of your alveoli to collapse."
2. "You have difficulty breathing in enough air."
3. "Your airways open wider on inspiration and trap air on expiration."
4. "Your lung compliance is decreased."

12 A client is admitted to the hospital with a medical diagnosis of viral pneumonia. The nurse assesses for which of the following most frequent manifestation?

1. Presence of Ghon tubercle on chest x-ray
2. Nonproductive cough
3. Elevated white blood cell count
4. High fever

13 The nurse would question an order for ipratropium bromide (Atrovent) ordered for a client with asthma if the client had a concurrent history of which of the following?

1. Glaucoma
2. Cushing's syndrome
3. Warfarin therapy
4. Fluid retention

PRACTICE TEST

14 For the client newly diagnosed with asthma who has infrequent acute episodes, the nurse teaches the client that which medication is most effective for providing quick relief in acute episodes?

1. Corticosteroid via metered-dose inhaler as needed
2. Beta-agonist via metered-dose inhaler
3. Anti-inflammatory via metered-dose inhaler
4. Daily use of a bronchodilator inhaler

15 The nurse caring for a client diagnosed with acute respiratory distress syndrome (ARDS) considers that, in this client, impaired gas exchange is mostly likely related to which of the following?

1. Air trapping in the alveoli
2. Accumulation of exudative fluid into the alveoli
3. Shunting of blood around nonventilated alveoli
4. Excessive alpha-1-antitrypsin

16 A child with laryngotracheobronchitis (LTB) is being treated in the emergency department. The nurse would plan to do which of the following to ease respiratory distress?

1. Turn the child onto his side.
2. Administer racemic epinephrine.
3. Administer corticosteroids.
4. Administer intravenous antibiotics.

17 The parents of an infant with bronchiolitis ask the nurse why their baby's room has a sign on the door that says "Contact Precautions" and why the nurses all wear gowns and gloves when they hold him. What is the nurse's best response?

1. "The virus that usually causes bronchiolitis can spread to other babies if extra precautions are not taken."
2. "Your baby is very ill, and we don't want to have another baby catch what he has."
3. "It's because your baby is in isolation."
4. "We always wear gowns when babies are coughing."

18 Which of the following would be a priority nursing intervention for a child with bronchiolitis?

1. Keep the child well stimulated.
2. Maintain strict intake and output.
3. Encourage visitors.
4. Encourage oral fluids if tachypneic.

19 When taking the nursing history of a child with cystic fibrosis, what piece of information about the child's newborn period would the nurse expect the mother to report?

1. That the child required resuscitation in the delivery room
2. That labor was longer than 24 hours
3. That the child had a meconium ileus
4. That labor was less than 4 hours

20 The nurse should counsel the parents of a child with asthma that before performing postural drainage exercises, they should do which of the following?

1. Administer her bronchodilator
2. Change her clothes
3. Administer her antibiotic
4. Suction her throat

21 If treatment for acute epiglottis is effective, the nurse would expect to record that the child

1. has pale lips and mucous membranes.
2. maintains tripod position.
3. is tachypneic and dysphonic.
4. has clear, equal breath sounds.

22 The parents of a child with bronchopulmonary dysplasia (BPD) are receiving home instructions on tracheostomy care. With regard to suctioning, the nurse should advise the parents that each suction pass should take no longer than how many seconds? Provide a numerical answer.

Answer: ______________________

23 A toddler is being discharged after an emergency admission for foreign body aspiration. The parents ask the nurse what they can do to prevent another accident. The nurse should advise the parents to

1. watch her very carefully.
2. teach her not to eat nonfood items.
3. keep small objects and toys out of her reach.
4. avoid leaving her with teen babysitters.

24 The nurse wears gloves when assessing a child with respiratory syncytial virus (RSV). After removing the gloves, what should the nurse do next?

1. Discard the gloves in the laundry basket.
2. Inspect the gloves for holes or fraying.
3. Remind the parents to wear gloves.
4. Wash hands.

25 A 6-year-old child is hospitalized following an acute asthmatic episode. Which statement by the parents indicates that further teaching is needed?

1. "Next time we'll be sure he takes his Cromolyn before soccer."
2. "After this episode, he will need to quit the swim team."
3. "We think this was an exercise-induced asthma episode."
4. "We need to make sure he has his inhaler at all times."

26 The nurse would anticipate administering respiratory medications to a child hospitalized with asthma by which of the following most frequently used routes?

1. Aerosol
2. Intravenous
3. Subcutaneous
4. Oral

27 The nurse anticipates using postural drainage as a treatment modality for which of the following conditions?

1. Epiglottitis
2. Foreign body aspiration
3. Cystic fibrosis
4. Bronchopulmonary dysplasia

28 The nurse teaches a mother how to attach a spacer to the metered-dose inhaler for a young child, explaining that a spacer

1. makes the device look less intimidating to a small child.
2. makes it unnecessary to shake the inhaler before administering the drug.
3. decreases the chances for undesired side effects of medication.
4. reduces the risk for oral yeast by depositing medication more deeply into the airways.

29 The nurse documents which of the following expected findings after auscultating the lungs of a child with bacterial pneumonia?

1. Wheezes
2. Crackles
3. Apnea
4. Retractions

30 An infant with respiratory syncytial virus (RSV) is receiving ribavirin. While caring for this infant, the nurse should not

1. plan to become pregnant for at least 1 year.
2. care for any other children.
3. wear contact lenses.
4. stay in the room with the door closed.

PRACTICE TEST

ANSWERS & RATIONALES

1 **Answer: 1** Clients with COPD are highly susceptible to respiratory infections such as influenza, so they should be immunized yearly. Clients with COPD should undergo a progressive rehabilitation program to increase their activity tolerance. Fluid restriction is not needed with COPD unless there is fluid retention from another etiology.
Cognitive Level: Application **Client Need:** Health Promotion and Maintenance **Integrated Process:** Nursing Process: Planning **Content Area:** Adult Health: Respiratory **Strategy:** The critical words in the stem of the question are *health maintenance.* This phrase indicates that you should focus on the option that prevents a health problem rather than diagnoses or treats it.

2 **Answer: 1** The impaired gas exchange occurring with COPD is caused by the loss of alveolar surface area available for gas exchange. Destruction of alveoli is not related to increased dead space air, pulmonary emboli, or chronic dilation of bronchioles. With COPD there is progressive narrowing of bronchioles.
Cognitive Level: Application **Client Need:** Physiological Integrity: Physiological Adaptation **Integrated Process:** Communication and Documentation **Content Area:** Adult Health: Respiratory **Strategy:** The core issue of the question is the nature of the pathophysiology of COPD. Use general nursing knowledge and the process of elimination to make a selection.

ANSWERS & RATIONALES

3 **Answer: 1** Symptoms of COPD typically appear in the fifth and sixth decades of life following chronic abuse to pulmonary tissues by smoking or environmental pollutants. Onset of the physiological changes compatible with COPD is most often associated with a hereditary deficiency of alpha-1-antitrypsin, an enzyme that protects lung tissue against loss of elasticity. Onset of heavy smoking during childhood and heavy secondary smoke exposure during childhood are not typically associated with early onset of physiological alterations of COPD. Use of smokeless tobacco during childhood is associated with development of oral cancer.
Cognitive Level: Application **Client Need:** Physiological Integrity: Physiological Adaptation **Integrated Process:** Communication and Documentation **Content Area:** Adult Health: Respiratory **Strategy:** The core issue of the question is sharing with a client and family the correct basis of the current health problem. Use nursing knowledge and the process of elimination to make a selection.

4 **Answer: 1** One of the primary alterations occurring with ARDS is the collapse of alveoli and therefore loss of ventilation in those areas. Perfusion may be normal, but gas exchange is impaired due to inadequate ventilation. Surfactant production decreases with ARDS, a factor that impairs adequate gas exchange. Air does not become trapped in hyperinflated alveoli in ARDS; instead alveoli collapse.
Cognitive Level: Application **Client Need:** Physiological Integrity: Physiological Adaptation **Integrated Process:** Nursing Process: Planning **Content Area:** Adult Health: Respiratory **Strategy:** The core issue of the question is an understanding of disease process and how to select appropriate concepts for family teaching. Use nursing knowledge and the process of elimination to make a selection.

5 **Answer: 3** Coughing, deep breathing, and adequate hydration are essential for achieving effective airway clearance. Insertion of a tracheostomy or O_2 therapy are not primary treatments to maintain airway clearance. Elevating the head of the bed may help the client to cough more forcefully, but head elevation alone is not an effective maneuver.
Cognitive Level: Analysis **Client Need:** Physiological Integrity: Physiological Adaptation **Integrated Process:** Nursing Process: Implementation **Content Area:** Adult Health: Respiratory **Strategy:** The critical word in the stem of the question is *priority,* which tells you that more than one option may be correct, and you must choose the most important one. Use nursing knowledge and the process of elimination to make a selection.

6 **Answer: 1** The nurse should help the client and family to approach the diagnosis of lung cancer from a realistic perspective. Symptoms of lung cancer usually appear late in the course of the disease. Tumor growth does typically begin in a bronchus and progress upward, but this information has no relation to the client's psychological adaptation to the disease.
Cognitive Level: Application **Client Need:** Psychosocial Integrity **Integrated Process:** Nursing Process: Planning **Content Area:** Adult Health: Respiratory **Strategy:** The core issue of the question is the knowledge of the interrelationship between prognosis and the communication approaches used by the nurse. Use nursing knowledge and the process of elimination to make a selection.

7 **Answer: 3** Administration of anticoagulants (option 3) is an effective intervention to prevent pulmonary embolism. Thrombolytic drugs (option 1) may be used to dissolve a clot that is already formed. Vitamin K (option 2) and protamine sulfate (option 4) facilitate clotting and counteract the effect of anticoagulants.
Cognitive Level: Application **Client Need:** Physiological Integrity: Pharmacological and Parenteral Therapies **Integrated Process:** Nursing Process: Implementation **Content Area:** Adult Health: Respiratory **Strategy:** The core issue of the question is knowledge of medication to reduce risk of pulmonary embolus. Use nursing knowledge and the process of elimination to make a selection.

8 **Answer: 4** Increased respiratory rate, tachycardia, and agitation are all early signs of respiratory distress. Cyanosis develops later in the progression of respiratory distress.
Cognitive Level: Analysis **Client Need:** Physiological Integrity: Physiological Adaptation **Integrated Process:** Nursing Process: Assessment **Content Area:** Adult Health: Respiratory **Strategy:** The critical word in the stem of the question is *worsening,* which tells you that the symptom will be a late sign, not an early one. Cyanosis is always a late sign. Use nursing knowledge and the process of elimination to make a selection.

9 **Answer: 3** Symptoms associated with pulmonary embolism typically have a sudden onset. The client often feels panic because of the sudden dyspnea. Increase in heart rate and respiratory rate is abrupt, not slow. Cyanosis of the upper torso is associated with embolism of a central vein other than the pulmonary vasculature. Bilateral wheezing is more often associated with asthma than with pulmonary embolism.
Cognitive Level: Application **Client Need:** Physiological Integrity: Physiological Adaptation **Integrated Process:** Nursing Process: Assessment **Content Area:** Adult Health: Respiratory **Strategy:** The critical words in the stem of the question are *symptom* and *pulmonary embolism.* They tell you that the question is seeking an answer that is a correct assessment. Use nursing knowledge and the process of elimination to make a selection.

10 **Answer: 2** The finding of crepitus at any time is associated with pneumothorax and should be immediately reported to the physician. Oozing of blood from the thoracentesis puncture site is not uncommon and does not require emergency intervention, as would crepitus. Diminished breath sounds on the affected side and fever may or may not be related to the thoracentesis. All of these findings should be noted and reported to the physician, but the finding of crepitus is clearly related to development of pneumothorax and signals immediate need for intervention by the physician.
Cognitive Level: Analysis **Client Need:** Physiological Integrity: Physiological Adaptation **Integrated Process:** Nursing Process: Assessment **Content Area:** Adult Health: Respiratory **Strategy:** The core issue of the question is the ability to recognize and prioritize complications that need to be reported to the health care provider. Use nursing knowledge and the process of elimination to make a selection.

11 **Answer: 3** The primary physiological alteration occurring with COPD is alveolar air trapping and alveolar hyperinflation, which lead to alveolar rupture and loss of area avail-

able for gas exchange. Decreased surfactant production is associated with ARDS and is not a primary alteration of COPD. Lung compliance is decreased but is due to the alveolar air trapping and hyperinflation.
Cognitive Level: Application **Client Need:** Physiological Integrity: Physiological Adaptation **Integrated Process:** Communication and Documentation **Content Area:** Adult Health: Respiratory **Strategy:** The core issue of the question is knowledge of the underlying changes associated with COPD and how to communicate that information effectively to a client or family. Use nursing knowledge and the process of elimination to make a selection.

12 **Answer: 2** Viral pneumonia is considered less serious for the client because symptoms are not as apparent compared to bacterial pneumonia. Viral pneumonia is associated with nonproductive cough, low-grade fever, normal white blood cell count, and normal or minimal chest x-ray findings. Ghon tubercles are seen on x-ray in clients with tuberculosis.
Cognitive Level: Application **Client Need:** Physiological Integrity: Physiological Adaptation **Integrated Process:** Nursing Process: Assessment **Content Area:** Adult Health: Respiratory **Strategy:** The critical words in the stem are *most frequent.* With this in mind, you must compare options in terms of their frequency. Use nursing knowledge and the process of elimination to make a selection.

13 **Answer: 1** Anticholinergics such as ipratropium are contraindicated in clients with angle-closure glaucoma because it can inhibit flow of aqueous humor and raise intraocular pressure. The other options do not address this concern.
Cognitive Level: Application **Client Need:** Physiological Integrity: Pharmacological and Parenteral Therapies **Integrated Process:** Nursing Process: Implementation **Content Area:** Adult Health: Respiratory **Strategy:** The core issue of the question is knowledge of contraindications to medication therapy. Use nursing knowledge and the process of elimination to make a selection.

14 **Answer: 2** Clients with mild and infrequent asthma symptoms are treated with regular daily administration of an anti-inflammatory inhaler and a short-acting beta-agonist inhaler for quick relief in acute episodes. Bronchodilators and corticosteroids as oral or inhaled medication are used for clients with more severe and frequent episodes of asthma.
Cognitive Level: Application **Client Need:** Physiological Integrity: Physiological Adaptation **Integrated Process:** Nursing Process: Planning **Content Area:** Adult Health: Respiratory **Strategy:** The core issue of the question is knowledge of the rapid management of symptoms in a client with asthma. Use nursing knowledge and the process of elimination to make a selection.

15 **Answer: 3** A primary physiological alteration occurring with ARDS is shunting of blood around nonventilated alveoli. Alveoli collapse in ARDS, and ventilation decreases. Blood perfusing to these areas cannot undergo adequate gas exchange.
Cognitive Level: Application **Client Need:** Physiological Integrity: Physiological Adaptation **Integrated Process:** Nursing Process: Analysis **Content Area:** Adult Health: Respiratory **Strategy:** The core issue of the question is knowledge of pathophysiology in the development of ARDS. Use nursing knowledge and the process of elimination to make a selection.

16 **Answer: 2** Epinephrine is a bronchodilator used to increase the diameter of the airways. The best position is semi- to high-Fowler's. Corticosteroids and antibiotics may be used but will not ease respiratory distress immediately.
Cognitive Level: Application **Client Need:** Physiological Integrity: Physiological Adaptation **Integrated Process:** Nursing Process: Implementation **Content Area:** Child Health: Respiratory **Strategy:** The core issue of the question is the expected plan of care for a client with laryngotracheobronchitis. Use nursing knowledge and the process of elimination to make a selection.

17 **Answer: 1** RSV is the cause of bronchiolitis in most cases; RSV can live for several hours on nonporous surfaces and can be transferred by the hands.
Cognitive Level: Analysis **Client Need:** Physiological Integrity: Physiological Adaptation **Integrated Process:** Nursing Process: Implementation **Content Area:** Child Health: Respiratory **Strategy:** The core issue of the question is the ability of the nurse to explain the rationale and use of isolation techniques. Use nursing knowledge and the process of elimination to make a selection.

18 **Answer: 2** Maintaining strict I & O will provide immediate notification of signs of dehydration; children with bronchiolitis may already have a history of poor fluid intake when initially seen by medical personnel. Because of respiratory difficulty, the child should be kept quiet with limited stimulation and visitors. If the child is tachypneic, oral fluids present a risk of aspiration.
Cognitive Level: Analysis **Client Need:** Physiological Integrity: Physiological Adaptation **Integrated Process:** Nursing Process: Implementation **Content Area:** Child Health: Respiratory **Strategy:** The core issue of the question is knowledge that a client with bronchiolitis has a priority need for hydration. Use nursing knowledge and the process of elimination to make a selection.

19 **Answer: 3** Meconium ileus in the newborn period is often the first indication of cystic fibrosis. The other options are unrelated to this question.
Cognitive Level: Application **Client Need:** Physiological Integrity: Physiological Adaptation **Integrated Process:** Nursing Process: Assessment **Content Area:** Child Health: Respiratory **Strategy:** The core issue of the question is knowledge of the association between meconium ileus and cystic fibrosis in the neonate. Use nursing knowledge and the process of elimination to make a selection.

20 **Answer: 1** Bronchodilators open the airways and afford easier removal of secretions. Options 2 and 3 are unnecessary. Option 4 could be done after the procedure if necessary.
Cognitive Level: Analysis **Client Need:** Physiological Integrity: Physiological Adaptation **Integrated Process:** Nursing Process: Implementation **Content Area:** Child Health: Respiratory **Strategy:** The core issue of the question is knowledge of proper sequence of actions when a client undergoes chest physiotherapy. Use nursing knowledge and the process of elimination to make a selection.

21 **Answer: 4** Clear breath sounds indicate effective airway clearance and decreased mucosal swelling and obstruction. Tripod position is a clinical manifestation of a child in distress caused by epiglottitis. Pale lips and mucous membranes

may indicate hypoxia. Tachypneic and dysphonic are symptoms of the disease.

Cognitive Level: Analysis **Client Need:** Physiological Integrity: Physiological Adaptation **Integrated Process:** Nursing Process: Evaluation **Content Area:** Child Health: Respiratory **Strategy:** The core issue of this question is correctly identifying when an appropriate outcome measure has been achieved. Use nursing knowledge and the process of elimination to make a selection.

22 **Answer: 5** Tracheostomy suctioning can be stressful to the child and increases risk for hypoxia, infection, and mucosal damage. Each pass of the suction catheter should be limited to no more than 5 seconds, and the child is allowed to rest between passes with supplemental oxygen if needed.

Cognitive Level: Application **Client Need:** Physiological Integrity: Physiological Adaptation **Integrated Process:** Nursing Process: Implementation **Content Area:** Child Health: Respiratory **Strategy:** The critical issue of this question is the appropriate length of time for suctioning without impairing the respiratory status of a child. Use nursing knowledge and the process of elimination to make a selection.

23 **Answer: 3** Toddlers are naturally inquisitive and explore things with their hands and mouths. It is developmentally inappropriate to attempt to teach a toddler to stop normal hand-to-mouth activity. Small objects and foods should be kept out of reach. Teen babysitters are unrelated.

Cognitive Level: Application **Client Need:** Safe Effective Care Environment: Safety and Infection Control **Integrated Process:** Nursing Process: Implementation **Content Area:** Child Health: Respiratory **Strategy:** The core issue of the question is the best method to provide a safe environment for a toddler. Use nursing knowledge and the process of elimination to make a selection.

24 **Answer: 4** Handwashing is the most important infection control practice and decreases spread of RSV and other organisms. Option 1 is unnecessary because gloves are discarded in the trash basket. Options 2 and 3 are not timely.

Cognitive Level: Application **Client Need:** Safe Effective Care Environment: Safety and Infection Control **Integrated Process:** Nursing Process: Implementation **Content Area:** Child Health: Respiratory **Strategy:** The core issue of the question is basic principles of infection control using medical asepsis. Use nursing knowledge and the process of elimination to make a selection.

25 **Answer: 2** Swimming is recommended for children with asthma because prolonged expiration under water is beneficial. Cromolyn sodium is used prophylactically to prevent exercised-induced asthma, and immediate access to rescue inhaler is also recommended.

Cognitive Level: Analysis **Client Need:** Physiological Integrity: Physiological Adaptation **Integrated Process:** Nursing Process: Evaluation **Content Area:** Child Health: Respiratory **Strategy:** The core issue of the question is an understanding of the relationship of exercise to episodes of asthma. Use nursing knowledge and the process of elimination to make a selection.

26 **Answer: 1** Aerosol therapy such as a nebulizer is frequently used during hospitalization to administer medications. An advantage is that this route delivers medication directly to the airways.

Cognitive Level: Application **Client Need:** Physiological Integrity: Pharmacological and Parenteral Therapies **Integrated Process:** Nursing Process: Implementation **Content Area:** Child Health: Respiratory **Strategy:** The core issue of the question is an understanding of medication routes used in children, specifically those with a respiratory problem. Use nursing knowledge and the process of elimination to make a selection.

27 **Answer: 3** Chest physiotherapy and postural drainage for children with cystic fibrosis help loosen pulmonary secretions and facilitate removal from airways. It is not used for epiglottitis and bronchopulmonary dysplasia because it may increase respiratory distress in those conditions. It will not remove the foreign body.

Cognitive Level: Application **Client Need:** Physiological Integrity: Physiological Adaptation **Integrated Process:** Nursing Process: Planning **Content Area:** Child Health: Respiratory **Strategy:** The core issue of the question is the purpose of doing chest physiotherapy in a child with cystic fibrosis. Use nursing knowledge and the process of elimination to make a selection.

28 **Answer: 4** Steroids given via metered-dose inhaler on oral mucosa increase risk for yeast infection. A spacer avoids the mucus membranes and works directly on the airways.

Cognitive Level: Application **Client Need:** Safe Effective Care Environment: Safety and Infection Control **Integrated Process:** Nursing Process: Implementation **Content Area:** Child Health: Respiratory **Strategy:** The core issue of the question is the rationale for using a spacer. Use nursing knowledge and the process of elimination to make a selection.

29 **Answer: 2** Excess fluid in the alveoli is a manifestation of bacterial pneumonia. The sound produced by fluid in the airways is crackles. Retractions are asymmetrical chest wall movements which are seen in any client having respiratory difficulty. Wheezes are often typical of pneumonia caused by RSV or conditions where the air passages are narrowed, such as asthma. Apnea is a pause in respirations, which is under the control of the central nervous system.

Cognitive Level: Analysis **Client Need:** Physiological Integrity: Physiological Adaptation **Integrated Process:** Communication and Documentation **Content Area:** Child Health: Respiratory **Strategy:** The core issue of the question is the type of adventitious breath sound that is expected in pneumonia. Eliminate apnea because the focus is respiratory, not central nervous system. Eliminate retractions next because they are seen rather than heard. Choose crackles over wheezes recalling that the infectious process leads to fluid accumulation, rather than bronchoconstriction.

30 **Answer: 3** Ribavirin is an antiviral drug that causes crystallization of soft contact lenses and is associated with conjunctivitis. The other options are satisfactory items in the care of this client.

Cognitive Level: Application **Client Need:** Safe Effective Care Environment: Safety and Infection Control **Integrated Process:** Nursing Process: Planning **Content Area:** Child Health: Respiratory **Strategy:** The core issue of the question is safe administration of ribavirin to a client. Use nursing knowledge and the process of elimination to make a selection.

Key Terms to Review

alveolar ventilation p. 1004
alveoli p. 1004
atelectasis p. 1015
barrel chest p. 1013
bronchopulmonary dysplasia (BPD) p. 1025
compliance p. 1005
diffusion p. 1005
digital clubbing p. 1024
dyspnea p. 1015
epiglottis p. 1027
expiration p. 1004
foreign body aspiration p. 1029
inspiration p. 1004
laryngotracheobronchitis p. 1026
oxygen saturation p. 1007
perfusion p. 1005
pulmonary ventilation p. 1004
respiration p. 1004
sweat test p. 1024
tachypnea p. 1015
trigger p. 1015
ventilation-perfusion mismatch p. 1015

References

Ball, J., & Bindler, R. (2006). *Child health nursing: Partnering with children and families*. Upper Saddle River, NJ: Pearson Education.

Black, J., & Hawks, J. (2005). *Medical surgical nursing: Clinical management for positive outcomes* (7th ed.). St. Louis: Elsevier Science.

Corbett, J. (2004). *Laboratory tests and diagnostic procedures with nursing diagnoses* (6th ed.). Upper Saddle River, NJ: Pearson Education.

Harkreader, H., & Hogan, M. (2004). *Fundamentals of nursing: Caring and clinical judgment* (2nd ed.). St. Louis: Elsevier Science.

Hockenberry, M., Wilson, D., Winkelstein, M., & Kline, N. (2003). *Nursing care of infants and children* (7th ed.). St. Louis: Mosby.

Ignatavicius, D., & Workman, L. (2006). *Medical-surgical nursing: Critical thinking for collaborative care* (5th ed.). Philadelphia: W. B. Saunders.

Kozier, B., Erb, G., Berman, A., & Snyder, S. (2004). *Fundamentals of nursing: Concepts, process, and practice* (7th ed.). Upper Saddle River, NJ: Pearson Education.

LeMone, P., & Burke, K. (2004). *Medical surgical nursing: Critical thinking in client care* (3rd ed.). Upper Saddle River, NJ: Pearson Education.

Lewis, S., Heitkemper, M., & Dirksen, S. (2004). *Medical surgical nursing: Assessment and management of clinical problems* (6th ed.). St. Louis: Elsevier Science.

Porth, C. (2004). *Pathophysiology: Concepts of altered health states* (7th ed.). Philadelphia: Lippincott Williams & Wilkins.

Smeltzer, S., Bare, B., & Boyer, M. (2007). *Brunner & Suddarth's textbook of medical surgical nursing:* (11th ed.). Philadelphia: Lippincott Williams & Wilkins.

Smith, S., Duell, D., & Martin, B. (2004). *Clinical nursing skills: Basic to advanced skills* (6th ed.). Upper Saddle River, NJ: Pearson Education.

57 Cardiovascular Disorders

Test Yourself

Are you ready for the NCLEX-RN® or course exams? Use the practice tests on the companion CD-ROM to check.

In this chapter

Cross reference

Other chapters relevant to this content area are

Cardiovascular Medications	**Chapter 38**
Common Laboratory Tests	**Chapter 47**
Common Diagnostic Tests and Procedures	**Chapter 48**

I. OVERVIEW OF ANATOMY AND PHYSIOLOGY OF THE CARDIOVASCULAR SYSTEM

A. Structures of heart

1. Hollow muscular organ enclosed in a protective sac, divided into 4 chambers—2 atria and 2 ventricles—divided by septum into right and left sides
2. Heart wall has three layers: *epicardium,* fibrous outside protective layer; *myocardium,* middle layer of specialized cardiac muscle; *endocardium,* endothelial lining of chambers
3. *Pericardium:* protective sac encasing heart
4. Valves of heart
   - **a.** Atrioventricular (AV) valves (tricuspid on right and mitral on left) separate atria from ventricles; control blood flow between atria and ventricles
   - **b.** Semilunar valves (pulmonic on right and aortic on left) separate ventricles from great vessels and control blood flow from heart
   - **c.** S_1, first heart sound ("lub"), is heard when AV valves close during systole
   - **d.** S_2, second heart sound ("dub"), is heard when semilunar valves close during diastole
5. Coronary circulation
   - **a.** Left anterior descending (LAD) artery supplies anterior left ventricle, anterior ventricular septum, and left ventricle apex; circumflex artery supplies left atrium and lateral and posterior left ventricle
   - **b.** Right coronary artery (RCA): supplies right atrium and ventricle, inferior left ventricle, posterior septal wall, and sinoatrial (SA) and atrioventricular (AV) nodes

B. Functions of heart

1. Circulation: right side circulates deoxygenated blood to lungs; left side pumps oxygenated blood throughout body to perfuse tissues
2. Coronary arteries branch off aorta to supply oxygenated blood to heart
3. Cardiac conduction system transmits electrical impulses, stimulates depolarization and cardiac muscle contraction; cells have electrophysiologic properties: *automaticity* (ability to initiate an electrical impulse), *excitability* (ability of a cell to respond to a stimulus), and *conductivity* (ability to transmit impulses from one cell to another)
   - **a.** Sinoatrial (SA) node: natural pacemaker; generates heart rate normally at 60 to 100 beats per minute (bpm)
   - **b.** Internodal pathways: carry impulse from SA node to AV node; depolarization results in myocardial contraction of both atria
   - **c.** AV node: slows electrical impulse; allows atria to fully empty before initiating depolarization of ventricles; when SA node is not functioning, AV node can initiate an impulse at rate of 40 to 60 bpm
   - **d.** Bundle of His: short branch of conductive cells connecting AV node to bundle branches at intraventricular septum
   - **e.** Bundle branches: right (RBB) and left (LBB) split off on either side of intraventricular septum; carry impulses to Purkinje fibers
   - **f.** Purkinje fibers: terminal branches of conduction system; initiate rapid depolarization wave throughout myocardium causing ventricular contraction; when SA and AV nodes fail, can initiate impulses at rate of 20 to 40 bpm
4. Cardiac cycle: one complete heartbeat; includes two parts—systole (ventricular contraction) and diastole (relaxation and ventricular refilling)
5. **Cardiac output (CO):** volume of blood in liters ejected by heart each minute; indicator of pumping function of heart; normal adult CO is 4 to 8 L/min

$$CO = HR \times SV$$

   - **a.** Heart rate (HR): number of complete cardiac cycles per minute
   - **b.** **Stroke volume (SV):** volume of blood ejected from left ventricle with each cardiac cycle; SV and ultimately CO are influenced by preload, afterload, and contractility

c. **Preload:** degree of myocardial fiber stretch at end of ventricular diastole; influenced by ventricular filling volume and myocardial compliance
d. **Afterload:** resistance that ventricles must overcome to eject blood into systemic circulation; directly related to arterial blood pressure (BP)
e. **Contractility:** strength of contraction regardless of preload; decreased by hypoxia and some drugs (e.g., beta-blockers and calcium channel blockers); increased by drugs (e.g., digoxin and dopamine)

6. Autonomic nervous system: responds to chemoreceptors, baroreceptors, and stretch receptors in body
   a. Sympathetic: produces norepinephrine; results in increased HR, myocardial contractility, peripheral vasoconstriction, and arterial BP
   b. Parasympathetic: produces acetylcholine, results in decreased HR and contractility

C. Fetal circulation

1. Ductus venosus
   a. Umbilical vein carries oxygenated blood from placenta to fetus; blood bypasses liver through ductus venosus
   b. At birth when umbilical cord is clamped and cut, blood flow from maternal circulation ceases and ductus venosus closes; blood flows into liver
2. Foramen ovale
   a. Oxygenated systemic blood enters right atrium; flows from right to left atria through foramen ovale
   b. Blood bypasses lungs, which are nonfunctional
   c. Blood flows from left atria to left ventricle and out to aorta
   d. Foramen ovale closes after birth with change in pressure in cardiac chambers
3. Ductus arteriosus
   a. A fistula that allows blood flowing through pulmonary artery to enter aorta; this is normal and desired in fetus
   b. Closes after birth with first few breaths so neonate's heart can circulate oxygenated blood to body

D. Structure and function of blood vessels

1. Distribute blood to body tissues
2. Walls of an artery or vein consist of three layers: tunica intima, tunica media, and tunica adventitia; amount of pressure in vessel determines thickness of walls and amount of connective tissue and smooth muscle
3. Arterial system consists of high-pressure vessels, beginning with aorta, then arteries, then arterioles, and ending with capillaries; delivers blood to various tissues for nourishment and contributes to tissue temperature regulation
4. Venous system begins after capillaries and consists of venules and veins (large-diameter, thin-walled vessels) under much less pressure; some veins, most commonly in legs, contain valves to regulate one-way flow; returns blood from capillaries to right atrium and acts as a reservoir for blood volume

E. Regulation of BP

1. Autonomic nervous system
2. Baroreceptors in aortic arch and carotid sinus; chemoreceptors
3. Antidiuretic hormone (ADH)
4. Renin-angiotensin-aldosterone system; angiotenisn I is converted to angiotensin II, a powerful vasoconstrictor
5. Others: temperature (cold results in vasoconstriction, heat results in **vasodilation**), substances such as nicotine (vasoconstrict) and alcohol (vasodilate), diet (sodium and fat intake), and factors such as age, gender, ethnicity, weight, physical health, and emotional state

II. DIAGNOSTIC TESTS AND ASSESSMENTS

A. Laboratory tests (see also chapter 47)

! 1. Serum cardiac enzymes: myoglobin, troponins, creatinine kinase (CK), and lactic dehydrogenase (LDH); increase with heart damage, such as myocardial

infarction (MI); serial testing over days detects trend and determines peak time and extent of injury

2. Serum drug levels:
   - a. Digoxin: therapeutic range is 0.5 to 2.0 ng/mL; early signs of toxicity include nausea, vomiting, anorexia; abdominal pain, bradycardia, other dysrhythmias, and visual disturbances (yellow to green halos) may occur
   - b. Quinidine: therapeutic range is 2 to 6 mcg/mL; signs of toxicity include tinnitus, hearing loss, visual disturbances, nausea, dizziness, widened QRS, ventricular dysrhythmias
3. Electrolytes: normal levels of sodium (135–145 mEg/L), potassium (3.5–5.1 mEg/L), calcium (8.6–10.2 mg/dL), and magnesium (1.8–2.6 mg/dL) are essential for proper cardiac function; cardiac disorders and medications can alter electrolyte balance; see Chapter 54 for detailed information
   - a. Potassium (K^+): hypokalemia such as with diuretic therapy increases risk of digitalis toxicity, ventricular dysrhythmias; hyperkalemia from renal disease or excess potassium supplements can lead to ventricular dysrhythmias and asystole;
   - b. Sodium (Na^+): hyponatremia with long-term diuretic therapy; hypernatremia could occur with excess saline IV infusion
   - c. Calcium: cardiac effects of hypocalcemia include ventricular dysrhythmias, prolonged QT interval and cardiac arrest; hypercalcemia shortens QT interval and causes AV block, digitalis hypersensitivity, and cardiac arrest
   - d. Magnesium: cardiac effects of decreased magnesium include ventricular tachycardia and fibrillation, while increased magnesium causes bradycardia, hypotension, prolonged PR and QRS intervals
4. Serum lipid profile: a measurement used to determine risk of developing atherosclerosis (see also Chapter 47)
   - a. Includes total serum cholesterol (< 200 mg/dL) triglycerides (10–190 mg/dL) and lipoproteins
   - b. High-density lipoproteins (HDL): transport cholesterol to liver for excretion ("good" cholesterol); normal is 30 to 70 mg/dL
   - c. Low-density lipoproteins (LDL): transport cholesterol to peripheral tissues ("bad" cholesterol) and increases risk of heart disease; normal is under 130 mg/dL

B. Electrocardiography (see also Chapter 48)

1. A graphic recording of electrical activity of heart; diagnoses myocardial ischemia, injury, and necrosis areas of cell death (MI); hypertrophy, electrolyte imbalance and effects of antidysrhythmic drugs
2. Resting electrocardiogram (ECG): represents a single recorded picture of electrical activity of heart
3. Holter monitoring: continuous ambulatory ECG monitoring over time (usual 24 hours) with small, timed, portable ECG recording device
4. Stress test: continuous multilead ECG monitoring during controlled and supervised exercise, usually on treadmill

C. Echocardiography: an ultrasound that evaluates structure and function of heart chambers and valves

D. Phonocardiography: a graphic recording of heart sounds with simultaneous ECG; is not painful

E. Coronary angiography and arteriography (see also Chapter 48); is an invasive procedure during which physician injects dye into coronary arteries and immediately takes a series of x-ray films to assess structure of the arteries

F. Cardiac catheterization:

1. Insertion of a catheter into heart and surrounding vessels to obtain diagnostic information about heart structure and function (see also Chapter 48)
2. Client preparation, nursing care during procedure, and postprocedure nursing care are summarized in Box 57–1

G. Radionuclide tests

1. Safe, nonpainful methods of evaluating left ventricular muscle function and coronary artery blood distribution; radionuclide contrast is injected via

Box 57-1

Care of the Client Undergoing Cardiac Catheterization

Client Preparation

- Obtain written consent.
- Assess client history of allergies to iodine, dye, or shellfish.
- Explain that client will be awake and may experience various sensations during the procedure, including flushing sensation as dye is injected or fluttering feeling as the catheter passes through the heart.
- Explain the postprocedure routine (see Postprocedure Nursing Care).
- Prepare insertion site by shaving and cleansing with antiseptic.
- Nothing by mouth (NPO) except sips of water with cardiac medications as indicated for 6 to 8 hours.
- Initiate IV site with fluids as ordered.
- Administer preprocedure medications as ordered.

Nursing Care During Procedure

- Procedure is performed in catheterization laboratory by cardiologist; nurse monitors ECG and vital signs continuously, administers conscious sedation as ordered, and provides emotional support.

Postprocedure Nursing Care

- Maintain client on bedrest, often for 4 to 6 hours.
- Keep affected extremity straight; after 1 to 2 hours, head may be elevated up to 30 degrees for those who had the femoral artery as the insertion site.
- Maintain pressure dressing at insertion site.
- Monitor BP, heart rate, distal pulses, color and temperature of extremity, and assess for signs of bleeding at the site (with leg site, check under client for bleeding) according to agency schedule, (routinely q 15 minutes for 1 hour, q 30 minutes for 2 hours, q hour for 4 hours, or q 8 hours for associated procedure of percutaneous transluminal coronary angioplasty [PTCA]).
- Report signs of chest pain, dysrhythmias, bleeding, hematoma formation, or other changes; significant changes in vital signs, pulses, color or temperature of extremity should be reported immediately to the physician. Bleeding may be reported by the client as a feeling of warmth in the insertion area.
- If bleeding occurs, restore manual pressure to site.
- Maintain IV and encourage oral fluids as ordered to eliminate dye as soon as possible; the contrast medium can be nephrotoxic.
- Monitor I & O to determine whether client is becoming dehydrated from increased urine output because of dye excretion.

venipuncture; encourage client to drink fluids postprocedure to facilitate excretion of contrast; assess venipuncture site for bleeding or hematoma; may be used in conjunction with stress testing

2. Allows visualization of ventricles through several cardiac cycles; calculate **ejection fraction** (EF), portion of blood ejected during systole compared to total ventricular filling volume, (normal EF = 55 to 65%)
3. MUGA (gated pool imaging or multigated acquisition) scan
4. Thallium imaging: used to assess myocardial **ischemia** (decreased supply of oxygenated blood) during stress testing
5. PET (positron emission tomography) scan: evaluates cardiac metabolism and assesses tissue perfusion

H. Electron beam computed tomtography (EBCT): easily detects calcium deposits, which correlate with heart disease but also occur in greater frequency with advancing age; is a controversial "screening" tool that may or may not be useful for any given individual

I. Hemodynamic monitoring

1. Measurement of pressures of heart and calculation of hemodynamic parameters
2. Central venous pressure (CVP) monitoring: monitors fluid volume status in those who are not candidates for more invasive pulmonary artery pressure monitoring
   a. Long catheter is inserted with tip lying in superior vena cava at juncture with right atrium
   b. Measures pressure that indicates right heart filling pressure; does not measure left heart pressures
   c. Normal CVP is 2 to 8 cm H_2O or 2 to 6 mmHg; decreased CVP indicates hypovolemia; increased CVP indicates hypervolemia or right heart failure
3. Pulmonary artery pressure (PAP) monitoring: appropriate for critically ill clients requiring more accurate assessments of left heart pressures (cardiac surgery, shock, serious MI)
   a. Pulmonary artery (Swan-Ganz) catheter has tip in pulmonary artery
   b. Pressure measurement obtained after catheter tip is wedged in small pulmonary artery (called pulmonary capillary wedge pressure, or PCWP); is a good indicator of left ventricular end diastolic pressure (LVEDP)
   c. Allows calculation of actual cardiac output and other hemodynamic parameters at frequent intervals in critically ill clients
4. Nursing responsibilities in hemodynamic monitoring: position transducer at level of right atrium (left midaxillary line, fourth intercostal space—phlebostatic axis); level CVP or pulmonary artery catheter (Swan-Ganz) transducer to this point each shift and before each measurement; maintain patency of catheter with a constant small amount of fluid delivered under pressure

J. Doppler ultrasound: a noninvasive test that measures velocity of blood flow through a vessel and emits an audible signal; can determine blood flow when arterial palpation is difficult or impossible because of occlusive disease; a palpable pulse and a Doppler pulse are not equivalent, so document clearly

K. Plethysmography: records volume changes in an extremity associated with cardiac contractions or in response to pneumatic venous occlusion; can detect and quantify vascular disease by changes in pulse contour, BP, or arterial and venous blood flow

L. Digital intravenous angiography: utilizing computer technology, visualizes blood vessels after IV injection of contrast medium; allows for small peripheral venous injections of contrast medium instead of large doses used with arterial cannulation

M. Venography: injection of radiopaque dye into veins, with serial x-rays taken to detect deep-vein thrombosis and incompetent valves

N. Angiography: injection of radiopaque dye into arteries to detect plaques, occlusions, injury, and so on; similar to care for postcardiac catheterization

O. Ankle-brachial index: most commonly used parameter for overall evaluation of extremity status; ankle pressure normally is same or higher than brachial systolic pressure

P. Computed tomography: allows for visualization of arterial wall and its structures; used to diagnose abdominal aortic aneurysm (AAA) and postoperative vascular complications such as graft occlusion and hemorrhage

Q. Magnetic resonance imaging (MRI): uses magnetic fields rather than radiation; used with angiography to detect abnormalities, especially in clients who cannot have dye injected

III. COMMON NURSING TECHNIQUES AND PROCEDURES

A. Dysrhythmia monitoring

1. Continuous ECG monitoring in one lead with portable telemetry unit; indicated for high-risk clients undergoing surgery, those with cardiac disease, and those undergoing procedures or receiving medications affecting heart
2. Lead placements (ECG continuous monitors have 3 leads or 5 leads)
   a. Placement of leads with 3-lead monitor are below right clavicle (right arm), below left clavicle (left arm), and at lowest rib, left midclavicular line (left leg)

b. Placement of leads with 5-lead monitor are same as 3-lead with fourth lead placed at lowest rib, right midclavicular line (right leg) and fifth lead on one of six chest leads (V leads) sites

! 3. Preparation of client: explain procedure and reassure client that he or she will not receive electrical impulses or shocks; identify proper placement, cleanse skin with soap and water, shave hairy areas, use alcohol or skin prep according to agency policy, dry with cloth or gauze, and apply fresh electrodes

! 4. Interpretations of ECG patterns originating in the sinus node (see Table 57–1 ■)
   a. Sinus rhythm is normal
   b. Sinus tachycardia (normal ECG complex with rate greater than 100)
   c. Sinus bradycardia (normal ECG complex with rate lower than 60)
   d. Sinus arrhythmia (normal ECG complex with irregular pattern)
   ! e. Nursing and therapeutic interventions: with sinus arrest, tachycardia, or bradycardia, assess for signs of inadequate cardiac output and tissue perfusion, including changes in blood pressure, activity tolerance, and level of consciousness (LOC); identify and treat cause of sinus tachycardia; atropine and possible pacemaker indicated for symptomatic or extreme low rates (<50)

5. ECG patterns originating in the atria (refer again to Table 57–1)
   a. Premature atrial contraction (PAC)
   b. Atrial tachycardia
   c. Atrial flutter
   ! d. Atrial fibrillation
   ! e. Nursing and therapeutic interventions: carotid massage, synchronized cardioversion, antidysrhythmia medications including beta-blockers, calcium channel blockers, and digoxin; anticoagulant therapy to reduce the risk of thrombus

6. ECG patterns originating from the AV node (refer again to Table 57–1)
   a. Junctional (nodal) tachycardia
   b. First-degree heart block
   c. Second-degree heart block, Mobitz type I (Wenckebach)
   d. Second-degree heart block, Mobitz type II
   e. Third-degree (complete) heart block
   ! f. Nursing and therapeutic interventions include monitoring and observation; atropine, isoproterenol or pacemakers for symptomatic heart block (external or transthoracic, temporary, or permanent)

7. ECG patterns originating from the ventricles (refer again to Table 57–1)
   ! a. Premature ventricular contraction (PVC)
   b. Ventricular tachycardia (VT)
   c. Ventricular fibrillation (VF)
   ! d. Nursing and therapeutic interventions: for PVCs monitor for signs of decreased cardiac output; instruct client to avoid caffeine and nicotine; with VT, assess immediately to determine LOC and if client has stable BP and pulse; if stable, treat with lidocaine, procainamide, and finally defibrillation; if client becomes unconscious or unstable or has pulseless VT or VF, immediate defibrillation is required

B. Percutaneous transluminal coronary angioplasty (PTCA)

1. Increases blood flow to coronary arteries by inserting a catheter with a balloon tip into narrowed segment of affected artery, inflating balloon to expand vessel lumen and removing catheter; may also include insertion of an expandable intracoronary stent, which is inserted over balloon and remains in place after balloon is removed
2. Client preparation, nursing care during procedure, and postprocedure nursing care are as outlined previously in Box 57–1
3. Administer anticoagulants as ordered to prevent thrombus formation, and monitor coagulation studies as indicated
! 4. Because of anticoagulants used during procedure, site may have a vice-type pressure device requiring a longer period of hourly site checks; monitor closely for any changes in ECG or signs of chest pain (even minor changes may indicate ischemia); obtain a 12-lead ECG and notify physician of any complications

Table 57-1 Selected Cardiac Rhythms and Dysrhythmias

Rhythm/ECG Appearance	ECG Characteristics	Management
Supraventricular Rhythms		
Normal sinus rhythm (NSR) 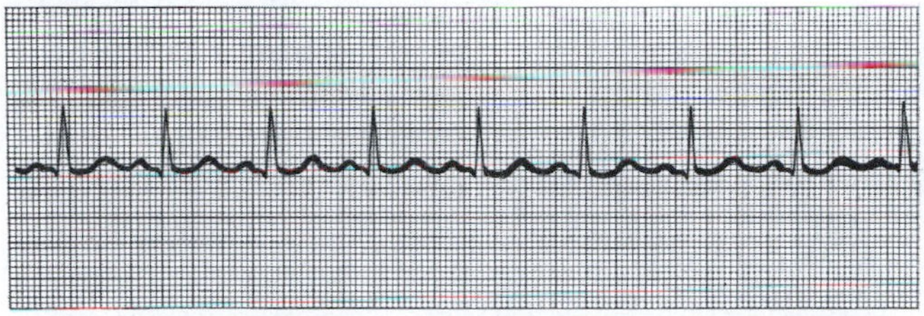	Rate: 60–100 bpm Rhythm: regular P:QRS ratio is 1:1 PR interval: 0.12–0.20 sec QRS complex: 0.06–0.10 sec	None; normal heart rhythm
Sinus arrhythmia 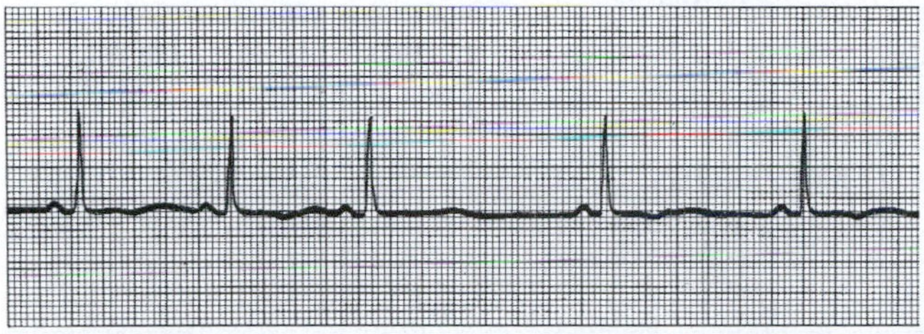	Rate: 60–100 bpm Rhythm: irregular, varying with respirations P:QRS ratio is 1:1 PR interval: 0.12–0.20 sec QRS complex: 0.06–0.10 sec	Generally none; considered a normal rhythm in the very young and very old
Sinus tachycardia 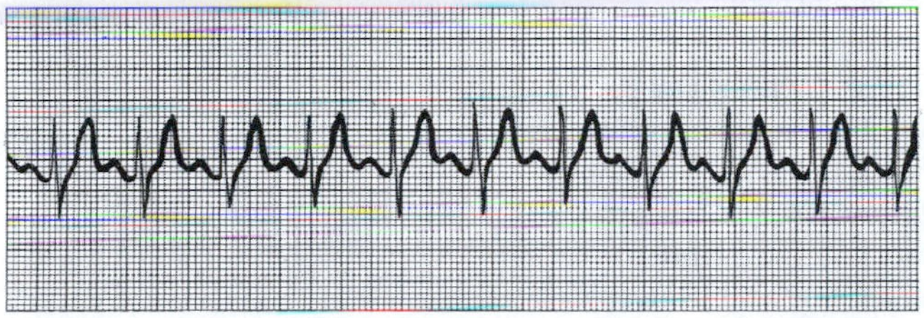	Rate: 101 to 150 bpm Rhythm: regular P:QRS ratio is 1:1 (with very fast rates, P wave may be hidden in preceding T wave) PR interval: 0.12–0.20 sec QRS complex: 0.06–0.10 sec	Treat only if client is experiencing symptoms or is at risk for myocardial damage; treat underlying cause (e.g., hypovolemia, fever, pain); beta-blockers or verapamil may be used
Sinus bradycardia 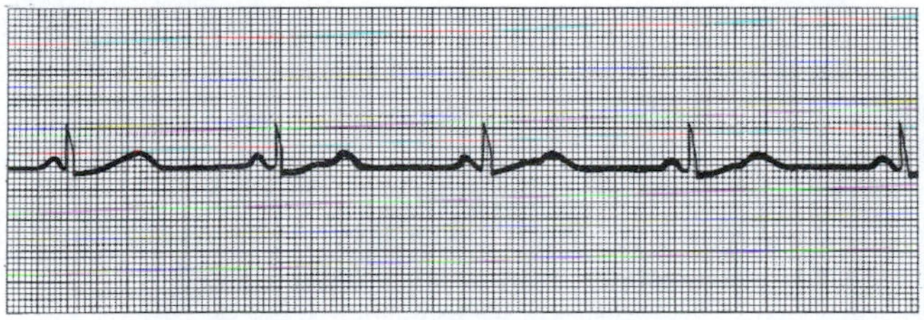	Rate: less than 60 bpm Rhythm: regular P:QRS ratio is 1:1 PR interval: 0.12–0.20 sec QRS complex: 0.06–0.10 sec	Treat only if client is experiencing symptoms; intravenous atropine and/or pacemaker therapy may be used
Premature atrial contractions (PAC) 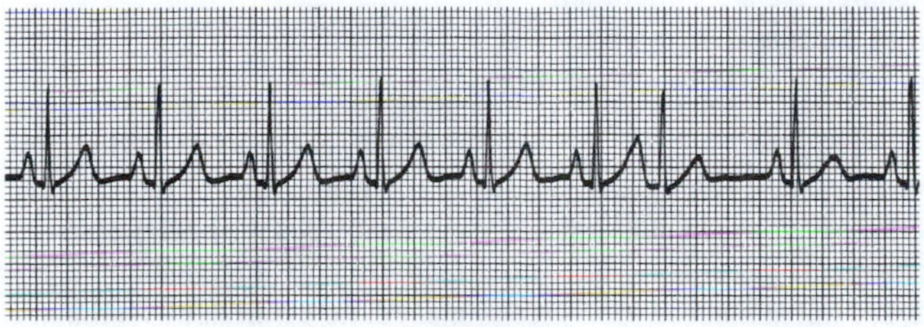	Rate: variable Rhythm: irregular, with normal rhythm interrrupted by early beats arising in the atria P:QRS ratio is 1:1 PR interval: 0.12–0.20 sec but may be prolonged QRS complex: 0.6–0.10 sec	Usually requires no treatment; advise client to reduce alcohol and caffeine intake, to reduce stress, and to stop smoking
Paroxysmal supraventricular tachycardia (PSVT) 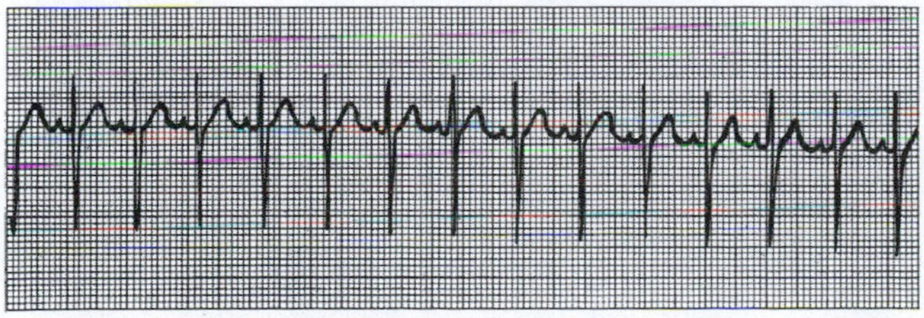	Rate: 100–280 bpm (usually 150–200 bpm) Rhythm: regular P:QRS ratio: P waves often not identifiable PR interval: not measured QRS complex: 0.06–0.10 sec	Treat if client is experiencing symptoms; treatment may include vagal maneuvers (Valsalva, carotid sinus massage); oxygen therapy; adenosine, verapamil, procainamide, propranolol, and esmolol; and synchronized cardioversion

Table 57-1 (continued)

Rhythm/ECG Appearance	ECG Characteristics	Management
Atrial flutter 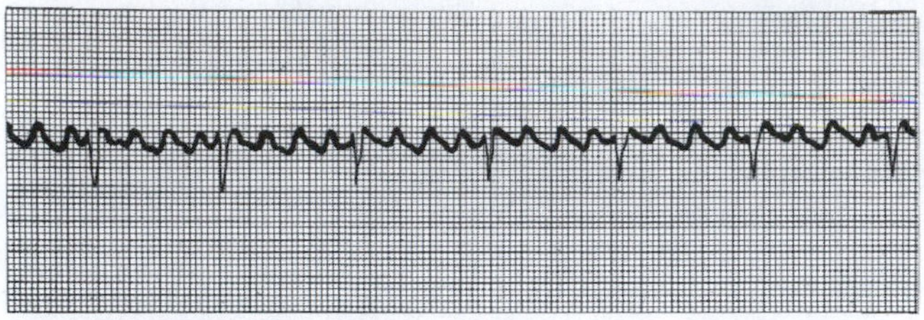	Rate: atrial 240–360 bpm; ventricular rate depends on degree of AV block and usually is less than 150 bpm Rhythm: atrial regular, ventricular usually regular P:QRS ratio may be 2:1, 4:1, 6:1 or may be variable PR interval: not measured QRS complex: 0.06–0.10 sec	Synchronized cardioversion; medications to slow ventricular response, such as beta-blocker or calcium channel blocker (verapamil), followed by quinidine, procainamide, flecainide, or amiodarone
Atrial fibrillation 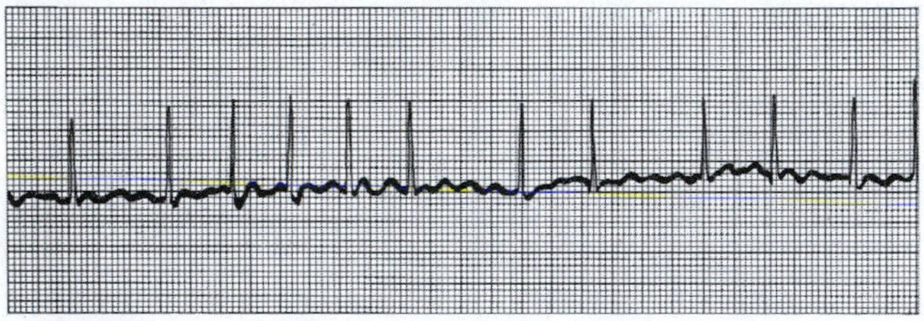	Rate: atrial 300–600 bpm (too rapid to count); ventricular 100–180 bpm in untreated clients Rhythm: irregularly irregular P:QRS ratio is variable PR interval: not measured QRS complex: 0.06–0.10 sec	Synchronized cardioversion; medications to reduce ventricular response rate: verapamil, propranolol, digoxin, anticoagulant therapy to reduce risk of clot formation and stroke
Junctional escape rhythm 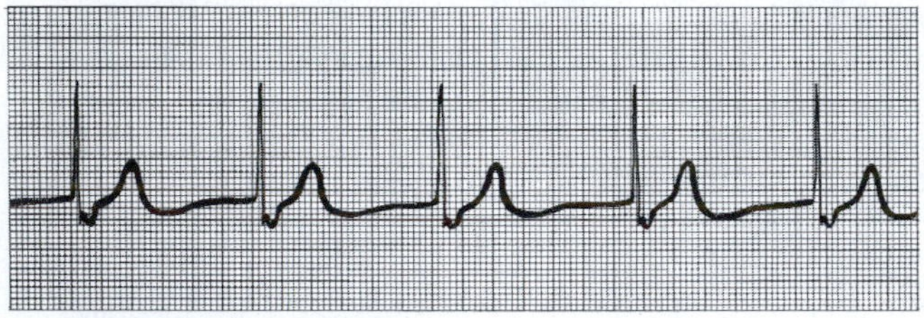	Rate: 40–60 bpm; junctional tachycardia 60–140 bpm Rhythm: regular P:QRS ratio: P waves may be absent, inverted, and immediately preceding or succeeding QRS complex or hidden in QRS complex PR interval: less than 0.10 sec if P wave is prior to QRS complex QRS complex: 0.06–0.10 sec	Treat cause if client is experiencing symptoms
Ventricular Rhythms		
Premature ventricular contractions (PVC) 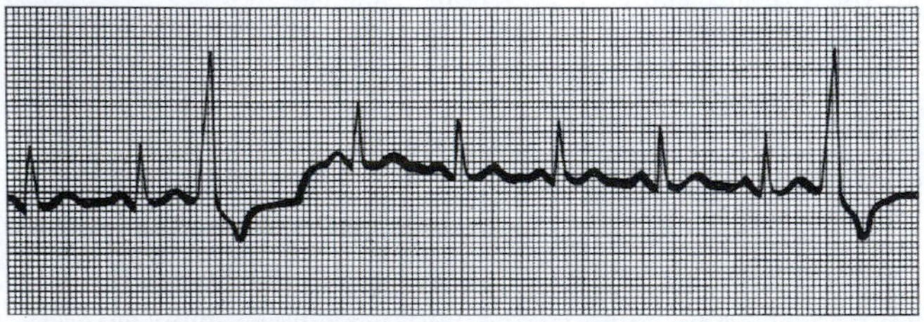	Rate: variable Rhythm: irregular, with PVC interrupting underlying rhythm and followed by a compensatory pause P:QRS ratio: no P wave noted before PVC PR interval: absent with PVC QRS complex: wide (greater than 0.12 sec), bizarre in appearance; differs from normal QRS complex	Treat if client is experiencing symptoms; advise against stimulant use (caffeine, nicotine); drug therapy includes intravenous lidocaine, procainamide, quinidine, propranolol, phenytoin, bretylium
Ventricular tachycardia (VT or V tach) 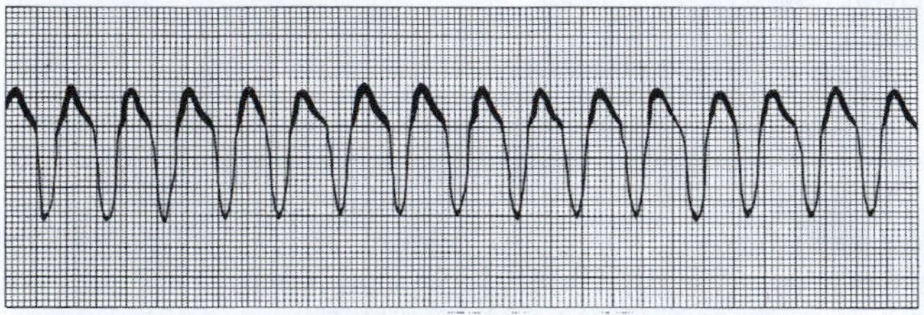	Rate: 100–250 bpm Rhythm: regular P:QRS ratio: P waves usually not identifiable PR interval: not measured QRS complex: 0.12 sec or greater; bizarre shape	Treat if VT is sustained or if client is experiencing symptoms; treatment includes intravenous procainamide or lidocaine and/or immediate defibrillation if the client is unconscious or unstable

Table 57–1 (continued)

Rhythm/ECG Appearance	ECG Characteristics	Management
Ventricular fibrillation (VF or V fib) 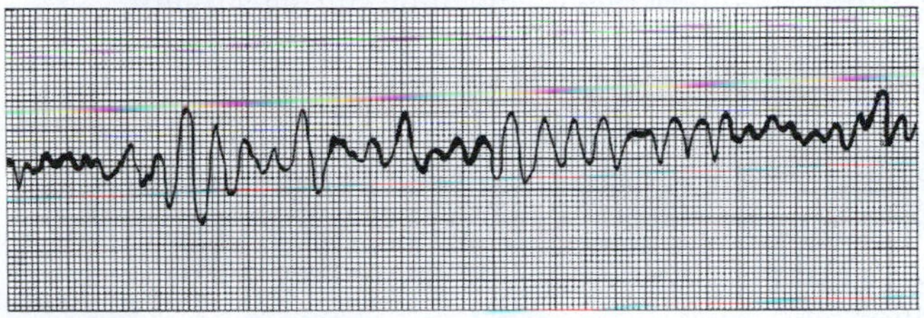	Rate: too rapid to count Rhythm: grossly irregular P:QRS ratio: no identifiable P waves PR interval: none QRS: bizarre, varying in shape and direction	Immediate defibrillation
Atrioventricular Conduction Blocks *First-degree AV block* 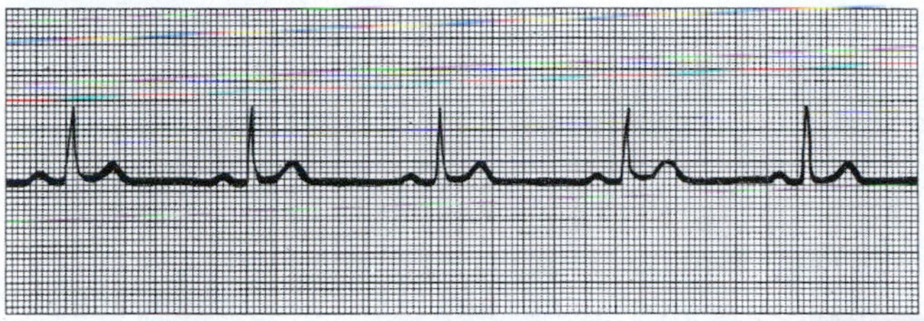	Rate: usually 60–100 bpm Rhythm: regular P:QRS ratio is: 1:1 PR interval: greater than 0.20 sec QRS complex: 0.06–0.10 sec	None required
Second-degree AV block, type I (Mobitz I, Wenckebach) 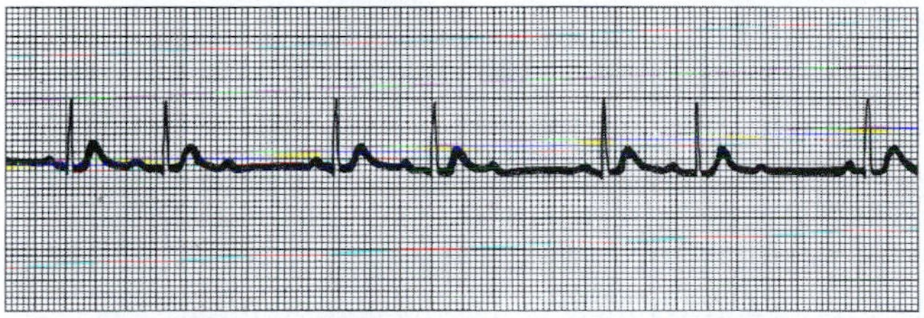	Rate: 60–100 bpm Rhythm: atrial regular; ventricular irregular P:QRS ratio is: 1:1 until P wave blocked with no subsequent QRS complex PR interval: progressively lengthens in a regular pattern QRS complex: 0.06–0.10 sec; sudden absence of QRS complex	Monitoring and observation; atropine or isoproterenol if client is experiencing symptoms
Second-degree AV block, type II (Mobitz II) 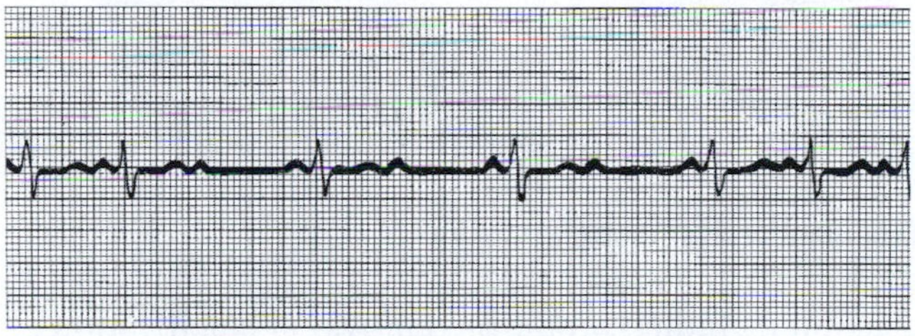	Rate: atrial 60–100 bpm; ventricular less than 60 bpm Rhythm: atrial regular; ventricular irregular P:QRS ratio is: typically 2:1, may vary PR interval: constant PR interval for each conducted QRS complex QRS complex: 0.06–0.10 sec	Atropine or isoproterenol; pacemaker therapy
Third-degree AV block (complete heart block) 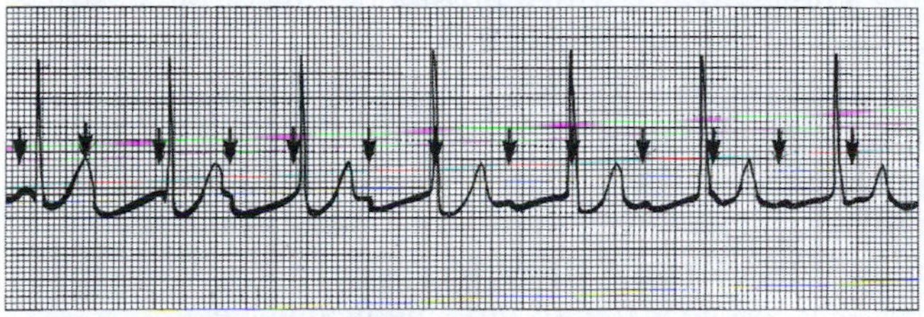	Rate: atrial 60–100 bpm; ventricular 15–60 bpm Rhythm: atrial regular; ventricular regular P:QRS ratio: no relationship between P waves and QRS complexes; independent rhythms PR interval: not measured QRS complex: 0.06–0.10 sec if junctional escape rhythm; 0.12 sec if ventricular escape rhythm	Immediate pacemaker therapy

Source: LeMone P., Burke, K. (2004). *Medical surgical nursing: Critical thinking for collaborative care* (3rd ed.). Upper Saddle River, NJ: Prentice Hall; pp. 845–847, Table 29-6.

C. Coronary artery bypass grafting (CABG)

1. Surgery is indicated for more than 50% occlusion in left main coronary artery or severe blockage in several vessels; diseased arteries are "bypassed" with saphenous veins, mammary arteries, or less frequently, artificial grafts; indicated for myocardial ischemia that cannot be managed by medical treatment; client is typically maintained on cardiopulmonary bypass machine during surgery
2. Client preparation
   a. Ensure that all consents are signed
   b. Perform routine preoperative teaching, including turning, coughing, and deep breathing (vigorous coughing is discouraged because increased intrathoracic pressure may cause instability in sternal area), use of incentive spirometer (IS) to prevent respiratory complications, and leg exercises to prevent emboli formation
   c. Explain postoperative course, including respiratory support on ventilator with an endotracheal tube; suctioning; surgical incisions, chest tubes, multiple IV lines, tubes, drains, and monitors with alarms and noises; pain management, communication techniques, visiting policies, and expected length of hospitalization and recovery period

!

3. Postprocedure nursing care: immediate postoperative care given in cardiac critical care units; within 1 to 2 days client is transferred to a step-down/telemetry unit where care includes the following:
   a. Monitor client for signs of decreased cardiac output, continuous ECG monitoring; I & O; full assessments with lung sounds and heart sounds at regular intervals (every 4 hours initially, then at least every 8 hours)
   b. Assess and treat postoperative pain
   c. Monitor indicators of cardiac output with client's increasing activity
   d. Monitor respiratory status and encouraging deep-breathing and IS
   e. Monitor surgical wounds and treat as needed
   f. Instruct client about new medication regime, activity plan for home, cardiac rehabilitation, resumption of sexual activity (usually allowed by surgeon when client can walk up 2 full flights of stairs without shortness of breath [SOB] or chest pain; client should be rested, not after a heavy meal or alcohol consumption)
   g. Instruct client about symptoms to report to physician after discharge including chest pain, SOB, decrease in activity tolerance, fever, redness, swelling or drainage from surgical incisions
   h. Instruct client that clinical depression occurs in about 20% of clients up to 6 months after cardiac surgery, and client should notify physician because antidepressants have been shown to be effective; include family in teaching and planning for discharge

D. Valvular surgery repair or replacement of dysfunctional valve

1. Repair
   a. *Valvuloplasty:* reconstruction including repair or removal of calcification or vegetation
   b. *Annuloplasty:* narrowing a dilated valve with a prosthetic ring or purse-string sutures, or enlarging a stenosed valve with a balloon
   c. Repair is the preferred option because of lower incidence of postsurgical complications and mortality than occur in valve replacement
2. Replacement: valve is completely replaced
   a. Mechanical valves: more durable and longer lasting; subject to mechanical failure; require lifetime anticoagulation with warfarin (Coumadin), and infections are harder to treat; an example is the St. Jude medical valve
   b. Tissue valves: may deteriorate; frequent replacement is required; not associated with thrombus formation, no long-term anticoagulation; infections are easier to treat

!

3. Client preparation and postprocedure nursing care: (same as for cardiac surgery, discussed previously); provide instructions for preventing infection, including precautions such as prophylactic antibiotic therapy prior to invasive procedures (e.g., dental care), gentle oral care to prevent bacteria from entering the blood-

stream through the gums; provide instruction on management of anticoagulation therapy if applicable

E. Pacemakers

1. Permanent pacemakers are inserted to treat permanent cardiac conduction defects; generator box is implanted under chest wall and wires are threaded into blood vessel through right atrium for implantation in right ventricle (commonly)
2. Client preparation: obtain informed written consent; bedrest is required for 24 hours and activity is gradually increased to prevent dislodging leads; daily one-minute pulse count will be required (should be equal to or higher than preset rate)
3. ! Postprocedure nursing care
   a. Monitor ECG continuously to ensure that pacing impulses are being captured (e.g., pacer spike is followed by ECG complex such as QRS) and that client heartbeats are sensed (pacemaker does not fire when client rhythm is present)
   b. Monitor pacemaker site for signs of bleeding or infection
   c. Dressing should remain clean and dry with no temperature elevation, swelling, redness, or tenderness
   d. Minimize right arm and shoulder movements immediately postprocedure to ensure that pacemaker wire remains in contact with ventricular wall
4. Temporary pacemakers are utilized for heart blocks that occur suddenly or may occur as a temporary reponse to cardiac surgery or myocardial infarction as examples
   a. May be placed transvenously with external pacemaker box used to set milliamps of energy and rate
   b. Monitor cardiac rhythm for lack of capture and watch for site infection as risks
   c. May also utilize external pacemaker as initial measure, which is noninvasive and easy to use but may be uncomfortable to client

F. Blood pressure (BP) measurement

1. Is primarily a function of cardiac output and systemic vascular resistance; arterial blood pressure equals cardiac output multiplied by systemic vascular resistance
2. Have client sit with arm bared, supported, and at heart level; ensure no smoking or caffeine intake 30 minutes prior
3. Take BP in both arms initially using appropriate-sized cuff (rubber bladder should at least encircle the arm by 80%)
4. If averaging two or more readings, separate measurements by at least 2 minutes
5. If both client's arms are inaccessible (from combination of IV lines, dialysis shunt, mastectomy, burns, etc.), obtain readings from thigh or calf, auscultating popliteal or posterior tibial arteries, respectively

IV. MYOCARDIAL INFARCTION

A. Overview

1. Myocardial injury from sudden restriction of blood supply to a portion of heart; is a life-threatening condition
2. Main cause is **coronary artery disease** (CAD), build up of atherosclerotic plaque in coronary arteries that restricts blood flow to heart
   a. Nonmodifiable risk factors include age, gender, family history, diabetes, and ethnic background
   b. ! Modifiable risk factors include smoking, obesity, stress, elevated cholesterol, and hypertension
3. Coronary artery blood flow is blocked by atherosclerotic narrowing, thrombus formation, or (less frequently) persistent vasospasm; myocardium supplied by arteries is deprived of O_2; persistent ischemia may rapidly lead to tissue death
4. ! **Angina pectoris** is chest pain resulting from this restricted blood flow; it may occur in the following forms:
   a. *Stable angina,* a predictable response to increased activity
   b. *Unstable angina* with unpredictability (at rest) and increasing severity
   c. *Prinzmetal angina* caused by arterial spasm often awaking client from sleep
5. Angina pectoris may change in character and may progress to MI

! **B. Nursing assessment**

1. Chest pain unrelieved by nitroglycerine or rest often indicates MI; may be crushing substernal pain; may radiate to jaw, neck, back, or left arm (some clients, especially diabetic clients and women, report no pain)
2. Other symptoms may include diaphoresis, nausea, fear, anxiety, dyspnea, dysrhythmias
3. ECG (12-lead): ST elevation, accompanied by T-wave inversion; and later, new pathologic Q wave
4. Lab findings: elevated troponins (early or late diagnosis); elevated CK-MB isoenzymes over 5% (early diagnosis); or elevated LDH with "flipped" isoenzymes (late diagnosis)

! **C. Therapeutic management**

1. Assess pain status frequently with pain scale or other appropriate tool to estimate changes in pain level; pain is usually first presenting sign of new or extended MI
2. Assess hemodynamic status including BP, HR, LOC, skin color, and temperature frequently (every 5 minutes during episodes of pain; every 15 minutes postpain) during the acute phase to evaluate CO; continue to monitor frequently (every 1 to 2 hours) for the first 24 hours post-MI
3. Monitor continuous ECG to detect dysrhythmias (PVCs and tachycardia common)
4. Perform 12-lead ECG immediately with new pain or changes in level or character of pain to identify ischemia and injury
5. Monitor respirations, breath sounds, and I & O to detect early signs of heart failure
6. Monitor O_2 saturation and administer O_2 (usually via nasal cannula at 2 to 4 L/min) as prescribed to increase oxygenation to heart
7. Provide for physiological rest to decrease O_2 demands on heart
8. Keep client NPO or progress to liquid diet as ordered; maintain IV access for medications as needed
9. Provide care in specialized cardiac critical care unit; provide a calm environment and reassure client and family to decrease stress, fear, and anxiety
10. Report significant changes immediately to physician to ensure rapid treatment of complications
11. Interventions in recovery phase: maintain bedrest (with bedside commode) for 24 to 36 hours and gradually increase activity as ordered while closely monitoring CO, ECG, and pain status; reinforce to client importance of reporting any new pain immediately; progress diet from NPO or liquids to soft diet as ordered
12. Administer nitroglycerine as prescribed to dilate coronary vessels and increase blood flow
13. Administer morphine sulfate as ordered to relieve chest pain
14. Administer anticoagulants (IV heparin) and aspirin (antiplatelet) as ordered to prevent additional clot formation; monitor PTT to maintain heparin at therapeutic level
15. Administer thrombolytic therapy if no contraindications (recent hemorrhagic stroke, surgery, childbirth, trauma); common drugs include alteplase recombinant (Activase), tissue plasminogen activator (TPA), or streptokinase (Streptase); they dissolve clot, stop progress of MI, and decrease myocardial damage; monitor frequently for signs of bleeding
16. Monitor neurological status frequently for changes; alteplase recombinant and streptokinase are not clot-specific and will dissolve other clots—can cause thrombolytic (hemorrhagic) CVA, a life-threatening complication
17. Administer beta-blockers post-MI as ordered to decrease cardiac work and decrease O_2 demands on heart
18. Administer antidysrhythmic drugs as prescribed or by emergency protocol for dysrhythmias
19. Surgical interventions: PTCA, CABG (see previous discussion)

D. Client teaching

1. Include appropriate family members whenever possible
2. Cardiac rehabilitation program if ordered

3. Explain modifiable risk factors and develop a plan with client, including supportive resources to change lifestyle to decrease these factors
4. Medication regime as prescribed; identify side effects to report (provide written instructions for later reference)
5. Importance of immediate reporting of chest pain or signs of decreased CO
6. ! Bleeding precautions if client is on anticoagulant therapy: use soft toothbrush, electric razor, avoid trauma or injury; wear or carry Medic-Alert identification

V. HEART FAILURE

A. Overview

1. Inability of heart to pump adequate blood to meet metabolic needs of body
2. Formerly called congestive heart failure
3. Multiple causes include myocardial damage from MI, incompetent valves, inflammatory conditions of the heart, cardiomyopathy, hypertension, and pulmonary hypertension (right-sided failure, called **cor pulmonale**)
4. Compensatory phase (early): CO falls → sensed by baroreceptors → stimulate sympathetic nervous system → release norepinephrine → increase in HR and vasoconstriction → increased in filling pressures → increase in SV and CO (because CO = HR × SV, CO is increased); compensatory mechanisms increase cardiac metabolic demands and in time decrease cardiac function and the ability to compensate
5. Depending upon cause, heart failure presents initially as right-sided failure or left-sided failure; other side becomes affected as it progresses
   a. Left heart failure: left ventricle has reduced capacity to pump blood into systemic circulation, causing decreased CO and stasis or "backup" of fluid into pulmonary circulation
   b. Right heart failure: right ventricle has reduced capacity to pump blood into pulmonary circulation, causing stasis or "backup" of fluid in venous circulation
6. Onset of heart failure
   a. Acute, with significant overload in lungs (**pulmonary edema,** characterized by acute restlessness, anxiety, increased crackles, tachypnea, tachycardia, pink frothy sputum, decreased SO_2 and PO_2)
   b. Chronic, with fatigue and activity intolerance as main features; clients with advanced chronic heart failure require careful management to prevent acute exacerbations

B. Nursing assessment !

1. Presenting symptoms
   a. Left failure: dyspnea on exertion (often first clinical sign), orthopnea, paroxysmal nocturnal dyspnea, crackles, new S_3 (ventricular gallop) as early sign; pulmonary edema is acute life-threatening left heart failure
   b. Right failure: lower extremity edema; **jugular venous distention (JVD)** is visible more than a few millimeters above clavicle with client supine with 45-degree head elevation; abdominal discomfort and nausea occur from fluid congestion in abdominal organs
   c. Both sides: unexplained fatigue or altered mental status, decreased exercise tolerance
2. Diagnostic findings
   a. Chest x-ray may show cardiomegaly or vascular congestion
   b. Echocardiogram shows decreased ventricular function and decreased ejection fraction
   c. CVP elevated in right-sided failure
   d. Pulmonary artery pressure monitoring may be used to guide treatment in serious case of pulmonary edema

C. Therapeutic management

1. Acute phase
   a. Monitor and record BP, pulse, respirations, ECG, and CVP or PCWP (if appropriate) to detect changes in CO
   b. ! Maintain client in sitting position to decrease pulmonary congestion and facilitate improved gas exchange

c. Auscultate heart and lung sounds frequently: increasing crackles, increasing dyspnea, decreasing lungs sounds, or new S_3 heart sound indicate worsening failure
d. Administer O_2 as ordered to improve gas exchange and increase oxygenation of blood; monitor SO_2 and arterial blood gases (ABG) as ordered to assess oxygenation
e. Administer prescribed medications on time
f. Monitor serum electrolytes to detect hypokalemia secondary to diuretic therapy
g. Monitor accurate I & O to evaluate fluid status (may require Foley catheter to allow for accurate measurement of urine output)
h. If fluid restriction is prescribed, spread fluid throughout day to reduce thirst
! i. Encourage physical rest and organized activities with frequent rest periods to reduce cardiac work
j. Provide a calm, reassuring environment to reduce anxiety, thereby decreasing O_2 consumption and demands on heart

2. Chronic heart failure
a. Educate client and family about rationale for therapeutic regime
b. Establish baseline assessment for fluid status and functional abilities: it is baseline "normal" for some clients with heart failure to have bilateral crackles in bases, or some level of peripheral edema, or to be unable to walk more than a specific number of feet before tiring
! c. Monitor daily weights to evaluate changes in fluid status
d. Assess at regular intervals for changes in fluid status or functional activity level

3. Angiotensin-converting enzyme (ACE) inhibitors such as lisinopril (Prinivil) to reduce afterload and consequently increase CO (primarily used in ongoing management); monitor for hypotension, especially orthostatic hypotension
! 4. Diuretics (often loop diuretics such as furosemide/Lasix) to decrease preload and pulmonary congestion, which decreases cardiac work and increases CO; carefully monitor potassium levels for hypokalemia or hyperkalemia, depending on whether potassium-losing or potassium-sparing diuretics are used
5. Vasodilators including nitroglycerine to reduce preload; monitor for hypotension
6. Morphine to sedate and vasodilate during acute pulmonary edema; decreases cardiac work; monitor for hypotension or respiratory depression
! 7. Digoxin (Lanoxin) to improve contractility and correspondingly increase stroke volume and CO; take apical pulse for 1 full minute and withhold if heart rate is less than 60 and notify prescribing physician
8. Other: inotropic agents such as dopamine (Intropin) and dobutamine (Dobutrex) are used in critical care settings to increase force of cardiac contraction when decompensation of CO includes hypotension; monitor BP and IV site frequently

D. Client teaching

1. Include family members or others in teaching as appropriate
! 2. Weight monitoring: measure and record daily weights (with same amount of clothing before breakfast but after voiding) and report unexplained increase of 3 to 5 pounds—most sensitive indicator of increased fluid overload
! 3. Diet: sodium restriction to decrease fluid overload; increase intake of potassium-rich foods if taking potassium-losing diuretics; restriction of high-potassium foods and salt substitutes if taking potassium-sparing diuretics; do not restrict water intake unless directed (this will not decrease fluid retention)
4. Medication regime: follow all medication instructions; although frequent urination is bothersome, regular diuretic therapy prevents fluid overload and acute exacerbation; take radial pulse for one full minute before taking digoxin; withhold dose and call prescriber if pulse is lower than 50 or 60 as instructed (variability exists) or is higher than 120
5. Activity: plan paced activity to maximize available CO
6. Symptoms: report to health care provider promptly any of the following: chest pain, new onset of dyspnea on exertion, paroxysmal nocturnal dyspnea
7. Other: report even minor changes to physician or homecare nurse because they may be early signs of decompensation

VI. ENDOCARDITIS (INFECTIVE, SUBACUTE BACTERIAL)

A. Overview

1. Inflammation of inner layer of heart; usually involves cardiac valves
2. Caused by microorganisms in blood: risk factors include IV drug use, structural defects in heart or valves (which increase number of platelet and fibrin strands in endothelium)
   a. Acute endocarditis: sudden onset with *Staphylococcus aureus* being most common organism
   b. Subacute endocarditis: gradual onset with *Streptococcus viridans* or other less virulent bacteria
3. Microorganisms in bloodstream colonize on fibrin and platelet strands in endothelium, multiply and develop new strands; seen as "vegetation" attached to endothelium, particularly valves, causing damage; segments of vegetation may break off and travel to extremities manifested as petechiae

! B. Nursing assessment

1. Acute: spiking fever and chills; signs of heart failure (see previous section); WBC elevation
2. Subacute: fever of unknown origin; cough; dyspnea; anorexia; malaise; normal WBC; anemia; and elevated erythrocyte sedimentation rate (ESR)
3. Both: positive blood cultures; new cardiac **murmurs** (abnormal heart sounds) or change in existing murmur; embolic complications from segments of vegetation circulating to organs and extremities, including petechiae; splinter hemorrhages in nail beds

! C. Therapeutic management

1. Manage IV therapy; assess for any signs of infection
2. Assess appropriateness of home infusion therapy; client may require inpatient treatment in a subacute care facility if home infusion therapy is contraindicated (as with an IV drug abuser)
3. Provide for periods of rest and moderate periods of exercise to prevent venous stasis
4. Use antiembolism stockings to prevent thrombus formation
5. Provide for diversional activity; client is restricted from resuming normal activity for 4 to 6 weeks
6. Antibiotics given by IV route are needed for 6 weeks

D. Client teaching

1. Role in home infusion therapy
2. After one episode of endocarditis, client is susceptible to repeated infections because of lesions on endocardium; tell future caregivers about infection
3. Symptoms to report to physician, such as fever, anorexia, malaise
4. Gentle, thorough, oral care because infectious organisms can easily enter bloodstream through gums with vigorous brushing or oral treatments
5. Prophylactic antibiotics prior to invasive procedures and routine dental care

VII. VALVULAR DISORDERS

A. Overview

1. Defects in cardiac valve structure or function that interfere with proper cardiac circulation
2. **Stenosis:** heart valve leaflets are fused together; opening is narrow, stiff, and unable to open or close properly
3. **Regurgitation:** there is improper or incomplete closure of heart valves, resulting in back flow of blood
4. Multiple causes including: rheumatic heart disease (most common), congenital, MI, endocarditis
5. Calcium deposits or scar tissue from endocarditis or MI may cause stiffening of valves in stenosis

! B. Nursing assessment

1. Heart sounds: valve dysfunctions have distinctive characteristic changes in heart sounds (see Table 57–2 ■)

Table 57–2

Heart Valve Disorders

Valve Disorder	Specific Assessment	Planning and Implementation
Mitral stenosis	Murmur: low-pitched rumbling diastolic Common in young women Atrial dysrhythmias, especially atrial fibrillation (A-fib)	Monitor closely during pregnancy Administer diuretics and digoxin as prescribed Maintain sodium-restricted diet Anticoagulant therapy if A-fib present Prepare for surgery
Mitral regurgitation (insufficiency)	Murmur: high-pitched blowing systolic Clients generally asymptomatic A-fib common with low incidence of embolization	Administer diuretics, nitrates and ACE inhibitors as prescribed Maintain sodium-restricted diet
Mitral prolapse	Murmur: systolic click Most clients asymptomatic May have PVCs and palpitations, syncope, weakness, and anxiety	Administer beta-blockers as prescribed for syncopy and palpitations Monitor for signs of infective endocarditis Administer prophylactic antibiotics with invasive procedures
Aortic stenosis	Murmur: harsh systolic Late course symptoms: angina; S_3 and S_4; syncope	In symptomatic client, restrict activity to decrease myocardial oxygen consumption Monitor for signs of infective endocarditis Administer prophylactic antibiotics with invasive procedures Prepare for surgery: symptomatic aortic stenosis has poor prognosis without surgical intervention
Aortic regurgitation (insufficiency)	Murmur: blowing diastolic Widened pulse pressure Palpitations; tachycardia and PVCs	Medical management same as aortic stenosis Prepare for surgery, which is the only effective long-term therapy for aortic regurgitation

2. Symptoms and severity depend on extent of valve dysfunction, from asymptomatic to severe heart failure, and on type of valve dysfunction (stenosis or regurgitation); see Table 57–2

! **C. Therapeutic management**

1. Refer again to Table 57–2
2. Monitor heart sounds to assess for changes
3. With signs of decreased CO, manage or restrict activity to decrease demands on heart
4. Monitor for signs of endocarditis
5. Report changes to healthcare provider
6. Medication therapy is determined by symptoms; may inlcude antidysrhythmic and anticoagulant therapy (atrial fibrillation), antibiotic therapy (endocarditis), and drugs to treat heart failure as needed
7. Surgical interventions: valve replacement

D. Client teaching

1. Management of anticoagulants (warfarin, Coumadin) to prevent thrombus formation, including monitoring PT/INR and regulation of vitamin K in diet (green leafy vegetables)
2. Relationships among valve disorders, surgical valves, and increased risk for bacterial endocarditis
3. Methods to prevent endocarditis

VIII. CARDIOMYOPATHY

A. Overview

1. An abnormality of heart muscle that leads to functional changes in heart
2. Cause is unknown; however, in some cases it is associated with viral infections, chronic alcohol abuse, or pregnancy
3. Three types: dilated, hypertrophic, and restrictive
   a. Dilated cardiomyopathy (most common): enlargement of all four chambers, starting with enlarged ventricles, followed by decreased contractility; CO progressively decreases
   b. Hypertrophic cardiomyopathy: unexplained progressive thickening of ventricular muscle mass causing increased pulmonary and venous pressures; CO progressively decreases
   c. Restrictive cardiomyopathy (least common): excessively rigid ventricular walls do not stretch during diastolic filling, creating back pressure and right heart failure as well as reduced SV and consequently, lowered CO

B. Nursing assessment

1. Fatigue with all types
2. Dilated: weakness, signs of left heart failure, S_3 (ventricular gallop heard immediately after S_2 with left ventricular failure or mitral regurgitation) and S_4 (atrial gallop heard immediately before S_1 with coronary heart disease, left ventricular hypertrophy, or aortic stenosis)
3. Hypertrophic: exertional dyspnea, syncope, angina, signs of heart failure, S_4, sudden death often first sign in asymptomatic individuals
4. Restrictive: dyspnea, right-sided heart failure, S_3 and S_4, emboli formation

C. Therapeutic management

1. ! Monitor indicators of level of heart failure (vital signs, lung sounds, edema, dyspnea, activity tolerance)
2. ! Encourage rest and minimize stressful situations to reduce workload on heart
3. Provide counseling and psychological support because of poor prognosis
4. Medications are used to treat signs of heart failure
5. Anticoagulation therapy is used with restrictive cardiomyopathy to prevent emboli

D. Client teaching

1. Instruct client to avoid alcohol consumption because of its cardiac-depressant effects
2. Assist clients in planning to pace activities to reduce cardiac workload
3. Instruct client in medication and dietary management of heart failure
4. Explain anticoagulation therapy and monitoring if appropriate to prevent emboli formation

IX. PERICARDITIS

A. Overview

1. Inflammation of pericardium
2. Acute pericarditis: may have multiple causes, including infection (viral most common), post-MI status (Dressler's syndrome), neoplasms, trauma, uremia, connective tissue diseases, or endocrine diseases
3. Chronic pericarditis: leads to fibrous thickening of pericardium, constricting movement of myocardium and restricting diastolic filling

! B. Nursing assessment

1. Acute: substernal pain, radiating to neck, aggravated by breathing (particularly during inspiration) or coughing; friction rub (scratchy, high-pitched sound on auscultation); elevated WBC; fever; malaise; ECG changes including ST and T wave elevations followed by inverted T waves when ST returns to baseline
2. Chronic restrictive pericarditis: increasing dyspnea, fatigue leading to progressive signs of heart failure

! C. Therapeutic management

1. Assess and manage pain
2. Administer O_2 as ordered and monitor SO_2

! 3. Monitor for complications, especially cardiac **tamponade** (medical emergency; excess fluid collection in pericardial sac that interferes with heart filling and function); signs include the following:
   a. JVD with clear lungs
   b. Elevated CVP
   c. Narrowing pulse pressure
   d. Decreased CO
   e. Muffled heart sounds
4. Report significant changes to physician immediately
5. Position client for comfort: high Fowler's, sitting, or side-lying
6. Provide for periods of rest and limit activity to decrease cardiac workload
7. Medication therapy: analgesics for pain, nonsteroidal anti-inflammatory drugs (NSAIDs) followed by steroids if needed, antibiotics if caused by infection; avoid anticoagulants because of risk of tamponade
8. Pericardiocentesis: removal of fluid from pericardial sac to determine cause or as emergency treatment for tamponade
9. Dialysis for inflammation caused by uremia
10. Radiation to treat neoplasms

D. **Client teaching**
1. Disease process and medication management
2. Take anti-inflammatory drugs with food, milk, or antacids to reduce gastric distress
3. Risk for repeated episodes of pericarditis; report similar pain or dyspnea promptly to physician

X. PRIMARY HYPERTENSION

A. **Overview**
1. BP that consistently exceeds 140/90, confirmed on at least two visits several weeks apart
2. Hypertension can be primary (essential) or secondary; risk factors for primary hypertension include family history, high sodium intake, obesity, inactivity, and excessive alcohol intake

! B. **Nursing assessment**
1. Past history of cardiovascular, cerebrovascular, renal, or thyroid diseases, diabetes, smoking, or alcohol use
2. Family history of hypertension or cardiovascular disease
3. Often silent with absence of symptoms
4. Possible fatigue, nocturia, dyspnea on exertion (DOE), palpitations, angina, headaches, weight gain, edema, muscle cramps, or blurred vision may be caused by target organ damage
5. Possible retinal vessel changes, diminished or absent peripheral pulses, bruits, murmurs, and S_3 and S_4 heart sounds
6. Possible cardiomegaly on x-ray or abnormal ECG showing left ventricular hypertrophy

! C. **Therapeutic management**
1. Tell client numeric BP readings for ongoing record-keeping
2. Accurately record I & O and daily weights of hospitalized clients
3. Medication therapy
   a. No single primary drug is used; medications used include diuretics, beta-blockers, calcium channel blockers, ACE inhibitors, and vasodilators
   b. Stepped care approach is often used to guide treatment; this protocol begins with lifestyle changes and adds medications based on response to previous therapy

D. **Client teaching**
1. Hypertension is usually asymptomatic, and symptoms will not reliably indicate BP levels

! 2. Lifestyle modification
   a. Sodium restriction
   b. Weight reduction and exercise

c. DASH (dietary approaches to stop hypertension) diet: includes prescribed number of servings of following foods: grains and grain products; vegetables; fruits; low-fat or nonfat dairy foods; meats, poultry, and fish; nuts, seeds, and legumes; fats and oils; and sweets
d. Moderation of alcohol intake
e. Relaxation techniques and stress management
f. No smoking

! 3. Prevent **orthostatic hypotension** (a drop in blood pressure of 10 to 20 mmHg with upright posture) by rising out of bed or chair slowly
4. Avoid hot baths and strenuous exercise within 3 hours of taking vasodilators
5. Adhere to treatment plan, even if asymptomatic, to reduce risk of target organ damage

XI. PERIPHERAL ARTERIAL DISEASE

A. Overview

1. Disorders that interrupt or impede arterial peripheral blood flow; primarily caused by **atherosclerosis** (local accumulation of lipid and fibrous tissue along intimal layer of artery), but also by trauma, embolism, thrombosis, vasospasm, inflammation, or autoimmunity
2. By the time symptoms appear, vessel is about 75% narrowed
3. Femoral-popliteal area is most common site in nondiabetics; clients with diabetes most often develop disease in arteries below knees
4. Chronic arterial obstruction leads to inadequate tissue oxygenation, causing **intermittent claudication,** ischemic muscle pain precipitated by a predictable amount of exercise and relieved by rest

! B. Nursing assessment

1. Intermittent claudication, an early sign of disease
2. **Rest pain,** which may even awaken client at night; pain is usually in distal extremity (toes, arch, forefoot, heel) and is relieved when foot is placed in dependent position; indicates more advanced disease
3. Extremities may be cool, pale, and numb with a cyanotic color on elevation
4. Bruits may be auscultated
5. Diminished or absent peripheral pulses
6. Thickened and opaque nails (trophic changes)
7. Skin on legs may be shiny with sparse hair growth (trophic change)
8. Ulcers may be present on lower extremities in areas affected by reduced circulation
9. Diagnostic testing: digital subtraction angiography (DSA), angiography, Doppler ultrasound, plethysmography
10. See Table 57–3 ■ for a comparison of arterial and venous vascular disease

! C. Therapeutic management

1. Assess and record strength of pulses
2. Encourage smoking cessation

Table 57–3

Comparison of Arterial and Venous Vascular Disease

Assessment	Arterial Disease	Venous Disease
Color	Pale	Ruddy; cyanotic if dependent
Edema	None or minimal	Usually present
Nails	Thick and brittle	Normal
Pain	Worse with elevation and exercise; may be sudden or severe; rest pain; claudication	Better with elevation; possible Homan's sign, dullness or heaviness
Pulses	Decreased, weak, or absent	Normal
Temperature of extremity	Cool	Warm
Ulcers	Dry and necrotic	Moist; malleolar

3. Change position at least hourly and avoid crossing the legs
4. Encourage client to exercise and walk to point of pain; stop walking when pain occurs and resume when pain stops to build exercise tolerance and stimulate growth of collateral circulation
5. Assess pain on a 1-to-10 scale and provide analgesics as ordered
6. If an ulcer develops, healing will be slow unless arterial blood flow is improved through surgery
7. If surgery is indicated, provide appropriate postoperative care
8. Angioplasty
   a. ! Monitor **neurovascular status** (color, motion, sensitivity, temperature, and presence of distal peripheral pulses) to affected extremity every 15 minutes for 4 hours, every 30 minutes for 4 hours, then every 1 to 4 hours after sheath removal
   b. Notify physician if client experiences weak or thready pulses, coolness, numbness, or tingling in extremity
   c. Monitor sheath site for external and subcutaneous bleeding
   d. Instruct client to notify nurse and apply manual pressure to site if warm or wet sensation is felt at site
   e. Maintain immobilization of affected extremity for at least 6 hours by reminding client to keep extremity still, or lightly immobilize ankle with sheet tucked under both sides of mattress
   f. Maintain a pressure dressing and sand bag at site
9. Bypass grafting
   a. Provide standard postoperative care
   b. Assess for occlusion of graft: severe ischemic pain, loss of pulses, decreasing ankle-brachial index, numbness or tingling in extremity, coolness of extremity
10. **Endarterectomy** (opening artery and removing obstructing plaque) or amputation in severe cases; use same principles of care as for other procedures
11. Medication therapy: aspirin inhibits platelet aggregation; pentoxifylline (Trental) decreases blood viscosity and increases blood flow; cilostazol (Pletal) inhibits platelet aggregation and enhances vasodilation; clopidogrel (Plavix) and ticlopidine (Ticlid) prevent thrombi formation with recent MI or stroke

D. Client teaching

1. ! See Box 57–2
2. Teach relaxation techniques because stress increases vasoconstriction

Box 57–2

Client and Family Education for Peripheral Arterial Disease

- Stop smoking.
- Lose weight and eat a low-fat diet.
- Do not cross legs while sitting.
- Elevate feet at rest, but not above heart level.
- Do not stand or sit for long periods of time.
- Do not wear restrictive clothing.
- Keep affected extremity warm but never apply direct heat.
- Inspect feet daily and keep them clean and dry.
- Avoid walking barefoot; wear proper-fitting shoes.
- Avoid mechanical or thermal injury to the legs and feet; have nail care performed by podiatrist.
- Begin and maintain an exercise and walking program.
- Notify healthcare provider of any changes in color, sensation, temperature, or pulses in extremities.

XII. ARTERIAL EMBOLISM

A. Overview

1. Arterial emboli usually develop in heart from atrial fibrillation, myocardial infarction, prosthetic valves, or heart failure
2. Thrombi become detached and are carried from left heart into arterial system where they may lodge and cause obstruction
3. Symptoms may be abrupt and depend on size and location of embolus
4. Ischemia will progress to necrosis and gangrene within hours if untreated

! B. Nursing assessment: the "six Ps"

1. Pain
2. Pallor (pale color)
3. Pulselessness (diminished or absent pulses)
4. Parasthesias (altered local sensation)
5. Paralysis (weakness or inability to move extremity)
6. **Poikilothermia** (body temperature that varies with environment, usually is decreased)

! C. Therapeutic management

1. Assess peripheral pulses and neurovascular status every 2 to 4 hours
2. Place affected extremity in a neutral position with no restrictive bedding or clothing
3. Assess level of pain using a 1-to-10 scale
4. Change position every 2 hours to improve collateral circulation
5. Assess for and report unusual bleeding from anticoagulant therapy
6. Monitor lab values, including APTT, PT, and INR levels
7. An emergency embolectomy should be performed within 4 to 5 hours of embolism to prevent permanent damage; if necrosis is present, surgical treatment is required
8. Medication therapy (if no necrosis present): thrombolytic therapy with streptokinase, TPA or heparin; warfarin therapy at home

D. Client teaching

1. Pre- and postoperative teaching if embolectomy is performed
2. Measures to promote peripheral circulation and maintain tissue integrity (refer back to Box 57–2)

XIII. BUERGER'S DISEASE (THROMBOANGIITIS OBLITERANS)

A. Overview

1. Inflammatory disease of small- and medium-sized veins and arteries accompanied by thrombi and sometimes vasospasm; may occur in upper or lower extremities but is most common in leg or foot
2. Etiology is uncertain but is currently thought to be autoimmune reaction to chemicals in cigarettes (occurs mostly in young men who are heavy smokers)
3. Inflammation occurs; microthrombi form; both can lead to vasospasm, and this process ultimately obstructs blood flow

! B. Nursing assessment

1. Initially, a bluish cast to a toe or finger and a feeling of coldness in affected limb is common
2. Rest pain, possibly severe
3. Excessive sweating in feet is possible from overactive sympathetic nerves, even though feet feel cold
4. Intermittent claudication and other symptoms similar to those of chronic obstructive arterial disease often appear gradually after occlusion
5. Ischemic ulcers and gangrene are common complications of progressive Buerger's disease

! C. Therapeutic management

1. Arrest progress of disease by smoking cessation
2. Take measures to promote vasodilation (similar to other arterial disorders)
3. Provide for pain relief
4. Provide emotional support

5. Medication therapy: analgesic pain medications, calcium channel blockers to ease vasospasm, pentoxifylline (Trental) to reduce blood viscosity

D. **Client teaching**

1. Stop smoking
2. Take measures to promote peripheral circulation and maintain tissue integrity (refer back to Box 57–2)

XIV. RAYNAUD'S DISEASE

A. **Overview**

1. Localized, intermittent episodes of vasoconstriction of small arteries of hands and, less commonly, feet, causing pallor, coolness, and cyanosis; primarily affects young women
2. Vasospastic attacks tend to be bilateral and symmetrical and usually begin at tips of digits, causing pallor, numbness, and sensation of cold
3. Attacks are triggered by exposure to cold, emotional stress, caffeine ingestion, and tobacco use

! B. **Nursing assessment**

1. Classic triphasic color changes (pallor, cyanosis, and rubor) in hands with accompanying reduction in skin temperature
2. Intensity of pain increases as disease progresses
3. Skin of fingertips may thicken, and nails may become brittle

C. **Therapeutic management**

1. ! Keep hands warm and free from injury
2. Avoid stressful situations
3. In severe cases, a **sympathectomy** (surgical dissection of nerve fibers to relieve symptoms) may be performed
4. Medication therapy: analgesics for pain and possibly vasodilators and calcium channel blockers (vasospasm)

! D. **Client teaching**

1. Keep hands warm: wear gloves when outdoors, in air-conditioned environments, or when handling cold food
2. Avoid injury to hands
3. Lifestyle changes: stop smoking; employ stress relief such as biofeedback

XV. AORTIC ANEURYSM

A. **Overview**

1. Localized dilation or outpouching of weakened area in aorta, classified by region as thoracic or abdominal, or as dissecting (layers of blood vessels separated by a layer of blood)
2. More common in abdominal aorta below level of renal arteries but can occur in thoracic area
3. Growth rate is unpredictable, and large aneurysms tend to rupture, a life-threatening emergency
4. Major risk factor is atherosclerosis

! B. **Nursing assessment**

1. Thoracic aneurysms are often asymptomatic, with first sign being rupture
   a. Symptoms may include pain in back, neck, and substernal area that may occur only when lying supine
   b. Possible dysphagia and dyspnea, stridor, or cough when pressing on esophagus or laryngeal nerve
2. Abdominal aneurysms may also be asymptomatic until rupture
   a. Client may report a "heartbeat" in abdomen when lying down
   b. ! Possible pulsating abdominal mass; do not palpate (risk of rupture)
   c. Moderate to severe abdominal or lumbar back pain may be present (severe pain may be a sign of impending rupture)
   d. Client may experience claudication
   e. Cool or cyanotic extremities may be noted
   f. Systolic bruit may be heard

3. Dissecting aneurysms present with sudden, severe, and persistent pain described as "tearing" or "ripping" in anterior chest or back
   a. Pain may extend to shoulder, epigastric area, or abdomen
   b. Pallor, sweating, and tachycardia are evidenced
   c. Initially, client may have an elevated BP that may be different in one arm than other
   d. Possible syncope and paralysis of lower extremities may be present

C. Therapeutic management

1. Diagnosis by chest x-ray, transesophageal echocardiography, aortography, ultrasound, and CT scan or MRI
2. Hematomas into scrotum, perineum, flank, or penis indicate retroperitoneal rupture
3. Surgery may be performed on an emergency or elective basis (not usually performed if less than 4 to 5 cm); involves excision of aneurysm with insertion of synthetic graft
4. Preoperatively mark and assess all peripheral pulses for comparison postoperatively
5. Postoperatively assess neurovascular status and assess for complications, such as graft occlusion, hypovolemia (renal failure), respiratory distress, cardiac dysrhythmias, paralytic ileus, and paraplegia (paralysis); use overbed cradle
6. Medication therapy
   a. Antihypertensives and diuretics to control blood pressure
   b. Postoperative anticoagulant therapy: heparin during hospitalization and warfarin (Coumadin) after discharge

D. Client teaching

1. If under medical care, get routine physical examinations to monitor status of aneurysm
2. Signs and symptoms of impending rupture (see assessment of dissecting aneurysms above)
3. Monitor BP and report any increases immediately; take medications as ordered
4. Postoperative teaching
   a. Do limited lifting for 4 to 6 weeks after surgery (no heavy lifting at all)
   b. Monitor incision site for bleeding and infection
   c. Understand how to assess neurovascular status of extremities and presence of pulses
5. Clients who receive a synthetic graft may require prophylactic antibiotics before invasive procedures

XVI. THROMBOPHLEBITIS

A. Overview

1. Formation of a thrombus (clot) associated with vein inflammation; classified as superficial or deep
2. Etiology: Virchow's triad (at least two of three conditions present for thrombosis to occur)
   a. Stasis of venous flow
   b. Damage to inner lining of vein (endothelial layer)
   c. Hypercoagulability of blood
3. If detachment occurs, emboli travel through venous system to heart and into pulmonary circulation

B. Nursing assessment

1. History of thrombophlebitis, pelvic or abdominal surgery, obesity, neoplasm (hepatic and pancreatic), CHF, atrial fibrillation, prolonged immobility, MI, pregnancy and/or postpartum period, IV therapy, hypercoagulable states (polycythemia, dehydration, or malnutrition)
2. Superficial
   a. Palpable, firm, subcutaneous, cordlike vein
   b. Surrounding area warm, red, tender to touch
   c. Edema may or may not be present
   d. Most common cause in arms is IV therapy; in legs it is often related to varicose veins

3. Deep
    a. Unilateral edema, pain, warm skin, and elevated temperature
    b. If inferior vena cava is involved, both legs will be edematous
    c. If superior vena cava is involved, both upper extremities, neck, back, and face may become edematous or cyanotic
    d. If calf is involved, **Homan's sign** may be present (pain on dorsiflexion of the foot, especially when leg is raised, nonspecific sign)
4. Diagnostic studies: venous duplex scanning; Doppler ultrasonic flowmeter, MRI, and lung scan

C. Therapeutic management

1. Provide analgesics for pain relief
2. Elevate affected leg higher than heart to promote venous drainage
3. Apply warm, moist compresses, intermittent or continuous, to affected extremity; never massage affected extremity to reduce risk of embolism
4. Measure and monitor limb circumference when edema is present
5. Monitor status of peripheral pulses
6. Keep bed covers from touching affected limb by using an overbed cradle to avoid skin breakdown
7. Maintain strict bedrest
8. Instruct client to report any pink-tinged sputum and monitor for tachypnea, tachycardia, shortness of breath, chest pain, and apprehension, which may indicate a pulmonary embolism
9. Medication therapy: anticoagulants, thrombolytics, analgesics (NSAIDs to reduce pain and relieve inflammation)

D. Client teaching

1. Prevention
    a. Early ambulation postoperatively
    b. Use of compression stockings or pneumatic compression boots
    c. Low-dose anticoagulant therapy
    d. Avoid prolonged standing or sitting and sitting with crossed legs
    e. Avoid restrictive clothing
    f. Stop smoking
2. Anticoagulant therapy

XVII. VENOUS INSUFFICIENCY

A. Overview

1. Inadequate venous return over time causes venous hypertension, which stretches veins and damages valves, reducing blood return
2. Risk factors include thrombus formation, prolonged standing or sitting (teachers, waitresses, nurses, office workers), pregnancy, and obesity

B. Nursing assessment

1. Past history of thrombophlebitis, hypertension, varicosities
2. Past history of long periods of sitting and/or standing
3. Edema of lower legs, may extend to knee
4. Thick, coarse, brownish skin around ankles and feet
5. Stasis ulcers, usually in malleolar area
6. See Table 57–3 for a general comparison of manifestations of arterial and venous disorders

C. Therapeutic management

1. Bedrest with legs elevated above heart level
2. Avoid long periods of standing
3. Wear elastic support or compression hose (apply *before* getting out of bed and placing leg in a dependent position); remove at night
4. Never push hosiery down around leg—will further impair circulation
5. Treat venous stasis ulcer(s)
    a. Open lesions: hydrocolloid dressing and compression wraps; possible topical ointment, such as low-dose hydrocortisone, zinc oxide, or an antifungal

b. Unna Boot or other compression wrap that is changed every 1 to 2 weeks and usually applied over a base dressing
c. Severe ulcers may need surgical debridement
6. Medication therapy
a. Topical agents to skin ulcers, such as hydrocortisone, antifungals, or zinc oxide
b. Oral or IV antibiotics may be prescribed (infected ulcer or cellulitis)

D. Client teaching
1. Elevate legs for at least 20 minutes four times a day
2. Keep legs above level of heart when in bed
3. Avoid prolonged sitting or standing
4. Do not cross legs when sitting
5. Do not wear tight, restrictive pants, socks, or boots; avoid girdles and garters that restrict circulation in upper leg
6. Wear support stockings as instructed

XVIII. VARICOSE VEINS

A. Overview
1. A vein or veins in which blood has pooled, producing distended, tortuous, and palpable vessels; valve leaflets become defective
2. Risk factors: women over 35, obesity, positive family history, prolonged standing
3. As vein swells, increased hydrostatic pressure pushes plasma through stretched vessel walls and edema may occur

! **B. Nursing assessment**
1. Reports of aching, heaviness, itching, swelling, and unsightly appearance to leg(s)
2. Dilated, tortuous, superficial veins along upper and lower leg
3. Superficial inflammation may develop along path of varicose vein
4. Positive Trendelenburg test (done to evaluate valve competence; veins fill from proximal rather than distal end after sitting up from supine position with legs raised)

! **C. Therapeutic management**
1. Analgesics as needed
2. Improve venous circulation as described for venous insufficiency
3. Assess pulses and neurovascular status of lower extremities
4. Apply support stockings
5. Elevate feet above heart level when lying down
6. Prevent skin breakdown; teach proper skin care and importance of avoiding trauma to legs
7. Sclerotherapy: injection of sclerosing agent into varicosed vein, usually in physician's office (palliative but not curative; elastic bandages often worn for several weeks)
8. Vein ligation surgery involves ligation (tying off) of entire vein (usually saphenous) and dissection and removal of incompetent tributaries
a. Perform hourly circulation checks postoperatively in postanesthesia area
b. Elevate extremity to a 15-degree angle to prevent stasis and edema
c. Apply compression-gradient stockings from foot to groin
9. Medication therapy: no specific medications are used

D. Client teaching: prevention as for venous insufficiency; lose weight if necessary

XIX. ACYANOTIC HEART DEFECTS

A. Heart conditions that do not cause deoxygenation or low O_2 levels; skin and mucous membrane color is usually normal pink

B. Atrial septal defect (see Figure 57–1 ■)
1. Defect in atrial septal wall allowing blood to flow from left atrium to right atrium, called a left-to-right shunt; caused by failure of foramen ovale to close
! 2. Assessment: often asymptomatic if defect is small; dyspnea, fatigue, poor growth, and soft systolic murmur in pulmonic area, splitting S_2
3. Diagnosis by echocardiogram (right ventricular overload and shunt size), cardiac catheterization (visualization of defect)

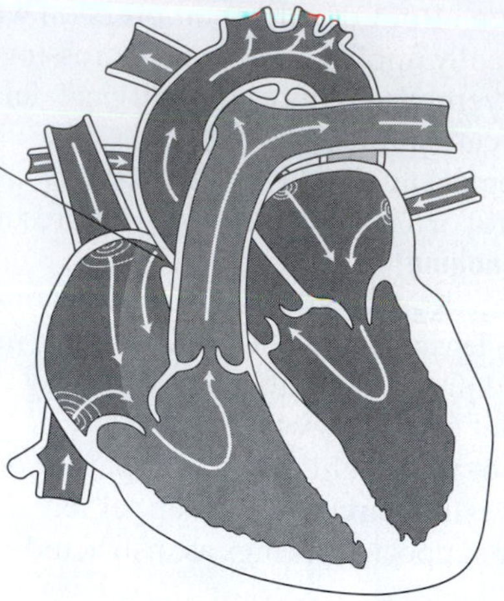

Figure 57–1

Atrial septal defect.

Source: Ball, J. & Bindler, R. (2006). Child health nursing: Partnering with children & families. *Upper Saddle River, NJ: Pearson Education, p. 911, Table 26-8.*

4. Therapeutic intervention includes surgical closure or patch of defect, transcatheter device closure during cardiac catheterization
5. Nursing management of child with acyanotic heart disease (see Table 57–4 ■)
6. Child and family education
   a. Purpose of tests and procedures
   b. Ways to support nutrition, reduce stress on heart, promote rest, and support growth and development during preoperative period
   c. Signs of CHF and infection
   d. Prepare parents and child for surgery by visiting intensive care unit, explaining equipment and sounds
   e. Prepare older child for postoperative experience, including coughing and deep breathing and need for movement
   f. Need for antibiotic prophylaxis to prevent subacute bacterial endocarditis

C. Ventricular septal defect (VSD) (see Figure 57–2 ■)

1. Defect in ventricle septal wall allowing blood to flow from left ventricle to right ventricle (**left-to-right shunt**) because of higher pressue in left ventricle
2. Shunting of blood causes an increased load on right ventricle and increases pulmonary blood flow

Table 57–4

Nursing Management of the Child with an Acyanotic Heart Defect

Problem	Nursing Management
Anxiety and inadequate coping	1. Assess coping mechanisms of family. 2. Provide family with information about condition. 3. Refer family to American Heart Association.
Possible delayed growth and development	1. Treat the child as normally as possible. Teach parents that children are more comfortable when they know what to expect. 2. Promote mental development activities as appropriate for age and condition.
Risk for infection	1. Limit exposure to individuals with infections. 2. Promote good pulmonary hygiene—change position, use percussion and postural drainage. 3. Use prophylactic antibiotics when undergoing surgical or dental treatments to prevent subacute bacterial endocarditis.
Inadequate nutrition	1. Offer small, frequent meals. 2. Use soft nipple for infant to ease the stress of sucking. 3. Organize nursing care to allow for rest.
Impaired gas exchange	1. Promote good pulmonary hygiene. 2. Monitor intake and output. Limit fluids as ordered. 3. Administer diuretics as ordered. 4. Change position every 2 hours.

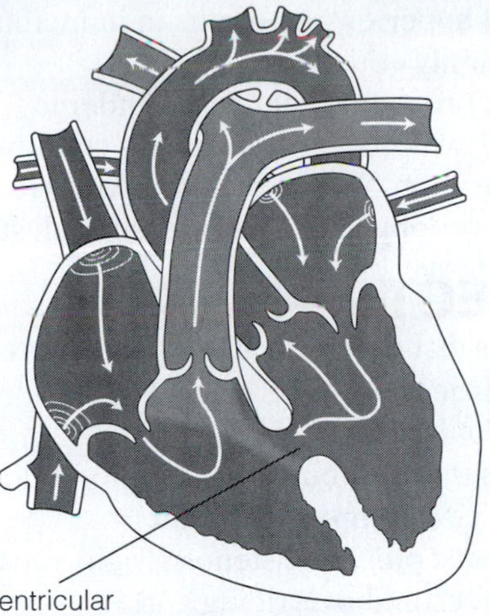

Figure 57–2

Ventricular septal defect.

Source: Ball, J. & Bindler, R. (2006). Child health nursing: Partnering with children & families. *Upper Saddle River, NJ: Pearson Education, p. 912, Table 26-8.*

3. Assessment: tachypnea, dyspnea, poor growth, reduced fluid intake, palpable thrill, systolic murmur at left lower sternal border; ECG and radiology detect larger septal defects; signs of heart failure
4. Therapeutic management (see Table 57–4)
   a. Occasionally spontaneous closure occurs
   b. Surgical patching if failure to thrive occurs
   c. Prophylactic antibiotics treatment to prevent endocarditis
   d. Preoperative nursing care involves promoting growth and development and promoting oxygenation (see Table 57–4)
   e. Postoperative nursing care continues with activities of preoperative care and providing analgesics for pain relief and use of sterile dressings on incision
5. Child and family education (same as for atrial septal defect)

D. Coarctation of aorta (see Figure 57–3 ■)

1. Narrowing of descending aorta that restricts blood flow leaving heart
2. Often near ductus arteriosus
3. Progressive disorder that leads to CHF
4. Assessment: may be asymptomatic; BP difference of 20 mm between upper and lower extremities, brachial and radial pulses full, femoral pulses weak, headache, vertigo, epistaxis, exercise intolerance, left ventricular hypertrophy, dyspnea, cerebrovascular accident (CVA) secondary to hypertension in upper circulation
5. Therapeutic management
   a. Balloon cardiac catheterization
   b. Surgical resection and patch of coarctation
   c. Prophylaxis for endocarditis when undergoing surgical or dental procedures
   d. Prior to correction, monitor BP in upper and lower extremities

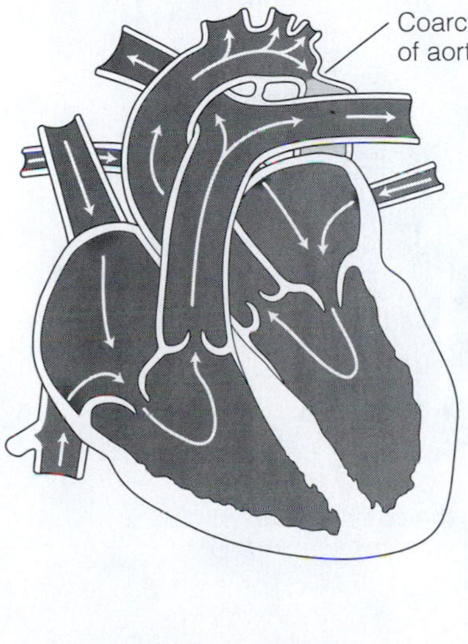

Figure 57–3

Coarctation of aorta.

Source: Ball, J. & Bindler, R. (2006). Child health nursing: Partnering with children & families. *Upper Saddle River, NJ: Pearson Education, p. 927, Table 26-11.*

e. Rebound hypertension occurs in immediate postoperative period
6. Child and family education
   a. Tests and procedures child will undergo
   b. Signs and symptoms of worsening condition
   c. Administration of cardiac and vasoactive drugs
   d. Need for prophylactic antibiotics for all surgical and dental procedures

XX. CYANOTIC HEART DEFECTS

A. **Heart conditions that cause blood to contain inadequate O_2**; skin and mucous membrane color is usually pale to blue

B. **Tetralogy of Fallot (see Figure 57–4 ■)**

1. Four defects that combine to allow blood flow to bypass lungs and enter left side of heart, called a **right-to-left shunt**
   a. Four defects: pulmonic stenosis, right ventricular hypertrophy, ventricular septal defect, and overriding aorta
   b. Atrial septal defect occurs at times
   c. Deficient O_2 in tissues leads to acidosis
   d. Hypercyanosis (TET) spells occur, which are transient periods when there is an increase in right-to-left shunting of blood
2. Unoxygenated blood enters systemic circulation, accounting for cyanosis
3. Assessment
   a. TET spells: hypoxia, pallor, and tachypnea; precipitated by crying, defecation, and feeding; older children assume a squatting position to decrease blood return from lower extremities; treatment involves placing child in knee-chest position and administering morphine or propranolol and oxygen

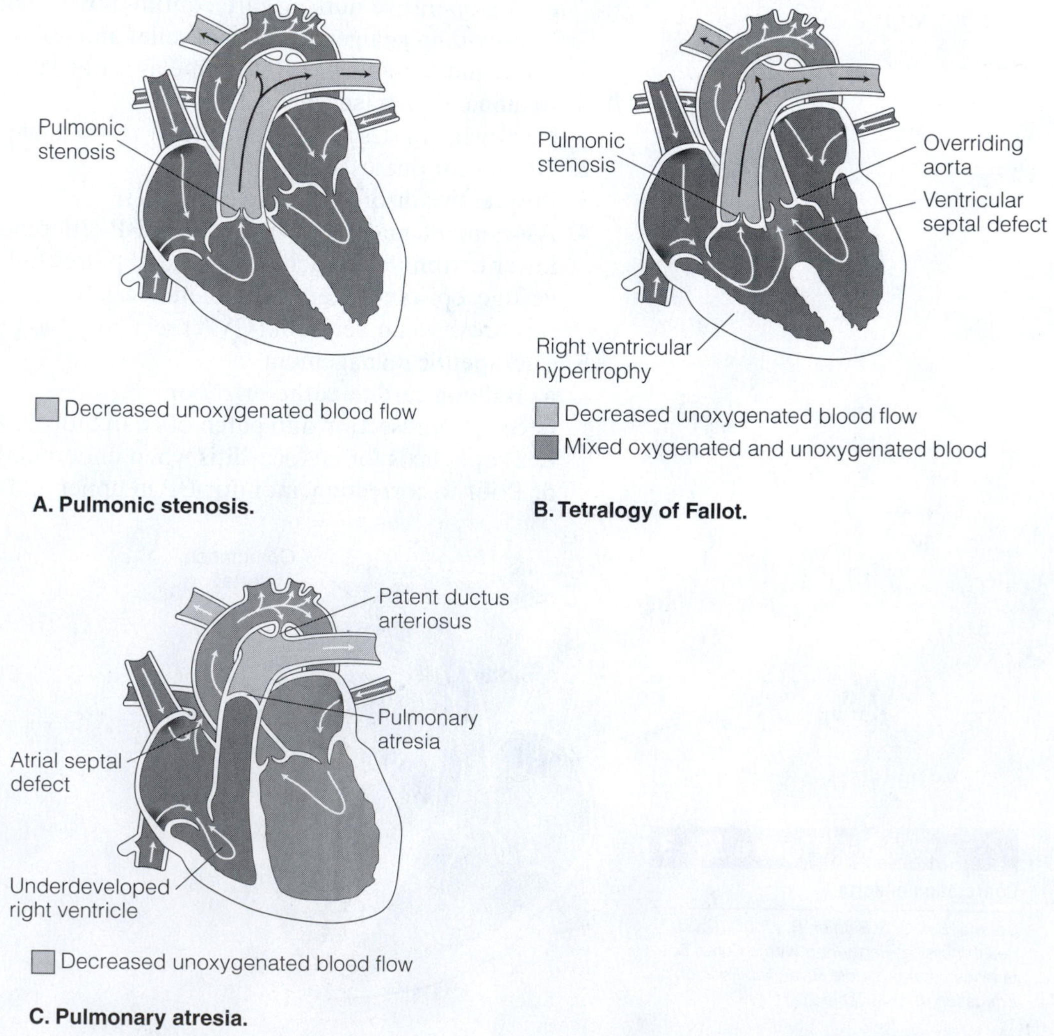

Figure 57–4

Heart Defects with Decreased Pulmonary Blood Flow.

Source: Ball, J. & Bindler, R. (2006). Child health nursing: Partnering with children & families. *Upper Saddle River, NJ: Pearson Education, p. 918, Table 26-9.*

b. Clubbing of digits
c. **Polycythemia** (excess number of RBCs), metabolic acidosis
d. Poor growth, exercise intolerance
e. Systolic murmur in pulmonic area
f. Right ventricular hypertrophy
g. Cardiac catheterization visualizes anomalous structures

4. Therapeutic management
   a. **Prostaglandin E1:** to maintain open ductus arteriosus
   b. Palliative surgery to improve oxygenation includes shunting procedures
   c. Corrective surgery includes patching VSD and relieving pulmonary stenosis
   d. See Table 57–5 ■ for associated nursing care
5. Child and family education
   a. Promote nutrition in light of weak suck
   b. Discuss activities to promote oxygenation
   c. Symptoms of respiratory infections
   d. Treatments and procedures child will undergo

C. Transposition of great vessels (see Figure 57–5 ■)

1. Pulmonary artery originates from left ventricle; blood travels from left ventricle to pulmonary artery, then to lungs, and then back into left atrium
2. Aorta originates from right ventricle; blood leaves right ventricle by aorta, travels to body cells, and returns to right atrium by way of vena cava
3. There are two closed circulation pathways
4. Survival depends on foramen ovale remaining open to mix oxygenated and deoxygenated blood

Table 57–5

Nursing Management of the Child with Cyanotic Heart Disease

Problem	Nursing Management
Inadequate tissue perfusion	1. Monitor hemoglobin and hematocrit levels. 2. Keep the child calm. Do not allow long periods of crying. 3. When hypercyanosis occurs, assist the child to squatting or knee-chest position. 4. Administer oxygen and morphine as ordered during these spells.
Risk for infection	1. Limit exposure to individuals with infections. 2. Promote good pulmonary hygiene—change position, percussion, and postural drainage. 3. Use prophylactic antibiotics when undergoing surgical or dental treatments to prevent subacute bacterial endocarditis.
Inadequate nutrition	1. Offer small, frequent meals. 2. Use soft nipple for infant to ease the stress of sucking. 3. Organize nursing care to allow for rest.
Possible impaired gas exchange	1. Limit activity. 2. Maintain clear airways. 3. Monitor electrolytes.
Possible decreased cardiac output	1. Assess vital signs. 2. Monitor for signs of congestive heart failure. 3. Note peripheral edema. 4. Weigh child daily. 5. Maintain strict I & O measurement. 6. Administer diuretics as ordered. 7. Administer oxygen as ordered. 8. Palpate liver every 4 to 12 hours (indicates right-sided failure). 9. Administer digoxin as ordered: a. Assess for apical pulse—monitor for bradycardia or arrhythmias. b. Be consistent in measurement of medication and time of administration. c. Do not repeat dose if child vomits.
Risk for injury	1. Monitor hemoglobin and hematocrit. 2. Observe for signs of thrombus formation.

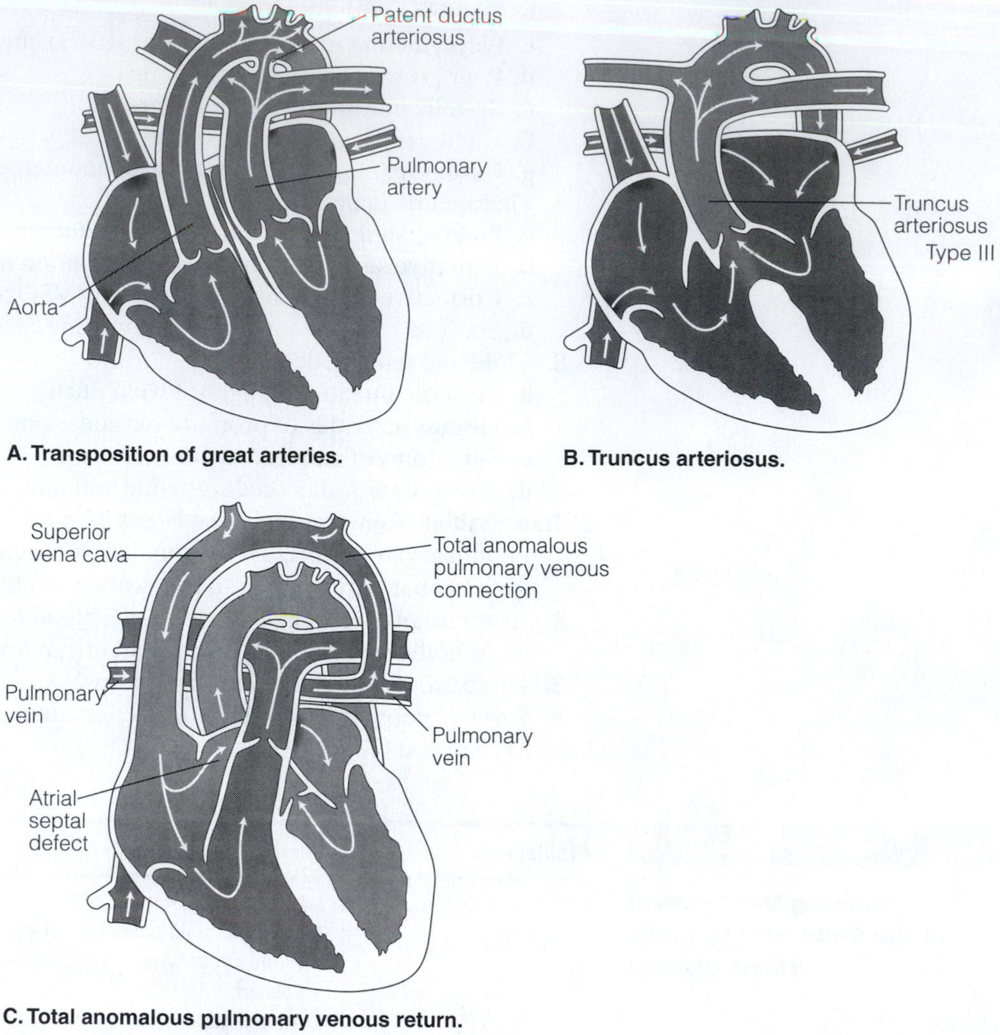

Figure 57–5

Mixed heart defects.

Source: Ball, J. & Bindler, R. (2006). *Child health nursing: Partnering with children & families.* Upper Saddle River, NJ: Pearson Education, p. 920, Table 26-10.

! 5. Assessment: progressive cyanosis leads to hypoxia and then acidosis; signs of heart failure, tachypnea, poor feeding, failure to grow; echocardiogram identifies misplacement of arteries

! 6. Therapeutic management
   a. Prostaglandin E1 to maintain open ductus arteriosus
   b. Palliative surgical interventions
   c. Corrective surgery
   d. Prophylactic antibiotic therapy to prevent endocarditis
   e. Nursing activities to promote nutrition and reduce respiratory congestion (see Table 57–5)
7. Child and family education
   a. Home care requirements related to nutrition, rest, and oxygenation
   b. Preparation for procedures and treatments
   c. Safe administration of cardiac drugs and diuretics

D. Hypoplastic left heart syndrome

1. Abnormally small left ventricle noted at birth, causing inadequate oxygen supply
2. Absent or stenotic mitral and aortic valves
3. Abnormally small left ventricle and aortic arch with major resistance to aortic blood flow
4. Hypertrophy of right ventricle
5. Prognosis poor
6. Assessment
   a. Tachypnea, chest retractions, dyspnea
   b. Cyanosis

c. Decreased pulses, poor peripheral perfusion
d. Increased right ventricular impulse
e. Echocardiogram indicates small and weak left ventricle
f. CHF

7. Therapeutic management
a. Prostaglandin E1 given to prevent closure of patent ductus arteriosus
b. Palliative surgery
c. Transplant may be performed
d. Survival rate is low

XXI. RHEUMATIC FEVER

A. Overview

1. Systemic inflammatory disease involving heart and joints and possibly CNS and connective tissue
2. Follows 2 to 6 weeks after a group A beta-hemolytic streptococcal infection
3. May be an autoimmune reaction against microorganisms; strep organisms cannot be cultured out of lesions of rheumatic fever
4. Acute phase lasts 2 to 3 weeks and is characterized by inflammation of connective tissue in heart, joints, and skin
5. Proliferative phase primarily affects heart, with Aschoff bodies developing on heart valves; cardiac valve leaflets scar and lead to valvular stenosis and regurgitation
6. Episode of rheumatic fever lasts up to 3 months and is self-limiting
7. ! Long-term consequence is rheumatic heart disease, which is often manifested in valvular damage
8. Difficult to diagnose because it mimics other diseases; diagnosis is usually based on **Jones criteria,** which lists major and minor manifestations according to likelihood of rheumatic fever infection; diagnosis is based on presence of two major or one major and two minor criteria

! B. Assessment using Jones criteria

1. Major criteria
a. Inflammation of multiple joints; most frequently large joints—knees, elbows, and wrists
b. Carditis (most severe criteria): a new murmur, pericardial friction rub, changes on ECG; tachycardia in form of a sleeping pulse greater than 100
c. CNS: chorea, which involves involuntary movement of limbs; emotional lability and slurred speech; tends to have a latent period of 2 months or more from strep infection
d. Erythema marginatum is a erythematous, macular rash that occurs primarily on trunk and proximal limbs; frequently associated with carditis
e. Subcutaneous nodules (nontender) on skin over flexor surfaces of joints and vertebrae
2. Minor criteria: fever (spiking temperature), arthralgia; elevated ESR, C-reactive protein, and decreased RBC count; prolonged PR and/or QT interval on ECG
3. Supporting evidence (of recent streptococcal infection): history of same, history of scarlet fever, positive throat culture for streptococcus, elevated antistreptolysin O (ASO) titer

C. Therapeutic management

1. Bedrest until ESR returns to normal
2. Aspirin and prednisone as ordered; anti-inflammatory agents to reduce inflammation; aspirin will also promote relief from painful joints
3. Monitor client for cardiac function
4. Give penicillin as ordered in either an oral daily dose or monthly long-acting injection after recovery from rheumatic heart disease to reduce risk of recurrence of strep infection; erythromycin given if client is allergic to penicillin
5. ! Design nursing activities to promote rest and to encourage diversional activities that do not stress heart; maintain bedrest with bathroom privileges
6. Child and family education
a. Pathology of disease and rationale for bedrest

b. Diversional activities that allow for mental stimulation without physical activity
c. Planning for home care of child

XXII. KAWASAKI'S DISEASE

A. Overview

1. A multisystem disorder involving **vasculitis** (inflammation of tunica intima lining of arteries and veins)
2. Also called mucocutaneous lymph node syndrome
3. Unknown cause but generally affects young children; most frequently affected are boys under age 2 years
4. Three phases of disease
   a. Acute phase characterized by fever, conjunctival hyperemia, swollen hands and feet, rash, and enlarged cervical lymph nodes
   b. Subacute phase is characterized by cracking lips, desquamation of skin on tips of fingers and toes, cardiac disease, and thrombocytosis
   c. Convalescent phase has lingering signs of inflammation
5. Significantly increased platelet count
6. Possible cardiac pathology, including dysrhythmias, CHF, and MI

! **B. Nursing assessment**

1. Phase one (days 1 to 10): fever lasting longer than 5 days and unresponsive to antipyretics, conjunctivitis, crusted and fissured lips, swelling of hands and feet, erythema, **lymphadenopathy** (a condition that causes swollen glands and can be caused by infection or cancer)
2. Phase two (days 10 to 25): fever diminishes, irritability, anorexia, desquamation of hands and feet, arthritis and arthralgia, cardiovascular manifestations
3. Phase three (days 26 to 40): drop in ESR and diminishing signs of illness

C. Therapeutic management

1. Administer aspirin 80 to 100 mg/kg/day as ordered while temperature is elevated
2. Administer intravenous immune globulin (IVIG) as ordered to reduce risk of coronary artery lesions and aneurysms
3. ! Nursing management
   a. Promote comfort
   b. Small, frequent feedings; encourage fluids
   c. Passive range of motion to extremities
   d. Cool baths and gentle oral care
   e. Monitor for complications: aneurysms; side effects of aspirin therapy (bleeding, GI upset); side effects of IVIG therapy (elevated BP, facial flushing, tightness in chest)
   f. Monitor temperature
   g. Monitor eyes for conjunctivitis

D. Child and family education

1. Safe administration of aspirin therapy
2. Keep skin clean and avoid soaps and lotions
3. Offer liquids high in calories, low in acids
4. Low-cholesterol diet
5. Call physician if child refuses to walk
6. Monitor temperature in morning and at night prior to giving aspirin

Check Your NCLEX-RN® Exam I.Q.

You are ready for testing on this content if you can

- Identify basic structures and functions of the cardiovascular system.
- Describe the pathophysiology and etiology of common cardiovascular disorders.
- Discuss expected assessment data and diagnostic test findings for selected cardiovascular disorders.
- Discuss therapeutic management of a client experiencing a cardiovascular disorder.
- Discuss nursing management of a client experiencing a cardiovascular disorder.
- Identify expected outcomes for the client experiencing a cardiovascular disorder.

PRACTICE TEST

1 The nurse has admitted a client to the emergency room with complaints of chest pain over the previous 2 hours. There are no clear changes on the 12-lead ECG. The nurse would expect which laboratory test to provide confirmation of a myocardial infarction (MI)?

1. Potassium of 5.2 mEq/L
2. Creatinine kinase (CK) of 545 with MB of 4%
3. CK of 320 with MB of 12%
4. WBC of 11,400/mm^3

2 The nurse is preparing to discharge a client after CABG surgery. The client is taking several new medications, including digoxin (Lanoxin), metoprolol (Lopressor), and furosemide (Lasix). The client complains of nausea and anorexia. The nurse is preparing to report this finding to the physician before discharging the client. Which laboratory result will the nurse check before calling the physician?

1. Potassium level
2. Sodium level
3. PT/INR
4. Digoxin level

3 The registered nurse has finished reviewing the 7:00 a.m. shift report on a telemetry unit. Which of the following clients would be the best for the RN to assign to the licensed practical nurse?

1. A 7-day postoperative CABG client with an infection in the sternal surgical incision, requiring dressings and irrigation
2. A client who has just arrived on the unit from the emergency room for observation to rule out a myocardial infarction
3. A client who has had successful valve replacement therapy and will be discharged this morning
4. A client who is scheduled for a percutaneous transluminal coronary angioplasty (PTCA) at 10:00 a.m.

4 The nurse is caring for a client with a history of hypertension. The client is being treated with metoprolol (Lopressor), hydrochlorothiazide (Hydrodiuril), and captopril (Capoten). The client has a blood pressure of 120/80 mmHg and a pulse rate of 48. Which of the following is the best action by the nurse?

1. Administer the metoprolol (Lopressor) and the hydrochlorothiazide (HydroDiuril), hold the captopril (Capoten), and notify the physician.
2. Administer the captopril (Capoten) and the hydrochlorothiazide (HydroDiuril), hold the metoprolol (Lopressor), and notify the physician.
3. Administer all the medications and notify the physician.
4. Withhold all the medications and notify the physician.

5 The nurse has finished reviewing the shift report on a cardiac unit. The nurse should plan to see which of the following assigned clients first?

1. A client with hypertrophic cardiomyopathy who is reporting dyspnea
2. A client who had a cardiac catheterization and will be ambulating for the first time
3. A client receiving antibiotics for bacterial endocarditis who is reporting anxiety and chest pain
4. A client who is recovering from coronary artery bypass grafting (CABG) surgery with a temperature of 101°F

6 The nurse is discharging a client to home with a new diagnosis of atrial fibrillation. The nurse explains that which of the following is the most important symptom to report to the physician?

1. Irregular pulse
2. Fever
3. Fatigue
4. Hemoptysis

7 The nurse is caring for a client with a history of renal failure and a new myocardial infarction. The nurse who is reviewing laboratory findings would call the doctor to report which of the following results?

1. Potassium level of 5.0 mEq/L
2. Sodium level of 145 mEq/L
3. Calcium level of 7.0 mg/dL
4. Digoxin/digitalis level of 0.8 ng/mL

8 The nurse is caring for a client who had a permanent pacemaker inserted because of a complete heart block. The nurse determines that which of the following client outcomes indicates a successful procedure?

1. Client ambulating in the hall within 4 hours of the procedure without dyspnea or chest pain
2. Client's ECG monitor demonstrates normal sinus rhythm
3. Heart rate of 80 beats per minute, blood pressure 120 systolic, and 80 diastolic
4. Client's ECG monitor shows paced beats at the rate of 68 per minute

9 The nurse is caring for a client with a diagnosis of aortic stenosis. The client reports episodes of angina and passing out recently at home. The client has surgery scheduled in 2 weeks. Which of the following would be the nurse's best explanation about activity at this time?

1. "It is best to avoid strenuous exercise, stairs, and lifting before your surgery."
2. "Take short walks three times daily to prepare for postoperative rehabilitation."
3. "There are no activity restrictions unless the angina reoccurs; then please call the office."
4. "Gradually increase activity before surgery to build stamina for the postoperative period."

10 The nurse is caring for a client who has just undergone cardiac angiography. The catheter insertion site is free from bleeding or signs of hematoma. The vital signs and distal pulses remain in the client's normal range. The intravenous fluids were discontinued. The client is not hungry or thirsty and refuses any food or fluids, asking to be left alone to rest. Which of the following is the nurse's best response?

1. "You are recovering well from the procedure and resting is a good idea."
2. "It is important for you to walk, so I will be back in 1 hour to walk with you."
3. "It is important to drink fluids after this procedure, to protect your kidney function. I will bring you a pitcher of water, and I encourage you to drink."
4. "You will need to do the leg exercises that you practiced before the procedure to keep good circulation to your legs. After your exercises, you can rest."

11 A client undergoes ligation of varicose veins. The nurse includes in the plan of care which of the following important interventions for the nursing diagnosis of ineffective tissue perfusion?

1. Teach client to remove compression stockings for at least 1 hour per day.
2. Teach client to flex lower extremities four times a day.
3. Teach client that numbness is common after vein ligation.
4. Encourage client to briskly scrub lower extremities to improve circulation.

12 A client's angiogram demonstrates the final stage of atherosclerosis. The nurse concludes that this client's pathophysiology includes which of the following elements?

1. The presence of atheromas
2. Fatty deposits in the intima
3. Lipoprotein accumulation in the intima
4. Inflammation of the arterial wall

13 When assessing a client with peripheral arterial disease, the nurse assesses the client for which of the following signs and symptoms that would be consistent with tissue ischemia?

1. Peripheral edema
2. Widened pulse pressure
3. Leg pain while walking
4. Brownish discoloration to the skin on the leg

14 In providing community education on prevention of peripheral arterial disease, the nurse is careful to include which of the following as a major risk factor?

1. Dysrhythmias
2. Low-protein intake
3. Exposure to cool weather
4. Cigarette smoking

15 When teaching a client with an aneurysm what signs and symptoms may indicate impending rupture, the nurse considers which of the following?

1. Medication therapy the client is receiving
2. Client's usual blood pressure
3. Age and gender of the client
4. Size and location of the aneurysm

16 An important outcome of care for a female client with hypertension has been met when the client is able to do which of the following?

1. Return to her usual activities of daily living
2. Identify actions to counteract two of her modifiable risk factors
3. Lower her blood pressure by 10%
4. Discontinue lifestyle modifications

17 Which of the following suggestions should the nurse include when conducting health teaching for clients with arterial insufficiency?

1. Avoid long periods of sitting and standing.
2. Keep the legs and feet in a raised position.
3. Decrease ambulation to decrease pain.
4. Apply moist heat twice a day.

18 A client with endocarditis develops sudden leg pain with pallor, tingling, and a loss of peripheral pulses. The nurse's initial action should be to

1. Elevate the leg above the level of the heart.
2. Wrap the leg in a loose blanket.
3. Notify the physician about the findings.
4. Perform passive ROM exercise to stimulate circulation.

19 In coordinating care for a client with venous stasis ulcers, the nurse explains to unlicensed assistive personnel that which of the following is the most important intervention in ulcer healing?

1. Surgical debridement
2. Meticulous cleaning of the ulcers to prevent infection
3. Performance of leg exercises to increase collateral circulation
4. Elevation of the extremities to increase venous return

20 Which of the following clients is most at risk for developing a deep-vein thrombosis?

1. A 30-year-old client who is 1 week postpartum
2. A 63-year-old client post-CVA on anticoagulant therapy
3. A 40-year-old woman who smokes and uses oral contraceptives
4. A 41-year-old female who underwent laparoscopic cholecystectomy

21 The nurse is caring for a 2-month-old child with transposition of the great vessels. Which of these interventions has highest priority?

1. Providing comfort for parents
2. Maintaining proper caloric intake
3. Reducing stressors for infant
4. Documenting vital signs

22 During the acute phase of rheumatic fever, which of the following is a priority action of the nurse?

1. Encourage ambulation at least four times per day.
2. Assess for early signs of endocarditis.
3. Maintain hydration by encouraging sips of water.
4. Manage pain with strong narcotic analgesics.

23 A 6-year-old child has been diagnosed with coarctation of the aorta. Lately, he has been complaining when he comes in from recess. The health nurse should question the child about which of the following?

1. Weakness and pain in legs
2. Blurred vision
3. Increased respiratory rate
4. Bruises on shins

24 A toddler with Kawasaki's disease is going home on salicylate (aspirin) therapy. Which is the priority teaching at the time of discharge?

1. Monitor the child for gastrointestinal bleeding.
2. Avoid contact with other children.
3. Report complaints of tingling extremities.
4. Maintain a low-calorie diet.

25 A toddler requires supplemental oxygen therapy for a cyanotic heart defect. In planning for home care, the nurse would discuss which of the following with the parents?

1. The need to maintain the child on bedrest
2. Means of promoting mobility while meeting the need for supplemental oxygen
3. Symptoms of oxygen toxicity
4. How to draw blood for blood gases

PRACTICE TEST

26 The nurse would assess for which of the following manifestations in a client with suspected arterial embolism to the left hand? Select all that apply.

1. Pain
2. Pale skin
3. Bounding radial pulse
4. Parasthesias
5. Pitting edema

ANSWERS & RATIONALES

ANSWERS & RATIONALES

1 **Answer: 2** A CK level above 150 with over 5% MB isoenzyme indicates myocardial damage from acute myocardial infarction. Elevated potassium is not indicative of myocardial infarction. Elevated WBC is an indicator of many conditions, including MI.
Cognitive Level: Analysis **Client Need:** Physiological Integrity: Physiological Adaptation **Integrated Process:** Nursing Process: Assessment **Content Area:** Adult Health: Cardiovascular **Strategy:** The core issue of the question is the ability to correlate indicators of myocardial damage with a client situation. Evaluate each option carefully, and use nursing knowledge and the process of elimination to make a selection.

2 **Answer: 4** Nausea and anorexia are signs of digitalis toxicity. The other laboratory values would not explain the client's symptoms and therefore are not priorities to assess before telephoning the physician.
Cognitive Level: Application **Client Need:** Physiological Integrity: Physiological Adaptation **Integrated Process:** Nursing Process: Analysis **Content Area:** Adult Health: Cardiovascular **Strategy:** The core issue of the question is the ability to correlate early signs of digoxin toxicity with a need to check digoxin level in a client with cardiac disease. Evaluate each option carefully, and use nursing knowledge and the process of elimination to make a selection.

3 **Answer: 1** A stable client with complex dressings is an appropriate assignment for a LPN because the task is appropriate for an LPN. Initial assessment (new admission from the ED), the assessment of a client before and after a complex procedure (PTCA), and discharge teaching are all responsibilities of the professional registered nurse and may not be delegated to the LPN.
Cognitive Level: Analysis **Client Need:** Safe Effective Care Environment: Management of Care **Integrated Process:** Nursing Process: Analysis **Content Area:** Adult Health: Cardiovascular **Strategy:** Evaluate each option carefully, and use nursing knowledge and the process of elimination to make a selection.

4 **Answer: 2** The client's heart rate is bradycardic, and metoprolol, a beta-blocker, decreases the heart rate. Neither the captopril nor the hydrochlorothiazide lower the heart rate, and either may be safely administered to maintain control of the hypertension. When a dose of medication is withheld, it is the responsibility of the nurse to notify the physician of the action and rationale.
Cognitive Level: Analysis **Client Need:** Physiological Integrity: Physiological Adaptation **Integrated Process:** Nursing Process: Planning **Content Area:** Adult Health: Cardiovascular **Strategy:** The core issue of the question is determining which medication is responsible for the adverse effect on client status and acting accordingly. Evaluate each option carefully, and use nursing knowledge and the process of elimination to make a selection.

5 **Answer: 3** A client with endocarditis is at risk for thrombus formation, and chest pain and anxiety are signs of pulmonary embolism (PE), which is a life-threatening complication requiring immediate attention. Dyspnea is a chronic symptom with hypertrophic cardiomyopathy, which requires assessment; a temperature of 101°F requires additional assessment, and a client who is ambulating for the first time will be assessed by the nurse. However, the client who needs to be assessed for PE is the most emergent.
Cognitive Level: Analysis **Client Need:** Safe Effective Care Environment: Management of Care **Integrated Process:** Nursing Process: Planning **Content Area:** Adult Health: Cardiovascular **Strategy:** The key to determining the answer to priority-setting questions is to evaluate which client is most unstable or has the greatest risk for developing a complication. Evaluate each option carefully using these methods, and use nursing knowledge and the process of elimination to make a selection.

6 **Answer: 4** A serious complication of atrial fibrillation is pulmonary embolism. Chest pain and hemoptysis are common symptoms of pulmonary embolism. Irregular pulse is expected with atrial fibrillation. Fatigue may accompany atrial fibrillation in some individuals. Fever is not associated with atrial fibrillation and is not necessarily included in discharge teaching. However, it could be a sign of illness that could increase the workload of the heart, and therefore it would be the second-most important item to report if it occurred.
Cognitive Level: Analysis **Client Need:** Physiological Integrity: Physiological Adaptation **Integrated Process:** Nursing Process: Implementation **Content Area:** Adult Health: Cardiovascular **Strategy:** The core issue of the question is knowledge of signs and symptoms of complications to report to the physician in the presence of atrial fibrillation. Evaluate each option carefully, and use nursing knowledge and the process of elimination to make a selection.

7 **Answer: 3** Renal failure is a common cause of hypocalcemia, and a value of 7.0 mg/dL is below the normal range of serum calcium. Options 1 and 2 are within the upper limits for potassium and sodium, and option 4 is within the therapeutic range of digoxin.
Cognitive Level: Application **Client Need:** Physiological Integrity: Physiological Adaptation **Integrated Process:** Nursing Process: Implementation **Content Area:** Adult Health: Cardiovascular **Strategy:** The core issue of the question is knowledge of normal and abnormal values that are important to report in a client with an acute cardiac problem and a history of renal failure. The best strategy in questions such as these is to pick

the value with the most abnormal number and/or one that relates to the underlying disorder(s).

8 **Answer: 4** The client is not allowed to ambulate for 24 hours to prevent dislodging of the electrodes. Normal sinus rhythm, heart rate of 80, and a BP of 120 over 80 do not reflect pacemaker function. Paced beats indicate that the pacemaker is functioning.
Cognitive Level: Application **Client Need:** Physiological Integrity: Physiological Adaptation **Integrated Process:** Nursing Process: Evaluation **Content Area:** Adult Health: Cardiovascular **Strategy:** Evaluate each option carefully, and use nursing knowledge and the process of elimination to make a selection.

9 **Answer: 1** Symptomatic aortic stenosis has a poor prognosis without surgery. Restricting activity limits myocardial oxygen consumption. Since the incidence of sudden death is high in this population, it is prudent to decrease the strain on the heart while awaiting surgery.
Cognitive Level: Analysis **Client Need:** Physiological Integrity: Physiological Adaptation **Integrated Process:** Nursing Process: Implementation **Content Area:** Adult Health: Cardiovascular **Strategy:** The core issue of the question is the level of activity that will minimize the client's risk of complications or sudden death until surgery. Evaluate each option carefully, and use nursing knowledge and the process of elimination to make a selection.

10 **Answer: 3** The dye used in angiography is nephrotoxic, and a client should have adequate fluids after the procedure to eliminate the dye. The client should lie with the affected leg extended for 6 to 8 hours. Leg exercises are not recommended because exercise could disrupt the clot that formed at the insertion site. Option 1 is incorrect because it gives false reassurance to a client who could be at risk if fluids are not taken in.
Cognitive Level: Analysis **Client Need:** Physiological Integrity: Physiological Adaptation **Integrated Process:** Communication and Documentation **Content Area:** Adult Health: Cardiovascular **Strategy:** The core issue of the question is knowledge of the correlation between lack of fluid intake and risk of kidney complications following angiography. Evaluate each option carefully, and use nursing knowledge and the process of elimination to make a selection.

11 **Answer: 1** Compression stockings exert pressure on the veins of the lower extremities, promoting venous return back to the heart. Stockings are removed for at least an hour per day to allow for inspection and ensure blood flow through small, superficial vessels. Flexing the extremities does not aid tissue perfusion, although it maintains joint range of motion. However, after this surgery clients are taught to either stand or lie down and avoid flexing at the hip and knee. Numbness is a temporary or rarely permanent complication of surgery. Briskly scrubbing the extremities will not aid tissue perfusion.
Cognitive Level: Application **Client Need:** Physiological Integrity: Physiological Adaptation **Integrated Process:** Nursing Process: Planning **Content Area:** Adult Health: Cardiovascular **Strategy:** The core issue of the question is a measure that will improve tissue perfusion for a client following vein ligation. Using principles of blood flow, choose the option that will aid circulation. Evaluate each option carefully, and use nursing knowledge and the process of elimination to make a selection.

12 **Answer: 1** The final stage of the atherosclerotic process is the development of atheromas, which are complex lesions consisting of lipids, fibrous tissue, collagen, calcium, cellular waste, and capillaries. The calcified lesions may rupture or ulcerate, stimulating thrombosis. The other options are not consistent with the ultimate or final changes in the atherosclerotic process.
Cognitive Level: Application **Client Need:** Physiological Integrity: Physiological Adaptation **Integrated Process:** Nursing Process: Analysis **Content Area:** Adult Health: Cardiovascular **Strategy:** Note the critical words *final stage.* Evaluate each option carefully, and use knowledge of pathophysiology and the process of elimination to make a selection.

13 **Answer: 3** Leg pain (also called intermittent claudication) is a primary manifestation of peripheral arterial disease. Intermittent claudication is muscle pain caused by interruption in arterial flow, resulting in tissue hypoxia. Peripheral edema and brownish discoloration to the skin on the leg would be consistent with venous disease, not arterial disease. Widened pulse pressure would be an unrelated finding.
Cognitive Level: Application **Client Need:** Physiological Integrity: Physiological Adaptation **Integrated Process:** Nursing Process: Assessment **Content Area:** Adult Health: Cardiovascular **Strategy:** The critical words in the question are *peripheral arterial disease,* which direct you to look for manifestations that are abnormal and that are consistent with arterial but not venous disease. Evaluate each option carefully, and use nursing knowledge and the process of elimination to make a selection.

14 **Answer: 4** Nicotine in cigarettes promotes vasoconstriction. The three most significant risk factors for development of peripheral arterial disease are smoking, hyperlipidemia, and hypertension. The presence of dysrhythmias, low-protein intake, and exposure to cool weather are not risk factors for the disease, although cool weather could worsen the symptoms when disease is already present.
Cognitive Level: Application **Client Need:** Physiological Integrity: Physiological Adaptation **Integrated Process:** Teaching and Learning **Content Area:** Adult Health: Cardiovascular **Strategy:** Note the critical word *prevention* to focus on the option that contains information that will affect the likelihood of whether the client will develop peripheral arterial disease. Evaluate each option carefully, using nursing knowledge and the process of elimination to make a selection.

15 **Answer: 4** Aneurysms vary by size and location. Signs of rupture depend on the location of the aneurysm. Dissection can occur anywhere but most often occurs in the ascending aorta where pressure is the highest. The medication the client is receiving is vague and is not directly related. The blood pressure relates to whether the aneurysm may rupture, not to the associated signs and symptoms. The age and gender of the client are unrelated to the size and symptoms of aneurysm rupture.
Cognitive Level: Analysis **Client Need:** Physiological Integrity: Physiological Adaptation **Integrated Process:** Nursing Process: Analysis **Content Area:** Adult Health: Cardiovascular **Strategy:** With the critical words *signs and symptoms* in mind, choose the option that most directly relates to the core issue of the question. Evaluate each option carefully, and choose

option 4 as the only one that could affect the specific list of signs and symptoms that the nurse would teach related to aneurysm rupture.

16 **Answer: 2** An important outcome in care of the hypertensive client is the ability to identify and counteract personal risk factors that the client has the ability to change. Modifiable risk factors for hypertension include smoking, hypercholesterolemia, diabetes mellitus, sedentary lifestyle, obesity, stress, and alcohol use. Option 1 is not likely to be an issue. Option 3 may or may not be sufficient. Option 4 is contraindicated.
Cognitive Level: Application **Client Need:** Physiological Integrity: Physiological Adaptation **Integrated Process:** Nursing Process: Evaluation **Content Area:** Adult Health: Cardiovascular **Strategy:** The core issue of the question is the ability to identify an indicator that is a positive effect of care for the hypertensive client. Evaluate each option carefully, and use nursing knowledge and the process of elimination to make a selection.

17 **Answer: 1** The client should avoid long periods of standing or sitting to promote adequate blood flow. The legs and feet should be below heart level to increase peripheral circulation. Regular exercise enhances development of collateral circulation, increases vascular return, and is recommended for clients with either arterial or venous insufficiency. Moist heat is helpful for venous problems.
Cognitive Level: Application **Client Need:** Physiological Integrity: Physiological Adaptation **Integrated Process:** Nursing Process: Implementation **Content Area:** Adult Health: Cardiovascular **Strategy:** A critical word in the stem of the question is *arterial,* which tells you that the correct answer is an option that is beneficial to the client with impaired circulation to the legs. Choose option 1 over the others because it is a generally helpful measure to increase circulation, while options 2 and 4 are helpful with venous problems. Option 3 does not help either arterial or venous circulatory problems.

18 **Answer: 2** The client is exhibiting symptoms of acute arterial occlusion. Without immediate intervention, ischemia and necrosis will result within hours. The nurse should first wrap the leg to maintain warmth and protect it from further injury, and should then quickly notify the physician. The leg should not be elevated above heart level because doing so would worsen the tissue ischemia, and passive range of motion will also increase ischemia by increasing tissue demand for oxygen.
Cognitive Level: Analysis **Client Need:** Physiological Integrity: Physiological Adaptation **Integrated Process:** Nursing Process: Implementation **Content Area:** Adult Health: Cardiovascular **Strategy:** The core issue of the question is recognizing the complication of acute arterial occlusion and then determining which action should be taken first. Choose an option that is client-focused rather than physician-notification focused, if one is available. In this case, the nurse can protect the client from further injury with option 2.

19 **Answer: 4** The client with venous ulcers must keep the legs elevated above the level of the heart as much as possible. Elevation of the extremities enhances venous return and improves circulation, providing oxygen and nutrients to the lower extremities. The client with a leg ulcer should avoid exercise to prevent further damage to tissues at risk. Option 1 may or may not be indicated. Asepsis is important, but no ulcer will heal unless the edema and stagnant tissue metabolites can be reduced through leg elevation.
Cognitive Level: Analysis **Client Need:** Physiological Integrity: Physiological Adaptation **Integrated Process:** Nursing Process: Planning **Content Area:** Adult Health: Cardiovascular **Strategy:** The critical words in the stem of the question are *most important intervention,* indicating that more than one option, or all options, may be correct, but one is better than the others. Look at the question carefully and note that the nurse is talking to an ancillary caregiver. Consider that the correct option is one that is within the scope of practice of that caregiver in making a selection.

20 **Answer: 3** A major risk factor for formation of thrombophlebitis is oral contraceptive use in women who smoke. Being 1-week postpartum does not place a client at risk since mobility is usually restored. Anticoagulant therapy is used to prevent development of thrombi. Laparoscopic surgical procedures are associated with more rapid recovery times with reduced immobility, keeping this client at lower risk than the client in option 3.
Cognitive Level: Application **Client Need:** Physiological Integrity: Physiological Adaptation **Integrated Process:** Nursing Process: Assessment **Content Area:** Adult Health: Cardiovascular **Strategy:** The critical words in the stem of the question are *most at risk,* telling you that the correct option is the one that contains the most severe or greatest number of risk factors for thrombophlebitis. With this in mind, evaluate each option and use the process of elimination to make a selection.

21 **Answer: 3** The open ductus arteriosus will allow a small amount of mixing of oxygenated and unoxygenated blood. Stress will increase the cardiac workload and therefore is a priority for the nurse to avoid. Maintaining caloric intake and comfort are the next priorities using Maslow's hierarchy. Documenting vital signs is a routine activity and not a priority when compared to actual care activities.
Cognitive Level: Analysis **Client Need:** Physiological Integrity: Physiological Adaptation **Integrated Process:** Nursing Process: Planning **Content Area:** Child Health: Cardiovascular **Strategy:** Use Maslow's hierarchy of needs to review each option and choose the one that most closely relates to the ABCs and thus cardiac workload. Use this knowledge and the process of elimination to make a selection.

22 **Answer: 2** The main complication of rheumatic fever is carditis. The nurse must assess for early signs of bacterial endocarditis. The client should be encouraged to rest during the acute phase, and hydration needs may not be sufficiently met with sips of water. Narcotic analgesics may not be necessary, although NSAIDs are likely to be ordered.
Cognitive Level: Application **Client Need:** Physiological Integrity: Physiological Adaptation **Integrated Process:** Nursing Process: Planning **Content Area:** Child Health: Cardiovascular **Strategy:** The core issue of the question is the ability to set priorities for a client with rheumatic fever. Omit option 1 because of the words *at least,* knowing that rest is encouraged. Likewise, eliminate option 3 because of the word *sips.* Choose option 2 over 4 knowing that NSAIDs are likely to be effective in managing pain and inflammation from rheumatic fever.

23 **Answer: 1** Decreased circulation to lower extremities would contribute to muscle fatigue and pain in the legs. Many of the children returning from recess will have increased respiratory rate secondary to play activities. Blurred vision and bruises are not related to coarctation.
Cognitive Level: Application **Client Need:** Physiological Integrity: Physiological Adaptation **Integrated Process:** Nursing Process: Assessment **Content Area:** Child Health: Cardiovascular **Strategy:** The core issue of the question is knowledge of signs of exercise intolerance in a 6-year-old client with a cyanotic heart defect. Use principles of gas exchange and knowledge of normal and abnormal findings after exercise to make a selection.

24 **Answer: 1** Salicylates prevent platelet agglutination. Gastrointestinal bleeding is often a side effect of aspirin therapy. It is not necessary to avoid other children. Tingling of extremities is not a concern, although ringing in the ears could be a sign of salicylate toxicity. A low-calorie diet is not indicated.
Cognitive Level: Application **Client Need:** Physiological Integrity: Pharmacological and Parenteral Therapies **Integrated Process:** Nursing Process: Implementation **Content Area:** Child Health: Cardiovascular **Strategy:** The core issue of the question is knowledge of adverse drug effects of salicylate therapy for the child with Kawasaki's disease. Use this knowledge and the process of elimination to make a selection.

25 **Answer: 2** Allowing mobility is helpful to promote growth and development in the toddler. Strategies should be discussed to promote mobility while maintaining the supplemental oxygen. Options 1 and 4 are unnecessary. Signs of oxygen toxicity are not the priority based on the information in the question.
Cognitive Level: Application **Client Need:** Physiological Integrity: Physiological Adaptation **Integrated Process:** Nursing Process: Planning **Content Area:** Child Health: Cardiovascular **Strategy:** The core issue of the question is home care needs of a toddler receiving oxygen therapy. Use principles of needs related to normal growth and development to help select the correct option.

26 **Answer: 1, 2, 4** The client would exhibit pain, pallor of the affected skin, diminished or absent radial pulse, parasthesias (altered local sensation), paralysis (weakness or inability to move extremity), and poikilothermia (cooler temperature). The client would not have a bounding radial pulse (opposite finding is true) or pitting edema, indicating a fluid volume excess or heart failure.
Cognitive Level: Analysis **Client Need:** Physiological Integrity: Physiological Adaptation **Integrated Process:** Nursing Process: Assessment **Content Area:** Adult Health: Cardiovascular **Strategy:** The core issue of the question is knowledge of assessment findings in arterial embolism. Visualize a clot in the local circulation and use that image to determine the effect of the blockage on circulation to the affected area.

ANSWERS & RATIONALES

Key Terms to Review

acyanotic heart defect p. 1063
afterload p. 1040
angina pectoris p. 1049
atherosclerosis p. 1057
cardiac output (CO) p. 1039
contractility p. 1040
coronary artery disease p. 1049
cor pulmonale p. 1051
cyanotic heart defect p. 1066
ejection fraction (EF) p. 1042
endarterectomy p. 1058
Homan's sign p. 1062
infarction p. 1041
intermittent claudication p. 1057
ischemia p. 1042
Jones criteria p. 1069
jugular venous distention (JVD) p. 1051
left-to-right shunt p. 1064
lymphadenopathy p. 1070
murmur p. 1053
neurovascular status p. 1058
orthostatic hypotension p. 1057
poikilothermia p. 1059
polycythemia p. 1067
preload p. 1040
prostaglandin E1 p. 1067
pulmonary edema p. 1051
regurgitation p. 1053
rest pain p. 1057
right-to-left shunt p. 1066
stenosis p. 1053
stroke volume (SV) p. 1039
sympathectomy p. 1060
tamponade p. 1056
vasculitis p. 1070
vasodilation p. 1040

References

Ball, J., & Bindler, R. (2006). *Child health nursing: Partnering with children and families*. Upper Saddle River, NJ: Pearson Education.

Black, J., & Hawks, J. (2005). *Medical surgical nursing: Clinical management for positive outcomes* (7th ed.). St. Louis: Elsevier Science.

Corbett, J. (2004). *Laboratory tests and diagnostic procedures with nursing diagnoses* (6th ed.). Upper Saddle River, NJ: Pearson Education.

Harkreader, H., & Hogan, M. (2004). *Fundamentals of nursing: Caring and clinical judgment* (2nd ed.). St. Louis: Elsevier Science.

Hockenberry, M., Wilson, D., Winkelstein, M., & Kline, N. (2003). *Nursing care of infants and children* (7th ed.). St. Louis: Mosby.

Ignatavicius, D., & Workman, L. (2006). *Medical-surgical nursing: Critical thinking for collaborative care* (5th ed.). Philadelphia: W. B. Saunders.

Kozier, B., Erb, G., Berman, A., & Snyder, S. (2004). *Fundamentals of nursing: Concepts, process, and practice* (7th ed.). Upper Saddle River, NJ: Pearson Education.

LeMone, P., & Burke, K. (2004). *Medical surgical nursing: Critical thinking in client care* (3rd ed.). Upper Saddle River, NJ: Pearson Education.

Lewis, S., Heitkemper, M., & Dirksen, S. (2004). *Medical surgical nursing: Assessment and management of clinical problems* (6th ed.). St. Louis: Elsevier Science.

Porth, C. (2004). *Pathophysiology: Concepts of altered health states* (7th ed.). Philadelphia: Lippincott Williams & Wilkins.

Smeltzer, S., Bare, B., & Boyer, M. (2007). *Brunner & Suddarth's textbook of medical surgical nursing* (11th ed.). Philadelphia: Lippincott Williams & Wilkins.

Smith, S., Duell, D., & Martin, B. (2004). *Clinical nursing skills: Basic to advanced skills* (6th ed.). Upper Saddle River, NJ: Pearson Education.

58 Neurological Disorders

Test Yourself

Are you ready for the NCLEX-RN® or course exams? Use the practice tests on the companion CD-ROM to check.

In this chapter

Cross reference

Other chapters relevant to this content area are

I. OVERVIEW OF ANATOMY AND PHYSIOLOGY OF THE NERVOUS SYSTEM

A. Cells in nervous system (NS)

1. Neurons: basic anatomical and functional units in NS; have 3 parts: cell body, axon, and dendrites; nerve cells are separated by a synaptic cleft; neurotransmitters are secreted into cleft by one neuron to stimulate dendrites of another neuron and conduct nerve impulses
2. Glial cells: structures of NS that nourish, support, and protect brain neurons; 4 main types of glial cells in brain are astrocytes, oligodendrocytes, ependymal cells, and microglia; Schwann cells are in peripheral nervous system (PNS)

B. Central nervous system (CNS)

1. Consists of cerebrum, cerebellum, brain stem, and spinal cord
2. Cerebrum, largest division of brain, enables individuals to reason, function intellectually, express personality and mood, and interact with environment
   a. Includes two hemispheres, each divided into a frontal lobe, temporal lobe, parietal lobe, and occipital lobe; each lobe has specific functions
   b. Right hemisphere generally controls left side of body and left controls right side of body; usually one hemisphere is considered dominant
   c. Frontal lobe performs high-level cognitive function, has memory storage, influences somatic motor control, controls voluntary eye movements, and controls motor aspect of speech in **Broca's area,** located in dominant hemisphere (usually left)
   d. Temporal lobe has primary auditory receptive areas and auditory association area (**Wernicke's area**), which is usually found on dominant side and is responsible for interpreting speech; interpretive area integrates somatic, auditory, and visual data (this impacts perception, learning, memory, emotions, and intellectual abilities)
   e. Parietal lobe holds primary sensory cortex and sensory association areas that define and localize sensations such as size, shape, weight, texture, and consistency; also processes visual–spatial information and controls spatial orientation
   f. Occipital lobe is visual center for eyes; controls eye reflexes and interpretation of sight
3. Diencephalons and hypophysis of brain have many functions, including temperature control, water metabolism, pituitary secretion, visceral and somatic activities, visible physical expressions in response to emotions, sleep–wake cycle, and hunger
4. Cerebellum is a double-lobed area posterior to pons responsible for muscle synergy and coordination and maintains balance through feedback loops
5. Brainstem is an integration system that also controls basic functions; has 3 major divisions: the midbrain, pons, and medulla; reticular activating system (RAS) is responsible for alertness; substantia nigra is affected in Parkinson's disease; most cranial nerves originate in brainstem
6. The spinal cord is an elongated mass of nerve tissue that runs most of length of vertebral column
   a. Divided into four areas: cervical area (C1 to C7) near neck; thoracic area (T1 to T12) near chest; lumbar area (L1 to L5) near lower back; sacral area (S1 to S4) is in sacrum
   b. Sensory tracts (dorsal roots) carry afferent impulses from periphery to dorsal root ganglia where they are sent to brain; general somatic afferent fibers carry pain, temperature, touch, and proprioception from body wall, tendons, and joints; general visceral fibers carry sensory input from body organs
   c. Motor tracts (ventral roots) convey efferent impulses from spinal cord to somatic fibers that innervate voluntary striated muscle, smooth muscle, cardiac muscle, and that regulate glandular secretions

C. The PNS

1. Consists of 31 pairs of spinal nerves, 12 pairs of cranial nerves, and autonomic NS divided into sympathetic and parasympathetic NS

2. Each pair of spinal nerves has dorsal and ganglion roots that exit spinal cord via an intervertebral foramina; they carry input between specific areas called dermatomes and spine
3. Cranial nerves (CN): 12 pairs arise from brain; there are three pure sensory nerves, five pure motor nerves, and four mixed (sensory and motor) nerves; olfactory nerve (CN I) and optic nerve (CN II) arise from cerebrum; CN III and IV arise in midbrain; CN V through VIII arise in pons; CN IX to XII arise in medulla (see Table 58–1 ■ for an overview of cranial nerves)
4. Autonomic NS: a collection of motor nerves that regulate activities of viscera, smooth muscles, and glands to maintain a stable internal environment; two parts of system (sympathetic and parasympathetic) work antagonistically
   a. Sympathetic nervous system (SNS) is active during times of stress, such as flight-or-fight response; it increases heart rate (HR) and blood pressure (BP) and vasoconstricts the peripheral blood vessels (BVs)
   b. Parasympathetic nervous system is a conservation, restoration, and maintenance system; it decreases HR and increases gastrointestinal (GI) activity

D. Blood supply

1. Brain is unique in that it can only use glucose for energy; a lack of glucose for 5 minutes results in irreversible brain damage; brain receives 750 mL/min of blood or 15% to 20% of resting cardiac output
2. Cerebral arteries are thinner, have more internal elasticity and less smooth muscle than arteries elsewhere in body; brain is supplied with blood by two sets of arteries: anterior and posterior circulation
   a. Anterior circulation, fed by internal and external carotids, delivers blood to a central area at base of cerebrum called circle of Willis; from there it feeds anterior cerebrum via anterior cerebral artery, middle of cerebrum via middle cerebral artery, and posterior cerebrum via posterior cerebral artery
   b. Posterior circulation, fed by vertebral arteries, delivers blood to posterior fossa; at bottom of posterior fossa, blood flows together into one basilar artery and delivers it to cerebellum, midbrain, pons, and medulla
   c. Meninges are supplied with blood from branches of external carotid arteries that ascend into brain at base of skull
3. Venous system of brain is unique
   a. Vessel walls are thinner than other veins of body; do not follow path of arteries but instead follow their own course
   b. There are no valves in brain's venous system and therefore drainage depends on venous pressure and gravity
   c. Dural sinuses collect blood from brain and empty it into jugular veins

Table 58–1
Overview of Cranial Nerves

Cranial Nerve Name	Type of Nerve	Physiological Functions
Olfactory (I)	Sensory	Ability to smell
Optic (II)	Sensory	Visual fields, visual acuity
Oculomotor (III)	Motor	Extraocular movements (EOM)
Trochlear (IV)	Motor	EOM
Trigeminal (V)	Mixed	Movement of eyelids, ability to clench jaw
Abducens (VI)	Motor	EOM
Facial (VII)	Mixed	Movement of eyelids, facial symmetry
Acoustic (VIII)	Sensory	Hearing ability
Glossopharyngeal (IX)	Mixed	Gag, swallow, and cough reflexes; voice quality
Vagus (X)	Mixed	Gag, swallow, and cough reflexes; voice quality
Spinal Accessory (XI)	Motor	Neck strength and shoulder shrug
Hypoglossal (XII)	Motor	Tongue movement

E. Blood–brain barrier

1. A network of endothelial cells in wall of capillaries and astrocyte projections in close proximity that do not have pores between them
2. This tight junction does not allow normal nonspecific filtering process that occurs in rest of body; therefore, molecules must enter brain by active transport, endocytosis and exocytosis, which creates a highly selective barrier that guards entrance to neurons
3. Movement of substances across this barrier depends on particle size, lipid solubility, chemical dissociation, and protein-binding potential
4. Barrier is very permeable to water, oxygen (O_2), carbon dioxide (CO_2), other gases, glucose, and lipid soluble compounds

F. Protective structures

1. **Meninges:** covers brain and spinal cord to protect and support; divided into 3 layers from outer to inner (dura mater, arachnoid, and pia mater)
   a. Dura is a tough, membranous tissue that surrounds and extends into the brain tissue
   b. Arachnoid membrane lies below dura and is a network of delicate, elastic tissue that contains BVs of varying sizes
   c. Pia mater is a vascular membrane that covers entire brain with tiny BVs that extend into gray matter of brain
   d. Within meninges, there are important potential spaces (epidural, subdural, subarachnoid) where bleeding can occur
2. Skull: bony structure of head that includes 8 fused cranial bones and 14 facial bones; encloses brain in a protective vault
3. Spine: flexible column that encloses spinal cord, formed from stacking of 7 cervical, 12 thoracic, 5 lumbar, and 4 sacral vertebrae
4. Cerebrospinal fluid (CSF) and ventricular system
   a. CSF is a clear, colorless, odorless solution that fills ventricular system and subarachnoid space of brain and spinal cord; acts as a shock absorber; also has electrolytes, glucose, protein, O_2, and CO_2 dissolved in solution
   b. Ventricular system is composed of two lateral ventricles (one in each hemisphere of cerebrum), a third that lies midline in thalamic area, and a fourth that lies below third, anterior to cerebellum and subarachnoid space

II. DIAGNOSTIC TESTS AND ASSESSMENTS OF THE NERVOUS SYSTEM

A. Assessment of NS

1. Assess circumstances of injury and admission, pertinent family and social history
2. Assess chief complaint: use mnemonic APQRST

Memory Aid

Remember the mnemonic APQRST to trigger recall of all important points to assess whenever a client has an acute onset symptom:
A—any associated symptoms with chief complaint
P—what provokes (makes worse) or palliates (makes better) symptoms
Q—quality of pain
R—region and radiation
S—severity of pain on a scale of 1 to 10
T—timing: when it stops and starts, whether it is intermittent or constant, its duration

3. Health information: including past medical history, current medications, recent surgeries or other treatments, alcohol or illegal drug use
4. Mental status exam
   a. A screening mental status examination includes orientation to person, place, and time; appearance and behavior; mood; speech pattern; and thought and perception including insight, thought, content, and judgment
   b. To conduct this exam, client must be awake, alert, and able to understand and respond to questions

Table 58–2

Terms Used to Describe Level of Consciousness

Term	Description
Full consciousness	Alert; oriented to person, place, and time; and comprehends written and spoken words
Confusion	Disoriented to person, place, and/or time; misinterprets environment; has poor judgment; unable to think clearly
Lethargic	Oriented but slow and sluggish in speech, mental processes, and motor activity
Obtundation	Readily arousable to stimuli; responds with one or two words; can follow simple commands when asked but quickly drifts back to sleep
Stupor	Lies quietly with minimal movement; responds with a groan or eye opening only to vigorous and repeated verbal with tactile stimuli; usually localizes painful stimuli
Coma	Unarousable to stimuli; nonverbal; may exhibit nonpurposeful response to stimuli
Light coma	Unarousable; withdraws nonpurposefully to pain; may decerebrate or decorticate; brainstem reflexes intact
Deep coma	Unarousable; unresponsive to painful stimuli; brainstem reflexes usually absent; decerebrate posturing usually noted
Delirium	Has rapid onset; brief impairment of cognitition including a clouding of consciousness and difficulty sustaining and shifting attention
Dementia	A generalized, long-term decline in cognitive abilities such as memory, language, and clear consciousness

Source: Adapted from LeMone, P., and Burke, M. (2004), *Medical surgical nursing: Critical thinking in client care* (3rd ed.). Upper Saddle River, NJ: Prentice Hall.

- **c.** A client with an altered **level of consciousness (LOC)** may have a range of behaviors; terms used to describe this include confusion, delirium, obtunded, stupor, and coma (unarousable to painful stimuli); see Table 58–2 ■
- **d.** Acute confusion or delirium should be recognized and treated by eliminating the cause; try to avoid confusing delirium with dementia (a chronic problem)

5. Cranial nerves: assessment can be performed as described in Table 58–3 ■; some methods test more than one cranial nerve at a time

6. Motor function
- **a.** Inspect all body muscles for size, tone, movement, and strength
- **b.** Compare left and right side for symmetry and equality
- **c.** Assess for tremors (rhythmic movements) and fasciculations (twitching)
- **d.** Criteria for grading muscle strength (see Box 58–1, p. 1084)

! **7.** Cerebellar examination: balance and coordination are under cerebellar control
- **a.** Gait: have client walk normally and then on heels and toes to assess coordination; perform a Romberg's test by having client stand with feet together and eyes closed while you stand close by to prevent falling; there should be minimal swaying for 20 seconds
- **b.** To assess coordination, observe client's ability to touch own nose and then touch one of your fingers, then his or her nose again; next observe client's ability to touch each finger to thumb of same hand; finally, observe client's ability to run heel down shin on each side while lying in supine position

8. Sensory function
- **a.** Have client close eyes while you touch client on all dermatomes with objects that are sharp, dull, light to touch, and that vibrate (over bony prominence); client should be able to discriminate location and type of touch
- **b.** To assess a client's sense of position (kinesthesia), have client close eyes and move client's finger or toe up or down and ask client to describe movement
- **c.** To assess for stereognosis, have client identify an object in his or her hand with eyes closed

Table 58–3
Cranial Nerve Assessment Tests

Cranial Nerve	Assessment
Cranial nerve I (olfactory)	Assess ability to identify common odors
Cranial nerve II (optic)	Use Snellen chart to assess vision
Cranial nerves III, IV, and VI (oculomotor, trochlear and abducens)	EOM: have client follow finger through cardinal fields of gaze Ptosis (III): a droopy eyelid PEARLA: assess pupils equal and reactive to light and accommodation Nystagmus: pupil movement is choppy Doll's eyes: in the comatose client, doll's eyes is present when eyes stay center while head moves left and right; absent when eyes move with the head
Cranial nerve V (trigeminal)	Jaw clench: palpate the masseter and temporal muscles when the client's jaw is clenched; note differences on left or right Compare light, dull, and sharp sensations on both sides of the face Corneal reflex: on an unconscious client, a wisp of cotton is touched to the cornea; normal response is to blink Lids (V, VII): stroke each lid to elicit a blink response
Cranial nerve VII (facial)	Facial symmetry: note droopiness of nasal labia fold, lower eyelid or corner of mouth when asking client to grin, raise eyebrows, and sniff; assess accuracy of tasting sweet, sour, and salty items on anterior two-thirds of the tongue
Cranial nerve VIII (acoustic)	Assess hearing of each ear with a ticking watch or whispering; cold caloric testing: irrigating ear in ice cold water causes a slow movement of the eyes toward the irrigated side with a rapid return to midline; this is called the oculovestibular reflex and indicates an intact brainstem
Cranial nerves IX and X (glossopharyngeal and vagus)	Swallow reflex: assess whether client can swallow water or has dysphagia (difficulty swallowing) Gag reflex: assess gag by touching the back of both sides of the throat; a unilateral loss may be noted Hoarseness: assess client's voice for hoarseness Cough reflex: assess whether client's cough is strong, weak or absent Assess sweet, salty, and sour taste on the posterior third of the tongue
Cranial nerve XI (spinal accessory)	Neck strength: have client turn head against resistance Shoulder shrug: have client shrug shoulders against resistance
Cranial nerve XII (hypoglossal)	Tongue deviation: have client stick out tongue and move it side to side against resistance; if there is a weakness, the tongue will go to the stronger side

d. To assess for graphesthesia, have client identify a number or letter traced on palm of hand

e. Test two-point discrimination by touching a client with two simultaneous pinpricks and asking how many pinpricks there were; use dull points on a caliper and begin on finger pads

9. Reflexes

a. Deep tendon reflexes (patellar, biceps, brachioradialis, triceps, and Achilles) are assessed with a reflex hammer and scored; see Box 58–2 for scoring criteria

b. Assess superficial abdominal reflex by lightly stroking abdomen from side to midline; normally, side stroked will contract

c. Assess cremasteric reflex by lightly stroking inside of thigh on a male client to raise testicle on that side

d. Assess Babinski reflex by stroking lateral aspect of sole of foot from heel to ball, curving medially in ball; its presence is noted with dorsiflexion of big toe and fanning of other toes; is considered normal in infants but abnormal in adults (normal adult response is curling of toes, called a negative Babinski)

Box 58–1

Criteria for Grading Muscle Strength

0 = No contraction

1 = Trace of contraction

2 = Active movement with gravity

3 = Active movement against gravity

4 = Active movement against gravity and resistance

5 = Normal power

Note: Findings are recorded as a fraction with 5 (highest possible score) as the denominator; for example, normal finding is 5/5.

10. Speech is usually described from interview
    a. Clear: normal, fluent speech
    b. **Dysarthria:** ineffective articulation of speech; may be a motor deficit of tongue and speech muscles
    c. **Aphasia:** a language disorder classified by type
    d. Expressive, motor, or nonfluent aphasia: sometimes called Broca's aphasia; it is an inability to express one's self using motor aspects of speech
    e. Receptive, fluent, or sensory aphasia: sometimes called Wernicke's aphasia; it is an inability to comprehend spoken words
    f. Global aphasia: a client can neither express nor comprehend language (mixed receptive and expressive)
11. Specialized tests for meningeal irritation
    a. **Kernig's sign:** positive or present when client's leg is raised with knee flexed and any resistance or pain is felt; this is a common finding indicating meningeal irritation in meningitis
    b. **Brudzinski's sign:** positive or present when head is flexed while in supine position, resulting in involuntary flexion of knees or hips; commonly found also in meningitis

Memory Aid

Recall that the words *Kernig's* and *knee* both begin with *K,* while *Brudzinski's* and *brain* both begin with *B.* This will aid in recalling how to conduct each test.

B. Diagnostic studies of NS

1. Lumbar puncture: collects CSF for analysis via needle aspiration; CSF is studied; normal CSF is colorless, clear, and without blood or bacteria (white cells 0 to 5 cells/mm^3), glucose 40 to 80 mg/dL, and protein 16 to 45 mg/dL; following lumbar puncture, position head elevated with water-based contrast and flat with oil-based contrast; assess site for leakage of CSF and for signs of infection
2. Cerebral angiography: outlines vascular structure of brain; detects arteriovenous (AV) malformations and/or aneurysms; use standard measures associated with use of contrast media (assess for allergy to iodine or shellfish; encourage fluids following procedure to aid in excretion)
3. Computed tomography (CT): helpful in detecting bleeding, hydrocephalus, and ischemic strokes older than 48 hours; may be done with or without contrast; see precautions noted above

Box 58–2

Standard Criteria for Grading Reflexes

0 = absent or no response

1 = hypoactive; weaker than normal (+)

2 = normal (++)

3 = stronger than normal (+++)

4 = hyperactive (++++)

4. Magnetic resonance imaging (MRI): detects soft tissue changes including necrotic tissue, tumors, edema, congenital disorders, and degenerative diseases; assess client for implanted sources of metal that would contradict use of this procedure
5. Electroencephalography (EEG): diagnostic procedure that measures brain waves with multiple scalp electrodes; patterns of brain waves may suggest epilepsy, herpes simplex, encephalitis, and dementia disorders; EEG is also an important criterion in determining brain death
   a. Teach client that test will not deliver electric shock
   b. Shampoo hair before procedure for cleanliness and after procedure to remove residual electrode gel or paste
   c. Withhold anticonvulsants and other medications as ordered for 12 to 24 hours prior
   d. Have client eat regular meals to avoid hypoglycemia that could affect results
6. Electromyography (EMG) and nerve conduction studies: differentiate between peripheral nerve and muscle disorders; measures conduction velocity of muscles between two points and measurements are recorded at rest, with movement, and with electrical stimulation
7. Ultrasound
   a. Carotid Doppler scan: a noninvasive ultrasound of carotids that detects occlusions and stenosis; cause no discomfort
   b. Transcranial Doppler ultrasonography (TCD): a portable, noninvasive technique that assesses intracranial circulation by measuring blood flow velocity; assesses vasospasm, transient ischemic attack (TIA), headache, subarachnoid hemorrhage (SAH), head injury, and AV malformations

III. ALTERED LEVEL OF CONSCIOUSNESS (LOC)

A. Overview

1. A change in arousal or alertness and/or a change in cognition or ability to solve complex problems (thought processes, memory, perception, problem solving, and emotion); often first sign of a change in neurologic status
2. Causes for unconsciousness vary from primary CNS disorders (such as damage to RAS or cerebrum) to dysfunction of other organ systems
3. In addition, metabolic disorders may alter cellular environment enough to inhibit neuronal activity
4. The term **coma** is reserved for those who have long periods of unconsciousness, lasting from hours to months; neurological origin of coma results from damage to both hemispheres of brain, damage to brainstem, or both

B. Nursing assessment

1. Except for cases of damage to brainstem, brain function deterioration and changes in LOC follow a predictable pattern from higher functions to primitive functions
2. Confusion; forgetfulness; disorientation to time, then person, then place; agitation; poor problem-solving abilities; or any change in behavior may be an early change in cerebrum function
3. Changes of lethargy, obtundation, and stupor result from greater cerebral deterioration
4. A change from purposeful movements to decorticate posturing (see Figure 58–1a ■), small reactive pupils, and positive doll's eyes are manifestations of midbrain deterioration
5. Decerebrate posturing (see Figure 58–1b ■), fixed pupils, and positive cold caloric tests show deterioration at level of pons
6. Fixed pupils, flaccidity, and negative cold caloric tests indicate involvement at level of medulla
7. Glasgow Coma Scale assessment includes components of eye opening (scored 1 to 4), best verbal response (scored 1 to 5), and best motor response (scored 1 to 6); total score ranges from 3 to 15; a score of 8 or lower usually indicates coma; see Table 58–4 ■

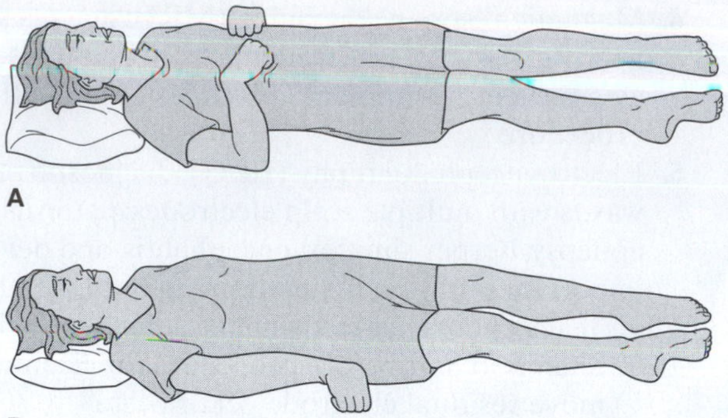

A

B

Figure 58–1

Abnormal posturing. A. Decorticate rigidity. B. Decerebrate rigidity.

Source: LeMone, P., & Burke, K. (2004). Medical surgical nursing: Critical thinking in client care (3rd ed.). Upper Saddle River, NJ: Pearson Education, p. 1304.

8. Diagnostic and laboratory test findings
   a. CT and MRI may detect hemorrhage, tumor, cysts, edema, or brain atrophy
   b. EEGs evaluate unrecognized seizures as a cause for an altered LOC
   c. Cerebral angiography evaluates cerebral circulation for aneurysm and AV malformations
   d. Transcranial Doppler study is a less invasive method to study blood flow
   e. A lumbar puncture with CSF analysis determines presence or status of infection
   f. Laboratory tests such as glucose, serum electrolytes, osmolarity, creatinine, liver function, complete blood count (CBC), arterial blood gases (ABGs), and toxicology screens may be ordered to rule out metabolic, toxic, or drug-induced disorders

C. Therapeutic management

1. Depends on cause of altered mental status; in addition to treating cause, ongoing care focuses on airway maintenance, skin integrity, preventing contractures, and maintaining nutrition

! **2.** Assess for ability to clear secretions; assess breath sounds; maintain patent airway in unconscious client; maintain client with ineffective airway in side-lying position; provide tracheostomy care every 4 hours if client has tracheostomy

! **3.** Assess swallowing and gag reflex; provide interventions to prevent aspiration (such as elevated head of bed); monitor for and report possible aspiration

4. Assess skin integrity every shift; reposition client every 2 hours; provide interventions to prevent skin breakdown; keep linens clean, dry, and wrinkle-free

Table 58–4

Glasgow Coma Scale

Assessment	Response	Score*
Eyes open (record C if eyes are closed by swelling)	Spontaneously To speech To pain No response	4 3 2 1
Best motor response (record best upper arm response)	Obeys commands Localized pain Flexion-withdrawal Abnormal flexion Abnormal extension No response	6 5 4 3 2 1
Best verbal response (record T if an endotracheal or tracheostomy tube is in place)	Oriented Confused Inappropriate words Incomprehensible sounds No response	5 4 3 2 1
Total Score:		—

*A higher score indicates a higher level of functioning.

Source: LeMone, P., & Burke, K. M. (2004). *Medical surgical nursing: Critical thinking in client care* (3rd ed.). Upper Saddle River, NJ: Prentice Hall, p. 1299.

5. Provide proper support devices to maintain extremities in functional condition; perform passive range of motion (ROM) regularly
6. Monitor nutritional status and assess daily weight; assess need for alternative methods of nutritional support
7. Provide emotional support to client and family
8. Provide for alternate means of communication as needed (such as questions with yes and no or other single-word answers)

D. Family teaching

1. Family anxiety is common when clients have altered mental status, especially if prognosis is uncertain
2. Reinforce information provided by physician
3. Encourage family to talk to client
4. Evaluate and provide information about client's care when family is ready
5. Offer support services as needed

IV. INCREASED INTRACRANIAL PRESSURE

A. Overview

1. Increased ICP is defined as a prolonged pressure greater than 15 mmHg measured in lateral ventricles; exerted by brain tissue, CSF, and blood within cranial vault
2. Coughing, sneezing, straining, and bending forward cause a transient increase in ICP that does not cause significant tissue ischemia
3. **Cushing's triad**/response: involves three classic signs or responses to increased ICP: increased systolic BP with unchanged diastolic BP, widening pulse pressure, and reflex bradycardia from stimulation of carotid bodies
4. A prolonged increase in ICP causes tissue ischemia because cerebral blood flow and perfusion are compromised
5. Autoregulation, a compensatory mechanism to maintain cerebral blood flow, is disrupted and can lead to cellular hypoxia and ischemia
6. Untreated increased ICP leads to herniation and ultimately death
7. Because brain is encased in a closed cavity, expansion of any contents of cavity can cause increased ICP
8. Cerebral edema is an increase in volume of brain tissue due to alterations in capillary permeability (vasogenic edema), changes in functional or structural integrity of cell membrane (cytotoxic edema), or an increase in interstitial fluids (interstitial cerebral edema); edema is usually proportional to size of injury and may be localized or generalized
9. Hydrocephalus is an increase in volume of CSF within ventricular system; it may be noncommunicating hydrocephalus in which drainage from ventricular system is impaired (such as tumor or mass) or communicating hydrocephalus, in which blood blocks CSF absorption, such as with subarachnoid hemorrhage

B. Nursing Assessment

1. Earliest signs of increased ICP may be blurred vision, decreased visual acuity, and diplopia because of pressure on visual pathways; headache, papilledema, or swelling of optic disk and vomiting are next signs; most significant sign of increased ICP is a change in LOC; as pressure increases from front to back of brain, the LOC deteriorates
2. Diagnostic and laboratory test findings are directed to identifying and treating underlying cause of increased ICP
   a. CT or MRI scanning is generally initial test
   b. LP is not usually performed because of possibility of brain herniation caused by sudden release of pressure
   c. Laboratory tests are performed to augment and monitor treatment approaches; serum osmolarity monitors hydration status and ABGs measure pH, O_2, and CO_2 (hydrogen ions and CO_2 are vasodilators that can increase ICP)

C. Therapeutic management

1. Increased ICP is a medical emergency with little time for lengthy diagnostic studies; it centers on restoring normal pressure and can be accomplished through medications, surgery, and drainage of CSF from ventricles

2. A drainage catheter, inserted via ventriculostomy into lateral ventricle, can monitor ICP and drain CSF to maintain normal pressure; if used, system is calibrated with transducer leveled 1 inch above ear (height of foramen of Munro); sterile technique is of utmost importance
3. Assess neurological status every 1 to 2 hours and report any deterioration; assessment areas include LOC, behavior, motor/sensory function, pupil size and response, vital signs with temperature
4. Maintain airway; elevate head of bed 30 degrees or keep flat as prescribed; maintain head and neck in neutral position to promote venous drainage
5. Assess for bladder distention and bowel constipation; assist client when necessary to prevent Valsalva maneuver
6. Plan nursing care so it is not clustered because prolonged activity may increase ICP; provide for a quiet environment (lights kept low also) and limit noxious stimuli; limit stimulants such as radio, TV, and newspaper; avoid ingesting stimulants such as coffee, tea, cola drinks, and cigarette smoke
7. Maintain fluid restriction as prescribed
8. Keep dressings over catheter dry and change dressings as prescribed; monitor insertion site for CSF leakage or infection; monitor clients for signs and symptoms of infection; use aseptic technique when in contact with ICP monitor
9. Medication therapy
   a. Osmotic diuretics such as mannitol (Osmitrol) and loop diuretics such as furosemide (Lasix) are mainstays used to decrease ICP; they draw water from edematous tissues into vascular system; they can also disturb glucose and electrolytes, so it is necessary to monitor their effect
   b. Corticosteroids may be effective in decreasing ICP, especially with tumors, although their mechanism of action is unclear
10. Client education
   a. Teach client at risk for increased ICP to avoid coughing, blowing nose, straining for bowel movements, pushing against bed side-rails, or performing isometric exercises
   b. Advise client to maintain neutral head and neck alignment
   c. Encourage family to maintain a quiet environment and minimize stimuli
   d. Educate family that upsetting client may increase ICP

V. HEAD INJURY

A. Skull fracture

1. Overview
   a. A break in skull that occurs with or without intracranial trauma; force of impact significantly increases risk of hematoma formation; disruption of skull can lead to infection and cranial nerve injury
   b. Occurs from trauma; may be labeled as open or closed, depending on whether or not skin is broken
   c. *Linear* fractures are most common of four types; risk of infection and CSF leakage is minimal because dura remains intact; hematoma formation is possible
   d. *Comminuted* and *depressed* skull fractures have a higher risk of brain tissue damage and infection, especially if overlying skin and dura is torn or damaged; risk of secondary brain injury is reduced because impact energy caused bone fracture instead of being transferred to brain tissue
   e. *Basilar* skull fractures involve base of skull and are usually secondary injuries; most are uncomplicated, but those that disrupt sinuses and middle ear bones can lead to infection and CSF leakage
2. Nursing assessment
   a. Clinical manifestations may give clues to area of fracture; basilar skull fracture may produce manifestations listed in Box 58–3
   b. Diagnostic and laboratory tests: plain x-ray films and CT or MRI scans; basilar skull fractures may be difficult to identify on plain x-ray

Box 58–3

Signs of Basilar Skull Fracture

- Battle's sign: ecchymosis over the mastoid process
- Hemotympanum: blood visible behind the tympanic membrane
- Raccoon eyes: bilateral periorbital ecchymosis
- Rhinorrhea: CSF leakage through the nose
- Otorrhea: CSF leakage through the ear

3. Therapeutic management: treatment depends on type and location of injury
   a. Linear skull fractures generally require bedrest and observation for underlying brain injury; no specific treatment is necessary
   b. Comminuted and depressed skull fractures require surgical intervention within 24 hours
   c. Basilar skull fractures do not require surgery unless there is persistent CSF leakage, but do require regular neurological assessments for meningitis
   d. Observe client for otorrhea or rhinorrhea
   e. ! Test clear ear drainage and sinus drainage for glucose; only CSF has glucose; mucous secretions do not
   f. ! Observe blood-tinged drainage for halo sign; glucose-containing CSF dries in concentric rings on gauze or tissues
   g. Keep nasopharynx and external ear clean; use sterile technique and supplies when cleaning drainage from nose and/or ears
   h. ! Instruct client not to blow nose, cough, or inhibit sneeze and to sneeze through an open mouth
   i. Use aseptic technique when changing head dressings
   j. Medication therapy: dexamethasone to decrease cerebral edema and antibiotics when there is a risk of infection
4. ! Client teaching: go to emergency department if client experiences drowsiness or confusion, difficulty waking, vomiting, blurred vision, slurred speech, prolonged headache, blood or clear fluid leaking from ears or nose, weakness in an arm or leg, stiff neck, or convulsions

B. Intracranial hemorrhage

1. Overview
   a. An escape of blood into cranium (often because of blunt trauma); hemorrhage may cause a very slow to very rapid neurological deterioration
   b. Results directly from trauma or from shearing forces on cerebral arteries and veins from acceleration-deceleration injuries; they are classified by location
   c. Bleeding can be epidural, subdural, or intracranial (see Box 58–4)
2. Assessment
   a. **Epidural hematoma:** client may initially lose consciousness then have a short period of lucidness, followed by rapid deterioration from drowsiness to coma; other manifestations include headache, fixed dilated pupil on affected side, hemiparesis, hemiplegia, and possible seizures; this condition is a surgical emergency
   b. **Subdural hematoma:** manifestations may develop slowly and may be mistaken for dementia in an elderly client; slow thinking, confusion, drowsiness, or lethargy are common; headaches, ipsilateral pupil dilation and sluggishness, and possible seizures are other signs
   c. Intracerebral hematomas vary in initial presentation depending on location; headache is common; as hematoma progresses, a decreased LOC, hemiplegia, and ipsilateral pupil dilation occurs; an expanding clot may lead to herniation
   d. Diagnostic and laboratory tests: CT and MRI; laboratory values do not establish diagnosis but provide baseline data for client's overall health status
3. Therapeutic management
   a. Small hematomas will reabsorb spontaneously and may be treated conservatively
   b. Surgical intervention is needed to drain epidural hematomas and larger subdural hematomas; surgery is less successful in intracerebral hematomas

Box 58-4

Types of Intracranial Bleeding

Epidural Hematoma

- Develops between the dura and the skull
- As the hematoma forms, it strips the dura away from the skull
- Usually develops from a tear in the meningeal artery
- Because this is an arterial bleed, it rapidly expands, leading to a rapid deterioration in neurological status

Subdural Hematoma

- Forms between the dura mater and the arachnoid–pia mater layers of the meninges
- Usually involves veins but may involve small arteries as well
- As blood collects, pressure is applied to the underlying brain tissue
- May be acute (develops within 48 hours after an acute injury), subacute (2 days to 3 weeks after lesser injury), or chronic (3 weeks to months after a minor injury), or may develop spontaneously

Intracerebral Hemorrhage

- Bleeding into the brain tissue
- Can occur anywhere in the brain but is most common in the frontal or temporal lobes
- May be the result of closed head trauma, where shearing forces are applied deep in the brain; this type of hemorrhage occurs, for example, in a motor vehicle accident in which an individual hits the head on the windshield, resulting in coup and contrecoup injury

because of widespread tissue damage; supportive care and preventing complications are goals of therapy

c. Assess neurological signs on a regular schedule; clear client's nose and mouth of secretions; suction airway as needed

d. Monitor respiratory pattern for rate, depth, and rhythm if client is not mechanically ventilated; prepare for O_2 administration and endotracheal (ET) intubation for respiratory distress

e. Prepare for cranial surgery for deteriorating neurological condition

f. Provide appropriate preoperative and postoperative care as needed

g. Provide previously discussed measures to manage increased ICP

! **h.** Medication therapy: none specific to hematomas; osmotic diuretics and steroids could reduce increased ICP; anticonvulsants could treat seizures if they occur as complications

4. Client education: family needs to be informed of possibility of surgery to evacuate hematoma

C. Contusion

1. Overview

a. Bruising of brain tissue as a result of blunt trauma or coup/contrecoup injuries

b. Usually involves damage to parenchyma with tears in vessels or tissue, pulling, and subsequent areas of necrosis or infarction

2. Nursing assessment: symptoms will vary depending on site of injury; may have decreasing LOC

3. Therapeutic management

a. Monitor neurological status

b. Monitor for signs of complications; can have sequelae specific to area of injury

4. Client and family education

a. Teach symptoms of complications that may occur after discharge

! **b.** Provide written instructions as well as explicit information about when to seek medical care (worsening neurological status, increasing headache)

D. Concussion

1. Overview
   - a. Concussion or "mild traumatic brain injury" involves some transient loss of consciousness, usually from blunt head trauma
   - b. Is usually related to stretching, compression, or shearing of nerve fibers
   - c. Postconcussion syndrome occurs after initial head injury; poor concentration and problems with memory may be noted; client may complain of headache, dizziness, and photophobia; subtle change in personality may be noted
2. Nursing assessment: symptoms include amnesia of event, headache, and nausea; clients are neurologically intact with a Glasgow Coma Score of 13 to 15; there are 3 levels of concussion severity
   - a. Grade 1: client has transient confusion with no loss of consciousness and a duration of abnormal mental status for less than 15 minutes
   - b. Grade 2: client has transient confusion with no loss of consciousness and a duration of abnormal mental status for more than 15 minutes
   - c. Grade 3: client has loss of consciousness for a few seconds or several minutes or longer
3. Therapeutic management
   - a. Treatment is supportive with close observation for 24 hours in an emergency room or at home under certain circumstances
   - b. Clients who had loss of consciousness for greater than 5 minutes or amnesia of event are usually admitted for observation to rule out any other potential injuries
4. Client and family education: client may be discharged home with caregivers who have received instructions to continue monitoring and what steps to take if complications arise; share information about postconcussion syndrome

VI. SPINAL CORD INJURY

A. Overview

1. Usually caused by trauma; young adults and adolescents are most commonly affected
2. Affects motor and sensory function at level of injury and below
3. Classified by complete versus incomplete cord injury, cause of injury, and level of injury; in clinical practice, these overlap
4. Perception, sexual function, and elimination are also affected
5. Usually results from excessive force applied to spinal cord and vertebral column; four types of injuries occur:
   - a. Hyperflexion compresses vertebral bodies and disrupts ligaments and discs
   - b. Hyperextension disrupts ligaments and causes vertebral fractures
   - c. Axial loading is an application of excessive vertical force and may cause compression fractures
   - d. Excessive rotation tears ligaments and fractures articular surfaces and causes compression fractures (see Figure 58–2 ■)
6. Risk factors include age, gender, and alcohol and drug abuse

B. Nursing assessment

1. Spinal shock, a temporary loss of reflex function, may occur following a spinal cord injury: symptoms include bradycardia; hypotension; flaccid paralysis of skeletal muscles; loss of pain, touch, temperature, pressure, visceral, and somatic sensations; bowel and bladder dysfunction; and loss of ability to perspire; spinal shock has resolved once spinal reflexes return
2. **Paraplegia** is paralysis of lower portion of body; occurs when injury level is in thoracic spine or lower
3. **Tetraplegia,** formally quadriplegia, is paralysis of arms, trunk, legs, and pelvic portions of body; occurs when level of injury is in cervical spine
4. **Autonomic dysreflexia** is an exaggerated sympathetic response that occurs in clients with T6 injuries or higher; response is seen after spinal shock occurs when stimuli cannot ascend cord; a stimulus such as urge to void or abdominal discomfort triggers massive vasoconstriction below injury, vasodilation above

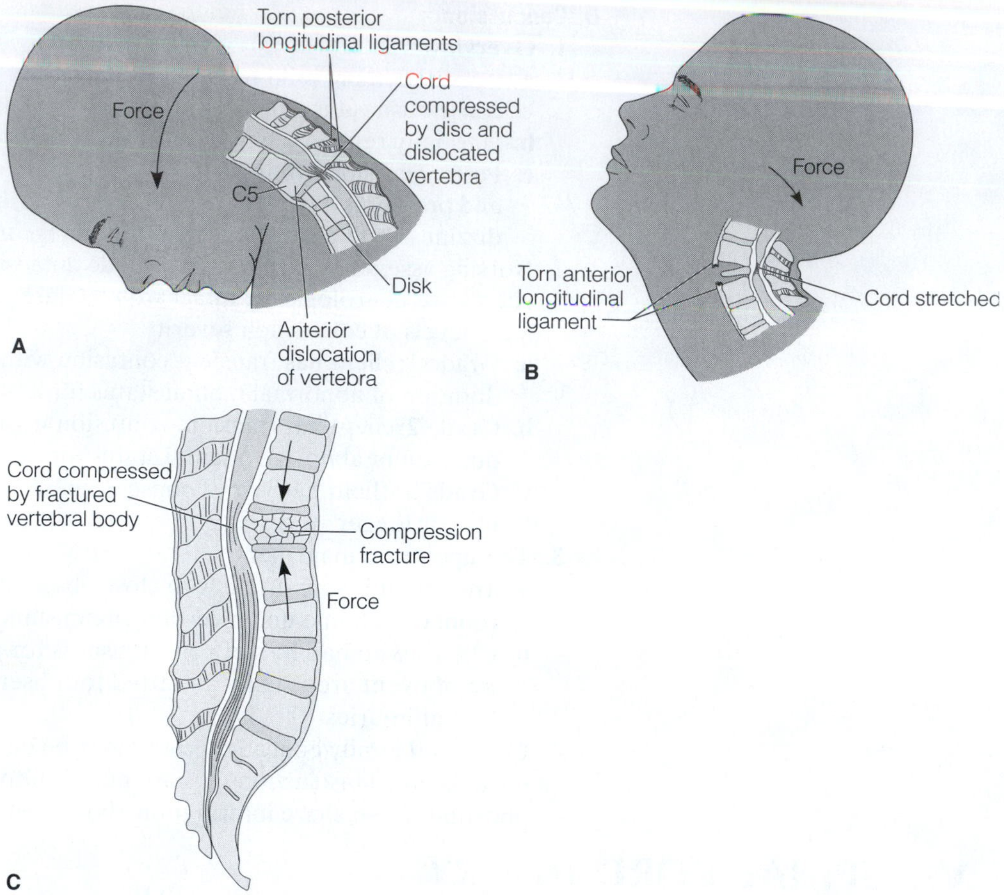

Figure 58–2

Spinal cord injury mechanisms.
A. Hyperflexion. B. Hyperextension.
C. Axial loading, a form of compression.

Source: LeMone, P., & Burke, K. (2004). Medical surgical nursing: Critical thinking in client care (3rd ed.). Upper Saddle River, NJ: Pearson Education, p. 1324.

injury, and bradycardia and rapidly occurring systolic hypertension with widening pulse pressure

5. Diagnostic and laboratory test findings: x-ray films are done to visualize fractures; CT and MRI scans show changes in the vertebrae, spinal cord, and tissues surrounding cord; an EMG is done after acute injury to locate level of injury

C. Therapeutic management

1. Acute management involves immobilizing injury and assessing and stabilizing client
2. Treat complications of respiratory distress, atonic bladder, paralytic ileus, and cardiovascular alterations
3. High-dose steroid protocol might be initiated to prevent secondary cord injury from edema and ischemia; this therapy is controversial at present because evidence has not supported its efficacy
4. Stabilization with devices such as halo traction and Gardner-Wells tongs or surgery is done when indicated
5. Monitor vital capacity and respiratory effectiveness; high cervical cord injuries (C6 or above) may inhibit respirations requiring mechanical ventilation
6. Monitor for signs of ascending edema; may cause respiratory compromise
7. Assist client with quad coughing by pushing in and up at xiphoid process when client is coughing
8. Treat autonomic dysreflexia immediately
   a. Elevate head of bed and remove antiembolism stockings
   b. Assess BP every 2 to 3 minutes while assessing for stimuli that initiated response; remove stimulus immediately when found
   c. With severe hypertension unresolved by removing offending stimulus, notify physician and administer antihypertensives as ordered per protocol
9. Encourage client to verbalize feelings about loss of function and care
10. Institute bowel and bladder training programs to restore a regular schedule for elimination

11. Encourage self-care and independent decision making
12. Include family and important others in discussions
13. Clients with spinal cord injury because of fracture or dislocated cervical vertebrae may benefit from a Halo brace; it is an external fixation device that allows earlier mobility because skeletal cervical traction by Gardner-Wells tongs or other apparatus is not needed
14. ! Medication therapy: corticosteroids (such as methylprednisolone, [Solu-Medrol]) may be used to decrease or control edema of cord; vasoactive drugs treat hypotension or hypertension due to spinal shock or autonomic dysreflexia; antispasmodics (baclofen [Lioresal] and diazepam [Valium]) treat spasticity in clients; analgesics and tricyclic antidepressants treat pain

D. Client education

1. Teach client and family to promote independence in self-care, such as self-catheterization technique, bowel evacuation, activities of daily living
2. Educate client and family about variety of community resources needed
3. ! If client has a Halo vest, teach that it raises center of gravity; avoid bending over to reduce risk of falls; neck is immobilized in midline so client must learn to turn entire body to scan environment; driving is prohibited; food is cut into small pieces, and a straw is used for liquids

VII. GUILLAIN-BARRÉ SYNDROME

A. Overview

1. An acute, rapidly progressive inflammation of peripheral motor and sensory nerves characterized by motor weakness and paralysis that ascends from lower extremities in a majority of cases
2. Occurs most frequently between ages of 30 and 50
3. Autoimmune reaction is suspected, because Guillain-Barré syndrome often develops after viral infection, immunizations, fever, injury, and sometimes surgery; antibody (IgM) formation targets peripheral nerve **myelin,** which damages myelin sheath and disrupts nerve conduction; nerve remyelinizes in opposite direction of demyelination
4. Outcome is generally excellent if care is appropriate

B. Nursing assessment

1. ! Weakness or paresis or partial paralysis progressing upward from lower extremities (paralysis in Guillain-Barré is "ground to the brain") and then to total paralysis requiring ventilatory support
2. Paresthesias (numbness and tingling) and pain
3. Muscle aches, cramping, and nighttime pain
4. ! Respiratory compromise and/or failure (dyspnea, diminished vital capacity and breath sounds), decreasing O_2 saturation, abnormal ABGs
5. ! Difficulty with extraocular eye movements, dysphagia, diplopia, difficulty speaking
6. ! Autonomic dysfunction (orthostatic hypotension), hypertension, change in HR, bowel and bladder dysfunction, flushing, and diaphoresis
7. Diagnostic and laboratory findings: nerve conduction test results are diminished, CSF examination shows elevated protein

C. Therapeutic management

1. Supportive care to maintain function of all systems, including respiratory, cardiac, GI, renal, and skin; medications as ordered
2. Plasmapheresis: plasma is removed and separated from whole blood; blood cells are then returned without plasma to removed antibodies that cause disorder; monitor for complications of this therapy, which include bleeding from loss of clotting factors and fluid and electrolyte imbalance
3. ! Monitor respiratory status: rate, depth, breath sounds; vital capacity; note secretions; check gag, cough, and swallowing
4. ! Monitor cardiac status: HR, BP, dysrhythmias
5. Administer chest physiotherapy and pulmonary hygiene measures
6. Maintain adequate nutrition as appropriate: administer enteral or parenteral nutrition as needed; if client can swallow, assist with small, frequent feedings of

soft foods; weigh client weekly; check electrolyte status; provide mouth care every 2 hours

7. Monitor bowel and bladder function: assess bowel sounds and frequency, amount, color of bowel movements; offer bedpan; check for distention and residuals in client who cannot void spontaneously; perform intermittent catheterization as needed; encourage fluid intake to 3500 mL/day
8. Prevent complications of immobility: encourage use of weak extremities as able; provide assistance with ROM and exercises prescribed by physical therapist; protect immobile extremities with use of air mattress or special bed and elbow and heel protectors; turn and reposition every 2 hours; elevate extremities to prevent dependent edema; use antiembolism compression devices/stockings
9. Provide eye care for client with inability to close eyelids completely; instill artificial tears, cleanse eyes as needed, use eye shields, and tape eyes closed if needed
10. Provide comfort and analgesics as needed
11. Promote communication with client and family, using alternative means of communication if client is on ventilator or cannot speak because of weak speech muscles
12. Initiate discharge planning at time of admission
13. Medication therapy: IV immunoglobulins (may result in low-grade fever, muscle aches, headache, or [rarely] acute renal failure or retinal necrosis); adrenocorticotropic hormone (ACTH) and corticosteroids or anti-inflammatory drugs; supportive medications include stool softeners, antacids or H_2 receptor antagonists, and analgesics

D. **Client education:** explain all care with rationales and provide information about disease progression; encourage client and family to express feelings and participate in care as much as possible

VIII. CEREBROVASCULAR ACCIDENT (CVA, BRAIN ATTACK, STROKE)

A. Overview

1. A condition in which neurological deficits result from decreased blood flow to a localized area of brain; onset may be rapid or gradual
2. ! Hypertension, diabetes mellitus, sickle cell disease, substance abuse, cardiac dysrhythmias, and atherosclerosis are risk factors for stroke
3. Ischemia followed by cell death results from severe and prolonged cerebral blood flow obstruction; resulting deficits predict location of stroke; there are four types of brain attacks
   a. ! Transient ischemic attack (TIA) is a brief period of neurological deficits that resolve within 24 hours; they are frequently precursors to a permanent CVA; causes of TIAs may be inflammatory arterial disorders, sickle cell anemia, or atherosclerotic changes in cerebral, jugular and/or carotid blood vessels, thrombosis, and emboli
   b. Thrombotic CVA is caused by a thrombus (blood clot) occluding a cerebral vessel; thrombi tend to form on atherosclerotic plaque in larger arteries while blood pressure is low (such as during sleep or rest); thrombosis occurs quickly but deficits progress slowly
   c. Embolic CVA is caused by a traveling blood clot; source of clot is elsewhere in body; CVA has a sudden onset with immediate symptoms; if embolus is not absorbed, deficits will be persistent
   d. Hemorrhagic CVA or intracranial hemorrhage occurs when a blood vessel ruptures; most often occurs in presence of long-term, poorly controlled hypertension; other factors that may cause a hemorrhagic CVA include a ruptured intracranial aneurysm, embolic CVA, tumors, AV malformations, anticoagulant therapy, liver disease, and blood disorders; this form of CVA is most often fatal because of rapidly increasing ICP; onset of symptoms is rapid; loss of consciousness occurs in about half of cases

B. Nursing assessment

1. Clinical manifestations: vary according to cerebral vessel involved

2. Internal carotid: contralateral motor and sensory deficits of arm, leg and face; in dominant hemispheric CVA, aphasia (loss of ability to use language); in non-dominant hemispheric CVA, **apraxia** (inability to perform known tasks), **agnosia** (inability to recognize), and unilateral neglect and homonymous **hemianopsia** (loss of one half of visual field in each eye)
3. Middle cerebral artery: drowsiness; stupor; coma; contralateral hemiplegia and sensory deficits of arm and face; aphasia; and homonymous hemianopsia
4. Anterior cerebral artery: contralateral weakness or paralysis and sensory loss of foot and leg, loss of decision-making and voluntary action abilities, and urinary incontinence
5. Vertebral artery: pain in face, nose, or eye; numbness or weakness of face on ipsilateral side; problems with gait; **dysphagia** (difficulty swallowing); and dysarthria (difficulty speaking)
6. Diagnostic and laboratory test findings: CT and MRI demonstrate hemorrhage, tumors, ischemia, edema, and tissue necrosis; cerebral angiography detects abnormal vessel structure, vasospasm, stenosis of the carotid artery, and loss of vessel wall integrity; ultrasound evaluates blood flow

C. Therapeutic management

1. Drug therapy is most common treatment for CVAs; if it is a thrombotic stroke, medications could include thrombolytics and/or heparin
2. It is imperative not to disrupt a clot that has formed following hemorrhagic CVA
3. Surgery is not usually indicated as a treatment modality
4. Rehabilitation is crucial to improve deficits
5. Encourage active ROM on unaffected side and passive ROM on affected side
6. Turn client every 2 hours
7. Monitor lower extremities for thrombophlebitis
8. Encourage use of unaffected arm for ADLs
9. Teach client to put clothing on affected side first
10. Resume diet orally only after successfully completing a swallowing evaluation; clients may need thickened liquids, foods with consistency of oatmeal, and to chew on unaffected side of mouth; this diet is sometimes called a dysphagia diet
11. Collaborate with occupational and physical therapy for rehabilitation
12. Try alternate methods of communication for clients with aphasia
13. Accept client's frustration and anger as normal to loss of function
14. Teach client with homonymous hemianopsia to overcome deficit by turning head side to side to be able to fully scan visual field
15. Medication therapy
    a. Antiplatelet agents are used to treat TIAs and previous CVA clients (except hemorrhagic CVAs)
    b. During acute phase of thrombotic and embolic stroke, thrombolytic therapy using tissue plasminogen activator may be administered within 3 hours to dissolve clot
    c. Anticoagulant therapy is provided with heparin initially and then continued with an oral anticoagulant after acute phase
    d. In clients with cerebral edema, hyperosmolar solutions (mannitol [Osmitrol]) or diuretics (furosemide [Lasix]) may be given
    e. In clients with seizures, anticonvulsants such as phenytoin (Dilantin), barbiturates, diazepam (Valium), and lorazepam (Ativan) may be given

D. Client teaching: CVA and CVA prevention, community resources, physical care, and need for psychosocial support, medications

IX. SEIZURE DISORDER

A. Overview

1. A seizure is an episode of excessive and abnormal electrical activity in brain
2. This abnormal electrical activity is manifested by disturbances in skeletal motor activity, sensation, autonomic dysfunction of viscera, behavior, or consciousness

3. Seizures are classified as partial or generalized; partial seizures begin in one area of cortex; generalized seizures involve both hemispheres and deeper brain structures
4. Risk factors in adults include acute febrile state, head injury, infection, metabolic or endocrine disorders, and exposure to toxins
5. Risk factors during infancy include perinatal hypoxia, congenital diseases, infections, metabolic or degenerative diseases, drug withdrawal, and neoplasms
6. Risk factors during childhood include febrile infections, head injury, lead toxicity, drugs, genetic disorders, and neoplasms
7. If seizure activity is chronic (i.e., they reoccur within minutes, days, or even years), a diagnosis of epilepsy is made
8. Metabolic needs, O_2 requirements, metabolic by-products, and cerebral blood flow increase dramatically during seizure
9. As long as cerebral blood flow can meet demands of seizure, brain is protected from cellular exhaustion and destruction

B. Nursing assessment

1. *Simple partial seizures* are limited to one hemisphere; manifestations include alterations in motor function, sensory signs, or autonomic or psychic symptoms
2. *Complex partial seizures* originate in temporal lobe and may be preceded by an aura; an impaired LOC and repetitive nonpurposeful movements such as lip-smacking, picking, or aimless walking are noted; amnesia is common
3. *Generalized partial seizure* is a partial seizure that has spread to both hemispheres and deeper structures of brain
4. *Absence seizure* is a generalized seizure that lasts 5 to 30 seconds; there is a sudden, brief cessation of motor activity and a blank stare; they may occur occasionally or up to 100 per day; they may be accompanied by eyelid fluttering or automatisms such as lip-smacking; more common in children than adults
5. **Tonic-clonic** seizures (grand mal) are most common type of seizure
   a. May be preceded by an aura but often occur without warning
   b. Typically start with a loss of consciousness and sharp muscle contractions
   c. Client falls to floor and may have urinary and/or bowel incontinence
   d. Breathing ceases and cyanosis develops during tonic phase (about 15 to 60 sec); see Figure 58–3a ■
   e. Clonic phase (60 to 90 sec) follows with alternating muscle contraction and relaxation in all extremities, hyperventilation, and eyes rolled back in head; see Figure 58–3b ■
   f. In next phase (postictal period), client is relaxed with quiet breathing and is unconscious and unresponsive; client gradually regains consciousness and may have transient confusion and disorientation; clients often complain of head and muscle aches, and fatigue and may sleep several hours
   g. Clients will have amnesia of seizure and events just prior to seizure

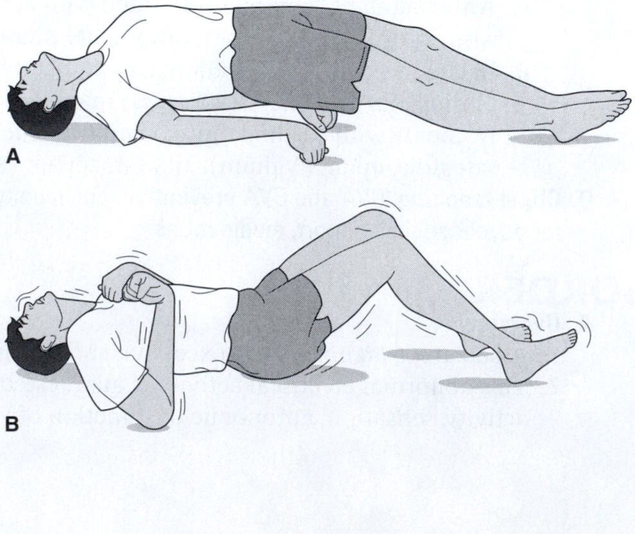

Figure 58–3

Tonic-clonic contractions in grand mal seizures. A. Tonic phase. B. Clonic phase.

Source: LeMone, P., & Burke, K. (2004). Medical surgical nursing: Critical thinking in client care *(3rd ed.). Upper Saddle River, NJ: Pearson Education, p. 1367.*

6. *Status epilepticus* is a life-threatening emergency that can occur during seizure activity; it is characterized by continuous cycles of tonic-clonic activity with short periods of calm between them; this cumulative effect can interfere with respiration; client is in great danger of developing hypoxia, hyperthermia, hypoglycemia, and exhaustion if seizure activity is not stopped
7. During actual seizure activity, observe order of events and duration of seizure; for tonic-clonic seizures, be certain to time length of seizure until jerking stops; tonic indicates continuous muscle contraction; clonic indicates alternating contraction and relaxation of muscles; for all other types of seizures, note duration from start of seizure to time that consciousness is regained; describe any precipitating events or unusual behavior; note parts of body involved and if it begins in any particular body part
8. Observe face for any color change, perspiration, and lack of expression; observe mouth for any deviation to one side or other, clenched teeth, tongue biting, frothing, and/or flecks of blood or bleeding; if able to access pupils, note any change in size, equality, reaction to light, and accommodation
9. Observe for presence or length of apnea; other general observations might be involuntary urination or defecation
10. Postictally, it is important to note duration of postictal period; level of consciousness; orientation to time, person, place; and any alterations in motor ability or speech
11. Diagnostic and laboratory tests: complete neurological examination, EEG, skull X-ray series, CT scan, lumbar puncture with CSF analysis, blood studies, and electrocardiogram

C. Therapeutic management

1. Provide interventions during seizure to maintain airway patency
   a. Turn client to side if necessary to maintain airway and promote drainage of secretions without aspiration
   b. Have O_2 and suction equipment at bedside for use following a seizure if needed
   c. Do not try to force an object, such as a bite stick, into mouth of client who is seizing, as this may break teeth or cause other injury
2. Provide interventions during a seizure to reduce the risk of injury; do not restrain client but provide an environment that will not create further injury; teach family members how to protect client during seizures
3. Document seizure activity promptly and report it as appropriate
4. Provide support to client that concerns are normal; help client identify leisure activities that are safe; provide information about resources and support groups; provide accurate information about hiring practices and legalities of driving or operating heavy/dangerous equipment
5. Medication therapy
   a. Antiepileptics that raise seizure threshold or limit spread of abnormal electrical activity are mainstay of epilepsy treatment
   b. Some commonly used antiepileptics are phenytoin (Dilantin), divalproex sodium (Depakote), valproic acid (Depakene), carbamazepine (Tegretol), gabapentin (Neurontin), and lamotrigine (Lamictal)
   c. Diazepam (Valium), lorazepam (Ativan), and phenobarbital are also used intermittently to stop seizure activity during acute episodes
6. When all attempts fail, then surgery for excision of tissue involved in seizure activity may be an alternative
7. Promote client's development of a positive self-image, especially if a child; talk with client about his or her feelings; plan strategies to promote acceptance and decrease fear among peers
8. Encourage client and family to express feelings

D. Client teaching

1. Correct misconceptions, fears, and myths about epilepsy
2. Provide information about community and national resources for epilepsy
3. Stress importance of follow-up care

4. Review any laws (such as driving a motor vehicle) that apply to people with epilepsy
5. Refer for employment or vocational counseling as needed
6. Stress importance of wearing a medical alert band
7. Emphasize aura alert so client is aware of impending seizure
8. Stress importance of medication compliance
9. Stress importance of avoiding physical and emotional stress
10. Avoid alcohol and limit caffeine; take showers instead of baths to avoid drowning
11. Discuss triggers for seizure activity: increased stress, lack of sleep, emotional upset, and alcohol use
12. Families need to know what to do when client has a seizure; teach safety measures and when to call emergency medical services
13. Do not use any over-the-counter medications prior to consulting with health care provider (for example, antihistamines since side effects are increased)
14. Educate adults and older children about type of seizure and past and present medication, and they should be able to give a history of seizure control or number of seizures experienced and their timing

X. PARKINSON'S DISEASE

A. Overview

1. A progressive, degenerative neurological disease characterized by **bradykinesia,** muscle rigidity, and nonintentional tremor
2. Commonly affects older adults and is usually diagnosed between age 50 to 60; as disease progresses, burden of care increases
3. Atrophy occurs in substantia nigra, which produces dopamine; as dopamine decreases, acetylcholine is no longer inhibited; this neurotransmitter imbalance is clinical basis for symptoms

B. Nursing assessment

1. Clinical manifestations begin subtly with fatigue and a slight resting tremor as initial symptoms; in a small population of clients, dementia may be presenting symptom
2. Bradykinesia is slow movements caused by muscle rigidity; may affect also eyes, mouth, and voice; some clients exhibit a staring gaze
3. Uncoordinated movements and postural disturbance, trunk tilted forward
4. Short-stepped, shuffling and propulsive gait, which leads to increased risk of falls
5. Seborrhea
6. Heat intolerance; excessive sweating of face and neck; absence of sweating on trunk and extremities
7. Constipation
8. Anxiety and depression, possible sleep disturbances
9. Dysphagia

C. Therapeutic management

1. Includes medications, surgery, and rehabilitation aimed at optimizing functional level; a team approach is essential to quality care of clients with Parkinson's disease
2. Client should perform active ROM twice a day; provide passive ROM when client is unable to do active ROM
3. Ambulate at least four times a day
4. Use assistive devices when recommended; consider velcro instead of buttons and slip-on shoes instead of those that tie
5. Assess communication skills, speech, hearing, and writing
6. Consult with a speech pathologist if necessary
7. Assess nutritional status and self-feeding abilities
8. Monitor diet to ensure foods high in bulk and fluids
9. Medication therapy: monoamine oxidase (MAO) inhibitors, dopaminergics, dopamine agonists, and anticholinergics; eventually all drugs lose effectiveness; a fluctuating response to drugs is called an on-off response; antidepressants, espe-

cially amitriptyline, are used to treat depression; propranolol may be used to treat tremors

D. Client education

1. Preventive measures for malnutrition, falls, and other environmental hazards, constipation, skin breakdown from incontinence, and joint contractures
2. Gait training and exercises for improving ambulation, swallowing, speech, and self-care

XI. MULTIPLE SCLEROSIS

A. Overview

1. Chronic CNS disorder in which myelin and nerve axons in brain and spinal cord are destroyed
2. There are four forms based on rate of progression: benign, relapsing-remitting, primary progressive, and secondary progressive
3. Unknown etiology, possibly an autoimmune or genetic basis or may be caused by childhood viral infections
4. Destruction of myelin and nerve axons causes a temporary, repetitive, or sustained interruption in nerve impulse conduction, which causes symptoms of multiple sclerosis (MS)
5. Plaque formation occurs throughout white matter of CNS, which also affects nerve impulses of optic nerves, cervical spinal cord, thoracic and lumbar spine
6. Inflammation occurs around plaques as well as around normal tissue
7. Astrocytes appear in lesions, and scar tissue forms, replacing axons and leading to permanent disability

B. Nursing assessment

1. Visual disturbances or blindness (retrobulbar neuritis)
2. Sudden, progressive weakness of one or more limbs
3. **Spasticity** of muscles, nystagmus, tremors, and gait instability
4. Fatigue
5. Bladder dysfunction (UTIs, incontinence)
6. Depression
7. Lumbar puncture for CSF reveals clonal IgG bands
8. MRI, CT scans, muscle testing show characteristic changes

C. Therapeutic management

1. No cure is available; supportive care is indicated
2. Overall goal of care is to maintain as much independent function as possible
3. Include rest periods to prevent fatigue, which is an exacerbating factor
4. Help client to recognize choices in care and set priorities on a day-to-day basis whenever possible to maintain sense of control and independence
5. Assist client with ADLs on an as-needed basis; provide adaptive utensils or other assistive devices as needed
6. Maintain fluid intake of at least 2000 mL/day to promote bowel and bladder function and prevent impaction and/or urinary tract infection (UTI)
7. Communicate with client about issues of concern, such as coping skills, sexuality, changing body image, or others identified by client
8. Avoid sources of infection; illness can act as a stressor and trigger an exacerbation
9. Medication therapy: immunosuppressant therapy, antiviral drugs, corticosteroids, antibiotics for UTI, interferon-alpha, glatiramer (Copaxone), anticholinergic drugs, and antispasmodics

D. Client education: medications, symptoms, bladder training, intermittent self-catheterization, sexual functioning, avoiding complications, and possible triggers (fatigue, temperature extremes, illness)

XII. MYASTHENIA GRAVIS

A. Overview

1. A chronic progressive disorder of peripheral NS affecting transmission of nerve impulses to voluntary muscles

2. Causes muscle weakness and fatigue that increases with exertion and improves with rest; eventually leads to fatigue without relief from rest
3. Causes include unknown etiology, family history of autoimmune disorders, and thyroid tumors
4. An autoimmune process triggers autoantibody formation that decreases numbers of acetylcholine receptors and widens gap between neuronal axon and muscle fiber in neuromuscular (myoneural) junction
5. Muscle contraction is hindered because IgG autoantibodies prevent acetylcholine from binding with receptors; destruction of receptors at neuromuscular junction occurs
6. Associated with continued production of autoantibodies by thymus gland in 75% of cases
7. Onset is usually slow but can be precipitated by emotional stress, hormonal disturbance (pregnancy, menses, thyroid disorders), infections and vaccinations, trauma and surgery, temperature extremes, excessive exercise, drugs that interfere with neuromuscular transmission (opioids, sedatives, barbiturates, alcohol, quinidine, anesthetics), and thymus tumor

B. Nursing assessment

1. Mild diplopia (double vision) and unilateral ptosis (eyelid drooping) caused by weakness in extraocular muscles; weakness may also involve face, jaw, neck, and hip
2. Complications arise when severe weakness affects muscles of swallowing, chewing and respiration; respiratory distress is manifested by tachypnea, decreased depth, abnormal ABGs, O_2 saturation under 92%, and decreased breath sounds
3. Bowel and bladder incontinence, paresthesias, and pain in weak muscles
4. Myasthenic crisis: sudden motor weakness; risk of respiratory failure and aspiration; most often caused by insufficient dose of medication or an infection
5. Cholinergic crisis: severe muscle weakness caused by overmedication; also cramps, diarrhea, bradycardia, and bronchial spasm with increased pulmonary secretions and risk of respiratory compromise
6. ABGs and pulmonary function tests may show respiratory insufficiency
7. Electromyography (EMG) shows decreased amplitude when motor neurons are stimulated
8. Tensilon test: diagnosis is confirmed when IV edrophonium chloride (Tensilon), which allows acetylcholine to bind with receptors, temporarily improves symptoms; weakness returns after effects of Tensilon are discontinued

C. Therapeutic management

1. Focuses on medication management with anticholinesterases (see also Chapter 39): neostigmine (Prostigmin), pyridostigmine (Mestinon); immunosuppressants: corticosteroids, azathiopirine (Imuran), and cyclosporine (Cytoxan); anti-inflammatory drugs; thymectomy (removal of thymus gland); plasmapheresis—removes IgG antibodies, atropine sulfate (Atropine) for cholinergic crisis
2. Maintain effective breathing pattern and airway clearance; thoroughly assess for respiratory distress
3. Monitor meals and teach client to bend head slightly forward while eating and drinking to improve swallowing
4. Teach client to avoid exposure to infections, especially respiratory
5. Teach client effective coughing, use chest physiotherapy and incentive spirometry; have oral suction available, teach client and family how to use it; be prepared to intubate if needed
6. Provide adequate nutrition: schedule medications 30 to 45 minutes before eating for peak muscle strength while eating; frequently offer small amounts of foods that are easy to chew and swallow—soft or semisolid as needed; administer IV fluids and nasogastric tube feedings if client is unable to swallow
7. Promote improved physical mobility with referrals to physical and occupational therapy
8. Provide eye care: instill artificial tears; use a patch over one eye for double vision (diplopia); wear sunglasses to protect eyes from bright lights

9. Promote positive body image and coping skills: encourage participation in treatment plan; plan time for active listening and encourage client to express feelings; reinforce progress and explain all care
10. Medication therapy: anticholinesterases such as neostigmine (Prostigmin), pyridostigmine (Mestinon); immunosuppressants such as corticosteroids, azathioprine (Imuran), and cyclosporine (Cytoxan); anti-inflammatory drugs; see also Chapter 39

D. Client teaching

1. Plan rest periods and conserve energy; plan major activities early in day; schedule activities during peak medication effect
2. Avoid extremes of hot and cold, exposure to infections, emotional stress and meds that may worsen or precipitate an exacerbation (alcohol, sedatives, local anesthetics)
3. Signs of myasthenic crisis (symptoms of disorder caused by inadequate medication related to need) and cholinergic crisis (over medication)
4. Encourage client to wear a Medic-Alert bracelet
5. Instruct in alternative methods of communication if necessary: eye blink, finger wiggle for yes or no; flash cards or communication board; teach to support lower jaw with hands to assist with speech

XIII. CRANIAL NERVE DISORDERS

A. Trigeminal neuralgia

1. Overview
   a. A chronic disease of trigeminal nerve (CN V) that causes severe facial pain
   b. Has an unknown cause; affects one or more of 3 divisions of trigeminal nerve—ophthalmic, maxillary, and mandibular—maxillary and mandibular divisions are affected most often
2. Nursing assessment
   a. Brief, intense, skin surface pain is characteristic symptom; episodes may occur as frequently as 100 times a day or as infrequently as a few times each year
   b. Pain typically starts peripherally and advances centrally
   c. Motor or sensory deficits do not occur; some clients may have trigger zones that initiate onset of pain; in others, pain may be triggered by light touch, eating, swallowing, talking, shaving, sneezing, brushing teeth, or washing the face
3. Therapeutic management
   a. Centered on controlling pain with antiepileptic medications such as carbamazepine (Tegretol)
   b. Surgical procedures include microvascular decompression (removal of blood vessel from posterior trigeminal root) or rhizotomy (surgical severing of nerve root)
   c. Encourage client to chew on unaffected side
   d. Monitor dietary intake, encouraging soft foods
   e. Avoid triggers for pain, which include firm toothbrush, very hot or cold foods or liquids, or mechanical pressure on cheeks
   f. Medication therapy: most useful drug for controlling pain is carbamazepine (Tegretol); when this is not effective, phenytoin (Dilantin) is tried
4. Client teaching: avoidance of triggers

B. Bell's palsy

1. Overview
   a. A unilateral paralysis of facial muscles
   b. Has an unknown cause, with inflammation of nerve and a viral cause suggested; 80% of clients recover completely within a few weeks to months; of those remaining, 15% recover some function but have permanent facial paralysis
2. Nursing assessment
   a. One-sided paralysis of facial muscles
   b. Paralysis of upper eyelid with loss of corneal reflex on affected side
   c. Loss or impairment of taste over anterior portion of tongue on affected side
   d. Increased tearing from lacrimal gland on affected side

3. Therapeutic management
   a. Assist with physiotherapy, including moist heat, gentle massage, and facial nerve stimulation with faradic current
   b. Protect cornea with artificial tears, sunglasses, eye patch at night, and gentle intermittent closure of eye
   c. Medication therapy: a corticosteroid such as prednisone (Deltasone) influences outcome by decreasing edema of nerve tissue; antivirals are also used
   d. Assist with body image disturbance, which is often temporary
4. Client teaching
   a. Wear an eye patch at night and protective glasses when outside
   b. Inspect inside of mouth on affected side for food that may collect between mouth and teeth

XIV. CEREBRAL PALSY

A. Overview

1. A nonprogressive motor CNS disorder resulting in alteration in movement and posture
2. Classified as spastic, athetoid, ataxic, or mixed
3. Topographic descriptions explain part(s) of body affected and include hemiplegia, diplegia, and quadriplegia (tetraplegia)
4. Causes include trauma, hemorrhage, anoxia, or infection before, during, or after birth
5. One third of children with cerebral palsy (CP) also have some degree of mental retardation

B. Nursing assessment

1. Abnormal muscle tone and coordination: child with spastic cerebral palsy presents with spasticity (hypertonicity of muscle groups); child with athetoid cerebral palsy presents with wormlike movements of extremities; ataxic form of cerebral palsy involves disturbed coordination
2. May display hypertonia or hypotonia and may have varying degrees of tonicity on different extremities
3. Absence of expected reflexes or presence of reflexes that extend beyond expected age suggest cerebral palsy
4. Failure to meet developmental norms may be first suggestion that "something is wrong"
5. Physical symptoms include altered speech and difficulty with swallowing; visual and hearing defects may be present; nurse may note scissoring of lower extremities when walking
6. Seizures may accompany CP and may be another indication of brain injury

C. Therapeutic management

1. Many individuals with CP require increased calorie intake because of spasticity or increased motor functioning
2. If motor involvement causes child to have poor coordination or if child has seizure activity, a safe environment and precautions such as protective headgear and a padded bed are needed
3. Communication can be a problem if there is oral involvement; child may need to use a communication board or computer-assisted communication; touch is an excellent means to communicate caring to a child
4. Self-care is a goal for all children; extensive collaboration with occupational therapists for strategies and devices to assist in this area may be necessary
5. Risk for aspiration is present if oral muscles are involved; use of adaptive feeding devices and positioning during feedings can decrease risk; for some clients with severe spasticity, a gastrostomy tube might be surgically placed for enteral feedings
6. Collaborate with multidisciplinary team for speech, nutrition, occupation, and physical therapies
7. Regional early-intervention consortiums conduct community-based developmental screenings to identify children at risk or who have developmental delays from disorders such as CP; referrals for further assessment help ensure that

early intervention is initiated; Denver II is most widely used developmental screening test

8. Provide adequate nutrition and rest
9. ! Maintain a safe environment
10. To control spasticity, traditional treatments have included surgery to release tendons to promote mobility, rehabilitation therapies, oral medications, and intramuscular injections of phenol and botulinum toxin
11. Newer treatment is use of a surgically implanted **intrathecal** pump, which administers a continuous infusion of baclofen (Lioresal); potential pump-related problems include infection and overdose; benefits include improved function, gait, and motor control and generally improved health

D. Client and family teaching

1. Teach parents use of physical therapy strategies such as ROM exercises to use at home
2. Child will need to learn self-care skills such as feeding and dressing self and performing hygiene activities
3. Teach parents special feeding techniques and use of adaptive devices such as special silverware and dishes, or how to do gastrostomy tube feedings if indicated

XV. NEURAL TUBE DEFECTS

A. Overview

1. Are also known as spina bifida or myelodysplasia, develop during first trimester of pregnancy; can occur at any place along spinal canal (see Figure 58–4 ■)
2. ! Etiology is uncertain and thought to be associated with maternal folic acid deficiency; degree of disability is determined by location of defect and number of spinal nerves encased in sac; higher defects are associated with greater neurologic dysfunction
3. There are several types of spina bifida or neural tube defects
4. Spina bifida occulta: posterior vertebral arches fail to fuse, but there is no herniation of spinal cord or meninges (fibrous membrane that covers brain and lines vertebral canal); no loss of function
5. Meningocele: posterior vertebral arches fail to fuse, and there is a saclike protrusion at some point along posterior vertebrae; sac contain meninges and CSF
6. Myelomeningocele: posterior vertebral arches fail to fuse; saclike herniation contains meninges, CSF, and a portion of spinal cord or nerve roots; sometimes leakage of CSF occurs
7. Encephalocele: brain and meninges herniate through defect in skull into a sac

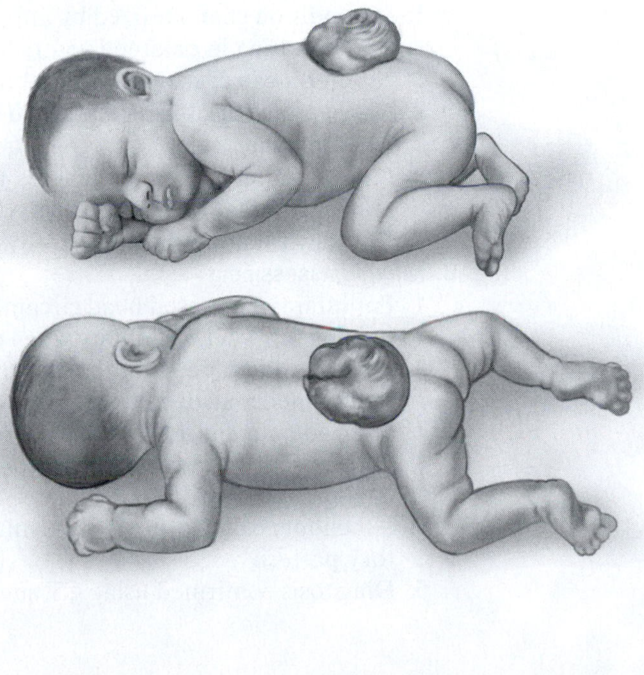

Figure 58–4

Infant with lumbarsacral myelomeningocele.

Source: Ball, J., & Bindler, R. (2006). Child health nursing: Partnering with children and families. *Upper Saddle River, NJ: Pearson Education, p. 1331.*

B. Nursing assessment

1. Prenatal diagnosis can be determined by elevated levels of alpha-fetoprotein (AFP) in fluid obtained by amniocentesis; defect can also be assessed on prenatal ultrasound
2. During postnatal period, monitor for leakage of CSF from sac and monitor skin integrity of sac; assess for infection around sac and possible systemic or CNS infection
3. Assess degree of sensation at or below level of lesion; this can be evidenced by lack of movement or sensation in legs, and a **neurogenic** (lacking innervation) bladder or bowel
4. Measure head circumference because there is a high risk of hydrocephalus

C. Therapeutic management

1. Collaborative management: defect/sac is surgically repaired during first 48 hours after birth
2. Focus preoperative care on maintaining skin integrity of sac and keeping it free of infection; position infant on side or abdomen to achieve this goal; keep sac moist with sterile, saline-soaked dressings; avoid contamination of sac area by urine or feces
3. Individuals with myelodysplasia have an increased incidence of latex allergies; monitor for this
4. Neurogenic bladder: frequent, clean, straight catheterization is preferred method of management; maintain home schedule as much as possible
5. Neurogenic bowel: work with family to develop a bowel management plan using control of high-fiber diet, adequate fluid intake, and pattern for evacuation of bowels; in some cases, laxatives and enemas are used as prescribed by physician
6. Collaborate with physical therapy to develop modes of transport, such as using braces with crutches or wheelchair
7. Since areas with altered sensation are prone to skin breakdown, teach child and family to reposition frequently and inspect affected areas on a regular basis
8. Medication therapy: low-dose anti-infectives may be prescribed to prevent UTI

D. Client and family education

1. Teach family about possibility of child developing hydrocephalus, signs and symptoms of increased ICP, and what to do if changes develop
2. Since most children with neural tube defects (except spina bifida occulta) have some neurogenic bladder, teaching about clean, intermittent, straight catheterization is important; work with family to develop bowel management program also

XVI. HYDROCEPHALUS

A. Overview

1. A condition characterized by imbalance between CSF production and absorption, resulting in enlarged ventricles and an increase in ICP; if untreated, this condition can cause permanent brain damage
2. Congenital causes include Arnold Chiari malformation associated with myelomeningocele
3. Can be acquired from meningitis, trauma, or intraventricular hemorrhage in premature infants
4. Etiology is idiopathic in up to 50% of cases

B. Nursing assessment

1. For infants, increased head circumference, split cranial sutures, high-pitched cry, bulging fontanel, irritability when awake, and seizures (see Figure 58–5 ■)
2. Toddlers and older children may also present with sunset eyes, seizures, irritability, papilledema, decreased LOC, and change in vital signs (increased systolic BP and widening pulse pressure)
3. Older children and adults may complain of headaches and have difficulty with balance and coordination
4. All clients can present with vomiting, lethargy, and Cheyne-Stokes respiratory pattern
5. Diagnosis confirmed using CT and MRI to reveal location of CSF obstruction

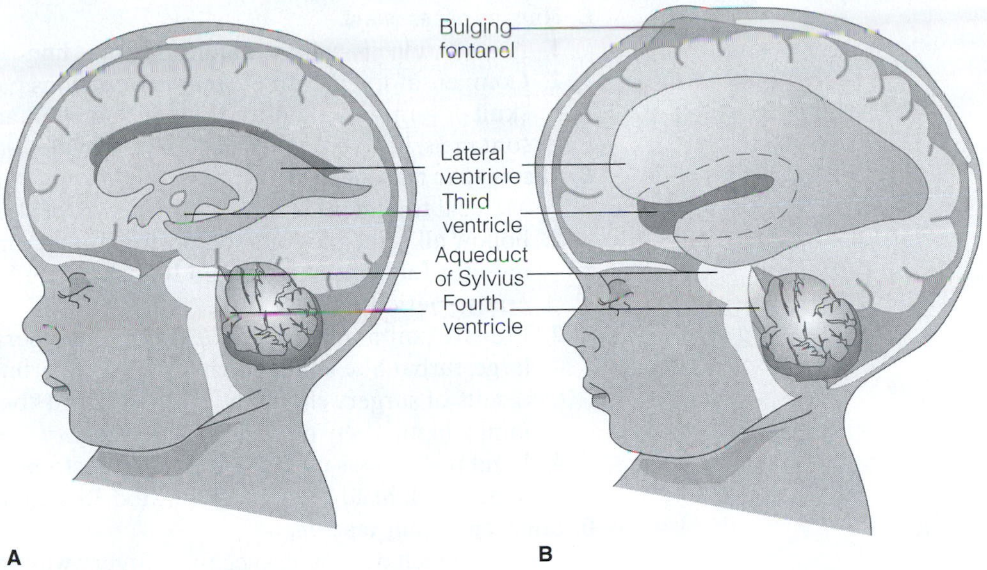

Figure 58–5

Development of hydrocephalus in a young child. A. Normal ventricles. B. Enlarged ventricles and bulging fontanel.

Source: Ball, J., & Bindler, R. (2006). Child health nursing: Partnering with children and families. *Upper Saddle River, NJ: Pearson Education, p. 1325.*

C. Therapeutic management

1. Surgical insertion of a tube (consistency of piece of cooked spaghetti) into ventricles with distal end in either the peritoneum or atrium
   a. Most common version of this shunt is ventriculoperitoneal
   b. Preoperatively monitor client for symptoms of increased ICP
   c. Postoperatively place client flat and on unoperative side; if an infant or child client is held by a caregiver, it is important not to allow head to be elevated
   d. Postoperatively, monitor client for symptoms of infection; notify physician if symptoms are present: fever, change in LOC, excessive redness at incision site or along shunt tract, elevated WBC count with leukocytosis or shift to left
2. Medication therapy: may receive prophylactic antibiotics before and/or after surgery

D. Client and family education

1. Symptoms of shunt infection and malfunction and what actions to take should symptoms develop
2. Signs of shunt malfunction
   a. Infant whose cranial suture lines have not fused; signs include increased head circumference, high-pitched cry, bulging fontanel, irritability when awake, and seizures
   b. Toddlers and older children display vomiting, irritability, and headache; as condition persists, sunset eyes, seizures, papilledema, decreased LOC, and change in vital signs (increased systolic BP and widening pulse pressure) occur
   c. Older clients have difficulty with balance and coordination
   d. All clients may have lethargy and Cheyne-Stokes respirations
3. Some children with hydrocephalus have brain damage that results in motor, language, perceptual, and intellectual disabilities; parents may need referrals to early-intervention professionals to provide long-term rehabilitation services
4. Children with hydrocephalus and myelomeningocele have an increased risk of latex allergies; teach parents to avoid nipples, pacifiers, and toys made of latex products

XVII. CRANIOSYNOSTOSIS

A. Overview

1. Premature closure of cranial sutures in young children
2. There is some relationship between craniosynostosis and several inherited syndromes
3. Etiology is unknown; can be diagnosed by clinical exam, and is confirmed with skull films, CT scan, and MRI
4. Premature closure of skull bones may lead to increased ICP and resulting brain damage

B. Nursing assessment

1. A bony ridge is palpated along a suture line
2. Compensatory growth of skull in directions parallel to closed suture line creates skull deformities; monitor fontanels in all infants for premature closure of fontanels; head circumference also provides data related to this diagnosis

C. Therapeutic management

1. Medical treatment is surgical correction of skeletal defect
2. ! Follow all principles of good postoperative care: keep incision dry and intact; monitor for signs of increased ICP, changing LOC, and infection during postoperative period
3. Prepare parents and child for child's postoperative appearance; in addition to large, turbanlike bandage, child will have orbital edema and bruising; long-term results of surgery should be discussed, and "before and after" pictures may assist family in mentally preparing for surgery
4. ! Fluid restrictions may be ordered in postoperative period; child may be maintained with head of the bed elevated 30 degrees

D. Client and family teaching

1. Should include reassurance that surgery will improve child's appearance and that most children postoperatively are healthy and have normal brain development
2. Instructions about how to change dressing at home

XVIII. MENINGITIS

A. Overview

1. Inflammation of meninges of brain and spinal cord
2. Frequently caused by infection of meninges and CSF (rarely, chemicals are a cause)
3. Besides infectious disease exposure, risk factors include basilar skull fracture, otitis media, sinusitis, mastoiditis, neurosurgery or other invasive procedures, systemic sepsis, and impaired immune function
4. Bacterial causative organisms include *haemophilus influenzae* (type B), *streptococcus pneumoniae,* and *neisseria meningitides* (meningococcal)
5. Bacterial meningitis may be complicated by hydrocephalus, cerebral edema, arthritis, and cranial nerve damage
6. Viral meningitis is usually less severe; course of disease is usually shorter and more benign

B. Nursing assessment

1. ! Clinical manifestations in adults
   a. Restlessness, agitation, and irritability
   b. Abdominal and back pain
   c. Nausea and vomiting
   d. Severe headaches
   e. Signs of meningeal irritation: **nuchal rigidity** (stiff neck), positive Brudzinski's sign (pain, resistance, and hip and knee flexion occur when neck is flexed to chest while lying supine), positive Kernig's sign (pain and/or resistance occurs with flexion of knee and hip and straightening of knee in supine position), and **photophobia** (sensitivity of eyes to light)
   f. Chills and high fever
   g. Confusion, altered LOC
   h. Seizures
   i. Signs and symptoms of increasing ICP
   j. Diagnostic and laboratory test findings: lumbar puncture with CSF analysis, including Gram stain and cultures, is definitive diagnostic measure for meningitis; cultures of blood, urine, throat, and nose are collected to identify possible source of infection
2. ! Bacterial meningitis in infants and toddlers: poor feeding, vomiting, high-pitched cry, bulging fontanel, fever or hypothermia depending on maturity of infant's neurological system, and poor muscle tone; children and adolescents present similarly to adults; **opisthotonus** posture (hyperextending head and neck) is believed to relieve some discomfort from meningeal irritation; petechial or purpuric rash will be seen if it is a meningococcal infection

3. Viral meningitis in infants and toddlers: irritability, lethargy, vomiting, and change in appetite; for older child and adult, usually preceded by a nonspecific febrile illness; presents with headache, malaise, muscle aches, nausea and vomiting, photophobia, and nuchal rigidity or spinal rigidity
4. Diagnosed by analysis of CSF obtained by LP; see Table 58–5 ■

C. Therapeutic management

1. Bacterial meningitis is a medical emergency that, if not treated, can be fatal within days
2. ! Treatment of bacterial meningitis focuses on eradicating bacterial infection with antibiotics
3. Surgical treatment may include placement of an Ommaya reservoir to allow intrathecal (into subarachnoid space) administration of antibiotics
4. ! Monitor respiratory status, administer O_2, and maintain artificial airway
5. Assess neurological status and vital signs (with temperature) regularly; report changes in neurological status or presence of cranial nerve dysfunction
6. Assess, prepare for, and report any seizure activity
7. ! Provide an environment that will minimize ICP elevation; this can include elevating head of bed 15 to 30 degrees, avoiding neck extension or flexion, and maintaining head in a neutral position; keep environment quiet and subdued, and handle client in a gentle manner; assess for signs of increased ICP
8. Administer prescribed medications and maintain fluid restrictions
9. Assess for fluid volume deficits; monitor I & O, daily weights, skin turgor, laboratory values, and urine concentration
10. Medication therapy
    a. Bacterial meningitis is treated for 7 to 14 days with IV antibiotics sensitive to causative organism
    b. ! Preventive care includes a vaccine currently available to protect all young children from haemophilus influenzae infection (Hib); medications for client also include ciprofloxacin (Cipro) or ceftriaxone (Rocephin); individuals who have close contact with clients diagnosed with meningococcal and *H. influenzae* meningitis may receive rifampin (Rifadin) prophylactically
    c. Antiepileptics (usually phenytoin [Dilantin]) to prevent or control seizures
    d. Antipyretic, antiemetic, and analgesic medications for symptom relief
    e. IV fluid replacement until client can resume oral intake
11. Assess for evidence of pain with all routine assessments; administer nonopioid pain medication as prescribed; however, narcotics (opioids) should be avoided because they mask neuro signs and increasing ICP; pain relief should promote rest and reduce risk of increased ICP
12. ! Clients with bacterial meningitis must be isolated on droplet precautions until at least 24 hours of antibiotic therapy have been completed
13. ! Monitor for complications of meningitis (seizures, hearing loss, visual alterations); neurologic sequelae such as mental retardation, CP, and hydrocephalus may occur in children; a complication of meningococcal meningitis is meningococcemia, an overwhelming septic infection that can lead to circulatory collapse and tissue necrosis
14. Viral meningitis is treated symptomatically; usually only infants are hospitalized for viral meningitis

Table 58–5

Comparison of Cerebrospinal Fluid in Meningitis

	Normal	Viral Meningitis	Bacterial Meningitis
Pressure	5–15 mm Hg	Normal or slightly elevated	Elevated
Appearance	Clear	Clear	Cloudy
Leukocytes (mm^3)	0–5	Slightly elevated	Elevated
Protein (mg/dL)	10–30	Slightly elevated	Elevated
Glucose (mg/dL)	40–80	Normal or decreased	Decreased

D. Client and family teaching

1. Importance of taking prescribed antibiotics until finished and other ordered medications as well
2. Recognize and report signs and symptoms of ear, throat, and upper respiratory infections so client can be assessed for meningitis
3. Information about disease and its transmission; provide information about need for possible droplet precautions and antibiotic therapy; also explain need for prophylactic treatment for those in contact with client
4. Provide family with information about possible development of sequelae from disease and possible side effects of medications
5. Share information about follow-up as well as rehabilitation services with family

XIX. ENCEPHALITIS

A. Overview

1. An inflammation of brain tissue
2. Presenting symptoms vary depending on causative organism and location of infection in brain; classic symptoms include an acute febrile illness accompanied by neurologic signs
3. Etiology is usually a viral organism; herpes simplex type 1 is most common cause during neonatal period; enteroviruses are frequently identified as causative agents; nonviral agents include bacteria, parasites, fungi, and rickettsiae
4. Infectious process usually begins elsewhere in body
5. Prognosis depends on degree of CNS involvement; permanent neurologic sequelae may result

B. Nursing assessment

1. In addition to fever, the client may have a severe headache, nausea, vomiting, and signs of an upper respiratory infection
2. Neurologic symptoms include those of nuchal rigidity, photophobia, and positive Kernig's and Brudzinski's signs
3. Other signs include disorientation, confusion with personality or behavior changes, speech disturbances, motor dysfunction, cranial nerve deficits, and focal or generalized seizures that alternate with periods of screaming, hallucinating, and bizarre movement; LOC can change from stupor to coma

C. Therapeutic management

1. Monitor client's vital signs, respiratory status, oxygenation, and urine output
2. Provide seizure precautions and have resuscitation materials close to bed; clients with encephalitis are best managed in an intensive care unit (ICU) during acute phase
3. Maintain skin integrity and prevent other complications of immobility through proper positioning, frequent turning, and chest physiotherapy
4. Work with family in planning for discharge; since many clients have neurologic sequelae, family will need support in giving physical and emotional care at home; parents will play an active role in child rehabilitation process; follow-up visits must be coordinated; families may need referral to home care, counseling, social services, and community support groups
5. Medication therapy: if suspected organism is bacterial, appropriate antibiotics will be ordered; acyclovir or other antiviral agents are administered for herpes virus infection

D. Client and family education

1. Information about causative agent and plan of treatment
2. Discharge plans must be started early; because of neurologic sequelae, plans for rehabilitation must be discussed

XX. REYE SYNDROME

A. Overview

1. An acute metabolic encephalopathy of childhood; fatty degeneration of liver leads to liver dysfunction
2. Characterized by five stages
   a. Vomiting and lethargy
   b. Combativeness and confusion

c. Coma, decorticate posturing
d. Decerebrate posturing
e. Seizures, loss of deep tendon reflexes, respiratory arrest

3. While exact etiology is unclear, Reye syndrome usually develops after a mild viral illness such as chickenpox
4. Research has linked development of Reye syndrome to use of aspirin; following the recommendation that parents use only acetaminophen or ibuprofen, incidence of Reye syndrome has significantly decreased

B. Nursing assessment

1. Child presents with an abrupt change in LOC; history reveals child is recovering from a viral disease with sudden onset of vomiting and mental confusion
2. Liver enzymes and ammonia levels are elevated; blood glucose levels are below normal and prothrombin time is prolonged; bilirubin levels remain normal; liver biopsy shows small fat deposits

C. Therapeutic management

1. Most children are monitored in an ICU; care is focused on support and on assessing child's physical status, such as monitoring for cerebral edema; enforce fluid restrictions (usually instituted); measure frequent vital signs and neurological assessments, which may include Glasgow Coma Scale
2. Monitor lab values for elevated ammonia, acidosis, or hypoglycemia; measure I & O
3. Provide all standard nursing measures to prevent complications of immobility
4. Provide emotional support to family; sudden onset and rapid deterioration in child's condition often overwhelm parents' ability to cope
5. Medication therapy
   a. Controlling cerebral edema is a primary concern; drug management may include corticosteroids to reduce swelling and barbiturates to induce a coma for severe cerebral edema; mannitol (Osmitrol; an osmotic diuretic) may be given
   b. Phenytoin may be used to control seizures
   c. Vitamin K may be given to aid in coagulation

D. Child and family teaching

1. Explanations of disease and its cause, treatment plan and prognosis, ICU environment and medical equipment in use; information helps parents to cope
2. Discharge planning will include rehabilitative needs of child as well as follow-up requirements
3. The public must be educated about Reye syndrome and its connection with viral illnesses and administration of salicylates; public needs to be aware that if a child displays symptoms, early medical intervention is associated with a better prognosis

Check Your NCLEX-RX® Exam I.Q.

You are ready for testing on this content if you can

- Identify basic structures and functions of the neurological system.
- Describe the pathophysiology and etiology of common neurological disorders.
- Discuss expected assessment data and diagnostic test findings for selected neurological disorders.
- Discuss therapeutic management of a client experiencing a neurological disorder.
- Discuss nursing management of a client experiencing a neurological disorder.
- Identify expected outcomes for the client experiencing a neurological disorder.

PRACTICE TEST

1 Which of the following assessment findings in a 35-year-old client with an intracranial hematoma should concern the nurse?

1. Hamstring pain when the hip and knee is flexed and then extended
2. Curling of the toes when the bottom of the foot is stroked in upward motion
3. Muscle aches and cramping, especially at night
4. Cogwheel and lead pipe rigidity

PRACTICE TEST

PRACTICE TEST

2. The nurse would prevent corneal abrasion in the client with myasthenia gravis by performing which of the following nursing interventions?
   1. Doing a saline eye irrigation every shift
   2. Instilling artificial tears in the eyes every 1 to 2 hours
   3. Ensuring the client's contact lenses are on while awake
   4. Providing sunglasses when client is outside

3. The client with newly diagnosed Parkinson's disease states, "I just don't think I can handle having Parkinson's disease." What is the nurse's best first response?
   1. "You sound overwhelmed. Can you tell me more?"
   2. "I am sure you can. A lot of other people do!"
   3. "What do you think will be the hardest thing to handle?"
   4. "The entire health care team will help you manage the disease."

4. The nurse caring for the client with myasthenia gravis would do which of the following as a priority to minimize the risk for complications of the disease?
   1. Inspect for hemorrhage.
   2. Assess for pneumonia.
   3. Offer to cut the client food as needed.
   4. Provide the client with a bedside commode.

5. A client calls the telephone triage nurse to report fever, nausea, chills, and malaise. The nurse instructs the client to come immediately to the emergency room when he relates he also has which of the following?
   1. A bad headache
   2. A stiff sore neck
   3. A heart rate of 106
   4. A roommate with the same symptoms

6. When assessing the client with meningitis, the nurse looks for which of the following as a frequent first sign of increased intracranial pressure?
   1. A rising systolic blood pressure
   2. Change in mood or attention level
   3. Irregular respiratory rate and depth
   4. A bounding radial pulse

7. The nurse is instructing the client who has been in the hospital with bacterial meningitis and will be going home soon. Which of the following will be of the highest priority?
   1. Take all of the antibiotics as directed until completely gone.
   2. Eat a high-protein, high-calorie diet
   3. Exercise daily, beginning with active ROM.
   4. Get at least 8 hours of sleep per night with frequent rest periods.

8. Which of the following instructions would the nurse give to a client with multiple sclerosis who has urinary retention?
   1. "Run water whenever you experience difficulty initiating urination."
   2. "Decrease your fluid intake to prevent urgency."
   3. "Drink a caffeinated beverage to promote the ability to form urine."
   4. "Catheterize your bladder according to the schedule we discussed."

9. The nurse advises the family of the client with Parkinson's disease that the best approach to helping the client maintain as much functional independence as possible will be to
   1. assist the client to take a warm bath every morning.
   2. perform passive ROM three times a day.
   3. display an unhurried manner that allows the client sufficient time to respond or act.
   4. obtain assistive devices that will make activities of daily living (ADLs) easier.

10. The nurse concludes that more teaching may be necessary when visiting a client post-CVA during the first home visit because
   1. The commode is observed to be at the bedside.
   2. A fluid restriction chart is on the refrigerator.
   3. Metamucil is on the kitchen counter.
   4. Hand weights are next to the couch.

11 The office nurse should encourage a client on the phone to go directly to the hospital emergency room based on which of the following statements?

1. "My legs are weak and now I'm having trouble getting a good breath."
2. "My shaky hand is no better than last visit. In fact, I think it's getting worse."
3. "The double vision went away when I put my eye patch on."
4. "My headache doesn't seem any better even though I gave up coffee."

12 A 76-year-old woman comes to the emergency room by ambulance because of a possible stroke. Vital signs are pulse 90, blood pressure 150/100, respirations 20. Thirty minutes later, vital signs are pulse 78, blood pressure 170/90, respirations 24 and irregular. The nurse should take which action at this time?

1. Ask the woman to describe how she's feeling.
2. Check the client's phenytoin (Dilantin) level.
3. Get an order to decrease the rate of IV fluids.
4. Offer the client clear liquids to prevent dehydration.

13 A client seen in the neighborhood clinic complains of "eye problems" and noticed generalized weakness that became markedly worse after visiting with a friend and using the friend's hot tub. The client gives considerably long, detailed answers during the history. The nurse's best response is:

1. "Was the weather the same each time you used the hot tub?"
2. "You'll feel better after getting this all off your mind."
3. "Please be brief in your answers so I can get you through this."
4. "Can you tell me more about the eye problems?"

14 An abnormal EEG indicates that a 2-year-old client has epilepsy, but the parents indicate that they have never observed a seizure. The pediatric nurse concludes that the child may be experiencing seizures of the following type?

1. Petit mal
2. Myoclonic
3. Jacksonian
4. Grand mal

15 The nurse provides care for a 13-year-old who was placed in a halo brace within the last 24 hours because of a spinal cord injury. Which of the following is the first priority of the nurse?

1. Loosen any connections on the vest to assess the skin
2. Assess the pin sites
3. Ask how the client is able to reposition self in bed
4. Encourage active range of motion to lower extremities

16 The rehabilitation nurse is admitting a client following spinal cord injury. The nurse concludes that the client has developed Brown-Séquard syndrome after assessing which of the following in the client?

1. Ipsilateral motor loss above the lesion
2. Contralateral loss of proprioception
3. Hyperanesthesia below the level of the lesion
4. Ipsilateral proprioception loss below lesion

17 While assessing airway and breathing, the client presenting with increased intracranial pressure would most likely exhibit which of the following vital signs?

1. BP 190/84, HR 150, and an irregular respiratory pattern
2. BP 80/50, HR 50, and Kussmaul respirations
3. BP 80/50, HR 150, and Cheyne-Stokes respirations
4. BP 190/84, HR 50, and an irregular respiratory pattern

18 In providing for the safety of the client during a grand mal seizure, the nurse performs which of the following interventions?

1. Positions the client on his back
2. Gently places a padded tongue blade between the teeth
3. Protects the client from injury
4. Applies oxygen immediately via mask

19 The community health nurse interprets that clients who live in a swampy bayou area in the southern United States might be at risk of contracting which of the following?

1. Meningitis
2. Parkinson's
3. Encephalitis
4. Multiple sclerosis

20 The client recently diagnosed with Guillain-Barré syndrome is drooling and having difficulty swallowing secretions. When the family asks why this occurs, the nurse indicates that the cause is

1. Obstructed blood flow to the midbrain.
2. Demyelination of cranial nerves responsible for swallow and gag reflex.
3. Enlargement of the parotid and salivary glands.
4. Deficiency in the thiamine and pyridoxine in the central nervous system.

21 A 1-year-old child has been diagnosed with cerebral palsy. The child has the spastic form that affects all extremities. Which of the following nursing diagnoses would be appropriate for a child at this age?

1. Urinary incontinence
2. Feeding self-care deficit
3. Impaired thought processes
4. Impaired verbal communication

22 The nurse observes a child starting to have a seizure. After assessing the airway, which the highest priority of the nurse?

1. Insert an artificial airway.
2. Observe and record seizure activity.
3. Administer diazepam (Valium).
4. Restrain the extremities to protect the child from injury.

23 The nurse has taught the parents of a 6-year-old child with a ventriculoperitoneal (VP) shunt to monitor the child for shunt malfunction. The nurse determines the parents understand the instructions if they state they will notify the physician if the child presents with

1. Bulging soft spot.
2. Expanding head size.
3. Sunset eyes.
4. Altered level of consciousness.

24 A child is admitted with a head injury after being in a motor vehicle accident. The nurse notes a clear drainage from the left ear. The nurse would suspect

1. Linear skull fracture.
2. Basilar skull fracture.
3. Subdural hematoma.
4. Epidural hematoma.

25 The nurse has formulated a nursing diagnosis of *ineffective family processes related to hospitalization of child with a potentially fatal condition* for the family of a child who sustained a brain injury during an automobile accident. Which of the following interventions would have the highest priority?

1. Teach the family the importance of using seatbelts.
2. Refer the family to support services in the community.
3. Encourage family to ask questions and express feelings.
4. Explain rules for visiting in the intensive care unit.

26 A client arrives at the Emergency Department following head injury and is diagnosed with a concussion. The client exhibits transient confusion with no loss of consciousness and a duration of abnormal mental status for less than 15 minutes. The nurse concludes that this client's symptoms are compatible with a concussion of what grade? Provide a numerical response.

Answer: ____________________

ANSWERS & RATIONALES

1 **Answer: 1** A positive Kernig's sign is common in intracranial hematomas, which is described in option 1. Option 2 is a negative Babinski; with a hematoma, the nurse should expect a positive Babinski (dorsiflexion of the toes in an adult). Option 3 is common in many illnesses; option 4 is specific to Parkinson's disease.
Cognitive Level: Application **Client Need:** Physiological Integrity: Physiological Adaptation **Integrated Process:** Nursing Process: Assessment **Content Area:** Adult Health: Neurological **Strategy:** The core issue of the question is knowledge of associated findings with intracranial hematoma. Use nursing knowledge and the process of elimination to make a selection.

2 **Answer: 2** Corneal abrasion in the client with myasthenia gravis is caused by dryness of the cornea from inability to close the eyelids and blink. It can be prevented by application of artificial tears every 1 to 2 hours. The other options do not address this need.
Cognitive Level: Application **Client Need:** Physiological Integrity: Physiological Adaptation **Integrated Process:** Nursing Process: Implementation **Content Area:** Adult Health: Neurological

Strategy: Use nursing knowledge and the process of elimination to make a selection.

3 **Answer: 1** The nurse should first encourage the client experiencing a loss to express his feelings. This answer acknowledges the client's feelings, is open-ended, and promotes further discussion. Option 2 provides false reassurance. Options 3 and 4 do not address the client's feelings as shared with the nurse.

Cognitive Level: Analysis **Client Need:** Psychosocial Integrity **Integrated Process:** Communication and Documentation **Content Area:** Adult Health: Neurological **Strategy:** The core issue of the question is a therapeutic communication. For communication questions, look first for the option that addresses the client's feelings or concerns.

4 **Answer: 3** When the muscles involved in chewing and swallowing as well as the diaphragm and intercostal muscles are weak, the client may aspirate or experience poor gas exchange; both increase the risk for pneumonia. Options that protect the airway always have highest priority. The client is not at risk for hemorrhage (option 1) or pneumonia (option 2). Option 4 may be an element of routine care.

Cognitive Level: Analysis **Client Need:** Physiological Integrity: Physiological Adaptation **Integrated Process:** Nursing Process: Assessment **Content Area:** Adult Health: Neurological **Strategy:** The core issue of the question is the ability to determine a priority complication of myasthenia gravis and to then select the intervention that reduces it. Use nursing knowledge and the process of elimination to make a selection.

5 **Answer: 2** A stiff sore neck is a sign of meningeal irritation and possible meningitis. The nurse may further inquire if flexion of the neck causes pain and the hip and knee to flex (Brudzinski's sign) and how high the fever is. The other symptoms are typical of influenza.

Cognitive Level: Analysis **Client Need:** Physiological Integrity: Physiological Adaptation **Integrated Process:** Nursing Process: Implementation **Content Area:** Adult Health: Neurological **Strategy:** The core issue of the question is the ability to recognize clients at risk for or showing early signs of meningitis. Use nursing knowledge and the process of elimination to make a selection.

6 **Answer: 2** The first signs of increased intracranial pressure are often subtle changes in level of consciousness. Other changes (including rising systolic BP, irregular respiratory rate, and bounding pulse) come later as intracranial pressure rises further.

Cognitive Level: Analysis **Client Need:** Physiological Integrity: Physiological Adaptation **Integrated Process:** Nursing Process: Assessment **Content Area:** Adult Health: Neurological **Strategy:** The core issue of the question is the ability to discriminate early signs of rising intracranial pressure from later ones. Use nursing knowledge and the process of elimination to make a selection.

7 **Answer: 1** It is essential that the client recovering from bacterial meningitis take all of the prescribed antibiotic as directed. Failure to do so puts the client at risk for a relapse of symptoms and contributes to development of bacterial resistance to antibiotics. Options 2, 3, and 4 are important aspects of self-care during recuperation but are not as essential as the completion of antimicrobial therapy.

Cognitive Level: Application **Client Need:** Physiological Integrity: Physiological Adaptation **Integrated Process:** Communication and Documentation **Content Area:** Adult Health: Neurological **Strategy:** The core issue of the question is the ability to prioritize completion of antibiotic therapy with bacterial meningitis as essential. Use nursing knowledge and the process of elimination to make a selection.

8 **Answer: 4** Urinary retention in the client with multiple sclerosis is a sequela of impaired conduction of nerves innervating the bladder. Performing self-catheterization will drain the bladder and help prevent urinary tract infection. The client with multiple sclerosis will be encouraged to increase fluid intake to prevent constipation. Because urinary retention is incomplete emptying of the bladder, neither running water nor caffeinated beverages would be useful.

Cognitive Level: Application **Client Need:** Physiological Integrity: Physiological Adaptation **Integrated Process:** Communication and Documentation **Content Area:** Adult Health: Neurological **Strategy:** The core issue of the question is knowledge of appropriate methods to manage urinary retention in a client with multiple sclerosis. Use nursing knowledge and the process of elimination to make a selection.

9 **Answer: 3** While options 1, 2, and 4 are all appropriate interventions for the client with Parkinson's disease, the essential approach to enhance and encourage self-care abilities will be an unhurried one that allows sufficient time for self-expression and for the client to do as much as possible for himself or herself.

Cognitive Level: Application **Client Need:** Physiological Integrity: Physiological Adaptation **Integrated Process:** Nursing Process: Implementation **Content Area:** Adult Health: Neurological **Strategy:** The critical word in the question is *approach,* which implies a manner of behaving rather than a specific or single action. Use nursing knowledge and the process of elimination to make a selection.

10 **Answer: 2** Fluid restriction may be needed in the period immediately following a stroke, but this is not necessary after discharge to home. Keeping urine dilute will help prevent urinary tract infection. A fluid intake of 2000 mL per day will also improve bowel elimination.

Cognitive Level: Analysis **Client Need:** Physiological Integrity: Physiological Adaptation **Integrated Process:** Nursing Process: Implementation **Content Area:** Adult Health: Neurological **Strategy:** The core issue of the question is knowledge of fluid needs in a client post-stroke who has been discharged from the acute care setting. Use nursing knowledge of rehabilitation and the process of elimination to make a selection.

11 **Answer: 1** What the client describes is a classic ascending progression of Guillain-Barré syndrome. The muscular weakness may ascend to include the diaphragm. Total respiratory paralysis can occur, requiring ventilatory support. The incorrect responses refer to chronic problems, not an acute one.

Cognitive Level: Analysis **Client Need:** Physiological Integrity: Physiological Adaptation **Integrated Process:** Nursing Process: Implementation **Content Area:** Adult Health: Neurological **Strategy:** Remember the ABCs and prioritize an answer that refers to a possible impaired airway. Use nursing knowledge and the process of elimination to make a selection.

12 **Answer: 3** The client is showing signs of rising intracranial pressure, and infusion of IV fluids leads to hypervolemia and worsens the intracranial pressure. Following Maslow's hierarchy, choose physiological before psychological answers. A Dilantin level would not be relevant to CVA status. The nurse would want to avoid adding to client's volume status by offering fluids, and dehydration is not a concern at this time.
Cognitive Level: Application **Client Need:** Physiological Integrity: Physiological Adaptation **Integrated Process:** Nursing Process: Implementation **Content Area:** Adult Health: Neurological **Strategy:** Use nursing knowledge and the process of elimination to make a selection.

13 **Answer: 4** A more detailed assessment is important in collecting data to meet client needs. A picture of multiple sclerosis may be unfolding. The nurse takes the time to be therapeutic without providing false reassurance or limiting responses. Open-ended, nonjudgmental responses are ideal.
Cognitive Level: Analysis **Client Need:** Physiological Integrity: Physiological Adaptation **Integrated Process:** Communication and Documentation **Content Area:** Adult Health: Neurological **Strategy:** The core issue of the question is selection of an appropriate communication that focuses on assessment. Use nursing knowledge and the process of elimination to make a selection.

14 **Answer: 1** Also known as absence seizures, petit mal seizures may be no more observable than brief staring instances. The mother should be instructed to note and report any change in the child's behavior, no matter how small.
Cognitive Level: Analysis **Client Need:** Physiological Integrity: Physiological Adaptation **Integrated Process:** Nursing Process: Assessment **Content Area:** Child Health: Neurological **Strategy:** The core issue of the question is the ability to discriminate different types of seizures based on presentation (or lack of manifestations). Use nursing knowledge and the process of elimination to make a selection.

15 **Answer: 2** The nurse would want to assess the pin sites for redness, edema, and drainage and would want to ensure that the vest fits snugly. Following the nursing process, an assessment answer would precede an implementation answer (options 3 and 4).
Cognitive Level: Application **Client Need:** Physiological Integrity: Physiological Adaptation **Integrated Process:** Nursing Process: Implementation **Content Area:** Adult Health: Neurological **Strategy:** The core issue of the question is knowledge of appropriate care for a client who is in a halo vest. Use nursing knowledge and the process of elimination to make a selection.

16 **Answer: 4** Hemisection of the anterior and posterior portions of the spinal cord results in loss of position sense (proprioception) on the same side of the body as the trauma, below the level of injury. Option 3 is seen in anterior cord syndrome; option 1 is incorrect.
Cognitive Level: Application **Client Need:** Physiological Integrity: Physiological Adaptation **Integrated Process:** Nursing Process: Assessment **Content Area:** Adult Health: Neurological **Strategy:** The core issue of the question is knowledge of characteristics of Brown-Sequard syndrome following spinal cord injury. Use nursing knowledge and the process of elimination to make a selection.

17 **Answer: 4** The brain stem's final effort to maintain cerebral perfusion is seen with an increased systolic blood pressure, bradycardia, and an irregular respiratory pattern know as Cushing's response.
Cognitive Level: Analysis **Client Need:** Physiological Integrity: Physiological Adaptation **Integrated Process:** Nursing Process: Assessment **Content Area:** Adult Health: Neurological **Strategy:** The core issue of the question is the ability to recognize patterns of change in vital signs that reflect increasing intracranial pressure. Use nursing knowledge and the process of elimination to make a selection.

18 **Answer: 3** The nurse's priority is to protect the client from injury. To promote drainage, it is more effective to secure an airway by turning the client onto the side (option 1). Inserting a tongue blade can cause trauma (option 2); the tongue blade may move during the seizure and obstruct the airway. Oxygen should be available but does not have to be applied (option 4).
Cognitive Level: Application **Client Need:** Safe Effective Care Environment: Safety and Infection Control **Integrated Process:** Nursing Process: Implementation **Content Area:** Adult Health: Neurological **Strategy:** The core issue of the question is priority concerns for a client experiencing a seizure. Use Maslow's hierarchy of needs, nursing knowledge, and the process of elimination to make a selection.

19 **Answer: 3** Mosquitoes, the vectors that transport encephalitis, are found in large numbers in swampy areas. Meningitis can be attributed to overcrowded conditions; Parkinson's has an uncertain etiology; and risk factors for multiple sclerosis include genetics and family history.
Cognitive Level: Application **Client Need:** Physiological Integrity: Physiological Adaptation **Integrated Process:** Nursing Process: Assessment **Content Area:** Adult Health: Neurological **Strategy:** The core issue of the question is knowledge of risk factors for encephalitis. Use nursing knowledge and the process of elimination to make a selection.

20 **Answer: 2** Guillain-Barré syndrome is an acute demyelinating disorder that less commonly may present with initial weakness in the cranial nerves that progresses downward. Impairment of cranial nerves IX and X will affect swallowing.
Cognitive Level: Application **Client Need:** Physiological Integrity: Physiological Adaptation **Integrated Process:** Nursing Process: Implementation **Content Area:** Adult Health: Neurological **Strategy:** The core issue of the question is the ability to explain pathophysiology underlying signs and symptoms of Guillain-Barré syndrome. Use nursing knowledge and the process of elimination to make a selection.

21 **Answer: 4** At this age, a 1-year-old is beginning speech. This child will have trouble developing language because of the spasticity. Urinary incontinence occurs in all 1-year-old children, as does feeding self-care deficit. Thought processes are difficult to evaluate in a 1-year-old.
Cognitive Level: Analysis **Client Need:** Physiological Integrity: Physiological Adaptation **Integrated Process:** Nursing Process: Analysis **Content Area:** Child Health: Neurological **Strategy:** The core issue of the question is the ability to determine appropriate nursing diagnoses for a client with cerebral palsy while taking into consideration growth and development. Use nursing knowledge and the process of elimination to make a selection.

22 **Answer: 2** Observation and documentation of seizure activity can provide valuable information to help in diagnosis and treatment. Once a seizure is in process, it would be dangerous to attempt to insert an airway. Administration of medication would require a physician's order. Actually restraining the extremities is more likely to inflict injury than prevent.
Cognitive Level: Application **Client Need:** Safe Effective Care Environment: Safety and Infection Control **Integrated Process:** Nursing Process: Implementation **Content Area:** Child Health: Neurological **Strategy:** The core issue of the question is the ability to provide safe care to a client experiencing a seizure. Use nursing knowledge and the process of elimination to make a selection.

23 **Answer: 4** In most children, by age 6, the cranial suture lines have fused and the fontanelles are closed, so the first three symptoms would not be common. An altered level of consciousness would be a symptom of shunt malfunction for the older child.
Cognitive Level: Application **Client Need:** Physiological Integrity: Physiological Adaptation **Integrated Process:** Nursing Process: Evaluation **Content Area:** Child Health: Neurological **Strategy:** The core issue of the question is knowledge of early signs of rising intracranial pressure, which is a sign of shunt malfunction. Use nursing knowledge and the process of elimination to make a selection.

24 **Answer: 2** Drainage of cerebrospinal fluid (a clear fluid) from the ear is a symptom of basilar skull fracture. Children with linear skull fractures are often asymptomatic. Subdural and epidural hematomas present with signs of increasing intracranial pressure.
Cognitive Level: Analysis **Client Need:** Physiological Integrity: Physiological Adaptation **Integrated Process:** Nursing Process: Analysis **Content Area:** Child Health: Neurological **Strategy:** The core issue of the question is the ability to correctly interpret signs of head injury. Use nursing knowledge and the process of elimination to make a selection.

25 **Answer: 3** While families may need education about seatbelts and sources of support, it is not the optimal time to implement such teaching at this point in the crisis. It is optimal to find out what the family's perception is of what is going on and what they feel their needs are. The best way to determine this is to encourage them to ask questions and express their feelings. Timelines for visitation are appropriate but of less priority than option 3.
Cognitive Level: Analysis **Client Need:** Psychosocial Integrity **Integrated Process:** Nursing Process: Planning **Content Area:** Child Health: Neurological **Strategy:** The core issue of the question is the ability to determine priorities for the family of a critically ill child. Select the option that will most closely address the family's current issues and concerns.

26 **Answer: 1** In a grade 1 concussion, the client exhibits transient confusion with no loss of consciousness and a duration of abnormal mental status for less than 15 minutes. Grades 2 and 3 concussion consist of more severe neurological symptoms, with increasing levels of loss of consciousness and more significant abnormalities of mental status.
Cognitive Level: Analysis **Client Need:** Physiological Integrity: Physiological Adaptation **Integrated Process:** Nursing Process: Analysis **Content Area:** Adult Health: Neurological **Strategy:** The core issue of the question is the ability to correctly interpret signs of head injury related to concussion. Use knowledge of the pathophysiology of concussion to determine an answer.

ANSWERS & RATIONALES

Key Terms to Review

agnosia p. 1095
aphasia p. 1084
apraxia p. 1095
autonomic dysreflexia p. 1091
bradykinesia p. 1098
Broca's area p. 1079
Brudzinski's sign p. 1084
coma p. 1085
Cushing's triad p. 1087
dysarthria p. 1084
dysphagia p. 1095
epidural hematoma p. 1089
hemianopsia p. 1095
intracranial pressure (ICP) p. 1087
intrathecal p. 1103
Kernig's sign p. 1084
level of consciousness (LOC) p. 1082
meninges p. 1081
myelin p. 1093
neurogenic p. 1104
nuchal rigidity p. 1106
opisthotonus p. 1106
paraplegia p. 1091
photophobia p. 1106
spasticity p. 1099
subdural hematoma p. 1089
tetraplegia p. 1091
tonic-clonic p. 1096
Wernicke's area p. 1079

References

Ball, J., & Bindler, R. (2006). *Child health nursing: Partnering with children and families*. Upper Saddle River, NJ: Pearson Education.

Black, J., & Hawks, J. (2005). *Medical surgical nursing: Clinical management for positive outcomes* (7th ed.). St. Louis: Elsevier Science.

Corbett, J. (2004). *Laboratory tests and diagnostic procedures with nursing diagnoses* (6th ed.). Upper Saddle River, NJ: Pearson Education.

Harkreader, H., & Hogan, M. (2004). *Fundamentals of nursing: Caring and clinical judgment* (2nd ed.). St. Louis: Elsevier Science.

Ignatavicius, D., & Workman, L. (2006). *Medical-surgical nursing: Critical thinking for collaborative care* (5th ed.). Philadelphia: W. B. Saunders.

Kozier, B., Erb, G., Berman, A., & Snyder, S. (2004). *Fundamentals of nursing: Concepts, process, and practice* (7th ed.). Upper Saddle River, NJ: Pearson Education.

LeMone, P., & Burke, K. (2004). *Medical surgical nursing: Critical thinking in client care* (3rd ed.). Upper Saddle River, NJ: Pearson Education.

Lewis, S., Heitkemper, M., & Dirksen, S. (2004). *Medical surgical nursing: Assessment and management of clinical problems* (6th ed.). St. Louis: Elsevier Science.

Porth, C. (2004). *Pathophysiology: Concepts of altered health states* (7th ed.). Philadelphia: Lippincott Williams & Wilkins.

Smith, S., Duell, D., & Martin, B. (2004). *Clinical nursing skills: Basic to advanced skills* (6th ed.). Upper Saddle River, NJ: Pearson Education.

59 Renal or Genitourinary Disorders

Test Yourself

Are you ready for the NCLEX-RN® or course exams? Use the practice tests on the companion CD-ROM to check.

In this chapter

Cross reference

Other chapters relevant to this content area are

Meeting Nutritional Needs	Chapter 26
Renal Medications	Chapter 40
Common Laboratory Tests	Chapter 47
Common Diagnostic Tests and Procedures	Chapter 48

I. OVERVIEW OF ANATOMY AND PHYSIOLOGY OF THE RENAL AND URINARY SYSTEMS

A. Renal structures

1. Kidneys: bean-shaped organs located on either side of spinal column behind peritoneal cavity; regulate fluid and acid-base balance
2. Adrenal glands: located atop each kidney; influence blood pressure (BP) and sodium (Na^+) and water retention

3. Renal cortex: outer region of kidneys; contains blood-filtering mechanisms
4. Renal medulla: middle region of kidneys; contains renal pyramids
5. Renal pyramids: triangular wedges containing tubular structures
   a. Apex: tapered section of each pyramid; empties into calyx (calyces)
   b. Calyces: channel urine from renal pyramids to renal pelvis
6. Renal pelvis: expansion of upper end of ureters, formed as calyces join together
7. **Nephron**: basic functional unit of kidneys; selectively secretes and reabsorbs ions; perform mechanical filtration of fluid, wastes, electrolytes, acids, and bases; contains a **glomerulus** surrounded by Bowman's capsule

B. Function of kidneys

1. Nephrons filter waste products as well as needed materials, such as electrolytes, from blood; necessary substances are returned to blood through reabsorption
2. Filtration: first step in blood processing; water and solutes move from plasma in glomerulus into Bowman's capsule; depends on pressure gradient between blood in glomeruli and filtrate in Bowman's capsule
3. Reabsorption: second step in urine formation; molecules move from tubules into blood through tubule cells; active and passive transport mechanisms are used in all parts of renal tubules
   a. Proximal tubules: reabsorb sodium (Na^+) and other major ions through active and passive transport
   b. Loop of Henle: reabsorbs through countercurrent mechanism (passive); contents flow in opposite directions
   c. Distal tubules: reabsorb Na^+ by active and passive transport in smaller amounts than proximal tubules
   d. Collecting ducts: prevent water from leaving filtrate; use active and passive reabsorption
4. Tubular secretion: movement of substances out of blood into tubular fluid; tubules secrete certain substances in addition to performing reabsorption
5. Regulation of urine volume: hormones play a central part in urine regulation
6. Osmolality: osmotic pressure of a solution expressed as a number of osmols of pressure per kg of water; active transport and reabsorption mechanisms are based on osmolality of solutions

C. Renal hormones and enzymes

1. *Antidiuretic hormone (ADH):* regulates urine volume by acting in distal tubule and collecting ducts to increase water reabsorption and urine concentration
2. *Atrial natriuretic hormone (ANH):* secreted by muscle fibers in atrium of heart; promotes loss of Na^+ via urine
3. *Aldosterone:* secreted by adrenal cortex; increases sodium absorption in distal and collecting tubules and controls potassium (K^+) secretion, leading to osmotic imbalance that causes reabsorption of water; works in conjunction with ADH
   a. Increased serum K^+ levels lead to increased aldosterone secretion
   b. Increased aldosterone secretion increases Na^+ and water retention and depresses formation of renin
4. Renin: enzyme secreted by kidneys; helps regulate Na^+ retention and therefore blood pressure (BP) and fluid volume
   a. Renin-angiotensin system: converts angiotensinogen to angiotensin I in liver
   b. Angiotensin II: formed in lungs from angiotensin I; vasoconstrictor that stimulates adrenal cortex to produce aldosterone
5. Erythropoietin: hormone produced by kidneys in response to low oxygen (O_2) levels in arterial blood; travels to bone marrow and stimulates increased red blood cell (RBC) production

D. Urinary excretion

1. Ureters: extend from renal pelvis of kidney to urinary bladder; conduct urine
2. Bladder: elastic sac located behind symphysis pubis; stores and excretes urine
3. Urethra: tube that carries urine from bladder to exterior of body
4. Urinary meatus: exterior opening of urethra
5. Urination: an involuntary or voluntary reflex allowing urine to leave body
   a. Micturition reflex: parasympathetic response that stimulates relaxation and contraction of external sphincter, allowing urine to pass

b. Internal sphincter muscle: helps control urine passage into urethra; relaxes in response to parasympathetic nerve fibers in bladder wall
c. External sphincter muscle: voluntary muscle that allows urine to pass into urethra; controlled by micturition reflex

! 6. Characteristics of normal urine
a. Color: clear, pale amber
b. Consistency: 95% water with many dissolved substances
c. Output: 1,000 to 2,000 mL per 24-hour period; kidneys produce a minimum of 30 mL/hour under normal circumstances
d. Specific gravity: commonly 1.015 to 1.025 (range 1.010 to 1.030)
e. Odor: faint ammonia

E. Renal system differences between child and adult
1. Fluid is more important to body chemistry of infants and small children because it constitutes a larger fraction of total body weight
2. During first 2 years of life, kidneys are less efficient at regulating electrolyte and acid-base balance; infants are more prone to fluid volume excess and dehydration
3. Bladder capacity increases from 20 to 50 mL at birth to 700 mL in adulthood
4. Innervation of "stretch" receptors in bladder wall, which initiates urination and control of bladder sphincters (does not occur before age 2); children under 2 cannot maintain bladder control
5. Urethra is shorter in children than in adults and may contribute to frequency of urinary tract infections (UTIs) in children
6. Kidneys are more susceptible to trauma in children because they do not have as much fat padding

II. DIAGNOSTIC TESTS AND ASSESSMENTS OF THE URINARY SYSTEM

A. Physical assessment
1. Appearance of meatus: normal position and lack of redness, swelling
2. Voiding pattern: frequency, amount, hesitancy, urgency, dysuria

B. Urine studies
1. Urinalysis: urinalysis for dipstick results, microscopic examination, or culture; refer to Chapter 47 for normal results and Table 59–1 ■ for significance of color changes
2. Clean-catch specimen: urine specimen collected in a clean specimen container following cleansing of the urinary meatus and surrounding tissue; in infants and toddlers, catheterization may be performed; parental assistance is needed for school-aged, toilet-trained children, and specimens are obtained individually by adolescents after careful instruction
3. Sterile urine specimen: obtained by urinary catheterization only

Table 59–1

Interpreting Changes in Urine Color

Color	Possible Meaning
Pale yellow	Normal
Yellow	Concentrated urine
Amber	Bile in urine
Orange	Alkaline or concentrated urine
Red-orange	Acidic urine, medication effect
Red	Blood, menses
Pink	Dilute blood
Burgundy	Laxatives
Tea	Melanin, hematuria
Dark gray	Medications, dyes
Blue	Dyes, medications

4. Urine culture: checks urine for bacteria; urine is normally sterile
5. Twenty-four-hour urine specimen: urine is collected over 24 hours for following tests:
   a. **Creatinine:** nitrogenous waste product excreted by muscle tissue; normally found in urine (normal = 15 to 25 mg/kg in 24 hours)
   b. Creatinine clearance: test to assess how well the kidneys remove creatinine from the blood (male = 95 to 135 mL/min; female = 85 to 125 mL/min)
   c. Protein: less than 150 mg/24 hours
   d. Urea nitrogen: end product of protein metabolism (normal 6 to 17 g/24 hours)
6. Urine osmolality: osmotic pressure (concentration) of urine; average is 500 to 800 mOsm/kg water, with an extreme range of 50 to 1,400 mOsm/kg water

C. **Renal scan:** intravenous (IV) radioactive substance (radionuclide) is injected, then observed passing through kidneys; evaluates renal blood flow, nephron and collecting system function, and renal structures

D. **Radiographic studies (see also Chapter 48)**
1. Kidney-ureter-bladder (KUB) radiography: shows kidney size, position, and structure; provides limited diagnostic information
2. Renal angiography: detects abnormalities such as cysts, renal artery stenosis, and renal infarction
3. Renal venography: detects renal vein thrombosis
4. Retrograde cystography: contrast medium instilled into bladder via a catheter, followed by x-ray examination; several films are taken and dye is then drained via catheter; a final picture is taken when bladder is emptied; helps diagnose ruptured or neurogenic bladder and other conditions
5. Voiding cystourethrography: same process as a cystogram except when bladder is filled with contrast dye, urethral catheter is removed; client is allowed to void when urge is felt; films are taken during bladder filling, during **micturition** (voiding) and after voiding

E. **Computerized tomography (CT) scan:** identifies masses and other lesions; contrast medium may be injected

F. **Magnetic resonance imaging (MRI):** produces three-dimensional images of renal tissue

G. **Ultrasonography:** evaluates kidney size, shape, and position

H. **Blood studies**
1. *Blood urea nitrogen (BUN):* measures nitrogenous urea in blood; urea is produced by protein metabolism; insufficient excretion causes levels to rise and may indicate renal disorders; also rises with dehydration and intake of high-protein diet or other conditions in which excess protein is metabolized
   a. Normal: 8 to 25 mg/dL
   b. BUN levels best evaluated in conjunction with serum creatinine levels
2. Serum creatinine: creatinine is a nitrogenous waste resulting from muscle metabolism of creatine; creatinine levels reflect glomerular filtration rate
   a. Measures renal damage more reliably than BUN, because severe renal damage is the only cause of significant elevation
   b. Normal: 0.6 to 1.5 mg/dL for adult males; 0.6 to 1.1 mg/dL for adult females

I. **Intravenous pyelography (IVP):** one or more x-rays of renal pelvis and ureters following injection of a contrast medium; special pre-procedure care may be necessary

J. **Cystoscopy or cystourethroscopy:** insertion of a cystoscope with a fiberoptic light source and telescopic lens into urethra for biopsy of bladder and prostate, lesion resection, calculi collection, or passage of catheter to renal pelvis

K. **Percutaneous renal biopsy:** client is positioned on abdomen while needle is inserted into kidney to remove tissue; x-ray may be used to guide needle; reveals renal disease, malignant tumors, and other conditions; risks include bleeding, hematoma, arteriovenous fistula, and infection

III. COMMON NURSING TECHNIQUES AND PROCEDURES

A. **Urinary catheterization:** introduction of a catheter into urinary bladder
1. Indwelling urinary catheter: a retention (Foley) catheter with balloon is inserted and remains in place; see Box 59–1

Box 59–1

Insertion of an Indwelling Urinary Catheter

- Explain procedure to client and ensure privacy
- *Female:* assist client to supine position with knees flexed and thighs externally rotated; drape the client
- Wearing disposable gloves, cleanse perineal area; remove gloves
- Prepare equipment and set up sterile field; don sterile gloves; drape client with sterile drape
- Lubricate sterile cotton balls with antiseptic solution (agency policy may differ concerning use of antiseptic) and lubricate insertion tip of catheter with water-soluble jelly
- Clean meatus with antiseptic (check agency policy)
- Use nondominant hand to separate labia minor and expose urinary meatus; assess meatus for swelling, discharge, or redness
- Grasp catheter near the insertion end with sterile, gloved hand; gently insert catheter into meatus and advance the catheter until urine flows; do not use forceful pressure; ask client to take deep breaths to relax external sphincter
- Advance the catheter farther into bladder (1 to 2 inches) and inflate balloon by injecting contents of prefilled syringe
- Apply slight tension by pulling back on catheter until resistance is felt to confirm that balloon is in the bladder
- Anchor catheter to client's thigh with nonallergic tape and secure drainage bag to bed frame in a dependent position
- *Male:* use same positioning except knees do not need to be flexed
- Wearing disposable gloves, wash penis and dry it well
- Follow catheter preparatory steps as described above
- Grasp insertion end of catheter with sterile, gloved hand; lift penis to 90-degree angle with body and exert slight traction
- Insert catheter steadily about 20 cm (8 inches) until urine begins to flow; ask client to take deep breaths to relax external sphincter; rotate catheter during insertion if slight resistance is met because of curvature of the urethra
- Advance catheter farther into bladder (1 to 2 inches) and inflate balloon by injecting contents of prefilled syringe; secure as described above

2. Intermittent catheterization: used for clients with neurogenic bladder dysfunction; may be done by nurse or at home by client after proper instruction on procedure (Box 59–2)

B. Urine collection

1. Twenty-four-hour urine collection
    a. Obtain specimen container with preservative from laboratory
    b. Provide clean receptacle to collect urine (bedpan, urinal, commode, or collection device on toilet) unless client already has an indwelling urinary catheter
    c. Post signs in client's room, on chart, and in bathroom alerting personnel to save urine
    d. ! Have client void and discard first urine at beginning of collection period; if indwelling catheter used, empty the collection bag at the start time
    e. During collection period, save all urine in container; place container on ice or refrigerate as indicated; don't contaminate urine with bathroom tissue or feces
    f. ! Instruct client to empty bladder at end of collection period and save this urine
    g. Send collected urine to laboratory with completed requisition
    h. Document collection of specimen, time started and completed, and any observations
2. Clean catch (midstream)
    a. Ask client to wash genital and perineal area with soap and water from front to back

Box 59–2

Client Instructions for Intermittent Urinary Self-Catheterization

- Catheterize as often as needed; may be every 2 to 3 hours at first, then every 4 to 6 hours
- Encourage client to void before procedure if appropriate; use catheter to obtain residual urine if amount voided is less than 100 mL
- Assemble all supplies and use good lighting
- Wash hands
- Clean urinary meatus with towelette or soapy washcloth, then rinse and dry; female clients should clean perineum from front to back
- Assume comfortable position, such as standing with one foot elevated, semireclining in bed, or sitting on chair or toilet
- Apply lubricant to catheter tip
- *Female:* locate meatus using a mirror or touch; separate labia with dominant hand; direct catheter through meatus, then forward and upward
- *Male:* hold penis with slight upward tension to 90-degree angle and insert catheter
- Hold catheter in place until all urine is drained, then withdraw slowly
- Wash catheter with soap and water; store in clean container
- Notify care provider of cloudy urine, sediment, bleeding, fever, or difficulty passing catheter
- Drink at least 2,000 to 2,500 mL of fluid daily; cranberry and prune juices help to acidify the urine to possibly reduce bacterial growth in the bladder

b. Instruct to clean meatus with antiseptic towelettes
c. Female clients: use three towelettes, clean perineal area from front to back; use each towelette only once
d. Male clients: clean meatus with circular motion and distal portion of penis; use each towelette only once
e. For client who needs assistance: nurse may don gloves, clean perineal area, assist client to a comfortable position, and open clean-catch kit
f. Instruct client to begin voiding, then place specimen container in stream of urine; collect 30 to 60 mL of urine
g. Cap container, touching only outside
h. Label container, place in biohazard bag along with requisition, and immediately send to laboratory
i. Document pertinent data, such as difficulty voiding, strong odor to urine, or sediment

C. Peritoneal dialysis: removes toxins from blood of client with acute or chronic renal failure; uses peritoneal membrane as semipermeable dialyzing membrane (see Figure 59–1 ■)

1. Hypertonic dialyzing solution (dialysate) is instilled through a catheter in peritoneal cavity
2. Excess concentrations of electrolytes and uremic toxins move by diffusion across peritoneal membrane into dialysis solution; excess water moves into solution by osmosis
3. Dialysate is drained after appropriate dwelling time
4. Procedure is performed manually or by use of a cycler machine; client may also perform continuous ambulatory peritoneal dialysis (CAPD)
5. ! Possible complications
   a. Peritonitis from bacteria entering peritoneal cavity (use surgical aseptic technique when handling catheter or tubing); peritonitis is critical to prevent because it could result in client having to change therapy to **hemodialysis** (removal of wastes in blood)
   b. Catheter obstruction from clots or kinking (keep all lines unobstructed; add heparin to dialysate per protocol)
   c. Insufficient outflow (reposition client as needed to bring fluid into contact with catheter; allow to ambulate if condition allows)

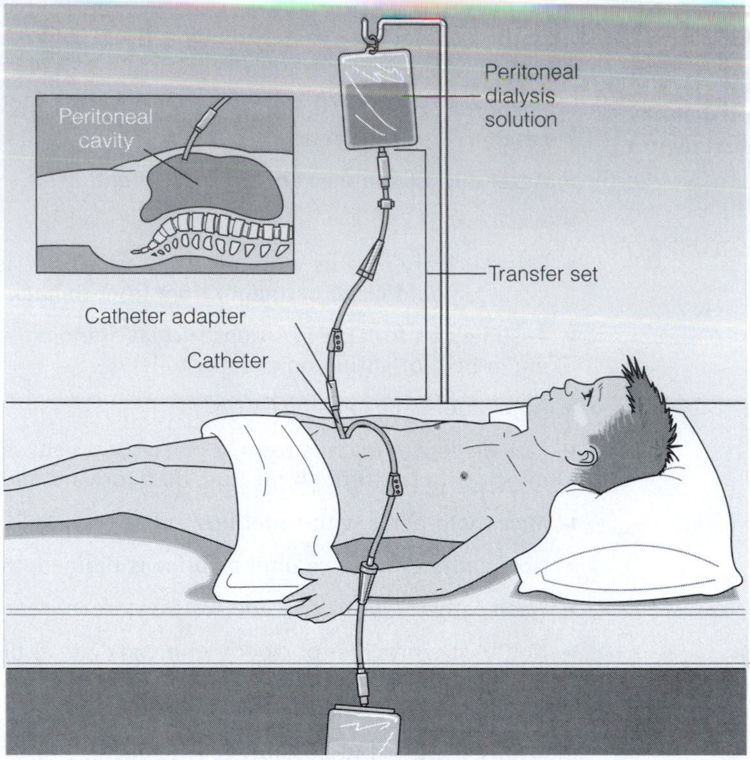

Figure 59–1

Peritoneal dialysis.

Source: Hogan, M., & White, J. (2002). Child health nursing: Reviews and rationales. *Upper Saddle River, NJ: Pearson Education, p. 179.*

d. Hypotension and hypovolemia from excess fluid removal (carefully monitor I & O records; report accordingly)
e. Hyperglycemia (from glucose in dialysate; monitor diabetic clients closely; do not allow fluid to dwell longer than ordered)

! 6. Peritoneal dialysis procedure (see Box 59–3)

D. Urinary diversion stoma care

! 1. Collection device should fit snugly around stoma; allow no more than 1/8-inch margin of skin between stoma and faceplate
2. Stoma should appear light or bright red; suspect a problem if it is deep red or bluish in color
! 3. Check peristomal skin for breakdown; main cause of irritation is urine leakage; change device and cleanse skin if leakage occurs
   a. Cleanse area with warm water and pat dry; apply light coating of karaya powder and thin layer of protective dressing
   b. Notify physician if severe skin excoriation occurs
4. Assess I & O; note changes in urine color, odor, or clarity
! 5. Home care by client
   a. Expect stoma shrinkage within 8 weeks after surgery; may require smaller pouch opening
   b. Encourage client to change appliance as needed in early morning when urine production is less following sleep
   c. Appliance is often a one-piece unit (faceplate and collection bag) and must be emptied regularly and changed according to product directions
   d. Instruct client to report fever, chills, flank pain, abdominal pain, and pus in urine (**pyuria**) or blood in urine (**hematuria**)
   e. Refer client to support group, such as United Ostomy Association

E. Care of an arteriovenous (AV) fistula

1. An AV fistula provides vascular access to a vein and an artery for hemodialysis; most common sites are radial or brachial artery and cephalic vein
! 2. Assess circulation at access site by auscultating for bruits and palpating for thrills; lack of bruit may indicate blood clot and requires immediate surgical intervention
! 3. Avoid using accessed arm for other procedures, such as IV insertion, BP monitoring, or venipuncture

Box 59–3

Peritoneal Dialysis Procedure

- ➤ Explain procedure and check vital signs and weight
- ➤ Have client urinate, if able, to avoid bladder puncture or discomfort; perform catheterization if client is unable to void
- ➤ Warm dialysate to body temperature in a warmer
- ➤ Use 1.5%, 2.5%, or 4.25% dextrose solution, usually with heparin added to prevent catheter clotting; dialysate should be clear and colorless; add prescribed medication as ordered
- ➤ Put on surgical mask and prepare dialysis administration set, maintaining strict sterile technique at all times
- ➤ Place drainage bag below client and connect outflow tubing
- ➤ Connect dialysis infusion line to dialysate bags and hang on IV pole
- ➤ Place client in supine position, prime the tubing with solution, close the clamps, and connect infusion line to abdominal catheter
- ➤ Test catheter by instilling 500 mL of dialysate into peritoneal cavity; clamp tubing; unclamp outflow line and drain fluid into collection bag; if outflow is brisk, the catheter is patent
- ➤ Unclamp infusion lines and infuse prescribed amount of dialysate; close clamps when bag is empty
- ➤ Allow solution to dwell for prescribed time (usually up to 4 hours)
- ➤ Open outflow clamps and allow solution to drain
- ➤ Repeat cycle according to prescribed number of times; when completed, clamp peritoneal catheter and disconnect inflow line while wearing sterile gloves
- ➤ Apply sterile dressing to catheter site
- ➤ During procedure, monitor vital signs every 10 minutes until stable, then every 2 to 4 hours
- ➤ Observe for signs of peritonitis: fever; persistent abdominal pain and cramping; slow or cloudy dialysate drainage; swelling, redness, or tenderness around catheter; increased WBC count
- ➤ Wear protective eyewear when draining or handling outflow solution
- ➤ Check outflow tubing periodically for clots or kinks; having client change position may increase flow
- ➤ Clients lose protein during peritoneal dialysis and require fewer or no dietary restrictions of protein
- ➤ Calculate fluid balance at end of each exchange (with manual dialysis), or at end of each session, or every 8 hours, depending on protocol; include oral and IV intake, urine output, and wound drainage in calculations

4. Monitor site for bleeding after completion of hemodialysis
5. Home care instructions for client
   a. Keep fistula area clean and dry
   b. Notify health provider of pain, swelling, redness, or drainage in accessed arm
   c. Exercise is beneficial and helps stimulate vein enlargement
   ! d. Don't allow any treatments or procedures on accessed arm
   ! e. Avoid excessive pressure to arm; don't sleep on it, wear constrictive clothing or jewelry, or lift heavy objects
   f. Avoid showering, bathing, or swimming for several hours after dialysis

F. ***Hemodialysis:*** **removes wastes from body by filtering client's blood using a machine**

1. Nurses who have undergone specialized instruction and training perform hemodialysis
2. ! Before procedure, weigh client and take vital signs (VS); check BP in lying and standing positions (orthostatic blood pressures); check for routine medications that should be withheld until dialysis is completed (i.e., antihypertensives that could lower BP or medications that would be dialyzed out of client's system)

3. Wear protective eyewear, gown, and gloves for protection during hemodialysis procedure
4. Dialysis is continued usually for 3 to 4 hours, depending on client's condition; monitor partial thromboplastin time (PTT) or other standard laboratory studies as ordered according to protocol (heparin is used as an anticoagulant during procedure)
5. At end of treatment, obtain blood samples as ordered, return blood remaining in dialyzer to client, and remove needles from vascular access device
6. Monitor access device for bleeding and maintain pressure on site as needed
7. Early in course of hemodialysis, assess for and report disequilibrium syndrome, a condition in which cerebral edema forms from less rapid excretion of wastes behind blood–brain barrier, and subsequent uptake of fluid by brain cells
   a. Assess client for headache, mental confusion, decreasing LOC, nausea, vomiting, twitching, and possible seizure activity
   b. Call physician to obtain necessary orders for anticonvulsant medication
   c. Is prevented by dialyzing for shorter times or at reduced blood flow rates early in course of therapy

IV. NURSING MANAGEMENT OF THE CLIENT HAVING RENAL OR BLADDER SURGERY

A. **Lithotripsy**: also called extracorporeal shock-wave lithotripsy (ESWL); uses high-energy shock waves to break up calculi, restoring normal passage of urine
1. Perform preoperative teaching about procedure and postoperative course and care
   a. Treatment takes 30 minutes to 1 hour
   b. Client will receive a general or epidural anesthetic
2. Postprocedure care
   a. Perform baseline assessment and check VS following agency policy
   b. Maintain patency of indwelling urinary catheter and monitor I & O
   c. Strain urine for calculi fragments and send these to laboratory for analysis
   d. Slight hematuria is common, but report persistent bleeding
   e. Encourage ambulation to aid passage of calculi fragments
   f. Increase fluid intake as ordered to aid passage of calculi fragments
   g. Give analgesics as needed; severe pain may indicate presence of new calculi—report such findings immediately
3. Home care instructions for client
   a. Drink 3 to 4 L of fluid daily up to 1 month after treatment
   b. Strain urine during first week and save any calculi fragments; bring these to first follow-up visit with physician
   c. Expect blood-tinged urine, mild GI upset, and pain in treated side as calculi fragments pass; bruising on affected side will disappear
   d. Report severe pain, persistent blood in urine, inability to void, fever and chills, or nausea and vomiting
   e. Review prescribed medications or dietary regimen

B. **Ureterolithotomy, pyelolithotomy, nephrolithotomy**: involve making an incision into ureter, renal pelvis, or renal calyx to remove urinary calculi
1. Preoperative period
   a. Explain procedure to client
   b. Explain postoperative care, including presence of a urinary catheter
   c. Administer pre-anesthetic medications as ordered
2. Postoperative period
   a. Perform baseline assessments as for all postoperative clients (VS, LOC, status of dressing)
   b. Monitor urine output (UO) for amount, color, and clarity; urine may be bright red initially, but amount of bleeding should diminish; cloudy urine may indicate infection
   c. Maintain placement and patency of urinary catheters; irrigate gently as ordered
   d. Assess for pain and administer analgesics as needed
   e. Increase client's fluid intake, as ordered, to aid passage of calculi fragments
   f. Strain urine for calculi fragments and send them to laboratory for analysis

3. Home care for client
   a. Follow agency policy for home incision care
   b. Drink 3 to 4 liters of fluid daily up to a month after treatment
   c. Report bloody, cloudy, or foul-smelling urine
   d. Report inability to void, fever, chills, redness, swelling, or purulent drainage from incision
   e. Strain urine during first week and save any calculi fragments; bring them to first follow-up visit with physician
   f. Avoid strenuous exercise, sexual activity, heavy lifting, or straining until advised otherwise by physician
   g. Mild activity aids passage of any retained calculi fragments
   h. Review prescribed medications or dietary regimen
   i. Explain catheter care if client is discharged with indwelling catheter

C. Cystectomy with urinary diversion

1. Complete radical **cystectomy** involves surgical removal of bladder plus adjacent muscles and tissues
   a. In men, prostate gland and seminal vesicles are removed, which results in impotence
   b. In women, uterus, Fallopian tubes, and ovaries are removed, resulting in sterility
   c. A urinary diversion is created to provide for urine collection and drainage
2. **Urinary diversion:** a procedure that provides an alternative route for urine excretion when normal channels are damaged or defective
   a. Ileal conduit: also called ileal loop; reroutes urine from kidneys to pouch in abdominal wall created from a segment of the ileum; urine drains continuously from the ileal pouch
   b. Nephrostomy: drains urine through a catheter placed directly into kidney; used when a ureter is blocked or damaged; may be temporary
3. Preoperative period
   a. Reduce anxiety through preoperative teaching about procedure and postoperative course and care
   b. Client may awaken with nasogastric tube, IV, indwelling urinary catheter, Penrose drain, or other drains
   c. Assess client's support systems and ability to care for self after surgery
   d. Address concerns about changes in body image and loss of sexual or reproductive function
   e. Administer preanesthetic medications as prescribed
   f. Administer antibiotics (usually erythromycin and neomycin) for 24 hours before surgery, as prescribed
   g. Begin bowel preparations about 4 days prior to surgery
   h. Administer enema on night before surgery to clear fecal matter from bowel as prescribed or per protocol
4. Postoperative period
   a. Perform baseline assessments as for all postoperative clients (VS, LOC, status of dressing, and patency of urinary catheter)
   b. Monitor amount and character of urine drainage every hour; report output less than 30 mL/hour; irrigate catheter as ordered
   c. Observe for signs of hypovolemic shock, such as pallor, hypotension, and tachycardia
   d. Inspect stoma and incision for bleeding and observe urine for frank bleeding and clots; expect slight hematuria for several days
   e. Observe incision for signs of infection (redness and purulent drainage); change dressing according to agency policy or surgeon's order
   f. Encourage frequent position changes, coughing and deep breathing, and early ambulation if appropriate
   g. Assess respiratory status frequently
   h. Administer prescribed analgesic and antispasmodic medications as needed

5. Home care instructions for clients
   a. Report signs of infection, including fever, chills, cloudy urine, purulent drainage, or redness of incision
   b. Report persistent blood in urine, inability to void, or painful urination
   c. Instruct in stoma care and provide supplies as needed; refer client to support organization such as the United Ostomy Association
   d. Weakness, incisional pain, and fatigue may persist for several weeks

D. Ureteral stent: catheter used to maintain patency and promote healing of ureters; may be temporary after surgery or used for long periods in clients with a damaged ureter

1. Stent is positioned during surgery or cystoscopy
2. Nursing care
   a. If stent has been brought to surface, secure it and maintain its position
   b. Monitor UO, including color, consistency, and odor
   c. Observe for signs of infection, obstruction, or bleeding, including fever, tachycardia, cloudy urine, pain, hematuria
   d. Maintain fluid intake
   e. If stent is semipermanent, instruct client and family in its care

E. Nephrectomy: removal of kidney

1. Preoperative period
   a. Reduce anxiety through preoperative teaching about procedure and postoperative course and care
   b. Client may awaken with nasogastric tube, IV, indwelling urinary catheter, Penrose drain, or other drains
   c. Assess client's support systems and ability to care for self after surgery
   d. Administer preanesthetic medications as ordered
   e. Assess baseline urinary status
2. Postoperative period
   a. Perform baseline assessments as for all postoperative clients (VS, LOC, status of dressing, and patency of urinary catheter)
   ! b. Assess client's fluid and electrolyte status, because significant amount of blood is lost during nephrectomy; monitor hemoglobin and hematocrit results and urine specific gravity
   ! c. Monitor amount and character of urine output every hour; report output less than 30 mL/hour; irrigate catheter as ordered
   d. Observe for signs of urinary infection: fever, redness at surgical site, cloudy urine, or discharge
   e. Assess patency of urinary or wound drainage tubes; reinforce or change dressing as needed
   ! f. Assess respiratory status frequently; encourage frequent position changes, coughing and deep breathing, and early ambulation if appropriate to reduce the risk of respiratory complications caused by pain from high abdominal/flank incision
   g. Administer analgesic medications as needed

F. Renal transplantation

1. Preoperative period
   a. Reduce anxiety by teaching about procedure and postoperative course and care; encourage client to express feelings and ask questions
   b. Assess support systems and ability to care for self after surgery and follow medical regime
   ! c. Instruct client that rejection of donated organ is the major obstacle in transplantation (see Table 59–2 ■); reassure client that rejection usually isn't life-threatening and client can resume dialysis if needed
   d. Begin administering immunosuppressant drugs; discuss purpose and possible adverse effects with client; monitor for increased BP and signs of anaphylaxis
   e. Plan for client to undergo dialysis the day before surgery, a cleansing enema, and many laboratory tests
2. Postoperative period
   a. Perform baseline assessments as for all postoperative clients (VS, LOC, status of dressing)

Table 59-2

Renal Transplant Rejection

Description	Manifestations	Management
Hyperacute Occurs within hours of surgery; results from antibody reaction to donor antigens; occurs rarely now because of better histocompatibility assessments	Urine output stops; examination of kidney shows a blue, flaccid appearance	Transplanted kidney must be removed; client must resume hemodialysis until (possibly) another kidney is available
Acute Occurs within days to months after surgery; body mounts an immune system defense against tissue in donor organ	Urine output drops sharply and BUN and creatinine rise; possible fever, graft tenderness, swelling	Increased dosage of immunosuppressant drugs, including steroids and monoclonal antibodies
Chronic Occurs from months to years after surgery; etiology is unclear but may involve immune response to donor tissue	More gradual decline in kidney function, including urine output, BUN, and creatinine; proteinuria may occur	No specific treatment; client must resume hemodialysis caused by loss of graft until or unless another donor kidney is transplanted

b. Encourage frequent position changes, coughing and deep breathing, and early ambulation if appropriate

! **c.** Use special infection control measures: strict aseptic technique when changing dressings or performing catheter care; limit client's contact with staff and visitors; wear a surgical mask when in client's room; monitor WBC count and notify physician of significant drop

! **d.** Observe for signs of tissue rejection: fever; redness, tenderness, and swelling at surgical site; elevated WBC count; decreased UO with increased proteinuria; sudden weight gain; hypertension; elevated BUN and creatinine

e. Provide analgesic medications as needed; pain should decrease after 24 hours

f. Monitor UO closely; report output less than 100 mL/hour; decreased urine may indicate thrombus formation at renal artery anastomosis site

g. Expect blood-tinged urine for several days; irrigate catheter as ordered, using strict aseptic technique

! **h.** With a living donor transplant, urine flow should begin immediately after revascularization and connection of ureter to client's bladder; with a cadaver transplant, expect **anuria** (complete or almost complete cessation of urine production by kidneys) for 2 days to 2 weeks, client will need dialysis during this period

i. Monitor daily renal function tests: creatinine clearance, and BUN; urine creatinine, electrolytes, urine pH, and specific gravity

j. Observe for signs of hyperkalemia (weakness and irregular pulse, tall peaked T-waves on cardiac rhythm strip)

k. Weigh client daily; rapid weight gain may indicate fluid retention

3. Home care for client

a. Carefully measure and record I & O; notify physician if UO falls below 600 mL for any 24-hour period

b. Instruct client how to collect 24-hour urine samples

! **c.** Advise client to weigh self at least twice weekly

d. Drink at least 1 to 2 liters of fluid daily unless advised otherwise

! **e.** Report signs of rejection: redness, warmth, tenderness, or swelling over the kidney; fever; decreased UO; elevated BP (obtain and use home BP measuring device)

! **f.** Avoid crowds and persons with known infections for 3 months after surgery

g. Practice regular, moderate exercise, but avoid heavy lifting or contact sports for at least 3 months; use shoulder but not lap-style seat belts

h. Wait at least 6 weeks before engaging in sexual activity

V. URINARY CALCULI

A. Overview

1. Presence of stones in urinary tract
2. Stones form when chemicals and other elements of urine become concentrated and form crystals; usually related to metabolic or dietary causes
3. Types of stones: calcium phosphate and/or oxalate (most common type), struvite, uric acid, and cystine (least common type)
4. Most stones form in kidneys, but bladder stones are common in clients with indwelling urinary catheters or those unable to empty bladder completely (see Figure 59–2 ■)
5. Stones may be single or multiple and vary in size; large calculi cause pressure necrosis and can also lead to obstruction
6. ! Risk factors
    a. Dehydration: concentrates calculus-forming substances
    b. Infection: damaged tissue and changing pH provide an environment for calculi to develop; bacteria may form the nucleus of calculi
    c. Obstruction: urine stasis allows solid materials to collect; also promotes infection, which worsens obstruction
    d. Metabolic factors: hypoparathyroidism, renal tubular acidosis, elevated uric acid levels, defective oxalate metabolism, and excessive vitamin D or dietary calcium intake

B. Nursing assessment

1. Severe pain is most common symptom
2. ! Renal calculi cause flank pain on side of affected kidney; may radiate to groin, called renal colic
3. ! Fluctuates in intensity and may be severe; nausea and vomiting sometimes accompany severe pain
4. Other symptoms: abdominal distention, fever, and chills
5. Urinalysis (may reveal hematuria, pyuria, and crystal fragments)
6. Twenty-four-hour urine levels for calcium, uric acid, and oxalate
7. Serum levels for calcium, phosphorus, and uric acid
8. Chemical analysis of stones passed for content and type
9. KUB, IVP, retrograde pyelography, renal ultrasound, CT scan, cystoscopy, and MRI

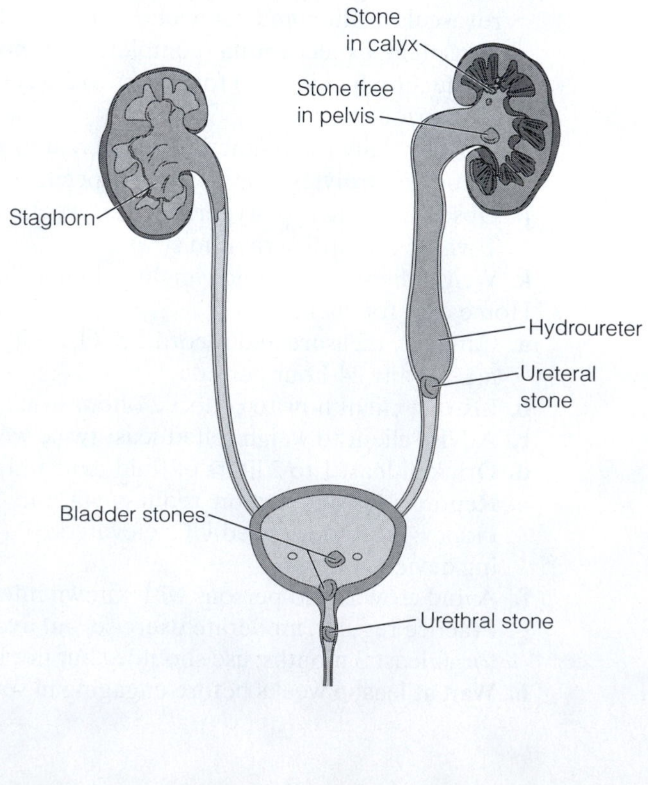

Figure 59–2

Development and location of calculi within the kidneys and urinary tract.

Source: LeMone, P., & Burke, K. (2004). Medical surgical nursing: Critical thinking in client care (3rd ed.). Upper Saddle River, NJ: Pearson Education, p. 715.

C. Therapeutic management

1. Stones that are too large to pass spontaneously (usually more than 5 mm in diameter), multiple stones, and those that obstruct urinary tract usually require surgical intervention
   a. Extracorporeal shock-wave lithotripsy (ESWL) uses externally generated waves to pulverize or shatter urinary stones and calculi, which are then excreted in urine
   b. Ureterolithotomy, pyelolithotomy, or nephrolithotomy: surgical removal of calculi from affected areas; requires a large flank incision and an extended recovery time
   c. Percutaneous nephrostomy: small incision in flank allows insertion of an endoscope to visualize renal pelvis; stones are removed with forceps or a basket device, or lithotripsy is used to crush stones
   d. Transurethral uroscopy: a ureteral catheter is passed via a cystoscope to drain urine proximal to a stone and dilate ureter, allowing stone to pass; a basket catheter passed through cystoscope can also remove calculus
2. ! Treatment for calcium phosphate and/or oxalate stones
   a. Acid-ash diet with limitations of foods high in calcium and oxalates (see Box 59–4)
   b. Increase hydration and exercise
3. ! Treatment for struvite stones: acid-ash diet
4. ! Treatment for uric acid stones: alkaline-ash and low-purine diet; increase hydration
5. ! Treatment for cystine stones: alkaline-ash diet; increase hydration
6. Goal of treatment is relief of symptoms, removal or destruction of calculi, and prevention of future stone formation
7. Most calculi (90%) pass out of urinary system without invasive treatment
8. Provide pain relief measures and treat other symptoms as they occur
9. Assess urinary function and monitor I & O
10. ! Strain all urine and save solid material for analysis
11. ! Encourage ambulation and large fluid intake to help client pass calculi
12. Record daily weight to assess fluid status and renal function
13. Medication therapy: antimicrobial therapy for infection; analgesics for pain; and diuretics to prevent urine stasis

! **D. Client teaching**

1. Proper diet is essential to prevent recurrence of stones; teach dietary needs related to type of calculus (refer again to Box 59–4)
2. Increase fluid intake to 2,500 to 3,500 mL/day
3. Maintain activity at level that will prevent urinary stasis and resorption of calcium from bone
4. If discharged prior to stone passage, collect and strain all urine and bring stones to follow-up visit; observe amount and character of urine and report to health care provider at follow-up visit also
5. Report increased pain, persistent blood in urine, inability to void, significant decrease in UO

Box 59–4

Dietary Considerations with Urinary Calculi

Acid-ash foods: Cranberries, plums, grapes, and prunes; tomatoes; eggs and cheese; whole grains; meat and poultry

Alkaline-ash foods: Legumes, milk and milk products, green vegetables, rhubarb, fruits except those acid-ash fruits noted above

Foods high in calcium: Milk and other dairy products, beans and lentils, dried fruits, canned or smoked fish (except tuna), flour, chocolate, and cocoa

Foods high in oxalates: Asparagus, beets, celery, cabbage, dark green leafy vegetables, rhubarb, fruits, tomatoes, green beans, chocolate and cocoa, beer, cola beverages, nuts, and tea

Foods high in purines: Organ meats, sardines and herring, venison, and goose; other meats also contain purines and should be limited in quantity

6. Report signs of infection: burning with urination, cloudy urine, or fever
7. Review specific drug information and procedures for self-administration

VI. URINARY RETENTION

A. Overview

1. Inability to empty bladder that leads to bladder distention, poor contractility of detrussor muscle, and further inability to urinate
2. Mechanical obstruction of bladder outlet is most often caused by benign prostatic hypertrophy or acute inflammation
3. Functional problems
   a. Surgery may disrupt function of detrussor muscle, leading to retention of urine
   b. Many medications can interfere with detrussor muscle function, including anticholinergics, antidepressant and antipsychotic agents, anti-Parkinson drugs, antihistamines, and some antihypertensives

B. Nursing assessment

1. ! Firm, distended bladder that may be displaced to one side of midline
2. ! Overflow voiding or incontinence may occur, with 25 to 50 mL of urine eliminated at frequent intervals
3. ! Residual urine (postvoiding catheterization) in amounts over 50 mL obtained from bladder catheterization
4. Positive urine culture indicates presence of urinary tract infection (UTI)
5. Elevated serum creatinine and BUN levels indicate disturbances in renal function
6. Elevated blood glucose may indicate diabetes
7. Cystometrography evaluates muscle function

C. Therapeutic management

1. Surgical correction of any condition causing mechanical obstruction of urine flow, including benign prostatic hyperplasia (BPH) and calculi
2. Palpate bladder for distention at regular intervals
3. Monitor I & O and observe urine characteristics
4. Attempt to stimulate relaxation of urethral sphincter by running water, providing warm water in which client can place fingers, pouring warm water over perineum, or providing warm sitz bath
5. Perform intermittent straight catheterization as ordered
6. ! Evaluate client's medication regime for drugs that cause urinary retention
7. ! Medication therapy: cholinergic medications to promote detrussor muscle contraction and bladder emptying; anticholinesterase drugs to increase detrussor muscle tone

D. Client teaching

1. How to perform straight catheterization at home if necessary
2. Recognize and report signs of UTI: burning with urination, cloudy urine, pelvic pain, fever, and strong urine odor
3. ! Moderate to high fluid intake and a diet that acidifies the urine; cranberry juice is one item that helps maintain acidity
4. Specific drug information and procedures for self-administration

VII. URINARY INCONTINENCE

A. Overview

1. Involuntary urination; five types according to North American Nursing Diagnosis Association International (NANDA-I)
   a. Stress incontinence: loss of urine with increased abdominal pressure
   b. Reflex incontinence: involuntary loss of urine at somewhat predictable intervals when a specific bladder volume is reached
   c. Urge incontinence: involuntary passage of urine soon after a strong urge to void
   d. Functional incontinence: involuntary, unpredictable passage of urine
   e. Total incontinence: continuous and unpredictable loss of urine
2. Incontinence is a symptom of other problems, not a disease in itself, although it has a significant impact on client's life

3. May be acute or chronic, and cause may be congenital or acquired
4. Occurs when pressure within bladder exceeds urethral resistance, allowing urine to escape; any condition causing higher than normal bladder pressure or reduced urethral resistance may lead to incontinence
5. Common causes: relaxation of pelvic musculature, disruption of cerebral and nervous system control, and disturbances of bladder musculature
6. Risk factors in older clients: decreased bladder capacity, laxity of pelvic muscles in females, immobility, chronic degenerative diseases, low fluid intake, diabetes, and stroke

B. Nursing assessment

1. Clinical manifestations: involuntary passage of urine
2. Weak abdominal and pelvic muscle tone in women
3. Enlarged prostate in men
4. Postvoiding residual urine greater than 50 mL
5. Cystometrography: reduced muscle function and tone
6. Ultrasonography and cystoscopy identify possible causes of the incontinence

C. Therapeutic management

1. Surgical suspension of bladder neck to treat stress incontinence associated with urethrocele
2. Prostatectomy to treat overflow incontinence due to enlarged prostate
3. Implantation of an artificial sphincter to treat clients with neurogenic bladder
4. Goal is to identify and correct cause of incontinence; if unable to correct underlying problem, client may learn techniques to manage UO
5. Monitor diagnostic tests to evaluate cause of incontinence
6. Employ behavioral techniques, such as bladder training, for clients who are cognitively and functionally intact
7. Insert urinary catheter as ordered and monitor client's UO
8. Medication therapy: anticholinergics for stress incontinence to increase bladder capacity and inhibit detrussor muscle contractions; antihistamines to enhance contraction of smooth muscles of bladder neck; estrogen therapy for incontinence associated with postmenopausal atrophic vaginitis

D. Client teaching

1. Care of indwelling urinary catheter at home
2. Recognize and report signs of UTI: burning with urination, cloudy urine, pelvic pain, fever; and strong urine odor
3. Moderate to high fluid intake and a diet that acidifies urine
4. Specific drug information and procedures for self-administration
5. Possible need to keep a voiding diary to help diagnose cause(s) of incontinence
6. Teach Kegel exercises to strengthen pelvic floor muscles (see Box 59–5)
7. Dietary and fluid intake modifications to reduce stress and urge incontinence; consume most fluids during times of day client is most able to remain continent
8. Wear clothing that is easily removed for ease in toileting
9. Use assistive devices, such as raised toilet seats, bedside commode, and urinal or bedpan as needed

Box 59–5

Teaching Kegel Exercises

- First, sit or stand with the legs apart.
- Tense your muscles to pull your rectum, urethra, and vagina up inside, and hold for a count of 3 to 5 seconds. The pull should be felt at the cleft of your buttocks.
- Try to stop and start your stream of urine.
- Develop a schedule that will help remind you to do these exercises.
- To control episodes of stress incontinence, brace the muscles and use the Kegel maneuver when doing any activity that increases intra-abdominal pressure, such as coughing, laughing, sneezing, or lifting.

VIII. URINARY TRACT INFECTIONS (UTI)

A. Overview

1. Presence of microorganisms in urinary tract leading to inflammation
2. Infections are classified according to region and primary site affected; infection in bladder is called **cystitis**
3. Urinary tract is sterile above urethra; pathogens enter by ascending from perineal area or are introduced from bloodstream; ascending route is most common
4. *Escherichia coli* is most frequent infective organism, causing about 80% of all cases; 5% to 15% are caused by *staphylococcus*
5. Free urine flow, large UO, and pH are antibacterial defenses
6. Microscopic examination identifies organism (especially important for chronic infections)
7. Females are prone to UTIs because female urethra is shorter than male urethra
8. Males are more likely to develop UTI with aging because of prostatic hypertrophy, which impedes urine flow and leads to incomplete bladder emptying and urinary stasis
9. Noninfectious cystitis results from exposure to radiation, chemical agents, or a metabolic disorder

B. Nursing assessment

1. ! Burning, frequency, fever, cloudy urine, strong odor to urine, and pain in pelvic area
2. ! Older clients may have nonspecific symptoms, such as nocturia, incontinence, confusion, lethargy, or anorexia
3. Urine cultures and Gram stain determine presence and number of bacteria
4. WBCs are elevated with an increase in neutrophils
5. Blood or urine tests are also performed to rule out sexually transmitted infections, which produce similar symptoms

C. Therapeutic management

1. Surgical intervention may be necessary if recurrent UTI is caused by structural abnormalities, including ureteroplasty (surgical repair of ureter) for stricture or placement of ureteral stent (catheter in ureter to provide free flow of urine)
2. ! Increase fluid intake to 3,000 mL per day
3. ! Administer urinary antimicrobials as ordered
4. Administer analgesic and antispasmodic medications as needed
5. Encourage client to void every 2 to 3 hours and to completely empty bladder to reduce urinary stasis
6. Monitor I & O and observe urine characteristics
7. Medication therapy
   - a. Antimicrobials to eradicate bacteria
   - b. Antispasmodics and analgesics to relieve pain, frequency, and burning

! D. Client teaching

1. Avoid beverages that irritate bladder: carbonated or caffeinated drinks and alcohol
2. Teach women about hygiene measures to prevent reoccurrence: wipe from front to back, keep perineum clean and dry, do not douche, avoid tight-fitting pants; void after sexual intercourse
3. Finish complete course of antibiotics, even if symptoms subside
4. Teach correct use, purpose, and effects of medication
5. Phenazopyridine (Pyridium), a urinary analgesic, turns urine reddish orange; protect clothing and do not mistake this discoloration for bleeding (hematuria)
6. Instruct in signs of infection: frequency, burning, cloudy urine, fever, and malodorous urine
7. Maintain acidic urine with acid-ash diet which may include drinking cranberry juice daily (helps prevent bacteria from clinging to bladder wall)
8. Maintain fluid intake of at least 8 to 10 glasses per day
9. Practice frequent voiding (every 2 to 4 hours) to flush bacteria from urethra
10. Avoid harsh soaps, bubble bath, powder, or sprays in perineal area
11. Take showers rather than baths if recurrent infection is a problem

IX. PYELONEPHRITIS

A. Overview

1. Infection of one or both kidneys that usually begins in renal pelvis; may be acute or chronic
2. Affects renal pelvis and parenchyma (functional portion of kidney)
3. Infection develops in scattered areas and spreads from renal pelvis to cortex; kidney becomes edematous and abscesses may develop; tissue destruction primarily affects tubules; with healing, scar tissue replaces normal tissue and affected tubules atrophy
4. *E. coli* causes 85% of cases; *Proteus* and *Klebsiella* bacteria are examples of less common causes
5. Acute form is a bacterial infection, usually caused by bacteria that ascend from lower urinary tract
6. Risk factors: pregnancy, urinary tract obstruction, congenital malformation, urinary tract trauma, calculi, and diabetes
7. Asymptomatic bacteriuria or cystitis may lead to acute pyelonephritis
8. Chronic form is associated with nonbacterial infections and noninfectious processes caused by metabolic, chemical, or immunologic disorders
   a. Often results from an autoimmune process leading to inflammation
   b. Acute episodes may contribute to the inflammation and scarring associated with chronic form
   c. Fibrosis and scarring lead to dilation of renal pelvis and gradual destruction of tubules
   d. May lead to chronic renal failure (CRF) and end-stage renal disease (ESRD)
9. **Vesicoureteral reflux** (urine moves from bladder back toward kidneys) is a common risk factor in children who develop pyelonephritis; is seen also in adults when bladder outflow is obstructed

! **B. Nursing assessment**

1. Clinical manifestations: urinary frequency, dysuria, flank pain, costovertebral tenderness, tachypnea, GI symptoms, muscle tenderness, fever, chills, malaise
2. Urine culture: hematuria, pyuria, bacteriuria, leukocyte casts in urine, and leukocytosis

! **C. Therapeutic management**

1. Maintain bedrest until symptoms subside
2. Encourage large fluid intake to maintain UO of 1,500 mL/day
3. Continue monitoring for presence of bacteria
4. Monitor urinalysis: concentration and electrolytes
5. If **oliguria** is present, maintain diet low in protein and high in calories and vitamins
6. Observe for edema and signs of renal failure
7. Medication therapy: antimicrobial therapy, urinary antiseptics, and analgesics for pain

D. Client teaching

1. Monitor UO and notify care provider if less than 1,500 mL/day
2. Methods to prevent chronic renal insufficiency
3. Take high-calorie, low-protein diet if oliguria is present
4. Hygiene to prevent further infections (see previous section on UTI)
5. ! Encourage bedrest during acute stage
6. ! Finish complete course of antibiotics, even if symptoms resolve

X. NEOPLASTIC DISEASE

A. Overview

1. Excessive and pathologic tissue growth that may be benign or malignant
2. Other classifications: solid, cystic, superficial, invasive, primary, or metastatic
3. Most urinary tract tumors arise from epithelial tissue that lines entire urinary tract
4. Even nonmalignant tumors may lead to obstruction, renal failure, hemorrhage, and invasion and inflammation of surrounding tissues
5. Tissue destruction may cause fistulas, which can allow urine to leak into pelvis, vagina, or bowel

6. Bladder cancer is fifth most common malignancy; occurs most often after age 50 and is more common in men than women
7. Major risk factors in bladder cancer are presence of carcinogens in urine and chronic inflammation or infection of bladder mucosa
8. Other risk factors: cigarette smoke, exposure to chemicals and dyes used in certain industries, chronic use of phenacetin-containing analgesic agents; carcinogenic agents from these materials are excreted in urine and stored in bladder between voidings, leading to abnormal cell development

B. Nursing assessment

1. Painless hematuria is presenting symptom in 75% of cases; hematuria may be gross or microscopic and is often intermittent
2. Inflammation surrounding tumor may cause signs of UTI, such as frequency, urgency, and dysuria
3. With ureteral tumors, observe for colicky pain from obstruction
4. Neoplasms cause few outward symptoms and may not be discovered until urinary obstruction occurs or a fistula develops
5. Urinalysis shows gross or microscopic hematuria
6. Urine cytology shows abnormal tumor or pretumor cells
7. Visualization of tumors via intravenous pyelography, ultrasound, CT scan, cystoscopy, or ureteroscopy

C. Therapeutic management

1. Radiation therapy
2. Surgical intervention for bladder tumors
   a. Tumor resection
   b. Partial cystectomy: resection of tumor
   c. Radical cystectomy: removal of the bladder and adjacent structures
3. Urinary diversion may also be created
   a. Cutaneous ureterostomy: one or both ureters excised from bladder and brought to a stoma
   b. Ileal conduit: portion of ileum is isolated from small intestine and formed into a pouch; ureters are attached to pouch; pouch has open stoma
   c. Colon conduit: same as ileal conduit but a portion of sigmoid colon is used
   d. Kock pouch: same as ileal conduit but nipple valves are formed preventing leakage and reflux (see Figure 59–3 ■)
   e. Indiana continent urinary reservoir: reservoir is formed from colon and cecum and portion of ileum is brought to surface
   f. Ileocystoplasty: section of ileum is used; this procedure is ideal for men because it allows client to void
4. Monitor urinary status, including I & O, signs of infection, hematuria, and BUN and creatinine levels

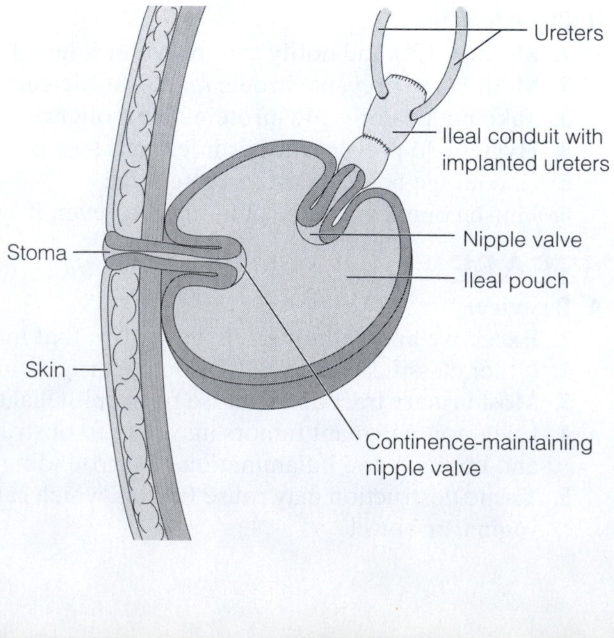

Figure 59–3

A continent urinary diversion. A segment of ileum is separated from the small intestine and formed into a pouch. Nipple valves are formed at each end of the pouch by intussuscepting tissue backward into a reservoir to prevent leakage.

Source: LeMone, P., & Burke, K. (2004). Medical surgical nursing: Critical thinking in client care *(3rd ed.). Upper Saddle River, NJ: Pearson Education, p. 725.*

5. Monitor UO from all catheters, stents, and tubes for amount, color, and clarity
6. Prepare client for invasive tests to confirm location and size of neoplasm
7. Follow guidelines for care before and after surgery, chemotherapy, and radiation treatments
8. Encourage increased fluid intake unless contraindicated
9. Provide analgesics as needed for pain
10. Encourage client to express feelings about potentially life-threatening illness and to ask questions
11. Medication therapy: chemotherapeutic agents may be given IV or administered by intravesical instillation (into bladder)

D. Client teaching

1. Explain all nursing and medical interventions, including benefits and possible adverse effects
2. Reinforce explanations from health care provider about diagnosis and client's specific neoplasm
3. Stress importance of compliance with long-term treatment plan and follow-up care
4. Instruct client in methods to prevent infection
5. For clients with a stoma or indwelling catheter, teach home care procedures and when to consult care provider
6. For clients with a continent ileostomy, teach how to catheterize pouch (approximately every 4 hours) and wear a small dressing to protect the stoma and clothing
7. Teach relaxation techniques and other coping mechanisms

XI. GLOMERULONEPHRITIS

A. Overview

1. A group of kidney diseases caused by inflammation of capillary loops in glomeruli of kidney
2. Caused by an immunologic reaction to an antigen
   a. Endogenous antigens are already present in glomerulus or other body tissues
   b. Exogenous antigens come from infections occurring in body
3. Antigen–antibody complexes trapped within glomeruli produce an inflammatory response that damages glomeruli
4. Most often follows infections with group A-beta-hemolytic streptococcus
5. Upper respiratory infection, skin infection, and autoimmune processes (systemic lupus erythematosus) predispose to glomerulonephritis
6. Symptoms appear 2 to 3 weeks after original infection
7. Has higher incidence in men than in women; may occur at any age

B. Nursing assessment

1. Early symptoms may be mild: pharyngitis, fever, and malaise; weakness and fatigue
2. Recent upper respiratory or skin infections, pericarditis, or lower UTI
3. Anorexia, nausea, and vomiting
4. Cocoa-colored urine; hematuria, proteinuria (most important indicator of glomerular injury)
5. Peripheral edema
6. Hypertension
7. Hypoalbuminemia
8. Pulmonary infiltrates
9. Positive antibody response test for streptococcal exoenzymes: elevated anti-streptinolysin O (ASO) titer
10. Elevated erythrocyte sedimentation rate (ESR)
11. Elevated BUN and creatinine; decreased creatinine clearance
12. Decreased serum sodium, elevated potassium, and decreased phosphate
13. Delayed uptake and excretion of radioactive dye in renal scan
14. Positive renal biopsy findings

C. Therapeutic management

1. Plasmapheresis: removal of harmful components in the plasma
2. Sodium (Na^+) restriction
3. Dialysis if the disease progresses to renal failure

4. Provide appropriate diet: protein restriction if oliguria is severe; high CHO to provide energy; K^+ usually restricted; Na^+ restriction for hypertension and edema
5. Maintain fluid restriction as needed
6. Encourage complete bedrest during acute stage
7. Monitor VS frequently; observe for hypertension
8. Monitor I & O and daily weight
9. Evaluate for signs of renal failure: oliguria, azotemia, and acidosis
10. Medication therapy: antimicrobials (such as penicillin) for infection; analgesics for pain relief; and vitamin and electrolyte replacement as needed

D. Client teaching

1. Maintain strict bedrest during acute phase
2. Dietary changes and importance of maintaining diet
3. Importance of fluid restriction if oliguria present
4. Purpose of laboratory tests and other procedures

XII. NEPHROTIC SYNDROME

A. Overview

1. Renal disease characterized by massive edema and albuminuria
2. Seen with any renal condition that damages glomerular capillary membrane: glomerulonephritis, lipoid nephrosis, syphilitic nephritis, amyloidosis, or systemic lupus erythematosus
3. Allows plasma proteins to escape into urine, resulting in hypoalbuminemia, with decreased oncotic pressure in plasma that causes fluid to shift from intravascular to interstitial spaces and subsequent edema
4. Salt and water retention also contribute to edema, which may be severe
5. Kimmelstiel-Wilson syndrome, a specific form of intercapillary glomerulosclerosis, is associated with diabetes mellitus
6. Thromboemboli (mobilized blood clots) are a common complication and may occlude peripheral veins and arteries, pulmonary arteries, and renal veins
7. Prognosis is poor for adults with this syndrome; less then 50% experience complete remission; at least 30% develop end-stage renal disease (ESRD)

B. Nursing assessment

1. Severe generalized edema
2. Symptoms of renal failure
3. Loss of appetite and fatigue
4. Amenorrhea
5. Pronounced proteinuria, hypoalbuminemia, and hyperlipidemia
6. Positive renal biopsy finding

C. Therapeutic management

1. No specific treatment
2. Since 30% of adults with nephrotic syndrome progress to ESRD, care may involve management of renal failure
3. Provide nursing care to control edema
   a. Na^+-restricted diet and avoidance of Na^+-containing drugs (such as several OTC products)
   b. Administer diuretics that block aldosterone formation (such as furosemide [Lasix])
   c. Administer salt-poor albumin to reduce fluid retention
4. Provide high-protein diet to restore body proteins, high-calorie diet, and a restricted Na^+ diet if edema is present
5. Administer drug therapy as prescribed
6. Maintain bedrest until edema begins to subside
7. Monitor laboratory results, including BUN, creatinine, serum electrolytes, urinalysis, hemoglobin, and hematocrit
8. Observe for signs of pulmonary edema: tachypnea, dyspnea, crackles in lungs
9. Record total I & O every 4 to 8 hours and weigh client daily
10. Maintain fluid restriction; offer ice chips and provide frequent mouth care
11. Provide for adequate rest and energy conservation

12. Be aware that immune system depression increases risk of infection
    a. Assess for signs of infection, such as purulent wound drainage and signs of UTI
    b. Monitor CBC, with close attention to WBC and differential
    c. Use good handwashing and infection control techniques
    d. Avoid or minimize invasive procedures
13. Medication therapy: immunosuppressive therapy with autoimmune disorders; angiotensin converting enzyme (ACE) inhibitors to reduce protein loss; NSAIDs to reduce proteinuria; penicillin or other broad-spectrum antibiotics to eradicate bacteria; and antihypertensives as needed to lower BP

D. Client teaching

1. Take measures to maintain general health, as disorder may persist for months or years
2. Avoid sources of infection such as people with upper respiratory infections
3. Nutritious diet (low-sodium, high-protein)
4. Activity as tolerated
5. Use and potential effects of medications
6. Signs, symptoms, and implications of improving or declining renal function

XIII. POLYCYSTIC KIDNEY DISEASE

A. Overview

1. Hereditary disease characterized by cyst formation and massive kidney enlargement, affecting both children and adults
2. Autosomal-dominant form affects adults, while autosomal-recessive form is usually diagnosed in childhood
3. Renal cysts are fluid-filled sacs affecting nephron; they develop in tubular epithelium of nephron and fill with glomerular filtrate or secreted solutes and fluid
4. Cysts range in size from microscopic to several centimeters
5. As cysts enlarge and multiply, kidneys also enlarge; renal blood vessels and nephrons are compressed and obstructed, and functional tissue is destroyed
6. Disorder is slow and progressive; adult symptoms usually manifest by age 30 to 40
7. Clients with this disorder often develop cysts elsewhere in body, including liver, spleen, pancreas, brain, and other organs

B. Nursing assessment

1. Flank pain
2. Polyuria and nocturia
3. Gross hematuria, proteinuria
4. Signs of UTI and renal calculi
5. Hypertension
6. Palpable, enlarged, and knobby kidney
7. Signs of chronic renal failure as the client approaches age 50 to 60
8. Positive findings in renal ultrasonography, IVP, and CT scan

C. Therapeutic management

1. Provide supportive care to help client cope with symptoms; no effective treatment is available
2. Encourage fluid intake of 2,000 to 2,500 mL/day to help prevent UTI and calculi
3. Administer antihypertensive agents as prescribed
4. Discuss that hemodialysis and possibly renal transplant will be indicated as disease progresses
5. Provide nursing care directed toward edema control
    a. Na^+-restricted diet
    b. Diuretics that block aldosterone formation
6. Medication therapy: ACE inhibitors to control hypertension; diuretics to control edema; and antibiotics if infection develops

D. Client teaching

1. Maintenance of general health status because disorder is chronic and progressive
2. How to avoid UTI and to recognize early signs of infection
3. Avoid medications that are potentially toxic to kidneys and check with care provider before taking any new drug

4. Need for genetic counseling and screening of family members for evidence of disease
5. Maintain fluid intake of at least 2,500 mL/day

XIV. ACUTE RENAL FAILURE

A. Overview

1. Sudden loss of kidney function caused by failure of renal circulation or damage to the tubules or glomeruli
   a. Usually reversible, with spontaneous recovery in a few days to weeks
   b. Ischemia is primary cause; when allowed to continue for more than 2 hours, it produces irreversible damage to tubules
2. Etiologic categories
   a. Prerenal: accounts for 55% of renal failure; caused by decreased blood flow to kidneys; readily reversible when recognized and treated early; may be caused by severe dehydration, diuretic therapy, circulatory collapse, hypovolemia, or shock
   b. Intrarenal: caused by a disease process, ischemia, or toxic conditions such as acute glomerulonephritis, vascular disorders, toxic agents, or severe infection
   c. Postrenal: caused by any condition that obstructs urine flow such as in benign prostatic hyperplasia (BPH), renal or urinary tract calculi, or tumors

B. Nursing assessment (see also Table 59–3 ■)

1. Clinical manifestations follow three phases: initiation, maintenance, and recovery; the initiation stage has very few manifestations; the maintenance phase is characterized by oliguria (UO <400 mL/24 hours); signs of improving UO and renal function characterize the recovery stage
2. Muscle weakness, nausea, vomiting, and diarrhea may occur
3. Neurologic symptoms such as confusion, agitation, disorientation, seizures, and coma may also be present
4. Hyperkalemia, hyperphosphatemia, and hypocalcemia
5. Metabolic acidosis
6. **Azotemia** (retention of excess nitrogenous waste in blood)

Table 59–3 Clinical Manifestations of Renal Failure

Body System	Clinical Manifestations	Cause of Manifestations
Cardiovascular	Hypervolemia, hypertension, tachycardia, arrhythmias, congestive heart failure, pericarditis	Increased fluid volume, build up of metabolic wastes, chronic hypertension, change in renin-angiotension mechanism
Hematologic	Anemia, leukocytosis, decreased platelet function, thrombocytopenia	Decreased production of erythropoietin and RBCs, decreased survival of RBCs, decreased platelet activity; blood loss through dialysis and bleeding
Gastrointestinal	Anorexia, nausea, vomiting, abdominal distention, diarrhea, constipation, bleeding	Build up of uremic toxins, electrolyte imbalances, changes in platelet activity, conversion of urea to ammonia by saliva
Neurologic	Lethargy, confusion, convulsions, stupor, coma, sleep disturbances, behavioral changes, muscle irritability	Uremic toxins, electrolyte imbalances, cerebral swelling caused by fluid shifts
Dermatologic	Pallor, pigmentation, pruritus, ecchymosis, excoriation, uremic frost	Anemia, decreased activity of sweat glands, dry skin, phosphate deposits on skin
Urinary	Decreased urine output, decreased specific gravity, proteinuria, casts and cells in the urine	Damage to the nephron
Skeletal	Osteoporosis, renal rickets, joint pain	Decreased calcium absorption, decreased phosphate excretion

7. Anemia
8. Elevated creatinine and BUN levels
9. **Proteinuria**
10. Urinalysis show specific gravity (SG) equal to SG of plasma; presence of casts, RBC, WBC, and renal tubular epithelial cells
11. Positive renal biopsy findings

C. Therapeutic management

1. Provide fluid and electrolyte management
2. Supportive therapy with dialysis
3. Monitor I & O
4. Observe for oliguria followed by **polyuria** (excess UO from diuresis)
5. ! Weigh daily and observe for edema
6. ! Monitor for complications of electrolyte imbalances, such as acidosis and hyperkalemia
7. Allow client to verbalize concerns regarding disorder
8. ! Encourage prescribed diet: moderate protein restriction, high in carbohydrates (CHO), restricted potassium (K^+) and sodium (Na^+)
9. Once diuresis phase begins, evaluate slow return of BUN, creatinine, phosphorus, and K^+ to normal
10. Medication therapy
    a. ! Avoid nephrotoxic drugs
    b. Use volume expanders as prescribed to restore renal perfusion in hypotensive clients and dopamine (Intropin) IV to increase renal blood flow
    c. Use loop diuretic to reduce toxic concentration in nephrons and establish urine flow
    d. Use ACE inhibitors to control hypertension
    e. Use antacids or histamine H_2-receptor antagonists to prevent gastric ulcers
    f. Use Kayexalate to reduce serum K^+ levels and sodium bicarbonate to treat acidosis

D. Client teaching

1. ! Dietary and fluid restrictions, including those that may be continued after discharge
2. Signs of complications, such as fluid volume excess, CHF, and hyperkalemia
3. ! Monitor weight, BP, pulse, and UO
4. ! Avoid nephrotoxic drugs and substances: NSAIDs, some antibiotics, radiologic contrast media, and heavy metals; consult health care provider prior to taking any OTC drugs
5. Recovery of renal function requires up to 1 year; during this period, nephrons are vulnerable to damage from nephrotoxins

XV. END-STAGE RENAL DISEASE (ESRD)

A. Overview

1. Loss of renal function characterized by a glomerular filtration rate (GFR) less than 20% of normal
2. Final stage of **chronic renal failure** (CRF; slow, progressive loss of kidney function and glomerular filtration); ends fatally with **uremia** (excess urea and other nitrogenous waste products in blood)
3. ! Most common causes of CRF are diabetes mellitus, hypertension, glomerulonephritis, systemic lupus erythematosus, and polycystic kidney disease
4. Progressive loss of renal function occurs in four stages; fourth stage ends with ESRD (uremia)
5. As 90% or more of nephrons are destroyed, BUN and creatinine clearance rise, and urine specific gravity is fixed at 1.010 (normal up to 1.025)
6. Uremia: means "urine in blood"; term used for symptoms associated with ESRD
7. Loss of erythropoietin leads to chronic anemia and subsequent fatigue
8. ! There is inadequate clearance of fluid and electrolytes, leading to fluid and Na^+ retention, as well as hyperkalemia, hypermagnesemia, hyperphosphatemia, and hypocalcemia; metabolic acidosis occurs because of impaired hydrogen ion excretion

B. Nursing assessment

1. Early: nausea, apathy, weakness, and fatigue; declining urine output
2. Late: possibly frequent vomiting, increasing weakness, lethargy, and confusion
3. Client may report "restless leg syndrome," paresthesia, and sensory loss
4. Personality changes, such as anxiety, irritability, and hallucinations; seizures and coma posible in late stages
5. Respirations may change to Kussmaul pattern, with deep coma following
6. Skin becomes pale and dry, with yellowish hue; metabolic wastes cause itching and uremic frost (crystallized deposits of urea on skin)
7. Urinalysis shows fixed specific gravity approximately 1.010, equivalent to plasma; abnormal proteins, blood cells, and casts are present.
8. Elevated creatinine and BUN and decreased creatinine clearance
9. Abnormal electrolyte values as noted above
10. Moderate anemia
11. Decreased platelets
12. Decreased renal size by ultrasonography
13. Positive renal biopsy if damage caused by cancer

C. Therapeutic management

1. Provide diet low in protein (such as 60 grams protein) with supplemented amino acids; restrict fluids as ordered
2. Provide electrolyte replacement or restriction
   - a. Na^+ restriction (such as 2 grams daily)
   - b. K^+ restriction (such as 2 grams daily)
   - c. Replacement of bicarbonate stores to treat acidosis
3. Monitor and plan nursing care for hypertension and heart failure
4. Prepare client for dialysis or kidney transplant
5. Monitor I & O and VS
6. Monitor laboratory results for BUN and serum creatinine, pH, electrolytes, and CBC
7. Provide symptomatic relief for nausea and vomiting
8. Observe for signs of infection
9. Provide rest periods to combat fatigue, which is chronic in nature
10. Help client learn about and adjust to diagnosis; support coping strategies and work with client to develop realistic goals
11. Medication therapy: limited by kidneys' inability to excrete
    - a. Diuretics to reduce volume of extracellular fluid
    - b. ACE inhibitors to maintain normal BP
    - c. Electrolyte replacement
    - d. Phosphate binding agents
    - e. Kayexalate to reduce serum K^+ levels
    - f. Folic acid, iron supplements, and possibly epoietin (Epogen) to combat anemia; multivitamins
    - g. Medications to manage other health problems may require reduced dosage if excreted via kidneys

D. Client teaching

1. Monitor weight, VS, and UO at home
2. Fluid and dietary restrictions (low-Na^+, low-K^+, low-protein) need to be followed carefully
3. Monitor symptoms of uremia
4. Avoid nephrotoxic drugs and substances: NSAIDs, some antibiotics, radiologic contrast media, and heavy metals
5. Teach strategies to avoid thirst, yet continue fluid restrictions, such as frequent mouth care, sugarless hard candy, using ice chips instead of liquids, or using a spray bottle instead of a cup to limit fluids ingested
6. Discuss hemodialysis or renal transplant therapies as indicated
7. Recommend methods to combat nausea: antiemetics; mouth care; small, frequent meals
8. Provide referral to mental health counseling or support group

XVI. HYPOSPADIAS AND EPISPADIAS

A. **Overview**

1. Hypospadias: congenital defect in which urinary meatus is not at end of penis but is located on lower or underside of shaft
   a. Meatus can be anywhere on underside of penis to base of penis; in epispadias, meatal opening can be anywhere along upper shaft; most frequent anomalies are minor with openings off-center but still on glans
   b. Hypospadias is more common anomaly, occurring in 1 out of 500 newborns
   c. Hypospadias is often accompanied by **chordee,** a downward curvature of penis
2. Epispadias: congenital defect in which urinary meatus is not at end of penis but on upper side of penile shaft; less common than hypospadias
   a. Epispadias is often associated with **exstrophy** of bladder
   b. Both males and females can be affected by hypospadias or epispadias; in most instances, female anomaly does not require surgical correction

B. **Nursing assessment:** noted on admission to the newborn nursery

C. **Therapeutic management**

1. Does not interfere with voiding but could interfere with reproduction if not repaired before adulthood
2. Document findings carefully and report to physician
3. **Circumcision** (operation to remove part or all of prepuce) is delayed because prepuce may be used in reconstruction
4. If chordee is present, curvature of penis may be released before hypospadias repair
5. ! Surgical correction is usually begun before age of 18 months
6. ! Postoperative care
   a. Penis may have a urethral stent in place and be wrapped with a pressure dressing
   b. Arm and leg restraints may be needed to prevent accidental removal of stent
   c. Encourage increased fluid intake to maintain UO and stent patency
   d. Call physician if no UO occurs for 1 hour because there could be kinks in system or occlusion by sediment
   e. Medication therapy includes antibiotics until stent falls out, acetaminophen (Tylenol) for pain, and anticholinergics such as oxybutynin (Ditropan) for bladder spasms

D. **Client and family teaching**

1. Parents need explanation of disorder and surgical repair
2. ! Postsurgical discharge teaching
   a. Double-diapering technique to protect stent
   b. Limit activity for approximately 2 weeks, restriction of activities that put pressure on site (riding toys, sitting on lap)
   c. Medication administration
   d. Maintain adequate fluid intake
   e. Monitor for signs of infection
   f. Call physician if urine leaks from anywhere but penis (urine will also be blood-tinged for several days)

XVII. EXSTROPHY OF THE BLADDER

A. **Overview**

1. Lower portion of abdominal wall and anterior bladder wall are missing, resulting in bladder being open and exposed on abdomen
2. Occurs more frequently in boys than in girls and is most frequently associated with epispadias
3. Bladder appears as an angry red mass glistening with urine
4. Continuous drainage of urine from ureters may lead to excoriation of skin surrounding bladder
5. Exstrophy of bladder can be life threatening and therefore must be corrected as soon after birth as possible

B. **Nursing assessment:** immediately obvious at birth; infant should be evaluated for other anomalies

C. **Therapeutic management**

1. Bladder closure is corrected during first 48 to 72 hours of life
2. Correction of exstrophy of bladder is usually a staged surgical correction, with epispadias repair at about 9 months of age (if present) and bladder neck reconstruction with ureteral reimplantation at 2 to 3 years
3. Preoperative nursing care involves covering bladder with sterile plastic wrap and maintaining skin integrity of surrounding area using skin sealant to protect it from excoriating effects of urine
4. Postoperative nursing care may involve Bryant's traction to facilitate healing, and avoiding abduction of legs (puts stress on surgical area); change dressings as ordered by surgeon; monitor UO and characteristics and watch for signs of obstruction, bladder spasms, and urine or blood draining from meatus
5. Emotional support of infant and parents is important; activities to support bonding as well as helping parents accept deformity are a major component of nurse's activities

D. Client and family teaching

1. Explanation of anomaly as well as instructions for care
2. As soon as possible, parents should participate in care of their infant

XVIII. CRYPTORCHIDISM

A. Overview

1. Failure of one or both testes to descend from inguinal canal into scrotum; normal descent of testes occurs late in gestation
2. More frequently seen in premature infants than in full-term infants
3. Failure to descend exposes testes to body heat, leading to low sperm counts at sexual maturity
4. Undescended testicles are also at greater risk for torsion (twisting of a testis on its blood supply) and trauma; undescended testes have a higher incidence of cancer
5. Frequently associated with an inguinal hernia

B. Nursing assessment: absence of one or both testes in scrotal sac at birth

C. Therapeutic management

1. Often testes descend on own during first year of life; monitor periodically
2. If testes do not descend, human chorionic gonadotropin hormone is given to induce descent
3. If testes remain undescended, an orchiopexy is performed during toddler years; if testes are damaged or absent, a prosthesis is placed in scrotum
4. Nursing care preoperatively is directed at preparing child and family for surgery
5. Postoperatively, nursing care includes putting ice on surgical area, giving analgesics for pain, and monitoring child for infection; bedrest is maintained

D. Client and family teaching

1. Explanations of surgical repair
2. How to care for child at home postoperatively, since child will likely go home after recovering from anesthesia
3. Symptoms of infection to report

Check Your NCLEX-RN® Exam I.Q.

You are ready for testing on this content if you can

- Identify basic structures and functions of the renal system.
- Describe the pathophysiology and etiology of common renal disorders.
- Discuss expected assessment data and diagnostic test findings for selected renal disorders.
- Discuss therapeutic management of a client experiencing a renal disorder.
- Discuss nursing management of a client experiencing a renal disorder.
- Identify expected outcomes for the client experiencing a renal disorder.

PRACTICE TEST

1 Which of the following statements made by a client with chronic renal failure and who is on hemodialysis indicates the need for further teaching?

1. "I will report any increase in my weight of 5 pounds in a 2-day period."
2. "I take my prescribed antihypertensive drugs daily."
3. "I am careful to take precautions in the arm with the AV fistula."
4. "I comply with salt restrictions in my diet by using salt substitutes."

2 What type of renal failure would the nurse expect to see in a client who overdosed accidentally on tobramycin (Nebcin)?

1. Prerenal failure
2. Postrenal failure
3. Extrarenal failure
4. Intrarenal failure

3 A client with urinary tract infection (UTI) is prescribed phenazopyridine (Pyridium). Which of the following instructions would the nurse give the client?

1. "This drug will take care of the infection causing your symptoms."
2. "Your urine may turn reddish orange and may cause staining of your clothes."
3. "Take the drug before meals to minimize GI symptoms."
4. "Always keep this drug and use it at the first symptom of a UTI."

4 A client with a urinary diversion device has the nursing diagnosis *risk for impaired skin integrity.* Which of the following interventions will the nurse use with this client?

1. Change urine collection device every other day.
2. Teach self-catheterization technique.
3. Empty the bag reservoir every 2 hours.
4. Monitor for foul-smelling urine.

5 A client with renal calculi is advised to restrict calcium in his diet. The nurse determines that the client understands the restrictions when he states he will avoid which of the following?

1. Chicken, beef, and salmon
2. Green vegetables, fruit, and legumes
3. Chocolate, smoked fish, and low-fat milk
4. Eggs, meat, and poultry

6 In conducting client teaching with a client who will undergo peritoneal dialysis at home, the nurse includes discussion of what common and significant complication of peritoneal dialysis?

1. Pulmonary embolism
2. Hypotension
3. Dyspnea
4. Peritonitis

7 The nurse is preparing to admit a client with urge incontinence. In writing the nursing care plan, the nurse writes interventions that target the client's

1. involuntary loss of urine without warning or stimulus.
2. loss of urine when coughing or sneezing.
3. inability to empty bladder.
4. inability to stop urine flow long enough to reach the toilet.

8 A male client who presents to the emergency department with coffee-colored urine and edema states that he had a bad sore throat a few weeks ago. His blood pressure is elevated, and urinalysis shows blood and protein in the urine. The nurse interprets that the client's clinical picture is consistent with which of the following?

1. Urinary tract infection
2. Urinary calculi
3. Acute glomerulonephritis
4. Acute prostatitis

9 A client in the intensive care unit develops prerenal failure following surgery. Which of the following causes should the nurse suspect?

1. Vascular disease
2. Urethral obstruction
3. Hypovolemia
4. Glomerulonephritis

PRACTICE TEST

10 Which of the following discharge instructions would the nurse give to a client who will receive aminoglycoside antibiotics at home?

1. Limit fluid intake to 1200 mL daily
2. Report sudden weight gain or puffy eyes
3. Edema is a normal side effect of the medication
4. Elevated blood pressure is an expected effect of the medication

11 The nurse caring for a client undergoing a hemodialysis procedure places high priority on evaluating the client frequently for what common complication during the treatment?

1. Hyperglycemia
2. Infection and fever
3. Dialysis dementia
4. Hypotension

12 The nurse is explaining the process of peritoneal dialysis to a client who recently developed renal failure. Which of the following statements would the nurse include in a discussion with the client?

1. "The solutes in the dialysate will enter the bloodstream through the peritoneum."
2. "The peritoneum is more permeable because of the presence of excess metabolites."
3. "The peritoneum acts as a semipermeable membrane through which wastes move by diffusion and osmosis."
4. "The metabolites will diffuse from the interstitial space to the bloodstream mainly through diffusion and ultrafiltration."

13 Which of the following laboratory data is the most accurate indicator that a client with acute renal failure has met the expected outcomes?

1. Decreasing blood urea nitrogen (BUN) levels
2. Decreasing serum creatinine
3. Decreasing neutrophil count
4. Decreasing lymphocyte count

14 Which of the following statements made by a client with polycystic kidney disease indicates that the desired outcome has been met?

1. "I know these drugs will make the cysts disappear."
2. "The development of renal failure with this disease is very rare."
3. "I will have my family seek genetic counseling and screening."
4. "I sure am glad that hemodialysis will shrink the cysts."

15 A client is scheduled for a partial nephrectomy. In teaching the client about postoperative care, the nurse uses which rationale to explain why aggressive measures are needed to prevent atelectasis and pneumonia?

1. Nephrectomy involves paralyzing the intercostal muscles.
2. Intraoperative surgical contamination of the pulmonary structures is unavoidable.
3. The client must be maintained in a flat position for 24 hours.
4. The surgery involves an upper abdominal incision.

16 Which of the following statements made by a client who has received a renal transplant indicates that the desired outcome of the discharge teaching plan has been met?

1. "I will double my prednisone dose if my urine output is less than 300 mL/day."
2. "I will need to avoid crowds and prevent infection."
3. "Now I can eat whatever I want as long as I watch how much salt I use."
4. "Since I have not yet rejected the transplant, I never have to worry about rejection anymore."

17 Which of the following statements by a female client indicates that instruction in ways to prevent urinary tract infection (UTI) was understood?

1. "I should limit intake of water so I won't need to urinate so often."
2. "I should drink 8 to 10 glasses of fluid per day."
3. "I should only wear nylon underpants."
4. "I should void every 6 hours while I am awake."

18 A client with chronic renal failure asks the nurse why he is anemic. Which of the following responses by the nurse is best?

1. "The increased metabolic waste products in your body depress the bone marrow."
2. "We will need to review your dietary intake of iron-rich foods."
3. "There is a decreased production by the kidneys of the hormone erythropoietin."
4. "It is most likely that you have hereditary traits for the development of anemia."

19 A client with end-stage renal failure is to be admitted to the hospital because of shortness of breath. The serum potassium level is 7.0 mEq/L. What appropriate hospital unit should this client be admitted to?

1. A semiprivate room in a medical surgical unit
2. A private room in a medical surgical unit
3. A nursing unit with continuous electrocardiographic monitoring
4. A nursing unit for ventilator-assisted clients

20 A client with chronic renal failure has excess fluid volume excess. The laboratory report indicates the sodium level to be 120 mEq/L. The nurse interprets this as which of the following?

1. An elevated sodium level that must be reported immediately to the physician
2. An error in the laboratory analysis
3. A possible hemodilution effect secondary to excessive water retention
4. An expected electrolyte abnormality in clients with chronic renal failure

21 A child has been admitted to the unit with nephrotic syndrome. In talking with the mother, she reports that a cousin had acute glomerulonephritis (AGN) last year. The mother asks how these two diseases compare, as they both affect the kidneys. The nurse's response would include the information that

1. both diseases produce smoky colored urine.
2. both diseases cause greatly reduced urine output.
3. both diseases have a genetic basis.
4. treatment for both involves antibiotic therapy.

22 A child is being treated for nephrotic syndrome. The nurse has told the mother that it is important to keep the child's skin clean and dry. The mother asks why. The nurse's response is based on the knowledge that

1. the skin is fragile secondary to electrolyte deficiency.
2. frequent urination may leave moisture on the skin that predisposes breakdown.
3. dietary restrictions make fighting infection hard.
4. the condition causes a reduction of gamma globulin in the body.

23 In a child with acute renal failure, the nurse would help to prevent hyperkalemia by limiting which of the following foods in the child's diet?

1. Grains, cheese, and citrus fruits
2. Potatoes, tomatoes, and oranges
3. Cereals, processed sugars, and wheat
4. Rice, leafy green vegetables, and carbonated beverages

24 A child has been admitted with acute glomerulonephritis (AGN). All of the following tests are positive for AGN. The nurse concludes that which laboratory test is most conclusive of this disease?

1. Elevated antistreptinolysin O (ASO) titers
2. Elevated erythrocyte sedimentation rate (ESR)
3. Presence of hematuria according to urinalysis
4. Elevated creatinine concentrations

25 The mother of a child at the renal clinic asks why a radiological evaluation is performed on all children who have had one documented UTI. The best explanation by the nurse will include the information that the x-ray

1. rules out structural abnormalities.
2. confirms the absence of bacterial colonies after antimicrobial therapy.
3. determines which kidney was infected.
4. determines the probability of the infection recurring.

26 The nurse is caring for a client with poor urine output. The nurse would report to the health care provider if the client had a urine output less than how many milliliters per hour for 2 consecutive hours? Provide a numerical response.

Answer: ______________________

ANSWERS & RATIONALES

1 **Answer: 4** Many salt substitutes use potassium chloride. Potassium intake is carefully regulated in clients with renal failure, and the use of salt substitutes will worsen hyperkalemia. Increases in weight (option 1) do need to be reported to the health care provider as a possible indication of fluid volume excess. The control of hypertension (option 2) is essential in the management of a client with renal failure. An AV fistula does need to be protected from injury that could be caused by constricting clothing, venipunctures, and other items (option 3).
Cognitive Level: Analysis **Client Need:** Physiological Integrity: Physiological Adaptation **Integrated Process:** Nursing Process: Evaluation **Content Area:** Adult Health: Renal/Genitourinary **Strategy:** The core issue of the question is the ability to determine accurate statements about self-care of clients with renal failure. Specifically, clients need to restrict both sodium and potassium, and salt substitutes are high in potassium. Use nursing knowledge and the process of elimination to make a selection.

2 **Answer: 4** Nephrotoxic drugs, such as aminoglycoside antibiotics (tobramycin), can damage the nephrons and cause intrarenal (within the kidneys) failure. There is no condition called extrarenal failure.
Cognitive Level: Application **Client Need:** Physiological Integrity: Physiological Adaptation **Integrated Process:** Nursing Process: Analysis **Content Area:** Adult Health: Renal/Genitourinary **Strategy:** The core issue of the question is the ability to associate causes of renal failure with their categories in specific client situations. Use nursing knowledge and the process of elimination to make a selection.

3 **Answer: 2** The drug makes the urine reddish orange in color, and the client should be advised that this might stain the underwear and other clothing. The client should also be reassured that it should not be confused with blood in the urine. The use of Pyridium in UTI is controversial because it does not target the cause of the infection. However, it offers relief of UTI symptoms such as pain, frequency, and urgency (option 1). Taking the drug after meals minimizes GI symptoms associated with the use of this drug (option 3). Option 4 is incorrect because the indiscriminate use of a urinary analgesic can mask symptoms and delay initiation of treatment.
Cognitive Level: Analysis **Client Need:** Physiological Integrity: Pharmacological and Parenteral Therapies **Integrated Process:** Communication and Documentation **Content Area:** Adult Health: Renal/Genitourinary **Strategy:** The core issue of the question is knowledge of expected adverse effects of Pyridium. Use nursing knowledge and the process of elimination to make a selection.

4 **Answer: 3** Emptying the reservoir bag every 2 hours prevents overfilling and possible leakage of urine into the skin surface. The urine collection device should be changed as needed to maintain integrity of the system. Self-catheterization is not appropriate for this nursing diagnosis. Monitoring for foul-smelling urine and monitoring for signs of infection are more appropriate interventions for the diagnosis risk for infection.
Cognitive Level: Application **Client Need:** Physiological Integrity: Physiological Adaptation **Integrated Process:** Nursing Process: Implementation **Content Area:** Adult Health: Renal/Genitourinary **Strategy:** The core issue of the question is knowledge of appropriate care for a client with a urinary diversion. Use nursing knowledge and the process of elimination to make a selection.

5 **Answer: 3** Chocolate, smoked fish, milk products, beans, lentils, and dried fruits are high in calcium. In calcium phosphate and calcium oxalate calculi, dietary management includes an acid-ash diet and limiting foods high in calcium and oxalate.
Cognitive Level: Analysis **Client Need:** Physiological Integrity: Physiological Adaptation **Integrated Process:** Nursing Process: Evaluation **Content Area:** Adult Health: Renal/Genitourinary **Strategy:** The core issue of the question is knowledge of foods that are high in calcium. Use nursing knowledge and the process of elimination to make a selection.

6 **Answer: 4** Peritonitis is a grave complication of peritoneal dialysis, caused by bacteria that may enter through the catheter or dialysate solution. Hypotension is a common complication of hemodialysis but not peritoneal dialysis (option 2). Pulmonary embolism and dyspnea are not common complications of peritoneal dialysis.
Cognitive Level: Application **Client Need:** Physiological Integrity: Physiological Adaptation **Integrated Process:** Nursing Process: Implementation **Content Area:** Adult Health: Renal/Genitourinary **Strategy:** The core issue of the question is knowledge of the complications associated with peritoneal dialysis and their relative frequency. Use nursing knowledge and the process of elimination to make a selection.

7 **Answer: 4** Urge incontinence is the unpredictable passage of urine soon after a strong urge to void is felt. Option 1 describes total incontinence, option 2 describes stress incontinence, and option 3 describes urinary retention. The pathophysiology, contributing factors, therapeutic and nursing interventions for the different types of incontinence differ.
Cognitive Level: Application **Client Need:** Physiological Integrity: Physiological Adaptation **Integrated Process:** Nursing Process: Planning **Content Area:** Adult Health: Renal/Genitourinary **Strategy:** Use nursing knowledge and the process of elimination to make a selection.

8 **Answer: 3** The symptoms are typical of acute glomerulonephritis. Hematuria and proteinuria are caused by a damaged glomerular capillary membrane, which allows blood cells and proteins to escape into the renal filtrate. A urinary tract infection usually manifests with signs of infection including fever, malodorous urine, frequency, and urgency. Clients with urinary calculi usually present with renal colic. Prostatitis, or inflammation of the prostate gland, also has presenting symptoms similar to a urinary tract infection.
Cognitive Level: Analysis **Client Need:** Physiological Integrity: Physiological Adaptation **Integrated Process:** Nursing Process: Assessment **Content Area:** Adult Health: Renal/Genitourinary **Strategy:** The core issue of the question is the ability to iden-

tify signs and symptoms of glomerulonephritis and associate it with a common etiology. Use nursing knowledge and the process of elimination to make a selection.

9 **Answer: 3** Prerenal failure is caused by factors such as hypovolemia and decreased cardiac output that affect renal blood flow and perfusion. Urethral obstruction (option 2) can cause postrenal failure. Vascular disease and glomerulonephritis may be factors in the development of intrarenal failure.
Cognitive Level: Application **Client Need:** Physiological Integrity: Physiological Adaptation **Integrated Process:** Nursing Process: Analysis **Content Area:** Adult Health: Renal/Genitourinary **Strategy:** The core issue of the question is the ability to identify causes of prerenal failure. Use nursing knowledge and the process of elimination to make a selection.

10 **Answer: 2** To reduce the risk of nephrotoxicity, the client who receives aminoglycoside antibiotics should report signs of edema or hypertension and maintain a fluid intake of 2,000 to 2,500 mL per day.
Cognitive Level: Analysis **Client Need:** Physiological Integrity: Pharmacological and Parenteral Therapies **Integrated Process:** Nursing Process: Implementation **Content Area:** Adult Health: Renal/Genitourinary **Strategy:** The core issue of the question is the ability to correctly institute client teaching with knowledge of nephrotoxicity as an adverse effect of aminoglycoside medications. Use nursing knowledge and the process of elimination to make a selection.

11 **Answer: 4** Hypotension is the most common complication during hemodialysis and is related to several factors, including changes in serum osmolality and rapid removal of fluid from the intravascular compartment. Dialysis dementia is a progressive, long-term complication. Infection and fever should be an ongoing assessment for a hemodialysis client. Hyperglycemia could occur in peritoneal dialysis because of the composition of the dialysate, but it is not of great concern unless the client has diabetes mellitus.
Cognitive Level: Application **Client Need:** Physiological Integrity: Physiological Adaptation **Integrated Process:** Nursing Process: Assessment **Content Area:** Adult Health: Renal/Genitourinary **Strategy:** The core issue of the question is the ability to identify important complications associated with hemodialysis. Use nursing knowledge and the process of elimination to make a selection.

12 **Answer: 3** The peritoneum acts as a semipermeable membrane, allowing substances to move from an area of high concentration (the blood) to an area of lower concentration (the dialysate). Metabolic waste products and excess water can be eliminated through osmosis and diffusion utilizing the peritoneum as the semipermeable membrane.
Cognitive Level: Application **Client Need:** Physiological Integrity: Physiological Adaptation **Integrated Process:** Communication and Documentation **Content Area:** Adult Health: Renal/Genitourinary **Strategy:** The core issue of the question is the ability to relate accurately the key elements of peritoneal dialysis. Use nursing knowledge and the process of elimination to make a selection.

13 **Answer: 2** Creatinine is the metabolic end product of creatine phosphate and is excreted via the kidneys in relatively constant amounts. BUN, a measurement of the nitrogen portion of urea, is also excreted in urine and is a good indicator of renal function. However, conditions that increase protein catabolism also cause a rise in BUN levels. Therefore, the serum creatinine levels are more appropriate to evaluate in determining the return of renal function. Neutrophils and lymphocytes are not used to monitor the return of renal function.
Cognitive Level: Analysis **Client Need:** Physiological Integrity: Physiological Adaptation **Integrated Process:** Nursing Process: Evaluation **Content Area:** Adult Health: Renal/Genitourinary **Strategy:** The critical words in the question are *most accurate.* This tells you that more than one response is technically correct, and you must prioritize to choose the option that best answers the question. Use nursing knowledge and the process of elimination to make a selection.

14 **Answer: 3** Adult polycystic kidney disease is an autosomal-dominant disorder, and the client should be advised to have family members screened for the disease. The management of clients with polycystic kidney disease is mainly supportive. Eventually, clients with this disease require dialysis or transplantation.
Cognitive Level: Analysis **Client Need:** Physiological Integrity: Physiological Adaptation **Integrated Process:** Nursing Process: Evaluation **Content Area:** Adult Health: Renal/Genitourinary **Strategy:** The core issue of the question is knowledge that this disorder has a genetic basis. Use nursing knowledge and the process of elimination to make a selection.

15 **Answer: 4** The upper abdominal incision site in clients with nephrectomy predisposes them to the development of respiratory complications, particularly atelectasis and pneumonia. The proximity of the incision to the muscles involved in breathing and coughing makes the client breathe shallowly and avoid coughing because of the fear of pain. Adequate pain control is necessary in the care of this client. The other options are not accurate statements.
Cognitive Level: Application **Client Need:** Physiological Integrity: Physiological Adaptation **Integrated Process:** Nursing Process: Implementation **Content Area:** Adult Health: Renal/Genitourinary **Strategy:** The core issue of the question is the ability to correlate location of incision with risks for postoperative complications following nephrectomy. Use nursing knowledge and the process of elimination to make a selection.

16 **Answer: 2** Clients with renal transplant need to be on long-term immunosuppressive drugs. This predisposes them to infection. The client must verbalize factors that potentially expose him to infection. Dietary restrictions must be discussed with the physician and the dietician. The client with renal transplant also needs to verbalize understanding of his medications to prevent rejection, including the use of immunosuppressants. However, he must adhere to the dose prescribed by the physician. The success of transplantation is not guaranteed.
Cognitive Level: Analysis **Client Need:** Physiological Integrity: Physiological Adaptation **Integrated Process:** Nursing Process: Evaluation **Content Area:** Adult Health: Renal/Genitourinary **Strategy:** The core issue of the question is the knowledge that clients who have had organ transplant are greatly at risk for

infection because of drug therapy needed to prevent organ rejection. Use nursing knowledge and the process of elimination to make a selection.

17 **Answer: 2** Maintaining an intake of 8 to 10 glasses of fluid daily will help prevent UTI. Cotton underpants are best, and nylon should be avoided because synthetic fibers dry and irritate the perineal area. Irritation of the perineal area can promote the growth of bacteria. The client should not delay voiding when the urge is felt. Emptying the bladder every 2 to 4 hours while awake is recommended to prevent urinary stasis.

Cognitive Level: Analysis **Client Need:** Physiological Integrity: Physiological Adaptation **Integrated Process:** Nursing Process: Evaluation **Content Area:** Adult Health: Renal/Genitourinary **Strategy:** The core issue of the question is knowledge of risk factors for UTIs that must be avoided by clients at risk. Use nursing knowledge and the process of elimination to make a selection.

18 **Answer: 3** Anemia is common in clients with renal failure. Among the factors causing the anemia are decreased production of erythropoietin by the kidneys and shortened RBC life. Erythropoietin is involved in the stimulation of the bone marrow to produce RBCs.

Cognitive Level: Application **Client Need:** Physiological Integrity: Physiological Adaptation **Integrated Process:** Communication and Documentation **Content Area:** Adult Health: Renal/Genitourinary **Strategy:** The core issue of the question is the pathophysiology underlying renal failure and associated changes. Use nursing knowledge and the process of elimination to make a selection.

19 **Answer: 3** Clients with potassium levels of 6.5 and greater are predisposed to develop cardiac arrhythmias, muscle cramps, and gastrointestinal symptoms. The client should be admitted to a nursing unit with telemetry or cardiac monitoring capabilities because of the risk of developing life-threatening cardiac dysrhythmias. Typical ECG abnormalities associated with hyperkalemia are prolonged PR interval; wide QRS; tall, tented T-wave; and ST segment depression. Major cardiac dysrhythmias common in clients with highly elevated potassium levels include heart block, ventricular standstill, and ventricular fibrillation.

Cognitive Level: Analysis **Client Need:** Physiological Integrity: Physiological Adaptation **Integrated Process:** Nursing Process: Planning **Content Area:** Adult Health: Renal/Genitourinary **Strategy:** The core issue of the question is knowledge of the significance of a high serum potassium level and the appropriate placement of the client to detect possible complications. Use nursing knowledge and the process of elimination to make a selection.

20 **Answer: 3** Clients with renal failure retain sodium, and any decrease in the serum level will most likely be caused by hemodilution from the excessive fluid retention. A sodium level of 20 mEq/L is lower than normal.

Cognitive Level: Analysis **Client Need:** Physiological Integrity: Physiological Adaptation **Integrated Process:** Nursing Process: Analysis **Content Area:** Adult Health: Renal/Genitourinary **Strategy:** The core issue of the question is the ability to make an accurate interpretation of laboratory data in a client with renal failure. Use nursing knowledge and the process of elimination to make a selection.

21 **Answer: 2** Typical symptoms of nephrotic syndrome are clear, frothy urine that is diminished in volume. AGN presents with smoky urine that is also diminished in volume. AGN is a postinfectious disease with no genetic basis. Antibiotics are not used in nephrotic syndrome. Oliguria is usually defined as 0.5 to 1.0 mL/kg/hr.

Cognitive Level: Analysis **Client Need:** Physiological Integrity: Physiological Adaptation **Integrated Process:** Nursing Process: Analysis **Content Area:** Child Health: Renal/Genitourinary **Strategy:** The core issue of the question is knowledge of the similarities and differences between nephrotic syndrome and glomerulonephritis. Use nursing knowledge and the process of elimination to make a selection.

22 **Answer: 4** Nephrotic syndrome involves the loss of protein in the urine. Gamma globulins, which help the body fight infections, are proteins. Skin that is not clean and dry is more prone to breakdown, which could lead to infection. The child is oliguric and therefore does not urinate frequently. The only restrictions on the child's intake are fluid and perhaps sodium. There is no electrolyte deficiency.

Cognitive Level: Analysis **Client Need:** Physiological Integrity: Physiological Adaptation **Integrated Process:** Nursing Process: Implementation **Content Area:** Child Health: Renal/Genitourinary **Strategy:** The core issue of the question is the ability to relate gamma globulin deficiency in nephrotic syndrome to situations that increase risk of infection, such as unclean or moist skin. Use nursing knowledge and the process of elimination to make a selection.

23 **Answer: 2** Potatoes, tomatoes, and oranges have a high level of potassium content. The others have less potassium in them.

Cognitive Level: Application **Client Need:** Physiological Integrity: Physiological Adaptation **Integrated Process:** Nursing Process: Implementation **Content Area:** Child Health: Renal/Genitourinary **Strategy:** The core issue of the question is knowledge of foods that are high in potassium to avoid in the client with renal failure. Use nursing knowledge and the process of elimination to make a selection.

24 **Answer: 1** An elevated ASO titer indicates a recent streptococcal infection, which is a precursor to AGN. The elevated ESR indicates inflammation in the body and is associated with many diseases. Hematuria is simply blood in the urine, which has many possible causes. Creatinine concentrations reflect the functioning of the kidney.

Cognitive Level: Analysis **Client Need:** Physiological Integrity: Physiological Adaptation **Integrated Process:** Nursing Process: Analysis **Content Area:** Child Health: Renal/Genitourinary **Strategy:** The critical words in the question are *most indicative.* This tells you that all options are correct, and you must select the response that uniquely identifies glomerulonephritis as the disorder. Use nursing knowledge and the process of elimination to make a selection.

25 **Answer: 1** Radiological evaluations done after a documented UTI in children reveal structural abnormalities in 1% to 2% of girls and 10% of boys. Radiological tests cannot confirm bacterial colonies, determine the site of an old infection, or help predict whether infection will reoccur.

Cognitive Level: Application **Client Need:** Physiological Integrity: Physiological Adaptation **Integrated Process:** Nursing Process: Implementation **Content Area:** Child Health: Renal/Genitourinary **Strategy:** The core issue of the question is knowledge that UTIs are uncommon in children and could result from structural abnormalities that are yet undiagnosed. With this in mind, use the process of elimination to make a selection from the available options.

26 **Answer: 30** The minimal urine output by the kidneys per hour is 30 mL. It is prudent for the nurse to report a drop below this amount if it persists for 2 hours or longer so that corrective treatment can be undertaken.

Cognitive Level: Application **Client Need:** Physiological Integrity: Physiological Adaptation **Integrated Process:** Nursing Process: Implementation **Content Area:** Adult Health: Renal/Genitourinary **Strategy:** The core issue of the question is knowledge of minimal hourly urine output based on normal kidney function. Use nursing knowledge to formulate an answer.

Key Terms to Review

acute renal failure p. 1138
anuria p. 1127
azotemia p. 1138
chordee p. 1141
chronic renal failure p. 1139
circumcision p. 1141
creatinine p. 1119
cryptorchidism p. 1142
cystectomy p. 1125
cystitis p. 1132
epispadias p. 1141
exstrophy p. 1141
glomerulonephritis p. 1135
glomerulus p. 1117
hematuria p. 1122
hemodialysis p. 1121
hypospadias p. 1141
intravenous pyelography (IVP) p. 1119
lithotripsy p. 1124
micturition p. 1119
nephrectomy p. 1126
nephron p. 1117
nephrotic syndrome p. 1136
oliguria p. 1133
peritoneal dialysis p. 1121
polycystic kidney disease p. 1137
polyuria p. 1139
proteinuria p. 1139
pyelonephritis p. 1133
pyuria p. 1122
uremia p. 1139
urinary diversion p. 1125
vesicoureteral reflux p. 1133

References

Ball, J., & Bindler, R. (2006). *Child health nursing: Partnering with children and families.* (3rd ed.). Upper Saddle River, NJ: Pearson Education.

Black, J., & Hawks, J. (2005). *Medical surgical nursing: Clinical management for positive outcomes* (7th ed.). St. Louis: Elsevier Science.

Corbett, J. (2004). *Laboratory tests and diagnostic procedures with nursing diagnoses* (6th ed.). Upper Saddle River, NJ: Pearson Education.

Harkreader, H., & Hogan, M. (2004).*Fundamentals of nursing: Caring and clinical judgment* (2nd ed.). St. Louis: Elsevier Science.

Hockenberry, M., Wilson, D., Winkelstein, M., & Kline, N. (2003). *Nursing care of infants and children* (7th ed.). St. Louis: Mosby.

Ignatavicius, D., & Workman, L. (2006). *Medical-surgical nursing: Critical thinking for collaborative care* (5th ed.). Philadelphia: W. B. Saunders.

Kozier, B., Erb, G., Berman, A., & Snyder, S. (2004). *Fundamentals of nursing: Concepts, process, and practice* (7th ed.). Upper Saddle River, NJ: Pearson Education.

LeMone, P., & Burke, K. (2004). *Medical surgical nursing: Critical thinking in client care* (3rd ed.). Upper Saddle River, NJ: Pearson Education.

Lewis, S., Heitkemper, M., & Dirksen, S. (2004). *Medical surgical nursing: Assessment and management of clinical problems* (6th ed.). St. Louis: Elsevier Science.

Porth, C. (2004). *Pathophysiology: Concepts of altered health states* (7th ed.). Philadelphia: Lippincott Williams & Wilkins.

Smith, S., Duell, D., & Martin, B. (2004). *Clinical nursing skills: Basic to advanced skills* (6th ed.). Upper Saddle River, NJ: Pearson Education.

60 Gastrointestinal Disorders

Test Yourself

Are you ready for the NCLEX-RN® or course exams? Use the practice tests on the companion CD-ROM to check.

In this chapter

Cross reference

Other chapters relevant to this content area are

Health and Physical Assessment	Chapter 16
Meeting Nutritional Needs	Chapter 26
Maintaining Function of Tubes and Drains	Chapter 28
Total Parenteral Nutrition	Chapter 34
Gastrointestinal Medications	Chapter 41
Common Laboratory Tests	Chapter 47
Common Diagnostic Tests and Procedures	Chapter 48

I. OVERVIEW OF ANATOMY AND PHYSIOLOGY OF THE GI SYSTEM

A. **Oral cavity and pharynx:** consists of mouth, oropharynx and laryngopharynx; passageway for food, fluids, and air

B. **Esophagus:** extends from pharynx to stomach; enters stomach at gastroesophageal sphincter (also called lower esophageal sphincter, or LES), which prevents reflux

C. **Stomach:** distensible organ located high on left side of abdomen; continues mechanical breakdown of food and mixes food with gastric secretions forming a mixture called chyme; divided into four regions (cardiac, fundus, body, and pyloric; digests food with assistance of pepsin and hydrochloric acid; produces intrinsic factor for vitamin B12 absorption in small intestine; churns gastric contents via peristalsis

D. **Small intestine:** begins at the pyloric sphincter and ends at the ileocecal valve; contains three regions: duodenum, jejunum, and ileum; pancreatic enzymes (trypsin, chymotrypsin, lipase, and amylase) and bile enter duodenum near pyloric sphincter to further digest chyme; most absorption occurs in villae of small intestine

E. **Large intestine:** also called colon; extends from ileocecal valve to anus; divided into five areas: cecum, appendix, colon (ascending, transverse, and descending), rectum, and anus; major function is to absorb water, salts, and vitamins formed by bacteria in large intestine and eliminate undigestible food and residue

F. **Hepatobiliary system**

1. Liver
   a. Located in the right upper quadrant (RUQ) of the abdomen, beneath diaphragm; produces bile, an alkaline, yellow-green fluid containing bile salts (conjugated bile acids), cholesterol, bilirubin (byproduct of red blood cell destruction), electrolytes, and water
   b. Stores vitamin B_{12} and fat-soluble vitamins (A, D, E, and K)
   c. Stores and releases blood during hemorrhage
   d. Synthesizes plasma proteins to maintain plasma oncotic pressure
   e. Synthesizes prothrombin, fibrinogen, and clotting factors I, II, VII, IX, X
   f. Converts amino acids to carbohydrates through deamination
   g. Stores and releases glucose and copper; stores iron as ferritin
   h. Detoxifies alcohol and certain drugs
2. Biliary tract: composed of gallbladder and associated ducts (cystic, hepatic, and common bile ducts); transports bile formed in liver to bile ducts and eventually to duodenum
3. Gallbladder: saclike organ located on inferior surface of liver; stores and concentrates bile; releases bile into cystic duct and common bile duct in response to presence of fat in duodenum, which leads to hormone secretion and relaxation of sphincter of Oddi
4. Pancreas: has exocrine and endocrine functions; head is located within curve of duodenum, tail touches spleen, and body lies behind stomach
   a. Pancreatic secretions flow into duodenum

b. Endocrine pancreas secretes insulin and glucagon hormones from islets of Langerhans; insulin is a protein hormone that promotes storage and utilization of food, primarily glucose and fats; glucagon stimulates glycogenolysis in liver
c. Exocrine pancreas secretes enzymes in response to hormonal and vagal stimuli; produces about 1 to 1.5 L of alkaline pancreatic juice/day, which neutralizes acidic chyme as it empties into duodenum; produces lipase (fat breakdown); amylase (carbohydrate breakdown); and trypsin, chymotrypsin, and carboxypeptidase (protein breakdown)

II. DIAGNOSTIC TESTS AND ASSESSMENTS OF THE GI SYSTEM

A. **Laboratory tests:** serum chemistry study, liver profile, lipid profile, gastrin levels, Schilling test, erythrocyte sedimentation rate (ESR), C-reactive protein (CRP), thyroid function (see Chapter 47)

B. **Upper GI series:** series of x-rays using contrast medium (barium sulfate or Gastrografin) to diagnose hiatal hernia, tumors, ulcerations, inflammation, varices, or obstruction
1. After client drinks barium, a series of x-rays document progression of contrast as client is placed in different positions
2. Gastroesophageal reflux (from stomach into esophagus) can be assessed with client in a flat or head-down position
3. Contraindications: complete bowel obstruction, esophageal or gastric perforation (may use Gastrografin), pregnancy, or unstable vital signs
4. ! Possible complications: aspiration of contrast medium, constipation (if barium used), or partial bowel obstruction; if Gastrografin is used, there may be significant diarrhea

C. **Lower GI series:** series of x-rays utilizing contrast medium (barium enema)
1. Visualizes colon, including appendix, for anatomic abnormalities, polyps, ulcers, tumors, inflammatory bowel disease, fistulas, and diverticula
2. ! Scheduling considerations: perform before an upper GI study to prevent residual barium remaining in colon, and colon should also be empty
   a. Clear liquid diet day before test
   b. Magnesium citrate or other bowel prep night before test
   c. NPO after midnight and continue until test is complete
   d. Cleansing enemas may be ordered before test
   e. Contraindications: perforated colon, uncooperative client
   f. Possible complications: colonic perforation or barium impaction

D. **Upper GI endoscopy:** ***esophagogastroduodenoscopy (EGD),*** gastroscopy
1. Allows direct visualization of esophagus, stomach, and duodenum through lighted endoscope; detects mucosal inflammations (gastroesophageal reflux, gastritis), tumors, varices, hiatal hernias, polyps, ulcers, and obstruction
2. Used also to directly sample tissues and fluids, to stop areas of active GI bleeding with injection of sclerosing agents or cautery, and to perform GI surgery using laser beams
3. Contraindications: perforated colon, fulminant ulcerative colitis, toxic megacolon, pregnancy, uncooperative clients
4. ! Possible complications: pulmonary aspiration of GI contents; perforation of esophagus, stomach, or duodenum; bleeding from biopsy site; and reactions to sedative medication given during test
5. ! Special nursing considerations postprocedure: NPO until client is completely alert and swallowing/gag reflexes have returned (2 to 4 hours); general safety precautions because of sedation; monitor for signs of bleeding, dyspnea, or dysphagia

E. **Colonoscopy:** fiberoptic direct visualization of colon from anus to cecum to detect tumors (benign or malignant), polyps, inflammation, ulcerations, and bleeding; suspicious tissue may be biopsied
1. Contraindications: suspected colon perforation, acute diverticulitis, peritonitis, or fulminant ulcerative colitis
2. ! Possible complications: perforation of colon, bleeding from biopsy sites, oversedation

3. Special nursing considerations: requires complete bowel prep; monitor vital signs postprocedure for signs of bleeding and colon perforation

F. **Sigmoidoscopy:** direct visualization of anus, rectum, and sigmoid colon with either a rigid or flexible sigmoidoscope; similar to colonoscopy in procedure, contraindications, complications, and nursing considerations, but is a less extensive study

G. **Ultrasonography:** non-invasive visualization of abdominal organs using high-frequency sound waves that penetrate organ and bounce back to a transducer where they are converted to an electronic pictorial image

1. Can detect organ size, cyst formation, tumors, and filling defects
2. No contrast medium or radiation is involved, so there are no contraindications and no complications

H. **Computed tomography (CT) scan:** radiologic procedure (with or without contrast medium) used to diagnose conditions such as tumors, cysts, abscesses, perforation, bleeding inflammation, aneurysms, and obstruction (see also Chapter 48)

1. Take usual precautions with use of iodinated contrast medium; contraindicated with pregnancy, unstable vital signs, morbid obesity, and claustrophobia
2. Special nursing considerations: encourage clients to drink fluids to promote contrast elimination and monitor client for delayed reaction to contrast medium

I. **Gastric analysis:** stomach contents are aspirated via NG tube; pH is measured at a basal rate (BAO—basal acid output) and also during a stimulated state (MAO—maximal acid output); may be done via tubeless gastric analysis whereby a resin dye (Diagnex Blue) is ingested, gastric acid displaces dye from resin, and dye is absorbed by bowel and excreted by kidneys

1. Differentiates causes of hypergastrinemia, including **Zollinger-Ellison syndrome** (elevated gastrin levels from pancreatic tumor), chronic antacid ingestion, and atrophic gastritis; direct measurement of gastrin levels is used most often for this purpose
2. Frequently used to assess effect of medical or surgical antiulcer therapy
3. Precautions: anyone with heart failure, carcinoid syndrome, or hypertension may have symptom exacerbation with this test because histamine is used to stimulate gastric acid

J. **Stool examination:** examines fecal specimen for obvious and occult blood and fat, assays it for clostridial toxin and cultures it for bacterial, viral, and parasitic pathogens

1. Stool culture, ova, and parasites: detects many bacterial pathogens and parasitic pathogens include such as (hookworm), *Strongyloides* (tape worm), and *Giardia* (protozoans)
2. Stool for occult blood: stool is tested with a reagent to detect blood that is not visible; caused by benign and malignant GI tumors, ulcers, inflammatory bowel disease, diverticulosis, and hemorrhoids; see Box 60–1 for substances that cause a false-positive or false-negative result for blood

Box 60–1

Stool for Occult Blood

Common Substances Causing False-Positive Results

- Red meat
- Fish
- Oral iron supplements
- Iodine
- Boric acid
- Colchicine
- Drugs irritating to gastric mucosa
  - Aspirin
  - NSAIDs
  - Corticosteroids

Common Substances Causing False-Negative Results

- Vitamin C
- Turnips
- Horseradish
- Beets
- Melons

3. Fecal fat: measures fat content of stool over 24 hours from conditions such as cystic fibrosis, celiac disease, sprue, Crohn's disease (regional enteritis), Whipple's disease, and maldigestion from pancreato-biliary tree obstruction; instruct client to abstain from alcohol and eat a diet that contains 100 grams of fat per day for 3 days before and during stool collection
4. Stool for clostridial toxin: *Clostridium difficile* bacteria release a toxin that causes necrosis of bowel epithelium; infection occurs in people who are immunocompromised or after taking broad-spectrum antibiotics

III. NURSING MANAGEMENT OF CLIENT HAVING GASTROINTESTINAL SURGERY

A. ***Colostomy:*** fecal diversion to an external collection device; named for portion of colon from which they are formed: ascending, transverse, descending, or sigmoid

1. Preoperative period
   a. Teach client and family about procedure and postoperative course, including pain relief, breathing exercises, and appearance of stoma; this information will reduce client anxiety and promote postoperative participation in care; encourage client to verbalize fears and concerns about lifestyle changes; provide appropriate referrals for support (such as United Ostomy Assoc.)
   b. Consult with enterostomal therapist, who will advise surgeon regarding optimal ostomy placement
   c. Carry out bowel preparation orders, which usually include low-residue day for 1 to 2 days before surgery; bowel cleansing with cathartics and enemas as well as oral or parenteral antibiotics (to reduce bacteria count)
   d. Complete usual preoperative activities and checklist
2. Postoperative period
   a. Routine care for surgical client: monitor vital signs (VS) and bowel sounds; assess I & O including wound drainage and drainage from tubes (NG, urinary drainage, etc.); evaluate incision(s) and perianal area; assess LOC and encourage deep breathing, use of incentive spirometer (IS), and splinting of incision
   b. Assess appearance and drainage from stoma, identify any changes, and notify surgeon if stoma becomes pale, darkened, cyanotic, sunken, stenosed (narrowed opening) or if bleeding increases
   c. Assess pouch system for proper fit (only 1/8 inch space between stoma and appliance) and any signs of leakage; empty when one third full; assess skin surrounding stoma to be sure it is intact when changing ostomy appliance
   d. Monitor pain control and take appropriate actions if pain is not controlled (check patency of IV access, notify physician, provide comfort measures)
   e. Encourage ambulation as ordered to stimulate peristalsis
   f. Resume oral intake as ordered and monitor for nausea, abdominal distension, and adequacy of bowel sounds
   g. Begin discharge teaching: possible postoperative complications and preventative measures (infection, bowel obstruction, abdominal abscess); colostomy care (irrigation depending on stoma location, pouch management, skin care)

B. ***Ileostomy:*** large intestine is completely removed and fecal diversion is created at level of the ileum

1. Preoperative period: same care as before colostomy surgery
2. Postoperative period
   a. Provide routine postoperative care as per colostomy surgery
   b. Apply ostomy appliance (pouch) over the stoma and teach client and family about procedure and nature of effluent (initially dark green, more liquid than colostomy, but will thicken over time and become yellow-brown)
   c. Protect skin around stoma with a skin barrier from irritating effects of effluent, which contains digestive enzymes and bile salts
   d. Begin educating client and family as soon as possible about how to manage stoma, appliance, and skin care, and when to report any abnormalities in the stoma, effluent, or abdomen

e. Emphasize importance of good nutrition and need for adequate fluid and electrolyte intake and the signs and symptoms of an imbalance; because of liquid effluent, clients are at high risk for dehydration and electrolyte imbalance, especially during hot weather, sustained exercise, or fever

C. **Gastrectomy:** removal of stomach with anastomosis of esophagus to jejunum (esophagojejunostomy); rarely performed, usually only for extensive gastric cancer or Zollinger-Ellison syndrome unresponsive to medical treatment

1. Preoperative period
   a. Reinforce physician teaching and obtain signed surgical consent form
   b. Advise client and family what to expect postoperatively, including pain relief, breathing exercises, expected tubes (nasogastric [NG], drains, jejunostomy feeding tube), and ambulation
2. Postoperative period
   a. Assess VS, lung and bowel sounds, I & O including drainage from NG tube, wound drainage (amount and character), effectiveness of pain-control measures
   b. Do not reposition, irrigate, or check placement of NG tube because of risk of disrupting esophagojejunostomy sutures (depending on surgeon's orders)
   c. Implement standard postoperative care (pain management, progressive activity to ambulation)
   d. Discuss limitations in oral intake and alternative methods to maintain nutrition; may require jejunostomy tube with an elemental (requires no digestion) enteral feeding
   e. Teach client about postoperative complications, including pernicious anemia, abdominal abscess or infection, and decreased nutrition

D. **Gastric resection:** portion of stomach removed for diseases such as cancer and peptic ulcer disease refractory to medical management (removing antrum eliminates most gastrin-producing cells)

1. Preoperative period
   a. Insert NG tube if ordered and connect to suction (may be inserted in operating room)
   b. Provide standard preoperative interventions as for any client undergoing abdominal surgery
2. Postoperative period
   a. Assess VS, lung and bowel sounds, I & O including drainage from NG tube, wound drainage (amount and character), effectiveness of pain-control measures
   b. Do *not* reposition, irrigate, or check placement of NG tube (unless there is a specific physician order to do so) because of risk of disrupting sutures inside stomach
   c. Encourage ambulation to promote peristalsis and prevent postoperative complications such as paralytic ileus and obstruction
   d. Implement standard postoperative care for clients with abdominal surgery
   e. Be alert for development of acute gastric dilation as a postoperative complication; signs and symptoms include epigastric pain, fullness, hiccups, tachycardia, and hypotension; this complication results from a malfunctioning NG tube and rapidly improves after tube is flushed (physician order) or replaced (by surgeon or designee)
3. **Dumping syndrome** is a common complication of gastric resection when pylorus is bypassed; after eating there is rapid dumping of food into jejunum without proper mixing and duodenal digestion
   a. Early manifestations: occur 15 to 30 minutes postprandial (after eating) and include vertigo, tachycardia, syncope, sweating, pallor, and palpitations; believed to be caused by a rapid shift of extracellular fluid into bowel to dilute hypertonic chyme, thereby decreasing blood volume
   b. Late manifestations occur 2 to 3 hours postprandial and include epigastric fullness, distension, diarrhea, abdominal cramping, nausea and high-pitched bowel sounds; caused by excessive release of insulin in response to a rapid rise in blood glucose due to high-carbohydrate (CHO) bolus entering jejunum

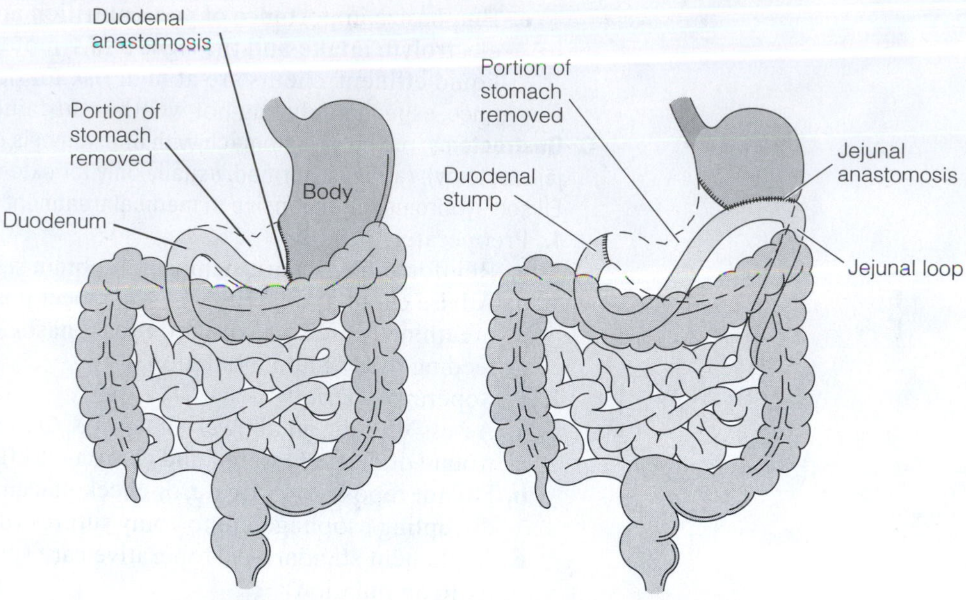

Figure 60–1

Partial gastrectomy.

A. Gastroduodenostomy or Billroth I.

B. Gastrojejunostomy or Billroth II.

Source: LeMone, P., & Burke, K. (2004). Medical surgical nursing: Critical thinking in client care (3rd ed.). Upper Saddle River, NJ: Pearson Education, p. 567.

c. Can be minimized by a low-CHO, high-protein, high-fat diet; suggest also that client avoid drinking fluids with meals and lie down after eating; prescribed antispasmodics or sedatives may delay gastric emptying

E. **Billroth I (gastroduodenostomy):** a partial gastrectomy in which distal portion of stomach (including antrum) is removed and remainder is anastomosed to duodenum (see Figure 60–1a ■); gastrin-producing cells in antrum, as well as some parietal cells (acid-pepsinogen secreting cells), are removed

1. Preoperative and postoperative care is same as for any client having gastric surgery
2. Dumping syndrome is a common complication of this procedure

F. **Billroth II (gastrojejunostomy):** a partial gastrectomy in which lower portion of stomach is removed and proximal remnant is anastomosed to jejunum (see Figure 60–1b); used to treat gastric and duodenal ulcers refractory to medical treatment

1. Preoperative and postoperative care is same as for any client having gastric surgery
2. ! Dumping syndrome is a common complication of this procedure

IV. MALNUTRITION

A. Overview

1. Insufficient amounts, improper proportions, malabsorption, or improper distribution of food substances necessary to provide body with energy for normal functions
2. Can also result from loss of nutrients as in vomiting
3. When more energy is expended than is consumed, body uses stored forms of energy in a certain order: first CHOs stored as glycogen, then fat stores, and finally protein stores in form of muscle tissue
4. ! Malnutrition can result from a variety of conditions and diseases
   a. Insufficient nutrients: liver failure (liver normally makes blood proteins), starvation, anorexia nervosa or bulimia, severe illness or trauma (increases protein and calorie requirements)
   b. Improper proportions: fad dieting, unavailability of variety of foods, maldigestion of certain foods because of a loss of enzymes, acid, or hormones
   c. Malabsorption: rapid GI transit time, gastric resection, partial gastrectomy, intestinal infections, absence of some enzymes as in celiac disease, decreased production or release of bile
   d. Improper distribution: in absence of insulin, glucose cannot enter cells to be used for energy
   e. Loss of nutrients: vomiting and severe diarrhea

B. Nursing assessment

1. Body mass index (BMI) estimates total body fat stores in relation to height and weight (weight in kg divided by body surface area)

2. Clinical manifestations include cheilosis, glossitis, stomatitis, muscle wasting, anemia, edema, alopecia, spongy bleeding gums, dry scaling skin, subcutaneous fat loss, bone pain, confusion, disorientation, paresthesia, heart failure, and decreased hair pigmentation
3. Diagnosed by history; physical exam; and laboratory evaluation of protein, iron stores, vitamin levels, serum cholesterol, and electrolytes

C. Therapeutic management

1. Ensure that client receives proper diet as ordered by health care provider (high-calorie, high-protein), and provide a pleasant dining environment, removing sources of unpleasant odors (bedpans, urinals, soiled dressings)
2. Encourage client to eat in a slow, relaxed manner
3. Provide enteral nutrition if ordered (see also Chapter 26)
4. Provide skin care and encourage activity to prevent skin breakdown
5. Assess for and instruct client about signs and symptoms of infection and to report them to health care provider if they occur
6. Medications generally include pancreatic enzymes, vitamins, minerals, antiemetics, antidiarrheals, antibiotics (for infectious diarrhea), insulin, and possibly, total parenteral nutrition (TPN)

D. Client teaching

1. Reinforce diet teaching provided by dietitian and emphasize importance of adhering to diet prescription; safe weight gain is 1 to 2 lbs/wk
2. Help client choose high-calorie, high-protein foods
3. Teach client about use of any prescribed medications for digestion, vomiting, diarrhea, or intestinal infections
4. Teach client about proper administration of enteral or parenteral feedings if prescribed

V. GASTROESOPHAGEAL REFLUX DISEASE (GERD)

A. Overview

1. Backward movement of stomach contents into esophagus without vomiting
2. Caused by relaxation of lower esophageal sphincter (LES), decreased LES tone, increased intra-abdominal pressure, increased gastric volume, or a combination (see Box 60–2 for factors influencing LES tone)
3. Reflux of gastric contents is irritating to esophagus and causes breakdown of mucosal barrier, leading to inflammation and erosion
4. Healing of esophageal erosion involves substitution of columnar epithelium (Barrett's epithelium) for normal squamous epithelium in lower esophagus
5. Barrett's epithelium resists acid (and thus supports healing) but is a premalignant tissue associated with an increased incidence of esophageal cancer
6. Occurs at any age but increases in individuals over age 50; availability of over-the-counter (OTC) H_2 receptor antagonists have decreased reporting of mild cases

B. Nursing assessment

1. Heartburn or substernal burning pain is most common symptom and is exacerbated by bending over, recumbent position, or straining

Box 60–2

Factors Decreasing Lower Esophageal Sphincter (LES) Tone

- Nicotine
- Caffeine (coffee, tea, cola)
- Chocolate
- Fatty foods
- Alcohol
- Peppermint, spearmint
- High levels of estrogen and progesterone
- Anticholinergic drugs
- Beta-adrenergic blockers
- Calcium channel blockers
- Nitrates
- Theophylline
- Diazepam
- Tight, restrictive clothing
- Bending, straining
- Hiatal hernia

2. Other clinical manifestations include regurgitation not associated with vomiting or nausea; bad or sour taste upon awakening; coughing, hoarseness, or wheezing at night; belching, and flatulence
3. Adult onset asthma is most often caused by GERD
4. Chronic GERD may cause dysphagia, indicating possible stricture or cancer
5. Diagnosis is most accurate through 24-hour pH monitoring
6. Esophagoscopy may be necessary in long-standing GERD to rule out malignancy

C. Therapeutic management

! 1. Avoid foods and medication that reduce LES tone (see Box 60–2)
! 2. Do not eat within 2 hours of bedtime or assume a recumbent position after eating
3. Avoid restrictive clothing that increases intra-abdominal pressure
! 4. Avoid large meals; eat smaller meals more frequently (such as 6 small meals per day)
! 5. Elevate head of bed for sleeping
6. Stop smoking
7. Medication and pharmacological intervention
   a. Antacids neutralize stomach acid and are used to treat mild to moderate symptoms
   b. H_2 receptor antagonists such as ranitidine (Zantac), famotidine (Pepcid), nizatidine (Axid), and cimetidine (Tagamet) are available by prescription or OTC and are advertised to public for treatment of GERD symptoms
   c. Proton pump inhibitors: omeprazole (Prilosec), lansoprazole (Prevacid), esomeprazole (Nexium), pantoprazole (Protonix), and rabeprazole (AcipHex)

D. Client teaching

1. Reinforce importance of smoking cessation and avoidance of caffeine
2. Avoid bending over, especially after eating
3. Take medications as prescribed
4. Lose weight if overweight to decrease intra-abdominal pressure
5. Raise head of bed by using concrete or wooden blocks to reduce nighttime reflux

VI. HERNIAS

A. Diaphragmatic hernia in children

1. Overview
   a. A **hernia** is a protrusion of bowel through an abnormal opening in abdominal wall
   b. Congenital diaphragmatic hernia (CDH) is rare and results when abdominal contents protrude into thoracic cavity through an opening in diaphragm
   c. CDH occurs when there is failure of transverse septum and pleuroperitoneal folds to completely develop and form the diaphragm
   d. Intestines and other abdominal structures enter thoracic cavity
   e. Lung growth may cease; after birth, respiration becomes further compromised by pulmonary hypoplasia and lung compression, including airways and blood vessels
2. Nursing assessment
   a. Clinical findings depend on severity of defect
   b. Fetal ultrasound shows abdominal organs in chest
   c. Postnatal diagnosis is confirmed by chest x-ray examination
   ! d. Diminished or absent breath sounds on affected side
   ! e. Bowel sounds may be heard over chest
   f. Cardiac sounds may be heard on right side of chest
   ! g. Dyspnea, cyanosis, nasal flaring, tachypnea, retractions
   h. Sunken abdomen, barrel-shaped chest
! 3. Preoperative therapeutic management
   a. Assess vital signs frequently with ongoing respiratory assessment
   b. Elevate head of bed and position on affected side
   c. Maintain patency of NG tube to decompress stomach
   d. Monitor IV fluids

e. Maintain mechanical ventilation, extracorporeal membrane oxygenator (ECMO), chest tubes
f. Provide minimal stimulation

4. Postoperative therapeutic management
a. Focuses on promoting lung function
b. Monitor for signs of infection and respiratory distress
c. Continue to support respirations by positioning in semi-Fowler's position on affected side; organize care to decrease exertion
d. Promote nutrition when feeding is resumed
e. Support family through crisis

5. Client and family teaching
a. Instruct parents on wound care, prevention of infection, and feeding techniques
b. Provide written and verbal information on growth and developmental needs
c. Provide information regarding long-term problems and necessity of regular follow-up visits

B. Hiatal hernia in adults

1. Overview
a. Diaphragmatic weakness through which a portion of stomach protrudes into thoracic cavity
b. Incidence may be as high as 40% of population but reaches 60% by the sixth decade of life; affects women more than men
c. Caused by congenital weakness of diaphragm, trauma, obesity, aging, increased intra-abdominal pressure, or a combination of these factors
d. Two major types: sliding hernia (90% of hernias), in which esophagogastric junction and portion of fundus move into thorax through esophageal hiatus; and rolling hernia (paraesophageal), in which only fundus and (less frequently) part of greater curvature roll into thorax

2. Nursing assessment
a. Most cases are asymptomatic
b. Symptoms include heartburn (pyrosis), substernal burning or pain, feeling of fullness, dysphagia, belching; these are usually worse when reclining
c. Diagnosed by upper GI series and symptom history

3. Therapeutic management
a. Conservative treatment: diet therapy and lifestyle modifications (same as discussed for GERD)
b. Avoid straining
c. Avoid excessive vigorous exercise
d. Sleep with head of bed elevated 8 to 12 inches
e. Assist client in decision making about surgical procedure (used only when conservative treatment has failed)
f. Nissen fundoplication (used for GERD as well) most common; fundus of stomach is wrapped 360 degrees around lower portion of esophagus
g. Hill repair: similar to Nissen repair but fundus is wrapped around esophagus only 180 degrees
h. Provide preoperative and postoperative care as discussed previously for client undergoing gastric surgery
i. Medication therapy: antacids and H_2 receptor antagonists (see treatment for GERD)

4. Client teaching
a. Report any increase in symptoms
b. Do not take antacids within 2 hours of other medications
c. Avoid alcohol, caffeine, NSAIDs, and any medication containing aspirin (such as Alka-Seltzer)
d. Reinforce diet and lifestyle modifications

C. Umbilical hernia

1. Overview
a. A soft, skin-covered protrusion of intestine and omentum (double fold of peritoneum) through a weakness in abdominal wall around umbilicus

b. In an umbilical hernia, incomplete closure of umbilical ring results in protrusion of portions of omentum and intestine through opening
c. Defect usually closes spontaneously by age 3 or 4 years; surgical correction is necessary if closure does not occur or if incarceration of herniated bowel occurs
d. Most common in low-birthweight infants or black infants and commonly occurs in children with Down syndrome, hypothyroidism, and Hurler syndrome

2. Nursing assessment
   a. Soft swelling or protrusion around umbilicus, usually reducible using a finger
   b. An incarcerated hernia is one that cannot be reduced and increases risk of bowel ischemia
   c. An incarcerated hernia produces such symptoms as irritability, tenderness at site, anorexia, abdominal distention, and difficult defecation
3. Therapeutic management
   a. Most umbilical hernias disappear spontaneously by 1 year of age
   b. No surgical repair is needed unless it causes symptoms, persists past 5 years of age, becomes strangulated, or continues to grow
   c. Binding is not effective in reducing or minimizing the protrusion
   d. Monitor for changes in size of hernia
   e. Assess for increased bowel sounds and irreducible mass, which may indicate strangulation
   f. Postoperatively, assess for wound infection, maintain hydration, assess and manage pain, allow for self-expression
4. Client and family education
   a. Signs of strangulation, such as vomiting, pain, and an irreducible mass at umbilicus; signs and symptoms of wound infection
   b. Avoid ineffective and potentially harmful home remedies such as "belly binders"
   c. Any precautions and restrictions, such as tub bathing or strenuous activity if surgery was performed

VII. PEPTIC ULCER DISEASE (PUD)

A. Overview

1. A generic term for ulcers or breaks in mucosal lining of GI tract that come in contact with gastric secretions; can occur in stomach (gastric ulcers, 15%), duodenum (duodenal ulcers, 80%), or rarely lower esophagus (esophageal ulcers)
2. Gastric ulcer
   a. Occurs most often on lesser curvature near pylorus
   b. Results from a disruption in normal protective mechanism that keeps gastric epithelial pH normal
   c. Prostaglandins in gastric mucosa increase resistance to acid; therefore, medications that reduce prostaglandins, (such as aspirin, NSAIDs, alcohol), will decrease gastric mucosal resistance
   d. Gastric ulcers are associated with *H. pylori,* gastritis, alcohol, smoking, use of NSAIDs, stress, and an increased incidence of gastric cancer
3. Duodenal ulcer
   a. A chronic break in duodenal mucosa to muscularis mucosae layer; is most common type of ulcer
   b. Results from increased gastric acid from increases in number of parietal cells, vagal activity, or secretion of gastrin
   c. Rarely associated with an increase in gastric cancer
   d. Associated with chronic *H. pylori* infection, alcohol, smoking, cirrhosis, and stress
4. Etiology and pathophysiology of PUD
   a. *H. pylori* is associated with 90% to 95% of clients with duodenal ulcers
   b. Chronic NSAID use (aspirin is worst) is associated with a fourfold increased risk for gastric ulcers
   c. Factors that increase risk for PUD include cigarette smoking, family history, blood group O (duodenal ulcer), alcohol use
   d. Incidence of ulcers increases steadily with age and peaks in sixth decade
   e. Men and women are affected equally

B. Nursing assessment

1. Pain: gnawing, burning, aching, hungerlike, in the epigastrium
2. Duodenal ulcers: pain relieved by eating
3. Gastric ulcers: pain not relieved by food and may be exacerbated by food
4. Upper GI series often done initially; diagnosis is made most conclusively by EGD
5. Tests for *H. pylori* usually positive
6. Observe for complications: perforation (pain, signs of peritonitis, shock), hemorrhage (hematemesis, tarry stool, stool positive for occult blood), or pyloric obstruction (vomiting, feeling of fullness)

C. Therapeutic management

1. Reinforce importance of following treatment plan in reducing symptoms
2. No foods have been determined to be ulcerogenic but some foods aggravate active PUD (coffee, cola, tea, chocolate, foods high in sodium, and spicy food), and they should be avoided during acute phase; even decaffeinated coffee stimulates gastrin release
3. Refer client to smoking cessation program
4. Medication therapy
   a. Antacids are used to neutralize acid
   b. H_2 receptor antagonists block histamine-stimulated gastric secretions; proton pump inhibitors suppress the production of hydrochloric acid
   c. Prostaglandin analogs: misoprostol (Cytotec) contributes to mucosal barrier preventing NSAID-induced ulcers
   d. Mucosal barrier fortifier: sucralfate (Carafate) forms protective barrier over ulcer crater and prevents further erosion by acid and pepsin
   e. Treatment for *H. pylori* changes frequently but generally includes antimicrobials such as metronidazole (Flagyl), proton pump inhibitors, and bismuth subsalicylate (Pepto-Bismol)

D. Client teaching

1. Take medications as prescribed
2. Learn signs of complications: blood in the stool, vomiting, increased pain
3. Follow diet recommendations restricting caffeine, alcohol, and nicotine

VIII. IRRITABLE BOWEL SYNDROME (IBS)

A. Overview

1. Common noninflammatory functional bowel disorder also known as spastic bowel, functional colitis, and mucous colitis; is a motility disorder of lower GI tract
2. Cause is unknown, but aggravating factors are stress, anxiety, depression, certain foods and food additives in some clients, drugs, toxins, and hormones
3. There is no change in physical characteristics of intestinal mucosa
4. Usually manifests in three patterns: predominantly diarrhea, predominantly constipation, or combination of diarrhea and constipation; each pattern may or may not include abdominal pain

B. Nursing assessment

1. Abdominal pain: relieved by defecation, intermittent and colicky, or continuous and dull
2. Change in bowel motility and character
   a. Diarrhea or constipation
   b. Presence of mucus
   c. Feeling of incomplete evacuation
   d. Possible bloating, flatulence, urgency
3. Diagnosis is made by excluding organic causes of clinical manifestations
4. Sigmoidoscopy may demonstrate spastic contractions that may be painful; mucosa is normal in appearance

C. Therapeutic management

1. Possibly tegaserod maleate (Zelnorm)
2. Dietary fiber 30 to 40 grams/daily may help in predominantly constipation type
3. Assist client to identify and eliminate foods that exacerbate problem

4. Common offenders: fruit, berries, lettuce, lactose, caffeinated drinks, preservatives (sodium sulfite), alcohol
5. Encourage a program of relaxation and stress reduction; regular exercise may help control symptoms
6. Medication therapy
   a. No standard pharmacologic treatment
   b. Bulk-forming agents (Metamucil, Fibercon) may help predominantly constipation-type IBS
   c. Antidiarrheal agents (Imodium, Lomotil) may be used for predominantly diarrhea-type IBS
   d. Antidepressants, anxiolytics, antispasmodics, or anticholinergics may be used

D. Client teaching

1. Provide information about fiber content of various foods
2. Follow prescribed regimen
3. Encourage bathroom privacy and a regular time for defecation
4. Provide information about programs of relaxation or support groups

IX. CHRONIC INFLAMMATORY BOWEL DISEASE (IBD)

A. Ulcerative colitis

1. Overview
   a. Area of chronic inflammation of mucosa and submucosa in colon and rectum
   b. Peak incidence is between 15 and 35 years of age with a second peak between age 50 and 70
   c. Characterized by periods of exacerbation and remission
   d. Cause is unknown but may be related to stress, genetics, infection, dietary factors (low fiber intake), or antibody formation
   e. Inflammation (at base of crypts of Lieberkuhn, usually in rectum) develops into abscesses that penetrate mucosa and spread laterally
   f. Begins in rectum and can progress proximally, but is usually limited to sigmoid colon and rectum
   g. Can range in severity from mild to severe
2. Nursing assessment
   a. Diarrhea; 10 to 20 liquid stools per day often containing blood and sometimes mucus; nocturnal diarrhea is common
   b. May complain of fatigue resulting from blood loss, lack of sleep, and/or fluid imbalance
   c. May affect quality of life; client may be afraid to leave house because of severe diarrhea
   d. Complications include hemorrhage, abscess formation, toxic megacolon, malabsorption, bowel obstruction, bowel perforation, increased risk of colon cancer, and extraintestinal symptoms (arthritis, uveitis)
   e. Diagnosed by sigmoidoscopy: characteristic edematous, friable mucosa with a granular appearance with evident crypt abscesses; lesions are contiguous
3. Therapeutic management
   a. Provide standard pre- and postsigmoidoscopy or colonoscopy care
   b. Rest is required to decrease intestinal activity
   c. Diet therapy may include a low-residue, high-protein, high-calorie diet with vitamins and iron; in severe cases, nothing by mouth to rest the bowel; TPN will be ordered in severe cases
   d. Surgery (proctocolectomy with colostomy or ileostomy) may be necessary if IBD not controlled by medical means
   e. Encourage client to talk about concerns related to disease process and its effect on lifestyle
   f. Medication therapy: corticosteroids during exacerbations to decrease bowel inflammation; salicylate compounds (sulfasalazine [Azulfidine], mesalamine [Asocol, Pentasa]) to decrease prostaglandin formation and bowel inflammation; immunomodulators such as azathioprine (Imuran) to alter immune response; antidiarrheals to provide symptom management

4. Client teaching
   a. Take medications as ordered
   b. Avoid foods that exacerbate symptoms: raw vegetables, raw fruits, whole-grain breads and cereals, seeds, nuts, popcorn, and any highly spiced or flavorful food
   c. Notify health care provider if symptoms increase or there is blood in stool
   d. Provide information about ulcerative colitis support groups
   e. Teach client importance of good perianal skin care to prevent complications
   f. Educate client about exacerbation and remission nature of the disease and symptom management
   g. Instruct postoperative client in stoma and incision care as described in earlier section

B. Crohn's disease (regional enteritis)

1. Overview
   a. Chronic inflammation of GI mucosa occurring anywhere from mouth to anus but most often in terminal ileum
   b. Characterized by exacerbations and remissions
   c. Cause is unknown, but possible factors are autoimmune, genetics, infectious agents, and environmental (stress)
   d. Lesions extend to all thicknesses of bowel wall and are prone to fistula formation
   e. Lesions have a "cobblestone appearance" with sections of normal mucosa between lesions called "skip" lesions
   f. Over time, chronic inflammation causes fibrotic changes in bowel wall, leading to obstruction
   g. Depending on severity and location of lesions, malabsorption may occur as well as losses of protein from lesions themselves
2. Nursing assessment
   a. Diarrhea (5 to 6 liquid to semiformed stools/day) is most common symptom (usually without blood); depending on location, steatorrhea (fatty stool) may occur
   b. Abdominal pain in RLQ that is unrelieved by defecation
   c. Systemic manifestations include fever, fatigue, malaise, weight loss
   d. Complications include abscess and fistula formation, intestinal obstruction, malnutrition, and bowel perforation; hemorrhage is uncommon
   e. Barium enema and upper GI series often show areas of ulceration, narrowing, strictures, and fistulas; upper GI tract shows classic "string sign" of terminal ileum
   f. Diagnosed by colonoscopy; characteristic aphthoid ulcers, strictures, and segmental involvement is visualized; lesion is biopsied
   g. Laboratory tests (serum albumin, folic acid, hemoglobin, and hematocrit) assess for complications and rule out other causes of diarrhea
3. Therapeutic management
   a. Provide prescribed diet: usually high-calorie, high-protein; involve client in making appropriate menu choices
   b. Encourage intake of prescribed nutritional supplements
   c. Weigh daily, maintain calorie count, and monitor I & O
   d. Allow client to express fears and anxiety about course of illness and possibility of surgical intervention (not as common as for ulcerative colitis because it is not necessarily curative)
   e. Medications are same as for ulcerative colitis (antidiarrheals, salicylate-containing compounds, corticosteroids, immunomodulators)
   f. Metronidazole (Flagyl), a broad-spectrum antimicrobial, may also be given
   g. Antispasmodics decrease abdominal cramping following eating
   h. TPN may be ordered during periods of severe exacerbation to provide total bowel rest
4. Client teaching
   a. Reinforce information about disease process, prescribed medications, and dietary needs

b. Teach client and family signs and symptoms of complications: increased pain, rectal bleeding, fever, chills, lethargy
c. If TPN is ordered, teach client and family about proper catheter care and administration techniques (see also Chapter 34)
d. Encourage intake of nutritional supplements, such as Ensure for optimum nutrition

X. DIVERTICULITIS

A. Overview

1. Inflammation of diverticula, which are outpouchings in intestinal wall (diverticulosis is presence of multiple diverticula)
2. Majority of diverticula occur in sigmoid colon (90% to 95%); incidence increases with age
3. Caused by increased pressure in intestinal lumen and herniation of mucosa through defects in bowel wall; decreased fecal bulk (low-fiber diet) contribute to bowel wall hypertrophy and result in increased intraluminal pressure
4. Diverticula become inflamed when undigested food or bacteria are trapped; abscess formation contributes to disease and diverticulum may rupture

B. Nursing assessment

! 1. Pain, usually in LLQ, ranging in severity from mild to severe and can be constant or cramping; if perforation occurs, abdominal pain is generalized
! 2. Most cases of diverticular disease are asymptomatic
! 3. May note constipation alternating with increased frequency bowel elimination pattern
! 4. Fever, chills, and tachycardia along with generalized abdominal pain may indicate perforation of diverticulum and onset of peritonitis
5. Diverticular disease is diagnosed with barium enema; however, this is contraindicated when diverticulitis is present because of risk of rupturing diverticulum when barium is instilled
6. CT scan or ultrasonography can diagnose acute diverticulitis

C. Therapeutic management

! 1. Reinforce dietary modifications to reduce complications of diverticulosis
   a. High-fiber diet after acute phase
   b. Bowel rest: NPO or low-residue diet during initial acute phase
   c. Addition of bran to everyday foods
   d. Common advice is to avoid intake of seeds and foods with small seeds such as berries and figs
2. Assess for signs of bleeding: check stool for occult blood
3. Prepare for possible surgical intervention; colon resection is done in 25% of cases of diverticulitis
! 4. Medication therapy includes antibiotics to decrease bowel flora and reduce infection, opioid analgesics to relieve pain, and stool softeners, although laxatives and enemas are contraindicated

D. Client teaching: fiber content of various foods, self-administration and side effects of medications, signs and symptoms of complications of diverticulitis

XI. INTESTINAL OBSTRUCTION

A. Overview

1. Failure of bowel contents to move forward; can be partial or complete
2. Mechanical obstruction results from forces outside of intestines, (adhesions, hernia, fibrosis); or blockage in lumen (fecal impaction, edema, tumor, stricture, volvulus, intussusception)
3. Nonmechanical obstruction or paralytic ileus results from impairment of muscle tone or nervous system innervation preventing forward movement of intestinal contents (anesthesia, abdominal surgery, spinal injuries, peritonitis, vascular insufficiency)
4. Obstructions occur most often in ileum where intestinal diameter is smallest

5. Peristalsis increases in intestine above blockage, leading to increased secretions, edema, and increased capillary permeability and resulting in fluid and electrolyte imbalances and hypovolemia

B. Nursing assessment

1. Early in bowel obstruction, bowel sounds may be high-pitched and tinkling proximal to obstruction and hypoactive or silent distal to obstruction
2. Late in bowel obstruction bowel sounds become absent
3. Abdominal pain can be colicky and increase in intensity as obstruction progresses
4. Vomiting is common and may have a fecal odor
5. Abdominal distension is common, and peristalsis may be visible in early stages of obstruction
6. Vital signs may be normal in early obstruction but client can demonstrate signs of shock as obstruction progresses (tachycardia, fever, tachypnea, hypotension)
7. Diagnosed by history, physical findings, and abdominal x-ray; dilated loops of bowel can be seen (barium studies are contraindicated)

C. Therapeutic management

1. Prepare client for possibility of surgery: exploratory laparotomy, colon resection, colostomy
2. Prepare client for insertion of nasogastric or nasointestinal tube
3. Provide mouth care to minimize effect of fecal-type secretions
4. Provide IV therapy as prescribed
5. Maintain NPO status until peristalsis returns
6. Provide comfort measures such as frequent position changes
7. Monitor vital signs including I & O; early detection of hypovolemic shock can prevent complications (bowel ischemia and necrosis)
8. Monitor level of pain; sudden change in nature of pain may indicate complications (ischemia and necrosis)
9. Monitor progression and drainage from intestinal tube
10. Medication therapy
    a. Analgesic medication is generally limited because opioid analgesics decrease GI motility which further compromise bowel; meperidine (Demerol) may be given in small amounts but is now controversial because of toxic metabolic (normeperidine)
    b. IV fluid with appropriate electrolyte replacement prevents hypovolemia and shock

D. Client teaching

1. Instruct client about insertion and maintenance of NG tube or intestinal tube
2. Reinforce instructions for postoperative use of incentive spirometer, coughing and deep breathing exercises, ambulation, activity, and wound care
3. Provide support to client and family in coping with possibility of a colostomy
4. Stress importance of maintaining a healthy lifestyle on discharge

XII. JAUNDICE

A. Overview

1. Yellow-orange discoloration of skin and mucous membranes; caused by a disturbance of bilirubin metabolism causing ***hyperbilirubinemia*** (serum bilirubin greater than 2.5 mg/dL); also known as icterus
2. Associated with diffuse hepatocellular disorders or present in newborns because of impaired bilirubin uptake and conjugation
3. Hyperbilirubinemia and jaundice can result from hemolysis or from disorders of bile ducts (obstruction) or liver cells
4. Caused by accumulation of bilirubin pigments in skin and can be classified as obstructive or hemolytic
5. Obstructive jaundice is classified as extrahepatic (gallstones or tumor, with increased direct bilirubin) or intrahepatic (drug reactions or hepatitis, with increased indirect bilirubin)

6. Hemolytic jaundice is caused by excessive breakdown of red blood cells (RBCs)
   a. Amount of bilirubin produced exceeds liver's ability to conjugate it, so level of unconjugated or indirect bilirubin in serum increases
   b. Unconjugated bilirubin is insoluble in water and is not found in urine; causes include blood transfusion reactions, membrane defects of RBCs, severe infection, or toxic substances

B. Nursing assessment

1. Recent appetite and color of urine and stool
2. Abdominal swelling, pain in the RUQ, and presence of hepatomegaly
3. Yellowish discoloration of skin and mucous membranes
4. Scleral icterus (yellowish discoloration of sclera)
5. Pruritus (severe itching) secondary to accumulation of bilirubin in skin
6. Elevation of conjugated bilirubin that causes urine to be dark (tea- or cola-colored); may be present before jaundice appears
7. Complete obstruction of flow of bile into duodenum causes light or clay-colored stools
8. Jaundice caused by an infectious process may be accompanied by fever and chills
9. Any client with liver dysfunction or injury may complain of nausea, anorexia, and/or fatigue
10. Laboratory findings (see also Chapter 47)
    a. Increased indirect bilirubin: hepatocellular failure, hemolytic jaundice
    b. Increased direct bilirubin: obstructive causes of jaundice
    c. An elevated level of bilirubin in the urine is always caused by an increased level of direct bilirubin (it is water-soluble, and indirect bilirubin is not)
    d. Alanine aminotransferase (ALT): elevation indicates damage to liver cells and helps rule out hemolysis as cause of jaundice
    e. Aspartate aminotransferase (AST): elevated, but levels vary depending on type of jaundice; with hepatitis, levels can be elevated 20 times above normal, gallstones can cause levels 10 times above normal
    f. ALT and AST ratios; used to help diagnose causes of liver dysfunction
    g. Alkaline phosphatase (ALP): increased with both extrahepatic and intrahepatic biliary obstruction
    h. Radiologic procedures can help confirm infiltrative or cholestatic processes; abdominal ultrasound and CT scans can detect tumors, stones, and other focal liver lesions that may be causing jaundice

C. Therapeutic management

1. Aimed at symptom management and includes keeping client comfortable
2. Often clients are kept NPO pending diagnostic testing and because food increases pain secondary to stimulation of GI tract
3. IV hydration and pain management are important aspects of care
4. Management is aimed at treating cause of jaundice
5. Cool or tepid baths containing colloidal substances (oatmeal, cornstarch, soybean powder) can reduce or ease pruritus
6. Cool room (68–70°F) with 30% to 40% humidity
7. Use an emollient lotion rather than one containing alcohol, which is too drying
8. Medication therapy: there is no specific medication therapy for jaundice
   a. Topical corticosteroids may provide some relief
   b. Bile-sequestering agents remove excess bile from the fat deposits under skin, decreasing pruritus

D. Client teaching

1. Educate client about required diagnostic tests
2. Once cause of jaundice is determined, educate client about disease process and future management
3. Causes of jaundice are usually correctable
4. Advise client with liver problems to avoid alcohol and acetaminophen, since both can cause further liver damage

XIII. HEPATITIS

A. Overview

1. An inflammation of liver; ranges greatly in severity and can be caused by several different viruses, toxins, or disease states
2. Hepatitis viruses cause local necrosis of parenchymal cells of liver; inflammatory response leads to swelling and blockage of liver's drainage system
3. Hepatitis occurs in varying levels of severity from asymptomatic or mild cases, in which the liver cells regenerate completely in 2 to 3 months, to more severe forms, in which hepatic necrosis and death may occur in 1 to 2 weeks
4. Hepatitis A
   a. Transmitted via GI tract (oral–fecal route), particularly in overcrowded and unsanitary conditions, and is vaccine preventable
   b. Sources include contaminated food, water, and shellfish; may also be contracted from contact with infected persons
   c. Incubation period is 15 to 50 days
   d. Highly contagious and easily spread throughout households and daycare centers
   e. Client is most contagious 10 to 14 days prior to onset of symptoms when fecal shedding of virus is greatest
   f. Is usually self-limiting
5. Hepatitis B
   a. Blood-borne, vaccine-preventable disease
   b. Transmitted through exchange of blood or body fluids; risk increases in heterosexuals with multiple sex partners, homosexual males, and IV drug users; health care workers comprise about 3% of all reported cases
   c. Transmitted also through contaminated blood or blood products or sharing of needles with persons infected with virus; clients who require hemodialysis are also at risk
   d. Incubation period is 30 to 160 days
   e. Can progress to a chronic form of disease; is a common cause of cirrhosis and hepatocellular carcinoma
6. Hepatitis C, also called posttransfusion hepatitis, is spread by blood and body fluids; most common cause of chronic hepatitis
   a. Previously known as non-A non-B
   b. Blood transfusions, sexual contact, sharing contaminated needles, and unintentional needlesticks account for a significant number of cases
   c. Up to 80% of clients develop chronic hepatitis, which is a risk factor for liver failure and hepatocellular carcinoma
   d. Incubation period is between 2 and 20 weeks postexposure
7. Hepatitis D
   a. Known as Delta-agent hepatitis, is transmitted by percutaneous route and occurs only in people infected with hepatitis B (depends upon HBV virus to replicate)
   b. Incubation period is 3 to 24 weeks
   c. Transmitted parenterally; there is a question of whether it can be transmitted via blood and body fluids
8. Hepatitis E is believed to be transmitted by the fecal–oral route, such as by infected water supply; uncommon in United States; incubation period is between 2 and 9 weeks
9. Acute fulminating hepatitis: bleeding problems, hepatic encephalopathy, ascites, acute liver failure, death; this complication is seen infrequently but quickly leads to liver decompensation that can result in death within a week

B. Nursing assessment

! 1. A range of symptoms occurs, including anorexia, nausea, vomiting, malaise, fever, jaundice, and abdominal pain secondary to liver swelling; client may show signs of dehydration if vomiting is severe

! 2. Course of acute viral hepatitis is divided into three phases
   a. Prodromal (preicteric) phase (most contagious) occurs before jaundice appears, about 2 weeks after exposure to virus, and includes flulike symptoms

(general malaise, GI complaints such as nausea, vomiting, diarrhea, and anorexia), headache, fatigue, myalgia, joint pain, and low-grade fever; food odors, smoking, or alcohol may trigger nausea

b. **Icteric** phase is marked by onset of jaundice; occurs about 2 weeks after prodromal phase and lasts 2 to 6 weeks; includes dark-colored urine and clay-colored stools prior to appearance of jaundice and pruritis; liver remains enlarged and may be tender to touch

c. Recovery (posticteric) phase begins with resolution of jaundice and lasts several weeks, during which symptoms improve, energy levels increase, and serum enzymes normalize

3. Acute infection with hepatitis C is generally asymptomatic, although 25% to 35% of clients develop malaise, weakness, and anorexia
4. Diagnostic and laboratory test findings
   a. Antibodies to specific virus (anti-HAV, HBsAg, HBsAb; HBcAg; HBcAb; anti-HCV, anti-HDV) may be found in blood from onset of symptoms, and some may persist indefinitely
   b. Alkaline phosphatase (ALP); nonspecific test to evaluate liver or bone dysfunction; can be elevated with hepatitis
   c. Gamma-glutamyl transferase (GGT); acutely elevated with alcohol consumption and hepatotoxic drugs
   d. Transaminases: ALT and AST; elevated to varying degrees with hepatitis caused by hepatocyte injury
   e. Bilirubin; both direct and indirect levels can be elevated secondary to liver cell injury
   f. Prothrombin time (PT); prolonged if liver is injured to point that it can no longer produce proteins necessary for blood coagulation

C. Therapeutic management

1. Includes both pre- and postexposure prophylaxis as well as symptom management
   a. With cases of hepatitis A, controlling spread of infection is a major nursing focus; includes reporting to local public health department; exposed individuals should receive immune globulin as soon as possible; those at risk should receive vaccine
   b. With cases of hepatitis B, prevention is major health focus; hepatitis B vaccines are begun during neonatal period and are recommended for all infants as part of well-child care
2. Use standard precautions and meticulous handwashing for all forms, but especially for hepatitis A (client, family, and staff)
3. Hepatitis A precautions include private bathroom and proper bagging, cleansing, and disposal of contaminated items
4. Provide antiemetic medications as ordered and encourage a diet high in CHO and low in fat
5. Abstinence from alcohol is essential
6. If liver function is compromised, protein and salt should be restricted
7. Encourage a good breakfast; clients tend to become more nauseous later in day
8. Initiate intravenous (IV) fluids as ordered
9. Assess for signs of dehydration and monitor electrolyte status
10. Encourage bedrest initially and very gradual increase of activity as tolerated
11. Plan nursing activities to allow for adequate rest
12. Inform clients they may never donate blood
13. Observe for blood in stool or urine, multiple ecchymosis, petechiae, or oozing of blood from gums or minor cuts, which may indicate a complication
14. Medication therapy
    a. Aimed at symptom relief; consists of antiemetics and analgesics; because most analgesics are metabolized in liver, their use must be limited
    b. IV fluids may be necessary if client is unable to tolerate oral fluids
    c. Prophylaxis may be considered if client has known HAV exposure and is early in incubation period

d. Vaccination for hepatitis B is available; given as a series of 3 intramuscular injections to adults, children, and infants; second and third injections are given at 1 and 6 months after initial injection; efficacy of vaccination approaches 95%
e. Postexposure vaccination for hepatitis B is recommended for clients in contact with infected blood or body fluids, those who have sexual contact with infected individuals, and infants exposed to a caregiver with known HBV infection or born to a mother with known HBsAg
f. Hepatitis C: combination therapy is used for 12 to 18 weeks or as long as 48 weeks with interferon alfa-2b and ribavirin therapy
g. Hepatitis D: there are no medications specific to treatment of HDV
h. Vitamin K is indicated if PT is prolonged
i. Antihistamines can be given for pruritis

D. Client teaching

1. Hepatitis A and E: detailed information about disease and prevention of transmission; meticulous handwashing must be used, and client must avoid sharing eating utensils, bath towels, and other personal care items that are in contact with body fluids
2. Educate client about safe sex practices as a general health measure (hepatitis B, C, D)
3. Avoid alcohol and any drugs that may be hepatotoxic (such as acetaminophen)
4. Instruct client about possibility of developing chronic active hepatitis and importance of follow-up
5. Reinforce use of vaccination and prevention of disease transmission according to type

XIV. CIRRHOSIS

A. Overview

1. Irreversible and chronic liver disease characterized by diffuse inflammation and fibrosis of liver tissue, which cause scarring and obstruction of hepatic blood flow
2. Three classifications: Laënnec's, biliary, and postnecrotic
   a. Laënnec's cirrhosis, also called alcoholic cirrhosis, is most prevalent type and is caused by prolonged, excessive alcohol intake with or without malnutrition; is directly related to toxic effects of alcohol on liver
   b. Biliary cirrhosis is caused by obstruction of bile canaliculi and ducts and results in necrosis and fibrosis; cause can be autoimmune or result tumors, gallstones, or chronic pancreatitis
   c. Postnecrotic cirrhosis results from a chronic, severe liver disease such as hepatitis; it is also caused by inherited metabolic liver disorders such as Wilson's disease
3. Regardless of cause, cirrhosis develops slowly; severity and rate of progression depend on cause and repeated injury to hepatocytes
4. Disruption of portal blood flow secondary to structural changes in liver results in edema, ascites, splenomegaly (caused by splanchnic venous congestion), portal hypertension (see next section), hemorrhoids, varicose veins, and esophageal varices (see section that follows)

B. Nursing assessment

1. See Box 60–3
2. Vital signs: orthostatic measurement of BP and pulse, temperature and weight
3. Nutritional status: muscle atrophy and wasting
4. Decreased ability to metabolize CHOs leads to hypoglycemia, decreased energy, and alterations in glycogenolysis, glyconeogenesis, and glycogenesis
5. Altered fat metabolism causes increased synthesis of fatty acids and triglycerides leading to fatty liver and hepatomegaly
6. Altered protein metabolism leads to low albumin levels and, with decrease in osmotic pressure and development of edema and ascites; decreased protein also decreases production of clotting factors, which increases risk of bleeding

Box 60-3

Signs and Symptoms of Cirrhosis

- General malaise
- Skin
  - Pruritis
  - Jaundice and scleral icterus
  - Spider angiomata and telangiectasia
  - Ecchymoses, petechiae, hematomas, and propensity for bleeding
  - Edema
- Gastrointestinal
  - Nausea and vomiting
  - Anorexia, weight loss/malnutrition
  - Pyrosis
  - Clay-colored stools
  - Constipation
  - Flatulence, hemorrhoids
- Abdomen
  - Change in bowel sounds
  - Pain or tenderness in RUQ
  - Hepatomegaly, splenomegaly
  - Ascites (increasing abdominal girth)
  - Abdominal pain (RUQ)
  - Positive fluid wave
  - Shifting dullness
  - Caput medusa
- Neurological
  - Fatigue
  - Disorientation
  - Decreased level of consciousness
  - Encephalopathy
  - Asterixis (flapping tremor of hand from increased ammonia levels)
  - Decreased deep-tendon reflexes (DTRs)
- Pulmonary
  - Decreased breath sounds in bases (may indicate pleural effusion)
  - Crackles (might indicate development of heart failure)
- Reproductive
  - Gynecomastia
  - Testicular atrophy
  - Erectile dysfunction
  - Menstrual irregularities
- Palmar erythema
- Anemia
- Loss of body hair
- Dark urine

7. Decreased metabolism of sex steroids (estrogen, progesterone, and testosterone) leads to gynecomastia, loss of body hair, development of palmar erythema and spider angiomata, erectile dysfunction, and menstrual disorders
8. Decreased metabolism of aldosterone results in sodium and water retention and worsens edema and **ascites**
9. ! Decreased metabolism of ammonia leads to increased serum ammonia levels and hepatic encephalopathy (manifests as lack of coordination, decreased memory, lack of orientation, and coma)
10. Decreased stores of vitamins and minerals leads to malnutrition, fatigue, and anemia
11. Obstruction of bile flow leads to hyperbilirubinemia and jaundice, clay-colored stools, dark-colored urine
12. Splenomegaly leads to pancytopenia
13. Fibrosis and scarring continue, resulting in increased portal pressure that causes ascites, hemorrhoids, esophageal varices, caput medusa (superficial abdominal veins)
14. ! Involuntary tremor or flapping of the hands is called liver flap or **asterixis**
15. ! Liver biopsy is only definitive way to diagnose type of cirrhosis; may not be necessary if client has clinical manifestations with supportive risk factors; may not be advisable because prolonged PT would place client at increased risk for bleeding; see also Chapter 48
16. No laboratory tests will diagnose cirrhosis, but ordered tests are similar to those discussed for hepatitis

17. Findings include varying degrees of increased transaminases, decreased albumin, prolonged PT, hyperbilirubinemia, hyponatremia from excess-free water, hypokalemia from diuretic therapy, and hypomagnesemia.
18. Complete blood count (CBC) reflects pancytopenia (anemia, thrombocytopenia, leukopenia)
19. Elevated serum ammonia level
20. Liver ultrasound may reveal an enlarged fibrofatty liver or a small fibrotic and nodular liver; highly dense areas may reflect possible hepatocellular carcinoma

C. Therapeutic management

1. Abdominal **paracentesis** for only severe ascites; is an invasive procedure that drains fluid from abdomen via a needle; fluid is often sent for culture
2. Surgical intervention to relieve portal hypertension and prevent reaccumulation of ascitic fluid: insertion of a LeVeen shunt or transjugular intrahepatic portosystemic shunt (TIPS)
3. Fluid-restriction to prevent further accumulation of ascitic fluid
4. Diet restrictions include low sodium intake to prevent further ascitic fluid accumulation and decreased protein intake
5. Provide small, frequent meals
6. Weigh daily, and monitor I & O
7. Measure abdominal girth each day or shift as ordered to monitor ascites
8. For respiratory support, use high Fowler's position and use supplemental O_2 as ordered; encourage deep-breathing; allow activity as tolerated; measure O_2 saturation and ABGs as ordered
9. Maintain skin integrity; remove moist linens promptly; keep skin clean and moistened with emollient; administer antihistamines as ordered; encourage activity as tolerated, or reposition every 2 hours
10. Institute bleeding precautions as needed: prevent constipation, avoid injections, observe for signs of bleeding, encourage use of soft toothbrush, monitor labs (CBC, PT)
11. Assess understanding of illness; identify support system; assess coping skills; offer clergy support; encourage Alcoholics Anonymous for those with cirrhosis secondary to alcohol dependence; provide substance abuse consultation as indicated
12. Medication therapy
    a. Diuretics are given cautiously to promote excretion of excess fluid to decrease ascites; most commonly used drugs are spironolactone (Aldactone), a potassium-sparing diuretic, and furosemide (Lasix), a loop diuretic
    b. Lactulose (Cephulac) is a disaccharide laxative that is not absorbed by GI tract; it pulls water into bowel and helps to decrease absorption of ammonia
    c. Other medications include vitamin K to treat prolonged PT, antihistamines, and antiemetics

D. Client teaching

1. Lifestyle changes include dietary restrictions, abstinence from alcohol, fluid restrictions; suggest nutrition consultation
2. Reduce intake of foods high in sodium; avoid canned and frozen foods, highly processed cheeses, potato chips, and other salty foods
3. Limit intake of foods high in protein: eggs, cheese, milk, and meats
4. Avoid taking any OTC medications without checking with health care provider first because many medications are hepatotoxic (such as acetaminophen)
5. Signs and symptoms that require medical attention after discharge: weight gain, increased abdominal girth, respiratory distress, bleeding gums, blood in the stool or urine, fever, abdominal pain
6. How to adjust dose of lactulose according to number of loose stools per day (usually three)
7. Involve family and other support persons in client's care

E. Complications of cirrhosis

1. **Portal hypertension**
    a. An abnormally high BP within portal venous system; most commonly caused by cirrhosis but also caused by hepatitis or infection, hepatic vein thrombus,

tumor, or right heart failure (any condition that impedes blood flow through portal venous system or vena cava)

b. Clinical manifestations include all findings described with cirrhosis

c. Other potentially fatal conditions that can develop as a result of portal hypertension are varices, ascites, hepatic encephalopathy leading to coma, and hepatorenal syndrome (see discussion of these conditions later in chapter)

! **d.** Most common clinical manifestation is vomiting of blood (**hematemesis**) secondary to rupture of esophageal varices; clients with oozing varices may present with anemia and melanotic stools

e. Splenomegaly can result from increased pressure within splenic vein, which branches off portal vein

f. Clients may complain of irritation from hemorrhoids or may present with bright red rectal bleeding secondary to hemorrhoids

g. Therapeutic management is same as treatment of cirrhosis and is based on symptomatic treatment of varices, ascites, encephalopathy, and hepatorenal syndrome

! **h.** Medication therapy: aimed at decreasing portal venous pressure without precipitating hypotensive crisis; diuretics and fluid restriction are treatments of choice; propranolol (Inderal), a beta-blocker, has also been used to decrease portal venous pressures

2. Esophageal varices

a. Develop from increased portal pressure; are distended and tortuous vessels that can rupture secondary to coughing, sneezing, vomiting, or ingestion of foods high in roughage; bleeding can be abrupt and painless with mortality reaching 50%; ruptured esophageal varices are considered a medical emergency

! **b.** Clinical manifestations: if bleeding is slow, melena and decreasing hemoglobin and hematocrit are present, but if bleeding is abrupt, severe hematemesis and signs of hypovolemic shock (tachycardia, hypotension) can occur

! **c.** Therapeutic management: includes stopping bleeding either by **sclerotherapy** or **esophageal tamponade,** which is direct pressure by use of Sengstaken-Blakemore or Minnesota tube with esophageal and gastric balloons; keep scissors at bedside to cut tube if tube position changes and airway is compromised; see also Chapter 28

! **d.** Sclerotherapy and banding are accomplished via endoscopy; physician locates bleeding vessel via endoscope and injects a sclerosing agent (causes thrombosis and hemostasis); may be done emergently or as an elective procedure

e. Maintain airway, breathing, and circulation and measure VS

f. Start two large-bore IVs with infusion of normal saline (NS) as ordered

g. Draw serum laboratory tests (CBC, type and cross-match, chemistries)

h. Begin gastric **lavage** if ordered

i. Keep clients NPO for both sclerotherapy and esophageal tamponade (if elective); explain procedure and give a mild pre-procedure sedative as ordered

j. Prepare client for transfer to a setting with cardiac monitoring capability

! **k.** Administer vasopressin via IV intermittent or continuous infusion, usually given once a cardiac monitor is in place; lowers portal pressure and controls bleeding by causing splanchnic vasoconstriction; use with caution in clients with cardiac disease

l. Administer propranolol (Inderal), a beta-blocker that reduces portal pressure, or sandostatin (Octreotide), which decreases splanchnic blood flow and subsequent bleeding from esophageal varices

3. Ascites

a. Accumulation of plasma-rich fluid within peritoneal cavity secondary to portal hypertension, increased aldosterone, and decreased oncotic pressure (**hypoalbuminemia**); cirrhosis is common cause; kidneys retain sodium and thus water, further increasing third-spaced fluid and anasarca (generalized body edema)

! **b.** Clinical manifestations: abdominal distention, weight gain, increased abdominal girth, dilated abdominal veins (caput medusa), generalized edema, and respiratory distress if accumulation of ascitic fluid is large

c. Therapeutic management includes paracentesis to remove fluid; diuretics; shunting devices (to treat portal hypertension)
d. Monitor fluid and electrolyte status; give fluids as ordered
e. Monitor daily weights and measure abdominal girth every 8 to 24 hrs
f. Restrict intake of dietary protein and sodium
g. Provide education about disease process and diagnostic tests
h. Assess for respiratory distress from upward pressure on diaphraghm; monitor vital signs for hypotension and/or tachycardia

4. **Hepatic encephalopathy**
a. A neurological complication caused by accumulation of toxic substances (primarily ammonia) in blood
b. Clinical manifestations: loss of memory, irritability, confusion, lethargy, sleep disturbances, stupor, coma, and asterixis
c. Therapeutic management: aimed at reducing production of nitrogenous wastes (urea) and ammonia, correcting fluid and electrolyte imbalances, and eliminating use of sedating drugs and drugs metabolized by liver
d. Perform frequent neurologic assessment to note progression of lethargy
e. Restrict dietary protein
f. Avoid sedating medications
g. Monitor for fluid and electrolyte imbalances and implement prescribed corrective measures
h. Treat cause of liver disease by implementing ordered therapies
i. Administer lactulose (Cephulac) as ordered, a hyperosmolar laxative that prevents absorption of ammonia and produces diarrhea
j. Neomycin is sometimes used to reduce bacteria in bowel, thus limiting further ammonia production; use with caution because of nephrotoxicity

5. **Hepatorenal syndrome**
a. Renal failure associated with advanced liver failure and caused by circulatory alterations without primary renal disease; most commonly found in Laënnec's cirrhosis and fulminant hepatitis; results in sudden renal failure possibly from diuretics, characterized by intrarenal vasoconstriction, oliguria, azotemia, anorexia, and fatigue; is associated with a poor prognosis
b. Clinical manifestations include decreased urine output (UO), hyponatremia, decreased urine osmolality, hypotension, jaundice, ascites, possible GI bleeding, increased BUN and creatinine
c. Treat fluid and electrolyte imbalances and encephalopathy with aim of restoring renal and liver function
d. Eliminate nephrotoxic or hepatotoxic drugs (such as neomycin sulfate)
e. Liver transplantation is definitive treatment
f. Hemodialysis is used to treat hyperkalemia and fluid overload
g. Carefully assess I & O and daily weights
h. Provide anticipatory teaching about all treatments and procedures

XV. CANCER OF THE LIVER

A. Overview

1. Most common types are metastases from lung, breast, kidney, and other forms of GI cancers
2. Primary liver cancer (hepatoma) is uncommon in United States and more prominent in areas with increased chronic liver disease (Africa, Asia)
3. Prognosis is poor; there is less than 20% survival rate for those with primary liver cancer
4. Tumors arise in liver cell (hepatocellular) or bile duct (cholangiocellular)
5. Tumor can be diffuse, nodular, or single nodule; compresses surrounding cells and can invade blood supply, causing necrosis or hemorrhage
6. Most primary hepatic cancers in United States result from Laënnec's cirrhosis or hepatitis B virus; other etiologic agents are nitrosamines, prolonged androgen therapy, pesticides, and contraceptive steroids

B. Nursing assessment

1. RUQ pain or mass; feeling of fullness in epigastric region
2. Fatigue and general malaise
3. Anorexia and weight loss
4. Later signs can include ascites, fever, jaundice, variceal bleeding, liver failure, and splenomegaly
5. Laboratory findings vary according to degree of liver damage
   a. CBC: anemia
   b. Hyperbilirubinemia
   c. Prolonged PT
   d. Elevated ESR due to liver inflammation
   e. Hypoalbuminemia when there is malnutrition, liver failure
   f. Elevated alkaline phosphatase, AST, ALT when there is liver failure or damage
   g. Alteration of blood glucose due to liver damage
   h. AFP (alpha-fetoprotein): high elevations in 70% of those with hepatocellular cancer
6. Ultrasound, CT scan, or MRI may reveal focal liver lesions
7. Definitive diagnosis is made through biopsy or aspiration of lesion

C. Therapeutic management

1. Partial hepatectomy for individuals with solitary lesions and without extrahepatic manifestations; serial AFPs are done post-procedure to assess effects of intervention
2. Liver transplantation may be done for those meeting established criteria for procedure
3. Radiation therapy (palliative measure) may shrink tumor or reduce pain or pressure on surrounding structures
4. Chemotherapy as a primary therapy has limited response; sometimes chemotherapy is infused via hepatic arterial pump
5. Provide pain control measures and evaluate effectiveness
6. Provide care as outlined for other complications of liver failure or other disorders
7. Medication therapy: chemotherapy and other medications commonly used to treat liver disease

D. Client teaching

1. Disease process, expected outcomes, and chemotherapy
2. Etiologic agents that cause or contribute to development of hepatic cancer
3. Refer to prior sections on liver disorders and complications for other teaching points related to liver disease

XVI. CHOLELITHIASIS

A. Overview

1. Cholelithiasis (gallstones) can occur anywhere within biliary tree, although most are located within gallbladder; 80% are composed of cholesterol, 20% are pigmented; may be asymptomatic
2. Cholesterol stones (usually several) develop slowly; are hard, white, or yellow-brown, radiolucent; can be up to 4 cm in size; are enhanced by production of mucin glycoprotein, which traps cholesterol and leads to stasis of bile
3. Pigmented stones form because of an increase in unconjugated bilirubin and calcium with a concurrent decrease in bile salts; usually develop within the intra- and extrahepatic ducts and are preceded by bacterial invasion
4. Increased bile concentration, bile stasis, and hypercholesterolemia contribute to stone formation
5. Risk factors associated with the formation of gallstones are listed in Box 60–4

B. Nursing assessment

1. Classic manifestations include severe and steady RUQ pain that radiates to right scapula or shoulder; sudden onset, lasting 1 to 3 hours
2. May occur after a high-fat meal
3. Other symptoms include nausea, vomiting, heartburn, and flatulence
4. Fever and chills occur with acute cholecystitis

Box 60-4

Risk Factors for Gallstones

- Female gender
- Family history (may be related to familial high dietary fat intake and sedentary lifestyle)
- Obesity
- Very-low-calorie diet with rapid weight loss
- Pregnancy
- Use of estrogen-containing medications (oral contraceptives, hormone replacement therapy)
- Crohn's disease
- Jejunal bypass surgery
- Type 1 diabetes mellitus
- Aging
- Congenital malformation of biliary duct
- Hyperlipidemia
- Cirrhosis
- Caucasian race

5. Biliary colic or cramping pain occurs when stone is lodged in cystic or common bile duct; if stone blocks duct, edema and inflammation of gallbladder (cholecystitis) occur and may be associated with jaundice
6. Physical exam findings include positive Murphy's sign (palpation of RUQ causes severe pain with inspiration); bowel sounds may be absent
7. Jaundice is not usually seen unless common bile duct is blocked
8. Laboratory findings include elevated WBC count (infection), increased serum bilirubin levels (stone in biliary ductal system causing obstruction), possible electrolyte depletion secondary to vomiting or anorexia; elevated liver function tests (LFTs) with hepatic involvement or damage caused by bile duct obstruction
9. Abdominal x-rays (flat plate) may reveal stones; however, most stones are not radiopaque
10. Ultrasonography is used to identify stones, gallbladder, and ductal dilatation in nonobese clients
11. Oral cholecystogram is not used as frequently as ultrasound for diagnosis of stones; involves ingestion of oral dye to assess ability of gallbladder to concentrate and excrete bile; outlines stones for visualization
12. Gallbladder scans: cholescintigraphy-nuclear medicine scan to evaluate for acute cholecystitis; also called HIDA (hepatobiliary iminodiacetic acid) scan

C. Therapeutic management

1. Oral ursodeoxycholic acid (UCDA) to dissolve cholesterol stones for clients who are poor surgical risks or refuse surgery; effective for stones under 2 cm in diameter; full treatment can take up to 3 years with 50% recurrrence rate within 5 years
2. ! Extracorporeal shock wave **lithotripsy** uses shock waves to disintegrate stones; oral dissolution therapy is used postprocedure to dissolve stone fragments; clients may experience biliary colic postprocedure when gallbladder is contracting to pass stone fragments
3. ! Endoscopic retrograde cholangiopancreatography (ERCP) uses a fiberoptic endoscope to visualize biliary tree, remove stones, drain bile sludge, and collect biopsies
4. ! Laparoscopic cholecystectomy is less invasive than ERCP and involves shorter hospital stay; abdomen is insufflated with CO_2; laparoscope is introduced through a small incision, and gallbladder is deflated and removed through small abdominal incision

5. Cholecystectomy: surgical removal of gallbladder; occasionally a T-tube is placed in common bile duct to assist passage of bile until edema has decreased; bile collects in a bag by gravity drainage
6. Implement comfort measures, including administering prescribed analgesics and antiemetics
7. Provide education regarding diagnostic tests and disease process
8. Maintain NPO status preprocedure as ordered; institute IV fluids as ordered
9. Provide diet instruction regarding low-fat diet, frequent small meals
10. Encourage obese individuals to lose weight
11. Monitor fluid and electrolyte balance
12. Also see discussion of surgical intervention for disorders of gallbladder
13. Medication therapy
    a. Symptomatic treatment of pain and nausea with analgesics and antiemetics as ordered
    b. Meperidine (Demerol) versus morphine as opioid analgesic
    c. Cholestyramine (Questran) is used for severe cases of pruritus; binds bile salts to hasten excretion through feces
    d. Chenodeoxycholic acid (CDCA): a bile acid taken orally to dissolve cholesterol stones
    e. Urodeoxycholic acid (UDCA): similar to CDCA but less hepatotoxic and does not cause fatty diarrhea as does CDCA

D. **Client teaching:** disease process and gallstone formation; diagnostic procedures and expected outcomes; diet instruction to limit high-fat foods

XVII. CHOLECYSTITIS

A. Overview
1. An acute or chronic disorder, cholecystitis most often caused by gallstones obstructing cystic duct, resulting in distention and inflammation of gallbladder; pain is similar to that of gallstones
2. Approximately 5% of clients develop acalculous cholecystitis precipitated by trauma, prolonged hyperalimentation, fasting, or surgery

! B. Nursing assessment
1. Clinical manifestations include all of those previously identified for cholelithiasis
2. Fever, leukocytosis, elevated serum bilirubin (possible jaundice) and alkaline phosphatase, elevated amylase with pancreatic duct involvement
3. Abdominal guarding, rigidity, and rebound tenderness suggest peritoneal involvement
4. Diagnostic and laboratory testing as outlined for cholelithiasis

! C. Therapeutic management
1. NPO with IV fluids for hydration until the pain subsides
2. Opioid analgesics are used for pain control
3. IV antibiotics are administered
4. Surgical intervention is postponed until acute infectious process has subsided

D. Client teaching
1. Preoperative teaching
2. Some clients will be discharged to home and return after a period of convalescence for elective cholecystectomy

E. Surgical intervention for disorders of gallbladder
1. Laparoscopic cholecystectomy: removal of gallbladder through a small abdominal incision guided by a fiberoptic endoscope
2. Cholecystectomy: surgical removal of gallbladder through a RUQ abdominal incision
3. Cholecystectomy with T-tube placement (less common): gallbladder is removed and a T-tube is placed within common bile duct to facilitate bile flow through edematous ducts postprocedure
4. ! Postoperative nursing care
    a. Prevent infection: administer IV antibiotics as ordered, keep incision clean and dry; perform abdominal assessment for peritonitis every 4 hours; monitor VS, report any temperature over 100°F

b. Prevent pain: administer pain medication as ordered; instruct client to request pain medication before pain becomes too intense; medicate for pain prior to postoperative exercise/ambulation; keep client comfortable to promote pulmonary hygiene because incision is near diaphragm
c. Prevent pulmonary infection: keep client comfortable to promote turning every 2 hours, coughing, deep breathing; reinforce the importance of incentive spirometry every 1 hr postoperatively
d. ! Maintain clients who have had T-tube placement in a Fowler's position to promote gravity drainage of bile; report bile drainage in excess of 500 mL in first 24 hours; should be less than 200 mL daily in 2 to 3 days
e. Instruct client that T-tube is removed when bile drainage has subsided and stools have returned to a normal brown color
f. Assess surrounding skin for inflammation secondary to bile leakage
g. Instruct client about proper handling of tube for turning and ambulating
h. Maintain NPO status as ordered; advance diet as tolerated
i. Monitor bowel sounds and encourage ambulation to promote peristalsis
j. Prevent deep-vein thrombosis with leg exercises, frequent ambulation, sequential compression devices, and elastic hosiery
k. Provide general postoperative instruction prior to discharge regarding wound care, analgesia, diet, and signs of infection

XVIII. ACUTE PANCREATITIS

A. Overview

1. Obstruction to flow of pancreatic enzymes results in inflammation of pancreas
2. Can be mild, severe, or fulminant
3. Alcohol abuse and gallbladder disease (obstructive cholelithiasis causing reflux of bile into pancreas) are major causes
4. Other causes are PUD, medications (thiazide diuretics, NSAIDs, estrogens, steroids, salicylates) and hyperlipidemia
5. Injury to pancreas or obstruction of pancreatic duct results in leakage of pancreatic enzymes into pancreatic tissue, leading to autodigestion of pancreas
6. Pain is caused by edema and stretching of pancreatic capsule and chemical irritation; pain may be referred to back because of retroperitoneal location of pancreas
7. Enzymes break down pancreatic tissue, causing inflammation, edema, damage to vasculature, hemorrhage, and necrosis of pancreatic tissue
8. Leakage of these enzymes into the bloodstream can cause further systemic complications, which can result in death
9. Excess hydrochloric acid secretion from chronic alcohol ingestion causes spasms of sphincter of Oddi and ampulla of Vater, which also obstruct flow of pancreatic enzymes
10. Fatty necrosis is normally present with fulminant disease and involves pancreas as well as thoracic and abdominal cavities
11. Necrotic tissue can form walled-off abscesses and lead to systemic complications
12. Types include acute interstitial pancreatitis, acute hemorrhagic pancreatitis, biliary pancreatitis, and alcoholic pancreatitis

B. Nursing assessment

1. Clinical manifestations vary with severity of attack
2. ! Acute epigastric pain, steady and severe, can occur in umbilical area and radiate to back; it may be temporally associated with ingestion of alcohol or a fatty meal
3. ! Pain is greater when lying supine and improves with sitting up and leaning forward, flexion of knee, or fetal positioning
4. ! Nausea and vomiting is common and is worse with any oral intake; vomiting does not relieve abdominal pain
5. VS: fever (rarely above 102°F), hypotension, and tachycardia
6. ! Leukocytosis, hyperglycemia (as high as 500–900 mg/dL), and elevated amylase (for 48 hours) and lipase (for 5–7 days); increased urinary amylase
7. Abdominal tenderness, rigidity, progressive distention, and decreased bowel sounds

8. Fulminant disease can progress to hypovolemic shock, ascites, jaundice, and renal failure
9. Grey Turner sign is a bluish discoloration over flank area and represents accumulation of blood in that area
10. Cullen sign is a bluish discoloration around umbilicus
11. Hypocalcemia if calcium is sequestered by fat necrosis in abdomen, sign of severe pancreatitis
12. Elevated C-reactive protein indicates severity of disease
13. Alcohol abusers may have hypomagnesemia and hypoalbuminemia
14. Pancreatitis with liver involvement; elevated bilirubin and LFTs
15. Abdominal x-ray: identifies ascites, gallstones
16. Abdominal ultrasound to identify gallstones, pancreatic mass, or pseudocyst
17. CT scan: gold standard to visualize size of pancreas and to identify fluid collections, abscesses, masses, and areas of hemorrhage or necrosis
18. Chest x-ray identifies pleural effusion resulting from enzymatic irritation from leaking pancreatic fluid

C. Therapeutic management

1. Treatment is aimed at supportive care, preventing further pancreatic autodigestion and preventing systemic complications
2. NPO status with NG tube if there is ileus or protracted vomiting or to decrease gastric secretions that stimulate pancreatic secretions
3. IV hydration to prevent hypotension and shock
4. TPN if needed for prolonged episodes; reverses catabolic state
5. Possible peritoneal lavage to remove toxic exudates from abdominal cavity
6. ERCP to remove retained or obstructing gallstones or to perform a sphincterotomy
7. Surgical removal of gallbladder for gallstones after acute pancreatitis is resolved
8. Surgical removal and drainage of pseudocyst or abscess may be necessary for recovery
9. Administer pain medications as ordered and on regular schedule
10. Monitor vs, daily weights, hourly UO, bowel sounds, and stool chart (frequency, color, odor, and consistency)
11. Assess respiratory function; provide pulmonary hygiene measures to prevent pneumonia
12. Provide diet instruction (several small meals with no alcohol allowed) when oral feeding is resumed (usually when amylase level returns to normal and abdominal pain subsides)
13. Maintain bedrest during acute phase and increase as tolerated
14. Medication therapy
    a. Opioids and antiemetics
    b. Gastric protection with IV H_2 blocker: ranitidine (Zantac) or proton pump inhibitiors such as pantoprazole (Protonix)
    c. Antispasmodics such as dicyclomine (Bentyl)
    d. Electrolyte replenishment as indicated by laboratory tests
    e. Insulin as required to regulate serum glucose levels
    f. Antibiotics as ordered for infection
    g. Some clients with chronic pancreatic involvement may require long-term treatment with pancreatic enzyme replacement pancrelipase (Lipancreatin)

D. Client teaching

1. Disease process and expected outcomes
2. Nutrition; explain necessity for NPO status during acute phase and rationale for several small meals with no alcohol allowed once diet resumes
3. Importance of taking enzyme replacement to prevent malnutrition and weight loss

XIX. CANCER OF THE PANCREAS

A. Overview

1. Most involve cancer of ductal epithelium and are adenocarcinomas; occurs most often after age 50

2. Is associated with cigarette smoking, environmental toxins, and a diet high in fat and/or meat
3. Other risk factors include diabetes mellitus, chronic pancreatitis, and hereditary pancreatitis
4. Usually located in head of pancreas, deep within tissue, often causing obstruction of common duct
5. Metastasis almost always occurs prior to symptoms with invasion of tumor into posterior wall of stomach, duodenal wall, colon, and common bile duct

B. Nursing assessment

1. Slow onset with anorexia, nausea, weight loss, flatulence, and dull epigastric pain
2. Later pain is severe, is worse when lying down, and is unrelated to meals
3. Jaundice, pruritis, clay-colored stools, and dark urine when bile duct is involved
4. Classic signs and symptoms when disease is far advanced include pain, jaundice, and weight loss
5. Some clients may have a palpable abdominal mass or ascites
6. Diarrhea and steatorrhea late in disease
7. Diabetes mellitus
8. Diagnostic tests same as for pancreatitis, jaundice, and cholelithiasis
9. MRI and CT scan reveal a mass, and CT-guided needle biopsy provides histological diagnosis

C. Therapeutic management

1. Most clients do not present for treatment until cancer is too advanced, and thus treatment is in most cases aimed at supportive or palliative care
2. Pancreatic cancer is usually fatal within 6 months regardless of treatment
3. ERCP may be performed to place stents within ductal system to facilitate bile drainage
4. Surgical management
    a. Gastrojejunostomy: bypasses duodenum
    b. Choledochojejunostomy: relieves biliary obstruction
    c. Pancreatoduodenectomy (Whipple's procedure): surgical removal of head of pancreas, entire duodenum, distal third of stomach, a portion of jejunum, and lower half of common bile duct
5. Chemotherapy and radiation therapy are usually adjuncts to surgical intervention
6. Provide supportive care and education regarding treatment options and assistance with educated decision making
7. Pain management is integral to quality of life; administer analgesics as ordered and assess effectiveness for appropriate discharge regimen
8. Provide preoperative teaching if client opts for surgical intervention
9. Provide information about support groups
10. Medication therapy
    a. No specific medications for treatment of pancreatic cancers
    b. All medications are aimed at controlling symptoms: pain, nausea, vomiting
    c. Chemotherapy is rarely effective and is used most often for palliative treatment

D. Client teaching: disease process and poor prognosis; importance of pain control and symptom relief; importance of abstinence from smoking and alcohol

XX. CLEFT LIP AND CLEFT PALATE

A. Overview

1. Cleft lip is a congenital anomaly involving one or more clefts in upper lip; degree of cleft varies from a small notch to a complete separation (see Figure 60–2 ■)
2. Cleft palate is a congenital anomaly consisting of a cleft ranging from soft palate involvement alone to a defect including hard palate and portions of maxilla in severe cases
3. Causes include hereditary, environmental, and teratogenic factors
4. Both anomalies occur during embryonic development; cleft lip results from failure of fusion of lateral and medial tissues forming upper lip around 7 weeks gestation; cleft palate is a failure of fusion of tissues forming palate around 9 weeks' gestation

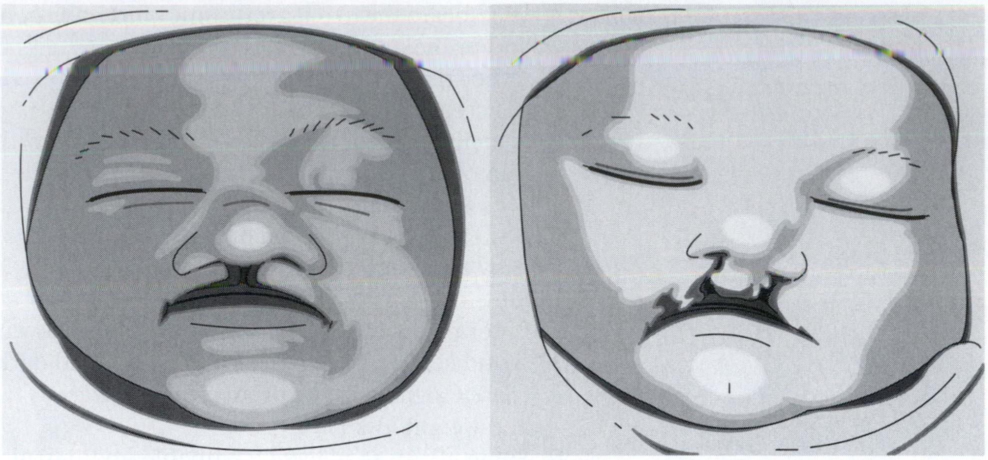

Figure 60–2

Cleft lip. A. Unilateral. B. Bilateral.

Source: Hogan, M., & White, J. (2002). Child health nursing: Reviews and rationales. Upper Saddle River, NJ: Pearson Education, p. 314.

B. Nursing assessment (defects are readily apparent at birth)

1. Cleft lip involves a notched upper lip border, nasal distortion, and may include unilateral or bilateral involvement
2. Cleft palate is a visible or palpable gap in uvula, soft palate, hard palate, and/or incisive foramen with exposed nasal cavities and associated nasal distortion
3. Perform careful physical assessment to rule out other midline birth defects

C. Therapeutic management

1. Depending on severity of defect and infant's general health, cleft lip is often surgically corrected at 1 to 3 months of age; cleft palate is generally repaired between 12 and 18 months; cleft palate may be corrected through several operations performed in stages
2. Early correction of cleft palate enables development of more normal speech patterns and proper dentition; delayed closure of large defects may require use of orthodontic devices
3. Preoperative nursing care
   a. Assess respiratory status continuously during feedings
   b. Feed infant in upright position
   c. Feed slowly and burp the infant frequently

Memory Aid

Use ESSR: *E*nlarged nipple, *S*timulate suck by rubbing nipple on lower lip, *S*wallow, *R*est after each swallow to allow for complete swallowing.

   d. Use alternate feeding devices such as elongated nipple (lamb's nipple) or breast shield
   e. Assess degree of cleft and ability to suck
   f. Provide postoperative feeding instructions
   g. Encourage parents to verbalize fears, concerns, negative emotions
   h. Facilitate grief responses of shock, denial, anger, and mourning
   i. Encourage touching, holding, cuddling, and bonding
   j. Provide parents with pictures of other children before and after surgical repair
   k. Discuss infant's positive characteristics
   l. Refer to community resources and parent support groups
4. Postoperative care
   a. Monitor for respiratory distress during postoperative period; monitor lung sounds and encourage deep breathing without placing stress on suture line
   b. No oral temperatures
   c. Advance feedings as tolerated
   d. No straws, pacifiers, spoons, or fingers in or around mouth for 7 to 10 days
   e. For cleft lip, resume preoperative feeding techniques; a metal appliance or adhesive strips may be used to prevent tension on surgical site

f. For cleft palate, liquids can be taken from a cup; no straws are allowed; soft foods can be taken from side of spoon; to reduce risk of injury, child is not allowed to feed self
g. Clean lip from suture line out after feedings and prn
h. Apply antibacterial ointment as ordered
i. Use elbow restraints to keep infant from putting fingers in mouth or touching surgical site
j. No tooth brushing for 1 to 2 weeks
k. Place infant in side-lying position on unaffected side to avoid excessive contact with bed linens
l. Monitor site for redness, swelling, excess bleeding, purulent drainage, or fever
m. Assess pain using appropriate tools
n. Provide comfort measures to decrease stress, such as crying, on suture line; encourage rocking, cuddling, and holding
o. Provide analgesics and sedatives on a scheduled basis
p. Provide age-appropriate activities for diversion

D. Client and family teaching

1. Precautions to prevent aspiration of formula and phone numbers in case of emergency
2. Provide information on CPR certification
3. Teach parents safety and care issues regarding use of restraints
   a. Do not apply restraints too tightly
   b. Remove at least every 2 hours and play games to encourage flexion
   c. Remove only one restraint at a time
4. Stress importance of follow-up care and referral appointments
5. Make appropriate and early referrals for speech and language disabilities
6. Encourage early speech attempts and arrange for speech therapy
7. Encourage good dental hygiene and orthodontic follow-up

XXI. PYLORIC STENOSIS

A. Overview

1. Occurs when circular areas of muscle surrounding pylorus hypertrophy and block gastric emptying
2. Exact cause remains unknown; heredity is thought to play an important role
3. Firstborn children and offspring of affected children are at highest risk; males are affected more than females and full-term infants more than premature infants
4. The pylorus narrows because of progressive hypertrophy and hyperplasia of circular pyloric muscle
5. This leads to obstruction of the pyloric sphincter, with subsequent gastric distention, dilatation, and hypertrophy
6. Pyloromyotomy (creation of an incision along anterior pylorus to split the muscle) is commonly performed to relieve obstruction

B. Nursing assessment

1. Previously healthy infant with progressive, projectile, nonbilious vomiting
2. Movable, palpable, firm, olive-shaped mass in RUQ
3. Visible, deep, peristaltic waves from LUQ to RUQ immediately before vomiting
4. Irritability, hunger, and crying
5. Sunken fontanels, poor skin turgor, dry mucous membranes, decreased urine output, constipation, jaundice, metabolic alkalosis
6. Ultrasonography and upper GI series may reveal delayed gastric emptying and an elongated pyloric canal
7. Laboratory findings: possible increased pH and bicarbonate level (metabolic alkalosis), decreased serum chloride, sodium, and potassium levels, and increased hematocrit and hemoglobin (hemoconcentration)

C. Therapeutic management

1. Assess skin turgor, mucous membranes, and fontanels at least every shift, monitor urine specific gravity, weigh daily

2. Maintain NPO status prior to surgery, monitor I & O hourly, administer IV fluids and electrolytes as ordered
3. Maintain NG tube patency and monitor NG output
4. Keep infant warm and quiet
5. Initiate small, frequent feedings of clear liquids within 4 to 6 hours after surgery; follow strict diet regimen of gradual advancement of feedings until normal formula feedings have been resumed
6. Continue IV hydration until age- or weight-appropriate amounts of formula are tolerated
7. Assess incision for redness, swelling, and drainage; immediately report signs of infection to physician
8. Monitor VS at least every 4 hours
9. Encourage parental involvement and rooming-in

D. Client and family teaching

1. Explain what pyloric stenosis is and how it is treated, including all equipment such as the NG tube and IV
2. Discharge instructions: report any vomiting, abdominal tenderness, fever, incisional redness, or drainage to the physician
3. Provide verbal and written feeding instructions if child has not returned to full-strength formula feedings prior to discharge
4. Importance of follow-up care with physician

XXII. OMPHALOCELE AND GASTROSCHISIS

A. Overview

1. Omphaloceles are congenital malformations in which intra-abdominal contents herniate through umbilical cord
   a. Results from failure of abdominal contents to return to abdomen when abdominal wall begins to close by tenth week of gestation
   b. Viscera is outside of abdominal cavity but inside translucent sac covered with peritoneum and amniotic membrane
   c. Often associated with other congenital anomalies such as cardiac defects, genitourinary anomalies, chromosomal defects, craniofacial abnormalities, and diaphragmatic abnormalities
2. Gastroschisis occurs when bowel herniates through abdominal wall defect, usually to right of umbilical cord, and through rectus muscle; there is no membrane covering exposed bowel
   a. Uncertain etiology; some suggest that at some point a tear occurs at base of umbilical cord, allowing intestine to herniate
   b. Viscera is outside of abdominal cavity and not covered with peritoneal sac
   c. Rarely associated with other major congenital anomalies, but jejunoileal atresia, ischemic enteritis, and malrotation may occur as a result of defect itself

B. Nursing assessment

1. Obvious protrusion of abdominal contents present at time of delivery
2. Size of sac varies depending on extent of protrusion
3. Rupture of sac results in evisceration of abdominal contents
4. Defect may be noted on prenatal ultrasound

C. Therapeutic management

1. Assess body temperature continuously using skin probe; place infant in warmer immediately after birth
2. Use sterile technique when handling or working with defect
3. Immediately cover with sterile gauze soaked with warm sterile normal saline for irrigation, and wrap in plastic to retain moisture and preserve heat
4. Minimize movement of infant and handling of intestines
5. Assess respiratory status continuously during immediate newborn period by placing on cardiac and apnea monitor with pulse oximetry
6. Monitor for circulatory compromise by monitoring temperature, pulses, capillary refill, skin color, and heart rate and respiratory rate

7. Assess mucous membranes for moisture and skin for elastic turgor; monitor I & O, weigh daily, assess fontanels, monitor electrolytes, maintain IV, and administer fluids and TPN as ordered
8. Maintain NG tube for decompression and NPO status
9. Monitor for signs of ileus by auscultating bowel sounds, measuring abdominal girth, assessing bowel movements
10. Assess parents' coping mechanisms and encourage them to verbalize feelings of loss of "perfect" child and guilt that may accompany congenital anomaly
11. Encourage parental participation in infant's care

D. Family teaching
1. Provide written and verbal information on growth and developmental needs
2. Teach parents appropriate techniques for developmental stimulation
3. Provide information regarding support groups and other community resources
4. Teach parents signs of bowel obstruction

XXIII. BILIARY ATRESIA

A. Overview
1. A progressive inflammatory process that causes both intrahepatic and extrahepatic bile duct fibrosis
2. Etiology is unknown; because problem originates during prenatal period, viruses, toxins, and chemicals are a few suspected causes
3. Obstruction of extrahepatic bile ducts causes obstruction of normal flow of bile from liver into gallbladder and small intestine
4. Bile plugs form and cause bile accumulation in liver
5. Inflammation, edema, and irreversible hepatic injury occur
6. Liver becomes fibrotic, and cirrhosis and portal hypertension develop, leading to liver failure
7. Because of lack of bile in intestines, fat and fat-soluble vitamins cannot be absorbed, resulting in malnutrition, deficiencies of fat-soluble vitamins, and growth failure
8. Without treatment, this disease is fatal
9. Treatment involves surgery (Kasai procedure) to temporarily correct obstruction and supportive care
10. Liver transplantation is eventually necessary

B. Assessment
1. Healthy-appearing infant at birth
2. Jaundice occurs within 2 weeks to 2 months
3. **Acholic** stools: puttylike, clay-colored stools
4. Abdominal distention and hepatomegaly
5. Increased bruising of the skin, prolonged bleeding time
6. Intense itching
7. Tea-colored urine
8. Increased bilirubin levels; ultrasound and liver biopsy confirm disorder

C. Therapeutic management
1. Weigh daily
2. Administer TPN with or without intralipids as ordered
3. Administer fat-soluble vitamins A, D, E, and K as ordered
4. Monitor stool pattern
5. Establish an open, caring relationship with family
6. Refer parents to support groups

D. Client and family teaching
1. Instruct the parents in meticulous skin care
2. Provide verbal and written information regarding nutritional needs
3. Provide instructions on home medication regimen and allow time for return demonstration
4. Inform parents of the signs and symptoms for which to call the physician
5. If a transplant is performed, include detailed instruction on post-transplant medications

XXIV. HIRSCHSPRUNG'S DISEASE

A. Overview

1. A congenital anomaly resulting from an absence of ganglion cells in colon; also known as megacolon and congenital aganglionosis
2. Believed to be a familial, congenital defect; incidence is higher in children with Down syndrome and genitourinary abnormalities
3. Rectosigmoid region is most commonly affected
4. Absence of autonomic parasympathetic ganglion cells in one portion of colon results in lack of innervation in that portion and absence of peristalsis
5. Lack of peristalsis causes accumulation of intestinal contents and distention of bowel proximal to defect

B. Nursing assessment

1. Clinical manifestations in newborns
   a. Failure to pass meconium stools
   b. Reluctant to ingest fluids
   c. Abdominal distention
   d. Bile-stained emesis
2. Clinical manifestations in infants
   a. Failure to thrive
   b. Constipation
   c. Abdominal distention
   d. Vomiting
   e. Episodic diarrhea
3. Clinical manifestations in toddlers and older children
   a. Chronic constipation
   b. Foul-smelling stools
   c. Abdominal distention
   d. Visible peristalsis
   e. Palpable fecal mass
   f. Malnourishment
   g. Signs of anemia and hypoproteinemia
4. Rectal examination typically reveals an absence of stool
5. Laboratory studies and diagnostic tests commonly reveal an enlarged portion of colon and a rectal biopsy confirms absence of ganglion cells

C. Therapeutic management

1. Involves removing aganglionic bowel; a temporary colostomy is created soon after diagnosis, which will be closed and the bowel reanastomosed at a later time, usually around age of 2 years
2. Preoperatively, assess bowel function and characteristics of stool; measure abdominal girth; monitor child for vomiting and respiratory distress
3. Monitor urine specific gravity; monitor electrolytes; assess hydration status
4. Prepare child for surgery and temporary placement of colostomy
5. Administer antibiotics as ordered
6. Monitor VS; measure abdominal girth; assess surgical site for redness, swelling, drainage after surgery
7. Assess stoma for color, bleeding, breakdown of surrounding skin
8. Assess anal area after pull-through for patency of any appliance that may be in place, presence of stool, redness, drainage
9. Provide meticulous skin care, use appropriately sized stoma supplies
10. Notify physician of any fever, unusual drainage, redness, or odor
11. Keep child NPO until bowel sounds return or flatus is passed; maintain NG tube, administer IV fluids as ordered; monitor daily weights; begin diet with clear liquids and progress as tolerated
12. Assess pain using age-appropriate scales; provide comfort measures and involve parents; provide pain medications on regular basis as ordered; notify physician if pain is not managed
13. Involve child in quiet, age-appropriate activities for diversion

14. Encourage parents to share feelings, anxieties, and concerns about disorder and post-surgical care
15. Refer to support groups and make appropriate referrals

D. Client and family teaching

1. Explain surgical repair and recovery process
2. Encourage preschool and early school-aged children to draw pictures, use dolls, and play to express concerns about bodily appearance, irrigations, and colostomy
3. Provide parents with instructions about how to complete rectal irrigations and allow time for return demonstration
4. ! Teach ostomy care in immediate postoperative period and encourage parents to participate and give return demonstration while in hospital; encourage child to learn and assume care as soon as appropriate
5. ! Teach parents how to assess for distention and obstruction and importance of reporting these findings to physician

XXV. APPENDICITIS

A. Overview

1. Inflammation and infection of vermiform appendix, a small lymphoid, tubular blind sac at end of cecum
2. Exact cause is poorly understood but results from obstruction of lumen by hardened fecal material (**fecalith**), foreign bodies, microorganisms, or parasites
3. Obstruction of lumen causes accumulation of normal mucous secretions and distension of appendix, which causes capillary and venous engorgement and increased intraluminal pressure
4. Ischemia occurs and can lead to necrosis and perforation of intestinal wall; if perforation occurs, bacteria from bowel contaminate peritoneum and may lead to peritonitis and sepsis
5. Appendicitis is most common reason for abdominal surgery in childhood; frequency increases with age with peak incidence between ages 15 and 30 years

B. Nursing assessment

1. ! Generalized abdominal pain progressively worsening and localizing in RLQ at **McBurney's point** (Figure 60–3 ■)
2. Nausea and vomiting, fever, and chills
3. Anorexia, diarrhea, or acute constipation
4. Elevated WBC count: 15,000 to 20,000 cells/mm^3
5. Ultrasound indicating an enlarged incompressible appendix

C. Therapeutic management

1. Surgical removal (appendectomy) is done as soon as diagnosis made
2. Preoperative nursing care
   a. Explain procedure and postoperative care to client and family
   b. Keep client NPO before surgery and prevent dehydration by administering IV fluids as ordered
   c. ! Place client in semi-Fowler's or right-side lying position to help localize and prevent spread of any infection (used both preoperatively and postoperatively)
   d. Assess for abdominal distention, auscultate bowel sounds, and observe elimination patterns
   e. ! Do nothing to stimulate peristalsis, which would hasten perforation; avoid laxatives, enemas, and heat applications
   f. Apply cold packs to client's abdomen to help relieve discomfort
   g. ! Sudden relief of pain usually indicates a ruptured appendix
3. Postoperative nursing care
   a. ! Monitor VS, assess for abdominal distention, and inspect surgical wound for signs of infection
   b. Encourage ambulation within 6 to 8 hours after surgery if not contraindicated
   c. Encourage client to turn, cough, and breathe deeply
   d. Monitor I & O and ensure that spontaneous voiding occurs
   e. Assess for pain and administer analgesics as ordered

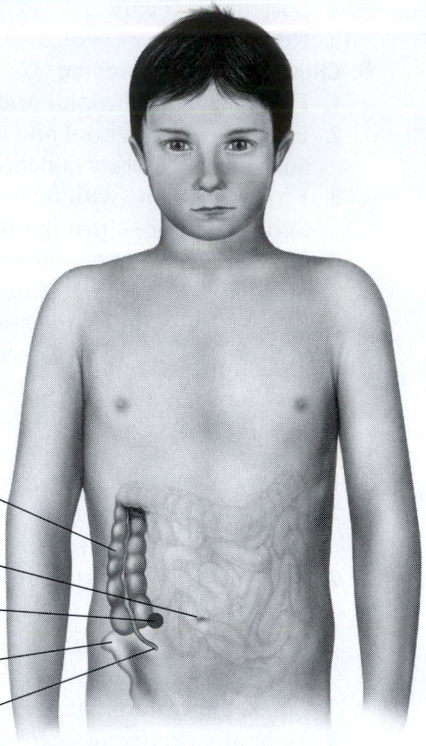

Figure 60–3

McBurney's point in right lower quadrant of abdomen with appendicitis.

Source: Ball, J. & Bindler, R. (2006). Child health nursing: Partnering with children and families. *Upper Saddle River, NJ: Pearson Education, p. 1135.*

! f. If appendix ruptures, postoperative recovery is slowed; child will probably have an NG tube to decompress stomach and a Jackson-Pratt or Penrose drain; antibiotics may be administered

D. Client and family teaching

1. Diagnostic procedures, cause of appendicitis, surgical treatment, and anticipated postoperative care
2. How to assess surgical incision for signs and symptoms of infection
3. Other problems to report to physician, such as fever, increased discomfort, and incision dehiscence (separation)
4. ! Instruct parents that child should avoid lifting, stretching, and strenuous activities until all follow-up care is completed
5. Provide information on fluids and nutrition during recovery process and advancement of diet; include signs and symptoms of which to notify physician, such as vomiting, abdominal distention, and increased pain

XXVI. CELIAC DISEASE

A. Overview

1. A genetic GI malabsorption condition also known as gluten-sensitive enteropathy
2. A chronic inability to tolerate foods containing gluten
3. ! Results from inability to fully digest gliadin and glutenin or protein components of certain grains like wheat, barley, rye, and oats
4. ! This deficiency in digestion requires lifelong dietary modifications
5. Exact cause is unknown; there may be a genetic predisposition possibly influenced by environmental factors and an immunologic abnormality
6. When exposed to gluten, intestinal mucosa becomes damaged; villi eventually atrophy and reduce absorptive surface of small intestine, which reduces absorption of ingested nutrients; chronic diarrhea results
7. ! Acute episodes (called celiac crises) are characterized by a general flare-up of symptoms and are precipitated by infections, prolonged fasting, ingestion of gluten, or exposure to anticholinergic drugs; can lead to electrolyte imbalance, rapid dehydration, and severe acidosis; clients may be at increased risk for developing lymphoma

B. Nursing assessment

1. Symptoms typically appear within 3 to 6 months after introduction of gluten (usually in form of grains) into child's diet
2. ! Frequent bulky, greasy, malodorous stools with frothy appearance due to fat in stool (**steatorrhea**)
3. Abdominal distention, vomiting, and anorexia
4. Growth retardation with lack of fat deposits and muscle wasting
5. Anemia, irritability, edema
6. ! In a celiac crisis, severe diarrhea and dehydration ensue; electrolyte imbalances and metabolic acidosis can create life-threatening disease
7. For unknown reasons, some children do not exhibit symptoms until after age 5 with growth retardation and delayed sexual maturation as predominant manifestations
8. Laboratory studies and diagnostic tests
   a. Flat mucosal surface, absence or atrophy of villi, and deep crypts visible on biopsy of small intestine
   b. ! Steatorrhea on analysis of 72-hour quantitative fecal fat study
   c. Presence of serum antigliadin antibody (AGA) and reticulin antibody levels are elevated

C. Therapeutic management

1. ! Nursing care focuses on supporting child and parents in maintaining a gluten-free diet; corn and rice become substitute grains (see Table 60–1 ■)
2. Assess child's growth at each routine visit using a standard growth chart
3. Administer fluids for hydration; serum electrolytes and serum osmolality may be used as lab indicators of hydration status
4. ! Monitor I & O, assess skin turgor, mucous membranes, and urine specific gravity
5. Encourage participation in age-appropriate activities
6. Inform parents of organizations such as the American Celiac Society, the Celiac Sprue Association/United States of America, and the Gluten Intolerance Group

D. Client and family teaching

1. Written and verbal instructions on gluten-free diet
2. ! Read labels of processed foods, because most contain gluten as a filler
3. Urgency of seeking medical care in the event of celiac crisis
4. ! Importance of lifelong compliance with dietary modifications and follow-up medical care

XXVII. NECROTIZING ENTEROCOLITIS (NEC)

A. Overview

1. An inflammatory disease of intestinal tract that occurs primarily in premature infants
2. Characterized by varying degrees of mucosal or transmural necrosis of intestine
3. Usual onset is in first 2 weeks of life but can be later in very low-birthweight infants
4. Caused by several factors, such as intestinal ischemia, bacterial or viral infection, and immaturity of gut; occurs most often in terminal ileum and colon
5. Pathology appears to begin when reduced blood flow to bowel leads to bowel wall ischemia; this ischemia allows bacteria to enter bowel wall and colonize
6. Damage to bowel can lead to perforation, which leads to need for bowel resection

Table 60–1

Suggestions for a Gluten-Free Diet

Unrestricted Food Items	Restricted Food Items
Beef, pork, poultry, fish	Items with bread coating using wheat, oats, rye or barley
Eggs	Any food made from wheat, rye, oats, or barley (bread, rolls, cookies, cakes, crackers, cereal, spaghetti, macaroni)
Milk, cream, cheese	Beer and ale, Ovaltine, instant tea mix, commercially prepared ice cream, malted milk, prepared puddings
Vegetables	Canned baked beans, commercially seasoned vegetable mixes or vegetables with sauce
Fruit	Salad dressings and mayonnaise, ketchup, gravy
Rice, corn, gluten-free wheat flour, puffed rice, corn flakes, corn meal	

B. Nursing assessment

! 1. History may include prematurity, small for gestational age, maternal hemorrhage, preeclampsia, cocaine exposure in utero, exchange transfusions, umbilical catheters, low Apgar scores, or asphyxia
2. Typically, suspected NEC (stage I) consists of nonspecific clinical findings that simply represent physiologic instability and may resemble other common conditions in premature infants; these findings include the following:
   a. Temperature instability
   b. Lethargy
   c. Recurrent apnea and bradycardia
   d. Hypoglycemia
   e. Poor peripheral perfusion
   f. Increased pregavage gastric residuals
   g. Feeding intolerance, vomiting, abdominal distention
   h. Guaiac positive stools
! 3. NEC (stage II) consists of nonspecific signs and symptoms plus the following:
   a. Severe abdominal distention
   b. Abdominal tenderness
   c. Grossly bloody stools
   d. Palpable bowel loops
   e. Edema of the abdominal wall
   f. Bowel sounds may be absent
! 4. NEC (stage III) occurs when the infant becomes acutely ill; signs and symptoms include the following:
   a. Deterioration of vital signs
   b. Evidence of septic shock
   c. Edema and erythema of abdominal wall
   d. Right lower quadrant mass
   e. Acidosis (metabolic and/or respiratory)
   f. Disseminated intravascular coagulopathy (DIC)
5. Diagnostic testing includes an abdominal x-ray revealing free peritoneal gas, dilated bowel loops, bowel distention, and bowel thickening

C. Therapeutic management

! 1. Nursing care focuses on early detection to minimize bowel necrosis
2. Measure abdominal girth frequently
3. Prepare feedings using aseptic technique
! 4. Observe toleration of feedings; assess and maintain optimal hydration status
5. Monitor cardiac and respiratory status
6. Promote and maintain adequate body temperature
7. Administer antibiotics as ordered
8. Encourage family interaction and promote attachment process
9. Provide developmentally appropriate activities

D. Client and family teaching

1. Encourage parents to express concerns about outcomes of surgery
! 2. Instruct parents on signs of intestinal obstruction, strictures, poor tolerance of feedings, and impaired healing processes
! 3. Instruct parents about care of ostomy and IV central line

XXVIII. FAILURE TO THRIVE (FTT)

A. Overview

1. Describes a child whose weight falls below 5th percentile on a standardized growth chart; growth measurements in addition to a persistent deviation from an established growth curve is generally a cause for concern
2. Organic FTT results from a physical cause; cystic fibrosis is leading cause of organic FTT; other physical causes include celiac disease, congenital heart defects, chronic renal failure, gastroesophageal reflux, malabsorption syndrome, or endocrine dysfunction
3. Nonorganic FTT is caused by psychosocial factors and is suspected in absence of history, physical, or laboratory findings of organic disease; lack of bonding to

primary caregiver is most common nonorganic cause; however, other factors include poverty, health beliefs, inadequate nutritional knowledge, family stress, feeding resistance, or insufficient breast milk

B. Nursing assessment

1. Physical findings
   - **a.** Weight below 5th percentile
   - **b.** Sudden or rapid deceleration in growth curve
   - **c.** Delay in developmental milestones
   - **d.** Decreased muscle mass
   - **e.** Abdominal distension
   - **f.** Muscular hypotonia
   - **g.** Generalized weakness and **cachexia** (malnutrition accompanied by wasting)
2. Behavioral indicators
   - **a.** Avoidance of eye contact or physical touch
   - **b.** Intense watchfulness
   - **c.** Sleep disturbances
   - **d.** Disturbed manner, such as apathy, extreme irritability, extreme compliance
   - **e.** Repetitive rocking, head banging, intense sucking, intense chewing of fingers or hands, or head rolling
3. Diagnostic tests
   - **a.** Developmental screening
   - **b.** Tuberculin skin test
   - **c.** Bone scan, chest x-ray, ECG, IV pyelogram, upper and lower GI series
   - **d.** Urinalysis, complete blood count, sweat chloride test, stool tests, T_4 test
   - **e.** Bowel and muscle biopsies

C. Therapeutic management

1. Document child's eating patterns
2. Document parent–child interaction
3. Encourage parents to discuss positive and negative feelings of care, procedures, and interaction with child
4. Feed on demand or increase intake as tolerated
5. Offer high-protein, high-calorie snacks
6. Offer frequent, small portions of a wide variety of foods
7. Monitor I & O, daily weights
8. Provide consistency in nursing care
9. Try to make mealtimes as stress-free as possible

D. Client and family teaching

1. Normal growth and development
2. Provide information on effective feeding practices and ways to make mealtimes less of a control issue

XXIX. VOMITING AND DIARRHEA

A. Overview

1. Vomiting is a forceful ejection of gastric contents through mouth
   - **a.** Is common and usually self-limiting
   - **b.** Requires no specific treatment unless complications occur (dehydration and electrolyte imbalances, malnutrition, and aspiration)
   - **c.** Can be an associated symptom of an acute infectious disease, increased intracranial pressure, toxic ingestion, food intolerance and allergy, mechanical obstruction of GI tract, metabolic disorder, or a psychogenic problem
   - **d.** Color and consistency of emesis suggests etiology: green bilious with bowel obstruction; coffee ground texture from blood mixing with stomach contents suggests GI bleeding; curdled stomach contents, mucus, or fatty foods several hours after eating suggest poor gastric emptying
   - **e.** Associated symptoms also help to identify etiology: fever and diarrhea with infection; constipation with obstruction; localized abdominal pain with appendicitis, pancreatitis, or PUD; change in level of consciousness or headache with a central nervous system or metabolic disorder; forceful or projectile vomiting with pyloric stenosis

2. **Diarrhea** is defined as frequent, watery, loose stools and is actually a symptom rather than a disease
   a. Accompanies many disorders, including respiratory infections and GI disorders, and can also be caused by stress, food intolerance or sensitivity, medications, and surgical procedures that reduce absorptive surface of intestine
   b. Can be acute or chronic, inflammatory or noninflammatory, or viral or bacterial in nature
   c. Can lead to dehydration, electrolyte imbalance, hypovolemic shock, and even death in pediatric clients
   d. Increased intestinal motility and rapid emptying results in impaired absorption of nutrients and excessive excretion of water and electrolytes, especially sodium and potassium

B. Nursing assessment

! 1. Assessment of hydration status is highest priority (see Table 60–2 ■ for signs of dehydration)
2. Assess amount, color, consistency, and time of stools and vomitus
! 3. Assess daily weights (best indication of fluid balance)
4. Assess I & O and client's activity level
5. Assess for abdominal cramping, fever, and other related symptoms
6. Stool culture for bacteria, ova, parasites, or rotaviruses; stool examination for pH, leukocytes, glucose, and presence of blood; serum electrolytes, BUN, creatinine, and glucose; x-rays, ultrasound, or endoscopy

C. Therapeutic management

1. Priority nursing interventions focus on assessing for dehydration

Table 60–2 Severity of Clinical Dehydration

	Mild	Moderate	Severe
Percent of body weight lost	Up to 5%	6%–9% (60–90 mL/kg)	10% or more (100+ mg/kg)
Level of consciousness	Alert, restless, thirsty	Restless or lethargic (infants and very young children); alert, thirsty, restless (older children, adolescents, and adults)	Lethargic to comatose (infants and young children); often conscious and apprehensive (older children and adults)
Blood pressure	Normal	Normal or low; postural hypotension (older children and adults)	Low to undetectable
Pulse	Normal	Rapid	Rapid, weak to nonpalpable
Skin turgor	Normal	Poor	Very poor
Mucous membranes	Moist	Dry	Parched
Urine	May appear normal	Decreased output (<1 mL/kg/hr); dark color, increased specific gravity	Very decreased or absent output
Thirst	Slightly increased	Moderately increased	Greatly increased unless lethargic
Fontanel	Normal (children)	Sunken (children)	Sunken (children)
Extremities	Warm; normal capillary refill	Delayed capillary refill (>2 sec)	Cool, discolored; delayed capillary refill (>3–4 sec)
Respirations	Normal	Normal or rapid	Changing rate and pattern

Modified slightly from: Ball, J., & Bindler, R. (2006). *Child health nursing: Partnering with children & families.* Upper Saddle River, NJ: Pearson Education, p. 730, Table 23-2.

2. Weigh client on admission and daily using same scale at same time of day in same amount of clothing
3. Monitor and document I & O hourly; weigh diapers in infants after voiding and bowel movements; monitor urine specific gravity
4. Monitor vital signs and avoid rectal temperatures
5. Client is usually NPO to allow bowel rest; administer IV fluids as ordered
6. Begin oral rehydration young children with frequent, small feedings
   a. Oral rehydration fluids (ORFs) include commercial preparations such as Pedialyte for children
   b. Offer frequent, small amounts of liquids—1 to 3 teaspoons every 10 to 15 minutes; for older children and adults, offer sips to total up to 8oz in an hour
   c. Infants progress from clear liquids to their typical diet, although soy protein formula rather than milk-based formula may be recommended for formula-fed infants
   d. A bland, milk-free BRAT diet (bananas, rice cereal, applesauce, and toast) is disfavored now because of low nutritional value; as vomiting and diarrhea improve, child may resume regular diet
7. Administer antidiarrheals, antibiotics, antiprotozoals as ordered
8. Monitor lab tests (electrolytes, hematocrit, pH, serum albumin)
9. Implement measures to reduce fever if needed
10. Cleanse diaper area (infants) or perianal skin with mild soap and water after each stool, avoid harsh astringent wipes that could further irritate reddened skin
11. Practice standard precautions

D. **Client and family teaching:** causes of vomiting and diarrhea, oral rehydration therapy, skin care, and signs and symptoms requiring medical attention

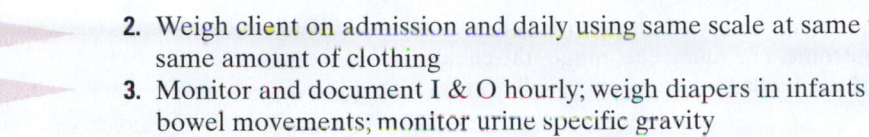

Check Your NCLEX-RN® Exam I.Q.

You are ready for testing on this content if you can

- Identify basic structures and functions of the gastrointestinal system.
- Describe the pathophysiology and etiology of common gastrointestinal disorders.
- Discuss expected assessment data and diagnostic test findings for selected gastrointestinal disorders.
- Discuss therapeutic management of a client experiencing a gastrointestinal disorder.
- Discuss nursing management of a client experiencing a gastrointestinal disorder.
- Identify expected outcomes for the client experiencing a gastrointestinal disorder.

PRACTICE TEST

1 A client has a total gastrectomy. The nurse explains to the client the need for long-term injections of which of the following vitamins?

1. Thiamine
2. Folic acid
3. Cyanocobalamin
4. Niacin

2 A client with diverticular disease undergoes a colonoscopy. When conducting an abdominal assessment, the nurse looks for which of the following as a sign of possible complication of the procedure?

1. Diarrhea
2. Nausea and vomiting
3. Guarding and rebound tenderness
4. Redness and warmth of the abdominal skin

3 The client who has ulcerative colitis is scheduled for an ileostomy. When the client asks the nurse what to expect related to bowel function and care after surgery, what response should the nurse make?

1. "You will be able to have some control over your bowel movements."
2. "The stoma will require that you wear a collection device all the time."
3. "After the stoma heals, you can irrigate your bowel so you will not have to wear a pouch."
4. "The drainage will gradually become semisolid and formed."

4 The nurse is conducting dietary teaching with a client who has dumping syndrome. The nurse encourages the client to avoid which of the foods that the client usually enjoys?

1. Eggs
2. Cheese
3. Fruit
4. Pork

5 A client is being evaluated for possible duodenal ulcer. The nurse assesses the client for which of the following manifestations that would support this diagnosis?

1. Epigastric pain relieved by food
2. History of chronic aspirin use
3. Distended abdomen
4. Positive fluid wave

6 The client returning from a colonoscopy has been given a diagnosis of Crohn's disease. The oncoming shift nurse expects to note which of the following manifestations in the client?

1. Steatorrhea
2. Firm, rigid abdomen
3. Constipation
4. Enlarged hemorrhoids

7 A client is scheduled for a fecal fat exam. In planning client education, the nurse includes that which dietary modification is necessary before the test?

1. Eat a fat-free diet the day before the exam.
2. Eat a high-fat meal right before the exam.
3. Eat a diet containing 35 grams of fat for 36 hours before the test.
4. Eat at least 100 grams of fat for 3 days before and during the test.

8 The client with diverticular disease is scheduled for a sigmoidoscopy. He suddenly complains of severe abdominal pain. On examination, the nurse notes a rigid abdomen with guarding. What action should the nurse take next?

1. Notify the physician.
2. Place the client in a more comfortable position.
3. Keep the client distracted until the procedure begins.
4. Tell the client that the test will show what is causing his problem.

9 The nurse is educating the client with gastroesophageal reflux disease (GERD) about ways to minimize symptoms. Which information in the client's history should the nurse address as an indicator that needs to be changed?

1. Lifting weights for exercise
2. Being a vegetarian
3. Having a body mass index of 23
4. Taking calcium carbonate tablets

10 The client with a duodenal ulcer asks the nurse why an antibiotic is part of the treatment regimen. Which information should the nurse include in the response?

1. Antibiotics decrease the likelihood of infection.
2. Many duodenal ulcers are caused by the *Helicobacter pylori* organism.
3. Antibiotics are used in an attempt to sterilize the stomach.
4. Many people have *Clostridium difficile,* which can lead to ulcer formation.

11 The nurse should evaluate results of which of the following laboratory tests for a client who has cirrhosis in order to plan for safe care?

1. Prothrombin time
2. Urinalysis
3. Serum lipase
4. Serum troponin

12 The nurse is caring for a client with a history of alcoholism. Which of the following findings would indicate that the client has possibly developed chronic pancreatitis?

1. Steady weight gain
2. Flank pain on left side only
3. Fatty stools
4. Excessive hunger

13 The nurse caring for a client with hemolytic jaundice anticipates which of the following findings on the laboratory results?

1. Elevated serum indirect bilirubin
2. Decreased serum protein
3. Elevated urine bilirubin
4. Decreased urine pH

14 A client was admitted to the hospital with cholelithiasis the previous day. Which of the following new assessment findings indicates to the nurse that the stone has probably obstructed the common bile duct?

1. Nausea
2. Elevated cholesterol level
3. Right upper quadrant (RUQ) pain
4. Jaundice

15 The nurse caring for a client with uncomplicated cholelithiasis anticipates that the client's laboratory test results will show an elevation in which of the following?

1. Serum amylase
2. Alkaline phosphatase
3. Mean corpuscular hemoglobin concentration (MCHC)
4. Indirect bilirubin

16 In caring for the client 4 days post-cholecystectomy, the nurse notices that the drainage from the T-tube is 600 mL in 24 hours. Which is the appropriate action by the nurse?

1. Clamp the tube q 2 hours for 30 minutes
2. Place the patient in a supine position
3. Assess drainage characteristics and notify the physician
4. Encourage an increased fluid intake

17 The post-cholecystectomy client asks the nurse when the T-tube will be removed. Which of the following responses by the nurse would be appropriate?

1. "When your stool returns to a normal brown color, the tube can be removed."
2. "The tube will be removed at the same time as your staples."
3. "When the tube stops draining, it will be removed."
4. "The tube is usually removed the day after surgery."

18 Which of the following assessments made by the nurse could indicate the development of portal hypertension in a client with cirrhosis?

1. Hemorrhoids
2. Bleeding gums
3. Muscle wasting
4. Hypothermia

19 The nurse is caring for a client who has ascites, and the health care provider prescribes spironolactone (Aldactone). The client asks why this drug is being used. Which is the best response by the nurse?

1. "This drug will help increase the level of protein in your blood."
2. "The drug will cause an increase in the amount of the hormone aldosterone your body produces."
3. "This medication is a diuretic but does not make the kidneys excrete potassium."
4. "This will help you excrete larger amounts of ammonia."

20 When caring for a client who has cirrhosis, the nurse notices flapping tremors of the wrist and fingers. How should the nurse chart this finding?

1. "Trousseau's sign noted."
2. "Caput medusa noted."
3. "Fetor hepaticus noted."
4. "Asterixis noted."

21 A mother arrives at the pediatric clinic with her 6-month-old infant. While the nurse is assessing the child, the mother points to the umbilicus and says: "What am I going to do about this? When he cries, it looks like it's going to burst." Which of the following is the best response by the nurse?

1. "It's best if you don't let him cry. Just let him do what he wants."
2. "It probably won't rupture unless he gets excessively upset. I wouldn't worry about it at this time."
3. "I know it looks frightening, but it really won't burst."
4. "Put a binder around it, and that will keep it from bursting when he gets mad."

22 A 9-year-old male client with severe esophagitis is 12 hours status/post Nissen fundoplication for gastroesophageal reflux. To implement appropriate nursing care, the nurse should do which of the following?

1. Encourage him to take small amounts of clear liquids every 4 hours.
2. Administer NG or gastrostomy feedings every 4 hours.
3. Ask him to choose a face on the Wong FACES pain rating scale.
4. Insert a pH probe to monitor esophageal acidity.

PRACTICE TEST

23. A 10-month-old female infant with biliary atresia is being discharged after a Kasai procedure. Which statement, if made by the parents, indicates that teaching with regard to prognosis has been understood?

1. "We are glad this problem was found so early; now everything will be fine."
2. "We will stop her liver medicine now that she is being discharged."
3. "We are happy to be able to stop that special formula and many of those vitamins."
4. "We know that even though surgery is over, she will likely need a liver transplant."

24. Which of the following diagnostic assessment methods would the nurse expect to be ordered for a child with dehydration as a result of vomiting and diarrhea?

1. Serum sodium and serum osmolality
2. Stool for ova and parasites
3. Upper-gastrointestinal series
4. Seventy-two-hour fecal fat collection

25. The nurse is caring for a child with a history of severe diarrhea. Which of the following notations in the medical record about acid-base imbalance would the nurse expect to find?

1. Respiratory acidosis
2. Respiratory alkalosis
3. Metabolic acidosis
4. Metabolic alkalosis

26. A nurse who floats to the infant and toddlers nursing unit asks the pediatric nurse about the notation "ESSR" on the care plan of a client. The nurse explains that this documentation refers to

1. the feeding method for children with gastroesophageal reflux.
2. the feeding method for children with cleft lip or palate.
3. the procedure for repair of pyloric stenosis.
4. the procedure for repair of Hirschsprung's disease.

27. A child with Hirschsprung's disease is being discharged after Soave endorectal pull-through procedure for colostomy closure. Which of the following items should the nurse include in the discharge teaching plan?

1. Stools may be infrequent and uncomfortable for the first few weeks.
2. It will be necessary to perform weekly rectal irrigations for approximately 6 weeks.
3. Report fever, increasing pain or discomfort, or redness of the incision to the surgeon.
4. Stools will be fatty for a week or so and then gradually return to normal.

28. The nurse is taking a history from the mother of a child being admitted with flare-up of celiac disease. What piece of information would the nurse expect the mother to report?

1. Stools that are fatty
2. An increased appetite with no weight gain
3. Episodes of abdominal pain that are wavelike just before meals
4. Soft, formed stools

29. The mother of a child undergoing an emergency appendectomy tells the nurse, "If I had brought him in yesterday when he complained of an upset stomach, this wouldn't have happened." Which of the following is the best response by the nurse?

1. "It's okay; you got him here just in time before it ruptured."
2. "It is often difficult to predict when a simple complaint will become more serious."
3. "Next time he seems sick, you should bring him in immediately."
4. "Sometimes parents can make a mistake without meaning to do so."

30. The nurse is teaching home feeding guidelines to the mother of a child with nonorganic failure to thrive. Essential information for the nurse to include would be the importance of

1. restricting eating except at mealtimes.
2. allowing the child to eat alone to minimize distraction.
3. allowing the child to snack on finger foods, such as Cheerios, french fries, and bananas.
4. a relaxed mealtime with few limits on behavior.

31 The nurse is admitting a child with a diagnosis of "rule out appendicitis." The nurse assesses this client for which of the following manifestations? Select all that apply.

1. Generalized abdominal pain
2. Pain localizing in right lower quadrant
3. Fatty stools
4. Elevated white blood cell count
5. Indigestion

ANSWERS & RATIONALES

1 **Answer: 3** The loss of parietal cells that secrete intrinsic factor results in vitamin B_{12} (cyanocobalamin) deficiency post-gastrectomy, because intrinsic factor is needed for absorption of vitamin B_{12}. For this reason, clients require vitamin B_{12} injections for life. The other options identify other B-complex vitamins.
Cognitive Level: Analysis **Client Need:** Physiological Integrity: Physiological Adaptation **Integrated Process:** Teaching and Learning **Content Area:** Adult Health: Gastrointestinal **Strategy:** The core issue of the question is knowledge that gastric surgery results in loss of ability to produce intrinsic factor and subsequent vitamin B_{12} deficiency. Use nursing knowledge and the process of elimination to make a selection.

2 **Answer: 3** Bowel perforation is a possible result of colonoscopy if the colonoscope accidentally pierces the bowel wall. Perforation could lead to symptoms of peritonitis, such as guarding and rebound tenderness. The other options are incorrect, because diarrhea (option 1), nausea and vomiting as signs of obstruction (option 2), and redness and warmth of abdominal skin (option 4) are not of concern.
Cognitive Level: Analysis **Client Need:** Physiological Integrity: Physiological Adaptation **Integrated Process:** Nursing Process: Assessment **Content Area:** Adult Health: Gastrointestinal **Strategy:** The core issue of the question is assessment data that correlates with complications of colonoscopy, such as peritonitis. Use nursing knowledge and the process of elimination to make a selection.

3 **Answer: 2** A client with an ileostomy has no control over bowel movements and must always wear a collection device. The drainage tends to be liquid but becomes pastelike with intake of specific foods.
Cognitive Level: Application **Client Need:** Physiological Integrity: Physiological Adaptation **Integrated Process:** Communication and Documentation **Content Area:** Adult Health: Gastrointestinal **Strategy:** The core issue of the question is knowledge of stool characteristics and associated stoma appliance needs following ileostomy. Use nursing knowledge and the process of elimination to make a selection.

4 **Answer: 3** Dumping syndrome, in which gastric contents rapidly enter the bowel, can occur following gastrectomy. Dietary fats and proteins are increased, and carbohydrates, especially simple carbohydrates such as fruits, are reduced. This helps slow the GI transit time and reduce the GI cramping, diarrhea, and vasomotor symptoms associated with dumping syndrome.
Cognitive Level: Application **Client Need:** Physiological Integrity: Physiological Adaptation **Integrated Process:** Nursing Process: Implementation **Content Area:** Adult Health: Gastrointestinal **Strategy:** The core issue of the question is knowledge of foods to avoid when the client has dumping syndrome. Use nursing knowledge and the process of elimination to make a selection.

5 **Answer: 1** The pain of a gastric ulcer is dull and aching, occurs after eating, and is not relieved by food as is the pain from duodenal ulcer. The pancreatic juices that are high in bicarbonate are released with food intake and relieve duodenal ulcer pain when the client eats. Chronic aspirin use is irritating to the stomach (option 2). The manifestations in options 3 and 4 are unrelated.
Cognitive Level: Application **Client Need:** Physiological Integrity: Physiological Adaptation **Integrated Process:** Nursing Process: Assessment **Content Area:** Adult Health: Gastrointestinal **Strategy:** The core issue of the question is expected assessment findings in duodenal ulcer. Recall the effect of pancreatic juices on the duodenal ulcer surface and use the process of elimination to make a selection.

6 **Answer: 1** Steatorrhea is often present in the client with Crohn's disease. Diarrhea is also key feature, but unlike ulcerative colitis, the loose stool usually does not contain blood and is usually less frequent in number of episodes.
Cognitive Level: Application **Client Need:** Physiological Integrity: Physiological Adaptation **Integrated Process:** Nursing Process: Assessment **Content Area:** Adult Health: Gastrointestinal **Strategy:** The core issue of the question is identification of common symptoms of Crohn's disease. Use nursing knowledge and the process of elimination to make a selection.

7 **Answer: 4** It is suggested that adults consume at least 100 grams of fat per day for 3 days before the test and throughout specimen collection. The other responses provide incorrect information.
Cognitive Level: Application **Client Need:** Physiological Integrity: Physiological Adaptation **Integrated Process:** Nursing Process: Planning **Content Area:** Adult Health: Gastrointestinal **Strategy:** The core issue of the question is the ability to provide correct information when teaching a client about proper preparation for fecal fat examination. Use nursing knowledge and the process of elimination to make a selection.

8 **Answer: 1** Perforation of an obstructed diverticulum can cause abscess formation or generalized peritonitis. The manifestations of peritonitis are abdominal guarding and rigidity and pain. Sigmoidoscopy is contraindicated in cases of perforation. Because treatment of this complication is beyond the scope of independent nursing practice, the physician must be notified.
Cognitive Level: Analysis **Client Need:** Physiological Integrity: Physiological Adaptation **Integrated Process:** Nursing Process:

Implementation **Content Area:** Adult Health: Gastrointestinal **Strategy:** The core issue of the question is the ability to identify the occurrence of peritonitis as a complication of diverticular disease and determine the appropriate course of action. Use nursing knowledge and the process of elimination to make a selection.

9 **Answer: 1** Lifestyle modifications can minimize symptoms of GERD. Anything that increases intra-abdominal pressure should be avoided, such as lifting weights. Obesity also aggravates symptoms, but a body mass index of 23 is normal. Being a vegetarian does not increase risk, and calcium carbonate tablets often aid in symptom relief.
Cognitive Level: Application **Client Need:** Physiological Integrity: Physiological Adaptation **Integrated Process:** Nursing Process: Analysis **Content Area:** Adult Health: Gastrointestinal **Strategy:** The core issue of the question is ability to identify risk factors that aggravate symptoms of GERD. Use nursing knowledge and the process of elimination to make a selection.

10 **Answer: 2** *H. pylori* infection is a major cause of peptic ulcers. Treatment includes eradicating *H. pylori* with antibiotics. The other responses are incorrect.
Cognitive Level: Application **Client Need:** Physiological Integrity: Physiological Adaptation **Integrated Process:** Nursing Process: Implementation **Content Area:** Adult Health: Gastrointestinal **Strategy:** The core issue of the question is knowledge of etiology of peptic ulcers, including duodenal ulcers. Use nursing knowledge and the process of elimination to make a selection.

11 **Answer: 1** Many clotting factors are produced in the liver, including fibrinogen (factor I), prothrombin (factor II), factor V, serum prothrombin conversion accelerator (factor VII), factor IX, and factor X. The client's ability to form these factors may be impaired with cirrhosis, putting the client at risk for bleeding. The prothrombin time will evaluate blood clotting ability; the others will not.
Cognitive Level: Application **Client Need:** Physiological Integrity: Physiological Adaptation **Integrated Process:** Nursing Process: Assessment **Content Area:** Adult Health: Gastrointestinal **Strategy:** The critical word in the question is *safe.* With this in mind, the correct answer is one that could detect a complication of cirrhosis. Use nursing knowledge and the process of elimination to make a selection.

12 **Answer: 3** Manifestations of chronic pancreatitis include nausea, vomiting, weight loss, flatulence, constipation, and steatorrhea (fatty stools) that result from a decrease in pancreatic enzyme secretion. Weight gain (option 1) is the opposite of what occurs with this disorder, while options 2 and 4 are unrelated.
Cognitive Level: Application **Client Need:** Physiological Integrity: Physiological Adaptation **Integrated Process:** Nursing Process: Assessment **Content Area:** Adult Health: Gastrointestinal **Strategy:** The core issue of the question is the ability to identify assessment findings that are consistent with the development of chronic pancreatitis. Use nursing knowledge and the process of elimination to make a selection.

13 **Answer: 1** Hemolytic jaundice is caused by excessive breakdown of red blood cells, and the amount of bilirubin produced exceeds the ability of the liver to conjugate it, so there is an increase in indirect bilirubin. Unconjugated bilirubin is insoluble in water and is not found in the urine.
Cognitive Level: Application **Client Need:** Physiological Integrity: Physiological Adaptation **Integrated Process:** Nursing Process: Assessment **Content Area:** Adult Health: Gastrointestinal **Strategy:** The core issue of the question is knowledge of clinical indicators of hemolytic jaundice. Use nursing knowledge and the process of elimination to make a selection.

14 **Answer: 4** Nausea and RUQ pain occur in cystic duct disease, but obstruction of the common bile duct results in reflux of bile into the liver, which produces jaundice. Alkaline phosphatase increases with biliary obstruction but cholesterol level does not increase.
Cognitive Level: Analysis **Client Need:** Physiological Integrity: Physiological Adaptation **Integrated Process:** Nursing Process: Assessment **Content Area:** Adult Health: Gastrointestinal **Strategy:** The core issue of the question is knowledge of clinical indicators of common bile duct obstruction. Think about the pathophysiology of blocked bile drainage and use the process of elimination to make a selection.

15 **Answer: 2** Obstructive biliary disease causes a significant elevation in alkaline phosphatase. Obstruction in the biliary tract causes an elevation in direct bilirubin, not indirect bilirubin (option 4). Options 1 and 3 are unrelated.
Cognitive Level: Application **Client Need:** Physiological Integrity: Physiological Adaptation **Integrated Process:** Nursing Process: Assessment **Content Area:** Adult Health: Gastrointestinal **Strategy:** Use nursing knowledge and the process of elimination to make a selection.

16 **Answer: 3** The T-tube may drain 500 mL in the first 24 hours and decreases steadily thereafter. If there is excessive drainage, the nurse should further assess the drainage to be able to describe it accurately and notify the physician immediately. Option 1 would be contraindicated; options 2 and 4 are of no help.
Cognitive Level: Application **Client Need:** Physiological Integrity: Physiological Adaptation **Integrated Process:** Nursing Process: Implementation **Content Area:** Adult Health: Gastrointestinal **Strategy:** The core issue of the question is knowledge of appropriate nursing action following notation of excessive T-tube drainage. Use nursing knowledge and the process of elimination to make a selection.

17 **Answer: 1** When T-tube drainage declines and stools return to a normal brown color, the tube can be clamped 1 to 2 hours before and after meals in preparation for tube removal. If the client tolerates clamping, the tube will then be removed.
Cognitive Level: Application **Client Need:** Physiological Integrity: Physiological Adaptation **Integrated Process:** Communication and Documentation **Content Area:** Adult Health: Gastrointestinal **Strategy:** The core issue of the question is the appropriate timeframe for use of a T-tube following gallbladder surgery. Use nursing knowledge and the process of elimination to make a selection.

18 **Answer: 1** Obstruction to portal blood flow causes a rise in portal venous pressure resulting in splenomegaly, ascites, and dilation of collateral venous channels predominantly in the paraumbilical and hemorrhoidal veins, the cardia of the stomach, and extending into the esophagus. Bleeding gums

would indicate insufficient vitamin K production in the liver. Muscle wasting commonly accompanies the poor nutritional intake commonly seen in clients with cirrhosis. Hypothermia is an unrelated finding.

Cognitive Level: Analysis **Client Need:** Physiological Integrity: Physiological Adaptation **Integrated Process:** Nursing Process: Assessment **Content Area:** Adult Health: Gastrointestinal **Strategy:** The core issue of the question is knowledge of associated findings in a client with portal hypertension. Use knowledge of the pathophysiology of the condition and the process of elimination to make a selection.

19 **Answer: 3** Spironolactone (Aldactone) is used in clients with ascites that show no improvement with bedrest and fluid restriction. It inhibits sodium reabsorption in the distal tubule and promotes potassium retention by inhibiting aldosterone. The other options do not address this rationale.

Cognitive Level: Application **Client Need:** Physiological Integrity: Pharmacological and Parenteral Therapies **Integrated Process:** Communication and Documentation **Content Area:** Adult Health: Gastrointestinal **Strategy:** The core issue of the question is knowledge of medication effects in a client with ascites. Use nursing knowledge related to pharmacology and the process of elimination to make a selection.

20 **Answer: 4** Asterixis, also called liver flap, is the flapping tremor of the hands when the arms are extended. Option 1 reflects hypocalcemia. Option 2 refers to spiderlike abdominal veins that are also commonly found in clients with cirrhosis who have portal hypertension as a complication. Option 3 is a specific odor noted in liver failure.

Cognitive Level: Application **Client Need:** Physiological Integrity: Physiological Adaptation **Integrated Process:** Nursing Process: Assessment **Content Area:** Adult Health: Gastrointestinal **Strategy:** The core issue of the question is knowledge of typical assessment findings in a client with cirrhosis. Use nursing knowledge and the process of elimination to make a selection.

21 **Answer: 3** It is a common finding that when the infant with an umbilical hernia cries, the hernia protrudes. It is not going to rupture. The family is instructed not to apply tape, straps, or coins to the umbilicus to reduce the hernia.

Cognitive Level: Application **Client Need:** Physiological Integrity: Physiological Adaptation **Integrated Process:** Communication and Documentation **Content Area:** Child Health: Gastrointestinal **Strategy:** The core issue of the question is knowledge of the consequences of umbilical hernia and knowledge of therapeutic communication techniques. Use this knowledge and the process of elimination to make a selection.

22 **Answer: 3** Pain management is a high priority following gastric surgery, and the nurse should use age-appropriate tools to assess for pain, such as the Wong FACES rating scale. A gastrostomy tube or nasogastric tube placed during surgery is kept in place to maintain gastric decompression. The child is kept NPO until bowel function returns. The use of a pH probe to measure gastric acidity is not necessary.

Cognitive Level: Application **Client Need:** Physiological Integrity: Physiological Adaptation **Integrated Process:** Nursing Process: Implementation **Content Area:** Child Health: Gastrointestinal **Strategy:** The core issue of the question is knowledge of appropriate interventions in the first 24 hours following gastric surgery. Use knowledge that the gastric tube should not be manipulated or used for feeding to eliminate some options. Use nursing knowledge of routine postoperative care and the process of elimination to make a final selection.

23 **Answer: 4** Kasai procedure is palliative, and prognosis is best if performed before 10 weeks of age. Its purpose is to achieve biliary drainage and avoid liver failure. A liver transplant is required in 80 to 90% of cases.

Cognitive Level: Analysis **Client Need:** Physiological Integrity: Physiological Adaptation **Integrated Process:** Nursing Process: Evaluation **Content Area:** Child Health: Gastrointestinal **Strategy:** The core issue of the question is knowledge of the typical success of surgery with Kasai procedure in an infant with biliary atresia. Use nursing knowledge and the process of elimination to make a selection.

24 **Answer: 1** Measuring urine specific gravity provides data about the concentration of urine and provides information regarding hydration. Urine specific gravity is elevated in dehydration and would be decreased with high fluid intake. The other tests listed are not indicated in the care of the dehydrated client.

Cognitive Level: Application **Client Need:** Physiological Integrity: Physiological Adaptation **Integrated Process:** Nursing Process: Implementation **Content Area:** Child Health: Gastrointestinal **Strategy:** The core issue of the question is dehydration and thus the correct option is one that addresses fluid balance in the body in some way. Use nursing knowledge and the process of elimination to make a selection.

25 **Answer: 3** In severe diarrhea, excess bicarbonate (base) is lost, which predisposes to metabolic acidosis. There is also carbohydrate malabsorption and depletion of glycogen stores, resulting in fat metabolism. Ketoacids are the byproducts of fat metabolism, which adds to the metabolic acidosis. It is not a respiratory problem.

Cognitive Level: Analysis **Client Need:** Physiological Integrity: Physiological Adaptation **Integrated Process:** Nursing Process: Analysis **Content Area:** Child Health: Gastrointestinal **Strategy:** The core issue of the question is the ability to correlate acid-base imbalance with a diagnosis of diarrhea. Recall that bicarbonate is a base and that the respiratory system is not directly involved to make a selection.

26 **Answer: 2** ESSR is the abbreviation for the four key steps in feeding the infant or child with cleft lip or palate. These steps are to *E*nlarge nipple; *S*timulate suck reflex; *S*wallow fluid; *R*est after each swallow. It does not refer to treatment of gastroesophageal reflux, pyloric stenosis, or Hirschsprung's disease.

Cognitive Level: Application **Client Need:** Physiological Integrity: Physiological Adaptation **Integrated Process:** Nursing Process: Analysis **Content Area:** Child Health: Gastrointestinal **Strategy:** The core issue of the question is knowledge of a feeding technique in cleft lip or palate that reduces the risk of aspiration. Use nursing knowledge and the process of elimination to make a selection.

27 **Answer: 3** It is important that any signs of infection be reported at once. After Soave procedure, the colostomy is usually closed and normal bowel function is expected (options 1 and 4). No rectal irrigations are necessary (option 2).

Cognitive Level: Application **Client Need:** Physiological Integrity: Physiological Adaptation **Integrated Process:** Nursing Process: Planning **Content Area:** Child Health: Gastrointestinal **Strategy:** The core issue of the question is knowledge of routine discharge teaching following an abdominal surgical procedure. Use nursing knowledge and the process of elimination to make a selection.

28 **Answer: 1** Acute episodes of celiac disease are characterized by bulky, frothy stools, anorexia, and irritability. Pain does not occur in waves prior to mealtimes.

Cognitive Level: Application **Client Need:** Physiological Integrity: Physiological Adaptation **Integrated Process:** Nursing Process: Assessment **Content Area:** Child Health: Gastrointestinal **Strategy:** The core issue of the question is knowledge of assessment findings in a client with celiac disease. Use nursing knowledge and the process of elimination to make a selection.

29 **Answer: 2** Parents often react to a child's illness with feelings of guilt for not recognizing the severity of the condition sooner. A response that provides emotional support and reduces parental anxiety encourages parents to feel confident in their abilities as caregiver. The other responses ignore the parent's feelings (option 1) or add to the parent's guilt or stress (options 3 and 4).

Cognitive Level: Application **Client Need:** Psychosocial Integrity **Integrated Process:** Communication and Documentation **Content Area:** Child Health: Gastrointestinal **Strategy:** The core issue of the question is the ability to formulate a therapeutic response to a parent who indicates distress about not seeking help earlier for an ill child. Use nursing knowledge of therapeutic communication skills and the process of elimination to make a selection.

30 **Answer: 3** Finger foods are helpful in encouraging children with failure to thrive to increase food intake. The parent should also be taught to encourage increased food intake and to make mealtimes regular, nonstressful, but structured family events.

Cognitive Level: Application **Client Need:** Physiological Integrity: Physiological Adaptation **Integrated Process:** Nursing Process: Planning **Content Area:** Child Health: Gastrointestinal **Strategy:** The core issue of the question is the intervention that will help to increase food intake in a child with nonorganic failure to thrive. Use nursing knowledge and the process of elimination to make a selection.

31 **Answer: 1, 2, 4** Manifestations of appendicitis often include generalized abdominal pain progressively worsening and localizing in the right lower quadrant at McBurney's point, nausea and vomiting, fever, chills, anorexia, diarrhea or acute constipation, and elevated WBC count: 15,000 to 20,000 cells/mm^3. Fatty stools and indigestion are not part of the clinical picture.

Cognitive Level: Application **Client Need:** Physiological Integrity: Physiological Adaptation **Integrated Process:** Nursing Process: Assessment **Content Area:** Child Health: Gastrointestinal **Strategy:** The core issue of the question is knowledge of manifestations that are consistent with appendicitis. Use knowledge that the affected area is the large intestine to eliminate indigestion (stomach area, too vague) and fatty stools (small intestine absorption problem).

ANSWERS & RATIONALES

Key Terms to Review

References

Ball, J., & Bindler, R. (2006). *Child health nursing: Partnering with children and families.* Upper Saddle River, NJ: Pearson Education.

Black, J., & Hawks, J. (2005). *Medical surgical nursing: Clinical management for positive outcomes* (7th ed.). St. Louis: Elsevier Science.

Corbett, J. (2004). *Laboratory tests and diagnostic procedures with nursing diagnoses* (6th ed.). Upper Saddle River, NJ: Pearson Education.

Harkreader, H., & Hogan, M. (2004). *Fundamentals of nursing: Caring and clinical judgment* (2nd ed.). St. Louis: Elsevier Science.

Ignatavicius, D., & Workman, L. (2006). *Medical-surgical nursing: Critical thinking for collaborative care* (5th ed.). Philadelphia: W. B. Saunders.

Kozier, B., Erb, G., Berman, A., & Snyder, S. (2004). *Fundamentals of nursing: Concepts, process, and practice* (7th ed.). Upper Saddle River, NJ: Pearson Education.

LeMone, P., & Burke, K. (2004). *Medical surgical nursing: Critical thinking in client care* (3rd ed.). Upper Saddle River, NJ: Pearson Education.

Porth, C. (2004). *Pathophysiology: Concepts of Altered Health States* (7th ed.). Philadelphia: Lippincott Williams & Wilkins.

Smith, S., Duell, D., & Martin, B. (2004). *Clinical nursing skills: Basic to advanced skills* (6th ed.). Upper Saddle River, NJ: Pearson Education.

Endocrine and Metabolic Disorders 61

In this chapter

Test Yourself

Are you ready for the NCLEX-RN® or course exams? Use the practice tests on the companion CD-ROM to check.

Cross reference

Other chapters relevant to this content area are

Meeting Nutritional Needs	Chapter 26
Endocrine Medications	Chapter 42
Common Laboratory Tests	Chapter 47
Common Diagnostic Tests and Procedures	Chapter 48
Fluid and Electrolyte Imbalances	Chapter 54

I. OVERVIEW OF ANATOMY AND PHYSIOLOGY OF THE ENDOCRINE SYSTEM

A. Basic structures of endocrine system

1. Exocrine glands secrete substances that reach their target tissue directly or by traveling through a duct; they include sebaceous, salivary, mammary, and sweat glands

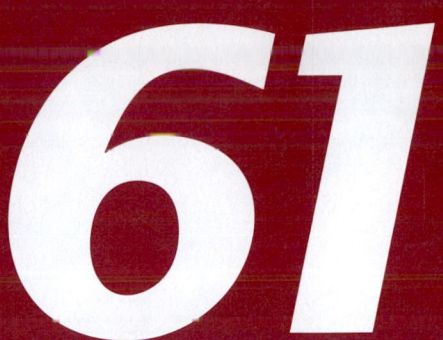

2. Endocrine glands secrete hormones directly into bloodstream to affect a variety of biological functions; neuronal stimulation, chemical substances, or hormones can control secretion of endocrine glands
3. A hormone is a biologically active substance secreted by an endocrine gland that circulates throughout body, affecting the function of one or more target organs, tissues, or bodily functions
4. Various conditions can cause endocrine glands to hypersecrete or hyposecrete, leading to altered body functions
5. **Hyposecretion** is a condition in which an insufficient amount of substance is secreted
6. **Hypersecretion** is a condition in which an excessive amount of substance is secreted

B. Basic functions of endocrine system

1. Endocrine glands: coordinate and regulate long-term changes in function of all body organs and tissues to maintain homeostasis
2. Hormones: chemical messengers that travel in circulatory system and alter cellular activities by changing enzymes and proteins in target cells
   a. **Receptor**: specially designed link on a target cell membrane or in cytoplasm for a specific hormone to contact and initiate an action response
   b. Regulation of secretion: effects on target tissue act as a negative-feedback mechanism to signal initiating gland to slow or stop secretion

C. Major endocrine system glands

1. Posterior pituitary gland: regulates fluid balance and facilitates childbirth and prostate gland function
   a. Releases antidiuretic hormone (ADH) and oxytocin, which are produced and stored in hypothalamus
   b. ADH stimulates kidneys to reabsorb water, decreasing urine output and supporting BP and blood volume; also stimulates peripheral blood vessels (BVs) to constrict
   c. Oxytocin stimulates uterus to contract for childbirth, mammary glands for milk ejection, and smooth muscles of prostate gland to contract and eject secretions
2. Anterior pituitary gland: major role is to produce and release 7 different hormones (most of which regulate secretion of other hormones): thyroid-stimulating hormone (TSH), adrenocorticotropic hormone (ACTH), follicle-stimulating hormone (FSH), luteinizing hormone (LH), prolactin (PRL), interstitial cell–stimulating hormone (ICSH), and growth hormone (GH), also called somatotropin
3. Thyroid gland: determines rate of cellular metabolism; in children, hormones are responsible for normal development of skeletal, muscular, and nervous systems
   a. Calcitonin targets bone and kidney cells to regulate calcium ion concentrations in body fluids
   b. Thyroxine (TX or tetraiodothyronine or T_4), and triiodothyronine (T_3) bind to mitochondria and nucleus of cells to increase rate of ATP production
4. Parathyroid glands: monitor and maintain circulating concentration of calcium (Ca^{++}) ions, by secreting parathyroid hormone (PTH), which increases serum Ca^{++} level; PTH stimulates osteoclasts, inhibits osteoblasts, promotes Ca^{++} absorption of calcium by intestines, and decreases renal excretion of calcium
5. Pancreas (islets of Langerhans): regulates blood glucose concentrations
   a. Alpha cells produce glucagon to break down stored fat and carbohydrate (CHO) into glucose in response to low glucose level
   b. Beta cells produce insulin to transport glucose across cell membranes
   c. Delta cells produce somatostatin that inhibits production of glucagons and insulin
6. Adrenal medulla: increases cellular energy use and muscular strength endurance, and mobilizes energy reserves
   a. Secretes epinephrine (adrenaline) and norepinephrine (noradrenaline); receptors are on skeletal muscle fibers, adipose tissues, and liver
   b. Mobilizes glycogen reserves, metabolizes glucose for ATP, and increases cardiac rate and force of contraction
7. Adrenal cortex: hormones play a vital role for survival and affect metabolism of many different tissues

a. Glucocorticoids: cortisol (hydrocortisone), corticosterone, and cortisone stimulate most cells to increase rate of glucose synthesis, glycogen formation, release of fatty acids, and break down fatty acids; exert an anti-inflammatory effect to suppress immune system
b. Mineralocorticoids: aldosterone stimulates kidneys to increase reabsorption of sodium (Na^+ and water, and reduces Na^+ and water loss by sweat glands, salivary glands, and digestive tract
c. Small amount of androgens

8. Female gonads (ovaries): regulate secondary sexual characteristics and reproduction
   a. Estrogens stimulate most cells to develop secondary sex characteristics and behaviors, follicle maturation, and growth of uterine lining
   b. Provide negative feedback to anterior pituitary gland to stop FSH secretion
   c. Progestins stimulate uterus to prepare for implantation and mammary glands for lactation
9. Male gonads (testes): regulate secondary sexual characteristics and reproduction
   a. Androgens, primarily testosterone, stimulate most cells for protein synthesis, maturation of sperm, secondary sexual characteristics and behaviors
   b. Inhibin secreted for negative feedback to anterior pituitary gland to stop secretion of FSH

II. DIAGNOSTIC TESTS AND ASSESSMENTS OF THE ENDOCRINE SYSTEM

A. **Computed tomography (CT) scan:** with or without contrast; see also Chapter 48

B. **Studies of pituitary gland**
1. Serum studies include GH or somatotropin, somatomedin C, GH release post-exercise, insulin-induced hypoglycemia, prolactin level, gonadotropin levels (FSH, LH), and water-deprivation test
2. Radiologic studies include skull x-ray to detect the integrity of the bone and tumors of the bone, CT scan, and magnetic resonance imaging (MRI) to outline organ structure, tumors, edema and infarcts, blood flow patterns, and blood vessel integrity

C. **Studies of thyroid gland**
1. ! Serum studies
   a. L-thyroxine (total T_4): measures both free and protein-bound thyroxine; normal is 4.5 to 10.9 mcg/dL in adults
   b. Free T_4 is amount of thyroxine not bound to globulins; normal values are 0.8 to 2.7 ng/ml by actual assay or 4.6 to 11.2 by calculated method
   c. Triiodothyronine (T_3) (normal value 60–181 ng/dL), also called T_3 RIA, T_3 resin uptake (T_3RU)
   d. Additional tests are TSH or thyrotropin (normal value 0.5–5.0 units/mL) and serum calcitonin
2. Radiologic studies include thyroid scan or radioactive isotope uptake study to determine uptake of radionuclide by thyroid gland, and whole body scan to detect metastasis from a known malignant thyroid tumor

D. **Studies of parathyroid glands**
1. Serum studies
   a. PTH, which regulates serum Ca^{++} and phosphorus
   b. Total Ca^{++} (including free Ca^{++} and Ca^{++} bound to plasma proteins)
   c. Phosphorus: reported as phosphorus (P) or phosphate (PO_4) and 1,25 Dihydroxyvitamin D
2. Radiologic studies include skeletal x-ray and CT scan

E. **Studies of adrenal glands**
1. Serum cortisol: secreted by adrenal cortex, a larger amount in morning, then decreasing during day
2. Serum and/or urinary aldosterone: a mineralocorticoid secreted by adrenal cortex
3. Serum ACTH stimulation to confirm suspected disease of adrenal cortex
4. Dexamethasone suppression and metyrapone suppression

5. Urinary 17-Ketosteroids (17 KS): 24-hour urine is collected to measure amount of 17 KS or metabolites of steroids produced by adrenal cortex and testes
6. Vanillylmandelic acid (VMA): a metabolite of catecholamines
   a. A 24-hour urine is collected in bottle containing HCL (a strong acid) obtained from lab
   b. Warn client about acid in bottle, to keep face away from opening when removing cap to add urine, and to avoid inhaling odor from bottle
   c. Instruct client to avoid exposure to stress or exercise
   d. Check with lab about specific foods to be avoided during testing period
   e. If possible client should not take any medication for 7 days before and during testing period
   f. Record BP, height, and weight on lab slip

F. **Studies of pancreas**
1. Fasting blood glucose (FBG) levels or fasting plasma glucose; withhold food and insulin for at least 8 hours, (water is permitted); adult reference value: 70 to 110 mg/dL (whole blood: 60–100 mg/dL), elderly 70 to 120 mg/dL
2. Oral glucose tolerance test (GTT): tests for transitional gestational glucose intolerance; medications, infection, trauma, bedrest, and stress can alter results; see Chapter 47
3. Capillary glucose monitoring
   a. Warm extremity to encourage vasodilation; select digit to be used
   b. Cleanse site with soap and water or 70% alcohol; dry with a gauze sponge
   c. Avoid squeezing site to enhance blood flow since squeezing causes dilution with tissue fluid
   d. Avoid touching skin with reagent strip; skin oils may affect results
   e. Elevate digit and apply gentle pressure with dry sterile gauze to site until bleeding stops
4. **Glycosylated hemoglobin:** prolonged **hyperglycemia** causes glucose to bind irreversibly to hemoglobin (Hgb) of red blood cell (RBC) for remaining life of RBC; HgbA1c determines diabetic control of blood glucose over past 3 to 5 weeks, generally; see Chapter 47, Table 47–3 for expected values
5. Urine studies
   a. Ketones: metabolic end-product of fatty acid metabolism; body uses fatty acids for energy when there is insufficient supply of glucose; ketones should be absent in urine (negative)
   b. Acetone: metabolite of fatty acid metabolism; should be absent in urine (negative)

III. GROWTH HORMONE DEFICIENCY (HYPOPITUITARISM)

A. **Overview:** a disorder caused by deficiency of growth hormone (GH) from pituitary gland; may be inherited or caused by infection, pituitary gland infarction (such as in sickle cell disease), tumor, cranial irradiation, and psychosocial deprivation

B. **Nursing assessment**
1. Normal weight and length at birth
2. Below third percentile on growth chart by 1 year of age
3. Infants: hypoglycemic seizures, hyponatremia, neonatal jaundice, pale optic discs, and in males, micropenis and undescended testicles
4. Children: overweight, hyperglycemia, high-pitched voice, delayed dentition, "ripply" abdominal fat, decreased muscle mass and skeletal maturation, and decreased sexual maturation
5. Low levels of IGF-1 (insulin-like growth hormone) on screening test

C. **Therapeutic management**
1. Treatment of underlying disorder if present
2. GH therapy by subcutaneous injection 3 to 7 times weekly until acceptable height is reached or growth velocity drops to less than 2 cm (1 in.) per year
3. Monitor growth and document on growth chart at periodic health checkups (every 3 to 4 months)

D. Client and family teaching

1. Medication therapy: how to administer injections and information about course of therapy
2. Close monitoring and follow-up is important
3. Medication therapy is expensive, but drug companies may provide assistance if insurance is insufficient
4. Child can experience disturbed body image; use age-appropriate communication and style of dress (rather than according to body size)

IV. HYPERPITUITARISM

A. Overview: excessive secretion of GH that leads to gigantism (in children before long bone epiphyseal closure) or acromegaly (in adults after epiphyseal closure)

! **B. Nursing assessment**

1. Tall stature if onset in childhood
2. Large hands and feet with prominent jawbone
3. Joint changes consistent with arthritis
4. Deep voice and possible dysphagia
5. Hypertension
6. Organomegaly
7. Skin changes leading to rough, oily texture

C. Therapeutic management

1. Assess for disturbed body image and provide emotional support to client and family
2. Provide measures to relieve joint pain
3. Possible radiation therapy to pituitary gland
4. Possible hypophysectomy (see next section)

D. Hypophysectomy

1. Transphenoidal hypophysectomy may be used to resect pituitary gland
2. Provide standard preoperative care
3. ! Teach client about measures used to prevent rises in intracranial pressure (ICP) following surgery (see also Chapter 58)
4. ! Postoperative care
   a. Monitor vital signs (VS), level of consciousness (LOC), and elements of neurological status
   b. Keep head of bed elevated to approximately 30 degrees
   c. Assess "mustache" dressing taped under nose for drainage and test drainage for glucose to rule out cerebrospinal fluid (CSF) leakage
   d. Assess for postnasal drip, which could also indicate CSF leakage
   e. Monitor intake and output (I & O) and assess for signs of diabetes insipidus (DI; water intoxication) as temporary postoperative complication; see next section
   f. Keep oral mucous membranes moist; drying can occur because nasal packing after transphenoidal surgery can lead to mouth-breathing
5. Client teaching
   a. ! Avoid activities that raise ICP, such as bending, lifting, sneezing, coughing, blowing nose, and any activity that closes glottis (Valsalva maneuver)
   b. Medication teaching, including analgesics and possible antibiotic postoperatively, and possible hormone replacement therapy if entire gland is surgically removed

V. SYNDROME OF INAPPROPRIATE ANTIDIURETIC HORMONE (SIADH)

A. Overview

1. An excessive amount of serum ADH resulting in water intoxication and hyponatremia (serum Na^+ less than 135 mEq/L)
   a. Usual feedback mechanism does not function to decrease posterior pituitary secretion of ADH with decreased serum osmolality
   b. Elevated ADH leads to renal reabsorption of water and suppression of the renin-angiotensin mechanism, causing renal excretion of Na^+

c. Renal excretion of Na^+ leads to water intoxication, cellular edema, and dilutional hyponatremia
2. Causes include certain hormone-secreting malignant tumors; injury, infection, and medications; increased intrathoracic pressure that stimulates aortic baroreceptors; and activation of limbic system from trauma, pain, stress, and acute psychosis

B. Nursing assessment

1. General manifestations of fluid volume excess, possibly including increased BP pressure, crackles auscultated in lung fields, distended jugular neck veins, taut skin, and intake greater than output
2. Clinical manifestations: headache, fatigue, anorexia, nausea, muscle aches, abdominal cramps, weight gain without edema, progressive altered LOC, seizures, coma, and small amounts of concentrated amber-colored urine
3. Diagnostic and laboratory test findings: high urine osmolality (>1200 mOsm/kg H_2O) and specific gravity higher than 1.032, low serum osmolality (<275 mOsm/kg), and decreased hematocrit, BUN and serum Na^+

C. Therapeutic management

1. Restrict oral fluids, including ice chips, to 80 mL/day to prevent further hemodilution
2. Supplement Na^+ intake orally or by hypertonic saline IV infusion
3. Flush all enteral and gastric tubes with normal saline instead of water to replace Na^+ and prevent further hemodilution
4. Monitor I & O accurately
5. Monitor for low serum Na^+, BUN, and urine osmolality and specific gravity
6. Weigh daily; a weight loss of 2.2 pounds (1 kilogram) indicates a loss of approximately 1 L of fluid
7. Assess for changes in LOC, mentation, cognition, nutrition, muscle twitching, and comfort
8. Medication therapy: IV hypertonic saline (3%) and demeclocycline (Declomycin) to replace electrolytes; diuretics to eliminate excessive fluid

D. Client teaching

1. SIADH and symptoms to report
2. Medication may be lifelong depending on cause
3. Identify hidden sources of water and fluids, such as ice and ice cream, to prevent accidental excessive intake
   a. Plan meal pattern and maintain fluid limitation and Na^+ prescription
   b. Weigh daily on same scale and report gain of 2 pounds in 1 day

VI. DIABETES INSIPIDUS (DI)

A. Overview

1. Results from excessive loss of water caused by hyposecretion of ADH or kidneys' inability to respond to ADH
2. Subsequent **polyuria** (excessive urine output ranging from 4 to 30 L in 24 hours) can lead to severe dehydration if client does not replace lost water
3. Causes can be neurogenic (insufficient ADH secretion by posterior pituitary gland), nephrogenic (kidneys unable to respond to ADH), and medications (lithium carbonate and demeclocycline can cause kidneys to alter response to ADH)
4. Primary DI results from an inherited or idiopathic malfunction of posterior pituitary gland
5. Secondary DI is caused by brain tumors, head trauma, infection, surgery on or near pituitary gland, metastatic tumors from lung or breast, cerebrovascular hemorrhage, granulomatous disease, or cerebral aneurysm

B. Nursing assessment

1. History of head injury, brain surgery, infection, or tumor
2. Obtain a list of current and past medications
3. Assess LOC, VS including orthostatic BP, skin turgor, I & O, weight, skin integrity, **polydipsia** (excessive thirst), tenting or sagging skin, bowel sounds, constipation

4. Clinical manifestations: polyuria; excessive thirst; dry, tented skin; dry mucous membranes; and severe hypotension leading to cardiovascular collapse (which can occur if the excessive water loss is not replaced)
5. Diagnostic and laboratory test findings: urine specific gravity less than 1.005, urine osmolality less than 300 mOsm/kg, positive water deprivation test, reduced serum ADH level in primary DI, serum sodium higher than 145 mEq/L

C. Therapeutic management

1. Water replacement orally is preferred or intravenous (IV) D_5W as needed to normalize lab values
2. For neurogenic DI, hormone replacement with desmopressin (DDAVP), a synthetic vasopressin; adjunctive medications, such as chlorpropamide (Diabinese), or carbamazepine (Tegretol), may increase ADH release or enhance effect of ADH on renal collecting duct
3. For nephrogenic DI, correct underlying disease or stop causative medication; begin a low-salt, low-protein diet to decrease net excretion of solute
4. Monitor I & O hourly; report urine output over 200 mL/hour for 2 consecutive hours or 500 mL over 2 hours; assess for continence and provide easy access to bathroom as appropriate
5. Weigh daily; report weight loss
6. Monitor urine specific gravity and report if it decreases; monitor serum osmolality and Na^+ for increases
7. Encourage fluid intake greater than urine output; provide fluids within reach at all times; provide IV fluid replacement as ordered
8. Use skin protective barriers with incontinence

D. Client teaching

1. Information about DI, self-administration of medication, and possible need for lifelong medication
2. Wear a Medic-Alert bracelet listing DI and treatments
3. Drink fluid equal to amount of urine output, keeping a log of I & O
4. Weigh self daily, on same scale at same time of day, and report weight loss
5. Consult practitioner before taking over-the-counter (OTC) medications

VII. HYPERTHYROIDISM (GRAVES' DISEASE)

A. Overview

1. Excessive secretion of thyroid hormone (TH) from thyroid gland leads to increased basal metabolic rate, cardiovascular function, GI function, neuromuscular function, weight loss, and heat intolerance; thyroid hormone affects metabolism of fats, carbohydrates (CHOs), and proteins
2. Hyperthyroidism can be caused by excess secretion of TSH from pituitary gland, autoimmune reaction (Graves' disease), thyroiditis (inflammation or viral infection of thyroid), tumor, and excessive dose of supplemental thyroid hormone

B. Nursing assessment

1. Clinical manifestations: range from very minimal to severe depending on amount and time period of hypersecretion
2. **Thyroid crisis** or **thyroid storm:** life-threatening emergency occurring in extreme hyperthyroidism; usually occurs in clients with long-term, untreated hyperthyroidism or in clients with hyperthyroidism experiencing a stressor such as infection, trauma, or manipulation of thyroid gland
3. Common manifestations of thyroid storm are temperature over 102°F (39°C), tachycardia, systolic hypertension, abdominal pain, nausea, vomiting, diarrhea, agitation, tremors, confusion, and seizures
4. Include in overall assessment: health history, vital signs, neck (for goiter), eyes (exophthalmos or bulging) tachycardia, possible hypertension, signs of hypermetabolism (hyperthermia, hunger, heat intolerance), diarrhea, weight loss over weeks, and fluid balance
5. Diagnostic and laboratory test findings: elevated serum T_3, T_4, free T_4; decreased TSH; positive RAI uptake scan and thyroid scan (depending on cause)

C. Therapeutic management

1. Consists of medical treatment or surgical removal of part of thyroid gland (partial or total thyroidectomy)
2. Ethionamide drugs for life to reduce secretion of thyroid hormone
3. Ablative therapy with radioactive Iodine 131: thyroid gland absorbs I-131, which destroys some thyroid cells over a period of 6 to 8 weeks
   a. Not recommended for pregnant women
   b. Radiation precautions are not required for small doses (<30 mCi) of I-131
   c. Instruct client to drink solution with straw to minimize exposure to buccal cavity
   d. Monitor lab values, report weight gain, fatigue, decreased pulse, and lowered BP
   e. Total or subtotal (partial) thyroidectomy may be indicated based on situation
4. Preoperative preparation for thyroidectomy
   a. Teach deep-breathing exercises and appropriate cough
   b. Instruct client to hold hands behind neck when coughing, sitting, turning, or getting up/back to bed to reduce postoperative pain and neck muscle strain
   c. Instruct client on self-administration of prescribed antithyroid drugs to decrease vascularity and size of thyroid and minimize risk of surgical hemorrhage
5. Postoperative care following thyroidectomy
   a. Provide comfort: analgesics, position client in semi-Fowler's position with neck and head supported by pillows to prevent muscle strain, ice collar to wound area for comfort and to prevent edema
   b. Monitor for hemorrhage: tightness of dressing; sanguineous exudate on anterior or posterior neck dressing or on skin of neck, upper chest and upper back, shoulders, and back of neck; auscultate trachea for stridor (indicating edema and narrowed airway); first 24 hours postoperative is time of greatest risk
   c. Promote patent airway: keep head of bed elevated 30 degrees; assess for respiratory distress; keep oral and sterile suction supplies and emergency tracheostomy tray (with tracheostomy kit and IV calcium gluconate or calcium chloride) within immediate access; maintain humidification of inspired air if ordered; encourage deep-breathing exercises and incentive spirometer hourly; cough only if needed to clear secretions
   d. Prevent tetany by early identification of hypocalcemia (serum calcium less than 8 mg/dL) evidenced by numbness or tingling of toes, extremities, and lips; muscle twitches; positive Chvostek's and Trousseau signs; see also Chapter 54
   e. Maintain patent IV site
   f. Assess for laryngeal nerve damage, noting ability to speak loudly, quality and tone of voice (hoarseness may be temporary after surgery)
   g. Analgesics to control surgical pain

D. Client teaching

1. Correct self-administration of medications and that medication use is lifelong with medical treatment
2. Hyperthyroidism, hypothyroidism, and symptoms to report
3. Conditions to report, including signs of hemorrhage, hypocalcemia, incisional infection, respiratory difficulty and discomfort
4. For exophthalmos, instruct client on methods to protect eyes and adapt to altered visual field
   a. Have regular eye exams
   b. Call practitioner immediately for any change in vision or appearance of eye; closure of eyelids; eye pain; eye exudate, or **photophobia** (sensitivity to light)
   c. Protect eyes with tinted glasses or eye shields because lids do not cover eyes completely and corneal/blink reflex may be delayed
   d. Moisten eyes frequently with artificial tears to prevent dry irritation and corneal infection; use caution not to contaminate eyedropper
   e. Soothe dry-eye irritation with cool, moist compresses
   f. Sleep with head of bed elevated to minimize pressure on optic nerve, and wear eye patches to protect eyes during sleep if lids do not close
5. Surgical client
   a. Surgical procedure and expected outcomes

! b. Support neck with hands; position neck and head with pillows and maintain semi-Fowler's position; avoid hyperextension and sudden quick movements of head and neck

c. Wound care

! d. Avoid/minimize talking and coughing until wound is healed to prevent strain on laryngeal nerve and vocal cords

6. Assist client to cope with lifestyle and self-image changes

VIII. HYPOTHYROIDISM

A. Overview

1. Insufficient amount of TH is secreted by thyroid gland, causing decreased metabolic rate, decreased heat production, and various effects on body systems
2. Primary hypothyroidism accounts for 99% of all cases, and 50% of cases are caused by cell-mediated and antibody-mediated destruction of thyroid gland
3. Other causes are thyroiditis, subacute postpartum, external irradiation of gland, iatrogenic (30% to 40%), infections, iodine deficiency, congenital or idiopathic
4. Secondary hypothyroidism, also called central hypothyroidism, is caused by insufficient secretion of TSH from pituitary gland or related to disease of hypothalamus
5. Thyroid gland gradually enlarges, forming a goiter (thickening of gland) in an attempt to secrete more thyroid hormone

! B. Nursing assessment

1. Lethargy and diminished reflexes
2. Periorbital edema
3. Bradycardia and possible dysrhythmias, hypotension, constipation
4. Reproductive problems (menorrhagia and infertility in females and decreased libido in males)
5. Coarse dry hair that is easily lost and coarse dry skin
6. Signs of slowed metabolism (hypothermia, fatigue, weight gain, anorexia)
7. Anemia and elevated serum lipids
8. Myxedema (a life-threatening crisis state of hypothyroidism): non-pitting edema in connective tissues throughout body, puffy face and tongue, severe metabolic disorders, hypothermia, cardiovascular collapse, and coma
9. Diagnostic and laboratory test findings: varies according to whether cause is thyroid gland or pituitary; may include decreased T_4 and free T_4, normal T_3, and increased TSH levels

! C. Therapeutic management

1. Medication therapy: thyroid hormone replacement, such as dessicated thyroid, thyroxine (Synthroid), or triiodothyronine (Cytomel)
2. Give medication in morning 1 hour before food intake or 2 hours after food intake to facilitate absorption
3. Adjust environmental temperature and use blankets as needed for comfort; chilling increases metabolic rate, cardiac workload, and O_2 demand
4. Pace activities with rest periods; instruct client to report shortness of breath, fatigue, dizziness, or any discomfort
5. Encourage intake of 2,000 mL water daily and a high-fiber diet to promote regular bowel movements

D. Client teaching

1. Disorder and its management
2. Importance of wearing a Medic-Alert bracelet
3. ! Medication is needed for life and should be taken at same time every morning, 1 hr before a meal or 2 hrs after a meal
4. Take same brand of medication because brands vary in chemical properties and bioavailability
5. ! Report weight gain or loss of 5 pounds, activity intolerance, chest pain, heat or cold intolerance, and sleep pattern disturbance
6. Report symptoms of hypothyroidism and hyperthyroidism

IX. HYPERPARATHYROIDISM

A. Overview

1. Results from increased PTH secretion from parathyroid gland
2. Primary hyperparathyroidism: hyperplasia or tumor of one of parathyroid glands, increasing absorption of Ca^{++} in GI tract
3. Secondary hyperparathyroidism: gland enlargement caused by chronic hypocalcemia in presence of elevated PTH
4. Increased reabsorption of calcium and increased excretion of phosphate lead to hypercalcemia and hypophosphatemia
5. Kidneys increase bicarbonate excretion and decrease acid excretion, leading to metabolic acidosis and hypokalemia
6. Bones increase rate of Ca^{++} and phosphorus release, leading to bone decalcification
7. Hypercalcemia causes Ca^{++} deposits in soft tissues, renal calculi, altered neurological function with muscle weakness and atrophy, altered GI function with constipation, abdominal pain, anorexia, and altered cardiovascular system

B. Nursing assessment

1. Polyuria (early sign) and renal calculi
2. Anorexia, constipation, nausea, vomiting, abdominal pain (from peptic ulcer disease)
3. Generalized bone pain, pathologic fractures, and muscle weakness and atrophy
4. ! CNS signs (depressed deep tendon reflexes, **paresthesias** [altered sensations], depression, psychosis)
5. Elevated serum Ca^{++} and PTH; decreased phosphate
6. Possible bone changes on skeletal x-rays and CT scan

C. Therapeutic management

1. ! Decrease serum Ca^{++} level with IV normal saline (NS) infusions, diuretics, and phosphate replacement
2. Possible surgery to remove involved parathyroid glands
3. Promote comfort and safety; client may need to use walker to prevent falls
4. Strain all urine to detect calcium-based urinary stones
5. ! Provide 2,000 to 3,000 mL of fluids daily as tolerated and a high-fiber diet
6. Encourage progressive activity as tolerated, pacing activity with rest periods
7. Promote nutrition and fluid and electrolyte balance; weigh daily
8. ! Assess for hypocalcemia to prevent tetany caused by surgery (removal of parathyroid gland) or aggressive excretion of Ca^{++}
   - **a.** Numbness and tingling around mouth and fingertips
   - **b.** Muscle twitching of extremities
   - **c.** Change in voice
   - **d.** Positive Chvostek sign (spasm of facial muscles when cheek touched) and Trousseau sign (spasm of hand when BP cuff inflated)
9. Medication therapy: analgesics to control pain; diuretics and NS by IV infusion to excrete excess calcium; phosphate and calcitonin (Miacalcin) may be used to inhibit bone reabsorption

D. Client teaching

1. Hyperparathyroidism and appropriate self-administration of medications
2. Symptoms to report, including those indicating hypocalcemia, activity intolerance, and infection

X. HYPOPARATHYROIDISM

A. Overview

1. Low PTH levels causing hypocalcemia, usually caused by surgical removal of all or part of gland
2. Hypocalcemia raises threshold for excitability in nerve and muscle fibers, causing fibers to be easily stimulated; could lead to life-threatening tetany

B. Nursing assessment

1. GI symptoms: abdominal pain, nausea, vomiting, diarrhea, anorexia
2. ! Signs of hypocalcemia (anxiety, headaches, paresthesia, neuromuscular irritability with tremors and muscle spasms); positive Chvostek's or Trousseau's sign

3. Possible difficulty swallowing or hoarse voice, sensation of tightness in throat
4. Dry thin hair, patchy hair loss, ridged finger nails
5. Decreased serum PTH, total calcium, free calcium; increased serum phosphate

C. Therapeutic management

1. Supplemental Ca^{++} and vitamin D
2. Promote comfort and safety; client may need to use walker to prevent falls
3. Encourage progressive activity as tolerated, pacing activity with rest periods
4. Promote nutrition and fluid and electrolyte balance
5. Medication therapy: Ca^{++} supplement orally or by IV infusion; vitamin D orally to promote intestinal absorption of Ca^{++}

D. Client teaching

1. Disorder and its management, to wear Medic-Alert bracelet listing disease and medications, and self-administration of medication
2. Symptoms to report (see again nursing assessment)
3. Diet high in Ca^{++} and vitamin D, identifying minimum daily intake; foods high in calcium are cheese, milk, turnip greens, almonds, collard greens, beans, peanuts, frankfurters, and bologna

XI. CUSHING'S DISEASE

A. Overview

1. Hyperfunction of adrenal cortex (AC) causing elevated serum cortisol or ACTH levels
2. Elevated serum cortisol causes life-threatening changes in physiological, psychological, and metabolic functioning
3. Incidence is greater in women; usual age of onset is 30 to 40 years
4. Primary Cushing's disease is caused by a tumor of adrenal cortex
5. Secondary Cushing's disease is caused by disorder of pituitary or hypothalamus (causing increased ACTH and hyperplasia of adrenal cortex) or by an ectopic tissue (such as an ACTH-producing cancer of lung, bronchus, or pancreas)
6. Iatrogenic: long-term use of glucocorticoid medication such as steroids

B. Nursing assessment

1. Generalized weakness with muscle wasting
2. Thin skin that bruises easily, striae, and hirsutism
3. Skin infections or poor wound healing
4. Emotional lability (mood swings)
5. Hypertension
6. Fluid overload and weight gain
7. Osteoporosis
8. Abnormal fat deposits (truncal obesity, moon facies, fat pad on back of neck)
9. Possible amenorrhea, impotence, or decreased libido
10. Elevated serum cortisol, Na^{+}, and glucose, and lowered Ca^{++} and potassium (K^{+})
11. Serum ACTH can be elevated or decreased; positive ACTH suppression test
12. Elevated urine 17 KS; normal BUN

C. Therapeutic management

1. Possible radiation therapy to pituitary gland
2. Single or bilateral adrenalectomy or hypophysectomy (removal of pituitary gland)
3. Assist client to achieve fluid, electrolyte, glucose, and calcium balance
4. Analyze daily weights and I & O
5. Promote safety: uncluttered walking area, adequate lighting, assistive walking devices to prevent falls as needed, and use of stable, nonskid shoes or slippers
6. Assist client to pace activities and rest to prevent fatigue
7. Prevent infection before and after surgery: use standard precautions, provide aseptic wound care, and promote optimal nutrition
8. Assist client to use effective coping strategies and encourage client to discuss feelings about change in physical appearance
9. Preoperative care: ensure that client understands planned surgical procedure, postoperative routines, and expected outcomes

10. Postoperative care
    a. Promote effective breathing pattern by encouraging hourly coughing and deep-breathing exercises (clients with pituitary removal should avoid coughing)
    b. Assist with turning and repositioning every 2 hours, and encourage ankle dorsiflexion exercises hourly
    c. Promote wound healing by minimizing stress on incision line
    d. After adrenalectomy, client should log roll to side to sit up at bedside and should do the reverse to recline
    e. Follow principles of postoperative care discussed previously if client underwent removal of pituitary gland
    f. Keep head of bed elevated 30 degrees, and use aseptic technique for wound care
11. Prevent Addisonian crisis: give NS by IV infusion bolus and cortisol per practitioner's order for following symptoms: dry, tenting skin; decreased BP; increased pulse; decreased LOC; anorexia; and weakness
12. Medication therapy: may include metapyrone (directly inhibits cortisol production and secretion by adrenal cortex); octreotide (Sandostatin), a somatostatin analog that suppresses ACTH secretion; and mitotane (Lysodren), which suppresses function of AC and decreases metabolism of corticosteroids, thus decreasing serum cortisol

D. Client teaching
1. The disorder of Cushing's disease and its management
2. To wear Medic-Alert bracelet listing disease and medications
3. Self-administration of medication
4. Eat a diet high in protein and vitamins B and C to support immune system, and also take supplemental K^+ and Ca^{++}
5. Wound care and postoperative cortisol replacement for surgical clients (temporary replacement for 1 year or less for unilateral adrenalectomy; lifelong if surgery is bilateral)

XII. ADRENAL INSUFFICIENCY (ADDISON'S DISEASE)

A. Overview
1. Insufficient level of cortisol resulting from autoimmune disorder, tuberculosis, septicemia, acquired immunodeficiency syndrome (AIDS), bilateral adrenalectomy, infiltrative diseases, and sudden cessation of long-term high-dose steroid medication
2. Decreased aldosterone and cortisol levels lead to hyponatremia, hyperkalemia (high serum K^+), decreased extracellular fluid, decreased intravascular volume, decreased gluconeogenesis, hypoglycemia, and stress intolerance
3. High ACTH level leads to hyperpigmentation

B. Nursing assessment
1. Hyperpigmentation of skin (eternal tan)
2. Delayed wound healing
3. Cardiovascular changes (tachycardia, dysrhythmias, postural hypotension)
4. Dehydration and hypovolemia, weight loss
5. Anorexia, nausea, vomiting, diarrhea
6. Depression, lethargy, emotional lability, confusion
7. Muscle weakness and tremors, and muscle and joint pain
8. Addisonian crisis: a life-threatening response to sudden withdrawal of steroids or exposure to any form of stress, manifested by severe hypotension, circulatory collapse, shock, and coma
9. Decreased serum cortisol, glucose, Na^+, and urine 17 KS
10. Increased serum K^+, BUN, and ACTH levels
11. No increase in cortisol with ACTH stimulation test
12. CT scan can be positive

C. Therapeutic management
1. Maintain fluid and electrolyte balance: analyze lab values, I & O, and daily weight; encourage 3,000 mL of daily oral fluid intake and added Na^+ in diet

2. Promote safety: appropriate walking assistive devices, adequate lighting, clear area for walking, and appropriate slippers or shoes
3. Medication therapy: hydrocortisone (Cortef) to replace cortisol; fludrocortisone (Florinef) to replace mineralocorticoids as needed

D. Client education

1. Addison's disease and symptoms to report (weight gain, easy bruising or bleeding, weakness, dizziness, lethargy, epigastric discomfort, and change in BP or pulse)
2. Need for lifelong medication and disease management
3. Need to consult practitioner before taking any OTC medications
4. Self-administration of medication, and plan for medication adjustment upward during times of stress
5. Wear Medic-Alert bracelet listing Addison's disease, medications, and contact numbers
6. Diet to promote immune system function and foods to high in Na^+ and low in K^+ (see also Chapter 54)

XIII. DIABETES MELLITUS (DM)

A. Overview

1. Disorder of pancreas characterized by insufficient or absolute lack of insulin production, causing hyperglycemia (elevated blood glucose) and resulting in multisystem changes in health status
2. Type 1: results from autoimmune destruction of beta cells; has a genetic predisposition; is more common in males; can occur at any age but usually occurs in children and adolescents; is also characterized by hyperglycemia and **ketosis** (ketones in blood resulting from gluconeogenesis from fats)
3. Type 2: exact cause remains unknown; several theories are presented, including compromised ability of beta cells to respond to hyperglycemia, abnormal insulin receptors on cells, and peripheral insulin resistance; it has a genetic predisposition, can occur at any age, and is more common in obesity, older adults, African Americans, Hispanic Americans, and Native Americans
4. Acute complications include hypoglycemia, diabetic ketoacidosis, and hyperglycemic hyperosmolar nonketotic (HHNK) coma, also called hyperosmolar coma (HOC) in type 2
5. Long-term or chronic complications
    a. Neurologic: somatic neuropathies (paresthesias, pain, and loss of sensation and motor control) and visceral neuropathies (pupil constriction, fixed heart rate, constipation or diarrhea, dysfunction of sweat glands, incomplete voiding, and sexual dysfunction)
    b. Sensory: cataracts, glaucoma, and diabetic retinopathy
    c. Cardiovascular: orthostatic hypotension, accelerated atherosclerosis leading to stroke, myocardial infarction (MI), and peripheral vascular disease (PVD), increased blood viscosity, and platelet disorders
    d. Renal: hypertension, edema, albuminuria, and chronic renal failure
    e. Integumentary: atrophic changes, foot ulcers or gangrene
    f. Immune: poor healing, periodontal disease, lung infections, chronic skin infections, urinary trac tinfections, vaginits

B. Nursing assessment

1. Type 1: polyuria, polydipsia (excess fluid intake), **polyphagia** (increased food intake), weight loss, malaise, and fatigue
2. Type 2: polyuria, polydipsia, blurred vision, fatigue, paresthesia (numbness, tingling, sensitivity), and skin infections
3. Elevated random and/or fasting blood glucose (BG)
4. Abnormal oral glucose tolerance test
5. Elevated glycosylated hemoglobin
6. Positive serum ketones and possible urine ketones or acetone with ketoacidosis

C. Therapeutic management

1. Diet

a. Follow diet recommended in MyPyramid or exchange system diet from American Diabetes Association
b. Caloric intake is based on individual needs, including possible weight loss needs for type 2 DM
c. CHO in amounts tailored to individual need, avoiding simple sugars
d. Protein at 10% to 20% of caloric intake
e. Saturated fat less than 10% of calories with cholesterol intake equal to or less than 300 mg/day
f. Sodium intake 2,400 to 3,000 mg/day (same as for general population)
g. Dietary fiber 20 to 35 gm/day
h. Tailor diet to individual and cultural preferences whenever possible to increase adherence

! 2. Oral antidiabetic medications
a. Used in type 2 DM only and indicated when diet and exercise alone fail to control BG levels
b. Consist of oral sulfonylureas, alpha-glucosidase inhibitor, biguanides, and a miscellaneous agent; see also Chapter 42
c. Instruct clients taking oral sulfonylureas that concurrent use of alcohol can cause a disulfiram-type reaction (hypoglycemia, flushing, headache, nausea, and abdominal cramps)
d. Instruct client about risk of metabolic acidosis and to discuss with primary care provider about need to discontinue medicine if severe diarrhea, infection, or dehydration occur
e. Instruct all clients about manifestations of both hyperglycemia and hypoglycemia, and appropriate corrective actions

! 3. Insulin therapy
a. Is used in type 1 DM or when diet, exercise, and oral agents are insufficient to control type 2 DM
b. Different insulin preparations are available to maintain near-normal blood glucose levels; insulin is classified according to source, onset, peak, and duration of action
c. Source: human insulin has a faster onset of action, a shorter peak, and a shorter duration than animal derived insulin; it is preferred to pork or beef insulin (higher incidence of allergic reaction)
d. Preparations: include rapid-acting (e.g., Insulin lispro [Humalog], aspart [Novolog], and glulisine [Apidra]), short-acting (e.g., regular [Humulin R or Novolin R]) intermediate-acting zinc [Lente], (e.g., NPH [Humulin N]), long-acting (e.g., zinc extended [Ultra lente], detemir [Levemir], glargine [Lantus]), mixtures of NPH and regular, and buffered insulin (e.g., Humulin BR); buffered preparations are used for external insulin pumps
e. Insulin preparations can be combined to mimic pancreatic response to variations in BG levels; for example, rapid- and short-acting preparations are usually given to cover mealtimes, while intermediate- and long-acting preparations are used to maintain basal insulin requirements between meals
f. Insulin regimens combine short-acting, intermediate-acting, and long-acting preparations to maintain target BG levels
g. Only regular insulin may be given IV; insulin preparations are usually given via the subcutaneous route; a continuous subcutaneous insulin infusion (insulin pump) is also available to deliver a basal rate of insulin and allow for additional bolus doses of insulin based on requirements (e.g., before a meal)

4. Encourage an exercise plan that meets needs of growing child or enhances fitness and euglycemia in adult

! 5. Promote safety: use appropriate lighting; have client wear protective slippers, socks, and shoes that do not rub or impinge on skin; analyze symptoms, activity tolerance, and coping effectiveness; monitor BG levels; give medication and appropriate food and fluids

! 6. Prevent infection through appropriate foot care, aseptic injection technique, and fingerstick glucose monitoring technique

7. Identify appropriate glucose-monitoring protocol and medication administration process depending on client's vision, finances, finger dexterity, living environment, resources, literacy, lifestyle, personal values, work/school environment, and coping status
8. Coordinate continuing care as appropriate for client's school, work, and other schedules, such as health club
9. Promote acceptance and effective coping while living with DM
10. Promote safety: explain early identification of hypoglycemia; check BG as scheduled; treat hypoglycemia with 15 gram CHO snack, such as 8 oz skim milk, 5 Lifesaver candies, 3 large marshmallows, 6 oz juice; and need to recheck BG after treatment of hypoglycemia
11. Maintain hydration and avoid hyperglycemia; develop sick-day protocol and exercise protocol with client
12. See Table 61–1 ■ for suggestions on promoting age-appropriate self-care for children with type 1 DM

D. Client teaching

1. Type of DM, symptoms to report, self-administration of medication, fingerstick glucose monitoring, plan for regular exam by practitioner, need to wear Medic-Alert bracelet indicating DM and medication prescription, need for lifelong medication management and lifestyle adjustments
2. Foot care: keep feet clean and dry; inspect feet daily using mirror to see soles; protect feet by wearing shoes (allow ½- to ¾-inch toe room) or slippers at all times; avoid snug fitting socks or stockings; use cotton socks because they wick perspiration away from skin
3. Sick-day management: maintain food and fluid intake, continue to take insulin; BG monitoring (up to q4h; report > 250 mg/dL); monitor urine for ketones
4. Diet plan, including considerations for traveling, attendance at parties, sports, and other reasons for altered daily routine
5. Provide these instructions to clients receiving insulin
   a. Storage: insulin in use should be stored at room temperature, away from direct sunlight, and should be replaced after 4 weeks; administration of cold insulin causes subcutaneous atrophy (lipoatrophy) or hypertrophy (lipodystrophy), which alters insulin absorption; extra vials of insulin not in use should be stored in refrigerator
   b. Preparation: note date of expiration; discard vial and use new one if regular insulin appears cloudy; do not shake—shaking may cause inactivation and/or formation of bubbles that lead to dosage errors; roll nonregular insulin gently between hands to evenly disperse suspended particles; draw regular (clear) insulin first when mixing it with other types of insulin; only mix insulins of same concentration (e.g., U100 regular and U100 NPH) and from same source

Table 61–1 Developmental Care for the Child with Type 1 Diabetes Mellitus

Infants and Toddlers	Preschoolers	School-Age	Teen
Allow toddler to make choices in food selection while monitoring CHO levels. The toddler may wish to help with the finger stick by cleaning his or her finger. Monitor temper tantrums as a possible sign of hypoglycemia.	Allow preschooler to make food choices while monitoring CHO levels. Be prepared to substitute snacks at birthday parties and at daycare. Encourage guided independence during blood glucose/fingerstick procedure. Have appropriate snacks available if needed during sports activities that require a high energy expenditure.	Encourage independence of school-aged child in food selection, glucose monitoring, and insulin injections. Assess level of knowledge. Assure that school personnel are available and knowledgeable if hypoglycemia should occur during school hours. Encourage exercise but have snacks available for the child. Discourage fast food or snack machine selections.	Assess teen's body image and sense of identity. Assess compliance with other tasks. Encourage independence with food selection, blood glucose monitoring, and insulin injections. Supervise diabetic tasks if teen is noncompliant. Discuss future plans with teen. Include diabetic issues, but promote a normal lifestyle.

c. Injection: rotate injection sites to prevent lipoatrophy and lipodystrophy; do not inject insulin in an area that will be involved in exercise, as it will increase rate of absorption, onset, and peak action

d. Monitor for signs of hypoglycemia; have candy or foods with simple carbohydrates available

e. Avoid alcohol while taking insulin because it lowers BG levels and can cause hypoglycemia

! 6. Teach symptoms of hypoglycemia (restlessness, irritability, weakness, hunger, nausea, pale diaphoretic skin, shakiness or trembling, headache, confusion, inability to concentrate, deteriorating LOC to coma, seizures), actions to take, causes of hypoglycemia, and methods to prevent

7. Instruct in prevention and management of acute complications of DM (hyperglycemia, hypoglycemia, diabetic ketoacidosis, and HHNK; and chronic complications of DM (diabetic retinopathy, nephropathy, and neuropathy); see Table 61–2 ■ for comparison of hypoglycemia and hyperglycemia with ketoacidosis

! 8. Develop with client a plan for wellness, including exercise

a. Daily cardiovascular exercise decreases risk for insulin resistance, reduces risk for complications, and improves glucose management

b. Check BG before exercise; check for urine ketones if fasting BG is 250 mg/dL; call practitioner if ketones are present and avoid exercise

c. Monitor for signs of hypoglycemia for up to 24 hours after extensive exercise

Table 61–2

A Comparison of Hypoglycemia and Hyperglycemia with Ketoacidosis

	Causes	Symptoms	Treatment
Hypoglycemia	Too much insulin; inadequate intake or missed meals; strenuous exercise without increased intake	1. Blood glucose levels drop below normal 2. Diaphoresis, tremors, hunger, weakness, pallor, dizziness, somnolence, coma and seizures, death	Depends on severity of symptoms but involves replacement of glucose. Mild or moderate: juice or milk, graham crackers, glucose tablets or gel. Severe: glucose paste; family may be taught to administer glucagon SC.
Hyperglycemia with ketoacidosis	Insufficient insulin; infection or other illness may contribute to its development	1. Blood glucose > 250 mg/dL 2. Blood pH of < 7.2; bicarbonate < 15 mEq/L 3. Glycosuria and ketonuria, elevated serum potassium and chloride levels; decreased serum sodium, phosphate, calcium, and magnesium 4. Kussmaul respirations, acetone breath, dehydration, weight loss, tachycardia, flushed facial skin, hypotension, decreased LOC, death 5. Complaints of stomach ache or chest pain are common; vomiting may occur	Intravenous insulin Fluid and electrolytes are replaced as needed in a timely fashion Normal saline is given IV until glucose decreases to 250–300mg/dL; then solution is changed to D5½ NS to prevent rebound hypoglycemia Potassium levels are monitored; initial hyperkalemia may change to hypokalemia following fluid and insulin therapy

XIV. DIABETIC KETOACIDOSIS (DKA)

A. Overview

1. Life-threatening metabolic acidosis resulting from persistent hyperglycemia and breakdown of fats into glucose, leading to presence of ketones in blood
2. Can be triggered by emotional stress, uncompensated exercise, infection, trauma, or insufficient or delayed insulin administration
3. Hyperglycemia causes uncompensated polyuria, hemoconcentration, dehydration, hyperosmolarity, and electrolyte imbalance; a significant accumulation of serum ketones leads to acidosis

! **B. Nursing assessment**

1. Thirst
2. Nausea and vomiting
3. Malaise and lethargy
4. Polyuria
5. Warm dry skin, flushed face
6. Acetone (fruity) odor to breath, Kussmaul respirations (deep, nonlabored, rapid respirations)
7. Serum glucose above 250 mg/dL; plasma pH under 7.35; plasma bicarbonate under 15 mEq/L; serum ketones present; urine positive for glucose and ketones; may have abnormal serum sodium and chloride levels and hyperkalemia

! **C. Therapeutic management**

1. Consists of IV fluids, electrolytes, and regular insulin to correct hyperglycemia and acidosis; supportive care as indicated such as NPO status, vasopressors, and possibly ventilator for respiratory support
2. Insulin
   a. A bolus of IV regular insulin is given followed by a continuous IV drip (0.1 unit/kg body weight) until BG level drops to 250 mg/100 mL or the pH is 7.30
   b. Once this blood level is reached, regular insulin is given on a sliding scale per BG results
   c. Bedside BG monitoring is done every 1 to 2 hours to evaluate effectiveness of this therapy
3. Fluid therapy is needed for excessive dehydration that accompanies DKA
   a. As much as 1 to 2 L normal saline solution may be given during first hour, then IV rate is decreased to 500 mL/hr as tolerated by cardiac and respiratory systems
   b. When the BG level reaches 250 to 300 mg/dL, a 5% glucose solution (such as D_5 ½ NS) is added to prevent hypoglycemia and cerebral edema
   c. Central venous pressure or hemodynamic monitoring may be necessary to evaluate the effectiveness of therapy
4. Potassium replacement is generally necessary in DKA
   a. The initial serum (K^+) level is usually elevated
   b. With reversal of acidosis and administration of insulin, the K^+ shifts into intracellular compartment and serum level can drop rapidly
   c. Institute replacement therapy based on serum K^+ level and urinary output
   d. Institute cardiac monitoring to detect cardiac changes due to hyper- and hypokalemia and to monitor effects of therapy on serum K^+ level
   e. Replace other electrolytes such as phosphate based on laboratory results; bicarbonate is not given routinely in DKA because rapid correction of acidosis can cause severe hypokalemia
5. Analyze I & O, blood glucose, urine ketones, vital signs, oxygenation, and breathing pattern
6. Maintain skin integrity; promote healing of impaired skin; prevent infection by turning and positioning client every 2 hours; provide pressure relief as indicated; manage incontinence and perspiration with skin protective barriers and cleansing; provide appropriate nutrition and oxygen support
7. Promote safety by analyzing vital signs, client communication, LOC and emotional response, and activity tolerance; implement measures to prevent falls
8. Assist client to verbalize concerns and cope effectively with illness and fears
9. Assist client to update Medic-Alert bracelet information as appropriate

D. Client education: nature and causes of DKA (excess glucose intake, insufficient medications, or physiological and/or psychological stressors) and any new medications

XV. HYPERGLYCEMIC HYPEROSMOLAR NONKETOTIC SYNDROME (HHNK)

A. Overview

1. Life-threatening metabolic disorder of hyperglycemia, usually occurring with type 2 DM and triggered by stressors such as medications, infection, acute illness, invasive procedure, or chronic illness
2. Increased insulin resistance (caused by one or more triggers) along with increased CHO intake leads to hyperglycemia
3. Polyuria and decreased plasma volume occur
4. Subsequent decreased glomerular filtration rate (GFR) leads to glucose retention and Na^+ and water excretion
5. Hyperosmolarity causes dehydration and reduced intracellular water (cell shrinkage)

! **B. Nursing assessment**

1. Symptoms gradually occur over 24 hours to 2 weeks
2. Decreased LOC, dry mucous membranes, polydipsia, hyperthermia, impaired sensory and motor function, positive Babinski sign, and seizures
3. Elevated serum Na^+, serum osmolality greater than 340 mOsm/L, serum glucose greater than 600mg/dL, abnormal serum K^+ and chloride, no serum ketones, and normal serum pH

! **C. Therapeutic management**

1. Determine and treat triggering situation; treat coexisting health deviations
2. Provide IV infusion of NS to replace fluids and Na^+, regular insulin IV to manage hyperglycemia, and K^+ to replace losses and shifts
3. Monitor I&O, weight, vital signs, lab values, sensory function, and cognitive function
4. Maintain intact skin by turning every 2 hours, use of pressure relief aids, nutritional support, use of skin moisturizers and barriers, and management of incontinence
5. Prevent aspiration by using appropriate feeding precautions, elevate head of bed (HOB) 15 to 30 degrees during and after feeding for 1 hour; if BP too unstable to elevate HOB with feeding, then withhold oral feedings

D. Client teaching: HHNK symptoms to report, and administration of new medications

XVI. DELAYED PUBERTY

A. Overview

1. A condition noted in girls if breast development has not occurred by age 13, pubic hair has not appeared by age 14, or menarche has not occurred within 4 years after onset of breast development, usually by age 16
2. In boys, delayed puberty is a concern if there is no testicular enlargement or scrotal changes by 13½ or 14 years of age, pubic hair has not appeared by age 15, or genital growth is not complete by 4 to 5 years after testicular enlargement
3. Delayed puberty can be hereditary: many family members may have constitutional delay (delay of overall growth and puberty)
4. May be caused by hypogonadism (ovaries and testicles are not secreting hormones—estrogen or testosterone); hypogonadism may result from abnormality of hypothalamus or pituitary gland (brain tumors, hypothyroidism, anorexia, and other chronic illnesses)
5. May also result from problem with testicle itself (Klinefelter's syndrome) or with ovary (Turner's syndrome); these syndromes are secondary to chromosomal abnormalities and can be evaluated by studying child's karyotype
   a. Klinefelter's syndrome is manifested by IQ scores below normal range, tall stature, and overly long arms and legs; boys with this disorder have one or more extra X chromosomes, commonly 47 chromosomes with an XXY karyotype; they are usually sterile
   b. Girls who have Turner's syndrome exhibit delayed puberty, short stature, webbed neck, and cubitus valgus (where forearm deviates laterally); kary-

otype demonstrates a female with a missing X chromosome (45XO); these girls are usually infertile

6. Many clients with delayed puberty have short stature and may be treated as a child by teachers, coaches, and community members; during adolescent years, they may have difficulty in social situations

B. Nursing assessment

1. Assessment of the family growth history (especially growth patterns of parents)
2. Complete examination including measurements of arm span and (in males) testicular size and penile length
3. X-ray of left hand and wrist for bone age for skeletal growth and status of epiphyseal growth plate closure; beginning of puberty better correlates with bone age than chronological age
4. MRI or CT scan may be needed to determine a CNS lesion if a brain tumor is suspected
5. Possible blood levels of FSH (follicle stimulating hormone), LH (leutinizing hormone), and sex hormones; a complete blood count, thyroid function tests, and chemistry panel
6. A karyotype (number and types of chromosomes) should be done if Turner's or Klinefelter's syndromes are suspected; the gonadotropin-releasing hormone (GnRH) stimulation test may be used for diagnosis also

C. Therapeutic management

1. Assure children with constitutional delay and delayed bone age that they usually do not require any treatment; medical intervention of low-dose injections of testosterone may be initiated if adolescent is over age 14
2. If hypogonadism is present and other conditions are ruled out, child may receive hormone therapy to stimulate development of secondary sexual characteristics; boys receive testosterone enanthate injections, and girls take oral ethinyl estradiol with a combination of medroxyprogesterone
3. Provide psychological support to the child, especially if he or she has social concerns

D. Client and family teaching

1. Information regarding different stages of puberty and causes of delayed puberty; use language appropriate to child's chronological age
2. Administration of hormones if ordered; arrange for home nursing care to provide injections if needed

XVII. PRECOCIOUS PUBERTY

A. Overview

1. A condition characterized by early onset of puberty, usually occurring before age 8 in girls and before age 9 in boys
2. Accompanied by appearance of secondary sexual characteristics and advanced growth rate and bone maturation, causing early fusion of epiphyseal plates and eventual short adult stature
3. Most cases of precocious puberty in both boys and girls are idiopathic; some cases are caused by benign hypothalamic tumors, other brain tumors, infection, cranial radiation, and head trauma
4. In normal puberty, the hypothalamus secretes GnRH; this hormone stimulates pituitary gland to secrete LH and FSH in male and female that result in development of secondary sexual characteristics
5. In precocious puberty, premature hormone secretion causes early onset of sexual characteristics; linear and skeletal growth is apparent because affected children appear very tall early on, but epiphyseal closure occurs because of hormone secretion, causing short stature as an adult

B. Nursing assessment

1. Signs of precocious puberty in female include breast development, pubic hair, axillary hair, acne, adult body odor, and onset of menstrual periods
2. Signs of precocious puberty in male include testicular enlargement, pubic hair, penile enlargement, axillary and chest hair, facial hair, acne, adult body odor, and deepening voice

3. The GnRH stimulation test stimulates secretion of FSH and LH; blood samples are obtained every 2 hours; if LH level is higher than FSH level, puberty has occurred
4. Bone age x-rays will aid in determining epiphyseal maturation and closure; if bone age is more advanced than chronological age, skeletal growth acceleration is apparent

C. Therapeutic management

1. ! Support children with precocious puberty by discussing their concerns about body image and sexuality
2. Offer support as family deals with sensitive issues such as premature appearance of secondary sexual characteristics and sexuality
3. ! Encourage clients to express feelings about body changes; role-playing may help children cope with issues of peer teasing
4. Assure children that friends will go through same body changes
5. If synthetic form of LH-releasing factor is used to slow down or arrest progression of puberty, plan for monthly or daily injections with family
6. ! Medication therapy: a synthetic form of LH-releasing factor (Lupron Depot and others) that slows or stops progression of puberty and skeletal growth, which will preserve adult height

D. Child and family education

1. Information about condition and possible referral to pediatric endocrinologist
2. If client is receiving synthetic LH, teach family subcutaneous or intramuscular injection technique, and provide child and family with information about drug side effects as per product literature

XVIII. PHENYLKETONURIA (PKU)

A. Overview

1. An inherited disorder that affects protein utilization and is caused by abnormal metabolism of essential amino acid phenylalanine, found in many natural protein foods
2. Autosomal-recessive trait or a mutation affecting mostly white children; PKU is rare in African Americans, Japanese, and the Jewish population
3. A deficiency in liver enzyme phenylalanine hydoxylase (which breaks down amino acid phenylalanine into tyrosine) causes serum phenylalanine metabolite levels to rise, leading to musty body and urine odor (excretion of phenol acids), seizures, hyperactivity, irritability, vomiting, and an eczema-type rash
4. Decreased levels of tyrosine cause a deficiency of pigment melanin, causing most children with PKU to have blond hair, blue eyes, and fair skin that is prone to eczema
5. Decreased levels of neurotransmitters dopamine and tryptophan, which affect protein synthesis and myelinization, cause degeneration of gray and white matter in brain; mental retardation and seizures occur if phenylalanine level is not decreased

B. Nursing assessment

1. Many infants with PKU appear healthy at birth; if treatment is not started to lower phenylalanine level immediately, infant's IQ can drop as many as 10 points within first month and will continue to decline
2. All 50 states require newborn screening using Guthrie blood test at 48 hours after birth
   a. Guthrie blood test is a bacterial inhibition assay for phenylalanine in blood; *Bacillus subtilis* is present in blood if increased levels of phenylalanine are present; normal value is 1.6 mg/dL
   b. The infant should ingest adequate protein (usually 24 hours of normal feedings of breast milk or formula) prior to test being performed
   c. ! Heel blood should be used for specimen; the heel stick sample should be collected after first 24 hours but no later than 7 days after birth

d. A normal level is under 2 mg/dL; Guthrie test detects levels greater than 4 mg/dL; if level is elevated, a repeat Guthrie test is performed to validate original results
e. If infant is discharged prior to 48 hours, test should be performed within 1 week after discharge from hospital or birthing center by a public health nurse, pediatrician, or pediatric nurse practitioner

3. Symptoms arise over time and include failure to thrive, vomiting, irritability, and unpredictable behavior in infant; the urine will have a musty odor; the child may experience myoclonic or grand mal seizures

C. Therapeutic management

1. Ensure that Guthrie blood test has been done correctly and results have been received; repeat blood test if phenylalanine levels are elevated on first test
2. Allow phenylalanines in diet based on weight of child and usually at a level of 20-30 mg/kg body weight or amount prescribed by physician; consult with registered nutritionist to aid in food calculations
3. Place child on protein-restricted diet
   a. Encourage use of mature breast milk or modified-protein, phenylalanine-free, hydrolysate formula as a source of infant nutrition to keep phenylalanine level at 2 to 6 mg/dL
   b. Use special protein foods that are free of phenylalanine
4. Monitor serum phenylalanine levels periodically throughout child's life
5. Maintain restricted phenylalanine diet at least through adolescence; current evidence suggests that diet should continue into adulthood, especially when pregnant or contemplating pregnancy (children of women with PKU may be born with congenital defects, including mental retardation, unless woman resumes a low phenylalanine diet before conception)
6. In young children inadequately screened after birth and who develop PKU, dietary modification at time of diagnosis usually improves behavioral and other symptoms; it prevents further mental retardation but does not raise IQ to previous level
7. Parents may be overwhelmed initially by diagnosis and dietary restrictions; emotional support is essential; suggest genetic counseling because each child born to this couple may have a 1 in 4 chance of having PKU
8. Medication therapy: antiepileptic medications if client is having seizures

D. Client and family teaching

1. Support parents and teach them disease and its management
2. Guthrie test may need to be repeated if initial test was done before 24 to 48 hours of age or if test was positive initially
3. Review low-phenylalanine diet, including preparation of low-phenylalanine formula; avoid giving child meats, dairy products, and products containing aspartame because they contain large amounts of phenylalanine
4. Encourage resumption of low-phenylalanine diet in adolescence if restriction was previously lifted if child is having difficulty with attention span, concentration, and school tasks
5. Offer emotional support and refer older child and parents to a support group for issues and problems related to chronic illness

Check Your NCLEX–RN® Exam I.Q.

You are ready for testing on this content if you can

- Identify basic structures and functions of the endocrine system.
- Describe the pathophysiology and etiology of common endocrine disorders.
- Discuss expected assessment data and diagnostic test findings for selected endocrine disorders.
- Discuss therapeutic management of a client experiencing an endocrine disorder.
- Discuss nursing management of a client experiencing an endocrine disorder.
- Identify expected outcomes for the client experiencing an endocrine disorder.

PRACTICE TEST

PRACTICE TEST

1 A client recently diagnosed with hypothyroidism demonstrates understanding of prescribed levothyroxine (Synthroid) medication when she makes which of the following statements?

1. "I should be able to become pregnant in a couple of months."
2. "This medication will help me lose all this excess weight."
3. "I should call the physician for nervousness, diarrhea, or increased pulse."
4. "This medication should be taken with food, preferably dairy products."

2 The client is post-transphenoidal hypophysectomy. The client demonstrates understanding of education when he states, "I know I need to be careful not to increase the pressure in my head by

1. Sitting in a soft chair and leaning over slowly to tie my shoes."
2. Holding my breath when I reach down to pick up something from the floor."
3. Bending my knees first before squatting down to reach something on the floor."
4. Holding my breath while I use mouthwash, then leaning my head down toward the sink to spit it out."

3 The client who is 80 hours post-transphenoidal hypophysectomy reports numbness on the upper lip and gum, a headache when reclining, and has a tendency to kick around small rugs in the room when walking. The home health nurse should do which of the following?

1. Inform the client that these are normal responses and will disappear over 2 to 3 weeks.
2. Assess neuromuscular function and incisional area and then report all findings to the surgeon.
3. Immediately arrange for the client to be transported to the hospital for treatment of increased intracranial pressure.
4. Assess vital signs, fluid volume status, bowel function and nutrition status.

4 The client with diabetes mellitus requests a medication for headache soon after returning from an early morning x-ray procedure. The nurse observes the client is upset about the headache, angry at missing breakfast, and has moist hands. The nurse should do which of the following as the priority action?

1. Administer the medication for headache and arrange for a breakfast tray.
2. Check the blood glucose level and be prepared to give 4 ounces of juice immediately.
3. Acknowledge his dissatisfaction, offer to obtain a snack, and give the medication.
4. Administer the headache medication and review the day's lab test results.

5 A 70-year-old client admitted a few hours ago with a blood glucose level of 750 mg/dL is being treated for hyperosmolar hyperglycemic nonketotic coma (HHNK) with intravenous regular insulin at 10 units/hour, normal saline with 40 mEq of potassium per liter infusing at 250 mL/hr, and oxygen at 2 L/min. The client is oriented when stimulated, and FBG has dropped to 400 mg/dL. The client starts demanding to get out of bed and the nurse notes the skin feels cool and moist. The nurse should do which of the following?

1. Interpret this as a sign of hypoglycemia and check his blood glucose.
2. Recognize that client is feeling better and is seeking control of his situation.
3. Auscultate breath sounds and assess oxygen saturation for signs of decreased cardiac output.
4. Assess the client for bladder distention or signs of imbalanced body temperature.

6 A client who underwent a colonoscopy after being premedicated with midazolam (Versed), returns to the nursing unit. The client is given morphine sulfate IV push after reporting abdominal pain associated with BP 140/80, pulse 78, RR 20. Twenty minutes later, the client is lethargic, has weak hand grasps, weak peripheral pulse of 88, BP 120/66, RR 14. The nurse makes which interpretation of these assessment findings?

1. The client is resting with pain relieved.
2. The client is now showing signs of dehydration because of the colon procedure preparation.
3. The client is now fatigued because of anxiety, pain, and fear of outcome of the procedure.
4. The client is experiencing impaired gas exchange because of hypoventilation.

7 The client is scheduled for bilateral adrenalectomy secondary to an adrenal cortex tumor. Which of the following is the nurse's highest priority for this client in the immediate postoperative period?

1. Assess fluid and electrolyte balance, signs of hypoglycemia, and hypotension.
2. Assess for signs of hypoxia, cardiac arrhythmias, and peripheral edema.
3. Monitor the incision integrity, peripheral pulses, and magnesium level.
4. Assess for hyperthermia, bed mobility, pupil reaction and eye movement.

8 A female client has been taking propylthiouracil (PTU) for 5 months to treat hyperthyroidism. After falling and spraining her ankle, she is treated in the emergency department and is given crutch-walking instructions. She states that she will never have enough energy to get around on crutches and is frustrated at the 10 pounds she gained this winter. The nurse's first action should be to

1. Document the client's complaints and consult the physician to order a serum T_4.
2. Discharge the client to home and encourage her to have a TSH level drawn.
3. Encourage the client to rest at home until the sprain is healed, then increase activity.
4. Investigate the availability of a walking splint instead of using the crutches.

9 The client with diabetes mellitus (DM) is going home following angioplasty. The nurse observes that the client walks to the restroom barefoot, although slippers are in reach. The priority nursing diagnosis for this client is which of the following?

1. Risk for injury related to potential for falls while walking barefoot
2. Risk for infection related to impaired tissue perfusion and walking barefoot
3. Deficient knowledge related to post angioplasty care
4. Risk for impaired cerebral perfusion related to potential for hypoglycemia

10 The client is 6 hours post-thyroid surgery. The nursing assistant reports that the client is upset because there is blood on the client's gown. Which of the following is the priority action of the nurse?

1. Assess the client's breath sounds and respiratory effort.
2. State that it is normal to have some bleeding and ask the nurse aide to change the gown.
3. Reassure the client that some bleeding is normal, and then assess the client's level of pain.
4. Reinforce the dressing, change the gown, and call the surgeon.

11 A client who was admitted with hyperglycemic hyperosmolar nonketotic coma (HHNK) asks how he can prevent recurrence of this illness. The nurse would instruct the client that which of the following are helpful prevention measures?

1. Use sliding-scale insulin to cover periodic snack of candy.
2. Maintain fluid balance by drinking 4 glasses of water daily.
3. Detect and treat infection early, maintain hydration, and use stress-management techniques.
4. Consult primary care provider when fasting blood glucose is elevated.

12 The client who has a long history of type 1 diabetes mellitus is being treated for bronchitis and sinusitis. The nurse observes deep, rapid, unlabored respirations, fruity odor on the client's clothes, and dry skin. Which of the following actions should the nurse take next?

1. Assess breath sounds for additional signs of response to treatment of the infection.
2. Assess blood glucose level for signs of hypoglycemia.
3. Encourage the client to rest frequently and to drink 8 to 10 glasses of fluids daily.
4. Assess blood glucose level for hyperglycemia and check urine for ketones.

13 A female client newly diagnosed with hypothyroidism indicates that she no longer wants to participate in evening social activities stating, "There is too much walking, and I prefer to go to bed early. I see enough of my friends at work every day." The nurse formulates which of the following as a priority nursing diagnosis for this client?

1. Social isolation related to sleep rest needs as evidenced by desire to go to bed early
2. Disturbed sleep pattern related to excessive work as evidenced by desire to go to bed early and avoid evening activities
3. Fatigue related to reduced metabolic rate as evidenced by desire to avoid evening activities after work
4. Decreased cardiac output related to weak myocardium as evidenced by desire to avoid walking

PRACTICE TEST

14 A recently retired client who lives alone is admitted with myxedema coma. It is determined that myxedema occurred after she stopped her thyroid medication because she could not afford to buy the medication. Which of the following is the highest priority of the nurse in this client's plan of care?

1. Assist the client to chair every 4 hours to promote oxygenation and prevent skin breakdown.
2. Prevent injury related to mental confusion and elevated BP.
3. Prevent skin breakdown and promote nutrition with low-fiber foods.
4. Monitor for signs of decreased cardiac output and airway obstruction.

15 A client with hyperparathyroidism is admitted to the critical care unit with cardiac dysrhythmias, including frequent premature atrial contractions, bursts of supraventricular tachycardia, and occasional premature ventricular contractions. The client asks why the cardiologist prescribed so much IV fluid and then furosemide (Lasix). The best explanation by the nurse is that these orders would

1. Improve cardiac output.
2. Eliminate metabolic wastes.
3. Replace missing electrolytes.
4. Promote excretion of calcium.

16 A client with hypoparathyroidism is to be discharged home after stabilization of fluid and electrolyte levels. Which of the following critical concepts does the nurse teach the client prior to discharge?

1. Importance of keeping follow-up appointments for lab and with primary health care provider
2. Strategies to prevent falling and how to plan meals high in calcium
3. Significant signs of hypoglycemia to monitor for and report
4. Signs and symptoms of renal calculi and urinary tract infections to monitor for and report

17 A client recently diagnosed with syndrome of inappropriate antidiuretic hormone (SIADH) is receiving continuous enteral nutrition via an enteral feeding tube. Considering the impact of the disorder on fluid balance, the nurse does which of the following when working with the enteral feeding tube?

1. Discard the 50 mL residual and replace it with 50 mL water.
2. Flush the tube with 50 mL normal saline.
3. Count the flush but not the feeding in planning the fluid limitation.
4. Flush the tube with 50 mL water to maintain patency.

18 A client with a history of Cushing's syndrome is being admitted for acute management of multiple contusions and lacerations following a motor vehicle accident. Morning serum laboratory values are BUN 30 mg/dL, creatinine 1.0 mg/dL, sodium 148 mEq/L, potassium 4.8 mEq/L, chloride 108 mEq/L, and cortisol 29 mcg/dL. This client's two high-priority nursing diagnoses are

1. Impaired urinary elimination and risk for fluid volume excess.
2. Risk for injury and risk for disuse syndrome.
3. Ineffective airway clearance and ineffective health maintenance.
4. Risk for infection and deficient fluid volume.

19 A client underwent adrenal gland radiation therapy for benign tumors. The client is being treated with fludrocortisone acetate (Florinef Acetate) for mineralocorticoid and glucocorticoid replacement. The high-priority nursing diagnosis for this client is

1. Risk for excess fluid volume.
2. Risk for infection related to radiation damage.
3. Risk for constipation.
4. Ineffective breathing pattern.

20 The client is being treated for Addison's disease with glucocorticoid replacement medication. The nurse evaluates that the client understandings medication therapy when the client makes which of the following statements?

1. "I should take this medication every evening at bedtime."
2. "My irregular pulse should convert to a regular rate and rhythm."
3. "This medication will help me control my increased blood pressure."
4. "I should call my doctor if I gain 2 pounds, feel weak, or have a cold."

21 An 8-month-old infant born outside the United States is brought to the endocrine clinic with symptoms of a musty body odor, seizures, and an eczema-like rash. The infant is tested for phenylketonuria (PKU) and the diagnosis is positive. In planning nursing care for this infant, the nurse will anticipate

1. The need for dietary information about a low-phenylalanine diet.
2. Admission to a long-term care setting for handicapped infants.
3. Preparing the family for the child's early demise.
4. roviding instruction on medication management of PKU.

22 A 15-year-old weighing 250 pounds has started to experience increased thirst, increased appetite, and frequent urination. When he is admitted to the hospital, he is given oral medication after being diagnosed with diabetes mellitus. What information should the nurse give the teenager about medication therapy?

1. "You might receive a pill now, but you'll get insulin injections later if you don't comply with diet and medication therapy."
2. "Overweight teenagers may develop type 2 diabetes, which can be treated with an oral medication. You may or may not need insulin in the future."
3. "Insulin is used when diabetics won't take oral pills, so you can avoid injections by taking your medication as ordered."
4. "Your diabetes is mild, so you don't need to take medication for long. You will probably only need to restrict sweets."

23 A mother is quite concerned about her 7-year-old daughter after noticing some breast development and the appearance of a small amount of pubic hair. The mother asks the nurse if this is a cause for concern. What would be the best response by the nurse?

1. "No. Some girls just develop earlier than boys."
2. "Yes. Your daughter may have precocious puberty. Let's talk to the pediatrician because she may need referral to an endocrinologist."
3. "Yes. She probably doesn't want the other children at school making fun of her."
4. "No. This early development may slow down when she reaches 9 years old."

24 The mother of a diabetic adolescent tells the nurse that her son likes to go out with his friends on Friday nights and eat burgers and french fries. The adolescent knows that he is exceeding the allowable carbohydrate exchanges on the diabetic diet, but he does so anyway. The nurse discusses with the mother that teens sometimes take chances that place health at risk because

1. They want to be just like their peers.
2. They have a self-destruction wish.
3. They often like french fries and can't eat them at home.
4. They want to show risk-taking behavior.

25 A 13-year-old girl is being evaluated for delayed puberty. The client says, "The doctor said he was going to do a karyotype. Will that hurt?" Which of the following is the best response by the nurse?

1. "A karyotype is just a microscopic picture of your chromosomes."
2. "The karotype test is an evaluation of your luteinizing hormone levels."
3. "The doctor has ordered an x-ray of your hand to determine your bone age."
4. "You don't need to worry about that because I will be with you."

26 The nurse is assessing a client with a tentative diagnosis of hyperpituitarism. What assessment findings should the nurse observe for in this client? Select all that apply.

1. Short stature if onset is in childhood
2. Large hands and feet with prominent jawbone
3. Joint changes consistent with arthritis
4. Soft, high-pitched voice
5. Hypertension

ANSWERS & RATIONALES

1 **Answer: 3** Side effects of thyroid hormone replacement medication may mimic symptoms of hyperthyroidism. After the client has reached normal serum T_4 levels, the normal metabolic rate may help the client lose the weight gained during the hypothyroid state, but this is not the purpose of the replacement medication. Usually, the medication should be taken on an empty stomach, 1 hour prior to a meal or 2 hours after a meal.

Cognitive Level: Analysis **Client Need:** Physiological Integrity: Pharmacological and Parenteral Therapies **Integrated Process:** Nursing Process: Evaluation **Content Area:** Adult Health: Endocrine and Metabolic **Strategy:** The core issue of the question is knowledge of side effects of medications used to manage hypothyroidism. Use nursing knowledge and the process of elimination to make a selection.

2 **Answer: 3** Bending the knees and squatting is preferred to bending at the waist to reach the floor as a means of preventing rises in intracranial pressure (ICP) following pituitary surgery. Holding the breath as well as leaning over will increase ICP. Clients should be taught to avoid holding the breath for any reason and to avoid leaning forward or bending at the waist to prevent an increase in intracranial pressure. To tie shoes, the client should sit on the couch or bed, bend the knee and place his or her foot on the couch or bed to reach the shoelaces; Alternatively, the client can sit on the floor to tie shoes or can avoid shoes that tie until there is no risk for increased ICP.

Cognitive Level: Application **Client Need:** Physiological Integrity: Physiological Adaptation **Integrated Process:** Nursing Process: Evaluation **Content Area:** Adult Health: Endocrine and Metabolic **Strategy:** The core issue of the question is knowledge of measures to prevent rises in intracranial pressure following pituitary surgery. Use nursing knowledge and the process of elimination to make a selection.

3 **Answer: 2** The numbness of the upper lip and gum near the incision as well as a decreased sense of smell are normal and should resolve in 3 to 4 months. The movement of the small rugs suggests an unsteady gait or foot drop; both this and the headache are signs of increased intracranial pressure. In-depth assessments of neuromuscular function and incision site are needed, and then the surgeon should be consulted immediately. The other responses are either excessive or insufficient.

Cognitive Level: Application **Client Need:** Physiological Integrity: Physiological Adaptation **Integrated Process:** Nursing Process: Assessment **Content Area:** Adult Health: Endocrine and Metabolic **Strategy:** The core issue of the question is the ability to accurately interpret the significance of client findings after pituitary surgery and then determine the next action. Use nursing knowledge and the process of elimination to make a selection, recalling that further assessments are often indicated when encountering abnormal data.

4 **Answer: 2** Headache, restlessness, anxiety, sweating, and increased pulse are signs of hypoglycemia. Resolution of symptoms should occur after the client drinks the juice. The other options either delay treatment (options 1 and 3) or fail to recognize the real problem (option 4).

Cognitive Level: Analysis **Client Need:** Physiological Integrity: Physiological Adaptation **Integrated Process:** Nursing Process: Implementation **Content Area:** Adult Health: Endocrine and Metabolic **Strategy:** The core issue of the question is recognition that the client is at risk for hypoglycemia and the corrective actions that need to be taken. Use nursing knowledge and the process of elimination to make a selection.

5 **Answer: 3** Increased preload caused by the intravenous infusion at 250 mL/hr may exceed the myocardium's workload capacity, leading to signs of decreased cardiac output and congestive heart failure. The other options focus on inappropriate information.

Cognitive Level: Analysis **Client Need:** Physiological Integrity: Physiological Adaptation **Integrated Process:** Nursing Process: Assessment **Content Area:** Adult Health: Endocrine and Metabolic **Strategy:** The core issue of the question is recognition that rapid infusion of fluid in a 70-year-old client could lead to circulatory decompensation. Use nursing knowledge and the process of elimination to make a selection.

6 **Answer: 4** Decreased level of consciousness, weak hand grasp, and peripheral pulses with increased heart rate and decreased BP result from acidosis. These are signs of respiratory acidosis secondary to hypoventilation from the midazolam. For this reason, option 4 is the appropriate diagnostic reasoning process.

Cognitive Level: Analysis **Client Need:** Physiological Integrity: Physiological Adaptation **Integrated Process:** Nursing Process: Analysis **Content Area:** Adult Health: Endocrine and Metabolic **Strategy:** The core issue of the question is accurate interpretation of a change in client status. A critical word in the stem of the question is *midazolam.* Recall the properties of this medication, and use nursing knowledge and the process of elimination to make a selection.

7 **Answer: 1** During the first 48 hours after adrenalectomy, clients are at risk for adrenal insufficiency and hypovolemic shock. The lack of cortisol production can cause fluid and electrolyte loss and hypoglycemia. Elevated cortisol does place the client at risk for delayed wound healing and infection, but adrenal insufficiency is more life threatening and more common in the first 2 days following surgery.

Cognitive Level: Analysis **Client Need:** Physiological Integrity: Physiological Adaptation **Integrated Process:** Nursing Process: Assessment **Content Area:** Adult Health: Endocrine and Metabolic **Strategy:** The core issue of the question is knowledge that clients are at risk for adrenal insufficiency following adrenalectomy and how to assess for its occurrence. Use nursing knowledge and the process of elimination to make a selection.

8 **Answer: 1** The client's complaints of lack of energy and weight gain are consistent with hypothyroidism, which is diagnosed with a serum T_4. Considering the client's complaints of energy deficit, the recent fall causing the sprain, and information about the thyroid medication, the nurse is obligated to consult the physician for T_4 evaluation to prevent further injury. Encouraging the client to rest and investigating the need for a walking splint are appropriate actions but not the first priority.

Cognitive Level: Application **Client Need:** Physiological Integrity: Physiological Adaptation **Integrated Process:** Nursing Process: Planning **Content Area:** Adult Health: Endocrine and Metabolic **Strategy:** The core issue of the question is the ability to correlate client reports with the underlying diagnosis of hypothyroidism. Use nursing knowledge and the process of elimination to make a selection.

9 **Answer: 2** Clients with either diabetic mellitus or other conditions that have arterial insufficiency as a component of the disorder must constantly protect their feet from injury; as-

sess the skin condition daily; prevent dry, cracked skin; and avoid crossing the legs in order to maintain tissue perfusion and prevent infection. These clients have delayed wound healing and poor sensation in their feet, increasing risk for injury and undetected injury with infection.
Cognitive Level: Analysis **Client Need:** Physiological Integrity: Physiological Adaptation **Integrated Process:** Nursing Process: Analysis **Content Area:** Adult Health: Endocrine and Metabolic **Strategy:** The core issue of the question is interpretation of behaviors that pose risk for complications to the client with diabetes mellitus. Use nursing knowledge and the process of elimination to make a selection.

10 **Answer: 1** Usually, with thyroid surgery, there is minimal bleeding postoperatively. Blood on the gown indicates excessive incisional bleeding. Breath sounds, including auscultating over the tracheal area, and respiratory effort should be assessed first to determine if edema is present in the tissues, thus compromising the airway. After thoroughly assessing the client and reinforcing or changing the dressing per protocol, the nurse should inform the surgeon of the amount of bleeding and all other assessment data. Options 2 and 3 do not protect the client from possible harm. Option 4 ignores the client's airway, a high priority following this surgery.
Cognitive Level: Analysis **Client Need:** Physiological Integrity: Physiological Adaptation **Integrated Process:** Nursing Process: Implementation **Content Area:** Adult Health: Endocrine and Metabolic **Strategy:** The core issue of the question is possible threat to the airway and breathing with excessive bleeding following thyroid surgery. Use nursing knowledge, the ABCs, and the process of elimination to make a selection.

11 **Answer: 3** HHNK is associated with hyperglycemic response to infection or other disease or illness, some medications, dehydration, stress-induced hyperglycemia, or a combination of these factors. HHNK occurs in clients with type 2 diabetes mellitus, primarily the elderly, and thus insulin is not part of the usual treatment plan (option 1). Option 2 is insufficient; 6 to 8 glasses of water are recommended for general health. Option 4 does not demonstrate an understanding of prevention of HHNK.
Cognitive Level: Application **Client Need:** Physiological Integrity: Physiological Adaptation **Integrated Process:** Nursing Process: Implementation **Content Area:** Adult Health: Endocrine and Metabolic **Strategy:** The critical work in the stem of the question is *prevent.* With this in mind, look for the option that will reduce the likelihood of the client experiencing a recurrence. Use nursing knowledge and the process of elimination to make a selection.

12 **Answer: 4** Diabetic ketoacidosis can occur in diabetic clients with infection and is characterized by elevated blood glucose and ketonuria. Deep, rapid, unlabored respirations are called Kussmaul respirations. Kussmaul respirations, fruity odor, and dry skin are signs of hyperglycemia. Option 2 represents the opposite problem, not than the hyperglycemia being displayed. Options 1 and 3 do not address hyperglycemia and ketoacidosis, which is the issue of the question.
Cognitive Level: Analysis **Client Need:** Physiological Integrity: Physiological Adaptation **Integrated Process:** Nursing Process: Assessment **Content Area:** Adult Health: Endocrine and Metabolic **Strategy:** The core issue of the question is recognition that a diabetic client with an infection is at risk for diabetic ketoacidosis and knowing how to assess for this complication. Use nursing knowledge and the process of elimination to make a selection.

13 **Answer: 3** Hypothyroidism is associated with fatigue, weight gain, and decreased activity tolerance. There is not enough data to conclude decreased cardiac output or sleep alterations. Client stated she is able to socialize during the day at work.
Cognitive Level: Analysis **Client Need:** Physiological Integrity: Physiological Adaptation **Integrated Process:** Nursing Process: Analysis **Content Area:** Adult Health: Endocrine and Metabolic **Strategy:** The core issue of the question is the etiology of the clinet's symptoms and applying a nursing diagnostic label to the problem. Use nursing knowledge and the process of elimination to make a selection.

14 **Answer: 4** Myxedema is characterized by severely decreased cardiac output, fluid and electrolyte imbalance, acidosis, decreased respiratory function, tongue edema, and hypothermia. Skin breakdown is a significant risk that needs to be managed concurrently with promotion of oxygenation, but airway and circulation have highest priority.
Cognitive Level: Analysis **Client Need:** Physiological Integrity: Physiological Adaptation **Integrated Process:** Nursing Process: Planning **Content Area:** Adult Health: Endocrine and Metabolic **Strategy:** The core issue of the question is assigning a priority to client needs during myxedema. Recall that physiological needs take priority before psychosocial needs. Use nursing knowledge about the condition and the process of elimination to make a selection.

15 **Answer: 4** Hyperparathyroidism causes hypercalcemia. Large doses of saline infusions concurrently with Lasix will stimulate a decrease in serum calcium through renal excretion. In acute situations requiring rapid reduction, clients can be given IV calcitonin and phosphates.
Cognitive Level: Application **Client Need:** Physiological Integrity: Physiological Adaptation **Integrated Process:** Nursing Process: Implementation **Content Area:** Adult Health: Endocrine and Metabolic **Strategy:** The core issue of the question is knowledge of methods used to manage hypercalcemia in hyperparathyroidism. Use nursing knowledge and the process of elimination to make a selection.

16 **Answer: 2** Clients with hypoparathyroidism have low serum calcium levels, paresthesia, mood disorders, muscle spasms, and hyperactive reflexes placing them at risk for falling. They must actively seek to increase their intake of calcium and vitamin D to maintain therapeutic serum levels in addition to taking their prescribed medication. The other options do not address safety as the critically important need.
Cognitive Level: Application **Client Need:** Physiological Integrity: Physiological Adaptation **Integrated Process:** Teaching and Learning **Content Area:** Adult Health: Endocrine and Metabolic **Strategy:** The core issue of the question is health teaching that is appropriate for a client with hypoparathyroidism. Use nursing knowledge about safety measures and altered calcium levels and the process of elimination to make a selection.

17 **Answer: 2** Clients with SIADH are usually on a strict fluid restriction to correct water overload; therefore, all fluids (including the enteral feeding and the flush solution) should be considered when planning the fluid restriction. Clients are also encouraged to drink fluids high in sodium, so clients being treated for SIADH should have their feeding tubes flushed with normal saline and not water. To prevent electrolyte loss, all of the residual that is aspirated from a feeding tube should be returned to the client.
Cognitive Level: Application **Client Need:** Physiological Integrity: Physiological Adaptation **Integrated Process:** Nursing Process: Implementation **Content Area:** Adult Health: Endocrine and Metabolic **Strategy:** The core issue of the question is proper fluid use and management in a client with SIADH. Use nursing knowledge about fluid imbalance in this disorder and the process of elimination to make a selection.

18 **Answer: 4** The BUN and sodium are elevated because of dehydration and deficient fluid volume, since the creatinine is normal, thus supporting normal renal function. The potassium and chloride are at the higher end of the normal range, which also supports dehydration and fluid volume deficit. Clients with Cushing's syndrome are at risk for infection because of an impaired immune function related to an elevated cortisol level.
Cognitive Level: Analysis **Client Need:** Physiological Integrity: Physiological Adaptation **Integrated Process:** Nursing Process: Analysis **Content Area:** Adult Health: Endocrine and Metabolic **Strategy:** The core issue of the question is the ability to determine priorities of care for a client with Cushing's syndrome who experiences trauma. Use knowledge of pathophysiology and the process of elimination to make a selection.

19 **Answer: 1** Florinef and other adrenal replacement drugs cause sodium and fluid retention. Clients are at risk for excess sodium and fluid retention leading to fluid volume excess. Risk for infection could apply but is not timely if the client has completed this course of therapy. Impaired gas exchange may result from extensive fluid volume excess that can lead to ineffective breathing pattern. The highest priority is the risk for fluid volume excess.
Cognitive Level: Analysis **Client Need:** Physiological Integrity: Physiological Adaptation **Integrated Process:** Nursing Process: Analysis **Content Area:** Adult Health: Endocrine and Metabolic **Strategy:** The core issue of the question is the ability to determine priority concerns for a client receiving mineralocorticoid and glucocorticoid therapy. Use nursing knowledge and the process of elimination to make a selection.

20 **Answer: 4** Glucocorticoid replacement medication can cause fluid and sodium retention, leading to weight gain and fluid volume excess. These medications need to be increased during times of stress and can impair the body's ability to recover from an infection. Therefore, the physician must be consulted for weight gain or signs of a cold or infection. These medications should be taken in the morning with food and will increase BP (thus are not safe for clients with hypertension), and the medication will not affect cardiac rhythm.
Cognitive Level: Application **Client Need:** Physiological Integrity: Pharmacological and Parenteral Therapies **Integrated Process:** Nursing Process: Evaluation **Content Area:** Adult Health: Endocrine and Metabolic **Strategy:** The core issue of the question is knowledge of adverse effects of drug therapy following client teaching. Use nursing knowledge and the process of elimination to make a selection.

21 **Answer: 1** A low-phenylalanine diet reduces the amount of toxic metabolites in the body, thus reducing or preventing additional damage. There is no indication of a need to admit the child to a long-term care facility, and babies with PKU have normal life expectancy. No medications are currently being used to treat PKU.
Cognitive Level: Application **Client Need:** Physiological Integrity: Physiological Adaptation **Integrated Process:** Nursing Process: Planning **Content Area:** Child Health: Endocrine and Metabolic **Strategy:** The core issue of the question is management of PKU in a newly diagnosed infant. Use nursing knowledge and the process of elimination to make a selection.

22 **Answer: 2** Some teens develop type 2 diabetes, especially those who are overweight. They might need to take an oral hypoglycemic with or without accompanying insulin. Insulin is not used for those who won't take oral medication. Sweets and complex carbohydrates still need to be restricted. Option 1 does not offer the information that the child needs about the treatment options.
Cognitive Level: Application **Client Need:** Physiological Integrity: Physiological Adaptation **Integrated Process:** Teaching and Learning **Content Area:** Child Health: Endocrine and Metabolic **Strategy:** The core issue of the question is correct information about medication therapy for overweight adolescents with new onset diabetes. Use nursing knowledge and the process of elimination to make a selection.

23 **Answer: 2** The child should be seen by the physician because there might be secretion of sex hormones, and precocious puberty may affect linear growth. Although she may be teased in school by the other children (option 3), the main reason for seeking treatment is health promotion. Options 1 and 4 are incorrect statements.
Cognitive Level: Application **Client Need:** Physiological Integrity: Physiological Adaptation **Integrated Process:** Nursing Process: Planning **Content Area:** Child Health: Endocrine and Metabolic **Strategy:** The core issue of the question is the priority need of a client with suspected precocious puberty. Use nursing knowledge and the process of elimination to make a selection.

24 **Answer: 1** Adolescents need to feel like part of their group, even if it means impairing their health. Displaying risk-taking behaviors is not likely the primary motivation, but rather a secondary event. Option 3 is true but is not likely to be the motivating factor. There is no information to support a self-destructive wish (option 2).
Cognitive Level: Analysis **Client Need:** Physiological Integrity: Physiological Adaptation **Integrated Process:** Nursing Process: Analysis **Content Area:** Child Health: Endocrine and Metabolic **Strategy:** The core issue of the question is knowledge of age-specific concerns of adolescents with diabetes mellitus. Use nursing knowledge and the process of elimination to make a selection.

25 **Answer: 1** A karyotype is simply a study of the chromosomes. A blood sample may be used to provide the cells for analysis. Options 2 and 3 are incorrect. Option 4 provides no information at all for the child and does not address the client's concern.
Cognitive Level: Application **Client Need:** Physiological Integrity: Physiological Adaptation **Integrated Process:** Communication and Documentation **Content Area:** Child Health: Endocrine and Metabolic **Strategy:** The core issue of the question is appropriate information about a karyotype test. Use nursing knowledge and the process of elimination to make a selection.

26 **Answer: 2, 3, 5** The client with hyperpituitarism will exhibit the following: tall stature if onset in childhood, large hands and feet with prominent jawbone, joint changes consistent with arthritis, deep voice and possible dysphagia, hypertension, organomegaly, and skin changes leading to rough, oily texture. The client would not have a soft voice or be short in stature.
Cognitive Level: Analysis **Client Need:** Physiological Integrity: Physiological Adaptation **Integrated Process:** Nursing Process: Assessment **Content Area:** Child Health: Endocrine and Metabolic **Strategy:** The core issue of the question is knowledge of assessment findings with hyperpituitarism. Recall the functions of the pituitary gland and then correlate the functions with the logical signs of excess to make the appropriate selections.

Key Terms to Review

glycosylated hemoglobin p. 1202
hyperglycemia p. 1202
hypersecretion p. 1200
hyperthyroidism (Graves' disease) p. 1205
hyposecretion p. 1200
ketosis p. 1211
paresthesia p. 1209
photophobia p. 1206
polydipsia p. 1204
polyphagia p. 1211
polyuria p. 1204
receptor p. 1200
thyroid crisis (thyroid storm) p. 1205

References

Ball, J., & Bindler, R. (2006). *Child health nursing: Partnering with children and families.* Upper Saddle River, NJ: Pearson Education.

Black, J., & Hawks, J. (2005). *Medical surgical nursing: Clinical management for positive outcomes* (7th ed.). St. Louis: Elsevier Science.

Corbett, J. (2004). *Laboratory tests and diagnostic procedures with nursing diagnoses* (6th ed.). Upper Saddle River, NJ: Pearson Education.

Harkreader, H., & Hogan, M. (2004). *Fundamentals of nursing: Caring and clinical judgment* (2nd ed.). St. Louis: Elsevier Science.

Ignatavicius, D., & Workman, L. (2006). *Medical-surgical nursing: Critical thinking for collaborative care* (5th ed.). Philadelphia: W. B. Saunders.

Kozier, B., Erb, G., Berman, A., & Snyder, S. (2004). *Fundamentals of nursing: Concepts, process, and practice* (7th ed.). Upper Saddle River, NJ: Pearson Education.

LeMone, P., & Burke, K. (2004). *Medical surgical nursing: Critical thinking in client care* (3rd ed.). Upper Saddle River, NJ: Pearson Education.

Porth, C. (2004). *Pathophysiology: Concepts of altered health states* (7th ed.). Philadelphia: Lippincott Williams & Wilkins.

Smith, S., Duell, D., & Martin, B. (2004). *Clinical nursing skills: Basic to advanced skills* (6th ed.). Upper Saddle River, NJ: Pearson Education.

62 Musculoskeletal Disorders

Test Yourself

Are you ready for the NCLEX-RN® or course exams? Use the practice tests on the companion CD-ROM to check.

In this chapter

Cross reference

Other chapters relevant to this content area are

Neurological and Musculoskeletal Medications	Chapter 39
Common Laboratory Tests	Chapter 47
Common Diagnostic Tests and Procedures	Chapter 48

I. OVERVIEW OF ANATOMY AND PHYSIOLOGY OF THE MUSCULOSKELETAL SYSTEM

A. **Skeleton:** consists of bones, joints, and cartilage; supports framework of body and protects soft tissue and vital organs; composed primarily of calcium (Ca^{++} phosphate and Ca^{++} carbonate; provides points of attachment for muscles

B. **Classification of bones**

1. Two major classifications of bones are based on structure: compact bone (dense) or cancellous bone (spongy)
2. A central shaft (**diaphysis**) and two end portions (**epiphyseals**) characterize long bones (e.g., humerus and radius)

3. Short bones are characterized by cancellous bone covered by a thin layer of compact bone (examples: carpals and tarsals)
4. Flat bones are characterized by two layers of compact bone separated by a layer of cancellous bone (e.g., skull, ribs, scapula, and sternum)

C. Bone marrow

1. Soft, spongy, highly cellular blood-forming tissue that fills the cavities of bones and is the site for hematopoiesis (RBC production) and storage of RBCs
2. Responsible also for production of WBCs, and platelets
3. Becomes predominantly fatty with age, particularly in long bones of limb

D. Axial section

1. Each vertebra is constructed like a ring, one on top of the next, with a padding of cartilage between; vertebral rings are studded with bony projections called processes, which function as attachments for muscles and points of articulation with bones
2. Twelve pairs of ribs attach to thoracic vertebrae; upper 7 opposing pairs attach at front to sternum; 3 of remaining 5 pairs attach to rib immediately above by cartilage, and the last 2 pairs are unattached

E. Appendicular section

1. Connected to axial skeleton by bones of upper and lower extremities
   a. Shoulder girdle supports arms; humerus is located in upper arm and ulna and radius in forearm
   b. Each innominate bone (hip bone) consists of 3 parts—ileum, ischium, and pubis; innominate bones unite with sacrum and coccyx of vertebral column to form pelvic girdle, which supports legs

F. Joint articulations

1. Result when two bones are joined together; categorized according to type of motion
2. Composed of fibrous connective tissue and cartilage (dense avascular connective tissue) that covers ends of bones making movement smooth
3. Joint cavity secretes synovial fluid, which lubricates joint and reduces friction

G. Ligaments: bands of rigid connective tissue that hold joints together, allowing for movement and stability; have a relatively poor blood supply, which significantly prolongs healing process after injury

H. Muscles

1. Primarily function as a source of power and pull against bones to move body
2. Three primary types of muscle: skeletal muscle (striated, voluntary) moves extremities and external areas of body; cardiac muscle (striated, involuntary) is found in heart; smooth muscle (nonstriated, involuntary) is found in walls of arteries and bowel

II. DIAGNOSTIC TESTS AND ASSESSMENTS

A. Radiologic tests: x-rays are widely used to assess musculoskeletal problems and effectiveness of treatment; radiological studies other than simple x-rays may be done with or without contrast

B. EMG (electromyogram or myogram): records and evaluates electrical activity of muscles during contraction

1. There are two different types of EMG: intramuscular (IM) EMG (more commonly used) and surface EMG (SEMG)
2. ! Long, small-gauge needles are inserted through the skin into muscle; client may feel mild to moderate discomfort during the procedure
3. Needles detect electrical activity of muscle and transmit data to electromyogram machine, which displays electrical activity on an oscilloscope or transmits through an audiotransmitter (microphone)
4. SEMG: electrodes are placed above muscle to detect electrical activity

C. *Arthroscopy:* surgical procedure done under local or general anesthesia to examine internal structure of a joint using an arthroscope (a pencil-sized device with optical fibers and lenses), which is inserted into very small skin incisions; device is connected to a video camera to allow for visualization of interior of joint

1. Procedure may diagnose or treat musculoskeletal disorders such as osteoarthritis, rheumatoid arthritis, infectious types of arthritis, and internal joint injuries like meniscus tears, ligament strains or tears, and cartilage deterioration
2. Arthroscopic surgery can be done during procedure to repair joint tissue; arthroscopic surgery creates less tissue trauma, less pain, and allows for more rapid recovery than traditional joint surgery
3. ! Client education: postprocedure
   a. Take analgesics for comfort and limit activity as directed
   b. Observe site for hematoma or bleeding
   c. Perform neurovascular self-assessment (temperature, color, capillary refill, movement, and sensation) on affected extremity
   d. Report signs and symptoms of infection: elevated temperature, warmth at surgical site, purulent discharge, and redness

D. **Arthrogram:** contrast media or air is injected into joint cavity for visualization of joint structures; client moves joint through a series of movements while a series of x-rays are taken; assess for allergy to contrast media
1. ! Client education preprocedure: if injected contrast dye is used, inform client that once dye is injected there may be a feeling of warmth, nausea, headache, salty taste in the mouth, itching, hives, and rash throughout body (symptoms are usually temporary and will be treated if necessary)
2. ! Client education postprocedure
   a. Inform client that temporary discoloration of skin and urine is normal after use of dye
   b. Perform neurovascular self-assessment on affected extremity
   c. Increase fluid intake to aid in dye excretion and protect kidneys from dye

E. **CT scan (computerized axial tomography):** combines x-rays with computer technology to produce a highly detailed, cross-sectional image of bones, joints, and other structures

F. **MRI (magnetic resonance imaging):** similar uses as CT Scan

G. **Bone scan:** technique used to create images of bones on a computer screen or on a film using a small amount of radioactive material that travels through bloodstream; increased radioisotope uptake is seen with osteomyelitis, osteoporosis, fractures, Paget's disease, and cancer of bone

H. **Bone densitometry (bone density):** measurement of bone mineral density (BMD) that aids in diagnosis of osteoporosis, predicts fracture risk, and aids in evaluating effectiveness of treatment
1. Noninvasive radiologic test that digitally images hip, spine, wrist, finger, tibia, or heel using photon energy beams
2. Takes 30 seconds to 4 minutes per site, and no preprocedure or postprocedure care is required
3. Client's scores include a T-score (compares client score with the score of a normal 30-year-old) and a Z-score (compares client normal to normal in a healthy, age-matched client)
4. Results are reported in standard deviations (SD) below normal and are expressed as negative numbers; scores within 1 standard deviation are considered normal; a score of -1 SD represents a 12% reduction in bone mass); treatment is initiated at -2.5 SD or lower
5. Results should be reassessed every 2 years

I. ***Arthrocentesis* (joint aspiration) and analysis:** fluid is removed from joint to reduce swelling and pain and/or obtain fluid for examination using a sterile needle and syringe
1. Postprocedure complications are uncommon but may include localized bruising, minor bleeding into joint cavity, and loss of pigment at injection site (septic arthritis is a rare but serious complication)
2. ! Client education
   a. If cortisone was injected into joint, teach client to monitor for inflammation of injected area, atrophy or loss of pigment at injection site, and increased blood glucose
   b. Instruct client to follow postprocedure activity restrictions as directed by health care provider and monitor for postprocedure complications; check dressing for excessive bleeding

III. LABORATORY STUDIES

A. Antinuclear antibodies (ANA): sensitive screening blood test used to detect autoimmune disease
1. ANAs destroy nucleus of cells
2. Test not definitive but suggests presence of autoantibodies (antibodies directed against body's own tissue)
3. Present in clients with a number of autoimmune diseases such as rheumatoid arthritis, systemic lupus erythematosus, scleroderma, and others

B. Calcium (Ca^{++}): an abundant electrolyte in body that causes neuromuscular irritability and contractions; adult normal reference value is 9 to 11 mg/dL; range varies slightly by laboratory; see also chapter 54
1. Decreased calcium levels may be found in osteomalacia, inadequate dietary intake of calcium, renal disease, and hypoparathyroidism
2. Increased calcium levels may be seen in bone neoplasm, multiple fractures, immobilization, renal calculi, and hyperparathyroidism

C. Phosphorus (2.5 to 4.5 mg/dL is normal reference range); may be measured and compared to calcium level
1. Decreased levels can be seen with hypercalcemia, starvation, malabsorption syndrome, osteomalacia, and vitamin D deficiency
2. Increased levels can be seen with healing fractures, metastatic bone tumors, and hypocalcemia

D. Rheumatoid factor (RF) (Normal is negative or <1:20): screening blood test used to detect antibodies (IgM, IgG, or IgA) in rheumatoid arthritis; elevated RF level may indicate diseases other than rheumatoid arthritis

E. Erythrocyte sedimentation rate (ESR): normal is under 20 mm/hr; gender variations exist; nonspecific serologic test that measures rate at which RBCs settle out of unclotted blood in mm/hr; elevated levels indicate inflammatory process in diseases such as rheumatoid arthritis and osteomyelitis

F. Uric acid (normal male 4.5–6.5 mg/dL, female 2.5–5.5 mg/dL)
1. Elevated uric acid level is seen in gout
2. ! Hyperuricemia (elevated urine or serum uric acid levels) occurs because of poor renal function, excessive purine metabolism, and/or excessive dietary intake of purine foods

IV. COMMON NURSING TECHNIQUES AND PROCEDURES

A. Crutch-walking
1. Crutch gaits: safe method of walking using crutches, alternating body weight on one or both legs and the crutches
2. ! See Box 62–1 for crutch-walking techniques
3. See Box 62–2 for transfer techniques (getting in and out of a chair) using crutches
4. ! See Box 62–3 for negotiating stairs while using crutches, 1283

> **Memory Aid**
> Use the phrase "good leg up; bad leg down" to help remember which leg to place first when going up and down stairs with crutches.

B. *Traction:* direct pulling force applied to a fractured extremity that results in realignment of bone; see Figure 62–1 ■, p. 1234
1. Reduces fracture, lessens muscle spasms, relieves pain, corrects deformities, promotes rest, and allows for exercise
2. Skin and skeletal traction are most commonly used; manual traction is used only briefly under physician direction
3. ! Skin traction (using tape, boots, splints)
   a. Generally used for short-term treatment (48 to 72 hours) and is applied directly to skin; used until skeletal traction or surgery are available to treat fracture
   b. Assists in reduction of a fracture (does not primarily achieve reduction) and helps decrease muscle spasms
   c. Weights range from 5 to 10 pounds

Box 62-1

Instructions for the Client on the Use of Crutches

Four-Point Gait

- Slow gait
- Requires good coordination
- Weight-bearing is on both legs
- Move each foot and crutch forward separately (right crutch, left foot; left crutch, right foot)

Two-Point Gait

- Faster than four-point gait
- Requires more balance
- There is partial weight-bearing on each foot
- Arm movements simulate arm movement when walking
- Move left crutch and right foot forward together; move right crutch and left foot forward together

Three-Point Gait

- Fast gait
- Two crutches and unaffected leg bear weight alternately
- Weaker leg and both crutches move together followed by stronger leg

Swing-To Gait

- Fast gait
- Used by clients with paralysis of legs and hips
- Prolonged use may lead to atrophy of unused muscles
- Advance crutches forward together, lift body using arms, then swing to meet crutches

Swing-Through Gait

- Fast gait
- Good balance, skill, coordination and strength required
- Move both crutches forward together
- Lift body using arms, then swing through and beyond crutches

!

4. Skeletal traction (using pins or wires inserted into bones)
   a. Indicated for long-term use
   b. Used to align injured bones and joints or to treat joint contractures and congenital hip dysplasia
   c. Weights are usually 15 to 30 pounds and amounts of weight may be adjusted initially until full fracture reduction is achieved as noted on x-ray
5. Balanced suspension (traction that is a hanging support to immobilize body part in a desired position)
   a. Used with skeletal traction to improve mobility while maintaining alignment of fracture
   b. Body part is suspended using splints, ropes, and weights
   c. Client can perform activities such as toileting and personal hygiene; bed linen can be changed without disturbing traction alignment
   d. Risk for skin breakdown exists over bony prominences that are in contact with sheets (including back of head)
6. **Countertraction:** pulling force exerted in opposite direction to prevent client from sliding to end of bed; examples include client's weight, elevating foot of bed (Trendelenburg), and elevating head of bed with cervical traction

Box 62–2

Transfer Techniques for Clients with Crutches

Getting Into a Chair

1. Use chair with armrests and support back of chair against a wall for stability.
2. Center the back of the unaffected leg against the chair.
3. Transfer crutches to the hand on the affected side.
4. Hold crutches by horizontal hand bars.
5. Grasp the arm of the chair with the hand on the unaffected side.
6. Lean forward, flex the knees and hips, and lower into the chair.

Getting Out of a Chair

1. Move forward to the edge of the chair.
2. Place unaffected leg slightly under or at the edge of the chair (this position helps the client to stand up from the chair and achieve balance, since the unaffected leg is supported against the edge of the chair).
3. Grasp the crutches by the horizontal hand bars using the hand on the affected side.
4. Grasp the arm of the chair using the hand on the unaffected side (the body weight is placed on the crutches and the hand on the armrest to support the unaffected leg when the client rises to stand).
5. Push down on the crutches and the chair armrest while raising the body out of the chair.
6. Assume a *tripod position* (crutches out laterally in front of feet, approximately 6 inches, with feet slightly apart creating a wide base of support) for balance before moving.

! 7. See Box 62–4 (p. 1235) for nursing care of client in traction

! C. **Cast care:** a cast is applied for immobilization to ensure stability of a fracture; see Box 62–5, p. 1236, for associated nursing care

D. **Splinting and immobilization:** like casts, splints are used to immobilize a fractured extremity to ensure stability after closed reduction and external fixation; teach client how to perform neurovascular assessment (color, temperature, capillary refill less than 3 seconds, and pulses)

Box 62–3

Instructions for Clients with Crutches: Negotiating Stairs

Going Up Stairs (stand behind client slightly to the affected side for support if needed)

1. Assume the tripod position.
2. Transfer the weight to crutches and move the unaffected leg onto the step.
3. Transfer weight to the unaffected leg on the step and move crutches and the affected leg up to the step.
4. Repeat steps 2 and 3 until client reaches the top of the stairs.

Going Down Stairs (stand one step below client on the affected side for support if needed)

1. Assume tripod position at the top of the stairs.
2. Shift weight to the unaffected leg.
3. Move crutches and the affected leg down onto the next step.
4. Transfer weight to the crutches and move the unaffected leg to that step.
5. Repeat steps 2 and 3 until the client reaches bottom step.

Figure 62–1

Types of traction. A. Skin traction (also called straight traction), such as Buck's traction for hip fracture. B. Balanced suspension traction, often used for fractures of the femur. C. Skeletal traction, in which pulling force is applied directly to bone, such as for a fracture of the humerus.

Source: LeMone, P., & Burke, K. (2003). Medical surgical nursing: Critical thinking for client care *(3rd ed.). Upper Saddle River, NJ: Pearson Education, p. 1199.*

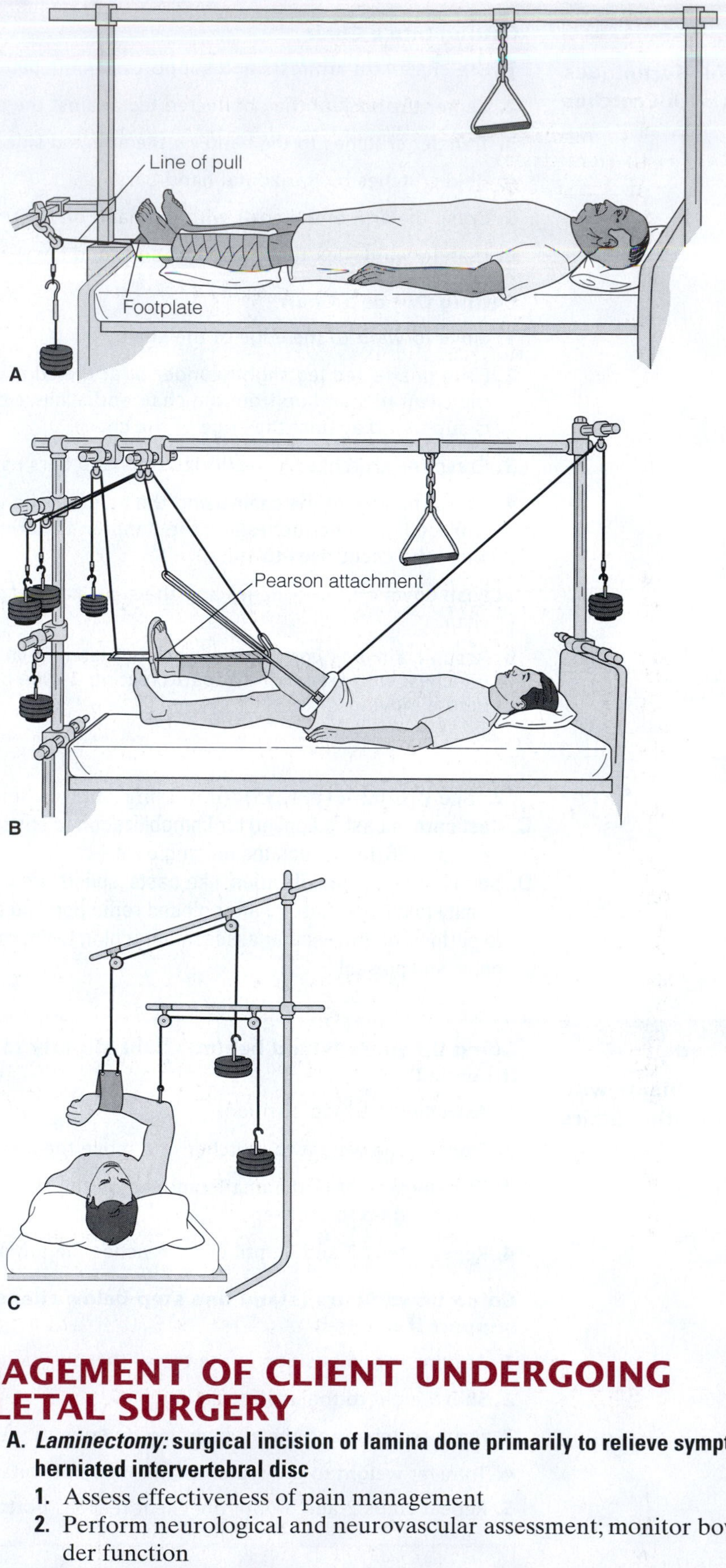

V. NURSING MANAGEMENT OF CLIENT UNDERGOING MUSCULOSKELETAL SURGERY

A. *Laminectomy:* surgical incision of lamina done primarily to relieve symptoms related to herniated intervertebral disc

1. Assess effectiveness of pain management
2. Perform neurological and neurovascular assessment; monitor bowel and bladder function
3. Assess client for complaints of severe headache or leakage of cerebrospinal fluid (CSF), nausea, abdominal discomfort, incontinence, amount and character of drainage on dressing

Box 62–4

Nursing Care of the Client in Traction

- ➤ Ensure that all ropes, weights, and pulleys are hanging freely, not shredded or torn, in a straight line.
- ➤ Bed linen should be kept off traction ropes.
- ➤ Teach client that weights should not be lifted for any reason (lifting of weights alters the line of pull and could potentially interfere with bone healing).
- ➤ Ensure that the ordered amount of weight is maintained at all times.
- ➤ Avoid jarring bed or equipment.
- ➤ Ensure that knots are not lying on or near the pulley.
- ➤ Perform neurovascular assessment to monitor for superficial nerve damage (radial, median, ulnar, femoral, sciatic, peroneal nerves).
- ➤ Teach client how to perform circulatory assessment on unaffected and affected limb, comparing observations (color, temperature, capillary refill, pulses).
- ➤ Teach client how to perform skin assessment to monitor and prevent skin breakdown on bony prominence and pressure areas.
- ➤ Ensure that body is always kept in proper alignment to prevent complications such as external rotation of the joint, increased pain, and poor healing of the fracture.
- ➤ Provide pin care as per agency policy, and teach client how to monitor for infection at pin sites (fever, localized warmth, redness, swelling, abnormal drainage, and odor).
- ➤ Inform client to avoid massaging calves or reddened areas to prevent clot dislodgment caused by venous stasis.
- ➤ Encourage client to increase fluid intake (2500 mL/day unless contraindicated) and roughage (fresh fruits and vegetables) in diet to prevent constipation, urinary tract infection, and renal calculi.
- ➤ Teach client how to perform deep-breathing and coughing exercises to prevent respiratory complications.
- ➤ Encourage client to use the overhead trapeze (and unaffected leg if possible) to reposition for comfort, shift weight to prevent skin breakdown, perform exercises, and assist with personal care, toileting, and bed linen changes.
- ➤ Encourage client to adhere to exercise regimen to maintain muscle tone, endurance, and prevent bone demineralization.
- ➤ Provide diversional activities and encourage social interaction with family and friends to prevent potential isolation.

4. Use *logroll* technique (turning a client as a unit) to turn and reposition client; maintain proper alignment of spine at all times
5. ! Inform client that bedrest may be maintained for first 24 to 48 hours after procedure; pillows may be used for comfort under thighs in supine position and between in the side-lying position
6. Help client to "rise as a unit" when getting out of bed (especially for first time)
7. Instruct client that paresthesia (numbness and tingling of extremities) may not be relieved immediately after procedure

B. *Internal fixation:* fracture immobilization with a metal device (made of screws, pins, and/or plates) that is surgically inserted to realign and maintain a fracture

1. Inform client that x-rays will be taken at regular intervals to ensure proper alignment of fixation device
2. Instruct client about signs and symptoms of infection to report: elevated temperature, localized pain and warmth, tenderness, chills, malaise, and changes in neurovascular status of affected extremity

C. Joint replacement, total hip replacement (THR)

1. THR is frequently performed for client with conditions such as rheumatoid arthritis, malignant bone tumors, arthritis associated with Paget's disease, juvenile rheumatoid arthritis, and hip fractures

Box 62-5

Nursing Care of the Client in a Cast

- ➤ Teach client that plaster cast should not get wet and that cast padding should not be removed; if cast becomes soiled with feces, clean with a damp cloth or rub baking soda on soiled area to limit odor.
- ➤ Teach client that no foreign objects should be inserted into the cast (sticks, food crumbs, etc.) to prevent skin breakdown; teach client how to smooth rough edges.
- ➤ Instruct client to avoid covering a new cast with blanket or plastic for extended periods (air cannot circulate, and heat builds up in the cast).
- ➤ Turn client from side to side (using palms, not fingertips) every 2 hours to facilitate drying for the first 24 to72 hours (use of fingertips causes indentation and pressure areas when cast is dry).
- ➤ Explain that casts made with newer synthetic materials dry more quickly and allow faster mobility (often can bear weight within 30 minutes)
- ➤ Instruct client to apply ice for the first 24 hours over fracture site to control edema, ensuring that ice is securely contained so cast does not become wet.
- ➤ Instruct client to elevate extremity above the level of the heart to promote venous return for the first 24 hours after application.
- ➤ Instruct client to perform active range of motion (AROM) to joints above and below immobilized extremity.
- ➤ Teach client about signs and symptoms to report to health care provider: increasing pain in immobilized extremity, excessive swelling and discoloration of exposed limb, burning or tingling, sores, or foul odor under cast.

2. Advantages of THR: substantial relief of pain, improved function and quality of life
3. Teach client about plan for effective pain management and side effects/adverse effects of pain medications
4. ! Teach client about dislocation precautions
    a. Avoid extremes of internal rotation, adduction, and 90-degree flexion of affected hip for at least 4 to 6 weeks after procedure
    b. Prevent adduction: use an abduction pillow, avoid crossing legs, avoid twisting to reach for objects behind, and avoid driving a car and taking tub baths for at least 4 to 6 weeks
    c. Modify equipment to avoid 90-degree hip flexion (raised toilet seats, platform under chair, use of reaches, long-handled shoe horns, and sock pullers)
5. Inform client that passive range of motion (ROM) and physical therapy exercises will begin on first postoperative day to restore and maintain ROM, muscle strength, and mobility and to prevent complications such as deep vein thrombosis (DVT)
6. ! Teach client about signs and symptoms to report to health care provider
    a. Infection: redness, swelling, abnormal drainage, foul odor, and elevated temperature
    b. DVT: pain, sudden swelling in affected extremity, enlargement of superficial veins, skin discoloration, and localized warmth
7. Instruct client that homecare management program will include:
    a. Ongoing nursing assessment of pain management
    b. Periodic dressing changes and monitoring for infection
    c. ! Monitoring and adjustment of coagulation status weekly if taking warfarin (Coumadin) and less often if taking enoxaparin (Lovenox), a low-molecular-weight heparin
    d. An exercise program assisted by a physical therapist to assess and restore muscle strength and range of motion
8. ! Instruct client to inform all health care providers (dentists, etc.) of history of joint replacement surgery so that prophylactic antibiotics can be prescribed as necessary
9. Inform client that periodic x-rays will be required as followup throughout lifetime
10. ! Note for clients undergoing knee replacement: continuous passive motion (CPM) machine may be put in place immediately after surgery and accompanies

client to surgical unit after postanesthesia recovery period; assess that client's limb is positioned correctly and that pain medication is adequate; device should be used at least 8 of every 24 hours and increased as client can tolerate it

D. Amputation

1. Provide client teaching about effective pain management techniques; signs and symptoms to report: redness, elevated temperature, and/or unusual, foul-smelling drainage; abrasions; and any other signs of skin breakdown
2. ! Teach client how to care for residual limb
   a. Wash daily using warm water and bacteriostatic soap
   b. Rinse and gently pat dry thoroughly
   c. Expose to air for at least 20 minutes after washing
   d. Avoid use of lotions, alcohol, powder, or oils unless prescribed by health care provider
   e. Change cotton or wool limb sock daily, wash sock using mild soap and dry flat, and discard sock that is in poor condition
3. Instruct client to perform upper extremity active range of motion (AROM) exercises daily
4. Instruct client to lay prone for 30 minutes 3 to 4 times/day (if client is able and if part of standard of care) and avoid elevating or sitting with residual limb on pillows to prevent flexion contractures
5. ! Tell client that phantom pain may persist in amputated extremity because of irritation of residual nerve endings; this is normal and real; discomfort will be treated with analgesics or other interventions

VI. OSTEOPOROSIS

A. Overview

1. Disease characterized by low bone mass and structural deterioration of bone tissue, causing bone (especially weight-bearing bones such as hip, spine, and wrist) to become fragile and more susceptible to fractures
2. Affects both women and men; however, women are at greater risk
3. As people age, bone resorption happens faster than bone formation, which causes bone to lose Ca^{++} and bone density; since most of body's Ca^{++} is stored in bones and teeth, this rapid bone resorption leads to porous bone or osteoporosis
4. When serum Ca^{++} decreases, body takes stored Ca^{++} from bone

! **B. Nursing assessment**

1. Risk factors include caucasian or Asian ethnicity; family history; inadequate dietary intake of Ca^{++}; sedentary lifestyle; smoking; excessive alcohol intake; steroid medications; chronic liver disease; anorexia; and malabsorption
2. Females are at a higher risk for osteoporosis than men
   a. Smaller body frames contribute to less bone density
   b. Bone resorption begins at an earlier age and is accelerated in menopause
   c. Breast-feeding and pregnancy deplete skeletal reserves unless Ca^{++} intake is increased to match demands
   d. Longevity increases the likelihood of osteoporosis (compared to men)

! **C. Therapeutic management**

1. Provide client teaching about prevention
   a. Take adequate amounts of Ca^{++} throughout lifetime to decrease the incidence of osteoporosis
   b. Proper nutrition for adequate Ca^{++} intake
   c. Weight-bearing exercises to force Ca^{++} back into the bone
   d. Safety measures to prevent falls that can result in fractures
   e. BMD tests to measure bone mass in clients at risk for developing osteoporosis
   f. Provide clients with information about recommended daily dietary intake of Ca^{++}: 1,000–1200 mg/day for premenopausal and postmenopausal women taking estrogen replacement therapy (ERT), and 1,500 mg/day for postmenopausal women who are not taking ERT
   g. Provide information about foods high in Ca^{++} and importance of Ca^{++} intake with vitamin D: dark, green leafy vegetables (such as broccoli, bok choy,

collard greens, spinach), sardines, salmon with bone, dairy products (such as milk, cottage cheese, cheese, yogurt, and ice cream); Ca^{++} supplements can also be added to dietary intake

2. Medication therapy (see also Chapter 39)
   a. ERT is generally used to prevent osteoporosis after menopause; usually given in form of a pill or skin patch; can increase risk for endometrial cancer (progesterone may be given with estrogen, called hormone replacement therapy or HRT, to decrease risk); client is also at risk for developing DVT
   b. Calcitonin (Micalcin, Calcimar): naturally occurring hormone secreted by thyroid gland; currently available as a nasal spray or injection; slows bone loss, increases spinal bone density, relieves pain from bone fractures, and reduces risk for spinal and hip fractures
   c. Alendronate (Fosamax): prevents bone resorption in men and women with glucocorticoid-induced osteoporosis; take with a glass of water at least 30 minutes before eating; remain standing or sitting for 30 minutes after dose
   d. Raloxifene (Evista): used to prevent or treat osteoporosis; selective receptor modulator (SERM) that prevents bone loss; side effects are rare but may include hot flashes or DVT; may be taken without regard to food
   ! e. Risedronate sodium (Actonel): biphosphonate, used to prevent and treat osteoporosis in postmenopausal women and glucocorticoid-induced osteoporosis in both men and women; take drug with a glass of water at least 30 minutes before first food or beverage of day and avoid eating for at least 30 minutes after taking medication; remain in an upright position for at least 30 minutes after taking medication

D. Client teaching

1. Reinforce importance of weight-bearing exercises (jogging, walking, hiking, stair climbing, tennis, dancing, and weight training)
2. Encourage client to stop smoking and avoid excessive intake of alcohol

VII. OSTEOMYELITIS

A. Overview

1. Acute or chronic infection of bone usually caused by *staphylococcus aureus* organism
2. Infection can occur from direct or indirect invasion of infectious organisms; see Figure 62–2
3. Direct invasion generally occurs from invasive procedures such as surgery (joint prosthesis, arthroplasty) and injuries such as fractures

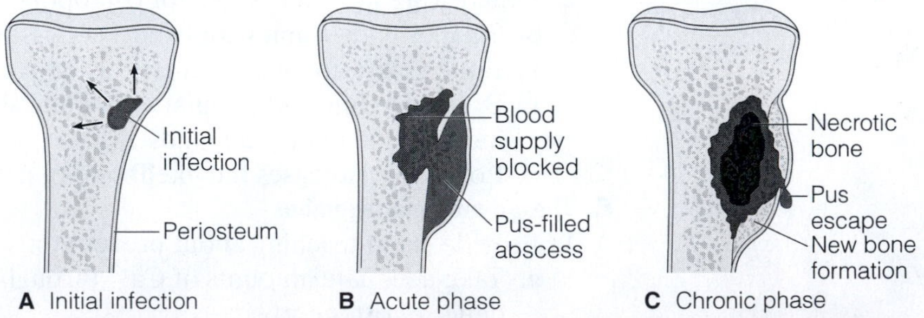

Figure 62–2

Osteomyelitis. A. Site of initial infection. Bacteria enter bone and multiply, initiating inflammatory response. B. Acute phase, with spread of infection to other parts of bone. Pus forms, edema occurs, and vascular supply is compromised. If infection reaches outer margin of bone, periosteum lifts, and ischemia and necrosis occur eventually. C. Chronic phase. Necrotic bone separates, a new layer of bone forms around necrotic bone, and sinus develops to allow wound to drain.

Source: LeMone, P., & Burke, K. (2003). Medical surgical nursing: Critical thinking for client care *(3rd ed.). Upper Saddle River, NJ: Pearson Education, p. 1268.*

4. Infection can also be caused by indirect invasion (also referred to as hematogenous dissemination), where infection of bone tissue or joint is caused by spread of organism through bloodstream from a preexisting site of infection; course and virulence of infection is influenced by blood circulation to affected bone
5. Long bones are common sites of infection in children, and spine, hip, and foot are common sites of infection in adults
6. At-risk populations include children, elderly, and individuals with weakened immune systems
7. Osteomyelitis warrants aggressive immediate treatment with antibiotics or surgery (wound debridement) if infection of bone is extensive

! **B. Nursing assessment**

1. Observe for symptoms of local and/or systemic infection: elevated temperature, chills, restlessness, severe bone pain unrelieved by analgesics or rest and aggravated by movement, swelling, redness, and warmth at the infection site
2. Wound culture, bone scan, CT scan, and MRI provide information for diagnosis and assess extent of infection

! **C. Therapeutic management**

1. Explain all therapies and interventions to client and family to decrease anxiety and enhance cooperation with plan of care
2. Use a rating scale to assess pain and evaluate effectiveness of pain management measures
3. Provide ongoing education and emotional support since seriousness of infection, duration and uncertainty about recuperation time, potential complications, and associated risk can be a very fearful experience for client and family
4. Teach client about risk factors for osteomyelitis, which include previous joint replacement surgery and implants
5. ! Use sterile technique for all dressing changes and manipulation of affected limb; handle extremity very gently
6. ! Avoid activities that increase circulation to affected area or cause edema, pain, and pathologic fractures, such as exercise, application of heat, or keeping extremity in dependent position
7. Immobilize affected extremity as prescribed and keep body in proper alignment
8. Monitor temperature at least every 2 hours
9. Provide cool environment, light clothing, antipyretic medication, antibiotics, and other therapies as prescribed and/or appropriate to keep temperature within client's baseline
10. Keep client well hydrated to prevent dehydration from insensible water loss
11. ! If long-term management is required, provide instructions about wound care using sterile technique, medication regimen (including instruction on venous access devices if needed), antibiotic administration, proper diet, rest, follow-up visits, and laboratory tests
12. Provide information about adverse effects of antibiotic therapy such as ototoxicity and nephrotoxicity (aminoglycosides) and hepatotoxicity (cephalosporins)
13. Instruct and assist client with interventions to prevent complications associated with immobility (turn and reposition every 2 hours, coughing and deep breathing exercises, etc.)
14. Medication therapy is indicated with or without surgical intervention; generally includes antibiotics and analgesics

D. Client teaching

1. Importance of taking antibiotic medications as prescribed (for full duration) and to report adverse medication effects to prescriber
2. Review medication regimen and have client verbalize an understanding of teaching
3. Reinforce importance of rest and proper diet to facilitate healing and prevent constipation and dehydration
4. ! Reinforce importance of limb immobilization during treatment

VIII. MUSCULAR DYSTROPHY (MD)

A. Overview

1. Group of genetic sex-linked childhood disorders characterized by progressive muscle weakness, muscle wasting of symmetrical groups of muscles, and increasing disability and deformity
2. Types of MD include Duchenne (most common), myotonic, Becker's, facioscapulohumeral, and limb girdle
3. Significant risk factor is family history
4. Each type differs in regard to muscle groups affected, age at onset, rate of progression, and pattern of inheritance
5. Each type of MD affects specific muscle groups

B. Nursing assessment

1. Muscle biopsy confirms diagnosis (shows degeneration of muscle fibers)
2. EMG is also used to identify origin of muscle weakness (destruction of muscle or nerve damage)
3. Progressive muscle weakness, hypotonia (loss of muscle mass), and delayed development of motor skills such as walking may be observed and reported by parent or caregiver
4. Ptosis (drooping of the eyelid), impaired chewing and swallowing, abnormal gait, fatigue with minimal activity, frequent falls may all be observed and reported by parent or caregiver
5. Delayed intellectual development is seen with some forms of MD
6. Muscle contractures and deformities common
7. Abnormal curvature of spine (scoliosis or lordosis)
8. Enlargement of calf muscle (pseudohypertrophy) caused by fatty infiltration causing muscular enlargement
9. Cardiomyopathy or arrhythmia may be present with some forms of MD

C. Therapeutic management

1. Provide support and assist family with decision-making process surrounding:
   a. Development of a homecare plan to support as much independence as possible
   b. Modifications in home environment to support client's maximal functional ability
2. Encourage family to actively involve client in care
3. Family members may experience a myriad of emotions, including fear, guilt, anger, and blame; support family to enhance coping with client's progressively worsening disease; refer to local support groups including the Muscular Dystrophy Association of America
4. Assist client and family to cope with progressive, incapacitating, and fatal nature of disease
5. Encourage family to interact with client based on developmental rather than chronological age
6. Teach family strategies to prevent skin breakdown (frequent skin care and linen changes if incontinent, turn and reposition at least every 2 hours, use of protective skin barrier ointments, and adequate fluid intake)
7. Perform passive ROM exercises to maintain function in unaffected extremities and prevent or delay contractures in affected extremities
8. Medication therapy: there is no effective drug therapy; corticosteroids are often used to increase muscle strength

D. Client teaching

1. Provide information about health care team members and roles, including those involved in homecare program for client
2. Instruct family to offer client soft foods and to cut into small pieces to prevent aspiration and choking
3. Encourage family members to seek genetic counseling (parents, female siblings, maternal aunts, and female offspring)
4. Assist family in decision-making about appropriate clothing and footwear because of contractures and wheelchair-bound status
5. Provide family with information on community support groups and agencies with respite services to prevent role strain

IX. PAGET'S DISEASE (OSTEITIS DEFORMANS)

A. Overview

1. Chronic skeletal bone disease with insidious onset often diagnosed around fourth decade of life
2. Results in enlarged, deformed bones but does not affect normal bones
3. Generally affects skull, long bones, spine, and ribs
4. Cause of disease unknown; however, viral infection has been hypothesized as a probable etiology
5. Hereditary factor: may be seen in more than one family member
6. Early diagnosis and treatment is important to prevent disease progression and deformity
7. Excessive bone resorption followed by bone formation leads to weakened bone, bone pain, arthritis, deformity, and potential pathologic fractures
8. Normal bone marrow is replaced by vascular, fibrous, connective tissue that leads to formation of larger, disorganized, and weaker bone tissue

B. Nursing assessment

1. X-ray is most definitive diagnostic test; serum alkaline phosphatase may be elevated
2. ! Bone scan may be done after positive serum alkaline phosphatase test (positive scan shows characteristic abnormally curved contours and thickened cortex); positive bone scan prompts x-ray for definitive diagnosis
3. Mild form of disease may be undetected because there may be no symptoms
4. ! Symptoms include bone pain (most common complaint) and other symptoms depending on which bones are affected
   - a. If skull is affected, headache and hearing loss may be reported as well as increasing head size
   - b. Hip pain may be present if pelvis or femur is involved
   - c. Bowing of lower extremities producing a waddling gait and curvature of spine may be seen in advanced stages
5. Arthritis may result because of damage to joint cartilage
6. Complications are pathologic fractures (may be first indicator of disease) and osteogenic sarcoma (form of bone cancer)

C. Therapeutic management

1. Prognosis is good especially if treatment is started before major deformity occurs
2. Provide analgesics and muscle relaxants for comfort
3. Administer medications as directed to control progression of disease (see medication section)
4. Encourage client to take medication as directed by health care provider because deformity and loss of bone strength will continue without prescribed medications
5. If skull is affected, assist with diet modification, dentures, and eating utensils because teeth may become weak from disease
6. Hearing aid may be recommended if hearing loss results from disease
7. Refer client and family to support group
8. Medication therapy: goal is to control progression of the disease; FDA–approved drugs include: biphosphonates, etidronate disodium (Didronel), pamidronate disodium (Aredia), alandronate sodium (Fosamax), tiludronate disodium (Skelid), risedronate sodium (Actonel), and calcitonin (Miacalcin)

D. Client teaching

1. Ensure that client has a good understanding of plan for pain management
2. Encourage client to take analgesics as prescribed
3. ! Teach client importance of a balanced diet, high in Ca^{++} (1,000–1,500 mg/day) and vitamin D (at least 400 units/day); vitamin D can be obtained from exposure to sunlight
4. Instruct client to inform health care provider of any history of kidney stones or disease before taking Ca^{++}
5. Encourage client to participate in an exercise program to maintain skeletal muscle health, ideal body weight, and joint mobility

6. Instruct client to sleep on a firm mattress if back discomfort is present; if back brace is needed, instruct client on prevention of skin breakdown under brace (undershirt) and safety measures (no driving with brace)
7. Encourage client to modify environment at home to prevent falls that may lead to subsequent fractures
8. Encourage client to participate in community support group

X. FRACTURES

A. Overview

1. A fracture is a break in continuity of a bone
2. May be classified as close/simple fracture (bone breaks but skin remains intact) or open/compound (broken ends of bone penetrate skin)
3. ! Other classification of fractures (see Figure 62–3 ■)
   a. Avulsion: a fracture resulting from tearing of supporting tendons and ligaments
   b. Comminuted: broken bone fragments into more than two pieces
   c. Compressed: bone is crushed
   d. Impacted: ends of broken bone are driven into each other
   e. Depressed: such as in skull fracture, where bone structure is broken and pressed inward
   f. Spiral: break spreads in a spiral fashion along bone shaft; is usually caused by sports injuries and child abuse
   g. Greenstick: an incomplete break in bone where one side splinters leaving other side bent or intact; more common in children
4. Fractures occur in all age groups, although elderly are more prone to fractures resulting from falls
5. When a bone breaks, healing process occurs in three phases
   a. A fracture initiates an inflammatory response (inflammatory phase)
   b. Ca^{++} eventually is deposited in area and osteoblasts promote new bone formation (reparative phase)
   c. Eventually ends of fracture reunite (remodeling phase)

B. Nursing assessment

!

1. Deformity: may be caused by break in continuity of bone itself and pull of muscles on fragmented bones
2. Edema and swelling caused by bleeding into surrounding tissues
3. Pain may be caused by muscle spasms and nerve pressure
4. Crepitus may also be present on palpation; **crepitation** is a popping or grating sound created by movement of broken bone fragments
5. Muscle spasms may be noted near fractured bone
6. Ecchymosis or a bluish discoloration of area caused by blood extravasation into surrounding subcutaneous tissues

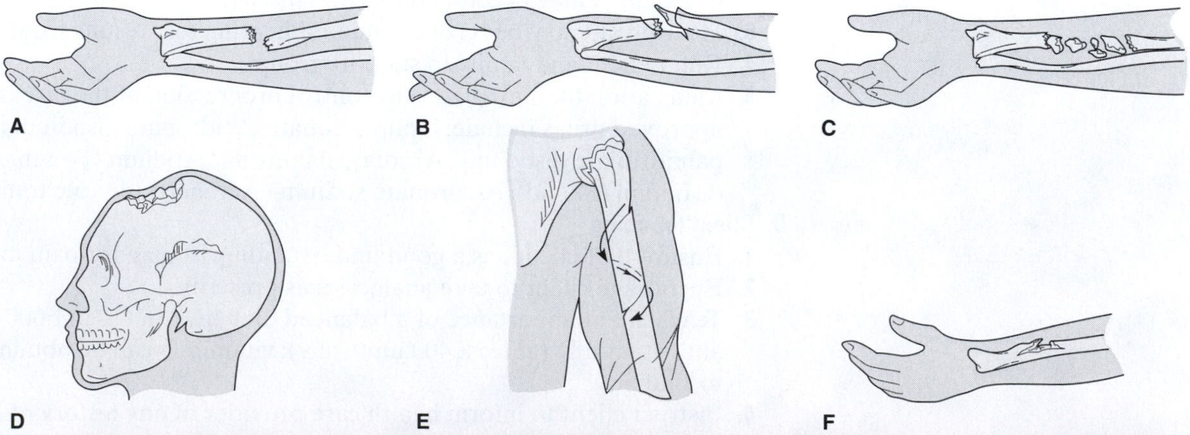

Figure 62–3

Types of fractures. A. Closed. B. Open. C. Comminuted. D. Depressed. E. Spiral. F. Greenstick.

Source: *Ball, J., & Bindler, R. (2006).* Child health nursing: Partnering with children and families. *Upper Saddle River, NJ: Pearson Education, p. 1444.*

7. Pain that may be intense and possibly shock if blood loss is severe

C. Therapeutic management

1. Perform frequent neurovascular assessment; note and report abnormal findings
2. Immobilize joints above and below fracture; movement of affected area may cause a closed fracture to become open; immobilization may be achieved by application of splints
3. Cover open wounds with sterile dressings
4. Manage fracture pain with prescribed analgesics
5. Elevate fractured extremity to reduce swelling and pain
6. Apply ice to affected extremity
7. Assist in fracture reduction: closed reduction involves external manipulation to realign bones; open reduction involves a surgical procedure to realign bones
8. Maintain traction as prescribed; see section on nursing care of client in traction
9. See also section on nursing care of a client in a cast

D. Complications

1. **Compartment syndrome**
   a. Impairment of circulation within inelastic fascia caused by external pressure (>30 mmHg) that results in tissue death and nerve injury
   b. External pressure can be created by casts, splints, or dressings
   c. Manifestations include unrelieved pain, diminished or absent pulses distal to injury, cyanosis of extremity, tingling or diminished sensation (paresthesia), loss of sensation, pallor, coolness of extremity, and weakness
   d. Bivalving (splitting cast lengthwise and resecuring with elastic wrap) may be necessary if cast is too tight
2. Infection: wound drainage, fever, pain, and odor
3. Fat embolism: an emergency situation in which client experiences chest pain, dyspnea, tachycardia, decreased O_2 saturation, apprehension, changes in LOC, petechiae on upper trunk and axilla; aggressive diagnosis and treatment is necessary to save client's life
4. DVT: calf pain and tenderness, swelling or edema

E. Client teaching

1. Exercise extremities not immobilized to prevent muscle atrophy
2. Cast care, splint, and/or traction (see previous discussions)
3. Neurovascular self-assessments that need to be done
4. Pin care procedure and methods of preventing wound infection

XI. HIP FRACTURE

A. Overview

1. Hip can fracture at different sites: head, neck, and trochanteric areas; see Figure 62–4 ■, p. 1244
2. Incidence of hip fracture increases with age; 90% of hip fractures are caused by falls
3. A hip fracture is a medical emergency

B. Nursing assessment

1. Hip fractures are generally sustained from falls; monitor LOC and assess for other injuries
2. Perform neurovascular assessment on affected extremity (assess adverse changes such as cool, pale skin and delayed capillary refill more than 3 seconds)

Memory Aid

Use the 5 P's to remember abnormal neurovascular assessment findings: pain, pallor, paresthesia, pulselessness (or decreased pulses), and paralysis (or weakness).

3. Extremity of affected hip will be shorter than unaffected extremity and is generally externally rotated

C. Therapeutic management

1. Prepare client for surgery (verify allergies, informed consent, etc.)
2. Instruct client that an abductor pillow or splint may be necessary to prevent disarticulation of femur

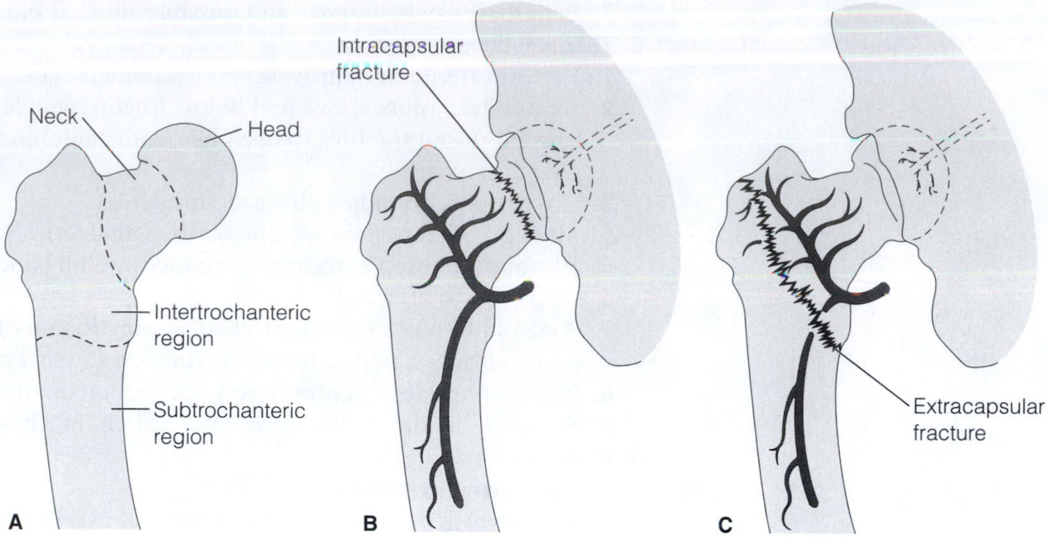

Figure 62-4

A. Hip fractures can occur in the head, neck, or trochanteric regions of the femur. B. An intracapsular fracture affects the femur head or neck. C. An extracapsular fracture occurs across the trochanteric region. All fractures disrupt the blood supply to the bone.

Source: LeMone, P., & Burke, K. (2003). Medical surgical nursing: Critical thinking for client care *(3rd ed.). Upper Saddle River, NJ: Pearson Education, p. 1206.*

3. Inform client that sandbags may be used along external border of affected limb to prevent external rotation
4. Inform client that pain medication will be available for comfort postoperatively (generally, patient-controlled analgesia [PCA] is used)
5. Teach client about pain rating scale to be used postoperatively and encourage client to report any discomfort
6. Teach client deep-breathing and coughing exercises preoperatively
7. Use aseptic technique for dressing changes and wound drainage
8. Provide information on therapies and equipment to expect postoperatively (indwelling urinary catheter, PCA, IV therapy, possible traction, incentive spirometer, etc.)
9. Monitor preoperative use of skin traction (Buck's traction) to immobilize limb until surgery is performed
10. Medication therapy: analgesics to manage pain

D. Client teaching

1. Reinforce deep-breathing and coughing exercises postoperatively
2. ! Preoperatively teach client about postoperative precautions to prevent hip dislocation (no hip flexion greater that 90 degrees, internal rotation of affected hip, or adduction of affected hip); these include such activities as avoiding low chairs, using raised toilet seat, no excessive bending
3. Reinforce teaching about postoperative course

XII. SPRAINS AND STRAINS

A. Overview

1. A **sprain** is a stretch and/or tear of a ligament
2. A **strain** is a twist, pull, and/or tear that may involve both muscles and tendons
3. Caused by direct or indirect trauma (caused by fall, blow to body, muscle exhaustion), overuse or prolonged repetitive motion of muscles and tendons, inadequate rest periods during intensive training
4. Ankles, knees, and wrist are most vulnerable
5. Frequently seen in athletes and individuals with poor physical conditioning or who are overweight

B. Nursing assessment

1. Sprains are classified based on degree of ligament injury
2. Pain is aggravated by continuous use and influenced by degree of injury
3. ! Assess for bruising, edema, joint swelling, muscle spasms, and inflammation at affected site
4. ! Assess for changes in neurovascular status (pulse, temperature, capillary refill, and movement) of affected extremity
5. Decreased mobility in affected extremity

C. Therapeutic management

1. Teach client about the RICE approach to recovery
   - **a.** *R*est affected extremity
   - **b.** *I*ce for 15 to 30 minutes at a time for 2 to 3 days
   - **c.** *C*ompression elastic support bandages or adhesive tape
   - **d.** *E*levation

Memory Aid Use RICE for musculoskeletal injuries (rest, ice, compression, and elevation).

2. Perform neurovascular assessment on affected extremity
3. Encourage client to wrap affected extremity with elastic support bandages before strenuous activities
4. Inform client that x-rays of injured extremity may be necessary
5. Administer analgesics as needed
6. Teach client about importance of stretching and warm-up exercises before athletic activities
7. Encourage client to adhere to exercise program to regain muscle tone and strength in collaboration with physical therapist
8. Medication therapy: analgesics, muscle relaxants, and anti-inflammatory agents as necessary

D. Client education: reinforcement of information previously discussed

XIII. GOUT

A. Overview

1. Primary form of disease is hereditary; secondary form is acquired
2. Laboratory findings show elevated serum uric acid (hyperuricemia); see norms at beginning of chapter
3. Characterized by recurring attacks of acute joint inflammation; frequent sites affected are great toe or knee
4. Is an inherited abnormality in uric acid metabolism
5. Hyperuricemia is caused by increased purine synthesis and/or decreased renal excretion of uric acid; may also be caused by prolonged fasting and excessive alcohol intake

B. Nursing assessment

1. Risk factors: obesity, excessive weight gain, excessive alcohol intake, impaired renal function, hypertension, chemotherapy for leukemia and certain lymphomas, certain thiazide diuretics, aspirin, and tuberculosis medications
2. Diagnosis includes analysis of synovial fluid, serum uric acid, and 24-hour urine
3. Joint inflammation is extremely painful and is caused by deposits of uric acid crystals in synovial lining and fluid
4. Assess for elevated temperature (may not always be present), tenderness and cyanosis of affected extremity, inflammation of small joints (commonly seen in great toe), and multiple joint involvement
5. Precipitating factors generally include dehydration, fever, injury to joint, and excessive ingestion of alcohol

C. Therapeutic management

1. Prevent any bed linen from touching affected extremity because of extreme tenderness (bed cradle and/or footboard can be used)
2. Instruct client to adhere to activity restriction such as bedrest and immobilization of affected extremity during periods of exacerbation
3. Monitor uric acid levels to prevent exacerbation and evaluate effectiveness of treatment
4. Instruct client about precipitating factors for disease
5. Avoid foods high in purines (such as herring, sardines, sweetbreads, yeast)
6. Medication therapy: usually includes anti-inflammatory agents (such as colchicine, NSAIDs, or corticosteroids), an antihyperuricemic (such as allopurinol [Zyloprim]), and uricosurics (such as probenecid [Probalan])

D. Client education

1. Reinforce teaching of therapeutic management above
2. Action, side/adverse effects of medication
3. Take medications with meals to avoid gastric irritation
4. Avoid use of alcoholic beverages when taking medication
5. Drink at least 2.5 to 3 liters of fluid per day when taking medication

XIV. DEGENERATIVE JOINT DISEASE (DJD) OR OSTEOARTHRITIS (OA)

A. Overview

1. Slowly progressive disorder of articulating joints, especially weight-bearing joints
2. Commonly affects hands and weight-bearing joints (knees, hips, feet, and back)
3. Breakdown of articular cartilage occurs
4. Injury is usually limited to joint and surrounding tissue
5. Disease ranges from very mild to very severe
6. Cartilage degeneration causes bones to rub against each other, causing pain and decreasing joint function
7. Risk factors
   a. Age (most significant): primarily affects middle-age to older adults
   b. Obesity (generally causes arthritis of the knees)
   c. Repetitive joint injuries caused by sports, accidents, or work-related injuries
   d. Genetics (especially seen with OA of hands): client may be born with defective cartilage or slight defect in how joint fits together, and as client ages, joint cartilage continues to progressively degenerate and enzymes (hyaluronidase) are released, which cause further breakdown

B. Nursing assessment

1. Disease is diagnosed with physical exam and a history of symptoms
2. X-ray confirms disease
3. Joint pain is present with movement and weight-bearing and is relieved by rest
4. There is limited range of motion with progressive loss of function
5. There is joint stiffness after rest
6. Crepitation (grating sensation caused by rough joint surfaces rubbing together) occurs
7. **Heberden's nodes** (raised bony growths over distal interphalangeal joints) are present
8. **Bouchard's nodes** (raised bony growths over proximal interphalangeal joint of hand) are noted

C. Therapeutic management

1. Encourage client to participate in an exercise program (approved by health care provider) to maintain joint flexibility and improve muscle strength
2. Encourage client to maintain ideal body weight to prevent excessive stress on joints
3. Instruct client to apply heat/cold therapy to affected joint for temporary pain relief
4. Assist client in planning scheduled rest periods to relieve stress on joints
5. Assist client with activities of daily living (ADL) as needed
6. Provide information about complementary therapies such as visual imagery and relaxation techniques for pain control
7. Medication therapy
   a. Acetaminophen is generally used to control mild pain without inflammation
   b. Therapy also includes anti-inflammatory agents such as NSAIDs and corticosteroids
   c. If NSAIDs are ineffective in controlling inflammation and pain, glucocorticosteroids may be injected directly into joint

D. Client education

1. Nature of and treatment for disease; principles of good body mechanics
2. Correct use of assistive devices; encourage use as needed
3. How to plan daily activities and tasks allowing for scheduled rest periods
4. Avoid activities that put excessive stress on joints and cause pain

XV. LOW BACK PAIN

A. Overview

1. Pain may result from acute or repeated stress on lower back over years
2. Pain occurs because of degeneration and/or acute or repeated injury to tissue of lower back
   a. Caused by sprain or strain of ligaments and muscles
   b. Pain may be felt at the site of the injury or referred
3. Overall health of lower back muscles determines degree of risk for injury as well as speed of recovery
4. Two most common causes of low back pain are mechanical strain (irritation or injury to disc causing degeneration) and herniation of nucleus pulposus (putting pressure on nerve roots)

! B. Nursing assessment

1. Risk factors include but are not limited to: degenerative disc disease, poor muscle tone of lower back, sedentary lifestyle, obesity, poor body mechanics, smoking, and stress
2. Client will report pain caused by a shift of one vertebra on another or pinching and irritation of nerve root
3. Muscle spasms are a common symptom
4. Pain does not appear at time of injury but is related to gradual increase of muscle spasms of paravertebral tissue
5. Straight leg raise test may not be positive with acute injury but pain is present with radiation to buttock and leg along path of sciatic nerve with chronic injury

! C. Therapeutic management

1. Goal of treatment is to improve symptoms and slow progression of degenerative process
2. Include client and family in plan of care and provide emotional support
3. Medication therapy: includes but is not limited to analgesics, NSAIDs, and muscle relaxants; epidural corticosteroid injections may be used if conservative treatment is ineffective

D. Client teaching

1. Expected therapeutic effects, side/adverse effects, and contraindications with medication use
2. Use of pain rating scale; use of heat/cold therapy for comfort
3. Importance of adhering to activity restrictions such as bedrest
4. Importance of adhering to exercise plan and gradual increase in activity
5. Importance of maintaining ideal body weight
6. Physical therapy will aid in maintaining muscle strength and flexibility as well as improving muscle tone
7. Importance of adhering to the principles of body mechanics to avoid excessive strain on the lower back
8. Sleep on a firm mattress
9. Have client demonstrate correct sleeping position using principles of body mechanics (side lying or supine with knees and hips flexed)
10. Avoid or stop smoking
11. Use of prescribed brace or corset (if needed) to prevent flexion and extension motions of lower back

XVI. CONGENITAL MUSCULOSKELETAL HEALTH PROBLEMS

A. *Clubfoot*

1. Overview
   a. Foot is twisted and fixed in an abnormal position; may be one or a combination of 4 deformities: plantar flexion (foot is lower than heel), dorsiflexion (heel is lower than foot), varus deviation (foot turns in), or valgus deviation (foot turns out)
   b. Involves bone deformity and malposition with soft tissue contracture
   c. May be unilateral or bilateral

d. Exact cause is unknown but may include abnormal intrauterine position or neuromuscular or vascular problems
e. Strong familial tendency, with 1 in 10 chance that a parent with clubfoot will have an affected offspring

2. Nursing assessment
a. Foot is twisted in a fixed abnormal position, which is easily recognized at birth; may be recognized on prenatal ultrasound
! b. Affected foot is usually smaller and shorter, with an empty heel pad and transverse plantar crease
c. When defect is unilateral, affected limb is usually shorter with possible calf atrophy

3. Therapeutic management
a. Correction is achieved best if begun in newborn period because small bones in foot begin to ossify shortly after birth
! b. Manipulation and serial casting is begun immediately and continued for 8 to 12 weeks, with foot placed in a cast in an overcorrected position; casts are changed every 1 to 2 weeks because of rapid growth
c. Parents need to perform passive ROM exercises of foot and ankle several times a day for several months once cast is off
d. Infant may need to sleep in Denis Browne splints (shoes attached to a metal bar to maintain position) or wear corrective shoes for up to 1 year
e. Surgery is performed when manipulative therapy does not achieve full correction with casting; most children have surgery between 4 to 12 months of age, which involves realigning foot bones holding them in place with steel pins; foot is casted for 6 to 12 weeks
! f. Nursing care of child postcasting and postsurgical repair of clubfoot includes neurovascular checks at least every 2 hours; assess for swelling around cast edges; elevate ankle and foot on pillows; monitor for cast drainage; pain management; and appropriate distraction

4. Client and family teaching
! a. Change diapers frequently to prevent soiled diapers from touching cast and causing soiling
! b. Sponge-bathe infant to keep cast dry
! c. Evaluate crying episodes carefully because they may be caused by tingling sensation of circulatory compression
d. Reinforce need for passive ROM exercises several times a day for several months
e. Reinforce use of Denis Browne splints or corrective shoes to maintain correction
f. Discuss options for clothing that accommodates casts
g. Teach child in a brace or cast (see Box 62–6)

B. Developmental dysplasia of hip (DDH) or congenital hip dysplasia

1. Overview
a. Refers to a variety of conditions in which femoral head and acetabulum are improperly aligned; DDH has been referred to as congenital hip dysplasia in past
b. Unilateral in 80% of affected children
c. Cause is unknown, though certain factors are known to increase risk
d. Family history increases risk ten-fold
e. Prenatal conditions may affect development of DDH, such as frank breech position, maternal hormones (relaxin and estrogen may cause laxity of hip joint and capsule, leading to joint instability), twinning, and large infant size
f. Sociocultural methods of childrearing, such as way infants are carried, may promote or decrease extent of involvement; infants held with hips abducted have decreased involvement

2. Nursing assessment in infancy
a. Diagnosis should be made in newborn period; treatment that is initiated before 2 months of age achieves highest rate of success
! b. Shortening of affected limb

Box 62-6

Child and Family Education for a Child in a Brace or a Cast

Perform Neurovascular Checks

- Observe the fingers or toes for swelling, discoloration, and temperature.
- Check movement and sensation.
- Notify health care professional with any changes in neurovascular status.
- Teach the parents how to blanch the nail bed and watch for capillary refill.

Observe for Infection

- Monitor for temperature increase.
- Assess for drainage through the cast or brace.
- Assess for odors coming from beneath the cast or brace.
- Notify health care professional of any of the above.

Assess and Maintain Skin around Cast or Brace Edges

- Perform frequent assessment of the skin around the cast or brace edge for irritation, rubbing, or blistering.
- Keep edges clean and dry, avoiding the use of lotions, powders, or oils near the cast or brace.
- Petal the cast edges as needed with tape to cover rough edges.
- Do not allow the child to put anything down the cast.
- If the child is incontinent, protect the cast edges with waterproof tape and plastic.
- Keep the cast or brace clean and dry.

Activity

- Follow the health professional's orders for activity level or restriction of activity.
- Avoid allowing the affected extremity to hang in a dependent position for more than 30 minutes.
- Encourage frequent rest for the first few days following brace or cast application, keeping the injured extremity elevated while resting.
- Keep a clear path for ambulation, removing toys, hazardous floor rugs, pets, or other items over which the child might stumble.
- If in a body cast or brace, assist the child to be mobile with the use of a wagon, cart, or large skateboard; do not move or reposition client using bar between lower extremities if present.

Comfort

- Assess for discomfort and medicate according to health professional's orders.
- Contact the health care provider if pain is not relieved by any comfort measures.

Follow-up

- Encourage compliance with follow-up.
- Take the child to the health care professional if the cast becomes too loose or becomes soft or cracked.

c. Allis sign: child in supine position, thighs flexed to a 90-degree angle toward abdomen, unequal knee height

! **d.** Uneven number and placement of skin folds on posterior thighs

e. Restricted abduction of hips after 6 to 10 weeks of age

f. Wide perineum in bilateral dislocation

! **g.** Positive Ortolani up to 2 to 3 months of age; to assess for this, lie infant supine and flex knees and hips to 90 degrees; place middle fingers over greater trochanter and thumb in internal side of thigh over lesser trochanter;

abduct hips while applying pressure over greater trochanter and listen for a clicking sound, which would indicate a positive Ortolani's sign; no sound will be heard with a normal hip
   h. Positive Barlow's sign: with fingers in same position, hold knees and hips at 90 degrees, apply backward pressure, and adduct hips; positive Barlow's sign is present if able to feel hips dislocate

! **3.** Nursing assessment in an older child
   a. Affected leg shorter than other
   b. Telescoping or piston mobility of affected leg
   c. History of delay in walking
   d. Limp and toe walking
   e. Trendelenburg's sign: when child bears weight on affected side, pelvis tilts downward on normal side instead of upward
   f. Waddling gait and lordosis with bilateral dislocation

4. Therapeutic management
   a. Correction involves positioning hip into a flexed, abducted (externally rotated) position to press femur head against acetabulum and deepen its contour
! **b.** For infants under 3 months, most common treatment is use of a Pavlik harness, an adjustable chest halter that abducts legs; soft plastic stirrups hold hips flexed, abducted, and externally rotated; may or may not be removed for bathing; usually worn for 3 to 6 months (see Figure 62–5 ■)
   c. For infants older than 3 months, skin traction followed by spica cast application may be required
   d. Correction in child older than 18 months requires traction, operative reduction, and rehabilitation

! **5.** Client and family teaching
   a. Pavlik harness: proper application, sponge bath, assess skin under straps daily for irritation or redness; t-shirt and knee socks should be worn under brace to prevent skin irritation; diaper should be placed under straps and changed without taking harness off
   b. For all abduction devices: modification of car seat, modification of positioning for nursing and eating
   c. Parents need to ensure child has adequate stimulation with toys and activities at appropriate eye level; encourage activities that stimulate upper extremities

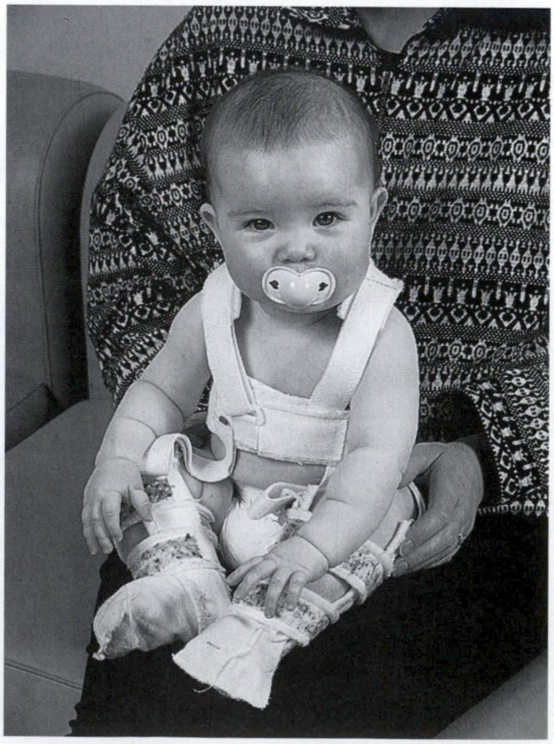

Figure 62–5

Pavlik harness.

Source: Ball, J., & Bindler, R. (2006). Child health nursing: Partnering with children and families. Upper Saddle River, NJ: Pearson Education, p. 1417.

d. Children will catch up with developmental milestones once abduction splint is off

C. Osteogenesis imperfecta (OI)

1. Overview
   a. Characterized by formation of pathologic fractures resulting from connective tissue and bone defects
   b. Occurs in several forms with variable degree of severity
   c. Bones are so fragile that fractures result from trauma but also from simple walking or pressure of birth
   d. A child with this diagnosis should not be confused with child with fractures because of abuse
   e. Children with OI have normal Ca^{++} and phosphorus levels and abnormal pre-collagen type I, which prevents formation of collagen, a major component of connective tissue
   f. Bone of children with OI consists of large areas of osseous tissue and increased numbers of osteoblasts
   g. Genetically transmitted, generally in an autosomal dominant inheritance pattern, although some types are transmitted in a recessive pattern
2. Nursing assessment
   a. Major clinical manifestations include multiple and frequent fractures, some of which may be present at birth
   b. As child grows older, multiple breaks tend to cause limb and spinal column deformities, interfering with alignment or growth
   c. Other clinical manifestations include blue sclera; thin, soft skin with easy bruising; increased joint flexibility; weak muscles; short stature; conductive hearing loss often by adolescence or young adulthood
   d. May have dentinogenesis imperfecta: hypoplastic teeth with opalescent blue or brown discoloration
3. Therapeutic management
   a. Keep floors dry; remove objects that could cause falls
   b. Handle children gently: avoid lifting by a single arm or leg; use a blanket for extra support when lifting and moving
   c. Never hold by ankles when being diapered, but gently lift by slipping a hand under buttocks
   d. Lightweight leg braces, splints, casting, and physical therapy may be helpful
   e. Intermedullary rods may be effective in strengthening bones
   f. Medication therapy: calcitonin possibly (aids bone healing), biphosphonates (to increase bone mass), possible growth hormone (stimulate growth)
4. Client and family teaching
   a. Encourage a lifestyle that promotes growth and development yet minimizes risk of trauma
   b. Teach how to support when bathing, dressing, and moving
   c. Encourage exercise, such as swimming, to improve muscle tone and prevent obesity
   d. Encourage realistic occupational planning
   e. Suggest genetic counseling
   f. Educational materials and information can be obtained from the Osteogenesis Imperfecta Foundation (www.oif.org)

XVII. ACQUIRED CHILDHOOD MUSCULOSKELETAL HEALTH PROBLEMS

A. Legg-Calve-Perthes disease

1. Overview
   a. A self-limiting disorder in which there is aseptic necrosis of femoral head
   b. Disease affects children between ages of 2 and 12 years but is most common in those 5 to 7 years of age
   c. Caucasian children are affected 10 times more often than African American children, and males more than females

d. Disease is bilateral in 10% to 15% of cases
e. Cause is unknown; familial predisposition present and possibly associated with preceding mild traumatic injury
f. There is a disturbance of circulation to femoral capitol epiphysis that produces an ischemic aseptic necrosis of femoral head
g. Stage I: avascular stage; aseptic necrosis of femoral capitol epiphysis with degenerative changes producing flattening of femoral head
h. Stage II: fragmentation or revascularization stage; old bone absorption and revascularization
i. Stage III: reparative stage; new bone formation
j. Stage IV: regeneration stage; gradual reformation of femoral head
k. Middle childhood is time when blood supply to femoral head is most tenuous, being supplied almost entirely by lateral retinacular vessels; these vessels can become obstructed by trauma, inflammation, coagulation defects, among other causes
l. Affected children may have delayed skeletal maturation and abnormal thyroid levels

! 2. Nursing assessment
   a. Mild pain in hip or anterior thigh and limp that are aggravated by increased activity and relieved by rest
   b. Stiffness in morning or after rest
   c. As disease progresses, there is limited ROM, weakness, muscle wasting, possible shortening of affected limb, and positive Trendelenburg sign

3. Therapeutic management
   a. Prepare child for x-ray (usual diagnostic test); there may be no radiological findings early in disease, but bone scans and MRIs are helpful to diagnose early disease
   b. Initial treatment includes rest to reduce inflammation and restore motion
   ! c. Goal is to keep head of femur in contact with acetabulum, which serves as a mold of spherical shape of head of femur
   ! d. Treatment may be conservative: rest; avoidance of weight bearing on lower extremities; traction and containment with abduction braces, leg casts, or leather harness slings
   e. Conservative therapy may be needed for 2 to 4 years
   f. Surgical correction may be done, which returns child to normal activities in 3 to 4 months
   ! g. Assist in selection of suitable activities for a child unable to maintain usual level of physical activity
   h. Ensure compliance with conservative devices
   ! i. If surgery is done, postoperative care includes frequent neurovascular checks, pain management, and activity based on surgeon's orders
   j. Assist family with appropriate activities for child during treatment

4. Client and family teaching
   a. Teach purpose, function, application, and care of corrective device, and importance of compliance to achieve desired outcome
   b. Stress importance of continuing school activities
   c. Promote normal growth and development with appropriate diversional activities

B. Slipped capitol femoral epiphysis

1. Overview
   a. A condition in which upper femoral epiphysis gradually slips from its functional position
   b. Incidence is greatest during rapid growth spurt during adolescence; 13 to 16 years of age for males and 11 to 14 years of age for females
   c. It is twice as frequent in African Americans as other races, and twice as frequent in males
   d. Etiology is unknown and thought to be multifactorial; genetic predisposition possible

e. Is more common in obese or rapidly growing children, suggesting that growth hormone or trauma from excessive weight may have an influence on etiology
f. Slippage of femoral head occurs at proximal **epiphyseal plate,** and femur displaces from **epiphysis** (rounded end portion of long bones); this is usually a gradual process, but may result from trauma

2. Nursing assessment
   ! a. Onset of symptoms may be gradual, with persistent hip pain that is aching or mild, and can be referred to thigh and/or knee, along with limp and decreased ROM and internal rotation of hip; child may hold leg in an externally rotated position to relieve stress and pain in hip joint
   ! b. Child with an acute slip presents with sudden, severe pain and cannot bear weight
   c. Prepare client for an x-ray, which will confirm diagnosis
3. Therapeutic management
   ! a. As soon as diagnosis is made, place client on strict bedrest until surgery; adolescent may use crutches as long as affected leg is non-weight-bearing, but should not sit in a wheelchair, as this may increase slippage
   b. Reinforce initial bedrest, as adolescents often do not see value of this measure
   c. Provide appropriate diversional activities
   d. Prepare for surgery with pinning or external fixation to stabilize femur head
   e. Provide postoperative care, including frequent neurovascular checks and pain management
   f. Provide adequate nutrition for healing
4. Client and family teaching
   a. Reinforce ambulation and weight-bearing as ordered by surgeon
   b. Contact sports are usually restricted until growth is complete
   c. Reinforce compliance with followup visits until epiphyseal plates are closed

C. *Scoliosis*

1. Overview
   a. Lateral curvature of spine; may be functional, which occurs as a compensatory mechanism in children who have unequal leg lengths, or poor posture; structural scoliosis is a permanent curvature of spine accompanied by damage to vertebrae
   b. Structural scoliosis occurs most often during rapid growth spurt in adolescence, 11 to 14 years for females, 13 to 16 years for males
   c. Female-to-male ratio is 5:1 for curves greater than 21 degrees
   d. Seventy percent of structural scoliosis is idiopathic; there is a familial predisposition
   e. Scoliosis is common in diseases in which there is unequal muscle balance, such as CP, MD, and myelomeningocele
2. Nursing assessment
   a. A painless and insidious onset is typical
   ! b. Parent may first notice that skirts hang unevenly, or that bra straps are adjusted unevenly
   ! c. On examination, there is unequal shoulder heights, waist angles, scapula prominences, rib prominences, and chest asymmetry
   d. Screening by school nurse begins in fifth grade as mandated by law in many states
   e. Scoliometer is used to document clinical deformity found on screening
3. Therapeutic management
   a. Prepare adolescent for x-ray, which will identify extent of curvature and give baseline information for followup
   ! b. If spinal curve is less than 15 to 20 degrees, teen is monitored every 3 to 6 months for change; exercises to improve posture and muscle tone and increase flexibility of spine are encouraged
   c. If curve is greater than 24 degrees, treatment is provided by an orthopedic surgeon; if less than 40 degrees, conservative, nonsurgical treatment is

indicated, with bracing, such as a Milwaukee brace; this brace, and others like it, are made of leather and plastic; it is worn until teen's spinal growth stops; see client teaching section

   d. Electrical stimulation may be used for mild to moderate curvatures to cause regular and frequent muscle contractions; possibly helping to straighten spine
   e. If curvature progresses or is greater than 40 degrees, surgery is warranted; instruments such as rods, screws, and wires are placed next to curvature; spine is then fused in correct position; bone from iliac crests may be used to strengthen fusion
   f. Preoperative teaching includes deep-breathing, coughing, turning every 2 hours, use of spirometry, pain medication, use of nasogastric (NG) tube and NPO status, ROM exercises, activity, possible ICU tour
   g. ! Postoperative care includes ROM exercises, logrolling every 2 hours, encouraging coughing and deep breathing and use of incentive spirometer, NPO, NG tube, strict I & O, frequent VS and neurological checks, monitoring hematocrit, blood transfusions, pain management, antibiotic administration, antiembolism stockings, and gradual resumption of activity as ordered
   h. Halo traction may be used for nonsurgical treatment of moderate curves or postoperatively in severe curves to provide stability for spine

4. Client and family teaching
   a. Use of a Milwaukee or other brace: worn for 23 hours a day; off to shower, bathe, and swim; wear T-shirt under brace next to skin for protection; do exercises (such as pelvic tilt and lateral strengthening) several times daily while in brace to correct thoracic lordosis
   b. Consistent use of brace will provide maximum benefit
   c. Slight muscle aches may be noticed when first wearing brace
   d. Encourage teens to be as active as possible while in brace
   e. ! Discharge teaching: must not slump in chairs, bend or twist torso, or lift over 10 pounds; maintain activity restrictions for 6 to 8 months as ordered; address self-esteem issues; comply with follow-up visits

Check Your NCLEX-RN® Exam I.Q.

You are ready for testing on this content if you can

- Identify basic structures and functions of the musculoskeletal system.
- Describe the pathophysiology and etiology of common musculoskeletal disorders.
- Discuss expected assessment data and diagnostic test findings for selected musculoskeletal disorders.
- Discuss therapeutic management of a client experiencing a musculoskeletal disorder.
- Discuss nursing management of a client experiencing a musculoskeletal disorder.
- Identify expected outcomes for the client experiencing a musculoskeletal disorder.

PRACTICE TEST

1 The nurse provides teaching to a client after the removal of a short leg cast. The nurse should include which of the following in discussions with the client?

1. Wash the skin with undiluted hydrogen peroxide.
2. Vigorously scrub the legs to remove dead skin.
3. Gently wash and lubricate the leg.
4. Avoid touching the leg for 2 weeks.

2 Which of the following nursing diagnoses would be the priority for a client with Paget's disease?

1. Risk for noncompliance
2. Disturbed sleep pattern
3. Impaired physical mobility
4. Disturbed body image

3 A client with a right arm cast for fractured humerus states, "I haven't been able to extend the fingers on my right hand since this morning." What action should the nurse take next?

1. Assess neurovascular status.
2. Ask the client to massage the fingers.
3. Encourage the client to take the prescribed analgesics as ordered.
4. Elevate the right arm on a pillow to reduce edema.

4 A client with an open fracture is at risk for developing osteomyelitis. Which of the following classic symptoms would the nurse assess for to detect development of this complication?

1. Low bone density
2. Elevated temperature
3. Acute respiratory distress
4. Shortening of the affected extremity

5 An obese client with degenerative joint disease is being managed pharmacologically with aspirin therapy. The nurse knows that additional client teaching is necessary when the client makes which of the following statements?

1. "I take my aspirin only when I have extreme pain and stiffness."
2. "I use heat sometimes to help decrease my pain and joint stiffness."
3. "I frequently examine my stools for bleeding."
4. "I started an exercise program to lose weight."

6 A client underwent a lumbar laminectomy today. Which nursing diagnosis has highest priority for this client?

1. Disturbed body image
2. Social isolation
3. Ineffective role performance
4. Impaired physical mobility

7 A client had a left above-the-knee amputation today. For the first 24 hours postoperatively, the nurse makes it a priority to do which of the following to properly manage the surgical site?

1. Elevate the residual limb on a pillow.
2. Loosen the stump dressing every 4 hours.
3. Maintain the residual limb in a dependent position.
4. Change dressings as often as needed.

8 A client with a femoral fracture is in Buck's traction. While making rounds, the nurse notices that the client's foot is flush with the footboard of the bed. Based on the nurse's knowledge of the principles of traction, an appropriate action is to do which of the following?

1. Wedge a pillow between the footboard and the client's foot.
2. Praise the patient for maintaining countertraction.
3. Center the client on the bed.
4. Ask the client to pull up in bed while holding the weights.

9 A truck driver presents to the primary care provider with complaints of persistent back pain. The nurse explains that which client activity documented during the nursing history may contribute to further back injury?

1. Lifting objects close to the body
2. Shifting positions often when sitting for prolonged periods
3. Providing back support with a pillow when sitting
4. Prolonged standing or sitting

10 A client underwent a lumbar laminectomy. Which of the following activities would be *best* 4 hours postoperatively?

1. Sitting up in a chair to watch television
2. Sitting at the side of the bed
3. Lying in bed in good alignment with the head of bed flat
4. Using the side-rails for support to get out of bed

11 The nurse provides teaching to a 50-year-old male caucasian client with chronic low back pain. The client weighs 200 pounds, works as a truck driver, sits for prolonged periods, and seldom participates in exercise activities. The client smokes one pack of cigarettes and drinks six cans of beer per day. What risk factors should the nurse include in the discussion?

1. Lack of exercise, obesity, sitting for long periods, smoking, sedentary occupation
2. Degenerative disk disease, gender, race, smoking
3. Degenerative disk disease, race, alcohol use, smoking, inactivity
4. Age, obesity, lack of exercise, genetic factors

PRACTICE TEST

12 The nurse is teaching a postmenopausal client about the use of calcium to prevent the effects of osteoporosis. The client asks: "Why do I have to take vitamin D with my calcium?" Which of the following is the nurse's best response?

1. "Vitamin D prevents osteoporosis."
2. "Vitamin D increases intestinal absorption of calcium."
3. "You are most likely to be deficient in vitamin D."
4. "Calcium and vitamin D supplementation is the only way to prevent osteoporosis."

13 The nurse is caring for a client with a week-old cast. The client asks why the nurse palpates the casted area when doing the assessment. Which of the following is the most appropriate response by the nurse?

1. "I am making sure that the cast has dried."
2. "I am evaluating the strength of the cast."
3. "I am feeling for hot spots that might indicate infection."
4. "I am making sure that the cast is not too tight."

14 A client is placed on continuous passive motion (CPM) machine postoperatively after a total knee replacement. The nurse observes that the client's knee is externally rotating during flexion. What should the nurse do next?

1. Move the client up in bed or move the CPM machine down toward the foot of the bed
2. Support the client's knee with sandbags to prevent external rotation
3. Assist the client to sit up in bed in a 45-degree position
4. Do nothing; the client's knee is properly aligned

15 A client in skeletal traction for a right femur fracture is complaining of pain in the affected limb. The nurse assesses that the right foot is pale without a pulse. What should the nurse do next?

1. Ensure that the leg is not raised above heart level
2. Administer analgesics as ordered
3. Release the traction
4. Document the observation and recheck the pulse in 5 minutes

16 A nurse receives a client from the emergency department in Buck's traction following a fracture of the right femur. The nurse documents which of the following as a priority in the client medical record?

1. Status of skin underneath the traction and over bony prominences
2. Type of pin, wire, or tongs used
3. The effectiveness of pain medication given in the field
4. Medications given in the emergency department

17 The nurse planning for the care of a client admitted with balanced suspension traction explains to the family that an advantage of balanced suspension is which of the following?

1. It eliminates the risk for skin breakdown.
2. It allows the client to raise the buttocks off the bed for bedpan use and skin care.
3. It is more effective in reducing hip contracture.
4. It requires only one weight to maintain traction.

18 A client is taking colchicine for gout. The client complains of weakness, abdominal pain, nausea, vomiting, and diarrhea for the past 2 days. The nurse interprets these complaints indicating which of the following?

1. Therapeutic effects of the medication
2. Signs of toxicity
3. Expected side effects
4. An allergic response

19 An 87-year-old client sustained a right hip fracture. The client asks the nurse about the length of time needed for the fracture to heal. The nurse's response includes consideration of which client factor that influences the rate of bone healing?

1. Frequency of physical therapy
2. Age of the client
3. Weight of the client
4. Early ambulation

20 A client is scheduled to have a closed reduction of a right ankle fracture. The nurse determines the client understands the procedure when the client states that the procedure involves which of the following?

1. Applying an endoscopic procedure to realign the bones
2. Realigning the bone using surgery
3. Correcting the bone alignment using manual manipulation
4. Inserting pins, rods, or other implantable devices

21. A child is admitted to the hospital with a diagnosis of osteomyelitis. Which of the following would the nurse likely find when gathering the nursing history?

1. History of an upper respiratory infection
2. History of gastroenteritis
3. History of Legg-Calve-Perthes disease
4. History of congenital hip dysplasia

22. Two hours after a child had a cast applied for a fractured radius, the nursing assessment reveals swelling in the hand, which is elevated higher than the heart. Ice has been applied continuously. The child does not complain of pain but does complain of numbness and tingling. Which should the nurse do first?

1. Medicate for pain.
2. Elevate the injured extremity even higher.
3. Call the physician.
4. Provide the child with diversional activities.

23. The pediatric nurse interprets that which of the following infants is the least likely to be diagnosed with developmental dysplasia of the hip?

1. The infant with a family history of developmental dysplasia of the hip
2. The infant who weighs over 10 pounds
3. The infant carried on the mother's hips
4. The infant who had breech position while in the uterus

24. Which of the following interventions would be essential for the nurse to implement to promote a stable respiratory status in the adolescent who recently had a spinal fusion for scoliosis?

1. Logrolling and repositioning every 4 hours
2. Coughing and deep breathing every 2 hours during the day
3. Assessing pain status and ensuring adequate pain relief
4. Encouraging use of incentive spirometry every 4 hours while awake

25. An 8-year-old child presents to the emergency department with complaints of his ankle hurting and difficulty walking. The triage nurse notes the following assessments: pain, redness, and swelling of the ankle. The ankle has decreased mobility and range of motion. The child has a temperature of 100.8°F and a heart rate of 140 beats per minute. The child does not recollect any injury to the ankle. Which of the following diagnoses would the triage nurse suspect?

1. Legg-Calve-Perthes disease
2. Slipped capitol femoral epiphysis
3. Fracture of the ankle
4. Osteomyelitis

26. The nurse is preparing to help a client get up from a chair using crutches. Place in order the steps that the nurse outlines to the client to do this procedure correctly.

1. Place unaffected leg slightly under or at the edge of the chair.
2. Grasp the arm of the chair using the hand on the unaffected side.
3. Grasp the crutches by the horizontal hand bars using the hand on the affected side.
4. Move forward to the edge of the chair.
5. Push down on the crutches and the chair armrest while raising the body out of the chair.

Answer: __________________

PRACTICE TEST

ANSWERS & RATIONALES

ANSWERS & RATIONALES

1. **Answer: 3** Dead skin and exudates often collect under the cast, and efforts to remove it should be done gradually. The client should be instructed to avoid any vigorous scrubbing of the skin to avoid breaks, which increase the risk for infection. The use of undiluted peroxide is too harsh for the skin. There is no reason why the leg cannot be touched after removal of the cast.
Cognitive Level: Application **Client Need:** Physiological Integrity: Physiological Adaptation **Integrated Process:** Nursing Process: Implementation **Content Area:** Adult Health: Musculoskeletal

Strategy: The core issue of the question is the knowledge of skin care following cast removal. Use nursing knowledge and the process of elimination to make a selection.

2 **Answer: 3** Impaired physical mobility is the appropriate priority nursing diagnosis for a client with Paget's disease. The client needs to remain active to decrease the complications associated with immobility and to maintain the ability to perform self-care activities. The other diagnoses, although appropriate, are not the priority in clients with Paget's disease.
Cognitive Level: Application **Client Need:** Physiological Integrity: Physiological Adaptation **Integrated Process:** Nursing Process: Planning **Content Area:** Adult Health: Musculoskeletal **Strategy:** The core issue of the question is the knowledge of priorities for the client with Paget's disease. Use nursing knowledge and the process of elimination to make a selection.

3 **Answer: 1** This symptom suggests neurological injury caused by pressure on nerves and soft tissue because of swelling. Other symptoms of neurovascular compromise should be assessed and reported to the physician.
Cognitive Level: Analysis **Client Need:** Physiological Integrity: Physiological Adaptation **Integrated Process:** Nursing Process: Implementation **Content Area:** Adult Health: Musculoskeletal **Strategy:** The core issue of the question is the knowledge of priority assessments in a client with possible compartment syndrome. Use nursing knowledge and the process of elimination to make a selection.

4 **Answer: 2** Elevated temperature is a classic symptom seen with this osteomyelitis as a systemic response to the invading organism. Pain, swelling, and tenderness may also accompany the fever. Acute respiratory distress (option 3) is more suggestive of embolism but not infection. The extremity does not shorten.
Cognitive Level: Application **Client Need:** Physiological Integrity: Physiological Adaptation **Integrated Process:** Nursing Process: Assessment **Content Area:** Adult Health: Musculoskeletal **Strategy:** The core issue of the question is the knowledge of manifestations of osteomyelitis. Use nursing knowledge and the process of elimination to make a selection.

5 **Answer: 1** Aspirin therapy for this condition is continuous and is effective only after a therapeutic level is reached. It should not be taken intermittently (option 1). The other options are correct statements about self-care measures when taking aspirin for degenerative joint disease.
Cognitive Level: Application **Client Need:** Physiological Integrity: Physiological Adaptation **Integrated Process:** Nursing Process: Evaluation **Content Area:** Adult Health: Musculoskeletal **Strategy:** The core issue of the question is the knowledge of appropriate self-management techniques for degenerative joint disease. Use nursing knowledge and the process of elimination to make a selection.

6 **Answer: 4** Immediately after surgery, the client will be inclined not to move because of pain and fear of disturbing the operative site. Minimal scarring results from this surgery, so body image disturbance is not likely to be appropriate (option 1). The psychosocial diagnoses in options 2 and 3 have less priority than option 4 because option 4 is a physiological concern.
Cognitive Level: Analysis **Client Need:** Physiological Integrity: Physiological Adaptation **Integrated Process:** Nursing Process: Analysis **Content Area:** Adult Health **Strategy:** The core issue of the question is the knowledge of priority nursing diagnoses following musculoskeletal surgery. Use nursing knowledge and the process of elimination to make a selection.

7 **Answer: 1** Elevating the limb on a pillow facilitates venous return, decreases swelling, and promotes comfort. The stump dressing is usually a compression type to mold the stump and to decrease the edema associated with inflammation, so option 2 is an inappropriate intervention. The other options are also inappropriate because option 3 increases risk of edema and option 4 is done as ordered.
Cognitive Level: Application **Client Need:** Physiological Integrity: Physiological Adaptation **Integrated Process:** Nursing Process: Implementation **Content Area:** Adult Health: Musculoskeletal **Strategy:** The core issue of the question is the knowledge of postoperative stump care and positioning. Use nursing knowledge and the process of elimination to make a selection.

8 **Answer: 3** Traction, to be effective, must have an opposing force (countertraction). The aim in traction is to maintain a constant force to align the distal and proximal ends of a fractured bone. Options 1, 2, and 4 violate this principle of traction in the treatment of fractures. Centering the client in bed maintains the line of pull and ensures that countertraction is maintained.
Cognitive Level: Application **Client Need:** Physiological Integrity: Physiological Adaptation **Integrated Process:** Nursing Process: Implementation **Content Area:** Adult Health: Musculoskeletal **Strategy:** The core issue of the question is the knowledge of proper use of traction. Use nursing knowledge and the process of elimination to make a selection.

9 **Answer: 4** Prolonged sitting or standing aggravates back injury because of the additional stress placed on the structures supporting the back. Lifting objects close to the body, shifting positions frequently, and providing back support are appropriate actions to maintain good body mechanics.
Cognitive Level: Analysis **Client Need:** Physiological Integrity: Physiological Adaptation **Integrated Process:** Nursing Process: Assessment **Content Area:** Adult Health: Musculoskeletal **Strategy:** The core issue of the question is the knowledge of risk factors and aggravating factors of low back pain. Use nursing knowledge and the process of elimination to make a selection.

10 **Answer: 3** The physician orders the client's activity after a laminectomy. After a laminectomy procedure, a client should be assisted to logroll from side to side. The principle is to maintain the alignment of the vertebral column at all times. Clients with lumbar laminectomy should be kept flat or with head of bed slightly elevated to minimize stress on the suture line. Using the side-rails to get out of bed causes shifting of the vertebral column. Sitting up in a chair or on the side of the bed is usually done the evening of the surgery or the first day following surgery, and it is for brief periods only.

Cognitive Level: Application **Client Need:** Safe, Effective Care Environment: Safety and Infection Control **Integrated Process:** Nursing Process: Implementation **Content Area:** Adult Health: Musculoskeletal **Strategy:** The core issue of the question is the knowledge of activity levels after surgery that will not cause harm to the surgical area following laminectomy. Use nursing knowledge and the process of elimination to make a selection.

11 **Answer: 1** Smoking has been found to contribute to disc deterioration. Lack of exercise predisposes the muscles of the back to strain. The extra weight of obese individuals imposes more strain on the back and also interferes in maintaining good body mechanics in lifting. Occupations that require prolonged sitting or standing predispose those individuals to exacerbation of back pain. Option 1 is the only answer that accurately reflects risk factors associated with chronic low back pain for the client described in the question.

Cognitive Level: Analysis **Client Need:** Physiological Integrity: Physiological Adaptation **Integrated Process:** Nursing Process: Planning **Content Area:** Adult Health: Musculoskeletal **Strategy:** The core issue of the question is the knowledge of factors that aggravate low back pain. Use nursing knowledge and the process of elimination to make a selection.

12 **Answer: 2** A combination of calcium and vitamin D is recommended for the prevention of osteoporosis. Vitamin D increases the intestinal absorption of calcium and mobilizes calcium and phosphorus into the bone. Vitamin D alone does not prevent osteoporosis (option 2). Whereas some elderly might be deficient in vitamin D, a postmenopausal state does not necessarily cause the deficiency (option 3). There are other interventions for the prevention of osteoporosis, including lifestyle modifications (e.g., smoking cessation), which makes option 4 inaccurate.

Cognitive Level: Application **Client Need:** Health Promotion and Maintenance **Integrated Process:** Communication and Documentation **Content Area:** Adult Health: Musculoskeletal **Strategy:** The core issue of the question is the knowledge of risk factors for and prevention of osteoporosis. Use nursing knowledge and the process of elimination to make a selection.

13 **Answer: 3** A complication of cast application is skin breakdown underneath the cast. If this occurs, infection can set in and can cause the area over the breakdown to be warmer than other areas. A bad odor coming from the area may also be noted. Option 1 is inaccurate because generally plaster casts dry in 48 hours or less and fiberglass casts in 30 minutes to 1 hour. If a cast is too tight, symptoms associated with neurovascular compromise will be noted, which include pain, paresthesia, pallor, diminished pulse distal to the cast, and paralysis (option 4).

Cognitive Level: Application **Client Need:** Physiological Integrity: Physiological Adaptation **Integrated Process:** Communication and Documentation **Content Area:** Adult Health: Musculoskeletal **Strategy:** The core issue of the question is the knowledge of various complications of casts. Use nursing knowledge and the process of elimination to make a selection.

14 **Answer: 1** The client's knee will externally rotate if there is insufficient space between the client's hip and the machine. The knee should be upright, facing the ceiling, as the machine moves the leg back and forth.

Cognitive Level: Application **Client Need:** Physiological Integrity: Physiological Adaptation **Integrated Process:** Nursing Process: Implementation **Content Area:** Adult Health: Musculoskeletal **Strategy:** The core issue of the question is the knowledge of appropriate assessment and care of the client in CPM. Use nursing knowledge and the process of elimination to make a selection.

15 **Answer: 1** Pain and absent pulse in the affected extremity are urgent signs requiring immediate intervention. Impairment of circulation in the affected limb initiates various pathophysiologic processes, including destruction of nerves and tissues. If this state is uninterrupted, loss of the limb may occur. The nurse needs to ensure that the leg is not above heart level so no further damage occurs. The physician needs to be notified immediately so medical interventions can be instituted before irreversible tissue and nerve damage occurs.

Cognitive Level: Application **Client Need:** Physiological Integrity: Physiological Adaptation **Integrated Process:** Nursing Process: Implementation **Content Area:** Adult Health: Musculoskeletal **Strategy:** The core issue of the question is the knowledge of adverse neurovascular changes to a client in a cast. Recall principles of gravity and blood flow to aid in answering the question. Use nursing knowledge and the process of elimination to make a selection.

16 **Answer: 1** It is essential to monitor the condition of the skin under traction, as well as bony prominences, because these areas are at risk for breakdown due to continuous friction and pressure from the skin traction device. Option 2 is incorrect because Buck's traction is a type of skin traction. Skeletal tractions use pins, wires, or tongs to aid in realignment. Option 3 is appropriate, but the most essential assessment to be documented for a client with skin traction is the condition of the skin underneath the straps.

Cognitive Level: Analysis **Client Need:** Physiological Integrity: Physiological Adaptation **Integrated Process:** Communication and Documentation **Content Area:** Adult Health: Musculoskeletal **Strategy:** The critical word in the question is *priority,* which tells you that all or more than one options are correct and that the most essential one is the correct answer. Use nursing knowledge about skin traction and the process of elimination to make a selection.

17 **Answer: 2** Balanced suspension allows for ease with bedpan use and skin care without disturbing the line of traction. In this type of traction, the client's injured extremity is lifted off the bed and a straight pull is accomplished by the application of several forces and several weights. Skin breakdown is not eliminated with this type of traction because any immobile client can be at risk.

Cognitive Level: Application **Client Need:** Physiological Integrity: Physiological Adaptation **Integrated Process:** Nursing Process: Implementation **Content Area:** Adult Health: Musculoskeletal **Strategy:** The core issue of the question is the knowledge of Buck's traction as a skin traction and the need to assess the underlying skin. Use nursing knowledge and the process of elimination to make a selection.

18 **Answer: 2** Colchicine is used in treating the acute attack of gout. The symptoms described are signs of toxicity. The client should be instructed to stop the medication and be seen for follow-up treatment. The expected effect of colchicine is to diminish the joint pain associated with the acute attack.
Cognitive Level: Application **Client Need:** Physiological Integrity: Pharmacological and Parenteral Therapies **Integrated Process:** Nursing Process: Analysis **Content Area:** Adult Health: Musculoskeletal **Strategy:** The core issue of the question is the knowledge of actions and adverse effects of colchicines in the client with gout. Use nursing knowledge and the process of elimination to make a selection.

19 **Answer: 2** Age, site of the fracture, and blood supply to the affected area all affect the rate of bone healing. Younger and healthy individuals prior to the injury will have faster bone healing than the elderly and those with chronic illnesses. Although physical therapy will assist in mobility, it does not directly enhance bone healing. The weight of the client, unless accompanied by malnutrition, does not have a direct bearing on bone healing.
Cognitive Level: Application **Client Need:** Physiological Integrity: Physiological Adaptation **Integrated Process:** Nursing Process: Implementation **Content Area:** Adult Health: Musculoskeletal **Strategy:** The core issue of the question is knowledge of possible threats to bone healing in an identified client. Use nursing knowledge and the process of elimination to make a selection.

20 **Answer: 3** In a closed reduction procedure, the physician applies traction and manipulates the bone until the broken ends are realigned. Open reduction is a realignment of bone with surgery (option 2), and internal fixation devices are surgically inserted during an open reduction to immobilize the fracture during the healing process (option 4). Endoscopy (option 1) is not a surgical modality for reducing fractures.
Cognitive Level: Application **Client Need:** Physiological Integrity: Physiological Adaptation **Integrated Process:** Nursing Process: Evaluation **Content Area:** Adult Health: Musculoskeletal **Strategy:** The core issue of the question is the knowledge of various approaches to correct bone fracture. Use nursing knowledge and the process of elimination to make a selection.

21 **Answer: 1** The history of a child with osteomyelitis may include a recent upper respiratory infection (which may include an ear infection or sinus infection), skin infection, or blunt trauma to a bone. Gastroenteritis would not be found in the recent history of this child that would lead to this illness. LCPD and CHD do not lead to osteomyelitis.
Cognitive Level: Analysis **Client Need:** Physiological Integrity: Physiological Adaptation **Integrated Process:** Nursing Process: Assessment **Content Area:** Child Health: Musculoskeletal **Strategy:** The core issue of the question is the knowledge of risk factors for osteomyelitis. Use nursing knowledge and the process of elimination to make a selection.

22 **Answer: 3** A very swollen hand despite application of ice and elevation is a grave concern, especially with the child complaining of numbness. Such swelling can lead to compartment syndrome, which can lead to neurological damage. This is a medical emergency, and the physician should be called immediately. The nurse can then provide diversional activities while waiting for definitive orders.
Cognitive Level: Analysis **Client Need:** Physiological Integrity: Physiological Adaptation **Integrated Process:** Nursing Process: Implementation **Content Area:** Child Health: Musculoskeletal **Strategy:** The core issue of the question is recognition of a complication, compartment syndrome, that can lead to neurological damage. The correct answer is the one that provides for definitive treatment of the problem, which in this case is in the practice realm of the physician.

23 **Answer: 3** The infant who is carried with the hips abducted is at decreased risk for developing developmental dysplasia of the hip. Options 1, 2, and 4 are all factors that would possibly increase the incidence of this defect.
Cognitive Level: Analysis **Client Need:** Physiological Integrity: Physiological Adaptation **Integrated Process:** Nursing Process: Analysis **Content Area:** Child Health: Musculoskeletal **Strategy:** The core issue of the question is recognition of which situation allows the infant to keep the hips abducted. Evaluate each option according to this criteria to make a selection.

24 **Answer: 3** Pain must be managed properly in the child after spinal fusion in order for the client to participate in respiratory exercises. Logrolling and repositioning, as well as coughing, deep-breathing, and use of incentive spirometry should be done every 2 hours around the clock with this postoperative client. Providing adequate pain relief will enable the client to carry out these important activities.
Cognitive Level: Analysis **Client Need:** Physiological Integrity: Physiological Adaptation **Integrated Process:** Nursing Process: Implementation **Content Area:** Child Health: Musculoskeletal **Strategy:** The core issue of the question is the ability to prioritize nursing activities. While the ABCs are quite important, the client cannot meet goals for the respiratory portion of ABCs unless pain relief is achieved. With this in mind, choose option 3 as the correct answer.

25 **Answer: 4** The symptoms described are symptoms of osteomyelitis. This disease can result from a penetrating wound, but it also may result from an infection elsewhere in the body that traveled to the bone. Osteomyelitis may follow an upper respiratory infection, which is common in school-aged children.
Cognitive Level: Analysis **Client Need:** Physiological Integrity: Physiological Adaptation **Integrated Process:** Nursing Process: Assessment **Content Area:** Child Health: Musculoskeletal **Strategy:** The issue of the question is the ability of the nurse to analyze assessment data and compare it to typical data of childhood musculoskeletal problems. Note that the temperature is elevated to help choose the option related to infection.

26 **Answer: 4, 1, 3, 2, 5** The proper procedure is as follows:

1. Move forward to the edge of the chair.
2. Place unaffected leg slightly under or at the edge of the chair (this position helps the client to stand up from the chair and achieve balance, since the unaffected leg is supported against the edge of the chair).
3. Grasp the crutches by the horizontal hand bars using the hand on the affected side.
4. Grasp the arm of the chair using the hand on the unaffected side (the body weight is placed on the crutches and

the hand on the armrest to support the unaffected leg when the client rises to stand).

5. Push down on the crutches and the chair armrest while raising the body out of the chair.
6. Assume a *tripod position* (crutches out laterally in front of feet, approximately 6 inches, with feet slightly apart for balance before moving; not part of original answer.

Cognitive Level: Analysis **Client Need:** Physiological Integrity: Physiological Adaptation **Integrated Process:** Nursing Process: Implementation **Content Area:** Child Health: Musculoskeletal **Strategy:** Visualize the procedure and think about principles of joint support and balance to complete the ordered steps.

Key Terms to Review

arthrocentesis p. 1230
arthroscopy p. 1229
Bouchard's nodes p. 1246
clubfoot p. 1247
compartment syndrome p. 1243
countertraction p. 1232
crepitation p. 1242
diaphysis p. 1228
epiphyseal plate p. 1253
epiphysis p. 1253
gout p. 1245
Heberden's nodes p. 1246
internal fixation p. 1235
laminectomy p. 1234
osteomyelitis p. 1238
osteoporosis p. 1237
scoliosis p. 1253
sprain p. 1244
strain p. 1244
traction p. 1231

References

Ball, J., & Bindler, R. (2006). *Child health nursing: Partnering with children and families.* Upper Saddle River, NJ: Pearson Education.

Black, J., & Hawks, J. (2005). *Medical surgical nursing: Clinical management for positive outcomes* (7th ed.). St. Louis: Elsevier Science.

Corbett, J. (2004). *Laboratory tests and diagnostic procedures with nursing diagnoses* (6th ed.). Upper Saddle River, NJ: Pearson Education.

Harkreader, H., & Hogan, M. (2004). *Fundamentals of nursing: Caring and clinical judgment* (2nd ed.). St. Louis: Elsevier Science.

Ignatavicius, D., & Workman, L. (2006). *Medical-surgical nursing: Critical thinking for collaborative care* (5th ed.). Philadelphia: W. B. Saunders.

Kozier, B., Erb, G., Berman, A., & Snyder, S. (2004). *Fundamentals of nursing: Concepts, process, and practice* (7th ed.). Upper Saddle River, NJ: Pearson Education.

LeMone, P., & Burke, K. (2004). *Medical surgical nursing: Critical thinking in client care* (3rd ed.). Upper Saddle River, NJ: Pearson Education.

Porth, C. (2004). *Pathophysiology: Concepts of altered health states* (7th ed.). Philadelphia: Lippincott Williams & Wilkins.

Smith, S., Duell, D., & Martin, B. (2004). *Clinical nursing skills: Basic to advanced skills* (6th ed.). Upper Saddle River, NJ: Pearson Education.

63 Integumentary Disorders

Test Yourself

Are you ready for the NCLEX-RN® or course exams? Use the practice tests on the companion CD-ROM to check.

In this chapter

Cross reference

Other chapters relevant to this content area are

Integumentary Medications,	Chapter 43
Common Laboratory Tests,	Chapter 47
Common Diagnostic Tests and Procedures,	Chapter 48

I. OVERVIEW OF ANATOMY AND PHYSIOLOGY OF THE INTEGUMENTARY SYSTEM

A. **Epidermis (see Figure 63–1 ■):** outer layer of skin made up of epithelial cells; protects body and internal structures from harm by providing a barrier to external environment

B. **Dermis:** second layer of skin made up of lymph vessels, blood vessels, and nerve fibers; papillary layer contains capillaries and receptor sites for touch and pain; reticular layer contains receptors for deep touch as well as sweat and sebaceous glands

C. **Subcutaneous tissue:** lies beneath dermis, is made up of adipose (fat) tissue, and assists in connecting skin to structures below subcutaneous tissue

Figure 63–1

Layers and structures of the skin.

Source: Sims, L., D'Amico, J., Stiesmeyer, J., & Webster, J. (1995). Health assessment in nursing. *Redwood City, CA: Addison Wesley, p. 126.*

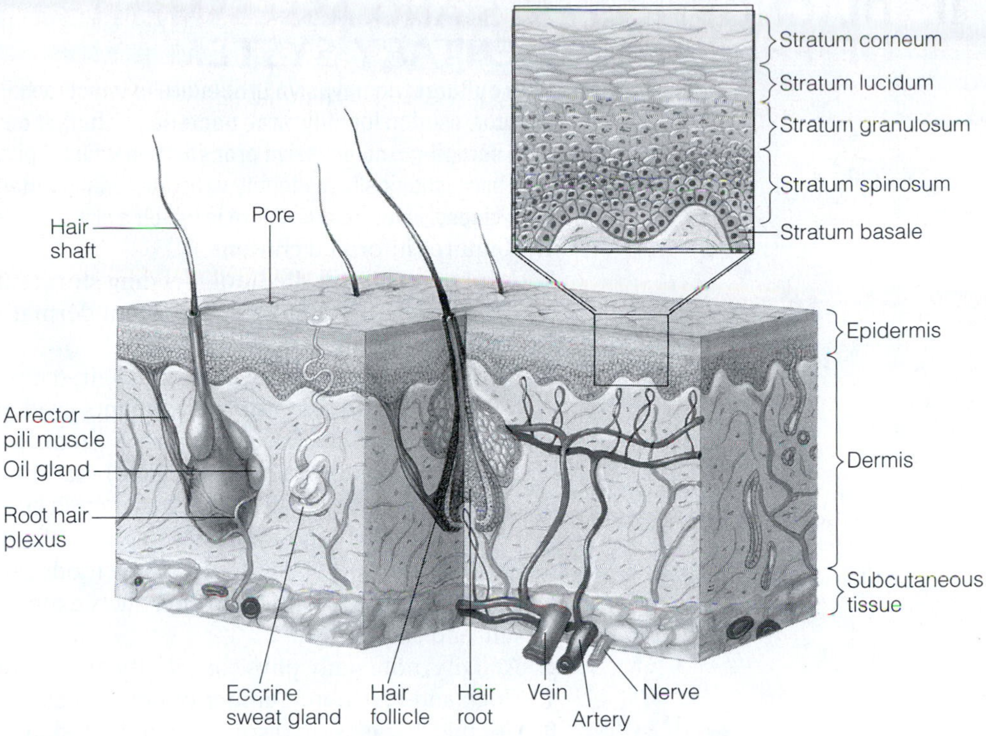

D. Appendages: include hair, nails, and glands

1. Hair
   - **a.** Composed of primarily dead cells; hair root begins in bulb of hair follicle and grows from dermis outward
   - **b.** Protects and pads scalp from external objects and helps to maintain body temperature
2. Nails: primarily made up of dead cells that cover nail bed; nail structure begins in epidermis and extends across and protects nail bed
3. Glands
   - **a.** Apocrine: sweat glands located in axilla, anus, and genital area; function unknown
   - **b.** Eccrine: sweat glands located on forehead, hands, and soles of feet; maintain a stable temperature for body through perspiration when body is overheated
   - **c.** Sebaceous: oil glands located throughout body that secrete sebum to lubricate skin, decrease water loss, and aid in killing bacteria on skin surface (see Figure 63–1);

E. Skin functions

1. Sensitivity to pressure, pain, touch, and temperature
2. First line of defense against infectious organisms
3. Thermoregulation through sweating, shivering, and subcutaneous insulation
4. Protects underlying tissues and organs from injury
5. Synthesizes vitamin D
6. Excretes water, salt, and electrolytes
7. Regenerates itself through shedding of old cells and replacing with new cells

F. Pediatric variations in skin

1. Newborns are covered by lanugo—fine, soft hair that is shed in first month of life
2. Newborns have thin skin with little subcutaneous fat that allows rapid heat loss and problems with thermoregulation
   - **a.** Leads to increased absorption of harmful chemical substances
   - **b.** Sweat glands not fully developed until middle childhood
3. Newborns' skin contains more water than does skin of older children
4. Dark-colored areas called Mongolian spots may be present on sacrum or buttocks of Native American, Asian, African American, or Latino infants

II. DIAGNOSTIC TESTS AND ASSESSMENTS OF THE INTEGUMENTARY SYSTEM

A. **Skin cultures:** noninvasive procedure in which a skin sample is obtained with a sterile applicator; used to identify viral, bacterial, or fungal causes of skin lesions

B. **Skin scrapings:** noninvasive procedure in which epithelial cells are scraped off and examined microscopically to identify viral, bacterial, fungal, or parasitic causes of skin lesion

C. **Skin biopsy:** invasive procedure in which a skin sample is removed for histological analysis
1. Requires informed consent
2. Apply pressure to site until bleeding stops; suture may be required
3. Used to identify tumors or persistent dermatitis

D. **Past medical history**
1. Note previous problems with skin, hair, scalp, or nails; discuss duration of symptoms, associated symptoms, treatments used and results
2. Medical disorders: discuss all body systems (cardiovascular, respiratory, hepatic, endocrine/metabolic, hematological) that may manifest as a skin disorder
3. ! Note allergies to medications, foods, environment, and so on; note allergies to tape, latex, povidone-iodine (Betadine), alcohol, and other substances
4. Nutrition: note dietary changes, new foods introduced, and fluid intake
5. External exposure: note new products exposed to skin, such as soaps, lotions, sun, and chemicals
6. Activity: note daily physical activity and exercise routine
7. Sleep and rest: note number of hours of sleep each night and any rest periods
8. Coping: discuss skin disorders and how skin is affected when stress is experienced; note coping behaviors used and results
9. Current medications: list current medications, onset and dose of medications
10. ! Recent surgeries or treatments: note any recent surgeries or treatment that may affect skin, such as phototherapy, radiation therapy
11. ! Current problem: elicit information regarding current problem; for skin rash, obtain detailed information such as date rash began, how it has changed, medications or ointments used and results of treatment

E. **Physical examination**
1. Note color (pink, yellow, white, purple, bruising, etc.)
2. For lesions, document color, size, shape, symmetry, and border (see Box 63–1)
3. Inspect hair for color, amount, distribution, lesions, and hygiene
4. Inspect nails for color, growth pattern, and thickness; inspect nail bed for inflammation or trauma
5. Note texture, temperature, and moisture of skin
6. Palpate skin turgor for hydration status
7. Palpate lower extremities (tibia and ankle) for edema
8. ! For lesions, note location and palpate texture, consistency, and mobility
9. Palpate hair for texture (coarse, fine); palpate nails for texture and check capillary refill

Box 63–1

Characteristics of Skin Lesions

Clients should be informed about how to monitor skin lesions. The ABCD rule is useful in teaching clients how to monitor changes in skin lesions and when to seek further assessment from the practitioner.

A = Asymmetry: Note any asymmetrical changes of the skin lesion. Lesions are normally symmetrical in shape. Any changes in the symmetry of the lesion need to be evaluated for possible removal.

B = Border: The border of the lesion should appear smooth. Note changes in the border that appear rough and jagged, and have the lesion evaluated for possible removal.

C = Color: The color of a lesion should stay the same. Lesions that get darker (brown or black) or have more than one color need to be evaluated for possible removal.

D = Diameter: The diameter or size of the lesion should be measured and documented. Lesions that change in size and enlarge need to be monitored and evaluated for possible removal.

III. SKIN PROBLEMS CAUSED BY VASCULARITY

A. Spider angioma

1. A flat, bright red spot with radiating blood vessels (BVs) at edges,
2. Commonly found on upper body; varies in size from a tiny dot up to 1.5 to 2 cm
3. Caused by vascular dilation of BVs commonly seen with high estrogen levels, pregnancy, liver disease, and/or vitamin B deficiency

B. Petechiae

1. Flat red spots, approximately 1 to 2 mm in diameter that do not change in color when blanched
2. Caused by tiny capillaries that have broken, possibly caused by thinning of blood (anticoagulant effect), liver disease, vitamin K deficiency, or septicemia

C. Purpura: purple or blue-appearing patch, varies in size and shape, caused by a bleeding disorder or broken BVs and may appear throughout body

IV. SKIN LESIONS

A. Primary skin lesions (see Figure 63–2 ■)

1. **Macule:** nonpalpable, flat lesion that has color and measures less than 1 cm; examples: freckles, chloasma
2. **Nodule:** elevated, firm lesion with a circumscribed border that measures approximately 1 to 2 cm
3. **Papule:** elevated, palpable mass, measuring less than 0.5 cm; examples include warts and moles
   a. Management depends on diagnosis, such as cryotherapy for wart removal
   b. Mole removal may be recommended if mole is considered premalignant; different methods of mole removal are available
   c. Excision of mole is one treatment that may be done in office setting; nursing care prior to treatment would be to explain procedure to client and obtain history of allergies (povidone–iodine, alcohol)
4. **Plaque:** elevated group of papules that have convalesced into one lesion larger than 0.5 cm; examples are actinic keratosis and psoriasis
5. **Pustule:** elevated, serous (pus)-filled vesicle that can measure any size; examples include acne and boils
6. **Vesicle:** fluid-filled, elevated mass that measures less than 0.5 cm; a fluid mass more than 0.5 cm, is called a bulla; examples of vesicles include chickenpox, small burns, and herpes virus lesion
7. **Wheal:** variable-sized, elevated **erythemic** (reddish) lesion with an irregular border that contains fluid in tissue of skin; examples include insect bites and hives

B. Secondary skin lesions

1. Atrophy: dry, thin, taut skin that appears wasted from loss of collagen; an example is aged skin; hydration with fluids and keeping skin well-moisturized with emollients such as Eucerin™ cream are helpful for this condition
2. Crusts: dried pus or blood on skin surface resulting from a vesicle that has ruptured; examples of crusts include final stages of chickenpox lesions or impetigo lesions

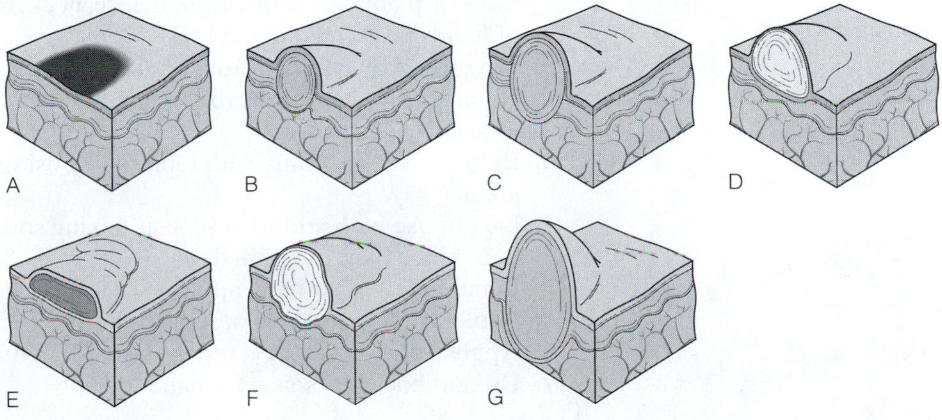

Figure 63–2

Primary skin lesions.

Source: LeMone, P., & Burke, K. (2003). Medical surgical nursing: Critical thinking for client care *(3rd ed.). Upper Saddle River, NJ: Pearson Education, p. 355.*

3. Erosion: superficial indentation of skin that results from a previous lesion; an example of erosion is a scratch mark that has not healed over time; therapeutic management includes warm, moist compresses to site for comfort; keep site clean and dry, cleaning with antibacterial soaps at least three to four times a day; may need to apply topical antibiotics if site gets secondary bacterial infection
4. Fissure: linear break in skin with sharp edges, extending into dermis; examples include athlete's foot or cracks in corner of mouth from chapped lips; therapeutic management for athlete's foot includes antifungal medications along with keeping feet cool and dry; encourage use of white, cool socks and avoid allowing feet to sweat; fissures of lips may be treated with topical ointments such as petroleum jelly or Blistex™ ointment
5. Scales: dry, dead skin that sloughs off skin surface and that may be dry or greasy; examples include dandruff or psoriasis
6. Scar: flat connective tissue resulting from healing over site of previous injury, which may vary in size, color, and shape; examples include healed surgery incisions or acne scars
7. Ulcers: deep excavations in skin; they may vary in size and shape and extend into dermis or subcutaneous tissue; examples include chancres and pressure ulcers

V. ATOPIC DERMATITIS (ECZEMA)

A. Overview

1. **Atopic dermatitis** is a superficial inflammatory skin disorder; sometimes called eczema (having a hereditary allergic tendency)
2. A chronic, superficial inflammatory skin disorder characterized by severe **pruritus** (itchiness)
3. Affects infants, children, adolescents, and adults
4. Sixty percent of affected children develop symptoms during infancy
5. Unknown etiology but occurs more frequently in children when one or both parents have allergies such as asthma, hay fever, or contact dermatitis
6. Infantile eczema is frequently related to food allergies
7. Eczema in older children is often related to allergies to dust mites
8. Intensified by dry skin, detergents, constricting clothing, or perfumed soaps and lotions

B. Assessment

1. In infancy, red papules (raised lesions) usually appear first on cheeks and then spread to forehead, scalp, and down extensor surfaces of arms and legs
2. ! Characterized by intense pruritus, which causes excoriation of skin that then leads to exudate and crust formation
3. Childhood stage may follow continuously from infancy, or eczema may make first appearance in toddler
4. ! Childhood eczema is characterized by dry, scaly, papular patches of skin on wrists, hands, ankles, antecubital and popliteal spaces
5. In adolescence, exudation is often caused by external irritation or secondary infection
6. ! Adolescent eczema is characterized by **lichenification** (large, dry, thickened lesions or plaques) on flexor folds, face, neck, back, upper arms, and dorsal aspects of hands, feet, fingers, and toes
7. Diagnosed by family history of allergies and inspection of skin
8. No diagnostic test exists for eczema

C. Therapeutic management

1. Bathe or shower daily with tepid water using mild soap only on nonaffected areas
2. ! Do not use bath additives such as baking soda, bubble bath, or bath oils
3. Pat, rather than rub, skin dry
4. Immediately after bath, apply emollient such as Eucerin or Lubriderm
5. ! Avoid use of perfumed or scented lotions
6. Apply wet wraps to severely affected skin after applying topical medications
7. Use antibacterial soaps for handwashing

8. Keep fingernails clean and short
9. Avoid wool or constricting clothing, which can promote itching or trap perspiration
10. Place cotton gloves or socks over the hands of infants or young children to prevent scratching
11. Provide support to child and family during flare-ups and reassurance that lesions do not produce scars unless excessively scratched and secondarily infected
12. Medication therapy includes topical steroids (hydrocortisone 1% or triamcinolone 0.1%) applied to lesions to reduce inflammation during flare-ups, tar preparations (sometimes used during flare-ups when symptoms are mild), antihistamines (control itching), and oral antibiotics (used only if there is widespread skin breakdown or infection)

D. Client teaching

1. Appropriate application of creams, ointments, or tar preparations
2. Proper application of soaks or compresses
3. Identify foods that exacerbate the rash and avoid them
4. Avoid getting sunburns
5. Avoid known or suspected contact allergens, pets, or environmental factors
6. Use antihistamines before naps or bedtimes if sleep deprivation occurs because of itching
7. Importance of following treatment plan to promote healing and prevent infections
8. Condition is not contagious
9. With infants, introduce one new food at a time to see if a flare-up occurs

VI. PSORIASIS

A. Overview

1. A chronic, inflammatory skin disorder in which lesions appear as whitish, scaly plaques on scalp, knees, or elbows
2. Psoriasis has no known etiology; is thought to be a multifactorial disease in which a T-lymphocyte–mediated dermal immune response occurs; most clients with psoriasis have a positive family history

B. Assessment: dry, scaly rash that may appear as silvery scales or plaques usually found on scalp, knees, or elbows

C. Therapeutic management

1. Direct sun exposure to skin or light therapy may be beneficial for some clients
2. Emollients: frequent use of emollients and keratolytic agents are beneficial for scalp psoriasis
3. Topical steroids may also be prescribed; antihistamines may be used for pruritus

VII. SEBORRHEIC DERMATITIS

A. Overview

1. A common, chronic skin condition occurring in areas of active sebaceous glands, such as face, scalp, body folds, sternal area, and axilla
2. Appears as an erythematous scaling lesion that may appear dry or greasy
3. Etiology is unknown, but possible causes are believed to be hormonal influence, nutritional deficiency, neurogenic influence, dysfunction of sebaceous glands, and/or fungal infection

B. Assessment

1. Erythemic, scaly lesions that appear in varying degrees (oily or flaky, dry skin), are pruritic, and may cause secondary bacterial infections
2. Common sites include scalp, eyebrows, nose, ears, sternal area, and axillae
3. Seborrheic dermatitis is seen more frequently in cold weather periods, and it is thought to be caused by decreased humidification and decreased exposure to sunlight

C. Therapeutic management: scalp treatment: selenium sulfide 2.5% suspension or coal tar shampoos and topical steroid creams

VIII. MALIGNANT NEOPLASMS

A. Actinic keratosis

1. Overview
   a. Premalignant macules found on skin surface of fair-skinned individuals who are 50 years or older, but can be seen in high-risk individuals at any age
   b. Occurs because of chronic sun exposure to skin
   c. Persons with light complexion are at highest risk for actinic keratosis
   d. Approximately 1% of these lesions will progress to squamous cell carcinoma
2. Assessment
   a. Erythematous, rough, and shiny-textured macules that may appear as a single macule or in groups
   b. Commonly seen on face, ears, scalp, lips, neck, and hands
3. Therapeutic management
   a. Prophylactic treatment is recommended to prevent development of these lesions
   b. Protection from ultraviolet (UV) rays of sun with use of clothing and sunscreens are recommended when exposed to sunlight
   c. Biopsy and removal of lesion is recommended if changes in lesion occur; these changes include color, border, size, and shape of lesions; refer back to Box 63–1

B. Basal cell carcinoma

1. Overview
   a. An abnormal cell growth of basal layer of epidermal skin
   b. Most common contributor is UV rays from sunlight exposure
   c. Basal cells do not mature appropriately into keratinocytes, which results in neoplastic growth surrounding tissue is also destroyed
   d. Basal cell carcinoma is least aggressive type of skin cancer and rarely metastasizes to other organs
2. Assessment: types and characteristics of the five types of basal cell carcinoma
   a. Nodular basal cell carcinoma: small, firm papule, which appears as pearly, white, pink, or flesh-colored and is commonly seen on face, neck, and/or head
   b. Superficial basal cell carcinoma: this papule or plaque is second-most common lesion and is commonly seen on trunk and extremities
   c. Pigmented basal cell carcinoma: is less common and usually found on head, neck, or face; has ability to concentrate melanin, which causes deeper pigmentation of center of tumor
   d. Morpheaform basal cell carcinoma: least common form; found on head and neck, appearing like a tumor with fingerlike projections (usually ivory or flesh-colored) and typically resembles a scar; has ability to invade and destroy adjacent tissue and structures
   e. Keratotic basal cell carcinoma: found on preauricular or postauricular area; contains both basal cells and squamous cells that keratinize; if removed, this tumor is likely to recur; also has a high risk of metastasizing to other structures
3. Therapeutic management
   a. Monitor progress of growth of all lesions; lesions that measure more than 2 cm have a high reoccurrence rate; suspicious lesions are excised and sent for pathological examination
   b. Educate clients regarding importance of monitoring lesions and early identification of new lesions; suggest monthly self-assessment of skin and periodic screening based on symptoms by health care provider
   c. Encourage protection from UV light exposure by using sunscreen products with SPF 15 or higher and wearing hats and and other protective clothing to protect skin
   d. Medication therapy: none

C. Cutaneous T-cell lymphoma

1. Overview: a type of lymphoma involving skin that rarely invades lymph nodes; it is a thymus-derived helper cell cancer
2. Assessment: three stages exist; however, stages may occur either in sequence or concurrently

a. Stage 1—erythematous stage: erythemic, well-defined border patch that is pruritic and may resemble psoriasis or eczema; patch may become diffuse with severe itching
b. Stage 2—plaque stage: erythemic, scaly patches that become indurated and/or elevated; center of plaque may appear healed with rough, ring-shaped borders; this stage may resemble tertiary syphilis or erythema multiforme perstans
c. Stage 3—tumor stage: terminal stage in which tumor growth of plaques occur, often seen with secondary bacterial infection

3. Therapeutic management
   a. Initial stages may only require a tar cream and treatment with UVB light therapy
   b. PUVA has also been effective in this treatment
   c. Nitrogen mustard treatment has also been beneficial when used in earlier stages
   d. Medication therapy: systemic corticosteroids are used for first two stages; radiation therapy and electron-beam radiation may be used at any point in disease; systemic chemotherapy has been used during plaque and tumor stage but may not always be successful

D. Kaposi's sarcoma

1. Overview
   a. A rare skin cancer of endothelial lining of small BVs, seen most commonly on face, nose, and ears
   b. May be related to an infective agent such as a retrovirus (e.g., HIV)
2. Assessment
   a. Vascular lesions (macules, papules, nodules) that can affect skin and viscera
   b. Over time, lesions enlarge and become confluent, forming large masses; as these masses enlarge, tissue below mass becomes involved and tumor then invades lymphatic tissue, which may result in varying degrees of lymphedema, primarily affecting genitalia and lower extremities
   c. As disease progresses, tumor may interfere with internal organ function and may even cause bleeding to point of hemorrhage (a late sign)
   d. Initially Kaposi's sarcoma may be symptom-free; however, pain maybe experienced in later stages
3. Therapeutic management
   a. Isolated lesions may be removed by excision, cryotherapy, and/or local radiation for comfort and/or cosmetic treatment
   b. Medication therapy: chemotherapy can be used as a single agent or a combination treatment

E. Nonmelanoma: Squamous cell carcinoma

1. Overview
   a. A cutaneous malignancy that arises from keratinocytes; most common type of skin cancer; fair-skinned males tend to have a higher incidence of nonmelanoma skin cancer, with majority occurring from 30 to 60 years of age
   b. Occurs on areas of skin frequently exposed to UV light, such as face, ears, nose, lips, and hands; of two nonmelanoma types of carcinoma, squamous cell carcinoma grows quicker, is more aggressive, and is more likely to metastasize than basal cell carcinoma
   c. Etiology of squamous cell carcinoma is multifactorial
   d. Environmental causes include UV radiation, chemicals, physical trauma, and pollution
   e. With exposure of UV light to skin, rays penetrate tissue and alter normal DNA and suppress body's T-cell and B-cell immunity, producing tumors of squamous epithelial or mucous membranes
   f. As tumor grows, cells increase in size and an irregular shape is formed
   g. Tumors may proliferate and invade dermal layer of skin
   h. Squamous cell carcinoma may also present from preexisting skin lesions, such as old scars; these tumors may proliferate into dermal structure and can cause metastasis via lymphatic tissue

2. Assessment
   - a. Squamous cell carcinoma may present as a small, flesh-colored papule that is firm to touch
   - b. As tumor grows, color may change and appear erythemic and sore, and may even bleed if touched
3. Therapeutic management
   - a. Recommended management is tumor removal by a variety of methods, including cryotherapy, surgical excision, electrodesiccation, or radiotherapy
   - b. Cure rate with these methods is approximately 90%
   - c. It is recommended to remove these tumors as soon as identified to prevent metastasis
   - d. Nursing management includes teaching methods to prevent further tumors from arising: minimize sun exposure, wear protective clothing, wear sunscreen with a SPF of 15 or higher, and avoid tanning booths
   - e. Medication therapy: none

IX. BACTERIAL INFECTIONS

A. Impetigo

1. Overview
   - a. A superficial skin infection that initially appears as an erythemic vesicle and later changes to a honey-colored crusted lesion
   - b. Is most commonly seen in children but occasionally affects adults
   - c. An alteration in skin integrity occurs, and bacteria invade epidermis and cause an infection
   - d. Most common organisms involved are *Staphylococcus aureas* and *group-A beta-hemolytic streptococcus*
2. Assessment
   - a. Commonly found on face, arms, legs, and buttocks
   - b. Appear as thin erythemic vesicles, which then become honey-colored crusts or erosions
   - c. May occur as a single lesion or several lesions that have coalesced and appear as a group of lesions
3. Therapeutic management
   - a. Eencourage good handwashing with hot soapy water to prevent spreading bacteria to others
   - b. For recurrent lesions, a culture of site is obtained to isolate pathogens
   - c. Medication therapy: topical antibiotics, or for severe cases, systemic antibiotics are recommended

B. Folliculitis

1. Overview
   - a. A superficial bacterial infection of hair follicle
   - b. Folliculitis can occur at any age and is seen more frequently in males
   - c. Can be aggravated by shaving, particularly skin on face (beard), legs, and axilla
   - d. Most common pathogens are *Staphyloccus aureus* and *Pseudomonas aeruginosa*
2. Assessment
   - a. Lesion appears as an erythemic, pruritic, mildly tender pustule located at hair follicle; various stages of folliculitis may occur, including a simple pustule, progressing to a furuncle or carbuncle
   - b. In severe cases, fever and chills may be present
3. Therapeutic management
   - a. Topical treatment includes cleaning site with warm soapy water 2 to 3 times a day
   - b. Warm compresses may be used for comfort as needed
   - c. If razors are being used, encourage client to use clean, sharp razors and to throw away old razors
   - d. Do not use irritating lotions or creams at site
   - e. Medication therapy: for simple folliculitis, topical mupirocon (Bactroban) applied to site 3 times a day is effective; for more severe cases, oral antibiotics are recommended

C. Furuncle

1. Overview
   a. An erythemic, warm, tender nodule of skin; commonly seen in children, teens, and young adults
   b. Common sites are nares, neck, axilla, and genital area
   c. *Staphylococcus* is most common infective organism and may be chronic in some cases
2. Assessment: warm, erythemic tender nodule of hair follicle
3. Therapeutic management
   a. Warm moist heat may be applied to site for comfort
   b. Occasionally, incision and drainage of site may be needed, in which case, Gram stain, culture, and sensitivity is obtained
   c. Medication therapy: oral antibiotics are not recommended except for immunocompromised clients

D. Furunculosis

1. Overview: an infection of an inflammatory nodule most commonly seen in children, adolescents, and young adults; hair follicle becomes inflamed, tender to touch, and warm at site
2. Assessment: an erythemic, hard, tender-to-touch nodule frequently found at site of a hair follicle
3. Therapeutic management: warm moist soaks to site; incision and drainage of site may be required; keep lesions clean by washing site with warm soapy water several times a day
4. Medication therapy: simple furunculosis does not require systemic antibiotics; topical antibiotics may be used; however, complicated furunculosis with cellulitis requires systemic antibiotics; recurrent furunculosis may be controlled with prophylactic antibiotic therapy

E. Carbuncle

1. Overview
   a. An inflammatory lesion formed when several furuncles coalesce to form one larger infected lesion of skin
   b. Carbuncles are frequently seen in children, teens, and young adults; males are affected more frequently; common sites are hair follicles in nose, neck, face, buttocks, and axilla; *Staphylococcus* is a common causative organism
2. Assessment: erythemic, tender nodule that develops at a hair follicle area with possible malaise and low-grade fever
3. Therapeutic management
   a. Warm moist heat may be applied
   b. Incision and drainage of site is recommended
   c. Frequent use of antibacterial soaps and frequent showers are recommended for preventation
   d. Medication therapy: antibiotics

F. Cellulitis

1. Overview
   a. A bacterial infection of dermal and subcutaneous tissues with lesions appearing in various stages, ranging from vesicles, bullae, abscesses, and plaques
   b. Most commonly seen in adults, with group-A beta hemolytic *Streptococcus pyogenes* and *Staphylococcus aureus* being most frequent organisms
   c. Cellulitis occurs because of a break in skin integrity (abrasion, laceration, etc.); may also occur secondary to a skin lesion
2. ! Assessment
   a. An erythemic, swollen, tender-to-touch area of skin at site of entry of bacteria
   b. Associated symptoms include fever, chills, malaise, and anorexia
   c. Regional lymphadenopathy
3. ! Therapeutic management
   a. Rest and elevation of affected part
   b. Moist heat to site for comfort
   c. Culture and sensitivity of tissue site for severe cases

d. For necrotic tissue, surgical excision and debridement are recommended along with antibiotic therapy
e. Hospitalization is needed if cellulitis is on face or covers a large area; otherwise, home management is done
f. Medication therapy: antibiotic therapy

X. VIRAL INFECTIONS

A. Herpes simplex virus (Type 1, Type 2)

1. Overview
   a. A viral infection manifested by vesicles on oral mucosa (mouth or lips), which is HSV Type I, or in genital mucosa (HSV Type II)
   b. Herpes simplex virus (HSV) can occur at any age
   c. Is spread by direct contact of contaminated body fluids and has an incubation period range of 2 to 14 days
   d. Primary infection: initial outbreak in which blisters occur on mucosa or lips; malaise and fever are also common symptoms
   e. Recurrent infections: outbreaks may occur at any time and are commonly precipitated by stress and illness; symptoms are usually milder than primary outbreak; recurrent infection is commonly present with a prodrome of tingling, itching, or a burning sensation at site prior to outbreak of lesions
   f. Latency period: virus remains dormant in body during this time
2. ! Assessment
   a. Primary symptoms include malaise, fever, and vesicles appearing on mucosa
   b. Secondary symptoms include prodrome of tingling, burning sensation prior to outbreak of vesicles on mucosa; latency period is asymptomatic
3. Therapeutic management
   a. Advise rest
   b. ! Encourage good handwashing technique to prevent spreading virus
   c. Comfort measures such as petroleum jelly or lip balm may be used for oral lesions
   d. ! To prevent spreading virus, teach client to avoid close contact with others while lesions are present; to prevent HSV Type 2, advise use of latex condoms to prevent spreading genital lesions
   e. Medication therapy: over-the-counter medications, such as acetaminophen (Tylenol) or camphophenique for comfort as needed; antiviral medications such as acyclovir (Zovirax), famciclovir (Famvir), or valacyclovir (Valtrex) may reduce further viral replication and diminish symptoms if started within 24 to 48 hours after initial onset of lesions

B. Herpes zoster

1. Overview
   a. A viral infection manifested by vesicles on skin and commonly seen in older adults and elderly
   b. Herpes zoster is a reactivation of varicella virus, which has been dormant for many years, in the dorsal root ganglia
2. ! Assessment
   a. A vesicular rash on skin that usually follows one dermatome
   b. Clusters of vesicles are common along with symptoms of tingling, itching, burning, and even pain at site of lesions
   c. May also experience fatigue, malaise, fever, and headache in addition to local discomfort of rash
3. Therapeutic management
   a. ! Comfort measures include wet dressings or soaks (Burow's solution) on lesions 2 to 3 times a day
   b. ! Oatmeal baths (Aveeno™) are soothing and help to dry lesions
   c. Rest is recommended
   d. To prevent viral spread to others, take care to avoid persons at risk
   e. Monitor lesions for secondary bacterial infections

f. Medication therapy: antiviral medications if therapy started within 24 to 48 hours after outbreak of vesicles; current medications include acyclovir (Zovirax), famciclovir (Famvir), and valacyclovir (Valtrex); acetaminophen (Tylenol) and ibuprofen (Motrin) may be used for discomfort

C. Warts

1. Overview
   - **a.** An elevation in epidermal skin layer, commonly seen in children and young adults; seen more common in women than in men
   - **b.** Caused by papillomavirus
   - **c.** A tumor develops on skin within epidermal layer
   - **d.** Virus may be transmitted from person to person by touch and is commonly seen on hands and feet
2. Assessment: a painless nodule on skin surface, which is flesh-colored and appears to have a rough surface with an irregular border; there are several types of warts
   - **a.** Common wart—flesh-colored nodule commonly seen on hands or extremities, but can occur anywhere on body; commonly appears to have a "black seed" in the center of lesion; these warts may come and go, usually lasting approximately 6 to 12 months without treatment
   - **b.** Flat wart—a tiny flesh-colored node, 1 to 3 mm in diameter, that may appear in clusters on dorsum of hand or forehead
   - **c.** Filiform wart—a tiny, thin, projected nodule commonly seen on face, nose, or eyelids
   - **d.** Plantar wart—a hard nodule found on bottom of foot; commonly projects into foot from constant pressure applied while walking on nodule; it measures approximately 2 to 3 cm and is frequently associated with discomfort or pain at site
3. Therapeutic management
   - **a.** Sometimes no treatment is necessary for warts because viral lesions will resolve on their own
   - **b.** Medication therapy: over-the-counter (OTC) therapy for wart removal includes salicylic acid (17%) and retinoic acid
   - **c.** Laser therapy may be used for selected warts, such as those that are large or located in certain body areas (e.g., genital)
   - **d.** Warts that are treated may reappear in same site or on other areas of skin

XI. FUNGAL INFECTIONS

A. Candidiasis

1. Overview
   - **a.** Infection caused by *candida albicans,* a yeast-like fungus that most often causes superficial cutaneous infections
   - **b.** Symptomatic infections occur on moist cutaneous sites and mucosal surfaces if local immunity is disturbed
   - **c.** Candida infections can affect all ages but are most often seen as a cause of diaper rash in infants, summertime inframammary rash in women, vaginitis in premenopausal women, oral candidiasis in immunocompromised clients, and buttock and perineal rash in incontinent clients
   - **d.** Risk factors include moist, warm, or altered skin integrity; systemic antibiotics; pregnancy; birth control use; poor nutrition; diabetes or chronic illnesses; and immunosuppression
2. Assessment: lesions are bright red, smooth macules with a macerated appearance and a scaling, elevated border; characteristic "satellite" lesions are small, similar-appearing macules outside main lesion
   - **a.** Oral candidiasis is also known as thrush and is characterized by white, milky plaques on oral mucosa; associated symptoms may include a burning sensation or decreased taste
   - **b.** Vulovaginitis is found on vaginal mucosa and can spread to perineum and groin; satellite lesions are usually present; other signs and symptoms include excessive itching and a thick, white, curdlike vaginal discharge

c. Perineal/diaper and skin-fold rash occurs on perigenital and perianal areas and can extend to inner thighs and buttocks; other areas affected include axilla, umbilical area, and under breasts; erythema, papules, pustules, and a scaling border are characteristic
d. Balanitis is an inflammation of glans and prepuce of penis that typically present as flattened pustules with edema, scaling, erosion, burning, and tenderness
e. Paronychial infection presents as erythema, edema, and tenderness of nail folds; a creamy, purulent discharge may be expressed with pressure on nail; nails usually become discolored and have ridging
f. Candida organisms may also be a causative agent in otitis externa and scalp disorders
g. Diagnosis is made by culture of scrapings or by microscopic examination of scaling with potassium hydrochloride (KOH) preparation

3. Therapeutic management
   - ! a. Avoid sharing linens or personal items
   - ! b. Use clean towel and washcloth daily
   - c. Dry all skin folds, avoid frequent immersion of hands in water
   - d. Wear clean cotton underwear daily
   - e. For vaginal candida, avoid tight clothing and pantyhose, bathe more frequently, and dry genital area thoroughly; may need to treat sexual partner at same time to avoid reinfection or have partner use condoms until resolved; avoid douching, and change perineal pads frequently
   - f. For balanitis, carefully retract foreskin and perform careful cleaning and drying of glans penis
   - g. Encourage weight loss for obese clients and maintenance of normal serum glucose levels in diabetics to decrease infection risk
   - ! h. Medication therapy: antifungal medications (topical, shampoo, or vaginal suppository depending on site) or nystatin powder or ointment; systemic medications require monitoring of liver function tests because of risk of hepatotoxicity

B. Tinea corporis

1. Overview
   - a. A fungal infection of face, trunk, and extremities with exclusion of palms of hands, soles of feet, and groin; also known as ringworm of body
   - b. All species of dermatophytes can be causative agent; generally more prevalent in hot and humid climates
   - c. Can affect all age groups, but children are more often affected
   - d. Can be spread human-to-human, animal-to-human, and soil-to-human by direct contact; other risk factors include prolonged use of topical steroids or immunosuppression
2. Assessment
   - ! a. Classic lesions are annular (ringlike) plaques with an elevated border, sharp margins, and a clearing center
   - b. May occur singly or in groups of 3 to 4
   - c. KOH preparation from these lesions is usually positive; woods lamp fluoresces yellow; dermatophyte test media changes medium from yellow to red
   - d. For most clinical purposes, classification by anatomic site is preferred
3. Therapeutic management
   - a. Avoid contact with suspected lesions
   - b. Topical creams are treatment of choice
   - c. Clean environment to remove fungal scales
   - d. Avoid sharing towels or other items that can transmit fungal scales
   - ! e. Search out infected animals/pets and treat appropriately
   - f. Apply creams after bathing and reapply after swimming and exercising
   - g. Keep skin dry
   - h. Monitor for superimposed bacterial infections
   - ! i. Medication therapy: topical drugs for superficial infections; eradication is slow and treatment may take 2 to 8 weeks; for added benefit, client should

wash with an antifungal shampoo such as ketoconazole (Nizoral) prior to using a cream

C. Tinea pedis

1. Overview
   - **a.** Also known as athlete's foot, is most common of all fungal infections; affects plantar surface of feet with mild to moderate erythema and scaly skin between toes
   - **b.** Caused by an infection by a dermatophyte (fungus that grows in nonliving, keratinized portions of skin)
   - **c.** Dermatophytes are commonly termed tinea and are named by affected location
   - **d.** Pustules may be present in severe cases with a foul odor, possibly indicating a secondary bacterial or yeast infection
   - **e.** Risk factors include communal showers and pools, occlusive footwear, excessive sweating, sharing of footwear, and hot, humid weather, immunocompromised status, and prolonged applications of topical steroids; both feet often are involved
2. Assessment
   - **a.** Interdigital scaling, crusting, and maceration; pruritis may or may not be present
   - **b.** Plantar and lateral surfaces of feet may also be affected
   - **c.** Vesicles, pustules, and interdigital blisters may provide an entry of secondary bacteria such as *Streptococcus* organisms
3. Therapeutic management
   - **a.** Keep involved areas clean, dry, and exposed to air when possible
   - **b.** Wear light cotton socks and change frequently throughout day
   - **c.** Wear sandals or open-toed shoes when possible; avoid plastic footwear and occlusive shoes
   - **d.** Carefully dry between toes after showering or bathing
   - **e.** Apply drying or dusting powers, topical antiperspirants
   - **f.** Put socks on before underwear to avoid spreading to groin
   - **g.** Instruct on signs and symptoms of bacterial infection such as pain, increased inflammation, pustules, or purulent exudates
   - **h.** Medication therapy: antifungal creams; powders may be used as an adjunct treatment and aid in keeping areas dry; for severe cases, Burow's solution soak for lesions that are oozing and oral antifungals such as griseofulvin, fluconazole, itraconazole, and tervinafine

XII. INFESTATIONS AND INSECT BITES

A. Bees and wasps

1. Stings that contain poison cause local tissue inflammation and destruction
2. Allergic reaction can occur from previous sensitization or toxic reaction from large inoculation of poison; IgE-mediated hypersensitivity to insect venom may be confirmed by skin testing with suitable dilutions of available venom, usually done by an allergist
3. Assessment
   - **a.** Local reactions include erythema, pain, heat, swelling, itching, blisters, secondary infection, necrosis, ulceration, and drainage
   - **b.** Toxic reactions include nausea, vomiting, headache, fever, diarrhea, lightheadedness, syncope, drowsiness, muscle spasms, edema, and/or convulsions
   - **c.** Systemic reactions include allergic/itching eyes, facial flushing, generalized urticaria, dry cough, chest/throat constriction, wheezing, dyspnea, cyanosis, abdominal cramps, diarrhea, nausea, vomiting, vertigo, chills/fever, stridor, shock, loss of consciousness, involuntary bowel/bladder action, frothy sputum, respiratory failure, cardiovascular collapse, and death
   - **d.** Delayed reactions include serum sickness–like reactions, fever, malaise, headache, urticaria, lymphadenopathy, polyarthritis
   - **e.** Unusual reactions include encephalopathy, neuritis, vasculitis, nephrosis, extreme fear/anxiety

4. Therapeutic management
   a. Outpatient or inpatient depending on individual response
   b. First-aid measures, local treatment, activate emergency services in severe reactions
   c. Remove stinger by scraping—do not squeeze with a tweezer—then cleanse wound
   d. Ice packs to bite or sting—alternate 10 minutes on and 10 minutes off
   e. Elevate and rest affected part
   f. Maintain adequate airway
   g. Persons with known sensitivity should wear medical ID tag
   h. Prevent reexposure in known hypersensitive persons; teach use of Epi-pen or anaphylactic kit
   i. Educate on risks of increasing severity of responses in future
   j. Instruct to use insect repellants when outdoors or in infested areas
   k. Medication therapy: local analgesics, diphenhydramine (Benadryl), or other antihistamines; topical or oral steroids; if severe systemic reaction, Epinephrine 1:1000 subcutaneous to combat urticaria, wheezing, angioedema; medications to treat shock if indicated; antivenom for black widow spider or scorpion
   l. Consider desensitization with immunotherapy in severe cases

B. Pediculosis

1. Overview
   a. An infestation of skin or hair by species of blood-sucking lice capable of living as external parasites on human host
   b. ***Pediculosis capitis*** is head louse, size of a sesame seed, clear in color when hatched but becomes grayish-white to red/brown after maturing
   c. Head lice infestation is very common among school-aged children of all socioeconomic backgrounds and is spread by sharing combs, hats, and scarves
   d. *Pediculosis pubis,* also known as "crabs," infests genital area and is a common sexually transmitted diseases
   e. Pubic lice can spread by sexual contact
   f. Nits/eggs attach to hair shaft by a cementlike or cocoonlike structure and are difficult to remove
   g. Lice live up to 30 days, and a female can lay up to 100 eggs
2. Assessment
   a. Intensive pruritis is most common symptom that may result in excoriations
   b. Head lice may resemble dandruff flakes; however, they are not easily brushed off
   c. Papular urticaria may be found at neck or pubic area
3. Therapeutic management
   a. Nits must be mechanically removed; a 50/50 white vinegar/water solution may loosen nits; olive oil may also be used; a nit comb is used to remove nits from hair shafts; lice may also be removed by fingers or tweezers; nits remove more easily by back-combing hair
   b. To treat eyelashes, apply petrolatum to lashes b.i.d. for 10 days; lice will either suffocate or slide off
   c. Educate children and parents about mode of transmission (person to person) and preventative measures, such as not sharing combs, brushes, hats, scarves, helmets, headphones, bedding, or sleeping bags
   d. Coats and hats should be hung separately and not touching each other
   e. Sleeping material should be labeled and kept separately in plastic bags, not stacked
   f. All family members need to be examined and treated at same time
   g. Soak personal hair items or any item in contact with hair in 2% Lysol or pediculocide for 1 hour
   h. Shaving hair is not found to be helpful
   i. Machine-wash all washable clothing used in last 48 hours and dry in hot dryer for at least 20 minutes
   j. Place unwashable items in airtight plastic bags for a period of 1 week to kill lice

k. Upholstered furniture or pillows may be ironed with a hot iron
l. Vacuum mattresses, rugs, upholstered furniture, and stuffed animals regularly
! m. For *pediculosis capitis:* permethrin (Nix), pyrethrin shampoo (Rid), or lindane (Kwell) shampoo left on 5 to 10 minutes and then washed off; lindane can be repeated in 1 week; due to neurotoxicity of lindane, it should not be used by children, nursing or pregnant women, individuals with known seizure disorders, or on open skin
n. For pediculosis pubis: treatment includes lindane, pyrethrin (Rid) or permethrin (Nix) as a shampoo left on for 10 minutes or as a lotion left on for several hours
o. Co-trimoxazole (Bactrim DS): b.i.d. for 3 days has been shown to be effective; a second therapy 10 days later may be necessary to kill emerging nits before they reproduce (non FDA–approved)

C. *Scabies*

1. Overview
   a. A contagious disease caused by infestation of skin by mite *Sarcoptes scabiei var hominis;* impregnated mite burrows into skin and remains there for life (approximately 30 days), laying 2 to 3 eggs per day; eggs hatch in 3 to 4 days and reach maturity in 4 days, migrate to skin surface, mate, and repeat cycle
   b. Is more common in people who don't have bathing facilities or access to clothes-washing facilities; mites can live in clothing fibers and can be transmitted by contact with infected clothing or bed linens
   c. Pathological findings by skin biopsy of a nodule will reveal portions of mite—although rarely performed; diagnosis is usually made by clinical presentation of burrows, vesicles, and nodules
2. Assessment
   ! a. Presents as a generalized pruritic rash particularly of hands, wrists, elbows, axillary areas, breasts, abdomen, or genitals
   b. Itching may become intense; increased warmth of skin and nocturnal itching is a classic symptom, since mites tend to have increased movment at night; exposure to hot water or steam also can increase pruritis
   c. Lesions may be erythematous, crusted papules, or purplish nodules, which may be accompanied by flesh-colored, raised burrows (threadlike linear ridges a few millimeters in length with a tiny black dot at one end); clients develop itch approximately 10 to 14 days after exposure
3. Therapeutic management
   a. Close family members and personal contacts must be treated as well, even if there are no apparent signs or symptoms
   ! b. All bed clothing, linens, unwashed worn clothing, and stuffed animals should be washed and dried in a hot dryer to kill mites
   ! c. Mites and eggs may be killed by placing items in airtight plastic bags for 7 days since mite cannot live away from host more than 3 days; mites can live 24 to 36 hours in room conditions and longer in humid environments
   d. Relief from itching may not occur for 3 to 6 weeks after treatment because of hypersensitivity of skin to debris left in burrow
   ! e. Lotions/creams should be applied from neck down, using a toothbrush to get under fingernails and toenails; lotion is showered off 8 to 12 hours later
   f. Permethrin 5% cream (Elimite) is treatment of choice; a second application in 48 hours is sometimes recommended
   g. Crotamiton 10% (Eurax) is less toxic but is also slightly less effective; therefore, application for 2 nights is advised
   ! h. Lindane 1% cream or lotion (Kwell) is least expensive but has potential for neurotoxicity and should not be used by children, nursing or pregnant women, people with a known seizure disorder, or any widespread excoriations/open skin; treatment may be repeated after 1 week
   i. Systemic antipruritics may be needed
   j. May require emollients and midpotency corticosteroids after using scabicide to suppress hyperreactivity caused by mites

XIII. ALLERGIC REACTIONS

A. *Contact dermatitis*

1. Overview
   a. An eruption of skin related to contact with an irritating substance or allergen; primary irritant dermatitis affects individuals exposed to specific irritants and produces discomfort immediately
   b. Common irritants include chemicals, dyes, metals, and latex gloves; allergic contact dermatitis affects only individuals previously sensitized; it represents a delayed hypersensitivity reaction; most common are poison ivy, sumac, and oak
   c. Contact dermatitis is an inflammation caused by an external irritant or allergic reaction mediated by IgE; epidermal reaction is caused by T-lymphocytes; location of rash helps provide clues to offending antigen; there is no specific age or sex affected, but black skin is less susceptible
2. Assessment
   ! a. Acute: papules, vesicles, bullae with surrounding erythema; crusting, oozing, and pruritis may be present
   b. Chronic: erythematous base, thickening with lichenification, scaling, and fissuring
3. Therapeutic management
   a. Identify and remove causative agents
   b. Topical emollients in combination with mid- to high-potency corticosteroids
   c. Drainage of large vesicles may be necessary without removing tops
   d. Apply wet dressings to oozing, pruritic lesions to aid in drying and debridement; cool tap water, Burow's solution 1 to 40, saline 1 tsp/pint water, and silver nitrate solution can be used
   e. Suppress inflammation with antibacterial solution
   ! f. May use topical steroid creams but do not use on face
   g. Aveeno (oatmeal) baths are helpful to decrease itching
   h. Antihistamines of choice may be used to decrease itching and edema
   i. Use calamine lotion to aid drying
   j. Midpotency topical corticosteroids
   k. High-potency topical corticosteroids such as amcinonide (Cyclocort) 0.1% or dexamethasone (Decaderm) 0.25%
   l. Systemic medications including prednisone, antibiotics, and antihistamines

B. *Urticaria*

1. Overview
   ! a. An itchy rash; single or multiple superficial raised pale macules with red halo; subsides rapidly, no scars or change in pigmentation; this condition may be recurrent
   b. Acute urticaria is a response to many stimuli; IgE-mediated histamine release from mast cells is sometimes seen in response to drug exposure and subsides over several hours
   c. Chronic urticaria persists over 6 weeks; it is not mediated by IgE; it is also associated with fever, chills, arthralgia, myalgia, and headache
   ! d. Urticaria is a response to massive release from mast cells in superficial dermis; can be caused by multiple agents such as drug reaction, food or food-additive allergy, inhalant, contact or ingestion allergy, transfusion reaction, insect bite or sting, bacterial, viral, fungal or helminthic infection, collagen vascular disease, lupus, heat, cold, sunlight, or emotional stress
   e. True urticarial lesions do not remain in same area of skin longer than 24 hours; lesions that are present 72 hours or longer suggest cutaneous vasculitis as a possible cause
2. Assessment
   ! a. Single or multiple raised, blanched, central wheals surrounded by red flare that is intensely pruritic
   b. May occur anywhere on the body
   c. Variable size of 1 to 2 mm to 15 to 20 cm or larger
   d. Resolves spontaneously in less than 48 hours

3. Therapeutic management
   a. Cool moist compresses help to control itching
   b. Avoidance if etiology is known
   c. Antihistamine if accidentally reexposed
   ! d. Instruct client that there is risk of life-threatening reaction on reexposure
   e. Subcutaneous administration of epinephrine 1:1000 for intense itching
   f. Antihistamines; histamine (H_2) receptor antagonists may enhance effectiveness of conventional antihistamines
   g. Cyprohepadine (Periactin) 4 mg every 6 hours for cold urticaria
   h. Corticosteroids for pressure urticaria
   i. Topical sunscreens and hydroxyzine (Vistaril) for solar urticaria

XIV. BENIGN CONDITIONS

A. *Acne*

1. Overview
   a. Androgenically stimulated, inflammatory disorder of sebaceous glands resulting in comedones, papules, inflammatory pustules, cysts, and occasional scarring; acne cannot occur without a hair follicle
   b. Has multifactorial causes including increased sebum production, abnormal keratinization of follicular epithelium, proliferation of proprioibacterium acnes, and inflammation
   c. Rate of sebum production is determined genetically and is increased by presence of androgens; earliest changes in acne may be seen in prepubescent years
2. Assessment
   a. Lesions may occur on forehead, cheeks, nose, and may extend over central back and chest
   b. Closed comedones—whiteheads
   c. Open comedones—blackheads
   d. Nodules or papules, pustules, with or without redness and edema, scars
   e. Grades of acne (see Box 63–2)
3. Therapeutic management
   a. Intended to control disease and is not curative
   b. Use a gentle antibacterial soap and wash affected areas with fingertips
   c. Avoid cosmetics containing oil and confine moisturizing lotions to dry patches of skin
   d. Instruct not to pick lesions, which would increase scarring
   e. Six to eight weeks of treatment is usual before obvious improvement occurs
   f. Diet does not cause acne
   g. Stress-management if acne flares with stress
   ! h. Topical retinoids are usually prescribed for all types of acne
   i. For mild acne, combination therapy of a topical retinoid plus one or more of the following: benzoyl peroxide, topical antibiotics, or azelaic acid

Box 63–2

Stages and Grades of Acne

Stages of Acne

Mild: few to several papules, no nodules, on face and neck only

Moderate: several papules to many papules and pustules; few to several nodules on face, back, chest, or upper arms

Severe: Numerous and extensive papules and pustules; many nodules with acne-induced scarring

Grades of Acne

Grade 1: comedonal—closed and open

Grade 2: papular—over 25 lesions on face and trunk

Grade 3: pustular—over 25 lesions with mild scarring

Grade 4: nodulocystic—inflammatory nodules and cysts with extensive scarring

j. For moderate acne, topical agents and oral antibiotics such as tetracycline for a specified period of time and then antibiotic is discontinued
k. For severe acne, isotretinoin (Accutane) 0.5 to 1.0 mg/kg daily
l. Antiandrogens such as birth control pills and spironolactone inhibit sebum production

B. Lentigo

1. Overview
   a. A brown macule resembling a freckle except that border is usually irregular
   b. Benign lentigo resembles a freckle; lentigo maligna (premelanoma) is a brown or black mottled, irregularly outlined, slowly enlarging lesion in which there are an increased number of scattered atypical melanocytes; it usually occurs on face; one third progress to melanoma but transition may take 10 to 15 years
   c. Senile lentigo (liver spot) occurs on exposed skin of older white individuals
2. Assessment
   a. Benign lentigo: freckle, pigmented, flat, or slightly elevated macule
   b. Lentigo maligna: brown/black uneven macule with irregular border which slowly extends
   c. Senile lentigo: pigmented flat areas usually on sun-exposed areas
3. Therapeutic management
   a. ! Instruct client to report changes in existing skin lesions: asymmetry, border, color, and diameter; these need evaluation by a health care provider

Memory Aid

Remember the alphabet—ABCD—to remember the adverse changes in skin lesions that need to be reported: asymmetry, border, color, and diameter!

   b. Teach to inspect skin routinely and seek professional advice for any noted changes
   c. ! Instruct clients to use sunscreens, hats, and protective clothing when out in sun to avoid overexposure
   d. No medication needed for lentigo
   e. Lentigo maligna: follow-up by a dermatologist is recommended

C. Seborrheic keratosis

1. Overview
   a. Benign plaques, beige to brown or even black in color, ranging in diameter from 3 to 20 mm with a velvety or warty surface
   b. Involves proliferation of immature keratinocytes and melanocytes totally within dermis; it affects mainly males 30 years and older
2. Assessment
   a. "Stuck-on" brown spots over trunk, which may bleed when irritated by clothing or picked
   b. Size varies from 1 to 3 cm
   c. May be skin-colored, tan, brown, or black and are usually oval-shaped with a warty, greasy feel
   d. Usually present on face, neck, scalp, back, and upper chest
3. Therapeutic management
   a. Sunscreens, decrease sun exposure, and avoid tanning
   b. Wear hats when outdoors
   c. ! Teach ABCD of skin lesions that indicate need for evaluation by a health care provider
   d. No medications indicated for seborrheic keratosis
   e. May be removed by electrocautery or frozen with liquid nitrogen; the area may be hypopigmented after removal

D. *Vitiligo*

1. Overview
   a. Totally white macules with an absence of melanocytes
   b. An acquired, slowly progressive depigmentation in small or large areas of skin caused by a decrease in active melanocytes

c. Type A: nondermatomal and widespread involvement in 75% of cases
d. Type B: dermatomal and segmental; 50% of cases begin between ages 10 to 30

2. Assessment
a. Loss of pigment with increased sunburning of areas; more often occurs around eyes, mouth, and anus
b. May be pruritic and associated with premature graying

3. Therapeutic management
a. Avoid sun exposure, which may increase differentiation between normal and abnormal skin
b. Skin dyes/cosmetics for blending purposes
c. Localized areas treated with midpotency steroids
d. Oral systemic steroids are effective in arresting disease progression
e. Depigmenting of normal skin with hydroquinone cream (Melanex)

XV. PRESSURE ULCERS

A. Overview

1. Ischemic lesions of skin and underlying tissue caused by external pressure that impairs flow of blood and lymph; formerly known as bedsores and decubitus ulcers
2. Pressure ulcers are a common and serious complication affecting frail, disabled, acutely ill, or immobile clients, usually in long-term care and rehabilitation settings
3. Most common sites are over bony prominences, such as elbows, hips, heels, outer ankles, and base of spine; over 95% of ulcers develop on lower part of body
4. Causes include an uneven application of pressure over a bony site: high pressure applied for 2 hours (produces irreversible tissue ischemia and necrosis), shearing forces that develop when a seated person slides toward floor or foot of bed if supine, frictional forces that develop when pulling a client across a bed sheet, and moisture from incontinence or perspiration

B. Assessment

! 1. Pressure ulcers are staged according to their characteristics; see Box 63–3
! 2. Risk factors (see Box 63–4)
3. Diagnostic and laboratory test findings: culture of wound, WBC with differential and sedimentation rate to diagnose primary or secondary infection; if no progression of ulcer, albumin levels may be obtained to determine dietary needs

C. Therapeutic management

! 1. Reposition client every 2 hours
! 2. Provide relief of pressure on wound; use support devices such as padding (gel pads), flotation pads, mattress overlays, and specialized (such as air-fluidized, oscillating, or kinetic) beds as indicated
3. Perform passive ROM and encourage active ROM exercises
! 4. Improve overall nutritional status—adequate protein intake; encourage oral high-calorie and high-protein supplements and oral zinc, vitamins A and C, and iron to aid in tissue healing
5. Clean wound each time dressing is changed to remove dead tissue, excess fluid, and debris; monitor healing and document
6. Maintain body temperature and acidic pH

Box 63–3

Pressure Ulcer Stages

Stage 1: Nonblanching erythema, warmth, and tenderness

Stage 2: Skin breakdown limited to the dermis, excoriation, blistering, drainage, more sharply defined erythema, variable skin temperature, local swelling, and edema

Stage 3: Ulcer formation into the subcutaneous tissues, crater formation, slough, eschar, and/or drainage

Stage 4: Ulcers extend beyond the deep fascia into the muscle or bone, decayed area may be larger than visibly apparent wound, osteomyelitis or sepsis may be present, granulation tissue and epithelialization may be present at wound margins

Box 63-4

Risk Factors for Pressure Ulcers

Immobility

Malnutrition and hypoalbuminemia

Low body weight

Fecal and/or urinary incontinence

Bone fracture

Vitamin C deficiency

Low diastolic blood pressure

Age-related skin changes such as diminished pain perception, thinning of epidermis, loss of dermal vessels, and altered barrier properties

Reduced immunity and slowed wound healing

Anemia

Infections

Peripheral vascular insufficiency

Dementia

Malignancies

Diabetes

CVA

Dry skin

Edema

7. Never use antiseptics and harsh skin cleansers that may harm tissue; provide gentle but thorough skin care and avoid drying
8. Avoid agents that delay wound healing such as topical corticosteroids, hydrogen peroxide, iodine, and hypochlorite
9. Control fecal and urine incontinence
10. Avoid massage over bony prominences
11. Use moisture barrier
12. ! Assess site every 8 to 12 hours; carefully document healing (e.g., state there is a "healing stage III ulcer" rather than "stage II ulcer" if ulcer was stage III and exhibits healing)
13. Use absorption dressing if wound has large amounts of exudate, and change frequently

D. Medication therapy

1. Clindamycin (Cleocin) or gentamycin (Garamycin) may be ordered for complications such as cellulitis, osteomyelitis, or sepsis
2. Vitamin C 500 mg twice daily and zinc sulfate supplements aid healing
3. Antibiotic prophylaxis will eradicate bacterial component
4. A 2-week trial of topical antimicrobials should be used only for a clean, superficial ulcer that is either not healing or is producing a moderate amount of exudates—cultures are necessary to determine whether antifungal or specific antibacterial agents are indicated
5. ! Enzymatic debriding agents such as collagenase (Santyl, Granulex), fibinolysin-desoxyribonuclease (Elase), papin (Panafil), or sutilains (Travase) are used with a moisture barrier to protect surrounding tissue
6. ! Recommended dressings include polyurethane films (Op-Site™, Tegaderm™), absorbent hydrocolloid dressings (Duoderm™)

E. Client education

1. Need for frequent evaluation of all clients with a history of pressure sores, especially if they have limited mobility
2. Nutritional requirements and meal planning

3. Early identification of skin redness to prevent breakdowns
4. Skin cleansing routine
5. Underpads to absorb moisture
6. Repositioning techniques and frequency
7. Need to evaluate and ensure continence and facilities
8. Use of mattress overlays, seat cushions or special mattresses
9. Ways to avoid injuries

XVI. BURN INJURY

A. Overview

1. An alteration in skin integrity resulting in tissue loss or injury caused by heat, chemicals, electricity, or radiation
2. ! There are several types of burn injury: thermal, chemical, electrical, and radiation
   a. Thermal burn: results from dry heat (flames) or moist heat (steam or hot liquids); is most common type; causes cellular destruction that results in vascular, bony, muscle, or nerve complications; thermal burns can also lead to inhalation injury if head and neck area is affected
   b. Chemical burn: caused by direct contact with either acidic or alkaline agents; alters tissue perfusion and leads to necrosis
   c. Electrical burn: severity depends on type and duration of current and amount of voltage; electricity follows path of least resistance (muscles, bone, blood vessels, and nerves); sources of electrical injury include direct current, alternating current, and lightning
   d. Radiation burn: usually associated with sunburn or radiation treatment for cancer; usually superficial; extensive exposure to radiation may lead to tissue damage and multisystem injury

B. Emergent/resuscitative stage: lasts from onset of injury through successful fluid resuscitation; during stage, it is determined whether client is to be transported to a burn center for complex intervention depending on onset of injury, identification of burn source, and complicating factors

1. ! Classification of burn depth: done according to depth of damaged tissue (Table 63–1 ■)
2. ! An estimate of burn size is calculated using Rule of Nines (see Figure 63–3 ■) or Lund and Browder method; each chart accounts for 100% of total body surface area (TBSA), although Lund and Browder method takes into account client's age when estimating body surface area
3. Severity of burn is classified using American Burn Association criteria as minor burn, moderate uncomplicated burn, and major burn; these categories help determine treatment

Table 63–1

Classification of Burn Injury by Depth of Burn

Superficial thickness (formerly first-degree)	Involves the epidermis only and is recognized by characteristics of erythema, absence of blisters for 24 hours, local pain; healing occurs spontaneously in 3 to 5 days with no scar formation
Superficial partial-thickness (formerly second-degree)	Involves the epidermis and dermis, characterized by moist areas that are red to ivory white in color, blisters form immediately; area is painful because touch and pain receptors are intact; area heals with greater or lesser amounts of scarring within 21 to 28 days
Deep partial thickness (formerly second-degree)	Involves possibly the entire layer of the dermis and is more severe than a superficial partial-thickness burn; skin appendages are left intact; area has a dry, waxy, whitish appearance and may be difficult to differentiate initially from full-thickness burns; may heal spontaneously in about 1 month, although skin grafting is often done to close the wound, accelerate healing, reduce scarring, and reduce risk of infection
Full-thickness (formerly third- or fourth-degree)	Involves destruction of all skin elements with coagulation of subdermal plexus; muscle and tendons may be involved

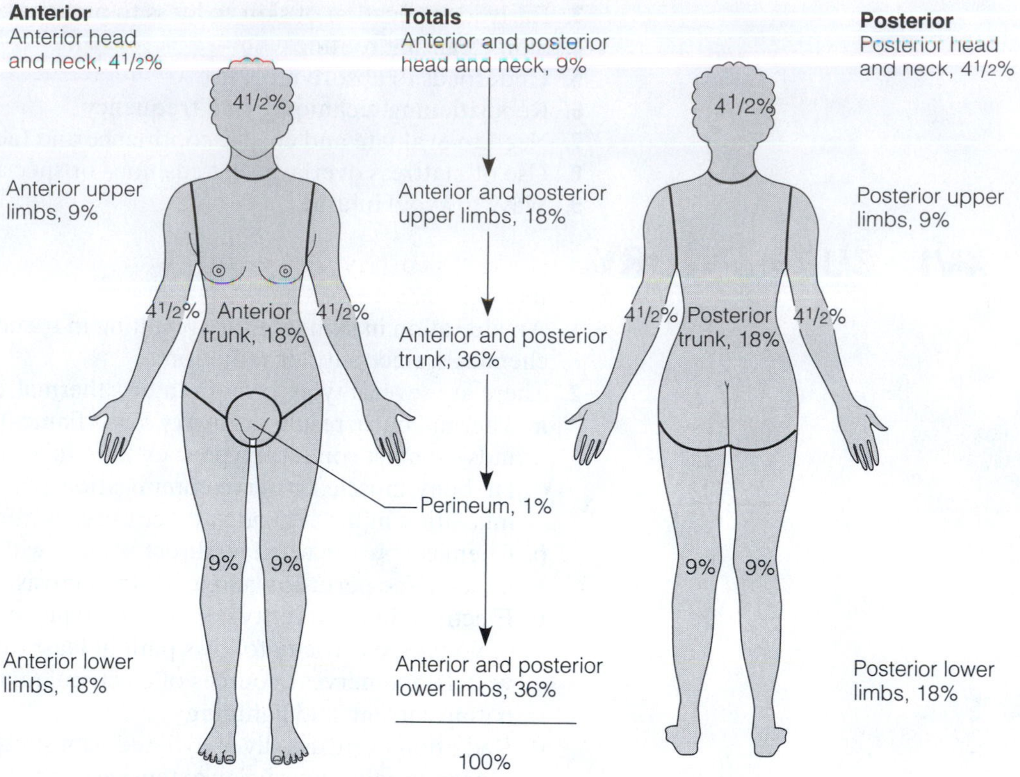

Figure 63–3

Calculating burn injury using the Rule of Nines.

Source: LeMone, P., & Burke, K. (2003). Medical surgical nursing: Critical thinking for client care (3rd ed.). Upper Saddle River, NJ: Pearson Education, p. 415.

a. Hands, feet, face, and perineal area burns have higher potential for functional impairment

b. Circumferential burns (those surrounding an extremity or trunk) are considered major burns

4. Nursing assessment: history of injury, estimate burn extent and depth, obtain past medical history and medication history including date of last tetanus prophylaxis; assess for other concurrent injuries

5. Systemic effects of severe burns include asphyxia from smoke inhalation that causes edema of respiratory passages; shock from fluid shifts; renal failure from shock; protein loss from open wound; potassium excess from tissue destruction and renal failure

6. Diagnostic and laboratory test findings: may have elevated hematocrit (Hct) and decreased hemoglobin (Hgb) caused by fluid shift, decreased sodium (Na^+) and increased potassium (K^+) caused by damage to capillary and cell membranes, elevated BUN and creatinine caused by dehydration, myoglobin in urine, and possible deterioration of arterial blood gases (ABGs) and oxygen (O_2) saturation readings depending on respiratory status

7. Therapeutic management

a. First aid: douse flames with water or smother them with a blanket, coat, or other similar object; cool a scald burn with cool water; flush chemical burns copiously with water or other appropriate irrigant after dusting away any dry powder if present; remove client from contact with an electrical source only after current has been shut off

b. Priority care is on ABCs: airway, breathing, and circulation; assess for smoke inhalation injury (singed nares, eyebrows or lashes; burns on face or neck; stridor, increasing dyspnea) and give O_2 (up to 100% as prescribed), being prepared for possible intubation and mechanical ventilation if severe inhalation injury or carbon monoxide inhalation has occurred; assess for signs of shock caused by fluid shifts (increased pulse, falling BP and urine output, pallor, cool clammy skin, deteriorating level of consciousness [LOC])

c. Fluid resuscitation: Brooke formula uses 2 mL/kg/% TBSA burned (3/4 crystalloid plus 1/4 colloid) plus maintenance fluid of 2,000 mL D_5W per

24 hours; Parkland (Baxter) formula uses 4 mL/kg/% TBSA burned per 24 hours (crystalloid only—lactated Ringer's); both formulas give half of 24-hour total in first 8 hours and second half over next 16 hours

d. Other considerations: remove all rings and jewelry to avoid tourniquet effect caused by swelling of burn site; provide cardiac monitoring for first 24 hours after an electrical burn

8. Medication therapy: analgesics—usually morphine sulfate IV, tetanus booster (> 5–10 years since last dose), topical antimicrobials, systemic antibiotics
9. Client education: focuses in this phase on brief explanations about injury, treatments, and ongoing nursing care

C. Acute phase of burn management: begins with start of diuresis (usually 48 to 72 hours postburn) and ends with closure of burn wound

1. Assessment: varies depending on cause, depth, and TBSA of burn; associated symptoms arising from other organ systems may include nausea and vomiting, pain, skin redness, chills, respiratory distress, and hypovolemia
2. Therapeutic management
   - **a.** Wound care management includes debridement, dressing changes, hydrotherapy, and possible escharotomy,
   - **b.** Mafenide (Sulfamylon) may be applied in thin layer over open wound and covered with dressing
   - **c.** Sulfadiazine (Silvadene) may applied in thin layer over open wound and covered with dressing; use with caution when impaired renal function exists; must be washed off and reapplied every 8 to 12 hours
   - **d.** Skin grafting may need to be done to achieve healing in full-thickness and large, deep partial-thickness burns
   - **e.** Nutritional therapies (high-calorie, high-protein diet with vitamins and minerals) and continue to maintain hydration status
   - **f.** Infection control with strict sterile technqiue
   - **g.** Maintain heated environment to prevent chilling
   - **h.** Phsyical therapy as needed
   - **i.** Psychosocial support
3. Medication therapy: topical and/or systemic antibiotic therapy; pain control with opioid analgesics is usually required; premedicate with analgesic 30 minutes prior to wound care

D. Rehabilitative phase of burn management: begins with wound closure and ends when client returns to highest level of health restoration

1. Assessment: depends on cause, TBSA affected, and depth; may have immobility or restriction of mobility of affected area; scarring is possible
2. Therapeutic management
   - **a.** Obtain psychosocial evaluation; provide support and management; arrange counseling if necessary
   - **b.** Prevent immobility contractures with exercises or ongoing physical therapy
   - **c.** Assist in returning to work, family, and social life
   - **d.** Use preventative measures for scar formation (such as burn garments)
   - **e.** Assess home environment for needs and accessibility
3. Medication therapy: ongoing pain management and antibiotic therapy as necessary
4. Client education
   - **a.** Environmental safety: use low temperature setting for hot water heater, ensure access to and adequate number of electrical cords/outlets, isolate household chemicals, avoid smoking in bed
   - **b.** Use of household smoke detectors with emphasis on maintenance
   - **c.** Proper storage and use of flammable substances
   - **d.** Evacuation plan for family
   - **e.** Care of burn at home
   - **f.** Signs and symptoms of infection
   - **g.** How to identify risk of skin changes
   - **h.** Use of sunscreen to protect healing tissue and other protective skin care measures soft tissue injuries; or deep chemical or electrical burns

Check Your NCLEX-RN® Exam I.Q.

You are ready for testing on this content if you can

- Identify basic structures and functions of the integumentary system.
- Describe the pathophysiology and etiology of common integumentary disorders.
- Discuss expected assessment data and diagnostic test findings for selected integumentary disorders.
- Discuss therapeutic management of a client experiencing an integumentary disorder.
- Discuss nursing management of a client experiencing an integumentary disorder.
- Identify expected outcomes for the client experiencing an integumentarydisorder.

PRACTICE TEST

1 A nurse is teaching a group of young adults about skin lesions. Which of the following would be inappropriate to include in discussions with these clients?

1. The benefits of suntanning
2. Importance of monthly skin self-inspections
3. Evaluation of skin lesions using the ABCD method
4. Need for seeking professional advice regarding lesions

2 A client with psoriasis receives a prescription from the primary physician. The nurse concludes that the client is not receiving first-line therapy after noting that the presciption is written for which of the following?

1. An emollient
2. Coal tar application
3. Topical corticosteroid
4. Methotrexate

3 The nurse practitioner documents in a client record that a client has closed comedones. The nurse explains to the client that this means the lesions are what type of skin eruption?

1. Whiteheads
2. Blackheads
3. Pustules
4. Cysts

4 The nurse evaluates that a client understands the therapeutic management of seborrheic keratosis if he mentions which of the following?

1. Antibiotics
2. Antifungal creams
3. Liquid nitrogen
4. Corticosteroids

5 A client with contact dermatitis asks the nurse how he could have developed the condition. The nurse includes in a response that contact dermatitis is caused by which of the following?

1. Allergic reaction mediated by IgE
2. Poor hygiene
3. Reactivation of IgA antibodies
4. Side effect of oral medication

6 When explaining the disorder to a client with tinea corporis, the nurse should include which of the following about this skin disorder?

1. It requires no treatment.
2. It can be passed human to human.
3. It should be exposed to sunlight.
4. It is a malignant skin condition.

7 A client asks the nurse about the meaning of the term "full-thickness burn." The nurse should respond that burns classified as full-thickness involve tissue destruction down to which of the following levels?

1. Epidermis
2. Subcutaneous tissue
3. Bone
4. Dermis

8 The client comes to the office for evaluation of a skin rash. What question would be included in obtaining a history?

1. "Have you ever had a skin rash like this before?"
2. "Do you smoke?"
3. "How long have you had that mole on your left arm?"
4. "Do you have a family history of skin cancer?"

9 The nurse is assessing the client's skin and wants to evaluate a site for petechiae. What technique can the nurse perform to help identify whether the site has petechiae?

1. Rub the site and watch for bleeding.
2. Apply pressure to the site to evaluate for blanching of the skin.
3. Look for other lesions that are similar to that lesion.
4. Apply a tourniquet in a limb and watch for the development of petechiae.

10 A client has been diagnosed with eczema. Which of the following statements made by the client indicates an understanding of the management of eczema?

1. "I will avoid excessive use of soap and water and keep my skin well-hydrated with emollients such as Eucerin."
2. "I will take daily baths and use strong antibacterial soaps to prevent skin infections."
3. "I will make sure to expose my skin to the sun at least 1 hour a day."
4. "I will wait 3 hours after bathing to apply lotion to my skin."

11 The client diagnosed with psoriasis has been prescribed an antihistamine. The client asks the nurse what this is used for because she does not have nasal allergies and congestion. What is the most appropriate response?

1. "Antihistamines are not used for psoriasis and should not have been prescribed."
2. "The insert on the package will tell you what the medication is for."
3. "Let me ask the doctor because I'm not really sure."
4. "Antihistamines are used to help relieve itching associated with the lesions."

12 Instructions for a client diagnosed with seborrheic dermatitis would include which of the following?

1. "Use any brand of shampoo because it does not make a difference in scalp therapy."
2. "Coal tar shampoos are recommended for seborrheic dermatitis of the scalp."
3. "Medicated shampoos are recommended because if not treated successfully, seborrheic dermatitis can cause permanent hair loss."
4. "Daily use of coal tar shampoos will cure seborrheic dermatitis."

13 In teaching clients about measures to reduce the risk of developing basal cell carcinoma, the nurse should include which of the following?

1. Limiting the use of tanning beds
2. Using sunscreen with protection SPF of 15 or greater when exposed to the sun
3. Only exposing the skin to the sun for 3 to 4 hours per day
4. The role of diet in prevention of skin cancer

14 The client with cellulitis is being discharged from the hospital. Discharge instructions for the client should include which of the following statements?

1. "If pustules develop, squeeze the lesion to remove the pus."
2. "If the lesion looks healed, stop taking the antibiotics so that you will not develop resistance to antibiotics."
3. "Monitor for signs of infection such as fever, chills, malaise, and redness or tenderness at the site."
4. "Drainage from the site is an expected finding and is no cause for concern."

15 Which of the following is a priority nursing diagnosis for a client experiencing the skin infection cellulitis?

1. Sleep pattern disturbance related to skin infection
2. Social isolation related to skin infection
3. Powerlessness related to inability to control the infection
4. Pain related to skin infection of cellulitis

16 The client receives a prescription to treat a skin infection affecting the scalp and neck. The medications prescribed are coal tar shampoo and topical steroids. The nurse concludes that which of the following is the probable diagnosis of this client?

1. Folliculitis
2. Cellulitis
3. Psoriasis
4. Furuncles

17 A client has just been diagnosed with herpes virus type 2. The nurse should share with the client which of the following pieces of information?

1. "The initial outbreak of herpes is usually the most uncomfortable. Recurrent infections usually present with a prodrome of tingling and burning sensation prior to the outbreak of the vesicle."
2. "Each outbreak of herpes is uncomfortable, with the amount of pain at the genital area worsening each time."
3. "You can only have one outbreak of herpes, so you will never experience another."
4. "You should never experience discomfort with herpes; therefore, if you have pain in the genital area, you probably have a sexually transmitted infection."

18 A client presents for removal of a skin lesion after it is determined that he meets all four criteria for removal according to the ABCD rule. The nurse interprets this to mean which of the following?

1. The lesion is symmetrical, with a smooth border, a single color, and the diameter has stayed the same.
2. The lesion is symmetrical with an irregular border, a single color, and the diameter has increased.
3. The lesion is asymmetrical with a regular border, two colors, and the diameter is smaller.
4. The lesion is asymmetrical with an irregular border, two colors, and has increased in diameter.

19 The nurse performing a skin examination of a client notes the client has vascular skin lesions that are flat, bright red in color, with tiny vessels that radiate out from the center of the lesion. The nurse concludes that the lesions are probably which of the following?

1. Petechiae
2. Spider angiomas
3. Venous stars
4. Port wine stains

20 A client presents on admission with pressure ulcers extending into the bone. The nurse documents this ulcer at what stage? Provide a numerical answer.

Answer: ____________________

21 A child was admitted to the emergency department with a thermal burn to the right arm and leg. Which of the following assessments requires immediate action?

1. Coughing and wheezing
2. Bright red skin with small blisters on the burn sites
3. Thirst
4. Singed hair

22 A school-aged child develops eczema secondary to food allergies. An appropriate nursing diagnosis for this child would be which of the following?

1. Imbalanced nutrition: less than body requirements
2. Disturbed body image
3. Risk for ineffective thermoregulation
4. Impaired tissue perfusion

23 An infant has a positive family history of allergies. To reduce the risk of the infant developing eczema, the nurse teaches the family to

1. Avoid synthetic clothing—use natural fibers like cotton and wool.
2. Keep up with the schedule of childhood immunizations.
3. Avoid contact with infected personnel.
4. Introduce only one new food a week so food allergies can be recognized and eliminated.

24 The parents of an 18-month-old with eczema are concerned that a secondary infection that has developed will permanently disfigure their child. How can the nurse best support the parents' feelings?

1. Divert the conversation to another topic.
2. Let them know that they are not being blamed for their feelings.
3. Encourage them to discuss their fears and concerns.
4. Tell them not to worry because scarring is unlikely with eczema.

25 The child has just been admitted to the pediatric burn unit. Currently, the child is being evaluated for burns to his chest and upper legs. He complains of thirst and asks for a drink. What is the most appropriate nursing action?

1. Give a small glass of a clear liquid.
2. Give a small glass of a full liquid.
3. Keep the child NPO.
4. Order a pediatric meal tray with extra liquids.

ANSWERS & RATIONALES

1 **Answer: 1** Tanning and sun exposure can increase susceptibility to skin cancers. This is a potentially harmful activity and should not be included in client teaching. The other items are important to discuss with clients who are trying to maintain healthy skin.
Cognitive Level: Application **Client Need:** Health Promotion and Maintenance **Integrated Process:** Nursing Process: Planning **Content Area:** Adult Health: Integumentary **Strategy:** The wording of the question tells you that the correct response is a false statement of fact. Use the process of elimination and nursing knowledge to make a selection.

2 **Answer: 4** Methotrexate is used for severe and nonresponsive cases of psoriasis. It is not a first-line form of therapy. Options 1, 2, and 3 are first-line treatments for psoriasis.
Cognitive Level: Application **Client Need:** Physiological Integrity: Physiological Adaptation **Integrated Process:** Nursing Process: Analysis **Content Area:** Adult Health: Integumentary **Strategy:** The core issue of the question is knowledge of the sequence of treatments for psoriasis. The wording of the question tells you that the correct response is also a true statement of fact. Use the process of elimination and nursing knowledge to make a selection.

3 **Answer: 1** Whiteheads are classified as closed comedones. Blackheads are open comedones. Options 3 and 4 are irrelevant.
Cognitive Level: Application **Client Need:** Physiological Integrity: Physiological Adaptation **Integrated Process:** Nursing Process: Assessment **Content Area:** Adult Health: Integumentary **Strategy:** The core issue of the question is knowledge of various skin eruptions. The wording of the question tells you that the correct response is also a true statement of fact. Use the process of elimination and nursing knowledge to make a selection.

4 **Answer: 3** No medication is indicated for seborrheic keratosis (options 1, 2, and 3). These lesions may be treated with electrocautery or liquid nitrogen for removal.
Cognitive Level: Application **Client Need:** Physiological Integrity: Physiological Adaptation **Integrated Process:** Nursing Process: Evaluation **Content Area:** Adult Health: Integumentary **Strategy:** The core issue of the question is knowledge of treatments for seborrheic keratosis. The wording of the question tells you that the correct response is also a true statement of fact. Use the process of elimination and nursing knowledge to make a selection.

5 **Answer: 1** Contact dermatitis is an inflammatory response following prior sensitization to an antigen with production of a specific IgE antibody. Skin manifestations occur with subsequent exposures. The other options are false.
Cognitive Level: Application **Client Need:** Physiological Integrity: Physiological Adaptation **Integrated Process:** Nursing Process: Assessment **Content Area:** Adult Health: Integumentary **Strategy:** The core issue of the question is the ability to correctly describe contact dermatitis. The wording of the question tells you the correct answer is also a true statement. Use the process of elimination and nursing knowledge to make a selection.

6 **Answer: 2** Fungal infections such as tinea corporis may be transmitted by direct contact with animals and other persons. Therefore, it is contagious from person to person. It does require treatment, is not malignant, and is not treatable by sunlight.
Cognitive Level: Application **Client Need:** Physiological Integrity: Physiological Adaptation **Integrated Process:** Nursing Process: Implementation **Content Area:** Adult Health: Integumentary **Strategy:** The core issue of the question is knowledge of the characteristics of infection with tinea corporis. The wording of the question tells you the correct statement is the correct answer. Use the process of elimination and nursing knowledge to make a selection.

7 **Answer: 2** A full-thickness burn involves all layers, including the epidermis and dermis, and may extend into the subcutaneous tissue and fat. The other options indicate varying depths of burn injury.
Cognitive Level: Application **Client Need:** Physiological Integrity: Physiological Adaptation **Integrated Process:** Nursing Process: Implementation **Content Area:** Adult Health: Integumentary **Strategy:** The core issue of the question is knowledge of the various depths of burn injury. The wording of the question tells you the correct statement is the correct answer. Use the process of elimination and nursing knowledge to make a selection.

8 **Answer: 1** The most important question for this office visit for evaluation of a skin rash would be to get information about the chief complaint. In this case, it would be to investigate additional information about the presenting rash. The other options are either unrelated or could be asked at a later time.
Cognitive Level: Application **Client Need:** Physiological Integrity: Physiological Adaptation **Integrated Process:** Nursing Process: Assessment **Content Area:** Adult Health: Integumentary **Strategy:** The issue of the question is appropriate questions to ask when obtaining a nursing history about a skin disorder. The wording of the question tells you the correct statement is the correct answer. Use the process of elimination and knowledge of health assessment to make a selection.

9 **Answer: 2** When assessing petechiae, pressure applied to the site will not produce blanching of the skin. For other lesions, blanching may occur. Options 1, 3, and 4 are false.

Cognitive Level: Application **Client Need:** Physiological Integrity: Physiological Adaptation **Integrated Process:** Nursing Process: Assessment **Content Area:** Adult Health: Integumentary **Strategy:** The issue of the question is knowledge of nursing assessment techniques for the skin. The wording of the question tells you the correct statement is the correct answer. Use the process of elimination and nursing knowledge to make a selection.

10 **Answer: 1** Skin care for eczema should include keeping the skin well hydrated and avoiding harsh soaps (option 2). This can be done by using mild bath soaps and applying emollients immediately after bathing (option 4). Option 3 is false. **Cognitive Level:** Application **Client Need:** Physiological Integrity: Physiological Adaptation **Integrated Process:** Nursing Process: Evaluation **Content Area:** Adult Health: Integumentary **Strategy:** The core issue of the question is knowledge of appropriate care to the skin when the client has eczema. The wording of the question tells you the correct statement is the correct answer. Use the process of elimination and nursing knowledge to make a selection.

11 **Answer: 4** Antihistimines are useful to help relieve itching. The other options do not explain the rationale for the use of this type of medication with psoriasis. **Cognitive Level:** Application **Client Need:** Physiological Integrity: Physiological Adaptation **Integrated Process:** Nursing Process: Implementation **Content Area:** Adult Health: Integumentary **Strategy:** An understanding of the nature of the condition and the client's symptoms are needed to make the correct response. The wording of the question tells you the correct statement is the correct answer. Use the process of elimination and nursing knowledge to make a selection.

12 **Answer: 2** Coal tar shampoos are recommended for seborrheic dermatitis of the scalp. Over-the-counter shampoos may not control symptoms. Seborrheic dermatitis cannot be cured. Symptoms can be controlled with proper treatment. **Cognitive Level:** Application **Client Need:** Physiological Integrity: Physiological Adaptation **Integrated Process:** Nursing Process: Implementation **Content Area:** Adult Health: Integumentary **Strategy:** The core issue of the question is knowledge of care and treatment for seborrheic dermatitis. The wording of the question tells you the correct statement is the correct answer. Use the process of elimination and nursing knowledge to make a selection.

13 **Answer: 2** The most common form of skin cancer is basal cell carcinoma, with approximately 400,000 new cases per year. Protecting the skin with sunscreen SPF 15 or higher, along with avoiding the sun during the peak hours of 10:00 a.m. to 2:00 p.m., is recommended to help prevent skin cancer. **Cognitive Level:** Application **Client Need:** Health Promotion and Maintenance **Integrated Process:** Nursing Process: Implementation **Content Area:** Adult Health: Integumentary **Strategy:** The core issue of the question is knowledge of behaviors that can reduce the risk of developing basal cell carcinoma. The wording of the question tells you the correct statement is the correct answer. Use the process of elimination and nursing knowledge to make a selection.

14 **Answer: 3** Infection may be manifested by fever, chills, erythema, tenderness, and drainage at the site, especially if it is cloudy or serous. The physician must be notified if these symptoms occur. **Cognitive Level:** Application **Client Need:** Physiological Integrity: Physiological Adaptation **Integrated Process:** Nursing Process: Implementation **Content Area:** Adult Health: Integumentary **Strategy:** The core issue of the question is the risk of infection and the need to notify the health care provider if signs of infection occur. The wording of the question tells you the correct statement is the correct answer. Use the process of elimination and nursing knowledge to make a selection.

15 **Answer: 4** Clients with cellulitis experience pain at the local site. Controlling the pain is the priority nursing diagnosis for this client. Option 1 may not apply unless the client is in pain. Options 2 and 3 may or may not apply, but would have lower priority than the physiological need (option 4). **Cognitive Level:** Analysis **Client Need:** Physiological Integrity: Physiological Adaptation **Integrated Process:** Nursing Process: Analysis **Content Area:** Adult Health: Integumentary **Strategy:** Recall that pain relief is high priority for many clients and is included in the physiological needs on Maslow's hierarchy. Use the process of elimination and nursing knowledge to make a selection, considering that physiological needs take priority over psychosocial needs in most cases.

16 **Answer: 3** Current treatments for psoriasis include coal tar shampoo and topical steroids. Folliculitis, cellulitis, and furuncles are bacterial infections of the skin and would be treated with antimicrobial therapy. **Cognitive Level:** Analysis **Client Need:** Physiological Integrity: Physiological Adaptation **Integrated Process:** Nursing Process: Analysis **Content Area:** Adult Health: Integumentary **Strategy:** The core issue of the question is knowledge of the uses of medication therapy for psoriasis. The wording of the question tells you the correct statement is the correct answer. Use the process of elimination and nursing knowledge to make a selection.

17 **Answer: 1** The initial outbreak of herpes is the most uncomfortable or painful. Recurrent episodes of herpes infection present with a prodome of symptoms, such as tingling and burning. Herpes is a virus that may lie dormant for periods of time, and repeated episodes may occur during periods of stress. **Cognitive Level:** Application **Client Need:** Physiological Integrity: Physiological Adaptation **Integrated Process:** Nursing Process: Implementation; **Content Area:** Adult Health: Integumentary **Strategy:** The core issue of the question is knowledge of the characteristics and presentation of this type of viral infection. The wording of the question tells you the correct statement is the correct answer. Recall that the first outbreak is the most severe to make a selection.

18 **Answer: 4** To meet all four criteria for removal of a lesion, the lesion will be asymmetrical (A) with an irregular border (B), have color change or more than one color (C), along with an increased diameter (D). **Cognitive Level:** Application **Client Need:** Physiological Integrity: Physiological Adaptation **Integrated Process:** Nursing Process: Assessment **Content Area:** Adult Health: Integumentary **Strategy:** The core issue of the question is knowledge of criteria that determine the need to remove a skin lesion. The

wording of the question tells you the correct statement is the correct answer. Use the process of elimination and nursing knowledge to make a selection.

19 **Answer: 2** Spider angiomas are red lesions with vessels radiating from the center. A venous star is a flat blue lesion with radiating linear veins. Petechiae appear as red "freckles" or dots. A port wine stain is a flat, irregular-shaped lesion that does not have radiating vessels.
Cognitive Level: Application **Client Need:** Physiological Integrity: Physiological Adaptation **Integrated Process:** Nursing Process: Assessment **Content Area:** Adult Health: Integumentary **Strategy:** The core issue of the question is knowledge of various types of skin lesions. The wording of the question tells you the correct statement is the correct answer. Use the process of elimination and nursing knowledge to make a selection.

20 **Answer: 4** Stage 4 ulcers result in full thickness skin loss with extensive damage to the muscle and bone.
Cognitive Level: Application **Client Need:** Physiological Integrity: Physiological Adaptation **Integrated Process:** Communication and Documentation **Content Area:** Adult Health: Integumentary **Strategy:** The core issue of the question is knowledge of various stages of ulcer development. The wording of the question guides you to a decision. Use nursing knowledge to make a selection.

21 **Answer: 1** Coughing and wheezing may indicate that the child has inhaled smoke or toxic fumes. Maintaining airway patency is the highest nursing priority in this situation. Skin color changes are expected. Thirst may be present but does not require immediate nursing action.
Cognitive Level: Analysis **Client Need:** Physiological Integrity: Physiological Adaptation **Integrated Process:** Nursing Process: Analysis **Content Area:** Child Health: Integumentary **Strategy:** The core issue of the question is the ability to determine that the client's airway could be in jeopardy. Use the ABCs whenever a question deals with burn injury as a first method to determine priority setting.

22 **Answer: 2** Eczema is a chronic inflammatory skin disorder. School-aged children are very aware of their own and others' skin appearance. Children with eczema will feel different from other children, and this may affect their body image. Food allergies do not relate to decreased nutrition. Eczema does not affect the skin's ability to maintain temperature, and it does not affect blood flow to the area.
Cognitive Level: Analysis **Client Need:** Psychosocial Integrity **Integrated Process:** Nursing Process: Analysis **Content Area:** Child Health: Integumentary **Strategy:** The core issue of the question is recognition of key concerns of a child with eczema. The wording of the question tells you the correct statement is the correct answer. Use the process of elimination and nursing knowledge to make a selection.

23 **Answer: 4** Infants with eczema frequently have food sensitivities. Slow introduction of new foods allows the parents to recognize food sensitivities and eliminate the offending item from the diet. The mother is taught to avoid scratchy clothing such as wool. Childhood immunizations would be given as scheduled but do not reduce risk. Eczema is not an infectious disease. Avoiding infectious personnel is appropriate for all children but does not prevent the development of eczema.
Cognitive Level: Application **Client Need:** Physiological Integrity: Physiological Adaptation **Integrated Process:** Nursing Process: Implementation **Content Area:** Child Health: Integumentary **Strategy:** The core issue of the question is appropriate client teaching to reduce risk of developing eczema. Recall the risk factors and use the process of elimination to make a selection.

24 **Answer: 3** The nurse should encourage parents to identify and discuss their feelings and concerns. Changing the topic or giving false reassurance is inappropriate. Merely not blaming parents does not give them the opportunity to discuss what is important to them.
Cognitive Level: Application **Client Need:** Psychosocial Integrity **Integrated Process:** Communication and Documentation **Content Area:** Child Health: Integumentary **Strategy:** The core issue of the question is the ability to use basic communication techniques in responding to the concerns of a parent. Choose the option that directly addresses the client's or family's issues and concerns.

25 **Answer: 3** Until a complete assessment and treatment plan are initiated, the child should be kept NPO. A complication of major burns is paralytic ileus, so until that has been ruled out, oral fluids should not be provided.
Cognitive Level: Analysis **Client Need:** Physiological Integrity: Physiological Adaptation **Integrated Process:** Nursing Process: Analysis **Content Area:** Child Health: Integumentary **Strategy:** The core issue of the question is the need to avoid fluid intake during the acute phase of burn injury when hemodynamics could be unstable. Use nursing knowledge to recall that fluid resuscitation needs to be done parenterally.

Key Terms to Review

acne p. 1279
actinic keratosis p. 1268
atopic dermatitis p. 1266
candidiasis p. 1273
cellulitis p. 1271
contact dermatitis p. 1278
dermis p. 1262
epidermis p. 1262
erythema p. 1265
lichenification p. 1266
macule p. 1265
nodule p. 1265
papule p. 1265
pediculosis capitus p. 1276
plaque p. 1265
pressure ulcers p. 1281
pruritus p. 1266
pustule p. 1265
scabies p. 1277
urticaria p. 1278
vesicle p. 1265
vitiligo p. 1280
wheal p. 1265

References

Ball, J., & Bindler, R. (2006). *Child health nursing: Partnering with children and families.* Upper Saddle River, NJ: Pearson Education.

Black, J., & Hawks, J. (2005). *Medical surgical nursing: Clinical management for positive outcomes* (7th ed.). St. Louis: Elsevier Science.

Corbett, J. (2004). *Laboratory tests and diagnostic procedures with nursing diagnoses* (6th ed.). Upper Saddle River, NJ: Pearson Education.

Harkreader, H., & Hogan, M. (2004). *Fundamentals of nursing: Caring and clinical judgment* (2nd ed.). St. Louis: Elsevier Science.

Ignatavicius, D., & Workman, L. (2006). *Medical-surgical nursing: Critical thinking for collaborative care* (5th ed.). Philadelphia: W. B. Saunders.

Kozier, B., Erb, G., Berman, A., & Snyder, S. (2004). *Fundamentals of nursing: Concepts, process, and practice* (7th ed.). Upper Saddle River, NJ: Pearson Education.

LeMone, P., & Burke, K. (2004). *Medical surgical nursing: Critical thinking in client care* (3rd ed.). Upper Saddle River, NJ: Pearson Education.

Porth, C. (2004). *Pathophysiology: Concepts of altered health states* (7th ed.). Philadelphia: Lippincott Williams & Wilkins.

Smith, S., Duell, D., & Martin, B. (2004). *Clinical nursing skills: Basic to advanced skills* (6th ed.). Upper Saddle River, NJ: Pearson Education.

Eye, Ear, Nose and Throat Disorders

64

In this chapter

Cross reference

Other chapters relevant to this content area are

Eye and Ear Medications	Chapter 44
Common Laboratory Tests	Chapter 47
Common Diagnostic Tests and Procedures	Chapter 48

Test Yourself

Are you ready for the NCLEX-RN® or course exams? Use the practice tests on the companion CD-ROM to check.

I. OVERVIEW OF ANATOMY AND PHYSIOLOGY OF THE EYE AND EAR

A. Eye structures

1. Outer protective layer, also called fibrous coat; consists of sclera and cornea
2. Middle vascular layer, also called uveal tract; contains pigmented iris surrounding pupil, which regulates amount of light entering eye, and ciliary body that surrounds lens and produces aqueous humor to maintain intraocular pressure (IOP) (flows from posterior to anterior chamber and drains into Schlemm's canal); also contains choroid that has blood vessels to supply eye tissues
3. Inner layer, the retina: thin, semitransparent layer containing rods and cones, responsible for vision in dim light and for perception of fine details, respectively

B. Eye functions

1. Eye receives light waves through cornea; waves are refracted by aqueous humor, lens, and vitreous humor as they are transmitted to retina; retinal images formed by light rays are inverted and reversed by biconvex lens
2. Rods and cones of retina translate light waves into neural impulses for relay to optic nerve and then to brain's occipital lobes for interpretation as vision
3. Fusion of images in brain from each eye into a single image is called binocular vision

! **C. Age-related changes of eye that affect vision**

1. Decreased ability of pupil to dilate, which reduces night vision and increases light needed for reading and small motor tasks, such as sewing
2. Development of **presbyopia,** a decreased elasticity of lens that makes focusing for near vision more difficult and results in farsightedness
3. Lens becomes discolored and opacified, which reduces color perception (especially green, blue, and violet)
4. Decreased eye motility and senile enophthalmos (sinking in) of eyes limits peripheral vision upward, downward, and to sides
5. Degenerative changes to choroid, retina, and optic nerve reduce depth perception and ability to see lines of demarcation (stair edges, doorframes)

D. Ear structures

1. External ear: outer visible ear or auricle and external auditory canal
2. Middle ear: tympanic membrane; malleus, incus, and stapes bones; and window membranes
3. Inner ear: semicircular canals, cochlea, distal portion of cranial nerve VIII (vestibulocochlear nerve)

E. Ear functions

1. Hearing: sound is transferred from tympanic membrane to malleus, incus, and stapes and through cochlea; vibrations are changed by transduction into action potentials that are sent to brain as neural impulses
2. **Proprioception** (balance): sensation about body's position in space is transferred to brain after changes in body position trigger fluid movement and bending of hair cells in vestibular structures

F. Age-related changes of ear that affect hearing

1. External auditory canal narrows; cerumen glands atrophy and produce thicker, drier cerumen
2. Tympanic membrane is less flexible, and ossicle joints calcify
3. Cochlear hair cell degeneration and loss of auditory neurons in organ of Corti lead to **presbycusis,** an age-related sensorineural hearing loss characterized by decreased ability to hear high-frequency sounds; results in difficulty hearing and localizing normal speech

II. DIAGNOSTIC TESTS AND ASSESSMENTS OF THE EYE AND EAR

A. Fluorescein angiography: injection of sodium fluorescein into arm blood vessel, (BV) followed by serial imaging and recording to detect disorders in retinal vessels, such as with diabetic retinopathy and eye tumors

1. Preprocedure care
   a. Assess for allergies and/or history of reactions to dye
   b. Ensure client has given informed consent
   c. Give prescribed mydriatic medication 1 hour prior to test to dilate pupil
2. Postprocedure care
   a. Encourage rest and increased fluid intake (aids in dye excretion)
   b. Teach client that dye causes temporary skin discoloration in injected area and temporary green discoloration of urine that resolves when dye is fully excreted
   c. Teach client to avoid sunlight or other bright light sources for several hours until pupil dilation returns to normal

B. Corneal staining: instillation of dye into conjunctival sac to highlight irregularities caused by trauma, abrasions, or ulcers; damaged corneal epithelium appears green when viewed through a blue filter

1. Ensure that contact lenses are removed prior to procedure, if worn
2. Tell client to blink to distribute dye evenly over cornea
3. Wipe excess dye from cheeks and instruct client not to rub eyes

C. Tonometry: measurement of IOP to detect glaucoma by determining resistance of eyeball to an applied force

1. Normal IOP ranges from 12 to 21 mmHg
2. Eye may be anesthetized, and client stares forward
3. Applanation: most accurate, measures force needed to flatten a small area of cornea; eye is anesthetized
4. Indentation: measures change in form of globe after standard weight (Schiøtz tonometer) is applied to cornea; eye is anesthetized
5. Noncontact: calculates IOP by measuring deflection of a puff of air applied to cornea; no anesthetic needed
6. Tell client not to rub eyes after test if anesthetic was used to avoid possible corneal scratches or injury

D. Physical assessment of eye and vision

1. Acuity of distance vision: measures vision using Snellen chart hung 20 feet away
   a. Client reads chart lines with one eye covered, moving downward from row that is most clear to last line that is completely read
   b. Findings are recorded as a fraction: numerator is client's distance from chart (20 feet), and denominator is number identified at end of smallest line read, which corresponds to distance at which normal eye can read that line; normal vision is 20/20; a larger denominator indicates myopia (nearsightedness)
   c. Red and green lines on Snellen chart can provide a quick test of color blindness
2. Acuity of near vision: measures vision using a Rosenbaum chart or a card with newsprint 12 to 14 inches from client's eyes; impairment indicates hyperopia (farsightedness) in a young client or presbyopia in an adult after approximately 45 years of age
3. Refraction test: uses Snellen chart to assess visual acuity while client reads through various strengths of corrective lenses; uses to prescribe correction for errors with *myopia* (nearsightedness), *hyperopia* (farsightedness), and *astigmatism* (irregularity of corneal surface that inhibits light rays from focusing clearly on retina)
4. Visual fields: measures peripheral vision, often called confrontation test
   a. Client and examiner face each other with client looking into examiner's eyes; both cover own eye on same side
   b. Examiner raises a finger or other small object at arm's length midway between client and examiner, and brings it in from periphery into line of vision; procedure is repeated from above and below on same side
   c. Client states "now" when able to see object; examiner should see object at about same time (test assumes examiner has normal peripheral vision); test is repeated on other eye
5. Color vision
   a. Tested for driver's license, employment requiring color discrimination, or with history of difficulty distinguishing colors; sensitive for red/green blindness, but not for blue

! b. Involves picking colored numbers or letters out of plates with multiple colors in background (such as an Ishihara chart) or noting green and red lines on Snellen chart; results recorded as a fraction of correct identifications divided by total number shown

6. Extraocular muscle movements
   a. Client's eyes follow a small object through six cardinal positions of gaze: to right (lateral), upward and right (temporal), down and right, left (lateral), upward and left (lateral), and down and left
   ! b. Client should have parallel eye movement and absence of **nystagmus,** involuntary rhythmic oscillating eye movements (vertical, horizontal, rotary, or mixed)
   c. As last step, client follows finger as it moves in to bridge of nose; eyes should sustain convergence to within 5 to 8 centimeters
7. Outer eye structures
   a. Sclera white in color, although dark-skinned clients may have slight yellow cast or pigmented dots; yellow discoloration (or heightened yellow) can indicate jaundice
   b. Cornea normally transparent, smooth, and shiny; opacities (cloudy areas) or specks may indicate prior injury
   c. Pupils should be round, equal in size, and constrict in response to direct light or to light shone in opposite pupil (consensual response); pupils should constrict and converge when looking at object over examiner's shoulder and then shifting gaze to an object 4 to 6 inches from own nose (accommodation)
8. Ophthalmoscopy
   a. Used to examine retina, optic disk, optic blood vessels, fundus, and macula
   ! b. As light shines on pupil, reflection of light on retina causes a red glare (red reflex); absence of red reflex may indicate lens opacity

E. Otoscopic examination

! 1. Tilt client's head slightly away, pull pinna up and back in an adult (down and back in a child) to straighten external auditory canal, and insert speculum while visualizing canal
2. Normal findings
   a. Pink, intact external canal with no lesions and variable amount of cerumen and fine hairs; absence of inflammation, deviations, or foreign bodies
   b. Tympanic membrane should be transparent, opaque, pearly gray, slightly concave, intact, and free of lesions or perforations

F. Whisper test

1. Have client occlude one ear at a time with a finger; stand 1 to 2 feet away from client on side of unoccluded ear
2. Whisper numbers or a statement and ask client to repeat; perform again with other ear; alternatively, a ticking watch can be held 5 inches from each
3. Note whether it is necessary to stand closer or raise voice to be heard

! **G. Rinne test**

1. Place stem of an activated tuning fork on mastoid bone and ask client to signal when sound is no longer heard
2. Quickly place vibrating end of tuning fork in front of ear close to ear canal and have client indicate when sound is no longer heard
3. With no conductive hearing loss, sound is heard twice as long by air conduction as by bone conduction
4. With conductive hearing loss, bone conduction is greater than air conduction in affected ear

! **H. Weber test**

1. Especially valuable when hearing in one ear is reported as better than other
2. Place stem of vibrating tuning fork on midline of forehead or vertex of head (skull) and ask whether sound is heard equally in both ears or if one side is better than other
3. Sound that lateralizes to one ear indicates conductive hearing loss in that ear or sensorineural hearing loss in opposite ear

I. **Audiometry:** quantifies hearing deficits by presenting various sound frequencies to each ear by either sound or bone conduction
J. **Speech audiometry:** identifies intensity at which speech is identifiable
K. **Tympanometry:** indirectly monitors compliance and impedance of middle ear to sound transmission after neutral, positive, and negative air pressure is applied to external auditory meatus
L. **Tests of vestibular function**
1. Romberg test: stand close to client to ensure safety; ask client to close eyes while feet are together and arms are resting at sides; observe for a normal slight sway; significant sway is a positive test
2. Past pointing test
   a. Client sits facing examiner, closes eyes, and points both index fingers at examiner; examiner places own index fingers under client's as a reference point; then client raises both arms and then lowers them to original spot with eyes closed
   b. With normal response, client can return to reference point easily; with vestibular dysfunction, fingers deviate to left or right
3. Gaze nystagmus test: observe client's eyes as they look straight ahead, 30 degrees to each side, upward, and downward; with vestibular problems, eyeballs exhibit nystagmus, (an involuntary, constant, and cyclical movement) in any direction
4. Hallpike maneuver: client lies supine and rotates head to side for 1 minute; is positive for positional vertigo or induced dizziness if nystagmus occurs

III. COMMON NURSING TECHNIQUES AND PROCEDURES FOR THE EYE AND EAR

A. **Ocular medications**
! 1. Eye drops
   a. Ensure that medication is sterile and treat each eye separately, if both are being medicated, to prevent cross-contamination
   b. Follow procedure as outlined in Chapter 30
   c. Wait 2 to 5 minutes between drops as per manufacturer's directions
2. Eye ointments: as per procedure outlined in Chapter 30
3. Medicated eye disk
   a. Position client with head tilted back and expose lower conjunctival sac
   b. Press tip of index finger of gloved hand against convex part of disk, place disk horizontally in sac between iris and lower eyelid
   c. Pull lower eyelid out and up over disk and ask client to blink until disk is not visible and have client press fingers against closed lids without moving eyes or disk to secure disk in position
   d. To remove disk, expose lower conjunctival sac and use thumb and index finger to pinch and lift disk from sac

B. **Ocular irrigation**
1. Position client with head tilted toward side to be irrigated and place waterproof pad and curved basin under affected side
2. Cleanse eyelids and lashes with gloved hand and moistened cotton ball, discarding each cotton ball after one wipe
3. Draw up ordered irrigant into sterile irrigation set or bulb syringe
4. Using nondominant hand to hold eyelids open, hold syringe 1 inch above eye and push fluid gently into conjunctival sac (fluid flows across eye from inner to outer canthus)
! 5. Avoid flushing directly onto eyeball to avoid damage to cornea

C. **Eye patches and shields**
1. Have client close both eyes during application of patch or shield
! 2. Position patch and secure with two strips of tape extending from midforehead to lateral cheekbone (medial top to lateral bottom) on same side
3. Do not use pressure unless specifically ordered, and then use two to three pads and extra tape
4. Change only with physician order

5. Apply shield alone or over an eye patch to protect eye from pressure or other type of irritation
6. ! Place shield on bony prominences of cheek, nose, and brow; secure with transparent tape in same manner as for eye patch

D. Eye prosthesis (artificial eye) care

1. Allow client to perform own artificial eye care if preferred; some prostheses are permanently implanted; others are removable
2. Remove prosthesis by retracting lower eyelid and exerting pressure just below eye to break suction and lift it from socket; can also use rubber bulb syringe or medicine dropper bulb to create suction effect
3. Cleanse with normal saline (NS) or tap water according to client's routine
4. Irrigate eye socket with NS using aseptic technique if ordered (such as for infection)
5. Cleanse edges of eye socket and surrounding area with moistened gauze
6. Reinsert by retracting upper and lower eyelids and slipping prosthesis into eye socket comfortably under upper eyelid
7. Store prosthesis in labeled container with NS or tap water

E. Otic medications

1. Use clean technique unless tympanic membrane is damaged, then use sterile technique
2. Follow procedure as outlined in Chapter 30

F. Otic irrigation

1. Assist client to a sitting or lying position with head tilted toward affected ear; place a waterproof pad and drainage receptacle under affected ear
2. Check that temperature of irrigant is 37°C or 98°F
3. Determine that tympanic membrane is intact before beginning an otic irrigation
4. ! Straighten ear canal and gently insert syringe tip into auditory meatus; direct solution slowly and steadily along wall of canal (not center, which could damage tympanic membrane); use no more than 50 to 70 mL at one time
5. After solution drains, dry outside of ear with cotton balls and place a dry one in auditory meatus lightly to absorb remaining excess fluid
6. Assist client to a side-lying position on affected side for further drainage, and assess client for discomfort

G. Hearing aid prosthesis care

1. There are several types of hearing aids available; they improve quality of hearing with conductive hearing loss but only intensify distortions heard with sensorineural hearing loss (they may be useful in signaling client of danger, enabling client to hear alarms, for example)
2. Wash hands before handling an external hearing aid
3. Make sure battery is working properly and is inserted correctly; have client keep an extra battery on hand
4. Do not drop hearing aid or twist cord
5. ! To insert a hearing aid: inspect to ensure it is intact, turn down volume, insert ear mold first into ear canal, then secure rest of device; once in place, turn up volume slowly until comfortable, and check for structural problems or placement problems if feedback occurs
6. Remove a hearing aid after turning it off and lowering volume; remove earmold by rotating it forward slightly and pulling outward
7. After removal, clean a detachable earmold with mild soap and water, rinse and dry well; avoid excessive wetting or use of alcohol, which can cause damage; wipe nondetachable earmolds with a damp cloth
8. ! Avoid using aerosol sprays, oils, or cosmetic products near hearing aid, because earmold opening could become clogged
9. Remove battery to prevent corrosion and leakage if aid will not be used for more than 24 hours; store in a safe place away from moisture and heat

IV. NURSING MANAGEMENT OF CLIENT HAVING EYE SURGERY

A. Preoperative care

1. Reduce anxiety by teaching about procedure and postoperative course and care

2. Assess client's support systems, ability to care for self after surgery, and environmental safety (such as hand rails, absence of throw rugs)
3. Shampoo or scrub around eyes if ordered; remove eye makeup; store contact lens or eyeglasses (needed to aid vision in other eye) so they are available after surgery
4. Administer preanesthetic medications and eyedrops as ordered, which commonly include **mydriatic** eye drops (to dilate pupils) and **cycloplegic** eye drops (to paralyze ciliary muscles); see Chapter 44 for overview of commonly ordered eye medications

B. Postoperative care

1. Perform baseline assessments as for all postoperative clients (vital signs (VS), level of consciousness (LOC), status of dressing); changes may be minimal if surgery done under local anesthesia
2. Maintain eye patch or eye shield in place to prevent eye injury, and instruct client not to rub or touch area
3. Elevate head to 30 to 45 degrees and have client lie on back or unaffected side (to reduce IOP) after surgery to treat cataracts or glaucoma; use small pillows at sides of head to immobilize head when lying on back
4. Position client with repair of detached retina as prescribed so that area of detachment is dependent/inferior (to maintain pressure on repaired retinal area and improve its contact with choroid)
5. Instruct and assist client to avoid activities that increase IOP, such as coughing, sneezing, vomiting, or straining at stool; if it is necessary to cough or sneeze, client should do so with mouth open and use tissues
6. Maintain client safety: orient to environment, keep articles and call bell on unaffected side, use side-rails with bed in low position, and assist with ambulation
7. Give antibiotic, anti-inflammatory, and other prescribed topical (eye) or systemic medications
8. Give analgesics as ordered, avoiding or using caution with opioids to prevent postoperative nausea, vomiting, and constipation; discomfort may be described as achy or scratching; avoid morphine, which can cause miosis
9. Assess for and report immediately possible surgical complications to preserve sight:
   a. Sudden sharp eye pain, possibly indicating hemorrhage; sudden rise in IOP; or other ocular emergency
   b. Hemorrhage, with blood noted in anterior chamber of eye
   c. Retinal detachment, noted by client sensations of flashes of light, floaters, or a curtain being drawn over the eye
   d. Corneal edema, noted by a cloudy appearance to cornea
10. Teach client and family about postdischarge care (see Box 64–1)
11. Refer to community health agency for assistance with home care if needed

V. NURSING MANAGEMENT OF CLIENT HAVING EAR SURGERY

A. Preoperative care: principles same as prior to eye surgery

1. Complete a baseline assessment of client's hearing ability to use as a comparison postoperatively
2. Shampoo or scrub around ear if ordered; complete usual preoperative activities and checklist; administer preanesthetic medications as ordered

B. Postoperative care

1. Perform baseline assessments as for all postoperative clients (VS, LOC, bleeding or drainage from dressing, pain, recovery from anesthesia)
2. Implement standard interventions for care of the postoperative client (pain control, mobility, prevention of postoperative complications)
3. Keep client on bedrest for 24 hours with head either elevated or flat (depending on surgeon's order) and lying on nonoperative side (operative ear upward) for 12 to 24 hours
4. Change internal or external dressings if ordered; wipe away discharge from ear with dry sterile dressing material

Box 64–1

Client Education Following Eye Surgery

The following points should be included in discharge instructions given to the client and family after eye surgery:

- Leave eye shield in place until the surgeon's office visit on the day after surgery; then use eye shield at night during sleep for eye protection as prescribed.
- Avoid rubbing, scratching, touching, squeezing, or putting pressure on surgical eye.
- Avoid activities that increase intraocular pressure, such as sneezing, coughing, vomiting, straining, moving rapidly, bending, or lifting more than 5 pounds.
- Maintain sedentary lifestyle for approximately 2 weeks or as prescribed by surgeon; avoid heavy work, such as gardening, mowing the lawn, or moving furniture.
- Avoid reading until allowed by surgeon, and then read in moderation during healing.
- Use measures to prevent constipation, such as adequate fiber and fluid intake, maintaining mobility as able, and possible use of stool softener.
- Wear sunglasses with side shields when out of doors (photophobia commonly occurs)
- New corrective lenses (if needed) will not be prescribed until vision stabilizes, which may take several weeks; make and keep all recommended follow-up appointments with physician.
- Use proper techniques for donning and removing eye patch or shield and for instillation of eye drops.
- Understand medication names, dose, schedule, side effects, purpose, and anticipated duration of use.
- Symptoms to report to physician include new, increased, or severe eye pain or pressure; decreased vision; redness; cloudiness; drainage; floaters or light flashes; and halos around brightly lit objects.

! 5. Assess for nausea and vomiting; medicate with antiemetics prn to prevent vomiting, which can disrupt surgical site by increasing pressure in middle ear

! 6. Assess for dizziness and vertigo postoperatively; avoid unnecessary movements or turning in bed; provide antivertigo medications; and provide assistance when client is allowed to ambulate to reduce falls

7. Assess client's hearing postoperatively and compare to baseline; use alternate communication means as needed

8. Remind client that decreased hearing immediately after surgery may be caused by edema and drainage at operative site; permanent hearing loss may be expected if cochlea is involved or no middle ear reconstruction is done

! 9. Teach client and family about post-discharge care (see Box 64–2)

VI. AMBLYOPIA

A. Overview

1. Reduction of central vision in an eye that is normal; also known as "lazy eye"
2. Results from untreated strabismus and causes decreased vision in one or both eyes; visual loss is caused by suppression of signals by brain

B. Assessment

1. Is diagnosed with assessment and vision testing by an optometrist or ophthalmologist
2. Nursing assessments depend upon age of child
3. ! Manifestations of visual impairment for infants include lack of tracking objects or lights with eyes and poor or no eye contact
4. Signs of visual impairment in toddlers and older children are excessive tearing, rubbing, and squinting of the eyes; frequent blinking; and holding objects close to eyes to see them or to read

C. Therapeutic management

1. ! Medical treatment options include corrective lenses in eyeglasses, occluding unaffected eye with a patch (occlusion therapy), eye muscle exercises

Box 64-2

Client Education Following Ear Surgery

The following points should be included in discharge instructions given to the client and family after ear surgery:

- Keep the outer ear dressing clean and dry; change it as ordered if needed; do not remove inner ear dressing until allowed by surgeon; do not insert small objects to clean external ear canal.
- Whenever possible, avoid activities that increase middle ear pressure, such as blowing nose, sneezing, coughing, straining.
- If it is necessary, cough or sneeze with mouth open; blow nose one nostril at a time with mouth open; avoid drinking through a straw for 2 to 3 weeks; avoid air travel until allowed by surgeon.
- Use measures to prevent constipation, such as adequate fiber and fluid intake, maintaining mobility as able, and possible use of stool softener.
- Do not shower or shampoo hair until allowed by surgeon (usually for 1 or more weeks).
- Keep ear dry for 6 weeks with use of petrolatum-coated cotton ball placed in external auditory canal as ordered; if used, change it daily; do not swim or dive until allowed by surgeon (when full healing occurs).
- Reduce risk of infection by avoiding those with respiratory infections.
- Understand medication names, dose, schedule, side effects, purpose, and anticipated duration of use (antibiotics, antiemetics, antivertigo agents).
- Symptoms to report to physician include persistent postoperative headache, increased drainage or bleeding from site, fever, new or increased ear pain or dizziness, and decreasing hearing.

2. Treatment is discontinued when vision has improved; however, 20/20 visual acuity is rarely attained
3. Treatment of amblyopia is most successful when accomplished by age 7 to 8 years of age
4. Untreated amblyopia can lead to permanent visual impairment
5. Nursing care involves educating parents and child about necessity of completing treatment

D. Client and family teaching: how to patch unaffected eye while maintaining skin integrity; therapy and long term benefits

VII. STRABISMUS

A. Overview

1. Misalignment of eyes; most common type is esotropia (crossed eyes)
2. Caused by lack of coordination of eye muscles
3. Positive family history occurs in about 50% of cases

B. Assessment:

1. **Cover-uncover test:** client fixes gaze straight ahead, focusing on a distant object; cover one eye with an opaque card while observing uncovered eye for movement; remove card while observing eye just uncovered for movement; this test screens for deviation in eye alignment and eye muscle weakness (weakness is seen as movement of "lazy eye" when it attempts to refocus during cover test)
2. **Corneal light reflex (Hirschberg test):** assesses parallel symmetry of eyes; examiner shines a penlight directly onto corneas of both eyes, holding penlight about 12 inches away from client's nasal bridge while client focuses on a distant object; light should be reflected at same spot in both eyes; an asymmetric light reflex indicates a deviation in alignment of client's eyes

C. Therapeutic management

! 1. Includes occlusion therapy ("good eye" is patched, forcing client to focus with weaker eye, thus strengthening eye muscles), corrective lenses in eyeglasses, eye drops to cause blurred vision in "good eye," eye muscle exercises

2. Surgical treatment
   a. Strabismus can be corrected surgically if conservative treatment fails; surgery on rectus muscles of eyes can achieve normal eye alignment
   b. Congenital strabismus should be corrected before 24 months of age to prevent amblyopia

D. Client and family teaching

1. Provide explanation of eye patching to parents
2. Preoperative teaching about maintaining NPO status prior to surgery and general preoperative and postoperative care

VIII. GLAUCOMA

A. Overview

1. Imbalance between aqueous humor production and drainage, leading to increased IOP
2. Can be of two types: open-angle or angle-closure (narrow-angle, closed-angle)
3. Usually exists as a primary condition without identified precipitating cause; most frequent in adults over 60 years of age
4. Open-angle glaucoma: most frequent form with unknown cause, although heredity is suspected; angle of anterior chamber between the iris and cornea is normal; flow of aqueous humor through trabecular network to canal of Schlemm is obstructed; it is usually a bilateral process
5. Angle-closure (narrow-angle, closed-angle) glaucoma: less common form, is often unilateral, although other eye can be affected at a later time
   a. Anterior chamber narrows because of corneal flattening or bulging of iris
   b. When iris thickens (pupil dilation) or lens thickens (during visual accommodation), angle can close completely, blocking outflow and causing sudden elevation of IOP
   c. Damage to neurons in retina and optic nerve can occur, rapidly lead to loss of vision if not treated quickly

B. Assessment

1. Open-angle
   a. Loss of peripheral vision, mild headaches, difficulty adapting to dark, seeing halos around lights, and difficulty focusing on near objects
   b. Symptoms may be vague with client unaware of them for a time; visual acuity deteriorates over time with rising IOP
2. Angle-closure
   a. Triggered by pupil dilation, such as with high emotions and darkness, among others
   b. Symptoms include severe eye and face pain, nausea and vomiting, malaise, colored halos around lights, and episodes of sudden decline in vision; possible reddened eye, cloudy cornea from edema, and pupil fixed at midpoint
3. Diagnosed by history; presenting symptoms; tonometry; ophthalmoscopy; **gonioscopy** (measurement of anterior chamber angle, differentiates open-angle from angle-closure glaucoma)

C. Therapeutic management

1. Acute glaucoma: medical emergency; vision loss can occur within 1 to 2 days if untreated; provide information to client and administer ordered therapies such as osmotic diuretics or carbonic anhydrase inhibitors to lower IOP (see Chapter 44); surgical intervention may be needed
2. Chronic glaucoma: interventions primarily consist of medication therapy and client education
3. Provide pre- and postoperative care as previously outlined if eye surgery is needed; surgical procedures to facilitate drainage of aqueous humor can include trabeculectomy, laser trabeculoplasty, iridectomy, or laser iridotomy
4. Medication therapy
   a. **Miotic** drugs that constrict pupils
   b. Carbonic anhydrase inhibitors to decrease production of aqueous humor
   c. Beta-adrenergic blockers to constrict pupils and reduce production of aqueous humor

D. Client teaching

1. Drug therapy is needed for life; noncompliance can lead to loss of vision that cannot be regained
2. Avoid mydriatic medications such as atropine that dilate pupils
3. Obtain Medic-Alert card or bracelet specifying type of glaucoma
4. Use safety precautions at night (lighting, hand rails) to compensate for reduced pupil dilation because of miotics, and remove obstacles in environment for safety
5. Follow general instructions following eye surgery; see previous discussion
6. Review specific drug information and procedures for self-administration

IX. CATARACTS

A. Overview

1. Progressive and gradual development of opacity in lens or lens capsule that results in loss of vision
2. Risk factors include age (most common), long-term exposure to ultraviolet light (UV-B rays), cigarette smoking, heavy alcohol use, eye injury or inflammation, congenital defect, diabetes mellitus, and some medications (such as systemic corticosteroids, chlorpromazine [Thorazine], busulfan [Myleran])
3. Fibers and proteins of lens degenerate with age or following insult; opacity often begins at periphery of lens and moves to center
4. Partial opacity is termed *immature cataract;* opacity of entire lens is termed *mature cataract*
5. Opacity tends to occur bilaterally but is asymmetric in development, with one maturing faster than other

B. Assessment

1. Decline in close and distance vision, blurred vision, changes in color vision (loss), glare, halos around lights, object distortion, white or cloudy gray pupil
2. Diagnosed by history and physical exam, results of visual acuity tests and slit-lamp exam; absence of red reflex with ophthalmoscopy

C. Therapeutic management

1. Provide emotional support because impaired vision is anxiety-producing for clients
2. Identify and correct safety concerns in environment related to impaired vision
3. Surgical removal of lens is sole treatment option and is accompanied by lens implant or is treated with corrective lenses
4. Assist client in decision making about surgery, which is indicated when vision or activities of daily living (ADLs) are affected or if cataract is causing secondary problems such as uveitis or glaucoma
5. Reinforce explanations about surgical extraction of lens
   a. Cryoextraction: forceps or supercooled probe used to extract lens after making small incision in cornea
   b. Phacoemulsification: ultrasound vibrations break lens into fragments that are aspirated (suctioned) from the eye
   c. Intracapsular extraction: removal of entire lens and surrounding capsule (see Figure 64–1a ■)
   d. Extracapsular extraction: removal of lens nucleus and cortex, leaving posterior capsule intact to support lens implant; currently most popular method (see Figure 64–1b)
6. Surgery is done on one eye at a time, usually on an outpatient basis and using local anesthesia
7. Lens implant rapidly restores binocular vision and depth perception
8. Provide preoperative and postoperative care as outlined in previous section
9. Medication therapy
   a. Indicated for temporary use after surgery
   b. Generally includes antibiotic and anti-inflammatory agents

D. Client teaching

1. Adaptive strategies to compensate for changes in vision and depth perception if surgery is not currently indicated or desired
2. Postoperative instructions as outlined in previous section on eye surgery

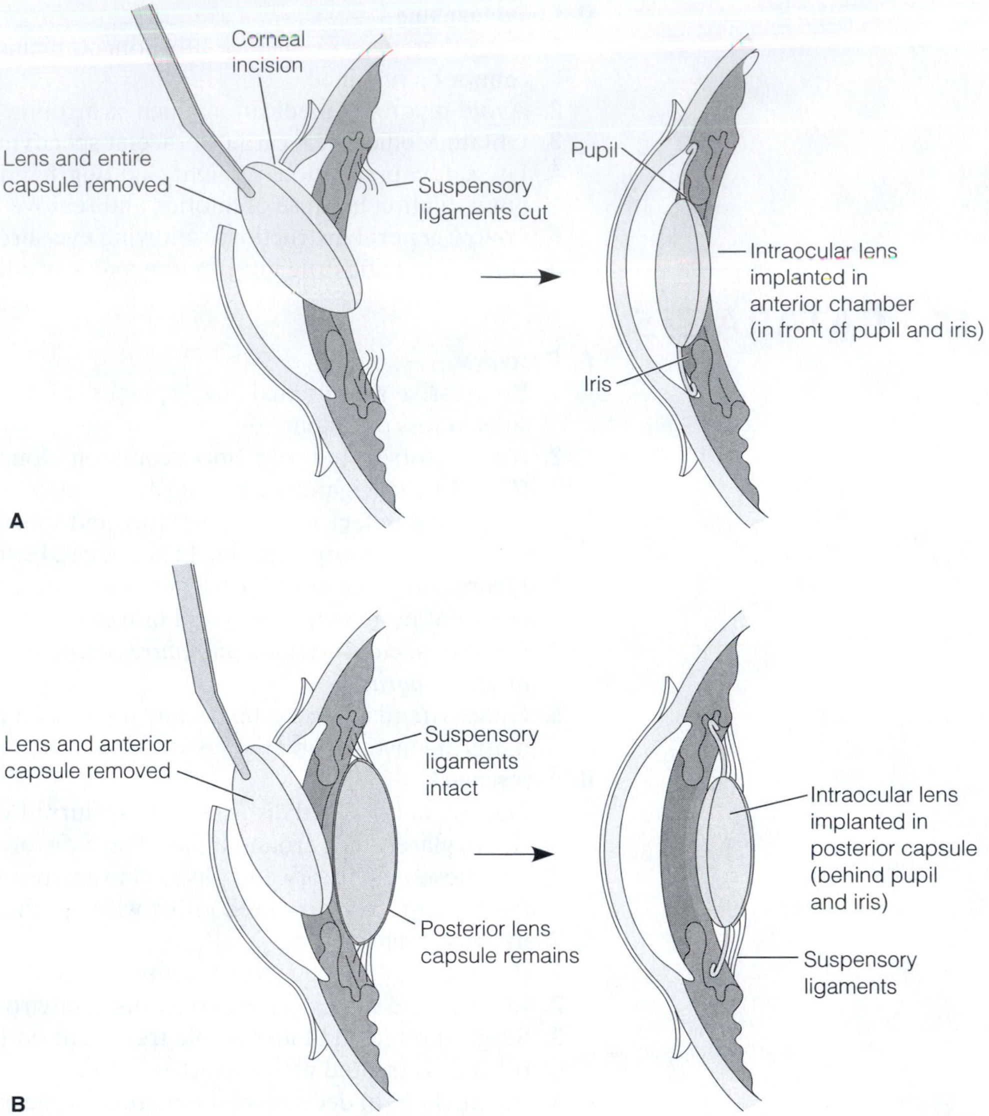

Figure 64–1

A. Intracapsular cataract extraction removes entire lens and capsule, with lens implantation in anterior chamber. B. Extracapsular cataract extraction removes lens and anterior capsule, with lens implantation within the intact posterior capsule.

Source: LeMone, P., & Burke, K. (2003). Medical surgical nursing: Critical thinking for client care *(3rd ed.). Upper Saddle River, NJ: Pearson Education, p. 1475.*

3. Leave eye patch or shield in place until changed or removed by surgeon at postoperative visit, usually within 24 to 48 hours
4. Eye protection may include sunglasses during day in bright light and eye shield at night
5. ! Information and procedures for medication use after surgery, such as acetaminophen for general discomfort, combination steroid (anti-inflammatory) and antibiotic eye drops, and others as needed by individual client
6. Insertion and care of postoperative contact lenses if prescribed
7. ! Permanent eyeglasses will be prescribed several weeks after surgery when healing is complete and vision has stabilized

X. DETACHED RETINA

A. Overview

1. Separation of sensory layer of retina from choroid (pigmented vascular layer)
2. Retina may tear and fold back onto itself or remain intact and be pulled away from choroid by shrinking of vitreous humor
3. Most frequently an age related condition with shrinkage of vitreous humor, which pulls on retina at points of attachment, such as the optic disk, macula, and periphery of eye
4. Can also be caused by trauma, inflammation, tumor, or complication of eye surgery (lens removal)

5. Corneal ulcer (local necrosis of cornea): caused by infection, trauma, or misuse of contact lenses; manifested by photophobia, discomfort ranging from gritty sensations to severe pain, excessive tearing; possible discharge; decreased visual acuity; inability to open eye or spasm of eyelid; visible area of ulceration
6. Keratitis (inflammation of cornea): similar to conjunctivitis; can lead to ulceration and blindness
7. Uveitis (inflammation of uveal tract, e.g., vascular layer): pupillary constriction, erythema around limbus, severe eye pain, photophobia, blurred vision

! **B. Therapeutic management**

1. Medication therapy with topical or systemic antibiotics or antiviral agents, antihistamines, and corticosteroids
2. Promote infection control through diligent handwashing; teach client and family that conjunctivitis can be highly contagious
3. Cleanse eye with warm water and remove any crusting or exudate before instilling eye drops or eye ointment
4. Reduce pain or discomfort with warm compresses, dark sunglasses, and analgesics (acetaminophen and/or codeine)
5. If corneal perforation is suspected, have client lie supine, close eye, and cover with dry, sterile dressing to avoid loss of eye contents until surgery is done

C. Client and family teaching

1. Teach client or caregivers to instill antibiotic drops or ointment into conjunctival sac
2. ! Give instructions on prevention measures to limit spread of infection to other eye or other people, including to not share face cloths or towels, not to rub eyes, discard eye makeup and purchase new after infection clears, refrain from wearing contact lenses during infection, and not to cross-contaminate infection to other eye

XIII. EYE INJURY

A. Overview and assessment

1. Corneal abrasion (disruption of superficial cornea from drying, contact lenses, eyelashes, or foreign bodies such as dust, dirt, or fingernails): pain, photophobia, tearing
2. Burns (from chemicals, heat, radiation, explosion): eye pain, decreased vision, swollen eyelids, burns, reddened and edematous conjunctiva, possible corneal haziness or cloudiness, ulcerations
3. Blunt trauma (caused by sports injuries, motor vehicle accidents, falls, physical assault): includes lid ecchymosis (black eye), conjunctival hemorrhage (painless erythema), hyphema (bleeding into anterior chamber with eye pain, decreased vision, and seeing a reddish hue), and orbital fractures (diplopia/double vision, pain with upward eye movement, limited eye movements, sunken appearance to eye, and decreased sensation on affected cheek)

! **B. Therapeutic management**

1. If chemical burn present, irrigate eye with copious amounts of normal saline (preferred) or water (if necessary) until pH of eye is in range of 7.2 to 7.4; use topical anesthetic to make irrigation easier; then evaluate vision with and without any corrective eyeglasses
2. Remove loose foreign bodies quickly using a sterile, moistened cotton-tipped applicator or by irrigation to prevent corneal abrasion
3. If no foreign substances are present, first evaluate vision with and without eyeglasses to provide data about extent of injury and for use as a baseline
4. Apply eye patches or sterile gauze dressings over both eyes if severe or penetrating eye injury occurs to reduce eye movements; stabilize any penetrating objects until surgery is done to help preserve vision; institute bedrest

C. Client education

1. Purpose, effects, and use of medications
2. Use eye patch or shield
3. Avoid activities that increase IOP during healing (lifting, bending, straining); teach how to avoid future injury

XIV. LEGAL BLINDNESS

A. Overview

1. Visual acuity that is no better than 20/200 even with correction in better eye, or a visual field of less than 20 degrees (instead of 180 degrees)
2. Common causes in United States are glaucoma and cataracts, macular degeneration, diabetic retinopathy, and congenital disorders

B. Therapeutic management

1. Assist client to move through grieving process that accompanies vision loss, because of loss of sight and interference with mobility, self-sufficiency, and possibly financial status
2. Support client who is experiencing changes in roles and relationships, communication patterns (through loss of ability to perceive nonverbal cues), and possibly sexual expression
3. ! Foster independence in hospital environment
   a. Verbally and physically orient client to room using bed as a reference point
   b. Keep room and hallway free of clutter
   c. Introduce self when entering client's room and state when leaving
   d. Use increased verbal communication: describe activities in environment and provide stimuli such as radio or television; ask client what assistance is needed
   e. Ensure that call bell and other needed articles are within client's easy reach and that client knows their location
   f. Describe location of food on plate using a clock face description (for a client who was previously sighted and knows what a clock face is)
   g. Assist with ambulation, walking slightly ahead and allowing client to hold your arm (not the reverse); describe environment that lies ahead, such as turns or stairs

! **C. Client teaching:** measures to minimize risk of injury in home setting and adapt to performing ADLs with impaired vision

XV. HEARING IMPAIRMENT

A. Overview

1. Condition that interferes with ability to receive auditory signals from environment
2. Three types: conductive hearing loss, sensorineural hearing loss, and mixed hearing loss
3. Conductive hearing loss: occurs when tympanic membrane cannot vibrate freely or when sounds cannot reach middle ear; common causes are otitis media, impacted cerumen, and foreign body in ear canal
4. Sensorineural hearing loss: occurs with damage to cochlea or auditory nerve; sensorineural hearing loss may be congenital (as in congenital rubella syndrome) or acquired (ototoxic drugs); hearing loss may also be genetic, such as with Tay-Sachs disease
5. Mixed hearing loss: involves a combination of conductive and sensorineural hearing losses

! B. Assessment of hearing impairment

1. In infants and young children with hearing loss, language development is affected; it should be diagnosed as early as possible to promote optimal development
2. Infancy: does not startle to loud noises, arouses to touch and not noise, does not turn head to sounds or localize sounds, little or no babbling or vocalizations
3. Toddlers and preschoolers: communicates through gestures; little or no speech, unintelligible speech; developmental delay; no response to doorbell, telephone
4. School-aged children and adolescents: sits close to speaker or turns up TV volume loudly, poor school performance, speech problems, cannot correctly respond except when able to view speaker's face
5. Adults or older adults: watches speaker's face during conversation; does not respond to noises if not in line of vision; uses loud volume with TV, radio, and other entertainment equipment
6. Diagnosed by otoscopic examination, tympanography, and audiography

C. Therapeutic management

1. Prevent acquired hearing loss by client education to avoid exposure to loud noises
2. Advocate prompt treatment of otitis media
3. Perform developmental assessment to aid in early identification of infants and children with hearing loss to prevent significant delays in developmental progress and school performance
4. If hearing loss is correctable in child, treatment of cause, such as removal of a foreign body in conductive loss, is therapeutic goal
5. If hearing loss cannot be corrected, a multidisciplinary team consisting of the otolaryngologist, audiologist, pediatrician, nurse, and speech-language pathologist work with child and family to obtain appropriate therapies and enhance communication
6. ! Hearing aids may be prescribed; see previous section on hearing aid care
7. Advocate for clients with hearing impairment and their families; provide support and appropriate referrals to child and family

D. Client teaching

1. Means of communicating with children or adults who have hearing loss
2. Encourage parents to enroll child in early intervention to promote speech development

XVI. OTOSCLEROSIS

A. Overview

1. Hereditary disorder of labyrinthine capsule in which abnormal bone growth occurs around ossicles
2. Causes fixation of stapes, leading to conductive hearing loss
3. Is an autosomal dominant hereditary disorder most common in Caucasians and females; onset is in adolescence or early adulthood; pregnancy exacerbates condition
4. Stapes do not vibrate as they should because of stiffening, which reduces sound transmission to inner ear

! **B. Assessment**

1. Bilateral conductive hearing loss that is progressive and asymmetrical, tinnitus, possible retention of bone conduction (so client has difficulty in ordinary conversation but can use telephone adequately)
2. Reddish or pinkish orange tympanic membrane from increased vascularity (Schwartz's sign)
3. Rinne test results: bone sound conduction equal to or longer than air conduction (abnormal finding) if hearing loss is greater than 25 decibels (dB)
4. Weber test results: lateralization to ear with greater conductive hearing loss

C. Therapeutic management

1. Encourage use of a hearing aid(s) to augment sound
2. Administer sodium fluoride as ordered to slow bone resorption and overgrowth
3. ! Implement strategies to enhance communication with a hearing-impaired client (see Box 64–4)

Box 64–4

Communication with a Hearing Impaired Client

- Approach client from within client's line of vision or tap client lightly on shoulder to get attention before speaking
- Reduce background noise, such as radio or TV, before beginning to speak
- Avoid covering mouth with hands or other objects while speaking
- Face the client and speak slowly and clearly—pronounce words clearly without overarticulating them; speak using low pitch and normal loudness
- Use nonverbal cues and written messages to enhance communication
- Repeat sentences using different words if client has difficulty understanding
- Ask client to repeat directions or teaching that was done to ensure client's understanding

4. Surgical intervention
   a. Stapedectomy with fenestration: microsurgical removal of diseased stapes, with drill or laser creation of a hole in footplate, followed by insertion of a steel or synthetic prosthesis to restore hearing
   b. Stapedotomy: insertion of a wire or platinum ribbon prosthesis into a small hole created in stapes footplate

D. Client teaching: referral to appropriate community agencies; postoperative care as previously outlined

XVII. EAR INFECTIONS

A. Overview

1. Otitis externa: infectious, inflammatory, or allergic response in external auditory canal or auricle; also called "swimmer's ear;" more frequent in warm, humid areas
2. **Otitis media**
   a. Infection or inflammation of middle ear; may be acute or chronic; greatest incidence is between 6 and 36 months of age during winter months
   b. Related to dysfunction of eustachian tube, which provides drainage and ventilation of middle ear; when blocked as a result of edema from an upper respiratory infection, fluid can accumulate in middle ear, providing a medium for bacterial growth and development of infection
   c. Children with facial malformations such as cleft palate and Down syndrome have anatomic variations of their eustachian tubes, making them more vulnerable to otitis media
   d. Causative organisms: most common are *Streptococcus pneumoniae, Haemophilus influenzae,* and *Neisseria catarrhalis*
3. Mastoiditis: infection of mastoid process (temporal bone adjacent to middle ear), usually a consequence of untreated or inadequately treated otitis media

! **B. Assessment**

1. Otitis externa: redness, swelling, and exudate in external auditory canal, earache, itching, sensation that ear is "plugged" or "blocked," hearing loss in affected ear
2. Otitis media
   a. Children (acute): ear pain, irritability, diarrhea, fever, and vomiting are common; pulling at the affected ear may be noted; some children are asymptomatic; diagnosis is based on examination of tympanic membrane using an otoscope; a red, bulging, nonmobile tympanic membrane indicates otitis media
   b. Adults (acute): severe earache or ear pain (classic), ear pressure, fever, malaise, diminished hearing, dizziness or vertigo, nausea and possible vomiting, possible tinnitus (ringing in ears), presence of fluid behind a bulging tympanic membrane
   c. Chronic: slight fever, diminished hearing, chronic ear discharge
3. Mastoiditis: fever, malaise, possible tinnitus and headache, persistent throbbing ear pain worsened by head movement, tenderness behind ear over mastoid process, local cellulitis of skin, drainage from ear, diminished hearing in affected ear

C. Therapeutic management in adults

1. ! Apply local heat 3 times per day for 20 minutes at a time as prescribed
2. Encourage bedrest as applicable to reduce head movements and pain
3. ! Administer prescribed antibiotics (otic or systemic), decongestants, antihistamines, analgesics (acetaminophen or aspirin), and antivertigo agents
4. Teach client to use caution while hearing is diminished
5. Provide care to clients undergoing ear surgery as previously outlined
6. Surgical procedures
   a. Myringotomy: surgically performed perforation of tympanic membrane to allow drainage of middle ear secretions and relieve pain and pressure (otitis media)
   b. Tympanocentesis: insertion of a 20-gauge spinal needle through inferior portion of tympanic membrane to drain secretions, possibly to obtain culture, and relieve pain and pressure (otitis media)

c. Mastoidectomy: surgical removal of infected mastoid air cells, bone, and pus; radical mastoidectomy involves removal of middle ear structures such as incus and malleus as well as diseased tissue (conductive hearing loss then occurs unless reconstructive surgery is done as well)
d. Tympanoplasty: surgical reconstruction of ossicles and tympanic membrane of middle ear to help restore hearing

D. Therapeutic management in children

!
1. Nursing management of child with tympanostomy tubes: usually surgery is accomplished in a day-surgery center, not an inpatient hospital setting
   a. Teach parents to give acetaminophen (Tylenol) for discomfort following myringotomy and insertion of tympanostomy tubes
   b. Parents should follow their physician's directions for postoperative care of the ear; eardrops are often prescribed
   c. Some physicians require parents to insert earplugs for bathing and swimming and avoid water in ear canal; others do not
   d. Teach parents that ear tubes will spontaneously extrude and fall out; they may note presence of spool-shaped tube in child's ear canal; ear tubes usually fall out in about 1 year
2. Medication therapy
   a. Antibiotic therapy for 10 to 14 days; first-line drugs are amoxicillin (Amoxil), and trimethoprim-sulfamethoxazole (Bactrim, Septra); both drugs are given orally
   b. Recurrent or chronic otitis media infections may require prophylactic antibiotic therapy as a 6-month trial
3. Surgical procedures: as described in previous section for adults
4. Client and family teaching: signs and symptoms of otitis media; need to monitor and treat temperature; how to administer medication safely and effectively (complete full course of antibiotic therapy even if feeling better; give doses on time)

XVIII. MENIERE'S DISEASE

A. Overview

1. A disorder of inner ear in which excessive endolymphatic fluid accumulates in membranous labyrinth; also called idiopathic endolymphatic hydrops
2. Has an unknown etiology; possibly heredity, viral influence, and immune dysfunction play a role; affects men and women equally with highest risk between ages 35 to 60
3. Impaired reabsorption of endolymph leads to dilation of lymph channels, which causes symptoms

!
B. Assessment

1. Recurrent severe attacks of vertigo accompanied by sense of fullness in ears, roaring or ringing tinnitus, nausea, headache, and gradual but progressive sensorineural hearing loss (often unilateral)
2. Attacks may last minutes to hours with possible associated symptoms of hypotension, diaphoresis, and nystagmus
3. Attacks may be triggered by increased sodium (Na^+) intake, vasoconstriction, premenstrual fluid retention, stress, or allergies, although sometimes no trigger is identified
4. Diagnosed by electronystagnography (including caloric testing), Rinne and Weber tests, X-ray, CT scan, evaluation of response to a test dose of an osmotic or loop diuretic

!
C. Therapeutic management

1. Low-Na^+ diet and, if symptoms are severe, fluid restriction
2. Avoid use of alcohol, caffeine, nicotine
3. Bedrest to control vertigo; assist with ambulation for safety
4. Medication therapy: atropine (to reduce parasympathetic response) or CNS depressant as an alternative to atropine, diuretics, antihistamines (if allergy present), antivertigo and antiemetic drugs

5. Endolymphatic decompression: relieves pressure in labyrinth and creates shunt between membranous labyrinth and subarachnoid space for fluid drainage (preserves hearing in most cases, relieves vertigo in approximately 70% of cases, relieves tinnitus and sensations of ear fullness in 50% of cases)
6. Vestibular neurectomy: severing of portion of CN VIII that controls balance and sensation of vertigo (relieves vertigo in up to 90% of cases)
7. Labyrinthectomy: complete removal of labyrinth, destroying cochlear function, relieving vertigo but causing loss of any minimal remaining hearing as well ("last resort")
8. Cochlear implant: for sensorineural hearing loss
   a. An electrode is implanted in cochlea to receive stimuli from a processor worn on body; used for a client with intact neurons capable of stimulation (see Figure 64–2 ■)
   b. A second type of device, used for clients with no excitable auditory fibers, amplifies and transmits a signal to a receiver implanted in brainstem
   c. Devices do not restore normal hearing but allow perception of sound to alert a client to conversation or dangers in the environment
9. Complications of all inner ear surgical procedures include infection and cerebrospinal fluid (CSF) leakage

D. Client teaching

1. ! Follow restrictions in Na^+, fluid, nicotine, alcohol, and caffeine
2. Take medications as prescribed
3. ! Learn signs of an impending attack: fullness in affected ear, increasing tinnitus, headache; lie down in bed in a dark quiet room if at home when an attack begins, or pull off the road for safety if driving
4. ! Avoid sudden movements or position changes; move head slowly, and do not get up unassisted during an attack
5. Wear a Medic-Alert identification
6. Learn stress reduction techniques of choice to help reduce severity of attacks
7. If tinnitus persists between attacks, use white noise or ambient sound machine to mask tinnitus and promote sleep; consider use of medication most commonly effective—oral antidepressant nortriptyline (Pamelor) taken at bedtime
8. Practice balance training exercises to help brain learn to compensate for damage to vestibular system; exercises consist of moving head up and down, side to side, and tilting head to left and right; repeated 10 times each twice a day

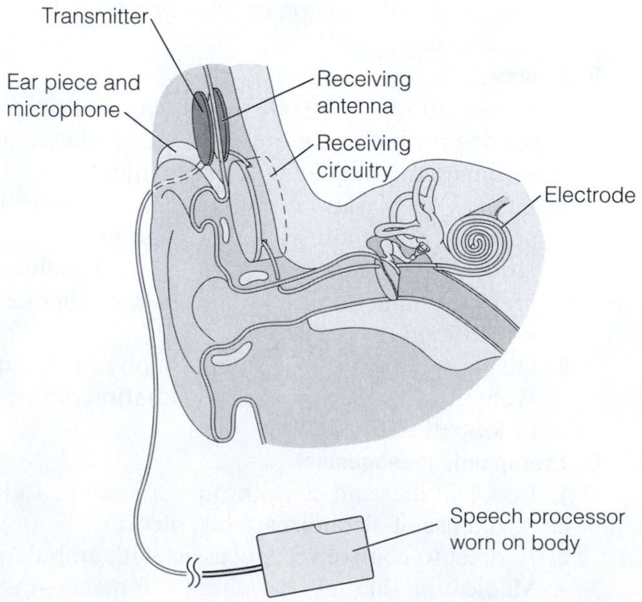

Figure 64–2

Cochlear implant used in sensorineural hearing loss in which excitable auditory neurons remain.

Source: LeMone, P., & Burke, K. (2003). Medical surgical nursing: Critical thinking for client care *(3rd ed.). Upper Saddle River, NJ: Pearson Education, p. 1504.*

XIX. EPISTAXIS

A. Overview

1. Also known as nosebleed; very common in children, especially boys
2. Superficial veins in nares are a common source of bleeding
3. Bleeding can occur from irritation, drying of mucosa from low humidity, increased blood pressure, or picking nose

B. Assessment

1. Assess vital signs of client brought to the emergency department or clinic with uncontrolled epistaxis while simultaneous efforts to control bleeding are being performed
2. If client has experienced significant blood loss, hemoglobin and hematocrit may be measured

C. Therapeutic managment

1. ! Teach client or parents to humidify air (especially during winter months and nighttime hours) and have child sleep with head elevated to prevent recurrence
2. ! Following an episode of nosebleed, client is prone to rebleeding; client should not bend forward, drink hot liquids, exercise excessively, or take hot baths or showers for 3 to 4 days following a significant nosebleed
3. If bleeding cannot be controlled by applying pressure, topical vasoconstrictive agents may be used, such as Neo-Synephrine, epinephrine, or thrombin
4. Cautery may be required with silver nitrate or electrocautery
5. If bleeding cannot be stopped, nose may be packed with absorbent packing material by health care provider to stop bleeding

D. Child and family education

1. ! Teach client or parents how to stop a nosebleed at home by applying steady pressure to both nostrils just below nasal bone for 10 to 15 minutes
2. Instruct client to sit upright and slightly forward to be best able to apply pressure to nostrils and prevent excessive swallowing of blood
3. Instruct client or parents to seek health care if bleeding cannot be stopped
4. Teach client to avoid picking at nose or forcefully blowing nose; teach to release sneezes through open mouth covered with tissues

XX. PHARYNGITIS

A. Overview

1. An infection of the pharynx, often involving tonsils
2. A common disorder in children 4 to 7 years of age, but rare in infancy
3. Approximately 80% of cases are of viral etiology, and relief of symptoms is indicated
4. Bacterial pharyngitis is most often caused by *group A beta-hemolytic streptococcus* and requires antibiotic therapy

! B. Assessment

1. Symptoms include sore throat, difficulty swallowing, drooling caused by sore throat, and inability to swallow saliva; inflammation of pharynx and enlargement of tonsils (with or without exudate), fever, vomiting, cough, lymphadenopathy, and headache; hoarseness or a change in voice quality may be noted
2. A throat culture is necessary to diagnose viral or bacterial etiology of pharyngitis; streptococcal infections can be diagnosed within minutes using a rapid strep test

! C. Therapeutic management

1. In viral pharyngitis, relief of symptoms is indicated; offer diet that is easy to swallow (soft or liquids) and soothing to sore throat (no citrus juices or other foods that could cause burning or increased irritation)
2. Saltwater gargles, throat lozenges, or anesthetic sprays can be used to promote pain relief
3. Medication therapy: analgesics (acetaminophen); antibiotics as ordered for bacterial infections

D. Client and family teaching

1. Stress importance of completing full course of antibiotic therapy to eradicate infectious organisms

2. Untreated or inadequately treated streptococcal infections can result in acute rheumatic fever, glomerulonephritis, or other serious sequelae

XXI. TONSILLITIS

A. Overview

1. Inflammation of tonsils located in posterior pharynx as a result of viral or bacterial infection
2. Causative organism in bacterial infection can be *group A beta-hemolytic streptococcus,* which is particularly virulent

! B. Assessment

1. Diagnosis of etiology is made by throat culture
2. Streptococcal infection can be diagnosed within minutes using a rapid strep test
3. Symptoms
   a. Enlarged, reddened tonsils, with or without exudate
   b. Sore throat, difficulty swallowing because of severe sore throat
   c. Drooling, caused by the inability to swallow saliva secretions
   d. Lymphadenopathy
   e. Mouth breathing

! C. Therapeutic management

1. Management for viral tonsillitis is symptom relief: promoting comfort, pain relief with acetaminophen (Tylenol); management is similar to that of viral pharyngitis
2. Management for bacterial tonsillitis is antibiotic therapy as well as symptom relief
3. Nursing management: offer diet that is easy to swallow (soft or liquids, including ice pops) and soothing to sore throat (no citrus juices or other foods that could cause burning or increased irritation)
4. Use of saltwater gargles, throat lozenges, or anesthetic sprays can promote pain relief
5. Medication therapy: analgesics (acetaminophen) for comfort and hyperthermia; administer antibiotics as ordered for bacterial infections

D. Child and family education: importance of completing full course of antibiotic therapy, how to manage symptoms

E. Tonsillectomy

1. Surgical removal of the tonsils, may be indicated for recurrent tonsillitis, peritonsillar abcess, or respiratory compromise from airway obstruction
2. Commonly performed in a day-surgery setting, ambulatory surgical setting, or may require an overnight hospital stay
3. Client should be free from symptoms of tonsillitis for at least 1 week prior to surgery
4. Preoperative nursing management: includes client and family preoperative teaching, baseline lab data, including bleeding and clotting times
5. ! Postoperative nursing management
   a. Provide pain control with analgesic medications and ice collar
   b. Most common complication is excessive bleeding or hemorrhaging from operative site; observe child for frequent or continual swallowing, vomiting bright red blood, and changes in vital signs
   c. Offer clear, chilled fluids or ice pops to relieve pain and reduce inflammation when awake and alert; red-colored fluids should be avoided because emesis of these fluids could be mistaken for blood
   d. Teach child and parents that a sore throat is to be expected for approximately 1 week postoperatively

F. Client and family education

1. Analgesic medications to be given at home
2. Assess child for signs of complications such as hemorrhage from operative site
3. Ensure adequate fluid intake to prevent dehydration; advance child's diet as tolerated to include soft, nonirritating foods, and avoid strenuous activity for about 1 week
4. Child may return to school in 10 days, when operative site is adequately healed

Check Your NCLEX-RN® Exam I.Q.

You are ready for testing on this content if you can

- Identify basic structures and functions of the eye and ear.
- Describe the pathophysiology and etiology of common eye and ear disorders.
- Discuss expected assessment data and diagnostic test findings for selected eye and ear disorders.
- Discuss therapeutic management of a client experiencing an eye and ear disorder.
- Discuss nursing management of a client experiencing an eye and ear disorder.
- Identify expected outcomes for the client experiencing an eye and ear disorder.

PRACTICE TEST

1 In order to communicate effectively with a client who has sensorineural hearing loss caused by presbycusis, the nurse should do which of the following to improve communication with the client?

1. Approach the client from behind.
2. Use the mouth to exaggerate word pronunciation.
3. Shout initially to get the client's attention.
4. Turn down background noise from radio or TV before speaking.

2 A client has completed a full course of antibiotics for acute otitis media. The nurse conducting a follow-up assessment determines whether medication therapy was effective by questioning the client about relief from which of the following most common presenting symptoms?

1. Dizziness
2. Impaired hearing
3. Nausea and vomiting
4. Ear pain

3 A client has undergone myringotomy. The nurse working in an ambulatory surgery center would instruct the client to avoid which of the following activities while healing is occurring?

1. Gardening
2. Swimming
3. Softball
4. Bowling

4 A 68-year-old female client tells the ambulatory care nurse during a routine visit that she has recently noticed a decline in her ability to hear. The nurse documents this information on the client's health record, suspecting that this client most likely is exhibiting which of the following?

1. Presbycusis
2. Otitis externa
3. Otalgia
4. Meniere's disease

5 After a client has undergone outpatient surgery for a right eye cataract removal, the nurse teaches the client to avoid which of the following when the client gets home?

1. Walking about the house unassisted
2. Lying on the right side
3. Picking up objects that are at waist level
4. Washing dishes in the sink

6 A client has hearing loss that is characterized by distortion of sounds that are heard. The client questions the nurse about the benefits of obtaining a hearing aid. The nurse would include in a response that a hearing aid will have which of the following effects for this client?

1. It will intensify the already distorted sounds.
2. It will improve the client's ability to distinguish words from background noises.
3. It will make sounds louder and clearer.
4. It will have no effect on hearing.

7 A client reports ongoing problems with vertigo. The nurse should question the client about which of the following accompanying manifestations to determine whether the client has developed Meniere's disease?

1. Purulent discharge from the ear and pain
2. Headache and double vision
3. Nausea, vomiting, and headache
4. Tinnitus, hearing loss, and a sense of fullness in the ear

8 The nurse prepares to initiate client teaching for which of the following medications commonly used to treat a client diagnosed with Meniere's disease?

1. Meclizine (Antivert)
2. Dexamethasone (Decadron)
3. Acetaminophen (Tylenol)
4. Propranolol (Inderal)

9 A client with glaucoma has been prescribed pilocarpine (Pilocar). The nurse explaining the use of this medication would state that it is useful because it works by

1. dilating the pupil.
2. constricting intraocular vessels.
3. constricting the pupil.
4. relaxing the ciliary muscles.

10 The initial nursing intervention for a client in the emergency department who suffered a chemical burn to the eyes is to

1. administer analgesics as prescribed.
2. evaluate vision with and without prescription eyeglasses.
3. administer antibiotics as prescribed.
4. irrigate the eyes with 0.9% saline solution or water.

11 The nurse is caring for a client who is in the recovery area following cataract surgery. The nurse would ask the client about which of the following manifestations that would indicate onset of retinal detachment as a postoperative complication?

1. Increased lacrimation
2. Flashing lights and loss of part of the visual field
3. Sudden, severe eye pain
4. Inability to move the eye and loss accommodation

12 A client who was diagnosed with chronic open-angle glaucoma has been started on medication therapy with timolol maleate (Timoptic). The nurse assesses for which of the following possible adverse systemic responses to the drug?

1. Tachycardia
2. Anxiety
3. Bradycardia
4. Hypertension

13 The daughter of an elderly client diagnosed with dry macular degeneration asks the nurse to explain this disorder. In formulating a response, the nurse would include information that this condition is characterized by which of the following?

1. Atrophy and degeneration of outer pigmented layer of the retina
2. Scar formation between the retina and the choroid
3. Rapid and severe loss of vision
4. Separation of the retina from the choroids

14 The nurse is evaluating the effectiveness of preoperative teaching done for a client who needs to have repair of a detached retina. The nurse evaluates that the client understands the procedure if the client indicates that scleral buckling involves

1. using a piece of silicone to indent the sclera to increase contact between the retinal layers.
2. injecting air into the vitreous humor to push the detached retina against the choroid.
3. removing the torn segment of retina.
4. replacing the torn segment of the retina with donor retinal tissue.

15 The nurse would take which of the following actions when the client first comes into the emergency department with blunt trauma to the eye?

1. Irrigate the eye to remove foreign substances.
2. Administer miotics.
3. Place the client in semi-Fowler's position.
4. Prevent loss of intraocular contents.

16 Which of the following statements indicates that the client has understood home care instructions following cataract surgery?

1. "I should not bend over to pick up objects from the floor."
2. "I can sleep on whichever side I want as long as my head is raised."
3. "I may not watch television for 6 weeks."
4. "I should keep the protective eye shield in place 24 hours a day."

17 The nurse is assessing a client's hearing using the Weber test. The nurse documents the client's result as normal if the client reports which of the following after placement of the vibrating tuning fork on the midline vertex of his head?

1. Sound lateralizes to the left ear.
2. Sound lateralizes to the right ear.
3. Sound is absent in both ears.
4. Sound is heard equally in both ears.

18 The nurse has an order to do an otic irrigation to the left ear of an assigned client. The nurse implements this procedure correctly by doing which of the following?

1. Direct the stream into the center of the ear canal.
2. Draw up 250 mL of solution.
3. Pack the external ear tightly with cotton balls after instilling the irrigant.
4. Help the client to lie on the left side after the irrigation is finished.

19 Which of the following would be least useful for the nurse to use as part of the collaborative management of a client who has conjunctivitis?

1. Cold eye compresses
2. Careful handwashing
3. Antibiotic therapy
4. Dark sunglasses

20 The nurse who is administering an ophthalmic medication to a client would do which of the following as correct procedure?

1. Drop the medication onto the eyeball.
2. Apply pressure to the inner canthus while administering the medication.
3. Rub the eye with a cotton ball after instillation.
4. Wait 10 seconds between drops.

21 The nurse has administered a dose of antibiotic intramuscularly to a 5-year-old client with tonsillitis. The child cries for a Band-Aid over the injection site. Which of the following is the best nursing action?

1. Apply a Band-Aid.
2. Ask the child why he wants the Band-Aid.
3. Explain to the child that a Band-Aid dressing is not necessary.
4. Show the child that the site is not bleeding.

22 Which is the most appropriate nursing intervention when caring for an infant with acute otitis media and 102.7°F fever?

1. Provide sponging with cool water to reduce fever.
2. Encourage the baby's intake of solids to maintain adequate caloric intake.
3. Swaddle the baby in layers of blankets to promote comfort and prevent chills.
4. Offer fluids frequently to prevent dehydration.

23 Which of the following would be the most appropriate nursing diagnosis for a child with pharyngitis?

1. Disturbed body image
2. Risk for ineffective airway clearance
3. Risk for deficient fluid volume
4. Impaired growth and development

24 The nurse recommends a humidified atmosphere for a child with recurrent epistaxis. When questioned by the parent, the nurse explains that which of the following is a benefit of humidity for the child?

1. Liquefies secretions
2. Improves oxygenation
3. Increases ventilation
4. Prevents drying of mucous membranes

25 A 9-month-old infant has been diagnosed with conjunctivitis. An antibiotic ointment has been prescribed. In teaching the mother to administer this drug, the nurse would recommend which of the following?

1. Wait until the child is asleep to instill the ointment.
2. Mummy the child to prevent accidental injury.
3. Place the ointment on a swab and spread across closed lids.
4. Use sterile gauze to apply the ointment to the lids.

26 The nurse would provide which of the following instructions to the client after fluorescein angiography? Select all that apply.

1. Encourage reduced fluid intake to limit intraocular pressure.
2. The dye causes temporary green discoloration to urine.
3. Avoid sunlight until pupil size returns to normal.
4. Lie down with eyes closed for 12 hours postprocedure after returning home.
5. Expect headache and blurred vision for approximately 24 hours after the procedure.

ANSWERS & RATIONALES

1 **Answer: 4** The best method to improve communication with the client is to eliminate background noises that could interfere with hearing. The client should be approached from the front so as not to frighten him or her. The nurse should use normal pronunciation of words, speak in normal tones, and refrain from shouting, which is demeaning and not helpful.
Cognitive Level: Analysis **Client Need:** Physiological Integrity: Physiological Adaptation **Integrated Process:** Communication and Documentation **Content Area:** Adult Health: Eye and Ear **Strategy:** The core issue of the question is the appropriate strategy for communicating with a client who is hearing impaired. Recall that clients rely on visual cues and can benefit from reduced background noise to aid in answering the question.

2 **Answer: 4** Ear pain is the most common symptom of otitis media that motivates clients to seek health care; secondary or associated symptoms include fever, nausea and vomiting, dizziness, and hearing impairment.
Cognitive Level: Analysis **Client Need:** Physiological Integrity: Physiological Adaptation **Integrated Process:** Nursing Process: Evaluation **Content Area:** Adult Health: Eye and Ear **Strategy:** The critical words in the question are *most common,* which tell you it is necessary to prioritize the options in terms of the frequency of their occurrence. Use nursing knowledge and the process of elimination to make this selection.

3 **Answer: 2** Myringotomy is a surgical procedure that perforates the tympanic membrane to allow drainage from the middle ear. Postoperatively, the client should avoid getting water into the ear canal, which could potentially enter the middle ear. The other activities are not risks to the client.
Cognitive Level: Application **Client Need:** Physiological Integrity: Physiological Adaptation **Integrated Process:** Nursing Process: Implementation **Content Area:** Adult Health: Eye and Ear **Strategy:** The core issue of the question is identification of activities that could be harmful to the client while healing is occurring after surgery. Recall that it is necessary to avoid getting the surgical area wet to make the appropriate selection.

4 **Answer: 1** Presbycusis is the most common form of sensorineural hearing loss in older adults. Otalgia is an earache; otitis externa is infection in the external auditory canal and can occur in clients of any age. Meniere's disease is an inner ear disorder that primarily affects middle-aged adults.
Cognitive Level: Application **Client Need:** Physiological Integrity: Physiological Adaptation **Integrated Process:** Nursing Process: Analysis **Content Area:** Adult Health: Eye and Ear **Strategy:** The core issue of the question is the ability to identify age-related changes in hearing in an older adult. Use nursing knowledge and the process of elimination to make a selection.

5 **Answer: 2** The client should avoid lying on the operative side following eye surgery in order to minimize edema and intraocular pressure. Options 3 and 4 pose no risk to the client. Option 1 is not a problem given the information in the question. Some clients with severe visual impairment or other health problems may need assistance to move about in the environment.
Cognitive Level: Analysis **Client Need:** Physiological Integrity: Physiological Adaptation **Integrated Process:** Nursing Process: Implementation **Content Area:** Adult Health: Eye and Ear **Strategy:** The core issue of the question is client teaching about safe and unsafe activities following cataract surgery. Recall that it is important to avoid positions in which gravity can lead to increased edema in order to make the correct selection.

6 **Answer: 1** When hearing loss is characterized by distortion of sounds, amplification of sound is of little help because it only increases the intensity of distorted sounds. The other options are incorrect.
Cognitive Level: Application **Client Need:** Physiological Integrity: Physiological Adaptation **Integrated Process:** Nursing Process: Implementation **Content Area:** Adult Health: Eye and Ear **Strategy:** The core issue of the question is the ability to correlate the types of hearing loss that can be improved with the use of a hearing aid. To do this, reflect on the types of hearing loss and the likely effect of a hearing aid for that condition. Use nursing knowledge and the process of elimination to make a selection.

7 **Answer: 4** Vertigo, tinnitus, hearing loss, and a sense of fullness in the ear are classic symptoms of Meniere's disease. Nystagmus also occurs with acute attacks. Headache, double vision, and pain are not part of this clinical picture. Purulent drainage suggests infection.
Cognitive Level: Application **Client Need:** Physiological Integrity: Physiological Adaptation **Integrated Process:** Nursing Process: Assessment **Content Area:** Adult Health: Eye and Ear **Strategy:** The core issue of the question is identification of signs and symptoms of Meniere's disease. Recall that this is a disorder of the inner ear, thus making symptoms related to balance as

well as hearing important to identify. Use nursing knowledge and the process of elimination to make a selection.

8 **Answer: 1** Antivertigo and antiemetic medications, such as meclizine, are used to control symptoms associated with Meniere's disease. Diuretics are used between acute attacks to reduce the volume of endolymph and prevent attacks. Glucocorticoids (option 2), beta-blockers (option 4), and analgesics (option 3) are not part of an effective treatment plan.
Cognitive Level: Analysis **Client Need:** Physiological Integrity: Physiological Adaptation **Integrated Process:** Nursing Process: Planning **Content Area:** Adult Health: Eye and Ear **Strategy:** The core issue of the question is the ability to anticipate medications that will be effective in relieving the symptoms associated with Meniere's disease. To answer correctly, it is necessary to have a core body of knowledge related to pharmacology. Use nursing knowledge and the process of elimination to make a selection.

9 **Answer: 3** Pilocarpine is a miotic agent, which constricts the pupil and thereby stimulates the ciliary muscles to pull on the trabecular meshwork surrounding the canal of Schlemm, which increases the flow of aqueous humor and decreases intraocular pressure.
Cognitive Level: Application **Client Need:** Physiological Integrity: Physiological Adaptation **Integrated Process:** Nursing Process: Implementation **Content Area:** Adult Health: Eye and Ear **Strategy:** The core issue of the question is the ability to anticipate medications that will be effective in relieving the symptoms associated with glaucoma. To answer correctly, it is necessary to have a core body of knowledge related to pharmacology. Use nursing knowledge and the process of elimination to make a selection.

10 **Answer: 4** The immediate priority for clients with chemical burns is flushing the affected eye with copious amounts of normal saline or water. Evaluation of visual acuity is an appropriate intervention after flushing. Analgesics, with the exception of topical anesthesia, are not indicated. Antibiotics may be administered after the initial actions have been taken.
Cognitive Level: Application **Client Need:** Safe Effective Care Environment: Safety and Infection Control **Integrated Process:** Nursing Process: Implementation **Content Area:** Adult Health: Eye and Ear **Strategy:** The critical word in the question is *initial,* which tells you that more than one or all options could be correct and that it is necessary to prioritize the most important or immediate action needed. Whenever there is an injury involving chemicals, the priority action is to remove the offending substance.

11 **Answer: 2** Clients with retinal detachment frequently report flashing lights and loss of vision, commonly described as a veil or curtain being drawn across the eye. Retinal detachment is not associated with increased lacrimation or tearing (option 1), eye pain (option 3), or change in ocular movements (option 4).
Cognitive Level: Application **Client Need:** Physiological Integrity: Physiological Adaptation **Integrated Process:** Nursing Process: Assessment **Content Area:** Adult Health: Eye and Ear **Strategy:** The core issue of the question is knowledge of complications of cataract surgery. Use nursing knowledge and the process of elimination to make a selection.

12 **Answer: 3** Medications that end in *-olol* are beta-adrenergic blocking agents. When taken as ophthalmic preparations, they can produce systemic effects such as bradycardia, hypotension, and bronchospasm. Beta-adrenergic blockers act as CNS depressants and may also be used to treat anxiety, but this does not relate to the issue of this question, which is glaucoma.
Cognitive Level: Application **Client Need:** Physiological Integrity: Physiological Adaptation **Integrated Process:** Nursing Process: Assessment **Content Area:** Adult Health: Eye and Ear **Strategy:** The core issue of the question is the ability to identify adverse effects of medication used to treat glaucoma. To answer correctly, it is necessary to have a core body of knowledge related to pharmacology. Use nursing knowledge and the process of elimination to make a selection.

13 **Answer: 1** Atrophic or dry macular degeneration results from atrophy and degeneration of the outer layer of the retina. In exudative or wet macular degeneration, blood leaks into the subretinal space and scar tissue gradually forms. The resulting loss of vision occurs rapidly and is more profound. Exudative macular degeneration accounts for 90% of all cases of legal blindness.
Cognitive Level: Application **Client Need:** Physiological Integrity: Physiological Adaptation **Integrated Process:** Nursing Process: Implementation **Content Area:** Adult Health: Eye and Ear **Strategy:** The core issue of the question is the ability to discriminate correct information to be used in teaching clients and/or families about disease processes. Thus, to answer this question, it is necessary to understand the two types of macular degeneration and how they present in terms of symptoms. Use nursing knowledge and the process of elimination to make a selection.

14 **Answer: 1** Scleral buckling is correctly described in option 1. It is used in conjunction with laser photocoagulation or cryothermy to achieve the best results. Option 2 defines pneumatic retinopexy. Options 3 and 4 are incorrect.
Cognitive Level: Application **Client Need:** Physiological Integrity: Physiological Adaptation **Integrated Process:** Nursing Process: Evaluation **Content Area:** Adult Health: Eye and Ear **Strategy:** The core issue of the question is evaluation of a client's understanding of a surgical procedure. To select correctly, it is necessary to be able to identify how the surgery will be performed. Use nursing knowledge and the process of elimination to make a selection.

15 **Answer: 3** Prevention or reduction of intraocular pressure (that may accompany blunt trauma to the eye) can be accomplished by the use of semi-Fowler's position and administration of a carbonic anhydrase inhibitor, such as acetazolamide (Diamox). Semi-Fowler's position also reduces edema formation at the site of injury when compared to lying flat. Constriction of the pupil with miotics is not indicated. Blunt trauma does not cause loss of intraocular contents; and no foreign body is present.
Cognitive Level: Application **Client Need:** Physiological Integrity: Physiological Adaptation **Integrated Process:** Nursing Process: Planning **Content Area:** Adult Health: Eye and Ear **Strategy:** The

core issue of the question is identification of a correct action in the treatment of eye trauma. Recall that injuries are characterized by formation of edema at the site, and therefore early actions for any injury may involve proper positioning of the client to reduce edema formation.

16 **Answer: 1** The client should avoid activities that raise intraocular pressure, such as bending over. The client should sleep on the nonoperative side. Activities involving the eyes are done at the advice of the surgeon. Typically, an eye shield is used at night, and dark protective glasses are worn during the day.
Cognitive Level: Application **Client Need:** Physiological Integrity: Physiological Adaptation **Integrated Process:** Nursing Process: Evaluation **Content Area:** Adult Health: Eye and Ear **Strategy:** The core issue of the question is the ability to evaluate client understanding of postoperative instructions following cataract surgery. Evaluate each of the options in terms of the truth of the statement, since the question contains the critical word *understood.*

17 **Answer: 4** To perform the Weber test, the nurse places a vibrating tuning fork on the midline vertex of the client's head. The sound should normally be heard equally in both ears. Sound that lateralizes to one side indicates either conductive hearing loss on that side or sensorineural hearing loss on the opposite side.
Cognitive Level: Analysis **Client Need:** Physiological Integrity: Physiological Adaptation **Integrated Process:** Nursing Process: Assessment **Content Area:** Adult Health: Eye and Ear **Strategy:** The core issue of the question is the ability to correctly analyze results of physical assessment techniques. Use nursing knowledge and the process of elimination to make a selection.

18 **Answer: 4** The client should lie on the affected side following the irrigation to allow gravity to further assist in draining the ear canal. The irrigant should be directed along the wall of the external canal, not the center (which could damage the tympanic membrane). Usually, 50 to 70 mL of solution are used, according to the size of the syringe used for the procedure. A single cotton ball is placed loosely into the external meatus to absorb any remaining irrigant after the procedure.
Cognitive Level: Application **Client Need:** Physiological Integrity: Physiological Adaptation **Integrated Process:** Nursing Process: Implementation **Content Area:** Adult Health: Eye and Ear **Strategy:** The core issue of the question is the ability to correctly perform the nursing procedure of eye irrigation. Use nursing knowledge and the process of elimination to make a selection.

19 **Answer: 1** Warm compresses, not cold, should be used as part of the management of conjunctivitis. Warm compresses help relieve discomfort and reduce inflammation by increasing circulation to the area. The other options contain items that are part of the standard collaborative management for conjunctivitis. Dark sunglasses are helpful in reducing photophobia.
Cognitive Level: Application **Client Need:** Physiological Integrity: Physiological Adaptation **Integrated Process:** Nursing Process: Implementation **Content Area:** Adult Health: Eye and Ear **Strategy:** The critical words in the stem of the question are *least useful,* indicating that the correct answer is an option that is either incorrect or lowest priority. Use nursing knowledge about care of the client with conjunctivitis and the process of elimination to make a selection.

20 **Answer: 2** The nurse should apply pressure to the inner canthus (nasolacrimal duct) during and for at least 30 seconds following instillation, according to agency procedure. Doing so will help prevent systemic absorption of the medication. The medication should be dropped into the lower conjunctival sac. The eye should not be rubbed after instillation of the medication. The nurse should wait from 1 to 5 minutes between drops, depending on the medication and manufacturer's recommendations.
Cognitive Level: Application **Client Need:** Physiological Integrity: Physiological Adaptation **Integrated Process:** Nursing Process: Implementation **Content Area:** Adult Health: Eye and Ear **Strategy:** The core issue of the question is the ability to administer eye medication correctly. Use nursing knowledge and the process of elimination to make a selection.

21 **Answer: 1** It is appropriate to comfort the child following a painful procedure. Option 1 provides support and comfort. By fulfilling the child's request, the nurse allows the child to regain some control over the situation. It is not appropriate to argue with the child.
Cognitive Level: Analysis **Client Need:** Psychosocial Integrity **Integrated Process:** Nursing Process: Implementation **Content Area:** Child Health: Eye and Ear **Strategy:** The core issue of the question is the best response to a 5-year-old client who is responding to a painful procedure such as an injection. Eliminate options 2 and 3 because these communications do not meet the client's immediate need for comfort following the injection, and option 4 is incorrect because the issue is a psychological/comfort issue, not a question of stopping bleeding.

22 **Answer: 4** A febrile infant is at risk for fluid volume deficit resulting from larger-than-normal insensible fluid losses and decreased fluid intake. It is contraindicated to sponge with cool water or add blankets. Intake of solid food is less important than preventing dehydration.
Cognitive Level: Analysis **Client Need:** Physiological Integrity: Physiological Adaptation **Integrated Process:** Nursing Process: Implementation **Content Area:** Child Health: Eye and Ear **Strategy:** The core issue of the question is an appropriate nursing intervention when a client has hyperthermia. Use nursing knowledge and the process of elimination to make a selection.

23 **Answer: 3** A symptom of pharyngitis is sore throat and difficult swallowing, which could lead to the refusal to drink. Thus, risk for deficient fluid volume is an appropriate diagnosis. Option 2 would apply when the client cannot clear secretions from the respiratory tract, which is not applicable to this question. Options 1 and 4 are not pertinent to this health problem.
Cognitive Level: Analysis **Client Need:** Physiological Integrity: Physiological Adaptation **Integrated Process:** Nursing Process: Planning **Content Area:** Child Health: Eye and Ear **Strategy:** The core issue of the question is the ability to determine priority

concerns for a client with pharyngitis by selecting a nursing diagnosis. Whenever the airway is involved, first think about the ABCs and then think about hydration/food intake as the next priority of physiological needs using Maslow's hierarchy.

24 **Answer: 4** Humidifying the air can prevent dry mucous membranes and recurrence of epistaxis. Other options do not correctly identify the benefit of humidity for a client with recurrent nosebleed.
Cognitive Level: Application **Client Need:** Physiological Integrity: Physiological Adaptation **Integrated Process:** Nursing Process: Implementation **Content Area:** Child Health: Eye and Ear **Strategy:** The core issue of the question is an understanding of the rationale for nursing actions for a client with recurrent epistaxis. Use nursing knowledge and the process of elimination to make a selection.

25 **Answer: 2** Children of this age cannot understand the necessity of cooperating with medication administration. Mummying the child reduces the risk of injury from the ointment tip and promotes adequate dosing. Applying ointment to the eyes of a sleeping child would increase the child's fears. The ointment is instilled in the lower conjunctival sac, not on the lids.
Cognitive Level: Application **Client Need:** Physiological Integrity: Physiological Adaptation **Integrated Process:** Nursing Process: Implementation **Content Area:** Child Health: Eye and Ear **Strategy:** The core issue of the question is identification of correct procedure for administering an ophthalmic medication to a child. Use nursing knowledge of this basic procedure and the process of elimination to make a selection.

26 **Answer: 2, 3** Typical instructions after fluorescein angiography include increased fluid intake to aid in dye excretion. The client should know that the dye causes temporary skin discoloration in the injected area and temporary green discoloration of urine that resolves when dye is fully excreted. The client should avoid sunlight or other bright light sources for several days until pupil dilation returns to normal. Although the client should rest after the procedure, it is not necessary to lie down with eyes closed for 12 hours. Headache and blurred vision are not expected.
Cognitive Level: Analysis **Client Need:** Physiological Integrity: Physiological Adaptation **Integrated Process:** Teaching and Learning **Content Area:** Adult Health: Eye and Ear **Strategy:** The core issue of the question is knowledge of post-procedure instructions to a client following fluorescein dye eye examination. Use nursing knowledge and general concepts of procedures that utilize contrast dye to make your selections.

Key Terms to Review

amblyopia p. 1300
cataract p. 1303
corneal light reflex (Hirschberg test) p. 1301
cover-uncover test p. 1301
cycloplegic p. 1299
epistaxis p. 1313
glaucoma p. 1302
gonioscopy p. 1302
Meniere's disease p. 1311
miotic p. 1302
mydriatic p. 1299
nystagmus p. 1296
otitis media p. 1310
otosclerosis p. 1309
pharyngitis p. 1313
presbycusis p. 1294
presbyopia p. 1294
proprioception p. 1294
strabismus p. 1301
tonometry p. 1295
tonsillitis p. 1314

References

Ball, J., & Bindler, R. (2006). *Child health Nursing: Partnering with children and families.* Upper Saddle River, NJ: Pearson Education.

Black, J., & Hawks, J. (2005). *Medical surgical nursing: Clinical management for positive outcomes* (7th ed.). St. Louis: Elsevier Science.

Corbett, J. (2004). *Laboratory tests and diagnostic procedures with nursing diagnoses* (6th ed.). Upper Saddle River, NJ: Pearson Education.

Harkreader, H., & Hogan, M. (2004). *Fundamentals of Nursing: Caring and clinical judgment* (2nd ed.). St. Louis: Elsevier Science.

Ignatavicius, D., & Workman, L. (2006). *Medical-surgical nursing: Critical thinking for collaborative care* (5th ed.). Philadelphia: W. B. Saunders.

Kozier, B., Erb, G., Berman, A., & Snyder, S. (2004). *Fundamentals of nursing: Concepts, process, and practice* (7th ed.). Upper Saddle River, NJ: Pearson Education.

LeMone, P., & Burke, K. (2004). *Medical surgical nursing: Critical thinking in client care* (3rd ed.). Upper Saddle River, NJ: Pearson Education.

Porth, C. (2004). *Pathophysiology: Concepts of altered health states* (7th ed.). Philadelphia: Lippincott Williams & Wilkins.

Smith, S., Duell, D., & Martin, B. (2004). *Clinical nursing skills: Basic to advanced skills* (6th ed.). Upper Saddle River, NJ: Pearson Education.

65 Hematological Disorders

Test Yourself

Are you ready for the NCLEX-RN® or course exams? Use the practice tests on the companion CD-ROM to check.

In this chapter

Cross reference

Other chapters relevant to this content area are

Meeting Nutritional Needs	Chapter 26
Blood and Blood Component Therapy	Chapter 33
Common Laboratory Tests	Chapter 47
Common Diagnostic Tests and Procedures	Chapter 48

I. OVERVIEW OF ANATOMY AND PHYSIOLOGY OF THE HEMATOLOGICAL SYSTEM

A. Blood components

1. Plasma: straw-colored liquid portion of blood; comprises 50% to 55% of a blood sample; consists of water (approximately 92%), amino acids, proteins, carbohydrates, lipids, vitamins, hormones, electrolytes, and cellular wastes
2. Serum is essentially the same as plasma only without fibrinogen and clotting factors
3. Blood cells (red blood cells [RBCs], white blood cells [WBCs]) and platelets comprise remaining blood sample; see Chapter 47 for detailed discussion of blood cells
4. Volume of blood is approximately 8% of total body weight

B. Normal clotting mechanisms

1. **Hemostasis** and coagulation are a series of reactions leading to clot formation in an injured or damaged area

2. Involves three mechanisms: vascular constriction and spasm, formation of platelet plug, and activation of clotting factors; fibrin clot is produced through either intrinsic or extrinsic pathway; both pathways end in common coagulation cascade
   a. Intrinsic pathway: stimulated by contact with foreign surfaces without tissue damage; initiated by activation of Hageman factor which, in presence of calcium (Ca^+) ions, triggers a series of changes leading to formation of prothrombin activator
   b. Extrinsic pathway: triggered by release of tissue thromboplastin from damaged tissues
3. After a clot forms, **fibrinolysis** (clot breakdown) occurs; plasminogen from blood clot is transformed into plasmin, which dissolves fibrin strands of clot; peak action is 7 to 10 days after clot formation

II. DIAGNOSTIC TESTS AND ASSESSMENTS OF HEMATOLOGICAL SYSTEM

A. RBC count (see Table 65–1 ■)

B. Hemoglobin and hematocrit
1. Hemoglobin (Hgb) measures oxygen-carrying capacity of an erythrocyte
2. Hematocrit (Hct) is ratio of RBC volume to volume of whole blood

C. RBC indexes
1. MCV (mean corpuscular volume): estimates size of RBC
2. MCH (mean corpuscular hemoglobin): measures content of Hgb in RBCs from a single cell
3. MCHC (mean corpuscular hemoglobin concentration): more accurate measurement of the Hgb content of RBC because it measures entire volume of RBCs

D. Serum ferritin, transferrin, and total iron-binding capacity (TIBC): evaluate iron levels; ferritin measures the iron in plasma, which is also a direct reflection of total iron stores; transferrin is major iron-transport protein

E. WBC count (see Table 65–2 ■)
1. Abnormal elevation of WBC count is referred to as **leukocytosis**
2. **Leukopenia** is a decrease in the number of WBCs
3. Differential count refers to breakdown of different types of cells

F. Coagulation studies
1. *Bleeding time:* normal range is 1 to 4 minutes; used in evaluation of platelet function; extended bleeding times are seen with **thrombocytopenia** (decrease or

Table 65–1

Normal Laboratory Values for Red Blood Cells and Platelets

Laboratory Test	Normal Value
Red blood cell count	
Men	4.2–5.4 million/mm^3
Women	3.6–5.0 million/mm^3
Reticulocytes	1.0–1.5% of total RBC
Hemoglobin (Hgb)	
Men	14–16.5 grams/dL
Women	12–15 grams/dL
Hematocrit (Hct)	
Men	40–50%
Women	37–47%
Mean corpuscular volume (MCV)	85–100 fL/cell
Mean corpuscular hemoglobin concentration (MCHC)	31–35 grams/dL
Mean corpuscular hemoglobin (MCH)	27–34 pg/cell
Platelet count	150,000–400,000/mm^3

Source: Adapted from Lemone, P., & Burke, K. (2004). *Medical-surgical nursing: Critical thinking in client care* (3rd ed.). Upper Saddle River, NJ: Pearson Education, p. 934.

Table 65-2

Normal Laboratory Values: White Blood Cells

Laboratory Test	Value
WBC count	5,000–10,000/mm^3
Differential	
Neutrophils	60–70% or 3,000–7,000/mm^3
Eosinophils	1–3% or 50–400/mm^3
Basophils	0.3–0.5% or 25–200/mm^3
Lymphocytes	20–30% or 1,000–4,000/mm^3
Monocytes	3–8% or 100–600/mm^3

Source: LeMone, P., & Burke, K. (2004). *Medical surgical nursing: Critical thinking in client care* (3rd ed.). Upper Saddle River, NJ: Pearson Education, p. 960.

cessation of platelet production) and aspirin therapy, as well anticoagulants and several other drugs

! 2. *Prothrombin Time (PT):* measures rapidity of blood clotting; normal range is 11 to 16 seconds; PT evaluates extrinsic coagulation pathway, which includes factors I, II, V, VII, X; International normalized ratio (INR) is often used instead of PT because it is a standardized value (therapeutic range often varies from 2 to 3 depending on condition)
3. *Partial thromboplastin time (PTT):* normal range is 60 to 70 seconds, which evaluates intrinsic coagulation pathway or fibrin clot formation

! 4. *Activated partial thromboplastin time (aPTT):* normal range is 30 to 45 seconds; is a modified PTT, preferred because it is quicker to perform; aPTT is used in heparin therapy and in the evaluation of hemophilia; aPTT is increased in anticoagulation therapy, liver disease, vitamin K deficiency, and disseminated intravascular coagulopathy (DIC)
5. *Fibrinogen:* normal range is 150 to 400 mg/dL; it is a soluble plasma protein necessary for clotting that is decreased in DIC and fibrinogen disorders and increased in acute infections, hepatitis, and oral contraceptive use
6. *Fibrin degradation products (FDP):* normal value is under 10 mcg/mL; FDP is increased in fibrinolysis, thrombolytic therapy, and DIC
7. *Fibrin D-dimer:* normal is 0 to 0.5 mcg/mL; D-dimer is the most sensitive indicator to differentiate DIC from primary fibrinolysis; it is elevated in DIC

G. Bone marrow examination

1. Specimens may be obtained by aspiration (most common) or biopsy

! 2. Sites for bone marrow aspiration may include sternum, iliac crest (most common), and tibia; the most common site for bone marrow biopsy is posterosuperior iliac spine; the sternum also is used
3. Position client based on site selected by physician; skin and periosteum are anesthetized to decrease pain with anesthetic such as procaine; marrow aspiration needle is then inserted; after marrow cavity is entered, marrow stylet is removed from needle and a sterile syringe is attached; syringe plunger is drawn back until marrow appears in syringe

! 4. During withdrawal of aspirate, client will experience sharp pain often described as burning

! 5. After needle is removed, apply pressure dressing over puncture site, where only minimal bleeding should occur; if client has thrombocytopenia, apply pressure for 3 to 5 minutes
6. Check agency procedure as to disposition of specimens
7. Most clients experience little, if any, pain or discomfort after procedure; some report tenderness and ache at aspiration site for a few days

! 8. Procedure for a bone marrow biopsy is essentially same as for aspiration; after procedure, assess clients for bleeding from puncture site

H. Lymphangiography: visualization of lymph system radiographically after injection of a dye; used primarily to stage Hodgkin's and non-Hodgkin's lymphoma

I. Lymph node biopsy: obtains lymph tissue for histologic analysis; a closed-needle biopsy can be done at the bedside, or an open biopsy can be performed in operating room

III. IRON-DEFICIENCY ANEMIA (IDA)

A. Overview: anemia that results when iron supply is inadequate for optimal RBC formation because of excessive iron loss from bleeding, decreased dietary intake, or malabsorption

1. Accounts for 60% of anemias in clients over age 65; most common cause is blood loss from GI or GU system
2. Normal iron excretion is less than 1 mg/day through urine, sweat, bile, feces, and from desquamated cells of the skin; an average woman loses 0.5 mg of iron daily or 15 mg monthly during menstruation (most common cause of iron deficiency in women); GI bleeding is most common cause in men
3. Anemia reduces O_2-carrying capacity of blood, producing tissue hypoxia
4. Iron is stored in body tissues (primarily in reticuloendothelial cells of liver, spleen, and bone marrow) as ferritin after being formed in intestinal mucosa
5. Anemia develops slowly through 3 phases: depletion of body stores of iron; insufficient iron transport to bone marrow, and onset of iron-deficient erythopoiesis
6. Average diet supplies body with 12 to 15 mg/day of iron, of which only 5% to 10% is absorbed; minimum daily needs are approximately 6 mg/day (infants under 6 months), 10 mg/day (6 months to adolescence, and over age 50), 12 mg/day (adolescent males), and 15 mg/day (females from adolescence to age 50)

! **B. Nursing assessment**

1. Fatigue and weakness
2. Shortness of breath
3. Pallor (ear lobes, palms, and conjunctiva)
4. Brittle spoonlike nails
5. **Cheilosis** (cracks in the corners of the mouth)
6. Smooth, sore tongue
7. Dizziness
8. Pica (craving to eat unusual substances such as clay or starch)
9. Blood sample shows **microcytic** and **hypochromic** anemia (small RBC diameter with decreased pigmentation) and an increase in red cell size distribution width (RDW)
   a. Decreased MCV, MCH, and MCHC; analyzed only when hemoglobin is low
   b. Low serum iron level and elevated serum iron-binding capacity or low serum ferritin levels

C. Therapeutic management

1. Assess history for cause
2. ! Examine stools for occult blood; endoscopic examination and other diagnostic procedures may be performed to detect possible sources of bleeding
3. ! Increase intake of iron-rich foods, such as organ meats, meat, beans, green leafy vegetables, molasses, and raisins
4. ! Administer iron supplements
   a. Give oral iron preparation with orange juice or vitamin C to increase absorption; antacids interfere with absorption of iron
   b. Oral liquid form of iron can stain teeth; clients should use a straw or place spoon at back of mouth to take supplement and rinse mouth thoroughly afterward
   c. Usual therapy is oral ferrous sulfate ($FeSO_4$) 300 to 325 mg t.i.d., given 1 hour before meals for 6 months; other oral forms may include ferrous gluconate (Fergon) and ferrous fumarate (Ircon, Femiron)
5. ! Administer parenteral iron dextran (InFed) by deep IM route via Z-track method
   a. Use separate needles for withdrawing and injecting medication
   b. There is risk of anaphylaxis with parenteral administration, so give small test dose before giving full dose
   c. Assess for systemic (allergic) reactions (flushing, nausea/vomiting, myalgias) and report promptly if they occur
6. Identify and implement energy-saving techniques (e.g., shower chair, sitting to perform tasks)
7. Promote quiet environment to facilitate sleep and rest
8. Monitor for dizziness; suggest position changes be made slowly

9. Provide assistance with activities and ambulation as needed, allowing patient independence as much as safely possible
10. Monitor laboratory studies (e.g., Hgb/Hct, RBC count)
11. Administer medications, blood, or blood products as indicated (see Chapter 33); monitor closely for transfusion reactions
12. Encourage and assist with good oral hygiene before and after meals, using soft-bristled toothbrush for gentle brushing of fragile gums
13. Determine stool color, consistency, frequency, and amount; may appear greenish black and tarry; caution client that iron supplements usually cause constipation and client should take preventive measures (fluids, fiber)
14. Encourage fluid intake of 2,500 to 3,000 mL day unless contraindicated by another medical condition, such as heart or renal failure
15. Discuss use of stool softeners, bulk-forming laxatives, mild stimulants, or enemas if indicated; monitor effectiveness
16. Refer to appropriate community resources when indicated (e.g., social services for food stamps, Meals on Wheels)
17. Transfusion of packed RBCs may be necessary if anemia is severe

D. Client teaching

1. Maintain good nutrition; older adults and those with limited economic means may have dietary deficiencies requiring referrals to appropriate agencies (e.g., Meals on Wheels)
2. Take iron on an empty stomach; absorption of iron is decreased with food; absorption may be enhanced when taken with an acidic beverage (such as one with vitamin C), but avoid grapefruit juice
3. Stools will appear black with oral iron intake
4. Report to health care provider persistent GI symptoms secondary to iron intake
5. Iron preparations cause constipation; use stool softeners and increase oral intake of fluids and fiber as preventive measures
6. Foods high in iron include organ meats (beef or calf liver, chicken liver), other meats, beans (black, pinto, and garbanzo), leafy green vegetables, raisins, and molasses

IV. MEGALOBLASTIC ANEMIA

A. Vitamin B_{12} deficiency anemia

1. Overview
   a. A type of anemia characterized by macrocytic RBCs
   b. Inevitably develops after total gastrectomy, 15% of clients develop pernicious anemia after partial gastrectomy or gastrojejunostomy
   c. Lack of vitamin B_{12} alters structure and disrupts function of peripheral nerves, spinal cord, and brain
   d. Lack of vitamin B_{12} impairs cellular division and maturation, especially in rapidly proliferating RBCs
   e. Pernicious anemia inhibits inability to absorb vitamin B_{12} because of lack of intrinsic factor, a substance secreted by parietal cells of gastric mucosa
2. Nursing assessment
   a. Pallor or slight jaundice with a complaint of weakness
   b. Smooth, sore, beefy red tongue (**glossitis**), and cheilosis (cracking of lips)
   c. Diarrhea
   d. Paresthesias (numbness or tingling in extremities)
   e. Impaired proprioception (difficulty identifying one's position in space, which may progress to difficulty with balance)
   f. Clients with this anemia tend to be fair-haired or prematurely gray
   g. Macrocytic (megaloblastic) anemia (RBC diameter >8) with increase in MCV and MCHC
   h. Gastric secretion analysis reveals achlorhydria: absence of free hydrochloric acid in a pH maintained at 3.5
   i. Twenty-four-hour urine for Schilling test (a vitamin B_{12} absorption test that indicates if client lacks intrinsic factor by measuring excretion of orally administered radionuclide-labeled B_{12}) confirms diagnosis of pernicious anemia

3. Therapeutic management
   a. Review required diet alterations to meet specific dietary needs; if deficiency is caused by vegetarian diet, fortified soy milk may be added, or oral supplements of B_{12} may be added
   b. Assess client carefully for neurologic deficits and assist client to prevent injury
   c. If deficiency is caused by gastric malabsorption such as deficiency of intrinsic factor, lifelong replacement therapy is required
   d. Medication therapy: parenteral vitamin B_{12}, 100 to 1000 mcg subcutaneously daily for 7 days, then once a week for 1 month, then monthly for lifetime is usually prescribed; a nasal form is now available also
4. Client teaching
   a. A burning sensation felt after a parenteral dose of vitamin B_{12} is temporary
   b. Dietary sources of vitamin B_{12} include dairy products, animal proteins, and eggs
   c. A regular schedule of replacement vitamin B_{12} and importance and necessity for continued treatment are important for clients who have pernicious anemia

B. Folic acid–deficiency anemia

1. Overview
   a. Anemia caused by a deficiency of folic acid resulting in interruption of DNA synthesis and normal maturation of RBCs; frequently accompanies iron-deficiency anemia
   b. Causative etiologies: poor nutrition, malabsorption syndrome, medications that impede the absorption (oral contraceptives, antiepileptics, methotrexate [MTX]), alcohol abuse, and anorexia
   c. Clients at risk include those with alcoholism, receiving total parenteral nutrition (TPN), pregnant women, infants, teenagers, and clients on hemodialysis
   d. Lack of folic acid causes formation of megaloblastic cells, which are fragile
2. Nursing assessment
   a. Pallor, progressive weakness, fatigue
   b. Shortness of breath
   c. Cardiac palpitations
   d. GI symptoms are similar to B_{12} deficiency but usually more severe (glossitis, cheilosis, and diarrhea)
   e. Neurological symptoms seen in B_{12} deficiency are not seen in folic acid deficiency and therefore assist in differentiating these two types of anemia
   f. RBC analysis shows macrocytic (megaloblastic) anemia (RBC diameter >8), high MCV with low hemoglobin, low serum folate level
3. Therapeutic management
   a. Includes dietary counseling and administration of folic acid
   b. Identify and implement energy-saving techniques (e.g., shower chair, sitting to perform tasks)
   c. Monitor for dizziness; suggest position changes be made slowly
   d. Provide assistance with activities and ambulation as needed, allowing client independence as much as safely possible
   e. Monitor laboratory studies (e.g., Hgb/Hct, RBC count)
   f. Encourage and assist with good oral hygiene before and after meals, using soft-bristled toothbrush for gentle brushing of fragile gums
   g. Refer to appropriate community resources when indicated (e.g., social services for food stamps, Meals on Wheels, Alcoholics Anonymous)
   h. Medication therapy: oral folate, 1 to 5 mg/day for 3 to 4 months; folate should be given along with vitamin B_{12} when both are deficient
4. Client teaching
   a. Dietary sources of folic acid such as green leafy vegetables, fish, citrus fruits, yeast, dried beans, grains, nuts, and liver
   b. Increase dietary intake through diet selection and supplementation for those at risk
   c. Strategies to decrease pain associated with glossitis such as eating bland and soft foods

V. APLASTIC ANEMIA

A. Overview

1. A form of anemia with decreased production of RBCs, WBCs, and platelets; may be congenital or acquired
2. Congenital aplastic anemia is caused by a chromosomal alteration
3. Acquired form may be caused by radiation, chemical agents and toxins, drugs, viral and bacterial infections, pregnancy, and idiopathic; in about 50% of cases, cause is unknown
4. There is a decrease or cessation of production of RBCs (**anemia**), WBCs (leukopenia), and platelets (thrombocytopenia); may result from damage to bone marrow stem cells, bone marrow itself, and replacement of bone marrow with fat; depending on causative factor, condition may be acute or chronic

! B. Nursing assessment

1. Pallor and fatigue
2. Palpitations and exertional dyspnea
3. Infections of the skin and mucous membranes
4. Bleeding from gums, nose, vagina, or rectum
5. Purpura (bruising)
6. Retinal hemorrhage
7. Blood counts reveal pancytopenia (decreased RBC, WBC, and platelets)
8. Decreased reticulocyte count
9. Bone marrow examination reveals decrease in activity of bone marrow or no cell activity

C. Therapeutic management

1. Identification of cause of bone marrow suppression
2. Bone marrow transplantation
3. Immunosuppression
4. Transfusion of leukocyte-poor RBCs
5. Splenectomy
6. ! Institute reverse isolation to protect client from infection
7. Limit visitors and potential sources of infection
8. ! Monitor for evidence of bleeding
9. ! Avoid invasive procedures including rectal temperatures
10. Provide frequent rest periods
11. Monitor tolerance to activities
12. Medication therapy: antilymphocyte globulin (ALG), antithymocyte globulin (ATG), and cyclosporine (Sandimmune), immunosuppresive agents such as prednisone and cyclophosphamide (Cytoxan)

D. Client teaching

1. ! Methods to prevent infection such as avoiding crowds, maintaining good hygiene, handwashing, and elimination of uncooked foods from the diet
2. ! Methods to prevent hemorrhage such as using a soft toothbrush, avoiding contact sports, and use of an electric razor
3. ! Avoid drugs that increase bleeding tendency, such as aspirin
4. Balance activity with adequate rest periods to avoid fatigue
5. Symptoms to report to health care provider, including signs of infection, bleeding, and increasing intolerance to activity

VI. SICKLE CELL DISEASE

A. Overview

1. A hereditary, chronic form of hemolytic anemia that predominantly affects clients of African descent
2. Sickle cell trait (heterozygous state) is a generally mild condition that produces few, if any, manifestations
3. Sickle cell anemia is caused by an autosomal genetic defect (one gene affected) that results in synthesis of hemoglobin S
4. Produced by a mutation in beta chain of hemoglobin molecule through a substitution of amino acid valine for glutamine in both beta chains

5. When there is decreased O_2 tension in plasma, hemoglobin S causes RBCs to elongate, become rigid, and assume a crescent, sickled shape; curved shape causes cells to clump together, obstructing capillary blood flow and leading to ischemia and possible tissue infarction
6. Conditions likely to trigger a sickle cell crisis include hypoxia, low environmental and/or body temperature, excessive exercise, high altitudes, and inadequate oxygen during anesthesia
7. Other causes of sickle cell crisis include elevated blood viscosity and decreased plasma volume, infection, dehydration, and increased hydrogen ion concentration (acidosis)
8. With normal oxygenation, sickled RBCs resume normal shape; repeated episodes of sickling and unsickling weaken cell membranes, causing them to hemolyze
9. Crisis is extremely painful and can last from 4 to 6 days

B. Nursing assessment

1. Pallor and jaundice
2. Fatigue and possible irritability
3. Large joints and surrounding tissue may become swollen during crisis
4. Priapism (abnormal, painful, continuous erection of penis) may occur if penile veins are obstructed
5. Severe pain
6. Anemia with sickled cells noted on a peripheral smear
7. Hemoglobin electrophoresis to detect presence and percentage of hemoglobin S is used for a definitive diagnosis
8. Elevated serum bilrubin levels
9. Elevated reticulocyte count

C. Therapeutic management

1. Bone marrow transplantation
2. Blood transfusions
3. Management of pain
4. Use of chemotherapy drug hydroxyurea (Droxia) to increase hemoglobin F and decrease sickling
5. Refer to appropriate agency for genetic counseling and family planning
6. Care of client in sickle cell crisis
   a. Recognize that client may have severe pain and medicate accordingly, usually with opioid analgesics
   b. Administer O_2 to increase oxygenation to cells
   c. Promote hydration to decrease blood viscosity; provide oral intake of at least 6 to 8 quarts daily or IV fluids of 3 liters daily
   d. Monitor for complications such as vaso-occlusive disease (thrombosis), hypoxia, CVA, renal dysfunction, priapism leading to impotence, acute chest syndrome (fever, chest pain, cough, pulmonary infiltrates, and dyspnea), and substance abuse
   e. Manage infection if appropriate
7. Medication therapy
   a. Nifedipine (Procardia) for priapism
   b. Hydroxyurea (Droxia) to increase hemoglobin F and decrease sickling
   c. Narcotic (opioid) analgesics during the acute phase of sickle cell crisis, often at large doses
   d. Broad-spectrum antibiotics to manage acute chest syndrome
   e. Folic acid supplements

D. Client teaching

1. Ways to prevent sickle cell crisis
   a. Maintain an oral intake of at least 4 to 6 quarts a day; avoid conditions that might predispose to dehydration
   b. Avoid high altitudes
   c. Prevent and promptly treat infections
   d. Use stress-reduction strategies
   e. Avoid exposure to cold
   f. Avoid overexertion

2. Importance of adhering to vaccination schedules for pneumococcal pneumonia, haemophilus influenza type B, and hepatitis B
3. Importance of regular medical follow-up

VII. POLYCYTHEMIA

A. Overview

1. An increased number of circulating RBCs and Hgb concentration in blood; also known as polycythemia vera (PV), or myeloproliferative red cell disorder; can be a primary or secondary disorder
2. Primary
   a. Neoplastic stem cell disorder characterized by increased production of RBCs, granulocytes, and platelets; more common in men of European Jewish descent over age 50
   b. With overproduction of RBCs, increased blood viscocity results in congestion of blood in tissues, liver, and spleen
   c. Thrombi form, acidosis develops, and tissue infarction occurs because of diminished blood flow caused by increased viscosity
3. Secondary
   a. Most common form; disturbance is not in RBC development but in excessive erythropoiesis as a physiologic response to hypoxia
   b. Chronic hypoxic states may be produced by prolonged exposure to high altitudes, pulmonary diseases, hypoventilation, and smoking
   c. Result of an increased RBC production is increased viscosity of blood, which alters circulatory flow

B. Nursing assessment

1. ! **Plethora:** a ruddy (dark, flushed) color of face, hands, feet, ears, and mucous membranes resulting from engorgement or distention of blood vessels
2. ! Symptoms associated with increased blood volume, including headaches, vertigo, blurred vision, and tinnitus
3. Distended superficial veins
4. Itching unrelieved by antihistamines
5. Symptoms associated with impaired tissue oxygenation, including angina, claudication, or dyspnea
6. Erythromyalgia, or burning sensation of the fingers and toes
7. Splenomegaly in majority of those with primary polycythemia vera
8. Epistaxis, GI bleeding
9. Elevated hemoglobin, hematocrit, RBC count, WBC count, basophils, and platelets
10. Decreased MCHC
11. Elevated leukocyte alkaline phosphatase, uric acid, cobalamin levels, and histamine levels
12. Bone marrow examination shows hypercellularity

C. Therapeutic management

1. ! Manage underlying condition (such as COPD) causing the chronic hypoxia
2. Repeated phlebotomy to decrease blood volume; goal is to keep hematocrit at 45% to 48% or lower
3. ! Hydration to decrease blood viscosity
4. Measures to relieve pruritus, including cool and tepid baths
5. Accurate monitoring of fluid intake and output
6. ! Nursing measures to prevent thrombotic events, including early ambulation, passive leg exercises when on bedrest, encouraging client to keep legs uncrossed and to maintain adequate hydration
7. Medication therapy
   a. Myelosuppressive agents to inhibit bone marrow activity including hydroxyurea (Hydrea), melphalan (Alkeran), and radioactive phosphorus
   b. Allopurinol to manage gout caused by increased uric acid levels (see also Chapter 62)
   c. Antiplatelet agents to prevent thrombotic complications

D. Client teaching

1. Maintain good hydration; drink at least 3 liters of fluid per day
2. Disease and methods of control, such as smoking cessation
3. Signs and symptoms of complications, including signs of vaso-occlusive states (MI, CVA) and bleeding, which require immediate medical attention
4. Prevent bleeding states such as by using electric razor and soft-bristled toothbrush, not flossing, and avoiding use of aspirin and aspirin-containing products
5. Importance of a regular medical check-up
6. Avoid products that contain iron
7. Ways to prevent thrombosis

VIII. THROMBOCYTOPENIA

A. Overview

1. Decrease in number of circulating platelets or platelet count of less than 100,000/mL blood
2. Decreased circulating platelets may result from three mechanisms: decreased production, increased destruction, or increased consumption
3. Cause of decreased platelet production may be inherited or acquired; inherited form is known as autoimmune or idiopathic thrombocytopenic purpura (ITP), and usually follows viral infection such as measles, rubella, or chicken pox
4. Causes of increased destruction of platelets include non–immune-related factors such as infection or drug-induced effects
5. A decrease in number of functional platelets leads to bleeding disorders; high risk for bleeding if platelet count is below 20,000/mm^3; cerebral and pulmonary hemorrhage can occur when platelet counts drop below 10,000/mm^3

B. Nursing assessment

1. Petechiae (pinpoint hemorrhages on skin and mucous membranes) and purpura (purplish discolored areas) most commonly found in mucous membranes, anterior thorax, arms, and neck
2. Epistaxis, gingival bleeding, menorrhagia, hematuria, and gastrointestinal bleeding (bloody or tarry stools)
3. Signs of internal hemorrhage
4. Decreased hemoglobin and hematocrit if bleeding is present
5. Decreased platelet count; platelet antibodies present if ITP
6. Prolonged bleeding time
7. Bone marrow examination may reveal decreased platelet activity or increased megakaryocytes

C. Therapeutic management

1. Treat underlying cause or remove causative agent in acquired thrombocytopenia
2. Platelet transfusions if there is active bleeding; little benefit in ITP
3. If medications are not successful, a splenectomy may be done in older child with 1 year of thrombocytopenia
4. Institute bleeding (thrombocytopenic) precautions
   a. Avoid intramuscular or subcutaneous injections
   b. Avoid indwelling catheters
   c. If absolutely necessary, use smallest gauge needles for injections or venipunctures; apply pressure on injection sites for 5 minutes or until bleeding stops
   d. Discourage straining at stool, vigorous coughing, and nose blowing
   e. Avoid rectal manipulation such as rectal temperatures, suppositories, or enemas
   f. Discourage the use of razors; use only electric shavers
   g. Use soft-bristled toothbrush or toothettes and avoid flossing
   h. Pad siderails if necessary and avoid tissue trauma
   i. Avoid use of aspirin and drugs that interfere with blood coagulation
5. Monitor for signs of bleeding; test stools for occult blood
6. Monitor CBC and platelet counts
7. Assess neurological status every shift and PRN
8. Medication therapy
   a. Steroids and immunoglobulins to suppress immune response in ITP

b. Immunosuppressive agents such as vincristine (Oncovin) and cyclophosphamide (Cytoxan)
c. Platelet growth factor such as oprelvekin (Neumega)

D. Client and family teaching

1. Monitor for signs of bleeding and when to contact primary care provider
2. Bleeding precautions such as using soft-bristled toothbrush, avoiding flossing, preventing tissue trauma and injury (including vigorous sexual intercourse), and using an electric razor for shaving
3. Methods of controlling bleeding and to seek medical assistance if severe
4. Avoid drugs that contain aspirin and others that interfere with coagulation
5. Medication dosing, schedule, and side effects
6. Importance of regular medical follow-up and platelet monitoring

IX. HEMOPHILIA

A. Overview

1. A group of hereditary clotting factor disorders characterized by prolonged coagulation time that results in prolonged and sometimes excessive bleeding
2. Hemophilia A and B are **X-linked recessive traits** transmitted by female carriers and displayed almost exclusively in males
   a. *Hemophilia A* (classic hemophilia) is a deficiency in factor VIII (an alpha-globulin that stabilizes fibrin clots; it is the most common form of hemophilia
   b. *Hemophilia B* (Christmas disease) is a deficiency in factor IX (a vitamin-dependent beta-globulin essential in stage 1 of the intrinsic coagulation system as an influence on the amount of thromboplastin available)
3. In clients with hemophilia A and B, platelet plugs are formed at site of bleeding, but clotting factor impairs coagulation response and capacity to form a stable clot
4. *Von Willebrand's disease* is a related disorder caused by deficiency of von Willebrand's factor (vWF) necessary for factor VIII activity and platelet adhesion

B. Nursing assessment

1. Persistent and prolonged bleeding from small cuts and injuries
2. Subcutaneous **ecchymosis** (black and blue mark) and subcutaneous hematomas
3. Gingival bleeding
4. GI bleeding, which may be manifested by hematemesis (vomiting blood), occult blood in stools, gastric pain, or abdominal pain
5. Urinary tract bleeding (hematuria)
6. Pain, paresthesia, or paralysis resulting from nerve compression by hematomas
7. **Hemarthrosis** (joint bleeding, swelling and damage)
8. APTT is increased in all types of hemophilia
9. Bleeding time is prolonged in von Willebrand's disease
10. Decreased factor VIII in hemophilia A, vWF in von Willebrand's disease, and factor IX in hemophilia B

C. Therapeutic management

1. Replacement of deficient coagulation factor(s)
2. Hemophilia A: cryoprecipitate containing 8 to 100 units of factor VIII per bag at 12-hour intervals until bleeding ceases; freeze-dried concentrate of factor VIII may also be given
3. Hemophilia B: plasma or factor IX concentrate given q 24 hours or until bleeding ceases
4. Von Willebrand's disease: cryoprecipitate containing 8 to 100 units of factor VIII per bag at 12-hour intervals until bleeding ceases; desmopressin (DDAVP) may also be used
5. Supportive treatment for hemarthrosis, including arthrocentesis and physiotherapy
6. Control of topical bleeding with hemostatic agents, pressure, and application of ice
7. Management of complications associated with hemorrhage
8. Refer for genetic counseling and family planning and to National Hemophilia Foundation for support and counseling
9. Monitor for signs of complications, including hemarthrosis and intracranial bleeding

10. Assist in managing pain associated with hemarthrosis; measures include joint immobilization, application of ice, and administration of analgesics; avoid aspirin and drugs affecting coagulation
11. Control bleeding and maintain hemostasis through direct pressure, application of topical hemostatic agents, and application of ice

D. Client teaching

1. Disease and therapeutic regimen
2. Signs and symptoms requiring immediate medical attention, such as severe joint pain, trauma or injury, and signs of uncontrolled internal bleeding
3. Precautions to prevent bleeding, including use of soft-bristled toothbrush, avoiding flossing, using electric razor, avoiding contact sports and other activities likely to cause injury, and avoiding aspirin and other drugs that interfere with coagulation
4. Wear a Medic-Alert bracelet indicating hemophilia; notify all health care providers of condition
5. Maintain good dental hygiene to decrease the necessity for invasive dental procedures
6. Importance of continued follow-up care with the primary health provider
7. Encourage genetic counseling if appropriate

X. DISSEMINATED INTRAVASCULAR COAGULOPATHY (DIC)

A. Overview

1. A syndrome characterized by abnormal initiation and acceleration of clotting and simultaneous hemorrhage; also called consumption coagulopathy
2. Precipitated by conditions such as widespread tissue damage, hemolysis, hypotension, hypoxia, and metabolic acidosis (see Box 65–1)
3. Clotting process initiated either through activation of factor XII, factors II and X, or release of tissue thromboplastin
4. Clotting factors II, V, VIII, fibrinogen, and platelets necessary for clotting are consumed more rapidly than they can be replaced
5. Body begins to break down clots with release of fibrin degradation products (FDPs), which are potent anticoagulants used to lyse the clots further; anticoagulants increase the bleeding state
6. With depletion of clotting factors and increase in FDPs, stable blood clots no longer form and hemorrhage occurs

B. Nursing assessment

1. Clinical manifestations (see Box 65–2)
2. Prolonged aPTT, PT, and thrombin time
3. Decreased fibrinogen and platelets
4. Elevated fibrin degradation products
5. Factor assays (factors V, VII, VIII, X, XIII): reduced
6. D-dimer (a cluster of above tests) elevated

C. Therapeutic management

1. Initiate treatment of underlying precipitating medical condition is a priority
2. Supportive treatment includes control of bleeding

Box 65–1

Risk Factors for DIC

- Venomous snakebite
- Tissue necrosis
- Sepsis
- Drug reactions
- Trauma
- Liver disease
- Obstetric complications
- Acute hemolysis
- Neoplasms
- Extensive burns
- Vascular disorders
- Prosthetic devices
- Hypoxia

Box 65-2

Clinical Manifestations of DIC

Integumentary
Decreased skin temperature
Pallor
Purpura
Ecchymosis
Hematomas
Acral cyanosis
Altered sensation
Superficial gangrene
Gingival bleeding
Bleeding from puncture sites

Gastrointestinal
Hemoptysis
Melena
Occult blood in stool or vomitus
Abdominal distention
Abdominal pain

Respiratory
Dyspnea
Tachypnea
Orthopnea
Decreased breath sounds
Chest pain

Cardiovascular
Decreased pulses
Decreased capillary filling time
Tachycardia
Venous distention

Genitourinary
Hematuria
Oliguria

Nervous System
Vision changes
Dizziness
Headache
Irritability
Anxiety
Confusion
Seizures

Musculoskeletal
Joint pain
Bone pain
Weakness

3. Life-threatening hemorrhage may be treated by administering platelets for thrombocytopenia; cryoprecipitate to replace fibrinogen, and factors V and VII; and fresh frozen plasma to replace all clotting factors except platelets; see Chapter 33 for administration of blood products
4. Assess client carefully for evidence of bleeding and altered tissue oxygenation
5. Institute thrombocytopenic/bleeding precautions (refer to previous discussion on thrombocytopenia)
6. Monitor intake and output (I & O) hourly
7. Monitor for signs of complications such as renal failure, pulmonary embolism, cerebrovascular accident, and acute respiratory distress syndrome
8. Provide emotional support to client and family
9. Medication therapy
   a. Heparin and antithrombin III, although their use is controversial; these drugs are usually indicated to manage thrombosis
   b. Epsilon aminocaproic acid (Amicar) to inhibit fibrinolysis
   c. Blood products (FFP, platelets, and cryoprecipitate)

D. Client teaching

1. Disorder, its treatments and interventions
2. Report symptoms of complications, including abdominal pain, headache, visual disturbances, and pain
3. Thrombocytopenic precautions (see previous client teaching section in thrombocytopenia)

XI. NEUTROPENIA

A. Overview

1. Neutrophils constitute about 70% of the total circulating WBCs
2. Neutropenia is a neutrophil count of less than 2,000/mm^3 (normal >2,000/mm^3)
3. Absolute neutrophil count (ANC) is determined using this formula:

$$\frac{\%\text{ neutrophils} + \%\text{bands}}{100} \times \text{total WBC count} = \text{ANC}$$

4. Caused by either decreased production or increased destruction of neutrophils
5. Because neutrophils play a major role in phagocytosis of microorganisms, neutropenia increases client's risk for infection
6. Neutropenia may occur as a primary hematologic disorder but may also be caused by drugs (such as cancer chemotherapy), autoimmune disorders, infections, and other medical conditions such as severe sepsis and nutritional deficiencies

B. Nursing assessment

1. Clinical manifestations: there are no real symptoms associated with neutropenia; it may not be discovered until client presents with signs of infection
2. Diagnostic and laboratory tests
   a. Absolute neutrophil count less than 1,000 to 1,500
   b. Bone marrow examination of cell morphology helps determine etiology of neutropenia

C. Therapeutic management

1. If etiology is drug-induced, medication should be discontinued whenever possible
2. Corticosteroids are used if etiology is immunologic
3. If etiology is decreased production, growth factors (granulocyte/macrophage colony–stimulating factor or GM-CSF) may be used
4. Monitor for signs of infection; monitor temperature elevations
5. Obtain cultures suspected as sites of infection
6. Infections are treated with antimicrobial therapy
7. Enforce strict hand hygiene by all individuals in contact with client
8. Institute reverse isolation (also called protective isolation); use private room with HEPA filtration if possible; do not allow those with infections to visit; use gloves and masks when entering client's room; prohibit known sources of microorganisms (plants, flowers, fresh unpeeled fruits and vegetables, standing water—such as water pitcher or vase)
9. Avoid invasive procedures whenever possible

D. Client teaching

1. What neutropenia is and rationale for therapeutic interventions
2. Report signs of fever
3. Strict hand hygiene and reverse-isolation procedure (for client and those who come in contact with client)
4. Maintain good personal hygiene to decrease microbes on skin

XII. LEUKEMIA

A. Overview

1. Malignancy of blood-forming tissues of bone marrow, spleen, and lymph system characterized by unregulated proliferation of WBCs and their precursors
2. Classified by type of WBC affected (granulocyte, lymphocyte, monocyte) and by cell differentiation (acute if majority of cells are primitive or poorly differentiated and chronic if mature or well differentiated)
3. Acute lymphocytic/lymphoblastic leukemia (ALL)
   a. Peak incidence at 2 to 4 years of age
   b. Immature granulocytes proliferate and accumulate in bone marrow
4. Chronic lymphocytic leukemia (CLL)
   a. More common in men and mainly between ages of 50 and 70
   b. Abnormal and incompetent lymphocytes proliferate and accumulate in lymph nodes and spread to other lymphatic tissues and spleen; most circulating cells are mature lymphocytes

5. Acute myelogenous/myelocytic leukemia (AML)
    a. All age groups are affected with a peak incidence at age 60
    b. There is uncontrolled proliferation of myeloblasts, which are precursors of granulocytes; they accumulate in bone marrow
6. Chronic myelogenous leukemia (CML)
    a. Uncommon in people under 20 years of age; incidence rises with age
    b. Uncontrolled proliferation of granulocytes results in increased circulating blast (immature) cells; marrow expands into long bones because of this proliferation and also extends into liver and spleen
    c. In most cases, Philadelphia chromosome, a characteristic chromosomal abnormality, is present
7. Abnormal or immature WBCs do not function properly; abnormal cells continue to multiply, infiltrate, and damage bone marrow, spleen, lymph nodes, liver, kidneys, lungs, gonads, skin, and CNS
8. Normal bone marrow becomes diffusely replaced with abnormal or immature WBCs, interfering with production of cells such as erythrocytes and thrombocytes; bone marrow becomes functionally incompetent with resulting bone marrow suppression
9. Acute leukemia has rapid onset and progression with a short clinical course; left untreated, death results in days or months; symptoms relate to depressed bone marrow, infiltration of leukemic cells into other organ systems, and hypermetabolism of leukemic cells
10. Chronic leukemia has more insidious onset and prolonged clinical course; usually asymptomatic early in disease; life expectancy may be more than 5 years; symptoms relate to hypermetabolism of leukemic cells infiltrating other organ systems; cells are more mature and function more effectively

B. Nursing assessment

1. Fever and night sweats
2. Bleeding such as ecchymoses, gingival bleeding, and epistaxis
3. Lymphadenopathy
4. Weakness and fatigue
5. Pruritic vesicular lesions
6. Anorexia and weight loss
7. Shortness of breath and decreased activity tolerance
8. Bone or joint pain
9. Visual disturbances
10. Pallor
11. Splenomegaly and hepatomegaly
12. Diagnostic and laboratory tests
    a. Increased WBC (in CLL and CML)
    b. A normal, decreased or increased WBC (in ALL and AML)
    c. Decreased reaction to skin sensitivity tests (**anergy**)
    d. Bone marrow tests reveal excessive blast cells in AML
    e. Philadelphia chromosome found in 90% to 95% of clients with CML; BCR/ABL gene is present in virtually all clients with CML
    f. Bone marrow biopsy and aspirate is the definitive diagnostic test

C. Therapeutic management

1. Induction of remission with chemotherapy and radiation therapy
2. Bone marrow and stem cell transplantation
3. Assist in bone marrow biopsy; apply pressure to site for 5 minutes or until bleeding stops; frequently assess site for signs of bleeding up to 4 hours after procedure
4. Institute neutropenic and bleeding precautions (see previous discussions)
5. Plan activities to prevent fatigue; provide measures for uninterrupted rest and sleep
6. Provide for diversionary activities
7. Maintain good nutrition; enlist assistance of a dietitian in maximizing and meeting nutritional needs of client
8. Assist client in maintaining good personal hygiene and promote good oral hygiene

9. Refer to appropriate agencies such as Meals on Wheels, American Cancer Society, and the Leukemia Society
10. Provide emotional support to client and family; refer to appropriate agency, organization, or professional for counseling and support
11. Administer prescribed drugs and monitor for side effects
12. Monitor laboratory results to evaluate effectiveness of interventions and therapy
13. Prepare client for bone marrow transplantation if part of treatment plan
14. Medication therapy: chemotherapeutic drugs include alkylating agents (Busulfan, Myleran), anthracyclines (Doxorubicin, Adriamycin), antimetabolites (Fludarabine, Fludara), corticosteroid (Prednisone), plant alkaloids (Vincristine, Oncovin), and others

D. Client teaching

1. Thrombocytopenic precautions; see previous discussion
2. Neutropenic precautions; see previous discussion
3. Maintain good oral hygiene; keep oral cavity moist: rinse mouth with saline, lubricate lips and oral mucosa with water-soluble lubricants every 2 hours; avoid alcohol-based mouthwash; use sponge-tipped applicators for oral hygiene if neutrophil and/or platelet counts are low
4. Measures to prevent perirectal complications: wash and clean perineal area thoroughly after each bowel movement
5. Therapeutic plans and interventions

XIII. MALIGNANT LYMPHOMAS

A. Overview

1. A group of malignant neoplasms that affect lymphatic system, resulting in proliferation of lymphocytes; can be classified as Hodgkin's lymphoma (Hodgkin's disease) and non-Hodgkin's lymphoma
2. Hodgkin's disease
   - a. More common in men than in women; has two peaks, at 15 to 35 and at 55 to 75 years of age; incidence is higher in whites than in African Americans
   - b. Etiology unknown but several identified factors contribute to development, including infection with Epstein-Barr virus (EBV), familial pattern, and exposure to toxins
   - c. Characterized by presence of Reed-Sternberg cell, a multinucleated and gigantic tumor cell thought to be of lymphoid origin
   - d. Originates in a lymph node (majority of cases in cervical nodes) and infiltrates spleen, lungs, and liver
3. Non-Hodgkin's lymphoma
   - a. Most common form of lymphoma; usually affects adults from 50 to 70 years old; is more common in men than in women and in whites than in other races
   - b. No known cause but incidence is linked to viral infections, immune disorders, genetic abnormalities, exposure to chemicals, and infection with *Helicobacter pylori*
   - c. Has a similar pathophysiology to Hodgkin's disease, although Reed-Sternberg cells are absent and method of lymph node infiltration is different
   - d. Often involves malignant B cells; usually originates outside lymph nodes; affected lymphoid tissues become infiltrated with malignant cells and crowd out normal cells

B. Nursing assessment

1. Hodgkin's disease
   - a. Often firm, painless enlargement of one or more lymph nodes on one side of neck
   - b. Fatigue and weakness
   - c. Anorexia and dysphagia
   - d. Dyspnea and cough
   - e. Pruritus and jaundice
   - f. Severe but brief pain at site after ingestion of alcohol
   - g. Abdominal pain and bone pain

h. Enlarged lymph nodes, liver, and spleen
i. B symptoms: fever without chills; night sweats, and unintentional 10% weight loss
j. Normocytic, normochromic anemia
k. Neutrophilia, monocytophilia, and lymphopenia
l. Presence of Reed-Sternberg cells in excisional bone biopsy
m. Mediastinal lymphadenopathy revealed by chest x-ray, CT scan, and radioisotope studies
n. Mediastinal mass and pulmonary infiltrates may be seen on chest x-ray
o. Absent or decreased response to skin sensitivity testing known as anergy

! 2. Non-Hodgkin's lymphoma
a. Painless lymph node enlargement
b. B symptoms (see above)
c. Abdominal pain, nausea, vomiting
d. Hematuria
e. Peripheral neuropathy, cranial nerve palsies, headaches, visual disturbances, changes in mental status, and seizures
f. Lymphocytopenia
g. X-ray may reveal pulmonary infiltrates
h. Lymph node biopsy helps to identify the cell type and pattern

C. Therapeutic management

1. Hodgkin's disease
a. Lymphangiography to evaluate abdominal nodes
b. Staging laparotomy to obtain specimen of retroperitoneal lymph nodes and remove spleen
c. Staging of disease to determine extent and appropriate therapy; stage I involves single lymph node region; stage IV (for Hodgkin's disease only) indicates diffuse or disseminated involvement of one or more extralymphatic organs, with or without lymph node involvement (liver, lung, marrow, skin)
! d. Treatment may include radiation therapy and/or chemotherapy

2. Non-Hodgkin's lymphoma
a. Staging of the disease is based on data obtained from CT scans and bone marrow biopsies
b. Combination chemotherapy
c. Radiation alone or in combination with chemotherapy for stage I and II
d. Biologic therapy with alpha-interferon, interleukin-2, and tumor necrosis factor
e. Administration of rituximab (Rituxan), a monoclonal antibody against the CD20 of malignant B lymphocytes, which causes cell lysis and death

! 3. Institute nursing interventions for clients on chemotherapy or radiation therapy
! 4. Assist in balancing activity with periods of rest
! 5. Provide and assist in maintaining good nutritional state
6. Provide measures to diminish the discomfort associated with pruritus
7. Help client to cope with body image changes such as alopecia, weight loss, and sterility
8. Refer client and family to appropriate agencies for support, such as the American Cancer Society
! 9. Plan interventions for the prevention of infection
! 10. Medication therapy: chemotherapy drugs and biologic therapy agents

D. Client teaching

1. Nature of disease, course of therapy, and associated interventions
2. Medications prescribed, precautions, and side effects
! 3. Symptoms necessitating immediate medical intervention, such as the occurrence of bleeding, infection, or fever

XIV. THALASSEMIA

A. Overview

1. Another of group of hereditary blood disorders of hemoglobin synthesis, characterized by mild to severe anemia

2. Most common type is beta-thalassemia, also known as Cooley anemia; there are three types of beta-thalassemia: thalassemia minor, thalassemia intermedia, and thalassemia major
   a. Thalassemia minor is also known as thalassemia trait and produces mild anemia
   b. Thalassemia intermedia produces severe anemia
   c. Thalassemia major produces anemia that requires transfusions; see Chapter 33 for blood transfusion procedure
3. Commonly seen in those of Mediterranean descent; however, they may also be seen among African, Asian, and Middle Eastern populations
4. Condition is autosomal recessive; when both parents carry gene, there is a 25% chance of passing disorder to child; if child acquires one gene, child will be a carrier
5. Thalassemia causes synthesis of defective hemoglobin; RBCs are fragile with shortened life span, which leads to anemia and chronic hypoxia
6. Body conserves iron from aged and broken down RBCs; when blood is administered, iron is retained also from transfused cells; this leads to high iron levels or **hemosiderosis,** which causes cellular damage and long-term complications, such as the following:
   a. Splenomegaly
   b. Cardiac complications
   c. Gallbladder disease
   d. Liver enlargement and cirrhosis
   e. Growth retardation and endocrine complications
   f. Jaundice and brown skin pigmentation
   g. Skeletal changes including enlarged head, thickened cranial bones, enlarged maxilla, and malocclusion of the teeth
7. If untreated, the child may die

!

B. Nursing assessment

1. Thalassemia can be diagnosed early in infancy when child presents with pallor, failure to thrive (FTT), hepatosplenomegaly, and severe anemia; see Box 65–3 for clinical manifestations of beta-Thalassemia

Box 65–3

Clinical Manifestations of Beta-Thalassemia

Anemia

Hypochromic and microcytic changes

Folic acid deficiency

Frequent epistaxis

Skeletal Changes

Osteoporosis

Delayed growth

Susceptibility to pathologic fractures

Facial deformities: enlarged head, prominent forehead due to frontal and parietal bossing, prominent cheek bones, broadened and depressed bridge of nose, enlarged maxilla with protruding front teeth, eyes with mongolian slant and epicanthal fold

Heart

Chronic congestive heart failure

Myocardial fibrosis

Murmurs

Liver/Gallbladder

Hepatomegaly

Hepatic insufficiency

Spleen

Splenomegaly

Endocrine System

Delayed sexual maturation

Fibrotic pancreas, resulting in diabetes mellitus

Skin

Darkening of skin

Source: Ball, J., & Bindler, R. (2006). *Child Health Nursing: Partnering with Children and Families.* Upper Saddle River, NJ: Pearson Education, p. 1021.

2. Signs and symptoms of chronic hypoxia such as lethargy, headache, bone pain, exercise intolerance, and anorexia
3. Hemoglobin electrophoresis shows decreased production of one hemoglobin chain; erythrocyte changes may be detected as early as 6 weeks of age
4. Decreased hemoglobin, hematocrit, and reticulocyte count
5. Folic acid deficiency may be present

! **C. Therapeutic management**

1. Administer blood products as ordered, observing for complications of multiple transfusions
2. Assess for signs of iron overload (hemosiderosis) and hepatitis
3. Observe for signs of infection and work to prevent infection through good handwashing, avoiding those with infection, proper rest and nutrition
4. Administer folic acid as ordered
5. Work toward fracture prevention by encouraging and providing opportunities for physical activities that do not increase risk of fractures, such as swimming and walking
6. Implement iron chelation therapy (desferoxamine) as ordered to aid in elimination of excessive iron
7. Provide support and opportunity for child and family to discuss feelings regarding chronic life-threatening illness
8. Encourage child and family to allow child to live as normal a life as possible
9. Bone marrow transplantation may be offered to cure disease

D. Child and family education

1. Nature of disease and its medical management
2. Possible complications, including iron overload, as well as signs of infection
3. Activity restrictions to reduce risk of fractures secondary to excessive iron stores
4. Encourage genetic counseling if appropriate

Check Your NCLEX-RN® Exam I.Q.

You are ready for testing on this content if you can

- Identify basic structures and functions of the hematological system.
- Describe the pathophysiology and etiology of common hematological disorders.
- Discuss expected assessment data and diagnostic test findings for selected hematological disorders.
- Discuss therapeutic management of a client experiencing a hematological disorder.
- Discuss nursing management of a client experiencing a hematological disorder.
- Identify expected outcomes for the client experiencing a hematological disorder.

PRACTICE TEST

1 The nurse is preparing a care plan for a client with polycythemia vera on ways to maintain nutrition. The nurse should include which of the following in the plan?

1. Increase intake of foods high in iron.
2. Encourage small, frequent meals rather than three big meals.
3. Increase the amount of red meats and organ meats in the diet.
4. Encourage the use of hot spices in foods to stimulate appetite.

2 A client with thrombocytopenia presents to the primary care center. During assessment, the nurse notices petechiae. The nurse interprets that which laboratory result best supports the presence of a disorder of hemostasis?

1. Decreased erythrocyte count
2. A platelet count below 150,000/uL
3. An elevated lymphocyte count
4. A hemoglobin value of 14 or more

3 A nurse is admitting a client with a diagnosis of aplastic anemia. Which of the following is the best room for the nurse to assign this client?

1. A semiprivate room with a client whose diagnosis is urosepsis.
2. A regular private room at the end of the hall.
3. A private isolation room equipped with a negative airflow.
4. A semiprivate room with a client whose diagnosis is thrombophlebitis.

4. The nurse is reviewing laboratory results of a client suspected of having disseminated intravascular coagulopathy (DIC). The nurse looks to the results of which test as the more specific marker for DIC?

1. Partial thromboplastin time (PTT)
2. Prothrombin time (PT)
3. Platelet count
4. Fibrin degradation products (FDP)

5. The husband of a client with disseminated intravascular coagulopathy (DIC) approaches the nurse and expresses his concern that his wife might be getting the wrong medication after he was told that the client was receiving heparin. What is the nurse's best response?

1. "I understand your concern, but the doctors know what they are doing."
2. "Let me make sure that I have not misread the physician's order."
3. "The drug is being used to stop the abnormal clotting in capillaries and arterioles."
4. "Please ask the physician why this medication is being given."

6. The nurse is administering oral care on a client with disseminated intravascular coagulopathy (DIC). Which if the following is the most appropriate for this client?

1. Limit flossing to once a day.
2. Use an alcohol-based mouthwash to prevent infection.
3. Use swabs to administer oral care.
4. Encourage tooth brushing at least once a shift.

7. A client with stomatitis and on neutropenic precautions is ordered to have mouthwashes every 2 hours. Which of the following choices of mouthwash solutions should the nurse question if ordered by the physician?

1. Viscous lidocaine (Xylocaine)
2. Normal saline solution
3. Hydrogen peroxide
4. Diluted baking soda

8. A client with acute myelogenous leukemia (AML) is scheduled for a bone marrow transplant (BMT). In teaching the client's family about BMT, which of the following statements by the nurse is best?

1. "The client will be in the operating room with the donor so that immediate transplantation can occur."
2. "The specially prepared marrow is infused intravenously to the client."
3. "The client will be brought to the radiology department to transplant the marrow."
4. "A large bore needle will be inserted into the client's bone marrow where the donor marrow will be infused."

9. A client has undergone a lymph node biopsy. The nurse anticipates that the report will reveal which of the following if the client has Hodgkin's lymphoma?

1. Reed-Sternberg cells
2. Philadelphia chromosome
3. Epstein-Barr virus
4. Herpes simplex virus

10. During physical examination, the nurse finds a nontender, moveable cervical node on a client. The nurse makes which interpretation of this finding?

1. Normal, since the node is moveable
2. Abnormal and may suggest the presence of a malignancy
3. Normal, since the node is nontender
4. Abnormal and a positive indicator of a malignancy

11. A client with thrombocytopenia has an order for neurological checks every hour. The nurse explains to a curious nursing assistant that the reason for frequent neurological assessment is which of the following?

1. To determine if the coagulopathy is related to a neurological disorder
2. To monitor for signs of intracranial bleeding
3. To evaluate the effectiveness of pharmacologic interventions
4. To correlate increasing platelet counts with the neurological status

12. During assessment, the nurse notices a systolic murmur on a client with anemia. The nurse interprets that this finding correlates with which of the following?

1. Increased quantity and speed of low-viscosity blood through valves
2. Structural abnormality of heart valves from the anemia
3. High viscosity of blood circulating through the cardiac structures
4. Decreased blood flow through the vascular system

PRACTICE TEST

13 A client with anemia has a nursing diagnosis of activity intolerance. Which of the following nursing interventions should the nurse implement?

1. Space interventions and encourage rest periods.
2. Teach client the basics of good nutrition.
3. Promote active or passive range of motion activities
4. Teach client to change position slowly to prevent dizziness

14 The nurse is teaching a client with hemophilia A about home management. Which of the following should the nurse include in the teaching plan?

1. Increase iron-rich foods in the diet
2. Avoid contact sports
3. Use aspirin when severe pain occurs
4. Minimize joint pain by walking and weight-bearing

15 The nurse is obtaining a health history on a client who is admitted with a diagnosis of "rule out aplastic anemia." Considering the diagnosis, which of the following data is most important for the nurse to elicit during the interview?

1. Recent travel outside the country
2. Exposure to chemicals and drugs
3. History of blood transfusion
4. Medication allergies

16 The nurse is teaching family members about precautions to take in visiting a client who has neutropenia. Which of the following instructions would not be included by the nurse in the discussion?

1. People who have colds or infectious diseases should not visit.
2. Visitors must wash their hands before and after a visit.
3. Face masks should be worn by all those who come in contact with the client.
4. Fresh flowers will help to provide a cheerful environment.

17 A client has a platelet count of 18,000/mm^3. What intervention must the nurse include in the plan of care?

1. Institute bleeding precautions.
2. Institute reverse isolation.
3. Schedule medications by intramuscular route when able.
4. Obtain temperatures rectally.

18 A nurse is assisting a physician with a bone marrow aspiration on a client with anemia. After the procedure, the nurse should take which of the following actions?

1. Apply pressure on the site to stop bleeding.
2. Massage the area to decrease pain.
3. Apply heat to the area to diminish the discomfort.
4. Cover the area with a light dressing.

19 The white blood cell (WBC) differential on a client indicates a shift to the left. The nurse makes which of the following accurate interpretations of this report?

1. There is an increase in the number of segmented neutrophils.
2. There is an increase in the number of bands released into the circulation.
3. The number of lymphocytes increased in number.
4. The number of lymphocytes exceeds the total WBC count.

20 A client with iron-deficiency anemia is scheduled for a complete blood count. The nurse anticipates that the report will show which characteristics of the red blood cells (RBCs)?

1. Normocytic, normochromic
2. Macrocytic, normochromic
3. Microcytic, hypochromic
4. Normocytic, hyperchromic

21 The nurse in the hematology clinic is reviewing laboratory findings for a 2-year-old being treated for anemia. Which finding is the best indication that the treatment is successful?

1. The child is no longer cyanotic.
2. The reticulocyte count is rising.
3. The child is more active.
4. Stools are black, indicating iron intake.

22 A pregnant woman tells the nurse that she has a family history of sickle cell anemia and is afraid her baby will be born with the disease. The nurse would provide which information during a discussion with this client?

1. Sickle cell anemia is a male disease and would be passed on through the man's family.
2. Genetic testing will be needed to determine if her fetus is affected.
3. Both mother and father must carry the defective gene for the child to have sickle cell anemia.
4. The child only needs one parent to be a carrier in order for the child to be affected.

23 A young child who was admitted to the hospital with a bleeding disorder has been diagnosed with idiopathic thrombocytopenic purpura (ITP). The mother of the child says to the nurse, "I have a friend who has a son with hemophilia. When he bleeds, they give him a 'factor,' which they keep in their home refrigerator. Can we just give my child this factor?" Which of the following is the best response by the nurse?

1. "Your friend's child has a natural deficiency in clotting factors; your child does not."
2. "Factor has a lot of negative side effects, and the doctors would rather not use it on your child."
3. "The amount of factor that would be required to treat your child would be excessive."
4. "That treatment may be tried later if your child does not respond to steroids."

24 The nurse has admitted a child newly diagnosed with anemia of unknown origin. Which of the following nursing diagnoses is most appropriate?

1. Insufficient cardiac output related to abnormal platelet count
2. Activity intolerance related to generalized weakness and fatigue
3. Imbalanced nutrition: less than body requirements
4. Risk for pain related to vaso-occlusion

25 The nurse is caring for a child with beta-thalassemia who has received many blood transfusions. The nurse assesses for which of the following as a priority at this time?

1. Neutropenia
2. Petechiae
3. Hemosiderosis
4. Hemoglobin S formation

26 A client with vitamin B_{12} deficiency needs to increase dietary intake of foods that are good sources of this vitamin. The nurse recommends that the client increase intake of which of the following foods? Select all that apply.

1. Apples
2. Spinach
3. Carrots
4. Oranges
5. Liver

ANSWERS & RATIONALES

1 **Answer: 2** Clients with polycythemia experience satiety and fullness resulting from hepatomegaly and splenomegaly. Frequent, small meals will help maintain adequate nutrition. Foods rich in iron are not appropriate because there is an increase in erythrocytes in this condition. Spicy foods will increase the gastrointestinal symptoms, which also include dyspepsia and increased gastric secretions.
Cognitive Level: Application **Client Need:** Physiological Integrity: Physiological Adaptation **Integrated Process:** Nursing Process: Planning **Content Area:** Adult Health: Hematological **Strategy:** The core issue of the question is knowledge of an appropriate diet for a client with polycythemia. Use nursing knowledge and the process of elimination to make a selection.

2 **Answer: 2** Clients with thrombocytopenia have decreased platelet counts below 150,000/uL. The usual presenting manifestation of this condition is the appearance of petechiae, purpura, and ecchymosis. The other laboratory values will not explain the petechiae or support the presence of a clotting disorder.
Cognitive Level: Analysis **Client Need:** Physiological Integrity: Physiological Adaptation **Integrated Process:** Nursing Process: Assessment **Content Area:** Adult Health: Hematological **Strategy:** The core issue of the question is the laboratory test results that best indicates a disorder of abnormal clotting ability. Use nursing knowledge and the process of elimination to make a selection.

3 **Answer: 2** Clients with aplastic anemia usually experience pancytopenia (decreased erythrocytes, leukocytes, and platelets). The client with this type of hypoplastic anemia should therefore have a room where reverse isolation can be instituted. The client with aplastic anemia is susceptible to infection as well as hemorrhage. Respiratory isolation requiring negative airflow (option 3) is not necessary in the care of clients with aplastic anemia.
Cognitive Level: Analysis **Client Need:** Physiological Integrity: Physiological Adaptation **Integrated Process:** Nursing Process: Planning **Content Area:** Adult Health: Hematological **Strategy:**

The core issue of the question is knowledge of the effects of aplastic anemia on the immune system, which then requires special intervention to prevent infection. Use nursing knowledge and the process of elimination to make a selection.

4 **Answer: 4** In DIC, there is abnormal initiation and formation of blood clots. As clots are formed and then begin to dissolve, more end products of fibrinogen and fibrin are also formed. These are called fibrin degradation products or fibrin split products. Although the PT and PTT are prolonged and the platelet count is reduced in DIC, they could also be a result of other coagulation disturbances. Only the increase is FDP would occur because of the widespread accelerated clotting present in DIC.
Cognitive Level: Analysis **Client Need:** Physiological Integrity: Physiological Adaptation **Integrated Process:** Nursing Process: Assessment **Content Area:** Adult Health: Hematological **Strategy:** The core issue of the question is knowledge of trends in changes of laboratory data in DIC. Use nursing knowledge and the process of elimination to make a selection.

5 **Answer: 3** Initially, there is an enhanced coagulation mechanism with resulting increase in fibrin and platelet deposition in arterioles and capillaries in DIC, resulting in thrombosis. Although it remains controversial in DIC, the use of heparin is aimed at preventing the formation of additional thrombotic clots that further complicate the bleeding disorder.
Cognitive Level: Analysis **Client Need:** Physiological Integrity: Physiological Adaptation **Integrated Process:** Communication and Documentation **Content Area:** Adult Health: Hematological **Strategy:** The core issue of the question is the possible role of heparin in the management of DIC. Use nursing knowledge and the process of elimination to make a selection.

6 **Answer: 3** Clients with DIC should be protected from injury that will result in bleeding. An oral swab is least likely to cause tissue injury to the oral cavity during the performance of oral care. Mouthwashes containing alcohol should be avoided because they may cause discomfort and because they tend to dry the mucous membranes. Toothbrushes may be used only if they are soft-bristled, but a swab or toothette is the best option.
Cognitive Level: Application **Client Need:** Physiological Integrity: Physiological Adaptation **Integrated Process:** Nursing Process: Implementation **Content Area:** Adult Health: Hematological **Strategy:** The core issue of the question is appropriate methods of providing mouth care to a client with stomatitis. Use nursing knowledge and the process of elimination to make a selection.

7 **Answer: 3** Hydrogen peroxide is not a good choice of mouthwash solution in clients with stomatitis because it tends to dry the oral mucosa and further aggravate the discomfort. The other three options are acceptable mouthwash solutions; diphenhydramine (Benadryl) or Maalox may also be used.
Cognitive Level: Application **Client Need:** Physiological Integrity: Physiological Adaptation **Integrated Process:** Nursing Process: Implementation **Content Area:** Adult Health: Hematological **Strategy:** The core issue of the question is a mouth care product that would be irritating to a client with stomatitis. Use nursing knowledge and the process of elimination to make a selection.

8 **Answer: 2** Harvested bone marrow is infused into the recipient intravenously. The transplantation is usually preceded by chemotherapy and radiation therapy. During this period and up to when the client's response to the transplantation has been successful, nursing interventions should focus on prevention of infection.
Cognitive Level: Application **Client Need:** Physiological Integrity: Physiological Adaptation **Integrated Process:** Teaching and Learning **Content Area:** Adult Health: Hematological **Strategy:** The core issue of the question is knowledge of bone marrow transplantation as a treatment method. Use nursing knowledge and the process of elimination to make a selection.

9 **Answer: 1** Histological isolation of Reed-Sternberg cells in lymph node biopsy examination is a diagnostic feature of Hodgkin's lymphoma. Philadelphia chromosome is attributed to chronic myelogenous leukemia. Viruses are much smaller than can be visualized with cytology.
Cognitive Level: Application **Client Need:** Physiological Integrity: Physiological Adaptation **Integrated Process:** Nursing Process: Analysis **Content Area:** Adult Health: Hematological **Strategy:** The core issue of the question is knowledge of characteristic findings in the diagnosis of lymphoma. Use nursing knowledge and the process of elimination to make a selection.

10 **Answer: 2** A nontender and moveable cervical node may suggest the presence of malignancy and even lymphoma. Palpable nodes do not confirm the diagnosis of a malignancy. Biopsy and histological examination will aid in interpreting the significance of enlarged nodes.
Cognitive Level: Analysis **Client Need:** Physiological Integrity: Physiological Adaptation **Integrated Process:** Nursing Process: Assessment **Content Area:** Adult Health: Hematological **Strategy:** The core issue of the question is the ability to interpret assessment data related to lymph nodes. Use nursing knowledge and the process of elimination to make a selection.

11 **Answer: 2** Clients with thrombocytopenia are at risk for altered cerebral perfusion from bleeding. Since a neurologic assessment can assist in determining the presence of occult bleeding in the cerebrovascular system, it is a necessary nursing intervention to include in the care of these clients.
Cognitive Level: Application **Client Need:** Physiological Integrity: Physiological Adaptation **Integrated Process:** Nursing Process: Implementation **Content Area:** Adult Health: Hematological **Strategy:** The core issue of the question is knowledge that a low platelet increases risk of bleeding, which includes the risk of intracranial bleeding. Use this nursing knowledge and the process of elimination to make a selection.

12 **Answer: 1** In anemia, there is a decrease in the viscosity of blood as a result of a decrease in the number of red blood cells. The increase in cardiac output and flow are compensatory mechanisms because of the decrease in the quantity of hemoglobin in circulating blood.
Cognitive Level: Analysis **Client Need:** Physiological Integrity: Physiological Adaptation **Integrated Process:** Nursing Process: Analysis **Content Area:** Adult Health: Hematological **Strategy:** The core issue of the question is knowledge of how pathophysiology relates to assessment data in a client with anemia. Use nursing knowledge and the process of elimination to make a selection.

13 **Answer: 1** Activity intolerance in clients with anemia results from the imbalance between oxygen demand and supply. Ac-

tivities should be planned to intersperse activity with periods of rest to decrease hypoxemic episodes and to decrease tissue demand for oxygen. All the other options are appropriate interventions for a client with anemia, but they do not relate to the nursing diagnosis of activity intolerance.
Cognitive Level: Application **Client Need:** Physiological Integrity: Physiological Adaptation **Integrated Process:** Nursing Process: Planning **Content Area:** Adult Health: Hematological **Strategy:** The core issue of the question is knowledge that anemia causes fatigue and that measures to prevent fatigue need to be incorporated in the plan of care. Use this knowledge and the process of elimination to make a selection.

14 **Answer: 2** Clients with hemophilia should be taught to participate in noncontact sports and to avoid any activities that increase the risk of tissue injury and bleeding. Clients with hemophilia should never use aspirin because of the risk for bleeding. Joint pain may be caused by hemarthrosis (bleeding in the joints), a situation in which the client should be taught to seek medical care immediately. Iron-rich foods are not appropriate in clients with this condition unless there is an accompanying anemia.
Cognitive Level: Application **Client Need:** Physiological Integrity: Physiological Adaptation **Integrated Process:** Teaching and Learning **Content Area:** Adult Health: Hematological **Strategy:** The core issue of the question is an appropriate element of client teaching with hemophilia. Use concepts related to prevention of bleeding and the process of elimination to make a selection.

15 **Answer: 2** Aplastic anemia may be congenital or acquired, but most cases do not have an identifiable etiology. It is known that aplastic anemia may follow exposure to chemicals (e.g., Benzene, DDT) or drugs (chloramphenicol, sulfonamides). It is therefore important that the nurse obtain exposure history on this client.
Cognitive Level: Analysis **Client Need:** Physiological Integrity: Physiological Adaptation **Integrated Process:** Nursing Process: Assessment **Content Area:** Adult Health: Hematological **Strategy:** The core issue of the question is knowledge of the possible etiologies of aplastic anemia. Use knowledge about the possible causes of this disorder and the process of elimination to make a selection.

16 **Answer: 4** A client with neutropenia has a compromised immune system and is predisposed to infections. Fresh fruits and flowers in the client's room are not allowed because they tend to harbor bacteria. All the other options are reasonable instructions to be given to visitors as well as health care personnel who come in contact with the client.
Cognitive Level: Application **Client Need:** Physiological Integrity: Safe, Effective Care Environment: Reduction of Risk Potential **Integrated Process:** Teaching and Learning **Content Area:** Adult Health: Hematological **Strategy:** The core issue of the question is knowledge of the components of neutropenic precautions. The wording of the question tells you the correct answer is an incorrect statement. Use nursing knowledge and the process of elimination to make a selection.

17 **Answer: 1** A platelet count below 20,000 indicates that the client is at risk for bleeding and necessitates the avoidance of activities and interventions that increase this risk. Nursing interventions such as the use of intramuscular injections, rectal temperatures, and shaving with a razor are activities that predispose the client to further injury. Reverse isolation is not appropriate for this client unless there is accompanying evidence of neutropenia.
Cognitive Level: Application **Client Need:** Physiological Integrity: Safe, Effective Care Environment: Reduction of Risk Potential **Integrated Process:** Nursing Process: Implementation **Content Area:** Adult Health: Hematological **Strategy:** The core issue of the question is appropriate interpretation of a low platelet count and interpreting the appropriate intervention to protect the client from bleeding. Use nursing knowledge and the process of elimination to make a selection.

18 **Answer: 1** Application of direct pressure and pressure dressing should follow the withdrawal of the aspiration needle after a bone marrow aspiration. If the client has thrombocytopenia, pressure should be applied on the site for at least 3 to 5 minutes or until hemostasis has been achieved. The other options are not appropriate following a bone marrow aspiration. Continued observation of the site should be made to assure that there is no bleeding.
Cognitive Level: Application **Client Need:** Physiological Integrity: Physiological Adaptation **Integrated Process:** Nursing Process: Implementation **Content Area:** Adult Health: Hematological **Strategy:** The core issue of the question is knowledge of specific care following bone marrow aspiration that will prevent complications of the procedure. Use nursing knowledge and the process of elimination to make a selection.

19 **Answer: 2** A shift to the left indicates an increase in immature neutrophils or bands. An increase in the number of bands indicates an increase in the production of granulocytes, which could be a compensatory mechanism in response to infection.
Cognitive Level: Analysis **Client Need:** Physiological Integrity: Physiological Adaptation **Integrated Process:** Nursing Process: Assessment **Content Area:** Adult Health: Hematological **Strategy:** The core issue of the question is the ability to make an accurate interpretation of findings on a laboratory report of WBC count and morphology. Use nursing knowledge and the process of elimination to make a selection.

20 **Answer: 3** The morphologic characteristics of RBCs in iron-deficiency anemia is microcytic and hypochromic. Vitamin B_{12} anemia produces a macrocytic and normochromic morphology. Aplastic anemia, hemolysis, and acute blood loss will reveal RBCs with normocytic and normochromic characteristics.
Cognitive Level: Application **Client Need:** Physiological Integrity: Physiological Adaptation **Integrated Process:** Nursing Process: Assessment **Content Area:** Adult Health: Hematological **Strategy:** The core issue of the question is the pathophysiological changes of RBCs in specific anemias. Use nursing knowledge and the process of elimination to make a selection.

21 **Answer: 2** Reticulocytes are immature RBCs. An increase in the number of reticulocytes indicates the body is producing new RBCs. Iron intake does not indicate an improvement in anemia status, and the child with anemia is not cyanotic but pale. An increase in activity is hard to measure subjectively and would be a late finding.
Cognitive Level: Analysis **Client Need:** Physiological Integrity: Physiological Adaptation **Integrated Process:** Nursing Process:

Evaluation **Content Area:** Child Health: Hematological **Strategy:** The core issue of the question is the ability to evaluate outcomes of care for a client with anemia. Use nursing knowledge and the process of elimination to make a selection.

22 **Answer: 3** Sickle cell is inherited as an autosomal recessive disorder. Both parents must carry the defective gene. The other statements are factually incorrect.
Cognitive Level: Application **Client Need:** Physiological Integrity: Physiological Adaptation **Integrated Process:** Teaching and Learning **Content Area:** Child Health: Hematological **Strategy:** The core issue of the question is the ability to teach a client about genetics as they relate to sickle cell disease. Use nursing knowledge and the process of elimination to make a selection.

23 **Answer: 1** Hemophilia is characterized by a deficiency in one or more clotting factors, while ITP is a platelet disorder. Because the child with ITP is not deficient in clotting factors, this treatment would not be beneficial.
Cognitive Level: Application **Client Need:** Physiological Integrity: Physiological Adaptation **Integrated Process:** Communication and Documentation **Content Area:** Child Health: Hematological **Strategy:** The core issue of the question is an understanding of the differences between hemophilia and bleeding disorders caused by platelet problems. Use nursing knowledge and the process of elimination to make a selection.

24 **Answer: 2** Clients with anemia will experience activity intolerance with even the simplest activities of daily living. There is no vaso-occlusion or abnormal platelet count with anemia. There may be insufficient cardiac output, but it will not be related to platelet count. There is no information in the question to indicate that the anemia is secondary to poor diet.
Cognitive Level: Analysis **Client Need:** Physiological Integrity: Physiological Adaptation **Integrated Process:** Nursing Process: Analysis **Content Area:** Child Health: Hematological **Strategy:** The core issue of the question is knowledge of typical pathophysiology and client assessments in anemia and using this information to identify the most important nursing diagnosis. Use nursing knowledge about anemia and the process of elimination to make a selection.

25 **Answer: 3** Frequent blood transfusion will lead to an overload of iron in the body. This iron is stored in tissues and organs and is called hemosiderosis. Blood transfusions do not lower the white count or cause petechiae or hemoglobin in the bile.
Cognitive Level: Analysis **Client Need:** Physiological Integrity: Physiological Adaptation **Integrated Process:** Nursing Process: Assessment **Content Area:** Child Health: Hematological **Strategy:** The core issue of the question is identification of a complication of chronic blood transfusion therapy. Note the critical word *priority* in the question, which tells you the correct option is the condition of most importance at the current time. Use nursing knowledge of thalassemia and the process of elimination to make a selection.

26 **Answer: 2, 4, 5** Clients with nutritional anemias require dietary sources of folic acid, such as green leafy vegetables, fish, citrus fruits, yeast, dried beans, grains, nuts, and liver. Apples and carrots are not as rich in folic acid as the other food sources listed.
Cognitive Level: Analysis **Client Need:** Physiological Integrity: Physiological Adaptation **Integrated Process:** Nursing Process: Implementation **Content Area:** Adult Health: Hematological **Strategy:** The core issue of the question is knowledge of foods that are rich in vitamin B_{12}. Use nursing knowledge and the process of elimination to make your selections.

Key Terms to Review

anemia p. 1328
anergy p. 1336
cheilosis p. 1325
ecchymosis p. 1332
fibrinolysis p. 1323
glossitis p. 1326
hemarthrosis p. 1332
hemosiderosis p. 1339
hemostasis p. 1322
hypochromic p. 1325
leukocytosis p. 1323
leukopenia p. 1323
microcytic p. 1325
plethora p. 1330
thrombocytopenia p. 1323
X-linked recessive trait p. 1332

References

Ball, J., & Bindler, R. (2006). *Child health nursing: Partnering with children and families*. Upper Saddle River, NJ: Pearson Education.

Black, J., & Hawks, J. (2005). *Medical surgical nursing: Clinical management for positive outcomes* (7th ed.). St. Louis: Elsevier Science.

Corbett, J. (2004). *Laboratory tests and diagnostic procedures with nursing diagnoses* (6th ed.). Upper Saddle River, NJ: Pearson Education.

Harkreader, H., & Hogan, M. (2004). *Fundamentals of nursing: Caring and clinical judgment* (2nd ed.). St. Louis: Elsevier Science.

Ignatavicius, D., & Workman, L. (2006). *Medical-surgical nursing: Critical thinking for collaborative care* (5th ed.). Philadelphia: W. B. Saunders.

Kozier, B., Erb, G., Berman, A., & Snyder, S. (2004). *Fundamentals of nursing: Concepts, process, and practice* (7th ed.). Upper Saddle River, NJ: Pearson Education.

LeMone, P., & Burke, K. (2004). *Medical surgical nursing: Critical thinking in client care* (3rd ed.). Upper Saddle River, NJ: Pearson Education.

Porth, C. (2004). *Pathophysiology: Concepts of altered health states* (7th ed.). Philadelphia: Lippincott Williams & Wilkins.

Smith, S., Duell, D., & Martin, B. (2004). *Clinical nursing skills: Basic to advanced skills* (6th ed.). Upper Saddle River, NJ: Pearson Education.

Oncological Disorders

66

In this chapter

Test Yourself

Are you ready for the NCLEX-RN® or course exams? Use the practice tests on the companion CD-ROM to check.

Cross reference

Other chapters relevant to this content area are

Promoting Healthy Lifestyle Choices	Chapter 17
Meeting Nutritional Needs	Chapter 26
Antineoplastic Medications	Chapter 45
Common Laboratory Tests	Chapter 47
Common Diagnostic Tests and Procedures	Chapter 48
Respiratory Disorders	Chapter 56
Gastrointestinal Disorders	Chapter 60
Hematological Disorders	Chapter 65

I. OVERVIEW OF CANCER

A. ***Cancer:*** mutation of normal cells into abnormally proliferating cells; a neoplasm is an abnormal growth or ***tumor*** (solid mass functioning independently and serving no useful purpose)
  1. **Benign neoplasms:** slow-growing, localized, and encapsulated nonmalignant growths with well-defined borders; are generally easily removed and do not cause tissue damage other than by compression of tissues and interfering with circulation
  2. **Malignant neoplasms:** aggressive growths that invade and destroy surrounding tissues; can lead to death unless aggressively treated
  3. Invasion occurs when cancer cells infiltrate adjacent tissues surrounding neoplasm
  4. **Metastasis** occurs when malignant cells travel through blood or lymph system and invade other tissues and organs to form a secondary tumor

B. **Characteristics of malignant cells**
  1. Rapid cell division and growth: regulation of the rate of mitosis is lost
  2. No contact inhibition: cells do not respect boundaries of other cells and invade their tissue areas
  3. Loss of differentiation: cells lose specialized characteristics of function for that cell type and revert back to an earlier, more primitive cell type
  4. Ability to migrate (metastasize): cells move to distant areas of the body and establish new site malignant lesions (tumors)
  5. Alteration in cell structure: cell membrane, cytoplasm, and overall cell shape
  6. Self-survival
     a. May develop ectopic sites to produce hormones needed for own growth
     b. Can develop a connective tissue stroma to support growth
     c. May develop own blood supply by secreting angiotensin growth factor to stimulate local blood vessels to grow into tumor

II. RISK FACTORS FOR DEVELOPMENT OF CANCER

A. **Age**
  1. Increased risk for people over age of 65
  2. Factors attributed to cancer in elderly include hormonal changes, altered immune responses, and accumulation of free radicals
  3. Age has been identified as single-most important factor related to development of cancer

B. **Gender**
  1. Certain cancers are more commonly seen in specific genders
  2. For example, breast cancer occurs more commonly in females

C. **Geographic location**
  1. Risks for cancer vary according to environment and location
  2. Rates for specific cancer sites, morbidity, and mortality vary from state to state, nation to nation, and in urban versus rural living

D. **Genetics**
  1. Accounts for approximately 15% of cancers
  2. Cancers demonstrating a familial relationship include breast, colon, lung, ovarian, and prostate
  3. Clients with a genetic predisposition to cancer should be counseled and screened according to American Cancer Society (ACS) guidelines

E. **Immune disturbance:** some viruses tend to increase risk, such as Epstein-Barr, genital herpes, papillomavirus, hepatitis B, and human cytomegalovirus (CMV)

F. **Chemical agents:** over 1,000 chemicals are known to be carcinogenic; exposure in some occupations heightens risk over decades

G. **Race**
  1. Cancer can affect any population
  2. Nonetheless African Americans experience a higher rate of cancer than any other racial or ethnic group and higher mortality rates, possibly because of more advanced state when seeking treatment

H. Tobacco

1. A strong correlation exists between smoking and lung cancer
2. Other cancers associated with tobacco use include bladder, esophageal, gastric, laryngeal, oropharyngeal, and pancreatic
3. Smokeless tobacco (snuff and chewing tobacco) increases risk of oral and esophageal cancers
4. Long-term exposure to secondhand smoke increases risk for lung and bladder cancers

I. Alcohol

1. Serves as a promoter in cancers of liver and esophagus
2. When combined with tobacco, risks for other cancers are even higher

J. Diet

1. Diet has been demonstrated in research to correlate with some cancers
2. Diets high in fat, low in fiber, and those containing nitrosamines and nitrosindoles (in preserved meats and pickled foods) promote certain cancers such as colon, breast, esophageal, and gastric

K. Miscellaneous factors studied that might correlate with increased incidence of cancer: stress, occupation involving exposure to carcinogens (such as miners and asbestos workers), viruses

III. AMERICAN CANCER SOCIETY RECOMMENDATIONS FOR EARLY CANCER DETECTION

! **A. American Cancer Society's seven warning signs of cancer (uses acronym CAUTION):**

1. *C*hange in bowel or bladder habits
2. *A* sore that does not heal
3. *U*nusual bleeding or discharge
4. *T*hickening or lump in breast or elsewhere
5. *I*ndigestion or difficulty in swallowing
6. *O*bvious change in wart or mole
7. *N*agging cough or hoarseness

Memory Aid

Remember to use CAUTION to recall risk factors for cancer.

! **B. Detection of breast cancer**

1. Beginning at age 20, routinely perform monthly breast self-examinations (BSEs)
2. Women ages 20 to 39 should have breast examination by a health care provider every 3 years
3. Women age 40 and older should have a yearly mammogram and breast examination by a health care provider

! **C. Detection of colon and rectal cancer**

1. All persons age 50 and older should have a yearly fecal occult blood test
2. Digital rectal examination and flexible sigmoidoscopy should be done every 5 years
3. Colonoscopy with barium enema should be done every 10 years

! **D. Detection of uterine cancer**

1. Yearly Papanicolaou (Pap) smear for sexually active females and any female over age 18
2. At menopause, high-risk women should have an endometrial tissue sample

! **E. Detection of prostate cancer**

1. Beginning at age 50, have a yearly digital rectal examination
2. Beginning at age 50, have a yearly prostate-specific antigen (PSA) test

F. Self detection of cancer: see Chapter 17 for breast and testicular self examinations

IV. DIAGNOSTIC METHODS, TESTS, AND ASSESSMENTS

A. Grading

1. Classifies cancer based on degree of abnormality of cells when examined under microscope

Box 66–1

Grading and Staging of Solid Tumors

Grading

Grade I: cells slightly different than normal, well differentiated (mild dysplasia)

Grade II: cells more abnormal, moderately well differentiated (moderate dysplasia)

Grade III: cells clearly abnormal, poorly differentiated (severe dysplasia)

Grade IV: cells anaplastic (immature) and undifferentiated (cell origin difficult to determine)

Staging

T indicates tumor size

T0: no evidence of tumor

Tis: tumor in situ

T1, T2, T3, T4: progressive degrees of tumor size and involvement

N indicates lymph node involvement

N0: no abnormal lymph nodes detected

N1a, N2a: regional nodes involved with increasing degree from N1a to N2a; no metastases detected

N1b, N2b, N3b: progressive regional lymph nodes involvement; metastasis suspected

Nx: inability to assess regional nodes

M indicates distant metastases

M0: no evidence of distant metastasis

M1, M2, M3: increasing degrees of distant metastasis and includes distant lymph nodes

2. Grading utilizes a Roman numeral rating of I through IV, with I being least abnormal and IV being most abnormal (see Box 66–1)

B. ***Staging:*** TNM system is utilized for classifying solid tumors (see Box 66–1)

C. ***Tumor markers***

1. Tumor markers are protein substances found in blood or body fluids
2. Are released either by tumor itself or by body as a defense in response to tumor (called host response)
3. Tumor markers are derived from tumor itself and include the following:
   a. *Oncofetal antigens,* present normally in fetal tissue, may indicate an anaplastic process in tumor cells; carcinoembryonic antigen (CEA) and alpha-fetoprotein (AFP) are examples
   b. *Hormones* at high levels may indicate a hormone-secreting malignancy; hormones that may be utilized as tumor markers include antidiuretic hormone (ADH), calcitonin, catecholamines, human chorionic gonadotropin (HCG), and parathyroid hormone (PTH)
   c. *Isoenzymes* normally present in a tissue may be released into bloodstream if tissue is experiencing rapid, excessive growth because of tumor; examples include neuron-specific enolase (NSE) and prostatic acid phosphatase (PAP)
   d. *Tissue-specific proteins* identify type of tissue affected by malignancy; an example is prostatic-specific antigen (PSA) utilized to identify prostate cancer
4. Host-response tumor markers include the following:
   a. C-reactive protein
   b. Interleukin-2
   c. Lactic dehydrogenase
   d. Serum ferritin
   e. Tumor necrosis factor

D. ***Biopsy*** **and cytology**

1. Histologic and cytologic examination of specimens are performed on tissues collected by needle aspiration of solid tumors, exfoliation from epithelial surface, or aspiration of fluid from blood or body cavities; examples include specimens from Pap smear, bone marrow, or tissue biopsy
2. Tissues for biopsy may be obtained by excisional, incisional, and needle biopsy methods
3. By examination of these tissues, the name, grade, and stage of tumor can be identified

E. Laboratory tests: see Table 66–1 ■

F. Diagnostic studies: include such tests as x-rays, radionuclide and nuclear imaging scans, CT scans, MRI

V. COMMON TREATMENT TECHNIQUES AND PROCEDURES

A. ***Radiation therapy***

1. Use of ionizing rays for therapeutic purposes in cancer therapy
2. Used to kill a tumor, reduce tumor size, relieve obstruction, or decrease pain
3. Causes lethal injury to DNA so it can destroy rapidly multiplying cancer cells; radiation therapy kills normal cells as well
4. Classified as internal radiation therapy (brachytherapy) or external radiation therapy (teletherapy)

B. Brachytherapy (internal radiation)

1. Sources of internal radiation
   - **a.** Implanted into affected tissue or body cavity
   - **b.** Ingested as a solution
   - **c.** Injected as a solution into bloodstream or body cavity
   - **d.** Introduced through a catheter into tumor
2. Side effects of internal radiation
   - **a.** Fatigue
   - **b.** Anorexia
   - **c.** Immunosuppression
   - **d.** Other side effects similar to external radiation (see section C2)
3. ! Client teaching
   - **a.** Avoid close contact with others until treatment is completed because of radioactivity
   - **b.** Maintain daily activities unless contraindicated, allowing for extra rest periods as needed
   - **c.** Maintain balanced diet; may tolerate food better if consumed in small, frequent meals
   - **d.** Maintain fluid intake to ensure adequate hydration (2–3 liters/day)
   - **e.** If implant is temporary, maintain bedrest to avoid dislodging the implant
   - **f.** Excreted body fluids may be radioactive; double-flush toilets after use
   - **g.** Radiation therapy may lead to bone marrow suppression (refer to precautions for anemia, thrombocytopenia, and immunosuppression later in chapter)
4. ! Nursing management of client receiving internal radiation
   - **a.** Exposure to small amounts of radiation is possible during close contact with persons receiving internal radiation; understand principles of protection from exposure to radiation: time, distance, and shielding
   - **b.** Time: minimize time spent in close proximity to radiation source; a common standard is to limit contact time to 30 minutes total per 8-hour shift; minimum distance of 6 feet used when possible
   - **c.** Distance: maintain maximum distance possible from radiation source
   - **d.** Shielding: use lead shields and other precautions to reduce exposure to radiation
   - **e.** Place client in private room
   - **f.** Instruct visitors to maintain at least a distance of 6 feet from client and limit visits to 10 to 30 minutes
   - **g.** Ensure proper handling and disposal of body fluids, assuring containers are marked appropriately

Table 66–1 Laboratory Tests Used in Diagnosing Cancer

Lab Test	Cancer-Related Abnormality
Acid phosphatase (ACP)	Elevated in bone, breast, and prostate cancers and in multiple myeloma
Alanine aminotransferase (ALT)	Elevated in liver cancer
Albumin	Decreased in metastatic liver cancer and malnutrition
Alkaline phosphatase (ALP)	Elevated in bone, breast, liver, and prostate cancers and in leukemia and multiple myeloma
Alpha-fetoprotein (AFP)	Elevated in testicular cancer and in germ cell tumors
Aspartate aminotransferase (AST)	Elevated in liver cancer
Bilirubin	Elevated in liver and gallbladder cancers
Bleeding time	Prolonged in leukemia and metastatic liver cancer
Blood urea nitrogen (BUN)	Increased in renal cancer; decreased in malnutrition
Calcitonin	Elevated in breast, lung, and thyroid medullary cancers
Calcium (Ca)	Elevated in bone cancer
C-reactive protein	Elevated in metastatic cancer and Burkitts's lymphoma
Creatinine	Decreased in malnutrition; elevated in most cancers
Dexamethasone suppression test	Nonsuppression in adrenal cancer and ACTH-producing tumors, severe stress
Estradiol-serum	Elevated in estrogen-producing tumors and testicular tumor
Gamma glutamyltransferase (GGT)	Elevated in liver, pancreas, prostate, breast, kidney, lung, and brain cancers
Haptoglobin	Elevated in Hodgkin's disease and lung, large intestine, stomach, breast, and liver cancers
Hematocrit (Hct)	Decreased in anemia, leukemia, Hodgkin's disease, lymphosarcoma, multiple myeloma, and malnutrition and as a side effect of chemotherapy
Hemoglobin (Hgb)	Decreased in anemia, many cancers, Hodgkin's disease, leukemia, and malnutrition and as side effect of chemotherapy
Human chorionic gonadotropin (HCG)	Elevated in choriocarcinoma
Lactic dehydrogenase (LDH)	Elevated in liver, brain, kidney, and muscle cancers, acute leukemia, anemia
Occult blood	Positive in gastric and colon cancers
Parathyroid hormone (PTH)	Increased in PTH-secreting tumors
Platelet count (thrombocytes)	Decreased in bone, gastric, and brain cancers, in leukemia, and as a side effect of chemotherapy
Prostate-specific antigen (PSA)	Elevated from 10 to 120+ in prostate cancer
Red blood cells (RBCs)	Decreased in anemia, leukemia, infection, multiple myeloma
Uric acid	Increased in leukemia, metastatic cancer, multiple myeloma, Burkitt's lymphoma, after vigorous chemotherapy
White blood cells (WBCs); Total leukocytes	Elevated in acute infection, leukemias, tissue necrosis; decreased as a side effect of chemotherapy
Neutrophils	Elevated in bacterial infection, Hodgkin's disease; decreased in leukemia and malnutrition and as a side effect of chemotherapy
Eosinophils	Elevated in bone, ovary, testes, and brain cancers
Basophils	Elevated in leukemia and healing stage of infection
Monocytes	Elevated in infection, monocytic leukemia, and cancer; decreased in lymphocytic leukemia and as a side effect of chemotherapy
Lymphocytes	Elevated in lymphocytic leukmemia, Hodgkin's disease, multiple myeloma; decreased in cancer and other leukemias, and as a side effect of chemotherapy

Adapted from: LeMone, P., & Burke, K. (2004). *Medical-surgical nursing: Critical thinking in client care* (3rd ed.). Upper Saddle River, NJ: Prentice Hall.

- **h.** Ensure proper handling of bed linens and clothing
- **i.** In event of a dislodged implant, use long-handled forceps and place implant into a lead container; never directly touch implant
- **j.** Do not allow pregnant women to come into any contact with radiation sources; screen visitors and staff for pregnancy
- **k.** If working routinely near radiation sources, wear a monitoring device to measure exposure
- **l.** Educate client in all safety measures
- **m.** Provide emotional support to client who may feel isolated because of necessary precautions and to family because of their concerns for client and inability to assist client at this time

C. External radiation therapy (teletherapy)

1. Radiation oncologist marks specific locations for radiation treatment using a semipermanent type of ink
   - **a.** Treatment is usually given 15 to 30 minutes per day, 5 days per week, for 2 to 7 weeks
   - **b.** Client does not pose a risk for radiation exposure to other people
2. Side effects of external radiation therapy
   - **a.** Tissue damage to target area (erythema, sloughing, hemorrhage)
   - **b.** Ulcerations of oral mucous membranes
   - **c.** Gastrointestinal effects such as nausea, vomiting, and diarrhea
   - **d.** Radiation pneumonia
   - **e.** Fatigue
   - **f.** Alopecia
   - **g.** Immunosuppression
3. ! Client teaching for external radiation
   - **a.** Wash marked area of skin with plain water only and pat skin dry; do not use soaps, deodorants, lotions, perfumes, powders or medications on site during duration of treatment; do not wash off treatment site marks
   - **b.** Avoid rubbing, scratching, or scrubbing treatment site; do not apply extreme temperatures (heat or cold) to treatment site; if shaving, use only an electric razor
   - **c.** Wear soft, loose-fitting clothing over treatment area
   - **d.** Protect skin from sun exposure during treatment and for at least 1 year after treatment is completed; when going outdoors, use sun-blocking agents with sun protection factor (SPF) of at least 15
   - **e.** Maintain proper rest, diet, and fluid intake as essential to promoting health and repair of normal tissues
   - **f.** Hair loss may occur; choose a wig, hat, or scarf to cover and protect head (refer to care of client with alopecia later in chapter)
4. ! Nursing management of client receiving external radiation
   - **a.** Monitor for adverse side effects of radiation (see preceding section)
   - **b.** Monitor for significant decreases in white blood cell (WBC) counts and platelet counts
   - **c.** Client teaching (refer to later sections for management of immunosuppression, thrombocytopenia, and anemia)

D. *Chemotherapy*

1. Chemotherapy: administration of cytotoxic medications and chemicals to promote tumor cell death; IV route is preferred, but drugs may also be administered by oral, intrathecal, topical, intra-arterial, intracavity, and intravesical routes
   - **a.** Chemotherapy disrupts cell cycle in various phases, interfering with cellular metabolism and reproduction
   - **b.** According to **cell-kill hypothesis,** during each cell cycle a fixed percentage of cells are killed by chemotherapy, leaving some tumor cells remaining; this necessitates repeated doses to reduce number of cells, allowing body's immune system to destroy any remaining tumor cells
2. Classified according to mechanism of action (see Chapter 45 for discussion of specific chemotherapeutic drugs by category)

a. *Alkylating agents* are non-phase-specific and act by interfering with DNA replication
b. *Antimetabolites* interfere with metabolites or nucleic acids necessary for RNA and DNA synthesis
c. *Cytotoxic antibiotics* disrupt or inhibit DNA or RNA synthesis
d. *Hormones and hormone antagonists* are phase-specific (G1 or first growth stage) and act by interfering with RNA synthesis
e. *Plant alkaloids* interfere with cell division
f. *Miscellaneous agents* may be cell-cycle phase-specific or non-phase-specific and interfere with DNA replication

! 3. Side effects of chemotherapeutic agents (see also Chapter 45)
a. **Bone marrow suppression**: decreased WBC count (immunosuppression), platelet count (thrombocytopenia), and hemoglobin and hematocrit (anemia)
b. Gastrointestinal effects: anorexia, nausea, vomiting, and diarrhea
c. **Stomatitis** (inflammation of mouth) and mucositosis
d. **Alopecia** (hair loss)
e. Fatigue
f. **Xerostomia** (dry mouth)
g. Other side effects specific to chemotherapeutic agent

! 4. Management and client teaching for immunosuppression
a. Risk for infection is high when WBC count is low
b. Avoid crowds, people with infections, and small children when WBC is low
c. Use meticulous personal hygiene to avoid infection
d. Wash hands before and after eating, after toileting, and after contact with other people and pets
e. Consume a low-bacteria diet; avoid undercooked meat and raw fruits and vegetables
f. Be aware of signs and symptoms of infection and report them immediately to primary care provider
g. Monitor laboratory values: CBC with differential, platelets, BUN, liver enzymes
h. Assess for infection; monitor vital signs for early indication of infection: fever, tachycardia, and tachypnea
i. Utilize neutropenic precautions: low-bacteria diet (no fresh/raw fruits or vegetables), no fresh plants or flowers in room, no pets, no visitors with infections when WBC level falls below predetermined level (such as 2,000 mm^3)

! 5. Management and client teaching for thrombocytopenia
a. Monitor stools and urine for bleeding; stools may be dark or tarry and urine will have pinkish to red tinge
b. Avoid use of razors; use electric shaver only
c. Avoid contact sports and other activities that may cause trauma
d. If trauma does occur, apply ice to area and seek medical assistance
e. Avoid dental work or other invasive procedures unless absolutely necessary
f. Inform all health care providers of chemotherapy and/or radiation treatments
g. Avoid aspirin and aspirin-containing products
h. Safety precautions for oral hygiene: use soft toothbrushes and do not floss; avoid alcohol-based mouthwashes
i. There is a high risk for spontaneous hemorrhage when platelet count is below 20,000; bleeding precautions are necessary for platelet count below 50,000
j. Assess for bleeding, monitor stools and urine for occult blood
k. Assess skin for ecchymosis, petechiae, and trauma
l. Educate client about ways to reduce risk of bleeding and measures that are part of bleeding precautions during times of high risk
m. Avoid intramuscular (IM) injections and limit venipunctures

! 6. Management and client teaching for stomatitis and mucositosis
a. Use a soft toothbrush; mouth swabs may be needed during acute episode
b. Avoid mouthwashes containing alcohol; do not use lemon glycerin swabs or dental floss

c. Consider using chlorhexidine mouthwash (Peridex) to decrease risk of hemorrhage and protect gums from trauma
d. Assess daily for lesions, infection, bleeding, or irritation
e. For xerostomia, apply lubricating and moisturizing agents to protect mucous membranes from trauma and infection
f. May consider using "artificial saliva" and hard candy or mints to help with dryness
g. Avoid smoking and alcohol, which can further irritate oral mucosa
h. Teach signs and symptoms of oral infection and to report to health care provider
i. Drink cool liquids, and avoid hot (very warm) and spicy or otherwise irritating foods
j. Assess oral mucous membranes every 4 hours
k. Teach and implement proper oral care (see client teaching above)

! 7. Management and client teaching for inadequate nutrition and fluid and electrolyte imbalance
a. Eat frequent, small, low-fat meals
b. Avoid spicy and fatty foods
c. Avoid extremely hot, spicy, or extremely cold foods
d. Perform oral hygiene before and after meals
e. Maintain fluid intake as prescribed
f. Take nutritional supplements as prescribed (vitamins, liquid nutrition)
g. Maintain a daily journal of food and fluid intake
h. Assess for adequate hydration; for duration of treatment, encourage daily fluid intake of 2 to 3 liters unless contraindicated
i. Administer antiemetics *prior* to chemotherapy
j. Weigh client routinely such as weekly, monitor for weight loss; daily weights are not necessary and could increase client anxiety or depression about weight loss
k. Monitor lab values indicative of nutritional status (hemoglobin, hematocrit, albumin, prealbumin)
l. Monitor for diarrhea or constipation and nausea or vomiting
m. Encourage adequate nutritional intake with meals that are served attractively and in an environment free of noxious stimuli (bedpan, urinal, perfumes, air fresheners, and other odors)

! 8. Management and client teaching for fatigue
a. Fatigue is a normal response to chemotherapy and doesn't necessarily indicate disease progression
b. Continue daily activities as much as possible, allowing for rest periods in between
c. Assist client in self-care needs when indicated
d. Allow for periods of rest; cluster activities

! 9. Nursing management and client teaching for alopecia (hair loss)
a. Chemotherapy and radiation therapy may cause hair loss; chemotherapy-induced hair loss is temporary and hair will grow back, usually beginning about a month after completion of chemotherapy, although texture and color of new hair growth may be different; hair loss during radiation therapy to head may be permanent
b. Encourage client to choose a wig *before* hair loss occurs in order to match texture and hair color; an alternative is to wear colorful scarf or turban if client wishes
c. Care of hair and scalp includes washing hair two to three times a week with a mild shampoo; pat hair dry, and do not use a blow dryer
d. Allow client to express feelings concerning altered body image

E. Bone marrow transplant (BMT)

1. BMT is used in treatment of leukemias, usually in conjunction with radiation or chemotherapy
a. *Autologous BMT:* client is infused with own bone marrow harvested during remission of disease

b. *Allogenic BMT:* client is infused with donor bone marrow harvested from a healthy individual
2. Bone marrow is usually harvested from iliac crests, then frozen and stored until transfusion
3. Before receiving BMT, client must first undergo a phase of immunosuppressive therapy to destroy immune system; infection, bleeding, and death are major complications during this conditioning phase
4. After immunosuppression, bone marrow is transfused IV through a central line
5. Side effects of BMT
   a. Malnutrition
   b. Infection related to immunosuppression
   c. Bleeding related to thrombocytopenia
6. Client teaching: refer to previous sections on client teaching for altered nutrition, immunosuppression, and thrombocytopenia
7. Nursing management of client undergoing a BMT
   a. Monitor for graft-versus-host disease
   b. Provide private room for client (will be hospitalized 6 to 8 weeks)
   c. Encourage contact with significant others by using telephone, computer, and other means of communication to reduce feelings of isolation
   d. Refer to nursing management for imbalanced nutrition, immunosuppression, and thrombocytopenia

F. Other therapeutic interventions

1. Immunotherapy/biologic response modifiers (BMR); see also Chapter 46
   a. Enhances client's immune responses to modify biologic processes resulting in malignant cells
   b. Currently considered experimental in use
   c. *Monoclonal antibodies:* antibodies are recovered from an inoculated animal with a specific tumor antigen, then given to person with that particular cancer type; goal is destruction of tumor
   d. *Cytokines:* normal growth-regulating molecules possessing antitumor abilities, such as interleukin-2, interferons, hematopoietic growth factors such as erythropoietin, and granulocyte colony–stimulating factors (GCSF)
   e. *Natural killer cells* (NK cells): exert a spontaneous cytotoxic effect on specific cancer cells; they also secrete cytokines and provide a resistance to metastasis
2. Gene therapy: investigational; increases susceptibility of cancer cells to destruction by other treatments; insertion of specific genes enhances ability of client's own immune system to recognize and destroy cancer cells
3. Photodynamic therapy
   a. Used to treat specific superficial tumors such as those of surface of bladder, bronchus, chest wall, head, neck, and peritoneal cavity
   b. Photofrin, a photosensitizing compound, is administered IV, where it is retained by malignant tissue
   c. Three days after injection, drug is activated by a laser treatment, which continues for 3 more days
   d. Drug produces a cytotoxic O_2 molecule (singlet oxygen)
   e. During IV administration, monitor for chills, nausea, rash, local skin reactions, and temporary photosensitivity
   f. Drug remains in tissues 4 to 6 weeks after injection; direct or indirect exposure to sun activates drug, resulting in chemical sunburn; educate client to protect skin from sun exposure

VI. ONCOLOGIC EMERGENCIES: DIAGNOSIS AND MANAGEMENT

A. Spinal cord compression

1. Occurs because of pressure in epidural space of spinal cord from expanding tumor (lung, breast, GI) or lymphoma
2. ! Early symptoms include back and leg pain, coldness, numbness, tingling, paresthesia; progression leads to bowel and bladder dysfunction, weakness, and paralysis

3. Early detection is essential: investigate all complaints of back pain or neurological changes
4. Treatment is aimed at reducing tumor size by radiation and/or surgery to relieve compression and prevent irreversible paraplegia; client may receive corticosteroids to reduce cord edema
5. Nursing interventions include early recognition of symptoms, monitoring vital signs, neurological checks, and medication administration

B. Superior vena cava syndrome

1. Compression or obstruction of superior vena cava (SVC) by a tumor
2. Usually associated with cancer of lung, non-Hodgkin's lymphomas, and Hodgkin's disease
3. Signs and symptoms result from blockage of venous circulation of head, neck, and upper trunk
4. Early signs and symptoms are periorbital edema, facial edema, and jugular vein distention (JVD)
5. Symptoms progress to edema of neck, arms, and hands; difficulty swallowing; shortness of breath
6. Late signs and symptoms are cyanosis, altered mental status, headache, hypotension, and possible seizures
7. Death may occur if compression is not relieved
8. Treatment includes high-dose radiation to shrink tumor and relieve symptoms and possible adjuvant chemotherapy
9. Nursing interventions include monitoring vital signs (VS), providing O_2 support, preparing for tracheostomy if necessary, initiating seizure precautions, and administering corticosteroids to reduce edema

C. Disseminated intravascular coagulopathy (DIC)

1. Severe disorder of coagulation, often triggered by sepsis, whereby abnormal clot formation occurs in microvasculature; this process depletes clotting factors and platelets, allowing extensive bleeding to occur; tissue hypoxia occurs from blockage of blood vessels from clots
2. Signs and symptoms are related to decreased blood flow to major organs (tachycardia, oliguria, dyspnea) and depleted clotting factors (abnormal bleeding and hemorrhage)
3. Treatment includes anticoagulants to decrease stimulation of coagulation and transfusion of one or more of the following: fresh frozen plasma (FFP), cryoprecipitate, platelets, and packed red blood cells (RBCs)
4. Nursing interventions include assessing client, monitoring for bleeding, applying pressure dressings to venipuncture sites, and preventing risk of sepsis
5. Mortality for clients experiencing DIC is greater than 70% despite aggressive treatment

D. Cardiac tamponade

1. Pericardial effusion secondary to metastases or esophageal cancer can lead to compression of heart, restricting heart movement and resulting in cardiac tamponade
2. Signs and symptoms are related to cardiogenic shock or circulatory collapse: anxiety, cyanosis, dyspnea, hypotension, tachycardia, tachypnea, impaired LOC, and increased central venous pressure
3. Pericardiocentesis is performed to remove fluid from pericardial sac
4. Nursing interventions include administering O_2, maintaining IV line, monitoring VS, hemodynamic monitoring, and administration of vasopressor agents

VII. NEUROBLASTOMA

A. Overview

1. Solid tumor outside cranium originating in primitive neurocrest cells, which give rise to adrenal medulla, paraganglia, and sympathetic nervous system cervical chain and thoracic chain
2. In children, most common tumor located outside cranium; usual age at onset is 22 months

3. Prognosis based on client age and staging of tumor; children under 1 year of age have a better prognosis
4. Cause unknown, although environmental factors, such as prenatal drug exposure, may be implicated
5. Oncogenes have been found in neuroblastoma cells; DNA sequence responsible for this is called *N-myc;* high *N-myc* level is associated with rapid disease progression and poorer prognosis
6. Tumor is often silent, leading to late diagnosis and poor prognosis

B. Nursing assessment

! 1. Symptoms represent location and stage of disease
   a. A peritoneal tumor may present as an abdominal mass or may be evidenced by bowel and bladder dysfunction
   b. Typical signs include weight loss, abdominal fullness, irritability, fatigue, and fever
   c. Mediastinal tumors cause dyspnea and lead to neck and facial edema if tumor is large
   d. Bone metastasis may lead to limp, fever, and malaise; ptosis and ecchymosis of eyes can also occur
2. CT of skull, neck, chest, abdomen, and bone locate tumor
3. Bone marrow aspiration helps to locate mass and determine metastasis
4. Urine testing detects breakdown products of adrenal catecholamines (epinephrine and norepinephrine), which some tumors secrete; these breakdown products are vanillylmandelic acid (VMA) and homovanillic acid (HVA)

C. Therapeutic management

1. Surgery is used for tumor removal following biopsy
2. Radiation therapy
3. Chemotherapy

! 4. If surgery is performed, monitor surgical site for hemorrhage and infection; use temperature as most accurate indicator of infection
5. Monitor skin integrity at radiation site

! 6. Monitor mucous membrane integrity; use appropriate nursing interventions to prevent and treat mouth ulcers
7. Minimize exposure to infection as previously discussed
8. Monitor bleeding as previously discussed

D. Client and family teaching

1. Disease process as well as treatment modalities
2. Blood dyscrasias and actions they can take to improve child's condition
3. Need for good nutrition and management of nausea

VIII. BRAIN TUMORS

A. Overview

1. Over half of brain tumors in children are **infratentorial** (below tentorium cerebelli in the posterior third of the brain), primarily in cerebellum and brainstem
2. Most adult tumors and some tumors in children are **supratentorial** (above tentorial notch in anterior part of brain) and are mainly in cerebrum
3. The terms benign and malignant are of little value; benign brain tumors can also be fatal because of solid skull that allows no room for expansion of tumor and thus causes increased intracranial pressure (ICP)
4. Cause is unknown, although radiation and environmental factors have been implicated
5. Supporting cells of brain, such as glias and astrocytes, frequently account for pediatric brain tumors

B. Nursing assessment

1. Symptoms depend upon location of tumor and age of client
2. Since an infant's sutures are open, symptoms may be found late

! 3. Increased ICP occurs with brain tumors because of presence of the tumor and obstructions in flow of CSF; symptoms related to increased ICP include headache, especially on awakening, and vomiting unrelated to eating

! 4. Visual symptoms include diplopia and papilledema

5. Supratentorial tumors give rise to symptoms that include personality changes and seizures
6. Infratentorial tumor symptoms include ataxia, visual disturbances, delayed or precocious puberty, and growth failures
7. Diagnosis is based on results of MRI, CT scans, and radiographic studies with IV contrast; angiography is done when CT scans are positive
8. Surgery is used for biopsy (diagnosis), to completely remove a tumor, or to **debulk** an unremovable tumor (palliative procedure to surgically remove part of a neoplasm when complete excision is impossible); surgery may also be performed to restore patency of ventricles
9. Laser surgery can be used for more sensitive areas, where greater precision is needed
10. Radiation therapy may be used at the site postoperatively
11. Chemotherapy is commonly used, sometimes intrathecally
12. Complications such as hydrocephalus, seizures, sensorimotor deficits, and endocrine disorders may also need management
13. Maintain nutritional support; if client vomits from increased ICP, provide hygiene and refeed
14. Monitor LOC and observe for signs of increased ICP (increasing systolic BP, widening pulse pressure, bradycardia, irregular respirations); regulate fluid status to prevent rises in ICP; observe for seizures and provide nursing care should they occur; protect client from injury and have suction and O_2 available at bedside
15. Monitor I&O and measure urine specific gravity (to detect diabetes insipidus [DI] or syndrome of inappropriate ADH [SIADH] from pituitary involvement)
16. Postoperatively, position of head is critical; with an infratentorial incision, head position is flat with neck slightly extended; with supratentorial incision, head is elevated; physician orders degree of head elevation, often 30 degrees; keep head and neck midline to promote arterial and venous blood flow
17. If a ventriculoperitoneal (VP) shunt has been placed to restore ventricle drainage, nursing care includes maintaining suture line and skin integrity over shunt
18. Provide eye care to prevent dryness if client cannot blink or close eyes because of postoperative orbital edema
19. Monitor pain and provide relief; avoid medications that sedate client, which could interfere with assessment of LOC
20. Assess sensory-perceptual status and assist with loss of function
21. Assess surgical site for hemorrhage and infection

C. Client and family teaching

1. Reinforce information provided by physician about diagnosis and treatment; prepare client and family for the surgical procedure, including need to shave head and to expect ecchymosis of eyes, which is common following craniotomy
2. Teach activities that can reduce client's pain preoperatively and postoperatively
3. Encourage client and family to talk honestly about diagnosis and their feelings
4. If DI occurs secondary to brain tumor, teach client and family about medication (desmopressin [DDAVP]) to control symptoms

IX. WILMS' TUMOR

A. Overview

1. Intrarenal tumor, also called a nephroblastoma
2. Common abdominal tumor during childhood, most frequently between 2 and 5 years of age
3. A small proportion of Wilms tumors show a genetic basis with family members being at increased risk of development
4. Tumor may be unilateral or bilateral; bilateral tumors have poorer prognosis
5. Tumor is often encapsulated until relatively late; it metastasizes to lungs and liver

B. Nursing assessment

1. Usually asymptomatic
2. Most frequent admitting symptom is abdominal mass, which parent often finds on one side of midline of abdomen
3. Pain and hematuria may be present in some children

4. Hypertension is present in approximately 25% of children because of increased renin production
5. Diagnosis is made by abdominal ultrasound and intravenous pyelogram (IVP)
6. CT scan and MRI of the lungs are done to detect metastasis
7. Avoid palpating abdomen preoperatively to reduce risk of rupturing capsule and causing tumor spillage; place a sign over child's bed with instruction "No abdominal palpations"

C. Therapeutic management

1. If unilateral tumor is present, surgery is performed to remove affected kidney and assess for metastasis
2. Radiation to abdomen and chemotherapy can be used before and/or after surgery
3. Postoperatively, monitor functioning of remaining kidney
   - a. Measure I&O
   - b. Monitor daily weight and urine specific gravity
   - c. Monitor fluid levels, IV infusions, and BP
4. Complete pain assessment with VS; provide pain relief with medications and nursing interventions; in addition to incisional pain, pain may result from postoperative shift of internal organs to compensate for loss of kidney
5. Assess bowel sounds, abdominal distention, and bowel movements
6. Monitor for infection, observing surgical wound and body temperature

D. Client and family teaching

1. Need to avoid unnecessary palpation of abdomen prior to surgical removal
2. Nature of disease, treatment options, and therapeutic and side effects of chemotherapy in use (to parents)
3. Need to protect remaining kidney; signs and symptoms of urinary tract infections; and avoid contact sports, during which injury to kidney might occur

X. BONE TUMORS

A. Osteogenic sarcoma

1. Tumor that arises from a bone cell, probably osteoblast
   - a. Most common bone cancer in children
   - b. Most frequently affects metaphysis of long bones
   - c. Osteogenic sarcoma usually occurs in adolescent boys; tumor growth is detected at time of rapid bone growth
   - d. Most frequently affects distal portion of femur; also affects humerus, tibia, pelvis, jaw, and phalanges
   - e. Malignant tumor that frequently metastasizes to lungs; metastasis may be present at time of diagnosis
   - f. Etiology is unknown, but increased incidence is noted in children who have had retinoblastoma; an abnormal gene may also be implicated, as familial tendency for osteogenic sarcoma has been noted
2. Nursing assessment
   - a. Pain and swelling are initial symptoms
   - b. X-rays following traumatic injury may be first indication of disease
   - c. Follow-up assessments include CT or MRI imaging to detect areas of metastasis
3. Therapeutic management
   - a. Treatment may include radical resection or amputation
   - b. Selected clients may have limb-salvaging procedures with prosthetic replacement
   - c. Thoracotomy may be performed for metastasis to lung
   - d. Chemotherapy may be administered pre- and postoperatively
   - e. Emotional support of child is important both pre- and postoperatively, as child and family deal with life-threatening disease and treatment affects body image and mobility
   - f. Employ a straightforward approach when amputation is indicated; allow for verbal expression of feelings
   - g. Postoperative care includes sterile stump care and special bandaging as ordered
   - h. Elevate stump for 24 hours, if prescribed, but avoid prolonged elevation
   - i. Maintain body alignment

j. Perform ROM to joints above amputation
k. Provide opioid analgesics to relieve postoperative pain as ordered; be aware that phantom pain can occur in amputated limb because of irritation of residual nerve endings; use opioid analgesics for this type of pain also
l. Assist with early ambulation; assist with temporary prosthesis use
m. Teach appropriate use of assistive devices
n. Encourage early interaction with peers

4. Client and family teaching
   a. Reinforce disease process and treatment options
   b. Stump care (wash daily; use clean cotton or woolen stump sock; examine daily for intact skin)
   c. Demonstrate safe use of prosthesis; teach child to monitor condition of stump
   d. Phantom limb pain and its management

B. Ewing's sarcoma

1. Overview
   a. A malignant, small, round cell tumor that usually involves diaphysial (shaft) portion of long bones; commonly found in femur, pelvis, tibia, fibula, ribs, scapula, humerus, and clavicle
   b. Tumor arises in marrow spaces of bone
   c. Tends to occur in individuals between ages of 4 and 25
   d. Is a highly malignant tumor that metastasizes to lung
2. Nursing assessment
   a. Pain
   b. Soft tissue mass
   c. Secondary symptoms of anorexia, malaise, fever, fatigue, and weight loss
   d. Diagnosed with x-rays of affected area
   e. Radionuclide bone scans and CT scans of chest assess for metastasis
3. Therapeutic management
   a. Amputation usually not recommended
   b. Treatment includes extensive radiation along with chemotherapy
   c. Emotional support of child is important, as radiation therapy can affect appearance and mobility of extremity
   d. Encourage mobility of extremity as tolerated
   e. Allow open communication with child and family about disease and its prognosis
4. Client and family teaching: disease process and treatment options; skin care related to radiation therapy

XI. COLON CANCER

A. Overview

1. Develops in bowel wall or begins as polyps in colon or rectum that deteriorate
2. Metastasizes via circulatory or lymphatic system or by direct extension to other areas of bowel or adjacent organs
3. Can cause abscesses or fistulas, bowel obstruction, hemorrhage or perforation of bowel, leading to peritonitis
4. Has third-highest incidence in men and women, with death rates same (10%) for both genders

B. Nursing assessment

1. Client may have no signs early in course of disease, making screening tests such as fecal occult blood and colonoscopy so important
2. Anorexia, vomiting, and weight loss; cachexia are late signs
3. Malaise
4. Anemia
5. Abdominal distention and possible guarding
6. Hematest positive or bloody stools with altered bowel pattern
   a. Tumor in ascending colon: diarrhea
   b. Tumor in descending colon: constipation or diarrhea; possible flat, ribbonlike stools from partial obstruction
   c. Tumor in rectum: alternating diarrhea and constipation
7. Abdominal mass (late sign)

C. Therapeutic management

1. Monitor for development of complications
   a. Bowel perforation: distended abdomen; fever; weak, rapid pulse; and hypotension
   b. Intestinal obstruction: abdominal pain and distention, constipation, vomiting (may be fecal), hyperactive bowel sounds early (attempt to push past obstruction) followed by hypoactive then absent bowel sounds
2. Preoperative or postoperative radiation therapy to shrink tumor and symptoms it causes or to prevent recurrence
3. Surgery: bowel resection, ileostomy or colostomy; see Chapter 60 for highlights of colostomy and ileostomy care
4. Note characteristics of stool following ostomy creation
   a. Ileostomy: liquid dark green stool progressing to yellow
   b. Ascending colostomy: liquid stool that is greenish then brown
   c. Transverse colostomy: liquid to semiformed brown
   d. Descending colostomy: semiformed to almost normal brown
5. Provide routine postoperative care including pain management and assessment of stoma and return of bowel function

D. Client teaching

1. Ostomy care
2. Dietary needs with ostomy (foods that loosen or thicken stool; foods that reduce or cause odor of stool)
3. Activity, medications, and follow-up care
4. Signs and symptoms of complications to report (such as infection, delayed wound healing)

XII. TESTICULAR CANCER

A. Overview

1. Unregulated growth of abnormal cells within testicles
2. Exact cause is unknown, but risk factors include cryptorchidism (undescended testicles at birth), maternal treatment with DES during pregnancy, mumps orchitis, trauma, environmental factors, and age
3. Most common cancer among males age 15 to 35, making sperm banking important to preserve ability to produce offspring
4. Testicular cancer is usually slow-growing and localized, with a good prognosis

B. Nursing assessment

1. Painless, hardened area or lump found during testicular self-examination (TSE) is common
2. Dull ache in pelvis or scrotum
3. Testicular pain may occur with associated infection, necrosis, or hemorrhage
4. Weight loss and fatigue
5. Metastatic signs such as respiratory symptoms, GI disturbances, lumbar back pain, lymphadenopathy, and gynecomastia
6. Scrotal ultrasound; CT or MRI scan of chest, abdomen, and pelvis may rule out metastasis
7. IVP to determine kidney involvement
8. AFP and beta unit of HCG are tumor markers; elevated levels strongly suggest testicular cancer; markers are measured after surgery to determine residual disease, possibly in lymph nodes
9. Serum lactic dehydrogenase (LDH) is elevated with testicular cancer

C. Therapeutic management

1. Prepare client for screening tests to determine type of cancer and stage
2. Provide emotional support for client and family; respond to questions and encourage client to express his feelings
3. Prepare client for surgery if indicated (orchiectomy and exploration of adjacent area to identify cancer cell type and stage disease; lymphadenectomy if indicated)
4. Prepare client for chemotherapy after surgery and possible radiation therapy if cancer has spread to lymph nodes

! 5. After surgery: provide analgesics, ice packs, and scrotal support to control pain and swelling; monitor for complications, such as bleeding or infection

D. Client teaching

1. Reinforce explanation of type of cancer found, extent of disease, and plans for treatment
2. Importance of monthly TSE, because malignancy may develop in remaining testis; see Chapter 17 for procedure
3. ! Possibility of preserving sperm in a bank before surgery to help relieve client's fears about infertility
4. Orchiectomy should have no lasting effects on client's sexual or reproductive function
5. Signs of complications: bleeding, gaping incision, or purulent drainage from incision
6. Methods to control pain, such as ice bags and scrotal support
7. Remain at home for about 5 days and avoid driving for 1 week
8. Avoid strenuous physical activity for 3 weeks
9. Follow health care provider's instructions for resuming sexual activity
10. Importance of follow-up, especially if retroperitoneal lymph nodes were not surgically explored; client will need periodic physical examinations, tumor markers, and CT scans of retroperitoneal nodes for 5 to 10 years after surgery

XIII. PROSTATE CANCER

A. Overview

1. Unregulated growth of abnormal cells in prostate gland
2. Adenocarcinoma is most common type; high levels of testosterone may play a role; is most common after 40 years of age
3. Usually begins in peripheral tissue on back and sides of gland
4. Metastasis via lymph and venous channels is common; bony tissue is major site of distant metastasis—especially pelvic bones and spine

B. Nursing assessment

1. Clients in early stages often show no symptoms; tumor may be found during digital prostate exam
2. ! Genitourinary: dysuria, frequency, reduced force of stream, hematuria, nocturia, abnormal prostate found on digital rectal exam
3. Musculoskeletal: back pain, migratory bone pain, bone or joint pain
4. Neurological: nerve pain, muscle spasms, bowel or bladder dysfunction, bilateral weakness of lower extremities
5. ! Systemic: fatigue and weight loss
6. ! Diagnostic and laboratory tests: elevated PSA levels, transrectal ultrasonography (obtained if PSA results are abnormal), tissue biopsy, bone scan; MRI, or CT scans to detect metastasis

C. Therapeutic management

1. Treatment options include hormone therapy, radiation therapy, brachytherapy (radioactive seeds implanted in the prostate), prostatic cryosurgery, and conventional surgery
2. Surgical procedures
   a. Orchiectomy decreases androgen production
   b. Radical prostatectomy procedures include removal of gland, capsule, ampulla, vas deferens, seminal vesicles, adjacent lymph nodes, and cuff of bladder neck
   c. Suprapubic prostatectomy: abdominal and bladder incisions to remove prostate tissue; abdominal dressing may leak copious urine; change dressing as needed and maintain continuous bladder irrigation (see next section); risk of hemorrhage and bladder spasms
   d. Retropubic prostatectomy: low abdominal incision without opening bladder; less bleeding and fewer bladder spasms than suprapubic route
   e. Perineal prostatectomy: incision between scrotum and anus (perineal area); minimal bleeding but increased risk of infection; urinary incontinence common; surgery causes sterility; avoid rectal tubes, enemas, and temperatures

f. Homium laser: laser treatment; less bleeding, fewer complications, and shorter hospital stay
3. Encourage annual prostate examination for men 40 years old and above
4. Medication therapy: estrogen therapy or luteinizing hormone antagonist (Lupron) given to slow rate of growth and extension of tumor

D. Care of client having prostate surgery

! 1. Monitor VS closely for 24 hours, observing for signs of hemorrhage (frank blood in urine, large blood clots, decreased hemoglobin and hematocrit, tachycardia, and hypotension)
2. Maintain usual postoperative assessments, including lung and bowel sounds, IV fluid infusions, pain, urine output
! 3. If dressings are present, monitor for drainage and change as needed
! 4. Clients have a urinary catheter following surgery; surgeon may apply traction against prostatic fossa to prevent bleeding; balloon at tip of catheter exerts pressure to prevent hemorrhage (surgeon positions external end of catheter by anchoring it tightly to client's inner thigh to maintain traction; do not reposition catheter)
5. A client who has a large indwelling catheter may feel urge to void, which results from stimulation of micturition center; explain to client this is a normal sensation; efforts by client to void or strain will increase risk of bleeding and aggravate pain
! 6. Continuous bladder irrigation (CBI) postoperatively
   a. Purpose is to prevent formation of blood clots
   b. If blood clots do form, urinary catheter will become plugged and prevent outflow of urine; obstruction will also cause bladder spasms and pain
   c. Titrate flow rate of irrigating solution to maintain outflow light pink (early) or pale yellow (later) in color and prevent blood clots from forming; it is essential to calculate both intake and output from catheter to determine true urine output; subtract CBI inflow from output for shift or 24-hour period to determine actual urine output
   d. Indications that irrigation rate is inadequate include decreased outflow from catheter; bladder spasms; and dark-colored, "punch-colored," or frankly bloody drainage
   e. Maintain sterile technique while changing irrigation bags
7. Monitor client for signs of hemorrhage; bladder spasms and frank bloody output may indicate bleeding
! 8. The irrigating solution used during and after surgery may be absorbed, causing fluid shifts and dilutional hyponatremia, referred to as TURP syndrome
   a. Monitor client for signs of hyponatremia and bradycardia, nausea, and vomiting
   b. Monitor serum sodium and hemoglobin and hematocrit (lowered with dilutional effect)
   c. Other signs of volume excess will also be evident, including hypertension and confusion
9. If manual irrigations are ordered, maintain sterile technique
! 10. Medicate as needed for surgical pain with opioids and use suppositories such as belladonna and opium (B&O) to relieve sudden severe pain caused by bladder spasm

E. Client teaching

1. Reinforce information about illness and treatment plan
2. Methods to deal with urinary incontinence, which occurs temporarily after surgery, but could be permanent if bladder sphincters have been permanently damaged
3. Care of urinary catheter
4. Teach methods of pain control
5. Impact of therapy on sexual function (temporary or permanent impotence, permanent infertility after radical prostatectomy)
6. Refer client to support groups, such as American Cancer Society
7. Importance of follow-up tests for recurrence of disease

C. Therapeutic management

1. Treatment options include surgery, radiation therapy, chemotherapy, and hormonal therapy
2. Explore treatment options with client and family; prepare client for treatment, which is based on stage of disease
3. Radiation therapy is used to destroy remaining cancer cells after surgery or to shrink tumor prior to surgery
4. Various types of mastectomy may be performed
   a. Segmental mastectomy or lumpectomy: removes tumor and a margin of breast tissue surrounding tumor
   b. Simple mastectomy: removal of complete breast but no other structures
   c. Modified radical mastectomy: removal of breast and axillary lymph nodes, but not chest wall muscles
   d. Radical mastectomy: removal of breast, axillary lymph nodes, and underlying chest wall muscles; seldom done anymore
   e. ! Breast reconstruction: may be performed at time of mastectomy or at a later time; can be accomplished through submuscular breast implant, placing an implant after using a tissue expander, using muscles with intact blood supply from back or abdomen, or creating a free muscle flap with gluteus maximus muscle
5. ! Assist client in dealing with psychological effects of illness; provide information and emotional support, including information about breast reconstruction surgery
6. Maintain skin and tissue integrity during radiation treatment and following surgery
7. Medication therapy: tamoxifen (Novadex) interferes with estrogen activity for treating advanced breast cancer, and chemotherapy when axillary nodes are involved

D. Nursing management of client undergoing a mastectomy

1. Maintain usual postoperative assessments
2. Begin emotional support before surgery and continue in postoperative period
3. Turn, cough, and deep-breathe to prevent respiratory complications; restrictive surgical dressing may decrease chest expansion
4. Position client on back or unaffected side
5. ! Maintain Jackson-Pratt drain or Hemovac to drain fluids that accumulate when lymph nodes are removed
6. Note signs of bleeding on dressing and reinforce pressure dressing as needed
7. ! Encourage early ROM exercise to prevent contractures and lymphedema
8. ! Use only unaffected arm to provide IV fluids and measure BP
9. ! Position affected arm with each distal joint higher than proximal one before it (shoulder, elbow, wrist, and fingers)

E. Client teaching

1. Reinforce all diagnostic tests and treatments, allowing client time to express feelings and ask questions
2. Information about mastectomy surgery and what to expect afterward
3. Wound care if surgery is performed, including care of short-term wound drains
4. ! Discharge instructions postmastectomy
   a. Use caution when lifting heavy objects with arm on affected side
   b. Avoid injury and infection on affected side; wear rubber gloves when washing dishes and garden gloves when working outside; use potholders and oven mitts when using warm or hot cooking items
   c. Don't allow procedures, such as BP or venipuncture, on affected side
   d. Availability of support groups for psychosocial support
   e. Avoid heavy lifting for at least 6 weeks or until approved by surgeon
5. Techniques for proper skin care if radiation therapy is performed
6. Encourage client to meet other women who have undergone treatment, if appropriate
7. Postoperative exercises and monthly SBE
8. Self-care during radiation and chemotherapy treatments
9. Importance of regular screening exams and follow-up after treatment is completed

PRACTICE TEST

Check Your NCLEX–RN® Exam I.Q. *You are ready for testing on this content if you can*

- Describe the pathophysiology and etiology of common oncological disorders.
- Discuss expected assessment data and diagnostic test findings for selected oncological disorders.
- Discuss therapeutic management of a client experiencing an oncological disorder.
- Discuss nursing management of a client experiencing an oncological disorder.
- Identify expected outcomes for the client experiencing an oncological disorder.

PRACTICE TEST

1 A 4-year-old child is receiving postoperative care for surgical resection of a Wilms tumor. In addition to urinary functioning, one of the most important postoperative assessments is

1. bowel function.
2. neurological status.
3. presence of bone pain.
4. activity level.

2 A child with a brain tumor has shown symptoms of diabetes insipidus. A nursing assessment to monitor this condition would include

1. blood glucose levels.
2. urine specific gravity.
3. adrenocorticotropic hormone (ACTH) levels.
4. blood urea nitrogen (BUN) levels.

3 The nurse determines that the client with Ewing's sarcoma understands instruction related to radiation therapy when the client reports that side effects include which of the following?

1. An increased risk of infection
2. Constipation
3. An increased appetite
4. Hemorrhagic cystitis

4 A 6-month-old infant is being treated for neuroblastoma. Because of the chemotherapy, the infant feeds poorly and vomits frequently. The nurse would use which of the following assessments to best determine the child's fluid status?

1. Daily weight
2. Urinary output
3. Specific gravity of urine
4. Hemoglobin and hematocrit

5 A child is being treated for acute lymphocytic leukemia (ALL). The laboratory report shows a white blood cell (WBC) count of 7,000/mm^3. The nursing care plan lists risk for infection as a priority nursing diagnosis, and measures are being taken to reduce the child's exposure to infection. The nurse determines that the plan has been successful when the

1. child's WBC count goes up.
2. child's WBC count goes down.
3. child's temperature remains within normal range.
4. parents demonstrate good handwashing technique.

6 A child with neuroblastoma will be started on total parenteral nutrition (TPN) because of cancer cachexia. The nurse would question which of the following newly written physician orders?

1. Add 10 units NPH insulin to the TPN solution
2. Monitor blood glucose level every four hours
3. Daily intake and output
4. Regular diet

7 A child has been diagnosed with a brain tumor, but surgery cannot be scheduled for several days. The mother asks what she can do to ease her child's headaches. The nurse suggests that the mother

1. help the child to drink plenty of liquids.
2. discourage the child from having a bowel movement.
3. encourage the child to sleep in a semi-Fowler's position.
4. encourage the child to blow the nose when headaches become severe.

8 A child is being treated with corticosteroids for acute lymphocytic leukemia (ALL). On a follow-up visit, the pediatric home health nurse assesses for side effects of steroid use, including

1. decreased blood pressure.
2. alopecia.
3. weight gain.
4. anorexia.

9 A client with squamous cell carcinoma of the lung comes to the emergency department reporting shortness of breath and respiratory difficulty. On assessment, the nurse notes generalized cyanosis and edema of the face and arms. Based on this assessment, the nurse suspects the client is probably experiencing which of the following?

1. Spinal cord compression
2. Syndrome of inappropriate antidiuretic hormone (SIADH)
3. Superior vena cava syndrome
4. Sepsis

10 The nurse reads in the medical record that a client's tumor is stage at T2, N0, M0. The nurse concludes that this staging indicates which of the following about the client's status?

1. There is an advanced tumor with metastasis.
2. The client has a measurable tumor with no indication of metastasis or involvement of nodes.
3. There is an advanced tumor with indication of involvement of lymph nodes but no indication of metastasis.
4. The client has an advanced tumor with indication of metastasis but no indication of involvement of lymph nodes.

11 A client with lung cancer is admitted to the oncology clinic to receive radiation therapy for treatment of spinal cord compression. The client's spouse asks why radiation is being done. The nurse's response would include that radiation therapy is used

1. to eradicate the tumor.
2. to reduce size of the tumor.
3. in the treatment of all oncological emergencies.
4. instead of chemotherapy to treat the lung cancer.

12 A client with esophageal cancer arrives in the emergency department with shortness of breath, tachycardia, hypotension, and cyanosis. The physician determines the client is experiencing cardiac tamponade. Which of the following interventions would the nurse expect to include in this client's care?

1. Administer a vasodilator agent intravenously.
2. Initiate oxygen and insert an intravenous catheter for IV access.
3. Prepare to assist physician with a thoracentesis.
4. Prepare the client for radiation therapy.

13 The nurse is discussing risk factors associated with cancer to a male client in the clinic. The client asks which cancers have the highest incidence in men. In order of occurrence, the nurse would explain that the client has greatest risk for which of the following cancers based on gender?

1. Lung, prostate, and colorectal cancers
2. Prostate, lung, and colorectal cancers
3. Colorectal, lung, and prostate cancers
4. Prostate, colorectal, and lung cancers

14 A new nurse on the unit is admitting a severely leukopenic client who is receiving radiation therapy. The preceptor determines that the new nurse understands precautionary measures necessary for this client when he or she admits this client to which of the following rooms?

1. A semiprivate room with a client who has pneumonia
2. A private room with contact isolation
3. A private room with protective isolation
4. A private room with no isolation precautions

15 After completing a health risk assessment on a client, you determine health teaching and education is necessary because of an increased risk for laryngeal cancer caused by which of the following risk factors?

1. Past infection with Epstein-Barr virus
2. Past exposure to asbestos
3. Smoking marijuana for recreational drug use
4. Smoking cigarettes and consuming large quantities of alcohol daily

16 A client newly diagnosed with breast cancer is scheduled for a lymph node biopsy and asks the nurse why it is necessary when a diagnosis of cancer has already been made. The nurse's response is based on which of the following?

1. A lymph node biopsy is necessary to determine what type of cancer cells are present.
2. A lymph node biopsy is performed on all females with cancer.
3. A lymph node biopsy is performed to determine if cancer has metastasized.
4. A lymph node biopsy is performed to determine what type of chemotherapy is indicated.

17 A 65-year-old postmenopausal client tells the nurse that she has recently experienced painless vaginal bleeding. The nurse should

1. Not be concerned because postmenopausal bleeding is normal.
2. Be concerned because painless uterine bleeding is a sign of uterine cancer.
3. Be concerned because the client may develop anemia.
4. Not be concerned because the client does not complain of pain.

18 A client is brought to the surgical unit after a suprapubic prostatectomy. He has a three-way Foley catheter. The nurse notices a very dark red output via the catheter. What is the appropriate nursing intervention?

1. Report the finding immediately to the physician.
2. Increase the irrigation flow rate.
3. Check the latest hemoglobin and hematocrit count.
4. Chart the observation in the medical record.

19 The nurse who is screening female clients for cancer anticipates which of the following in relation to the early signs of ovarian cancer?

1. Painful urination is a common complaint.
2. Pelvic pain radiating to thighs may occur.
3. Usually no symptoms are seen.
4. Low back pain is a common complaint.

20 A client has stage II ovarian cancer documented as a diagnosis on the medical record. The nurse plans care based on which characteristic of this tumor at this stage?

1. Tumor growth is limited to the ovaries.
2. Tumor growth involves one or both ovaries, with pelvic extension.
3. Tumor growth involves the ovaries and peritoneum, with positive lymph nodes.
4. Tumor growth involves distant metastasis.

21 A client is scheduled for a radical mastectomy. When reinforcing the surgeon's explanation of the procedure, the nurse would include that the surgery involves which of the following?

1. Removal of breast tissue and lymph nodes under the arm
2. Removal of the entire breast, underlying chest muscles, and lymph nodes
3. Removal of the complete breast only
4. Removal of the tumor and surrounding tissues

22 A client returns to the medical unit following transurethral resection of the prostate (TURP). The client states to the nurse that he wants the three-way Foley catheter to be removed because it is causing him to have bladder spasms. Which of the following is the best response by the nurse?

1. "Spasms are painful but expected because of the wide diameter of the catheter and the retention balloon in the bladder."
2. "This must be a complication because the Foley catheter is supposed to evacuate clots that cause the spasms."
3. "The spasm is an unexpected finding because the procedure does not invade the urethra."
4. "Foley catheters in general have the tendency to cause bladder spasms because of the silicone used in the catheter."

23 The client who underwent prostate surgery is approaching the time of discharge from the hospital. Which of the following instructions should the nurse provide to this client as part of discharge teaching?

1. "Reduce your fluid intake so you won't need to void as often."
2. "Call the doctor immediately if you notice blood in your urine."
3. "You may drive yourself home."
4. "Avoid strenuous activity and heavy lifting for 4 to 8 weeks."

24 The nurse would write which of the following interventions in the care plan of a client following mastectomy for breast cancer?

1. Use warm, moist compresses on affected arm for comfort.
2. Start intravenous lines on the affected side only in the antecubital area.
3. Wait for the third postoperative day to begin any arm exercises.
4. Keep the affected arm elevated above heart level.

25 A client has a continuous bladder irrigation running after prostatectomy. During the shift, 600 mL of one bag of irrigant has infused and 1,500 mL of the next has also infused. Upon draining the urine bag three times during the shift, the nurse measures the volumes to be 800 mL, 1,050 mL, and 950 mL. What is the client's true urine output? Provide a numerical answer.

Answer: ____________________

ANSWERS & RATIONALES

1 **Answer: 1** There is great potential for alteration in bowel function (adynamic ileus) because of surgery and radiation to the abdominal area and the use of chemotherapeutic agents. This is an intrarenal tumor, so neurological status and bone pain are not related manifestations. Activity level would not be a specific assessment to make with this diagnosis.
Cognitive Level: Analysis **Client Need:** Physiological Integrity: Physiological Adaptation **Integrated Process:** Nursing Process: Assessment **Content Area:** Child Health: Oncology **Strategy:** The core issue of the question is knowledge that Wilms tumor affects the kidney, and therefore principles related to care following abdominal surgery apply to this client. Use nursing knowledge and the process of elimination to make a selection.

2 **Answer: 2** Diabetes insipidus presents with symptoms of increased urinary output and very dilute urine. Urinary specific gravity will measure the concentration of the urine. Blood glucose and BUN are unrelated to the issue of the question. ACTH levels are not routinely monitored in any client.
Cognitive Level: Analysis **Client Need:** Physiological Integrity: Physiological Adaptation **Integrated Process:** Nursing Process: Assessment **Content Area:** Child Health: Oncology **Strategy:** The core issue of the question is knowledge of diabetes insipidus and methods to assess the status of this complication. Use nursing knowledge and the process of elimination to make a selection.

3 **Answer: 1** Bone marrow suppression occurs with radiation therapy, which can lead to risk of infection when white blood cells are affected, bleeding when platelets are affected, and anemia when red blood cells are affected. Constipation and hemorrhagic cystitis occur after chemotherapy. If appetite is affected, it decreases rather than increases.
Cognitive Level: Application **Client Need:** Physiological Integrity: Physiological Adaptation **Integrated Process:** Nursing Process: Evaluation **Content Area:** Child Health: Oncology **Strategy:** The core issue of the question is knowledge of bone marrow suppression in a client receiving radiation therapy. Use basic nursing knowledge and the process of elimination to make a selection.

4 **Answer: 1** Because infant kidneys do not concentrate urine as well as the kidneys of adults, urine volume and specific gravity may not indicate fluid volume as accurately as will daily weight. Weight loss can be directly tied to fluid loss. Hemoglobin and hematocrit could rise and fall because of hemodilution or hemoconcentration, depending on fluid status, but these levels would be indirect indicators with large changes in fluid status and therefore not specific fluid balance measurements.
Cognitive Level: Analysis **Client Need:** Physiological Integrity: Physiological Adaptation **Integrated Process:** Nursing Process: Analysis **Content Area:** Child Health: Oncology **Strategy:** The core issue of the question is the most reliable method of determining fluid balance in an infant that is not feeding well because of neuroblastoma. Use nursing knowledge of fluid balance measurement and the process of elimination to make a selection.

5 **Answer: 3** In leukemia, the WBCs that are present are immature and incapable of fighting infection. Increases or decreases in the number of WBCs can be related to the disease process and treatment and not related to infection. The only value that indicates the child is infection-free is the temperature. The use of proper handwashing technique is a measure or intervention used to meet a goal but is not a goal itself.
Cognitive Level: Analysis **Client Need:** Physiological Integrity: Physiological Adaptation **Integrated Process:** Nursing Process: Evaluation **Content Area:** Child Health: Oncology **Strategy:** The core issue of the question is knowledge of an indicator of infection in a client who is immunosuppressed from leukemia. Recall that temperature and WBC counts are frequently used as indicators of infection. Recall that in leukemia the WBCs are abnormal to choose the option related to temperature.

6 **Answer: 1** Only regular insulin is administered in solutions administered by the IV route. Monitoring blood glucose and I&O is appropriate. The child is usually anorexic but will be allowed to eat any food that appeals to him or her.
Cognitive Level: Analysis **Client Need:** Physiological Integrity: Physiological Adaptation **Integrated Process:** Nursing Process: Implementation **Content Area:** Child Health: Oncology **Strategy:** The core issue of the question is knowledge of total parenteral nutrition as a means of providing nutritional support to a client with cancer. Use nursing knowledge about the uses of various preparations of insulin and the process of elimination to make a selection.

7 **Answer: 3** When a client is lying flat, the blood flow to the brain is greater, increasing the intracranial pressure. If the client sleeps in semi-Fowler's position, less pressure will develop, which in turn should ease headaches. Excess liquids and blowing the nose could aggravate headache. Discouraging bowel movements will reduce straining but is not a helpful measure from a gastrointestinal perspective.
Cognitive: Analysis **Client Need:** Physiological Integrity: Physiological Adaptation **Integrated Process:** Nursing Process: Implementation **Content Area:** Child Health: Oncology **Strategy:** Recall principles of gravity to answer this question. When a client lies flat, blood can accumulate to a greater extent in the cranium, resulting in vasodilation, increased pressure, and worsening headache. Placing the client's head in an elevated position allows gravity to drain blood to the heart and thereby keeps intracranial pressure rises to a minimum.

8 **Answer: 3** A person taking steroids may have increased blood pressure, increased appetite, and weight gain. Alopecia is related to chemotherapeutic agents that may be used to treat the leukemia.
Cognitive Level: Application **Client Need:** Physiological Integrity: Physiological Adaptation **Integrated Process:** Nursing Process: Assessment **Content Area:** Child Health: Oncology **Strategy:** The core issue of the question is knowledge of adverse effects of

combination agents, specifically steroids in this case, needed to treat cancer in a child. Use nursing knowledge and the process of elimination to make a selection.

9 **Answer: 3** While all of the above are potential risks to clients with cancer depending on site, edema of the face and arms results from obstruction of blood flow, which is indicative of superior vena cava syndrome. Spinal cord compression would give rise to neurological symptoms. SIADH would result in general fluid overload, and sepsis would be noted by signs of infection.
Cognitive Level: Analysis **Client Need:** Physiological Integrity: Physiological Adaptation **Integrated Process:** Nursing Process: Assessment **Content Area:** Adult Health **Strategy:** The core issue of the question is knowledge of various oncological emergencies. Use nursing knowledge about which body systems are affected by each and then use the process of elimination to make a selection.

10 **Answer: 2** T2 indicates a measurable tumor, N0 indicates no regional node involvement, and M0 indicates no evidence of distant metastasis. Options 1, 3, and 4 are either partially or totally incorrect.
Cognitive Level: Analysis **Client Need:** Physiological Integrity: Physiological Adaptation **Integrated Process:** Nursing Process: Analysis **Content Area:** Adult Health: Oncology **Strategy:** The core issue of the question is knowledge of staging for solid tumors. Recall that for an option to be correct, all of the parts of the option must be correct. Note the numeric zeros by the N and the M to choose the option that does not contain metastasis or lymph node involvement.

11 **Answer: 2** Radiation is palliative treatment for spinal cord compression to reduce the tumor size and relieve compression. Options 1, 3, and 4 are incorrect statements.
Cognitive Level: Application **Client Need:** Physiological Integrity: Physiological Adaptation **Integrated Process:** Teaching and Learning **Content Area:** Adult Health: Oncology **Strategy:** The core issue of the question is the rationale for using radiation therapy in a client with spinal cord compression secondary to cancer. Recall that radiation therapy is often used as a supplement to shrink tumors to aid in making a selection.

12 **Answer: 2** Oxygen and IV access are immediate interventions for the client with cardiac tamponade. Vasopressor agents will be administered to manage hypotension (option 1); a pericardiocentesis is performed, not a thoracentesis (option 3); and radiation therapy is not indicated for cardiac tamponade (option 4).
Cognitive Level: Analysis **Client Need:** Physiological Integrity: Physiological Adaptation **Integrated Process:** Nursing Process: Planning **Content Area:** Adult Health: Oncology **Strategy:** The stem of the question indicates that the client has an ineffective airway (shortness of breath and cyanosis). Look for the option that first addresses airway (oxygen) as the correct answer.

13 **Answer: 2** Prostate cancer has surpassed lung cancer in order of occurrence; colorectal cancer is the third-most common cancer. Options 1, 3, and 4 are incorrect.
Cognitive Level: Application **Client Need:** Physiological Integrity: Physiological Adaptation **Integrated Process:** Teaching and Learning **Content Area:** Adult Health: Oncology **Strategy:** Specific knowledge of the risks associated with various cancers in men is needed to answer the question. Use nursing knowledge related to epidemiology of cancer and the process of elimination to make a selection.

14 **Answer: 3** Because of the immunosuppression, the client is at severe risk of infection. Precautionary measures such as a private room and protective isolation must be instituted to protect the client from sources of infection. The client with pneumonia (option 1) poses a risk of infection, contact isolation (option 2) is not necessary, and option 4 does not provide the client with the necessary isolation precautions.
Cognitive Level: Analysis **Client Need:** Physiological Integrity: Physiological Adaptation **Integrated Process:** Nursing Process: Evaluation **Content Area:** Adult Health: Oncology **Strategy:** The core issue of the question is knowledge of room accommodations required by a client who needs neutropenic precautions. Recall that infection is the risk and use process of elimination to make a selection.

15 **Answer: 4** Smoking and drinking large quantities of alcohol daily increase the risk of oral and esophageal cancers. Options 1 and 2 are risk factors of development of other types of cancers. Option 3 is unrelated.
Cognitive Level: Analysis **Client Need:** Physiological Integrity: Physiological Adaptation **Integrated Process:** Nursing Process: Assessment **Content Area:** Adult Health: Oncology **Strategy:** The core issue of the question is a risk factor for laryngeal cancer. Note the word *smoking* in one of the options and associate it with the word *laryngeal* (referring to airway) to make a word connection between the stem and the correct option.

16 **Answer: 3** The lymph node biopsy is performed to assess any metastasis from the primary site of cancer, and a common metastatic site for breast cancer is regional lymph nodes. Options 1, 2, and 4 are incorrect statements.
Cognitive Level: Analysis **Client Need:** Physiological Integrity: Physiological Adaptation **Integrated Process:** Communication and Documentation **Content Area:** Adult Health: Oncology **Strategy:** The core issue of the question is knowledge that a biopsy procedure is used to diagnose a primary tumor or to evaluate lymph node involvement or metastasis. Use nursing knowledge and the process of elimination to make a selection.

17 **Answer: 2** The nurse should be concerned because painless bleeding not related to the menstrual cycle is often the only symptom of uterine cancer. Postmenopausal bleeding is not normal, with or without pain. Anemia is not an immediate concern. Pain is often considered to be a late sign related to the diagnosis of cancer.
Cognitive Level: Analysis **Client Need:** Physiological Integrity: Physiological Adaptation **Integrated Process:** Nursing Process: Assessment **Content Area:** Adult Health: Oncology **Strategy:** The core issue of the question is the significance of painless vaginal bleeding in a client who is postmenopausal. Use nursing knowledge and the process of elimination to make a selection.

18 **Answer: 2** A very dark red output character following prostatectomy may indicate venous bleeding or inadequate dilution of the urine. The Foley catheter is at risk for occlusion. Increasing the irrigation flow will prevent the formation of blood clots and occlusion of the catheter. If the urine does not clear, then it would be appropriate to notify the physi-

cian. Although reviewing the latest hemoglobin and hematocrit may be appropriate, it is not the most pressing intervention the nurse must do following prostate surgery.
Cognitive Level: Analysis **Client Need:** Physiological Integrity: Physiological Adaptation **Integrated Process:** Nursing Process: Implementation **Content Area:** Adult Health: Oncology **Strategy:** The core issues of the question are interpreting the significance of dark red urine flow following prostatectomy and the ability to choose a corrective action. Interpret that the dark color is due to clots and then select the answer on the basis of which intervention will reduce clot formation.

19 **Answer: 3** Ovarian cancer generally causes no warning signs or symptoms in the early stages, which is why screening is important. Painful urination, pelvic pain radiating to the thighs, and low back pain are not associated with this health problem.
Cognitive Level: Application **Client Need:** Physiological Integrity: Physiological Adaptation **Integrated Process:** Nursing Process: Assessment **Content Area:** Adult Health: Oncology **Strategy:** The core issue of the question is knowledge of early signs of ovarian cancer. Use nursing knowledge and the process of elimination to make a selection.

20 **Answer: 2** Option 2 describes stage II ovarian cancer. Option 1 describes stage I, option 3 describes stage III, and option 4 describes stage IV.
Cognitive Level: Application **Client Need:** Physiological Integrity: Physiological Adaptation **Integrated Process:** Nursing Process: Analysis **Content Area:** Adult Health: Oncology **Strategy:** The core issue of the question is knowledge of the staging system for ovarian cancer. Use nursing knowledge and the process of elimination to make a selection.

21 **Answer: 2** Option 2 describes a radical mastectomy. Option 1 describes a modified radical mastectomy; option 3 is a simple mastectomy; and option 4 is a lumpectomy.
Cognitive Level: Application **Client Need:** Physiological Integrity: Physiological Adaptation **Integrated Process:** Teaching and Learning **Content Area:** Adult Health: Oncology **Strategy:** The core issue of the question is the ability to discriminate among various types of mastectomy procedures. Use nursing knowledge and the process of elimination to make a selection.

22 **Answer: 1** Clients with three-way Foley catheters usually complain of sensations of having to void despite the presence of the catheter. This urge to void is caused by the pressure exerted by the balloon in the internal sphincter of the bladder and the wide diameter of the catheter that is used for the purpose of irrigation. Antispasmodics may be prescribed for the client with a three-way irrigation catheter. A TURP involves the insertion of a resectoscope via the urethra. The complaint of having the urge to void is common with clients undergoing bladder irrigation. Local reactions to the catheter usually do not include bladder spasms.
Cognitive Level: Analysis **Client Need:** Physiological Integrity: Physiological Adaptation **Integrated Process:** Communication and Documentation **Content Area:** Adult Health: Oncology **Strategy:** The core issue of the question is knowledge of the significance of bladder spasms following prostate surgery. Recall that spasms are not expected findings to help narrow the plausible options. Then use nursing knowledge and the process of elimination to make a selection.

23 **Answer: 4** The healing period after prostate surgery is 4 to 8 weeks, and the client should avoid strenuous activity during this period. Blood in the urine is fairly common after surgery. Continued increased fluid intake will help the urine to remain dilute and reduce the risk of clot formation. The client should not drive for 2 weeks, except for short rides.
Cognitive Level: Application **Client Need:** Physiological Integrity: Physiological Adaptation **Integrated Process:** Teaching and Learning **Content Area:** Adult Health: Oncology **Strategy:** The core issue of the question is knowledge of postdischarge care to a client following prostate surgery. Use nursing knowledge and the process of elimination to make a selection.

24 **Answer: 4** The arm should be elevated above heart level following mastectomy to reduce the risk of edema after lymph node removal on the affected side. Warm, moist compresses could enhance edema formation, and IV lines should not be used on the affected side at any location (lab draws and injections and blood pressure readings should also be avoided). Gentle, simple range of motion exercises can be started immediately after surgery.
Cognitive Level: Application **Client Need:** Physiological Integrity: Physiological Adaptation **Integrated Process:** Nursing Process: Planning **Content Area:** Adult Health: Oncology **Strategy:** The core issue of the question is knowledge that edema is a risk following mastectomy and of nursing measures that can reduce this risk. Use nursing knowledge and the process of elimination to make a selection.

25 **Answer: 700 mL** The total infused is 600 + 1500 = 2,100 mL. The total drained was 800 + 1050 + 950 = 2,800 mL. Subtract 2,100 from 2,800 to obtain 700 mL, the true urine output for the shift.
Cognitive Level: Application **Client Need:** Physiological Integrity: Physiological Adaptation **Integrated Process:** Nursing Process: Implementation **Content Area:** Adult Health: Oncology **Strategy:** The principles for intake and output calculation are the same as for any other client. Tally first the intake, then the output, and subtract the difference to determine how much of the output is actually because of urinary drainage. Use knowledge of basic nursing procedures to calculate the answer.

Key Terms to Review

alopecia p. 1354
benign neoplasm p. 1348
biopsy p. 1351
bone marrow suppression p. 1354
cancer p. 1348
cell-kill hypothesis p. 1353
chemotherapy p. 1353
debulk p. 1359
infratentorial p. 1358
malignant neoplasm p. 1348
metastasis p. 1348
radiation therapy p. 1351
staging p. 1350
stomatitis p. 1354
supratentorial p. 1358
tumor p. 1348
tumor markers p. 1350
xerostomia p. 1354

References

Ball, J., & Bindler, R. (2006). *Child health nursing: Partnering with children and families.* Upper Saddle River, NJ: Pearson Education.

Black, J., & Hawks, J. (2005). *Medical surgical nursing: Clinical management for positive outcomes* (7th ed.). St. Louis: Elsevier Science.

Corbett, J. (2004). *Laboratory tests and diagnostic procedures with nursing diagnoses* (6th ed.). Upper Saddle River, NJ: Pearson Education.

Harkreader, H., & Hogan, M. (2004). *Fundamentals of nursing: Caring and clinical judgment* (2nd ed.). St. Louis: Elsevier Science.

Ignatavicius, D., & Workman, L. (2006). *Medical-surgical nursing: Critical thinking for collaborative care* (5th ed.). Philadelphia: W. B. Saunders.

Kozier, B., Erb, G., Berman, A., & Snyder, S. (2004). *Fundamentals of nursing: Concepts, process, and practice* (7th ed.). Upper Saddle River, NJ: Pearson Education.

LeMone, P., & Burke, K. (2004). *Medical surgical nursing: Critical thinking in client care* (3rd ed.). Upper Saddle River, NJ: Pearson Education.

Porth, C. (2004). *Pathophysiology: Concepts of altered health states* (7th ed.). Philadelphia: Lippincott Williams & Wilkins.

Immunological Disorders

67

In this chapter

Test Yourself

Are you ready for the NCLEX-RN® or course exams? Use the practice tests on the companion CD-ROM to check.

Cross reference

Other chapters relevant to this content area are

Blood and Blood Component Therapy	Chapter 33
Immunological and Anti-infective Medications	Chapter 46
Common Laboratory Tests	Chapter 47
Common Diagnostic Tests and Procedures	Chapter 48
Respiratory Disorders	Chapter 56

I. OVERVIEW OF ANATOMY AND PHYSIOLOGY OF IMMUNE SYSTEM

A. Basic structures of the immunologic system

1. Lymphoid system
   a. Lymphoid system consists of lymphoid organs (lymph nodes, spleen, thymus, and tonsils), lymphoid tissues (lymphocytes and plasma cells in mucosa and connective tissues) and *bone marrow,* a myeloid tissue involved in blood cell formation
   b. Lymphatic system consists of a communication network of vessels, lymph nodes, lymph node clusters, and circulating and resident lymphocytes that function as a primary component in immune system response
2. Central lymphoid organs
   a. *Thymus gland,* which assists in T lymphocyte formation, is located in superior mediastinum behind sternum
   b. Bone marrow sources can be found in iliac crest, sternum, and in bone cavities throughout body

3. Peripheral organs
   a. Tonsils are a group of lymphoid tissue found in palatine area of oropharynx
   b. A lymph node is a small rounded mass of tissue from which lymph fluid drains; lymph nodes are found throughout body
   c. Mucosa-associated lymph tissue (MALT) consists of a group of lymph tissue found in many organs of body that work together to promote an immune response; specific locators identify source of tissue; for example: bronchial-associated lymph tissue (BALT), gut-associated lymph tissue (GALT), skin-associated lymph tissue (SALT)
   d. Spleen, located in left upper quadrant of abdomen, is composed of white and red pulp; white pulp is composed of B and T lymphocytes; red pulp is composed of erythrocytes
4. Mononuclear phagocyte system (MPS)
   a. Monocytes are largest component of the white blood cells (WBCs) and have one nucleus and very little cytoplasm; they are considered to be agranulocytes
   b. Macrophages are mature cells of the MPS; they migrate to different areas of body, becoming specialized cells to perform function of defense
   c. MPS protects body by participating in immune response; it secretes chemical components and factors (enzymes, complement proteins, and interleukins)

B. Basic functions of immunologic system

1. Thymus gland produces T lymphocytes, which are involved in **cell-mediated immunity;** secretes thymic hormones such as thymosin (stable from birth to age 25 and then gradually decreases because gland atrophies with age)
2. Bone marrow
   a. Serves as a diagnostic predictor for immunologic, hematologic, and oncologic disorders
   b. Provides for analysis of chemical markers that identify specific disease processes
   c. Is a primary lymphoid action that helps to initiate and maintain immune response; marrow gives rise to cellular components of blood and stores stem cells
   d. Gives rise to B lymphocytes and humorally mediated responses (**humoral immunity**) that involve production of **antibodies,** specific substances produced in response to specific antigens
3. Spleen
   a. Site of destruction of RBCs, a storage site for blood, and a reservoir for B lymphocytes to develop into mature plasma cells
   b. Filters and removes foreign material and worn-out cells and forms of cellular debris

II. NORMAL IMMUNE RESPONSE

A. Defense

1. Communication network of protection that involves both nonspecific and specific forms of defense
2. Nonspecific defense relates to external reactions that include anatomic and chemical barriers such as skin and mucous membranes; nonspecific defenses are activated against any foreign substance that body encounters
3. Specific defense relates to internal physiological reactions that include both cell-mediated and humorally mediated antibodies; antibodies are unique substances that require activation
4. Immune response is activated in presence of an **antigen,** a protein substance that triggers antibody production

B. Homeostasis: body seeks to maintain a balanced response of circulating and resident lymphocytes to maintain adequate protection

C. Surveillance

1. Body's ability to use memory and recognition to maintain an immune response
2. Body remembers activation response even if person doesn't remember a specific insult

III. TYPES OF IMMUNITY

A. Acquired immunity

1. Long-term response that leads to development of antibodies that offer protection
   a. Individual develops antibodies in response to having a disease process or by a response to artificial antigens such as a vaccine or toxoid
   b. Response can be boosted and maintained via repeated injections
   c. Titer serum levels can be monitored to indicate whether or not immunity is present
2. ! Passive acquired immunity requires an antibody be introduced to individual, either by maternal transfer (placenta and/or colostrum) or immune serum antibody injection, to promote a specific antigen response

B. Natural immunity

1. Related to a species, race, or genetic trait
2. An individual is born with natural immunity

C. Humoral immunity

1. Involves recognition of antigens by B lymphocytes
2. B lymphocytes differentiate into plasma cells and memory cells
3. Memory cells lead to a more rapid response by remembering an original insult
4. Plasma cells secrete **immunoglobulins,** a group of glycoproteins, each of which has four polypeptide chains (two heavy and two light chains); the FAB fragment, which is different in each immunoglobulin, denotes specific antigen-binding sites
5. Immunoglobulins are identified as IgA, IgD, IgE, IgG, and IgM; see Table 67–1 ■ for listing and characteristics of immunoglobulins

D. Cell-mediated immunity

1. T lymphocytes recognize a specific **major histocompatibility complex (MHC),** a group of proteins that participate in autoimmune recognition and tissue rejection, and bind to them to elicit an immune response
2. Protein markers on surface of T-cell help define specific function receptor sites; these are called CD antigens or clusters of differentiation; CD markers serve as an important prognostic indicator of immune function and are used to diagnose and manage human immunodeficiency virus (HIV) and acquired immunodeficiency syndrome (AIDS)
3. ! Humoral immunity is considered a long-term process whereby T lymphocytes help protect body against bacterial, viral, and fungal infections
4. ! Cell-mediated immunity is also responsible for mediation of transplant rejection

E. Other immune system participants

1. Natural killer cell (null cell, NK cell) activity is present at birth, increases as individual reaches adulthood and decreases gradually in old age; null cells do not require prior sensitization and are not considered T or B lymphocytes

Table 67–1

Types of Immunoglobulins

Class	Location	Characteristic
IgA	Body secretions Tears, saliva Colostrum and breast milk	Lines mucous membranes Protects body surfaces
IgD	Plasma	Present on lymphocytes
IgE	Plasma Interstitial fluids Exocrine secretions	Allergic/anaphylaxis Bound to mast cells
IgG	Plasma Interstitial fluid	Crosses placenta Complement fixation Secondary immune response
IgM	Plasma	Complement fixation Primary immune response Involved in ABO antigens

2. Cytokines (also referred to as lymphokines and monokines) are soluble protein mediators of immune response; interleukins, tumor necrosis factor, and interferon are examples of these chemical messengers, which are treatment options in boosting immune response

F. **Complement system**
1. Group of glycoproteins activated in sequential order; provide a link to humoral response
2. IgG and IgM are responsible for activating complement cascade; once activated, complement has been fixed or **complement fixation** has taken place
3. Complement assays are used to diagnose immunodeficiencies and autoimmune diseases
4. There is a classic pathway and an alternate pathway whereby complement system can be activated

G. **Biological response modifiers (BRMs)**
1. Group of substances that can elicit, modify, and restore biological response between an individual and a tumor cell
2. Examples
   ! a. **Monoclonal antibodies,** (produced by a specific group of identical cells) may be used to treat tumors because of their specific targeting effect
   ! b. **Colony-stimulating factors,** (a group of proteins that stimulate growth of either RBCs or WBCs) prevent or help reduce a client's adverse response to disease; these types of BRMs are used in a variety of hematologic and immunologic diseases

IV. COMMON TESTS AND PROCEDURES OF THE IMMUNE SYSTEM

A. **Skin testing**
1. A small quantity of allergen is introduced into skin by scratching or intradermal (ID) injection
2. A scratch test is used to test many antigens at a single time; it is of lower sensitivity than injection, but many allergens can be tested at once and results can be obtained in 30 minutes
3. ID injection is more accurate but leads to higher incidence of systemic reactions
4. Patch test evaluates contact allergens by applying allergen directly to skin and covering with a dressing
5. ! Antihistamines that could impair immune response should be discontinued 72 hours prior to skin testing
6. ! Immediate positive reaction usually occurs within 10 to 30 minutes and consists of wheal formation and erythema formation greater than 3 millimeters of a positive control (histamine)
7. ! Minor itching at site can be relieved by cool compresses, topical steroids, and topical or oral antihistamines

B. **Radioallergosorbent test (RAST)**
1. Reveals elevated levels of IgE associated with **atopy** (allergic reactions stemming from hereditary disposition)
2. Allergen is usually planted on a surface such as a paper disk
3. Client blood is then applied to surface and incubated
4. Antibodies specific to an allergen bind to allergen, but others wash away, and level of IgE can be measured
5. More sensitive than skin testing but also more time consuming and expensive

C. **Pulmonary function tests to diagnose asthma; see Chapter 56**

D. **Blood assays reveal increased circulating IgE in presence of allergic disease**

E. **Eosinophilia may be present with allergic disease**

V. HYPERSENSITIVITY REACTIONS

A. ***Hypersensitivity*** is an abnormal exaggerated immune response to a specific substance

B. **The Gell and Coombs Classification of Hypersensitivity Reactions** categorizes a reaction according to type, class, and immunity (see Table 67–2 ■)

Table 67-2
Gell and Coombs Classification

Type	Class	Immunity
I	Immediate hypersensitivity	Humoral
II	Cytotoxic reactions	Humoral
III	Immune complex related	Humoral
IV	Delayed hypersensitivity	Cell-mediated

C. Type I: anaphylactoid reactions

1. Involves an immediate response; however, potential responses can be cumulative; for example, initial or sensitizing dose may not elicit a strong response, but subsequent contacts, even if not long term in nature, may cause a stronger response
2. Involves characteristic activation of IgE bound to mast cells, with release of histamine
3. Clinical manifestations range from bronchospasm, wheezing, rhinorrhea, and urticaria to angioedema and finally anaphylaxis; there may be progression from local to systemic reactions; characteristic allergic "gape" and allergic "shiner" can be seen in individuals with atopy
4. Diagnostic and laboratory test findings: immunoglobulin titers are predictive of potential allergen response; skin and patch testing are performed to determine potential allergens
5. Therapeutic management
   a. **Antihistamine** medications such as diphenhydramine (Benadryl) are used to block chemical release of mediators (histamines)
   b. Mast cell degradation inhibitors such as cromolyn sodium (Intal) also are used to block chemical response
   c. Decongestants and corticosteroids help minimize immune response; however, in potential anaphylactic reactions, use of epinephrine is warranted; an Epipen may be prescribed as appropriate therapy for individuals at profound risk for hypersensitivity reactions; they are available in both adult and pediatric dosages
   d. Immediately withdraw offending allergen in presence of documented or suspected reaction
   e. Manage client according to ABC (airway, breathing, and circulation) protocol

D. Type II: cytotoxic and cytolytic reactions

1. Involves activation of complement and is considered a form of humoral immunity
   a. Involves production of autoantibodies that result in destruction of own cells or tissues
   b. IgA and IgM are involved with this type of response, and complement system is activated
2. Clinical manifestations: range from hemolytic reactions (such as transfusion, erythroblastosis fetalis, hemolytic anemia, and drug-induced hemolysis) to target cell destruction as in Goodpasture's syndrome (autoimmune disease affecting pulmonary and renal systems) and other autoimmune disease processes such as myasthenia gravis and Graves' disease
3. Diagnostic and laboratory test findings: Coombs blood test can define presence of hemolytic anemia and identify potential ABO incompatibility
4. Therapeutic management
   a. Use proper identification during blood product administration to prevent exposure and sensitization
   b. Recognize that certain blood types and potential drug interactions can cause antigen complex activation to detect reactions early
   c. Remain in the room during first 15 minutes of any blood product administration because clients are more likely to experience a reaction during this time frame
   d. Make sure to follow agency policy and procedure for the administration of any and all blood products; see also Chapter 33

E. Type III: immune complex reactions

1. Involves formation of **antigen–antibody complexes** (a binding together of an antibody and an antigen)
    a. Leads to activation of serum factors, causing inflammation and leading to activation of complement cascade
    b. Rheumatoid arthritis (RA) and systemic lupus erythematosus (SLE) are examples of Type III reactions
    c. Deposits of antigen–antibody complexes in body tissues are not localized and can result in extensive tissue or organ destruction
2. Complement activation impacts vulnerable organs and leads to intravascular changes
3. Clinical manifestations
    a. Arthrus reaction involves a localized inflammatory response with excess IgG causing edema and necrotic lesions
    b. Serum sickness involves a systemic response leading to deposit and activation of complement throughout body manifested as joint pain, pyrexia, and/or lymphadenopathy
    c. Reactions can be acute or chronic in nature
4. Diagnostic and laboratory test findings: complement assays indicate acute and/or chronic process; erythrocyte sedimentation rate (ESR) is elevated; proteinuria may be found on urinalysis
5. Therapeutic management
    a. Analgesics, antihistamines and topical steroids may provide symptom relief; disease process is usually self-limiting because of use of human antitetanus serum and availability of antibiotics
    b. Assess for localized inflammatory reactions that may develop at site of serum injections after 1 week; this can be followed by a more systemic response involving both regional as well as generalized lymphadenopathies
    c. If symptoms arise, monitor client for potential complications; this is especially important because organ damage can occur and the kidneys can be compromised

F. Type IV: delayed hypersensitivity reactions

1. A form of cell-mediated immunity involving T lymphocytes; considered a delayed response
2. Involve recognition and response of T lymphocytes to foreign substances
3. Clinical manifestations
    a. Wide range of presentations from tuberculin response, poison ivy, and contact dermatitis to transplant or graft rejection; edema, ischemia, and eventual tissue destruction may ensue
    b. Pyrexia, pain, edema, and failure of transplanted organ characterize transplant rejection
4. Diagnostic and laboratory test findings: purified protein derivative (PPD) test result of induration more than 5 mm identifies type IV hypersensitivity to tubercle bacillus; abnormal test results indicating declining function of transplanted organ are used to diagnose transplant rejection
5. Therapeutic management
    a. Monitor client for evidence of potential transplant rejection
    b. Medicate client with immunosuppressive protocol drugs to prevent tissue rejection
    c. Identify potential irritants that can cause contact dermatitis and avoid exposure
    d. Teach client to avoid offending irritant if a past exposure has been documented
    e. Use topical and oral medications as indicated to alleviate many symptoms and increase client comfort

VI. ANAPHYLAXIS

A. Overview

1. Sudden and severe allergic reaction mediated by massive histamine release from cells

2. Common causes are drugs, foods (especially nuts and shellfish), latex exposure, insect bites, and stings
3. Can lead to shock state and death if not treated immediately
4. Onset of symptoms can be within minutes to an hour, with more rapid onset associated with severe episode

B. Nursing assessment

1. Hives and urticaria (itching)
2. Angioedema (swelling of face, lips, neck, and/or tongue)
3. Dyspnea and wheezing
4. Syncope and hypotension
5. Difficulty swallowing
6. Skin flushing
7. Respiratory obstruction
8. Shock
9. Circulatory collapse and possible death

C. Therapeutic management

1. Maintain patent airway
2. Subcutaneous epinephrine injection
3. Remove or discontinue causative agent
4. Administer oxygen
5. Place in modified Trendelenburg position for shock
6. Give IV fluids such as normal saline or lactated Ringer's to support circulation
7. Provide antihistamines or corticosteroids as ordered
8. Provide supportive care to stabilize client and emotional support

D. Client teaching

1. Avoid future contact with allergen
2. Wear Medic-Alert identification listing allergy
3. Tell all future caregivers about allergy and symptoms
4. Learn how to use epinephrine auto-injector pen

VII. AUTOIMMUNE DISORDERS

A. Overview

1. Concept of autoimmunity
   a. An abnormal response of body's immune system whereby it perceives "self" as a threat
   b. Several mechanisms of action can affect autoimmune process, such as cell-mediated, antibody-mediated, and immune complex reactions
2. Genetic component of autoimmune response: **Human leukocyte antigens (HLAs),** genetic markers found on chromosome 6, are involved with diagnosis of many autoimmune diseases and are also used for tissue typing
3. Cell-mediated autoimmunity
   a. Associated with an abnormal T-cell response
   b. Overabundance of T-cytotoxic (killer) cells or deficiency of T-suppressor (helper) cells may occur
4. Antibody-mediated autoimmunity
   a. Associated with development of autoantibodies that affect specific receptor sites, causing tissue and organ damage
   b. Complement activation causes inflammatory reactions and leads to cell damage
   c. Graves' disease and myasthenia gravis are examples of antibody-mediated autoimmunity
5. Immune complex disease
   a. Associated with deposition of immune complexes at serum level
   b. Complement activation causes inflammatory reactions and leads to further damage
6. Diagnostic testing for autoimmunity
   a. Autoantibody assays, complement fixation, and complement assays provide diagnostic information
   b. Identification of HLA antigens provides indication of genetic inheritance

7. Treatment for autoimmunity
   a. Immunosuppressive agents and corticosteroids are given to suppress abnormal immune response
   b. Symptom management can be achieved with anti-inflammatory agents to minimize pain from tissue damage caused by immune complex deposits
   c. **Plasmapheresis** is used to remove circulating immune complexes; in this treatment, plasma is removed from body, sent through a machine membrane that traps immune complexes, and returned to body
8. Progression of disease
   a. Autoimmune diseases are characterized by acute exacerbation of a chronic condition
   b. They affect a large percentage of average population and, depending on specific disease, can be seen across the lifespan, affecting both children and adults
   c. In many cases, splenectomy has been performed as part of therapeutic management of many autoimmune diseases; while an individual can live without a spleen, its removal is no longer always guaranteed as a form of therapeutic management; current therapeutic regimens being explored are chemotherapy and use of biological response modifiers, instead of splenectomy

B. Systemic lupus erythematosus (SLE)

1. Overview
   a. Multisystem autoimmune disease with a fluctuating, chronic course
   b. Multiple organ involvement results in eventual major organ system failure
   c. Two forms: systemic and discoid; systemic involves entire system response of individual, and discoid involves characteristic skin rash without systemic disease
   d. Specific HLA antigens indicate this type of disease (HLA-B8, HLA-DR2, HLA-DR3); C_2 and C_4 complement deficiencies are also seen
   e. Estrogen inhibits suppressor T-cell function leading to an abnormal immune response; primarily affects women of childbearing age (30 to 50 years of age being most common)

! 2. Nursing assessment
   a. Environmental triggers such as ultraviolet (UV) light, infection or other stressor, and/or drugs
   b. Arthritis (joint pain) is most common symptom presentation
   c. Butterfly rash (malar rash) or erythema of face is most common dermatologic expression; palmar erythema also possible
   d. Weakness, fatigue, and general malaise; anorexia and weight loss
   e. Pleural manifestations such as pleuritis and pleural effusions
   f. Renal involvement may lead to renal failure
   g. Central nervous system (CNS) involvement: photosensitivity, subtle behavioral changes, possible stroke or seizure activity
   h. Hematologic involvement: altered immune responses with anemia (decreased RBC count), leukopenia (noted by infection and fever), thrombocytopenia (low platelet count), and even hemolytic anemia (positive Coombs test)
   i. Pregnancy and use of oral contraceptives can affect a client's estrogen level and therefore may pose an increased risk for disease flare-ups
   j. A positive ANA titer
   k. During flare-ups, complement (C_3 and C_4) may be decreased and ESR and C reactive protein (CRP) may be elevated
   l. A positive rheumatoid factor (+RF) may be seen with a titer of higher than 1:40
   m. Urinalysis may reveal presence of casts and sediment; creatinine levels may rise as renal involvement progresses

! 3. Therapeutic management
   a. Aimed at recognizing flare-ups and preventing further complications
   b. Adjusted to disease activity; client receives individualized care
   c. Conservative measures include rest and general supportive pharmacotherapy; aggressive measures include splenectomy and chemotherapy
   d. Collaborate with dietitian to support immune functions and maintain integrity of body systems

e. Plan for rest periods to avoid fatigue and lessen client's stress levels
f. Avoid environmental triggers such as prolonged UV light exposure that may cause client to develop skin eruptions; client can be photosensitive, so consider this possibility when planning care
g. Monitor client for symptom presentation and medicate as ordered to promote symptom relief
h. Institute with other health care providers a long-term treatment plan that offers anticipatory guidance and emotional support
i. Monitor for potential complications resulting from treatment measures (glucocorticoids) or disease progression
j. Clients with this disease should try to have a planned pregnancy; alternative birth control methods such as diaphragm and condoms should be utilized because oral contraceptives can affect a client's estrogen level
k. Nonsteroidal anti-inflammatory drugs (NSAIDs) and acetylsalicylic acid (aspirin, ASA) are used to control joint pain experienced by most clients
l. Hydroxychloroquine (Plaquenil) is used to treat dermatologic symptoms
m. Glucocorticoids are used to suppress disease activity and for symptom management; dosing can be adjusted in response to flare-ups; oral or IV route is preferred; tapered dose therapy (pulse dose) is usually initiated to achieve best results to arrive at lowest possible dosage and to prevent side effects of steroid therapy
n. Immunosuppressive agents such as cyclophosphamide (Cytoxan) and azathiopine (Imuran) can be given to effectively modulate an immune response; however, client will be at increased risk for **myelosuppression** (inhibition or destruction of bone marrow) with this treatment regimen and therefore must be monitored accordingly
o. Gamma globulin can be given IV to client to promote specific immune function
p. Plasmapheresis can be used to remove immune complexes to help relieve client's symptoms

4. Client teaching
   a. Likelihood of flare-ups and chronic nature of disease
   b. Self-monitoring of condition to identify potential health problems more quickly
   c. Potential dynamic life changes such as pregnancy and childbearing that may influence disease activity
   d. Medication therapy

C. Rheumatoid arthritis (RA)

1. Overview
   a. Systemic disorder involving symmetrical inflammation of synovial membranes and joints that leads to deformities and loss of joint function
   b. Clinical course has periods of remission and exacerbation, but underlying disease process is chronic
   c. Stage 1: disease present but no disability
   d. Stage 2: disease beginning to interfere with ADLs
   e. Stage 3: major compromise in function
   f. Stage 4: incapacitation
   g. Thought to be associated with deposits of antigen–antibody complexes and development of rheumatoid nodules
   h. RA has a bimodal appearance: there is a juvenile form (JRA) as well as more common adult form

! 2. Nursing assessment
   a. Fatigue, general malaise, and anorexia and weight loss
   b. Persistent joint pain lasting more than 3 months that is more evident on motion, but pain at rest can occur
   c. Characteristic morning stiffness lasting more than 1 hour is also an indication of progression and severity of the disease; if present, note onset, duration, and joints involved
   d. Tenderness, swelling, and restricted range of motion in the affected joints early in disease process

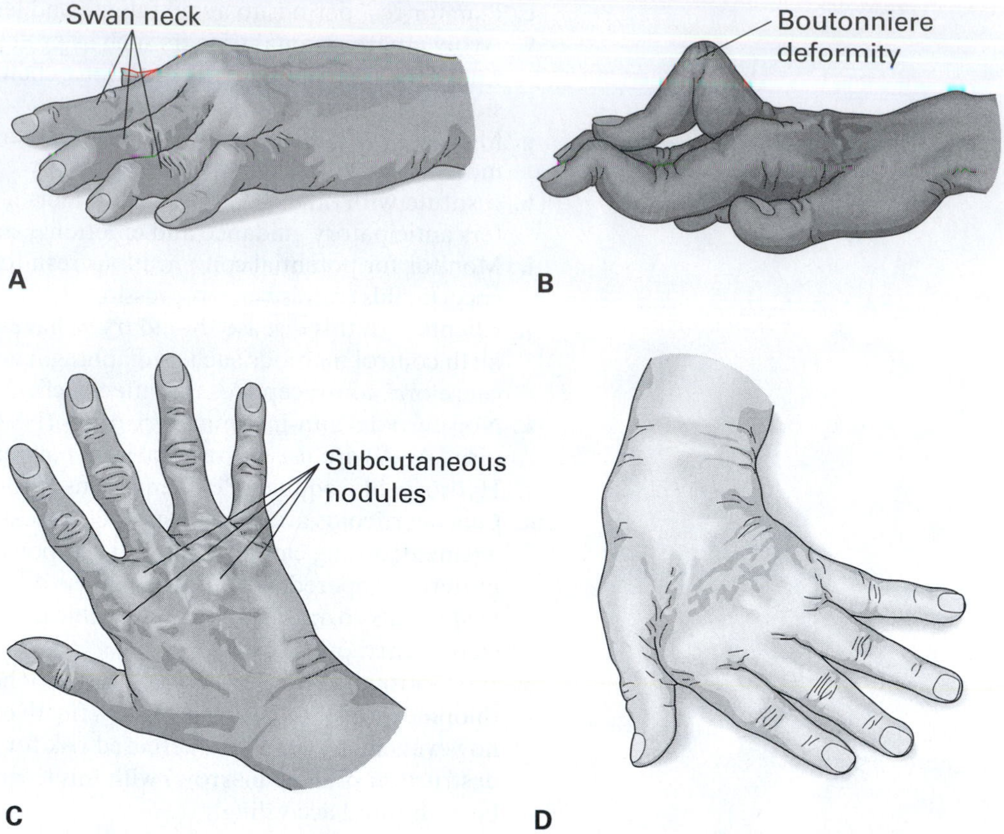

Figure 67–1

Characteristic hand deformities in rhematoid arthritis. A. Swan neck deformity. B. Boutonniere deformity. C. Subcutaneous nodules. D. Ulnar deviation.

Source: Hogan, M., & Madayag, T. (2004). Medical surgical nursing: Reviews and rationales. *Upper Saddle River, NJ: Pearson Education, p. 433.*

- **e.** With disease progression and less stable joints, characteristic deformities such as swan neck deformity, Boutonniere deformity, subcutaneous nodules, and ulnar deviation or drift (see Figure 67–1 ■) develop
- **f.** Systemic complaints range from fever to splenomegaly and reflect extra-articular findings
- **g.** Possible joint effusions
- **h.** +RF is a nonspecific finding because it may be found in healthy population as well
- **i.** Elevated ESR, CRP, and serum complement
- **j.** CBC with differential may reveal anemia as well as leukocytosis
- **k.** X-rays reveal a narrowing of joint spaces and erosive changes at bone margins as the disease progresses
- **l.** Aspiration of synovial fluid reveals characteristic findings such as turbidity, elevated cell counts, and formation of a poor mucin clot

! **3.** Therapeutic management
- **a.** Major treatment goal: help client maintain ability to function
- **b.** Treatment measures are aimed at decreasing joint pain and swelling
- **c.** Support client as diagnosis of disease is made and as disease progresses
- **d.** Identify assistive devices needed in client's environment to aid function
- **e.** Modify client's schedule as needed to incorporate rest periods
- **f.** Include nonpharmacologic measures such as use of imagery and biofeedback to provide alternate forms of pain relief
- **g.** Use heat and cold applications to affected joints to provide relief; these measures should be individualized to afford maximum client comfort
- **h.** Include foods high in omega-3 fatty acids, since current research shows that these are beneficial to clients who have RA as well as other diseases such as heart disease; suggested food items include fish oils and salmon
- **i.** ASA and NSAIDS are used to decrease joint inflammation and control symptoms

j. Disease-modifying antirheumatic drugs (DMARDS) are used to alter the rate of disease progression; examples include gold salts, antimalarial agents (Plaquenil), sulfasalazine (Azulfidine), D-pencillamine (Cuprimine), and immunosuppressive agents
k. Immunosuppressive agents such as azathioprine (Imuran), cyclophosphamide (Cytoxan), and methotrexate (Rheumatrex) are used in severe, disabling RA or RA refractory to other treatments
l. Methotrexate is widely used in the treatment of RA; onset of action is similar to other DMARDs; dosage is adjusted to get maximum response at lowest dose; relief effect continues during course of treatment
m. The FDA has approved etanercept (Enbrel), a tumor necrosis factor, in combination with methotrexate to treat RA

4. Client teaching
   a. Refer to a rheumatologist to coordinate management of care
   b. Occurrence of flare-ups and chronic nature of disease process
   c. Importance of adequate symptom management for optimal level of function
   d. Importance of client self-monitoring and compliance with treatment and medication therapy
   e. Potential dynamic life changes that might occur as a result of progression of deformity and loss of function

D. Scleroderma: progressive systemic sclerosis (PSS)

1. Overview
   a. A multisystem disease with fibrosis (hardening) of visceral organs and skin; leads to inability of involved organs to function with normal motility
   b. CREST syndrome is a specific, more limited form of disease

Memory Aid

C = Calcium deposits
R = Raynaud's syndrome
E = Esophageal dysmotility
S = Sclerodactyly (scleroderma digits)
T = Teleangiectasia (spider nevi)

   c. Systemic sclerosis morphea is a specific disease form that affects only skin
   d. Mild disease may go unrecognized unless it progresses or other medical issues bring it to forefront
   e. Has unknown etiology with underlying common factors: inflammation, vasoconstriction, and abnormal immune function and connective tissue
   f. Usually presents during third to fifth decade and affects females more than males

! 2. Nursing assessment
   a. Skin changes exist in two phases; painless, symmetrical and edematous changes occur first; then indurative changes lead to hardening and thickening of skin
   b. GI tract changes can lead to dysphagia, esophageal reflux, malabsorption, and bowel obstruction
   c. Cardiovascular changes: Raynaud's phenomenon (vasospastic disease), secondary bacterial endocardititis, myocardial fibrosis, left ventricular (LV) dysfunction, and heart failure
   d. Respiratory changes can result from lung restriction caused by fibrosis
   e. Renal changes lead to development of uremia, malignant hypertension, and eventually renal failure
   f. Often seen in conjunction with *Sjögren's syndrome,* an autoimmune disease affecting lacrimal and salivary glands, causing dryness of mucous membranes
   g. Low ANA titers are found in most clients with PSS
   h. SCL-70 antibody is highly specific for disease
   i. Anticentromere antibodies indicate a good prognosis because they are associated with a more limited form of disease
   j. ESR is usually elevated; positive RF is usually seen

k. Mild hypochromic, microcytic anemia can be seen in some clients
l. Imaging and other studies may be indicated to detect specific organ system involvement, such as GI, pulmonary, heart, kidney, and skin

3. Therapeutic management
a. Treatment is aimed at supportive and palliative measures
b. Long-term follow up is indicated to monitor for disease progression
c. Dialysis may be indicated if renal function deteriorates
d. If end-organ failure develops, renal or lung transplant may be indicated
e. Develop a support system for client and family members to help them cope with stressors of chronic disease
f. Identify potential complications as they affect client, and coordinate health care team approach to manage developing risk situations
g. Protect client's extremities from temperature changes that can exacerbate Raynaud's syndrome; encourage client to use gloves during activities that can affect temperature changes (such as washing dishes)
h. Calcium channel blockers and peripheral alpha$_1$-adrenergic blocking agents are used to treat symptoms of Raynaud's
i. Anti-inflammatory agents are used to treat joint pain
j. H_2 receptor antagonists and proton pump inhibitors are used to treat esophageal reflux
k. Angiotensin converting enzyme (ACE) inhibitors are used to treat hypertension and prevent development of resultant renal crisis
l. Antibiotics are used to treat potential secondary infections of the bowel caused by decreased motility
m. O_2 therapy is used to support pulmonary function

4. Client teaching
a. Importance of adequate symptom management
b. Chronic nature of disease process
c. Support client and family members with diagnosis and impact that no known cause exists; provide anticipatory guidance
d. Client may be referred to a rheumatologist to coordinate care management

E. Polyarteritis nodosa

1. Overview
a. Collagen disease that leads to inflammation of arteries and subsequent thickening with impaired circulation
b. Etiology is unknown and often affects middle-aged men
c. Cardiac and renal sequelae are most serious complications

2. Nursing assessment
a. Low-grade fever
b. Weakness and fatigue
c. Weight loss
d. Abdominal pain
e. Bloody diarrhea
f. Elevated ESR

3. Therapeutic management
a. Provide supportive care
b. Provide emotional support and anticipatory guidance
c. Initiate support services depending on need
d. Corticosteroids and analgesics are used to manage inflammation and pain

4. Client teaching
a. Importance of well-balanced diet
b. Need for follow-up care
c. Medication therapy
d. Energy conservation measures

F. Pemphigus

1. Overview
a. Skin disorder beginning with lesions on oral mucosa that spread to generalized body areas

b. Rare with unknown etiology
c. Occurs mostly in middle-aged and older adults
2. Nursing assessment
a. Bullae that are fragile and appear flaccid
b. Rupturing of bullae leads to partial thickness lesions that weep, form crusts, and may bleed
c. Malaise
d. Pain
e. Impaired chewing and swallowing
f. Nikolsky's sign: when skin is rubbed, epidermis separates from underlying skin
g. Foul-smelling skin discharge
h. Leukocytosis and eosinophilia
3. Therapeutic management
a. Oral hygiene and measures to soothe oral lesions
b. Baths with oatmeal or potassium permanganate for relief of skin symptoms
c. Medication therapy including topical or systemic antibiotics (secondary infections), and corticosteroids or cytotoxic agents (as immunosuppressants)
d. Provide general supportive care
4. Client teaching
a. Need for follow-up care
b. Medication therapy

VIII. PRIMARY IMMUNODEFICIENCY DISORDERS

A. Overview

1. Caused by a primary defect or deficiency involving B lymphocytes, T lymphocytes, complement or phagocytic cells that results in severe recurrent or chronic infection (see Table 67–3 ■ for a listing of selected primary immunodeficiency diseases)
2. Involve specific genetic alterations in immune response that are seen in infants and young children

B. Nursing assessment

1. Overall immune response is abnormal, leading to infections by opportunistic agents that cause tissue and organ damage of heart and lungs over time because immune response cannot be supported
2. Signs and symptoms of infection and inflammation: fever, chills, cough (nonproductive or productive), respiratory complaints associated with difficulty swallowing or breathing, erythema, edema, or drainage
3. Diarrhea either due to overwhelming infection caused by offending agents or as a response to antimicrobial therapy
4. CBC with differential, ESR, antibody titers, ANA, ANC (absolute neutrophil count), and culture and sensitivity of pertinent areas may all provide a baseline and allow for identification of potential source(s) of infection
5. Testing for immunoglobulins and complement assay levels provide an overview of immune system function

C. Therapeutic management

1. Therapy is most effective when aimed at infection prophylaxis, early treatment of infections, and replacement of immunologic factors
2. Bone marrow transplant (BMT) and/or thymus transplant may be indicated depending on the severity of presentation

Table 67–3
Selected Primary Immunodeficiency Disorders

Disorder	Immune Cell Problem
Bruton's X-linked disorder	B lymphocytes
DiGeorge's syndrome	T lymphocytes
Graft-versus-host disease	B, T lymphocytes
Wiskott-Aldrich syndrome	B, T lymphocytes

3. Identify clients who present with repeated infections
4. Support family members with impending diagnosis of chronic medical condition
5. Offer assistance in obtaining collaborative health care team management to establish treatment goals
6. Assist client and family members in decisions regarding lifestyle changes to reduce infection and ADLs
7. Refer clients of childbearing families for genetic counseling
8. Collaborate with health care team members to support the client's ADLs and lifestyle changes during this hospitalization and after discharge
9. Antimicrobial therapy may be initiated to prevent infection or treat current infection
10. Depending on nature of organism, antifungals may be warranted
11. Gamma globulins may be needed to support and maintain deficient immunoglobulin levels
12. Colony-stimulating factors may be used to boost immune response

D. Client teaching

1. Genetic counseling
2. Antimicrobial therapy, including treatment, response, and need for long-term compliance
3. Importance of prevention and protection from high-risk environments that could lead to further infection

IX. HUMAN IMMUNODEFICIENCY VIRUS (HIV)

A. Overview

1. An RNA retrovirus attacks immune system at CD4 antigen, causing cell mutation that leads to eventual disease progression
2. HIV infection involves a process whereby course of disease progresses
3. Primary infection is followed by a clinical latency period during which time individual may appear asymptomatic
4. Infecting virus is transmitted through contact with blood and/or body fluids

B. Assessment

1. Primary HIV can manifest with flulike symptoms
2. Symptomatic HIV presentation leads to decreased CD4 cell counts and progressive weight loss
3. Systemic constitutional symptoms such as fatigue, fever, night sweats, and skin lesions may become apparent with further viral progression; once latency period ends, HIV infection progresses to acquired immunodeficiency syndrome (AIDS)
4. History of "high-risk" exposures (IV drug use, sexual contact, contaminated blood products, and perinatal transmission—in utero, during delivery and/or breastfeeding)
5. Enzyme-linked immunosorbent assay (ELISA) is screening test used to detect development of antibodies to HIV; this test is described as positive or negative
6. Western blot is used to confirm HIV infection because it detects both HIV antibodies and individual viral components that cause reactive bands; this test is described as positive or negative
7. Polymerase chain reaction (PCR) is used to detect proviral DNA by identifying specific gene sequences of HIV proviral DNA molecule
8. Nonspecific markers of disease progression include blood counts, albumin levels, and ESR
9. Specific markers include CD4 and viral load (VL) levels to indicate client's current status and response to treatment
10. Other lab and diagnostic tests, such as skin biopsy, serum chemistries, and imaging studies, may be indicated depending on organ or system involvement and disease progression

C. Therapeutic management

1. Periodic clinical reevaluation of client: physical examination and laboratory testing
2. Vaccination against preventable illnesses
3. Assist client to manage life issues that will be affected by disease process

4. Maintain awareness of current CDC recommendations, which affect client during course of treatment
5. Establish an early working relationship with a dietitian to deal with client's altered taste perception, and prevent or delay **wasting syndrome** (unexplained weight loss of more than 10% ideal body weight [IBW] associated with a cycle of malnutrition and subsequent wasting) later in disease process
6. Monitor for potential fluid and electrolyte imbalances during course of disease process or in response to therapy
7. Antiretroviral therapy is used to attack virus at a basic level
8. Nucleoside analogue reverse transcriptase inhibitors are aimed at specific processes to prevent the replication process
9. Protease inhibitors are aimed at specific processes to prevent replication process
10. Nonnucleoside analogues are used to treat emerging viral mutations
11. Fusion inhibitor (enfuvirtide [Fuzeon]) inhibits ability of HIV to bind to CD4 cells
12. Prophylactic medications are recommended based on CDC guidelines to provide primary and secondary prophylaxis of opportunistic infections
13. Oral progesterones (Megace, Winstrol) stimulate appetite, thereby assisting with treatment of weight loss and loss of taste perception

D. Client teaching

1. Disease progression and progression
2. ! Importance of compliance with long-term treatment regimen and adherence to drug regimen; noncompliance could lead to drug resistance over time
3. Need for follow-up physical examination and diagnostic tests to monitor response to treatment and disease progression
4. Risk of increased infection caused by disease-related immunodeficiency
5. Confidentiality and issues in release of information concerning health matters in business and personal relationships
6. Importance of nutritional support and maintaining IBW in early phase of treatment
7. ! Importance of balanced nutrition to support immune system function
8. ! Measures to prevent transmission, such as use of latex condoms and any measures that prohibit blood and body fluid contact with others

X. ACQUIRED IMMUNODEFICIENCY SYNDROME (AIDS)

A. Overview

1. AIDS is a progression of HIV
2. ! CD_4 count is under 200/mm^3 in presence of an AIDS-defining disease, such as opportunistic infections, malignancies, and/or neurologic diseases; pulmonary TB, recurrent pneumonia, and invasive cervical cancer are also considered AIDS-defining diseases (see Table 67–4 ■ for a listing of AIDS infections and malignancies)
3. Since AIDS affects total individual, all body organs and tissues are affected
4. ! **Opportunistic infections** are nonpathogenic infections that become pathogenic as a result of an individual's baseline immunosuppressive state; refer to Table 67–4 again for testing for opportunistic infections

B. Nursing assessment

1. Depending on organ and system affected, there can be a wide range of presentations
2. Non-Hodgkin's lymphoma, Kaposi's sarcoma, and invasive cervical cancer are secondary malignancies often associated with AIDS
3. ! Wasting syndrome is seen in all individuals who have AIDS; aggressive nutritional support at time of HIV-positive diagnosis may prevent or deter possible effects of wasting and malnutrition
4. ! Continued observation of client's skin and mucous membranes reveals early signs and symptoms of infection
    a. Clients with HIV are at risk for oropharyngeal candida infections, leading to stomatitis
    b. Clients can experience pain when eating and benefit from soft foods and beverages that are neither too warm nor too cold

Table 67-4
AIDS Infections and Malignancies

Classification	Type
Bacterial infection	Mycobacterium avium complex (MAC)
Fungal infection	Candidiasis Cryptococcus neoformans Histoplasmosis
Protozoan infection	Pneumocystic carinii Toxoplasmosis Cryptosporidium
Viral infection	Cytomegalovirus (CMV)
Dementia	HIV encephalopathy
Nutritional/malnutrition	Wasting syndrome
Cancer	Kaposi's sarcoma Associated lymphomas

5. Assess client's nutritional status and hydration level, carefully noting baseline weight changes and alterations in taste perceptions
6. Monitor for potential fluid and electrolyte imbalances, especially hyponatremia
7. Obtain CD4, VL, and PCR levels
8. Obtain pertinent imaging studies as determined by client's presentation
9. Biopsies and other invasive procedures are done to diagnose secondary malignancies

C. Therapeutic management

1. Provide ongoing coordination of health care team to provide optimal assistance to client during this time of stress and crisis
2. Have dietitian analyze client's nutritional requirements and make recommendations to maintain IBW
3. Provide specific nutrition-related measures, such as small, frequent meals, fluids between meals, and dry crackers to help with mealtime nausea
4. Premedicate with antiemetics to reduce risk of nausea
5. Use sorbets as palate cleansers, zinc supplementation, and plastic instead of metal utensils to reduce altered taste perception
6. Dairy products, fish, and poultry are tolerated better than red meat when client experiences altered taste
7. Provide counseling and guidance for both client and immediate support systems
8. Assess total impact of disease on client and family support group
9. Allow for expression of feelings relative to life situation
10. Maintain client advocacy
11. Provide prescribed antibiotic therapy if client develops an infection
12. Chemotherapy and/or surgery may be indicated if secondary malignancies are identified
13. Pain management may be required as disease progresses
14. Antiemetics and appetite stimulants may be relieve nausea and vomiting and loss of appetite
15. Antifungal medications may be used to treat active or chronic opportunistic infections; topical medications may be used for palliative care

D. Client teaching

1. Measures to maintain nutrition
2. Energy conservation measures
3. Continue to emphasize how new symptoms will be managed and how client is active member of health care team
4. Discuss life issues with client and support system members as disease progresses and prognosis worsens

Check Your NCLEX-RN® Exam I.Q.

You are ready for testing on this content if you can

- Identify basic structures and functions of the immunological system.
- Describe the pathophysiology and etiology of common immunological disorders.
- Discuss expected assessment data and diagnostic test findings for selected immunological disorders.
- Discuss therapeutic management of a client experiencing an immunological disorder.
- Discuss nursing management of a client experiencing an immunological disorder.
- Identify expected outcomes for the client experiencing an immunological disorder.

PRACTICE TEST

1 Which one of the following suggestions by the nurse would be most helpful to an human immunodeficiency virus (HIV) positive client who has altered taste perception?

1. Drink plenty of salty broths and other fluids to stimulate taste buds.
2. Try zinc supplementation to improve taste perception.
3. Increase intake of meat to at least one serving per day.
4. Avoid using plastic eating utensils.

2 Which of the following suggestions would the nurse give to a client with human immunodeficiency virus (HIV) infection to best alleviate nausea?

1. Drink liquids with meals.
2. Eat high-fat foods.
3. Eat small, frequent meals.
4. Lie down after eating.

3 To enhance meeting the psychosocial needs of a client on transmission-based precautions, the nurse should place highest priority on which of the following?

1. Letting the client sleep to build up stamina
2. Maintaining strict precautions when entering and leaving the room so that the client feels he or she is getting the best care
3. Providing client care within a limited time frame to maintain isolation and keep client safe
4. Providing the client with diversional activities to enhance sensory input

4 A client diagnosed with scleroderma is complaining of painful fingers that change colors (pale to red) when washing dishes. Which suggestion by the nurse might help the client with this symptom?

1. Increase the water temperature.
2. Use gloves during dishwashing.
3. Start physical therapy to increase blood flow to the hands.
4. Take over-the-counter H_2 receptor antagonist medications.

5 The white blood cell (WBC) count of a client with systemic lupus erythematosus (SLE) shows a shift to the left. Which nursing diagnosis reflects the highest priority for this client?

1. Ineffective health maintenance
2. Impaired skin integrity
3. Ineffective individual coping
4. Ineffective protection

6 A client is to start taking prednisone for the treatment of rheumatoid arthritis (RA). Which client statement indicates that medication teaching was successful?

1. "I will take the medication on an empty stomach to maximize absorption."
2. "I will take the specific dose ordered at the same time every day."
3. "I will not have to limit my sodium intake."
4. "I will not have to adjust my insulin regimen."

7 The nurse assesses the client with rheumatoid arthritis for which of the following characteristic joint changes?

1. Swan-neck deformity and ulnar deviation
2. Heberden's and Bouchard's nodes
3. Tophi
4. Charcot's joints

PRACTICE TEST

8. In establishing a plan of care to manage pain for a client with rheumatoid arthritis, what intervention would the nurse use to increase the client's mobility?

1. Have the client work through pain by continuing exercise in order to establish endurance.
2. Have the client use pain medication only when pain is present.
3. Teach the client that both heat and cold applications may help to relieve pain.
4. Teach the client to flex muscle groups when pain is felt in an extremity.

9. Which of the following information will the nurse use when explaining therapeutic measures to a client taking methotrexate (Rheumatrex) for rheumatoid arthritis?

1. Relief of symptoms will be assessed for within 1 week of starting medication.
2. Fluids should be restricted to prevent possible edema formation.
3. Drug doses will be adjusted for optimum effect at lowest dose once relief has been established.
4. Six months of therapy will be adequate stop the disease process from progressing.

10. The nurse looks for results of which laboratory measurement that provides a reliable indicator of lymphocyte status in a client with HIV infection?

1. B lymphocytes
2. T-helper cells (CD4)
3. Natural killer cells (NK)
4. T-cytotoxic cells

11. The nurse who is providing care to a group of clients concludes that the client with which of the following problems exhibits a type III immune-complex–mediated hypersensitivity reaction?

1. Transfusion reaction
2. Goodpasture's syndrome
3. Transplant rejection
4. Systemic lupus erythematosus

12. A male client who has acquired immunodeficiency syndrome (AIDS) asks why oral progesterone (Megace) is being prescribed for treatment. What is the nurse's best response?

1. "Megace is used to treat the nausea associated with this infection."
2. "Megace is used as an appetite stimulant to boost nutritional support."
3. "Megace provides symptomatic relief of constipation."
4. "Megace is used as an antineoplastic agent for palliative treatment."

13. The nurse would assess for which of the following electrolyte imbalances as a common finding in a client with AIDS?

1. Hyponatremia
2. Hypernatremia
3. Hyperkalemia
4. Hypocalcemia

14. Which of the following assessments by the nurse warrants further investigation to determine if the client has rheumatoid arthritis (RA)?

1. Negative family history
2. Complaints of prolonged morning stiffness lasting for 1 hour
3. Occasional use of NSAIDs for aches and pains
4. Complaints of pain with movement

15. The nurse teaches a client that which of the following factors might increase risk of developing an exacerbation of systemic lupus erythematosus (SLE)?

1. Pregnancy
2. Hypotension
3. Fever
4. GI upset

16. A client will undergo scratch tests for allergies. In teaching the client about the planned tests, the nurse should include which of the following information?

1. This test allows us to rule out one or two specific antigens.
2. The scratch test is the most sensitive allergy test.
3. Results can be obtained in 30 minutes.
4. The scratch test involves drawing a small amount of blood from the client.

17 The nurse would expect which of the following findings in a client with an immunologic disorder associated with an HLA antigen?

1. Acute course
2. Frequent effects on reproductive capacity
3. Genetic determination
4. Chronic and possibly subacute course

18 A client presents with dyspnea, pruritis, and localized swelling of the forearm after being stung by a bee. What is the priority intervention?

1. Remove the stinger from the client's arm
2. Keep the client warm with soft blankets
3. Check the tongue for swelling and listen for stridor
4. Place client in the Trendelenburg position

19 Medication instruction for the client with rheumatoid arthritis (RA) should include which the following teaching points?

1. Injection of gold salts requires monitoring for anaphylactic reactions every half-hour.
2. Treatment with sulfasalazine requires fluid restriction to avoid nausea and vomiting.
3. NSAIDs, acetaminophen, and aspirin maybe used interchangeably to decrease inflammation associated with RA.
4. Penicillamine may be safely used during pregnancy.

20 The nurse writing a care plan determines that which of the following is a priority nursing diagnosis early in the care of a client with scleroderma?

1. Impaired skin integrity
2. Disturbed body image
3. Activity intolerance
4. Hopelessness

21 An infant is admitted to the pediatric unit with a diagnosis of sepsis. The nurse is completing a nursing assessment. The priority assessment for this infant would be

1. skin integrity.
2. temperature.
3. jaundice.
4. respiratory function.

22 The nurse is caring for a pediatric client with acquired immunodeficiency syndrome (AIDS). Which activity by the nurse should be reported to the employee health department as an exposure for the nurse?

1. While flushing out the used bedpan, fluid splashes in the nurse's eyes.
2. The nurse does not wear a mask while in the client's room.
3. During the bath, the nurse removes gloves when giving a backrub on intact skin.
4. The nurse is stabbed with a sterile syringe to be used to draw up the client's medications.

23 The pediatric nurse would suspect severe combined immunodeficiency disorder (SCID) when which of the following children is admitted to the hospital nursing unit?

1. A 2-month-old with thrush and low white blood cell counts
2. A 2-year-old with history of recent repeated infections
3. A newborn with positive TORCH titer
4. A newborn admitted with positive ELISA test

24 A 5-year-old child is brought into the clinic after being stung by an insect. The child appears to be going into anaphylactic shock. Which of the following nursing action is of highest priority?

1. Assess urinary output to determine renal perfusion
2. Apply cold wet compresses to the site
3. Position the child's head to maintain an open airway
4. Establish intravenous access for medication delivery

25 A 12-year-old boy is hospitalized and diagnosed with the recent development of human immunodeficiency virus (HIV) infection secondary to factor transfusions for hemophilia. The family is very concerned about their ability to manage his care, risk of infection to family members, and whether the child should remain in the home. Which action by the nurse will best promote family coping at this time?

1. Explain to the family that the infection cannot be spread by casual contact.
2. Demonstrate positive acceptance of the child with each contact.
3. Explain that prophylactic drugs will prevent the virus from spreading.
4. Show the family how to wash their hands properly.

26 A client must undergo skin testing for allergies. The nurse determines during client history that the client takes an antihistamine to control symptoms. The nurse explains that the client must discontinue use of the antihistamine for how many days before the skin testing in order to avoid false negative results? Provide a numerical answer.

Answer: ______________________

ANSWERS & RATIONALES

1 **Answer: 2** Zinc deficiency is associated with taste changes; therefore, supplementation may benefit a client experiencing altered taste perception. Drinking salty broth and fluids will not help with taste changes but may help restore electrolyte balance in clients experiencing diarrhea. Dairy products, fish, and poultry are better food choices than meat when taste is altered. Substitution of plastic utensils for metal ones is suggested to decrease possibility of taste perception of "metal."
Cognitive Level: Application **Client Need:** Physiological Integrity: Physiological Adaptation **Integrated Process:** Nursing Process: Implementation **Content Area:** Adult Health: Immunological **Strategy:** The core issue of the question is knowledge of measures to minimize taste alterations in a client with HIV infection. Use nursing knowledge and the process of elimination to make a selection.

2 **Answer: 3** Small, frequent meals help lessen nausea because they require less work of digestion and do not overwhelm the client with food odors from a lengthy meal. High-fat foods are more difficult to digest and may distend the stomach. Lying down after eating can encourage reflux. Drinking liquids can give a sensation of fullness. High-fat foods, reclining after meals, and drinking large quantities of liquid all increase the risk of nausea and vomiting.
Cognitive Level: Application **Client Need:** Physiological Integrity: Physiological Adaptation **Integrated Process:** Teaching and Learning **Content Area:** Adult Health: Immunological **Strategy:** The core issue of the question is the ability to provide teaching to minimize nausea in a client with HIV. Use nursing knowledge and the process of elimination to make a selection.

3 **Answer: 4** It is important to assess the psychosocial needs of a client on transmission-based precautions and to intervene to provide sensory stimulation for the client. Isolation procedures can cause clients to become depressed and withdrawn and to sleep excessively. Although it is important to maintain isolation precautions as ordered, attention must be given to include the client's psychosocial needs as part of the plan of care. Limiting contact time may be indicated for infection control, but it does not provide psychosocial support.
Cognitive Level: Application **Client Need:** Physiological Integrity: Physiological Adaptation **Integrated Process:** Nursing Process: Planning **Content Area:** Adult Health: Immunological **Strategy:** The critical word in the question is *psychosocial.* With this word in mind, focus on the intervention that best meets nonphysical needs of the client. Use nursing knowledge and the process of elimination to make a selection.

4 **Answer: 2** Clients who have scleroderma usually have Raynaud's phenomenon. Raynaud's can be triggered by temperature changes, and prolonged water contact may cause activation. Use of gloves when washing dishes may prevent temperature changes yet still allow the client to participate in ADLs. Hotter water may increase the risk of scalding and so is not suggested. Physical therapy and H_2 receptor blockers are indicated for treatment of esophageal problems associated with scleroderma.
Cognitive Level: Analysis **Client Need:** Physiological Integrity: Physiological Adaptation **Integrated Process:** Nursing Process: Implementation **Content Area:** Adult Health: Immunological **Strategy:** The core issue of the question is recognition of Raynaud's syndrome and the ability to select an appropriate intervention for that problem. Use nursing knowledge and the process of elimination to make a selection.

5 **Answer: 4** All identified nursing diagnoses are of concern for a client with SLE. However, the results of the laboratory test demonstrate an increased risk for infection that is due to the disease process and/or possible treatment measures such as steroids and immunosuppressive agents. A shift to the left in a WBC differential indicates an increased number of immature cells, suggesting infection.
Cognitive Level: Analysis **Client Need:** Physiological Integrity: Physiological Adaptation **Integrated Process:** Nursing Process: Planning **Content Area:** Adult Health: Immunological **Strategy:** The core issue of the question is the ability to analyze WBC differential count data to determine risk of infection. Use nursing knowledge and the process of elimination to make a selection.

6 **Answer: 2** Steroid therapy is usually done as part of a tapered-dose treatment plan. It is important to take this medication at the same time each day and to become aware of tapered-dose effect. Steroids are usually taken with foods to minimize GI upset. Steroids cause fluid retention, and therefore sodium intake may be restricted. Steroids also increase blood glucose, so insulin therapy dosages may have to be adjusted.
Cognitive Level: Application **Client Need:** Physiological Integrity: Pharmacological and Parenteral Therapies **Integrated Process:** Nursing Process: Evaluation **Content Area:** Adult Health: Immunological **Strategy:** The core issue of the question is knowledge of client teaching related to steroid therapy. Use nursing knowledge and the process of elimination to make a selection.

7 **Answer: 1** Swan-neck deformity occurs at the proximal interphalangeal (PIP) joint and ulnar deviation occurs as a result of joint destruction with disease progression. Heberden's

and Bouchard's nodes are commonly found in clients with osteoarthritis. Tophi (firm moveable nodules) are associated with gout. Charcot's joint is considered a neuropathic disorder that falls under the broader category of rheumatism. It is not specific to RA and is more likely to be seen as a complication in clients with diabetes.
Cognitive Level: Application **Client Need:** Physiological Integrity: Physiological Adaptation **Integrated Process:** Nursing Process: Assessment **Content Area:** Adult Health: Immunological **Strategy:** The core issue of the question is identification of signs and symptoms or RA. Use nursing knowledge and the process of elimination to make a selection.

8 **Answer: 3** Heat and cold applications can provide analgesia and relieve muscle spasms. The individual client will have to determine whether heat, cold, or alternation of both is most effective. Pain medication should be taken on a regular schedule if the client has chronic pain so that the pain threshold can be raised and pain relief maintained at a constant level. Exercising in the presence of pain may only further exacerbate pain. Flexing of muscle groups is not related to effective pain control.
Cognitive Level: Application **Client Need:** Physiological Integrity: Physiological Adaptation **Integrated Process:** Nursing Process: Planning **Content Area:** Adult Health: Immunological **Strategy:** The core issue of the question is knowledge of measures that relieve the symptoms of RA. Use nursing knowledge and the process of elimination to make a selection.

9 **Answer: 3** Methotrexate treatment takes several weeks to effect relief. Once relief is obtained, the dose is adjusted to achieve maximum response at the lowest dose. If the drug is discontinued, then symptoms of the disease do return.
Cognitive Level: Application **Client Need:** Physiological Integrity: Physiological Adaptation **Integrated Process:** Nursing Process: Implementation **Content Area:** Adult Health: Immunological **Strategy:** The core issue of the question is knowledge of management principles for RA. Use nursing knowledge and the process of elimination to make a selection.

10 **Answer: 2** CD4 cells are indicative of a client's HIV status. As the disease progresses, the T-helper cells decrease in number and lose their ability to function effectively, leading to an overaggressive immune response. B lymphocytes indicate the status of humoral immunity and are not directly associated with HIV infection. NK cells and T-cytotoxic cells are not directly related to HIV infection and as such are not considered to be reliable indicators of HIV status.
Cognitive Level: Application **Client Need:** Physiological Integrity: Physiological Adaptation **Integrated Process:** Nursing Process: Assessment **Content Area:** Adult Health: Immunological **Strategy:** The core issue of the question is knowledge of which laboratory measure will provide information about the status of the immune system of a client with HIV. Use nursing knowledge and the process of elimination to make a selection.

11 **Answer: 4** Transfusion and Goodpasture's are examples of type II cytotoxic hypersensitivity reactions and are involved with the activation of complement. Lupus is an example of a type III hypersensitivity reaction, which involves IgG and IgM with the activation of complement.
Cognitive Level: Application **Client Need:** Physiological Integrity: Physiological Adaptation **Integrated Process:** Nursing Process: Analysis **Content Area:** Adult Health: Immunological **Strategy:** The core issue of the question is the ability to associate various types of hypersensitivity reactions with their etiologies. Use nursing knowledge and the process of elimination to make a selection.

12 **Answer: 2** While Megace is used as a palliative treatment for clients with advanced cancers, this is not the rationale for its use with AIDS. In AIDS clients, it provides appetite enhancement. Side effects of Megace can include nausea and constipation.
Cognitive Level: Application **Client Need:** Physiological Integrity: Pharmacological and Parenteral Therapies **Integrated Process:** Communication and Documentation **Content Area:** Adult Health: Immunological **Strategy:** The core issue of the question is the purpose of oral progesterone in a client with AIDS. Use nursing knowledge about anorexia as a symptom of AIDS and the process of elimination to make a selection.

13 **Answer: 1** Hyponatremia is a common finding in clients with AIDS. The incidence of opportunistic infections may contribute to this decrease in sodium. Hypernatremia, hyperkalemia, and hypocalcemia are not usually seen in clients who have AIDS.
Cognitive Level: Analysis **Client Need:** Physiological Integrity: Physiological Adaptation **Integrated Process:** Nursing Process: Analysis **Content Area:** Adult Health: Immunological **Strategy:** The core issue of the question is identification of an electrolyte disturbance that is more common to clients with AIDS. Use nursing knowledge and the process of elimination to make a selection.

14 **Answer: 2** Prolonged morning stiffness is associated with RA. Occasional use of NSAIDS is not by itself a direct link to the development of RA. Complaints of pain with movement are more likely to be associated with degenerative joint disease (osteoarthritis).
Cognitive Level: Analysis **Client Need:** Physiological Integrity: Physiological Adaptation **Integrated Process:** Nursing Process: Assessment **Content Area:** Adult Health: Immunological **Strategy:** The core issue of the question is the ability to identify symptoms that are possibly associated with RA. Use nursing knowledge and the process of elimination to make a selection.

15 **Answer: 1** Pregnancy can be associated with an exacerbation because of increased estrogen levels. Hypotension, fever, and GI upset do not exacerbate SLE.
Cognitive Level: Application **Client Need:** Physiological Integrity: Physiological Adaptation **Integrated Process:** Teaching and Learning **Content Area:** Adult Health: Immunological **Strategy:** The core issue of the question is risk factors and triggers for SLE. Use nursing knowledge and the process of elimination to make a selection.

16 **Answer: 3** A scratch test tests many allergens at once. It is of low sensitivity, but many allergens can be tested at once, and the results can be obtained in 30 minutes.
Cognitive Level: Application **Client Need:** Physiological Integrity: Physiological Adaptation **Integrated Process:** Nursing Process: Implementation **Content Area:** Adult Health: Immunological

Strategy: The core issue of the question is identification of appropriate concepts to teach a client about scratch tests for allergies. Use nursing knowledge and the process of elimination to make a selection.

17 **Answer: 4** Diseases with HLA associations have poorly understood etiologies, are usually chronic or subacute in nature, and have limited effect on reproductive capacity. **Cognitive Level:** Analysis **Client Need:** Physiological Integrity: Physiological Adaptation **Integrated Process:** Nursing Process: Analysis **Content Area:** Adult Health: Immunological **Strategy:** The core issue of the question is knowledge of diseases associated with the HLA antigen. Use nursing knowledge and the process of elimination to make a selection.

18 **Answer: 3** The priority intervention is to maintain a patent airway in a potential anaphylactic reaction. Therefore, the nurse should assess for swelling of the tongue and stridor, which could indicate impending respiratory obstruction. The other interventions are supportive measures that can be used during an allergic response. **Cognitive Level:** Analysis **Client Need:** Physiological Integrity: Physiological Adaptation **Integrated Process:** Nursing Process: Implementation **Content Area:** Adult Health: Immunological **Strategy:** Remember in emergency or near-emergency situations to use the ABCs (airway, breathing, and circulation) to plan priorities of care. Use the process of elimination to make a selection.

19 **Answer: 1** Gold salts may cause anaphylaxis. Sulfasalazine may cause nausea and vomiting, but fluids should be encouraged (option 2). Acetaminophen does not provide the same anti-inflammatory effects as ASA and NSAIDs (option 3). Penicillamine cannot be used during pregnancy (option 4). **Cognitive Level:** Application **Client Need:** Physiological Integrity: Pharmacological and Parenteral Therapies **Integrated Process:** Nursing Process: Analysis **Content Area:** Adult Health: Immunological **Strategy:** The core issue of the question is knowledge of appropriate client teaching related to medications used to treat rheumatoid arthritis. Use nursing knowledge and the process of elimination to make a selection.

20 **Answer: 1** Skin manifestations are a common finding in clients with scleroderma and therefore require preventative and supportive nursing care as the priority. As the disease progresses, dermatologic effects may lead to disturbances in body image. In addition, with disease progression, there may be an impact on respiratory and musculoskeletal function, leading to activity intolerance. Similarly, hopelessness can develop with new and worsening symptoms. Therefore, the nursing diagnoses in options 2, 3, and 4 are of lesser priority in the early phase of the disease process. **Cognitive Level:** Application **Client Need:** Physiological Integrity: Physiological Adaptation **Integrated Process:** Nursing Process: Planning **Content Area:** Adult Health: Immunological **Strategy:** The core issue of the question is knowledge that scleroderma is primarily a skin disorder in many cases and that therefore the primary nursing diagnosis needs to address loss of skin as a protective barrier. Use nursing knowledge and the process of elimination to make a selection.

21 **Answer: 4** Altered temperature, jaundice, and respiratory distress are all symptoms of sepsis in infants. Respiratory function is the highest priority because without an adequate airway and breathing, the client cannot maintain life. **Cognitive Level:** Analysis **Client Need:** Physiological Integrity: Physiological Adaptation **Integrated Process:** Nursing Process: Analysis **Content Area:** Child Health: Immunological **Strategy:** Use the ABCs and the process of elimination to make a selection. Airway and breathing typically take priority in situations of high acuity, such as sepsis.

22 **Answer: 1** Body fluid–contaminated liquids may contain the human immunodeficiency virus (HIV) and can be absorbed through the eye mucosa. The other activities do not expose the nurse to blood and/or body fluids of the client and therefore pose no risk of contracting HIV. **Cognitive Level:** Application **Client Need:** Safe Effective Care Environment: Safety and Infection Control **Integrated Process:** Nursing Process: Evaluation **Content Area:** Child Health: Immunological **Strategy:** The core issue of the question is the ability to identify a breach in standard precautions. Use nursing knowledge about transmission of HIV via body fluids and the process of elimination to make a selection.

23 **Answer: 1** The first infection often seen in these children is oral candidiasis (thrush). That symptom, along with the low WBC count, would be warning symptoms of SCID. A 2-year-old is unlikely to have survived this long undiagnosed. ELISA tests evaluate HIV infection, and a TORCH titer is unrelated. A newborn is too young for symptoms to have manifested. **Cognitive Level:** Analysis **Client Need:** Physiological Integrity: Physiological Adaptation **Integrated Process:** Nursing Process: Analysis **Content Area:** Child Health: Immunological **Strategy:** The core issue of the question is the ability to identify signs and symptoms of SCID. Use nursing knowledge and the process of elimination to make a selection.

24 **Answer: 3** Maintaining an open airway is always the highest priority. With anaphylactic shock, the airway may constrict, mucous membranes swell, and air trapping occurs. The second priority would be airway access, followed by renal assessment, and finally site care. **Cognitive Level:** Analysis **Client Need:** Physiological Integrity: Physiological Adaptation **Integrated Process:** Nursing Process: Planning **Content Area:** Child Health: Immunological **Strategy:** Use the ABCs—airway, breathing, and circulation to answer questions related to anaphylaxis. Airway is always the first priority in life-threatening situations.

25 **Answer: 2** The family has stated multiple concerns, and demonstrating acceptance of the child is the best way to foster acceptance of the child and development of further coping skills. Prevention of transmission, handwashing, and drug therapy are all important, but none of these individually targets the global concerns of the family. **Cognitive Level:** Analysis **Client Need:** Psychosocial Integrity **Integrated Process:** Nursing Process: Implementation **Content Area:** Child Health: Immunological **Strategy:** The core issue of the question is the best action of the nurse to model acceptance of the child and lead to enhanced coping skills by the family. Select the option that is the most global in nature because the family has multiple concerns, and use the process of elimination to make a selection.

26 **Answer 3** The client needs to discontinue use of antihistamines for 72 hours (3 days) prior to allergy testing to avoid false negative readings.
Cognitive Level: Application **Client Need:** Physiological Integrity: Reduction of Risk Potential **Integrated Process:** Nursing Process: Implementation **Content Area:** Adult Health: Immunological **Strategy:** The core issue of the question is knowledge of the time frame that antihistamine drugs need to be withheld so as not to interfere with the results of allergy testing. Use specific nursing knowledge to determine the correct answer.

Key Terms to Remember

antibody p. 1376
antigen p. 1376
antigen–antibody complexes p. 1380
antihistamine p. 1379
atopy p. 1378
cell-mediated immunity p. 1376
colony-stimulating factors p. 1378
complement fixation p. 1378
human leukocyte antigens (HLA) p. 1381
humoral immunity p. 1376
hypersensitivity p. 1378
immunoglobulins p. 1377
major histocompatibility complex (MHC) p. 1377
monoclonal antibodies p. 1378
myelosuppression p. 1383
opportunistic infection p. 1389
plasmapheresis p. 1382
wasting syndrome p. 1389

References

Ball, J., & Bindler, R. (2006). *Child health nursing: Partnering with children and families.* Upper Saddle River, NJ: Pearson Education.

Black, J., & Hawks, J. (2005). *Medical surgical nursing: Clinical management for positive outcomes* (7th ed.). St. Louis: Elsevier Science.

Corbett, J. (2004). *Laboratory tests and diagnostic procedures with nursing diagnoses* (6th ed.). Upper Saddle River, NJ: Pearson Education.

Harkreader, H., & Hogan, M. (2004). *Fundamentals of nursing: Caring and clinical judgment* (2nd ed.). St. Louis: Elsevier Science.

Ignatavicius, D., & Workman, L. (2006). *Medical-surgical nursing: Critical thinking for collaborative care* (5th ed.). Philadelphia: W. B. Saunders.

Kozier, B., Erb, G., Berman, A., & Snyder, S. (2004). *Fundamentals of nursing: Concepts, process, and practice* (7th ed.). Upper Saddle River, NJ: Pearson Education.

LeMone, P., & Burke, K. (2004). *Medical surgical nursing: Critical thinking in client care* (3rd ed.). Upper Saddle River, NJ: Pearson Education.

Porth, C. (2004). *Pathophysiology: Concepts of altered health states* (7th ed.). Philadelphia: Lippincott Williams & Wilkins.

68 Communicable or Infectious Diseases

In this chapter

Test Yourself

Are you ready for the NCLEX-RN® or course exams? Use the practice tests on the companion CD-ROM to check.

Cross reference

Other chapters relevant to this content area are

Preventing and Controlling Infection	Chapter 8
Providing Immunizations	Chapter 15
Immunological and Antiinfective Medications	Chapter 46

I. CHICKENPOX (VARICELLA)

A. Overview

1. Organism: varicella zoster virus
2. Mode of transmission: airborne and direct contact with contaminated objects (fomites)
3. Source: respiratory secretions and vesicular skin lesions (scabs not infectious)
4. Incubation period: often 13 to 17 days
5. Communicability: from 1 day before lesions erupt to crusting of all lesions

B. Nursing assessment

1. Fever
2. Malaise and anorexia for first 24 hours
3. Rash beginning on scalp and trunk and spreading to extremities; may involve oral mucous membranes or genital and rectal areas
4. Rash rapidly progresses to papules and vesicles that break and form crusts

C. Therapeutic management

1. Prevention: **Immunization** with varicella vaccine (see Chapter 15)
2. Maintain airborne and contact precautions in hospital
3. Isolate child in home until vesicles have crusted over and dried
4. Skin care: bathe and change clothes and bed linens daily; use oatmeal soaps, soaks, or lotions, and calamine lotion or topical antihistamines to prevent scratching of pruritic lesions; encourage child not to scratch; use mittens on young child
5. Administer acetaminophen for fever; avoid aspirin to prevent Reye syndrome

D. Complications

1. Encephalitis
2. Varicella pneumonia
3. Secondary bacterial infections (abscesses, cellulitis, sepsis)

II. DIPHTHERIA

A. Overview

1. Organism: *Corynebacterium diphtheriae*
2. Mode of transmission: direct contact with infected client, carrier, or contaminated objects
3. Source: nasal and respiratory secretions, skin, other lesions
4. Incubation period: 2 to 5 days, possibly slightly longer
5. Communicability: variable until virulent bacilli absent in 3 negative cultures; usually 2 to 4 weeks

B. Nursing assessment

1. Low-grade fever, sore throat, malaise, anorexia
2. Foul mucopurulent nasal discharge (as in common cold); may have epistaxis
3. Smooth, adherent, white or gray membrane on tonsils and pharynx
4. Hoarseness, cough, apprehension, dyspnea with retractions, possible airway obstruction and cyanosis

C. Therapeutic management

1. Prevention: diphtheria **vaccine** (see Chapter 15)
2. Maintain strict isolation and bedrest in hospital
3. Administer antibiotic therapy and antitoxin as prescribed (do skin or conjunctival test first to rule out sensitivity to horse serum)
4. Provide suction and oxygen as needed to maintain airway
5. Be prepared for emergency tracheostomy if airway obstruction occurs

D. Complications

1. Myocarditis
2. Neuritis
3. Toxemia and septic shock; death possible

III. ERYTHEMA INFECTIOSUM (FIFTH DISEASE)

A. Overview

1. Organism: human parvovirus B19 (HPV)
2. Mode of transmission: unknown; possibly respiratory secretions and blood
3. Source: infected individuals
4. Incubation period: 4 to 14 days, but possibly up to 20 days
5. Communicability: uncertain, but usually before onset of symptoms

B. Nursing assessment

1. Rash that occurs in three stages
   a. Erythema of face (mainly cheeks, giving a "slapped cheeks" appearance); disappears in 1 to 4 days
   b. Symmetrical, maculopapular red spots on upper and lower extremities (proximal to distal); lasts 1 week or longer
   c. Rash subsides but can reappear with skin irritation or trauma, as with sunlight, heat, cold, or friction
2. With aplastic crisis, rash is often absent but child has prodromal signs of fever, lethargy, myalgia, and GI symptoms including nausea, vomiting, and abdominal pain

C. **Therapeutic management**
1. Place hospitalized child on respiratory precautions
2. Provide antipyretics, analgesics, anti-inflammatory drugs as ordered
3. Provide supportive care and transfuse blood to clients with aplastic anemia as ordered

D. **Complications**
1. Self-limited or chronic arthritis
2. Aplastic crisis in clients with hemolytic disease or immune deficiency
3. Rarely myocarditis or encephalitis
4. Possible low risk of fetal death if mother is infected during pregnancy

IV. INFECTIOUS MONONUCLEOSIS

A. **Overview**
1. Organism: Epstein-Barr virus (EBV)
2. Mode of transmission: direct contact with infected blood or secretions
3. Source: oral secretions
4. Incubation period: 4 to 6 weeks
5. Communicability: unknown; viral shedding occurs before onset of symptoms until 6 months or longer after recovery

B. **Nursing assessment**
1. Fever, sore throat, headache
2. Malaise and fatigue
3. Nausea and abdominal pain
4. Lymphadenopathy and hepatosplenomegaly

C. **Therapeutic management**
1. Supportive care including rest
2. Assess for abdominal pain, left upper quadrant or left shoulder pain (signs of ruptured spleen)

D. **Complication: ruptured spleen**

V. MUMPS (PAROTITIS)

A. **Overview**
1. Organism: paramyxovirus
2. Mode of transmission: direct contact or via droplets from infected client
3. Source: saliva
4. Incubation period: 2 to 3 weeks
5. Communicability: greatest immediately before and after swelling begins

B. **Nursing assessment**
1. First 24 hours: fever, headache, malaise, and anorexia
2. Jaw pain and/or ear pain aggravated by chewing
3. Unilateral or bilateral swelling of parotid glands associated with pain and tenderness

C. **Therapeutic management**
1. Prevention: mumps vaccine (see Chapter 15)
2. Institute respiratory precautions during hospitalization
3. Maintain bedrest
4. Encourage fluids and soft, bland foods that require little chewing
5. Comfort measures: analgesics, antipyretics, warm or cool compresses to neck, warmth and local support (snug-fitting underwear) for orchitis

D. **Complications**
1. Sensorineural deafness, meningitis, or encephalitis
2. Myocarditis or arthritis
3. Hepatitis
4. Epididymo-orchitis and possible sterility

VI. PERTUSSIS (WHOOPING COUGH)

A. **Overview**
1. Organism: *Bordetella pertussis*

! 2. Mode of transmission: direct contact or droplet; contact with freshly contaminated articles
3. Source: respiratory tract secretions
4. Incubation period: range of 5 to 21 days, usually 10 days
5. Communicability: greatest during catarrhal stage before paroxysms of coughing begin and may extend to fourth week after paroxysms begin

! **B. Nursing assessment**
1. Catarrhal stage: sneezing, runny nose, lacrimation, low-grade fever, and cough that gradually worsens over 1 to 2 weeks
2. Paroxysmal stage: coughing occurs frequently at night, with a series of short rapid coughs followed by inspiration with a high-pitched "whooping" sound; cheeks become flushed or cyanotic; attack often followed by vomiting; lasts 4 to 6 weeks, then convalescent stage begins

! **C. Therapeutic management**
1. Prevention: pertussis vaccine (see Chapter 15)
2. Maintain bedrest during fever
3. Encourage small amounts of fluids frequently, especially after vomiting
4. Provide humidity via humidifier or tent; also humidify any oxygen given
5. Place on respiratory precautions
6. Administer antimicrobial such as erythromycin and also give pertussis immune globulin

D. Complications
1. Atelectasis and pneumonia
2. Otitis media
3. Dehydration
4. Hemorrhage (subarachnoid, epistaxis, subconjunctival)
5. Hernia and/or prolapsed rectum
6. Seizures

VII. POLIOMYELITIS

A. Overview
1. Organism: three types of enterovirus—abortive or unapparent, nonparalytic, and paralytic—each associated with varying severity of paralysis
! 2. Mode of transmission: direct contact or transmission by fecal–oral or oropharyngeal routes
3. Source: feces and oropharyngeal secretions
4. Incubation period: usually 1 to 2 weeks, with range of 5 to 35 days
5. Communicability: uncertain; virus present in throat and feces shortly after infection and lasts about 1 week in throat and 4 to 6 weeks in feces

! **B. Nursing assessment**
1. Abortive or unapparent type: fever, uneasiness, sore throat, headache, anorexia, vomiting, abdominal pain (lasts a few hours to a few days)
2. Nonparalytic type: similar to abortive poliomyelitis, but more severe, with pain and stiffness in back, neck, and legs
3. Paralytic type: initially similar to nonparalytic type, followed by recovery and then CNS paralysis

! **C. Therapeutic management**
1. Maintain complete bedrest
2. Assess for impending respiratory paralysis: shallow rapid respirations, dyspnea, difficulty talking, ineffective cough
3. Mechanical ventilation for respiratory paralysis, manual resuscitation bag at bedside, tracheostomy insertion tray at bedside
4. Care of immobilized client: range of motion exercises, proper positioning for body alignment, use footboard; prevent skin breakdown
5. Physical therapy for muscles after acute stage; moist heat to muscles

D. Complications
1. Kidney stones from bone demineralization during immobility
2. Hypertension

3. Respiratory arrest
4. Permanent paralysis

VIII. ROCKY MOUNTAIN SPOTTED FEVER

A. Overview

1. Organism: *Rickettsia rickettsii*
2. Mode of transmission: bite of infected tick
3. Source: tick; mammal source such as dog or rodent
4. Incubation period: 2 days to 2 weeks
5. Communicability: contact with tick or infected animal

B. Nursing assessment

1. Chills, fever, malaise, myalgia
2. Anorexia, nausea
3. Headache, mental confusion
4. Maculopapular or petechial rash often on extremities (ankles or wrists) that may spread over trunk, and face; characteristic locations are palms and soles

C. Therapeutic management

1. Prevention: avoid contact with ticks or infected animals; use of insect repellents and protective clothing; immunization of children at risk; inspection of skin for ticks (do not crush on skin if found; remove with tweezers)
2. Provide supportive care
3. Administer antimicrobials (doxycycline or tetracycline) as prescribed

D. Complications: can be fatal

IX. ROSEOLA (EXANTHEMA SUBITUM)

A. Overview

1. Organism: human herpesvirus type 6
2. Mode of transmission: unknown
3. Source: unknown
4. Incubation period: 5 to 15 days
5. Communicability: unknown, but usually occurs between 6 months and 3 years of age

B. Nursing assessment

1. Fever above 102°F for 3 to 4 days in child who appears well
2. Sudden drop in fever accompanied by appearance of rose-pink macules or maculopapules
3. Nonpruritic rash begins on trunk, then spreads to neck, face, and extremities; lasts 1 to 2 days
4. May be associated with lymphadenopathy in cervical area and behind ears, cough, runny nose, and injected pharynx

C. Therapeutic management

1. Supportive care
2. Antipyretics to control fever
3. Seizure precautions for child at risk of recurrent febrile seizures

D. Complications

1. Recurrent febrile seizures
2. Meningitis and rarely encephalitis
3. Hepatitis

X. RUBEOLA (MEASLES)

A. Overview

1. Organism: virus
2. Mode of transmission: direct contact with droplets
3. Source: respiratory secretions, blood, and urine
4. Incubation period: 10 to 20 days
5. Communicability: 4 days before to 5 days after appearance of rash but mainly communicable during prodromal (catarrhal) stage

B. Nursing assessment

1. Prodromal stage
   a. Fever, malaise, coryza, cough, and conjunctivitis
   b. Appearance of Koplik spots (small, irregular red spots with tiny bluish white center) on oral mucosa that last from 2 days before rash appears until about 2 days after
2. Rash
   a. Onset is 3 to 4 days after prodromal stage; erythematous maculopapular rash appears on face and spreads downward
   b. Original or earlier sites have more extreme and confluent rash (blending together), while later (lower) sites have less severe, discrete rash (rash that affects separate or unconnected skin areas)
   c. Rash becomes brownish 3 to 4 days later, and moist desquamation occurs over areas extensively involved

C. Therapeutic management

1. Prevention: measles vaccine (see Chapter 15)
2. Isolate child at home until fifth day of rash; institute respiratory precautions for hospitalized child
3. Maintain bedrest with quiet activity during prodromal stage
4. Provide supportive care: antipyretics for fever (no aspirin, to prevent Reye syndrome), seizure precautions if prone to febrile seizures, cool-mist vaporizer, and adequate fluid intake; tepid baths for skin care and warm saline to remove eye crusts; dim lights if photophobia present

D. Complications

1. Otitis media
2. Pneumonia, bronchiolitis, obstructive laryngitis, or laryngotracheitis
3. Encephalitis

XI. RUBELLA (GERMAN MEASLES)

A. Overview

1. Organism: rubella virus
2. Mode of transmission: direct contact or contact with objects freshly contaminated with nasopharyngeal secretions, urine, or feces
3. Source: respiratory secretions, virus also present in urine, stool, and blood
4. Incubation period: 2 to 3 weeks
5. Communicability: 7 days before to about 5 days after appearance of rash

B. Nursing assessment

1. Low-grade fever, headache, malaise, anorexia, mild conjunctivitis, coryza, sore throat, and lymphadenopathy lasting 1 to 5 days in adolescents and adults until 1 day after appearance of rash; often children do not have this prodromal stage
2. Discrete pinkish red maculopapular rash on face and spreading downward to neck, arms, trunk, and legs within 1 day
3. Rash disappears in the order it began and is usually gone by third day

C. Therapeutic management

1. Prevention: rubella vaccine (see Chapter 15)
2. Antipyretics for fever and analgesics for comfort
3. Comfort measures since illness is benign in children
4. Isolate child from pregnant women

D. Complications

1. Rare, but include arthritis, encephalitis, or purpura
2. Greatest risk is teratogenic effect on fetus (fetal deformity)

XII. SCARLET FEVER

A. Overview

1. Organism: group A beta-hemolytic streptococci
2. Mode of transmission: direct contact, droplets, indirect contact with contaminated objects, ingestion of contaminated milk or food
3. Source: respiratory secretions

4. Incubation period: 2 to 4 days with range of 1 to 7 days
5. Communicability: approximately 10 days during incubation period and clinical illness; also during first 2 weeks to perhaps months in carrier phase

B. Nursing assessment

1. Sudden-onset high fever, headache, chills, malaise, vomiting, abdominal pain
2. Pharyngeal or tonsillar redness, swelling and enlargement, tonsils are covered with gray-white exudate
3. Tongue is coated, and papillae become red and swollen (white strawberry tongue) followed by sloughing of white after 4 to 5 days
4. Red, pinhead-sized rash appears 12 hours after prodromal stage, which rapidly progresses to generalized rashes in axillae, groin, and neck; desquamation begins at end of first week and may last for 3 weeks or longer
5. Rash is characteristically absent on face, which has flushed appearance with circumoral pallor

C. Therapeutic management

1. Respiratory precautions for 24 hours after beginning antibiotic therapy (penicillin or erythromycin if allergic to penicillin)
2. Provide supportive care, including bedrest with quiet environment, and comfort measures for sore throat (gargles, lozenges, cool mist, throat sprays)
3. Increase fluid intake while avoiding irritating citrus juices; provide soft diet (no rough foods) during acute phase

D. Complications

1. Otitis media, sinusitis, or peritonsillar abscess
2. Glomerulonephritis
3. Carditis
4. Polyarthritis (uncommon)

XIII. SMALLPOX

A. Overview

1. Organism: variola major or variola minor virus
2. Mode of transmission: droplets and contact with contaminated objects
3. Source: frozen stores in U.S. Centers for Disease Control and Prevention; other sources unknown but is a potential agent for biological warfare

B. Nursing assessment

1. Fever and malaise
2. Vomiting
3. Headache
4. Vesicular, pustular rash initially on face and extremities that develops 2 days after onset of symptoms

C. Therapeutic management

1. Prevention: immunization with vaccinia (a related poxvirus) for laboratory workers or those at risk for exposure (such as military)
2. Supportive care

D. Complications: death

XIV. ANTHRAX

A. Overview

1. Organism: *Bacillus anthracis* (spore-forming bacteria usually seen in cattle, sheep, and goats)
2. Mode of transmission: direct skin contact, inhalation, digestive system
3. Source: infected animal hides that come in contact with broken skin, airborne spores, or spores impregnated in carrier agent such as a powder (biological warfare); ingestion of contaminated undercooked meat
4. Incubation period: 2 to 60 days
5. Highly contagious

B. Nursing assessment

1. Cutaneous form: reddish brown lesion ulcerates and forms scab surrounded by brawny edema; toxin destroys surrounding tissue

2. GI: internal hemorrhage, abdominal pain, headache, fever, nausea, and vomiting, severe diarrhea
3. Pulmonary form: fever, muscle aches and fatigue, rapidly developing respiratory distress and shock

C. Therapeutic management

!
1. Ciprofloxacin or erythromycin for all types
2. Clean contaminated surfaces with 5% hypochlorite solution
3. Provide vaccine to those at occupational high risk (animal workers)
4. Mechanical ventilation as needed and supportive treatment for shock
5. Institute contact and respiratory precautions because of resistant spores

D. Complications: respiratory form more likely to be fatal

Check Your NCLEX-RN® Exam I.Q.

You are ready for testing on this content if you can

- Identify basic structures and functions of the immunological system.
- Describe the pathophysiology and etiology of common infectious diseases.
- Discuss assessment data and diagnostic test findings for selected infectious diseases.
- Discuss therapeutic and nursing management of a client experiencing an infectious disease.
- Identify expected outcomes for the client experiencing an infectious disease.

PRACTICE TEST

1 The nurse has conducted client teaching with the mother of a 4-year-old child who has been exposed to chickenpox. In evaluating the effectiveness of the instruction, the nurse determines that the mother needs additional information after the mother makes which statement?

1. "I should monitor my child for Reye syndrome, which is a complication of chickenpox."
2. "My child should not visit my pregnant sister at this time."
3. "During the prodromal period, my child will have pox all over his body."
4. "Chickenpox is a viral infection that can be spread to other children."

2 A mother overhears two nurses discussing the incubation period for a measles outbreak. The mother asks the nurses why it is important to know the incubation period. The nurse's reply would include which of the following statements about the incubation period?

1. It describes a period when the child might be contagious.
2. It determines the severity of the infection.
3. It varies depending on the age of the child.
4. It is a time when medications can prevent the development of symptoms.

3 A mother brings her child to clinic with reports of malaise and low-grade temperature. In reviewing the child's medical history, the nurse notes the child is behind on immunizations. The nurse notes the presence of Koplik spots when assessing the mouth of the child. Based on this finding, the nurse suspects that the child has which childhood communicable disease?

1. Mumps
2. Measles
3. Chickenpox
4. Rubella

4 A 2-year-old child in the hospital for a fractured femur breaks out with chickenpox. Which nursing intervention will best prevent secondary skin infections?

1. Caladryl lotion to lesions
2. Acetylsalicylic acid
3. Immunoglobulin for the first 3 days
4. Nubaine every 4 hours as needed for pain

5 A child is being treated at home for chickenpox. The home-health nurse is visiting and notes an elevated temperature. To prevent a common complication of an elevated temperature, the nurse recommends which of the following?

1. Tepid sponge baths
2. Aspirin as needed for fever control
3. Keep child well covered to prevent chilling
4. Antibiotics as ordered

PRACTICE TEST

6 A child has been diagnosed with mumps, and the mother has been given instructions on caring for the child during the acute period. Which statement by the mother indicates a need for additional education?

1. "I can give my child acetaminophen for fever."
2. "My child will be more comfortable if I give him fluids and soft foods."
3. "I should watch my child for headache and vomiting."
4. "I will give my child antibiotics every four hours around the clock."

7 A 2-year-old child with rubeola (measles) is brought to the hospital with a rash covering the entire body, photophobia, and stuffy nose that interferes with breathing. The nurse utilizes which of the following nursing diagnoses as a priority for care when administering care to this child?

1. Impaired skin integrity
2. Disturbed body image
3. Risk for impaired gas exchange
4. Risk for disturbed sleep pattern

8 A child is exposed to a playmate who contracted chickenpox. Two days later, the child is admitted to the hospital for another problem, and the parents inform the nurse of the exposure on admission. How long after the exposure should the child be watched for signs of upper-respiratory illness?

1. 5 to 10 days
2. 10 to 21 days
3. 21 to 25 days
4. One month

9 The home-health nurse sees a child with mumps. The mother says that the child is not eating well and asks for suggestions. The nurse most appropriately suggests which of the following?

1. Provide warm, chopped foods.
2. Provide cool table foods with spices.
3. Provide cool fluids with minimum of acids.
4. Provide a regular diet tray at frequent intervals.

10 The mother of a 3-year-old child with measles calls the nurse at the clinic and asks what she can do to help decrease the redness and itching. The nurse responds that which of the following actions is likely to be helpful?

1. Overdress the child and cause him to perspire.
2. Keep the child out of drafts.
3. Bathe the child in an oatmeal (Aveeno) bath.
4. Provide adequate oral fluids.

11 The clinic nurse is working with a toddler who has been diagnosed with roseola (exanthema subitum) after being seen for fever and a skin rash. The nurse makes which response to the mother who asks how to reduce the risk of infecting other children at home?

1. "There is no way to reduce risk because the route of transmission is unknown."
2. "Do not allow the child to cough or sneeze in the presence of others whenever possible."
3. "Use disposable dishes and eating utensils, and dispose of them in a separate trash bag."
4. "Select one bathroom to be used exclusively by the toddler until the rash clears."

12 A college student was hospitalized following onset of a severe case of pertussis. In preparing for discharge, the nurse would correct which client statement that indicates a misconception about postdischarge care?

1. "Irritants that I breathe, such as smoke or dust, could make me have coughing spells again."
2. "I will try to avoid being around people for a full week after going home so I don't spread this to others."
3. "I will be very careful to wash my hands often."
4. "It will still be important to try to drink a lot of fluids when I go home."

13 A child who may have scarlet fever is being evaluated in the urgent care clinic. The nurse concludes that the client's presentation is not consistent with scarlet fever after noting which of the following during assessment?

1. Rash in the axillae and groin
2. Pharyngeal redness and swelling
3. Koplik spots in the oral mucosa
4. Red strawberry tongue

14 The nurse is assessing a child in the outpatient clinic who has fever, lethargy, nausea, and vomiting. The nurse notes that the child's cheeks have the appearance of being wind-burned or slapped. The nurse suspects which of the following childhood communicable diseases?

1. Chickenpox
2. Measles
3. Diphtheria
4. Fifth disease

15 The spouse of a postal worker who contracted cutaneous anthrax asks the nurse whether this communicable disease can be treated. Which of the following responses by the nurse is most appropriate?

1. "No, there is only supportive care available for the itching associated with skin lesions."
2. "No, although we will be ready to provide aggressive respiratory support measures if needed."
3. "Yes, the infection can be treated with antiviral agents and immune globulin."
4. "Yes, the infection can be treated with antibiotics such as ciprofloxacin or erythromycin."

16 The nurse is providing health teaching to a group of high school students regarding infectious mononucleosis. When discussion the incubation period as part of disease transmission, the nurse explains that the incubation period for this infection is how many weeks? Provide a numerical answer.

Answer: ____________________

ANSWERS & RATIONALES

1 **Answer: 3** The prodromal period is the time between the initial symptoms and the presence of the full-blown disease. The rash would not be apparent during this time. All the other statements are correct.
Cognitive Level: Analysis **Client Need:** Physiological Integrity: Physiological Adaptation **Integrated Process:** Nursing Process: Evaluation **Content Area:** Child Health: Communicable Disease **Strategy:** The core issue of the question is knowledge of client teaching points related to chickenpox, particularly related to the timing of symptoms. Use nursing knowledge and the process of elimination to make a selection.

2 **Answer: 1** The incubation period is the time between exposure and outbreak of the disease. It is often a period when the child can be contagious without others being aware of the possible exposure.
Cognitive Level Application **Client Need:** Physiological Integrity: Physiological Adaptation **Integrated Process:** Nursing Process: Implementation **Content Area:** Adult Health: Communicable Disease **Strategy:** The core issue of the question is knowledge of the significance of the prodromal period in a communicable disease. Use nursing knowledge and the process of elimination to make a selection.

3 **Answer: 2** Koplik spots are associated with measles (rubeola) and appear on the buccal mucosa 2 days before and after the onset of the rash. Mumps, chickenpox, and rubella are not associated with the presence of Koplik spots.
Cognitive Level: Application **Client Need:** Physiological Integrity: Physiological Adaptation **Integrated Process:** Nursing Process: Assessment **Content Area:** Child Health: Communicable Disease **Strategy:** The core issue of the question is the significance of Koplik spots in a child with a communicable disease. Use nursing knowledge and the process of elimination to make a selection.

4 **Answer: 1** Caladryl will reduce itching and discomfort and therefore diminish scratching and skin breakdown. Acetylsalicylic acid should not be given to young children with a viral disease because of the relationship to Reye syndrome. Immunoglobin will not decrease skin eruptions. Nubaine is a narcotic analgesic.
Cognitive Level: Application **Client Need:** Physiological Integrity: Physiological Adaptation **Integrated Process:** Nursing Process: Implementation **Content Area:** Child Health: Communicable Disease **Strategy:** The core issue of the question is knowledge of various products used in the care of children and which one will reduce the likelihood of itching or pruritus with skin lesions. Use nursing knowledge and the process of elimination to make a selection.

5 **Answer: 1** Tepid baths allow heat to be removed from the body. Aspirins are avoided because of the risk of Reye syndrome. The child should wear only light clothing to allow heat to escape. Antibiotics are not usually ordered for this viral infection.
Cognitive Level: Application **Client Need:** Physiological Integrity: Physiological Adaptation **Integrated Process:** Nursing Process: Implementation **Content Area:** Child Health: Communicable Disease **Strategy:** The core issue of the question is an effective measure to prevent febrile seizures as a complication of fever in a child. Use nursing knowledge and the process of elimination to make a selection.

6 **Answer: 4** Mumps is a viral infection and thus antibiotics will not be effective. The other statements are true. Acetaminophen, fluids, and soft foods are helpful, and the mother should watch for vomiting and headache.

Cognitive Level: Analysis **Client Need:** Physiological Integrity: Physiological Adaptation **Integrated Process:** Nursing Process: Evaluation **Content Area:** Child Health: Communicable Disease **Strategy:** The core issue of the question is knowledge of supportive measures for a child with mumps. Use nursing knowledge and the process of elimination to make a selection.

7 **Answer: 3** The child has a stuffy nose, which can impair air exchange. Nursing care involves use of a cool-mist vaporizer and gentle suctioning of the nose. The rash does not cause skin impairment. A 2-year-old will not have a disturbed body image. Disturbed sleep pattern would have less priority than gas exchange if this problem developed.
Cognitive Level: Analysis **Client Need:** Physiological Integrity: Physiological Adaptation **Integrated Process:** Nursing Process: Planning **Content Area:** Child Health: Communicable Disease **Strategy:** The core issue of the question is the ability to set appropriate priorities of care for a child with a communicable disease. Use nursing knowledge and the process of elimination to make a selection.

8 **Answer: 2** The upper-respiratory symptoms may be early prodromal symptoms of chickenpox. The incubation period of chickenpox is 10 to 21 days. The other responses are either too short (option 1) or too long (options 3 and 4).
Cognitive Level: Application **Client Need:** Physiological Integrity: Physiological Adaptation **Integrated Process:** Nursing Process: Assessment **Content Area:** Child Health: Communicable Disease **Strategy:** The core issue of the question is knowledge of the incubation period for chickenpox. Use nursing knowledge and the process of elimination to make a selection.

9 **Answer: 3** Cool fluids will help decrease the swelling of the glands around the mouth and neck. Acidic foods are too irritating and difficult to swallow. Warm, chopped foods may be difficult to swallow (option 1), and spices are also likely to be irritating (option 2). The child should be given small, frequent meals with soft foods rather a regular diet (option 4).
Cognitive Level: Application **Client Need:** Physiological Integrity: Physiological Adaptation **Integrated Process:** Nursing Process: Implementation **Content Area:** Child Health: Communicable Disease **Strategy:** The core issue of the question is knowledge of foods and beverages that will be helpful to the child with mumps. Use principles of diet therapy that utilize cool, soft, and nonirritating food items to make a selection.

10 **Answer: 3** Soothing the skin with an oatmeal-based substance will decrease the itching and redness. Overdressing the child will increase perspiration and thereby increase the itching. Although drinking adequate fluids is helpful, it does not directly affect the itching.
Cognitive Level: Application **Client Need:** Physiological Integrity: Physiological Adaptation **Integrated Process:** Nursing Process: Implementation **Content Area:** Child Health: Communicable Disease **Strategy:** The core issue of the question is an effective measure to treat itching caused by a communicable disease such as measles. Use nursing knowledge and the process of elimination to make a selection.

11 **Answer: 1** The route of transmission of roseola is unknown. It is not known to be transmitted by the respiratory tract (option 2), contact with contaminated articles (option 3), or body secretions such as urine or stool (option 4).
Cognitive Level: Analysis **Client Need:** Physiological Integrity: Physiological Adaptation **Integrated Process:** Teaching and Learning **Content Area:** Child Health: Communicable Disease **Strategy:** The core issue of the question is knowledge of transmission of roseola. The wording of the question tells you the correct answer is also a true statement. Use nursing knowledge and the process of elimination to make a selection.

12 **Answer: 2** Pertussis is most infectious early in the course of the disease, so it is not necessary for the client to self-isolate following discharge from the hospital. Coughing bouts may be still triggered by irritants, so these should be avoided. Frequent handwashing and increased fluid intake are generally helpful measures that should also be continued in the home setting.
Cognitive Level: Analysis **Client Need:** Physiological Integrity: Physiological Adaptation **Integrated Process:** Teaching and Learning **Content Area:** Adult Health: Communicable Disease **Strategy:** The core issue of the question is knowledge of care to a client recovering from pertussis. Note that the client is nearing discharge and is not in an acute state to choose the item that does not need to continue. The wording of the question tells you the correct answer is an incorrect client statement. Use nursing knowledge and the process of elimination to make a selection.

13 **Answer: 3** Koplik spots are seen with rubeola, not scarlet fever. Reddened edematous pharynx, red strawberry tongue, and rash in the axillae and groin are findings consistent with scarlet fever.
Cognitive Level: Analysis **Client Need:** Physiological Integrity: Physiological Adaptation **Integrated Process:** Nursing Process: Assessment **Content Area:** Adult Health: Communicable Disease **Strategy:** The core issue of the question is the ability to discriminate between clinical findings associated with scarlet fever and rubeola. The wording of the question tells you the correct answer is an incorrect client statement. Use nursing knowledge and the process of elimination to make a selection.

14 **Answer: 4** Fifth disease is characterized by flulike symptoms such as fever, malaise, nausea, and vomiting, and by the characteristic "slapped cheeks" appearance. This finding is not characteristic of chickenpox, measles, or diphtheria.
Cognitive Level: Analysis **Client Need:** Physiological Integrity: Physiological Adaptation **Integrated Process:** Nursing Process: Assessment **Content Area:** Adult Health: Communicable Disease **Strategy:** The core issue of the question is the ability to discriminate the classic sign of Fifth disease from other childhood communicable diseases. Use nursing knowledge and the process of elimination to make a selection.

15 **Answer: 4** Anthrax is caused by a bacterium and is therefore amenable to treatment with antibiotics. Antivirals and immune globulin play no role in treating this disease, and the statements in options 1 and 2 are incorrect because they indicate no treatment is available.
Cognitive Level: Analysis **Client Need:** Physiological Integrity: Physiological Adaptation **Integrated Process:** Communication and Documentation **Content Area:** Adult Health: Communicable Disease **Strategy:** The core issue of the question is knowledge of available treatment methods for anthrax. Use

nursing knowledge and the process of elimination to make a selection.

16 **Answer: 6** The incubation period for infectious mononucleosis is up to 6 weeks (with a minimum of 4 weeks). This has important implications for the nurse and the client, since the source of the exposure may be difficult to determine after several weeks.
Cognitive Level: Analysis **Client Need:** Physiological Integrity: Safe, Effective Care Environment: Safety and Infection Control **Integrated Process:** Teaching and Learning **Content Area:** Adult Health: Communicable Disease **Strategy:** The core issue of the question is knowledge of the incubation period for infectious mononucleosis. Specific knowledge is needed to answer this type of question. Note that the question asks for the number of *weeks,* which suggests that the number to be typed in is not excessively large.

Key Terms to Remember

immunization p. 1399 **vaccine** p. 1399

References

Ball, J., & Bindler, R. (2006). *Child health nursing: Partnering with children and families.* Upper Saddle River, NJ: Pearson Education.

Black, J., & Hawks, J. (2005). *Medical surgical nursing: Clinical management for positive outcomes* (7th ed.). St. Louis: Elsevier Science.

Harkreader, H., & Hogan, M. (2004). *Fundamentals of nursing: Caring and clinical judgment* (2nd ed.). St. Louis: Elsevier Science.

Ignatavicius, D., & Workman, L. (2006). *Medical-surgical nursing: Critical thinking for collaborative care* (5th ed.). Philadelphia: W. B. Saunders.

Kozier, B., Erb, G., Berman, A., & Snyder, S. (2004). *Fundamentals of nursing: Concepts, process, and practice* (7th ed.). Upper Saddle River, NJ: Pearson Education.

LeMone, P., & Burke, K. (2004). *Medical surgical nursing: Critical thinking in client care* (3rd ed.). Upper Saddle River, NJ: Pearson Education.

69 Basic Life Support

Test Yourself

Are you ready for the NCLEX-RN® or course exams? Use the practice tests on the companion CD-ROM to check.

In this chapter

Cross reference

Other chapters relevant to this content area are

I. OVERVIEW OF BASIC LIFE SUPPORT (BLS)

A. BLS consists of a set of guidelines for use with respiratory or cardiac arrest

B. Commonly called cardiopulmonary resuscitation (CPR)

1. Is a mechanical attempt to supply oxygen and blood flow to vital organs, especially brain
2. ! Follows a series of steps often called ABCs: airway, breathing, circulation

Memory Aid

Remember the ABCs of basic life support!

A—Airway
B—Breathing
C—Circulation

Also use this mnemonic to remember the key sequence for assessment whenever a client's status becomes unstable or deteriorates.

II. BARRIER MASKS AND DEVICES

A. Purpose: provide a barrier against contracting communicable disease such as HIV or hepatitis during resuscitation efforts

B. Face shield

1. A clear plastic or silicon sheet that can be placed over victim's mouth
2. Has an opening or tube in center sheet to permit air flow into airway during ventilations
3. Advantage: small and portable; fits on a key ring

C. Face mask

1. Rigid plastic device that fits over mouth and nose; more effective than face shield
2. Is bulky, costs more than face shield, and may not always be available

D. Bag-valve-mask ventilation

1. Utilizes a combination of a rigid plastic mask with manual resuscitation bag (Ambu bag)
2. Can be attached to oxygen (O_2) source for more effective oxygenation
3. Eliminates risk of communicable disease transmission
4. Is preferred method for providing respiratory support during respiratory insufficiency or arrest
5. Ensure that mouth and nose are covered completely and firmly with mask to make an effective seal

III. ADULT BLS FOR HEALTH CARE PROVIDERS

A. Used for resuscitating individuals at age of puberty or adolescence (12–14 years) and older when following American Heart Association healthcare provider guidelines; BLS for laypersons includes using adult CPR guidelines for adults and children age 8 and older

B. Airway

1. Assess client to determine unresponsiveness by tapping or gently shaking shoulder and asking loudly, "Are you okay?"
2. Call for help or activate emergency medical system (EMS); dial 911 if outside a health care facility; use institutional policy for calling a code or inhouse response team if inside a health care agency
3. Place client on flat firm surface in supine position
4. Use gloves and barrier device if available
5. Open airway using **head tilt-chin lift** method by lifting chin with two fingers while pushing down on forehead with other hand; kneel parallel to client's sternum
6. If head or neck (cervical spine) injury is suspected or has occurred, use **jaw thrust maneuver** to open airway by lifting mandible on both sides with fingertips while positioning hands on sides of client's face; kneel at client's head

C. Breathing

1. Place ear near client's mouth and nose and check for adequate breathing: observe whether chest rises and falls; listen for air movement from client's lungs, and feel for air movement on own cheek
2. Inadequate or absent breathing
   a. If client is not breathing adequately, maintain head tilt-chin lift and give two rescue breaths at rate of 1 second/breath; use breath sufficient to produce a rise in chest
   b. If chest does not rise with breath, reposition airway and try again (incorrect airway position is most common cause of obstructed rescuer ventilations)
   c. If chest still does not rise and fall, perform finger sweep of mouth to check for foreign body; clear airway and try again; remove dentures only if obstructing the airway
   d. Provide one breath every 5 to 6 seconds or 10 to 12 breaths per minute; allow time for client to exhale between ventilations; this is called rescue breathing
3. Breathing client
   a. If client is breathing adequately and has suspected or actual head or neck trauma, do not move client
   b. If client is breathing adequately and does not have suspected head or neck trauma, logroll client onto side as a unit (maintaining alignment of spine) and continue to monitor; this position is also called recovery position
4. Improper ventilation technique could lead to ineffective ventilations or gastric distention
5. Use mouth-to-nose ventilation if mouth cannot be sealed, has serious injuries, or cannot be opened for any reason
6. Use mouth-to-stoma ventilation after temporary tracheostomy or laryngectomy; seal client's mouth and nose to ensure adequate ventilation

D. Circulation

1. Maintain head tilt to keep airway patent
2. Place two or three fingers on Adam's apple and slide fingers into groove between Adam's apple and neck muscle

3. Palpate for carotid pulse for minimum of 5 seconds but not longer than 10 seconds
4. If pulse is present, continue rescue breathing at rate of 10 to 12 breaths per minute; continue to assess client
5. If no pulse is present, begin external cardiac compressions
   a. Using hand closest to client's feet, locate lower margin of ribcage and slide upward to locate sternal notch
   b. Place middle finger on notch and index finger next to middle finger
   c. Place heel of opposite hand next to index finger (hand position is now on lower half of sternum); proper positioning is critical for success of CPR and to avoid injuring client
   d. Position own body directly over hands, with shoulders above hands, and elbows straight
   e. ! Provide compressions at rate of 100/minute and at depth of 1.5 to 2 inches; 2005 AHA guidelines state to "push hard, push fast," and allow chest to recoil after each compression (AHA, 2005, p. 14).
   f. Use a 30:2 compression to ventilation ratio for either 1- or 2-rescuer CPR; change positions for "switch" as needed after 5 cycles of 30:2
   g. After first 5 cycles (about 2 minutes), check pulse; if no pulse, continue CPR and recheck pulse every few minutes
   h. If pulse returns, stop compressions but continue to provide rescue breathing as needed
6. Do not interrupt chest compressions for more than 10 seconds at a time except for defibrillation or intubation; interruptions for rescue breaths or pulse checks should take less than 10 seconds; "switches" during 2-person CPR should take less than 5 seconds
7. Do stop CPR to administer automated external defibrillation when EMS responders arrive, if pulse and respirations resume, or if a physician pronounces client deceased

IV. PEDIATRIC BLS FOR HEALTH CARE PROVIDERS

A. Overview

1. Principles are same as for adult CPR; differences relate to smaller body size and needs of client
2. ! Use child CPR if client is age 1 to 8
3. ! Use infant CPR for clients less than 1 year old
4. Activate EMS after performing 5 cycles of CPR; for sudden, witnessed collapse, activate EMS after determining that victim is unresponsive

B. Airway: open airway using head tilt-chin lift method for both infant and child

C. Breathing

1. After checking breathing, and if needed, provide two rescue breaths initially for both infant and child CPR with visible chest rise (same as for adult client); cover mouth and nose with infant breaths
2. ! After initial two breaths, provide 2 breaths after each 30 compressions for both child and infant with single rescuer
3. ! Deliver a breath every 3 to 5 seconds for a total ventilation rate of 12 to 20 breaths per minute

D. Circulation

1. ! Check carotid or femoral pulse for child and brachial or femoral pulse for infant (health care providers only, not lay rescuers)
2. Provide compressions at ratio of 30 compressions to 2 breaths for both child and infant CPR; when there are 2 healthcare provider rescuers, may use a 15:2 ratio
3. ! Maintain rate of 100 compressions per minute for both child and infant CPR; same as for adult
4. Use heel of one hand for compressions to child with compression depth of ⅓ to ½ of the depth of the chest; use same hand placement as adult
5. Use middle and ring fingers for compressions to infant at a depth of ⅓ to ½ the depth of the chest
6. Determine correct hand placement for infant by placing index finger of hand furthest from infant's head on sternum just below an imaginary line between

nipples; lower middle and ring fingers onto sternum and then lift index finger; provide compressions with middle and ring fingers

V. AUTOMATED EXTERNAL DEFIBRILLATOR (AED) USE

A. Overview

1. AED is a computerized defibrillator that analyzes cardiac rhythm of client, recognizes rhythm amenable to shock, and uses synthesized voice and flashing lights to indicate if shock is warranted
2. ! Apply AED when client has signs of cardiac arrest: unresponsive, absence of respirations, absence of pulse (or signs of circulation for laypeople)
3. Place AED machine near client's left ear, to allow room for reaching AED controls easily, applying pads without excessive reaching, and performing CPR without interference

B. Steps of AED operation

1. Turn power on
2. Apply AED electrode pads to client's chest
   a. Attach connecting cables to electrode pads (if not preconnected) before applying to client's chest
   b. Attach electrodes to chest as indicated on pad backing or packaging; placement does not have to be exact but should be within an inch or two of placement shown on diagram
   c. Apply first pad to upper right side of chest (to right of sternum between nipple and clavicle)
   d. Apply second pad to outside of left nipple, with top margin of pad several inches below left axilla
3. Analyze rhythm
   a. ! Do not touch client in any way, and do not allow others to do so; announce loudly to stand clear of client
   b. Do not push button to analyze rhythm until all contact with client has stopped; some machines analyze automatically without activation by button
4. Charge AED and, if indicated, deliver shock
   a. ! Stay clear of client while charging; most models charge automatically
   b. Look to see that no one is touching client; announce to stand clear
   c. Push button to deliver shock when instructed to do so unless machine delivers it automatically
   d. Allow machine to follow shock sequence programmed by manufacturer (new AHA CPR guidelines state 1 shock compared to 3 previously used for ventricular fibrillation or pulseless ventricular tachycardia; newer biphasic defibrillators have high first-shock success rates than older monophasic defibrillators
   e. If shock is ineffective, leave AED paddles attached and perform CPR for 2 minutes or 5 cycles of CPR; then reanalyze
   f. If shock is effective, follow the ABCs of CPR according to client need

C. Special circumstances

1. Do not use an AED on a child less than 1 year of age; use child pads and child system for children ages 1 to 8 if available, if not available, use adult AED and pads
2. ! Do not use AED on client lying in standing water until client is removed and chest is dried
3. Avoid placing AED electrodes directly over an implantable defibrillator
4. Remove transdermal medication before placing an AED electrode on that site; wipe skin dry and then position electrode
5. Use a prep razor if needed for hairy chest to ensure good contact between client's skin and AED electrodes

VI. FOREIGN BODY AIRWAY OBSTRUCTION

A. Adult or child who is choking

1. Conscious
   a. Ask client, "Are you choking?" (will not be able to cough or speak if choking with severe or complete airway obstruction; will also have increasing respiratory distress and developing cyanosis)

b. Encourage client to cough if crowing noise is heard (partial obstruction)
c. Use **Heimlich maneuver** (see Box 69–1) until client becomes unconscious or blockage is relieved

2. Unconscious (health care provider directions)
   a. Place client on back
   b. Open airway using head tilt-chin lift method (not tongue jaw lift) and look in mouth; remove object if seen but do *not* do blind finger sweep
   c. Attempt to ventilate; if chest does not rise, reposition head and attempt to ventilate again
   d. If chest still does not rise, straddle victim and give up to 5 quick abdominal thrusts for adults and children (not infants) (see Box 69–1)
   e. Repeat sequence until obstruction is cleared

B. Infant who is choking

1. Conscious
   a. Observe respiratory difficulty in infant
   b. Use series of five back blows and five chest thrusts on infant (positioned with head lower than trunk) until relieved
   c. Check mouth of infant for foreign object after each series, but avoid blind finger sweeps that could push obstruction further into airway
2. Unconscious
   a. Assess unconsciousness of infant
   b. Open airway using head tilt-chin lift
   c. Assess breathing and observe for foreign object; remove if seen
   d. Attempt ventilation
   e. Reposition head if unable to ventilate; attempt again to ventilate
   f. Relieve obstruction using 5 back blows and 5 chest thrusts in infants
   g. Finger sweep mouth only if object is seen
   h. Repeat sequence until successful or EMS personnel arrive

C. Pregnant or obese client who is choking

1. Conscious
   a. Stand behind client and put own arms around client's chest
   b. Place fist on middle of sternum between nipples (be sure to avoid xiphoid process)
   c. Grasp fist with other hand and deliver firm backward thrusts until object is removed or victim becomes unconscious
2. Unconscious
   a. Position victim lying on back; use a small pillow or wedge under right hip of pregnant client to shift uterus to left side of abdomen
   b. Open airway and observe for obstruction; and perform finger sweep with index finger of second hand if seen
   c. Attempt to give rescue breaths
   d. If unsuccessful, reposition head and try again
   e. Perform chest thrusts by kneeling at side of client and placing heel of one hand on top of the other; place heel of lower hand at nipple line; position body directly over hands (as for CPR)
   f. Deliver up to five chest thrusts
   g. Repeat sequence until obstruction is relieved

Box 69–1

Heimlich Maneuver

1. Stand behind client and encircle client's waist with own arms.
2. Make a fist with one hand.
3. Place thumb side of fist on abdomen above umbilicus but below xiphoid process of sternum.
4. Grasp fist with other hand and give five quick inward and upward thrusts.
5. Repeat until victim becomes unconscious or obstruction is expelled.
6. For unconscious client, straddle client facing the head; place heel of one hand above umbilicus but below xiphoid process; place second hand on top of first, and give up to five abdominal thrusts, pushing inward and upward toward chest.

Check Your NCLEX–RN® Exam I.Q. *You are ready for testing on this content if you can*

- Recognize and intervene when client requires cardiopulmonary resuscitation or Heimlich maneuver/abdominal thrusts.
- Evaluate and document response to resuscitation efforts.
- Explain emergency interventions to client and family when necessary.

PRACTICE TEST

1 A client is brought to the emergency department awake and alert following a fall from a ladder from a height of 15 feet. While the nurse is conducting an initial assessment, the client becomes unresponsive and stops breathing. Which method should the nurse use to open the airway?

1. Head tilt-chin lift
2. Jaw thrust
3. Tongue-jaw lift
4. None; client needs emergency intubation

2 The nurse has begun CPR on a 5-year-old child. The nurse times the rate of ventilation to achieve how many breaths per minute?

1. 8
2. 10
3. 20
4. 30

3 A nurse has begun to resuscitate a 10-month-old infant. After delivering breaths, the nurse next checks the pulse at which of the following locations?

1. Brachial
2. Radial
3. Carotid
4. Temporal

4 The nurse on a surgical nursing unit has just called a code blue using the telephone in the room of an unresponsive client who had abdominal surgery. Which of the following actions would be appropriate during initiation of CPR?

1. Open the airway using the jaw thrust method.
2. Deliver one deep breath before checking for a pulse.
3. Depress the sternum 1.5 to 2 inches during cardiac compressions.
4. Reevaluate status every 2 to 3 minutes until the code team arrives.

5 The nurse who is doing the documentation during a code blue on an adult client observes an unlicensed assistive personnel (UAP) doing CPR. The nurse interprets that the UAP is performing CPR correctly after noting that the UAP is depressing the sternum how many inches?

1. 2.5 to 3.5
2. 2 to 2.5
3. 1.5 to 2
4. 1 to 2

6 The nurse is performing CPR on a 10-month-old infant. The nurse times the rate of compressions to achieve a total number of approximately how many compressions per minute?

1. 180
2. 120
3. 100
4. 80

7 A nurse witnesses an adult male collapse at the airport and an automated external defibrillator (AED) is brought to the scene. The nurse should do which of the following in utilizing the device?

1. Press the electrodes down firmly, because the client has a hairy chest.
2. Instruct another person at the scene to keep the airway open during delivery of the electric shock.
3. Initiate CPR after 5 minutes if the AED has not restored a perfusing cardiac rhythm.
4. Quickly wipe up the spilled coffee under the victim's chest before using the AED.

8 A nurse is eating in a restaurant when a woman who is 8 months pregnant at the next table begins to choke. Which of the following hand placements should the nurse use to perform the Heimlich maneuver?

1. Midsternum
2. Lower sternum
3. Midway between umbilicus and xiphoid process
4. Midway between umbilicus and symphysis pubis

9 The long-term care nurse has been called to the aid of a resident who has become unconscious after choking in the dining room. After positioning the client on the back, which of the following actions should the nurse take next?

1. Attempt to ventilate the client
2. Observe the oral cavity; carry out a finger sweep of the mouth
3. Perform five abdominal thrusts
4. Perform five chest thrusts

10 A nurse enters an adult client's room and says, "Good morning!" while doing initial shift rounds after receiving report. The client does not respond. Put the nurse's actions in order of priority.

1. Call for someone to announce a code blue.
2. Open the airway.
3. Shake the client's shoulder and ask, "Are you okay?"
4. Take the manual resuscitation bag from the head of the bed and give two breaths.

Enter the numbers without spaces or commas in the box.

ANSWERS & RATIONALES

1 **Answer: 2** The jaw thrust maneuver is used whenever head or cervical spine injury is suspected to avoid causing further physiological damage. The head tilt-chin lift method (option 1) is the standard method for opening the airway when there is no suspected cervical spine injury. The tongue-jaw lift (option 3) aids in visualizing foreign bodies in the airway. The client does not need emergency intubation (option 4). **Cognitive Level:** Application **Client Need:** Physiological Integrity: Physiological Adaptation **Integrated Process:** Nursing Process: Implementation **Content Area:** Adult Health/Cardiovascular **Strategy:** Note key information in the stem, which indicates the client has suffered a traumatic injury and is therefore at risk of cervical spine injury. Next use knowledge of basic CPR procedures to select the option for opening the airway in a client with suspected head or neck injury.

2 **Answer: 3** The proper ventilation rate for a child or infant is 12 to 20 breaths per minute, which is the same as delivering one breath every 3 to 5 seconds. Ventilation rates of 8 (option 1) or 10 (option 2) do not provide sufficient oxygenation for the child during cardiopulmonary arrest. A rate of 30 breaths/min (option 4) is excessive and could be harmful. **Cognitive Level:** Application **Client Need:** Physiological Integrity: Physiological Adaptation **Integrated Process:** Nursing Process: Implementation **Content Area:** Adult Health/Cardiovascular **Strategy:** Use the process of elimination and knowledge of basic CPR procedures to make the proper selection. Remember that compressions and ventilation rates need to be higher in children than in adults to help you choose correctly.

3 **Answer: 1** The brachial artery is the correct location for determining whether an infant under one year of age has a pulse. The radial artery would not generate enough pulsation in an infant to be reliable (option 2) and is also more difficult to palpate. The carotid pulse is not as easily located in an infant with a small neck and neck folds (option 3), while the temporal pulse is not used in CPR for an individual of any age. **Cognitive Level:** Application **Client Need:** Physiological Integrity: Physiological Adaptation **Integrated Process:** Nursing Process: Implementation **Content Area:** Child Health/Cardiovascular **Strategy:** Eliminate options 2 and 4 first because they are not used in CPR. Choose option 1 (brachial) over option 3 (carotid) using knowledge of infant anatomy and accessibility of the site.

4 **Answer: 3** In an adult, the sternum should be depressed during CPR to a depth of 1.5 to 2 inches. The head tilt-chin lift method of opening the airway is used for the client who has no head or neck injury (option 1). The nurse should deliver two breaths to initiate ventilation (option 2). The nurse should reevaluate the client's status after approximately 1 minute (option 4). **Cognitive Level:** Application **Client Need:** Physiological Integrity: Physiological Adaptation **Integrated Process:** Nursing Process: Implementation **Content Area:** Adult Health/Cardiovascular **Strategy:** Use knowledge of basic CPR procedures to answer the question. Eliminate options 1 and 2 because they indicate incorrect procedure. Eliminate option 4 because the time frame is excessively long.

5 **Answer: 3** On an adult client, chest compressions should be done to a depth of 1.5 to 2 inches to be effective. Options 2 and 4 are excessively deep and could lead to injury, while option 4 is not deep enough to provide effective circulation. **Cognitive Level:** Application **Client Need:** Physiological Integrity: Physiological Adaptation **Integrated Process:** Nursing Process: Implementation **Content Area:** Adult Health/Cardiovascular

Strategy: Use the process of elimination and knowledge of basic CPR procedures to answer the question. Recall that compressions are never deeper than 2 inches to eliminate options 1 and 2. Recall that there is only a half inch variability in compression depth to choose option 3 over 4.

6 **Answer: 3** The rate of compressions for an infant during CPR is at least 100 per minute. Options 1 and 2 are higher than the minimum number of compressions per minute, while option 4 does not deliver a sufficient number of compressions per minute.
Cognitive Level: Application **Client Need:** Physiological Integrity: Physiological Adaptation **Integrated Process:** Nursing Process: Implementation **Content Area:** Child Health/Cardiovascular
Strategy: Use knowledge of basic CPR procedures to answer the question. Eliminate options 1 and 2 because they are too excessive for any client. Note that if the client in the question is an infant to choose option 3 over 4.

7 **Answer: 4** The client should not be lying in water or other liquid, which could lead to burns or to defibrillating another individual who comes in contact with the liquid during AED shock delivery. The electrodes should not be placed on hairy areas, or the site should be shaved (option 1). All people should stand clear of the individual during an AED shock to avoid being defibrillated themselves (option 2). CPR is initiated after 1 minute or whenever the series of shocks is terminated, as indicated by client condition. However, 5 minutes is too excessive and could lead to permanent brain damage if the client survives (option 3).
Cognitive Level: Application **Client Need:** Physiological Integrity: Physiological Adaptation **Integrated Process:** Nursing Process: Implementation **Content Area:** Adult Health/Cardiovascular
Strategy: First eliminate option 1 because hair interferes with good skin contact of any type of electrode. Next eliminate option 3 because brain death can occur within 4 to 6 minutes if CPR is not initiated. Use general principles of electrical safety to choose option 4 over option 2.

8 **Answer: 1** In a pregnant client, the Heimlich maneuver is performed in a manner that avoids causing injury to the fetus. For this reason, the hand placement is at the midsternum rather than at the abdomen (options 3 and 4). The lower sternum (option 1) should be avoided to prevent accidental fracture of the xiphoid process, which could lead to internal injury.
Cognitive Level: Application **Client Need:** Physiological Integrity: Physiological Adaptation **Integrated Process:** Nursing Process: Implementation **Content Area:** Adult Health/Cardiovascular
Strategy: Note key information in the question that the client is pregnant. Then use knowledge of basic CPR procedures to answer the question. Eliminate options 3 and 4 first because they involve the abdomen, and eliminate option 2 next as possibly unsafe.

9 **Answer: 2** There is a specific sequence of actions that is performed as part of basic life support when a client is choking. After positioning the client on the back, the nurse would observe the oral cavity to detect any foreign body that may be removed immediately. Next, the nurse would open the airway and attempt to ventilate (option 1). If unsuccessful, this process would be repeated. Finally the nurse would perform abdominal thrusts (option 3). Chest thrusts (option 4) are performed in the adult only for pregnant or obese clients.
Cognitive Level: Analysis **Client Need:** Physiological Integrity: Physiological Adaptation **Integrated Process:** Nursing Process: Implementation **Content Area:** Adult Health/Cardiovascular
Strategy: Remember the ABCs of life support to answer this question. Choose the option that attempts to clear the airway before taking any other actions.

10 **Answer: 3124** The first action of the nurse is to establish unresponsiveness. This can be done by shaking the shoulder and asking if the client is okay. The subsequent actions of the nurse would be to call for help (option 1), open the airway (option 2), and ventilate the client (option 4).
Cognitive Level: Analysis **Client Need:** Physiological Integrity: Physiological Adaptation **Integrated Process:** Nursing Process: Implementation **Content Area:** Adult Health/Cardiovascular
Strategy: Specific knowledge of the sequence of events is needed to answer the question. Using the ABCs (airway, breathing, circulation) will be of assistance once unresponsiveness has been determined.

Key Terms To Review

automated external defibrillator (AED) p. 1413
basic life support (BLS) p. 1410
cardiopulmonary resuscitation (CPR) p. 1410
head tilt-chin lift p. 1411
Heimlich maneuver p. 1414
jaw thrust maneuver p. 1411

References

American Heart Association (Winter 2005–2006). *Currents in emergency cardiovascular care.* 6(4), p. 128.

Ball, J., & Bindler, R. (2006). *Child health nursing: Partnering with children and families.* Upper Saddle River, NJ: Pearson Prentice Hall.

Harkreader, H., & Hogan, M. (2004). *Fundamentals of nursing: Caring and clinical judgment* (2nd ed.). St. Louis, MO: Elsevier Science, pp. 908–912.

Kozier, B., Erb, G., Berman, A., & Snyder, S. (2004). *Fundamentals of nursing: Concepts, process, and practice* (7th ed.). Upper Saddle River, NJ: Pearson Education, p. 1347.

LeMone, P., & Burke, K. (2004). *Medical-surgical nursing: Critical thinking in client care* (3rd ed.). Upper Saddle River, NJ: Pearson Education, pp. 864–866.

Comprehensive Exam

1. A client exposed to *Mycobacterium tuberculosis* starts on chemoprophylaxis. The nurse provides what instruction to the client?

   1. "You will take a single drug such as isoniazid (INH) by mouth every day for 6 to 12 months."
   2. "You will be on at least two drugs effective against the tubercle bacillus for three months."
   3. "You will be on combination therapy in order to prevent development of drug resistance."
   4. "You will need to learn to give yourself subcutaneous injections."

2. The nurse delegates an unlicensed assistive person (UAP) to assist a client with a clean urinary catherization procedure. The client had formerly been able to do the procedure but because of arthritis, he has been unable to perform the catheterization. Although the UAP has done this procedure before, which of the following must the nurse emphasize to the UAP?

   1. Let the client do most of the procedure and report the expected output.
   2. Report immediately any unusual observations, such as bleeding.
   3. Complete in proper order the steps of the procedure.
   4. Perform health teaching while performing the procedure.

3. The client is in the operating room for a surgical procedure. The nurse in the operating room is monitoring the physiological integrity of the client. Which of the following activities is most appropriate?

   1. Determine client satisfaction with care received.
   2. Assess client's emotional status.
   3. Monitor asepsis in the environment.
   4. Calculate fluid loss and its effects.

4. The clinic nurse is conducting health screenings. Which of the following client assessment findings indicates that client teaching is needed about the risk for stroke? Select all that apply.

   1. ____ Weight 205 lbs and height 5 feet 4 inches
   2. ____ Blood pressure 164/92 mmHg
   3. ____ Eats bran for breakfast daily
   4. ____ Smokes ½ pack cigarettes per day
   5. ____ Serum cholesterol level is 172 mg/dL

5. Which of the following actions would the nurse take to maintain medical asepsis when caring for a client with diabetes mellitus on the medical nursing unit who requires irrigation of a leg ulcer and insulin injections? Select all that apply.

   1. ____ Wash hands before and after client care.
   2. ____ Wear personal protective equipment during the dressing change.
   3. ____ Recap a needle after administering insulin.
   4. ____ Change the dressing for a diabetic ulcer using sterile gloves.
   5. ____ Wipe the rubber stopper on the insulin vial before withdrawing dose.

6. Laboratory test results indicate a client is in the nadir period that follows administration of a chemotherapy drug. Which drug should the nurse avoid administering to this client at this time?

   1. Acetaminophen (Tylenol)
   2. Ibuprofen (Motrin)
   3. Diphenhydramine (Benadryl)
   4. Guanefesin (Robitussin)

7. The newborn nursery has recently formed a unit policy and procedure committee. The nurse, while attending and participating in the meetings, determines that which nurse exemplifies a situational leader?

1. The nurse who offers suggestions, asks questions, and guides the group toward achieving group goals.
2. The nurse who recognizes the group's need for autonomy and abdicates responsibility.
3. The nurse who relies on the organization's rules, policies, and procedures to direct the group's work.
4. The nurse who recognizes that leadership style depends on the readiness and willingness of the group or the individuals to perform the assigned tasks.

8. The nurse places highest priority on taking which of the following actions to reduce the spread of microorganisms when caring for a client at risk for infection?

1. Wash hands before and after client care.
2. Use clean gloves when implementing client care.
3. Institute transmission-based precautions.
4. Place the client in a private room.

9. The nurse would report to the physician which of the following abnormal laboratory values for a 58-year-old client newly admitted to the nursing unit with fever and diarrhea? Select all that apply.

1. ____ White blood cell count 12,260/mm^3
2. ____ Sodium 142 mEq/L
3. ____ Potassium 3.9 mEq/L
4. ____ Blood urea nitrogen 38 mg/dL
5. ____ Serum creatinine 0.9 mg/dL

10. The mental health nurse working with children anticipates that unrealistic expectations or a sense of failure to meet standards would cause a 10-year-old child to develop a sense of which of the following?

1. Shame
2. Guilt
3. Inferiority
4. Role confusion

11. A postoperative client who has an order for 5,000 units of heparin SubQ for three doses wants to know why this drug is being ordered. What information would the nurse provide to the client to best answer the question?

1. "Heparin is used as a common medication in many clients who have surgery."
2. "Heparin is essential during the postoperative period to maintain adequate blood clotting levels."
3. "The injections will be given in the abdomen and are not usually associated with discomfort."
4. "Heparin is being used to prevent blood clots from forming as a result of surgery or decreased mobility."

12. The Emergency Department has recently experienced a significant increase in client visits. The year-to-date census reveals a 20% increase in admissions from the same period last year. In an effort to reduce staff stress and burnout by empowering the staff, the nurse manager uses which of the following approaches to demonstrate shared leadership?

1. Encourages the formation of self-directed work teams.
2. Encourages the group to try out nursing approaches that are evidence-based.
3. Suggests that staff who have demonstrated charting excellence be given opportunities for professional development activities.
4. Provides constructive criticism and facilitates the group to meet their goals.

13. A 56-year-old client reports to the nurse that his sleep patterns are different than when he was younger. The nurse anticipates that this client is likely to be experiencing which normal developmental pattern?

1. 6 to 8 hours of sleep per night with about 20 to 25% of rapid eye movement (REM) sleep and a marked decrease in Stage IV non-REM (NREM) sleep.
2. 6 to 8 hours of sleep per night with about 20% REM sleep and a decrease in Stage IV NREM sleep.
3. Erratic sleep because of work schedule with about 30% of REM sleep and no marked decrease in Stage IV NREM sleep.
4. Light sleep with equal amounts of REM sleep and NREM sleep.

14. The nurse concludes that teaching has been effective when the laboring client's partner shouts, "She's crowning!" as:

1. The nurse first starts to see a little of the baby's head.
2. The baby's head recedes upward between pushing contractions.
3. The perineum is thin and stretching around the occiput.
4. The mouth and nose are being suctioned.

15. A client questions the surgical nurse about the personnel in the operating room. Which of the following initial responses by a nurse to the client's concern is most therapeutic?

1. "The nurses are well-qualified for the job they do."
2. "Have you had a bad experience in the OR?"
3. "You're concerned about the personnel, but you have no need to worry."
4. "Can you tell me about why you are interested in the personnel?"

16. After three defibrillation attempts, the client continues to be in a pulseless ventricular tachycardia. A lidocaine bolus of 100 mg IV is administered. The nurse would expect to see which of the following as a therapeutic response to lidocaine?

1. Conversion from a ventricular tachycardia to a ventricular fibrillation
2. Slowing of heart rate to 80 beats per minute
3. Conversion to supraventricular rhythm
4. An increase in the level of consciousness

17. The nurse is assigned to a client diagnosed with head and neck cancer who is receiving enteral feedings via gastrostomy tube. When the nurse is called away to care for another client, which task for this client could most appropriately be delegated to the unlicensed assistive person (UAP)?

1. Determining the amount of residual for the tube feeding
2. Giving mouth care and assessing the oral cavity
3. Exploring how the client is currently coping with the diagnosis
4. Administering a bath and changing bed linens

18. A client with metabolic acidosis is admitted. Which of the following laboratory values would the nurse expect to find in this client?

1. pH 7.40; serum potassium 3.8 mEq/L
2. pH 7.36; serum potassium 3.1 mEq/L
3. pH 7.2; serum potassium 6.2 mEq/L
4. pH 7.0; serum potassium 5.5 mEq/L

19. A client has a BUN of 68 mg/dL and a creatinine level of 6.0 mg/dL. The IV fluid is 5% dextrose in 0.9% sodium chloride with 40 mEq KCL @ 100 mL/hour. Which action would be most appropriate for the nurse to take?

1. Encourage more protein in the diet.
2. Ambulate the client more to increase circulation.
3. Take vital signs every hour.
4. Question the use of potassium in the IV fluids.

20. The nurse concludes that a child is in Piaget's concrete operations stage after observing which of the following traits in the child?

1. Conservation
2. Egocentrism
3. Animism
4. Preconventional thought

21. A 60-year-old client has been prescribed rabeprazole (Aciphex) for symptoms of gastroesophageal reflux disease (GERD). He has trouble swallowing pills. What alternate medication should the nurse plan to request for this client?

1. Omeprazole (Prilosec)
2. Pantoprazole (Protonix)
3. Lansoprazole (Prevacid)
4. There is no substitute for Aciphex

22. At the start of the shift there were only three newborns in the nursery, so staffing consisted of one RN and one LPN. Within two hours, three more newborns were admitted to the nursery, one requiring Level II care, and the parents of two newborns needed discharge teaching so they could go home. The RN was needed full time in the Level II nursery as the newborn was stabilized. What staffing is needed to provide appropriate care in this situation?

1. The LPN can complete the admission assessments and discharge teaching for the five Level 1 newborns.
2. An UAP from the postpartum unit can be reassigned to the nursery to do the discharge teaching.
3. The RN can complete the admission assessments while continuing to stabilize the Level II newborn.
4. Another RN needs to be assigned to the nursery to implement the admission assessments and discharge teaching.

23. The nurse is working with a client suffering from chronic diarrhea. In teaching ways to reduce diarrhea, the nurse would encourage the client to avoid which of the following that contribute to the development of diarrhea?

1. Excessive intake of cheese and eggs
2. Habitually ignoring the urge to defecate
3. Anxiety or anger
4. Lack of exercise

24. The fetal head is determined to be presenting in a position of complete extension. After learning of this, the nurse anticipates which of the following?

1. Precipitous labor and delivery
2. Prolonged labor and possible cesarean delivery
3. Normal labor and spontaneous vaginal delivery
4. Forceps-assisted vaginal delivery

25. The nurse notices that an elderly nursing home resident has not been eating or drinking as much as usual. Which assessment finding would best indicate the presence of fluid volume deficit?

1. Clear lung fields with unlabored respirations
2. Tenting and dry, flaky skin
3. Increased drowsiness, mild confusion, and concentrated urine
4. Hand veins that fill within 3 to 5 seconds of being lowered below the heart

26. Following a liver transplant the client is taking prednisone among other medications to prevent organ rejection. The nurse should instruct the client to make it a priority to report which of the following signs and symptoms to the health care provider?

1. Moon face
2. Diminished pigmentation
3. Dysphagia
4. Bleeding

27. The nurse would place highest priority on which of the following nursing interventions when planning to prevent atelectasis in the newly admitted postoperative client?

1. Hourly coughing and deep breathing
2. Assisting the client out of bed
3. Administration of bronchodilators
4. Supplemental oxygen

28. A 14-year-old client has been diagnosed with bipolar disorder. The nurse would expect to see which of the following problems?

1. Intense mood swings lasting only 1 to 2 hours
2. Inflated self-esteem
3. Spending sprees
4. Fire-setting and gang behavior

29. A client's hemoglobin level is 14 grams/dL. Which interpretation of the laboratory value by the nurse is most accurate?

1. Client has a low value and is malnourished.
2. Client has a normal laboratory value and has no nutritional risk.
3. Client has a low to normal value indicative of a nutritional risk.
4. Client has an elevated value indicative of polycythemia.

30. Which of the following care measures should the nurse include in the discussion when teaching home care measures to the parents of a child who has bilateral bacterial conjunctivitis?

1. Use of warm, moist, disposable compresses to remove crusting
2. Use of oral antihistamine medication to relieve eye itching
3. Use of ophthalmic corticosteroids to decrease inflammatory response
4. Use of topical anesthetics applied to relieve discomfort

31. After a client has experienced a seizure, what is the most appropriate position in which the nurse should place the client?

1. On back with head raised 15 degrees
2. On the side
3. On abdomen
4. Upright in chair

32. After correctly positioning a client for a wound dressing change, the nurse sets up a sterile field, placing the wound supplies in the field. The nurse hears a page to respond to another client who has fallen in the hallway. Which of the following is the most appropriate nursing action for the nurse to take?

1. Ensure the client's safety, cover the field with a sterile towel, and respond to the other client.
2. Continue quickly with the procedure, and then assist the other client, checking back with the first client as soon as possible.
3. Ensure the client's safety, discard the sterile equipment, and respond to the other client.
4. Explain the situation to the client needing wound dressing change, leave the sterile supplies in place, and attend to the other client.

33. A client recently diagnosed with type 1 diabetes mellitus is learning to use the American Diabetes Association exchange lists. The nurse determines that the teaching has been effective if the client chooses which of the following as an appropriate exchange for white rice?

1. Egg
2. Tomato
3. Orange
4. Bread

34. The nurse is teaching a group of adults about health screenings for cancer. The nurse would include in the discussion which of the following points? Select all that apply.

1. _____ Genetic screening is helpful in identification of cancer risks.
2. _____ Annual medical exams uncover most tumors.
3. _____ Men need to perform breast and testicle exams monthly.
4. _____ Annual mammograms are recommended after a total mastectomy.
5. _____ Inspection of the skin for cancer becomes less important as one ages.

35. During a coffee break, the nurse notices two coworkers arguing about how to handle a difficult client. Their voices are raised and body postures are tense and defensive. Which would be the most appropriate approach for the nurse to use to address this conflict between staff members?

1. Let it pass because the coworkers probably did not intend to be critical.
2. Speak privately to the coworkers, telling them about personal reactions to this public encounter.
3. Confront and reprimand the coworkers publicly.
4. Inform each coworker privately that it would be most helpful not to display this behavior again.

36. The school nurse is assessing a muscular 17-year-old female who is coming to the high school health service for complaints of edema, voice changes, and hair loss. The nurse's *primary* analysis based on the subjective and objective data is that the student:

1. Is going through a stage of puberty.
2. May be using steroids.
3. May be abusing barbiturates.
4. Is using marijuana regularly.

37. A 4-year-old child has been exposed to chickenpox. After the nurse has provided information about chickenpox, the nurse asks the mother to repeat the information. Which statement by the mother indicates a need for additional information?

1. "During the prodomal period, my child will have pox all over his body."
2. "Chickenpox is a viral infection that can be spread to other children."
3. "I should monitor my child for Reye syndrome, which is a complication of chickenpox."
4. "My child should not visit my pregnant sister at this time."

38. The school health nurse is interested in promoting safety in the high school population. In planning safety education for this age group and their parents, the nurse would recognize that which of the following is the greatest developmental risk factor for adolescents?

1. Substance abuse as a lifestyle means of dealing with stress
2. Feelings of immortality related to perception of being invulnerable to risks that affect others
3. Sports-related injuries that are usually related to not obeying rules and/or intense competition
4. Polypharmacy, which results in mixing of multiple medications

39. When giving directions to a 24-year-old female with abdominal pain who is about to undergo a pelvic sonogram, which statement should the nurse make to the client?

1. "Drink nothing for several hours prior to the exam."
2. "You will be given an enema to cleanse the bowel."
3. "Drink plenty of liquids so you will have a full bladder."
4. "Do not take any medications prior to the exam."

40. The nurse is conducting an initial interview with a 10-year-old boy who has been brought to the mental health clinic by his parents. The nurse can establish rapport and credibility with the child by asking the child about his:

1. Behavioral symptoms.
2. Interests and hobbies.
3. Relationships with friends and family members.
4. Medical problems in the past.

41. The nurse is providing medication instructions to a client. The nurse informs the client that persistent gynecomastia can result from taking which of the following newly prescribed diuretics?

1. Hydrochlorothiazide (HCTZ)
2. Furosemide (Lasix)
3. Spironolactone (Aldactone)
4. Indapamide (Lozol)

42. As the nursing unit representative member serving on the hospital quality management committee, the nurse has been asked to evaluate the quality of nursing services on the unit. What would be an appropriate quality improvement activity for the nurse to ask team members to participate in?

1. Track the number of accidents or incidents on the unit.
2. Document nursing time and activities spent on direct client care.
3. Administer a client and family satisfaction survey.
4. Assess clients and report acuity to shift managers daily.

43. When a female client preparing for surgery suddenly bursts into tears, the preoperative holding unit nurse should take which of the following actions?

1. Pull the curtain closed and leave the area to provide privacy.
2. Be silent as a sign of compassion.
3. Ask the client to share what she is feeling.
4. Continue with the physical preparation of the client.

44. After reviewing the client's health history, the nurse concludes that which of the following is the most significant factor related to the development of bronchogenic carcinoma for this client?

1. Asthma
2. Smokeless tobacco
3. Cigarette smoking
4. Air pollution

45. The nurse is setting up the breakfast tray for a client with gastroesophageal reflux disease (GERD) and notices one food that the client should not eat. Which food should the nurse remove from the meal tray?

1. Poached egg
2. Dry toast
3. Coffee with cream
4. Skim milk

46. The nurse is assessing a 30-year-old client with a prior history of smoking who takes theophylline (Theo-Dur) for chronic obstructive pulmonary disease. Additional diagnoses include liver disease and congestive heart failure. The client is experiencing tremors, dizziness, tachycardia, and nausea. The nurse explains to the client that these symptoms may be the result of:

1. A history of smoking cigarettes.
2. Liver disease.
3. The client's age.
4. The client's weight.

47. The nurse has admitted to the surgical unit a client who just underwent open reduction and internal fixation of a severely fractured right radius and ulna. Which nursing care activities would be appropriate for the nurse to delegate to the Licensed Practical/Vocational Nurse (LPN/LVN)? Select all that apply.

1. _____ Measure vital signs every 30 minutes.
2. _____ Report drainage on the cast if it appears.
3. _____ Assess neurovascular status of the fingers of the casted arm hourly.
4. _____ Elevate the casted arm above heart level.
5. _____ Administer the prescribed intramuscular analgesic as ordered.

48. Which of the following actions would the nurse institute that is specific to the care of the assigned client who has tuberculosis?

1. Wearing a particulate respirator mask when taking vital signs.
2. Instructing the client to cover the mouth with the sheet from the stretcher when transported to other hospital departments.
3. Wearing sterile gloves when collecting a sputum specimen.
4. Keeping the client's door open to promote ventilation.

49. A client has a potassium level of 6.8 mEq/L. Which sign or symptom would the nurse expect to find when assessing this client?

1. Peaking of T wave on the telemetry monitor
2. The absence of bowel sounds, such as in an ileus
3. Muscle cramping of the lower extremities
4. Somnolence with early changes

50. The nurse is preparing to take a client to the electroconvulsive therapy (ECT) treatment suite. The nurse must ensure that which of the following pretreatment processes has been completed?

1. The client's husband has signed the consent form.
2. The client is wearing snug-fitting clothing.
3. The client is NPO.
4. The client has been given ample liquids before the procedure.

51. To minimize the pain related to intramuscular injection of 2 mL of penicillin G benzathine (Bicillin LA) in an adult client, the nurse would take which of the following actions?

1. Apply cold compress to site after injection.
2. Divide the dose and inject half into each deltoid.
3. Limit prolonging the time taken to administer the drug by not aspirating.
4. Administer the drug deep IM slowly into a large muscle such as the gluteus.

52. The nurse is assigned to the care of an obese client who has gastroesophageal reflux disease (GERD). Which of the following activities could the nurse appropriately delegate to the unlicensed assistant person (UAP)?

1. Teach the client about the need for weight loss.
2. Explore any concerns about the prescribed regimen for managing GERD.
3. Explain why it is important to eat several small meals per day.
4. Instruct the client to remain upright for at least 2 hours after eating.

53. The nurse is admitting a client with thermal burns to both arms and anterior trunk. The client asks for a drink of water. What is the most appropriate response for the nurse to make?

1. "I'm sorry, you cannot drink anything right now; let me moisten your mouth instead."
2. "I can only give you juice to drink, not water."
3. "I'll get you a drink as soon as I'm finished."
4. "Would you also like me to order you a meal tray?"

54. A mother brings a 3-year-old child to the clinic for a well-child checkup. The child has not been to the clinic since 6 months of age. The nurse determines that which of the following is the priority of care for this child?

1. Assess growth and development.
2. Begin dental care.
3. Complete hearing screening.
4. Update vaccinations.

55. A client who has pancreatitis is experiencing pain. After administering an analgesic, the nurse should place the client in which of the following positions to promote comfort?

1. Supine
2. Prone
3. Left lateral decubitus
4. Sitting up and leaning forward

56. The nurse would be most careful to assess for stomatitis in a client receiving which of the following chemotherapeutic agents?

1. Fluorouracil (5-FU)
2. Cisplatin (Platinol)
3. Bleomycin (Blenoxane)
4. Vincristine (Oncovin)

57. The nurse will be working with an unlicensed assistive person (UAP) for the work shift. Prior to delegating care to the UAP, the nurse places high priority on which of the following?

1. Determining that the UAP is competent to perform the required task
2. Providing written directions to the UAP
3. Making sure all the necessary supplies are available at the client's bedside
4. Informing clients that an unlicensed staff member will be assigned to them

58. The nurse believes a client has slight one-sided weakness and further tests the client's muscle strength. The nurse asks the client to hold the arms up with hands supinated, as if holding a tray, and then asks the client to close the eyes. The client's right hand moves downward slightly and turns. The nurse documents and reports that the client has which of the following findings on assessment?

1. Pronator drift
2. Nystagmus
3. Hyperreflexia
4. Ataxia

59. When a client has arterial blood gases drawn from the radial artery, the nurse should plan to do which of the following?

1. Hold the site for up to 1 minute.
2. Transfer the blood sample to a heparinized test tube.
3. Pack the sample in ice for transporting to the laboratory.
4. Obtain a second specimen after 10 minutes for comparison.

60. The nurse knows that a client in the long–term care unit suffers from dysthymia. The *most* important nursing intervention to include in the nursing care plan is:

1. Provide at least 2 hours of quiet time every morning for the client.
2. Encourage the client to eat in the main dining room with other clients.
3. Include at least three regular meals per day and no snacks.
4. Include at least 2 liters of clear liquids per day in the diet regime.

61. A client who is receiving intravenous heparin by protocol orders has an activated partial thromboplastin time (aPTT) level of 140 seconds (control time is 36 seconds). What is the priority action that the nurse should institute?

1. Increase the heparin dose as the aPTT level is not therapeutic. Obtain a repeat aPTT in 6 hours.
2. Stop the heparin therapy for 6 hours, then restart the therapy at the same unit dose and obtain a repeat aPTT in 6 hours.
3. Stop the heparin therapy for 1 hour. Decrease the rate of infusion per protocol and restart the medication in 1 hour. Obtain a repeat aPTT in 2 to 3 hours from the restart of the infusion.
4. Obtain an additional aPTT in 1 hour and continue to monitor the client.

62. The nurse has admitted to the intermediate care unit a client who sustained a spinal cord injury at T1 in a motor vehicle accident. Which of the following nursing care activities can the nurse delegate to the unlicensed assistive person (UAP) when working with this client? Select all that apply.

1. _____ Measure oxygen saturation level every hour.
2. _____ Listen to breath sounds.
3. _____ Provide mouth care.
4. _____ Teach use of incentive spirometer.
5. _____ Assess for Homan's sign while bathing client.

63. The nurse has been instructed to have a surgical consent form signed by a client who will be undergoing a surgical procedure. What is the most essential information to include in the discussion prior to the client signing the permission?

1. The client's diagnosis
2. Treatment proposed and the cost
3. The technical aspects of the procedure
4. Right to withdraw consent

64. The pregnant client is 7 centimeters dilated, 100% effaced, and at a +1 station. The fetus is in a face presentation. The nurse concludes that teaching has been effective when the client's husband states:

1. "Our baby will come out face first."
2. "Our baby will come out facing one hip."
3. "Our baby will come out buttocks first."
4. "Our baby will come out with the back of the head first."

65. A client is scheduled to have a transverse colostomy performed. While doing client teaching, the nurse points to which stoma on the diagram to show the client the location of the stoma? Select the correct stoma.

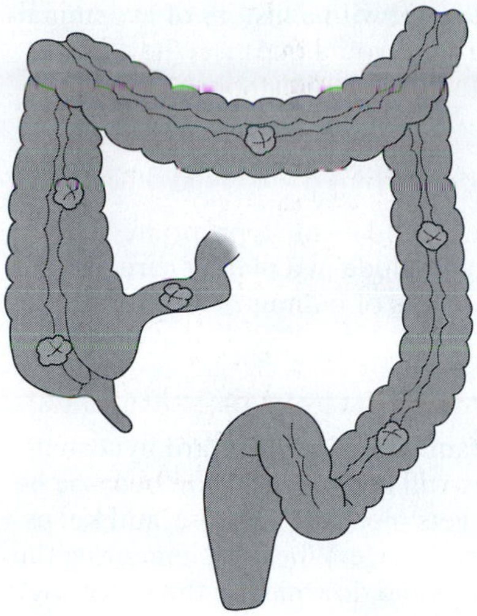

66. A child diagnosed with deficiency of growth hormone who needs replacement drug therapy comes to the clinic for treatment. Which one of the following nursing diagnoses would be most appropriate for this client?

1. Imbalanced nutrition: More than body requirements
2. Disturbed body image
3. Diversional activity deficit
4. Decreased cardiac output

67. The nursing unit is understaffed and a nurse from the surgical intermediate care unit has been floated to the unit for the day shift. Which of the following two clients should the nurse assign to this RN float nurse?

1. _____ A client newly admitted with exacerbation of heart failure
2. _____ A client newly diagnosed with type 2 diabetes mellitus
3. _____ A client who underwent emergency appendectomy during the night
4. _____ A client with nephrolithiasis scheduled for lithotripsy later in the morning
5. _____ A client admitted with thyrotoxicosis

68. The nurse would conclude that hypomagnesemia has not resolved if which of the following neuromuscular signs is still present after treatment?

1. Paralysis
2. Tetany
3. Flaccidity
4. Decreased reflexes

69. A client presents to the Emergency Department with a complaint of chest pain. Which serum laboratory test does the nurse check off on the laboratory slip as part of a protocol order to rule out an acute myocardial infarction?

1. LDH^4
2. Troponin
3. Amylase
4. CK-MM

70. The nurse is planning for a multidisciplinary team meeting concerning a client with bipolar disorder. In discussing the client's safety needs, the nurse would be sure to include:

1. Placement of the client in a four-bed room.
2. The client's risk level for self-harm.
3. Unrestricted visitors.
4. The need of the client to participate daily in many concentrated activities.

71. A nurse is teaching a female client newly diagnosed with *Helicobacter pylori* infection. The nurse anticipates that which of the following medications will not be used after learning the client is pregnant?

1. Metronizadole (Flagyl)
2. Amoxicillin (Amoxil)
3. Clarithromycin (Biaxin)
4. Ciprofloxacin (Cipro)

72. The nurse admitting a client with a history of trigeminal neuralgia (tic Douloureux) would question the client about which of the following manifestations?

1. Facial droop accompanied by numbness and tingling
2. Stabbing pain that occurs with twitching of part of the face
3. Aching pain and ptosis of the eyelid
4. Burning pain and intermittent facial paralysis

73. Which of the following would be an appropriate intervention for the nurse to include in a plan of care for a client with clinical diagnosis of bulimia?

1. Assess for laxative and diuretic possession.
2. Supervise mealtimes to ensure eating.
3. Observe for ritualistic eating patterns.
4. Reward nonpurging behavior with a favorite snack.

74. A client has a strong family tendency toward hypertension. He denies that he will get hypertension because he watches what he eats, gets plenty of exercise, and keeps his weight within normal range. When implementing the plan of care, the nurse would do which of the following?

1. Praise the client and reassure him that these actions will prevent him from becoming hypertensive.
2. Emphasize that no matter what he does, the client will eventually develop hypertension because of his family history.
3. Recognize the client's efforts towards a healthy lifestyle and emphasis that early detection is essential to prevent complications.
4. Recommend that the client request antihypertensive medications prophylactically because of his family history.

75. A parent asks the nurse what to do with rough edges of her child's cast, which are beginning to cause excoriation on the child's skin. Which of the following responses by the nurse describes the appropriate action to take?

1. "Perform good skin care to the skin around the cast edges, with a protective barrier like Vaseline."
2. "Call the physician to have the rough edges of the cast cut away."
3. "Tape a soft towel to the edge of the cast to provide some protection from the rough edges."
4. "Petal the cast edges with strips of adhesive tape, placing the tape from just inside the cast over the edge to outside the cast."

76. A 3-month-old infant is diagnosed with leukemia. Which of the following does the nurse anticipate will be part of the plan of care for this infant?

1. The baby will be placed in isolation.
2. Leukemia is familial and other children should be assessed.
3. All immunizations will be withheld during exacerbations.
4. The baby will be NPO during chemotherapy.

77. The registered nurse (RN) is assigned to the postpartum unit. Which task could the RN safely delegate to a beginning student nurse?

1. Ambulate a client who delivered by cesarean 2 days ago.
2. Complete the admission assessment on a newly delivered client.
3. Call the physician to report a low hemoglobin level.
4. Verify a unit of blood prior to transfusion.

78. A client presents to the Emergency Department with a stab wound to the right upper abdominal quadrant. The client's vital signs are BP 85/60, pulse 125, and respiratory rate of 28 breaths/minute. The nurse should immediately suspect damage to what organ?

1. Stomach
2. Liver
3. Large intestine
4. Kidney

79. The client is scheduled for a barium enema and is expressing concern that the barium will not be evacuated and a bowel obstruction will occur. What would be the best response for the nurse to make to the client?

1. "Don't worry. The physicians will make sure that all of the barium is out of your bowel before you return to the unit."
2. "You will be given extra fluids, laxatives, and an enema if you have not expelled the barium within 24 hours."
3. "The barium they are using will not cause an obstruction."
4. "Should I have the test rescheduled for when you are less concerned about it?"

80. The nurse is conducting an educational group on an inpatient unit. One of the clients has not spoken during the group. An effective therapeutic response by the nurse would include:

1. Allowing the client to remain present but nonparticipative.
2. Explaining to the client that everyone in the group needs to participate.
3. Asking the rest of the group members how they feel about this member not sharing.
4. Stopping the group and asking the client to leave.

81. A client is experiencing seizure activity. The nurse should prepare to administer which of the following medications according to protocol?

1. Selegilene (Eldepryl)
2. Diclofenac sodium (Voltaren)
3. Phenytoin (Dilantin)
4. Sumatriptan (Imitrex)

82. As part of the ongoing assessment of a client who has an electrical burn, a complete blood count (CBC), electrolyte panel, and renal panel were ordered. The nurse would expect to find which of the following results?

1. Potassium level of 5.9 mEq/L
2. Potassium level of 2.8 mEq/L
3. Hematocrit of 28 mg/dL
4. White blood cell count of 4,000/mm^3

83. A client with congestive heart failure (CHF) has been advised to follow a low-sodium diet. Which statement by the client indicates to the nurse that diet teaching has been effective?

1. "If I stop adding table salt, I shouldn't have any problems."
2. "I need to avoid eating processed foods and canned meats and vegetables."
3. "I can still use a small amount of table salt in cooking."
4. "I only have to worry about salty-tasting foods like potato chips."

84. After delivery, a Chinese client states she needs to restore the balance between hot and cold forces in her body and refuses to bathe. The most appropriate nursing intervention is to:

1. Show her a videotape on postpartum self-care.
2. Recognize her cultural beliefs and respect her wishes.
3. Discuss postpartum complications related to poor personal hygiene.
4. Request a psychiatric consult for this client.

85. While talking with a client the nurse notes that the client rapidly becomes more uncomfortable and anxious. What action should the nurse take?

1. Ask specific, focused questions to elicit detailed information about the source of the client's stress.
2. Encourage the client to try to relax by using guided imagery or other means preferred by the client.
3. Refocus the conversation on a less threatening topic.
4. Stop the interview at this time.

86. The nurse is preparing a client for discharge who will be taking lithium carbonate. Which of the following statements indicates that the client is feeling comfortable with being discharged on an antimanic medication?

1. "I don't want to take the medicine you will give me, but you said I have to."
2. "I know that if I take my lithium every day I won't have to come to the hospital again."
3. "I have a hard time taking this medicine and I don't like the shaking, but I will take it every day with meals, and have my blood tests done, and come back to the clinic next month for my check-up like you said."
4. "Even though I don't like taking medicine, I will take lithium daily with meals and have my blood tests on the dates I marked on my calendar. I should be able to do my normal things every day, and in a few weeks I won't feel shaky anymore."

87. A client has just finished a dose of intravesicular chemotherapy as treatment for bladder cancer. When giving instructions to the unlicensed assistive personnel (UAP) who will give routine care to this client, what statement should the nurse make?

1. "Be sure the client flushes the toilet after each use."
2. " Cleanse the toilet with bleach after each use for the next 6 hours."
3. "Ask the client to wipe the toilet seat with tissue after each bathroom use."
4. "Assist the client to the bathroom and wear sterile gloves for pericare."

88. The nurse is caring for a young child who has mitt restraints. Which of the following priority actions needs to be done regularly to ensure that the child's needs are met?

1. Check adequacy of circulation and skin condition.
2. Check that the tongue blades in pockets are intact and ends are covered or padded.
3. Ensure that the straps are tied to nonmovable parts of the crib.
4. Check that the call bell is pinned to the child's gown.

89. The client is to undergo an extensive process of allergy testing as an outpatient. The nurse would complete which of the following as a priority intervention during the initial testing?

1. Have emergency equipment available in the event of an anaphylactic reaction.
2. Instruct the client to wear a t-shirt to assure easy access to the skin testing sites.
3. Give discharge instructions prior to testing since the client will be able to go home immediately after the testing.
4. Set up the room before the client enters the examination area.

90. A client who has been experiencing panic attacks asks why the physician has ordered several laboratory tests. The nurse's answer should incorporate which of the following pieces of information?

1. Laboratory tests can differentiate between true anxiety and the anxiety associated with depression.
2. Laboratory tests can determine the specific cause of the panic attacks.
3. Physiologic symptoms associated with panic disorders often mimic medical disorders.
4. Symptoms of panic disorders are usually related to hypochondriasis.

91. A female client has been taking norethindrone (Micronor) oral contraceptive pills. Which of the following items is most likely to be found in her health history?

1. Superficial phlebitis
2. Currently breastfeeding
3. Dysmenorrhea
4. Menarche at age 18

92. The nurse in the emergency department is caring for a client who has fallen 20 feet from a roof. While performing the primary assessment, the most important nursing intervention will be which of the following?

1. Maintain cervical spine precautions.
2. Assess for facial lacerations.
3. Remove clothing.
4. Perform a mental status exam.

93. Which breakfast option indicates to the nurse that the client with coronary artery disease requires further diet instruction?

1. Orange juice, shredded wheat, skim milk, toast with jelly
2. Grapefruit juice, oatmeal, 1% milk, bagel with jelly
3. Canned peaches, egg omelet, whole milk, fruited yogurt
4. Applesauce, bagel with margarine, egg-white omelet, skim milk

94. The nurse would encourage the new mother to use which breast-feeding position to enable the mother to have optimal control of the newborn's head while giving the mother a full view of the infant's cheeks and jaw?

1. Lying-down position
2. Cradle position
3. Clutch (football) position
4. Across-the-lap position

95. The nurse observes a sinus rhythm pattern on the cardiac monitor of a client admitted with diarrhea and vomiting. On physical assessment, the nurse is unable to palpate a central pulse. The nurse would suspect that the client is demonstrating which of the following?

1. Pulseless electrical activity (PEA)
2. Ventricular fibrillation
3. Asystole
4. Ventricular tachycardia

96. While teaching a client about the proper administration of dipivefrine (Propine), the nurse would provide which of the following instructions?

1. Gently squeeze eyes closed for 30 seconds immediately after instillation of medication.
2. Close, but do not squeeze, eyes immediately after instillation of medication.
3. Do not blink for 30 seconds after instillation of medication.
4. Close the eyes for 1 full minute after instillation of medication.

97. The nursing unit is short-staffed for the shift and a registered nurse (RN) from the pediatric unit has been floated to the nursing unit. Which of the following clients should the nurse assign to the float nurse?

1. A 32-year-old client newly diagnosed with diabetes who needs dietary and medication teaching
2. A 56-year-old client newly admitted with Guillain-Barre syndrome who has severe leg weakness
3. An 86-year-old client with dementia who will be transferred to a skilled nursing facility during the shift
4. A 59-year-old client who will be returning from surgery following transurethral resection of the prostate

98. A client has experienced a near-drowning event in salt water. The nurse anticipates that one of the complications this client may experience is:

1. Heart block.
2. Renal failure.
3. Pulmonary edema.
4. Respiratory alkalosis.

99. The nurse has just read the results of a client's tuberculin (TB) test at a health fair. An induration is apparent. The client asks what this means. The nurse's best response would be:

1. "A positive test means that you have been exposed to the TB organism. It does not mean that you currently have active bacteria. Further testing will be needed."
2. "A positive TB test means that you currently have active TB, and you will need to be isolated immediately."
3. " Many false positives occur. You can expect to be retested in 6 months."
4. "A positive TB test means that you are currently infectious and will need to be started on medication immediately."

100. An anxious client begins to yell and interrupt other clients. The client's speech is rapid and pressured. What action should the nurse take?

1. Ask the client to speak more slowly and softly.
2. Instruct the other clients to ignore this client's behavior.
3. Point out to the client that the behavior is a sign of anxiety.
4. Remind the client of the need to use good manners when talking with other people.

101. The nurse suspects that hepatotoxicity is developing in a dark-skinned client who is on an antibiotic. In what area of the body should the nurse assess for jaundice?

1. Palms of the hands or soles of the feet
2. Hard palate of oral cavity
3. Sclera
4. Conjunctivae

102. The nurse on the oncology unit has received intershift reports on 4 clients. In what order should the nurse assess these clients? Place in numerical order of priority.

1. A client receiving radiation therapy who has a white blood cell (WBC) count of $4{,}500/mm^3$
2. A client receiving chemotherapy who has a platelet count of $50{,}000/mm^3$
3. A client who is crying because she has newly learned that her cancer has metastasized
4. A client who has questions about upcoming chemotherapy

103. Which nutritional measure would help a client with gastroesophageal reflux disease (GERD) to minimize the risk of symptoms?

1. Eating 3 large meals a day with no snacks
2. Using a lot of garlic to season food rather than salt
3. Limiting intake of coffee drinks to 2 or fewer cups a day
4. Using peppermint candies to take away the bitter taste in the mouth

104. A client who is 20 weeks gestation is concerned about how to tell her 3-year-old son about her pregnancy. Which of the following would be the best statement when counseling this client?

1. "If he is not pleased with the news of a new baby, you should tell him that you are disappointed in him."
2. "Tell him that he is going to have a lot of responsibilities in helping care for the baby."
3. "Try to provide extra attention to him and include him in plans for the baby."
4. "Tell him that he will have to stay with his grandparents when the baby is born because you will be busy with the baby."

105. A nurse is caring for a client with pneumonia. ABG results are pH 7.49, $PaCO_2$ 32 mmHg, HCO_3^- 28 mEq/L, PaO_2 89 mmHg. This nurse analyzes these results as:

1. Metabolic acidosis, uncompensated
2. Metabolic alkalosis, uncompensated
3. Mixed respiratory and metabolic alkalosis
4. Respiratory acidosis, uncompensated

106. A client experiences severe nausea for up to 2 weeks following her chemotherapy treatment. Which statement indicates a need for further instruction on management of nausea?

1. "I need to call my doctor if I lose more than 10 percent of my body weight."
2. "I should try to eat bland chilled foods, and drink liquids separate from my meals."
3. "I need to lie down for an hour after each meal."
4. "I should call the doctor if my nausea doesn't go away, to see if a different anti-emetic could provide better relief."

107. While assessing the chest tube drainage system of a client, the nurse observes a slight rise and fall in the water level in the water seal. The nurse should take which of the following actions?

1. Notify the physician immediately.
2. Have the client cough.
3. Continue to monitor the system.
4. Reposition the chest tube.

108. During which of the following procedures should the labor and delivery nurse wear protective goggles in addition to gloves?

1. Changing a soaked disposable bed pad
2. Assisting during an amniotomy
3. Starting an intravenous line
4. Washing dirty instruments

109. A client with cancer has a calcium level of 11.8 mg/dL. Which of the following symptoms would indicate a need for the nurse to call the physician for treatment orders?

1. Increased gastric motility
2. Peaked T waves on 12-lead ECG
3. Muscle spasms
4. Muscle weakness

110. When evaluating the effectiveness of nursing care plans used for an anxious client, it is important to validate that the client understands that:

1. Defense mechanisms should not be used.
2. Some anxiety can be helpful.
3. He should strive to never experience anxiety.
4. He should try to avoid the fight or flight response.

111. In assessing a hospitalized client 1 hour after receiving hydralazine (Apresoline) 20 mg PO, the nurse notes that the BP is 68/42. The client has been taking this medication for several years at home without difficulty. Which of the following factors most likely contributed to this episode of hypotension?

1. Dose is excessive for this medication.
2. Total intake for the previous 24 hours is 1,000 mL.
3. Serum potassium is 5.8 mEq/L.
4. Heart rate is 145 beats per minute.

112. A client with a history of heart failure suddenly exhibits shortness of breath, a respiratory rate of 30, crackles auscultated bilaterally, and frothy sputum. After telephoning the physician for medical orders, which action should the nurse delegate to the Licensed Practical/Vocational Nurse (LPN/LVN)?

1. Start an intravenous line and cap it with a saline lock.
2. Monitor vital signs every 15 minutes.
3. Administer morphine sulfate 2 mg IV push immediately.
4. Insert a urinary catheter.

113. An 86-year-old client will be undergoing a surgical procedure. Which of the following changes would the nurse make in the informed consent process for this elderly client?

1. Providing adequate time for the client to process the information
2. Encouraging the family members to make the decision for the client
3. Encouraging the client to sign immediately before the client forgets the purpose of the surgery
4. Providing the client with reading material about the surgery and the postoperative instructions

114. The labor and delivery nurse would make it a priority to assess which of the following two newborn body systems immediately after birth?

1. Gastrointestinal and hepatic
2. Urinary and hematologic
3. Neurologic and temperature control
4. Respiratory and cardiovascular

115. The nurse is caring for the client who is recovering from partial thickness burns. Which of the following breakfast options indicates client understanding of the recommended diet?

1. Two slices of toast with butter, orange juice, skim milk
2. Two poached eggs, hash brown potatoes, whole milk
3. Three pancakes with syrup, two slices of bacon, apple juice
4. One cup of oatmeal with skim milk, 1/2 grapefruit, coffee

116. An adult client with diabetes insipidus who has been taking desmopressin (DDAVP) intranasally comes to the clinic for a regularly scheduled appointment. The nurse assesses the client's mental status and notes some disorientation and behavioral changes. Significant pedal edema is also present. What should be the nurse's next action?

1. Check vital signs and notify the physician.
2. Have the client return in the morning for reevaluation.
3. Instruct the client to limit salt intake for a few days.
4. Suggest that the client change the route of administration to subcutaneous injections.

117. The nurse is assigned to the care of a client receiving radiation therapy for cancer. Which of the following activities needed in the care of a client receiving external beam radiation therapy could be safely delegated to an unlicensed assistive person (UAP) working on the nursing unit? Select all that apply.

1. _____ Observe the skin site following a treatment session.
2. _____ Document intake from the meal trays.
3. _____ Assess variations in level of fatigue during the shift.
4. _____ Explore how the client is coping with treatment.
5. _____ Assist the client to ambulate in the hall.

118. A 76-year-old woman visits the ambulatory clinic with reports of having difficulty reading and doing needlework because of visual distortions with blurring of images directly in the line of vision. The peripheral vision assessment by the nurse yields normal findings. The nurse suspects that this client is experiencing which of the following visual problems?

1. Glaucoma
2. Detached retina
3. Cataracts
4. Macular degeneration

119. A female client states that she will not undergo any invasive testing for her "stomach pain." The nurse explains that which of the following tests could be completed to assess the abdomen and still meet the client's wishes?

1. Abdominal ultrasound
2. Barium swallow
3. Colonoscopy
4. CT scan with contrast

120. Certain that her stomach pain is a symptom of cancer, a female client with somatization disorder exhibits pressured, rapid speech; elevated pulse and blood pressure; palpitations; and preoccupation with her pain, despite negative results from a gastroscopy. The nurse formulates which of the following as the priority nursing diagnosis?

1. Pain
2. Anxiety
3. Hopelessness
4. Disturbed body image

121. A client is taking an over-the-counter preparation containing bismuth subsalicylate (Pepto-Bismol) for diarrhea. Which of the following side effects would a nurse monitor for that is unique to the bismuth portion of this drug?

1. Darkening of the tongue
2. Dyspepsia
3. Abdominal pain
4. Diarrhea

122. The nurse is taking a nursing history from the mother of a child being admitted with flare-up of celiac disease. What piece of information would the nurse expect the mother to report?

1. Steatorrhea
2. Increased appetite
3. Vomiting
4. Soft, formed stools

123. A nurse is discussing the home maintenance regimen with a client who has irritable bowel syndrome. Which of the following statements indicates client understanding?

1. "I'll take a walk after dinner each evening."
2. "I'll have a cigarette after meals to relax."
3. "I'll chew gum between meals to curb my appetite."
4. "I'll eat a lot of fresh vegetables and fruits."

124. A primigravida client of 16 weeks gestation states that she has not yet felt fetal movement. The nurse's best response is:

1. "Your fetus will move any day now. Call me in a week if you don't feel it."
2. "Your fetus will begin moving at about 20 weeks gestation."
3. "You should have been feeling the movement already."
4. "Your fetus has been moving for the past 9 weeks without you feeling it. You will feel it within a month."

125. The mother of an infant who underwent surgery to repair hypospadias asks the nurse why the infant is diapered as shown. The nurse would respond that this method of diapering will help to:

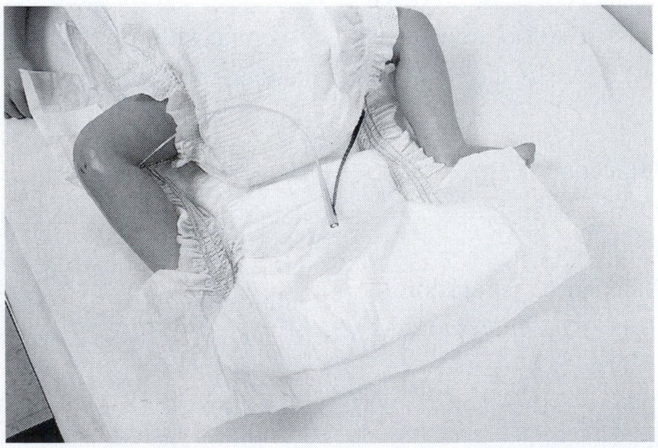

1. Protect the urinary stent that has been put in place.
2. Adequately measure the urinary output.
3. Provide for maximum absorption of urine.
4. Provide optimal protection of perineal skin from infected urine.

126. Following the administration of a diphtheria/pertussis/tetanus (DPT) immunization the nurse notes that the infant has inspiratory stridor. The nurse should take which of the following actions?

1. Administer epinephrine as per protocol orders.
2. Evaluate for pulmonary edema.
3. Inspect for periorbital edema.
4. Assess the baby again in 15 minutes.

127. The nurse is talking with the unlicensed assistive person (UAP) about time management skills and techniques. Which of the following statements would the nurse make if intending to act as a coach?

1. "You must get the vital signs taken on time or you will be disciplined."
2. "You never report morning blood glucose levels on time."
3. "Your timely response to clients' call lights is exemplary."
4. "It may be helpful if you bring in linens to the client rooms when you restock the gloves."

128. A nurse is explaining to a woman considering pregnancy how rubella is transmitted. The nurse determines that the teaching session had the desired outcome if the client states that rubella is transmitted by:

1. The airborne route.
2. Contaminated food.
3. The droplet route.
4. Direct contact.

129. A female client has been successfully resuscitated after cardiac arrest. Her arterial blood gas reveals a pH of 7.6. The nurse attributes this result to which of the following?

1. Anaerobic metabolism, which caused lactic acid production
2. Excess sodium bicarbonate, which was administered during the resuscitation
3. Repeat blood gases, which are performed during a code, frequently show acidosis
4. Normal blood gas results

130. The nurse would anticipate finding which of the following client characteristics when working with a client who has a pain disorder?

1. A preference to handle pain without medication
2. A lack of understanding of the relationship between pain and stress
3. Adequate role performance
4. Structural damage at the site of pain

131. Which of the following should be the highest priority of the education plan for a client being treated with medication therapy for a generalized seizure disorder?

1. Take medication even if there is no seizure activity.
2. Physical dependency may result from extended use of medications.
3. Urine may turn pink to brown but is not harmful.
4. Therapeutic effects of medications may not be seen for 2 to 3 weeks.

132. The pediatric nurse needs to rearrange room assignments of clients to accommodate three additional clients who will be admitted during the day. Which two of the following clients would be best for the nurse to place together in the same room? Provide a numerical response.

1. An 8-year-old who has encephalitis
2. A 10-year old who has a white blood cell count of $2{,}800/mm^3$
3. A 12-year-old who had an appendectomy
4. An 11-year-old with scarlet fever
5. A 9-year-old receiving chemotherapy for cancer

133. A 32-year-old female client who is HIV-positive is receiving treatment at an outpatient clinic. The nurse reviewing the dietary assessment record notes that the client has been skipping meals and progressively losing weight. What dietary interventions would be best for the nurse to suggest to promote weight gain?

1. Have the client keep a food diary and submit it at the next visit so that more information can be obtained regarding food preferences and usual dietary pattern.
2. Tell the client that her weight may fluctuate in response to her menstrual cycle so there is no need to worry for now.
3. Tell the client that additional salt in the diet will help to increase weight.
4. Tell the client that the use of nutrient-dense food and fortified protein shakes will help promote weight gain.

134. The nurse would assess a 76-year-old client for which common problem that most increases the risk for major complications of heart and lung disease?

1. Taking over-the-counter meds with prescription meds
2. Sharing medications with family and friends
3. Following directions exactly and taking medications on a regular basis
4. Polypharmacy resulting from visits to multiple doctors

135. A client with acute respiratory distress syndrome (ARDS) shows no improvement despite increases in the concentration of oxygen administered. What intervention should the nurse attempt which may improve ventilation-perfusion matching?

1. Transfusion of packed red blood cells
2. Infusion of albumin
3. Positioning supine with head elevated 30 to 45 degrees
4. Prone positioning

136. The nurse is giving general information about antihypertensive medications to a young female client with a history of hypertension. The nurse includes that which of the following types of antihypertensives should not be used if the client becomes pregnant?

1. Vasodilators
2. Diuretics
3. Angiotensin converting enzyme (ACE) inhibitors
4. Calcium channel blockers

137. A nurse from the pediatric intensive care unit has floated to the cardiovascular intermediate care unit for the shift. Which of the following clients would the nurse assign to the float nurse for the shift?

1. A client who experienced myocardial infarction 36 hours ago
2. A client in heart failure receiving digoxin (Lanoxin) and bumetanide (Bumex)
3. A client who just underwent coronary atherectomy
4. A client scheduled for cardiac stent placement later in the day

138. A client is admitted to the pre-surgical area before undergoing surgery to repair a detached retina. The admitting nurse would take which of the following actions first?

1. Position the client properly.
2. Darken the bedside area of the client.
3. Administer the prescribed preoperative analgesic.
4. Cover the affected eye.

139. A client has been admitted to the nursing unit with a three-day history of severe nausea and vomiting with diarrhea. The client is experiencing fatigue, anorexia, and muscle weakness. Based on this history, which laboratory findings should the nurse expect to find?

1. Calcium 11.6 mg/dL
2. Sodium 144 mEq/L
3. Potassium 2.9 mEq/L
4. Calcium 7.4 mEq/L

140. The nurse would select which of the following as a priority nursing diagnosis for a client who has many physical complaints that are not supported by diagnostic test evidence?

1. Ineffective individual coping
2. Impaired adjustment
3. Impaired verbal communication
4. Pain

141. A client presents to the Emergency Department with inspiratory and expiratory wheezes and intercostal retractions. A diagnosis of acute bronchospasm secondary to acute bronchitis is made. Epinephrine (Bronkaid) is ordered to be given subcutaneously. The nurse would anticipate seeing the intended effect of the medication in:

1. 1 minute.
2. 5 minutes.
3. 10 minutes.
4. 15 minutes.

142. During a scheduled exam the client's glycosylated hemoglobin was found to be 9%. The client has had diabetes mellitus for 3 years. The nurse should do which of the following?

1. Explore the client's general dietary pattern for the past 4 months.
2. Assess for signs of infection and client's intake for the past 24 hours.
3. Review the client's understanding of diabetic foot care.
4. Immediately give sliding scale insulin medication.

143. A client is admitted to the hospital with a primary diagnosis of hip fracture and a secondary diagnosis of Sjögren's syndrome. Which one of the following orders would be of most concern with regard to the nutritional status of the client?

1. NPO after midnight for surgery with a 7:30 a.m. case
2. IV of lactated Ringer's at 125 mL/hr
3. Maintain diet as tolerated
4. Restrict oral fluids to 1,000 mL/day

144. The nurse notes on the antepartal history that the client has an android pelvis. The nurse plans to assess this client carefully because of the increased risk of which of the following?

1. Occiput posterior position
2. Prolonged labor
3. Precipitous delivery
4. Developing postpartum complications

145. The nurse would utilize which of the following interventions when caring for a client with chronic pain disorder to help that client cope with the disorder?

1. A program of physical exercise
2. Music therapy for expression
3. Patient-controlled analgesia pump
4. Complete bed rest

146. A client receiving hydroxyamphetamine (Paredrine) for open-angle glaucoma demonstrates an understanding of the medication's serious side effects when informing the health care provider of which of the following symptoms?

1. Stinging on instillation
2. Occasional headache
3. Occasional brow ache
4. Confusion

147. The nurse is seeking employment in a hospital that uses a shared governance model. The nurse should accept a job offer in the hospital that has which of the following attributes?

1. Staff nurses delegate activities to certified nursing assistants (CNAs).
2. A unit manager seeks advice from her supervisor.
3. Staff nurses and CNAs make their own schedules.
4. Procedure manuals are written by a committee of nurse managers.

148. The nurse observes an unlicensed assistive person (UAP) in the room of a client with severe acute respiratory syndrome (SARS). Which of the following actions by the UAP indicates intervention and further teaching by the nurse is needed?

1. The UAP wears a protective gown, gloves, N95 respirator, and eye protection when entering the room.
2. The UAP does not remove the stethoscope, blood pressure cuff, and thermometer being kept in the room.
3. The UAP removes all personal protective equipment and washes the hands right before leaving the client's room.
4. The UAP visits with the client for 25 minutes.

149. The nurse examines the white blood cell (WBC) differential for a client who experienced a severe allergic reaction. The nurse anticipates that which of the following values will be elevated?

1. Neutrophils
2. Monocytes
3. Eosinophils
4. Lymphocytes

150. The partner of a client who has dissociative identity disorder with several alters is puzzled about why the children are included in family therapy. Which of the following would be the best explanation for the nurse to offer?

1. "Children need to have their experiences confirmed—and to learn to deal with the different personalities."
2. "There is probably a mistake in the referral; your partner is the one who has the problem."
3. "You and your partner should be seen, but it could be traumatizing to the children."
4. "It would be best to ask the children if they would like to participate, and bring them if they want."

151. The nurse assesses the results of a vancomycin (Vancocin) blood level drawn just prior to the next scheduled intravenous (IV) dose. The nurse would collaborate with the prescriber after drawing which of the following correct conclusions about the result?

1. There is a high serum level, indicating the peak level is too high.
2. This test measures the highest therapeutic concentration and it is low.
3. Toxicity is evident, suggesting the drug's half-life is too short with the frequency prescribed.
4. The drug level is low, indicating the drug dosage and/or frequency should be increased.

152. In a child with acute renal failure, the nurse would help to prevent hyperkalemia by limiting which of the following foods in the diet?

1. Potatoes, tomatoes, and oranges.
2. Grains, cheese, and citrus fruits.
3. Cereals, processed sugars, and wheat.
4. Rice, leafy green vegetables, and carbonated beverages.

153. A 28-year-old female client has recently been diagnosed with systemic lupus erythematosus (SLE). Which of the following would be most helpful for the overall management of care?

1. Have the client institute advance directives immediately.
2. Discuss with the client lifestyle modifications that will be needed as the disease progresses.
3. Ascertain information about the client's working environment and suggest limiting work schedule to minimize potential stress.
4. Establish the multidisciplinary health care team to help client identify goals.

154. The nurse is leading a support group for adult children of aging parents who have come to live in their home because of deteriorating health. Which of the following principles does the nurse encourage the group members to follow to promote quality of life for all concerned?

1. Do as much as possible for aging parents to prevent problems from occurring.
2. Allow independence in those things that are safe or with minimal risk of harm.
3. Let the parents do whatever they want as a means to maintain their self-esteem.
4. Take over responsibility for making important decisions to avoid major financial losses.

155. A client of 26 weeks gestation experiences a partial placenta abruptio. She asks, "Will this harm my baby?" The nurse responds that this may:

1. Decrease the amount of nutrients the fetus receives.
2. Cause a build up of urine in the fetus, causing kidney damage.
3. Cause the fetus to develop hydrops.
4. Cause a fetal anomaly.

156. The nurse writes on the worksheet for the shift to assess a client taking cholestyramine (Questran) for signs of possible deficiency of which vitamins?

1. Niacin and thiamine
2. Folic acid and vitamin C
3. Vitamins A and D
4. Thiamine and cyanocobalamin

157. Case management has become an important nursing care model in the 21st century. Which of the following clients would most likely be selected for case management?

1. A 21-year-old male with a gunshot wound in the ER
2. A 32-year-old male with a fractured pelvis
3. A 75-year-old female awaiting a hip replacement
4. A 41-year-old male coming in for outpatient tonsillectomy

158. While making rounds, the nurse observes a client receiving oxygen by this mode. The nurse concludes the client is using this mode of oxygen therapy because of which primary benefit?

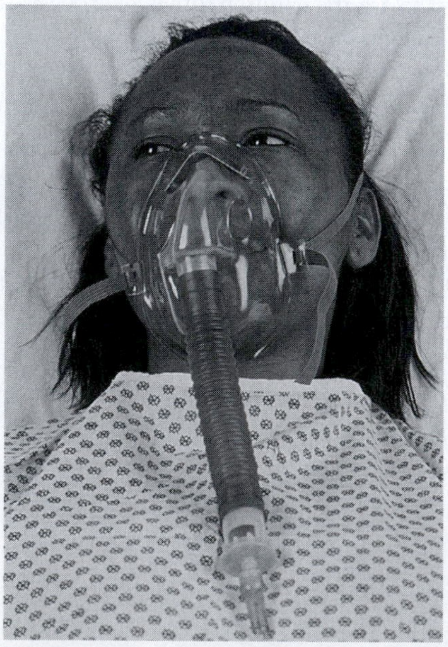

1. The ability to prevent rebreathing of exhaled carbon dioxide.
2. Oxygen concentration can be regulated.
3. Constant humidity can be administered to liquefy pulmonary secretions.
4. The ability to deliver up to 100% oxygen concentration for clients with COPD.

159. A client diagnosed with hypochondria states an allergy to the dyes used in diagnostic tests and "all" radioisotopes. The nurse explains that the client could undergo which diagnostic procedure without risk of possible allergic response?

1. Magnetic resonance imaging (MRI)
2. Myelogram
3. Ventilation/perfusion (VQ) scan
4. Computed tomography (CT) scan with contrast

160. A client had assumed a new identity and gained employment when he was found 400 miles away from his home. The mental health nurse interprets that this client's behavior is characteristic of:

1. Amnesia.
2. Akathisia.
3. Confabulation.
4. Fugue state.

161. The client is receiving a loading dose of lidocaine (Xylocaine) 100 mg IV for treatment of ventricular tachycardia. The nurse prepares to take which action next?

1. Start a continuous IV infusion at 1 to 4 mg/minute.
2. Repeat the dose every 10 minutes for 1 hour or PRN.
3. Begin oral procainamide (Pronestyl) therapy.
4. Prepare for pacemaker insertion to override the dysrhythmia.

162. The nurse on a cardiac medical unit has an unlicensed assistive person (UAP) assigned to the nursing team. The nurse would delegate which of the following client care activities to the UAP?

1. Assist the client to choose low fat and low sodium food selections from the dietary menu.
2. Measure client's pulse, blood pressure, and oxygen saturation after ambulation.
3. Explain the need to alternate activity periods with rest.
4. Help the client use nitroglycerin left at the bedside if chest pain occurs.

163. A client recovering from Guillain-Barré syndrome is admitted to the rehabilitation unit for general rehabilitative care. The nurse anticipates that which of the following methods will most likely be used to provide nutritional support for the client during this time?

1. Using a gastrostomy tube for feedings due to high incidence of malabsorption
2. Maintaining oral intake with adequate calories to maintain positive nitrogen balance
3. Limiting fresh fruit in the diet
4. Using thickened liquids to prevent aspiration

164. Based on the highest risks during this period of life, what would be the focus of the nurse who is setting up a health promotion booth for healthy adults in their thirties?

1. Screenings for breast, cervical, uterine, and prostate cancers
2. Chest x-rays for lung cancer
3. Bone density test for osteoporosis
4. Safety education for accident prevention

165. A client admitted with exacerbation of chronic obstructive pulmonary disease (COPD) has a respiratory rate of 18, a dry cough, and arterial blood gases that reveal a pH of 7.29, CO_2 of 50 mmHg, and O_2 of 72 mmHg. The nurse identifies which nursing diagnosis as the priority?

1. Impaired gas exchange
2. Activity intolerance
3. Risk for infection related to impaired respiratory defenses
4. Ineffective breathing pattern

166. The nurse is caring for a client who has just been diagnosed with Graves' disease. Client education regarding medication therapy needs to include which of the following?

1. Atropine
2. Thyroxine
3. Insulin
4. Propylthiouracil (PTU)

167. The nurse has delegated to an unlicensed assistive person (UAP) the care of a client who had a right hemisphere thrombotic stroke with hemiplegia. The nurse would give further direction to the UAP after noting that the UAP did which of the following?

1. Provided passive range of motion exercises to the affected arm and leg
2. Placed a chair for a visitor to the left of the bed
3. Placed the overbed table to the right side of the bed
4. Sat the client up slowly

168. The nurse determines that a client who has an infection with which of the following antibiotic-resistant microorganisms requires transmission-based droplet precautions?

1. Methicillin-resistant *Staphylococcus aureus*
2. Penicillin-resistant *Streptococcus pneumoniae*
3. Vancomycin-resistant *enterococci*
4. Vancomycin-intermediate-resistant *Staphylococcus*

169. The nurse is reviewing the results of a male client's recent lipid profile. The nurse notes that the client is experiencing beneficial effects of a heart healthy diet and exercise after noting elevations in which laboratory value?

1. High-density lipoprotein (HDL)
2. Low-density lipoprotein (LDL)
3. Total cholesterol
4. Triglycerides

170. The nurse concludes that client education about dissociation is effective when the dissociative client states:

1. "When I want to get out of a situation, I choose to space out."
2. "When I have to cope with problems, I imagine I am somewhere else."
3. "When I'm under stress, I have a tendency to dissociate."
4. "When I think about my life, I pretend I am someone else."

171. A client is advised to take an antiemetic to prevent nausea and vomiting. The nurse explains that anticipatory dosing should be done how long prior to activities that generally cause nausea?

1. 24 hours
2. 3 to 5 hours
3. 1/2 to 1 hour
4. 12 hours

172. The nurse working on a neuroscience unit has just received an intershift report. Which of the following assigned clients should the nurse assess first?

1. A client with Parkinson's disease who is crying because she cannot get up easily
2. A client with multiple sclerosis who is having noticeable leg spasms
3. A client who had a hemorrhagic stroke and is complaining of headache
4. A client scheduled for a craniotomy in 4 hours

173. Which of the following statements made by a client regarding human immunodeficiency virus (HIV) and acquired immunodeficiency syndrome (AIDS) would the nurse seek to further clarify?

1. "I can get the disease from eating contaminated food products."
2. "Blood tests will tell me if I have a nutritional anemia."
3. "Maintaining adequate fluid and fiber intake will help me."
4. "If I feel sick to my stomach, I should not drink liquids."

174. The registered nurse is assigned to the postpartum unit. Which task could the RN safely delegate to an unlicensed assistive person (UAP)?

1. Ambulate a client who had a vaginal delivery yesterday.
2. Complete the admission assessment on a newly delivered client.
3. Call the physician to report a low hemoglobin level.
4. Verify a unit of blood prior to transfusion.

175. The client has undergone hypophysectomy using a transphenoidal approach. You change the mustache dressing, noting clear exudate with a pale yellow colored ring at the edge of the drainage on the dressing. You should do which of the following next?

1. Document this as serous drainage and continue to monitor the client.
2. Assess for headache and check the glucose level in the drainage.
3. Apply an ice pack to the nasal bridge and a large fluffy dressing.
4. Lower the head of the bed to decrease the gravity pressure on the wound.

176. The client is experiencing severe itching with a skin disorder. Which of the following drugs, if ordered, would the nurse administer as an appropriate oral preparation to decrease the itching?

1. Cimetidine (Tagamet)
2. Lorazepam (Ativan)
3. Hydroxyzine (Atarax)
4. Bupivacaine (Sensorcaine)

177. A client who is legally blind has been admitted to the nursing unit. Which of the following activities should the nurse delegate to the unlicensed assistive person (UAP)? Select all that apply.

1. _____ Assist the client with meals.
2. _____ Complete the admission interview form.
3. _____ Assess the impact of the lost vision on the client's daily life.
4. _____ Assist the client to ambulate in the hall.
5. _____ Ask the client what community services are being utilized.

178. A client who has a history of Graves' disease accompanied by exophthalmos is arriving from surgery. Based on the observations as you note the photo, what should you educate the unlicensed assistive person (UAP) to do?

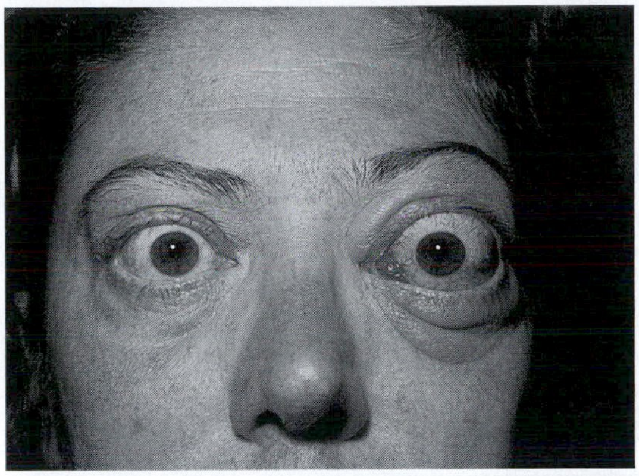

1. Keep the client's room warm to promote comfort.
2. Obtain fingerstick blood glucose every 2 hours twice.
3. Keep the head of the bed flat for 4 hours.
4. Provide eye protection measures for the client.

179. A client with bone cancer receiving chemotherapy has developed bone marrow suppression. Which laboratory report is of highest priority for the nurse to monitor at this time?

1. Calcium
2. Phosphorus
3. White blood cell (WBC) count
4. Serum prostate-specific antigen (PSA)

180. Which of the following behaviors would the nurse conclude is expected in a client who suffers from localized amnesia?

1. Wandering about in his neighborhood using a new name.
2. Forgetting about what happened during an assault.
3. Awareness of only a few of many alters.
4. Feelings of separation from his body.

181. The client will be discharged to home tomorrow on an antidepressant medication that will be taken once daily in the morning. He asks, "Do I have to take medicine every day? How will I be able to sleep when I go home? Do you think I'll be able to work, too, even though I have been in the hospital this long?" The nurse's best response is:

1. "The best approach is to take it one step at a time, so that everything will work out."
2. "I understand you're worried, but you and your wife will decide tomorrow when you get home."
3. "You seem to be worried about when you get home and how you will function. Would you like to sit and discuss a plan for your daily activities?"
4. "I'll do my best to set up a plan for discharge that you can take home with you and refer to later."

182. The client is admitted with all of the following orders to treat diabetic ketoacidosis (DKA) with severe metabolic acidosis. Which order would the nurse determine to be the first priority in managing this client?

1. Start IV fluid infusion for rehydration.
2. Insert an indwelling urinary catheter.
3. Administer NPH insulin.
4. Initiate continuous pulse oximetry.

183. The nurse would include which of the following statements when discussing nutritional status with a client who is infected with human immunodeficiency virus (HIV) and is progressing toward acquired immunodeficiency syndrome (AIDS)?

1. Clients who are asymptomatic have adequate nutritional stores of nutrients.
2. The HIV wasting syndrome is seen in the latter stages of the disease process.
3. Malnutrition is seen as a consequence of the immune disease.
4. Vitamin and mineral deficiencies occur in the latter stages of the disease process.

184. The nurse is taking the health history of a 77-year-old man. Which of the following symptoms reported by the client would the nurse consider to be an abnormal finding?

1. Delay of urination, hesitation, and decreased flow of urine stream
2. Increased tolerance to spicy foods
3. Increased isolating behaviors after his wife's death
4. Slight dizziness when getting up too quickly after lying down for a while

185. In planning care for a client with an axis II personality disorder, the nurse anticipates that the client will differ from clients with axis I disorders in that the client will:

1. Tend to experience symptoms as ego-syntonic.
2. Usually display clinical symptoms.
3. Tend to experience symptoms as ego-dystonic.
4. Seldom experience addictive behaviors.

186. The home health care nurse is visiting an elderly client who is taking a prescribed calcium channel blocker. In conducting dietary teaching, the nurse instructs the client that what food is contraindicated to take with a calcium channel blocker?

1. Oranges
2. Grapefruit
3. Bananas
4. Grapes

187. The client is admitted with thyroid storm. Assessment reveals: BP 188/102, HR 132 regular, RR 28 full depth and symmetrical, no urine output since admission to the Emergency Department 3 hours ago, alert, and anxious. Which of the following would be the high priority nursing diagnosis for this client?

1. Deficient fluid volume related to decreased absorption as evidenced by no urine output since admission
2. Anxiety related to fear as evidenced by client's appearance
3. Ineffective breathing pattern related to increased metabolism as evidenced by RR 28.
4. Decreased cardiac output related to increased ventricular workload as evidenced by adverse vital signs

188. The nurse must assess the temperature and blood pressure of a client on contact precautions for wound infection every shift. Which is the appropriate nursing action to minimize the spread of microorganisms?

1. Keep the equipment in the client's room.
2. Store the equipment in the soiled utility room between uses.
3. Cleanse the equipment after each use.
4. No special action is required with the equipment.

189. A client presents to the clinic with a chief complaint of a swollen and painful great toe. He states that his brother has it, and he has the same symptoms. The physician suspects gout. What specific laboratory test would the nurse expect to be ordered for this client?

1. Calcium
2. Hematocrit
3. Uric acid
4. Sodium

190. A female client has been diagnosed with a dependent personality disorder. Which statement is likely to be her response to the nurse's suggestion that she complete her morning care?

1. "I'll have no problem in deciding what to wear."
2. "I think you should wear more makeup."
3. "I think this outfit looks good on me."
4. "What do you think I should wear?"

191. The nurse should question an order for which beta agonist used to treat respiratory disease in a client with a history of atrial fibrillation accompanied by intermittent heart rates of 100/minute or greater?

1. Terbutaline (Brethine)
2. Pirbuterol (Maxair)
3. Isoproterenol (Isuprel)
4. Metaproterenol (Alupent)

192. A client with osteoporosis who has experienced fractures in the past is now admitted for dizziness and shortness of breath and has been determined to be at risk for falls. Which nursing intervention to assist this client can the nurse delegate to the unlicensed assistive person (UAP)? Select all that apply.

1. _____ Clear the room of unnecessary objects.
2. _____ Inquire if the dizziness has led to any recent falls.
3. _____ Remain with the client during ambulation.
4. _____ Ask physical therapy to evaluate the client for a walker.
5. _____ Advise the client about the benefits of calcium in the diet.

193. A client is receiving radiation to the head and neck area for treatment of cancer. What interventions would you use to help the client's complaint of a dry mouth?

1. Have client eat prior to radiation therapy.
2. Encourage the client to eat larger portions of food.
3. Advise the client to use mouthwash.
4. Suggest the use of sugar-free candies.

194. The client experienced an 18-hour labor with a second stage that lasted 2 hours. When the nurse brings the infant into the room 1 hour after delivery, the client tells the nurse to leave the infant in the crib and shows no interest in holding the newborn. The nurse should record which of the following nursing diagnoses in the chart?

1. Ineffective individual coping related to assuming parental role
2. Powerlessness related to loss of individual choices
3. Fatigue related to prolonged labor
4. Anxiety related to feelings of incompetence in parenting role

195. The nurse would expect to find a diminished pCO_2 level in the assigned client who has which of the following physical assessment findings?

1. Hyperventilation
2. Hypoventilation
3. Prolonged expiration
4. Stridor

196. A client is scheduled for an ophthalmic examination. Before administering the prescribed epinephrine solution, the nurse would assess for which of the following conditions?

1. Hypotension
2. Wide-angle glaucoma
3. Angle-closure glaucoma
4. Brow ache

197. The nurse is working on an orthopedic unit. After receiving intershift report, which client should the nurse assign to the unlicensed assistive person (UAP)?

1. A client with a newly applied cast who has increasing pain despite medication
2. A client with osteoporosis admitted 2 hours ago who fell and fractured the vertebra at L1
3. A client with a below-knee amputation who is anxious because "the leg feels like it's still there"
4. A client who had surgical repair of a fractured left hip 6 days ago and will be discharged to a rehabilitation facility near the end of the day

198. An adult client arrives to the Emergency Department with complaints of chest pain and shortness of breath. The nurse concludes that which of the following points, if present in the client's history, would indicate that this pain may be related to cardiac disease? Select all that apply.

1. _____ History of diabetes and smoking
2. _____ Recent travel out of the country
3. _____ The pain increases with activity
4. _____ The pain is reproducible when taking a deep breath
5. _____ The client is experiencing sweating and nausea when the pain is severe

199. A client asks the nurse to repeat what the physician explained about the anesthesia planned for an upcoming procedure. The nurse understands the procedure will be performed under moderate sedation. Which statement should the nurse make to the client concerning moderate sedation?

1. "You will be able to breathe and respond appropriately to physical stimuli and words that are spoken."
2. "Your pain threshold will be decreased so you can tolerate the pain."
3. "You will have a patent airway and will be able to remember and comprehend what is happening."
4. "You will not be awake but you will still feel slight pain during the surgical intervention."

200. A client is diagnosed with paranoid personality disorder. Which of the following assessment data does the nurse conclude are consistent with this diagnosis?

1. Delusions and hallucinations
2. Passivity and compliance with rules
3. Jealousy and secretiveness
4. Respect for authority

201. The nurse is administering nitrogen mustard (Mustargen) and notes swelling at the intravenous (IV) site. The nurse should take which of the following actions initially?

1. Continue with infusion after trying to aspirate for a blood return.
2. Stop administration and attempt to aspirate.
3. Flush the line with saline.
4. Obtain a new site for drug administration.

202. The nurse working on adult medical-surgical unit would assign which of the following clients to the licensed practical/vocational nurse (LPN/LVN) under the supervision of the RN?

1. A 62-year-old client admitted 8 hours ago with exacerbation of COPD
2. A 25-year-old client with a concussion from an auto accident the prior evening
3. An 81-year-old client with chronic heart failure and emphysema admitted 3 days ago
4. A 54-year old client newly diagnosed with diabetes mellitus who will be discharged today

203. A client has been referred for dietary teaching regarding the management of hepatitis. The nurse would base development of nutritional goals on which of the following pieces of information?

1. The type of hepatitis that the client has, as this will affect the treatment
2. The need for tube feedings to allow the liver to rest and regenerate
3. That dietary fats should be limited
4. That the diet should be high in calories and high in protein

204. The nurse is caring for a 15-year-old primipara who delivered yesterday. The nurse identifies the following nursing diagnosis for this client: risk for altered parenting related to knowledge deficit in newborn care. Which is the most appropriate intervention when planning this client's discharge teaching?

1. Have the client watch a video on newborn care.
2. Give her information about a support group for adolescent mothers.
3. Demonstrate how to care for the newborn and have the client return the demonstration.
4. Give the client printed instructions on newborn care.

205. To decrease skin irritation in children with the condition illustrated, the nurse instructs the parents to do which of the following?

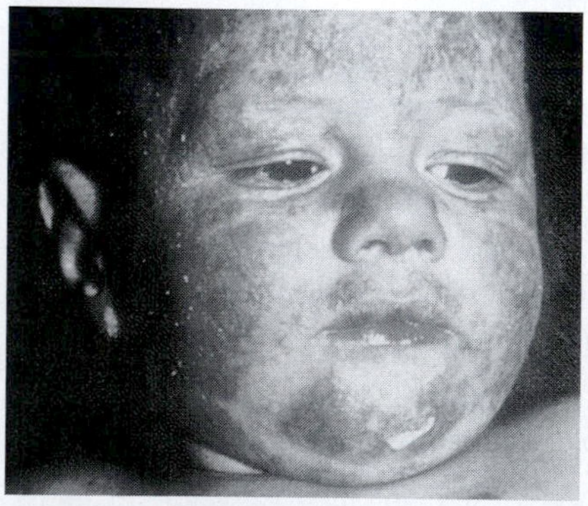

1. Take hot baths (not showers) daily.
2. Liberally apply a lotion of choice over entire body.
3. Use fabric softener for all clothes.
4. Use mild soap only as needed.

206. A client who is taking warfarin (Coumadin) therapy comes to the office for a follow-up visit and states that he has taken propoxyphene with aspirin (Darvon Compound 65) for aches and pains related to an old back injury. How should the ambulatory care nurse respond to this information?

1. Ask the client how long his back been hurting him and assess the need for a referral for pain management.
2. Tell the client that it is important to prevent the pain cycle from starting and to continue to take Darvon as ordered by the physician.
3. Advise the client that Darvon contains aspirin, which may interfere with Coumadin therapy, and consult with the physician for an alternate pain medication.
4. Instruct the client that continued daily use of Darvon would help to relieve back pain, but would require an increase in the dose of the Coumadin.

207. Which of the following is an assessment finding with developmental dysplasia of the hip in a 5-year-old child?

1. Asymmetry of gluteal and thigh fat folds
2. Positive Ortolani-Barlow maneuver
3. Telescoping of the femoral head into the pelvis
4. Limited abduction of the affected hip

208. The nurse would intervene after noting another nursing staff member take which of the following actions in the care of a child who has had surgery for clubfoot?

1. Applying ice bags to the foot and keeping the ankle and foot elevated on a pillow
2. Checking for drainage or bleeding and observing for swelling around cast edges
3. Administering pain medication immediately when it is due and covering the cast with blankets
4. Performing neurovascular status checks every 2 hours and providing diversional activities

209. An adolescent is undergoing a spinal fusion for scoliosis. Which of the following would not need to be included in the preoperative teaching completed by the nurse?

1. Deep-breathing and coughing exercises, use of incentive spirometry
2. Use of postoperative pain medications
3. The procedure for the spinal fusion and bone grafting
4. Placement of a urinary catheter to drain urine after surgery

210. The nurse interprets that which of the following statements made by a coworker is a typical staff response when working with a client diagnosed with a paranoid personality disorder?

1. "He constantly criticizes his care. I'm so frustrated."
2. "He is so pleasant but so shy."
3. "He has a wonderful sense of humor but he doesn't let it show often."
4. "I am pleased he was so helpful with his roommate. He can be so irritable at times."

211. A client has been admitted to the hospital with chest pain. The pain has not been relieved after one dose of nitroglycerine (NTG) sublingually. Upon monitoring the vital signs (VS), the nurse notices that the blood pressure has dropped to 126/84 from 130/90. Which of the following actions should the nurse take next?

1. Notify the physician.
2. Obtain an electroencephalogram (EEG).
3. Give another dose of nitroglycerine.
4. Add a dose of nitroglycerine paste.

212. The nurse working on an adult medical-surgical unit would assign which of the following clients to the licensed practical/vocational nurse (LPN/LVN) under the supervision of the RN?

1. A 45-year-old client admitted yesterday after a nephrectomy
2. A 78-year-old client with diabetes mellitus and osteoarthritis
3. A 32-year-old client with a fractured pelvis from an auto accident 3 days ago
4. A 62-year old client who underwent pelvic exenteration receiving medication via patient-controlled analgesia

213. The nurse anticipates which of the following regarding sodium restriction for a client diagnosed with ascites secondary to cirrhosis?

1. Sodium restriction is critical in managing the occurrence of ascites; therefore, the client should not receive any sodium.
2. There is no need to restrict sodium as paracentesis can be used to remove excess fluid.
3. If the client experiences resistance to diuretic therapy, there may need to be more stringent sodium restrictions.
4. Diets with sodium restriction are unpalatable; therefore, the client will likely be noncompliant with therapy.

214. A mother calls a clinic nurse to state that a letter had come home with her child from school stating she should examine her child for the nits from pediculosis capitus. She asks where she should look for these nits. The nurse would tell the mother to examine:

1. The forehead and scalp.
2. In the webs of the fingers.
3. The hair shafts at the nape of the neck.
4. In the folds of elbows.

215. Which of the following instructions would be appropriate for the nurse to include in the discharge teaching of an adolescent following a spinal fusion?

1. No contact sports will be allowed again.
2. The adolescent should not bend at the waist.
3. Walking is limited to only one half mile per day.
4. The adolescent should not climb stairs.

216. The physician has prescribed vitamin D for a client. The client asks the nurse what the medication is for. Which of the following is the best response by the nurse?

1. "Vitamin D decreases intestinal absorption of calcium and phosphorus and decreases their mobilization from bone."
2. "Vitamin D helps regulate calcium and phosphorus balance."
3. "Vitamin D helps the kidneys rid the body of excess calcium and phosphorus."
4. "Vitamin D decreases blood levels of calcium and phosphorus."

217. The nurse working on an adult medical-surgical unit would assign which of the following clients to the licensed practical/vocational nurse (LPN/LVN) under the supervision of the RN?

1. A 45-year-old client who underwent bilateral adrenalectomy the previous day
2. A 66-year-old client being discharged to home following arthroscopy
3. A 24-year old with hemophilia who fractured a leg after falling from a horse yesterday
4. A 53-year-old client with hypertension and chronic renal insufficiency

218. A client with acquired immunodeficiency syndrome (AIDS) who has *Pneumocystis carinii* is being admitted to the nursing unit. The nurse should institute which of the following?

1. Standard precautions
2. Airborne precautions
3. Droplet precautions
4. Contact precautions

219. A family member is sitting at bedside and observes the nurse admitting the client from the postanesthesia care unit (PACU) following a surgical procedure. The family member asks why the area around the surgical wound is orange. Which of the following statements about surgical skin preparation is the best response to the family member?

1. "It reduces the risk of all postoperative complications."
2. "It reduces the risk of postoperative wound infection."
3. "It lessens the chance for decreased tissue perfusion."
4. "It decreases the possibility for dermatitis."

220. The nurse is planning care for a client recently admitted with paranoid ideation. The nurse determines that it would be counterproductive to do which of the following when working with this client?

1. Ensure that a consistent program schedule be followed.
2. Confront and challenge inaccuracies in the client's ideation.
3. Orient the client to the unit and introduce him to the other staff.
4. Establish clearly defined expectations of the client.

221. Following the administration of a measles-mumps-rubella (MMR) vaccine, the nurse should make a priority assessment for which of the following client manifestations?

1. Wheezing
2. Pain
3. Anxiety
4. Vomiting

222. The nurse working on an adult medical-surgical unit would assign which of the following clients to the licensed practical/vocational nurse (LPN/LVN) under the supervision of the RN?

1. A 46-year-old client with COPD who will be seen by the pulmonary rehabilitation specialist in 2 hours
2. A 26-year-old client who is in sickle cell crisis
3. A 59-year-old client with Paget's disease who also has hypertension
4. A 75-year-old client who fractured a hip and is awaiting surgical repair scheduled for mid-morning

223. When assessing the genitourinary system of a 75-year-old male client, the nurse questions the client about symptoms of which of the following conditions that is common in older men?

1. Testicular cancer
2. Benign prostatic hyperplasia
3. Testicular torsion
4. Gonorrhea

224. The nurse is teaching a class on newborn care to a group of expectant parents. In explaining why the parents need to protect the infant from heat loss, the nurse should discuss that the characteristic of the infant's skin that is responsible for heat loss is:

1. Lanugo.
2. Nonfunctioning sebaceous glands.
3. Nonfunctioning apocrine glands.
4. Thinner skin.

225. Which of the following statements indicates that a client understands appropriate information about premenstrual syndrome (PMS)?

1. "I have PMS all month long."
2. "My husbands says if we had sex more often it would help my PMS."
3. "PMS starts about 10 days before my period."
4. "I should drink more coffee when I have PMS."

226. Which of the following symptoms would the nurse assess for in a client with the most common generalized seizure disorder?

1. Periods of inattention and daydreaming
2. Sudden loss of muscle tone and falling
3. Repetitive small muscle group activity
4. Tonic and clonic activity of the extremities

227. The nurse must assess the temperature and blood pressure of a client on contact precautions every shift. Which is the appropriate nursing action to minimize the spread of microorganisms?

1. Keep the equipment in the client's room.
2. Store the equipment in the soiled utility room between uses.
3. Cleanse the equipment after each use.
4. No special action is required with the equipment.

228. The nurse would implement which of the following as the most important measure on the surgical unit on the first postoperative day following surgical repair of an abdominal aneurysm?

1. Administer anticoagulant therapy.
2. Position the legs in Trendelenburg position.
3. Apply elastic stockings to both legs.
4. Palpate peripheral pulses every 2 to 4 hours.

229. The nurse is preparing a client for surgery. Prior to completing the skin preparation, the nurse assesses the surgical site for which of the following?

1. Presence of pustules or abrasions
2. Absence of hair growth
3. Presence of lanugo
4. Absence of pulsation

230. A client with schizophrenia is admitted to the psychiatric unit. As the nurse approaches the client with medication, he refuses it, accusing the nurse of trying to poison him. The nurse's *best* response would be to tell him that:

1. "It is not poison, and you must take the medication."
2. "If you won't take this, I will give you an injection."
3. "I'm sorry you think that this medication is poison. You don't have to take it right now if you don't want to."
4. "You may decide if you want to take the medication by mouth or injection, but this medication will help you."

231. The nurse is making a plan of care for a client who is prescribed fluphenazine (Prolixin) 1 mg daily at bedtime. The nurse will include which of the following to monitor for side effects of the medication?

1. Remind him frequently to rise slowly when getting out of bed or from a chair.
2. Assess for dizziness or lightheadedness frequently during the day.
3. Make sugarless hard candy, gum, and water available during the day.
4. Monitor for confusion frequently.

232. The nurse working on an adult medical unit would assign which of the following clients to the licensed practical/vocational nurse (LPN/LVN) under the supervision of the RN?

1. A 46-year-old client who will undergo cardiac catheterization later in the morning
2. A 54-year-old client who has osteoarthritis and low back pain
3. A 62-year-old client admitted the previous evening with chest pain
4. A 79-year-old client who has chronic bronchitis and early Alzheimer's disease

233. A client with venous stasis ulcers is being treated with an Unna boot. The nurse should include which of the following additional interventions in the plan of care?

1. Elevating legs and assessment of peripheral pulses
2. Keeping legs dependent for pain relief and improved circulation
3. Wet to dry dressings to ulcer twice daily
4. Elevating legs and standing as much as possible

234. A priority nursing action needed following a full body scan would include which of the following actions by the nurse?

1. Pain assessment due to discomfort of the actual procedure
2. Vital signs to assess for possible bleeding
3. Prophylactic antiemetic due to radiation exposure causing nausea
4. Therapeutic communication to reduce possible anxiety caused by outcomes

235. The nurse is teaching a client and family about health maintenance with chronic obstructive pulmonary disease (COPD). The nurse explains to the family that nutrition is important in managing this condition using which rationale?

1. COPD clients have an adequate immune response.
2. COPD clients are at increased risk of suffering from malnutrition.
3. COPD clients are likely to experience weight gain due to fluid retention.
4. Decreased energy requirements lead to weight gain.

236. The nurse provides discharge instructions to the client taking an antihypertensive medication. The nurse should include in the teaching plan that a hypertensive crisis will exist if the diastolic blood pressure (BP) is greater than which of the following?

1. 100 mmHg
2. 120 mmHg
3. 130 mmHg
4. 140 mmHg

237. Which of these statements if made by a client receiving dietary instruction for atherosclerosis would indicate a need for further discussion?

1. "Margarine has less fat than butter, so I will no longer use butter."
2. "I will steam, bake, or broil my foods."
3. "American cheese has 76 percent fat calories."
4. "I will increase my consumption of fruits and vegetables."

238. The nurse would choose to use medical aseptic technique when collecting which of the following specimens?

1. C & S from an abdominal wound
2. Sputum specimen via a tracheostomy
3. Stool specimen for ova and parasites
4. Urine specimen via straight cath

239. Following placement of a central venous line, which information should the nurse report immediately to the physician?

1. Pain at the insertion site
2. Fever
3. Increased heart rate and respiratory rate
4. Diminished breath sounds in lung bases

240. A client diagnosed with schizophrenia has improved and is playing a card game with peers. The group begins laughing at a joke told to them. The client jumps up and shouts, "You are all making fun of me." The nurse concludes that the client is displaying:

1. Hallucinations.
2. Ideas of reference.
3. Delusions.
4. Loose association.

241. A 70-year-old client with chronic obstructive pulmonary disease (COPD) is taking theophylline (Theo-Dur). A blood level is drawn and the result is 25 mg/dL. What explanation by the nurse helps the client understand this lab result?

1. "Your dose of theophylline needs to be increased."
2. "Your blood level is low because the dose was based on total body weight instead of lean body weight."
3. "The lab value could be high because of your age. We may have to decrease the dosage of your medication."
4. "I am sure that lab value is incorrect. Theophylline levels are never that high."

242. The mother of a 2-month-old receiving immunizations for the first time will also be a beginning nursing student when the next semester starts. When the mother asks the nurse to relate the immunizations to what she learned in the microbiology class, the nurse states that administering childhood immunizations interrupts the chain of infection at what link?

1. Mode of transmission
2. Portal of entry
3. Susceptible host
4. Portal of exit

243. A 9-year-old child is being treated with methimazole for Graves' disease. She has not responded to the drug therapy as quickly as the physician expected so a thyroidectomy is being considered. The child's mother asks the nurse, "Why would the physician seem hesitant to encourage the surgery?" Which response by the nurse is best?

1. "The surgery will leave a scar on the child's neck and will cause problems with her self-esteem."
2. "Removal of the thyroid gland may result in permanent hypothyroidism, which will require lifelong hormone replacement therapy."
3. "The convalescent time for this surgery is 6 months."
4. "Removal of the thyroid gland causes a change in thermoregulation."

244. The nurse doing health promotion in an ambulatory women's health clinic would plan to teach Kegel exercises to a woman with which of the following conditions?

1. Menopause
2. Uterine prolapse
3. Urinary tract infection
4. Premenstrual syndrome

245. A client with a diagnosis of paranoid schizophrenia who threatened his parents with a knife was placed on a 48-hour hold by the courts and the psychiatrist. The nurse explains to the family that once the 48-hour hold is expired, the psychiatrist and court must determine if the client is:

1. A danger to himself.
2. A danger to himself and others.
3. Agreeable to take his medications.
4. Willing to remain in outpatient treatment.

246. Which of the following statements made by a client receiving ophthalmic corticosteroids indicates a need for further teaching?

1. "I remove my contact lenses before instilling the medication, then put them back in after 30 minutes."
2. "I am not wearing my contact lenses for the duration of the corticosteroid treatment."
3. "I will take my medication for the length of time prescribed by my physician."
4. "I will return to my physician to have my eyes examined after my treatment is completed."

247. A nurse is teaching a new group of hospital teen volunteers about the chain of infection. Which of the following items would the nurse include as an example of how an infection would spread through droplets?

1. Nonsterile surgical instruments
2. Soiled linens
3. Contaminated dressings
4. Sneezing and coughing

248. A 12-year-old boy has signs of precocious puberty. He is 5 feet 7 inches tall, has a deep voice, and has started to shave his facial hair. His friends are envious of his tall stature and basketball skills. The boy comments on the fact that he expects to be over 6 feet tall and become a professional basketball player. What will the nurse use as information in explaining that the client will probably not reach that height?

1. Neither of the child's parents is 6 feet tall.
2. The child doesn't eat enough nutritious food.
3. The early presence of sex hormones stimulates closure of the epiphyseal growth plates, resulting in short stature in the future.
4. Few children attain heights above 6 feet and become professional basketball stars.

249. The client was taught calf-pumping exercises prior to surgery to decrease the possibility of thrombophlebitis developing postoperatively. The nurse observes the client performing the procedure and notes that client correctly understands the technique when the client is observed doing which of the following?

1. Alternately contracting and relaxing the leg muscles
2. Alternately flexing and extending the knees
3. Raising and lowering the legs
4. Alternately dorsiflexing and plantar flexing the feet

250. The nurse determines that the *highest* priority action when caring for a client who has alcohol-withdrawal delirium would be:

1. Reality orientation.
2. Restraint application.
3. Referral to Alcoholics Anonymous.
4. Replacement of fluids and electrolytes.

251. The nurse working the evening shift on an adult surgical unit would assign which of the following clients to the licensed practical/vocational nurse (LPN/LVN) under the supervision of the RN?

1. A 24-year old client who underwent extraction of four wisdom teeth earlier in the day
2. A 54-year-old client who had a laparoscopic cholecystectomy the previous day and will be discharged
3. A 62-year-old client who underwent open reduction, internal fixation of a fractured femur 3 days ago
4. A 48-year-old client returning from PACU following partial gastrectomy

252. The nurse should implement contact precautions with the client with which of the following health problems?

1. Scarlet fever
2. Pertussis
3. A wound infection
4. Rubella

253. The nurse is caring for a 68-year-old male diagnosed with benign prostatic hyperplasia (BPH). Which of the following statements by the client indicates the need for further teaching?

1. "The enlarged prostate gland causes me to get up three times every night to urinate."
2. "The enlarged prostate gland may produce blood in my urine."
3. "I can get urinary tract infections because of the enlarged prostate gland."
4. "I should cut down on the fluids I drink so I won't have to urinate so often."

254. Parents of a 10-year-old boy with mild cerebral palsy ask the nurse about having their son join a Boy Scout troop that meets after school. The boy attends a regular grade school class. The nurse considers which of the following when formulating a response?

1. The rigors of most scout events would be physically beyond this child's capability.
2. Scouting can provide children of all abilities with opportunities for recreation and socialization.
3. It would be embarrassing for the child to be different from the other boys and lower his self-esteem.
4. It is more important that the child conserve his energy for doing schoolwork.

255. The nurse should assess carefully a 79-year-old client who has been frequently sedated with haloperidol (Haldol) for signs of which of the following?

1. Tardive dyskinesia
2. Fecal impaction
3. Respiratory depression
4. Restlessness

256. A new staff nurse wants to clarify her responsibilities regarding delegation. To which of the following documents would the nurse mentor refer this nurse?

1. Policy manual
2. Job description
3. ANA standards of care
4. State nurse practice act

257. The nurse is preparing to enter the room of a client with pneumonia caused by penicillin-resistant *Streptococcus pneumoniae* (PRSP). The client has a tracheostomy and requires suctioning. Put the following personal protective equipment in order of donning:

1. Eye protection
2. Gloves
3. Mask
4. Gown

258. A school-age child has recently been diagnosed as having a seizure disorder. The parents express a concern about what will happen if the child has a seizure at school. The parents are afraid other children will make fun of their child. Which of the following responses by the nurse would be most helpful?

1. The child should always wears a Medic Alert bracelet.
2. The parents should talk with the teacher about how to handle the situation.
3. The child should learn about the pathophysiology of seizures so his self-esteem will not be affected.
4. The parents make an appointment with a psychiatrist to talk about their concerns.

259. The nurse is preparing to administer a purified protein derivative (PPD) tuberculin skin test to a client. Before administration, the nurse should take which of the following actions?

1. Cleanse the area thoroughly with soap and water.
2. Ensure that the client has not had a positive test result in the past.
3. Determine whether the client can return to the office in 24 hours for the test to be read.
4. Instruct the client not to wash the area for 48 hours.

260. The nurse determines that an appropriate outcome criterion for the *initial* nursing care of a client with acute delirium would be which of the following?

1. The client will verbalize dependence on drugs.
2. The client will demonstrate adaptive coping strategies for dealing with stress.
3. The client will be oriented to person, place, and time during lucid periods.
4. The client will explore reasons for addictive behaviors.

261. A child is admitted to the nursing unit with acute renal failure (ARF). When reviewing the nursing history, the nurse notes a history of all of the following health problems. The nurse concludes that which item in the child's history most likely precipitated the onset of ARF?

1. Chickenpox
2. Influenza
3. Dehydration
4. Hypervolemia

262. The nurse concludes client teaching about infection control measures has been effective when a client with tuberculosis states,

1. "I need to wear a particulate respiratory mask when I go to x-ray."
2. "Nurse, can you give me some gloves so I can blow my nose?"
3. "I will need to use paper plates and cups to eat."
4. "I will flush the toilet twice after urinating."

263. An 18-year-old client is seen in the Emergency Department with sudden onset of severe scrotal pain, nausea, and an absent cremasteric reflex. The nurse should suspect which of the following conditions?

1. Hydrocele
2. Prostatitis
3. Varicocele
4. Testicular torsion

264. Evidence that the outcome of "restore tissue integrity" has been met in a client with a venous stasis ulcer includes:

1. Absence of bleeding.
2. No reports of pain.
3. Increased activity tolerance.
4. No signs of inflammation or infection.

265. A 58-year-old client reports to the nurse during a health history that the physician recently diagnosed a type of dementia. The nurse checks in the medical record for documentation related to which of the following most likely disorders?

1. Senile dementia
2. Presenile dementia
3. Pseudodementia
4. Vascular dementia

Comprehensive Exam Answer Key

1. **Answer: 1** To prevent active tuberculosis after exposure, the client is initiated on a single agent regimen, usually isoniazid (INH). For newly diagnosed active disease (option 2), a combination of antitubercular agents is used for at least the first several weeks: isoniazid (INH), rifampin (Rifadin), and pyrazinamide (Tebrazid). The combination therapy lessens the risk of drug resistance (option 3). Except for streptomycin, which is for IM use, the antitubercular agents are administered orally (option 4).
Cognitive Level: Application **Client Need:** Physiological Integrity: Pharmacological and Parenteral Therapies **Integrated Process:** Teaching and Learning **Content Area:** Pharmacology **Strategy:** The critical words in the stem of the question are *exposed* and *chemoprophylaxis.* Differentiate exposure from infection as the key concept being tested. Recall that if active infection requires multi-drug therapy, exposure can be managed with a single agent alone.
2. **Answer: 2** The nurse ensures that the UAP understands the importance of reporting immediately any difficulties during the procedure such as bleeding. This provides for safe and effective care. Option 1 is incorrect because the client cannot do the procedure because of arthritis. Option 3 is unnecessary if the UAP is qualified to do the procedure. Option 4 is a function of the nurse, not the UAP.
Cognitive Level: Application **Client Need:** Safe Effective Care Environment: Management of Care **Integrated Process:** Nursing Process: Implementation **Content Area:** Leadership/Management **Strategy:** The core issue of the question is the appropriate procedure for the nurse to use when delegating care to a UAP. Eliminate option 4 first because it is the role of the nurse. Eliminate options 1 and 3 next, because they are not indicated or unnecessary, respectively.
3. **Answer: 4** Only option 4 relates to the client's physiological integrity. Options 1 and 2 pertain to the psychological aspects of client care, while option 3 relates to the safety in the environment.
Cognitive Level: Application **Client Need:** Physiological Integrity: Reduction of Risk Potential **Integrated Process:** Nursing Process: Assessment **Content Area:** Fundamentals **Strategy:** The core issue of the question is knowledge of physiological assessment priorities in the perioperative client. Fluid loss directly relates to cardiovascular status, which is one of the ABCs (airway, breathing, and circulation). Use nursing knowledge and the process of elimination to make a selection.
4. **Answer: 1, 2, 4** Obesity, hypertension, and smoking are modifiable risk factors for stroke. Hypercholesterolemia (cholesterol level greater than 200 mg) would also be a risk factor, but this client's level is less than 200 mg/dL. Eating a diet containing fiber helps keep cholesterol levels low and is not a risk factor for stroke.
Cognitive Level: Analysis **Client Need:** Health Promotion and Maintenance **Integrated Process:** Nursing Process: Assessment **Content Area:** Adult Health: Cardiovascular **Strategy:** The core issue of the question is knowledge of risk factors for stroke. Recall that these are similar to the risk factors for cardiac disease to help make your selections.
5. **Answer: 1, 2, 5** Options 1, 2 and 5 are core principles of medical asepsis. Option 3 violates principles of medical asepsis. Option 4 uses principles of surgical asepsis but the question asks specifically about medical asepsis.
Cognitive Level: Application **Client Need:** Safe Effective Care Environment: Safety and Infection Control **Integrated Process:** Nursing Process: Implementation **Content Area:** Fundamentals **Strategy:** Use knowledge of medical versus surgical asepsis as essential core concepts. Eliminate options that utilize surgical asepsis or are unrelated to the needs of the client.
6. **Answer: 2** Red blood cells, white blood cells, and platelet counts may be decreased during the nadir period following administration of chemotherapy that has hematological toxicity. Medications that inhibit platelet aggregation should be avoided during the nadir period following antineoplastic therapy. Aspirin, ibuprofen, and indomethacin are examples of some of these agents. Tylenol is the drug of choice for mild pain and fever. Benadryl is often used for sinus drainage or as an antihistamine and Robitussin is used to manage cough.
Cognitive Level: Analysis **Client Need:** Physiological Integrity: Pharmacological and Parenteral Therapies **Integrated Process:** Nursing Process: Implementation **Content Area:** Pharmacology **Strategy:** The core issue of the question is the ability to determine which drugs could increase the risk of bleeding when a client's blood counts may be low. Use the process of elimination and knowledge of drug actions and adverse effects to make a selection.
7. **Answer: 4** A situational leader recognizes that leadership style depends on the readiness and willingness of the group or the individuals to perform the assigned tasks. The democratic or participative leader offers suggestions, asks questions, and guides the group toward achieving the group

goals. The laissez-faire leader recognizes the group's need for autonomy and abdicates responsibility. A bureaucratic leader relies on the organization's rules, policies, and procedures to direct the group's work.

Cognitive Level: Application **Client Need:** Safe, Effective Care Environment: Management of Care **Integrated Process:** Nursing Process: Analysis **Content Area:** Leadership/ Management **Strategy:** The core issue of the question is knowledge of various leadership styles. Use this knowledge and the process of elimination to make a selection.

8. **Answer: 1** Hand hygiene is a core principle of standard precautions. Using gloves is appropriate when there is a risk of exposure to blood, body fluids, secretions, and excretions. However, handwashing should be done after removal of gloves. Not all clients require transmission-based precautions (option 3) or a private room (option 4).
Cognitive Level: Application **Client Need:** Safe Effective Care Environment: Safety and Infection Control **Integrated Process:** Nursing Process: Implementation **Content Area:** Fundamentals **Strategy:** Use the process of elimination based on nursing knowledge of standard precautions. Elements of transmission-based precautions are not initiated with all clients.

9. **Answer: 1, 4** The white blood cell count is elevated (normal 5,000–10,000/mm^3), as is the BUN (8–22 mg/dL). These changes would be expected with infection (noted by fever) and possibly accompanying dehydration from diarrhea. The sodium (135–145 mEq/L), potassium (3.5–5.1 mEq/L), and serum creatinine (0.8–1.6 mg/dL) are all within normal limits.
Cognitive Level: Analysis **Client Need:** Physiological Integrity: Reduction of Risk Potential **Integrated Process:** Nursing Process: Analysis **Content Area:** Adult Health: Immunological **Strategy:** The core issue of the question is the ability to discriminate between normal and abnormal laboratory values. Note the critical symptoms fever and diarrhea, which could lead to you select elevated white count for infection and elevated BUN with fluid loss from diarrhea.

10. **Answer: 3** According to Erikson's stages of development, a 10-year-old child is experiencing industry vs. inferiority. Shame (option 1), guilt (option 2), and role confusion (option 4) occur at other developmental levels.
Cognitive Level: Application **Client Need:** Psychosocial Integrity **Integrated Process:** Nursing Process: Analysis **Content Area:** Mental Health **Strategy:** The core issue of the question is the ability to anticipate levels of growth and development in a 10-year-old child. Use knowledge of Erikson's theory to make a selection.

11. **Answer: 4** Low-dose heparin therapy is indicated in many postoperative clients to prevent the development of thromboembolic episodes. It is not used in every postoperative situation (option 1), but it is usually used for clients who have orthopedic surgery or are anticipated to be immobilized for a time following surgery. Short-term therapy is not given to maintain adequate blood clotting levels (option 2) but merely to intervene as a preventative measure. While the statement that heparin is given SubQ in the abdomen and is not usually painful is factual, it is not the reason for the medication being given to the client (option 3).
Cognitive Level: Application **Client Need:** Physiological Integrity: Pharmacological and Parenteral Therapies **Integrated Process:** Communication and Documentation **Content Area:** Pharmacology **Strategy:** The critical words in the stem of the question are *best answer the question.* This tells you that the correct answer is one that responds to the client's concern, rather than just reciting a fact about the medication. Use nursing knowledge and the process of elimination to answer the question.

12. **Answer: 1** Shared leadership recognizes that there are many leaders within a group so the leader encourages the formation of self-directed work teams. In transformational leadership, the leader encourages risk taking such as trying out nursing approaches that are evidence-based or research-based. A transactional leader uses incentives to promote productivity such as giving rewards for excellent performance. A democratic leader provides constructive criticism and facilitates the group to meet their goals.
Cognitive Level: Application **Client Need:** Safe, Effective Care Environment: Management of Care **Integrated Process:** Nursing Process: Implementation **Content Area:** Leadership/ Management **Strategy:** The core issue of the question is knowledge of various leadership styles. Use this knowledge and the process of elimination to make a selection.

13. **Answer: 2** Middle-aged adults have a decrease in deep sleep, stage IV NREM. Option 1 is an expected pattern in older adults; option 3 is expected in young adults, and option 4 is expected in neonates.
Cognitive Level: Analysis **Client Need:** Physiological Integrity: Basic Care and Comfort **Integrated Process:** Nursing Process: Assessment **Content Area:** Fundamentals **Strategy:** The core issue of the question is knowledge of age-related changes in sleep pattern. Use this knowledge and the process of elimination to make a selection.

14. **Answer: 3** Crowning is the point in time when the perineum is thin and stretching around the fetal head both between and during contractions. Delivery is imminent when crowning occurs. Crowning occurs later than the first sight of the infant's head. A head that recedes upward between contractions is not crowning. The mouth and nose cannot be suctioned during crowning because they are not accessible, nor is it timely.
Cognitive Level: Analysis **Client Need:** Health Promotion and Maintenance **Integrated Process:** Nursing Process: Evaluation **Content Area:** Maternal-Newborn **Strategy:** The critical word in the stem of the question is *crowning.* Use knowledge of what occurs during crowning and the process of elimination to make a selection. Visualize the word *crown* and select the answer that matches the part of the head that a crown would sit on.

15. **Answer: 4** Option 4 gives the client an opportunity to explain to the nurse the reason for asking the question. This helps the nurse understand the client's frame of reference and allows the nurse to best address the client's concern. Options 1 and 3 offer false reassurance and can give the impression that the nurse did not listen to or address the

client's concerns. Option 2 is a close-ended question and may not help the nurse explore the client's concerns.
Cognitive Level: Analysis **Client Need:** Physiological Integrity: Reduction of Risk Potential **Integrated Process:** Communication and Documentation **Content Area:** Fundamentals **Strategy:** The core issue of the question is knowledge of communication techniques that are effective when working with a client who will undergo surgery. Use knowledge of communication theory and the process of elimination to make a selection.

16. Answer: 3 Lidocaine is the primary medication used to treat ventricular dysrhythmias. Lidocaine suppresses automaticity in the His-Purkinje system by elevating electrical stimulation threshold of the ventricle during diastole, thus decreasing ventricular irritability. Ventricular fibrillation (option 1) is a worsening dysrhythmia. Slowing the heart rate (option 2) without converting the rhythm to an atrial or sinus rhythm is not therapeutic. An increase in level of consciousness (option 4) would only occur once the ventricular rhythm is terminated.
Cognitive Level: Application **Client Need:** Physiological Integrity: Pharmacological and Parenteral Therapies **Integrated Process:** Nursing Process: Evaluation **Content Area:** Pharmacology **Strategy:** The core issue of the question is knowledge that Lidocaine is an antidysrhythmic that should reduce the irritability of the ventricle, thus making it more amenable to shock therapy. The reduction in ventricular irritability could manifest as a conversion to a supraventricular rhythm.

17. Answer: 4 The UAP is qualified to complete simple procedures, such as bathing a client and changing bed linens. While the UAP could possibly administer mouth care to this client, the nurse must assess the oral cavity (option 2) and should be the one to assess tube feeding residual (option 1). UAPs are not trained in therapeutic communication skills and techniques (option 3).
Cognitive Level: Analysis **Client Need:** Safe Effective Care Environment: Management of Care **Integrated Process:** Nursing Process: Implementation **Content Area:** Leadership/Management **Strategy:** The core issue of the question is an appropriate activity to delegate to an unlicensed assistant. Keep in mind that any activity that involves assessment is retained by the RN, so eliminate options 1 and 2. Choose option 4 over 3 because it is procedural in nature.

18. Answer: 3 A client in metabolic acidosis may also be hyperkalemic. As the hydrogen ions shift from the ECF to the ICF, potassium enters the ECF, leading to an increased serum potassium. pH values of < 7.35 are associated with acidosis (option 2). Options 3 and 4 have K^+ levels above 5.5 mEq/ L that are associated with acidosis, but option 3 contains the higher value. Option 1 has a normal pH and serum potassium level.
Cognitive Level: Analysis **Client Need:** Physiological Integrity: Physiological Adaptation **Integrated Process:** Nursing Process Assessment **Content Area:** Adult Health: Endocrine and Metabolic **Strategy:** Note the critical word *acidosis* in the question. Use this to eliminate options 1 and 2 because the pH is not low in either option. Focus on the critical word *metabolic* to pick the option that contains a cation with the highest value since hydrogen ions can enter the cell, which in this case is option 3.

19. Answer: 4 Potassium (KCL) is contraindicated in clients with renal dysfunctions. It can not be filtered out if there is decreased renal filtration. With increased damage in tissues additional potassium is released, causing an even greater level of potassium that can be life-threatening. Encouraging protein, ambulation, and taking vital signs do not safeguard the client from the danger of this potential electrolyte imbalance.
Cognitive Level: Analysis **Client Need:** Physiological Integrity: Reduction of Risk Potential **Integrated Process:** Nursing Process: Implementation **Content Area:** Adult Health: Renal and Genitourinary **Strategy:** *Protein* creates more wastes in the body and the lab shows that the kidneys are not filtering as they should. Additional potassium from protein metabolism may cause death. Activities, such as *ambulation,* will not change the BUN or creatinine since they reflect filtration of the renal system and not the rate of circulation of the blood. *Taking the vital signs every hour* only tells you information about the circulatory status and does not explain or improve the renal function. Action needs to be taken immediately to discontinue the IV with the potassium to minimize the build-up of potassium to toxic levels that could be life-threatening.

20. Answer: 1 In Piaget's theory on development, conservation is a hallmark sign in the concrete operational stage. Options 2, 3, and 4 are not characteristic of this stage.
Cognitive Level: Application **Client Need:** Psychosocial Integrity **Integrated Process:** Nursing Process: Analysis **Content Area:** Mental Health **Strategy:** The core issue of the question is knowledge of characteristics of various cognitive developmental levels according to Piaget. Use this knowledge and the process of elimination to make a selection.

21. Answer: 3 Omeprazole, pantoprazole, and rabeprazole must be swallowed whole. Lansoprazole and esomeprazole capsules may be opened and sprinkled on applesauce or dissolved in 40 mL of juice.
Cognitive Level: Application **Client Need:** Physiological Integrity: Pharmacological and Parenteral Therapies **Integrated Process:** Nursing Process: Planning **Content Area:** Pharmacology **Strategy:** The core issue of the question is knowledge of which medications used for GERD can be opened because they come in capsule form. Use knowledge of pharmacology to answer this question, which tests specific nursing knowledge of drug forms.

22. Answer: 4 It is an RN's responsibility to do assessments, analyze the data, plan and implement care and teaching, and evaluate the outcomes. A second RN needs to be assigned to the nursery to safely manage the care of the Level I newborns.
Cognitive Level: Analysis **Client Need:** Safe Effective Care Environment: Management of Care **Integrated Process:** Nursing Process: Implementation **Content Area:** Leadership/Management **Strategy:** Recognize that assessment and client education are part of the professional scope of practice. The

correct answer would be the option that safely retains these functions for the RN given the change in unit census.

23. **Answer: 3** Anxiety or anger increases peristalsis leading to subsequent diarrhea. Excessive intake of cheese or eggs, ignoring the urge to defecate, and lack of exercise can lead to the development of constipation.
Cognitive Level: Application **Client Need:** Physiological Integrity: Basic Care and Comfort **Integrated Process:** Nursing Process: Implementation **Content Area:** Fundamentals **Strategy:** The core issue of the question is knowledge of ordinary factors that can contribute to diarrhea. Evaluate each of the options in turn and determine whether it is likely to aggravate diarrhea. Note that anxiety and anger stimulate the sympathetic nervous system, which then increases peristalsis; this will help you to choose correctly.

24. **Answer: 2** The normal attitude of the fetal head is one of moderate flexion. Changes in fetal attitude, particularly the position of the head, present larger diameters to the maternal pelvis, which contributes to a prolonged and difficult labor and increases the likelihood of cesarean delivery.
Cognitive Level: Analysis **Client Need:** Health Promotion and Maintenance **Integrated Process:** Nursing Process: Analysis **Content Area:** Maternal-Newborn **Strategy:** The core issue of the question is the significance of moderate flexion of the fetal head. Recognize that changes in the position of the fetal head affect delivery to choose the correct option.

25. **Answer: 3** Mental status changes and concentrated urine are common signs of dehydration in the elderly. Tenting and dry flaky skin are consistent changes seen with normal aging. Hand veins that fill within 3 to 5 seconds and clear lungs sounds with unlabored breathing are normal findings.
Cognitive Level: Application **Client Need:** Physiological Integrity: Physiological Adaptation **Integrated Process:** Nursing Process: Assessment **Content Area:** Adult Health: Cardiovascular **Strategy:** Note the critical words in the question are *not eating or drinking* and *deficit.* With this in mind, look for a physical assessment finding that is consistent with dehydration. Eliminate options 1 and 2 first because of the words *clear* and *dry* respectively. Choose option 3 over 4 recalling that neurological symptoms are often present with altered fluid balance because sodium imbalance may occur simultaneously.

26. **Answer: 4** Liver function includes the regulation of blood clotting and corticosteroids can impair wound healing and irritate the GI tract. Thus, the client should be instructed to report signs and symptoms of bleeding. Option 1 is a side effect of corticosteroids but is not the priority from a physiological basis. Options 2 and 3 do not reflect the associated risk of bleeding with corticosteroid medications.
Cognitive Level: Analysis **Client Need:** Physiological Integrity: Physiological Adaptation **Integrated Process:** Nursing Process: Implementation **Content Area:** Adult Health: Immunological **Strategy:** The core issue of the question is knowledge that the liver is a vascular organ and that some medications used to suppress the immune system to prevent rejection, such as corticosteroids, can lead to bleeding.

27. **Answer: 1** Frequent coughing and deep breathing is an easy maneuver that has great benefit to optimize ventilation in the postoperative client. Good pain management facilitates effective coughing and deep breathing. Getting the client out of bed and administering oxygen and bronchodilators are all appropriate interventions for preventing or treating atelectasis, but clearly the best option is to prevent its occurrence by simple maneuvers such as coughing and deep breathing.
Cognitive Level: Analysis **Client Need:** Physiological Integrity: Physiological Adaptation **Integrated Process:** Nursing Process: Planning **Content Area:** Adult Health: Respiratory **Strategy:** Note the client in the question has newly arrived to the nursing unit following surgery. The critical words "nursing interventions" help you to eliminate options 3 and 4, which require a medical order. Choose option 1 over 2 because of the word "hourly" and because there is not enough information in the stem to determine whether the client can safely get out of bed at this time.

28. **Answer: 4** Children with bipolar disorders are often misdiagnosed as having conduct disorder or ADHD. Intense mood swings (option 1), inflated self-esteem (option 2), and spending sprees (option 3) occur more often in adults.
Cognitive Level: Analysis **Client Need:** Psychosocial Integrity **Integrated Process:** Nursing Process: Assessment **Content Area:** Mental Health **Strategy:** The core issue of the question is knowledge of how bipolar disorders may present in a child that is in early adolescence. Use nursing knowledge and the process of elimination to make a selection.

29. **Answer: 2** The laboratory value given is within normal limits (12–16.5 grams/dL). All the other statements are inaccurate. The client is not malnourished (option 1), at nutritional risk (option 3), and does not have polycythemia (high level) as indicated by option 4.
Cognitive Level: Analysis **Client Need:** Physiological Integrity: Reduction of Risk Potential **Integrated Process:** Nursing Process: Analysis **Content Area:** Adult Health: Hematological **Strategy:** The core issue of the question is knowledge of normal and abnormal hematological laboratory values. Use specific nursing knowledge and the process of elimination to make a selection. Note that option 1 and 3 are somewhat similar so you may eliminate both of those initially.

30. **Answer: 1** Crusting of dried exudate is common with bacterial conjunctivitis and it is important for the child's vision and safety that the crusts are removed. Warm moist wipes aid in comfort and they need to be disposable to reduce the risk of transmitting the infection to others in the home. Oral antihistamines, ophthalmic corticosteroids, and topical anesthetics are not indicated in the management of bacterial conjunctivitis.
Cognitive Level: Application **Client Need:** Physiological Integrity: Physiological Adaptation **Integrated Process:** Teaching and Learning **Content Area:** Child Health: Eye, Ear, Nose and Throat **Strategy:** Note the critical word *conjunctivitis* in the stem of the question. Recall that this infectious is highly contagious. Then determine the correct option by associating the word *disposable* in the correct option with the concept of infection in the stem of the question.

31. **Answer: 2** After the seizure, the client will be postictal, which is a deep sleeping state. She/he could aspirate secre-

tions unless side-lying to promote drainage from the upper airway. Positioning the client on the back (option 1) increases risk of aspiration. Positioning the client on the abdomen (option 3) or upright in chair (option 4) is unrealistic given the client's postictal state.
Cognitive Level: Application **Client Need:** Safe Effective Care Environment: Safety and Infection Control **Integrated Process:** Nursing Process: Implementation **Content Area:** Adult Health: Neurological **Strategy:** The core issue of the question is knowledge of a position that will reduce the risk of aspiration following seizure activity. Use nursing knowledge and the process of elimination to make a selection. Recall that the side-lying position is commonly used in any situation in which aspiration is a risk.

32. **Answer: 1** A client fall is a potential medical emergency; however, the nurse's responsibility is ensuring the safety of the client being attended to. Option 2 ignores the safety of the potentially injured client. Option 3 wastes supplies. Option 4 could lead to a contaminated sterile field.
Cognitive Level: Analysis **Client Need:** Safe Effective Care Environment: Management of Care **Integrated Process:** Nursing Process: Implementation **Content Area:** Leadership/Management **Strategy:** Option 1 and 4 are incorrect, sterile equipment is considered contaminated if left unattended and therefore must be thrown away. Option 2 is incorrect; the nurse needs to prioritize care appropriately. Thus the nurse needs to respond to the client who fell rather than continue with the wound dressing change.

33. **Answer: 4** The American Diabetes Association Exchange Lists divide food into groups with similar content (milk, vegetables, fruit, starch/bread, meat, and fat). All foods within a list are similar in calories, protein, fat, and carbohydrates if eaten in a certain size portion. Foods may be exchanged within the same list. Rice and bread are starches, egg is meat, tomato is vegetable, and orange is fruit.
Cognitive Level: Analysis **Client Need:** Physiological Integrity: Basic Care and Comfort **Integrated Process:** Nursing Process: Evaluation **Content Area:** Foundational Sciences: Nutrition **Strategy:** First recall the basic food groups that are part of the American Diabetes Association Exchange Lists. Then compare each food choice identified with the list. Eliminate options 2 and 3 first as vegetables and fruits, then pick option 4 over 1 because it is a starch/bread.

34. **Answer: 1, 3** Genetic screening can identify markers for several types of cancer. One method to remind men to perform self-checks for cancer is to mark a calendar to check monthly for changes. Self exams as well as regular medical tests and exams uncover tumors. After a total mastectomy, women do not need mammograms. Skin cancer risk increases with age.
Cognitive Level: Application **Client Need:** Health Promotion and Maintenance **Integrated Process:** Teaching and Learning **Content Area:** Adult Health: Oncology **Strategy:** Elimination of number 4 and looking suspiciously at the phrase *most tumors* will help to discriminate between the options. When in doubt, identify alternatives with *most* or *all* in the answer as false.

35. **Answer: 2** The nurse should speak privately to the coworkers about their behavior and the impact on the nurse overhearing them. It does not help the climate of the unit to let it pass (option 1). The nurse is not in a position to confront and reprimand coworkers (option 3). Option 4 is somewhat plausible but option 2 personalizes the discussion between the nurse and the coworkers, and thus is best to diffuse the situation.
Cognitive Level: Application **Client Need:** Safe Effective Care Environment: Management of Care **Integrated Process:** Communication and Documentation **Content Area:** Leadership/Management **Strategy:** Options 1, 3, and 4 are incorrect. To effectively manage conflict between staff members, address the conflict within an appropriate timeframe; do not let it pass unattended. Do not openly and publicly reprimand staff in front of other staff members or clients. Finally, address staff members privately but keep in mind what behavior is acceptable on the unit.

36. **Answer: 2** The student's age, along with symptoms of hair loss and edema indicate that this is not a stage of puberty. The symptoms are not indicated in abuse of barbiturates or marijuana use. By the process of elimination, the correct answer is option 2. In order to answer this correctly you need to have noted the muscular build of the student and know the signs and symptoms of illegal steroid use.
Cognitive Level: Application **Client Need:** Physiological Integrity: Pharmacological and Parenteral Therapies **Integrated Process:** Nursing Process: Analysis **Content Area:** Pharmacology **Strategy:** The core issue of the question is knowledge of adverse effects of steroid use. Use this information and the process of elimination to make a selection.

37. **Answer: 1** The prodomal period refers to the period of time between the initial symptoms and the presence of the full-blown disease. The rash would not be apparent during this time. All the other statements are correct.
Cognitive Level: Analysis **Client Need:** Physiological Integrity: Physiological Adaptation **Integrated Process:** Nursing Process: Evaluation **Content Area:** Child Health: Immunological **Strategy:** The critical words in the stem of the question are *need for additional information.* This tells you that the correct option is an incorrect statement. Use knowledge of this communicable viral infection and the process of elimination to make a selection.

38. **Answer: 2** Adolescents tend to feel that they are invulnerable and that if anything bad will happen, it will affect others but not themselves. They also tend to feel immortal, as it is difficult for them to comprehend their own death. Option 1 is a factor often related to the adult, option 3 is related to school-age children, and option 4 is related to the elderly.
Cognitive Level: Application **Client Need:** Nursing Process: Analysis **Integrated Process:** Safe Effective Care Environment: Safety and Infection Control **Content Area:** Fundamentals **Strategy:** Focus on the developmental level of the client. To answer this question correctly, it is necessary to understand growth and development and apply this knowledge to the needs of the adolescent for safety.

39. **Answer: 3** A full bladder is necessary to bounce the sound waves off to compare other tissues or structures are being

assessed. If done during pregnancy, the fetus must be over 26 weeks to not have the restriction for the full bladder, since the amniotic fluid would be used at that point. It would not be helpful to be NPO, because this would deprive the client of fluids. Enemas and refraining from medications are unnecessary.
Cognitive Level: Application **Client Need:** Physiological Integrity: Reduction of Risk Potential **Integrated Process:** Teaching and Learning **Content Area:** Adult Health: Gastrointestinal **Strategy:** Fluids are needed to fill the bladder and are not withheld prior to testing. Bowel structures do not interfere with the assessment of structures and an enema is not required. Medications do not impact on sound waves and holding medications is not necessary for any reason.

40. **Answer: 2** Children at 10 years of age are egocentric and concerned with themselves. Asking about interests and hobbies is likely to foster establishment of rapport. Focusing on behavioral symptoms (option 1) could lead to an adversarial relationship. Children often are uncomfortable talking about friends and family (option 3) until they get to know a person better. Most children are unconcerned about past medical problems (option 4); they are focused on the here-and-now.
Cognitive Level: Application **Client Need:** Psychosocial Integrity **Integrated Process:** Nursing Process: Assessment **Content Area:** Mental Health **Strategy:** The core issue of the question is knowledge of communication strategies that are likely to be effective in developing a therapeutic relationship. Focus of the age of the child and cognitive developmental level to make a selection.

41. **Answer: 3** Spironolactone is a potassium-sparing diuretic used to treat hypertension. Gynecomastia is one of its adverse reactions. Adverse reactions usually disappear after the drug is discontinued; however, gynecomastia may persist after discontinuing spironolactone.
Cognitive Level: Application **Client Need:** Physiological Integrity: Pharmacological and Parenteral Therapies **Integrated Process:** Teaching and Learning **Content Area:** Pharmacology **Strategy:** The core issue of the question is knowledge of adverse drug effects of spironolactone. Use specific drug knowledge and the process of elimination to make a selection.

42. **Answer: 3** Client and family satisfaction surveys are a formal set of activities that can be used to remedy deficiencies identified in the quality of direct patient care, administrative, and support services. Incident reports (option 1) serve as an indicator of risk. Documentation of time and activities related to direct care may be done as part of time and motion studies. Acuity relates to the need for nursing staff on the unit.
Cognitive Level: Application **Client Need:** Safe Effective Care Environment: Management of Care **Integrated Process:** Nursing Process: Planning **Content Area:** Leadership/Management **Strategy:** Note the critical word *services* in the stem of the question. With this in mind, the correct option is one that gathers data from the recipients of services. Options 1, 2, and 4 are not quality service measures.

43. **Answer: 3** Option 3 is best because it represents a communication with the client and is open-ended. Options 1 and 2 are not the most appropriate initial approaches since the client is not encouraged to share her concerns, although later on in the interaction these may be appropriate. Option 4 ignores the client and does not address the client's concerns.
Cognitive Level: Application **Client Need:** Physiological Integrity: Reduction of Risk Potential **Integrated Process:** Communication and Documentation **Content Area:** Fundamentals **Strategy:** The core issue of the question is the ability of the nurse to care for the emotional needs of a perioperative client. Since this is potentially an anxiety-producing time for clients, choose the option in which the nurse provides a therapeutic response to the client.

44. **Answer: 3** Cigarette smoking is the leading cause of lung cancer. Smokeless tobacco is more often associated with oral cancer. Air pollution may also be a contributing factor to development of lung cancer. History of asthma is not associated with greater risk of lung cancer.
Cognitive Level: Analysis **Client Need:** Health Promotion and Maintenance **Integrated Process:** Nursing Process: Assessment **Content Area:** Adult Health: Respiratory **Strategy:** Eliminate option 1 first because it is a health problem, not a risk factor. From there, choose cigarette smoking over the other options because it is highly associated with lung cancer.

45. **Answer: 3** Foods that reduce lower esophageal sphincter (LES) pressure will increase reflux symptoms. These include coffee, fatty foods, alcohol, chocolate. All the other items can be given to the client.
Cognitive Level: Analysis **Client Need:** Physiological Integrity: Basic Care and Comfort **Integrated Process:** Nursing Process: Analysis **Content Area:** Foundational Sciences: Nutrition **Strategy:** The core issue of the question is knowing that certain types of foods lower LES pressure, and then being able to take it a step further and identify what types of foods those are. Eliminate each option systematically by reasoning that any foods high in fat (such as the cream in the coffee) can have this effect.

46. **Answer: 2** Theophylline is a xanthine that causes bronchial dilation due to smooth muscle relaxation. Increased levels of theophylline occur with liver disease and congestive heart failure. Option 3 is incorrect because the client is young and therefore the age is insignificant. The smoking history (option 1) is not an issue; in fact, smokers metabolize theophylline more quickly and may need increased doses. There is no data about the client's weight (option 4) in the stem.
Cognitive Level: Analysis **Client Need:** Physiological Integrity: Pharmacological and Parenteral Therapies **Integrated Process:** Nursing Process: Analysis **Content Area:** Pharmacology **Strategy:** The core issue of the question is knowledge that adverse effects of xanthine medication such as theophylline are increased in liver disease. Use specific knowledge of drug adverse effects and the process of elimination to make a selection.

47. **Answer: 1, 2, 4, 5** The LPN/LVN is trained to collect data that is then reported to the registered nurse (RN). However, assessment remains the responsibility of the RN. For these reasons, the LPN/LVN can be expected to take vital signs, report drainage, administer medication, and elevate

the casted limb. The RN should retain the responsibility for assessing neurovascular status to the casted extremity in the immediate postoperative period.
Cognitive Level: Analysis **Client Need:** Safe Effective Care Environment: Management of Care **Integrated Process:** Nursing Process: Implementation **Content Area:** Leadership/ Management **Strategy:** Recall that procedures and simple data collection can be delegated to the LPN/LVN. With this in mind, eliminate each of the incorrect options systematically.

48. **Answer: 1** Tuberculosis is a respiratory infection, transmitted via airborne droplet nuclei less than 5 microns in size.
Cognitive Level: Application **Client Need:** Safe Effective Care Environment: Safety and Infection Control **Integrated Process:** Nursing Process: Planning **Content Area:** Fundamentals **Strategy:** Specific knowledge of the mode of transmission of *Mycobacterium tuberculosis* and the types of transmission-based precautions is needed to select the correct answer. Eliminate 2 and 3 as tuberculosis is transmitted via air currents. Choose option 1 over option 4 because tuberculosis is transmitted via airborne droplet nuclei less than 5 microns in size.

49. **Answer: 1** The potassium level is abnormally high (normal 3.5–5.1 mEq/L). Since potassium is an intracellular ion, higher levels will alter the electrical pattern of the EKG. "Peaking of a T wave" is an indication that potassium is too high. With *hyperkalemia* (higher than normal potassium levels), muscle weakness, flaccidity of muscles, diarrhea, abdominal cramping, cerebral irritability/restlessness are present. Therefore, *bowel sounds* would be *hyperactive* and not *silent,* such as with an ileus. Muscles are weak and flaccid, not in a *cramping* state. Cerebral functions are stimulated and *somnolence* (sleeping, sluggishness) is not present.
Cognitive Level: Analysis **Client Need:** Physiological Integrity: Reduction of Risk Potential **Integrated Process:** Nursing Process: Assessment **Content Area:** Adult Health: Cardiovascular **Strategy:** The core issue of the question is accurate interpretation of the potassium level and its significance. From there, associate the symptoms of hyperkalemia to make a selection.

50. **Answer: 3** The client should be NPO before the procedure in order to be given anesthesia for the procedure (option 3 and 4).The client, not the husband, should sign the consent form (option 1). The client should be wearing loose-fitting clothing (option 2).
Cognitive Level: Application **Client Need:** Physiological Integrity: Reduction of Risk Potential **Integrated Process:** Nursing Process: Implementation **Content Area:** Mental Health **Strategy:** The core issue of the question is knowledge that ECT requires anesthesia, which leads to loss of airway protective reflexes. Use this knowledge to reason that the client must be NPO to prevent the risk of aspiration during the procedure.

51. **Answer: 4** Administering very thick preparations such as penicillin G with benzathine (Bicillin LA) can be painful. To lessen the pain, intramuscular injection into a larger gluteal muscle should be administered over 12 to 15 seconds to separate the muscle fibers more gradually. Cold compresses to the injection site would delay absorption of the drug (option 1). Aspiration for blood return with all IM injections is necessary for safety since muscles contain larger blood vessels (option 3). Injection into the deltoid may also result in prolonged discomfort resulting in limited motion of the upper extremities (option 2). Rotating sites, light massage, and warm compress to site may also be employed to limit discomfort.
Cognitive Level: Application **Client Need:** Physiological Integrity: Pharmacological and Parenteral Therapies **Integrated Process:** Nursing Process: Implementation **Content Area:** Pharmacology **Strategy:** The core issue of the question is knowledge of proper administration technique for thick liquid parenteral medications. Use knowledge of intramuscular injection techniques and knowledge of drug absorption principles to make a selection.

52. **Answer: 4** Teaching and assessment are within the domain of the registered nurse (RN) and cannot be delegated to a UAP. The UAP is also not trained in therapeutic communication or counseling techniques. These ancillary caregivers can complete tasks under the supervision and direction of the nurse, and report simple data when asked to do so. With this in mind, the only activity that can be delegated is the simple direction to the client to remain upright after eating.
Cognitive Level: Analysis **Client Need:** Safe Effective Care Environment: Management of Care **Integrated Process:** Nursing Process: Implementation **Content Area:** Adult Health: Gastrointestinal **Strategy:** The core issue of the question is knowledge of the appropriate tasks to delegate to a UAP. Recalling that teaching, counseling and assessment remain the RN's responsibility assists in eliminating each of the incorrect options.

53. **Answer: 1** Clients should remain NPO upon admission to the clinical setting with a major burn. Initial fluid replacement is started via the parenteral route. NPO status is maintained because the client may be in shock with blood flow directed away from the digestive organs to more vital tissues. In addition it is possible that the client suffered burn injuries that could cause internal damage to body structures, and aspiration is also a risk initially. Options 2, 3, and 4 are incorrect—fluids and food via the mouth would be restricted at this time.
Cognitive Level: Application **Client Need:** Physiological Integrity: Basic Care and Comfort **Integrated Process:** Nursing Process: Implementation **Content Area:** Foundational Sciences: Nutrition **Strategy:** The core issue of the question is knowledge that the client who has experienced burn injury is under severe physiological stress, and as such, blood flow is directed away from the digestive tract. Focus on the need to stabilize the client physiologically and provide fluids by the IV route to help you choose correctly.

54. **Answer: 4** Every time a child enters the healthcare system, the immunization status should be checked. Some children have uncertain history of immunization because of parental noncompliance or special circumstances such as being refugees. Once immunization status has been determined, the nurse can go on to assess growth and development and hearing, and to teach the parents about dental care as necessary.

Cognitive Level: Application **Client Need:** Health Promotion and Maintenance **Integrated Process:** Nursing Process: Planning **Content Area:** Child Health: Immunological **Strategy:** The critical word in the stem of the question is *priority.* This tells you that more than one option is likely to be a correct nursing action, but that one is more important than the others. Note the age of the child to help you choose immunizations as the priority, especially noting that the child has not received health care for 2.5 years, during a time when vaccinations should be kept up to date.

55. Answer: 4 The pain in pancreatitis is usually aggravated by lying in a recumbent position, but improved by sitting up and leaning forward or in the fetal position with the knees pulled up to the chest. This position reduces pressure caused by contact of the inflamed pancreas with the posterior abdominal wall.

Cognitive Level: Application **Client Need:** Physiological Integrity: Physiological Adaptation **Integrated Process:** Nursing Process: Implementation **Content Area:** Adult Health: Gastrointestinal **Strategy:** The core issue of the question is knowledge of proper positioning techniques to reduce the pain of inflammation that can be aggravated by movement. Use the process of elimination to select the position in which the pancreas is not as likely to be compressed against other body structures.

56. Answer: 1 Although many chemotherapy agents can cause stomatitis, the antimetabolites are commonly known for causing this side effect. Fluorouracil is the only drug listed in this class. Cisplatin is an alkylating agent; bleomycin is an antitumor antibiotic; and vincristine is a plant (vinca) alkaloid.

Cognitive Level: Analysis **Client Need:** Physiological Integrity: Pharmacological and Parenteral Therapies **Integrated Process:** Nursing Process: Analysis **Content Area:** Pharmacology **Strategy:** The core issue of the question is knowledge of which antineoplastic agents cause stomatitis as an adverse effect. Use nursing knowledge and the process of elimination to answer the question.

57. Answer: 1 Safe and effective delegation is based on knowledge of the laws governing nursing practice and knowledge about job duties and responsibilities. Nurses must understand the competencies and training of unlicensed assistive personnel.

Cognitive Level: Application **Client Need:** Safe Effective Care Environment: Management of Care **Integrated Process:** Nursing Process: Implementation **Content Area:** Leadership/Management **Strategy:** Option 2 is incorrect; it is not necessary to give written directions when delegating tasks to UAPs as long as verbal directions are clear and expectations are understood. Option 3 is incorrect; your responsibility is not preparing the supplies for a delegated task but rather to ensure the delegated task is completed safely and correctly. Option 4 is incorrect; it is not necessary to inform the client about the tasks or assignments delegated to non-staff members. It is however, the responsibility of the staff member to inform the client prior to the assigned task what will be accomplished.

58. Answer: 1 This assessment may be done to detect small changes in muscle strength that might not otherwise be noted. Pronator drift occurs when a client cannot maintain the hands in a supinated position with the arms extended and eyes closed. Nystagmus is the presence of fine, involuntary eye movements. Hyperreflexia is an excessive reflex action. Ataxia is a disturbance in gait.

Cognitive Level: Application **Client Need:** Physiological Integrity: Physiological Adaptation **Integrated Process:** Communication and Documentation **Content Area:** Adult Health: Neurological **Strategy:** Specific knowledge of physical assessment techniques is needed to answer the question. Note the association between the terms *supinated* in the question and *pronator* in the correct answer, in response to the client's change in hand position.

59. Answer: 3 Packing the sample in ice will minimize the changes in gas levels during the transportation of the specimen to the lab. The arterial site should be held for 5 minutes or longer if the client is receiving anticoagulant therapy. The blood is drawn originally in a heparinized syringe and does not need to be transferred to one. A second specimen is not necessary.

Cognitive Level: Application **Client Need:** Physiological Integrity: Reduction of Risk Potential **Integrated Process:** Nursing Process: Implementation **Content Area:** Adult Health: Respiratory **Strategy:** The wording of the question tells you that the correct answer is also a true statement of fact. Eliminate option 1 first as being factually incorrect. Next, eliminate option 2 because the syringe is *heparinized* and the blood is not transferred to a test tube. Finally, eliminate option 4 because it is unnecessary.

60. Answer: 2 For clients with dysthymia, a major concern is social isolation. Option 1 is contraindicated, as is option 3. If the client has a poor appetite, assigning 2 liters of liquid intake (option 4) is not therapeutic, nor is planning three regular meals per day (option 3).

Cognitive Level: Analysis **Client Need:** Psychosocial Integrity **Integrated Process:** Nursing Process: Planning **Content Area:** Mental Health **Strategy:** The core issue of the question is knowledge of strategies to reduce the risk of isolation in a client with dysthymia. Use nursing knowledge and the process of elimination to make a selection.

61. Answer: 3 The effectiveness of a heparin protocol is monitored by trending aPTT results to achieve a therapeutic level. An aPTT of 140 is above the therapeutic level of anticoagulation and therefore the infusion should be stopped per protocol, and resumed at a decreased dose in one hour's time with a repeat aPTT ordered in 2–3 hours per protocol. The dose should not be increased, as this would cause serious consequence to the client. Stopping the medication for a total of 6 hours would undermine the anticoagulation control that the physician is trying to achieve. Ordering another aPTT and continuing to run the infusion could also cause serious consequences to the client.

Cognitive Level: Analysis **Client Need:** Physiological Integrity: Pharmacological and Parenteral Therapies **Integrated Process:** Nursing Process: Implementation **Content Area:** Pharmacology **Strategy:** The core issue of the question is recognition that this is a critically high value for the aPTT and that the action that will maintain client safety is to turn off the heparin for a period of time. Use the process of elimination and knowledge of the effects of heparin on aPTT times to answer the question.

62. **Answer: 1, 3** The UAP can perform tasks or nursing care activities under the direct supervision of the registered nurse (RN). The nurse retains responsibility for assessment (options 2 and 5) and teaching (option 4).
Cognitive Level: Analysis **Integrated Process:** Nursing Process: Implementation **Client Need:** Safe Effective Care Environment: Management of Care **Content Area:** Leadership/Management **Strategy:** The core issue of the question is the ability to discriminate between what the RN may delegate and what he or she may not. Evaluate each option and either choose it because it is a simple procedure or task, or choose not to select it because it involves assessment or teaching.

63. **Answer: 4** The client's right to withdraw consent is necessary to be part of the consent and it means that coercion was not utilized in obtaining the signature. It is the physician's responsibility, not the nurse's, to explain the diagnosis (option 1) and the need for the surgical procedure (option 2). Cost (option 2) is not an important aspect for informed consent. The technical aspects of the procedure are not needed by the client, although an overview of the procedure should be included (option 3), but again this is the role of the physician. All preparation for the procedure should include information about what the client will see, feel, and hear.
Cognitive Level: Analysis **Client Need:** Physiological Integrity: Reduction of Risk Potential **Integrated Process:** Nursing Process: Implementation **Content Area:** Fundamentals **Strategy:** The core issue of the question is knowledge of the nurse's role in obtaining informed consent. Keep in mind that the nurse reinforces explanations already given by the physician and use the process of elimination to make a selection.

64. **Answer: 1** Presentation refers to the part of the fetus that is coming through the cervix and birth canal first. Thus a face presentation occurs when the face is coming through first.
Cognitive Level: Analysis **Client Need:** Health Promotion and Maintenance **Integrated Process:** Teaching and Learning **Content Area:** Maternal-Newborn **Strategy:** Associate the word *face* in the question with the word *face* in the correct response. The word *presentation* helps you to choose option 1 over option 2, which also contains the word *face,* but in an inappropriate context to this question.

65. **Answer:** The correct area is the center stoma, not the distal one that is nearer to the distal colon and rectum. Coming from the small bowel in the center of the diagram, the stomas represent, in anatomical order, an ileostomy, cecostomy, ascending colostomy, transverse colostomy, descending colostomy, and sigmoidoscopy.
Cognitive Level: Analysis **Client Need:** Physiological Integrity: Basic Care and Comfort **Integrated Process:** Teaching and Learning **Content Area:** Adult Health: Gastrointestinal **Strategy:** To answer this question correctly, recall the names of the anatomic portions of bowel. It will also help you to choose correctly if you recall that the prefix *trans* means *across.* This might help you select the stoma that is halfway across the abdomen.

66. **Answer: 2** Children with growth hormone deficiency are smaller than their peers and frequently experience problems with self-esteem and body image. Option 1 would be the opposite problem of what the client is experiencing. The nursing diagnoses in options 3 and 4 are unrelated to the client in this question.
Cognitive Level: Analysis **Client Need:** Physiological Integrity: Physiological Adaptation **Integrated Process:** Nursing Process: Analysis **Content Area:** Adult Health: Endocrine and Metabolic **Strategy:** The core issue of the question is knowledge that deficiency of growth hormone leads to short stature and often disturbed body image in the child. Use nursing knowledge and the process of elimination to make a selection.

67. **Answer: 3, 4** The intermediate care surgical nurse should be most comfortable assuming the care of surgical clients. Heart failure and diabetes are medical problems, and the client with diabetes will also require extensive teaching. The client with nephrolithiasis may also require teaching about the procedure, but since the client will undergo moderate sedation, the nurse would be completing typical preoperative care.
Cognitive Level: Analysis **Client Need:** Safe Effective Care Environment: Management of Care **Integrated Process:** Nursing Process: Implementation **Content Area:** Leadership/Management **Strategy:** Note the critical word *surgical* in the description of the work setting of the float nurse. With this in mind, choose the two clients that have procedures that are surgical in nature.

68. **Answer: 2** Effects of hypomagnesemia are mainly due to increased neuromuscular responses. Paralysis, flaccidity and decreased reflexes may be present with hypermagnesemia.
Cognitive Level: Application **Client Need:** Physiological Integrity: Physiological Adaptation **Integrated Process:** Nursing Process: Evaluation **Content Area:** Adult Health: Neurological **Strategy:** Recall that options that have similarities are not likely to be correct. Examine the options from the viewpoint of neurological stimulation. Eliminate each of the incorrect responses because they reflect abnormally low activity of the nervous system.

69. **Answer: 2** Troponin is a sensitive test that indicates damage to the myocardial cells. A CK-MM isoenzyme elevation would indicate skeletal muscle damage. The LDH^4 isoenzyme is utilized to determine hepatic function and amylase is a digestive enzyme.
Cognitive Level: Application **Client Need:** Physiological Integrity: Reduction of Risk Potential **Integrated Process:** Nursing Process: Assessment **Content Area:** Adult Health: Cardiovascular **Strategy:** Specific knowledge is needed to answer this question. Recall that troponin is a newer enzyme that can be measured very early during myocardial damage and is an indicator of myocardial damage and thus myocardial infarction.

70. **Answer: 2** The client's level of risk for self-harm is a major concern. The client may need a private room (option 1) and

restricted visitors (option 3) if in a manic state. The client should not be overstimulated (option 4).
Cognitive Level: Application **Client Need:** Psychosocial Integrity **Integrated Process:** Nursing Process: Planning **Content Area:** Mental Health **Strategy:** Critical words in the stem of the question are *safety* and *bipolar disorder.* Use nursing knowledge to associate depression as part of bipolar disorder with the threat to safety with suicide as a form of self-harm. This will lead you to the correct answer.

71. **Answer: 4** Ciprofloxacin is not recommended for *Helicobacter pylori* infection during pregnancy. The other medications can be used after consulting with the physician.
Cognitive Level: Application **Client Need:** Physiological Integrity: Pharmacological and Parenteral Therapies **Integrated Process:** Nursing Process: Planning **Content Area:** Pharmacology **Strategy:** The core issue of the question is knowledge of the pregnancy categories of the specific drugs listed. Use the process of elimination to make a selection, realizing that specific drug knowledge is needed to answer the question.

72. **Answer: 2** Trigeminal neuralgia is manifested by spasms of pain that begin suddenly and last anywhere from seconds to minutes. Clients often describe the pain as stabbing or similar to an electric shock. It is accompanied by spasms of facial muscles, which cause closure of the eye and/or twitching of parts of the face or mouth.
Cognitive Level: Application **Client Need:** Physiological Integrity: Physiological Adaptation **Integrated Process:** Nursing Process: Assessment **Content Area:** Adult Health: Neurological **Strategy:** Note the critical word *neuralgia* in the question, which tells you the pain is of nervous system origin. Recalling that this type of pain is usually sharp, stabbing and possibly burning may help you to eliminate some incorrect options. Distinguish between spasm associated with this disorder and paralysis (an opposite finding) to discriminate between options 2 and 4.

73. **Answer: 1** Abuse of laxatives and diuretics is a frequent *purging* behavior for bulimic clients. Options 2 and 3 pertain to anorexia nervosa clients. In regard to option 4, food should never be used as a reward.
Cognitive Level: Application **Client Need:** Physiological Integrity: Basic Care and Comfort **Integrated Process:** Nursing Process: Planning **Content Area:** Foundational Sciences: Nutrition **Strategy:** The critical word in the question is *bulimia.* Recall that this disorder has the classic features of binging and purging to guide you to the correct answer, which in this question is one that signifies agents that help one to purge.

74. **Answer: 3** Lifestyle modifications and recognition of risk factors are important parts of prevention of long-term complications. Family history is a very strong risk factor but encouraging the client to maintain his current lifestyle and following up with health screening would be the best plan of action. False reassurance that he will never be hypertensive and prophylactic antihypertensive medications are inappropriate.
Cognitive Level: Analysis **Client Need:** Health Promotion and Maintenance **Integrated Process:** Communication and Documentation **Content Area:** Adult Health: Cardiovascular **Strategy:** The core issue of the question is lifestyle management to reduce the risk of developing hypertension. Select the option that focuses on prevention while addressing the continued risk that the client faces.

75. **Answer: 4** When a cast is dry, edges that are not smooth or covered by a piece of stockinette should be covered to prevent skin irritation. This can be done by petaling the cast edges with strips of adhesive tape, beginning each strip on the inside of the cast, and folding over the edge to the outside of the cast.
Cognitive Level: Application **Client Need:** Physiological Integrity: Physiological Adaptation **Integrated Process:** Communication and Documentation **Content Area:** Child Health: Musculoskeletal **Strategy:** The wording of the question indicates that the correct response is a true statement. Eliminate options 1 and 3 first as least plausible after visualizing these options, then discard option 2 as unrealistic, since the procedure would be completed at the time of application.

76. **Answer: 3** Immunizations should be withheld during leukemia exacerbations because the immune system is compromised and the client cannot manage an appropriate response to the immunization. There is no need to place the client in isolation without added evidence of immunosuppression (option 1). Options 2 and 4 are irrelevant to the issue of the question.
Cognitive Level: Application **Client Need:** Physiological Integrity: Physiological Adaptation **Integrated Process:** Nursing Process: Planning **Content Area:** Child Health: Immunological **Strategy:** The core issue of the question is knowledge that leukemia adversely affects the immune system. With this in mind, the nurse needs to be mindful that immunizations will need to be withheld during an exacerbation. Use nursing knowledge and the process of elimination to make a selection.

77. **Answer: 1** The RN is responsible for delegating tasks appropriately and is responsible for the actions of unlicensed personnel. Ambulating a postoperative client is the only task from those listed that the RN could delegate to a novice student. The other tasks require higher level assessment and critical thinking skills and should be performed by the RN.
Cognitive Level: Analysis **Client Need:** Safe Effective Care Environment: Management of Care **Integrated Process:** Nursing Process: Implementation **Content Area:** Leadership/Management **Strategy:** Note the critical word *beginning* to describe the student nurse. With this mind, select the delegation assignment that is simple and procedural in nature, and does not require assessment, teaching, or advanced knowledge in nursing.

78. **Answer: 2** The primary organ in the right upper quadrant of the abdominal cavity is the liver. Because of the early shock symptoms, which are presented, it would be expected that this organ has possibly been lacerated, causing extensive uncontrolled internal bleeding. The other organ systems would not be located in this area.
Cognitive Level: Analysis **Client Need:** Physiological Integrity: Physiological Adaptation **Integrated Process:** Nursing Process: Assessment **Content Area:** Adult Health: Gastrointestinal **Strategy:** First analyze the client's vital signs to determine

that the client's status is consistent with a shock state. Then determine which organs are located in the right upper quadrant. Associate the liver, which is a vascular organ, and the location to determine the correct option.

79. Answer: 2 The client will, in most cases, return to the unit with barium still present in the bowel. The physician will order laxatives or enemas if the client is potentially not able to expel the barium on his or her own. The nurse should encourage the client to increase fluid intake if possible as well. This is a common concern for many clients undergoing this procedure, and their feelings should not be ignored or belittled.
Cognitive Level: Analysis **Client Need:** Physiological Integrity: Reduction of Risk Potential **Integrated Process:** Communication and Documentation **Content Area:** Adult Health: Gastrointestinal **Strategy:** Note the critical words *best response* in the stem of the question. This tells you that the correct response is a true statement of fact. Recall that this test can cause constipation from residual barium to aid in selecting the correct option.

80. Answer: 1 The only respectful therapeutic response here is option 1. The others are contraindicated for any group process. Everyone does not need to participate in every session (option 2). It is inappropriate to focus the group's attention on one individual because of level of participation (option 3). The client should be allowed to remain part of the group until the client is ready to participate (option 4).
Cognitive Level: Application **Client Need:** Psychosocial Integrity **Integrated Process:** Communication and Documentation **Content Area:** Mental Health **Strategy:** The core issue of the question is knowledge of group process and conduct of a group meeting. Use knowledge of this treatment modality and the process of elimination to make a selection.

81. Answer: 3 Phenytoin is a first-line anticonvulsant medication that is used to control seizure activity. Selegilene (option 1) is used to treat Parkinson's disease. Diclofenac (option 2) is an NSAID, while sumatriptan (option 4) is used to treat headaches.
Cognitive Level: Application **Client Need:** Physiological Integrity: Pharmacological and Parenteral Therapies **Integrated Process:** Nursing Process: Implementation **Content Area:** Pharmacology **Strategy:** The core issue of the question is knowledge of medications that are effective against seizure activity. Use specific drug knowledge and the process of elimination to make a selection.

82. Answer: 1 After burn injuries, an elevated potassium level (normal 3.5–5.1 mEq/L) is expected because of cellular tissue damage with release of intracellular potassium into the bloodstream. The hematocrit will be elevated (not decreased as in option 4) due to hemoconcentration, and the white blood cell count will be elevated as part of the inflammatory response to injury.
Cognitive Level: Analysis **Client Need:** Physiological Integrity: Physiological Adaptation **Integrated Process:** Nursing Process: Assessment **Content Area:** Adult Health: Integumentary **Strategy:** First visualize what happens when cells are destroyed—intracellular contents are released into the circulation. Secondly, with burn injury fluid is lost through the burn surface and can lead to hemoconcentration. With this in mind, eliminate each option except potassium, which increases for both of the reasons just stated.

83. Answer: 2 In a 2-gram sodium diet, foods high in sodium content should be eliminated. It is not enough to stop adding salt or to go only by taste; clients should also be taught to read food labels for hidden sodium content. Added salt while cooking is allowed in a 4-gram sodium diet, not a 2-gram sodium diet.
Cognitive Level: Analysis **Client Need:** Physiological Integrity: Basic Care and Comfort **Integrated Process:** Nursing Process: Evaluation **Content Area:** Foundational Sciences: Nutrition **Strategy:** The critical words in the question are *low-sodium.* With this in mind, eliminate options 3 and 4 first because they are the least restrictive. Then eliminate option 1 because it is less comprehensive than option 2 and because option 2 addresses other sources of hidden sodium.

84. Answer: 2 Chinese clients may perceive an imbalance in the hot and cold forces in the body after delivery. They will avoid sources of cold, such as wind, cold beverages, and water (even if warmed) to regain a sense of balance between these extremes. A client's culture plays a very important part in who they are, and nurses should respect the client's wishes as long as it will not result in harm to the client or others.
Cognitive Level: Application **Client Need:** Health Promotion and Maintenance **Integrated Process:** Nursing Process: Implementation **Content Area:** Maternal-Newborn **Strategy:** Use principles of culturally competent care to answer this question. If using a multicultural perspective rather than one centered in a Western health care approach, you will be able to eliminate each incorrect response easily.

85. Answer: 3 When a client's level of anxiety markedly increases the nurse can relieve the anxiety by altering the focus of the discussion. Asking the client more details or abruptly stopping the interview will probably increase the client's anxiety level. Asking the client to relax may or may not be effective in reducing the client's anxiety.
Cognitive Level: Application **Client Need:** Psychosocial Integrity **Integrated Process:** Nursing Process: Implementation **Content Area:** Mental Health **Strategy:** The core issue of the question is the ability to recognize escalating anxiety in a client and determining the best means to effectively reduce it. Use knowledge of therapeutic measures for anxious clients and the process of elimination to make a selection.

86. Answer: 4 Option 4 is correct because the client is honest, has an understanding of how to take the medication and what the side effects are, and knows that the side effect will subside eventually. Options 1 and 2 indicate that the client is feeling forced to take the medication but has no desire or understanding of the benefits of the daily routine and dosages. Option 3 indicates that the client has memorized the actions but does not understand the benefits or side effects of the medications.
Cognitive Level: Analysis **Client Need:** Physiological Integrity: Pharmacological and Parenteral Therapies **Integrated Process:** Communication and Documentation **Content Area:** Pharmacology **Strategy:** The core issue of the question is

which statement indicates correct understanding of lithium as a medication. Use specific drug knowledge and the process of elimination to make a selection.

87. **Answer: 2** For 6 hours following intravesicular chemotherapy, the toilet should be disinfected after each use. This will help ensure that the biohazard of excreted chemotherapy drug is contained. The toilet may also be double-flushed. Options 1 and 3 are insufficient, while option 4 is unnecessary and does not address the biohazardous aspect of chemicals remaining in the toilet.
Cognitive Level: Application **Client Need:** Safe Effective Care Environment: Management of Care **Integrated Process:** Nursing Process: Implementation **Content Area:** Adult Health: Oncology **Strategy:** The core issue of the question is how to prevent unintentional exposure of other people to biohazardous chemicals in the client's urine following intravesicular chemotherapy. With this principle in mind, eliminate options 1 and 3 first because they are ordinary measures that do not provide additional protection. Eliminate option 4 next because of the word *sterile.* Clean gloves are needed only.

88. **Answer: 1** It is important that circulation is checked regularly. Typically the restraints are removed, one at a time, every 2 hours to evaluate skin condition and circulation. Although options 3 and 4 are correct, they are not the best response as they do not have to be checked as regularly as the circulation and skin condition. Option 2 applies to an elbow restraint.
Cognitive Level: Application **Client Need:** Safe Effective Care Environment: Safety and Infection Control **Integrated Process:** Nursing Process: Implementation **Content Area:** Child Health **Strategy:** Focus on the work *priority* in the stem of the question. Recalling that many aspects of restraint care are important, use the ABCs (airway, breathing, and circulation) to focus on the correct option—which addresses the child's circulation to the restrained limb.

89. **Answer: 1** Emergency airway and resuscitation equipment should be readily accessible whenever allergy testing is administered because of the potential for hypersensitivity response and anaphylactic reaction. Because of the potential for a serious reaction, the client will be asked to wait in the office for a period of time so he or she can be monitored for any untoward responses. Visibility of the tested areas is important but not immediately essential. The room should be set up prior to the arrival of the client but it is not a priority.
Cognitive Level: Analysis **Client Need:** Physiological Integrity: Reduction of Risk Potential **Integrated Process:** Nursing Process: Planning **Content Area:** Adult Health: Integumentary **Strategy:** Note the critical word *priority* in the stem of the question. This tells you that the correct answer is the most important option and that more than one may be technically correct. Recall that allergic reaction is a risk with skin testing to guide you to the correct answer.

90. **Answer: 3** Symptoms associated with a number of medical conditions are very similar to the symptoms associated with panic attacks. When a medical condition is present, it should be identified and treated. The other options are inaccurate responses to the client's question.
Cognitive Level: Application **Client Need:** Psychosocial Integrity **Integrated Process:** Communication and Documentation **Content Area:** Mental Health **Strategy:** The core issue of the question is knowledge that physiological symptoms need to be ruled out as having a medical basis before they can be attributed strictly to psychological origins. Use this information and the process of elimination to choose correctly.

91. **Answer: 2** Norethindrone (Micronor) contains only progestin and no estrogen. Because estrogen may decrease lactation, progestin-only pills are commonly used in lactating women. The other options do not address the issue of contraception during lactation.
Cognitive Level: Application **Client Need:** Physiological Integrity: Pharmacological and Parenteral Therapies **Integrated Process:** Nursing Process: Assessment **Content Area:** Pharmacology **Strategy:** The core issue of the question is which oral contraceptive is safe to use while breastfeeding. Use knowledge of the estrogen component of norethindrone and the process of elimination to make a selection.

92. **Answer: 1** It is essential that the client's spinal cord be immobilized to prevent further injury and loss of function. Assessing for lacerations, exposure of the client, and performing a full mental status exam are all part of the secondary assessment.
Cognitive Level: Analysis **Client Need:** Nursing Process: Implementation **Integrated Process:** Safe Effective Care Environment: Safety and Infection Control **Content Area:** Adult Health: Neurological **Strategy:** Focus on the critical words *most important.* Whenever a client has suffered a traumatic injury, the nurse must first address the ABCs and then address neurological status and needs. With this in mind, select option 1 over 4 as the priority because it safeguards the client.

93. **Answer: 3** The American Heart Association recommends a diet with reduced saturated fats and cholesterol for clients with coronary artery disease. Canned peaches are high in concentrated sugars, which increase triglyceride levels. Egg yolks are high in cholesterol and whole milk is high in saturated fats. The other options reflect appropriate food selections that are low in saturated fat and cholesterol content.
Cognitive Level: Analysis **Client Need:** Physiological Integrity: Basic Care and Comfort **Integrated Process:** Nursing Process: Evaluation **Content Area:** Foundational Sciences: Nutrition **Strategy:** The wording of the question tells you that the correct answer to the question is the one that contains incorrect items. Correlate the words *coronary artery disease* with fat-containing foods to begin the elimination process. Choose option 3 because it contains eggs and whole milk, two sources of fat and cholesterol.

94. **Answer: 3** The football, or clutch, position provides the mother with more control of the newborn's head and full view of face. The lying-down position is usually done in bed (option 1). The cradle position often causes the newborn's head to wobble around on the mother's arm (option 2). Options 1, 2, and 4 do not allow full view of the infant's face.
Cognitive Level: Application **Client Need:** Health Promotion and Maintenance **Integrated Process:** Nursing Process: Implementation **Content Area:** Maternal-Newborn **Strategy:**

Visualize each of the options and systematically eliminate those that do not promote visualization of the face while maintaining control of the head.

95. Answer: 1 PEA is associated with what appears to be a normal electrical conduction pattern but there is no mechanical pumping of the myocardium. Ventricular fibrillation, ventricular tachycardia, and asystole will not demonstrate an effective electrical conduction pattern on the cardiac monitor.
Cognitive Level: Application **Client Need:** Physiological Integrity: Physiological Adaptation **Integrated Process:** Nursing Process: Assessment **Content Area:** Adult Health: Cardiovascular **Strategy:** Associate the words *unable to palpate* in the stem of the question with the word *pulseless* in the correct option. Otherwise, it is necessary to understand the pathophysiology involved in this question.

96. Answer: 3 To promote absorption, the client should not blink for 30 seconds after the administration of dipivefrine. Options 1, 2, and 4 are incorrect for the administration of dipiveprine.
Cognitive Level: Application **Client Need:** Physiological Integrity: Pharmacological and Parenteral Therapies **Integrated Process:** Teaching and Learning **Content Area:** Pharmacology **Strategy:** The core issue of the question is knowledge of proper administration technique for dipivefrine. Use specific drug knowledge and the process of elimination to make a selection.

97. Answer: 1 Pediatric clients can be diagnosed with diabetes and the float nurse should be familiar with this health problem and could do client teaching. The nurse is not as likely to have recent experience in working with clients with Guillain-Barré syndrome or who have had prostate gland surgery. The client with dementia who is being transferred will require transfer paperwork to be completed, and the pediatric nurse may not be as familiar with these types of forms because of the pediatric population usually worked with.
Cognitive Level: Analysis **Client Need:** Safe Effective Care Environment: Management of Care **Integrated Process:** Nursing Process: Implementation **Content Area:** Adult Health: Endocrine and Metabolic **Strategy:** Review the diagnoses of each of the possible clients and choose the one that the pediatric nurse is most likely to have experience working with.

98. Answer: 3 Pulmonary edema occurs as a result of fluid shifts caused by the ingestion of the hypertonic salt water. The result is fluid collecting in the interstitial spaces causing pulmonary edema. Hypoxia, hypovolemia, and acidosis occur as a result of near-drowning incidents.
Cognitive Level: Application **Client Need:** Physiological Integrity: Physiological Adaptation **Integrated Process:** Nursing Process: Analysis **Content Area:** Adult Health: Respiratory **Strategy:** Note the critical words *salt water* and consider concepts and dynamics of fluid movement in the body. Because of the hypertonic water entering the client's lungs, envision that the client's own body fluid would move into the alveoli to equalize the tonicity.

99. Answer: 1 A positive TB test means that the organism is present in the body in either an active or a dormant state. It should not be ignored nor should further testing be deferred for several months. The client can expect to be scheduled for sputum tests for the presence of the bacillus and a chest x-ray to determine the presence of lesions or active disease. Medications and isolation are not instituted until a probable or definitive diagnosis has been made.
Cognitive Level: Application **Client Need:** Physiological Integrity: Reduction of Risk Potential **Integrated Process:** Communication and Documentation **Content Area:** Adult Health: Respiratory **Strategy:** Note the presence of the critical word *best.* This tells you that the correct answer is a true statement of fact. Use knowledge of this test and the process of elimination to make a selection.

100. Answer: 1 Speaking slowly and softly reduces stress-related emotions. Instructing the clients to ignore the behavior will not assist them in reducing anxiety. A client experiencing severe or panic anxiety will be unable to focus on identifying behaviors of anxiety. Reminding a client of the need to use good manners when talking with other clients ignores the client's anxiety and may only increase the symptoms of anxiety.
Cognitive Level: Application **Client Need:** Psychosocial Integrity **Integrated Process:** Nursing Process: Implementation **Content Area:** Mental Health **Strategy:** The core issue of the question is knowledge of therapeutic communication techniques with a client whose anxiety is escalating. Select the option that is most likely to have a calming effect on the client from a behavioral perspective.

101. Answer: 2 Jaundice in the dark-skinned client can best be observed by assessing the hard palate. Normally fat may be deposited in the layer beneath the conjunctivae that can reflect as a yellowish hue of the conjunctivae and the adjacent sclera in contrast to the dark periorbital skin. In these clients, palms and soles may appear jaundiced, but calluses on the surface of their skin can also make the skin appear yellow.
Cognitive Level: Application **Client Need:** Physiological Integrity: Pharmacological and Parenteral Therapies **Integrated Process:** Nursing Process: Assessment **Content Area:** Pharmacology **Strategy:** The core issue of the question is how to assess for jaundice in a client with dark skin. Keep in mind that the oral cavity is a good choice to help guide you to a correct response.

102. Answer: 2, 1, 4, 3 The nurse should assess first the client who has the low platelet count (normal 150,000–450,000/mm^3), and then the client who has the borderline low WBC count, because these represent greater and then lesser threat to physiological status. From there, the nurse should answer the questions for the client going for chemotherapy, and finally see the client who is upset so that the nurse can plan to spend time with this client.
Cognitive Level: Analysis **Client Need:** Safe Effective Care Environment: Management of Care **Integrated Process:** Nursing Process: Planning **Content Area:** Adult Health: Oncology **Strategy:** Remember that physiological needs take priority over psychosocial and learning needs. Choose the client with the most serious physiological need first (which is the client with the most abnormal labs) followed by the other client with a physiological concern. Then use time as a

means of setting priorities for the remaining clients, since the client who is in psychological distress would benefit from greater interaction time with the nurse.

103. Answer: 3 A client with GERD should limit (or possibly eliminate) the intake of coffee because this can relax LES pressure and lead to symptoms. The other options would not be warranted because all would contribute to the development of symptoms: large meals, spicy foods (extra garlic), and peppermint (which would relax LES pressure).
Cognitive Level: Application **Client Need:** Physiological Integrity: Basic Care and Comfort **Integrated Process:** Nursing Process: Planning **Content Area:** Foundational Sciences: Nutrition **Strategy:** Recall that coffee, chocolate, and fatty foods lower LES pressure and therefore increase the risk of reflux. Knowing that these types of food choices need to be limited help guides you to select option 3. As an alternative, eliminate options that would aggravate symptoms, which in this case are options 1, 2, and 4.

104. Answer: 3 The child should be included in planning for the new baby. Children may feel threatened by a new sibling and so may need extra time and attention. Parents should avoid putting too much responsibility on the child.
Cognitive Level: Application **Client Need:** Health Promotion and Maintenance **Integrated Process:** Communication and Documentation **Content Area:** Maternal-Newborn **Strategy:** Use knowledge of growth and development principles and communication skills to make a selection. The correct answer is the option that includes the needs of the child as a client as well as the parents.

105. Answer: 3 The pH is elevated, HCO_3 is elevated, and $PaCO_2$ is low. This indicates that there is a mixed respiratory and metabolic alkalosis. Clients with pneumonia are prone to develop respiratory alkalosis. Option 1 is incorrect because the HCO_3^- level alone would be decreased. Options 2 and 4 are incorrect because the ABG values do not reflect these conditions.
Cognitive Level: Analysis **Client Need:** Physiological Integrity: Physiological Adaptation **Integrated Process:** Nursing Process: Analysis **Content Area:** Adult Health: Respiratory **Strategy:** Note the critical word *pneumonia* in the question. With this in mind, reason that the disorder is likely to be respiratory in origin, which allows you to eliminate options 1 and 2. Choose option 3 over 4 because the high pH is associated with alkalosis.

106. Answer: 3 A client at risk for nausea should not lie down for at least 30 minutes after meals to avoid aspiration. The physician should be notified of excessive weight loss (option 1). Foods and beverages are better tolerated when they are neither hot nor cold (option 2). Option 4 is a good client action if other measures fail (option 4).
Cognitive Level: Analysis **Client Need:** Physiological Integrity: Pharmacological and Parenteral Therapies **Integrated Process:** Nursing Process: Evaluation **Content Area:** Pharmacology **Strategy:** The core issue of the question is knowledge of factors that will relieve or aggravate nausea caused by cancer chemotherapeutic agents. Use knowledge of the effect of gravity upon digestion as well as general measures of managing nausea to make a selection.

107. Answer: 3 The movement of the fluid, also referred to as tidaling, in the water indicates normal lung expansion. The physician should not be called unless the movement ceases. Coughing will increase the movement and repositioning the chest tube will have no effect on the oscillation.
Cognitive Level: Analysis **Client Need:** Physiological Integrity: Physiological Adaptation **Integrated Process:** Nursing Process: Assessment **Content Area:** Adult Health: Respiratory **Strategy:** To answer this question it is necessary to have a basic understanding of chest tube function. Beyond that, note the critical word *slight* in the stem of the question, which helps to eliminate option 1. Eliminate option 4 because it is not within the scope of nursing practice. Choose option 3 over 2 because there is no reason to ask the client to cough.

108. Answer: 2 According to standard precautions, the caregiver should wear goggles when contamination from splashing is possible, as when the membranes are artificially ruptured (amniotomy). The other options place the nurse at risk for contamination from skin contact, necessitating the use of gloves.
Cognitive Level: Analysis **Client Need:** Safe Effective Care Environment: Safety and Infection Control **Integrated Process:** Nursing Process: Planning **Content Area:** Maternal-Newborn **Strategy:** The core issue of the question is knowledge of when to use various personal protective equipment items. Recall that amniotomy refers to rupture of the amniotic membrane and then reason that this could involve splash and require the use of goggles.

109. Answer: 4 The normal calcium level is 9.0–11.0 mg/dL, making this client hypercalcemic. Muscle weakness is a key feature of hypercalcemia due to alterations in excitable membranes. This occurs as a complication in some clients with cancer. Peaked T waves, muscle spasm, and increased gastric motility are signs of hyperkalemia.
Cognitive Level: Analysis **Client Need:** Physiological Integrity: Reduction of Risk Potential **Integrated Process:** Nursing Process: Planning **Content Area:** Adult Health: Oncology **Strategy:** The core issue of the question is knowledge of electrolyte imbalance (hypercalcemia in this case) and the associated manifestations. Recall that calcium plays a key role in nervous system function to help guide you to the correct option.

110. Answer: 2 Anxiety can be a healthy protective response to an actual threat. Defense mechanisms are unconscious psychological responses designed to diminish or delay anxiety. Anxiety, at times, cannot be avoided and is a healthy adaptive reaction when it alerts the person to impending threats.
Cognitive Level: Analysis **Client Need:** Psychosocial Integrity **Integrated Process:** Nursing Process: Evaluation **Content Area:** Mental Health **Strategy:** The core issue of the question is knowledge that anxiety can exist to a greater or lesser state at any given time, and that some anxiety may be helpful as it increases alertness and performance. Use this background knowledge to select the correct option.

111. Answer: 2 Apresoline is a vasodilator and if the client becomes dehydrated, hypotension will result. In other words, during dehydration both preload and afterload are reduced, causing the *tank* to get larger with less volume. The

normal dose of hydralazine is 5 to 25 mg PO. Serum potassium is high but unrelated to apresoline. The increased heart rate is a reflexive response to the low cardiac output to compensate with decreased preload and afterload.
Cognitive Level: Application **Client Need:** Physiological Integrity: Pharmacological and Parenteral Therapies **Integrated Process:** Nursing Process: Assessment **Content Area:** Pharmacology **Strategy:** The core issue of the question is knowledge of factors that will compound or worsen a low blood pressure in a client taking an antihypertensive medication. Recall that factors that cause vasodilation or reduce the circulating volume (such as dehydration) can cause a drop in blood pressure. Use the process of elimination to systematically discard options that do not have this causative influence.

112. **Answer: 4** In a client whose condition is deteriorating, the RN should delegate the task that is most procedural in nature (in this case the urinary catheter). The LPN is able to collect data to report to the RN, but in a client whose acuity is changing, it is better for the RN to make the assessments (option 2). The RN should also insert the IV line and immediately administer the IV medication.
Cognitive Level: Analysis **Client Need:** Safe Effective Care Environment: Management of Care **Integrated Process:** Nursing Process: Implementation **Content Area:** Adult Health: Cardiovascular **Strategy:** Use knowledge of the principles of delegation. Eliminate the options that address IV and IV medication, because these should be retained by the RN. Choose the catheter over vital signs because the RN would need to interpret the significance of the vital signs, not merely measure them.

113. **Answer: 1** Older clients need time to digest the information and ask questions. Option 2 is incorrect because most older clients are able to make decisions for themselves. Option 3 can be considered coercion, while option 4 can be appropriate but is not the best option since clients need more than reading material for an informed consent.
Cognitive Level: Application **Client Need:** Physiological Integrity: Reduction of Risk Potential **Integrated Process:** Nursing Process: Implementation **Content Area:** Fundamentals **Strategy:** The core issue of the question is the need for the older adult undergoing surgery to have sufficient time to process information. Choose the option that takes into consideration age-related changes of older adults.

114. **Answer: 4** To begin life, the infant must make the adaptations to establish respirations and circulation. These two changes are crucial to life. All other body systems become established over a longer period of time (options 1, 2, 3).
Cognitive Level: Analysis **Client Need:** Health Promotion and Maintenance **Integrated Process:** Nursing Process: Assessment **Content Area:** Maternal-Newborn **Strategy:** Use the ABCs—airway, breathing, and circulation—as the strategy for answering this question.

115. **Answer: 2** The eggs provide 24 grams of protein and the whole milk adds calories. The other options are lower in protein and calories. A client recovering from burns requires a high-protein, high-calorie diet. Option 1 does not reflect an adequate protein source. Option 3 reflects an increased carbohydrate source and bacon is considered a fat, not protein. Option 4 does not reflect a high-protein, high-calorie meal but rather a low-calorie meal selection with a greater carbohydrate content.
Cognitive Level: Analysis **Client Need:** Physiological Integrity: Basic Care and Comfort **Integrated Process:** Nursing Process: Evaluation **Content Area:** Foundational Sciences: Nutrition **Strategy:** First recall that clients with burn injury need to take in foods that are high in protein and calories. With this in mind, compare each option against this need to eliminate each of the incorrect options systematically.

116. **Answer: 1** Signs of overdosage of desmopressin, an antidiuretic hormone, include blood pressure and pulse elevation, mental status changes, and water and sodium retention. Because the medication therapy needs to be interrupted, the nurse should notify the physician. Option 2 would place the client at risk because of lack of timely treatment. Options 3 and 4 would not address the current complication.
Cognitive Level: Analysis **Client Need:** Physiological Integrity: Pharmacological and Parenteral Therapies **Integrated Process:** Nursing Process: Implementation **Content Area:** Pharmacology **Strategy:** The core issue of the question is knowledge that fluid retention is an adverse drug effect and that this client is showing signs of excessive drug therapy. Use drug knowledge and the process of elimination to answer the question.

117. **Answer: 2, 5** Simple activities and nursing procedures can be delegated to the UAP. For this client, this would include ambulation and documentation of intake and output. The RN retains responsibility for assessment, teaching and counseling the client. For this reason, the nurse should not delegate assessment of the skin at the treatment site, patterns of fatigue, or how the client is coping with the diagnosis and treatment.
Cognitive Level: Analysis **Client Need:** Safe Effective Care Environment: Management of Care **Integrated Process:** Nursing Process: Implementation **Content Area:** Adult Health: Oncology **Strategy:** Recall that the RN does not delegate assessment, teaching and counseling and evaluate each of the options in relation to these guidelines.

118. **Answer: 4** Visual difficulty caused by distortions and impairment of central vision is common with macular degeneration. Peripheral vision in most cases is normal. The symptoms are not characteristic of glaucoma (loss of peripheral vision), cataracts (gradual deterioration of vision with opacity of lens), or detached retina (sudden change in vision with a sense of a curtain falling over the field of vision).
Cognitive Level: Application **Client Need:** Physiological Integrity: Physiological Adaptation **Integrated Process:** Nursing Process: Analysis **Content Area:** Adult Health: Eye and Ear **Strategy:** Specific knowledge of the various visual disorders is needed to answer the question. Eliminate options 2 and 4 first because of the client's description. Then choose correctly from the remaining two options because of the nature of the disorder.

119. **Answer: 1** An ultrasound is the only noninvasive procedure listed. The others require swallowing (option 2) or injecting (option 4) contrast, or insertion of an endoscope (option 3).

Cognitive Level: Application **Client Need:** Physiological Integrity: Reduction of Risk Potential **Integrated Process:** Teaching and Learning **Content Area:** Adult Health: Gastrointestinal **Strategy:** The core issue of the question is knowledge of noninvasive diagnostic tests for the gastrointestinal system. Eliminate each of the incorrect options because of the words or suffixes *swallow* in option 2, *-oscopy* in option 3, and *contrast* in option 4. These all imply that the test will be intrusive to the body.

120. **Answer: 2** When a client with a somatization disorder does not receive symptom relief, anxiety increases (as evidenced by her current symptoms). Although the client may experience pain, hopelessness, and disturbed body image, the major issue is anxiety.

Cognitive Level: Analysis **Client Need:** Psychosocial Integrity **Integrated Process:** Nursing Process: Planning **Content Area:** Mental Health **Strategy:** The core issue of the question is the ability to determine that the basis for the client's agitation is anxiety. The critical words in the stem of the question are *somatization disorder.* Review this topic area if this question was difficult.

121. **Answer: 1** Bismuth-containing preparations, such as Pepto-Bismol, can cause all the listed side effects, but transient darkening of the tongue and stool is a specific side effect to bismuth.

Cognitive Level: Application **Client Need:** Physiological Integrity: Pharmacological and Parenteral Therapies **Integrated Process:** Nursing Process: Assessment **Content Area:** Pharmacology **Strategy:** The critical word in the stem of the question is *unique.* With this in mind, use the process of elimination and knowledge of drug components to determine which side effect is caused by bismuth. As an alternative strategy, select option 1 because it is the only one that is located in the very upper GI tract.

122. **Answer: 1** Acute episodes are characterized by bulky, frothy stools and steatorrhea because of malabsorption, anorexia, and irritability. The client would not exhibit increased appetite (option 2), vomiting (option 3), or soft formed stools (option 4).

Cognitive Level: Application **Client Need:** Physiological Integrity: Physiological Adaptation **Integrated Process:** Nursing Process: Assessment **Content Area:** Child Health: Gastrointestinal **Strategy:** The core issue of the question is the manifestations of celiac disease that occur because of the underlying pathophysiology. Recall that this disorder is characterized by malabsorption of key nutrients to help eliminate incorrect options.

123. **Answer: 1** Regular exercise can help to normalize bowel function. Cigarette smoking and gum chewing increase swallowed air; fresh vegetables are gas-producing.

Cognitive Level: Analysis **Client Need:** Physiological Integrity: Basic Care and Comfort **Integrated Process:** Nursing Process: Evaluation **Content Area:** Adult Health: Gastrointestinal **Strategy:** Use knowledge of healthy lifestyle habits that stimulate normal bowel function as a means of answering this question. Eliminate options 2 and 3 first as least helpful in health promotion. Choose option 1 over 4 because excessive fresh fruits and vegetables could aggravate irritable bowel syndrome.

124. **Answer: 4** The embryo's muscles spontaneously contract beginning at 7 weeks. The mother perceives sensations of movement of the fetus from 16 to 20 weeks gestation. A primigravida usually perceives movement closer to 20 weeks.

Cognitive Level: Application **Client Need:** Health Promotion and Maintenance **Integrated Process:** Communication and Documentation **Content Area:** Maternal-Newborn **Strategy:** The core issue of the question is knowledge of fetal growth and development. An easy way to remember this information is to equate 4 weeks to be one month and then remember movements are felt at 4 to 5 months (16 to 20 weeks).

125. **Answer: 1** A double-diapering technique will help to protect a urinary stent following repair of hypospadias or epispadias. The inner diaper collects the infant's stool, while the outer one collects urine.

Cognitive Level: Application **Client Need:** Physiological Integrity: Physiological Adaptation **Integrated Process:** Teaching and Learning **Content Area:** Child Health **Strategy:** The core issue of the question is the rationale for a specific diapering technique following surgery to correct hypospadias. Eliminate option 2 first as least realistic and choose the correct option after determining which option best reflects safety considerations and protection of the surgical area.

126. **Answer: 1** An inspiratory stridor is indicative of a hypersensitivity reaction to the DPT immunization and epinephrine should be administered to counteract the symptoms of the allergic response. Options 2 and 3 are irrelevant, and option 4 places the infant at risk for injury or death.

Cognitive Level: Application **Client Need:** Physiological Integrity: Pharmacological and Parenteral Therapies **Integrated Process:** Nursing Process: Implementation **Content Area:** Pharmacology **Strategy:** The core issue of the question is recognition that stridor following immunization is a sign of hypersensitivity to the drug. With this in mind, use the process of elimination to select option 1 as the answer, since epinephrine is the drug treatment of choice.

127. **Answer: 4** To coach is to give direction and suggestions for improvement. Option 4 illustrates this concept. Option 1 is threatening rather than coaching. Option 2 is a criticism without a suggestion for improvement. Option 3 is helpful as a statement of positive reinforcement but does not specifically give direction for future actions.

Cognitive Level: Analysis **Client Need:** Safe Effective Care Environment: Management of Care **Integrated Process:** Communication and Documentation **Content Area:** Leadership / Management **Strategy:** The critical word in the stem of the question is *coach.* Use the ordinary definition of the word and choose the option that gives suggestions or advice to improve performance.

128. **Answer: 3** The nurse would determine that the client understood the information if the client stated rubella is transmitted by the droplet route. Clients with rubella are placed in droplet precautions, as the causative agent is transmitted by particle droplets larger than 5 microns. The other responses are factually incorrect.

Cognitive Level: Application **Test Plan:** Safe Effective Care Environment: Safety and Infection Control **Integrated Process:** Nursing Process: Implementation **Content Area:** Adult Health: Immunological **Strategy:** Knowledge about the transmission of rubella and the elements of each type of transmission-based precautions is required. Select an option based on nursing knowledge.

129. Answer: 2 A pH of 7.6 indicates an alkalotic state. The administration of bicarbonate would be the best answer. Anaerobic metabolism and the production of lactic acid lead to an acidotic state, explaining why blood gases drawn during a code usually show acidosis. This pH is not within normal limits.

Cognitive Level: Analysis **Client Need:** Physiological Integrity: Reduction of Risk Potential **Integrated Process:** Nursing Process: Evaluation **Content Area:** Adult Health: Respiratory **Strategy:** First recall that a pH of 7.6 is alkalotic to eliminate options 1 and 3. Next eliminate option 4 because the result is not normal. Alternatively associate the high pH with the drug sodium bicarbonate, which raises pH.

130. Answer: 2 Characteristics of a client with pain disorder include believing there is a physical cause for distress when there is no organic basis, the need to use analgesics or drugs to reduce pain, and impaired role performance.

Cognitive Level: Analysis **Client Need:** Nursing Process: Assessment **Integrated Process:** Psychosocial Integrity **Content Area:** Mental Health **Strategy:** The critical words in the stem of the question are *anticipate* and *pain disorder.* With this in mind, determine that the core issue of the question is characteristics that are compatible with this disorder. Use nursing knowledge and the process of elimination to make a selection.

131. Answer: 1 The client must understand the medication information as a priority item. Option 2 is a false statement. Effective medication dosing should control seizure activity (option 4). Teaching that urine may turn pink to brown may be included if appropriate, but is not the highest priority.

Cognitive Level: Application **Client Need:** Physiological Integrity: Physiological Adaptation **Integrated Process:** Nursing Process: Planning **Content Area:** Adult Health: Neurological **Strategy:** The critical words in the stem of the question are *highest priority.* This tells you that more than one option may be factually correct and that you must choose the most important item. Recall that insufficient drug therapy may lead to seizure recurrence to help you select appropriately.

132. Answer: 2, 5 The child with the low white blood cell count (normal 5,000–10,000/mm^3) and the child receiving chemotherapy are at risk for infection and could be cohorted together because they should both be on neutropenic precautions. The child who underwent appendectomy should be separated from the children with viral encephalitis and scarlet fever. The children with infections should not be cohorted because one is viral (encephalitis) and one is bacterial (scarlet fever) in origin.

Cognitive Level: Analysis **Client Need:** Safe Effective Care Environment: Management of Care **Integrated Process:** Nursing Process: Implementation **Content Area:** Leadership/Management **Strategy:** Examine the clients in the question and determine similarities and differences among them. The two that are the most similar and that have the most similar needs from an infection control perspective are the ones who should be placed together.

133. Answer: 4 A client who is HIV-positive (regardless of sex) is likely to lose weight due to repeated cycle of wasting and malnutrition. The client, who may be unable to merely increase caloric intake, should be instructed in dietary techniques that maximize quality of intake. Option 1 is incorrect—even though a food diary would provide pertinent information, the response allows for a delay in treatment that could result in further weight loss for the client. The priority is to intervene early on to prevent the onset of wasting. Option 2 is incorrect because it provides the client with a false belief that fluid retention changes associated with the menstrual cycle may have an impact on nutritional status. Option 3 is incorrect—even though increased salt in the diet can lead to fluid retention and weight, it does not address the underlying issue of nutritional balance.

Cognitive Level: Analysis **Client Need:** Physiological Integrity: Basic Care and Comfort **Integrated Process:** Nursing Process: Implementation **Content Area:** Foundational Sciences: Nutrition **Strategy:** Analyze each of the options and choose the one that has the most direct and positive impact on weight gain. Using this strategy, you can systematically eliminate each of the incorrect options.

134. Answer: 4 Rationale: Polypharmacy is using multiple doctors and multiple pharmacies to get the health care needed often from a variety of specialists. The overall problem is that different doctors may not know what other doctors had ordered. Some drugs may interact with others and others may be the same drug in a different form. Overdosing and interactions become more common with this problem.

Cognitive Level: Analysis **Client Need:** Health Promotion and Maintenance **Integrated Process:** Nursing Process: Assessment **Content Area:** Pharmacology **Strategy:** Although taking medications on one's own in combination with prescriptive meds can lead to problems, a greater problem is the polypharmacy issue. Sharing meds is also done in some adults when they want to assist another by offering them a medication that helped in their case. Financial issues may come into play as adults share meds, but this is also a smaller issue than polypharmacy. Taking the medications as ordered will not increase the risk of complications; it should reduce that risk.

135. Answer: 4 Placing the client with ARDS in a prone position allows for expansion of the posterior chest wall, which may be effective in enhancing oxygenation. Transfusing red blood cells or albumin does not increase oxygenation in ARDS. Option 3 should have been done as an initial measure.

Cognitive Level: Application **Client Need:** Physiological Integrity: Physiological Adaptation **Integrated Process:** Nursing Process: Implementation **Content Area:** Adult Health: Respiratory **Strategy:** The core issue of the question is an intervention that may increase oxygenation in a client with ARDS. Note the critical words *nursing intervention* to eliminate options 1 and 2, which require a physician's order. Choose option 4 over 3 because it allows for expansion of the back side of the client's lungs, and redistribution of blood flow using gravity.

136. **Answer: 3** Because ACE inhibitors can cause fetal harm or death, they should be discontinued as soon as pregnancy is detected. Its effect on breastfeeding infants is unknown. The effect of other medications is unknown during pregnancy.
Cognitive Level: Application **Client Need:** Physiological Integrity: Pharmacological and Parenteral Therapies **Integrated Process:** Teaching and Learning **Content Area:** Pharmacology **Strategy:** The core issue of the question is knowledge that ACE inhibitors need to be avoided during pregnancy because they are harmful to the fetus. Use knowledge of drug therapy and the process of elimination to make a selection.

137. **Answer: 2** The pediatric intensive care nurse is more likely to have experience working with heart failure, since children can experience heart failure secondary to cardiac defects. Myocardial infarction, stent placement, and coronary atherectomy are problems and procedures done for adult clients.
Cognitive Level: Analysis **Client Need:** Safe Effective Care Environment: Management of Care **Integrated Process:** Nursing Process: Implementation **Content Area:** Leadership/Management **Strategy:** Note the critical words *pediatric intensive care* in the stem of the question. Then determine which client has the health problem that could also be experienced in the pediatric population.

138. **Answer: 1** The priority nursing intervention is one that maintains contact of the retina with the choroid by positioning the client so the detached area falls against the choroid. It is unnecessary to darken the client's immediate environment. A preoperative medication may be ordered, but has lesser priority than maintaining proper position of the head to protect the eye. Both eyes, not just the affected eye, are patched to minimize eye movement.
Cognitive Level: Analysis **Client Need:** Safe Effective Care Environment: Safety and Infection Control **Integrated Process:** Nursing Process: Implementation **Content Area:** Adult Health: Eye and Ear **Strategy:** The critical words in the question are *actions* and *first.* This indicates that more than one option may be correct but that one is more important than the others. Use knowledge of pathophysiology to make the correct selection.

139. **Answer: 3** Loss of potassium caused by vomiting and diarrhea, in addition to lack of replacement intake, will lead to a risk for hypokalemia (normal range is 3.5–5.1 mEq/L). Calcium levels (normal 9–11 mg/dL) are not affected by vomiting and diarrhea and the sodium level (normal 135–145 mEq/L) will be elevated with the loss of potassium.
Cognitive Level: Analysis **Client Need:** Physiological Integrity: Reduction of Risk Potential **Integrated Process:** Nursing Process: Analysis **Content Area:** Adult Health: Gastrointestinal **Strategy:** Critical words in the question are *vomiting and diarrhea.* With this in mind, recall that potassium may be lost from the GI tract. Eliminate option 2 first because it is within normal range, and then eliminate the calcium levels as less relevant to the question than potassium.

140. **Answer: 1** The client who has many physical complaints with no organic basis is not conscious of conflicts and stressors, and is, therefore, unable to use other means to cope with anxiety. There is no evidence of impaired adjustment or verbal communication. Nothing in the stem of the question specifically states that the client is in pain.
Cognitive Level: Analysis **Client Need:** Psychosocial Integrity **Integrated Process:** Nursing Process: Planning **Content Area:** Mental Health **Strategy:** A key phrase is *many physical complaints* and a critical word is *priority.* With these in mind, use the process of elimination to select the nursing diagnosis that is compatible with the client information as stated. It is important not to read into the question.

141. **Answer: 2** Epinephrine is a beta-adrenergic agent that that has beta 1 adrenergic action, causing increased heart rate and increased force of myocardial contraction. The results of subcutaneous epinephrine should be seen in 5 minutes. The effects may last up to 4 hours. The other options are incorrect.
Cognitive Level: Application **Client Need:** Physiological Integrity: Pharmacological and Parenteral Therapies **Integrated Process:** Nursing Process: Planning **Content Area:** Pharmacology **Strategy:** The core issue of the question is knowledge of the timeframe for the onset of action with epinephrine. Use specific drug knowledge and the process of elimination to make a selection.

142. **Answer: 1** Glycosylated hemoglobin is elevated due to long-term hyperglycemia. Values greater than 8 percent indicate consistently poor control of blood glucose and the need to assess the client's dietary pattern for the past several months in relation to the treatment plan. The other options do not apply.
Cognitive Level: Analysis **Client Need:** Physiological Integrity: Physiological Adaptation **Integrated Process:** Nursing Process: Implementation **Content Area:** Adult Health: Endocrine and Metabolic **Strategy:** Recall that this test is a general indicator of diabetic control over several weeks. With this in mind, eliminate options 2 and 3 first. Choose option 1 over 4 because it relates to long-term control, not immediate control.

143. **Answer: 4** Sjögren's syndrome is an autoimmune disease that destroys exocrine glands in the body, and leads to a generalized "dryness" of body systems. The restriction of fluids is a concern because the use of fluids helps to keep the oral cavity moist. There is no information to suggest that the client has a need for fluid restriction due to other disease processes so this order should be clarified. All of the other options are reasonable for this client.
Cognitive Level: Analysis **Client Need:** Physiological Integrity: Basic Care and Comfort **Integrated Process:** Nursing Process: Planning **Content Area:** Foundational Sciences: Nutrition **Strategy:** To answer this question correctly, it is necessary to know the underlying pathophysiology of Sjögren's syndrome. From there, analyze each of the options that could exacerbate or worsen the underlying disease state.

144. **Answer: 2** An android pelvic structure is narrow in both the anterior-posterior diameter and the lateral diameter, and can cause a prolonged labor with a large fetus or a malpositioned fetus.

Cognitive Level: Application **Client Need:** Health Promotion and Maintenance **Integrated Process:** Nursing Process: Analysis **Content Area:** Maternal-Newborn **Strategy:** First determine the significance of the critical word *android* in the stem of the question. Eliminate options 3 and 4 first because they relate least to risks during labor caused by bone structure. Choose option 2 over 1 because the prefix *andr-* refers to males and from there determine that it indicates a narrower pelvis.

145. Answer: 1 Physical exercise, within the client's ability level, reduces muscle tension and pain. Additionally, exercise creates a feeling of greater self-efficacy. Verbal expression of conflicts and minimal use of analgesics are also indicated. Complete bedrest would not be indicated unless required by incapacitating conditions, but there is no evidence that this is the case in this question.
Cognitive Level: Application **Client Need:** Psychosocial Integrity **Integrated Process:** Nursing Process: Implementation **Content Area:** Mental Health **Strategy:** Note that critical words in the question are *chronic pain* and *cope.* This indicates that the correct answer is an activity that will help the client tolerate the pain to a greater extent. Eliminate options 3 and 4 first as most extreme, and then choose option 1 over 2 because of the physiological benefits.

146. Answer: 4 Confusion and increased heart rate are signs of toxicity or adverse side effects of hydroxyamphetamine. Stinging, headache, and brow ache are usual side effects of hydroxyamphetamine.
Cognitive Level: Analysis **Client Need:** Physiological Integrity: Pharmacological and Parenteral Therapies **Integrated Process:** Nursing Process: Evaluation **Content Area:** Pharmacology **Strategy:** The core issue of the question is knowledge of adverse drug effects. Use specific drug knowledge and the process of elimination to make a selection.

147. Answer: 3 Shared governance is based on the philosophy that nursing practice is best determined by nurses. Option 1 represents standard nursing practice. Option 2 is unrelated to governance. Option 4 represents leadership input into decision-making for the organization.
Cognitive Level: Application **Client Need:** Safe Effective Care Environment: Management of Care **Integrated Process:** Nursing Process: Analysis **Content Area:** Leadership/Management **Strategy:** The critical words in the question are *shared governance.* Choose the option that gives the best evidence of some kind of sharing.

148. Answer: 4 The employee should limit the amount of time in the client's room to minimize exposure. In option 1, the employee is wearing the correct combination of personal protective equipment. In option 3, the employee has followed the correct procedure for exiting the client's room. Equipment required for the care of the isolation client should remain in the client's room to limit exposure to other clients on the nursing unit.
Cognitive Level: Application **Test Plan:** Safe Effective Care Environment: Safety and Infection Control **Integrated Process:** Nursing Process: Evaluation **Content Area:** Adult Health: Respiratory **Strategy:** The wording of the question indicates that something was done incorrectly. Use the process of elimination after noting that options 1, 2, and 3 are correct actions. Only option 4 identifies an incorrect action.

149. Answer: 3 Eosinophils are responsible for responding to allergic reactions. Neutrophils and monocytes are primary responders to infection and tissue injury and inflammation. Lymphocytes assist in immune responses.
Cognitive Level: Application **Client Need:** Physiological Integrity: Reduction of Risk Potential **Integrated Process:** Nursing Process: Assessment **Content Area:** Adult Health: Immunological **Strategy:** The core issue of the question is knowledge of the various components of the WBC differential and their significance. Specific knowledge is needed to answer the question so take time to review if you have the need.

150. Answer: 1 All family members are affected by dissociative identity disorder. Children must also find ways to understand and deal with what is occurring to a parent, rather than denying what is obvious or proceeding on incorrect assumptions that are not challenged by accurate information.
Cognitive Level: Analysis **Client Need:** Psychosocial Integrity **Integrated Process:** Communication and Documentation **Content Area:** Mental Health **Strategy:** The core issue of the question is an understanding of the purposes and benefits of family therapy. Use knowledge of family dynamics to choose the correct answer.

151. Answer: 4 A serum specimen for peak level is drawn 15 to 30 minutes after IV administration to test for toxicity. Trough drug levels are drawn just prior to administration of the next IV dose to measure whether satisfactory therapeutic levels are being maintained. If the peak is too high, toxicity can occur and the dose needs to be reduced and/or the frequency of administration extended. If the trough is too low, then the dosage and/or frequency of administration need to be increased.
Cognitive Level: Analysis **Client Need:** Physiological Integrity: Pharmacological and Parenteral Therapies **Integrated Process:** Nursing Process: Analysis **Content Area:** Pharmacology **Strategy:** The core issue of the question is the ability to draw correct conclusions about the significance of serum drug level results. Focus on the words *just prior to* in the stem of the question, which tells you that it is the trough level that is being described. With this in mind, use the process of elimination to find the conclusion that is true of a need to collaborate about the trough level.

152. Answer: 1 Potatoes, tomatoes, and oranges have a high level of potassium content. The others have lesser amounts of potassium in them, when considering the groupings of foods in each option.
Cognitive Level: Application **Client Need:** Physiological Integrity: Physiological Adaptation **Integrated Process:** Nursing Process: Implementation **Content Area:** Child Health: Renal and Genitourinary **Strategy:** The core issue of the question is knowledge of foods that are high in potassium. Eliminate options 3 and 4 first because of the carbonated beverages and sugars, respectively. Choose option 1 over 2 because these foods have a greater potassium content.

153. Answer: 4 A client who receives a diagnosis of SLE will be profoundly affected by the chronic nature of this autoimmune disease process. The establishment of a healthcare team using a multidisciplinary approach will help the client to identify and realize individual goals. Even though the initiation of advance directives is important, it is not the priority concern at this point in time—there is no information provided to suggest that the client requires immediate activation of advance directives. Even though it is important to discuss the progressive effects of the disease, the priority is to establish a multidisciplinary team to assist the client. Option 3 is incorrect—telling the client to limit her work pattern may not be financially feasible or physically indicated at this time.

Cognitive Level: Analysis **Client Need:** Physiological Integrity: Physiological Adaptation **Integrated Process:** Nursing Process: Planning **Content Area:** Adult Health: Immunological **Strategy:** The core issue of the question is what are initial priorities of care when a client is diagnosed with a chronic illness in which the client's condition is expected to worsen over time. With this in mind, choose the option that calls together the interdisciplinary team so that the client has the fullest range of resources at hand.

154. **Answer: 2** Allowing independence as long as possible gives dignity and self-worth to clients. Option 1 is not helpful because it does not foster independence within the scope of remaining abilities. Option 3 could result in harm to the parents. Option 4 could be degrading and does not foster maintaining independence within limits of current ability.
Cognitive Level: Application **Client Need:** Health Promotion and Maintenance **Integrated Process:** Teaching and Learning **Content Area:** Fundamentals **Strategy:** Completely taking over all aspects of an adult's life does not give value or worth to those adults, especially if done too prematurely. Allowing them to do whatever they want to do may not be safe for them and harm may be done despite saving some self-esteem. Financial issues are the most worrisome issues that must be dealt with, and taking them over also removes the independence of the client. A plan of care needs to be clarified when the adult is thinking clearly and can delegate or make an advanced directive.

155. **Answer: 1** One of the major functions of the placenta is provision of nutrients to the fetus across the placenta membrane. An interference with the placenta circulation, such as abruptio placentae, impairs this ability. Another important function is removing metabolic waste from the fetus. While this takes place metabolically the fetus produces and excretes urine independently of the placenta. Hydrops is gross fetal edema related to hemolytic action, not placenta dysfunction. Anomalies usually occur in the first trimester when organogenesis occurs.
Cognitive Level: Application **Client Need:** Physiological Integrity: Physiological Adaptation **Integrated Process:** Teaching and Learning **Content Area:** Maternal-Newborn **Strategy:** To answer this question correctly, it is necessary to recall the function of the placenta to deliver oxygen and nutrients to the fetus. Focus on the critical word *partial* to aid in selecting the correct option.

156. **Answer: 3** Clients who are taking cholestyramine (which is a bile resin) should be monitored for fat soluble vitamin deficiencies (vitamins A, D, E, and K), as the gastrointestinal side effects of the medication can lead to reduced absorption. Niacin, thiamine, folic acid, cyanocobalamin, and vitamin C (options 1, 2, and 4) are all examples of water-soluble vitamins.
Cognitive Level: Application **Client Need:** Physiological Integrity: Pharmacological and Parenteral Therapies **Integrated Process:** Nursing Process: Assessment **Content Area:** Pharmacology **Strategy:** The core issue of the question is knowledge that cholestyramine places the client at risk for deficiency of fat-soluble vitamins. Use the process of elimination and reason that this answer is correct because the action of cholestyramine is to bind onto cholesterol (fat) and prevent its absorption into the GI tract.

157. **Answer: 3** Clients with less complex and more common diagnoses are selected for case management. The clients in the remaining options have problems that are more likely to have variation in their conditions (options 1 and 2) or have a less common diagnosis (option 4).
Cognitive Level: Analysis **Client Need:** Safe Effective Care Environment: Management of Care **Integrated Process:** Nursing Process: Analysis **Content Area:** Leadership/Management **Strategy:** Focus on the critical words *case management.* Use the common definition of this method to eliminate each option systematically.

158. **Answer: 2** The client in the photograph is receiving oxygen through a Venturi mask. Oxygen administered by a Venturi mask can be regulated to deliver between 24% and 50%, which is a benefit for clients who require higher oxygen supplement without mechanical ventilation. The Venturi mask does not prevent rebreathing of carbon dioxide, as does a non-rebreather mask. Oxygen concentration of 100% would be administered to COPD clients only in rare circumstances via mechanical ventilation.
Cognitive Level: Application **Client Need:** Physiological Integrity: Basic Care and Comfort **Integrated Process:** Nursing Process: Analysis **Content Area:** Adult Health: Respiratory **Strategy:** Specific knowledge is needed to answer the question. Reflect on the various modes of oxygen delivery and note that this type of device can be regulated easily because it is a mask and because the percentage of oxygen can be manipulated easily.

159. **Answer: 1** MRI is the only diagnostic examination listed that does not possibly require the ingestion or administration of contrast or radioactive material. Options 2 and 4 involve the use of contrast dyes or agents, while option 3 uses a radioisotope.
Cognitive Level: Application **Client Need:** Physiological Integrity: Reduction of Risk Potential **Integrated Process:** Communication and Documentation **Content Area:** Adult Health: Immunological **Strategy:** The core issue of the question is knowledge of which tests do and do not require use of some form of contrast media. With this in mind, eliminate each of the incorrect options using basic knowledge of diagnostic tests. Take time to review this material if you had difficulty selecting.

160. **Answer: 4** Fugue states are characterized by wandering or moving away from one's familiar place with an amnesia for the complete past, including self. The person often assumes

a new identity for the duration of the fugue. Amnesia is simply a loss of memory owing to brain damage or to severe emotional trauma. Akathisia is an abnormal condition characterized by restlessness and agitation. Confabulation is replacement of gaps in memory with imaginary information.
Cognitive Level: Analysis **Client Need:** Psychosocial Integrity **Integrated Process:** Nursing Process: Analysis **Content Area:** Mental Health **Strategy:** The core issue of the question is the ability to correctly interpret a client's behavior as characteristic of a fugue state. Use knowledge of characteristics of this mental health disorder and the process of elimination to make a selection.

161. Answer: 1 Lidocaine is given via IV push in doses of 1 to 1.5 mg/kg. The initial loading dose (bolus) is intended to achieve adequate blood levels to suppress ventricular dysrhythmias and is followed by an infusion of 1 to 4 mg/min via infusion pump. The initial bolus lasts approximately 10 minutes so the infusion must not be delayed. The dose may be repeated 1 time under certain conditions, but the total dose should not exceed 3mg/kg. Oral therapy and pacemaker insertion are not indicated at this time.
Cognitive Level: Application **Client Need:** Physiological Integrity: Pharmacological and Parenteral Therapies **Integrated Process:** Nursing Process: Planning **Content Area:** Pharmacology **Strategy:** The core issue of the question is knowledge of therapeutic protocols for intravenous antidysrhythmic medications such as Lidocaine. Use drug knowledge and the process of elimination to answer the question.

162. Answer: 2 The nurse should delegate the activity that is procedural in nature, which is within the scope of training of the UAP. The nurse does not delegate teaching (options 1 and 3) or interventions for chest pain (option 4).
Cognitive Level: Analysis **Client Need:** Safe Effective Care Environment: Management of Care **Integrated Process:** Nursing Process: Implementation **Content Area:** Leadership/Management **Strategy:** Keep in mind the principles of delegation. Recall that the nurse does not delegate assessment, teaching, or medication administration to a UAP.

163. Answer: 2 A client who is recovering from Guillain-Barré syndrome will need a diet that promotes positive nitrogen balance in order to counteract the effects of long periods of immobility on the body. Option 1 is incorrect—there is no evidence to support that the client is experiencing malabsorption at this time. Option 3 is incorrect because there is no clinical reason to limit fresh fruit. Even though the client may experience difficulty in chewing and swallowing, this is usually in the acute phase of the disease process. There is nothing to suggest that the client is experiencing problems in this area or is at risk for aspiration (option 4).
Cognitive Level: Application **Client Need:** Physiological Integrity: Basic Care and Comfort **Integrated Process:** Nursing Process: Planning **Content Area:** Foundational Sciences: Nutrition **Strategy:** The key words in the stem of the question are *general rehabilitative care.* This tells you that the client has no specific deficits that would affect nutritional status. With this in mind, choose the option that promotes the best nutrition for this client. Avoid reading into the question.

164. Answer: 4 A healthy 30-year-old has the greatest risks of safety related to lifestyle behaviors: multiple sexual partners, "on the edge" lifestyle (thrill seekers), haphazard dietary intake, speeding, not sleeping enough.
Cognitive Level: Application **Client Need:** Health Promotion and Maintenance **Integrated Process:** Nursing Process: Planning **Content Area:** Fundamentals **Strategy:** Cancers of the breast, uterus, lung, or prostate are not the mindset of a 30-year-old. This problem is the center of thinking for the older adult. Bone density testing for osteoporosis is often not recommended nor tested for the female in her thirties. Most women will test for this near menopause.

165. Answer: 1 All of these nursing diagnoses are appropriate for the client with COPD; however, the primary alteration is related to impaired gas exchange because of the abnormal blood gas results. The breathing pattern is satisfactory because the rate is within normal limits, and there is no data to support activity intolerance, although it is plausible. The client is at risk for infection but actual problems take priority over potential ones.
Cognitive Level: Analysis **Client Need:** Physiological Integrity: Physiological Adaptation **Integrated Process:** Nursing Process: Planning **Content Area:** Adult Health: Respiratory **Strategy:** Compare the data in the question and use that as a means of selecting the priority nursing diagnosis.

166. Answer: 4 Graves' disease is caused by elevated levels of thyroid hormone. Clients experience tachycardia, nervousness, insomnia, increased heat production, and weight loss. Medication therapy with an agent such as propylthiouracil will help control the disorder. Option 1 is irrelevant, while option 2 is indicated for hypothyroidism. A client with this disorder does not need insulin, because the pancreas is not affected by Graves' disease (option 3).
Cognitive Level: Analysis **Client Need:** Physiological Integrity: Pharmacological and Parenteral Therapies **Integrated Process:** Teaching and Learning **Content Area:** Pharmacology **Strategy:** The core issue of the question is that Graves' disease is characterized by excessive function of the thyroid gland. From there, you need to determine which medication will reduce the function of the thyroid. Eliminate options 1 and 3 as irrelevant first, then choose option 4 over 2 by its action.

167. Answer: 2 A client with right hemisphere stroke has left-sided paralysis or paresis and may have unilateral neglect. The UAP should keep all items on the right side so that the client is aware they exist in the environment.
Cognitive Level: Analysis **Client Need:** Safe Effective Care Environment: Management of Care **Integrated Process:** Nursing Process: Evaluation **Content Area:** Adult Health: Neurological **Strategy:** Recall that the manifestations of stroke appear on the opposite side of the body from the lesion. Use this principle to eliminate the incorrect responses after eliminating actions that are carried out correctly.

168. Answer: 2 Transmission-based precautions are required for all these organisms. Only penicillin-resistant *Streptococcus pneumoniae* is transmitted via respiratory droplets. The organisms specified in options 1, 3, and 4 are transmitted by direct contact.

Cognitive Level: Analysis **Client Need:** Safe Effective Care Environment: Safety and Infection Control **Integrated Process:** Nursing Process: Assessment **Content Area:** Adult Health: Respiratory **Strategy:** Knowledge of droplet precautions is necessary to answer the question. Penicillin-resistant *Streptococcus pneumoniae* suggests a microorganism that causes a type of pneumonia. Clients with pneumonia have increased respiratory secretions and coughing. Using the process of elimination, choose the microorganism that sounds as though it would cause a respiratory infection—option 2.

169. **Answer: 1** HDL is felt to be a beneficial lipoprotein because of its protective function against coronary artery disease. An elevation in this level is healthy and indicates compliance with diet and exercise recommendations. LDL and HDL are fractions of the total cholesterol level. Triglycerides and LDL have proven to be major contributors to and predictors of coronary artery disease, making elevations in all three remaining options threats to cardiovascular health in the future.

Cognitive Level: Analysis **Client Need:** Physiological Integrity: Reduction of Risk Potential **Integrated Process:** Nursing Process: Assessment **Content Area:** Adult Health: Cardiovascular **Strategy:** The core issue of the question is knowledge of which lipid levels should be raised and lowered to achieve cardiovascular health. Recall that HDL has the letter *H* and associate this with the word *healthy* to make the positive association between these.

170. **Answer: 3** When the client realizes the connection between stress, anxiety, and dissociation, he becomes able to modify his stressors or his response to them, thus preventing the dissociative process. The other responses in options 1, 2, and 4 do not reflect this concept.

Cognitive Level: Analysis **Client Need:** Psychosocial Integrity **Integrated Process:** Nursing Process: Evaluation **Content Area:** Mental Health **Strategy:** The core issue of the question is the ability to recognize triggers to a dissociative state. Recall that stress and anxiety can trigger this state to make the appropriate selection.

171. **Answer: 3** Anticipatory prevention of nausea with antiemetics is effective if medication is taken 30 to 60 minutes before any activity causing nausea. The other options indicate incorrect timeframes.

Cognitive Level: Application **Client Need:** Physiological Integrity: Pharmacological and Parenteral Therapies **Integrated Process:** Nursing Process: Assessment **Content Area:** Pharmacology **Strategy:** The core issue of the question is knowledge of how soon to take medication prior to activities that cause nausea. Recall that many oral drugs act in 30 to 60 minutes to help you make a selection.

172. **Answer: 3** The client who had a hemorrhagic stroke and has a headache could be about to have another bleed. Headache is a classic sign with intracranial bleed, and a second bleed carries a higher mortality rate than the first. The other clients have less severe needs that can be attended to after the client who is at risk for a fatal complication is seen.

Cognitive Level: Analysis **Client Need:** Safe Effective Care Environment: Management of Care **Integrated Process:** Nursing Process: Implementation **Content Area:** Adult Health: Neurological **Strategy:** When trying to decide priorities among clients who are acutely ill, it may help to analyze the complications each is at risk for or the consequences that could result from the current condition or complaint. The client with the most serious issue or who could experience the most severe complication is the one that takes priority.

173. **Answer: 1** Contaminated foods are not a source of HIV/AIDS infection. While contaminated foods may cause GI symptoms and food poisoning due to various etiologic agents, they do not cause the transmission of this disease. The nurse should clarify this statement by the client in order to provide accurate information. All of the other client statements reflect information that is appropriate for the management of client with HIV/AIDS.

Cognitive Level: Application **Client Need:** Physiological Integrity: Basic Care and Comfort **Integrated Process:** Physiological Integrity: Basic Care and Comfort **Content Area:** Foundational Sciences: Nutrition **Strategy:** The critical word in the stem of the question is *clarify.* This tells you that the correct answer is an incorrect statement on the part of the client. Use nursing knowledge and the process of elimination to make a selection.

174. **Answer: 1** The RN is responsible for delegating tasks appropriately and is responsible for the actions of unlicensed employees. Ambulating a postoperative client is the only task that the RN could delegate from those listed. The other tasks require higher level assessment and critical thinking skills and should be performed by the RN.

Cognitive Level: Analysis **Client Need:** Safe Effective Care Environment: Management of Care **Integrated Process:** Nursing Process: Implementation **Content Area:** Leadership/Management **Strategy:** Use principles of delegation and select the care activity that is the simplest and requires the least amount of high-level judgment, especially since the level of the student is not identified.

175. **Answer: 2** The presence of a halo effect indicates cerebrospinal fluid (CSF). Glucose present in the nasal drainage also suggests that the drainage is CSF. A persistent headache indicates a CSF leak. The physician needs to be informed of these assessment findings and the client must be maintained on bedrest to stop the leak. A spinal tap may be done to decrease CSF pressure. Option 1 is incorrect because it does nothing for the client. Options 3 and 4 do not address the real problem, a probable CSF leak.

Cognitive Level: Analysis **Client Need:** Physiological Integrity: Physiological Adaptation **Integrated Process:** Nursing Process: Implementation **Content Area:** Adult Health: Endocrine and Metabolic **Strategy:** To answer this question correctly, analyze the significance of the findings. Eliminate each of the incorrect responses systematically after noting that a risk after this type of surgery is CSF leak.

176. **Answer: 3** Hydroxyzine hydrochloride is an antihistamine that is a competitive inhibitor of the H_1 receptor. It is used to treat various reactions that are mediated by histamine. It will decrease the pruritus produced by the release of hista-

mine. Cimetidine is an H_2 histamine antagonist and these agents are not effective against hypersensitivity reactions. Lorazepam is a short-acting benzodiazepine that is indicated for anxiety. Bupivacaine is a local anesthetic for nerve blocks.
Cognitive Level: Analysis **Client Need:** Physiological Integrity: Pharmacological and Parenteral Therapies **Integrated Process:** Nursing Process: Planning **Content Area:** Pharmacology **Strategy:** The core issue of the question is knowledge of which drug relieves itching. Use specific drug knowledge and the process of elimination to make a selection.

177. Answer: 1, 4 The UAP can perform procedures and nursing care activities. Client care that requires assessment (options 2, 3, and 5) are not within the scope of the functions of the UAP.
Cognitive Level: Analysis **Client Need:** Safe Effective Care Environment: Management of Care **Integrated Process:** Nursing Process: Implementation **Content Area:** Adult Health: Eye and Ear **Strategy:** Recall that UAPs are trained and educated to perform simple care procedures. Use this framework to eliminate each of the incorrect options systematically.

178. Answer: 4 With exophthalmos, the eyelids may not cover and protect the cornea of the eye. Thus, eye protection from the sheets or preventing the hands from accidentally touching the eyes is needed while the client is in bed. With Graves' disease, clients usually experience heat intolerance, thus less covering and a cool room are preferred (option 1). Hyperglycemia is not usually associated with Graves' disease. The head of the bed should be elevated 30 degrees to minimize eye pressure (option 3).
Cognitive Level: Analysis **Client Need:** Safe Effective Care Environment: Management of Care **Integrated Process:** Nursing Process: Implementation **Content Area:** Leadership/Management **Strategy:** The core issue of the question is which need of the client with Graves disease can be met by the UAP. The need of the client with respect to eye safety can be met using ordinary nursing procedures, so this is the task that may be delegated to the UAP with education.

179. Answer: 3 Most chemotherapeutic agents cause some degree of bone marrow suppression. This results in a decrease in leukocyte and erythrocyte counts, both components of a hematology testing. Calcium, phosphorus, and serum PSA levels are not specifically affected by bone marrow suppression. The calcium level could change because of the underlying bone cancer, and this in turn could affect phosphorus, but this is not the focus of the question.
Cognitive Level: Analysis **Client Need:** Physiological Integrity: Reduction of Risk Potential **Integrated Process:** Nursing Process: Assessment **Content Area:** Adult Health: Oncology **Strategy:** The critical word in the question is *priority.* With this in mind, you need to determine which lab value has greatest importance in terms of monitoring. The core issue of the question is bone marrow suppression, which could affect production of red blood cells, white blood cells, and platelets. Choose the option that best correlates with this risk.

180. Answer: 2 All of the options are dissociative responses. However, only localized amnesia is the inability to recall events in a circumscribed time period.
Cognitive Level: Analysis **Client Need:** Psychosocial Integrity **Integrated Process:** Nursing Process: Assessment **Content Area:** Mental Health **Strategy:** Focus on the critical words *expected* and *localized amnesia.* These words indicate that the correct option is one that is consistent with what is assessed in this state. Focus on the word *localized* in the question and the time-bound nature of option 2 to choose correctly.

181. Answer: 3 Option 3 is correct because it acknowledges the client's feelings and addresses his concerns while still allowing him to make decisions for his present and future. Options 1 and 2 disregard and negate the client's feelings. Option 4 acknowledges his concern but takes away his decision-making options by having someone else (the nurse) make a plan for his daily activities, rather than have him participate and make decisions for himself with help.
Cognitive Level: Application **Client Need:** Psychosocial Integrity **Integrated Process:** Communication and Documentation **Content Area:** Mental Health **Strategy:** The best answer to communication questions is to choose the response that addresses the client's issue or concern. Use the process of elimination and this principle of communication to make a selection.

182. Answer: 1 Fluid and electrolyte replacement is the highest priority. Hyperglycemia is treated with regular insulin rather than NPH insulin (option 3). Concurrent administration of IV regular insulin would also be done as a priority. The items in the other options can be done after definitive treatment for dehydration is done.
Cognitive Level: Analysis **Client Need:** Physiological Integrity: Physiological Adaptation **Integrated Process:** Nursing Process: Planning **Content Area:** Adult Health: Endocrine and Metabolic **Strategy:** To answer this question correctly, it is necessary to understand the underlying pathophysiology. Determining that dehydration is a key issue will help you to focus on rehydration. Attend to regular care measures and monitoring after acute manifestations have been addressed.

183. Answer: 3 Malnutrition is seen as a consequence of the HIV/AIDS virus because the disease process has a progressive effect on client's nutritional status. Option 1 is incorrect—even clients who are asymptomatic may already have nutrient deficiencies and could be experiencing subclinical signs of malnutrition. Option 2 is incorrect because wasting syndrome occurs early in the disease process; current clinical research states that the maintenance and preservation of nutritional status is a priority in the clinical management of this condition. Option 4 is incorrect—clients can experience vitamin and mineral deficiencies early on during the disease process.
Cognitive Level: Application **Client Need:** Physiological Integrity: Basic Care and Comfort **Integrated Process:** Teaching and Learning **Content Area:** Foundational Sciences: Nutrition **Strategy:** The wording of the question tells you that the correct answer is a true statement of fact. Use nursing knowledge and the process of elimination to make a selection.

184. Answer: 3 Bladder and sphincter weakness are normal with the aging process. Decreased tolerance to spicy foods also is reflected by decreased acidity and motility of the digestive processes that are common in the aging process. Circulatory instability can occur when getting up too quickly since the vasoconstriction process of the legs can be slower as one ages. Also dehydration can also lead to slight dizziness when moving about. Increasing the process of isolation from others is not a healthy adaptation although it is common when one spouse dies that the other seems totally lost since most events include whole couples rather than newly singled again individuals.
Cognitive Level: Analysis **Client Need:** Health Promotion and Maintenance **Integrated Process:** Nursing Process: Assessment **Content Area:** Fundamentals **Strategy:** Understanding the expected changes at the various age brackets will allow you to anticipate what is within the normal range of changes and what is not.

185. Answer: 1 Clients who are diagnosed with a personality disorder most frequently perceive their personality patterns as ego-syntonic or a natural part of themselves rather than as ego-dystonic (option 3). This is one reason it is difficult to motivate individuals with personality disorders to try to change their maladaptive behavioral patterns. Individuals with personality disorders display problems living rather than clinical symptoms. Personality disorders are associated with concomitant disorders including substance abuse.
Cognitive Level: Application **Client Need:** Psychosocial Integrity **Integrated Process:** Nursing Process: Analysis **Content Area:** Mental Health **Strategy:** The core issue of the question is the ability to discriminate among various types of mental health disorders using DSM-IV criteria. Use this knowledge and the process of elimination to make a selection.

186. Answer: 2 Calcium channel blockers should be administered with a high-fat meal; grapefruit should be avoided before and after dosing due to its ability to alter drug effects. The foods listed in the other options will not have a dose-altering effect.
Cognitive Level: Application **Client Need:** Physiological Integrity: Pharmacological and Parenteral Therapies **Integrated Process:** Nursing Process: Implementation **Content Area:** Pharmacology **Strategy:** The core issue of the question is knowledge that grapefruit juice affects the availability of some drugs, such as calcium channel blockers, because of their action on enzyme systems. Use this knowledge and the process of elimination to make a selection.

187. Answer: 4 Tachycardia, hypertension, and tachypnea increase stroke volume and tissue demand for oxygen, leading to increased cardiac workload and possible heart failure. If fluid volume deficit is present, there is an additional risk for decreased cardiac output. There is insufficient data to determine fluid volume status. The tachypnea is a symptom of the increased metabolic rate.
Cognitive Level: Analysis **Client Need:** Physiological Integrity: Physiological Adaptation **Integrated Process:** Nursing Process: Analysis **Content Area:** Adult Health: Endocrine and Metabolic **Strategy:** Recall that physiological needs take priority over psychosocial needs. Also remember that the ABCs (airway, breathing, and circulation) are of highest priority in many cases.

188. Answer: 1 Equipment for client care is dedicated to the client on contact precautions and kept in the client's room. Any other action does not uphold principles of infection control.
Cognitive Level: Application **Integrated Process:** Nursing Process: Implementation **Client Need:** Safe Effective Care Environment: Safety and Infection Control **Content Area:** Adult Health: Integumentary **Strategy:** The key word *appropriate* suggests there is only one correct answer. Look for the nursing action that would limit the spread of pathogenic microorganisms.

189. Answer: 3 Clients with gout will usually have elevated serum uric acid levels. Laboratory findings as well as physical assessment will confirm the diagnosis. The joint of the great toe is usually involved in initial attacks of acute gouty arthritis as seen in the accompanying figure. There are many other factors that will affect the results of hematocrit, serum calcium, and sodium levels. Erythrocyte sedimentation rate (ESR or sed rate) and white blood cell (WBC) counts will also be elevated in cases of gout.
Cognitive Level: Application **Client Need:** Physiological Integrity: Reduction of Risk Potential **Integrated Process:** Nursing Process: Plananing **Content Area:** Adult Health: Endocrine and Metabolic **Strategy:** The core issue of the question is knowledge of diagnostic testing for gout. Recall that the word gout contains the letter *u* to associate this with measurement of uric acid, which begins with *u*.

190. Answer: 4 It is difficult for individuals diagnosed with dependent personality disorder to make decisions on their own (options 1 and 3); rather, they try to get others to make decisions for them. This characteristic is reflected in DSM-IV diagnostic criteria. They would be disinclined to make critical remarks (option 2) related to their need for support from others.
Cognitive Level: Analysis **Client Need:** Psychosocial Integrity **Integrated Process:** Nursing Process: Implementation **Content Area:** Mental Health **Strategy:** The critical word in the stem of the question is *dependent.* Focus on this word and look for an association between that word and the nature of the statement in each option. The option that most closely simulates a response that relies on another is the correct answer to the question.

191. Answer: 3 Terbutaline, pirbuterol, and metaproterenol are all beta 2 stimulants. Isoproterenol stimulates beta 1 and beta 2 receptors and therefore is contraindicated and should not be used with clients with tachydysrhythmias.
Cognitive Level: Analysis **Client Need:** Physiological Integrity: Pharmacological and Parenteral Therapies **Integrated Process:** Nursing Process: Implementation **Content Area:** Pharmacology **Strategy:** The core issue of the question is knowledge that isoproterenol is contraindicated because it is a cardiac stimulant. Use specific drug knowledge and the process of elimination to make a selection.

192. Answer: 1, 3 The nurse can delegate procedures to the UAP and retains responsibility for the outcomes of those tasks that are delegated. Clearing the room of unnecessary objects and remaining with the client during ambulation are among those that can be delegated. The nurse needs to retain responsibility for assessment (option 2), teaching (option 5), and collaborating with the interdisciplinary team (option 4).

Cognitive Level: Analysis **Client Need:** Safe Effective Care Environment: Management of Care **Integrated Process:** Nursing Process: Implementation **Content Area:** Adult Health: Musculoskeletal **Strategy:** Use the principles of delegation to answer the question. Eliminate those options that represent assessment, teaching or interdisciplinary communication or collaboration.

193. Answer: 4 Dry mouth can be a common complaint of clients undergoing radiation therapy. Using sugar-free candies or gum will help to stimulate the flow of saliva and ease the discomfort that the client is experiencing without contributing to dental caries or lack of appetite from sugar intake. Option 1 is incorrect—eating meals prior to radiation therapy may lead to increased nausea because the client would be lying down after eating the meal. It has no effect on complaints of a dry mouth. Option 2 is incorrect—eating larger portions of food will not help to ease complaints of a dry mouth. Furthermore, the client may not be able to increase the size of meals due to side effects experienced as a result of radiation therapy. Option 3 is incorrect—the use of mouthwash can further cause the mouth to be dry and intensify the client's symptoms.

Cognitive Level: Application **Client Need:** Physiological Integrity: Basic Care and Comfort **Integrated Process:** Nursing Process: Implementation **Content Area:** Foundational Sciences: Nutrition **Strategy:** The core issue of the question is determining a strategy to relieve dry mouth for a client with cancer that will not contribute to anorexia. Use general principles of nutrition and knowledge of the disease process to make a selection.

194. Answer: 3 Although this client is not demonstrating positive signs of bonding at this time, it is important to look at her history before concluding that she is not bonding well with her infant. This client just experienced a long labor and the influence of fatigue on the attachment process should be considered. It is important to continue to assess infant bonding with this client throughout her hospitalization to reach a nursing judgment based on evidence.

Cognitive Level: Analysis **Client Need:** Health Promotion and Maintenance **Integrated Process:** Nursing Process: Analysis **Content Area:** Maternal-Newborn **Strategy:** Compare the nursing diagnoses with the information in the stem of the question. Eliminate each incorrect option based on lack of supporting data in the question.

195. Answer: 1 Carbon dioxide is eliminated from the body as exhaled gas. The faster the rate of breathing, the greater the quantity of carbon dioxide eliminated.

Cognitive Level: Application **Client Need:** Physiological Integrity: Physiological Adaptation **Integrated Process:** Nursing Process: Assessment **Content Area:** Adult Health: Respiratory **Strategy:** Note the stem of the question contains the words *diminished* pCO_2, which indicates that the client is blowing off excessive CO_2. Use knowledge of respiratory disorders to select the option that is consistent with excessive respiration, which is option 1.

196. Answer: 3 Ophthalmic epinephrine is used to produce mydriasis for ocular examination. Dilation of pupil further constricts ocular fluid outflow, possibly causing an acute attack of glaucoma in a client with narrow-angle glaucoma. Systemic absorption also causes hypertension and tachycardia. Brow ache is a typical side effect of adrenergic agonists such as epinephrine (option 4).

Cognitive Level: Application **Client Need:** Physiological Integrity: Pharmacological and Parenteral Therapies **Integrated Process:** Nursing Process: Assessment **Content Area:** Pharmacology **Strategy:** The core issue of the question is knowledge that angle-closure glaucoma is a contraindication to use of epinephrine for mydriasis during an ocular examination. Use specific drug knowledge and the process of elimination to make a selection.

197. Answer: 4 The client that is the most stable and with the fewest needs that the nurse must attend to is the client who is 6 days postoperative and awaiting placement in a rehabilitation facility. The nurse could attend to this client's discharge paperwork later in the shift. The nurse needs to assess the pain and neurovascular status of the client in option 1, since the client could be experiencing a complication of an overly tight cast. The nurse also needs to assess the client with the new spinal fracture. The nurse would need to teach and counsel the client who has phantom limb sensation.

Cognitive Level: Analysis **Client Need:** Safe Effective Care Environment: Management of Care **Integrated Process:** Nursing Process: Implementation **Content Area:** Adult Health: Musculoskeletal **Strategy:** Recall the principles of delegation and that clients who need assessment or teaching need to remain under the direct responsibility of the nurse.

198. Answer: 1, 3, 5 Knowledge of the cardiovascular disease risk factors and associated symptoms can assist in determining the origin of chest pain and direct the nurse to prioritize and implement appropriate care. Diabetes, smoking, and hypertension are known modifiable and non-modifiable risk factors to cardiac disease. Chest pain that occurs during activity may indicate cardiac ischemia due to the increased oxygen demand. Associated symptoms of nausea and diaphoresis are known warning signs of cardiac ischemia. Chest pain that increases with breathing, especially taking a deep breath, is most likely pleuritic pain and travel out of the country is an unrelated factor.

Cognitive Level: Application **Test Plan:** Physiological Integrity: Physiological Adaptation **Integrated Process:** Nursing Process: Assessment **Content Area:** Adult Health: Cardiovascular **Strategy:** The core issue of the question is knowledge of risk factors of cardiac disease leading to chest pain. Eliminate option 2 as unrelated because of the critical word *recent,* recalling that chest pain from cardiac origin is not related to travel. Eliminate option 4 next because cardiac pain does not correlate with the respiratory cycle.

199. Answer: 1 The definition of moderate sedation is that there is a minimal depression of the level of consciousness in which the client is able to maintain a patent airway and respond appropriately to verbal and physical stimuli. The pain threshold is increased so that the client can tolerate pain (option 2). Amnesia is induced partially with conscious sedation (option 3). Option 4 is false because the client is awake.

Cognitive Level: Application **Client Need:** Physiological Integrity: Reduction of Risk Potential **Integrated Process:** Communication and Documentation **Content Area:** Fundamentals **Strategy:** The core issue of the question is knowledge of moderate sedation and communication techniques that explain this clearly and accurately. Use knowledge of key features of moderate sedation and the process of elimination to make a selection.

200. **Answer: 3** These characteristics are reflected in DSM-IV diagnostic criteria for paranoid personality disorder. They must be considered in planning and implementing care. Delusions and hallucinations are consistent with schizophrenia or other psychotic disorders. Options 2 and 4 describe behavior traits but they are not consistent with paranoid personality disorder.

Cognitive Level: Application **Client Need:** Psychosocial Integrity **Integrated Process:** Nursing Process: Assessment **Content Area:** Mental Health **Strategy:** The core issue of the question is knowledge of characteristics of paranoid personality disorder. Use nursing knowledge and the process of elimination to make a selection. Note the word *paranoid* in the stem and *secretiveness* in the correct option to help make an association between the two.

201. **Answer: 2** The question indicates that extravasation may be occurring. Prompt nursing action in general will minimize tissue damage; therefore nursing actions should be initially directed towards the suspicious site. The drug administration should be stopped, since failure to do so will further disperse drug into the tissue. Clients can experience extravasation without pain, but not without swelling. Flushing the line with saline or dextrose is not advised, since there may still be vesicant drug remaining in the tubing.

Cognitive Level: Application **Client Need:** Physiological Integrity: Pharmacological and Parenteral Therapies **Integrated Process:** Nursing Process: Implementation **Content Area:** Pharmacology **Strategy:** The core issue of the question is knowledge that nitrogen mustard is an antineoplastic agent and that these drugs may be vesicants. From there, you need to determine what action will reduce the risk of further damage, which is stopping the drug and trying to aspirate it out of tissue.

202. **Answer: 3** The nurse should delegate the care of the 81-year-old client with heart failure and emphysema. This client was admitted 3 days ago and has a stable medical status. The nurse would want to assess the client recently admitted with exacerbation of COPD and the 25-year-old with a concussion less than 24 hours ago. The newly diagnosed diabetic client would require teaching that should not be delegated to the LPN/LVN.

Cognitive Level: Analysis **Client Need:** Safe Effective Care Environment: Management of Care **Integrated Process:** Nursing Process: Implementation **Content Area:** Leadership/Management **Strategy:** Recall the principles of delegation. The nurse should not delegate the care of clients who require assessment due to changes in acuity or status and clients who require teaching. Stable clients may be delegated to the LPN/LVN under the RN's supervision.

203. **Answer: 4** Nutritional goals for a client with hepatitis are aimed at providing a diet that is high in calories (3,000–4,000 kcal) and high in quality protein (1.5–2.0 g/kg). The diet should also be adequate in carbohydrates to spare protein and fat, provide concentrated calories, and improve the taste of food. Option 1 is incorrect—the nutritional management of hepatitis is the same for all types. Option 2 is incorrect—there is no clinical indication to place the client on tube feedings given the information that is provided. If the gut works, then the usual clinical model is to use it. Option 3 is incorrect because dietary fat should not be limited unless the client is experiencing problems with malabsorption (steatorrhea) and there is no evidence to support this.

Cognitive Level: Application **Client Need:** Physiological Integrity: Basic Care and Comfort **Integrated Process:** Nursing Process: Planning **Content Area:** Foundational Sciences: Nutrition **Strategy:** The critical word in the stem of the question is *hepatitis.* From this point, analyze that the client recovering from hepatitis needs a high-calorie, high-protein diet for healing to make the correct selection.

204. **Answer: 3** Although all of the options may be appropriate, demonstrating newborn care will allow the client to ask questions and gain confidence as she cares for her baby. Having her return the demonstration will allow the nurse to evaluate the teaching.

Cognitive Level: Application **Client Need:** Health Promotion and Maintenance **Integrated Process:** Teaching and Learning **Content Area:** Maternal-Newborn **Strategy:** Recall principles of teaching and learning, and recall that active participation leads to most effective learning outcomes.

205. **Answer: 4** The illustration shows the typical appearance of skin that has eczema. Use of a mild soap such as Dove® or Tone® prevents the skin from excessive dryness. Hot water is drying to the skin so should be avoided. Fabric softeners and many lotions contain perfumes that are irritating to the skin so should also be avoided.

Cognitive Level: Application **Client Need:** Physiological Integrity: Physiological Adaptation **Integrated Process:** Teaching and Learning **Content Area:** Child Health: Integumentary **Strategy:** To answer this question correctly, it is necessary to be familiar with the skin disorder in the picture. Beyond that, eliminate the incorrect options because of the words *hot* and *daily* in option 1, *liberally* and *entire* in option 2, and *all* in option 3. Although option 4 contains the word *only,* note that it is tempered when combined into the phrase *only as needed.*

206. **Answer: 3** Clients who are taking Coumadin should be alerted to the potential for drug interactions when they are on long-term anticoagulation therapy. Aspirin can potentiate the effect of Coumadin and interfere with the ability to maintain a therapeutic level. The use of Darvon, although previously prescribed, is not in the best interest of the client at this time due to Coumadin therapy. Telling the client to

keep taking Darvon would lead to drug interactions (option 2). While a further assessment of the client's back pain may be necessary (option 1), it is not the primary action that the nurse should be addressing at this time. Option 4 is a false statement, because the two drugs together could enhance bleeding.
Cognitive Level: Application **Client Need:** Physiological Integrity: Pharmacological and Parenteral Therapies **Integrated Process:** Nursing Process: Implementation **Content Area:** Pharmacology **Strategy:** The core issue of the question is knowledge that drugs containing aspirin can have an interactive effect with warfarin, which increase the risk of bleeding. With this in mind, use the process of elimination to select the option that results in stopping pain therapy with an aspirin-containing drug.

207. Answer: 3 All symptoms listed are clinical manifestations of developmental dysplasia of the hip, although the only one that would be found in a 5-year-old would be the telescoping of the femoral head into the pelvis. Other clinical signs in an older child would be lordosis and a waddling gait with a marked limp. A positive Ortolani-Barlow maneuver is found in the infant younger than 2 to 3 months of age. Limited abduction is the sign most often used for an infant older than 3 months, along with asymmetry of thigh and gluteal folds.
Cognitive Level: Application **Client Need:** Physiological Integrity: Physiological Adaptation **Integrated Process:** Nursing Process: Assessment **Content Area:** Child Health: Musculoskeletal **Strategy:** Specific knowledge about this disorder is needed to answer the question. Take time to review this disorder if you had difficulty with this question.

208. Answer: 3 The postoperative care of the child undergoing repair of clubfoot would not include administering pain medication immediately when due and covering the cast with blankets. Medication for pain should be administered as needed, and the cast should not be covered with blankets because this will interfere with the cast drying and could enhance swelling if excessive heat is retained under the blanket. Use of ice bags, elevation, diversional activities, and assessment of neurovascular status, swelling, and drainage or bleeding are all appropriate interventions.
Cognitive Level: Analysis **Client Need:** Safe Effective Care Environment: Management of Care **Integrated Process:** Nursing Process: Implementation **Content Area:** Leadership/Management **Strategy:** The core issue of the question is knowledge that a client who underwent repair of clubfoot will have a cast in place. After determining this, evaluate each of the options in terms of their appropriateness as part of management of the client in a cast.

209. Answer: 3 All of the information above is needed by the adolescent undergoing a spinal fusion but the physician, not the nurse, should explain the actual procedure. The nurse should focus on the care of this child following surgery, the exercises for breathing, turning, moving extremities, the tubes that will be placed—the nasogastric tube, urinary catheter, and intravenous lines. Ways that pain will be dealt with should also be explained in the preoperative period.
Cognitive Level: Application **Client Need:** Physiological Integrity: Reduction of Risk Potential **Integrated Process:** Nursing Process: Planning **Content Area:** Child Health: Musculoskeletal **Strategy:** The core issue of the question is knowledge of which information is within the domain of nursing practice and which information needs to be given by the physician to obtain informed consent. Choose the option that is not included by selecting the option that is within the surgeon's scope of practice.

210. Answer: 1 Individuals diagnosed with paranoid personality disorder frequently are critical or argumentative to maintain a safe distance between themselves and others related to their inability to trust others. Nursing staff may need to remind themselves that criticism of nursing care may be a manifestation of a personality disorder. The other statements listed do not reflect behavior that is typical of a client with this disorder.
Cognitive Level: Analysis **Client Need:** Psychosocial Integrity **Integrated Process:** Nursing Process: Analysis **Content Area:** Mental Health **Strategy:** The core issue of the question is knowledge of the behavioral characteristics of a client with paranoid personality disorder. Reflect on the common meaning of the word *paranoid* and evaluate each option for consistency to make an appropriate selection.

211. Answer: 3 The standard protocol is to administer up to three doses of NTG 5 minutes apart as long as the vital signs remain stable. After three doses, the physician should be called if pain is unrelieved. An electrocardiogram (ECG) may be ordered, but not an EEG (to measure brain waves). Using NTG paste, a longer acting form of the medication, is not appropriate at this time.
Cognitive Level: Application **Client Need:** Physiological Integrity: Pharmacological and Parenteral Therapies **Integrated Process:** Nursing Process: Implementation **Content Area:** Pharmacology **Strategy:** The core issue of the question is knowledge that nitroglycerine can be repeated up to 3 doses as long as the pain continues and the blood pressure is stable. Use the process of elimination and safe drug action to answer the question.

212. Answer: 2 The nurse should delegate the care of the 78-year-old client with diabetes and osteoarthritis. This client has a stable medical status. The nurse would want to assess the client recently admitted following nephrectomy and the 32-year-old who fractured the pelvis. Since pelvic exenteration is done to treat cancer, the nurse would want to assess this client and also address this client's psychosocial needs in coping with the diagnosis and surgery.
Cognitive Level: Analysis **Client Need:** Safe Effective Care Environment: Management of Care **Integrated Process:** Nursing Process: Implementation **Content Area:** Leadership/Management **Strategy:** Recall the principles of delegation. The nurse should not delegate the care of clients who require assessment due to changes in acuity or status, and clients who require teaching. Stable clients may be delegated to the LPN/LVN under the RN's supervision.

213. Answer: 3 The development of ascites (third spacing) is a common complication of cirrhosis. With the development of ascites, sodium restriction is instituted. Depending on the

extent and response to clinical treatment, the restrictions may be 500 to 1,000 mg per day if the client does not respond to customary diuretic therapy. Option 1 is incorrect—sodium is necessary for all individuals and the development of hyponatremia carries its own metabolic consequences. Option 2 is incorrect—even though paracentesis may sometimes be indicated, it is not the primary solution to the problem. It is important to look at the underlying fluid and electrolyte disturbances and correct them in order to prevent the recurring problem of ascites. While low-salt diets are often unpalatable, there is nothing to suggest that the client would be noncompliant with sodium restriction therapy. In addition, other seasonings can be used to provide taste to the client's diet.
Cognitive Level: Application **Client Need:** Physiological Integrity: Basic Care and Comfort **Integrated Process:** Nursing Process: Analysis **Content Area:** Foundational Sciences: Nutrition **Strategy:** The core issue of the question is the ability to correlate collection of ascitic fluid in the abdomen with an aggravating factor, sodium. Use this information and the process of elimination to choose correctly.

214. Answer: 3 *Pediculosis capitus* is head lice. The nits (eggs) are usually found at the nape of the neck or behind the ears. Head lice do not move away from the scalp to lay eggs; therefore, other choices are not appropriate.
Cognitive Level: Application **Client Need:** Physiological Integrity: Physiological Adaptation **Integrated Process:** Communication and Documentation **Content Area:** Child Health: Integumentary **Strategy:** Note that the word *capitus* refers to the head to eliminate options 2 and 4. Discriminate between the other two options by selecting the one where the nits would be harder to detect and to remove.

215. Answer: 2 Activity restrictions should be followed for 6 to 8 months following a spinal fusion. Lying, standing, sitting, walking, normal stair climbing, and gentle swimming are generally allowed following spinal fusion. Bending and twisting at the waist is not recommended, along with lifting more than 10 pounds, household chores such as vacuuming, mowing the lawn, physical education classes, and any sports besides walking.
Cognitive Level: Application **Client Need:** Physiological Integrity: Physiological Adaptation **Integrated Process:** Teaching and Learning **Content Area:** Child Health: Musculoskeletal **Strategy:** To answer this question correctly, it is important to understand the disorder and the limitations in the postoperative period. Eliminate option 1 because the restriction is so extreme. Next, evaluate each of the options and choose the one that protects the spine immediately after discharge.

216. Answer: 2 Vitamin D regulates calcium and phosphorus levels by increasing blood levels, increasing intestinal absorption and mobilization from bone, and reducing renal excretion of both elements. The statements in the other options are the opposites of the actions of vitamin D.
Cognitive Level: Application **Client Need:** Physiological Integrity: Pharmacological and Parenteral Therapies **Integrated Process:** Teaching and Learning **Content Area:** Pharmacology **Strategy:** The core issue of the question is the purpose and intended effect of vitamin D. Use basic knowledge of nutrition and vitamin therapy and the process of elimination to make a selection.

217. Answer: 4 The nurse should delegate the care of the 53-year-old client with hypertension and chronic renal insufficiency. This client has a stable medical status. The nurse would want to assess the client recently admitted following adrenalectomy and the 24-year-old who has hemophilia and fractured a leg the previous day. The nurse would want to provide teaching to the client being discharged to home following arthroscopy about pain management, limitations in activity, and followup care.
Cognitive Level: Analysis **Client Need:** Safe Effective Care Environment: Management of Care **Integrated Process:** Nursing Process: Implementation **Content Area:** Leadership/Management **Strategy:** Recall the principles of delegation. The nurse should not delegate the care of clients who require assessment due to changes in acuity or status, and clients who require teaching. Stable clients may be delegated to the LPN/LVN under the RN's supervision.

218. Answer: 1 Standard precautions are used with all clients, regardless of the medical diagnosis. Clients with AIDS or *Pneumocystis carinii* pneumonia are not contagious and do not require transmission-based precautions.
Cognitive Level: Application **Client Need:** Safe Effective Care Environment: Safety and Infection Control **Integrated Process:** Nursing Process: Implementation **Content Area:** Fundamentals **Strategy:** Use the process of elimination based on nursing knowledge of standard precautions and the route of transmission for AIDS.

219. Answer: 2 Wound infection is decreased by skin preparation when debris and transient microbes from the skin are removed. The other possibilities are all incorrect since skin preparation will not prevent complications such as positioning injury or pressure ulcers. Dermatitis does not result if surgical skin preparation is omitted.
Cognitive Level: Application **Client Need:** Physiological Integrity: Reduction of Risk Potential **Integrated Process:** Communication and Documentation **Content Area:** Fundamentals **Strategy:** The core issues of the question are recognition of the family question as relating to surgical skin preparation and knowledge of the purposes and expected results of that prep. Use nursing knowledge and the process of elimination to make a selection.

220. Answer: 2 It would be counterproductive to confront and challenge a client's paranoid ideation until trust has been developed. A consistent program schedule will cut down on the number of surprises for the client and help develop trust in the staff (option 1). Orienting the client to the unit and introducing him to the staff will enable the client to start developing therapeutic relationships (option 3). Communicating clear expectations will prevent the client from being confused (option 4).
Cognitive Level: Analysis **Client Need:** Psychosocial Integrity **Integrated Process:** Nursing Process: Analysis **Content Area:** Mental Health **Strategy:** The core issue of the question is knowledge of therapeutic communication techniques with a client who is paranoid. Note the word *counterproductive* in the stem and the word *challenge* in the correct option. It

will help you to choose correctly if you can make an association between these words.

221. Answer: 1 The nurse should assess for signs and symptoms of hypersensitivity reaction following the administration of all vaccines. Wheezing is a sign of hypersensitivity reaction and warrants immediate further assessment and emergency action to prevent possible death. Local discomfort (option 1) may be expected and is treated if necessary with acetaminophen. Anxiety and vomiting (options 3 and 4) are not associated with administration.
Cognitive Level: Application **Client Need:** Physiological Integrity: Pharmacological and Parenteral Therapies **Integrated Process:** Nursing Process: Assessment **Content Area:** Pharmacology **Strategy:** The core issue of the question is knowledge that the MMR vaccine may cause allergic reaction in clients who have hypersensitivity to egg yolks. Use specific drug knowledge and the process of elimination to make a selection.

222. Answer: 3 The nurse should delegate the care of the 59-year-old client with hypertension and Paget's disease. This client has a stable medical status. The nurse would want to assess the client awaiting surgery and complete preoperative care and the preoperative checklist. The nurse would also want to assess and care for the client in sickle cell crisis because of the acuity of the client's condition. The nurse would want to collaborate and communicate with the pulmonary rehabilitation specialist to formulate the ongoing plan of care.
Cognitive Level: Analysis **Client Need:** Safe Effective Care Environment: Management of Care **Integrated Process:** Nursing Process: Implementation **Content Area:** Leadership/ Management **Strategy:** Recall the principles of delegation. The nurse should not delegate the care of clients who require assessment due to changes in acuity or status, and clients who require teaching. Stable clients may be delegated to the LPN/LVN under the RN's supervision.

223. Answer: 2 Benign prostatic hyperplasia (BPH) is the most common disorder of the aging male client. Testicular cancer is the most common cancer in men between the ages of 15 and 35. Testicular torsion occurs at any age and gonorrhea is highest in occurrence during the sexually active years. Women 15 to 19 years old and men 20 to 24 years old have the highest rate.
Cognitive Level: Application **Client Need:** Physiological Integrity: Physiological Adaptation **Integrated Process:** Nursing Process: Assessment **Content Area:** Adult Health: Renal and Genitourinary **Strategy:** The critical words in the stem of the question are *older men.* Recall that the prostate gland undergoes changes in later life to help select the correct option.

224. Answer: 4 At birth, the infant's skin is thin with little subcutaneous fat. In addition, the infant has a greater proportion of body surface area relative to the amount of water present in the skin. Lanugo is shed within a few weeks of birth and has no relationship to heat loss. Sebaceous glands and apocrine glands are immature in the infant but are not related to heat loss or temperature regulation.
Cognitive Level: Application **Client Need:** Health Promotion and Maintenance **Integrated Process:** Teaching and Learning **Content Area:** Maternal-Newborn **Strategy:** Specific information on the functions of the skin is needed to answer the question. Look at the critical word *newborn* and think about the characteristics of newborn skin to help make a selection.

225. Answer: 3 PMS occurs only during the luteal phase of the menstrual cycle (7 to 10 days before menstrual flow begins). Increasing sexual activity doesn't prevent PMS, and caffeine can worsen the symptoms.
Cognitive Level: Analysis **Client Need:** Physiological Integrity: Physiological Adaptation **Integrated Process:** Nursing Process: Evaluation **Content Area:** Adult Health: Renal and Genitourinary **Strategy:** The critical word in the question is *understands.* This tells you that the correct option is one that contains a true statement. Use knowledge of PMS and that caffeine aggravates it to successfully eliminate incorrect options.

226. Answer: 4 Tonic-clonic seizures are the most common generalized seizures. Periods of inattention and daydreaming characterize an absence seizure. Sudden loss of muscle tone and falling characterize an atonic seizure. Repetitive small muscle group activity characterizes a partial seizure.
Cognitive Level: Analysis **Client Need:** Physiological Integrity: Physiological Adaptation **Integrated Process:** Nursing Process: Assessment **Content Area:** Adult Health: Neurological **Strategy:** The core issue is knowledge of the characteristics of the most common seizure disorder. Use the process of elimination and specific nursing knowledge to answer the question.

227. Answer: 1 Equipment for client care is dedicated to the client on contact precautions and kept in the client's room.
Cognitive Level: Application **Client Need:** Safe Effective Care Environment: Safety and Infection Control **Integrated Process:** Nursing Process: Implementation **Content Area:** Fundamentals **Strategy:** The key word *appropriate* suggests there is only one correct answer. Look for the nursing action that would limit the spread of pathogenic microorganisms.

228. Answer: 4 Pulses are assessed frequently to ensure adequate circulation is present and an occlusion or leakage of the graft has not occurred. Pulses should be marked preoperatively so the nurse has a comparison point postoperatively. Pulses may be absent for a short-term postoperatively due to vasospasm or hypothermia. Anticoagulant therapy is not indicated. Trendelenburg position could reduce blood flow to the affected lower extremities. Elastic stockings may or may not be ordered because they could interfere with neurovascular assessment of the lower extremities; however, pneumatic boots would help to prevent deep vein thrombosis and allow visualization of lower extremities.
Cognitive Level: Application **Client Need:** Physiological Integrity: Physiological Adaptation **Integrated Process:** Nursing Process: Implementation **Content Area:** Adult Health: Cardiovascular **Strategy:** Note the critical words *first postoperative day.* This tells you that the client condition could change and that diligent assessment and ongoing monitoring is required. Use knowledge of the surgical procedure and routine postoperative care to make a selection.

229. Answer: 1 Abrasions, pustules, or other skin conditions have to be assessed and documented because these may interfere

with wound healing. Hair growth—lack of it or presence of lanugo or fine hair—will not interfere with the skin preparation. Pulsation is not always visible or available to assess depending upon the part of the body being operated on.
Cognitive Level: Analysis **Client Need:** Physiological Integrity: Reduction of Risk Potential **Integrated Process:** Nursing Process: Assessment **Content Area:** Fundamentals **Strategy:** The core issue of the question is knowledge that broken areas of skin are at risk for infection and need to be reported to the surgeon. Knowing that this is an important item helps to prioritize this as the item to assess.

230. Answer: 4 Option 4 provides the client with the choice of how he would like to take the medication, while being firm that he must take it; the choice gives the client a sense of control and helps to reduce the power struggle. Simply telling the client that the medication is not poison (option 1) would do little to persuade him to adhere. Option 2 provides no choice and implies punishment. The client should take the medication; therefore, option 3 would be inappropriate.
Cognitive Level: Analysis **Client Need:** Psychosocial Integrity **Integrated Process:** Communication and Documentation **Content Area:** Mental Health **Strategy:** The core issue of the question is knowledge of therapeutic communication techniques when working with a client who has schizophrenia. Use nursing knowledge of this disorder and the process of elimination to make a selection.

231. Answer: 3 Dry mouth occurs from the anticholinergic effects seen with fluphenazine. Options 1 and 2 are incorrect because orthostatic hypotension is not a major side effect of fluphenazine. Confusion (option 4) is not a side effect of this agent.
Cognitive Level: Application **Client Need:** Physiological Integrity: Pharmacological and Parenteral Therapies **Integrated Process:** Nursing Process: Planning **Content Area:** Pharmacology **Strategy:** The core issue of the question is knowledge of drug adverse effects and how to prevent them. Recall that anticholinergic effects are of concern with this medication and use the process of elimination to make a selection.

232. Answer: 4 The nurse should delegate the care of the 79-year-old who has chronic bronchitis and early Alzheimer's disease. This client has a stable medical status. The nurse would want to assess the client undergoing cardiac catheterization and complete the preparation activities for the procedure. The nurse would also want to assess the client with low back pain. The nurse would want to assess and monitor the client who had chest pain the previous evening because of the nature of the problem.
Cognitive Level: Analysis **Client Need:** Safe Effective Care Environment: Management of Care **Integrated Process:** Nursing Process: Implementation **Content Area:** Leadership/Management **Strategy:** Recall the principles of delegation. The nurse should not delegate the care of clients who require assessment due to changes in acuity or status, and clients who require teaching. Stable clients may be delegated to the LPN/LVN under the RN's supervision.

233. Answer: 1 Elevation of the extremities promotes venous return. Pulses are assessed to ensure adequate circulation. Option 3 is unnecessary because the Unna boot is treating the ulcer and is changed every 1 to 2 weeks.
Cognitive Level: Application **Client Need:** Physiological Integrity: Physiological Adaptation **Integrated Process:** Nursing Process: Implementation **Content Area:** Adult Health: Cardiovascular **Strategy:** The core issue of the question is knowledge of the type of condition that requires the use of an Unna boot and then determining an intervention that meets the same need. To answer correctly, you need to determine that the underlying problem is venous in nature and that leg elevation aids in relieving symptoms of venous disease.

234. Answer: 4 Anxiety reduction is needed when the client is waiting for the outcome of tests to assist them in processing their feelings and exploring their options based upon the results of the test.
Cognitive Level: Application **Client Need:** Physiological Integrity: Reduction of Risk Potential **Integrated Process:** Nursing Process: Implementation **Content Area:** Adult Health: Oncology **Strategy:** The purpose of the test is to identify a possible problem and the client's greatest fear is that the test will validate that something is wrong. Therefore, communication is the first priority in care of a post-test client. Pain is a possibility of a problem since the test does require the client to lie still for a while. But fear will intensify pain even more if not addressed first. Only minimal radiation exposure does occur during a scan and not enough to cause any radiation sickness (nausea). Bleeding is not a possible outcome from the scan since the procedure is not invasive.

235. Answer: 2 COPD places a client at risk to develop malnutrition due to reduction in muscle mass and fat reserves. Option 1 is incorrect because COPD clients are more likely to suffer from respiratory infections due to altered immune response (decreased cell-mediated immunity, altered immunoglobulin production, and impaired cellular resistance). Options 3 and 4 are incorrect because COPD clients usually present with weight loss and are hypermetabolic (require additional calories due to increased energy requirements as a result of increased work of breathing).
Cognitive Level: Application **Client Need:** Physiological Integrity: Basic Care and Comfort **Integrated Process:** Teaching and Learning **Content Area:** Foundational Sciences: Nutrition **Strategy:** The wording of the question tells you the correct answer is a true statement of fact. Use general knowledge of nutritional concepts and COPD to eliminate each of the incorrect options.

236. Answer: 3 In hypertensive urgencies, clients present with a systolic BP greater than 240 mmHg and diastolic BP greater than 120 mmHg. In hypertensive emergencies, the client's diastolic BP is greater than 130mmHg.
Cognitive Level: Application **Client Need:** Physiological Integrity: Pharmacological and Parenteral Therapies **Integrated Process:** Teaching and Learning **Content Area:** Pharmacology **Strategy:** The core issue of the question is knowledge of the parameters of hypertensive crisis. Use this knowledge and the process of elimination to make a selection.

237. Answer: 1 Atherosclerosis indicates the need to adopt a low-fat diet. Both butter and margarine have 4 grams of fat per serving, making the client's statement incorrect and in need of further clarification. The responses in the other options are correct.

Cognitive Level: Analysis **Client Need:** Health Promotion and Maintenance **Integrated Process:** Nursing Process: Evaluation **Content Area:** Adult Health: Cardiovascular **Strategy:** The critical words in the question are *further discussion.* With this in mind, evaluate each of the options in terms of how they relate to a low-fat diet.

238. Answer 3 Medical asepsis requires clean, not sterile, technique. Only option 3 requires medical aseptic technique. Collecting a wound culture (option 1), suctioning a tracheostomy (option 2), and catheterizing the client (option 4) all require the nurse to use sterile asepsis.

Cognitive Level: Application **Client Need:** Safe Effective Care Environment: Safety and Infection Control **Integrated Process:** Nursing Process: Planning **Content Area:** Fundamentals **Strategy:** Knowledge of medical versus surgical asepsis is essential. Look for similarities in the choices. Options 1, 2, and 4 require sterile technique. Option 3 is the only choice that requires medical aseptic technique.

239. Answer: 3 Increased heart rate and/or respiratory rate within minutes to several hours following central venous line insertion are symptoms of a pneumothorax caused by puncture of the pleura. The client will require a chest x-ray to determine if a pneumothorax is present. If the client does have a pneumothorax, placement of a chest tube is likely. Pain at the central line insertion site, fever, and diminished breath sounds in lung bases will require intervention, but the etiology of these symptoms is not likely to be potentially life threatening as is the development of a pneumothorax.

Cognitive Level: Analysis **Client Need:** Physiological Integrity: Reduction of Risk Potential **Integrated Process:** Nursing Process: Implementation **Content Area:** Adult Health: Respiratory **Strategy:** Consider an acute complication of central line insertion, which would include pneumothorax. Then consider how pneumothorax would manifest in the client to make a selection. Pain (option 1) might be expected to some degree. Fever (option 2) could occur with infection but this could not happen that quickly. Eliminate option 4 because of the qualifier *bases* with lung sounds, which indicates atelectasis, not pneumothorax.

240. Answer: 2 Ideas of reference or misinterpretation occurs when the client believes that an incident has a personal reference to one's self when, in fact, it is not at all related. A hallucination is the occurrence of a sight, sound, touch, smell, or taste without any external stimulus to the corresponding sensory organ; they are real to the person (option 1). Delusions are false beliefs that cannot be changed by logical reasoning or evidence (option 3). Loose association is a vague, unfocused, illogical flow or stream of thought (option 4).

Cognitive Level: Application **Client Need:** Psychosocial Integrity **Integrated Process:** Nursing Process: Assessment **Content Area:** Mental Health **Strategy:** The core issue of the question is the ability to draw correct conclusions from the behavior of a client with schizophrenia. Use knowledge of the features of this diagnosis and the process of elimination to make a selection.

241. Answer: 3 With increased age, there is an increased sensitivity to xanthines. Also, there could be other disease processes that may lead to this elevated value. The dose of theophylline should be decreased to get the blood level to the 10 to 20 mg/dL range. Theophylline doses should be based on lean body weight to prevent entering the medication into the adipose tissue.

Cognitive Level: Analysis **Client Need:** Physiological Integrity: Pharmacological and Parenteral Therapies **Integrated Process:** Nursing Process: Analysis **Content Area:** Pharmacology **Strategy:** The core issue of the question is knowledge that the drug level is high and knowledge of what factors can increase the drug level. Use concepts of the effects of age on pharmacokinetics and the process of elimination to make a selection.

242. Answer: 3 Immunizations interrupt the chain of infection by generating immunity in a susceptible host by introducing a weakened or killed antigen into the body. Immunizations do not affect the portal of entry, portal of exit, or the mode of transmission of a pathogenic organism.

Cognitive Level: Application **Test Plan:** Safe Effective Care Environment: Safety and Infection Control **Integrated Process:** Teaching and Learning **Content Area:** Fundamentals **Strategy:** Knowledge of the chain of infection is required. Immunizations change the immunity status of the person receiving them. Option 3 is the only choice where that is possible.

243. Answer: 2 The thyroidectomy is the third alternative treatment used when medication and iodine-based radiation therapy are unsuccessful. There is a great concern of causing hypothyroidism in the client. The other statements are not reflective of the underlying concern with performing a thyroidectomy in a child.

Cognitive Level: Application **Client Need:** Physiological Integrity: Physiological Adaptation **Integrated Process:** Communication and Documentation **Content Area:** Child Health: Endocrine and Metabolic **Strategy:** Determine the core issue of the question, which is a disadvantage of performing a thyroidectomy in a child. Use knowledge about hyperthyroid state and age-related concepts to eliminate each of the incorrect responses.

244. Answer: 2 Uterine prolapse is caused by weakened pelvic muscles, which can be strengthened by Kegel exercises. The other conditions are not treated with Kegel exercises.

Cognitive Level: Application **Client Need:** Health Promotion and Maintenance **Integrated Process:** Nursing Process: Planning **Content Area:** Adult Health: Renal and Genitourinary **Strategy:** The core issue of the question is knowledge that Kegel exercises can strengthen the pelvic floor. Evaluate each of the options to determine which condition could be improved by the use of these exercises.

245. Answer: 2 With this client, being a danger only to himself (option 1) isn't enough, he may not be a danger to himself but he still may want to harm his parents (others). Although the goal is for the client to continue to take his

medication (option 3) and remain in treatment (option 4), safety is a priority. Depending on state law, the length of hold may be either 48 or 72 hours.
Cognitive Level: Analysis **Client Need:** Safe Effective Care Environment: Safety and Infection Control **Integrated Process:** Nursing Process: Analysis **Content Area:** Mental Health **Strategy:** The core issue of the question is safety of all possible clients in the question. Note the association between the word *knife* in the stem and the word *danger* to narrow the possibilities to options 1 and 2. Choose option 2 over 1 because it is the most comprehensive option.

246. Answer: 1 Clients receiving ophthalmic corticosteroids have an increased risk of infection. Contact lenses should not be used during ophthalmic corticosteroid therapy. Options 2, 3, and 4 indicate an appropriate understanding of ophthalmic corticosteroid therapy.
Cognitive Level: Analysis **Client Need:** Physiological Integrity: Pharmacological and Parenteral Therapies **Integrated Process:** Nursing Process: Evaluation **Content Area:** Pharmacology **Strategy:** The core issue of the question is knowledge that corticosteroids increase risk of infection and how to reduce this risk when taking ophthalmic corticosteroids. Use nursing knowledge and the process of elimination to make a selection.

247. Answer: 4 Sneezing and coughing are examples of modes of transmission, whereby droplet nuclei can be transmitted directly to a susceptible host.
Cognitive Level: Application **Test Plan:** Safe Effective Care Environment: Safety and Infection Control **Integrated Process:** Teaching and Learning **Content Area:** Fundamentals **Strategy:** Look for commonalities among the options in order to eliminate choices. Options 1, 2, and 3 are inanimate objects that serve as vehicles to transmit infectious microorganisms. Choose option 4, as direct transmission of microorganisms occurs.

248. Answer: 3 The premature secretion of testosterone promotes the closure of the epiphyseal growth plates. Many of these children appear very tall around sixth grade, but their friends eventually catch up and surpass them in linear growth.
Cognitive Level: Application **Client Need:** Physiological Integrity: Physiological Adaptation **Integrated Process:** Teaching and Learning **Content Area:** Child Health: Endocrine and Metabolic **Strategy:** To answer this question, it is necessary to have an understanding of the underlying pathophysiology. Take time to review this information if you have the need.

249. Answer: 1 Calf pumping exercises involve contracting and then relaxing the leg muscles in an alternating fashion. Options 2, 3, and 4 do not exercise the calf muscles, including the gastrocnemius muscles.
Cognitive Level: Analysis **Client Need:** Physiological Integrity: Reduction of Risk Potential **Integrated Process:** Nursing Process: Evaluation **Content Area:** Fundamentals **Strategy:** The core issue of the question is knowledge of correct implementation of leg exercises in the perioperative period. Use this knowledge and the process of elimination to make a selection.

250. Answer: 4 When intervening in delirium, highest priority is given to nursing interventions that will maintain life. Fluid and electrolyte loss caused by nausea and vomiting can be a life-threatening condition during alcohol withdrawal, requiring replacement by intravenous therapy.
Cognitive Level: Analysis **Client Need:** Physiological Integrity: Physiological Adaptation **Integrated Process:** Nursing Process: Planning **Content Area:** Mental Health **Strategy:** The core issue of the question is knowledge that a state of delirium is characterized by some type of metabolic imbalance. Recall that questions that address priorities of care in unstable clients often focus on physiological needs first. With this in mind, eliminate options 1 and 3 first. Choose option 4 over 2 because it assists in correcting the client's internal metabolic state, and thus meets a physiological need. Option 2 addresses a safety need.

251. Answer: 3 The nurse should delegate the care of the 62-year-old who had surgery 3 days ago to repair the fractured femur. This client has a stable medical status. The nurse would want to assess the client returning to the unit following gastric surgery and the client who had wisdom teeth extraction. The nurse would want to complete discharge teaching with the client who had the cholecystectomy.
Cognitive Level: Analysis **Client Need:** Safe Effective Care Environment: Management of Care **Integrated Process:** Nursing Process: Implementation **Content Area:** Leadership/Management **Strategy:** Recall the principles of delegation. The nurse should not delegate the care of clients who require assessment due to changes in acuity or status, and clients who require teaching. Stable clients may be delegated to the LPN/LVN under the RN's supervision.

252. Answer: 3 A wound infection can be spread by direct contact with the wound. Scarlet fever, pertussis, and rubella involve the spread of infection by respiratory particle droplets larger than 5 microns.
Cognitive Level: Application **Test Plan:** Safe Effective Care Environment: Safety and Infection Control **Integrated Process:** Nursing Process: Implementation **Content Area:** Fundamentals **Strategy:** Look for commonalities among the options in order to eliminate choices. Options 1, 2, and 4 are contagious infections characterized by coughing. Choose option 3, as direct transmission of microorganisms occurs by direct contact with the client.

253. Answer: 4 The statements in the first three options correctly describe signs of BPH. Option 4 indicates the need for further teaching because the client should increase his fluid intake (unless contraindicated) to prevent urinary tract infections and lessen dysuria.
Cognitive Level: Analysis **Client Need:** Physiological Integrity: Physiological Adaptation **Integrated Process:** Nursing Process: Evaluation **Content Area:** Adult Health: Renal and Genitourinary **Strategy:** The critical words in the stem of the question are *need for further teaching.* This tells you that the correct answer is an incorrect statement made by the client. Use the process of elimination and knowledge of the disorder to make a selection.

254. Answer: 2 While work or industry is the primary developmental task of children this age, emphasis should not be placed exclusively on school. Recreational activities are an integral part of growing up, and all efforts should be made to provide access to such programs. Scouting programs provide recognition of individual successes and strengths and can do much to enhance a child's self-esteem.

Cognitive Level: Application **Client Need:** Physiological Integrity: Physiological Adaptation **Integrated Process:** Nursing Process: Analysis **Content Area:** Child Health: Neurological **Strategy:** Consider the word *mild* in the stem of the question and choose the response that is the broadest and most encompassing.

255. **Answer: 1** Elderly clients have slower metabolism and elimination of drugs, causing an increased susceptibility to side effects. Extrapyramidal side effects are most common with haloperidol, a high-potency antipsychotic. Frequent sedation of this elderly client with haloperidol can lead to the development of tardive dyskinesia, and requires careful monitoring by the nurse.

Cognitive Level: Application **Client Need:** Physiological Integrity: Pharmacological and Parenteral Therapies **Integrated Process:** Nursing Process: Assessment **Content Area:** Mental Health **Strategy:** The core issue of the question is knowledge of adverse effects of the drug haloperidol. Use specific nursing knowledge and the process of elimination to make a selection.

256. **Answer: 4** The state nurse practice act defines the scope of nursing practice in each state. Although there are general principles that apply to all, each state retains the right to formulate its own regulations about nursing practice, including delegation. The ANA standards of practice apply to care given to clients. Job descriptions and policy manuals are agency-specific and do not address the state regulations directly.

Cognitive Level: Application **Client Need:** Safe Effective Care Environment: Management of Care **Integrated Process:** Nursing Process: Implementation **Content Area:** Leadership/ Management **Strategy:** Use knowledge of the source of various regulations to answer the question. If needed, review concepts related to legal governance of nursing practice.

257. **Answer: 4, 3, 1, 2** The gown is applied first, as it takes the most time to don. The mask is donned next, followed by eye protection. These items can be more securely applied with ungloved hands. Gloves are donned last, so the gloves can be pulled up to cover the cuffs of the gown.

Cognitive Level: Application **Test Plan:** Safe Effective Care Environment: Safety and Infection Control **Integrated Process:** Nursing Process: Implementation **Content Area:** Fundamentals **Strategy:** Rationalize the ordering based on nursing knowledge of standard precautions and surgical asepsis.

258. **Answer: 2** The teacher is most aware of the varied reactions of the classmates and together the parents and teacher can plan strategies to promote acceptance of this child. A Medic Alert bracelet is appropriate but will not improve self-esteem. A psychiatrist might be consulted if the child shows symptoms of altered self-esteem, but this is not required now.

Cognitive Level: Application **Client Need:** Physiological Integrity: Physiological Adaptation **Integrated Process:** Communication and Documentation **Content Area:** Child Health: Neurological **Strategy:** The focus of the question is on how to maintain the client's self-esteem and the location of the concern centers around being at school. With this in mind, select the option that directly addresses the concern.

259. **Answer: 2** The client who has had a positive PPD test in the past should be evaluated with a chest x-ray, which would then be the screening test of choice. The arm should be cleansed with alcohol and allowed to air dry prior to the administration of the test. The test is usually read in 48 to 72 hours and the client may wash the area as usual.

Cognitive Level: Analysis **Client Need:** Physiological Integrity: Reduction of Risk Potential **Integrated Process:** Nursing Process: Assessment **Content Area:** Adult Health: Integumentary **Strategy:** The core issue of the question is knowledge of proper procedure and concerns when administering a PPD test. Recall that this is a skin test for tuberculosis to help you recall that assessment of a client's past reaction is a key first action.

260. **Answer: 3** Initially, the delirious client is dazed, drowsy, and perceptions will be disturbed, making it difficult for the client to sustain attention to any mental task. Delirium is characterized by alternating periods of confusion with lucidity; therefore, option 3 is an appropriate initial outcome criterion. Options 1, 2, and 4 may or may not be appropriate outcome criteria once the client has been stabilized.

Cognitive Level: Application **Client Need:** Psychosocial Integrity **Integrated Process:** Nursing Process: Planning **Content Area:** Mental Health **Strategy:** The core issue of the question is understanding of the condition of delirium. The critical word in the stem of the question is *initial.* With this in mind, choose the option that shows the beginnings of return of neurological status to normal.

261. **Answer: 3** Dehydration results in hypovolemia, which can precipitate acute renal failure in infants and children. The other responses are incorrect because they don't directly impact renal perfusion.

Cognitive Level: Analysis **Client Need:** Physiological Integrity: Physiological Adaptation **Integrated Process:** Nursing Process: Assessment **Content Area:** Child Health: Renal and Genitourinary **Strategy:** Consider the various etiologies of acute renal failure. Recall that the kidneys need a minimum glomerular filtration rate to function properly. Use this concept to choose correctly.

262. **Answer: 1** A client with tuberculosis must wear a particulate respiratory mask if transportation to another hospital department is unavoidable. This is an element of airborne precautions necessary to limit the transmission of the microorganism. Tuberculosis is not transmitted via eating utensils (option 3) or urine (option 4). Removal and disposal of respiratory secretions is important but does not require the client to wear gloves.

Cognitive Level: Application **Test Plan:** Safe Effective Care Environment: Safety and Infection Control **Integrated Process:** Nursing Process: Implementation **Content Area:** Fundamentals **Strategy:** Knowledge of how tuberculosis is transmitted is essential. Eliminate options 3 and 4 because they do not address transmission via the respiratory tract.

Select option 1 over 2 as the client would not wear gloves to protect themselves from their own infection.

263. **Answer: 4** Severe scrotal pain, nausea, and absent cremasteric reflex are characteristic of testicular torsion. Severe pain and an absent cremasteric reflex are not typical symptoms of the disorders listed in the other options.

Cognitive Level: Analysis **Client Need:** Physiological Integrity: Physiological Adaptation **Integrated Process:** Nursing Process: Analysis **Content Area:** Adult Health: Renal and Genitourinary **Strategy:** Note the critical word *sudden* in the stem of the question. Eliminate options 1 and 3, which are not as sudden in onset. Choose between Options 2 and 4, noting that the word *torsion* indicates twisting, which is compatible with the symptoms described by the client.

264. **Answer: 4** A goal of venous ulcer care is for the client to experience no signs of inflammation or infection. This is the goal directly related to tissue integrity. The other options are good outcomes but do not relate directly to the question as stated.

Cognitive Level: Analysis **Client Need:** Physiological Integrity: Physiological Adaptation **Integrated Process:** Nursing Process: Evaluation **Content Area:** Adult Health: Cardiovascular **Strategy:** Focus on the term *skin integrity* to compare the options. Eliminate options 2 and 3 first because they are not associated with skin integrity. Choose option 4 over option 1 because it is a more global or encompassing item, which is typical when determining an outcome.

265. **Answer: 2** The onset of dementia symptoms for this client was at or before 58 years of age. When Alzheimer's disease occurs in people under the age of 65, it is called presenile dementia.

Cognitive Level: Application **Client Need:** Psychosocial Integrity **Integrated Process:** Nursing Process: Assessment **Content Area:** Mental Health **Strategy:** The core issue of the question is the association of the age of 58 with the appropriate type of dementia. Use nursing knowledge of the types of dementia and the process of elimination to make a selection.

Index

Page numbers followed by b indicate box; those followed by f indicate figure; those followed by t indicate table.

D

H

M

U

Pearson Education, Inc.

YOU SHOULD CAREFULLY READ THE TERMS AND CONDITIONS BEFORE USING THE CD-ROM PACKAGE. USING THIS CD-ROM PACKAGE INDICATES YOUR ACCEPTANCE OF THESE TERMS AND CONDITIONS.

Pearson Education, Inc. provides this program and licenses its use. You assume responsibility for the selection of the program to achieve your intended results, and for the installation, use, and results obtained from the program. This license extends only to use of the program in the United States or countries in which the program is marketed by authorized distributors.

LICENSE GRANT

You hereby accept a nonexclusive, nontransferable, permanent license to install and use the program ON A SINGLE COMPUTER at any given time. You may copy the program solely for backup or archival purposes in support of your use of the program on the single computer. You may not modify, translate, disassemble, decompile, or reverse engineer the program, in whole or in part.

TERM

The License is effective until terminated. Pearson Education, Inc. reserves the right to terminate this License automatically if any provision of the License is violated. You may terminate the License at any time. To terminate this License, you must return the program, including documentation, along with a written warranty stating that all copies in your possession have been returned or destroyed.

LIMITED WARRANTY

THE PROGRAM IS PROVIDED "AS IS" WITHOUT WARRANTY OF ANY KIND, EITHER EXPRESSED OR IMPLIED, INCLUDING, BUT NOT LIMITED TO, THE IMPLIED WARRANTIES OR MERCHANTABILITY AND FITNESS FOR A PARTICULAR PURPOSE. THE ENTIRE RISK AS TO THE QUALITY AND PERFORMANCE OF THE PROGRAM IS WITH YOU. SHOULD THE PROGRAM PROVE DEFECTIVE, YOU (AND NOT PRENTICE-HALL, INC. OR ANY AUTHORIZED DEALER) ASSUME THE ENTIRE COST OF ALL NECESSARY SERVICING, REPAIR, OR CORRECTION. NO ORAL OR WRITTEN INFORMATION OR ADVICE GIVEN BY PRENTICE-HALL, INC., ITS DEALERS, DISTRIBUTORS, OR AGENTS SHALL CREATE A WARRANTY OR INCREASE THE SCOPE OF THIS WARRANTY.

SOME STATES DO NOT ALLOW THE EXCLUSION OF IMPLIED WARRANTIES, SO THE ABOVE EXCLUSION MAY NOT APPLY TO YOU. THIS WARRANTY GIVES YOU SPECIFIC LEGAL RIGHTS AND YOU MAY ALSO HAVE OTHER LEGAL RIGHTS THAT VARY FROM STATE TO STATE.

Pearson Education, Inc. does not warrant that the functions contained in the program will meet your requirements or that the operation of the program will be uninterrupted or error-free.

However, Pearson Education, Inc. warrants the diskette(s) or CD-ROM(s) on which the program is furnished to be free from defects in material and workmanship under normal use for a period of ninety (90) days from the date of delivery to you as evidenced by a copy of your receipt.

The program should not be relied on as the sole basis to solve a problem whose incorrect solution could result in injury to person or property. If the program is employed in such a manner, it is at the user's own risk and Pearson Education, Inc. explicitly disclaims all liability for such misuse.

LIMITATION OF REMEDIES

Pearson Education, Inc.'s entire liability and your exclusive remedy shall be:

1. the replacement of any diskette(s) or CD-ROM(s) not meeting Pearson Education, Inc.'s "LIMITED WARRANTY" and that is returned to Pearson Education, or
2. if Pearson Education is unable to deliver a replacement diskette(s) or CD-ROM(s) that is free of defects in materials or workmanship, you may terminate this agreement by returning the program.

IN NO EVENT WILL PRENTICE-HALL, INC. BE LIABLE TO YOU FOR ANY DAMAGES, INCLUDING ANY LOST PROFITS, LOST SAVINGS, OR OTHER INCIDENTAL OR CONSEQUENTIAL DAMAGES ARISING OUT OF THE USE OR INABILITY TO USE SUCH PROGRAM EVEN IF PRENTICE-HALL, INC. OR AN AUTHORIZED DISTRIBUTOR HAS BEEN ADVISED OF THE POSSIBILITY OF SUCH DAMAGES, OR FOR ANY CLAIM BY ANY OTHER PARTY.

SOME STATES DO NOT ALLOW FOR THE LIMITATION OR EXCLUSION OF LIABILITY FOR INCIDENTAL OR CONSEQUENTIAL DAMAGES, SO THE ABOVE LIMITATION OR EXCLUSION MAY NOT APPLY TO YOU.

GENERAL

You may not sublicense, assign, or transfer the license of the program. Any attempt to sublicense, assign or transfer any of the rights, duties, or obligations hereunder is void.

This Agreement will be governed by the laws of the State of New York.

Should you have any questions concerning this Agreement, you may contact Pearson Education, Inc. by writing to:

Director of New Media
Higher Education Division
Pearson Education, Inc.
One Lake Street
Upper Saddle River, NJ 07458

Should you have any questions concerning technical support, you may contact:

Product Support Department: Monday–Friday 8:00 A.M. –8:00 P.M. and Sunday 5:00 P.M.-12:00 A.M. (All times listed are Eastern). 1-800-677-6337

You can also get support by filling out the web form located at http://247.prenhall.com

YOU ACKNOWLEDGE THAT YOU HAVE READ THIS AGREEMENT, UNDERSTAND IT, AND AGREE TO BE BOUND BY ITS TERMS AND CONDITIONS. YOU FURTHER AGREE THAT IT IS THE COMPLETE AND EXCLUSIVE STATEMENT OF THE AGREEMENT BETWEEN US THAT SUPERSEDES ANY PROPOSAL OR PRIOR AGREEMENT, ORAL OR WRITTEN, AND ANY OTHER COMMUNICATIONS BETWEEN US RELATING TO THE SUBJECT MATTER OF THIS AGREEMENT.